W9-AQU-017

CLINICAL PHARMACOLOGY AND NURSING

SECOND EDITION

CLINICAL PHARMACOLOGY AND NURSING

SECOND EDITION

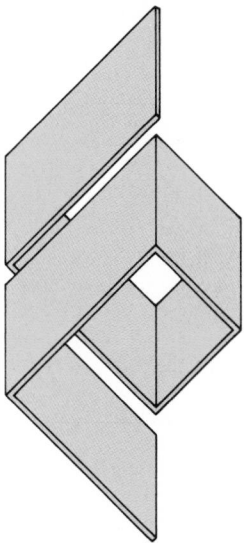

Charold L. Baer, RN, PhD, FCCM, CCRN
Professor, Department of Adult Health
and Illness, Oregon Health Sciences
University, School of Nursing,
Portland, Oregon

Bradley R. Williams, PharmD
Associate Professor of Clinical Pharmacy
and Clinical Gerontology, University of
Southern California, School of
Pharmacy and Andrus Gerontology Center,
Los Angeles, California

Springhouse Corporation
Springhouse, Pennsylvania

STAFF

Executive Director, Editorial
Stanley Loeb

Director of Trade and Textbooks
Minnie B. Rose, RN, BSN, MEd

Art Director
John Hubbard

Drug Information Editor
George J. Blake, RPh, MS

Editor
Nancy Priff

Copy Editor
Elizabeth Kiselev

Editorial Assistant
Mary Madden

Designers
Stephanie Peters (associate art director), Elaine Ezrow (book designer), Maria Errico, Kristina Gabage

Illustrators
Will Davidson, John Gist, Bob Jackson, Bob Newmann, Judy Newhouse, Mary Stangl

Art Production
Robert Perry (manager), Nancy Frazier, Donald Knauss, Anet Oakes, Ann Raphun, Thomas Robbins, Robert Wieder

Typographers
David Kosten (director), Diane Paluba (manager), Elizabeth Bergman, Joy Rossi Biletz, Phyllis Marron, Robin Rantz, Valerie L. Rosenberger

Manufacturing
Deborah Meiris (manager), T.A. Landis, Jennifer Suter

Production Coordinator
Caroline Lemoine

The drug selections and dosages in this textbook are based on research and current recommendations by medical and nursing authorities. These selections and dosages comply with currently accepted standards, although they cannot be considered conclusive. For each patient, any drug or dosage recommendation must be considered in conjunction with clinical data and the latest package-insert information. This is particularly essential with new drugs. The authors and the publisher disclaim responsibility for any untoward effects caused by these suggested selections and dosages or from the reader's misinterpretation of this information.

Authorization to photocopy items for internal or personal use, or the internal or personal use of specific clients, is granted by Springhouse Corporation for users registered with the Copyright Clearance Center (CCC) Transactional Reporting Service, provided that the base fee of $00.00 per copy, plus $.75 per page, is paid directly to CCC, 27 Congress St., Salem, MA 01970. For those organizations that have been granted a photocopy license by CCC, a separate system of payment has been arranged. The fee code for users of the Transactional Reporting Service is 0874343798/92 $00.00 + $.75.

PHAR-031091

Library of Congress Cataloging-in-Publication Data
Clinical pharmacology and nursing/[edited by] Charold L. Baer, Bradley R. Williams — 2nd ed.
p. cm.
Includes bibliographical references and index.
1. Pharmacology.   2. Nursing.   I. Baer, Charold Lee Morris, 1946-   II. Williams, Bradley R.
[DNLM: 1. Drug Therapy — nurses' instruction. 2. Pharmacology, Clinical — nurses' instruction. QV 38 C6413]
RM301.C53 1992
615′.1 — dc20
DNLM/DLC   91-5078
ISBN 0-874234-379-8   CIP

CONTENTS

UNIT ONE: GENERAL PHARMACOLOGY

UNIT TWO: THE NURSING PROCESS AND DRUG ADMINISTRATION

UNIT FIVE: DRUGS TO PREVENT AND TREAT PAIN

UNIT SIX: DRUGS TO ALTER PSYCHOGENIC BEHAVIOR AND PROMOTE SLEEP

UNIT SEVEN: DRUGS TO IMPROVE CARDIOVASCULAR FUNCTION

UNIT EIGHT: DRUGS AFFECTING THE HEMATOLOGIC SYSTEM

UNIT NINE: DRUGS TO IMPROVE RESPIRATORY FUNCTION

APPENDICES AND INDEX

ADVISORY BOARD

CONSULTANTS

Senior Consultants

Marlene Ciranowicz, RN, MSN, CDE
Independent Consultant, Philadelphia

Lisa E. Kerr Knauss, RN, MSN, CCRN
Assistant Professor, West Chester (Pa.) University,
West Chester

Cindy Tryniszewski, RN, MSN, CS
Independent Consultant, Springhouse Corporation, and Critical
Care Nurse, Albert Einstein Medical Center, Northern
Division, Philadelphia

Bruce H. Livengood, PharmD, RPh
Associate Professor of Clinical Pharmacy, Duquesne
University, School of Pharmacy, Pittsburgh

Steven R. Abel, PharmD, RPh, Assistant Director of Pharmacy, Clinical and Educational Services, Indiana University Medical Center, Indianapolis

Anita L. Applegate, RN, MSN, Nurse Educator-Coordinator, Helene Fuld School of Nursing, Trenton, NJ

Alan D. Barreuther, PharmD, RPh, Clinical Associate Professor, University of Arizona, College of Pharmacy, Tucson; Manager, Drug Information, Tucson Medical Center

John M. Benson, PharmD, Assistant Professor of Pharmacy, University of Georgia, College of Pharmacy, Medical College of Georgia, Augusta

Bruce C. Carlstedt, PharmD, RPh, Associate Professor of Clinical Pharmacy, Purdue University, West Lafayette, Ind.

Peggy L. Carver, PharmD, Clinical Pharmacist, Infectious Diseases Service, and Assistant Professor of Pharmacy, University of Michigan, College of Pharmacy, Ann Arbor

N. Michael Davis, RPh, MS, Coordinator, Drug Information Center, University of Miami, Jackson Memorial Medical Center, Miami, Fla.

Lois S. Ellis, RN, EdD, CRNA, Director, Graduate Nursing and Professor, Indiana Wesleyan University, Marion

Melissa M. Furio, PharmD, Assistant Director for Clinical Services and Quality Assurance, Bryn Mawr (Pa.) Hospital, Department of Pharmacy

Douglas R. Geraets, PharmD, RPh, Assistant Professor of Clinical and Hospital Pharmacy, College of Pharmacy, University of Iowa, Iowa City

Bridget A. Haupt, PharmD, Assistant Director of Pharmacy, Thomas Jefferson University Hospital, Philadelphia

David W. Hawkins, PharmD, Professor and Assistant Dean, University of Georgia, College of Pharmacy, Athens

Martin D. Higbee, PharmD, Clinical Associate Professor, University of Arizona, College of Pharmacy, Tucson

Charles M. Karnack, PharmD, Clinical Pharmacy Specialist, Mercy Hospital of Pittsburgh; Instructor in Clinical Pharmacy, Duquesne University, School of Pharmacy

Patricia A. Keys, PharmD, Assistant Professor of Clinical Pharmacy, Duquesne University, School of Pharmacy, Pittsburgh

Mary Mirch, RN, MS, Assistant Professor, Glendale (Calif.) Community College

Anita Norton, RN, MSN, Instructor in Nursing, and Chair, Department of Nursing, Jefferson State Community College, Birmingham, Ala.

Robert B. Parker, PharmD, Assistant Professor, University of Georgia, College of Pharmacy, Medical College of Georgia, Augusta

David Piper, PharmD, RPh, Assistant Director for Clinical Services, Forbes Regional Health Center, Monroeville, Pa.

Theresa R. Prosser, PharmD, Assistant Professor, St. Louis (Mo.) College of Pharmacy

Lilliam Sklaver, PharmD, Clinical Pharmacist, Memorial Hospital, Hollywood, Fla.

Gary D. Smith, PharmD, RPh, Vice President, Planning and Development, Clinical Pharmacy Advantage, Minneapolis

Joseph F. Steiner, PharmD, RPh, Professor of Clinical Pharmacy, University of Wyoming, Schools of Human Medicine and Pharmacy, Casper

James A. Sterchele, PharmD, Clinical Specialist, Drug Information, Allegheny General Hospital, Pittsburgh

Raymond C. Stierer, PharmD, Clinical Specialist, Internal Medicine, Allegheny General Hospital, Pittsburgh

Robert L. Talbert, PharmD, FCCP, Professor, College of Pharmacy, University of Texas, Austin; Departments of Medicine and Pharmacology, University of Texas Health Science Center, San Antonio

Christine Vourakis, RN, DNSc, Associate Professor, Samuel Merritt College, Department of Nursing, Oakland, Calif.

Roberta J. Wong, PharmD, FASHP, Investigational Drug Pharmacist, UCLA Medical Center, Los Angeles

CONTRIBUTORS

Steven R. Abel, PharmD, RPh, Assistant Director of Pharmacy, Clinical and Educational Services, Indiana University Medical Center, Indianapolis

Kathleen G. Andreoli, RN, DSN, FAAN, Vice President, Nursing Affairs and The John L. and Helen Kellogg Dean, College of Nursing, Rush-Presbyterian-St. Luke's Medical Center, Rush University, Chicago

Charold L. Baer, RN, PhD, FCCM, CCRN, Professor, Department of Adult Health and Illness, Oregon Health Sciences University, School of Nursing, Portland

Naomi R. Ballard, RN, MA, MS, CNRN, Associate Professor, Department of Adult Health and Illness, Oregon Health Sciences University, School of Nursing, Portland

Carol L. Beck, PharmD, RPh, Doctoral Candidate, Vanderbilt University, Department of Pharmacology, Nashville, Tenn.

Rebecca E. Boehne, RN, PhD, Education Program Specialist, Portland VA Medical Center, Portland, Ore.

Karna Bramble, RN, MS, CGNP, Assistant Professor of Nursing, California State University, Department of Nursing, Long Beach

Barbara Gross Braverman, RN,CS, MSN, CS, Psychotherapist and Consultant, Private Practice, Philadelphia

Linda P. Brown, RN, PhD, FAAN, Associate Professor, University of Pennsylvania, School of Nursing, Philadelphia

Kathleen C. Byington, RN, MSN, Pediatric Clinical Specialist, Vanderbilt Children's Hospital, Vanderbilt University, Nashville, Tenn.

James D. Carlson, PharmD, RPh, Director, PRACS Institute, Fargo, N.D.

Bruce C. Carlstedt, PhD, RPh, Associate Professor of Clinical Pharmacy, Purdue University, Pharmacy Dept., Wishard Memorial Hospital, Indianapolis

Vivian Hayes Churness, RN, DNSc, Clinical Assistant Professor, University of Southern California, Department of Nursing, Los Angeles

Teresa Lyon Coluccio, RN, MN, Clinical Nurse Specialist, Oncology, Providence Medical Center, Seattle

N. Michael Davis, MS, RPh, Coordinator, Drug Information Center, University of Miami-Jackson Memorial Medical Center, Miami

Robin Donohoe Dennison, RN, MSN, CS, Critical Care Clinical Nurse Specialist, Central Baptist Hospital, Lexington, Ky.

Patricia A. Diehl, RN, BSN, MA, Associate Professor, West Virginia University, School of Nursing, Morgantown

Patricia Dillon, RN, MSN, Nursing Instructor, Gwynedd Mercy College, Gwynedd Valley, Pa.

Laura D'Oria, PharmD, RPh, Pharmacist, Community Medical Center, Toms River, N.J.

Belle Erickson, RN, PhD, Assistant Professor, Villanova (Pa.) University, College of Nursing

Carmel A. Esposito, RN, MSN, Educational Consultant and Coordinator of Continuing Education, Ohio Valley Hospital, School of Nursing, Steubenville

Janet M. Farahmand, CRN, MSN, EdD, Associate Professor, Neumann College, Aston, Pa.

Corre J. Garrett, RN, EdD, CCRN, Former Assistant Professor, East Carolina University, School of Nursing, Greenville, N.C.

Anna Gawlinski, RN, MSN, CCRN, Cardiovascular Clinical Nurse Specialist, University of California Medical Center, Los Angeles

Douglas R. Geraets, PharmD, RPh, Assistant Professor of Clinical and Hospital Pharmacy, College of Pharmacy, University of Iowa, Iowa City

Martin R. Giannamore, PharmD, RPh, Clinical Specialist, Riverside Methodist Hospitals, Columbus, Ohio

Richard K. Gibson, RN, MN, JD, CCRN, CS, Clinical Nurse Specialist, Veterans Administration Medical Center, San Diego

Barbara Given, RN, PhD, FAAN, Director of Nursing Graduate Program, College of Nursing, Michigan State University, East Lansing

Dean E. Goldberg, PharmD, Manager, Clinical Pharmacy Programs, United HealthCare Corporation, Minneapolis

Kathleen Whittaker Groves, RN, MS, Personnel Recruiter, The Visiting Nurse Association of Baltimore

Anne Myers Gudmundsen, RN, PhD, Director, Craniofacial Research and Publications, Humana Hospital, Medical City, Dallas

Bridget A. Haupt, PharmD, Assistant Director of Pharmacy, Thomas Jefferson University Hospital, Philadelphia

David W. Hawkins, PharmD, Professor and Assistant Dean, University of Georgia, College of Pharmacy, Athens

Marcia J. Hill, RN, MSN, Manager, Dermatologic Therapeutics, Methodist Hospital, Houston

Phyllis G. Hummel, RN, MSN, Chairman, Department of Nursing, North Dakota State University, Fargo

Sande Jones, RN, MSN, MSEd, Nursing Education Specialist, Mount Sinai Medical Center, Miami Beach

Lynne Kreutzer-Baraglia, RN, MS, Assistant Professor, Concordia University, West Suburban College of Nursing, Oak Park, Ill.

Eileen Hayes Lantier, RN, MSN, Assistant Professor, Syracuse (N.Y.) University, College of Nursing

Jan L. Lee, RN,CS, PhD, Assistant Professor of Nursing, University of Southern California, School of Nursing, Los Angeles

Colleen Lucas, RN,CS, MN, Medical-Surgical Clinical Nurse Specialist, Good Samaritan Hospital and Medical Center, Portland

Brenda L. Lyon, RN, DNS, Associate Professor and Chairperson, Department of Nursing of Adults, Indiana University, Indianapolis

Mary Y. Ma, PharmD, Associate Clinical Professor, University of Southern California School of Pharmacy; Assistant Professor, Clinical Pharmacy, University of Southern California at San Francisco

FOREWORD

The first responsibility of the authors, contributors, and reviewers of *Clinical Pharmacology and Nursing, Second Edition* is to use their extensive experience and knowledge to provide comprehensive, accurate, and current pharmacologic information and present that information in a practical format. This edition goes beyond that responsibility to show its information applied to patient care, which it does by using the steps of the nursing process. In 73 clearly formatted chapters that are grouped into 16 units and in 10 valuable appendices, this Second Edition does what earlier pharmacology texts have never been able to do — that is, forge an understandable link between theory and application. It does this by repeatedly underscoring clinical application of the drug information.

The text is divided into sixteen units. Unit One, General Pharmacology, provides a framework for understanding all aspects of pharmacology. The first chapter defines pharmacology and describes its scope and branches. Successive chapters address a specific pharmacology branch or topic: pharmacokinetics, pharmacodynamics, pharmacotherapeutics, and adverse drug reactions.

Unit Two, The Nursing Process and Drug Administration, provides the basic information that the nurse needs to become knowledgeable and competent in safe, therapeutic drug administration. Its first chapter describes the nursing process as a framework for delivering care, discussing each step of the nursing process in relation to drug therapy. This chapter sets the stage for the nursing process application information that appears in Units Three through Sixteen. Unit Two also presents general nursing responsibilities, such as using safeguards to prevent errors during drug administration, measuring and calculating dosages accurately, and administering drugs using the appropriate routes and techniques. After providing information about general responsibilities, the unit addresses specific nursing care for pediatric, geriatric, pregnant, and lactating patients.

Units Three through Sixteen, which cover individual drug classes, are organized according to the drugs' uses or effects.

Units Three through Six include drugs with widespread effects. Unit Three provides a brief overview of the autonomic nervous system and then describes the drugs that affect it — cholinergic, adrenergic, and neuromuscular blocking agents. After reviewing the central and peripheral nervous systems, Unit Four details skeletal muscle relaxing, antiparkinsonian, and anticonvulsant agents. Unit Five reviews the theories of pain and explores drugs used to prevent and treat pain, including general and local anesthetics. Unit Six covers central nervous system (CNS) drugs that alter behavior or promote sleep.

Units Seven through Ten investigate drugs used to treat dysfunctions in specific body systems: cardiovascular, hematologic, respiratory, and gastrointestinal. Unit Eleven emphasizes drugs used for fluid, electrolyte, and nutritional balance, which may be necessary for patients with dysfunctions in any body system.

Unit Twelve presents a wide range of drugs used to treat endocrine system disorders. Unit Thirteen provides an overview of immune and inflammatory responses in chapters that address drugs used to control inflammation, allergy, and organ rejection. Unit Fourteen includes seven chapters on drugs that prevent or treat infection, ranging from antibacterial and antitubercular agents to urinary anti-infective agents. Unit Fifteen reviews the pathophysiology of malignant neoplasms and describes drugs used to treat them. Unit Sixteen presents other major drugs, including ophthalmic, otic, and other agents.

The chapters in Units Three through Sixteen have consistent formats that assist the reader in learning and recalling information. Each chapter begins with learning objectives and a chapter introduction, presents information about one or more drug classes, and concludes with a chapter summary, study questions, and selected references. All information has been restudied in this Second Edition. *For each drug class,* the text provides detailed information about pharmacokinetics, pharmacodynamics, pharmacotherapeutics, adverse drug reactions, and nursing process application.

Useful appendices provide answers to study questions, commonly used — and commonly misinterpreted — abbreviations in drug therapy, and the taxonomy of the North American Nursing Diagnosis Association. They also cover emergency drugs, agents used for integumentary system diseases, agents that promote active and passive immunity, as well as how to deal with poisons and substance abuse. A thorough index makes all topics easily available to the reader.

Many features of this text make it an excellent resource. Its opening emphasis on pharmacologic fundamentals prepares the reader to understand and retain information in the drug chapters. Theory that is interwoven throughout helps establish and reinforce the strong conceptual framework. Use of the nursing process in the drug chapters aids in clinical application of drug information, narrowing the gap between knowing and doing. Up-to-the-minute drug information ensures that the student or nurse can know the most recent advances in drug therapy.

These features produce a resource that encourages critical thinking and promotes safe, therapeutic patient care. Written for nursing students, faculty, and practitioners by nurses, academicians, and pharmacists with outstanding credentials and experience, *Clinical Pharmacology and Nursing, Second Edition* is the newest and finest authoritative reference in its field. No nurse should practice without it.

Kathleen G. Andreoli, RN, DSN, FAAN
Vice President, Nursing Affairs
and the John L. and Helen Kellogg Dean
of the College of Nursing
Rush-Presbyterian-St. Luke's Medical Center,
Rush University, Chicago

PREFACE

Many factors make drug therapy a complex part of a nurse's responsibilities. The nurse who is to be well-prepared for this major activity must know:

- which drugs the patient is receiving
- the dosage and frequency for each drug
- each drug's probable interactions
- each drug's therapeutic and adverse effects.

Additionally, the nurse must:

- know or be able to verify the pharmacokinetics, pharmacodynamics, and pharmacotherapeutics for each drug a patient receives
- apply the nursing process by assessing the patient's response to the drug therapy, formulating appropriate nursing diagnoses, planning and implementing care (including patient teaching), and evaluating the patient's response to care.

Clinical Pharmacology and Nursing, Second Edition prepares the reader by providing extensive pharmacology information and a full understanding of nursing process application in drug therapy. Specifically, it includes:

- detailed coverage of all drug classes and of more than 900 generic drugs
- newly approved drugs
- updated information on all drugs included in the first edition
- a new chapter on uncategorized drugs
- several new drug-related appendices
- key points in each section, identified in **boldface italicized** type, that the reader can use when preparing care plans
- a set-off alphabetized list in each drug chapter of representative diagnoses (including problem and etiology statements) appropriate for patients receiving the drugs covered
- the complete list of diagnostic categories grouped by functional pattern, as approved by the North American Nursing Diagnosis Association (NANDA)
- single-answer, multiple-choice study questions and updated references in each chapter.

This text distinguishes itself by integrating the nursing process throughout and applying it to clinical practice. For each drug class, the text sequences nursing care through steps of the nursing process.

Because of its emphasis on pharmacologic principles and nursing process application, *Clinical Pharmacology and Nursing, Second Edition* can be used by the student nurse in a basic pharmacology course or in integrated pharmacology studies and in subsequent clinical courses or set-tings. It also can serve as a general reference book for the experienced clinician.

Organized in sixteen units, *Clinical Pharmacology and Nursing, Second Edition* provides a conceptual framework for organizing the information for clinical application. Unit One covers the fundamentals of pharmacology. Unit Two presents the nursing process as it relates to drug administration. Units Three through Sixteen discuss individual drug classes and related nursing care. Consistently structured, each chapter presents the following in-depth information for each drug class: pharmacokinetics; pharmacodynamics; pharmacotherapeutics, including drug interactions; adverse drug reactions; and nursing process application.

The text consistently uses highly effective pedagogical devices. Each chapter begins with objectives that focus the reader's attention and an introduction that establishes a context for the information that follows. The text promotes critical thinking in its systematic presentation and in its study questions. A chapter summary pulls together vital information and reinforces learning and recall. The summary and study questions provide a comprehensive review apparatus for the student. The chapter concludes with up-to-date selected references that are suitable for further exploration.

To highlight important themes and types of information and to promote access to and use of the information, the text includes the following recurring features.

- *Selected nursing diagnoses,* an alphabetized list of appropriate nursing diagnoses based on the chapter's content and the NANDA taxonomy.
- *Selected major drugs,* a ready reference chart that presents the major indications, usual adult dosages, contraindications, and precautions for each major drug currently in clinical use.
- *Drug interactions,* a chart including drugs that may interact with the prescribed medication, possible effects from this interaction, and appropriate nursing interventions or implications.
- *Unit Glossary* that defines important terms.

Throughout *Clinical Pharmacology and Nursing, Second Edition* charts, illustrations, bulleted lists, and other set-off treatments focus the reader's attention, promote deeper understanding, and summarize data for easy review and recall. These elements are intended for frequent reuse.

Supplementary materials support teaching and learning with this text. For each text chapter, the *Instructor's Resource Manual and Test Bank* includes a chapter overview, suggested lecture topics, student critical-thinking activities, selected nursing diagnoses for patients who receive drugs addressed in the chapter, and a test bank with answers and rationales. Particularly noteworthy are separate pages of test questions suitable for photocopying and overhead transparency masters on anatomy, physiology, and administration techniques. The *Student's Manual* presents extensive self-test materials, such as matching related elements, fill-in-the-blank completion exercises, and clinical simulations with study questions. It also provides answers for all of these self-tests. In addition, *Dosage Calculations Manual, Second Edition* contains pre-tests, post-tests, extensive reviews of key mathematical principles, and numerous practice exercises with answers. This easy-to-use workbook accommodates the student's need to review or learn in small increments, practice calculations and conversions, and become more proficient in preparing medications for administration.

To provide the most current, accurate, and clinically appropriate information, the text and its supplements were written by practicing clinicians, academicians, and pharmacists — all of whom are at least master's-degree prepared. All materials were reviewed extensively by nurses and pharmacists from appropriate specialty areas. The combined efforts of these experts have produced a resource that is fully in step with today's nursing curriculum.

GENERAL PHARMACOLOGY

Today, many people use pharmacotherapeutic agents (drugs) rather liberally. Their drug use may encompass a wide range of products, from over-the-counter substances such as aspirin to controlled substances such as morphine.

The nurse must consider routine drug use—and the accompanying drug interactions and toxic effects—a major health problem for patients. As a result, the nurse must know the physiologic and psychological alterations produced by specific drugs and their interactions. Furthermore, the nurse must know how certain patient traits influence pharmacokinetics, pharmacodynamics, and pharmacotherapeutics. Such information is as necessary for providing optimum patient care as knowing the name, classification, onset and duration of action, dosage range, route of administration, contraindications, potential adverse drug reactions, drug interactions, and predicted outcomes of a specific drug.

OVERVIEW OF CHAPTERS

The information in Unit One provides a framework for understanding all of these aspects of pharmacology. Each chapter introduces a concept fundamental to drug therapy to provide a basis for understanding the drugs discussed later in the text.

Chapter 1
Introduction to Pharmacology

Chapter 1 defines pharmacology, describes its scope, and graphically depicts its five branches: pharmacokinetics, pharmacodynamics, pharmacotherapeutics, toxicology, and pharmacognosy. It introduces terminology and drug nomenclature that the nurse needs to know to make drug therapy decisions. Then the chapter provides a brief history of events significant to the evolution of pharmacology. After explaining pharmacognosy, it concludes with an overview of the development process for a new drug and the legal regulations and standards governing drug use.

Chapter 2
Pharmacokinetics

Chapter 2 presents the pharmacokinetic properties of a drug, including drug absorption, distribution, metabolism, and excretion. It also examines the onset of action, peak concentration, and duration of action as well as drug bioavailability and blood concentration levels. Throughout this discussion, it emphasizes the significance of these principles to nursing care.

Chapter 3
Pharmacodynamics

Chapter 3 describes drug pharmacodynamics, or the mechanisms by which drugs produce biochemical or physiologic changes in the body. It begins by discussing the mechanisms of action, highlighting drug action (interaction at the cellular level between a drug and cell components) and drug effect (the response resulting from the drug action). Next it describes the interaction between drugs and receptors and the outcome of drug action. Then the chapter graphically depicts various dose-response curves and relates drug potency and efficacy to those curves. It concludes by discussing the therapeutic index, a concept vital to safe drug therapy.

Chapter 4
Pharmacotherapeutics

Chapter 4 explores the pharmacotherapeutics of drugs, or the use of drugs to treat disease. After describing the different types of therapy, it explores the use of drugs to prevent, diagnose, and treat diseases. It continues by discussing factors that influence the choice of therapy and the patient's response to drugs during therapy. It concludes with an overview of drug interactions with other drugs, food, and laboratory tests.

Glossary

Absorption: process by which a drug leaves an administration site, passes through or across tissue into the general circulation, and becomes biologically available.

Active transport: use of cellular energy to move a drug from an area of low concentration to one of higher concentration.

Adverse drug reaction: undesirable patient response ranging from mild effects to severe, life-threatening hypersensitivity reactions. These reactions can be dose-related or patient-sensitivity-related.

Agonist: drug that has an affinity for a receptor and enhances or stimulates the receptor's functional properties.

Antagonist: drug that occupies a receptor and inhibits the receptor's functional properties.

Bioavailability: extent to which a drug's active ingredient is absorbed and transported to its site of action.

Distribution: degree to which an absorbed or intravenous drug is delivered to various body fluids and tissues.

Drug: pharmacologic agent or medication capable of interacting with living organisms to produce biological effects.

Drug action: interaction between a drug and cellular constituents.

Drug effect: response from a drug's action.

Drug excretion: process of drug elimination from the body.

Drug interactions: relationships between concurrently administered drugs that result in alterations in the therapeutic effects of any or all of the drugs.

First-pass effect: process by which orally administered drugs progress from the intestinal lumen to the hepatic system and undergo partial metabolism before entering the general circulation.

Half-life: time required to metabolize or inactivate the total amount of a drug in a person's body by 50%.

Ligands: endogenous substances, such as hormones, neurotransmitters, or autocoids, that interact with a receptor to produce a response.

Metabolism: biological process of altering or converting a drug from its present form to an inactive substance. Also called biotransformation.

Nonprescription drug: drug considered safe and effective when used according to proper direction by consumers without a physician's supervision. Also called over-the-counter (OTC) drug.

Orphan drug: drug useful for treating disease but undeveloped by a company, usually because of a limited market (such as a drug for a rare disease) or high-risk adverse effects.

Passive transport: movement of a drug from an area of high concentration to one of lower concentration without expending cellular energy.

Peak concentration level: point at which drug absorption and elimination are equal.

Pharmacodynamics: study of the biochemical and physical effects and mechanisms of action of drugs in living organisms.

Pharmacognosy: study of the natural sources of drugs, such as plants, animals, and minerals, and their products.

Pharmacokinetics: study of a drug's alterations as it is absorbed into, distributed through, metabolized in, and excreted from a living organism.

Pharmacology: scientific study of the origin, nature, chemistry, effects, and uses of drugs.

Pharmacotherapeutics: use or clinical indications of drugs to prevent, diagnose, and treat disease in living organisms.

Pinocytosis: movement of a drug by cellular engulfment.

Prescription drug: drug safely used only under the supervision of a person licensed to prescribe and dispense in accordance with a state's laws.

Pro-drug: precursor of a drug that becomes dissociated (separated into molecular fragments) and forms the parent drug.

Receptor: specialized reactive substance or large group of molecules that interlocks with a drug molecule. The interaction of a drug and its receptor should result in a drug effect, or pharmacologic response.

Therapeutic index: relationship between a drug's therapeutic effects and adverse effects. Also called margin of safety.

Tolerance: decreased response or sensitivity of a receptor to a drug at the same dose over a period of time.

Toxicity: condition caused by excess drug in the body.

Volume of distribution: concept that relates the amount of a drug in the body to the concentration of the drug in the blood.

Chapter 5
Adverse Drug Reactions

Chapter 5 discusses key concepts related to adverse drug reactions. It presents information about predisposing factors related to the patient, such as age, genetic variations, and disease state; to the drug, such as bioavailability, administration routes, and multiple drug therapy; and to exogenous factors, such as diet and environment. Then it describes the two classifications of adverse drug reactions: dose-related and patient-sensitivity-related adverse reactions.

INTRODUCTION TO PHARMACOLOGY

OBJECTIVES

After reading and studying this chapter, the student should be able to:

1. Differentiate among the five branches of pharmacology: pharmacokinetics, pharmacodynamics, pharmacotherapeutics, toxicology, and pharmacognosy.

2. Briefly define prescription, nonprescription, controlled, and recreational drugs.

3. Explain the differences among a drug's chemical, generic, and trade names.

4. Trace the history of drug research from traditional natural materials—plants, animals, minerals—to chemicals, enzymes, and hormones.

5. Describe the four phases required by the Food and Drug Administration (FDA) for approval and marketing of a new drug.

6. Explain why orphan drugs can be unprofitable, even though they may be needed.

7. Describe two consequences of the Federal Food, Drug, and Cosmetic Act (FFDCA) of 1906.

8. Define the five schedules of controlled drugs.

9. Explain these six drug properties: purity, bioavailability, potency, efficacy, safety, and toxicity.

10. List several sources of relevant drug information, including pharmacopeias and compendia, available to nurses.

INTRODUCTION

Chapter 1 defines pharmacology and describes its scope. Beginning with the historical evolution of pharmacology as a science, the chapter presents important terminology and drug nomenclature (names), sources, types, development, regulations, and standards. All cover vital information that nurses must have to fulfill major responsibilities.

The increasing numbers, kinds, and complexities of new drugs require that every clinician's knowledge of pharmacology be updated continually.

DEFINITION AND SCOPE

Pharmacology—one of the most dynamic aspects of nursing—represents the scientific study of the origin, nature, chemistry, effects, and uses of drugs. (For an illustration of the different categories that constitute this science, see *Five branches of pharmacology,* page 4.)

Pharmacokinetics refers to the absorption, distribution, metabolism, and excretion of a drug in a living organism. *Pharmacodynamics* is the study of the biochemical and physical effects of drugs and the mechanisms of drug actions in living organisms. *Pharmacotherapeutics* (clinical pharmacology) is a general term covering the use of drugs (clinical indications) in the prevention and treatment of disease. Most of a nurse's drug-related functions fall under this heading. *Toxicology* represents the study of poisons, including the adverse effects of drugs on living organisms. Detailed discussions of pharmacokinetics, pharmacodynamics, pharmacotherapeutics, and toxicology appear in Chapters 2, 3, 4, and 5 respectively. A discussion of poisons (a branch of toxicology) appears in the Appendix. *Pharmacognosy* deals with natural drugs—that is, plants, animals, or minerals and their products. It is discussed later in this chapter.

Pharmacology is an interdisciplinary science. Although most students traditionally associate chemistry with pharmacology, the physical, biological, and social sciences also contribute information on using drugs to achieve and main-

Five branches of pharmacology

An extensive science, pharmacology includes absorption, distribution, metabolism, and excretion (pharmacokinetics); biochemical and physical effects, and mechanism of action (pharmacodynamics); clinical indications or uses (pharmacotherapeutics); toxicity and adverse reactions (toxicology); and natural sources of drugs (pharmacognosy).

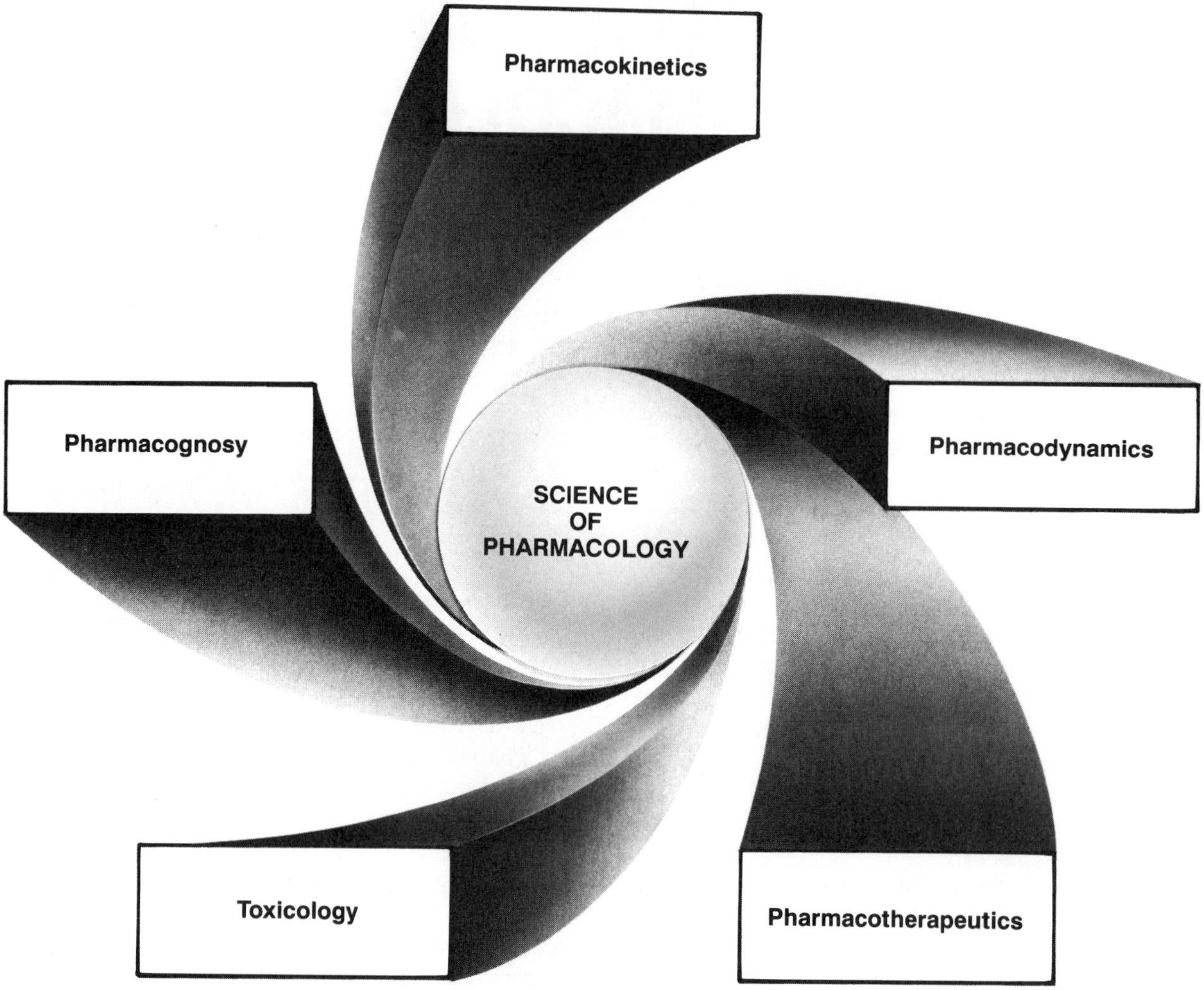

Pharmacokinetics

Pharmacognosy

Pharmacodynamics

SCIENCE OF PHARMACOLOGY

Toxicology

Pharmacotherapeutics

tain optimum health without causing toxicity or patient dependence.

TERMINOLOGY

Nurses must know the following terminology to enhance their own understanding and to enable them to interpret information for patients.

A *drug* (medication) is a pharmacologic agent that is capable of interacting with living organisms to produce biological effects.

A *prescription drug* can only be used safely under the supervision of a health care professional who is licensed to prescribe or dispense drugs according to state laws.

A *nonprescription drug* (over-the-counter, or OTC, drug) can be used by consumers safely without the supervision of a licensed health care practitioner, provided consumers follow the directions.

A *controlled drug* may lead to drug abuse or drug dependence and therefore its use is controlled by federal, state, and local laws.

Drug abuse describes the self-directed use of drugs for nontherapeutic purposes, a practice that does not comply with a culture's sociocultural norms.

Drug dependence results when a person cannot control drug intake. Drug dependence may be physiologic, psychological, or both.

Drug misuse, the improper use of common drugs, can lead to acute and chronic toxicity with such problems as gastrointestinal bleeding, kidney damage, or liver damage.

A *recreational drug* is one used for its pleasant psychological or physical effects with no therapeutic intent.

DRUG NOMENCLATURE

A drug's *chemical name* precisely describes its atomic and molecular structure. When a manufacturer wishes to market a promising new drug, the United States Adopted Names (USAN) Council selects a *generic name.* (The USAN is sponsored by the American Medical Association, American Pharmaceutical Association, and the United States Pharmacopeial Convention, Inc.) Typically derived from a drug's chemical name, its generic name usually is shorter—abbreviated for simplicity. The drug company selling the product selects its *trade name* (also known as the brand name or proprietary name). Trade names are protected by copyright. The symbol ® after the trade name indicates that the name is registered by and restricted to the drug manufacturer. Because pharmacies stock various trade-name drugs, nurses can avoid confusion by always using the generic name when speaking or writing about a drug. In 1962, the federal government mandated the use of *official names* so that only one official name would represent each drug. The official names are listed in the United States Pharmacopeia (USP) and National Formulary (NF). (For examples of various names assigned to drugs, see *Drug nomenclature.*)

Drugs that share similar characteristics are grouped together as a pharmacologic class (family), such as beta blockers. A second grouping is the therapeutic classification, which groups drugs by therapeutic use and is illustrated by antihypertensives. Thiazides and beta blockers are both antihypertensives, but they share few characteristics as the discussions in later chapters show.

Another way to group drugs is by using a prototype (representative) drug for each drug class. This grouping is used primarily as a method for teaching pharmacology. Some authorities claim that focusing on a prototype drug improves understanding of the drug class and recognition of the occasional drug with unique properties. However, the prototype system has two disadvantages. First, a particular drug may be retained as the prototype although a new drug in that class is clinically superior. For example, in the cardiac glycoside class, digitalis serves as the prototype, but the newer drug digoxin has proven to be more

Drug nomenclature

A drug has at least three names: chemical, generic, and trade. The surest way to avoid confusion is to use the generic name. Note that a drug may have several trade names. The ones listed here are examples only, not inclusive.

CHEMICAL NAME	GENERIC NAME	TRADE NAME
6-chloro-2*H*-1,2,4- benzothiadiazine-7-sulfonamide 1,1-dioxide	chlorothiazide	Diuril®
7-chloro-1,3-dihydro-1-methyl-5-phenyl-2H-1,4-benzodiazepin-2-one	diazepam	Valium®
ethyl 1-methyl-4-phenylisonipecotate hydrochloride	meperidine	Demerol®
[2,3-dichloro-4-(2-methylene-butyryl)- phenoxy] acetic acid	ethacrynic acid	Edecrin®
acetylsalicylic acid	aspirin	Ecotrin®
17,21-dihydroxypregna-1,4-diene-3,11,20-trione	prednisone	Deltasone® Meticorten®
magnesium hydroxide Mg(OH)$_2$	magnesium salts	Phillips Milk of Magnesia®

clinically significant. This may give the student the false impression that the prototype is the major drug in clinical use. Second, the student may assume that the drug characteristics and administration concerns for the prototype apply to all drugs in the class, which may not be true.

HISTORICAL PERSPECTIVE

History can help nurses see the development and uses of drugs in religious, social, and political contexts. (For a chronological list of important contributions in this branch of pharmacology and the names of the people responsible for the contributions, see *Historical development of pharmacotherapeutics,* pages 6 and 7.) The following discussion reviews important developments chronologically.

(Text continues on page 8.)

Historical development of pharmacotherapeutics

Interest in and experiments with plants, animals, and minerals as drugs began early in our history. Much later, in the 19th century, drug research shifted from traditional natural materials to chemical synthesis and manipulation of enzymes and hormones.

PERIOD OF HISTORY	DEVELOPERS	CONTRIBUTIONS
Before 3000 B.C.	Early physician figures known in various cultures as shamans, witch doctors, medicine men	Toxins to kill animals for food Cathartics and emetics Alcohol for anesthesia Bark of willow tree to relieve joint stiffness Salt as an essential ingredient for health
From 2700 B.C. through the beginning of the Christian era		
2700 B.C.	Chinese	Textbook of medicine recommending plants, such as rhubarb and senna, as laxatives
2100 B.C.	Inhabitants of the Euphrates River Valley (now Iraq)	Clay tablets written in cuneiform script containing medical prescriptions
2000 B.C.	Inhabitants of Babylonia, also located along the Euphrates River	Hammurabi's code of law protecting patients from medical malpractice
2000 B.C.	North American Indians (Iroquois)	Herbs used to stimulate the sense of taste
2000 B.C.	South American Indians (Incas of Peru)	Herbs used for diuretics, to relieve respiratory distress
1500 B.C.	Egyptian medical papyrus, known today as Ebers's Medical Papyrus	Scroll containing prescriptions for over 700 drugs, including aloe, castor oil, vinegar, opium, and peppermint; remedies were prepared as pills, powders, gargles, salves, and poultices
1500 B.C.	Hebrew priest-physicians and health inspectors living in what was then known as Palestine, now divided between Israel and Jordan	Wine and vinegar used for medicine Fig poultices Mosaic Health Code
600 B.C	Zoroastrian priest-physicians of Persia (now Iran)	Drugs used to stimulate uterine contractions; specialized medical practice divided among three groups—one specialty group used herbs for treatment
400 B.C.	The Greek physician, Hippocrates (father of medicine)	Mentions 400 drugs in his writings; however, used drugs selectively
200 B.C.	Hindu priests in India	Recognized colchicum, castor beans, and digitalis

PERIOD OF HISTORY	DEVELOPERS	CONTRIBUTIONS
From the 1st century through the 19th century A.D.		
100	Dioscorides, a Greek living in Rome	Wrote *De Materia Medica,* a textbook on medical materials
200	A Greek living in Rome named Galen (disciple of Hippocrates)	Originated many preparations from vegetables (galenicals), such as cold cream
500	Arabs living in Palestine, Egypt, North Africa, and Spain	Spread their knowledge of many drugs such as musk, myrrh, tamarind, and cloves Originated syrups, juleps, and aromatic water Pharmacy practiced separately from medicine
610	The Arab physician Avicenna	Wrote *Canon of Medicine*
1000 to 1500	Monastery gardeners of Europe	Cultivated herbs, such as clover, primrose, and belladonna, for medicinal purposes
1500 through 1700	Scientists working during the Renaissance in Europe	Beginnings of empirical chemistry—plants were classified; relationship of drug dose to toxicity was recognized
1526	German physician and alchemist Paracelsus	Investigated use of metals for medicinal purposes
1618	English scientists	First London pharmacopeia was published
1785	English, William Withering	Described medicinal uses of foxglove
1815	German, Frederick Sertürner	Isolated the alkaloid of morphine from opium
1842	American, Crawford Long	Used ether as a general anesthetic agent
In the 20th century		
1907	German, Paul Ehrlich	Discovered Salvarsan as a treatment for syphilis
1908	German, Gelmo	Discovered sulfanilamide
1922	Canadians, Banting, Best, and Macleod	Discovered insulin for treatment of diabetes mellitus
1929	English, Sir Alexander Fleming	Discovered penicillin
1955	American, Jonas Salk	Discovered poliomyelitis vaccine with inactivated (killed) virus
1970s and 1980s	Scientists worldwide	Purified drugs prepared from traditional natural materials; drugs include oral contraceptives, synthetic analogues of human sex hormones Chemical synthesis of drugs and manipulation of biological products, such as enzymes and hormones

Before 3000 B.C.

Early in the development of pharmacotherapeutics, people relied primarily on empirical methods (trial and error) when dealing with illness. Observations of animals and their eating habits helped primitive people conclude that what they ate provided nutritional or medicinal benefits, or both. Hunters learned to smear vegetable substances, such as ouabain, on arrowheads to stun or kill animals. Others learned how to ferment carbohydrate substances, such as grapes, potatoes, or rice, to yield alcohol, which they then used for its anesthetic effects.

At times, illness became so severe that tribes or settlements needed an expert to provide therapy. Thus emerged the physician figure, called in various societies a shaman, medicine man, or witch doctor. Because illness was equated with possession by evil spirits, the physician figure commonly gave his patients a vile-tasting concoction (often purgatives or laxatives) to drive out the evil spirits. Such "magical remedies" were passed on verbally from generation to generation.

From 2700 B.C. through the beginning of the Christian era

The earliest known written accounts of mixtures used for medicinal purposes appeared in Sumeria in 2100 B.C. The Sumerians, who lived in the Valley of the Euphrates River (now Iraq), preserved their prescriptions in cuneiform script on clay tablets. Although the Sumerians are credited with the first written prescriptions, the Chinese compiled a textbook dated about 2700 B.C. that documented the medicinal uses of plants and other natural substances. Some of the textbook's suggestions, such as the effectiveness of rhubarb and senna as laxatives, are still used today. Less effective remedies, such as the use of rhinoceros horn as an aphrodisiac, also appear in the text.

During his reign, the Babylonian ruler Hammurabi developed a code of laws used in the courts. Some of the laws in Hammurabi's code protected citizens from unskilled physicians and unnecessary medical procedures. The laws specified penalties and rewards for unsuccessful or successful treatments of disease.

Around the same time, Indian civilizations in North and South America were using herbs for ceremonial and medicinal purposes. For example, in North America, the Iroquois tribe chewed herbs to stimulate the sense of taste. In South America, the Incas used herbs as diuretics and to relieve respiratory distress.

In 1874, Georg Ebers, a German Egyptologist, edited a medical papyrus that he had discovered on an expedition to Egypt. Ebers's Medical Papyrus, a scroll about 22 feet long, indicates that some drug preparations had been standardized as early as 1500 B.C. Although Ebers's Medical Papyrus primarily contains information about substances that prevent decay of a body after death, it also gives many

prescriptions for substances used to treat the living. Additionally, it indicates that remedies were prepared in various forms, including tablets, powders, gargles, salves, and poultices.

By 1500 B.C., the Hebrew civilization in Palestine had developed remarkable hygienic and sanitary practices. The Mosaic Health Code addressed many aspects of life in the society, from personal hygiene to environmental protection.

The Persians, a group of Iranian tribes welded into a nation by Cyrus the Great in 600 B.C., practiced a religion known as Zoroastrianism. The Zoroastrians' sacred book, the Avesta, contains ceremonial rites relating to birth and death that were performed by Zoroastrian priests. Besides the priests, three types of physicians practiced medicine in Persia: those who healed with the knife, with herbs, and with holy words.

The Greeks were leaders in many creative areas including art, architecture, philosophy, and medicine. Hippocrates, commonly known as the father of medicine, practiced an early form of patient-centered (holistic) medicine. Hippocrates mentioned many drugs in his writings, but his clinical studies indicate that he used only a few of what we consider important drugs. For example, he prescribed opium for pain relief.

Around 200 B.C. in India, Hindu priests wrote about pharmacology, citing such preparations as colchicum, gentian, castor beans, and digitalis.

From the 1st century through the 19th century A.D.

Greeks who emigrated to Rome from the 1st to the 3rd centuries A.D. took the practice of medicine with them. Galen, a Greek physician living in Rome, pioneered the preparation of vegetables as medicinal aids (galenicals). Dioscorides, another Greek physician who journeyed to Rome, specialized in botany and wrote a text on drugs and their uses, *De Materia Medica*.

For several hundred years after the fall of the Roman Empire, Arabs settled throughout the Holy Land, Egypt, North Africa, and Spain. The Arabs were especially interested in medicine, chemistry, and pharmacy. They blended the scientific knowledge of the Greeks, Romans, and Jews with the ancient astrology of Egypt and India. The Arabs concocted many new drugs, using musk, myrrh, tamarind, and cloves and originated syrups, juleps, and aromatic water. In the Arab culture, pharmacy was practiced separately from medicine, and Arab pharmacists developed the prototype for the London Pharmacy.

The Middle Ages, a term commonly applied to the period between the 5th century and the middle of the 15th century, saw little advancement in the science of pharmacology, which returned to a primitive empiricism. Priests in monasteries throughout Europe were almost solely responsible for the preservation of ancient texts and prescriptions. In the monastery gardens (particularly those of the Benedictine order), the monks perpetuated the ancient practice of growing herbs for medicinal purposes.

With the Renaissance in the 15th century came a renewed interest in the accomplishments of the past. The revival applied to the visual arts, architecture, and literature, as well as to science, including pharmacology. Paracelsus, the son of a German physician and chemist, traveled widely throughout Europe, studying folk medicine and investigating the use of metals for medicinal purposes.

In the years after the Renaissance, pharmacologic advancements occurred frequently. In London, the first pharmacopeia was published in 1618. The London College of Physicians sponsored the pharmacopeia, with King James I mandating its use throughout the British realm. In the late 18th century, William Withering described the medicinal uses of foxglove.

In the 19th century, pharmacology started to become a highly specialized science. The first great pharmaceutical discovery occurred in 1815 when Frederick Sertürner isolated the alkaloid morphine from opium. This led to considerable research into the isolation of active components of drugs. Researchers conducted enthusiastic studies on vegetable drugs. Research in the 19th century also focused on the effects of chemicals on organs and tissues. In 1842, in the United States, Crawford Long first used ether to produce general anesthesia.

The 20th century

During the 20th century, drugs have become more chemical than botanical. In 1907, the German Paul Ehrlich introduced Salvarsan to treat syphilis; in 1922, Banting, Best, and Macleod discovered insulin. Both developments represent landmarks in the history of the 20th century. Gelmo's discovery of sulfanilamide in 1908 provided a breakthrough for other researchers who had hoped that chemotherapeutic agents would effectively combat infectious diseases. Still, the therapeutic effect of sulfanilamide was not fully recognized until 1932. Likewise, Sir Alexander Fleming's discovery of penicillin in 1929 did not immediately lead to use of the drug in therapy. Finally, penicillin was used to treat patients in 1942, when Dr. Howard Florey of Oxford University came to the United States and asked for the assistance of the National Research Council in studying penicillin. In 1955, the new poliomyelitis vaccines were hailed as providing relief from that dreaded disease.

In 1962, the Kefauver-Harris drug amendment was passed. The amendment requires proof of a drug's efficacy as well as its safety. Since passage of the amendment, the introduction of new drugs has required more time for clinical trials, yet new drugs valuable to the prevention and treatment of diseases continually become available.

The basic approach to drug development has changed since the middle of the 20th century. Although scientists still use the traditional natural materials as ingredients for drugs, theys increasingly develop drugs through chemical synthesis or the manipulation of biological products, such as enzymes and hormones. Indeed, 20th-century pharmacology has grown into a complex science involving a vast drug-manufacturing industry.

At the same time, many people have remained or become interested in natural products, including the commonly referred to "natural" foods and herbal remedies. The administration of and experimentation with herbal medicines may lead to the discovery of new and valuable drugs, although not without risk. For example, impurities in a newly discovered natural drug may cause adverse physical reactions. Therefore, the manufacturers of new natural drugs should identify all of the active ingredients and reliably produce purified drugs.

The future of pharmacology necessitates a balance between technology and the natural order. While promoting technology to improve the quality of life, scientists and manufacturers must take care to avoid toxic effects on patients and the environment. The readily available drug supply also creates a tremendous potential for drug abuse and misuse, which drains human productivity, increases crime, and overburdens law enforcement agencies.

Research constantly adds to the body of drug information recorded. (For a list of major information sources available to health care professionals, see *Sources of drug information,* page 10.)

PHARMACOGNOSY

Traditionally, *pharmacognosy* refers to the study of natural drug sources, such as plants, animals, or minerals and their products. Today, however, chemicals developed and used in the laboratory allow researchers to increase the number of drug sources. For example, oral contraceptives, which are synthetic analogues of human sex hormones, are manufactured chemically. Chemically developed drugs are free of the impurities found in natural substances.

Researchers and drug developers also can now manipulate the molecular structure of substances, such as antibiotics, so that a slight change in the chemical structure makes the drug effective against different organisms. The first-generation cephalosporins, produced by an organism cultured in seawater, were effective against the organisms *Streptococcus, Staphylococcus, Escherichia coli, Proteus mirabilis,* and *Shigella.* Subsequent chemically altered structures of cephalosporins (second and third generation) effectively treat infections caused by *Bacteroides fragilis*

Sources of drug information

Many types of publications help fulfill the need of physicians, nurses, and pharmacists for up-to-date and detailed drug information. The nurse in a clinical situation may need to consult various references to obtain all of the necessary information. The following are reliable sources:

Pharmacopeia – Official
• The United States Pharmacopeia (USP) and National Formulary (NF)
• The British Pharmacopeia (BP)
• The British National Formulary (BF)

Compendia – Nonofficial
• Martindale: The Extra Pharmacopeia
• Drug Information – American Hospital Formulary Service, published by authority of American Society of Hospital Pharmacists
• Facts and Comparisons
• USP Dispensing Information

Pharmaceutical Firms
• Physicians' Desk Reference (PDR)
• Package inserts – brochures required by law. Content is approved by the FDA.

Journal
• The Medical Letter on Drugs and Therapeutics

and *Haemophilus influenzae* (second generation) and *Pseudomonas* (third generation).

The hormone insulin, used to treat diabetes mellitus, was customarily obtained from the pancreata of slaughtered animals, mainly cattle and pigs. Although animal insulin is not chemically identical to human insulin, it is physiologically active in humans. Porcine insulin (derived from pigs) most nearly resembles human insulin. The chemical alteration of three amino acids in porcine insulin makes it identical to human endogenous insulin. The chemically altered porcine insulin is marketed and usually referred to as "human insulin." Drug developers also can manufacture human insulin from bacteria.

Plant sources of drugs

In most cases, the earliest concoctions using plants as drug sources consisted of the entire plant, including leaves, roots, bulb, stem, seeds, buds, and blossoms. Much extraneous material, some of it harmful to human tissues, found its way into the mixture. The active components in the crude mixture caused the drug's effect. As the understanding of plants as drug sources became more sophisticated, researchers sought to isolate the active components and avoid the extraneous material.

The active components consist of several types and vary in character and effect. The most important are alkaloids (one of the largest groups of active components), which act as alkali. The organic alkaloids react with acids to form a salt. This salt, a neutralized or partially neutralized form, is more readily soluble in body fluids. The names of alkaloids and their salts usually end in *-ine;* examples include atropine, caffeine, and nicotine.

Other active components include glycosides, gums, resins, and oils. As glycosides decompose, they yield sugars and an aglycon, or the noncarbohydrate group of a glycoside molecule. Names of glycosides usually end in *-in,* as in digitoxin and digoxin. Gums, usually polysaccharides producing viscous solutions, constitute another group of active components. Gums give products the ability to attract and hold water. Examples include seaweed extractions and seeds with starch. Resins, of which the chief source is pine tree sap, commonly act as local irritants or as laxatives and caustic agents. Oils, thick and sometimes greasy liquids, are classified as volatile or fixed. Examples of volatile oils include peppermint, spearmint, and juniper. Fixed oils, not easily evaporated, include castor oil and olive oil.

Animal sources of drugs

The body fluids or glands of animals can act as sources of drugs. The drugs obtained from animal sources include hormones, such as insulin; oils and fats (usually fixed), such as cod-liver oil; and enzymes, produced by living cells, which act as catalysts. Enzymes include pancreatin and pepsin. Vaccines (suspensions of killed, modified, or attenuated microorganisms) also are obtained from animal sources.

Mineral sources of drugs

Metallic and nonmetallic minerals provide various inorganic materials not available from plants or animals. The mineral sources are used as they occur in nature or are combined with other ingredients to yield acids, bases, or salts. For example, coal tar, an acid, yields salicylic acid, aluminum hydroxide (a base), and sodium chloride (a salt).

Laboratory-produced (chemical) sources of drugs

Today's researchers produce an ever-increasing number of drugs in the laboratory. The new drugs may be organic (from animal or vegetable life forms) or inorganic substances or a combination of the two. Examples of drugs produced in the laboratory include penicillin (organic), sulfonamides and oral contraceptives (inorganic), and propylthiouracil (combination organic and inorganic). Recombinant deoxyribonucleic acid (DNA) research has led to another chemical source of organic compounds: the reordering of genetic information enables scientists to develop bacteria that produce insulin for humans.

NEW DRUG DEVELOPMENT

In the past, drugs were found by trial and error. Now, they are developed primarily by systematic scientific research. Scientists still search for new organic and inorganic sources; however, they now focus most of their attention on the laboratory to discover needed drugs.

The Food and Drug Administration (FDA) carefully monitors new drug development, which can take many years to complete. Testing of new drugs begins with animals to determine the drug's pharmacologic use, dosage ranges, and possible toxic effects. Only after reviewing extensive animal studies and data on the safety and effectiveness of the proposed drug will the FDA approve the application for an Investigational New Drug (IND).

Four phases of clinical evaluation involving human subjects follow approval of the IND. The clinical studies are intended to provide information on purity, bioavailability, potency, efficacy, safety, and toxicity. Depending on the results of testing, the studies can be stopped at any phase.

Phase I

In phase I, a clinical pharmacologist supervises studies involving a small number of healthy volunteers. All effects of the drug on the volunteers are recorded. The recorded clinical data determine the need for further testing.

Phase II

A small number of individuals who have the disease for which the drug is purported to be diagnostic or therapeutic are then given the drug. Supervisors carefully document toxic effects and adverse reactions to determine the drug's proper dosage. Researchers then review and compare data from the animal studies and human studies, closely monitoring drug effects on animal and human fertility and reproduction.

Phase III

In phase III, large numbers of patients in medical research centers receive the drug. This larger sampling provides information about infrequent or rare adverse effects. Information collected during this phase helps determine any risks associated with the new drug. Researchers also must perform various tests that take into account those patients who are so emotionally involved that they experience relief of symptoms based on suggestion. The administration of a placebo, a medically inert substance, to some patients provides control for such psychological responses. In one frequently used procedure, one-half of the patients receive the drug and one-half receive the placebo. To remove all bias, neither the patients nor the physician knows who has received the drug and who has received the placebo until completion of the study, known as a double-blind study. In another type of study (crossover study), patients receive the drug for part of the time and a placebo for the rest of the time.

After the first three phases, the FDA evaluates the results. If the FDA announces a favorable evaluation, the company developing the drug then completes a New Drug Application (NDA). FDA approval of the company's NDA means that the new drug has been accepted and can be marketed exclusively by its sponsoring company.

Phase IV

After the NDA is approved, the drug company begins surveillance or post-market surveillance. It receives from physicians reports about the therapeutic results of the drug. The company must communicate adequately with the FDA and with the public during the drug's use. Some medications, such as benoxaprofen (Oraflex), have been found to be toxic and have been removed from the market after their initial release. At times, manufacturers have contended that a drug's benefits for a certain segment of the population outweigh its risks. Such was the manufacturer's response when the antidepressant tranylcypromine was withdrawn from the market. Eventually but with certain restrictions, the FDA reinstated tranylcypromine in the market for use by severely depressed patients.

Expedited drug approval

Although most INDs undergo all four phases of clinical evaluation, a few can receive expedited approval. For example, because of the public health threat posed by acquired immune deficiency syndrome (AIDS), the FDA and drug companies have agreed to shorten the IND approval process, allowing physicians to give qualified AIDS patients so-called Treatment INDs not yet approved by the FDA. Sponsors of drugs that reach Phase II or III clinical trials can apply for FDA approval of Treatment IND status. When approved, the sponsor supplies the IND to physicians whose patients meet appropriate criteria.

ORPHAN DRUGS

Some drugs useful to treat various diseases never reach the market. Drug companies do not adopt and develop the drugs, appropriately referred to as "orphans." The reasons vary. Some orphan drugs useful for rare diseases have a limited market; others produce high-risk adverse drug reactions that make insurance costs prohibitive. Many useful drugs remain orphans because manufacturers cannot hope to recover the huge amounts of money spent in developing a new drug.

In 1983, Congress signed the Orphan Drug Act, which offers substantial tax credits to companies that develop

Federal drug legislation

Since 1906 when Congress passed the Federal Food, Drug, and Cosmetic Act, the federal government has legislated drug manufacture, sales, and use. The following list gives the major legislative acts and their significance.

YEAR	LEGISLATION	SIGNIFICANCE TO THE PUBLIC
1906	Federal Food, Drug, and Cosmetic Act (FFDCA)	Designated official standards for drugs (United States Pharmacopeia and National Formulary)
1912	Federal Food, Drug, and Cosmetic Act—Sherley Amendment	Prohibited drug companies from making fraudulent claims about their products
1914	Harrison Narcotic Act	Classified certain habit-forming drugs as narcotics and regulated their importation, manufacture, sale, and use
1938	Federal Food, Drug, and Cosmetic Act—Amendment	Provided for governmental approval of new drugs before they enter interstate commerce; defined labeling requirements
1945	Federal Food, Drug, and Cosmetic Act—Amendment	Provided for certification of certain drugs through testing by the Food and Drug Administration
1952	Federal Food, Drug, and Cosmetic Act—Durham-Humphrey Amendment	Distinguished between prescription and over-the-counter drugs; specified procedures for the distribution of prescription drugs
1962	Federal Food, Drug, and Cosmetic Act—Kefauver-Harris Amendment	Provided assurance of the safety and effectiveness of drugs and improved communication about drugs
1970	Comprehensive Drug Abuse Prevention and Control Act (Controlled Substances Act)	Outlined controls on habit-forming drugs; established governmental programs to prevent and treat drug abuse; assisted with the campaign against drug abuse by developing a classification that categorized drugs according to their abuse liability; placed drugs into schedules
1983	Orphan Drug Act	Offered substantial tax credits to companies to develop drugs that are used to treat rare diseases or that have a limited market.

orphan drugs. Small companies may receive federal financial grants to help them research and develop orphan drugs. As a result, thousands of patients now may use drugs that until recently were unavailable. Despite the legislation, many orphan drugs remain without developers.

LEGAL REGULATIONS AND STANDARDS

As a society develops and uses drugs, it needs to establish controls regulating the manufacture, distribution, and use of those drugs. Religious and social mores may provide informal controls on drug use. In most cases, a society's attitudes and values more strictly determine the acceptable limits of drug use than formal controls. Formal drug controls range from individual institutional policies to governmental legislation.

International controls

The United Nations, through its World Health Organization, attempts to influence international health by providing technical assistance and encouraging research for drug use. One committee has been established to cope with the problems associated with habit-forming drugs. Drug enforcement agencies in various nations cooperate, but no administrative or judicial structures enforce controls. As a result, control of international drug trade depends largely on the voluntary cooperation of nations.

Controls in the United States

Legislative drug control in the United States began in 1906 with the passage of the FFDCA. Although the FFDCA primarily addressed the issue of food purity, it also designated the USP and the NF as the official standards for drugs. (For a summary of laws and amendments adopted since 1906, see *Federal drug legislation*.)

In 1912, the Sherley Amendment to the FFDCA increased federal involvement in drug control by prohibiting the use of fraudulent claims by drug companies. Because of a less than rigorous enforcement of the Sherley Amendment, drug companies continued to advertise wide-ranging claims for their products.

In 1914, Congress passed the Harrison Narcotic Act. The act classified certain drugs, such as marijuana, opium, cocaine, and their derivatives, as habit-forming narcotics. It also placed regulations on the importation, manufacture, sale, and use of habit-forming narcotics. The Harrison Narcotic Act was the first narcotic control legislation passed by any nation.

In the 1930s, the need for more stringent drug regulations became apparent when more than 100 people died from ingesting sulfanilamide, an antibacterial drug. Researchers discovered that the sulfanilamide had been prepared with a previously uninvestigated toxic substance called diethylene glycol. After the sulfanilamide incident, Congress passed the 1938 amendment to the FFDCA that established regulations for approval by the federal government of all new drugs and specified requirements for drug labeling. According to the amendment, drug labels were to consist of the following elements before the products could enter interstate commerce:

• A statement accurately describing the package's contents
• The usual names of the drugs, for official drugs (preparations listed in the pharmacopeia and adopted by the government as meeting pharmaceutical standards) and nonofficial drugs (those drugs not listed in the pharmacopeia)
• Indication of the presence, quantity, and proportion of certain drugs (such as alcohol, atropine, digitalis, and bromides) in the product
• A warning of habit-forming drugs in the product and of their effects
• The names of the manufacturer, packager, and distributor
• Directions for use and warnings against unsafe use, including recommendations for dosage levels and frequency (For information on unlabeled uses of drugs, see *Unlabeled uses of drugs.*)
• A statement on all new drugs not yet approved for interstate commerce, for example: "Caution: New Drug—Limited by Federal Law to Investigational Use." Finally, no false or misleading statements were to appear on the label.

In 1945, the FFDCA was amended further to provide for direct governmental supervision and inspection of pharmaceuticals during production. According to the 1945 amendment, governmental certification of certain drugs, such as antibiotics, could not be granted until each batch of the drug produced was tested. The Durham-Humphrey Amendment to the FFDCA in 1952 distinguished between prescription and over-the-counter drugs. It also specified procedures for the distribution of prescription drugs.

Unlabeled uses of drugs

When approving a new drug, the Food and Drug Administration (FDA) accepts it *only* for the indications for which phase II and III clinical studies have shown it to be safe and effective. These indications are approved (labeled); all others are not approved (unlabeled).

For example, the FDA may approve a new drug to treat hypertension if phase II and III studies showed that it was safe and effective in patients with hypertension. If the drug also works well as an antianginal agent, the FDA cannot approve it for this indication unless formal studies in patients with angina pectoris are completed successfully. Such a drug is unapproved for treatment of angina pectoris. Yet, it may be used for this unlabeled indication, based on empirical evidence. Here is how this may occur.

After prescribing a new drug approved to treat hypertension, a physician may discover that it also decreases the patient's angina. Then the physician may share this finding with colleagues in medical journals or at meetings, and they may prescribe it for unlabeled uses, too.

The FDA recognizes that a drug's labeling does not always contain the most current information about its usage. Therefore, after the FDA approves a drug for one indication, a physician legally may prescribe it, a pharmacist may dispense it, and a nurse may administer it for any labeled—or unlabeled—indication.

Although clinicians are *not* prohibited from prescribing, dispensing, or administering a drug for an unlabeled use, the FDA forbids the manufacturer from promoting a drug for any unlabeled indications. That is why drug package inserts and the *Physicians' Desk Reference* (a collection of drug manufacturers' product labeling) contain no information about unlabeled uses, and pharmaceutical sales representatives cannot discuss such uses.

Nevertheless, many drugs commonly are prescribed for unlabeled uses. One famous example is tretinoin (Retin-A), which is approved to treat acne—its only labeled use. However, because independent studies have shown that tretinoin helps eliminate skin wrinkles, many dermatologists prescribe it for this unlabeled use.

In the 1960s, the public became aware of the potential dangers of drugs when 200 cases of poliomyelitis developed from hastily prepared batches of poliomyelitis vaccine. Birth defects in some European countries that were linked to the ingestion by pregnant women of the drug thalidomide also caused great public concern. Media exposure of the poliomyelitis and thalidomide incidents and of the huge profits earned by many drug companies triggered the 1962 passage of the Kefauver-Harris Amendment. The amendment attempted to control the safety and effectiveness of drugs and to assure the public of necessary and timely drug information. As a result, several drugs and drug combinations have been taken off the market.

In 1970, Congress passed the Comprehensive Drug Abuse Prevention and Control Act (CSA or Controlled Substances Act), designed to contain the rapidly increasing problem of drug abuse. The Controlled Substances Act promoted drug education programs and research into the prevention and treatment of drug dependence. It also provided for the establishment of treatment and rehabilitation centers and strengthened drug enforcement authority. Further, the act designated categories, or schedules, that classified controlled drugs according to their abuse liability. (For examples of drugs in each of the five schedules, see *Schedules of controlled drugs.*)

Schedule I contains drugs that have a high abuse potential, have no currently accepted medical use in the United States, or pose unacceptable dangers. Clearance from the FDA is necessary to obtain Schedule I drugs. Heroin is an example of a Schedule I drug.

Schedule II represents drugs with high abuse potential, but with currently acceptable therapeutic use. The use of Schedule II drugs may lead to physical or psychological dependence, or both. Most common narcotics are Schedule II drugs.

Schedule III drugs have a lower abuse potential than those in Schedules I or II. They also have currently acceptable therapeutic use in the United States. Abuse of Schedule III drugs may lead to moderate or low physical or psychological dependence, or both. Some drugs in Schedule III are compounds containing limited amounts of certain narcotic and nonnarcotic drugs. Schedule III also includes certain depressants and barbiturates not listed in another schedule.

Schedule IV drugs have a low abuse potential compared to the drugs in Schedule III. They also have an acceptable therapeutic use in the United States. Chloral hydrate is an example of a Schedule IV drug.

Schedule V includes drugs with a lower abuse potential and with currently acceptable therapeutic use in the United States. Abuse of the drugs in Schedule V leads to more limited physical or psychological dependence compared to the drugs in Schedule IV. A common example of a Schedule V drug is cough syrup that contains codeine.

State, local, and institutional controls

Although state drug controls must conform to federal laws, states usually impose additional regulations, such as those determining the legal age for drinking alcohol. Local drug regulations imposed by counties or municipalities usually involve restrictions on the sale or use of alcohol or tobacco.

Institutional drug controls must conform to federal, state, and local regulations. Public and private institutions adopt and impose drug controls primarily to prevent health problems and legal violations by people within the institution.

Legislation in Canada

Drug control in Canada falls under the direct supervision of the Department of National Health and Welfare. The 1953 Canadian Food and Drugs Act (amended yearly) provides regulations for drug manufacture and sale. In 1965, the Canadian Narcotic Control Act restricted the sale, possession, and use of narcotics. It further restricts narcotic possession to authorized personnel. Under the law, legal possession of narcotics by a nurse is limited to occasions when the nurse administers the drug to a patient under a physician's order, when the nurse serves as a custodian of narcotics in a health care agency, or when the nurse personally uses the narcotic as part of a prescribed treatment. (For examples of controlled substances in Canada, see *Schedules of controlled drugs.*)

DRUG STANDARDS

The federal government establishes and enforces drug standards to ensure the uniform quality of drugs. The standards pertain to the following drug properties:

• *Purity* refers to the uncontaminated state of a drug containing only one active component. In reality, a drug consisting of only one active component rarely exists because manufacturers usually must add other ingredients to facilitate drug formation and to determine absorption rate. Extraneous substances from the manufacturing plant also may contaminate the pure drug. As a result, standards of purity do not demand 100% pure active ingredients but specify the type and acceptable amount of extraneous material.

• *Bioavailability* describes the degree to which a drug becomes absorbed and transported to its target site in the body. Factors affecting bioavailability include the particle size, crystalline structure, solubility, and polarity of the compound. The blood or tissue concentration of a drug at a specified time after administration usually determines bioavailability.

• *Potency* of a drug refers to its strength or its power to produce the desired effect. Potency standards are set by testing laboratory animals to determine the definite measurable effect of an administered drug.

• *Efficacy* refers to the effectiveness of a drug used in treatment. Objective clinical trials attempt to determine efficacy, but absolute measurement remains difficult.

• *Safety and toxicity* are determined by the incidence and severity of reported adverse reactions to the use of a drug. Some harmful effects may not appear for a considerable time. Safety and toxicity standards are being refined constantly as past experiences illuminate deficiencies in the standards.

The modern laboratory testing procedures of bioassay significantly help to determine drug standards and assure adherence to the standards. Still, much remains to be improved in testing procedures, some of which remain expensive and unreliable.

Schedules of controlled drugs

In the United States, the Controlled Substances Act of 1970 classified drugs into categories (schedules) according to their abuse liability. In Canada, the Food and Drug Act (amended yearly) and Narcotic Control Act of 1965 provide similar classifications, although the specific drugs in each class may differ. Health care professionals must be aware of these schedules to ensure the proper handling of controlled substances. The following list provides examples of representative controlled drugs in the United States and Cananda.

UNITED STATES		CANADA	
Schedule	**Examples**	**Schedule**	**Examples**
Schedule I Research use only.	**Narcotics** • Heroin **Hallucinogens** • LSD • Mescaline **Depressants** • Methaqualone	**Schedule H** Restricted drugs. No recognized medicinal properties.	**Hallucinogens** • Peyote • LSD • Mescaline
Schedule II Written prescriptions required. No telephone renewals. In an emergency, a health care professional who is licensed to prescribe may order over the telephone.	**Narcotics** • Codeine • Morphine • Meperidine • Opium poppy **Stimulants** • Amphetamine • Phenmetrazine **Depressants** • Secobarbital	**Narcotics Schedule** Stringently restricted drugs. The letter *N* must appear on all labels and professional advertisements.	**Coca leaf derivatives** • Cocaine **Opiates and opiate derivatives** • Morphine • Codeine • Methadone • Hydromorphone • Meperidine **Other drugs** • Phencyclidine • Cannabis
Schedule III Prescriptions required to be rewritten after 6 months or 5 refills. Health care professional who is licensed to prescribe may order over the telephone.	**Narcotics** • Codeine of less than 1.8 g/100 ml • Opium 25 mg/5 ml **Stimulants** • Benzphetamine • Mazindol **Depressants** • Butabarbital • Glutethimide • Methyprylon • Talbutal **Anabolic steriods** • Ethylestrenol • Fluoxymesterone • Methyltestosterone • Nandrolone decanoate	**Schedule G** Controlled drugs. Prescriptions are cotrolled because of the abuse potential of these drugs. The symbol ◈ must appear on all labels and professional advertisements	**Narcotic analgesics** • Nalbuphine • Butorphanol **Stimulants** • Amphetamines **Barbiturates** • Phenobarbital • Amobarbital • Secobarbital
Schedule IV Prescription required to be rewritten after 6 months or 5 refills.	**Narcotics** • Pentazocine • Propoxyphene **Stimulants** • Fenfluramine • Phentermine **Depressants** • Benzodiazepines • Chloral hydrate	**Schedule F** Prescription drugs. Although not controlled drugs, agents in this category include some with a relatively low abuse potential. The symbol *Pr* must appear on their labels.	**Anxiolytics** • Benzodiazepines

(continued)

Schedules of controlled drugs (continued)

UNITED STATES		CANADA	
Schedule	**Examples**	**Schedule**	**Examples**
Schedule V Dispensed as any other (non-narcotic) prescription drug. Some Schedule V drugs also may be dispensed without prescription unless additional state regulations apply.	Primarily small amounts of narcotics, such as codeine, dihydroco-deine, and diphenoxy-late, when used as antitussives or antidi-arrheals in combination products.	**Nonprescription Drug Schedule (Group 3)** Drugs available only in the pharmacy and used only on the physician's recommenda-tion. Limited public access.	**Analgesics** • Low-dose codeine prepara-tions **Other drugs** • Insulin • Nitroglycerin • Muscle relaxants

CHAPTER SUMMARY

Chapter 1 defined the science of pharmacology and identified and explained its five branches: pharmacokinetics, pharmacodynamics, pharmacotherapeutics, toxicology, and pharmacognosy. Here are the chapter highlights.

• Nurses must know drug terminology to enhance their own understanding and to help them interpret information for patients.

• Based on drug nomenclature, each drug has at least three names: a chemical name, which precisely describes the drug's atomic and molecular structure; a generic name, a shortened form of the chemical name that is selected by the USAN Council; and a trade name, which is a copyrighted brand name selected by the company that sells the drug.

• Drugs that share similar characteristics can be categorized by families or pharmacologic classes, such as beta blockers. Drugs also can be categorized by therapeutic classification, as illustrated by antihypertensives, or by prototype drug.

• A historical perspective of pharmacotherapeutics shows its development from early societies to modern times and helps the nurse understand the evolutionary development of drugs in religious, social, and political contexts. Historical perspective also explains how some natural sources of early medicinal products have evolved into today's modern drugs prepared by chemical synthesis and biological manipulation.

• A discussion of pharmacognosy, the study of the natural sources of drugs, reveals that active components in drugs traditionally were found in plants, animals, and minerals. Today, chemical sources produced in laboratories provide active components in most drugs. Laboratory methods also provide means to purify, alter, or synthesize active components found in nature.

• The process whereby a newly developed drug reaches the market is discussed. The FDA approves an application for an Investigational New Drug (IND). After the manufacturer has conducted extensive animal studies, phase I of the new drug development involves testing the drug on healthy volunteers. Phase II involves trials with human subjects who have the disease for which the drug is thought to be effective. The tests determine the proper dosage as well as effects of the drug on fertility and reproduction. Phase III involves large numbers of patients in medical research centers, using unbiased research methods to detect infrequent or rare adverse reactions. The FDA will approve a New Drug Application (NDA) if phase III studies are satisfactory. Phase IV involves post-market surveillance of the drug's therapeutic effects at the completion of phase III.

• The chapter also explored the difficulties in researching and developing orphan drugs that offer little financial gain. The Orphan Drug Act of 1983 has helped, providing tax incentives and monies for research to drug companies.

• Drug regulations and standards have been developed to control drug use and promote public safety. The passage of the Federal Food, Drug, and Cosmetic Act (FFDCA) in 1906 designated the United States Pharmacopeia (USP) and the National Formulary (NF) as the official standards for drugs. In 1912, the Sherley Amendment to the FFDCA attempted to prohibit the use of fraudulent claims. The Harrison Narcotic Act of 1914 regulated the importation, manufacture, sale, and use of habit-forming narcotics. The 1938 amendment to the FFDCA established regulations whereby the federal government approved the development and marketing of all new drugs.

• The 1938 amendment also established the elements of drug labeling. Labels had to give the package contents and the usual names of the drugs, as well as the presence, quantity, and proportion of certain drugs (alcohol, atropine, digitalis, bromides). Labels also had to include a warning of habit-forming drugs in the product and their effects; names of manufacturer, packager, and distributor; directions for use, including recommended dosages; and a warning statement on all new drugs not approved for interstate commerce. No false or misleading statements could appear on the label.

• The 1945 amendment to the FFDCA mandated the federal government to supervise and inspect the production of certain drugs by testing each batch. The Durham-Humphrey Amendment in 1952 distinguished between prescription and over-the-counter drugs. In 1962, the Kefauver-Harris Amendment gave assurance to the public concerning drug safety and effectiveness. The Kefauver-Harris Amendment attempted to ensure that the public would receive pertinent information about drug safety and effectiveness.

• In 1970, the Comprehensive Drug Abuse Prevention and Control Act (CSA, the Controlled Substances Act) attempted to control drug abuse. The CSA aided drug education, research, treatment, and enforcement. It also classified controlled drugs (Schedules I through V) according to their abuse liability.

• Drug control in Canada falls under the direct supervision of the Department of National Health and Welfare. Canadian laws mandate that nurses legally may possess narcotics only when administering a narcotic to a patient under a physician's order, acting as custodians of narcotics in a health care agency, or receiving the narcotic as prescribed treatment for themselves.

• Drug standards help achieve uniform quality with respect to purity, bioavailability, potency, efficacy, safety, and toxicity.

• Sources of drug information for physicians, nurses, and pharmacists who need current data include pharmacopeias (official), compendia (nonofficial), pharmaceutical firms, and journals.

STUDY QUESTIONS

See Appendix 1 for answers.

1. After back surgery, Charles Grisholm, age 49, receives pentazocine as prescribed for constant, moderate pain. The nurse wants to learn more about this drug's absorption, distribution, metabolism, and excretion. Which branch of pharmacology provides this information?
(a) pharmacokinetics
(b) pharmacodynamics
(c) pharmacotherapeutics
(d) pharmacognosy

2. Pentazocine is a controlled drug. How does a controlled drug differ from a drug that is not controlled?
(a) Controlled drugs are regulated by state laws only.
(b) Controlled drugs may lead to drug abuse or dependence.
(c) Controlled drugs can be used safely without supervision.
(d) Controlled drugs produce little or no adverse effects.

3. Pentazocine may be called by various names. Which name should the nurse use to minimize confusion?
(a) generic name
(b) chemical name
(c) brand name
(d) proprietary name

4. For hundreds of years, medicinal substances were discovered by trial and error. Which century marks the beginning of pharmacology as a specialized science?
(a) 17th century
(b) 18th century
(c) 19th century
(d) 20th century

5. Which of the following definitions best describes pharmacognosy?
(a) study of natural drug sources
(b) study of toxic drug effects
(c) study of clinical indications
(d) study of drug actions

6. All Investigational New Drugs must successfully complete four phases of testing to obtain FDA approval. During which phase are large numbers of patients tested to determine risks associated with a new drug?
(a) phase I
(b) phase II
(c) phase III
(d) phase IV

7. For a serious cough, Scott Harrison, age 34, is taking a Schedule V cough preparation that contains codeine. Which law established schedules of controlled drugs according to their abuse liability?
(a) Harrison Narcotic Act
(b) Durham-Humphrey Amendment
(c) Federal Food, Drug, and Cosmetic Act
(d) Controlled Substances Act

8. The federal government has established drug standards to ensure uniform quality of drugs. Which standard refers to the amount of active component of a drug?
(a) bioavailability
(b) potency
(c) efficacy
(d) purity

SELECTED REFERENCES

Aikman, L. (1977). Nature's healing arts: From folk medicine to modern drugs. In *Folk medicine: An enduring art.* Washington, DC: National Geographic Society.

Austin, A. (1957). *History of nursing source book.* New York: G.P. Putnam.

Compendium of pharmaceuticals and specialties (25th ed.). (1990). Ottawa, Ontario: Canadian Pharmaceutical Association.

DeMarco, C. (1984). *Pharmacy and the law* (2nd ed.). Rockville, MD: Aspen Systems.

Evans, W.E., et al. (1986). *Applied pharmacokinetics: Principles of therapeutic drug monitoring* (2nd ed.). Vancouver, WA: Applied Therapeutics.

Goodman and Gilman's *The pharmacological basis of therapeutics* (8th ed.). Elmsford, NY: Pergamon Press.

Koda-Kimble, M., and Young, L. (1988). *Applied therapeutics: The clinical use of drugs* (4th ed.). Vancouver, WA: Applied Therapeutics.

Leake, C. (1975). *An historical account of pharmacology to the twentieth century.* Springfield, IL: Charles C. Thomas Publishing Co.

Reiss, B., and Melick, M. (1987). *Pharmacological aspects of nursing care* (3rd ed.). Albany, NY: Delmar.

Remington's pharmaceutical sciences (17th ed.). (1987). Easton, PA: Mack Publishing.

Speight, T.M. (1987). *Avery's drug treatment: Principles and practice of clinical pharmacology and therapeutics* (3rd ed.). Baltimore: Williams & Wilkins.

Thorwald, J. (1963). *Science and secrets of early medicine.* New York: Harcourt, Brace and World.

Tyler, V. (1981). *Pharmacognosy* (8th ed.). Philadelphia: Lea & Febiger.

USPDI. (1991). *Drug information for the health care professional* (Vol. I, 11th ed). Rockville, MD: United States Pharmacopeial Convention.

USPDI. (1991). *Advice for the patient* (Vol. II, 11th ed.). Rockville, MD: United States Pharmacopeial Convention.

2

PHARMACOKINETICS

OBJECTIVES

After reading and studying this chapter, the student should be able to:

1. Describe how the different oral formulations, including compressed tablets, sustained-release formulations, and the osmotic pump, release active drug for absorption.

2. Describe how drug dosage forms—including orally administered drugs (tablets, capsules, sublingual, and buccal formulations) and parenteral drugs, such as intravenous injections—affect drug absorption.

3. Describe passive drug absorption, active transport, and pinocytosis.

4. Describe the effect of the following variables on drug absorption: surface area, blood flow, pain and stress, first-pass effect, enterohepatic recycling, drug solubility, gastrointestinal (GI) motility, dosage form, and drug interactions.

5. Compare the absorption rates for the enteral, parenteral, and topical routes.

6. Discuss how decreased binding between plasma proteins and an active drug can cause an excess of free active drug in the body.

7. Explain how a large volume of drug distribution can cause a lower blood concentration level of the drug and how a small volume of distribution can cause a higher blood concentration level.

8. Describe the general purpose of drug metabolism and the various kinds of metabolites that can result.

9. Explain the significance of a drug's half-life in terms of the frequency of a dosing schedule and the patient's clinical responses.

10. Describe the significance of a drug's onset of action, peak concentration, and duration of action.

11. Explain how a drug's minimum effective concentration level, toxic concentration level, and therapeutic range relate to each other.

INTRODUCTION

Chapter 2 focuses on pharmacokinetics, defining terminology and describing related concepts. Pharmacokinetics deals with a drug's actions as it is absorbed into, distributed to, metabolized within, and excreted from a living organism. The chapter explores the variables that affect drug absorption, onset of action, time of peak action, duration of action, ability to maintain an effective blood concentration level, and dosage schedule. All of these variables have an impact on the patient's response to drug therapy.

The discussion of pharmacokinetics in Chapter 2 encompasses two additional disciplines: pharmaceutics and biopharmaceutics. Pharmaceutics describes different dosage formulations, such as tablets and syrups, and their components. Biopharmaceutics describes the interactions between the biological system and the dosage formulation that result in a biologically available drug for therapeutic use. The concept of pharmacokinetics will help the nursing student understand pharmacokinetic application and related disciplines involved in drug administration.

DRUG ABSORPTION

Drug absorption encompasses a drug's progress from its pharmaceutical dosage form to a biologically available substance that can then pass through or across tissues. The transformation from dosage form to a biologically available substance must occur before the active drug ingredient reaches the systemic circulation. After a tablet or capsule disintegrates in the stomach or small intestine, enough liquid must be available for the active drug ingredients to dissolve before systemic absorption. The body requires a solution of the drug's active ingredients because tissues cannot absorb dry powders or dry crystals. (Pinocytosis, the exception to the rule, is explained on page 21. Because syrups and suspensions occur in dosage form as solutions, their progress from drug administration to drug absorption is more rapid, leading to a quicker onset of drug action.

ORAL DRUG ABSORPTION

A brief account of the most common types of drug formulations and their components provides a useful base for the study of drug absorption. A discussion of commonly used formulations also will help the student understand why certain tablets and capsules may not provide the anticipated response in selected situations.

Formulations

A *compressed tablet*, the most frequently dispensed form of a drug, provides a readily administered, standard dosage form. Compressed tablets, which may be engraved with a company symbol and code number for identification, usually have a thin, shiny coating that reduces dust during manufacturing and helps the patient swallow by decreasing the tablet's tendency to stick to the mouth or throat. The tablet may or may not be scored for dividing the dose. An unscored tablet should not be broken. Leaving an unscored tablet intact can protect the patient's stomach from a potentially irritating drug and protect the drug from stomach acid. Leaving the tablet intact also prevents too-rapid release of the drug from an otherwise sustained-release tablet.

Sustained-release formulations release drugs in a controlled, predictable manner, providing safe and effective drug absorption throughout the entire alimentary tract. Under normal circumstances, the nurse should never break or divide a sustained-release tablet or capsule formulation to provide a lower dose for a patient.

Manufacturers employ several processes to produce the many sustained-release formulations on the market. The oldest method involves applying an enteric coating to a tablet. By not dissolving in the stomach or upper intestinal tract, the enteric coating creates a barrier between the drug and the acids in the stomach or intestinal mucosa. The coating allows the tablet to pass undisturbed through the stomach to the lower small intestine, where a more basic pH safely dissolves it.

Another process uses beads or granules with varying thicknesses of protective coating over the different particles. The various coatings dissolve at different times, thereby releasing the drug at different rates over an extended time. (Spansules from Smithkline Beecham and Sequels from Lederle Laboratories represent such formulations.) Capsules containing coated granules should never be opened, nor should the product be chewed, because doing so immediately releases active drug into the body. Release of a total dose can cause severe adverse reactions.

Manufacturers also produce sustained-release formulations by embedding the drug in a slowly eroding matrix.

Both drug and matrix are formulated together in tableting machines. The matrix slowly breaks down during intestinal transit, releasing the drug. (Slow-K tablets from CIBA Pharmaceutical Company represent a drug in an eroding matrix.) Manufacturers sometimes embed the drug in an insoluble plastic matrix. The drug is then slowly leached from (absorbed through) the insoluble plastic matrix, and the intact plastic matrix passes through the alimentary tract. (Fero-Gradumet Filmtabs from Abbott Laboratories use the plastic matrix process.)

Repeat-action tablets carry an initial dose in an outer shell and a second dose within an inner shell. The inner shell of a repeat-action tablet disintegrates later in the intestinal tract. (Chlor-Trimeton Repetabs from Schering Corporation are repeat-action formulations.)

The newest process for manufacturing sustained-release formulations produces the *osmotic pump*. Osmotic pumps usually are tablets with special semipermeable membrane coverings. The tablet's covering allows water to enter. The drug in solution can then leave the tablet, but only through a single small hole made by a laser beam during formulation. The osmotic pump formulation provides controlled release of a drug for several hours. (Acutrim from CIBA Consumer Pharmaceuticals uses the osmotic pump formulation.)

Other novel formulations can improve patient compliance with oral tablets. Chewable tablets were developed for a few products, such as children's aspirin and acetaminophen, to simplify administering the products to children. Cardiac patients can take sublingual or buccal tablets. The soft compression of sublingual and buccal tablets combined with a sufficient lactose content causes rapid, almost instantaneous disintegration of the drug when the patient places the tablet sublingually or buccally. Nitroglycerin sublingual tablets produced by various manufacturers provide good examples of the method. Sublingual and buccal formulations are especially useful for drugs requiring a rapid patient response. By dissolving in the mouth, the drug quickly passes through the mucosa into the patient's bloodstream, avoiding the destructive effects of stomach acid and various other barriers, such as food in the stomach.

Inert ingredients

Tablets and capsules contain multiple inert ingredients, including diluents, lubricants, disintegrating agents, binders, and coloring agents. The inert ingredients assist the pharmaceutical manufacturer by (1) forming a powder that readily flows through the manufacturer's tableting equipment, (2) increasing the dimensions of a finished tablet to a manageable size for the patient, (3) binding the tablet to avoid crumbling in shipment, (4) enhancing the tablet's disintegration in the stomach or small intestine, and (5) providing an aesthetically pleasing product. Furthermore, combinations of inert ingredients in a tablet or capsule stimulate disintegration, dissolution, and drug availability in the body.

Although inert ingredients normally do not produce a biological effect, some patients experience allergic reactions to them. For example, tartrazine (FD&C Yellow #5), a common coloring agent used in prescription and over-the-counter drugs, may precipitate an acute asthma attack in sensitive, asthmatic individuals. Therefore, some manufacturers are removing tartrazine from all medications.

PARENTERAL DRUG ABSORPTION

Fewer formulation variables affect the release of a parenteral drug into the system. Clear liquid solutions for direct entry into the venous or arterial circulatory system usually pose no absorption problems because they rapidly become available to the appropriate target tissue. Differences in absorption occur, however, depending on the parenteral route selected. For example, intravenous (I.V.) administration requires no absorption time, whereas intramuscular (I.M.) and subcutaneous (S.C.) injections do.

Parenteral drugs indicated for any route other than intravenous or intrathecal, however, can pose absorption problems, although such problems occur rarely. For example, I.M. injections that provide a "long-acting" effect may be formulated in an oil or as microfine crystals. The nurse should never administer either formulation into a vein or an artery because the crystals or oil diluent may create emboli. The general principle regarding formulations is: *If the formulation looks cloudy or "thick," do not inject it into a vein or an artery.* The oral route of drug administration remains the preferred route for drug therapy, especially because it promotes patient comfort, safety, and ease of use.

THE PHYSIOCHEMICAL BASIS OF DRUG ABSORPTION

Drug absorption varies, depending on the absorptive surface. Damaged, impaired, or surgically removed absorptive surfaces can increase or decrease the amount of drug absorbed into the body and alter a patient's response. To predict the result of drug activity accurately, the health care professional should consider the drug absorption site, whether it is the intestinal lumen or a target cell wall. Drug absorption may occur by passive drug absorption, active transport, or pinocytosis. (For illustrations of these types of drug absorption, see *Cellular drug absorption,* page 22.)

Passive drug absorption requires no cellular energy because the drug moves from an area of higher concentration to one of lower concentration. It occurs when small molecules diffuse across membranes or, to a lesser degree, through pores. Diffusion ceases when drug concentration on both sides of the membrane is equal.

Drug molecules can pass through a cell membrane only if they are nonionized, that is, if they are not positively or negatively charged at that site. Because most drugs exist in the body partially ionized and partially nonionized, local pH can help determine if a drug will move across a membrane at a particular site. For example, weakly acidic drugs such as theophylline and phenytoin are ionized less in the low (acidic) pH of the stomach than in the high (alkaline) pH of the intestine. Therefore, absorption of these drugs is enhanced in the stomach. Conversely, weakly alkaline, or basic, drugs, such as quinidine, are ionized more in the acidic stomach than in the alkaline intestine. Therefore, absorption of quinidine is inhibited in the stomach and enhanced in the intestine.

Passive drug absorption occurs via three mechanisms: simple diffusion, convective absorption, and carrier-mediated diffusion. In simple diffusion, a drug moves (diffuses) from an area of higher concentration to one of lower concentration. This mechanism accounts for the absorption of most drugs from the alimentary tract into the bloodstream and from the bloodstream into target cells.

During convective absorption, small drug molecules, like those of some electrolytes, move along with fluid through the pores in cell walls.

In carrier-mediated diffusion, or facilitated transport, passive drug absorption also occurs without using cellular energy. The classic example is dietary vitamin B_{12}, which binds with intrinsic factor produced by the stomach wall. The vitamin B_{12}-intrinsic factor complex is carried selectively but passively from an area of higher concentration to one of lower concentration (gut lumen).

Active transport for drug absorption requires cellular energy to move the drug from an area of lower concentration to one of higher concentration. Active transport is the cellular mechanism used during the absorption of the electrolytes sodium and potassium as well as some drugs, such as levodopa.

Pinocytosis, the third method of drug absorption, is a unique form of active transport that occurs when a cell engulfs a drug particle in a manner comparable to phagocytosis. During pinocytosis, the drug need not be dissolved because the cell forms a vacuole or vesicle for drug transport across the cell membrane and into the inner cell. Cells commonly employ pinocytosis to transport fat-soluble vitamins (vitamins A, D, E, and K).

OTHER VARIABLES AFFECTING DRUG ABSORPTION

Besides the type of drug formulation, the condition of the absorptive surface, and the mechanism of absorption, other variables affect the rate of absorption as well as the amount of drug absorbed.

Cellular drug absorption

In most cases, drug absorption follows the same pathways as nutrient absorption. Passive mechanisms of absorption, including simple diffusion, convective absorption, and carrier-mediated diffusion, require no energy and involve drug movement from an area of higher concentration to one of lower concentration. Active transport for drug absorption requires energy to move drugs against a concentration gradient. Pinocytosis facilitates absorption by engulfing the drug particles and moving them across the cell membrane.

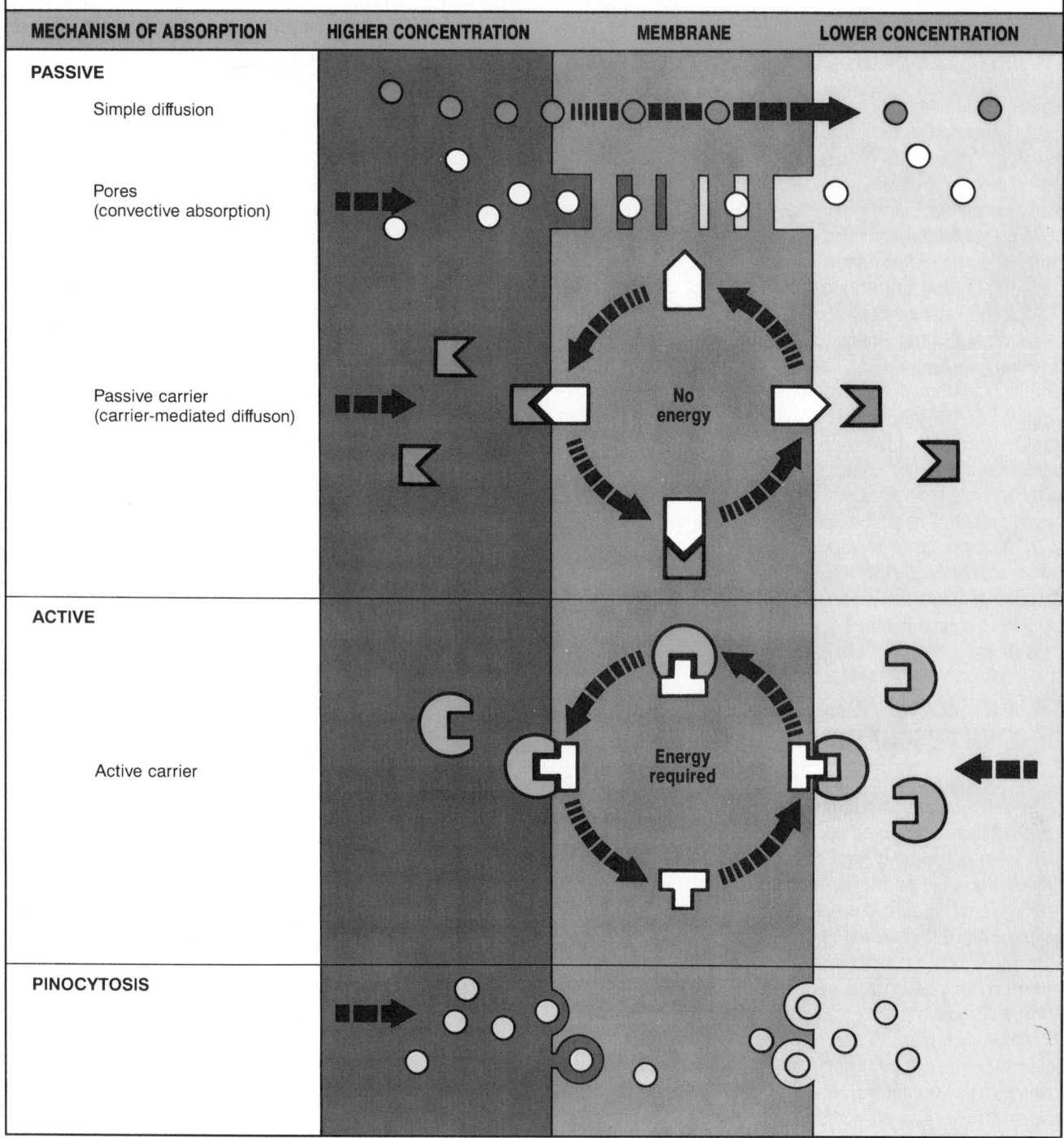

MECHANISM OF ABSORPTION	HIGHER CONCENTRATION	MEMBRANE	LOWER CONCENTRATION
PASSIVE			
Simple diffusion			
Pores (convective absorption)			
Passive carrier (carrier-mediated diffuson)		No energy	
ACTIVE			
Active carrier		Energy required	
PINOCYTOSIS			

Surface area. Most absorption of orally administered drugs occurs in the small intestine, where the mucosal villi provide extensive surface area. If large sections of the small intestine have been surgically resected, drug absorption decreases because of the reduced surface area. In some cases, the shortened intestine reduces intestinal transit time, which in turn diminishes the time that a drug is exposed to the intestinal lumen for absorption. Furthermore, not all areas of the intestine absorb drugs well. For example, the decreased number of villi in the distal small intestine and the absence of villi throughout the large intestine reduce the amount of absorption possible in these locations.

Blood flow. Drug absorption also depends on blood flow to the absorption site. During normal oral drug absorption, the drug moves rapidly from the blood capillary side of the intestinal lumen. A slow rate of oral drug absorption probably indicates a low availability of the drug at the intestinal lumen wall. Food stimulates blood flow (splanchnic blood flow) to the GI viscera and may enhance drug absorption. Strenuous physical exercise diminishes splanchnic blood flow by diverting blood to the muscles and, therefore, slows drug absorption.

With intramuscular drug absorption, drugs administered in the deltoid muscle are absorbed faster than drugs administered in the larger gluteal muscle because of the increased blood flow in the deltoid muscle. The more rapid absorption leads to a quicker onset of drug action.

Pain and stress. Pain, such as that with a migraine headache, can decrease the total amount of drug absorbed. Although the exact cause of the decreased absorption remains unknown, it probably results from a change in blood flow, reduced GI motility, or gastric retention triggered by autonomic nervous system activity that causes pyloric sphincter contraction. Decreased drug absorption also can occur during periods of stress, possibly from similar causes.

First-pass effect. Orally administered drugs do not go directly into the systemic circulation after absorption. They move from the intestinal lumen to the mesenteric vascular system to the portal vein and into the liver with its elaborate enzyme system before passing into the general circulation. During this passage, part of a drug dose may be metabolized. (For the progress of an orally administered drug, see *Oral drug absorption,* page 24.) Enzymes in the intestinal wall, liver, and terminal portal vein may metabolize a significant portion of the drug to an inactive form before it passes into the circulatory system and to the site of action.

The metabolic change of a drug before it reaches the systemic circulation is referred to as the first-pass effect. (For a list of some drugs susceptible to this process, see *First-pass effect drugs,* page 25.) Many orally administered drugs may undergo some metabolism during the first pass through the liver. For drugs undergoing a significant first-pass effect, the orally administered dose required for a therapeutic response is much greater than the dose for a route that bypasses the portal circulation (such as the vaginal, parenteral, and sublingual routes). Although such routes avoid the first-pass effect, they are not always preferred.

Propranolol hydrochloride represents a classic example of a first-pass effect drug. The usual recommended *oral* antiarrhythmic dose is 40 to 120 mg; the *intravenous* dose, 1 to 3 mg. The disparity between these dose ranges points out how knowing which drugs are susceptible to the first-pass effect can help the nurse avoid drug administration errors.

Enterohepatic recycling. After absorption, a drug moves through the bloodstream and eventually reaches the liver. From there, such drugs as digoxin and digitoxin leave the circulation and enter the biliary tract. The drug is excreted in bile intact and travels along the biliary tract, eventually returning to the intestine. From there, the drug is reabsorbed into the bloodstream. This process is known as enterohepatic recycling. Enterohepatic recycling becomes important when the patient experiences drug toxicity and requires rapid reduction in drug blood levels. For example, the body typically removes digoxin and digitoxin very slowly, partly because of enterohepatic recycling. However, orally administered cholestyramine binds digoxin and digitoxin in the GI tract, permanently removing the drugs from the bile and facilitating their excretion in the feces. By interrupting enterohepatic recycling, orally administered cholestyramine helps to reduce digoxin or digitoxin levels within hours rather than days.

Drug solubility. To facilitate drug absorption, the solubility of the administered drug must match the cellular constituents of the absorption site. Lipid-soluble (fat-soluble) drugs can penetrate lipoid (fat-containing) cells; water-soluble drugs cannot. For example, a water-soluble drug, such as penicillin, cannot penetrate the highly lipoid cells that act as barriers between the blood and brain. However, a highly lipid-soluble drug, such as thiopental, can penetrate the lipoid cells, cross into the brain, and induce an effect, such as anesthesia.

GI motility. High-fat meals and solid food affect alimentary transit time by delaying gastric emptying, which in turn delays initial drug delivery to intestinal absorption surfaces. The administration of anticholinergics, such as atropine, scopolamine, and the belladonna alkaloids, may slow intestinal motility and prolong intestinal transit time. The prolonged intestinal transit time may increase total drug absorption. Cathartics and diarrhea shorten a drug's contact

Oral drug absorption

Oral drugs absorbed in the gastrointestinal tract are exposed to the first-pass effect of metabolism. A drug that is not metabolized by the enzyme system in the terminal portal vein may pass into the systemic circulation and the biliary system. Drugs in the bile may be reabsorbed from the intestine and eventually into the systemic circulation.

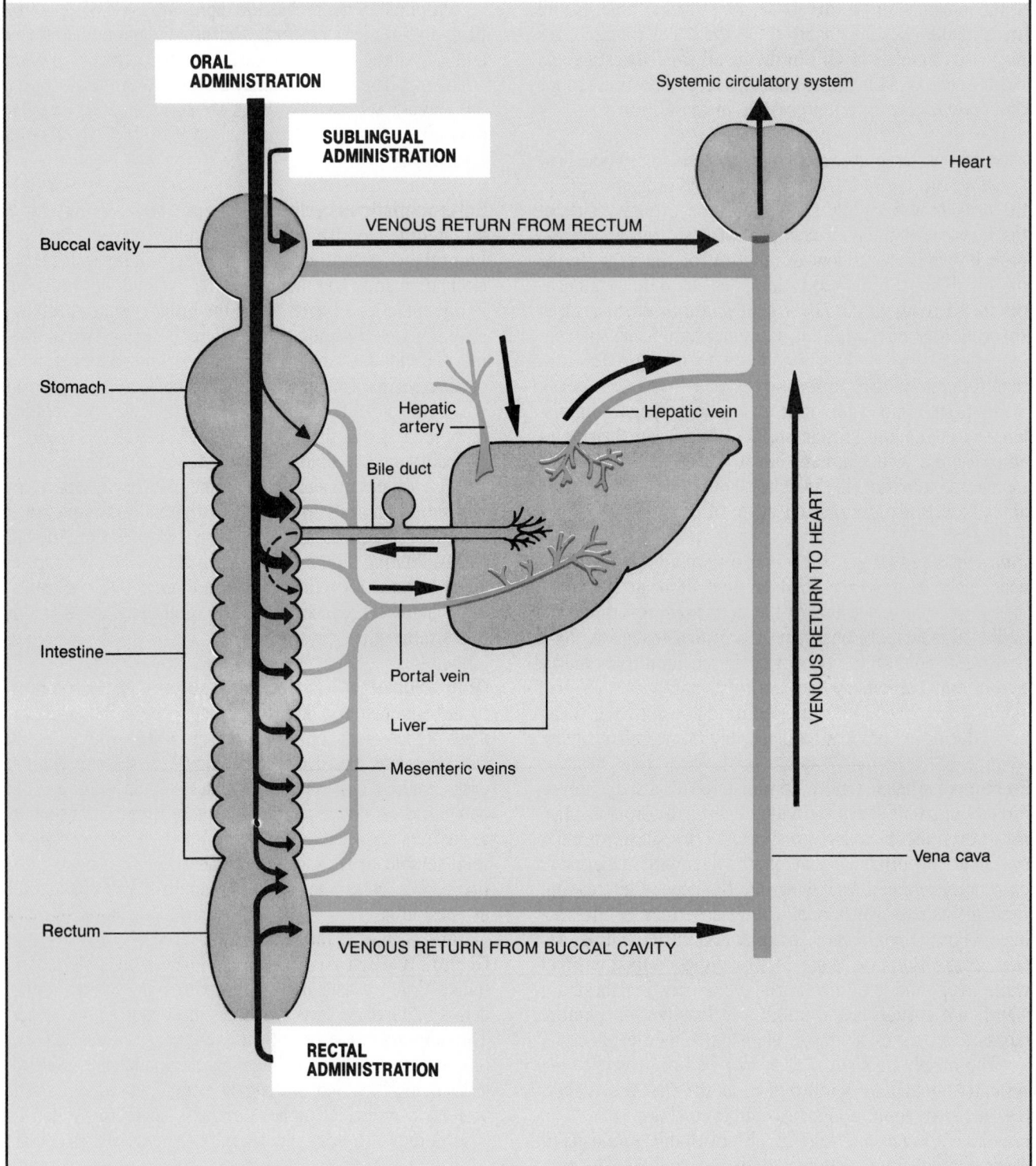

First-pass effect drugs

The following drugs are examples of agents susceptible to the first-pass effect, which reduces the amount of orally administered drug that reaches the circulatory system:

- dopamine
- imipramine
- isoproterenol
- lidocaine
- morphine
- nitroglycerin
- propranolol
- reserpine
- warfarin

time with small intestine mucosa, and this shortened contact time may decrease drug and nutrient absorption.

Dosage form. The drug absorption rate and the time needed to reach peak blood concentration levels depend on the dosage form used. Tablets and capsules dissolve at different rates. The time needed to reach peak effect for sublingual tablets is less than that needed for compressed tablets and sustained-release tablets.

Drug interactions. Combining one drug with another drug or with food can cause interactions that affect drug absorption. For instance, administering tetracycline with an antacid reduces the amount of tetracycline available for absorption. Similarly, tetracycline administered with milk undergoes reduced availability. To avoid undesirable interactions between drugs (drug-drug interactions) or between drugs and food (drug-food interactions), the nurse should consult the appropriate current compendia or the pharmacist before administering a new drug or educating the patient about that drug.

ROUTES FOR DRUG ABSORPTION

The three routes of drug administration discussed here are the enteral, parenteral, and topical. The enteral route is used when drugs are administered by mouth or rectum or directly into the intestinal system (such as through a gastrostomy tube). The parenteral route is used for drugs administered as injections into a vein, an artery, a muscle, a joint, or a skin layer or into the spinal column. The topical route is used for drugs administered onto the skin or the mucous membranes. Each drug administration route presents advantages and disadvantages that affect the drug's pharmacokinetics. (For a detailed discussion of these administration routes, see Chapter 9, Routes and Techniques of Administration.)

Enteral route. Drug absorption after enteral administration can occur in the oral mucosa, gastric mucosa, small and large intestine, or rectum. Drug administration for absorption through the oral mucosa usually is restricted to small

quantities of sublingual and buccal preparations. The preparations themselves also are restricted to water-soluble drugs, drugs with little flavor, and drugs requiring a rapid onset of action.

The gastric mucosa usually is not important to drug absorption because of the small gastric surface area (1 m^2) and the unremarkable capillary blood flow (150 ml/minute). The gastric region is, however, an important site for disintegrating and dissolving tablets or capsules in preparation for their absorption in the small intestine. Physical activity and body position may slow or hasten gastric emptying time, which will lengthen or shorten the time the drug is in contact with the gastric mucosal layers. A patient lying on the left side has a slower gastric emptying time because the body position causes the pyloric sphincter to lie above the stomach contents. In contrast, lying on the right side hastens gastric emptying time. Stomach fluid volume, viscosity, and contents also can affect gastric emptying time. For example, fat slows gastric emptying; liquids and carbohydrates hasten it. Strongly hypertonic solutions slow gastric emptying because the body is attempting to remove the hypertonic substance through emesis or to dilute the stomach contents with body fluids. Gastric acidity, which typically ranges from a pH of 1 to 2, may enhance or impair drug absorption, depending on the effect of pH on ionization, as discussed previously.

The major site of drug absorption for drugs administered by enteral routes is the small intestine. From there, the active drug passes into the systemic circulation. The relatively large surface area (about 200 m^2) and rapid intestinal capillary blood flow (estimated at 1 liter/minute) facilitate efficient, rapid absorption of most drugs. Furthermore, the pH of the acidic gastric secretions increases in the intestines to about 4 or 5 because of the alkalinizing secretions of the pancreas and the neutralizing capacity of the bile. The large intestine primarily reabsorbs water and electrolytes rather than drugs.

Rectal drug absorption advantageously circumvents the first-pass effect, but only if the drug is administered in the lower rectum. Administration in the lower rectum is an alternative enteral route if oral administration poses a problem because of potential emesis or mechanical obstacles. Rectal absorption may be erratic because of varied retention of the dosage form by the patient. Furthermore, the lack of fluid in the rectum can inhibit a drug's disintegration and dissolution and retard its transfer across the intestinal mucosal layer, further delaying absorption. Another problem with administering drugs in the lower rectum is local drug-induced irritation.

Parenteral route. The administration routes for parenteral drugs include intradermal, S.C., I.M., intrathecal, intraarticular, and I.V. The nurse usually does not administer drugs by the intrathecal and intraarticular routes. Compared with orally administered drugs, parenteral drugs must overcome fewer barriers between the sites of drug administration and drug action. Parenteral drugs, however, still must be absorbed into the tissues or cells to exert an effect on the system.

Using the intradermal route usually involves administering parenteral drugs between the skin layers just below the surface stratum corneum. The drugs diffuse slowly from the injection site into the local microcapillary system. In most cases, the intradermal route is limited to allergens of various strengths used in diagnostic allergy testing. A faster introduction of an allergen into a sensitive person could cause a life-threatening allergic reaction.

Using the S.C. route involves administering drugs in the region below the epidermis. Subcutaneous administration facilitates drug diffusion to the capillary vascular system at a rate much faster than that achieved by the intradermal route. Adding vasoconstrictors will slow the uptake of the drug by the circulation. The administration of mixtures, such as a combination of epinephrine (a vasoconstrictor) and lidocaine hydrochloride (a local anesthetic), prolongs the local anesthetic effect of lidocaine by slowing the removal of the drug from the blood. In contrast, gently massaging the area or applying warm compresses increases drug uptake by improving the blood flow and facilitating drug absorption from the injection site.

Parenteral drug absorption from I.M. sites depends on whether an I.M. solution, suspension, or emulsion is used. Solutions, which are clear preparations containing one or more substances dissolved in a fluid, provide a rapid therapeutic effect. Suspensions, which contain crystalline particles causing a cloudy appearance, and emulsions, which have an oil-like base, prolong drug activity by slowing active drug absorption from the I.M. injection site. The muscle area selected for I.M. administration also may make a difference in the drug absorption rate. For example, blood flows faster through the deltoid muscle than through the gluteal muscle; however, the gluteal muscle can accommodate a larger volume of drug than can the deltoid muscle.

Intrathecal administration places the parenteral drug directly into the cerebrospinal fluid, thereby avoiding the absorption barrier between the blood and the brain. The drug is absorbed directly into the target brain tissue. Bypassing the blood-brain barrier necessitates omitting stabilizers and buffers routinely used in injectables. Such stabilizers and buffers may produce serious adverse reactions, such as seizures, when placed directly in the patient's central nervous system. Intrathecal administration is used only for those drugs compatible with the intrathecal route and clearly specified on the product label "For Intrathecal Use Only."

Intraarticular drug administration involves placing the solution directly into the synovial joint fluid to provide a local effect. Systemic drug absorption after intraarticular drug administration usually is negligible.

Administering drugs by the I.V. route bypasses the absorption barriers and provides an immediate systemic response. Intravenous administration is prescribed for an immediate response or for drugs not tolerated or absorbed by other administration routes. The nurse always must read the product brochure before administering an I.V. drug to determine the method and diluent for reconstitution, the rate of administration, and any restrictions. I.V. drugs should not be administered too rapidly because sensitive target tissues can absorb an excess, possibly resulting in such effects as fatal heart block.

Topical route. Using topical routes of drug administration involves applying drugs to various body surfaces. In recent years, the transdermal drug delivery system (TDDS) has gained popularity. With this system, the nurse usually applies a multilayered laminate to the skin, covering an area about the diameter of a U.S. quarter. A protective film from the contact adhesive is removed and applied to an unshaven, preferably hairless, skin area. (Shaving alters the skin's integrity and allows the drug to penetrate faster.) Some TDDS formulations rely on intact skin to help slow drug entry into the body.

The TDDS provides continuous drug delivery to achieve a constant, steady blood concentration level. The continuous but regulated drug delivery should help avoid high blood concentration levels and the associated potential adverse reactions sometimes experienced by the patient during systemic therapy with oral or parenteral drugs. A disadvantage of TDDS application, however, is the slow onset of drug action from initiation until a steady blood concentration level is attained (up to several hours). The drug used for TDDS is available as a gel solution in a reservoir and migrates from the reservoir across the skin. The nurse should rotate application sites to avoid tissue irritation, which could change the drug absorption rate as well as damage the skin. The nurse also should review the manufacturer's recommendations for positioning the transdermal patch before application, because different areas of the skin have different permeabilities.

Topical ointments, creams, and gels typically provide local rather than systemic effects. Ointments, usually occlusive-type topical preparations, are used to treat chronic dry skin conditions. They resist removal by water and readily attain and maintain hydrated skin; however, systemic absorption from ointments usually is poor. Creams, sometimes called "vanishing creams," are easier to apply and remove with water than ointments. Gels contain large amounts of water for easy spreading of the drug. Topical preparations can cause some systemic adverse reactions, and adequate skin hydration for optimal drug absorption may be difficult to maintain without a protective covering over the applied ointment, cream, or gel. Because drug absorption of topical ointments, creams, and gels to treat systemic disorders is unreliable, the topical route seldom is used for this purpose.

Ophthalmic preparations administered in solution usually are absorbed rapidly. However, ophthalmic drugs can be administered as solutions, ointments, or inserts (small elliptic disks placed directly on the eyeball behind the lower eyelid). Ophthalmic solutions and ointments usually are applied two to four times a day. However, ophthalmic inserts provide a sustained-release preparation for drug absorption; some (Pilocarpine Ocuserts from Alcon Laboratories) can remain on the eye for several days. Application frequency depends on the disease or condition, the drug, and the type of formulation. Systemic drug absorption of ophthalmic solutions can occur, causing adverse reactions. For example, timolol maleate ophthalmic drops can exert a beta blocker effect on a patient's cardiac system.

Drugs instilled into the ears usually result in negligible absorption. An otic preparation is used primarily for its local effect, to soften and solubilize earwax and ease its removal or to treat a superficial ear canal rash or infection. Warming otic preparations before application helps prevent earaches.

The skin behind the ear (postauricular) provides an area for rapid drug absorption. Used to prevent motion sickness, a scopolamine patch for transdermal administration is an example of a drug that is absorbed rapidly in the postauricular area.

Drug absorption from nasal instillation or inhalation may cause local or systemic effects. Although nasal decongestant drops and sprays act locally to induce vasoconstriction, excessive use or abuse may result in systemic absorption. For example, use of nasal products with phenylephrine or pseudoephedrine can elevate blood pressure. Other intranasal agents, like beclomethasone dipropionate, can ease seasonal rhinitis with only negligible systemic effects. In contrast, the desired systemic effects of vasopressin can best be achieved by its nasal administration for some conditions.

Drug administration by inhalation demands the delivery of micron-size particles that can navigate the bronchial tree and reach the affected portions of the lung. The small particle size also enhances drug absorption because only a thin membrane separates the air and the drug in each pulmonary alveolus from the capillary blood flow. Drug administration by inhalation provides local effect in the bronchial tree (isoproterenol administered by oral inhalation to asthmatics) or systemic effect (vasopressin administered by nasal inhalation to treat diabetes insipidus).

RATE OF DRUG ABSORPTION

Absorption rate determines when peak concentration levels of a drug will be reached. Although a dosage form (such as a solution) may make a drug immediately available, the onset of drug activity may be rapid, intermediate, or slow, depending on the administration route and the number of barriers between the drug and the site of action. If only one or a few cells separate the active drug from the systemic circulation, rapid absorption will occur. Hence, a predicted rapid onset of action usually means that drug absorption occurs within seconds or minutes of administration via the sublingual, I.V., or inhalation route. Drugs with an intermediate absorption rate usually demonstrate an onset of action within 1 to 2 hours. In most cases, they are administered by the oral, I.M., or S.C. route. The onset of action occurs at a slower rate by the oral, I.M., or S.C. route because the complex membrane systems of GI mucosal layers, muscle, and skin delay drug passage. The slowest absorption rate may cause the drug to take several hours or days to reach peak concentration levels. A slow rate usually occurs with rectally administered or sustained-release drugs. Using a solution to disperse a rectally administered drug to the intestinal mucosae can accelerate onset of action. With sustained-release drugs, onset usually depends on the release rate from the system used, not on the drug.

In summary, drug absorption depends on the drug dosage form, the site of drug administration, the patient's condition, and the physiochemical barriers between the drug and the circulatory system, especially the portal circulation.

DRUG DISTRIBUTION

Distribution of an absorbed drug within the body depends on several factors: blood flow, the drug's affinity for lipoid or aqueous tissue, and protein binding. How efficiently a drug is distributed throughout the body affects the concentration level of the drug remaining in the circulatory system and at the site of action. Evaluating the blood concentration level of a drug helps determine the efficiency of drug absorption, the achievement of therapeutic blood concentration levels, and the time that the drug will remain in the body.

STORAGE SITES

In the body, a drug may be stored in various sites. During drug distribution through the vascular or lymphatic system, the drug comes in contact with proteins and remains free or binds to plasma carrier protein, storage tissue, or receptor protein. As soon as a drug binds to plasma carrier protein or storage tissue protein, it becomes inactive, rendering it unavailable for binding to a receptor protein and incapable of exerting therapeutic activity. However, a bound drug can free itself rapidly to maintain a balance between the amounts of free and bound drug. Only the free, or unbound, percentage of the drug remains active.

The percentage of drug that remains free and available for activity depends on the amount of plasma protein available for binding. The major intravascular source for carrier protein binding is plasma albumin.

The percentage of free drug usually is constant for a single drug but differs between drugs. For example, about 90% of the total gentamicin sulfate in the plasma usually remains free, whereas only about 1% of the total warfarin sodium in the plasma remains free. Administering a single dose of aspirin to a patient on long-term warfarin therapy causes competition for storage protein binding between the two drugs. As a result, the amount of free warfarin in the plasma increases from about 1% to 2%. Although the 1% increase appears minuscule, the amount of free warfarin available to exert a therapeutic effect increases by approximately 100%, with possible life-threatening consequences.

The amount of free drug in the plasma also differs among patients, depending on their medical conditions. For example, malnutrition, which directly affects the liver, deprives the body of protein building blocks and decreases plasma albumin production. This decrease in plasma albumin and the consequent decrease in protein-binding sites boosts the amount of free drug in the plasma, which may be undesirable. The nurse must note any changes in the patient's status that could alter the percentage of free drug in the patient's plasma. Unfortunately, the procedure for distinguishing between free and bound drug is too detailed and expensive to use routinely in the clinic or hospital, so it is performed only in selected cases.

VOLUME OF DISTRIBUTION

This concept represents body areas or compartments (such as blood, total body water, or fat) in which drugs distribute and localize. Although it is mathematically determined, volume of distribution does not refer to real volume. Rather, it is a convenient way to measure the size of a compartment that would be filled by the amount of a drug in the same concentration as that found in the blood or plasma. The nurse must keep in mind, however, that drug volume of distribution is unrelated to a drug's effectiveness or duration of action.

A highly water-soluble drug possesses a small volume of distribution and has a high blood concentration level, whereas a highly fat-soluble drug possesses a large volume of distribution and has a low blood concentration level. Factors that tend to keep a drug in the circulatory system, such as high water solubility and high serum protein binding, result in a lower volume of distribution and a higher blood concentration level. Conversely, factors that promote the movement of a drug from the blood to other compartments, such as high lipid solubility (promoting storage of the drug in fat) or high degrees of binding to body tissues, result in a higher volume of distribution and lower blood concentration levels.

Other factors also can influence a drug's volume of distribution, such as blood flow through different types of tissues that absorb a drug or a drug's ability to cross different barriers, such as the blood-brain barrier. The blood-brain barrier refers to a network of capillary endothelial cells in the brain. These cells have no pores and are surrounded by a sheath of glial connective tissue that makes them impermeable to water-soluble drugs. The network excludes most ionized drug molecules, such as dopamine, from the brain. However, it allows nonionized, unbound drug molecules, such as barbiturates, to pass readily and enter the brain.

The health care professional never should assume that a drug distributes well throughout the body system. Abscesses, exudates, glands, and tumors can affect drug distribution adversely. For example, antibiotics typically do not distribute to abscesses and exudates. Glands, such as the prostate, tend to be impermeable to most antibiotics, rendering a prostatic infection difficult to treat effectively.

Variable drug concentrations among different organs and sometimes different tissues within a single organ also can complicate drug distribution. The differences in tissue drug concentration levels result from such variables as tissue affinity for the drug, blood flow, and protein-binding sites.

DRUG METABOLISM

Drug metabolism, or biotransformation, refers to the body's ability to change a drug biologically from its dosage or parent form to a more water-soluble form. The resulting metabolite usually is an inactive form of the parent drug; however, the metabolism of some drugs results in the ability of one or all of the metabolites to demonstrate some degree of drug activity.

Through metabolism, the body detoxifies and disposes of foreign substances. Because drugs are unnatural to the body, they are disposed of as are other toxins. In most cases, the enzyme system increases the water solubility of a drug so that the renal system can excrete it. The lipid solubility of some drugs may be altered enzymatically so that the end products enter into and are excreted through the biliary system. Using the renal or the biliary pathway for disposal, the body usually transforms the drug into a readily eliminated, pharmacologically inactive product.

The metabolism of some parent drugs may, however, result in metabolites capable of drug activity. For example, the liver metabolizes imipramine to inactive metabolites and the active metabolite desipramine. (Discovery of the active desipramine led to its commercial marketing as a drug.) In a few cases, the body metabolizes an inactive parent drug to an active metabolite. For example, dopamine hydrochloride is the drug of choice for treating parkinsonism; however, it cannot cross the blood-brain barrier. Levodopa, a pro-drug (inactive precursor) of dopamine, readily crosses the blood-brain barrier into the central nervous system, where it is metabolized to dopamine with therapeutic results. (For a list of some other parent drugs and their active metabolites, see *Drug metabolism*.)

Not all drugs are metabolized to the same extent or by the same mechanisms. Some drugs, such as the aminoglycosides, are not metabolized; they pass through the body and are excreted in unchanged form. Other drugs, such as barbiturates, stimulate or induce enzyme metabolic activity, thus reducing the amount of active drug in the body. For example, repeated administration of phenobarbital induces metabolic enzyme activity, which increases drug metabolism. In such cases, the drug may stimulate its own metabolism, a process referred to as autoinduction. In a related process, called foreign induction, one drug stimulates the metabolism of another. For example, if theophylline therapy were added to an existing phenobarbital regimen, the phenobarbital-induced enzyme activity would stimulate the metabolism of the theophylline.

In contrast, some drugs inhibit or compete for enzyme metabolism, which may cause the accumulation of concurrently administered drugs. The accumulation increases the potential for an adverse reaction or drug toxicity. Cimetidine, for example, inhibits the enzyme system that metabolizes theophylline in the liver, causing an elevated theophylline level within the vascular system. The increased theophylline may cause such adverse reactions as tachycardia or seizures. (For some drugs that produce autoinduction and foreign induction and some drugs that inhibit enzyme metabolism, see *Common drugs affecting metabolism,* page 30.) Before interpreting a drug response or altering therapy because of an inappropriate blood concentration level of an active drug, the physician usually

Drug metabolism

Drug metabolism usually changes active parent drugs into inactive metabolites. Many drugs, however, are biologically transformed from an inactive parent drug to an active metabolite. Metabolism changes still other drugs from active parent drugs into more active metabolites. Some examples of parent drugs that are biologically transformed into active metabolites include the following.

PARENT DRUG	ACTIVE METABOLITE
acetohexamide	hydroxyhexamide
allopurinol	alloxanthine
amitriptyline	nortriptyline
chloral hydrate	trichloroethanol
cortisone acetate	hydrocortisone
diazepam	desmethyldiazepam
flurazepam hydrochloride	N-desalkyl-flurazepam
imipramine	desipramine
mephobarbital	phenobarbital
prednisone	prednisolone
procainamide hydrochloride	N-acetylprocainamide
propranolol hydrochloride	4-hydroxypropranolol
spironolactone	canrenone

investigates the possibility of drug-induced changes in drug metabolism.

Disease-induced physiologic changes can affect drug metabolism negatively. When end-stage cirrhosis damages the liver enough to reduce or alter liver blood flow, the supply of a drug to liver enzyme metabolic sites decreases. When congestive heart failure decreases the patient's cardiac output, drug metabolism decreases because the drug delivery to liver metabolic sites becomes inefficient. Genetics also may affect the efficiency of drug metabolism, as evidenced by the ability of some individuals to metabolize drugs rapidly while others metabolize them more slowly. Slowed metabolism of a drug may cause it to accumulate to toxic levels. Environment, too, may alter drug metabolism. For example, cigarette smokers metabolize theophylline much more rapidly than nonsmokers do. Developmental changes, particularly during infancy and old age, also can affect drug metabolism. (For more information about these changes, see Chapter 10, The Pediatric Patient, and Chapter 11, The Geriatric Patient.)

Common drugs affecting metabolism

Drug metabolism may be affected by autoinduction (a drug induces its own metabolism), foreign induction (one drug stimulates the metabolism of another), and enzyme inhibition (a drug inhibits enzyme metabolism, possibly leading to drug accumulation). The following chart provides examples of drugs that affect metabolism by each of these mechanisms.

Drugs producing autoinduction

glutethimide	nitroglycerin	probenecid
meprobamate	phenobarbital	tolbutamide

Drugs producing foreign induction

INDUCER	DRUGS WITH INDUCED METABOLISM
alcohol	pentobarbital sodium tolbutamide
antihistamines	hydrocortisone phenobarbital
DDT and chlordane	barbiturates warfarin
ethchlorvynol	warfarin sodium
glutethimide	barbiturates warfarin
griseofulvin	warfarin
haloperidol	warfarin
meprobamate	warfarin
phenobarbital and other barbiturates	androstenedione bilirubin chloramphenicol digitoxin doxorubicin hydrochloride estradiol griseofulvin hexobarbital and other barbiturates phenytoin progesterone testosterone thyroxine tolbutamide
phenytoin	hydrocortisone
tolbutamide	barbiturates

Drugs causing enzyme inhibition

ENZYME INHIBITORS	DRUGS WITH INHIBITED METABOLISM
allopurinol	mercaptopurine
aspirin	chlorpromazine
chloramphenicol	hexobarbital
chlorpromazine	hexobarbital
cimetidine	benzodiazepines theophylline warfarin
codeine	hexobarbital
cyclophosphamide	chloramphenicol
desipramine hydrochloride	amphetamines
disulfiram	alcohol
meperidine hydrochloride	oral contraceptives
6-mercaptopurine	allopurinol
MAO inhibitors	barbiturates tyramine sympathomimetic amines
morphine	hexobarbital
nortriptyline	hydrocortisone

In summary, drug metabolism varies for different types of drugs. Health care professionals are mindful of the way in which the body removes a drug, to drugs that may affect hepatic metabolic function, and to drugs that may affect the metabolism of concurrently administered drugs. Finally, physiologic, genetic, environmental, and developmental factors also may alter drug metabolism.

DRUG EXCRETION

The body eliminates drugs by metabolism (usually hepatic) and excretion (usually renal). Drug excretion refers to movement of a drug or its metabolites from the tissues back into the circulation and from the circulation into the organs of excretion. Physiologically, drugs can be eliminated via the lungs, exocrine glands (sweat, salivary, or mammary glands), kidneys, liver, skin, and intestinal tract. Drugs also may be removed artificially by direct interventions, such as peritoneal dialysis or hemodialysis.

HALF-LIFE

To predict the frequency of the drug dosage schedule, the physician must determine how long a drug will remain in the body. Usually, the rate of drug loss from the body can be estimated by determining the drug's half-life. Drug half-life represents the time required for the total amount of a drug in the body to diminish by one half. The half-life of a drug can be determined from a drug concentration-time curve. (For more information, see *Determining drug half-life*.)

If a patient receives a single dose of a drug with a half-life of 5 hours, the total amount of the drug in the patient's body would diminish by one half after 5 hours. The drug amount would continue to decrease accordingly with each subsequent half-life. Most drugs essentially are eliminated after five half-lives because the amount remaining is probably too low to exert any beneficial or adverse effect. (For more information, see *Amount of drug remaining,* page 32.) This concept is useful in many situations. For example, if a drug overdose occurs and the excretion rate of the drug is not compromised, about 97% of the original dose will be eliminated after five half-lives.

Determining drug half-life

Drug half-life can be determined from a drug concentration-time curve by measuring the time required for a drug blood concentration level to decrease by one half. As an example, the graph below shows a drug's concentration of 100 mcg/ml at 2 hours and a concentration of 50 mcg/ml at 4 hours (a half-life of 2 hours).

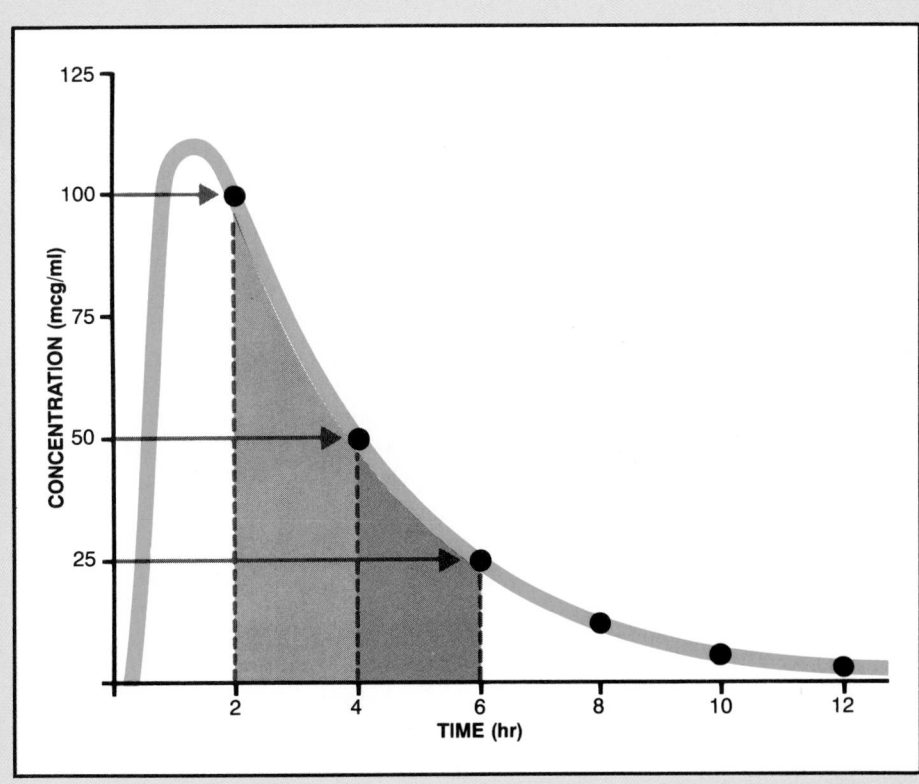

Amount of drug remaining

Drug half-life can be used to estimate the amount of drug remaining in the body after the last dose. With the discontinuation of drug therapy, all drug activity usually ceases after a period of five half-lives.

NUMBER OF HALF-LIVES	TOTAL AMOUNT OF DRUG REMAINING	PERCENT OF ORIGINAL DOSE
Dose	100 mg	100
1	50 mg	50
2	25 mg	25
3	12.5 mg	12.5
4	6.3 mg	6.3
5	3.1 mg	3.1
6	1.6 mg	1.6
7	0.8 mg	0.8

ACCUMULATION

Drug half-life also proves to be a useful tool when assessing drug accumulation. A drug that is not readministered is eliminated almost completely after five half-lives, but a regularly administered drug reaches a "constant" total body amount, or steady state, after about five half-lives.

Having once reached a steady state, the blood concentration levels of the drug will fluctuate above and below the "average" concentration level. This means that, although the drug was once at steady state, its concentration levels do not remain uniform; rather, they increase, peak, and decline, although within a constant range. (For a discussion of the range of blood concentration levels that can occur after successive doses of a drug, see *Steady-state dosing and drug concentrations*.)

For some drugs, the time required to reach therapeutic blood concentration levels may be too long. For example, when using digoxin, with a half-life of about 1.6 days, the physician would not be able to wait 8 days (1.6 days times 5 half-lives) to achieve steady-state blood concentration levels to control a life-threatening arrhythmia, such as atrial fibrillation. Therefore, an initial large dose, called a loading dose, would be rapidly administered to reach the desired therapeutic blood concentration level. Subsequently, smaller "maintenance dosages" would be given daily to replace the amount of drug eliminated since the last dose. These dosages maintain a therapeutic blood concentration level in the body at all times.

CLEARANCE

Drug clearance refers to removal of a drug from the body. A drug with a low clearance rate is removed from the body slowly; one with a high clearance rate is removed rapidly. A drug with a high clearance may require more frequent administration and higher doses than a comparable drug with a low clearance. A drug with a low clearance can accumulate to toxic concentration levels in the body unless it is administered less frequently or at lower doses.

Health care professionals must consider drug clearance when assessing dosing regimens. If a drug normally is removed by a metabolic process, determining the efficiency of the metabolic system before administering the first dose is difficult. As a result, the maintenance dosage and dosing frequency calculations may be based on a "best estimate," which correlates with information gained from similar cases involving patients with comparable diseases or disorders.

If the kidneys eliminate the drug, an estimate of the drug's renal clearance can be determined with simple bedside formulas that account for the patient's body size and creatinine clearance, or renal function. For example, if the kidneys normally eliminate 100% of a drug and the patient's renal function decreases by 50%, the drug dose can be decreased appropriately by 50% or the dosing interval can be doubled to maintain safe and effective blood concentration levels.

ONSET, PEAK, AND DURATION

Besides absorption, distribution, metabolism, and excretion, three other factors play an important role in a drug's pharmacokinetics: onset of action, peak concentration, and duration of action.

The onset of action refers to the time when the drug is sufficiently absorbed to reach an effective blood level and sufficiently distributed to its site of action to elicit a therapeutic response.

As the body absorbs more drug, the blood concentration level rises, more drug reaches the site of action, and the therapeutic response increases. These occurrences characterize the peak concentration level for the drug dose administered.

As soon as the drug begins to circulate in the blood, it also begins to be eliminated. Eventually, drug elimination exceeds its absorption rate because less of the dose remains to be absorbed. At this point, the blood concentration level — and the drug's effect — begin to decline. When the blood concentration falls below the minimum needed to produce an effect, drug action ceases although some drug

Steady-state dosing and drug concentrations

Drugs accumulate in the body during multiple dosing until they reach a plateau, or a steady state. Drug input then equals drug output during the dosing interval. In the following example, a drug is administered every half-life. If this hypothetical drug is given in 100-mg doses and is completely absorbed, the total amount in the body is 100 mg at 2 hours. At the next dose, one half-life later and 4 hours after the first dose, the amount has decreased to 50 mg. The next dose of 100 mg increases the amount in the body to 150 mg. At the next dose, one more half-life, the 150 mg has decreased by 50% to 75 mg. A third dose increases the amount in the body to 175 mg. This continues until steady state is reached, as shown in the table. The maximum and minimum amounts listed show the fluctuations of drug levels after a dose.

DOSE NUMBER	DOSE AMOUNT	MAXIMUM AMOUNT IN BODY (2 HOURS AFTER DOSE)	MINIMUM AMOUNT IN BODY (IMMEDIATELY BEFORE NEXT DOSE)
1	100 mg	100 mg	50 mg
2	100 mg	150 mg (50 mg + 100-mg dose)	75 mg (½ of 150 mg)
3	100 mg	175 mg (75 mg + 100-mg dose)	88 mg (½ of 175 mg)
4	100 mg	188 mg	94 mg (½ of 188 mg)
5	100 mg	194 mg	97 mg (steady state)
6	100 mg	197 mg	99 mg (½ of 197 mg)
7	100 mg	199 mg	100 mg (½ of 199 mg)
8	100 mg	200 mg	100 mg (½ of 200 mg)
9	100 mg	200 mg	100 mg (½ of 200 mg)

To illustrate differences in drug accumulation, the following curves compare the maximum and minimum drug concentrations that result from a constant dosing regimen (shown as a solid line) and the concentrations that result from a regimen that begins with a loading dose (shown as a dotted line). In this example, the patient receives the same dose (100 mg) every 4 hours in the constant dosing regimen. This yields a drug concentration of 100 mg at 2 hours and 50 mg at 4 hours (a half-life of 2 hours). After about five half-lives, the constant dosing regimen produces a steady-state drug concentration (peak and trough levels that remain constant after each dose), indicated by shading. This concentration level can be achieved much more rapidly by giving a calculated loading dose followed by maintenance dosages.

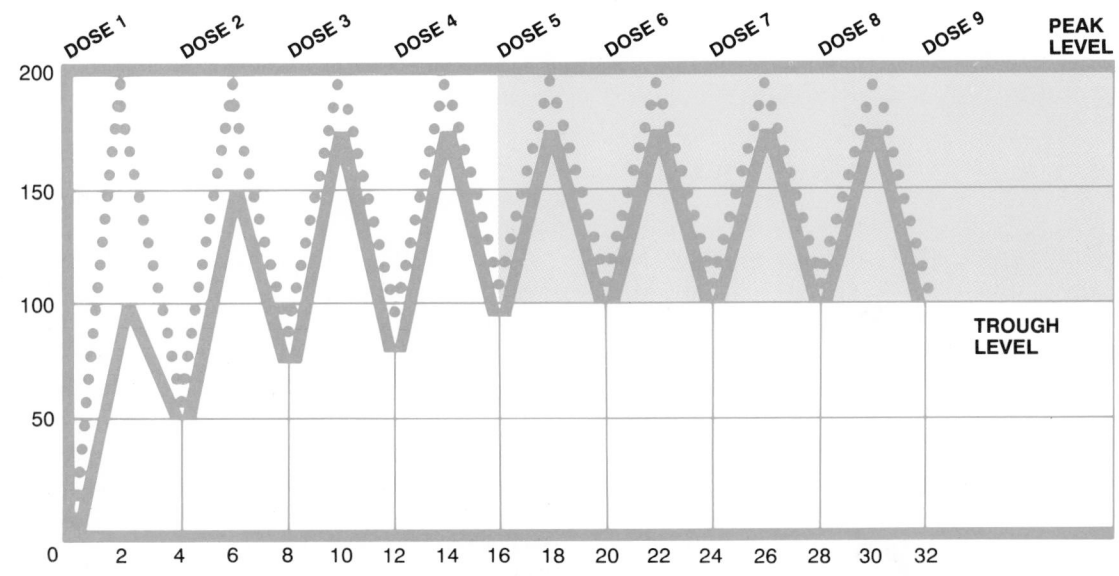

Therapeutic range

The minimum effective concentration (MEC) and the minimum toxic concentration (MTC) represent the lower and upper borders of the blood concentration level-time curve. Drug blood level concentration determinations help the physician and clinical pharmacist make drug therapy decisions. The peak drug level is represented by the square on the graph; the trough level is represented by the triangle. The time during which the drug concentration curve remains between the MEC and the MTC represents the duration of drug activity.

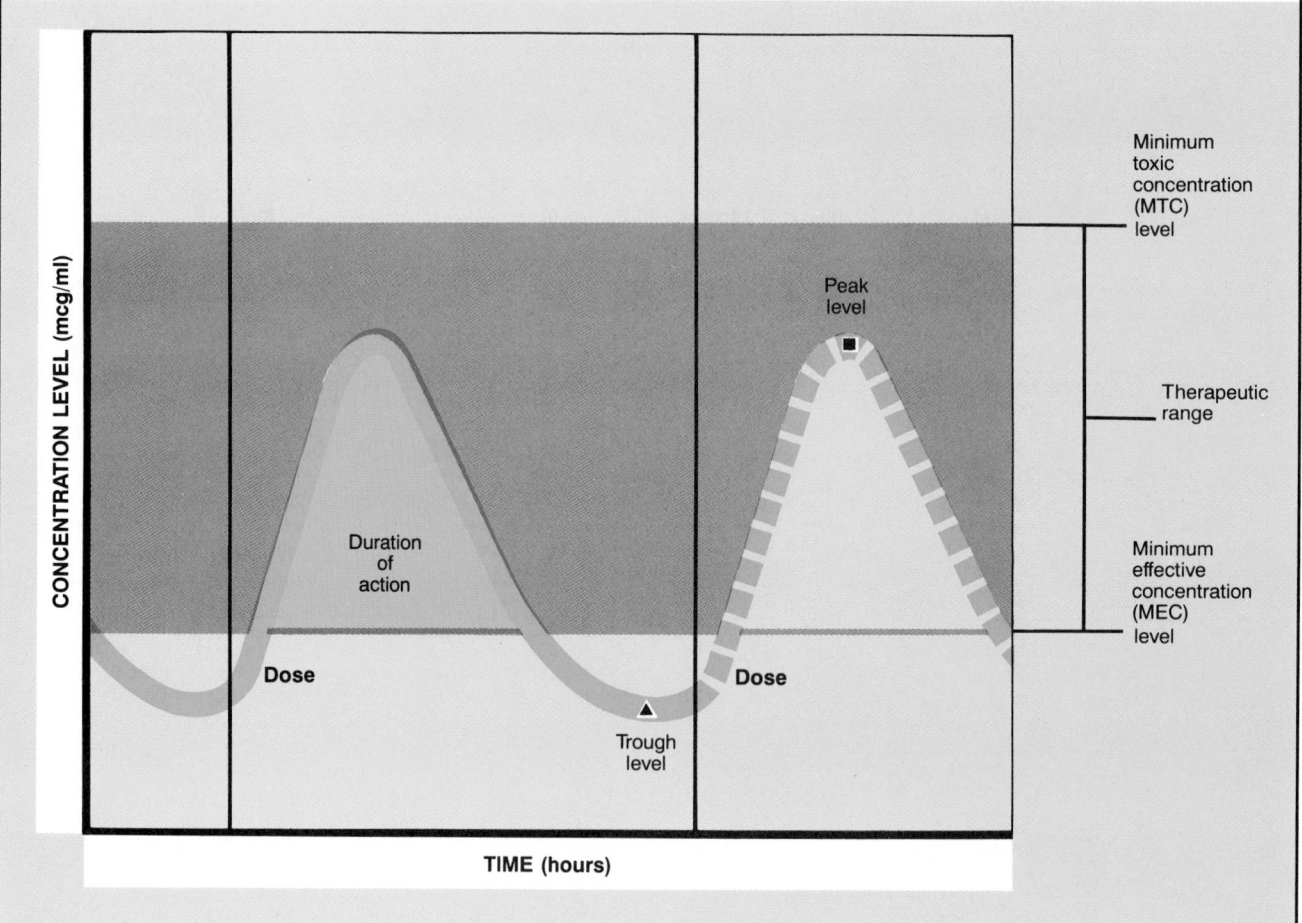

remains in the blood. Therefore, the duration of action is the length of time that drug concentration is sufficient in the blood to produce a therapeutic response.

A drug's onset, peak, and duration are determined primarily by its bioavailability and blood concentration level.

BIOAVAILABILITY

Bioavailability refers to the extent to which a drug's active ingredient is absorbed and transported to its site of action. It can be affected by the drug's solubility, crystalline structure, particle size, and polarity. When administering a drug, the nurse should be aware of bioavailability because different drug brands may contain the same active ingredient in the same dose, yet the amount absorbed may vary greatly.

Because of this, different brands of a drug may reach different concentrations at the site of action and may produce different degrees of therapeutic response.

Bioavailability is particularly important when administering an extremely potent drug, such as digoxin. In such cases, substitution of a generic drug for a brand name drug may lead to toxicity because of overdose or to inadequate therapy because of underdose. In other cases, substitution may be appropriate because many drugs that vary greatly in cost demonstrate similar bioavailability.

Drug bioavailability typically is measured by drug blood (or tissue) concentration level at a specific time after administration. Although bioavailability tests have not been well standardized, scientists and others now are working to develop reliable ones, such as mass spectrometry.

BLOOD CONCENTRATION LEVEL

The blood concentration level of a drug helps determine whether the dosing has achieved the therapeutic goals. (For a more detailed discussion of drug blood levels, see Chapter 4, Pharmacotherapeutics.) A drug concentration level usually is measured in plasma or serum; however, the same principles apply whether the level is measured in the blood or any other fluid, such as cerebrospinal fluid or saliva.

By correlating the blood concentration level-time curve with a patient's response, the physician and clinical pharmacist can gain valuable information about the minimum effective concentration (MEC), minimum toxic concentration (MTC), and therapeutic range for a drug. (For a typical blood concentration level-time curve, see *Therapeutic range*.) The MEC represents the necessary blood concentration level for the drug to be effective in most patients. The MTC represents the lowest blood concentration level at which significant adverse reactions to the drug usually occur. The therapeutic range is bordered at the low end by the MEC and at the high end by the MTC. The time during which the drug concentration remains between these values represents the drug's duration of action.

One goal of therapy is to extend the duration of action while avoiding the MTC. Regular monitoring of the drug concentration level is useful in achieving this goal. Shortly after a drug is administered, the highest, or "peak," level of the drug in the system can be measured. Just before administration of the next dose, the lowest, or "trough," level of the drug can be measured. For a drug like theophylline, the therapeutic range is between 8 and 20 mcg/ml. This means that the drug's peak level needs to be less than 20 mcg/ml and the trough level greater than 8 mcg/ml.

For many drugs, the blood concentration level correlates with the anticipated therapeutic response. Unfortunately, commercial assay methods have not been developed for most drugs.

CHAPTER SUMMARY

Chapter 2 explored the concepts of pharmacokinetics, explaining the ways in which drug absorption, distribution, metabolism, and excretion affect a patient's response to drug therapy. The chapter also described the importance of drug onset, peak, and duration to a therapeutic drug regimen. Here are the chapter highlights.

• Drug absorption depends on several variables, including the dosage form, the site and route of administration, physiochemical factors affecting drug transport into the circulatory system, and the physiologic status of the patient.

• Orally administered drugs include compressed tablets, sustained-release formulations, osmotic pumps, and other formulas. They disintegrate and are absorbed at different rates. Although parenteral drugs administered by I.V. and other routes present few drug absorption problems, oral drugs remain the preferred dosage form.

• Physiochemical factors influence the ways in which drug absorption occurs. Drugs may be absorbed by passive absorption, active transport, or pinocytosis.

• Other variables affecting drug absorption include the surface area at the absorption site, blood flow to the absorption site, pain and stress, first-pass effect, enterohepatic recycling, drug solubility, GI motility, dosage form, and drug interactions.

• The major routes for drug absorption include enteral, parenteral, and topical. Drugs administered by enteral routes are absorbed by the oral mucosa, gastric mucosa, small intestine, and rectum. Parenteral routes include the intradermal, subcutaneous, intramuscular, intrathecal, intraarticular, and intravenous. Topical routes are used for transdermal drugs, ophthalmic preparations, otic preparations, and drugs used for nasal instillation.

• Drug distribution within the body depends on blood flow, the drug's affinity for lipoid or aqueous tissue, and protein binding.

• When absorbed, many drugs bind to plasma proteins (albumin) for distribution, which can be affected by the patient's medical condition. For example, a patient with malnutrition will possess fewer protein "building blocks," lowering the body's protein levels. When adequate protein binding cannot occur, the excess free drug may magnify the drug response.

• Drug volume of distribution represents body areas or compartments in which drugs distribute and act locally. It does not refer to real volume, but to the size of a compartment that would be filled by the amount of a drug in the same concentration as that found in the blood or plasma. A large volume of drug distribution causes a lower blood concentration level. Conversely, a small volume of distribution causes a higher blood concentration level.

• Drug metabolism occurs as the body changes a drug from the dosage or parent form to a more water-soluble form. It creates metabolites, which may or may not demonstrate drug activity. Drug metabolism transforms a drug so that the renal and biliary systems can excrete it more readily.

• Various illnesses can alter drug metabolism. For example, cirrhosis can result in adverse drug reactions because the liver cannot remove the drug, leaving it in the blood for prolonged periods.

• Excretion of metabolized drugs typically occurs via the renal system. Drugs also can be eliminated via the lungs, exocrine glands, liver, skin, and GI tract. Direct intervention, such as peritoneal dialysis, removes drugs artificially.

• Drug half-life represents the time required for the total amount of a drug in the body to diminish by one half. Knowing a drug's half-life can help in predicting the frequency of drug dosing and in assessing drug accumulation.

• Besides absorption, distribution, metabolism, and excretion, three other factors help determine a drug's pharmacokinetics: onset of action, peak concentration, and duration of action. These factors are determined primarily by the drug's bioavailability and blood concentration level.

• Drug bioavailability refers to the extent to which a drug's active ingredient is absorbed and transported to its site of action. It is important because different brands of a drug may contain the same active ingredient in the same dose, yet the amount absorbed may vary greatly, producing different concentrations at the site of action and different degrees of therapeutic response.

• The health care professional can gain valuable information by reviewing the blood concentration level-time curve and the patient's response. The curve indicates the minimum effective concentration (MEC), the minimum toxic concentration (MTC), and the therapeutic range for a drug. The therapeutic range falls between the MEC and the MTC.

STUDY QUESTIONS

See Appendix 1 for answers.

1. Ronald Bolton, age 42, takes a drug orally for hypertension, as prescribed by his physician. The oral route allows relatively slow drug absorption. Which route allows the most rapid absorption?
(a) transdermal
(b) subcutaneous
(c) intramuscular
(d) intravenous

2. Which mechanism of cellular drug absorption requires energy to move a drug from an area of lower concentration to one of higher concentration?
(a) passive absorption
(b) convective absorption
(c) active transport
(d) pinocytosis

3. Which factor determines when the peak concentration level of a drug will be reached?
(a) the dose
(b) absorption rate
(c) metabolism
(d) first-pass effect

4. Through distribution, an absorbed drug moves to its site of action. What must a drug do to be active at this site?
(a) bind with plasma carrier proteins
(b) bind with albumin
(c) bind with lipids
(d) remain unbound

5. Which of the following statements accurately characterizes a drug with poor water solubility?
(a) It produces a low volume of distribution and high blood level
(b) It produces a high volume of distribution and high blood level
(c) It produces a low volume of distribution and low blood level
(d) It produces a high volume of distribution and low blood level

6. What is the purpose of drug metabolism?
(a) to initiate a physiologic response
(b) to break down the drug for distribution throughout the body
(c) to break down the drug into active metabolites
(d) to transform the drug for renal and biliary elimination

7. To predict the optimal dosing frequency for a drug, the health care professional would need to determine which of the following?
(a) drug half-life
(b) patient's age
(c) drug potency
(d) patient's need for the drug

SELECTED REFERENCES

Bourne, D., et al. (1986). *Pharmacokinetics for the non-mathematical.* Hingham, MA: Kluwer Academic Publishers.

DiPiro, J., et al. (1988). *Concepts in clinical pharmacokinetics.* Bethesda, MD: American Society of Hospital Pharmacists.

Kroboth, P.D., et al. (1988). *Pharmacokinetics and pharmacodynamics, Vol. 2: Current problems, potential solutions.* Cincinnati: HW Books.

Notari, N. (1986). *Biopharmaceutics and clinical pharmacokinetics: An introduction* (4th ed.). New York: Marcel Dekker.

Peck, C., et al. (1989). *Bedside clinical pharmacokinetics: Simple techniques for individualizing drug therapy.* Vancouver, WA: Applied Therapeutics.

Ritschel, W. (1986). *Handbook of basic pharmacokinetics, including clinical applications* (3rd ed.). Bethesda, MD: Drug Intelligence Publications.

Van Rossum, J., and Maes, A. (Eds.). (1986). *Pharmacokinetics: Classic and modern.* New York: VCH Publications.

Winter, M. (1988). *Basic clinical pharmacokinetics* (2nd ed.). Vancouver, WA: Applied Therapeutics.

3

PHARMACODYNAMICS

OBJECTIVES

After reading and studying this chapter, the student should be able to:
1. Describe the relationship between a drug's pharmacodynamic properties and the patient's response to the drug.
2. Differentiate between drug action and drug effect.
3. Explain how drugs cause physical and chemical modifications of the cell environment.
4. Describe how drugs modify cell function by drug-receptor interactions or drug-enzyme interactions.
5. Compare the actions of agonistic and antagonistic drugs.
6. Describe up-regulation and down-regulation as these terms apply to receptors.
7. Identify the factors that determine outcome of drug action.
8. Identify the characteristics of an ideal dose-response curve.
9. Differentiate between drug potency and drug efficacy.
10. Describe the significance of a drug's therapeutic index.

INTRODUCTION

Pharmacodynamics is the study of the mechanisms by which specific drug dosages produce biochemical or physiologic changes in the body. The pharmacodynamic phase is one of the four phases involved in the disposition of a drug. (For a depiction of the four phases of drug activity, see *Drug disposition*.) The pharmacodynamic phase of drug action progresses concurrently with the pharmacokinetic processes of (1) drug absorption from the administration site, (2) drug distribution throughout the body via body fluids, (3) metabolism of the parent drug to inactive, active, or more active metabolites, and (4) drug excretion.

After a drug penetrates the cellular barriers and reaches its site of action within the target cell, tissue, or body organ system, the resulting drug action is effected by one or more mechanisms. The drug action, or physiologic change, in turn leads to an overall response, or pharmacologic effect. The response observed represents the outcome of what may

be a complex sequence of physical and chemical interactions between the drug and specific cellular components at the site of action. The cellular components affected at the site of action usually are referred to as the *drug receptors*. As the final result, the function of the target cell changes to produce the desired pharmacologic response.

Attaining the objectives of drug therapy depends on an understanding of the pharmacodynamics of the administered drug, including the mechanisms of action, the expected pharmacologic responses, and any adverse reactions. To assess a patient's responses and to maximize the role of drug therapy in a treatment plan, the nurse must know the pharmacodynamics of the drugs administered.

MECHANISMS OF ACTION

To understand pharmacodynamics, the nurse must differentiate between drug action and drug effect. The interaction at the cellular level between a drug and cellular components, such as the complex proteins that make up the cell membrane, enzymes, or target receptors, represents *drug action.* The response resulting from drug action represents the *drug effect,* which may affect total body function. For example, when insulin is administered, the expected drug action is glucose transport across the cell membrane. The lowering of the blood glucose level represents the expected drug effect.

By modifying cell function, a drug causes a response that may lead to a positive therapeutic outcome or an adverse drug effect. Remember that a drug may modify cell function or the rate of function, but *a drug cannot impart a new function to a cell or target tissue.* Therefore, the drug effect or response depends on what the cell should be capable of accomplishing.

An alteration in cell function to cause a response in the target tissue may be initiated by one of two mechanisms

Drug disposition

The phases between drug administration and drug effect include pharmaceutical, pharmacokinetic, pharmacodynamic, and pharmacotherapeutic. The activities involved in each of the phases as well as the various factors that influence those activities are illustrated below.

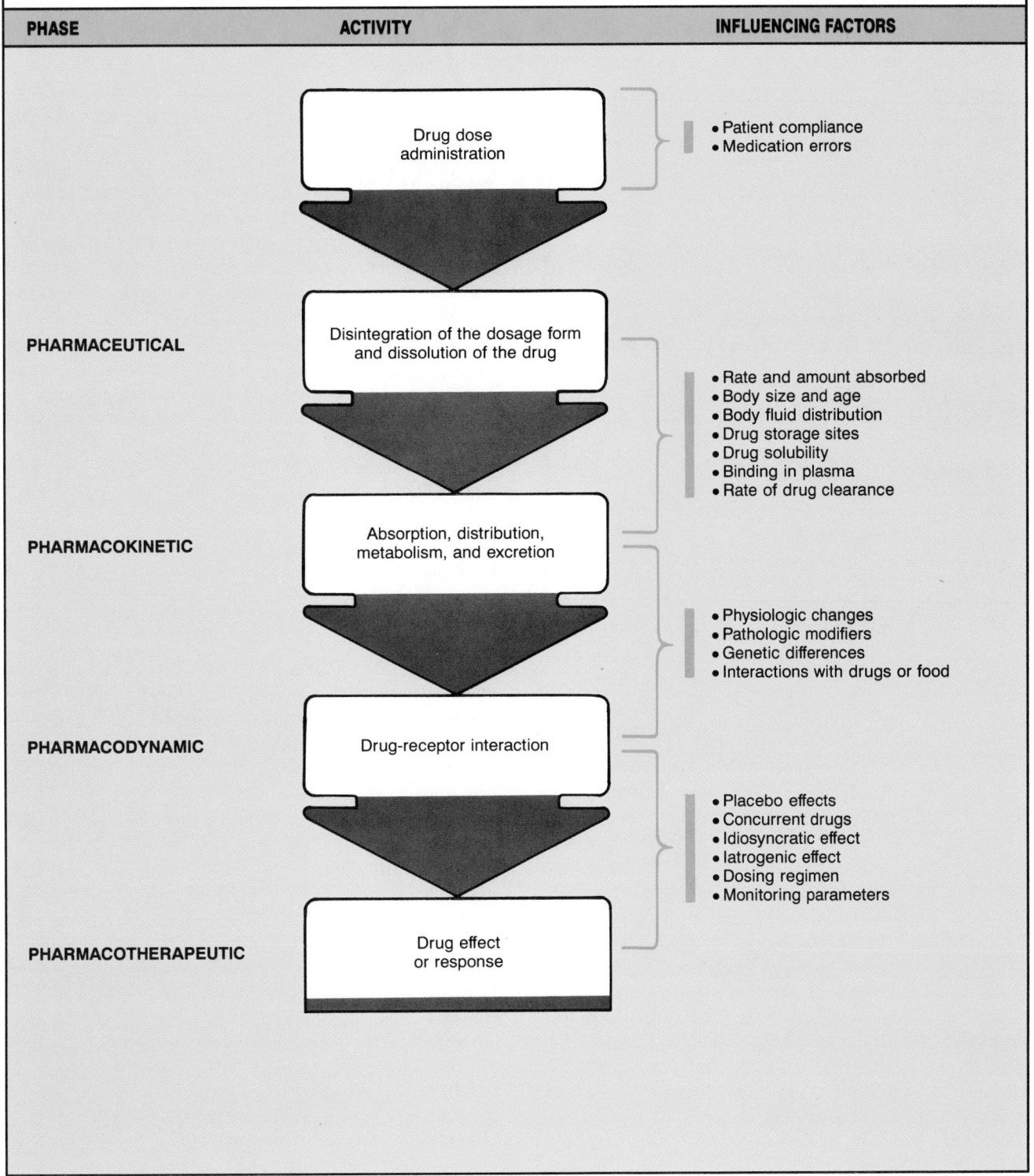

PHASE	ACTIVITY	INFLUENCING FACTORS
	Drug dose administration	• Patient compliance • Medication errors
PHARMACEUTICAL	Disintegration of the dosage form and dissolution of the drug	• Rate and amount absorbed • Body size and age • Body fluid distribution • Drug storage sites • Drug solubility • Binding in plasma • Rate of drug clearance
PHARMACOKINETIC	Absorption, distribution, metabolism, and excretion	• Physiologic changes • Pathologic modifiers • Genetic differences • Interactions with drugs or food
PHARMACODYNAMIC	Drug-receptor interaction	• Placebo effects • Concurrent drugs • Idiosyncratic effect • Iatrogenic effect • Dosing regimen • Monitoring parameters
PHARMACOTHERAPEUTIC	Drug effect or response	

Drug-receptor interaction

The two receptors in the following illustration are structurally compatible with drug A. Drug B will not interact with these receptors.

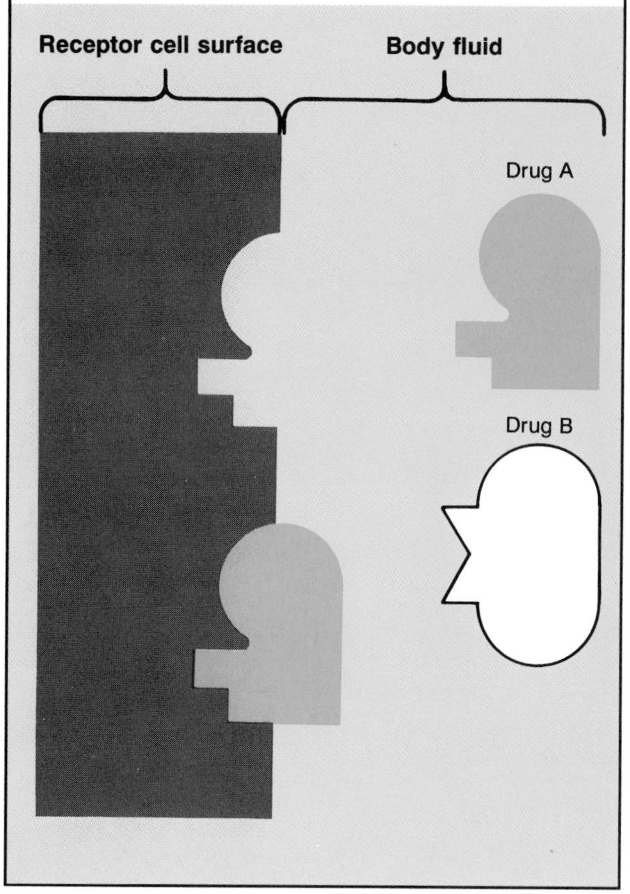

of action. A drug may alter the target cell's function by modifying the cell environment or the cell function.

A modification of the cell environment results from drugs that produce their therapeutic responses by affecting the cells externally. The mechanism of drug action occurs through a physical or chemical change in the cell environment. Drugs that produce responses by affecting the cell externally are considered to be structurally nonspecific. Some of these drugs act by biophysical means that do not change cell or enzyme functions.

By contrast, modification in cell function occurs when a drug molecule interacts with macromolecules within the target tissue. These macromolecules consist of a receptive substance or a configuration of molecules that acts as a receptor. Regardless of the target area, the process, referred to as a drug-receptor interaction, may accelerate or slow cell function in the target tissue.

NONSPECIFIC MODIFIERS OF CELL ENVIRONMENT

Drugs that modify the cell environment do not specifically attach to the cell. Such drugs, however, accumulate on or pass through cell membranes, where they physically or chemically interfere with some of the cell's metabolic processes. Because nonspecific modifiers do not demonstrate any structural attachment to the cell or drug receptors, they seem to act nonspecifically on cell membranes and the cellular processes. Thus, the drug effects are induced externally by changing the physical or chemical environment of the cells.

Physical modification of cell environment

Various drugs with structurally nonspecific mechanisms of action act by biophysical means that do not change cell or enzyme functions. Rather, the drugs physically modify the cell environment. The modification of cell environment may create a barrier, reduce surface tension, or lubricate. For example, applying petrolatum reduces diaper rash by providing a barrier between the skin and ammoniacal urine. Sunscreen lotion acts by providing a barrier between the skin and damaging ultraviolet sun rays. Surfactant stool softeners, such as docusate calcium or docusate sodium, reduce the surface tension of fecal matter. Such stool softeners allow water to penetrate the feces to promote stool softening and regularity. The administration of mineral oil facilitates the passage of feces by lubricating the contents of the bowel.

Chemical modification of cell environment

Although structurally nonspecific drugs usually do not alter cell function, chemical modification of the cell environment by nonspecific modifiers may alter cell function if the drug reacts with other chemicals or invokes changes in the components of the body fluids. For example, the intravenous administration of sodium bicarbonate in a patient with severe diabetic ketoacidosis results in improved cell function when the body pH approaches normal. A less dramatic chemical change in the cell environment may be induced when antacids, administered orally to neutralize increased gastric acid levels, promote ulcer healing.

Cell environment also can be changed by altering vascular osmolality. For example, intravenous mannitol administration increases the intravascular osmotic load, which in turn draws water into the vascular system to dilute the mannitol. The dilution of mannitol leads to an osmotic diuresis that removes excess water from the body and changes the cell environment.

Another example of chemical modification at the cell level involves lipid-soluble (fat-soluble) drugs, including some general anesthetics, hypnotics, and sedatives. The fat-soluble drugs enter the lipoid nerve cell membrane and inhibit nerve conduction. However, the drugs are not structurally specific to any receptor; their presence merely overwhelms the cell and alters cell function.

A deleterious change in the cell environment also may be induced by alcohol, detergents, certain disinfectants, and hydrogen peroxide. These agents act by irreversibly destroying the functional integrity of the living cell.

SPECIFIC MODIFIERS OF CELL FUNCTION

The drug-receptor interaction is the second major mechanism of drug action. A receptor consists of a specialized reactive substance or a macromolecule (a large group of molecules, such as a cell membrane, protein, or enzyme) that will interlock with a drug molecule. The interaction of the drug and its receptor should result in a drug effect, or pharmacologic response. The binding of a drug to a receptor can involve many different types of binding forces and may or may not be reversible. The drug-receptor interaction can be visualized as a key fitting a lock. (For an illustration of this mechanism of action, see *Drug-receptor interaction*.)

Drug-receptor interactions. These interactions occur within the target cell, tissue, or organ. The receptor primarily consists of protein. The molecular structure of protein allows each specific receptor to assume a different shape. The differing shapes among receptors support the theory of a structure-specificity relationship between the receptor and the drug. The structure-specificity relationship demonstrates the tendency of receptors to interact only with those drugs that are exactly compatible structurally.

The structure-activity relationship between a drug and a receptor is more complex. According to this relationship, if the structure of the drug is changed even slightly, the receptor still may interact with the drug, but the response elicited from the altered drug will differ from the response to the unaltered drug. The modified response could be a positive therapeutic outcome or an adverse reaction. (For a depiction of this kind of binding, see *Structure-activity relationship*.)

Drug-enzyme interactions. These interactions also may result in a drug response. An enzyme is a protein-based substance whose catalytic action can promote or accelerate a biochemical reaction with a substrate (substance acted on by an enzyme) molecule. Sometimes, the enzyme mistakenly identifies the drug as the usual substrate, and a drug-enzyme interaction occurs. This interaction could be the source of a drug response that increases or decreases the rate of a cellular biochemical reaction. For example, neostigmine, an anticholinesterase, interacts with the enzyme acetylcholinesterase and inhibits the destruction of acetylcholine released from the parasympathetic nerves.

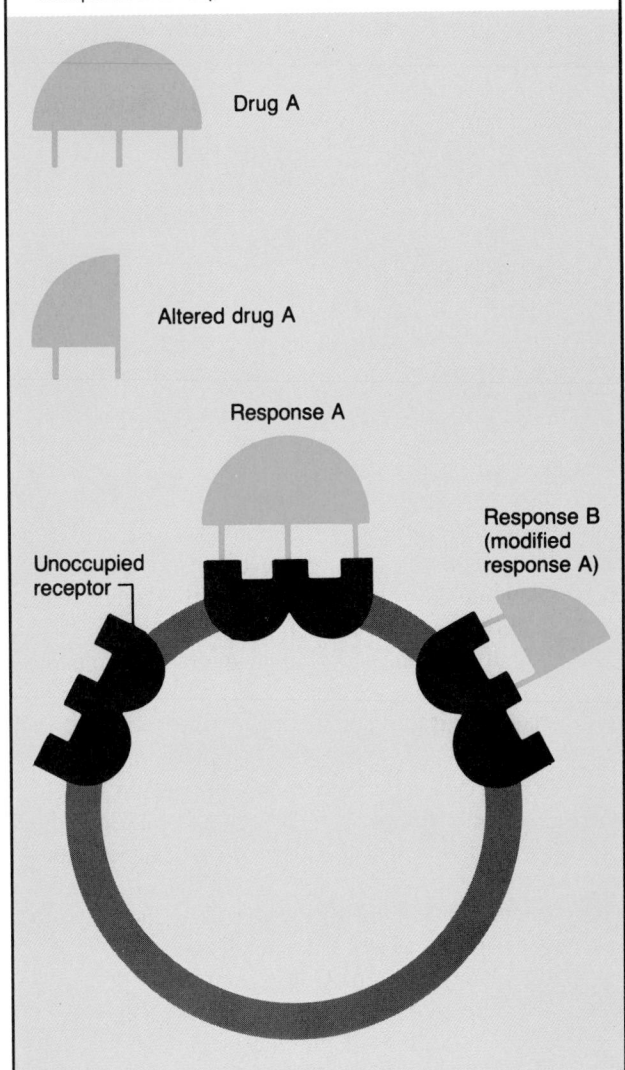

Structure-activity relationship

Some receptors are less selective of the drugs with which they will interact. Therefore, a receptor may interact with a drug that has been structurally altered. The response to the altered drug, however, will usually differ from the original drug response. Also, all of the receptors need not be occupied for a response to occur.

Drug A

Altered drug A

Response A

Response B (modified response A)

Unoccupied receptor

Thus, acetylcholine accumulates and increases the activity in the target tissue. The response may lead to increased gastric contractions or gastric acid secretion.

Nutrient effect on cell function. Nutritional substances, such as vitamins and trace elements, can modify cell function. As a result, they must be considered pharmacologically active. Vitamins and trace elements in small quantities promote daily cell function, but excessive amounts may cause deleterious effects. For example, proper amounts of vitamin A promote the homeostasis of multiple organ systems, including the eyes, skin, liver, pancreas, and lungs; however, excessive doses may induce papilledema, dry skin, headache, fatigue, vomiting, irritability, and other adverse reactions.

DRUG RECEPTORS

Several basic concepts help explain the action of drugs at receptor sites. A drug attracted to a receptor displays an affinity for that receptor. The drug's ability to initiate a response after binding with the receptor is referred to as intrinsic activity. When a drug displays an affinity for a receptor and then enhances or stimulates the functional properties of the receptor, the drug acts as an *agonist*. A drug that is not an agonist can compete with an agonist for a receptor by occupying the receptor, thereby preventing the action of the agonist. Such a drug, called an *antagonist*, does not initiate an effect. Instead, the antagonist prevents a response from occurring.

Antagonists consist of two types. The first, a competitive antagonist, competes with the agonist for receptor sites. If the concentration of the competitive antagonist increases without a change in the amount of agonist available, the affinity of the competitive antagonist for the receptor will displace the agonist. Eventually, the competitive antagonist will inhibit receptor activity completely. For example, naloxone is a competitive antagonist with an affinity for the opioid receptor. The parenteral administration of naloxone reverses opioid respiratory depression in 1 to 2 minutes, thereby reversing the effects of opioid overdose. The opposite result may occur when the concentration of a competitive antagonist remains constant. In such circumstances, receptor activity slowly resumes, and increasing amounts of agonist displace the antagonist.

The second type of antagonist, the noncompetitive antagonist, inhibits agonist response regardless of agonist concentration. The affinity of the noncompetitive antagonist for the receptor is so high that the receptor essentially becomes unavailable for the agonist or normal substrate. For example, the noncompetitive antagonist phenoxybenzamine protects the patient from the intermittent release of large amounts of catecholamines from adrenal tumors.

FUNCTION OF RECEPTORS

Receptors can change the rate of body functions or initiate an activity. Ligands (endogenous substances, such as hormones, neurotransmitters, or autacoids) interact with a receptor, binding with it to cause a response. A drug will mimic a ligand when the drug's structure resembles the ligand's or when the receptor is not appropriately selective. When ligand binding occurs, the activity rate of bodily functions is enhanced or inhibited.

CLASSIFICATION OF RECEPTORS

Drug receptors usually are classified by the effects produced. However, a nonselective drug may interact with more than one receptor type, thereby causing multiple effects. Also, some receptors are classified further by their specific effects. For example, the *beta receptors* usually produce increased heart rate and bronchial relaxation, besides other systemic effects.

Beta receptors, however, can be subdivided into $beta_1$ receptors (act primarily on cardiac tissue) and $beta_2$ receptors (act primarily on smooth muscles and gland cells). $Beta_1$ receptors predominate in the heart; $beta_2$ receptors, in the lungs. Administering a nonselective beta antagonist, or beta blocker, such as propranolol, to a patient with tachycardia will decrease the heart rate. Unfortunately, the nonselectivity of propranolol also will block $beta_2$ receptors, which could precipitate an asthmatic attack in a susceptible patient. Administering a selective $beta_1$ antagonist, such as metoprolol or atenolol, will reduce the risk of receptor nonselectivity and specifically decrease heart rate, but should not affect pulmonary function.

Epinephrine is a nonselective beta agonist used to treat acute asthmatic disorders. Unfortunately, when administered subcutaneously, epinephrine will interact with $beta_1$ and $beta_2$ receptors and further increase the asthmatic patient's accelerated heart rate. Therefore, terbutaline, administered parenterally, is a preferred drug: it is more selective for $beta_2$ receptors. The physician assesses the patient's responses to selective versus nonselective drugs before determining the most appropriate drug for each patient.

RECEPTOR NUMBERS AND RESPONSE

The number of receptors and their affinity for binding with a ligand may increase or decrease in some situations. An increased number of receptors, termed up-regulation, is associated with receptors that are triggered by hormones and neurotransmitters. For example, thyroid hormone is thought to increase the number of selective cardiac receptors, which would explain why in thyrotoxicosis the number of $beta_1$ receptors in the heart increases, and why propranolol, a $beta_1$ antagonist, is effective in treating tachycardia. In contrast, a decreased number of receptors, or their decreased affinity for the ligand, is termed down-regulation. The concepts of up-regulation and down-regulation help explain the sometimes mysterious changes in patient response that may occur during routine drug therapy.

Besides a patient's receptors varying in their affinity for ligand binding, a patient's overall responsiveness to a drug can vary considerably. (For more information about patient responsiveness, see Chapter 4, Pharmacotherapeutics.) A patient also may exhibit different responses to the same drug at different times during treatment. This variable can range from a heightened response to virtually no response. Hyperreactivity refers to a more magnified response to a drug dose than the response seen in most patients. (Do not confuse hyperreactivity with hypersensitivity, an immediate, possibly life-threatening, allergic drug response.)

Hyporeactivity refers to the less-than-usual response to a normal drug dose, which usually necessitates an unusually large drug dose to produce the usual drug effect. The resistance to drug therapy of patients with hypothyroidism typically reflects hyporeactivity. The condition resolves with thyroid hormone supplements that return the patient to normoreactivity.

Tolerance refers to a decreased response or sensitivity of the receptor to a drug. Although the mechanisms for this modification in response are not completely clear, tolerance seems to occur when a patient has had previous exposure to a drug. Tolerance also may result from increased rates of drug metabolism or from the receptor's adaptation to the local drug action. For example, hypnotics and sedatives used over a long period commonly become ineffective in producing sleep; that is, a tolerance to sedative induction at initial doses develops. Other examples of tolerance-producing agents include barbiturates, alcohol, nitrates, tobacco, and opiates. A cross-tolerance between drugs also can develop, as demonstrated by alcohol and general anesthetics. The tolerance that develops from chronic alcohol use increases the usual required dose of an anesthetic.

Immunity describes a reduced response only when the modification results from antibody formation. For example, tetanus toxoid initiates a low-grade immune response that later will protect the human body from the life-threatening response that follows exposure to the tetanus bacterium.

Occasionally, a patient demonstrates an idiosyncratic, or unusual, response to a drug. Idiosyncratic responses, which occur infrequently, usually are associated with genetic differences in enzyme activity or immunologic mechanisms.

OUTCOME OF DRUG ACTION

The major factors determining the outcome of drug action include the location and function of the receptors with which the drug interacts and the drug concentration at the receptor site. If the drug interacts with common receptors located throughout the body, the drug effects will be widespread. The use of drugs exhibiting such widespread response can be particularly dangerous because potential toxicity may affect many organ systems. The margin of safety for such drugs can be narrow, as in chemotherapeutic drugs. (For more information about margins of safety, see the "Therapeutic index" section later in this chapter.)

If the drug interacts with specific receptors that are unique for highly differentiated cells, the response should be quite predictable. For example, the careful use of controlled doses of radioactive iodine, which has a strong affinity for receptor sites within the thyroid gland, effectively treats hyperthyroidism.

The drug treatment outcome also may depend on whether the drug affects the target organs and tissues directly or indirectly. For example, in the treatment of asthma, theophylline directly modifies the bronchodilator receptors in the lung to improve ventilation. This direct effect provides a rapid onset of action and allows the physician to use theophylline blood concentration levels to correlate the therapeutic outcomes and drug dosages. In contrast, levodopa indirectly affects the target tissue in the central nervous system. Dopamine, the active metabolite of levodopa, cannot cross the blood-brain barrier and bind with the target tissue to elicit a response. Therefore, levodopa, which freely crosses the blood-brain barrier, must be used to produce dopamine in the central nervous system.

Outcome also depends on the drug concentration at the receptor site. The amount of drug at the site usually affects the intensity of the drug-induced response. The effect of drug concentration at the receptor site on outcome is best reflected in the dose-response curve.

DOSE-RESPONSE CURVE

As its name implies, a dose-response curve graphically represents the relationship between the dose of a drug and the response elicited. (For an illustration of the following discussion, see *The dose-response curve,* page 44.)

The dose-response curve

Most drugs demonstrate a high correlation between the dose and the response (effect A). All drugs, however, usually exert more than one effect. Unfortunately, with some drugs, the occurrence of adverse effects does not permit the use of a wide dosage range to achieve the desired effect (effect B). In fact, with some drugs, the onset of adverse effects may preclude using the drug even to obtain effect B.

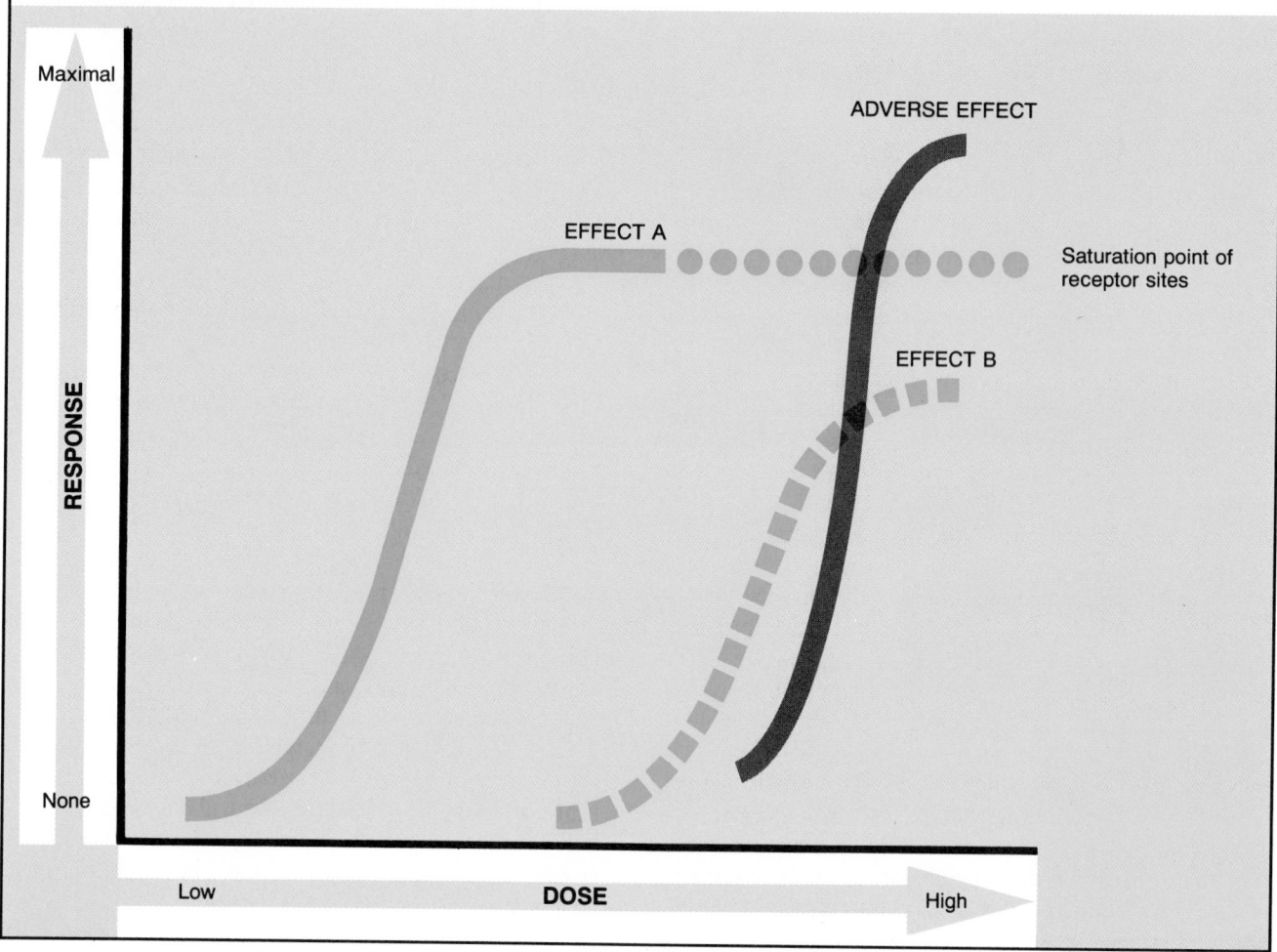

On a dose-response curve, an initial low dose usually corresponds with a low response. As the dose increases incrementally, the corresponding response usually increases. A high correlation between the dose and the response indicates that the dose regimen can be increased to reach a point where receptor sites are saturated without causing adverse reactions. At this point, further increase in dose will not increase response. In short, the maximal response to the drug has been attained.

The administration of theophylline reflects a high correlation between dose and response. The incremental increase in dose corresponds to an incremental increase in the blood concentration of the drug. Furthermore, the theophylline regimen can be increased without adverse reactions until the pulmonary function of the asthmatic patient improves. Eventually, however, the maximal response is attained; the pulmonary bronchi can dilate no further. At this point, any increase in theophylline dose will not improve ventilation.

All drugs elicit more than one response. Morphine at low doses may calm an irritable bowel; higher doses of the drug can serve as a narcotic analgesic. Unfortunately, some adverse reactions commonly occur at normal therapeutic doses. On a dose-response curve, the curve representing the doses of morphine used as a narcotic analgesic would overlap the curve representing the drug's adverse effects. In the case of morphine, respiratory depression may preclude the continual increase in dose to achieve pain relief.

Ideally, a drug will possess a low-dose-response curve, a high-dose-response curve, and an adverse effect-dose-

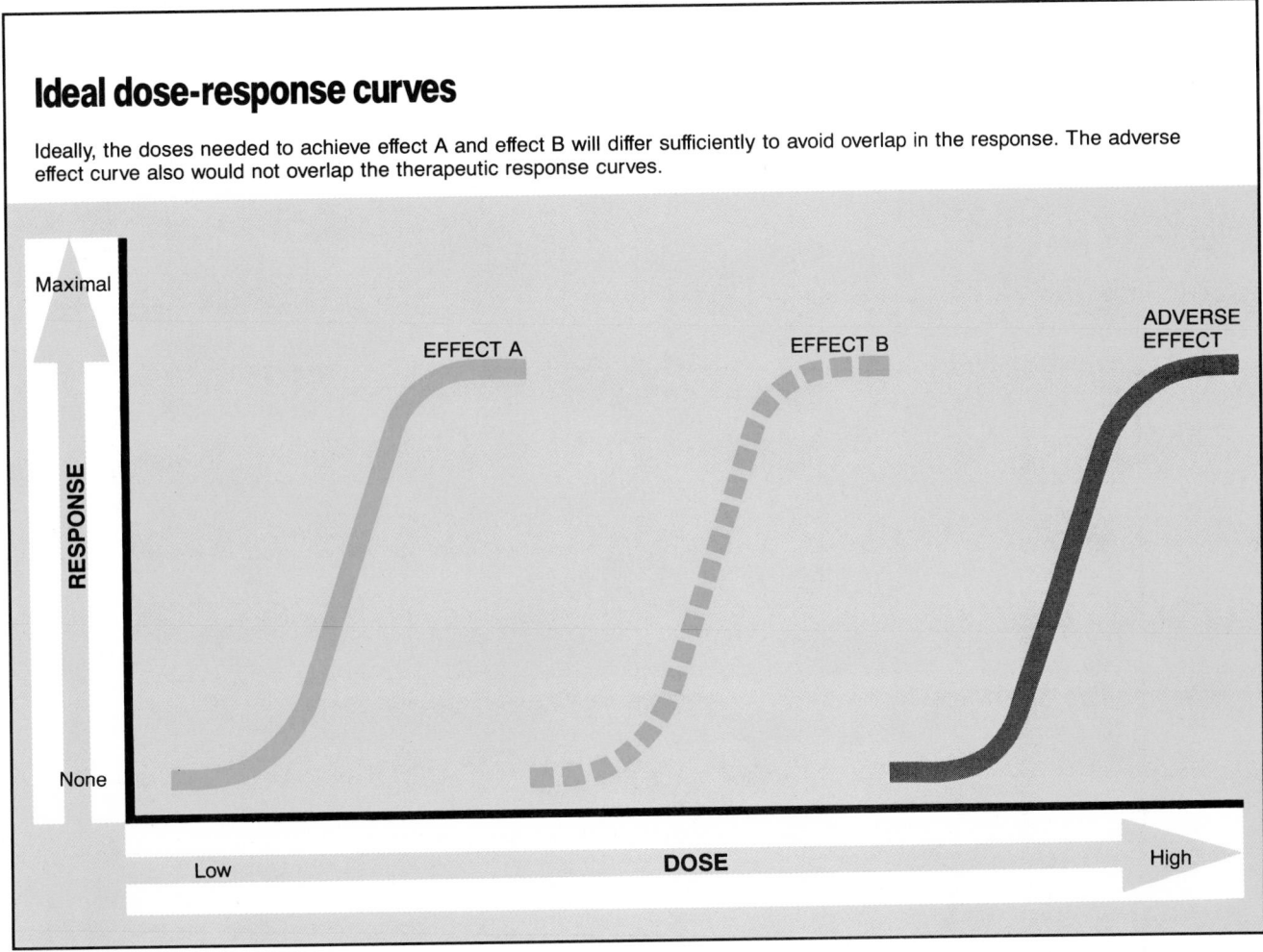

Ideal dose-response curves

Ideally, the doses needed to achieve effect A and effect B will differ sufficiently to avoid overlap in the response. The adverse effect curve also would not overlap the therapeutic response curves.

response curve, none of which overlaps the other. The three curves would be separated adequately, thus reducing exposure of the patient to any risk of an adverse drug reaction. (For an illustration of this concept, see *Ideal dose-response curves*.) Unfortunately, this treatment goal has yet to be achieved for most drugs.

DRUG POTENCY

Drug potency, a frequently used and misunderstood term, refers to the relative amount of a drug required to produce the desired response. Comparing the drug potency of one drug with that of another drug can reveal the more potent drug. For example, comparing the usual doses of two diuretics shows that chlorothiazide requires 500 to 1,000 mg daily to achieve a therapeutic effect, whereas hydrochlorothiazide requires only 50 to 100 mg daily. Because hydrochlorothiazide achieves comparable effects at a lower dose, it is the more potent of the two diuretics. (For an illustration of the differences in dosages needed between drug A and drug B to attain the desired effect, see *Drug potency and efficacy,* pages 46 and 47.) The drug potency

is relatively unimportant in clinical practice unless the quantity required for administration is unpalatable.

DRUG EFFICACY

Drug efficacy differs from drug potency in that it relates to the maximal response or effect achieved when the dose-response curve reaches its plateau. For example, compare the use of morphine and aspirin to treat pain. Aspirin is effective for mild to moderate pain only; morphine is effective for all pain levels. (For the dose-response curves of morphine and aspirin, see *Drug potency and efficacy,* pages 46 and 47.) Unfortunately, other factors may affect this dose-response-plateau relationship. For instance, the incidence and severity of adverse reactions before the plateau is attained can reduce a drug's efficacy. Furthermore, a drug's plateau may fall short of the maximal amount needed for effective therapeutic treatment.

(Text continues on page 48.)

Drug potency and efficacy

Potency and efficacy are commonly confused. A more potent drug achieves effects comparable to those of another drug but at smaller doses. Ideally, a drug should exhibit potency, a high efficacy, and a low incidence of adverse effects.

DRUG POTENCY

Drug potency is the relative difference between the doses of two drugs necessary to achieve a comparable drug response.

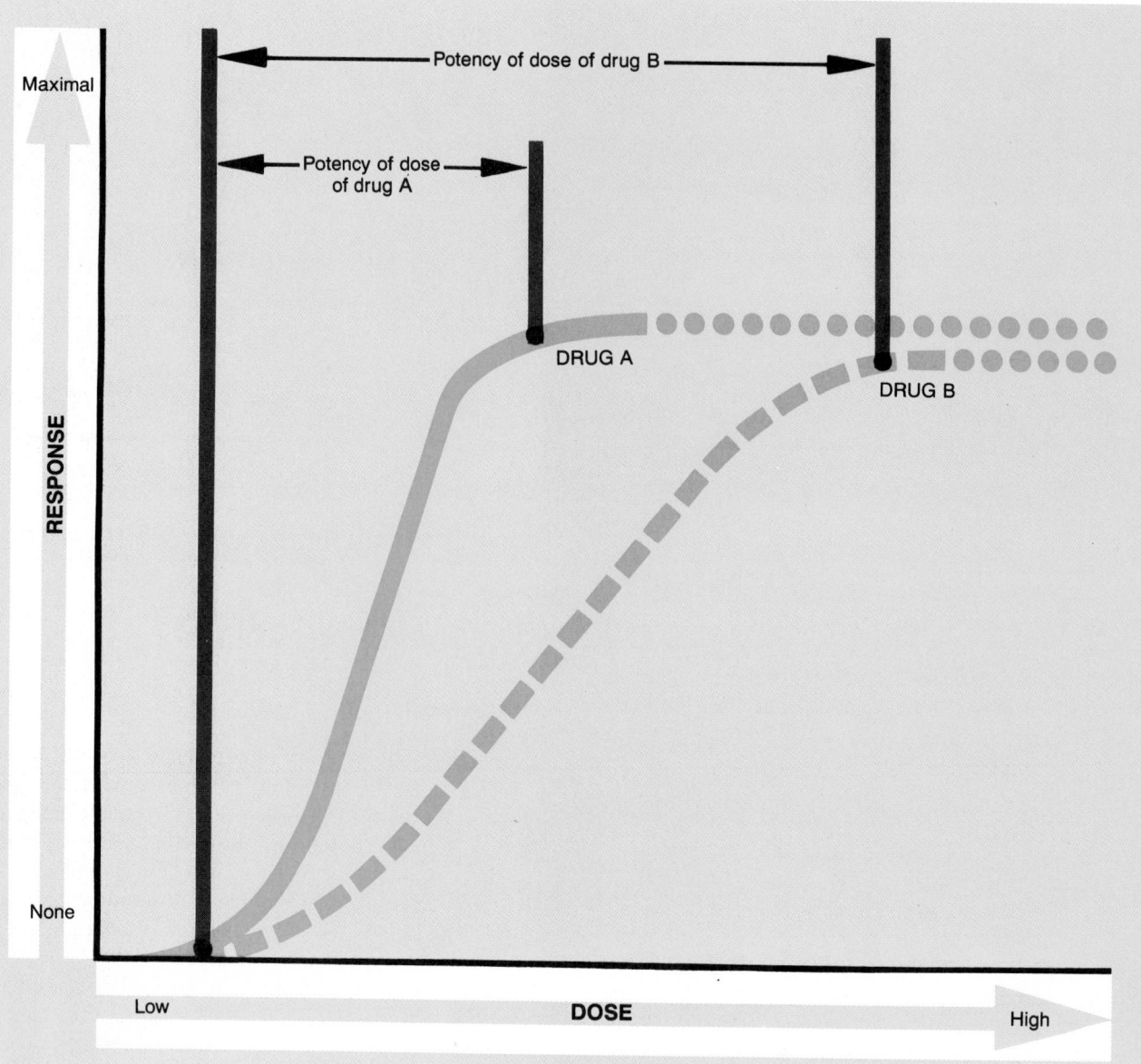

DRUG EFFICACY

Drug efficacy reflects the comparative differences in the maximal responses of two drugs. The physician must evaluate the incidence and severity of the patient's adverse reactions in determining the efficacy of a drug.

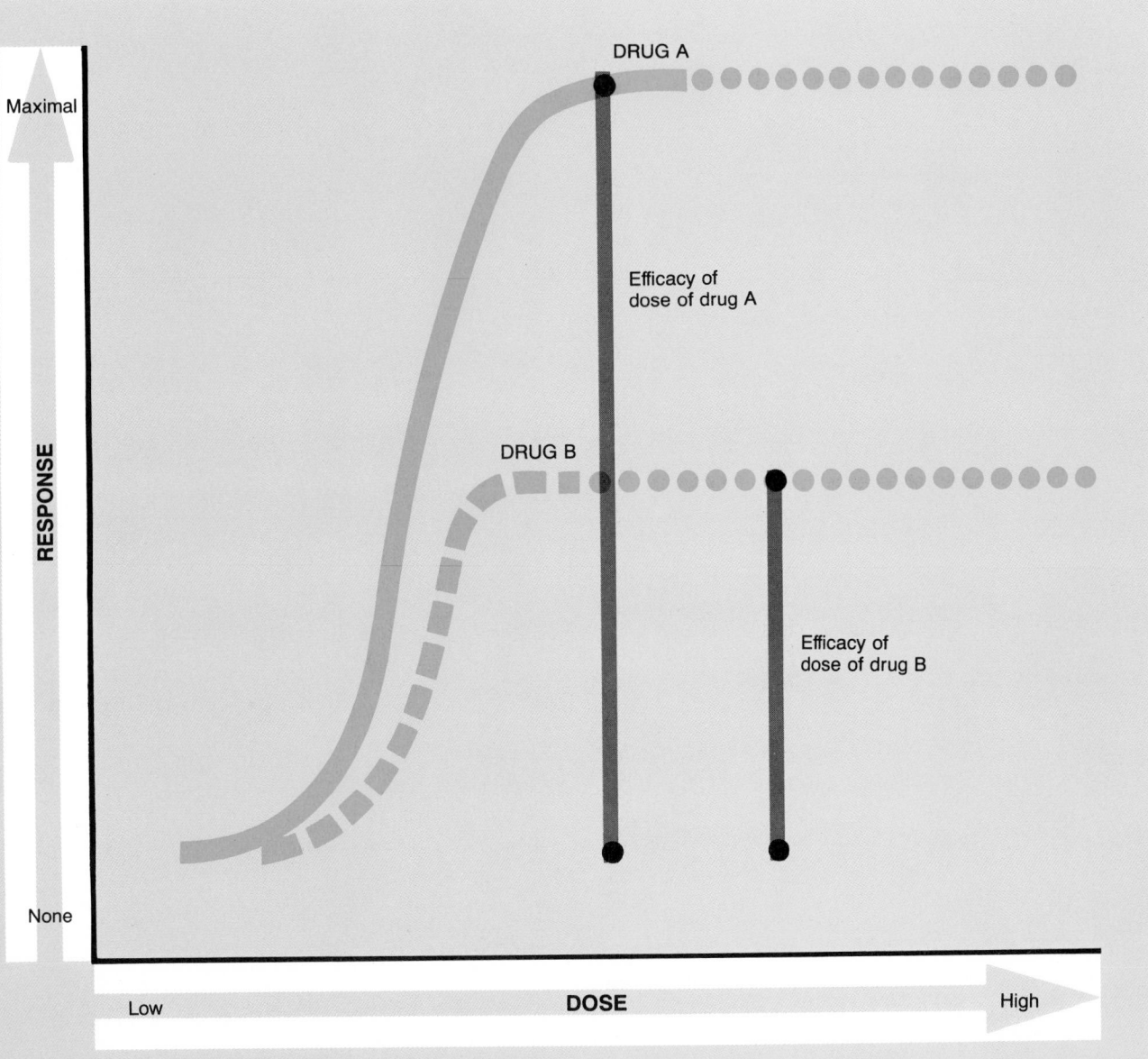

THERAPEUTIC INDEX

Most drugs produce multiple effects. For example, morphine acts as an analgesic, cough suppressant, and sedative, and also causes respiratory depression, constipation, and other adverse reactions. The relationship between a drug's desired therapeutic effects and its adverse effects is termed the drug's therapeutic index, its selectivity, or its margin of safety.

A review of how the therapeutic index is determined in animals illustrates the concept. In animal experiments, researchers compare the effective treatment dose for 50% of the animals to the dose that resulted in 50% of the animals succumbing to the drug's adverse effects. If the difference between the two doses is significant, the therapeutic index is wide. If the difference between the two doses is narrow, the therapeutic index is narrow. A narrow therapeutic index probably precludes the drug's use in humans.

Obviously, using this method to determine the therapeutic index in humans is not acceptable. Therefore, the human therapeutic index usually represents a measure of the difference between an effective dose for 50% of the patients treated and the minimal dose at which adverse reactions occur. All drugs with a narrow therapeutic index should be monitored routinely and thoroughly.

CHAPTER SUMMARY

Chapter 3 presented pharmacodynamics—the mechanisms of action by which drugs produce biochemical or physiologic changes in the patient's body. Here are the highlights of the chapter.
• Drug action represents the interaction between a drug and cellular components; drug effect describes the responses from the interaction. Drug action occurs at the cellular level; drug effect may affect total body function.
• A drug cannot impart a new function to a cell or target tissue. However, it can alter cell function by modifying the cell environment or altering the rate of cell functions.
• Receptors are specialized reactive substances or macromolecules (large groups of molecules, such as a cell membrane, a protein, or an enzyme). The drug-receptor interaction may be represented by the analogy of a lock and key.
• Drugs that display affinity for receptors and enhance or stimulate the receptors' functional properties are called

agonists. Drugs that occupy receptor sites and prevent the action of agonists are called antagonists. Agonists stimulate a drug response; antagonists inhibit such a response. Antagonists may be competitive or noncompetitive. When an agonist and a competitive antagonist are present simultaneously, the one in the highest concentration causes the response. The noncompetitive antagonist inhibits agonist response regardless of agonist concentration.
• Drug receptors usually are classified by the effects they produce.
• The major factors determining the outcome of drug action include the location and function of the receptors with which the drug interacts and the drug concentration at the receptor site.
• A dose-response curve graphically represents the relationship between the dose of a drug and the response it elicits.
• Drug potency refers to the relative amount of a drug required to produce a response. Drug efficacy relates to the maximal response achieved when the dose-response curve reaches its plateau. Ideally, a drug should exhibit potency, a high efficacy, and a low incidence of adverse effects.
• The therapeutic index, selectivity, and margin of safety all refer to the relationship between a drug's desired therapeutic effects and its adverse effects.

STUDY QUESTIONS

See Appendix 1 for answers.

1. Harold Melman, age 62, has just received a prescription for a drug to treat his angina pectoris. The nurse explains its pharmacodynamics to Mr. Melman. Which phrase best describes drug action?
(a) the interaction between a drug and cellular components
(b) the response that results from interaction between a drug and cellular components
(c) the new functions imparted to target cells or tissues by a drug
(d) the drug's ability to stimulate function of a receptor

2. Which of the following accurately describes a drug's effect or response?
(a) development of a new target tissue function
(b) modification of cell function
(c) stimulation of new target tissue growth
(d) development of new cell function

3. Before going outdoors, Bridget Nieman, age 22, applies a sunscreen to block damaging ultraviolet sun rays. How does a sunscreen produce this effect?
(a) by physically modifying the cell environment
(b) by chemically modifying the cell environment
(c) by internally modifying the cell function
(d) by developing a new cell function

4. A major mechanism of drug action is drug-receptor interaction. Which type of drug stimulates the functional properties of a receptor?
(a) antagonist
(b) competitive antagonist
(c) noncompetitive antagonist
(d) agonist

5. Jane Ergot, age 44, has been using a sedative for 6 months. Now she reports that it no longer helps her to sleep. Which term best describes this reaction?
(a) hyporeactivity
(b) tolerance
(c) immunity
(d) idiosyncrasy

6. After surgery, Harold Farber, age 55, receives a narcotic analgesic to relieve pain. On a dose-response curve, the drug's dose curve overlaps its adverse effects curve. Which statement best explains this action?
(a) Higher than usual doses are needed to obtain therapeutic effects.
(b) Adverse reactions may occur with therapeutic doses.
(c) Adverse reactions do not occur even with high doses.
(d) Lower than usual doses are needed to obtain therapeutic effects.

7. Before administering the narcotic analgesic, the nurse considers its potency. Which of the following best describes drug potency?
(a) the amount of drug needed to produce the desired response
(b) the maximal response produced by the drug
(c) the amount of drug at which adverse reactions occur
(d) the amount of drug needed to reach the plateau of the dose-response curve

8. What is the relationship between a drug's therapeutic effects and its adverse effects?
(a) drug potency
(b) drug efficiency
(c) therapeutic index
(d) dose response

SELECTED REFERENCES

Clayton, B., and Stock, Y. (1989). *Basic pharmacology for nurses* (9th ed.). St. Louis: C.V. Mosby.

DiPiro, J., Talbert, R., Hayes, P., et al. (Eds.). (1989). *Pharmacotherapy: A pathophysiologic approach.* New York: Elsevier.

Herfindal, E., Gourley, D., and Lloyd-Hart, L. (1988). *Clinical pharmacy and therapeutics* (4th ed.). Baltimore: Williams & Wilkins.

Johnson, G., and Hannah, K. (1988). *Pharmacology and the nursing process* (2nd ed.). Philadelphia: Saunders.

Karb, V. (1989). Drug information sources for practicing nurses. *Journal of Neuroscience Nursing,* 21(4), 261-264.

Mathewson-Kuhn, M. (1990). *Pharmacotherapeutics: A nursing process approach* (2nd ed.). Philadelphia: F.A. Davis.

PHARMACOTHERAPEUTICS

OBJECTIVES

After reading and studying this chapter, the student should be able to:

1. Describe the types of drug therapy and explain the factors that determine which types a patient receives.

2. Give examples of drugs used to prevent, diagnose, and treat diseases.

3. Explain the concept of the therapeutic index and its importance in drug therapy.

4. Discuss the effects of gastrointestinal (GI), renal, hepatic, thyroid, and cardiovascular diseases on drug action.

5. Describe how age, genetics, sex, body build, and circadian variations affect a patient's response to drugs.

6. Differentiate between drug tolerance and dependence.

7. Discuss three kinds of drug interactions and their effects on the patient.

8. Explain how incompatibilities among parenteral drugs can alter a drug's pharmacologic activity.

INTRODUCTION

This chapter presents an overview of pharmacotherapeutics, or the use of drugs to treat disease, and an examination of factors that may alter a patient's response to drug therapy.

Therapeutics describes the science and art of treating disease. It begins with the assessment of the nature and extent of the patient's health problem. This assessment is based on a patient history obtained by the health care professional, as well as on diagnostic procedures, laboratory tests, and careful clinical observation. Assessing the options and selecting appropriate therapies are based on a knowledge of the patient, related socioeconomic factors, and the risks and benefits of the applicable therapies.

During treatment, the nurse monitors the patient for adverse and therapeutic drug effects, recording expected and unexpected reactions. The frequency of assessment depends on the severity and urgency of the patient's condition. Therapy is adjusted if the patient's problem resolves or progresses, if unacceptable adverse reactions occur, or if the therapy proves unsuccessful. (For a summary of the activities involved, see *Steps of therapeutics*.)

TYPES OF THERAPY

The required therapy depends on the severity, urgency, and prognosis of the patient's condition. The patient's therapy may be acute, empiric, supportive, palliative, maintenance, supplemental, or replacement.

Critically ill patients require acute intensive therapy. For example, a trauma patient may require antibiotics to prevent or treat infection, pressor agents to treat hypotension, volume expanders to treat blood loss, and analgesics to relieve pain.

Empiric therapy is based on practical experience rather than on pure scientific data. Fever spikes in hospitalized patients commonly are treated initially with empiric antibiotic therapy, selecting the antibiotic from a deduction about the microorganisms the patient is most susceptible to—basing their deduction on the patient's general health, hospital stay, or chronic diseases instead of waiting for the results of culture and sensitivity tests.

Some diseases require supportive therapy, which does not treat the cause of the disease but maintains other threatened body systems until the patient's condition resolves. For example, no antiviral agents are available to treat acute viral gastroenteritis, which causes nausea, vomiting, and diarrhea. Instead, patients with this virus receive fluid and electrolyte replacements to prevent dehydration until the condition resolves.

Palliative therapy typically is used for patients with end-stage or terminal diseases, to make the patient as comfortable as possible. For example, high-dose continuous infusions of narcotic analgesics may be used to manage pain in a terminal cancer patient, or home oxygen may be supplied for a patient with end-stage pulmonary disease.

Steps of therapeutics

The steps of therapeutics resemble those of the nursing process.

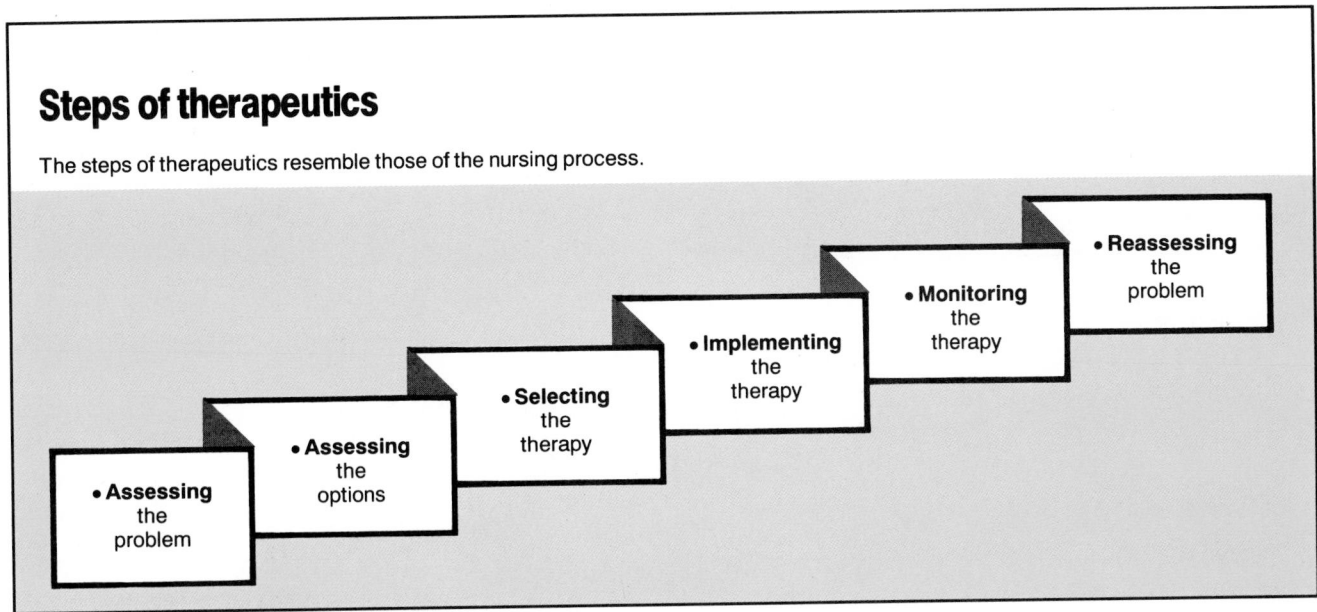

- **Assessing** the problem
- **Assessing** the options
- **Selecting** the therapy
- **Implementing** the therapy
- **Monitoring** the therapy
- **Reassessing** the problem

Maintenance therapy is used for patients with chronic conditions that do not resolve. This therapy seeks to maintain the patient's level of well-being while preventing further progression of the disease, if possible. An example is hypertension, in which the long-term effects can include decreased renal function, impaired vision, cerebrovascular accident, myocardial infarction, cardiac enlargement, and cardiac failure if maintenance therapy is not instituted.

Supplemental or replacement therapy may be short- or long-term. A patient with iron-deficiency anemia, for example, may receive iron supplements until hemoglobin and hematocrit levels are corrected and the body stores of iron are replenished, which may take about 6 months. However, a patient with diabetes mellitus who cannot produce adequate amounts of insulin may require lifelong injections that substitute for the missing hormone.

Other medical conditions may require continual supplemental or replacement therapies. A patient taking a potassium-depleting diuretic, such as furosemide, usually requires daily potassium replacement, and a patient with a hypoactive thyroid gland needs daily replacement of thyroid hormones.

USES OF DRUGS

Therapeutics includes all forms of medical therapy; pharmacotherapeutics is the study of drug use to prevent, diagnose, and treat diseases. Some drugs are used to prevent, diagnose, and treat; others are used for only one or two of these purposes. (For examples, see *Specific drug uses,* page 52.)

Drugs for prevention

Vaccinations are administered to prevent infectious diseases, either before or after patient exposure to the disease. School systems in the United States require that children be immunized against common infectious diseases. Some vaccines consist of weakened infectious agents or antigens that stimulate the body to produce its own antibodies (active immunity). Other vaccines provide the body with antibodies against the infectious agent (passive immunity).

Hepatitis B immune globulin (HBIG) is given to health care professionals to prevent hepatitis B after accidental needle sticks or close contact with patients with hepatitis B viral infections. The injections of HBIG contain antibodies isolated from the blood plasma of hepatitis B patients. Thus, a vaccination of HBIG provides passive immunity to and nearly instant protection from hepatitis B. Heptavax-B, a vaccine for hepatitis B, consists of inactivated viral antigens that stimulate the immune system to manufacture antibodies, thus providing active immunity.

Antibiotics commonly are prescribed to prevent infections. For example, patients may receive antibiotic injections before surgery to decrease the risk of postoperative infections. The antibiotic rifampin, which prevents meningitis, may be given prophylactically to patients with a high susceptibility to meningitis who have been exposed to *Haemophilus influenzae.*

Drugs for diagnosis

Radiologic studies using iodine-based dyes are used to diagnose abnormalities in organ function. For example, intravenous pyelography using iodine-based dyes allows

Specific drug uses

Drugs are used to prevent, diagnose, and treat diseases. Here are specific examples of these different uses.

DRUG	CONDITION
Prevention	
hepatitis B vaccine	• Hepatitis B
amantadine	• Influenza
antibiotics	• Postoperative infection • Urinary tract infections • Otitis media
estrogens	• Contraception • Osteoporosis
Diagnosis	
iodine dye	• Organ system abnormalities
purified protein derivative (PPD)	• Tuberculosis
technetium 99	• Bone alterations
Treatment	
methyldopa	• Hypertension
digoxin	• Arrhythmias • Heart failure
iron	• Anemia
thiamine	• Deficiency • Wernicke-Korsakoff syndrome
folate	• Megaloblastic anemia
quinidine	• Arrhythmias
insulin	• Diabetes mellitus
estrogens	• Menopause

visualization of the kidneys, ureters, and bladder, enabling the physician to check for structural abnormalities and obstruction.

Substances like barium that are clearly visible on X-rays are used in radiographic diagnostic studies. In one such test, the patient swallows a barium-containing suspension that outlines the inner lining of the upper GI tract on X-rays. This test can reveal ulcerations and structural abnormalities in the upper GI tract and the esophagus.

Radiopharmaceuticals, drugs labeled with radioactivity, are used in diagnostic studies of the liver, heart, spleen, bones, and other organs to determine functional alterations that may result from organ damage or disease.

Cosyntropin (Cortrosyn), a synthetic hormone that stimulates the adrenal glands to produce cortisol, is used to diagnose adrenal abnormalities. Cortisol levels are measured immediately before and 30 or 60 minutes after the cosyntropin injection. In patients with normal adrenocortical function, the adrenal cortex responds by secreting cortisol. Patients with adrenal insufficiency do not respond with increased cortisol levels and will require exogenous corticosteroids in periods of stress or illness.

Drugs for treatment

Physicians prescribe drugs to treat the causes of diseases or to alleviate symptoms if the causes are unknown, undetermined, or untreatable. Antineoplastic agents are used, in most cases in combination, to treat malignant neoplasms. Cisplatin (Platinol), chlorambucil (Leukeran), and doxorubicin (Adriamycin) are antineoplastic agents used to treat many kinds of malignant neoplasms.

Laxatives, such as milk of magnesia and bisacodyl, are used to treat constipation, a frequent symptom of unknown origin or of a specific disease or drug therapy. Antibiotics used prophylactically to prevent disease also are used to treat microbial infections.

FACTORS INFLUENCING THE CHOICE OF THERAPY

Several factors help a physician choose a patient's therapy, including an analysis of a drug's potential risks and benefits, the likelihood of patient compliance, and the cost of the therapy.

Analyzing risks and benefits

The physician and the patient must weigh the therapeutic value of a drug against its inherent risks. The physician considers the seriousness of the disease and the availability of less toxic and more reliable drugs. The physician or nurse should inform the patient that every beneficial therapy involves risks.

For example, a physician may consider using cyclosporine, which helps prevent patient rejection of transplanted organs, with a patient about to have such an operation. The drug's benefits, which could lead to a longer, more productive life after transplantation surgery, may outweigh the risks of its nephrotoxicity.

Patient compliance

Compliance describes the degree to which a patient follows the prescribed treatment regimen. Patient compliance is extremely important to a therapy's success or failure. Compliance can be improved by using drugs that simplify the regimen, such as those that require only one or two daily doses, come in palatable liquid dosage forms, dissolve easily, or are available as transdermal patches.

Cost

The physician needs to consider the cost to the patient when selecting a drug because the cost of drugs may interfere with patient compliance.

CLINICAL RESPONSE TO DRUGS

Several drug-related factors, including adverse and cumulative effects, influence the patient's response to drugs during therapy. The nurse must consider these factors when planning and implementing the patient's care.

The therapeutic index of a drug represents the ratio between its effective and toxic plasma concentrations. The therapeutic index is a quantitative measure of a drug's safety. A low therapeutic index indicates a narrow range between a therapeutically active dose and a toxic dose. Examples of drugs with low therapeutic indices include phenytoin, theophylline, and lidocaine. When administering any medication with a low therapeutic index, the nurse must check the dosage and monitor the patient closely. Monitoring activities include assessing the patient's response and laboratory tests (including drug levels) to evaluate the drug's effects. Although the nurse usually includes monitoring and teaching activities in every nursing care plan, these elements are especially important for the patient taking a drug with a low therapeutic index.

A drug is prescribed to benefit the patient; however, adverse reactions do occur. Recognizing them and knowing their effects on the patient are integral components of monitoring drug therapy. (For more information about adverse reactions to drugs, see Chapter 5, Adverse Drug Reactions.) A drug also may produce undesirable responses because of cumulative effects, sometimes resulting in toxicity. Cumulative effects may occur when the drug is excreted more slowly than it is absorbed or when another dose of the drug is administered before the previous dose is metabolized, or cleared from the body.

Toxic drug concentration levels may result when standard drug doses normally eliminated by the kidneys are administered to patients with decreased renal function. Be-

Factors affecting a patient's response

Because no two people possess identical physiologic or psychological compositions, drug response varies greatly, depending upon the following factors:

- Disease
- Infection
- Immunization
- Occupational exposure
- Drug interactions
- Circadian variations
- Diet
- Cardiovascular function
- GI function
- Immunologic function
- Hepatic function
- Renal function
- Albumin concentration
- Genetic constitution
- Enzyme induction
- Stress
- Fever
- Starvation
- Alcohol intake
- Age
- Sex
- Pregnancy
- Lactation
- Exercise
- Sunlight
- Barometric pressure
- Smoking
- Hypersensitivity
- Trauma

cause diseased or damaged kidneys cannot effectively remove the drug from the body, the drug accumulates and leads to toxicity. For example, normal doses of aminoglycoside antibiotics administered at normal intervals to patients with decreased renal function may result in nephrotoxicity and ototoxicity. The physician will need to decrease the drug dosage to prevent toxicity.

Drugs that undergo extensive hepatic metabolism may become toxic in patients with impaired or immature hepatic function. Neonates, for example, must receive reduced doses of the antibiotic chloramphenicol. If given normal adult doses of chloramphenicol, a neonate might develop concentration-related toxic effects, such as bone marrow suppression, because the neonate's immature hepatic enzyme system cannot metabolize the drug sufficiently to avoid the toxic effects.

Although a new drug undergoes extensive testing before receiving Food and Drug Administration (FDA) approval, its adverse effects cannot be predicted reliably until it has received widespread exposure in the general population. In recent years, some new FDA-approved drugs have been withdrawn from the market after some unpredicted, serious adverse effects had become evident.

Other factors, many related to the patient's overall health, can alter the patient's response to a drug. As a result, a physician must consider a patient's concurrent diseases and other medical conditions when selecting an appropriate drug therapy. (For more details, see *Factors affecting a patient's response*.)

DISEASES AND DISORDERS

Diseases and disorders of the major body systems or glands will alter a patient's response to drugs. Altered pharmacokinetic properties (absorption, distribution, metabolism, and excretion) can influence a drug's effect and necessitate alterations in its dosages.

Gastrointestinal system

Drugs are absorbed primarily from the small intestine. Consequently, alterations in gastric emptying or in the environment of the small intestine may affect the absorption of many orally administered drugs.

Hypomotility, or decreased GI movement, can slow or delay drug absorption. Several diseases are associated with hypomotility. In the long-term diabetic patient, for example, hypomotility is secondary to autonomic neuropathy of the GI tract. A patient with the eating disorder anorexia nervosa may exhibit delayed gastric emptying of a standard meal.

Achlorhydria, a condition characterized by the absence of hydrochloric acid in the gastric juices, may lead to decreased absorption of drugs like ketoconazole that require an acidic pH.

GI surgery, particularly gastrectomy and vagotomy, can result in decreased absorption of nutrients and deficiencies of iron, folic acid, and vitamin B_{12}. For example, subtotal gastrectomy (partial removal of the stomach) and vagotomy (severing of the nerves that stimulate acid production in the stomach) lead to decreased acid production and increased pH. This decreases iron absorption because dietary iron cannot be converted to a more absorbable form when the stomach has reduced acidity. The inability to absorb dietary iron eventually leads to iron deficiency.

Drug absorption also is altered in patients with inflammatory bowel disease (Crohn's disease and ulcerative colitis).

Renal system

Because most drugs are excreted at least partially by the kidneys, decreased renal function can influence significantly the therapeutic and toxic effects of a drug. Renal insufficiency can result from disorders, such as acute tubular necrosis, drug-induced renal failure, and diabetes mellitus. It also may result from aging. On average, the glomerular filtration rate decreases 35% to 45% between ages 20 and 90. Creatinine clearance, estimated from 24-hour urine collections or formulas, is used to gauge the glomerular filtration rate. The physician determines dosages for a patient with decreased renal function based on the creatinine clearance.

Hepatic system

Because the liver is involved extensively in drug metabolism, impaired hepatic function can alter drug metabolism and excretion. Impaired hepatic function may result from acute or chronic inflammatory or degenerative disease or neoplastic processes. Because the liver synthesizes protein, its function can affect drug distribution, particularly of highly protein-bound drugs. Patients with cirrhosis or ascites may experience alterations in the volume of distribution.

Unlike renal insufficiency, hepatic dysfunction does not lend itself to reliable guidelines for adjusting drug dosage, partly because no noninvasive methods for estimating hepatic function exist (as compared to using creatinine clearance to estimate renal function) and partly because the liver has an enormous reserve capacity. Large amounts of liver tissue can be destroyed before physiologic changes appear.

As a basic principle, the half-life of a drug that is metabolized extensively in the liver will increase in a patient with hepatic disease, depending on the extent of damage to the hepatic cells and blood flow in the liver. A patient with liver disease will require closer monitoring during the first few days of drug therapy.

Thyroid gland

Abnormal functioning of the thyroid gland can affect drug metabolism. A patient with hypothyroidism or hyperthyroidism metabolizes drugs at slower and faster rates, respectively. As drugs, surgery, or radiation brings patients to the euthyroid (normal thyroid function) state, metabolic rates adjust. For example, a hyperthyroid patient may require large doses of digoxin to maintain a therapeutic level. As the hyperthyroid state is treated, the patient's metabolism slows, as does clearance of the digoxin. When the patient becomes euthyroid, the digoxin dose must be decreased. Throughout the process, the nurse must monitor the patient closely.

Circulatory system

Alterations in circulatory system integrity can affect drug availability in the body. For a drug to act therapeutically, it must reach the site of action. Drug transport is hampered in a patient with peripheral vascular disease, which can develop secondary to diabetes mellitus, and atherosclerosis.

Shock, characterized by hypoperfusion throughout the body, can compromise circulation and significantly affect the administration and pharmacokinetics of emergency drugs. Emergency drugs should not be given intramuscularly to a hypotensive patient because of the unpredictable muscle perfusion and consequent erratic absorption of the drug.

OTHER FACTORS

Physiologic factors that most determine and modify drug activity in a patient include age, genetics, sex, body build, and circadian variations.

Age

The level of organ function changes throughout life. Premature neonates (less than 36 weeks' gestational age), neonates (first month after birth), and infants (age 1 month to 12 months) are extremely susceptible to the effects of drugs because of immature organ systems (especially the liver and kidneys), which significantly affect drug metabolism and excretion. Elderly patients, with decreased organ function secondary to aging, also are susceptible to drug effects. The decline in renal function is one example of the effect of aging on normal physiologic functioning.

The percentage of total body water varies from about 85% in a premature neonate to about 75% in a full-term neonate, decreases to the adult value of about 55% by age 12, and progressively decreases thereafter. Changes in total body water affect drug distribution and necessitate dosage adjustments. For example, neonates and infants require larger mg/kg doses of water-soluble aminoglycoside antibiotics than adults do.

Although total body water decreases with age, the percentage of body fat increases. A younger patient with less body fat obtains a higher blood concentration of a fat-soluble drug and a more rapid response than an older patient does. In a patient with increased body fat, fat-soluble drugs are distributed more to tissues and less to plasma, resulting in delayed responses because of redistribution from tissue to plasma. Fat-soluble drugs include benzodiazepines, phenothiazines, and barbiturates.

The physician and the pregnant patient must give special consideration to the effects of drugs on the fetus. Highly fat-soluble drugs may cross the placenta to the fetus in significant amounts, sometimes producing undesirable effects or even birth defects (teratogenicity). A pregnant patient should avoid all unnecessary drugs, especially during the first 3 months.

Children. Because of immaturity and incomplete development of certain functions, children under age 12 metabolize some drugs in ways that cause unusual effects. For example, the adult stimulant methylphenidate (Ritalin) calms hyperactive children. Also, children metabolize phenobarbital at a faster rate than adults do, thus requiring larger doses to achieve the same effects. Theophylline is metabolized to caffeine in neonates, but very little is so metabolized in adults. (For further discussions of the effects of drugs on children, see Chapter 10, The Pediatric Patient.)

Elderly patients. Disease or aging can decrease organ function in elderly patients, altering a drug's pharmacokinetic properties (absorption, distribution, metabolism, and excretion). For example, because of altered pharmacokinetics, an elderly patient may demonstrate increased sensitivity to the effects of depressants on the central nervous system (CNS). Such sensitivity can lead to oversedation and paradoxical psychotic reactions when an elderly patient receives a usual adult dose of a sedative-hypnotic instead of a reduced dose. Similar effects occur with other sedatives and CNS depressants. (For further discussions of the effects of drugs on elderly patients, see Chapter 11, The Geriatric Patient.)

Genetics

Genetically determined variability in rates of acetylation (one of several drug metabolic pathways) can affect the therapeutic effects and adverse reactions produced by a drug. Procainamide (Procan SR, Pronestyl), an antiarrhythmic drug, is reduced to a metabolite that contributes to the drug's effects. Thus, the physician must consider procainamide and its metabolite to calculate drug concentrations accurately, because a patient with a rapid acetylation rate may have low procainamide levels but adequate combined levels of procainamide and its metabolite.

A patient with a slow acetylation rate may be at risk for developing toxic reactions to some drugs. For example, a patient receiving the antihypertensive hydralazine may develop antinuclear antibodies and a drug-induced form of systemic lupus erythematosus.

Lack of enzymes or coenzymes also can cause toxicity and alter therapeutic effects. For example, drugs that require glucose-6-phosphate dehydrogenase (G6PD) for metabolism can cause hemolytic anemia if given to a patient lacking the enzyme. (G6PD deficiency is a hereditary defect commonly affecting Mediterranean peoples and about 10% of American blacks.) Drugs requiring G6PD for metabolism include quinidine, an antiarrhythmic agent; sulfa antibiotics; and antimalarial agents such as primaquine and quinacrine.

Sex

Females generally possess a greater percentage of adipose tissue and a smaller percentage of total body water than males. As a result, they may require drug dosage alterations.

Body build

A patient's body build directly influences the drug dosage required. Muscle mass and fat content significantly affect drug activity.

Muscle. A decreased muscle mass leads to decreased production of creatinine from muscle breakdown. An overestimation of creatinine clearance in a debilitated or elderly patient could lead to overdosing.

Fat. Lean body weight is important in determining doses of highly fat-soluble drugs; some drugs may require adjustments for obesity greater than 20% above ideal body weight. For example, doses of a highly fat-soluble anesthetic may require adjustment in an obese patient. The need for adjusted dosing of theophylline and aminoglycoside antibiotics in an obese patient is controversial; at the least, the nurse should monitor carefully the blood levels of such a patient to ensure adequate therapy.

Circadian variations

Variations caused by circadian or daily rhythms may affect a patient's metabolic processes and responses to drug therapy. Researchers have noted recently that the pharmacokinetics of the hypnotic triazolam differed significantly in the daytime as compared to the evening, when the drug usually is administered; administered in the evening, it had a slower absorption rate and a longer half-life.

Concentration levels of cortisol vary according to the time of day. The highest concentration levels occur in early to mid-morning. This fact is clinically significant for hormone drugs, such as corticosteroids and thyroid drugs. For example, one daily corticosteroid dose given in early to mid-morning will minimize adrenal suppression and most closely mimic normal physiologic activity.

DRUG ADMINISTRATION

The route and timing of drug administration affect drug activity. (For a discussion of how routes influence drug activity, see Chapter 2, Pharmacokinetics.)

The timing of drug administration is an important nursing responsibility, whether the nurse administers the drug or teaches the patient to self-administer it.

The dosing schedule of a drug can influence significantly the patient's response to therapy. Therapeutic serum levels of antibiotics, antiarrhythmics, and anticonvulsants must be maintained to achieve therapeutic effects. When these drugs are prescribed four times a day, the nurse should administer doses every 6 hours (q6h) to maintain therapeutic levels. If more time separates the last dose of the day from the first dose of the next day, the patient may experience breakthrough effects during the night. Evenly spaced dosing intervals are not as essential for a drug with an extremely long half-life, such as digoxin or levothyroxine; however, the nurse should encourage the patient on long-term therapy with such a drug to take the dose at the same time each day. Observing a regular dosing schedule also improves patient compliance.

Onset and duration of action

A drug's onset and duration of action depend largely on the drug's pharmacologic characteristics, such as lipid solubility. The drug's formulation and route of administration can, however, alter the onset of action. (For more information about onset and duration of action, see Chapter 2, Pharmacokinetics.)

STABILITY OF PHARMACEUTICAL PREPARATIONS

To ensure that a drug is as potent and therapeutically effective as intended, the nurse must carefully observe expiration dates and follow storage recommendations provided by the manufacturer or pharmacy.

Federal regulations require that expiration dates appear on all drug containers. The regulations stipulate that at least 90% of the active ingredient must be available up to the expiration date, ensuring that a patient does not receive a drug that is no longer therapeutically active or that has degraded to toxic compounds. Hospital pharmacists relabel expiration dates on oral drugs that are repackaged for hospital administration. Parenteral drugs are given new expiration dates after being reconstituted or mixed with intravenous (I.V.) fluids.

Drug storage can affect stability and, ultimately, therapeutic effectiveness. Drugs degrade more rapidly in warm, humid conditions. Tablets and capsules usually can be stored safely at room temperature, unless otherwise specified. Liquid dosage forms and injectable drugs sometimes require refrigeration. Some drugs also must be protected from light. For example, nitroglycerin should be stored in light-resistant bottles. The nurse always should check the label for storage requirements.

PSYCHOLOGICAL AND EMOTIONAL FACTORS

Besides the physiologic factors that affect drug activity, psychological and emotional factors also are at work. These include the placebo effect, patient compliance, and health beliefs. The nurse must consider these factors during drug therapy.

Placebo effect. A placebo is an inert or inactive substance sometimes administered in place of a drug. Because it can satisfy the patient's psychological need for a drug, a placebo may elicit a therapeutic response.

Patient compliance. The nurse must monitor compliance carefully, particularly in the ambulatory adult patient with little supervision. Many factors influence a patient's conscious or unconscious decision to take drugs as prescribed. Patient education about drug therapy (preferably by the nurse, pharmacist, *and* physician) can promote patient compliance significantly.

Health beliefs. A patient's health beliefs reflect what the patient considers a normal healthy state and what the patient believes can be accomplished by medical care. A patient who does not perceive abdominal upset and cramping after every meal as abnormal probably will not seek medical attention. Health beliefs vary among cultures, age-groups, and regions of the country and affect compliance, especially in patients with long-term diseases like hypertension who may never feel sick. The nurse should consider health beliefs when assessing a patient's condition and counseling the patient and family members.

TOLERANCE AND DEPENDENCE

Tolerance, a patient's decreased response to a repeated drug dose, differs from dependence. A drug-dependent patient displays a physical or psychological need for the drug. For example, an alcohol-dependent patient not only needs increasing quantities of alcohol to achieve the same effects, but also risks physical and psychological withdrawal symptoms if alcohol use is discontinued.

A cancer patient using a narcotic analgesic for severe pain can display tolerance and dependence. However, the psychological aspects differ from those of the substance abuser. The cancer patient usually is concerned with maintaining a reasonable level of pain relief; the substance abuser desires the euphoric effects of the drug. (For more information about this subject, see the appendix on substance abuse.)

DRUG INTERACTIONS

Drug interactions may occur between drugs or between drugs and foods. They may involve prescribed drugs or over-the-counter (OTC) products. The nurse always should ask the patient specifically about the use of OTC products when obtaining the patient history because the patient may not realize that many OTC products contain drugs.

Drug interactions may interfere with the results of a laboratory test or produce physical or chemical incompatibilities. The more drugs a patient receives, the greater the probability of a drug interaction. The nurse particularly should monitor an elderly patient, who typically has increased sensitivity to drug effects and receives several medications. The average ambulatory patient over age 65 takes 2 to 3.4 medications each day, and approximately 25% of patients over age 65 are discharged from the hospital with 6 or more prescription drugs. (For more information about drug effects on elderly patients, see Chapter 11, The Geriatric Patient.)

INTERACTIONS BETWEEN DRUGS

Interactions involving two drugs usually produce a combined effect equal to the single most active component of the mixture. Such an interaction, called indifference, does not alter the therapeutic effects of either drug, nor does it produce any unpredictable adverse reactions.

Two or more drugs administered to a patient also can produce additive effects that usually are equivalent to the sum of the effects of either drug administered alone in higher doses. The concept of additive pharmacologic response is illustrated by the two analgesics acetaminophen and codeine. Acetaminophen 325 mg and codeine 30 mg are equal in analgesic effect. When combined, as in Codeine #3, their analgesic effect is the same as either acetaminophen 650 mg or codeine 60 mg. Giving the combination drug has these advantages: lower doses of each drug, decreased probability of adverse effects, and greater decrease in pain intensity than from one of these drugs alone (probably because of different mechanisms of action).

A synergistic effect occurs when two drugs producing the same qualitative effect together produce a greater response than either drug alone. For example, ethanol depresses the CNS, leading to sedation and drowsiness. When ethanol and other drugs that have a CNS-depressant effect are combined, the sedative effect is enhanced and psychomotor skills are impaired. Therefore, a patient taking a barbiturate, benzodiazepine, or other drug that causes drowsiness or sedation is cautioned against ingesting moderate to heavy amounts of ethanol.

An antagonistic drug interaction occurs when the combined response of two drugs is less than the response produced by either drug singly. For example, a physician who prescribes levodopa to decrease a patient's stiffness, rigidity, and other symptoms of Parkinson's disease must know that pyridoxine (vitamin B_6) combined with levodopa reverses (or antagonizes) levodopa's effects. Pyridoxine may enhance the metabolism of levodopa, making less drug available to action sites within the brain.

Pharmacokinetic interactions
Many drug interactions alter the pharmacokinetic characteristics of the drugs involved, including absorption, distribution, metabolism, and excretion.

Alterations in absorption. Two drugs given concurrently may change the rate or extent of absorption of one or both of the drugs. For example, the combination of an antacid and the nonsteroidal anti-inflammatory drug naproxen slows the absorption rate of naproxen, but produces no effect on the total amount absorbed. This interaction does not require any dosage adjustments.

In contrast, an antacid administered with the antibiotic tetracycline will decrease the extent, or total amount, of tetracycline absorbed. To prevent this interaction, the nurse should space doses and avoid giving tetracycline within 1 to 2 hours of an antacid.

Alterations in distribution. Concurrent administration of two drugs can alter the volume of distribution by changes in protein binding. For example, the oral anticoagulant warfarin (Coumadin) is highly protein-bound (greater than 97%), and the nonsteroidal anti-inflammatory drug phenylbutazone (Butazolidin) successfully competes with warfarin for protein-binding sites. Combining these two drugs increases the amount of active warfarin available, which significantly increases the risk of bleeding in a patient receiving both drugs.

Alterations in metabolism and excretion. Drug interactions can alter the metabolism and excretion of the drugs. For example, in the antagonistic interaction between pyridoxine and levodopa, pyridoxine increases the metabolism of levodopa.

Barbiturates stimulate the hepatic microsomal enzymes, increasing the metabolism and excretion and decreasing the therapeutic effects of other drugs that are metabolized significantly in the liver. Tobacco smoke also stimulates the hepatic enzymes, causing faster theophylline metabolism and excretion in smokers than in nonsmokers. Propoxyphene (Darvon), a weak narcotic analgesic, also is metabolized faster in smokers than in nonsmokers. Rifampin is another drug noted for inducing hepatic metabolism.

Drug interactions affecting metabolism and excretion commonly lead to toxic levels of the inhibited drug. For example, the antiulcer drug cimetidine inhibits the hepatic metabolism of the bronchodilator theophylline, thereby decreasing theophylline metabolism and excretion and increasing theophylline's half-life and serum concentration levels. This interaction can result in toxic theophylline serum concentration levels if the theophylline doses are not adjusted.

Alterations in hepatic blood flow resulting from drug interactions and disease also affect drug metabolism and excretion. The antiulcer drug cimetidine reduces hepatic blood flow, as do chronic liver disease and cirrhosis. Decreased hepatic blood flow affects drugs, such as propranolol (Inderal), whose metabolism and excretion depend more on blood flow than on enzyme activity. Conversely, drugs whose metabolism and excretion depend on intrinsic enzyme activity generally are not affected by changes in hepatic blood flow.

Some drug interactions affect excretion only. For example, the interaction between the uricosuric drug pro-

benecid (Benemid) and penicillin can produce therapeutic effects. Combining probenecid and penicillin decreases the renal excretion of penicillin and increases the drug's half-life and blood concentration levels.

When therapy with the antiarrhythmic drug quinidine is initiated in a patient on digoxin, quinidine reduces digoxin excretion (primarily renal clearance) and also may displace digoxin from tissue binding sites. The interaction will increase the serum digoxin level and therefore must be monitored closely to determine if dosage adjustments are necessary.

Pharmacodynamic interactions

Drug interactions also produce pharmacodynamic alterations. The synergistic interaction and the enhanced sedation produced by combining ethanol and a barbiturate is an example of such a pharmacodynamic alteration.

Administered concurrently, the bronchodilator theophylline may sensitize pulmonary beta-adrenergic receptors, increasing response to a beta-adrenergic agonist, such as terbutaline or albuterol.

When combined with an opiate, the narcotic antagonist naloxone (Narcan) competes with the opiate for opiate receptor sites. As a result, naloxone can reverse opiate-induced respiratory depression.

DRUG INTERACTIONS AND LABORATORY TESTS

Drug interactions can alter laboratory tests. Health care professionals assess renal function by using a laboratory test that measures serum creatinine levels. The test uses a colorimetric method. Many cephalosporins, such as cefazolin (Kefzol) and cefoxitin (Mefoxin), contain noncreatinine chromogens that are not differentiated among by the colorimetric method. As a result, the laboratory test may overestimate the creatinine levels, possibly leading to inadequate drug dosages.

Guaiac tests of feces for the presence of occult, or unseen, blood can show false-positive results in a patient who takes large amounts of iron supplements.

Blood glucose testing is the preferred method of monitoring diabetes. However, some stable diabetic patients monitor their diabetes using urine testing for glucose. Drugs that interfere with urine glucose testing include cephalothin (Keflin), isoniazid, levodopa (Larodopa), probenecid (Benemid), and large amounts (1 to 2 grams/day) of ascorbic acid. False-positive results indicating high glucose levels could cause a patient to decrease food intake or to increase insulin doses when, in fact, the blood glucose level is stable.

Drug effects on the ECG

Some drugs, particularly cardiac drugs, produce visible effects on the electrocardiogram (ECG) that can lead to misinterpreted results. For example, the antiarrhythmic drug quinidine can widen the QRS complex and prolong the QT interval. The prolongation of the QT interval can be up to 35% greater than the baseline value without representing toxicity. ECG changes of this significance require medical attention in a patient not taking quinidine. The ECG also provides information about electrolyte imbalances that may be related to drug therapy.

DRUG AND FOOD INTERACTIONS

Interactions between drugs and food can produce alterations in the therapeutic effects of the drug or in the use of nutrients.

Alterations in bioavailability. Food can alter the rate and amount of drug absorbed from the GI tract. These alterations affect the bioavailability — that is, the amount of a drug dose available to the systemic circulation. (For further discussion of bioavailability, see Chapter 2, Pharmacokinetics.) For example, the bioavailability of the antifungal drug griseofulvin increases when the drug is administered with a high-fat meal, and the bioavailability of theophylline increases with a low-protein, high-carbohydrate diet.

Drugs also can bind with foods and impair vitamin and mineral absorption. For example, cholestyramine (Questran), used to treat hyperlipidemia, forms a complex with folate, thereby decreasing the amount of folate available to the body. Absorption of vitamins A, D, and K also is lowered, and some patients may require vitamin supplements. Mineral oil, an emollient laxative, forms an insoluble complex with the fat-soluble vitamins A, E, D, and K. The insoluble complex passes through the gut before absorption can occur. Because fat-soluble vitamins help maintain skin integrity, the long-term excessive use of mineral oil eventually can interfere with wound healing.

Induction of enzymes. Some drugs induce, or stimulate, enzyme production, and this induction increases metabolic rates and the demand for vitamins that are enzyme cofactors. For example, in an alcoholic patient, the increased demand for thiamine, a cofactor in alcohol metabolism, decreases serum levels and places the patient at high risk for thiamine deficiency and associated neurologic complications.

Alterations in sites of action. Broad-spectrum antibiotics interfere with vitamin K synthesis by altering the GI flora. Microorganisms in the colon are the normal sites for the GI production of vitamin K, important for coagulation. Prolonged use of a broad-spectrum antibiotic kills the synthesizing microorganisms and can result in bleeding problems, especially in a debilitated or elderly patient, if not accompanied by vitamin K supplements.

Increased toxicity. The antiacne drug isotretinoin (Accutane) is a structural isomer of vitamin A. Therefore, a patient taking isotretinoin must avoid taking vitamin A supplements or increasing dietary vitamin A because vitamin A overdose is a risk.

Many foods also produce pharmacologic activities. For example, aged cheddar cheese and wine contain tyramine. A patient taking a monoamine oxidase inhibitor (an antidepressant) should avoid foods containing tyramine because they could cause a release of catecholamines that are present in large amounts in nerve endings and the adrenal medulla, precipitating a hypertensive crisis.

PARENTERAL DRUG INCOMPATIBILITIES

The nurse must carefully consider drug incompatibilities when administering drugs via parenteral (intravenous, intramuscular, or subcutaneous) routes. Drug incompatibility can produce a physical reaction or a chemical inactivation.

Physically incompatible drugs interact before the drugs reach the site of action, usually interfering with the pharmacologic activity of one or both drugs. Mixing incompatible drugs can form precipitates or change a drug's color. Precipitate formation is especially dangerous for the patient if the solution is to be infused intravenously.

The anticonvulsant phenytoin is administered intravenously to control seizures caused by status epilepticus as well as those of unknown origin. The drug remains stable in an I.V. solution of normal saline (0.9% sodium chloride). However, when phenytoin is mixed with I.V. solutions of dextrose 5% in water, a cloudy, white precipitate forms. The precipitate also forms if the line from the dextrose-containing I.V. fluid is not flushed with saline solution before the nurse starts the phenytoin infusion.

Some light-sensitive drugs may change color if they are not protected. Whether the changed color indicates decreased drug activity is not known. Usually, the nurse should not administer drugs that have changed color.

Exposing an aminoglycoside antibiotic (amikacin, gentamicin, tobramycin) to a penicillin for a prolonged time inactivates the aminoglycoside. This chemical inactivation can occur: (1) if the two drugs are combined in the same I.V. administration bag, (2) if both drugs are being given to a patient with severe renal failure, and (3) if aminoglycoside blood levels in a patient with renal failure are not assayed promptly. In the third instance, the inactivation by the penicillin results in lowered blood levels of aminoglycoside that could be misinterpreted.

Obtaining blood samples for drug concentration levels

The nurse may be responsible for drawing blood samples from the patient for drug level analysis. The following represents therapeutic and toxic levels for some commonly administered drugs. Values may differ among health care facilities.

DRUG	HALF-LIFE	TIME REQUIRED TO ACHIEVE STEADY STATE	TIME TO DRAW SAMPLE	ADULT THERAPEUTIC RANGE	POTENTIALLY TOXIC LEVELS
Antibiotics					
amikacin gentamicin tobramycin	0.5 to 3 hours	2.5 to 15 hours	*Trough:* before dose *Peak concentration level:* 15 to 30 min after I.V. dose; 1 hour after I.M. dose	Amikacin: 7.5 to 10 mcg/ml gentamicin, tobramycin: 0.5 to 2 mcg/ml	*Trough:* Amikacin, >10 mcg/ml; gentamicin, tobramycin, >2 mcg/ml *Peak concentration level:* Amikacin, >30 mcg/ml; gentamicin, tobramycin, >10 mcg/ml
Anticonvulsants					
carbamazepine	5 to 27 hours	>2 weeks	*Trough:* before dose *Peak concentration level:* 3 hours after dose	4 to 12 mcg/ml	*Single drug regimen:* >12 mcg/ml *Multiple drug regimen:* >8 mcg/ml
phenobarbital	50 to 120 hours	10 to 25 days	4 hours after dose	15 to 40 mcg/ml	>40 mcg/ml
phenytoin (Dilantin only)	20 to 40 hours	1 to 2 weeks	*Trough:* before dose *Peak concentration level:* oral, 3 to 9 hours; I.V., 2 to 4 hours	10 to 20 mcg/ml	>20 mcg/ml
Cardiovascular drugs					
digoxin	1.6 days	1 to 2 weeks	5 to 8 hours after dose	0.8 to 2 ng/ml	>2 ng/ml
lidocaine	75 to 140 min	6 to 12 hours	12 hours after starting I.V. drip or toxicity suspected	1.5 to 5 mcg/ml	>5 mcg/ml
quinidine	6 to 8 hours	30 to 35 hours	*Trough:* before next dose	2.3 to 5 mcg/ml	>5 mcg/ml
Respiratory drugs					
theophylline	4.4 hours (smoker) 8.7 to 16 hours (nonsmoker)	1 to 2 days	*Peak concentration level:* 2 hours (solution/solid dosage); 4 to 6 hours (slow-release dosage); 12 hours after start of I.V. infusion, then every 24 hours	10 to 20 mcg/ml	>20 mcg/ml

MONITORING RESPONSE

The nurse can maintain an effective therapeutic drug regimen by understanding the prescribed drug and closely monitoring the patient. Knowing the biological half-life of a drug and the physiologic factors that may alter the half-life enables the nurse to understand the appropriate dosing interval for a patient.

When developing a drug therapy that will not interfere with the patient's life-style, the nurse also must consider the drug's adverse effects, which can lead to noncompliance. For example, a hypertensive patient who operates a vehicle or heavy machinery on the job may choose not to take an antihypertensive that causes drowsiness and CNS disturbances. Knowledge of adverse reactions also is necessary for accurate patient monitoring and effective patient education.

Therapeutic drug monitoring. For drugs with low therapeutic indices, toxic and therapeutic levels are close. When the therapeutic response and toxicity of a drug can be related to blood concentration levels, the nurse uses those levels to monitor drug therapy.

Drug level analysis. When samples need to be drawn for monitoring drug concentration levels, the nurse should refer to a current laboratory manual for appropriate procedures and therapeutic levels. Such specifics as when to draw blood or infuse drugs and how to draw blood for monitoring after I.V. infusion are covered there. (For a summary of this information as it relates to some commonly administered drugs, see *Obtaining blood samples for drug concentration levels*.)

To interpret drug levels accurately, the nurse must understand peak concentration (time when drug absorption and drug elimination are equal), blood level of a drug, and steady-state duration of action. (For more details, see Chapter 2, Pharmacokinetics.)

CHAPTER SUMMARY

Chapter 4 explored pharmacotherapeutics, the study of drug use to treat diseases. Here are the chapter highlights.
- The steps of therapeutics include assessing the problem, assessing the options, selecting the therapy, implementing the therapy, monitoring the therapy, and reassessing the problem.
- A patient may receive acute, empiric, supportive, palliative, maintenance, supplemental, or replacement therapy — depending on the severity, urgency, and prognosis of the patient's condition.
- Drugs are used to prevent, diagnose, or treat diseases; some have more than one purpose.
- A physician considers many factors when selecting a drug for a patient, including an analysis of the drug's potential risks and benefits, the likelihood of patient compliance, and the cost of the drug.
- The therapeutic index of a drug represents the ratio between its effective and toxic blood concentration levels.
- Certain diseases of the GI, renal, hepatic, and circulatory systems and of the thyroid gland can affect the absorption, distribution, metabolism, and excretion of drugs. These diseases may necessitate dosage adjustments. Age, genetics, sex, body build, and circadian variations also affect a patient's response to a drug. Very young and elderly patients are most susceptible to compromising alterations.
- The route and timing of drug administration can affect drug activity, as can drug stability. The nurse always should check the expiration date before administering any drug. The nurse and patient should follow the manufacturer's suggestions for drug storage.
- The placebo effect, patient compliance, and health beliefs significantly affect the results of drug therapy.
- A patient who develops drug tolerance requires more of the drug to produce the same effect. A drug-dependent patient displays a physical or psychological need for the drug.
- The nurse should monitor the patient carefully for all drug interactions involving other drugs or food because they can affect laboratory test results. Interactions between drugs can alter the absorption, distribution, metabolism, and excretion of the drug. Interactions between a drug and food can alter the bioavailability of the drug.
- Incompatibilities between parenteral drugs can interfere with the pharmacologic activity of one or both drugs or chemically inactivate the drugs.

STUDY QUESTIONS

See Appendix 1 for answers.

1. Ken Fowler, age 23, is admitted to the emergency department with a diagnosis of drug overdose. To maintain this patient's threatened body systems, the physician prescribes intravenous therapy. Which type of drug therapy maintains threatened body systems but does not treat the cause of the problem?
(a) empiric therapy
(b) supportive therapy
(c) maintenance therapy
(d) palliative therapy

2. Jessica Harrow, age 46, takes furosemide (Lasix) for hypertension, as prescribed. Because this drug depletes potassium, she also takes potassium daily. Which type of therapy is her potassium replacement?
(a) empiric therapy
(b) supportive therapy
(c) maintenance therapy
(d) supplemental therapy

3. Drugs like furosemide are used to treat disease. Others are used to prevent or diagnose it. Which of the following drugs is used to prevent disease?
(a) hepatitis B immune globulin
(b) purified protein derivative
(c) radioactive iodine
(d) cosyntropin

4. Throughout Ms. Harrow's therapy, the nurse monitors her closely for adverse reactions and their effects. Which effect may occur if a drug is excreted more slowly than it is absorbed?
(a) cumulative effect
(b) synergistic effect
(c) idiosyncratic effect
(d) antagonistic effect

5. Before Ms. Harrow began drug therapy, the nurse assessed her for diseases or disorders that would require a dosage adjustment. An abnormality in which system typically requires a dosage adjustment?
(a) renal
(b) respiratory
(c) gastrointestinal
(d) cardiac

6. The physician prescribes diazepam (Valium) for Ken Greenwald, age 40, to treat back muscle spasms. The nurse assesses Mr. Greenwald's drug history for use of CNS depressants because diazepam may interact with these drugs and produce a greater response than either drug given alone. Which of the following describes this effect?
(a) cumulative interaction
(b) additive interaction
(c) synergistic interaction
(d) antagonistic interaction

7. Ellen Drake, age 37, is receiving warfarin (Coumadin) and phenylbutazone (Butazolidin). If these drugs are administered concurrently, she runs an increased risk of bleeding because both drugs compete for protein-binding sites. Which pharmacokinetic characteristic is altered by this interaction?
(a) absorption
(b) distribution
(c) metabolism
(d) excretion

8. Which of the following statements is true for drugs administered parenterally?
(a) All drugs are compatible.
(b) All drugs are incompatible.
(c) Drug incompatibility may cause a physical reaction.
(d) Mixing drugs enhances their therapeutic effects.

SELECTED REFERENCES

Abrams, A. (1987). *Clinical drug therapy: Rationale for nursing practice* (2nd ed.). Philadelphia: Lippincott.

AHFS drug information 90. (1990). Bethesda, MD: American Society of Hospital Pharmacists.

American Health Research Institute Staff. (1987). *Drug therapy in health, medicine, and disease.* Annandale, VA: ABBE Publishers Association.

Chernow, B. (1988). *Pharmacologic approach to the critically ill patient* (2nd ed.). Baltimore: Williams & Wilkins.

DiPiro, J. (1988). *Pharmacotherapy: A pathophysiologic approach.* New York: Elsevier.

Wilson, J., et al. (Eds.). (1990). *Harrison's principles of internal medicine* (12th ed.). New York: McGraw-Hill.

CHAPTER

5

ADVERSE DRUG REACTIONS

OBJECTIVES

After reading and studying this chapter, the student should be able to:

1. Discuss how patient, drug, and exogenous factors can combine to cause an adverse drug reaction.

2. Provide examples of each predisposing factor.

3. Differentiate between dose-related and patient sensitivity-related adverse reactions.

4. Describe three types of dose-related adverse reactions.

5. Describe two types of patient sensitivity-related adverse reactions.

INTRODUCTION

With the growing use of drugs that improve life and health has come an increasing incidence of adverse drug reactions. This increase has occurred because every drug has the potential to affect a patient adversely.

Most drugs produce a spectrum of effects that range from the desired and routinely anticipated response to the unexplained and potentially life-threatening response. In all drug therapy, the physician and patient must weigh the drug's beneficial effects against its possible adverse effects.

A drug's desired effect is the expected therapeutic response. An adverse drug reaction, also called a side effect or adverse effect, is a harmful, undesirable response, which may result from any clinically useful drug. Adverse drug reactions can range from mild ones that disappear when the drug is discontinued to debilitating diseases that become chronic. Some adverse reactions are related to the drug dose and may be preventable with careful prescription and administration or may be inseparable from the drug's primary therapeutic effects. Others are related to patient sensitivity and may not be predictable.

In this era of sophisticated, complex pharmacotherapy, physicians and nurses must be able to identify and respond to adverse drug reactions. (For a list of adverse reactions to some widely used drugs and drug classes, see *Common adverse drug reactions,* page 64.)

Determining if an effect is desired or adverse may depend on the disorder being treated. For the common cold, for instance, diphenhydramine reduces nasal stuffiness and rhinorrhea. Unfortunately, the drug causes drowsiness, which may interfere with the patient's safe driving of a vehicle. In this case, the reduced nasal stuffiness represents the desired effect, and drowsiness represents the adverse reaction. In contrast, when diphenhydramine is used to treat insomnia, its ability to induce drowsiness is the desired effect. The adverse reaction in using diphenhydramine for insomnia is dry mucous membranes.

Although physicians, nurses, and pharmacists cannot always predict who will experience an adverse drug reaction, they can identify factors that increase the patient's risk and may prevent or minimize the patient's adverse response. To prepare the student for this responsibility, Chapter 5 discusses factors that lead to adverse drug reactions and classifies those reactions.

FACTORS THAT LEAD TO ADVERSE DRUG REACTIONS

A patient's therapeutic responses to a drug result from the interplay among patient characteristics, drug characteristics, and exogenous (external) factors. Patient, drug, and exogenous factors can alter that interplay to produce adverse drug reactions.

PREDISPOSING PATIENT FACTORS

Patient factors include extremes of age, extremes of body weight, genetic variations, the patient's temperament and attitudes, circadian rhythms, changes associated with disease, and changes associated with pregnancy.

Common adverse drug reactions

This chart correlates certain adverse reactions and examples of drugs or drug groups that cause those reactions.

ADVERSE REACTIONS	DRUGS INVOLVED
Rashes, hives, lesions	penicillin, sulfonamides, thiazide diuretics
Hemolytic anemia, thrombocytopenia, agranulocytosis	quinidine, meprobamate, chlorpromazine, phenylbutazone
Hepatitis, biliary obstruction, hepatic necrosis	tetracycline, halothane, acetaminophen
Glomerulonephritis, acute and chronic renal failure	aminoglycoside antibiotics, aspirin
Blurred vision, blindness, cataract development, corneal and retinal changes	chloroquine, phenothiazines, corticosteroids
Deafness, dizziness, loss of balance, tinnitus	salicylates, quinine, aminoglycoside antibiotics
Delirium, disorientation, lethargy	hypnotics, sedatives, antidepressants
Psychomotor retardation, subjective feelings of loss and sadness	reserpine, corticosteroids, methyldopa, indomethacin
Birth defects, fetal and neonatal functional abnormalities	antineoplastic drugs, narcotics, isotretinoin

Extremes of age

The absorption, distribution, metabolism, and excretion of drugs are different in infants and elderly patients than in young adults. Infants lack certain drug-metabolizing enzymes and have decreased renal blood flow. These physiologic factors increase drug and metabolite blood levels. The breast-feeding infant also may develop adverse reactions to drugs that pass into the mother's breast milk. (For specific drugs that pass into breast milk, see Chapter 12, The Pregnant or Lactating Patient.) Elderly patients have decreased blood flow to all organs, especially the liver and kidneys. These conditions result in increased drug concentration levels as well as changes in drug distribution and greater risk of toxicity.

Extremes of body weight

Recommended dosages typically are based on the average-sized adult. Therefore, the extremely thin or obese patient requires an individualized dosage calculation to prevent overdosing or underdosing. Abnormal thinness or obesity may alter drug distribution, resulting in higher- or lower-than-expected drug concentration levels in tissues and at receptor sites.

Genetic variations

Genetic variations that alter enzyme activity or cause enzyme deficiency affect drug metabolism or drug action. For example, isoniazid, hydralazine, and procainamide are metabolized in the liver by a pathway known as acetylation, a process that proceeds at a partially genetically determined rate. Most patients are either fast or slow acetylators. A slow acetylator will display a higher blood level of a given drug dose than a fast acetylator and may experience an adverse drug reaction as a result. Glucose-6-phosphate dehydrogenase (G6PD) plays a vital role in red blood cell stability. A deficiency of this enzyme, which is common in individuals of African, Mediterranean, or Asian descent, is an inherited defect that alters the action of drugs. In a patient with G6PD deficiency, aspirin and other drugs can precipitate hemolysis.

Various other genetic variations may produce adverse reactions to specific drugs. An autosomal recessive disorder that causes pseudocholinesterase in the plasma can lead to apnea when the patient receives succinylcholine. An unknown mechanism may lead to glaucoma and increased intraocular pressure when corticosteroids are administered. A similar mechanism may result in malignant hyperthermia (with severe hyperpyrexia, muscle rigidity, and possibly death) when the patient receives an anesthetic such as halothane, methoxyflurane, cyclopropane, ether, or succinylcholine. Some rare genetic variations include warfarin insensitivity, unstable hemoglobin Zurich, and unstable hemoglobin H, which cause adverse hematologic reactions to certain drugs.

An inherited predisposition to allergies increases the patient's risk of an allergic response to a drug. Especially at risk is the patient with a history of eczema, angioedema, asthma, hay fever, or hives. (For more information on allergic responses to drugs, see the discussion of drug allergy later in this chapter.)

Temperament and attitudes

Psychological factors and personal values and beliefs can predispose a patient to adverse drug reactions. For example, a patient who exhibits emotional, excitable, and hypochondriacal behavior may report adverse drug reactions more frequently than one without these psychological factors. Attitudes can shape a patient's patterns of drug taking and can lead to erratic and unsafe self-medication. The patient also may feel community and cultural pressures when interpreting drug effects and reporting undesirable reactions. Patient expectations of a drug's action also can affect response. These patient characteristics can affect the incidence of self-diagnosed adverse reactions and the frequency and thoroughness of reporting patterns.

Circadian rhythms

Normal physiologic rhythms can influence drug action and lead to adverse drug reactions. Research suggests that normal human biological rhythms can alter the absorption, metabolism, and excretion of certain drugs. Researchers are studying the contribution of sleep rhythms, hormone secretion, urinary excretion, and other regulatory processes to drug effectiveness and adverse drug reactions.

Changes associated with disease

Pathophysiologic changes associated with various diseases may cause adverse drug reactions. Diseases of organs responsible for drug absorption, metabolism, and excretion can alter drug actions and effects. For instance, cirrhosis of the liver may alter a drug's pharmacokinetic properties, especially its metabolism, thereby leading to abnormal drug concentration levels.

Diseases also can alter physiologic states unfavorably. For example, hypoalbuminemia can alter the availability of protein-binding drugs by decreasing the number of available plasma protein-binding sites. As a result, the drug's distribution, binding, and excretion are altered.

Changes associated with pregnancy

Although numerous physiologic changes occur during pregnancy, the pregnant patient is not necessarily at higher risk for adverse drug reactions. However, a pregnant patient may have a decreased blood concentration level of a drug, such as an anticonvulsant, necessitating dosage adjustments. Changes in drug distribution and excretion rates probably produce the decrease in blood concentration levels.

During a patient's pregnancy, health care professionals are concerned with the potential adverse effects of drugs on the fetus. Although many drugs cross the placenta, the type of drug, its concentration level, and fetal age determine the potential for adverse reactions in the fetus. (For more information on this subject, see Chapter 12, The Pregnant or Lactating Patient.)

PREDISPOSING DRUG FACTORS

Several drug factors influence adverse reactions, including bioavailability, additives, degradation, dosage, administration, and the number of drugs administered.

Bioavailability, additives, and drug degradation

Among different brands of the same drug, bioavailability may vary because of differences in manufacturing. Differences in onset of action, peak concentration levels, and duration of action among different products may lead to adverse drug reactions. The physician and pharmacist must exercise caution when substituting different forms of such drugs as anticonvulsants, anticoagulants, digitalis, and endocrine agents.

Dyes, buffering preparations, stabilizing agents, and other additives can produce adverse drug reactions in certain patients. When an additive produces widespread problems, the manufacturers may reformulate the product, removing the offending substance or substituting a less toxic compound.

Although uncommon, adverse drug reactions can occur when a patient uses a drug after its expiration date or uses one that has been stored in an unfavorable environment.

Drug dosage factors

A patient receiving higher dosages for prolonged periods may have an increased probability for an adverse reaction. For example, a patient taking the antihypertensive hydralazine may be more likely to develop drug-induced systemic lupus erythematosus when the dosage is greater than 200 mg P.O. daily and the therapy lasts longer than 6 months.

Administration routes and techniques

Parenteral drug treatment, especially administered intravenously, causes more frequent adverse reactions because a parenterally administered drug does not have to be absorbed through the gastrointestinal (GI) tract before distribution into the blood, which makes it more quickly available at receptor sites. Toxicity (a condition caused by excess drug in the body) and hypersensitivity occur more commonly in these circumstances.

Drugs are manufactured for administration via designated routes. Administration via unrecommended routes may cause adverse drug reactions. For example, instilling an otic solution into the eye may cause pain and irritation because the otic solution is not formulated to the pH of the eye. Suspensions intended for intramuscular or subcutaneous injections may be lethal if administered intravenously (I.V.).

Even when the appropriate route is used, improper administration can cause adverse drug reactions. For example, administering some intravenous drugs too rapidly can alter distribution and produce a toxic response. Administering an excessive amount intramuscularly may cause tissue necrosis.

Number of drugs administered
The risk of adverse drug reactions increases in direct relationship to the number of drugs administered to the patient. Complex interactions between drugs also may minimize some therapeutic effects and enhance others. (For the specific dynamics of drug interactions, see Chapter 4, Pharmacotherapeutics.)

PREDISPOSING EXOGENOUS FACTORS

Dietary and environmental factors also influence a patient's predisposition to adverse drug reactions.

Dietary factors
Substances in foods may interfere with the activity of certain drugs. For example, tyramine in some cheeses, beer, and red wine can precipitate a hypertensive crisis when ingested while a patient is taking monoamine oxidase inhibitors. Green leafy vegetables may interfere with oral anticoagulants because of their high vitamin K content.

Dietary factors also can influence the pharmacokinetics of a drug. Certain foods, such as charcoal-broiled meats, vegetables from the *Brassica* family (cabbage and broccoli), and those containing caffeine, can stimulate the activity of liver enzymes, increasing the drug metabolism rate.

The presence of food in the patient's stomach can alter drug absorption. Tetracycline absorption is decreased by food; carbamazepine absorption is increased. Foods can bind drugs and delay gastric emptying times.

Environmental factors
A patient's environment may influence the relationship between physiologic function and drug effects and contribute to adverse reactions. Pesticides, tobacco, and alcohol may alter the pharmacokinetics of certain drugs and increase the patient's risk of adverse drug reactions.

CLASSIFICATION OF ADVERSE DRUG REACTIONS

Adverse drug reactions can be classified as dose-related or patient sensitivity-related.

DOSE-RELATED ADVERSE REACTIONS

Most adverse drug reactions result from the known pharmacologic effects of a drug and typically are dose-related. Therefore, they can be predicted in most cases.

Excessive therapeutic effect
Such effects occur most commonly from miscalculations and overdose of a drug that requires precise, individualized dosage calculation. For example, a diabetic patient being treated with insulin may experience hypoglycemia from even a slight miscalculation of the insulin dose.

Secondary reactions
A drug typically produces not only a major therapeutic effect, but also additional and inseparable secondary pharmacologic actions that can be adverse. For example, morphine for pain control may lead to two undesirable secondary effects: constipation and respiratory depression. A physician may prescribe a drug for its secondary pharmacologic effects. For example, the physician may prescribe an antihistamine, typically used for allergies, to induce sleep because the secondary action of an antihistamine is drowsiness from central nervous system depression.

Hypersusceptibility to pharmacologic actions
A patient may be extremely susceptible to the primary or secondary pharmacologic actions of a drug. Even when given a usual therapeutic dose, a hypersusceptible patient can experience an excessive therapeutic response or augmented secondary effects. Hypersusceptibility typically results from altered pharmacokinetics, which leads to higher-than-expected blood concentration levels. Increased receptor sensitivity also may increase the patient's response to therapeutic or adverse effects.

Overdose toxicity
Most drugs produce toxicity if given in large enough doses, or when drug concentration levels exceed the threshold needed for therapeutic effect. Dose-related toxic effects may result from the local accumulation of a drug, as when chemotherapeutic agents accumulate in and damage hair follicle cells, which leads to alopecia (hair loss). Systemic drug effects also can produce toxicity. For example, rapid I.V. administration of aminophylline can precipitate severe hypotension and circulatory collapse. (For more information, see the appendix on poisons.)

Toxic effects may seriously damage tissues and organs and precipitate drug-induced diseases. Such conditions result from treatment with various drugs and can lead to serious, chronic health problems. Toxic effects may cause only transient changes in affected organs or more serious, irreversible changes, such as the tardive dyskinesias as-

Drug allergies

Drug allergies are categorized into four basic groups: Types I, II, III, and IV.

TYPE	RESPONSE	EXAMPLES
I	Immediate reactions to stings and drugs	Anaphylaxis, urticaria, angioedema
II	Drug-induced autoimmune disorders	Sulfonamide-induced granulocytopenia, quinidine-induced thrombocytopenic purpura, hydralazine-induced systemic lupus erythematosus
III	Reactions to penicillins, sulfonamides, iodides; antibody targeted against tissue antigens	Urticarial skin eruptions, arthralgia, lymphadenopathy, fever
IV	Reexposure to an antigen	Poison ivy and its resulting contact dermatitis

sociated with antipsychotic therapy. Such effects can be more serious than the original illness.

Iatrogenic drug effects
Some adverse drug effects induced by the prescribed drug, known as iatrogenic effects, may mimic pathologic disorders. For example, some drugs, such as antineoplastics, aspirin, corticosteroids, and indomethacin, commonly cause GI irritation and bleeding. Other examples of iatrogenic effects include propranolol-induced asthma, methicillin-induced nephritis, gentamicin-induced deafness, and thiazide-induced dizziness. Obtaining complete medical and drug histories from the patient helps reduce the risk of iatrogenic effects.

SENSITIVITY-RELATED ADVERSE REACTIONS

A less common type of adverse reaction is unrelated to dosage and results from a patient's unusual and extreme sensitivity to a drug or its components. These adverse reactions arise from unique tissue response rather than from an extension or alteration of the expected pharmacologic action. Extreme patient sensitivity may be manifested as a drug allergy or as an idiosyncratic response.

Drug allergy
Occasionally, a patient's immune system identifies a drug, a drug metabolite, or a drug contaminant as a dangerous foreign substance that must be neutralized or destroyed. Previous exposure to the drug or to one with similar chemical characteristics sensitizes the patient's immune system, and subsequent exposure mobilizes the system and causes an allergic reaction (hypersensitivity). An allergic reaction not only directly injures cells and tissues, but also produces broader systemic damage by initiating cellular release of vasoactive and inflammatory substances.

A drug allergy can be categorized according to the underlying immunologic mechanism it provokes. The adverse reaction may vary in intensity from an immediate, life-threatening anaphylactic reaction to penicillin, to a contact dermatitis secondary to topical application of neomycin cream. (For more information about these categories, see *Drug allergies*.)

Idiosyncratic response
Patient sensitivity-related adverse reactions that do not result from known pharmacologic properties of a drug or from patient allergy but are peculiar to the patient are called idiosyncratic responses. For example, a patient may experience nervousness and excitability after ingesting phenobarbital, normally a tranquilizing agent. A patient's idiosyncratic response sometimes has a genetic cause.

CHAPTER SUMMARY

Chapter 5 covered adverse drug reactions, addressing their predisposing factors and classifications. Here are the chapter highlights.
• An adverse drug reaction is a harmful, undesirable patient response to a specific drug therapy.
• Adverse drug reactions may result from any clinically useful drug. Some are dose-related, anticipated, and preventable with careful prescription and administration, or unavoidable if primary therapeutic effects are to be achieved. Others are patient sensitivity-related and may not be predictable.
• A patient's therapeutic responses to drugs result from the interplay among patient characteristics, drug characteris-

tics, and exogenous factors. The interplay can alter a drug's action or the patient's response, producing adverse drug reactions.

• Factors that predispose the patient to adverse drug reactions include extremes of age, extremes of body weight, genetic variations, the patient's temperament and attitudes, circadian rhythms, and changes associated with disease or pregnancy. Drug-related factors include bioavailability, additives, degradation, dosage, administration, and the number of drugs administered. Exogenous factors, such as diet and environment, also may predispose the patient to adverse reactions.

• Adverse drug reactions can be classified as dose-related or patient sensitivity-related. Most dose-related adverse reactions result from excessive therapeutic effect, secondary reactions, hypersusceptibility to pharmacologic actions, overdose toxicity, or iatrogenic drug effects. Patient sensitivity-related adverse reactions stem from drug allergy or idosyncratic response.

STUDY QUESTIONS

See Appendix 1 for answers.

1. Benjamin Briggs, age 21, is taking penicillin G potassium, as prescribed, for a streptococcal upper respiratory tract infection. The nurse should inform Mr. Briggs that penicillin may cause which of the following adverse drug reactions?
(a) rashes
(b) disorientation
(c) blurred vision
(d) deafness

2. Patient, drug, and exogenous factors may predispose Mr. Briggs to an adverse reaction to penicillin. Which of the following is a patient factor?
(a) genetic variation
(b) drug dosage
(c) dietary factors
(d) number of drugs taken

3. Which of the following is a drug factor?
(a) circadian rhythms
(b) disease status
(c) drug temperature
(d) drug dosage

4. Although Mr. Briggs may develop adverse reactions with oral administration of penicillin, which route is *most* likely to cause adverse drug reactions?
(a) transdermal
(b) subcutaneous
(c) intravenous
(d) intramuscular

5. Nelda Calvados, age 62, takes aspirin every day for arthritis. Aspirin may produce an adverse reaction that mimics pathologic GI bleeding. Which type of effect is this?
(a) iatrogenic effect
(b) idiosyncratic effect
(c) toxic effect
(d) allergic response

6. Aspirin also may cause a patient's immune system to identify it as a dangerous foreign substance that must be neutralized or destroyed. Which type of effect is this?
(a) iatrogenic effect
(b) idiosyncratic effect
(c) toxic effect
(d) allergic response

SELECTED REFERENCES

Basu, T. (1988). *Drug-nutrient interactions.* New York: Routledge, Chapman, & Hall.

Davis, N., and Cohen, M. (1989). Today's poisons: How to keep them from killing your patients. *Nursing89,* 19(1), 49-51.

Griffin, J., et al. (1988). *A manual of adverse drug interactions* (4th ed.). Woburn, MA: Butterworth.

Harrison's principles and practices of internal medicine (12th ed.). (1991). New York: McGraw Hill.

Mathewson, M. (1989). Drug interactions. *Critical Care Nurse,* 9(4), 84-93.

Tse, C., and Madura, A. (1988). An adverse drug reaction reporting program in a community hospital. *Quality Review Bulletin,* 14(11), 336-340.

Westfall, L., and Paulis, R. (1987). Why the elderly are so vulnerable to drug reactions. *RN,* 50(11), 39-43.

2

THE NURSING PROCESS AND DRUG ADMINISTRATION

Most nurses will agree that medication administration is the most challenging, and sometimes most frightening, new experience for a nursing student. It is challenging because safe therapeutic medication administration requires technical competence, sound judgment, and meticulous attention to detail. It can be frightening because it is a complex activity that can harm the patient if not implemented properly.

Nurses are legally responsible for maintaining patient safety, ethically responsible for making moral nursing decisions, and professionally responsible for facilitating the therapeutic effects of medications. To meet these responsibilities, the nurse must apply a broad knowledge base to all aspects of care and must be aware of the related legal and ethical implications of nursing care.

OVERVIEW OF CHAPTERS

Unit Two provides the basic information necessary for the nurse to become knowledgeable and competent in safe, therapeutic drug administration. It not only presents general nursing responsibilities, such as dosage calculations and administration techniques, but also describes specific nursing care for pediatric, geriatric, pregnant, and lactating patients. Although learning to administer medications is a complex task, the information contained in Unit Two should help the nurse successfully meet the challenge.

Chapter 6
The Nursing Process and Drug Therapy
Chapter 6 describes the nursing process as a framework for delivering nursing care. It discusses each step of the nursing process — assessment, diagnosis, planning, implementation, and evaluation — in relation to drug administration. It details the use of drug history and other information in assessing the patient and formulating nursing diagnoses. Then it describes planning, including the development of outcome criteria and interventions, such as patient teaching and promotion of patient compliance. The chapter concludes with a discussion of implementation and evaluation and the importance of documenting nursing activities related to drug therapy.

Chapter 7
Responsibilities in Drug Administration
Chapter 7 describes the essential components of a medication order and the seven types of medication orders typically used in hospitals. To help the nurse prevent medication errors, the chapter explores the five rights of medication administration and procedural safeguards. Then the chapter explores four types of drug delivery systems. It concludes with a discussion of the nurse's legal responsibilities and ethical obligations related to drug administration.

Chapter 8
Dosage Measurements and Calculations
After discussing factors that influence drug dosages, Chapter 8 surveys various systems of drug weights and measures, highlighting the metric, apothecaries', and household systems. Then the chapter introduces the fraction and ratio methods for conversions between systems of measurement. It illustrates the use of these methods and the "desired-available" method for computation of drug dosages. It concludes with special considerations for dosage calculations for pediatric and geriatric patients.

Chapter 9
Routes and Techniques of Administration
Chapter 9 begins by discussing drug forms and packaging. Then it details techniques for administering drugs by various routes, including the oral, sublingual, buccal, rectal, parenteral, intrathecal, epidural, intra-articular, dermal, ophthalmic, otic, nasal and sinus, respiratory, urethral, and vaginal routes. Throughout, the chapter emphasizes the rationales underlying nursing decisions about medication administration routes and techniques.

Glossary

Ampule: small, sterile, sealed glass or plastic container that holds a single drug dose.

Buccal route: oral medication administration in tablet form on the inside of the cheek.

Capsule: gelatin shell that dissolves in the stomach and contains drug in a powder, sustained-release bead, or liquid form.

Compliance: degree to which a patient follows the advice of a health care professional.

Cream: thick emollient (substance that softens tissue) that contains a paste-drug mixture of oil and water; designed for topical use.

Dermal route: topical medication administration by application to the skin.

Drops: medicated liquid administration in minute spheres.

Drug delivery system: institutional mechanism for obtaining medications from a general stock pharmacy for administration to patients in a clinical unit; also refers to dosage forms.

Elixir: flavored, sweetened hydroalcoholic (water and alcohol) liquid that contains a medicinal agent.

Enteric-coated tablet: tablet with a thin coating that prevents release and absorption of its contents until it reaches the small intestine.

Epidural route: medication administration through a catheter inserted into the space around the dura mater of the spinal column.

Ethical responsibility: duty that a nurse has to use fundamental moral values when making nursing decisions.

Evaluation: part of the nursing process in which the nurse judges the effectiveness of care based on preestablished criteria.

Goal: statement of the objective or aim of directed nursing care efforts.

Inhalant: medicinal vapor administered through the nose, trachea, or respiratory system.

Injection: introduction of a liquid into the body using a syringe; a solution of a medication suitable for injection.

Intra-articular route: medication administration by instillation or injection into a joint.

Intradermal route: medication administration by injection of small amounts of solution, usually antigens, between the epidermal and dermal (skin) layers.

Intramuscular route: medication administration by injection of a solution into a muscle.

Intraosseous route: medication administration by infusion into the medullary cavity of a long bone.

Intrathecal route: medication administration by direct injection through the theca (enclosing sheath) of the spinal cord into the subarachnoid space.

Intravenous route: medication administration by injection or infusion into a vein.

Intrauterine growth retardation: slowed growth of cells and part or all of the fetus, which may result from drug administration during gestation.

Legal responsibility: duty that a nurse has to abide by nursing practice acts and court decisions.

Lotion: medicated liquid applied topically to protect the skin or treat a dermatologic disorder.

Lozenge or **troche:** tablet containing a drug, flavoring, sweetener, and mucilage that is made to dissolve in the mouth.

Malpractice: wrongful conduct, improper discharge of duties, or failure of a professional to meet standards of care that causes harm to another. Negligence is a form of malpractice.

Milliequivalent: number of grams of a solute in one milliliter of a normal solution.

Negligence: failure to do something that could reasonably be expected to be done by an individual in a given situation or the performance of an act that a reasonable and prudent person would not do.

Nurse practice act: state (or Canadian provincial) legislation that describes educational requirements for professional licensure and professional scope of nursing practice.

Nursing care plan: written plan that includes prioritized goals, nursing interventions, and outcome criteria for a specific patient.

Nursing diagnosis: part of the nursing process in which the nurse uses a standard nomenclature to describe actual and potential patient care problems, their etiologies, and their signs and symptoms.

Nursing process: framework for nursing care that includes assessment, diagnosis, planning, implementation, and evaluation.

Ointment: semisolid, oil-based preparation that contains a medication for topical application.

Outcome criteria: statement of desired results that contains a content area, an action verb, a time frame, and criterion modifiers.

Over-the-counter (OTC) drug: drug available without a prescription.

Parenteral route: medication administration by injection, such as intradermal, intramuscular, and intravenous injection.

Patch: thin membrane or gel base applied to the skin that releases a measured dose of medication over an extended period.

Percentage solution: solution in which the solute (solid) represents a percentage of the solution's total weight. For example, *0.9% saline solution* means that every 100 milliliters of solution contains 0.9 grams of sodium chloride (or every liter of solution contains 9 grams of sodium chloride).

Placebo: inactive substance, such as normal saline solution, or a less-than-effective dose of a substance, such as a vitamin, prescribed as if it were an effective medication dose.

Powder: small particles of medication obtained by grinding a solid drug.

Prescription: order for medication, therapy, or a therapeutic device given by a properly authorized person to a person properly authorized to dispense or perform the order.

Professional responsibility: duty that a nurse has to the standards of practice established by the profession as its code of ethics.

Glossary *(continued)*

Rectal route: medication administration by insertion or infusion into the rectum.

Subcutaneous route: medication administration by injection of a substance under the skin into the layer of loose connective tissue.

Sublingual route: medication administration by placement of a tablet on the floor of the mouth under the tongue.

Suppository: medicated semisolid substance, usually cone-shaped, that melts or dissolves after insertion into a body cavity.

Suspension: preparation in which small particles of a solid drug are dispersed—but not dissolved—in a liquid for administration. Stirring or shaking the mixture maintains dispersal.

Syrup: concentrated solution that contains a medication, flavoring, sugar, and water.

Tablet: solid preparation in which medication is combined with inert ingredients and compressed into a shape.

Teratogenesis: development of physical defects in an embryo or fetus.

Tincture: liquid preparation that contains a medication and alcohol (alcoholic solution) or a medication, water, and alcohol (hydroalcoholic solution).

Vaginal route: medication administration by insertion or injection into the vagina.

Vial: small, glass, multidose medication container sealed with a rubber diaphragm.

Wax matrix tablet: wax, honeycomb structure that contains medication slowly released as the comb dissolves.

Chapter 10
The Pediatric Patient

Chapter 10 examines the special considerations for medication administration to pediatric patients. First the chapter describes age-related changes that affect a drug's pharmacokinetics, pharmacodynamics, and pharmacotherapeutics in pediatric patients. It illustrates these variations with specific examples and discusses the effects of drugs on normal growth and development. Next the chapter presents special pediatric dosage calculations and administration techniques. Lastly, it discusses family education and drug therapy.

Chapter 11
The Geriatric Patient

Chapter 11 presents special considerations for geriatric patients. It discusses the effects of aging and their influence on pharmacokinetics and pharmacodynamics in geriatric patients. Next it explores common drug related problems in elderly patients by body system. Then it discusses the nurse's role in reviewing medication regimens for geriatric patients and reviews ways to help cognitively impaired patients self-administer medication.

Chapter 12
The Pregnant or Lactating Patient

Chapter 12 explores the pharmacokinetic changes that occur when a drug is given to a pregnant woman. It explains placental transport and the relationship between teratogenicity and drug administration at different gestational ages of the fetus. It also discusses medications used to treat pregnancy-related symptoms, such as heartburn, nausea and vomiting, constipation, and headache. It briefly touches on drugs used during labor and delivery.

For the lactating patient, the chapter describes breast-milk formation and factors that influence drug transport to this milk—and to the breast-feeding infant. It concludes with guidelines to help the nurse counsel the pregnant or lactating patient who needs drug therapy.

THE NURSING PROCESS AND DRUG THERAPY

OBJECTIVES

After reading and studying this chapter, the student should be able to:

1. Explain the steps of the nursing process as they relate to drug therapy.

2. Collect appropriate data during assessment to serve as the basis for subsequent decisions about the patient's drug regimen.

3. Identify the critical components of a drug history.

4. Apply two diagnostic labels in developing a nursing care plan for a patient's drug therapy.

5. Write outcome criteria that contain the content area, an action verb, a time frame, and (if appropriate) criterion modifiers.

6. Identify the components of a teaching plan.

7. Explain how patient characteristics, the nurse-patient relationship, and the therapeutic regimen affect patient compliance.

8. Describe how the nurse uses outcome criteria during evaluation.

9. Explain how to evaluate therapeutic effects, adverse drug reactions, drug interactions, patient teaching, and patient compliance.

10. Explain the importance of documentation of nursing care and patient responses to care.

INTRODUCTION

This chapter investigates the nursing process in relation to drug therapy. The nursing process, a framework that aids in the development, implementation, and evaluation of patient care, consists of five essential steps: assessment, formulation of a nursing diagnosis (identifying a patient's health need), planning, implementation of the nursing plan of care, and evaluation. (For an illustration of the five steps and their relation to one another, see *The nursing process.*)

Since it is dynamic, the nursing process allows the nurse to develop and modify a total plan of care in a logical sequence for a particular patient.

Chapter 6 provides general information about application of the nursing process as it relates to drug therapy. It serves as a foundation for Chapter 13 through 73, which illustrate specific nursing care—in the nursing process framework—related to each drug class.

ASSESSMENT RELATED TO DRUG THERAPY

During the assessment step of the nursing process, the nurse gathers information that helps guide the patient's drug therapy. One important information source is the patient's drug history, which the nurse obtains from data given by the patient, spouse or partner, parent, or others who know that patient well. The nurse also obtains information by performing a physical assessment to detect any potential adverse reactions to the patient's drug regimen and by consulting the patient's previous medical records. Furthermore, the nurse examines the laboratory or diagnostic test results, noting any unusual findings that may indicate a possible adverse reaction, such as a toxic level of digoxin, or document drug efficacy, such as a therapeutic increase in clotting time secondary to the use of anticoagulants.

The nurse continually updates the assessment data by collecting information during interaction with the patient. Assessment represents a crucial step in the nursing process because all subsequent steps depend on the information collected.

COMPONENTS OF A DRUG HISTORY

The nurse must obtain a thorough drug history upon the patient's admission to the health care facility. Currently, instead of depending on one family physician for overall medical care, a patient may have numerous specialists, such as an internist, cardiologist, or pulmonologist. This increases the potential for conflicting or incompatible drug regimens, which makes obtaining a thorough drug history essential.

The nurse compiling a comprehensive drug history should ask specific questions that cover the patient's background—for example, allergies and socioeconomic status, prescription drugs, and OTC drugs. (For more information, see *Critical components of a drug history,* page 74.)

General information

General information covers background data related to the patient. The major components are allergies, medical history, habits, socioeconomic status, life-style and beliefs, and sensory deficits.

Allergies. To obtain a comprehensive profile of a patient's drug and food allergies, the nurse should investigate the patient's reactions to prescription and OTC drugs and various foods. While discussing allergic reactions to drugs, the nurse must inquire about the type of drug, when the reaction occurred, the situation and setting at the time of the reaction, the type of reaction, and any other contributing factors. Examples of contributing factors might include a change in eating or nutritional habits, exposure to environmental agents (such as pollens or poison oak), and initiation of a new drug regimen. The patient's responses may provide insight into the factors and circumstances that contributed to the allergic reaction.

The patient's description of an allergic reaction can help the nurse determine whether the patient actually reacts adversely to a particular drug or simply dislikes the drug. For example, one patient may report an allergic reaction to all major pain medications because they cause an "out of control" feeling. Another patient may develop a body rash and have difficulty breathing after receiving certain pain medications. The first patient does not have a true drug allergy and may need education about the effects of the different drugs. The second patient has experienced an allergic reaction. When a patient has a drug allergy, the nurse needs to document the specific drug and reaction in the patient's chart and other pertinent patient records.

The nurse also needs to assess for allergies to foods because such allergies also can affect a patient's drug regimen and care. For example, chick embryo tissue cultures sometimes are used to prepare mumps vaccines. A patient's information regarding allergic reactions to eggs will help ensure proper treatment.

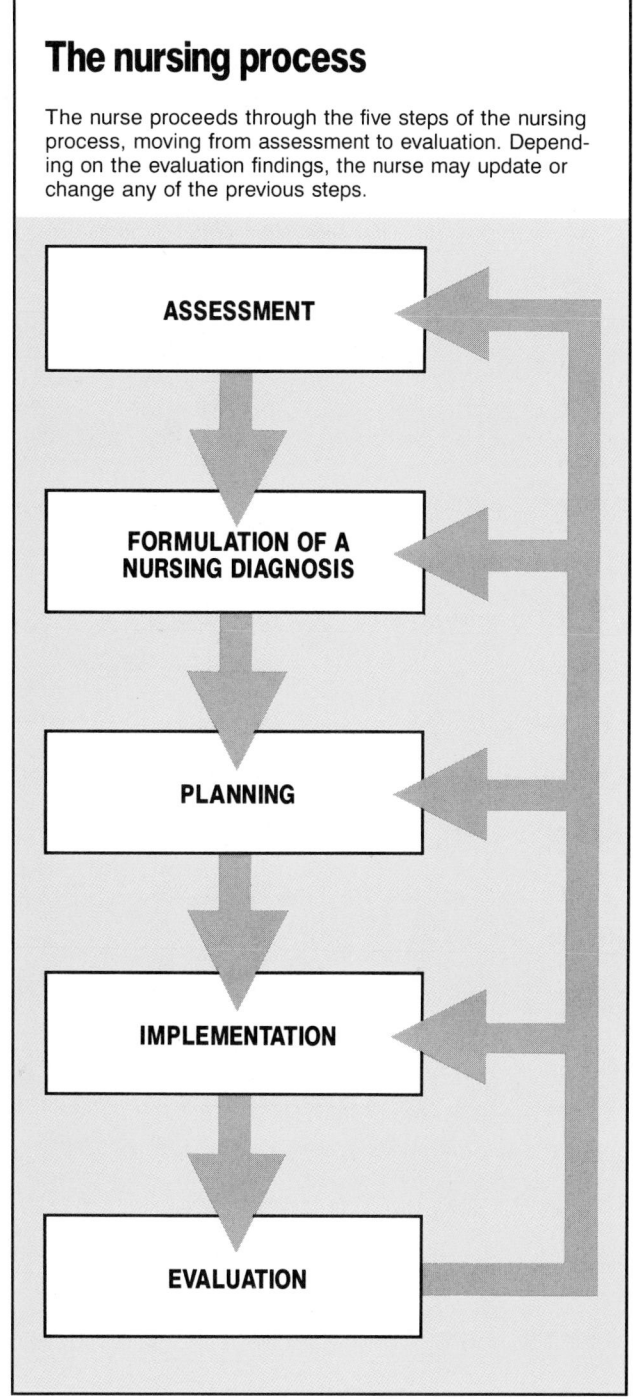

The nursing process

The nurse proceeds through the five steps of the nursing process, moving from assessment to evaluation. Depending on the evaluation findings, the nurse may update or change any of the previous steps.

ASSESSMENT

FORMULATION OF A NURSING DIAGNOSIS

PLANNING

IMPLEMENTATION

EVALUATION

Medical history. Examining a patient's medical history helps the nurse understand any particular drug regimen the patient may be following. When gathering data, the nurse should note any chronic or long-term diseases or disorders the patient may have, the drug regimen for each, and the frequency of consultation with a physician on each drug regimen.

Critical components of a drug history

When obtaining the patient's drug history, the nurse must gather general information on certain components essential to proper nursing practice as well as specific information on prescription and over-the-counter (OTC) drugs. The following list serves as a guide for obtaining a drug history.

GENERAL INFORMATION

Allergies
- Drugs
- Food

Medical history
- Associated illnesses and diseases

Habits
- Dietary
- Recreational drug use
  - alcohol
  - tobacco
  - stimulants, such as caffeine
  - illegal drugs

Socioeconomic status
- Age
- Educational level
- Occupation
- Health insurance coverage

Life-style and beliefs
- Support systems
- Marital status
- Childbearing status
- Attitudes toward health and health care
- Use of the health care system
- Daily activities pattern

Sensory deficits

PRESCRIPTION AND O.T.C. DRUGS

Reason for use

Knowledge of drugs

Frequency or dosage

Effectiveness or reactions

Pattern and route of administration

The nurse also should record any acute episodes of illnesses or disorders and the treatment for each. Treatments include home remedies as well as prescription and OTC drugs. The nurse also should record those remedies the patient found successful.

Habits. Documenting certain habits directly related to drug therapy represents another important step in compiling a patient's drug history. Two major areas that the nurse should

consider are the patient's dietary habits and use of recreational drugs, including alcohol, tobacco, stimulants, and illegal drugs, such as marijuana, cocaine, and heroin.

Dietary intake can alter the effectiveness of many drugs. For example, a person taking calcium supplements must maintain a diet that meets the daily requirements of vitamin D, which aids in the absorption and use of calcium.

The use of recreational drugs can inhibit the effectiveness of a particular drug regimen. For alcohol intake, the nurse needs to note the frequency of use as well as the type and amount of alcohol consumed. The nurse must quantify the amount of alcohol consumed when the patient uses such descriptive phrases as "social drinker," "weekend drinker," "occasional drinker," or "heavy drinker." The nurse also should note whether the patient primarily drinks beer, wine, cocktails, or hard liquor because equal amounts of the various types of alcoholic beverages contain different amounts of alcohol and affect each person differently.

For tobacco use, the nurse should note whether the patient smokes or chews tobacco. Then the nurse should identify how long the patient has been using tobacco and determine the type and amount used per day.

Next the nurse must document the intake of stimulants, such as caffeine, because stimulants can mimic such adverse drug reactions as palpitations or tremor. Finally, the nurse must document the use of illegal drugs because each type can produce a different and profound effect on a person, depending on the drug, the route of administration, and the individual. (For specific reactions to different illegal drugs, see the appendix on Substance Abuse.)

Socioeconomic status. The factors related to a patient's socioeconomic status include age, educational level, occupation, and health insurance coverage. Knowing the patient's age can help the nurse determine whom to include in the plan, such as parents or other family members, and what level of information to provide.

Knowing the patient's educational background helps the nurse focus selected interventions at an appropriate level and determine specific strategies to use in the nursing plan of care. Determining the patient's occupation can help the nurse plan a drug regimen that fits the patient's schedule, thus minimizing the chances of disrupting the patient's daily routine. Identifying the patient's health insurance coverage can help the nurse identify the need for extra funds or financial counseling.

Life-style and beliefs. In assessing a patient's life-style, the nurse should obtain information about the following subjects: support systems, marital status, childbearing status, attitudes toward health and health care, use of the health care system, and pattern of daily activities. Positive, strong support systems at home and in other areas of life can help a patient adhere to a specific drug regimen. Noting the type of support systems available to the patient is critical.

Marital status also is important because married patients exhibit a positive correlation with increased patient compliance. Information on the female patient's childbearing status and use of contraception is useful in determining appropriate teaching about the potential for some medications to cause fetal damage.

Numerous research studies also have shown that a patient's attitudes toward health and health care have a significant effect on compliance. For example, if the patient believes that the physiologic, psychological, or economic benefits of the prescribed health care regimen outweigh the disadvantages, the patient will be more likely to comply with the drug regimen.

The nurse also must consider how each patient uses the health care system. For example, a patient may be seeing a specialist for each body system, consulting regularly with the different specialists. Contacting the physican in charge can help the nurse avoid implementing conflicting drug regimens.

The last factor related to life-style is the patient's daily activities pattern. The nurse can address this issue by asking the patient to describe what occurs during a typical day and using that information to teach the patient and establish the least disruptive health care regimen for home use. Considering all the factors related to the patient's life-style and beliefs can help the nurse decrease the complexity of a drug regimen and increase patient compliance.

Sensory deficits. The presence or absence of sensory deficits significantly can shape the development of an appropriate health care plan for the patient. Besides noting obvious deficits, the nurse should explore such things as diseases or decreased sensations in the extremities, any of which can interfere with the patient's ability to give self-administered injections, break scored tablets, and open medication containers.

Prescription and OTC drugs

The nurse also must determine the patient's knowledge about previously prescribed drug regimens and the type of OTC drugs the patient is taking. In assessing a patient's history of drug use, the nurse should explore the following: the reason for using the drug; the patient's knowledge of when the drug should be taken, the dosage, and its efficacy; and the route of administration.

The nurse needs to know if the patient understands the reason for taking a particular drug, the type of adverse reactions the drug might cause, and when to contact a physician. The nurse also should note any special monitoring that the patient must perform in relation to the drug regimen, such as comparing the apical pulse rate with specified parameters before digoxin administration.

The nurse should find out if the patient knows the dosage and the particular schedule for taking each drug. The nurse should discuss the effectiveness of the drug regimen with the patient, noting any symptoms or adverse reactions that have occurred since the regimen began. Many OTC drugs can inhibit or potentiate the effects of a prescribed drug. For instance, a patient taking an anticoagulant, such as warfarin, should not take aspirin or any drug containing aspirin because aspirin potentiates the anticoagulant effects.

The nurse also should determine the patient's knowledge about the route of administration and note the pattern of administration that the patient follows at home because this information may provide insight into reasons why a particular drug regimen succeeds or fails. Information about the pattern of administration also can aid the physician and nurse in developing a realistic plan for the patient.

CLINICAL BEHAVIORS

Besides obtaining a drug history during assessment, the nurse needs to consider two other important matters that affect drug administration: the patient's cognitive abilities and the body systems that may be affected by the prescribed drugs.

A patient with intact cognitive abilities should be able to understand and implement the actions necessary for compliance. If a patient's cognitive abilities are not intact, the nurse must determine the probable cause, which can range from a drug-related effect to a pathophysiologic condition. Whatever the cause, the nurse must determine if the patient can to carry out the prescribed drug regimen. If the patient's cognitive abilities are impaired, the nurse may need to teach a family member or friend to administer the drug, obtain a visiting nurse referral, use a day-care setting, or consider admitting the patient to an extended-care facility.

Having completed the drug history, the nurse needs to assess those body systems that may be affected by the patient's prescribed drug regimen. Every drug produces a particular effect on a specific body system or systems. Some of the effects may represent the desired action of the drug. At the same time, however, every drug potentially can affect other body systems in adverse ways. For instance, chemotherapeutic drugs destroy cancerous cells, yet they also destroy normal cells and lead to nausea, loss of appetite, hair loss, and diarrhea. The nurse must monitor closely a drug's adverse effects to ensure that the patient does not become seriously compromised.

NURSING DIAGNOSES RELATED TO DRUG THERAPY

A nursing diagnosis represents an "actual or potential health problem, which nurses, by virtue of their education and experience, are capable and licensed to treat" (Gordon, 1976).

Formulating a nursing diagnosis occurs after the assessment or data collection step in the nursing process. Analysis of essential assessment data and identification of the specific signs or symptoms (defining characteristics) and probable cause (etiology) helps the nurse develop a particular nursing diagnosis.

Nursing diagnoses provide a common language to convey the nursing management needed for each patient among the many nurses involved in that patient's care. To help ensure standardized nursing diagnosis terminology and use, the North American Nursing Diagnosis Association (NANDA) has formulated and classified a series of nursing diagnosis categories based on nine human response patterns (NANDA, 1990). These patterns include:
- Exchanging (mutual giving and receiving)
- Communicating (sending messages)
- Relating (establishing bonds)
- Valuing (assigning worth)
- Choosing (selecting alternatives)
- Moving (activity)
- Perceiving (receiving information)
- Knowing (meaning associated with information)
- Feeling (subjective awareness of information)

Within each pattern are NANDA-approved nursing diagnostic categories specific to that topic. For example, the human response pattern devoted to *choosing* includes such diagnostic categories as *noncompliance* and *health-seeking behaviors*. The complete list of NANDA diagnostic categories, arranged by human response pattern, is called the nursing diagnosis taxonomy. (For the complete list, see the appendix on the NANDA Taxonomy of Nursing Diagnoses.)

Knowledge deficit and *noncompliance* are the two most common diagnostic labels used by the nurse to develop care plans for managing a patient's drug regimen. The nurse also may identify other nursing diagnoses depending on the potential risks or adverse effects of drug therapy. (For examples of nursing diagnoses appropriate for each drug category, see *Selected nursing diagnoses* in Chapters 13 through 73.)

KNOWLEDGE DEFICIT RELATED TO DRUG THERAPY

A *knowledge deficit* can occur for various reasons. The specific nursing diagnosis depends on the etiologies and defining characteristics that the nurse identifies. (For NANDA-approved etiologies and defining characteristics applicable to the *knowledge deficit* diagnostic label, see *Parameters for knowledge deficit*.)

The nursing diagnosis also depends on the assessment data and drug regimen of each patient. The following case illustrates how a knowledge deficit can result from several causes.

Mrs. Kaminsky, age 71, entered the hospital with shortness of breath and difficulty walking because of edema and pain in her legs. The attending physician diagnosed Mrs. Kaminsky's condition as congestive heart failure and started her on the following medications: digoxin 0.25 mg P.O. daily, furosemide (Lasix) 40 mg P.O. daily, and potassium chloride (K-Tab) 2 P.O. twice a day. The only significant item in Mrs. Kaminsky's medical history is hypertension for the past 2 years, which her family internist monitors. She takes no other drugs except for a calcium supplement and daily vitamins.

Currently, she can perform her activities of daily living (ADLs) without shortness of breath. Her legs remain slightly swollen, although greatly decreased in size from the time of admission, and her weight remains 3 pounds (1.5 kg) above her expected dry weight. She is to be discharged in about 3 days if no complications arise.

Mrs. Kaminsky lives alone, although her son and his family live nearby. She wants to return to her home and asks questions about her drugs, diet, disease, and activity levels.

In Mrs. Kaminsky's case, the defining characteristic is her request for information. However, the etiology may be one of several possibilities. The nurse may be dealing with a diagnosis of *knowledge deficit related to the new drug regimen, knowledge deficit related to the prescribed diet*, or *knowledge deficit related to the self-management of congestive heart failure*.

NONCOMPLIANCE RELATED TO DRUG THERAPY

Noncompliance is another diagnostic label that can occur when the nurse deals with a patient and a specified drug regimen. Some defining characteristics of *noncompliance* include:
- behavior indicating failure to follow a regimen, supported by direct observation or statement by the patient or an informed observer

---

Parameters for knowledge deficit

The nurse must be able to differentiate among the various diagnostic labels. The differentiating parameters usually consist of the defining characteristics and etiologies. The following shows a diagnostic label, its defining characteristics, and its associated etiologies.

DIAGNOSTIC LABEL
- Knowledge deficit

DEFINING CHARACTERISTICS
- Statement of misconception
- Verbalization of the problem
- Request for information
- Inaccurate follow-up on instructions
- Inadequate test performance
- Inappropriate or exaggerated behaviors

ETIOLOGIES
- Lack of exposure
- Information misinterpretation
- Unfamiliarity with information resources
- Lack of recall
- Cognitive limitation
- Lack of interest in learning or obtaining information

- failure on objective tests
- evidence of the development of complications
- exacerbations of the symptoms
- failure to keep appointments
- failure to progress
- inability to set or maintain mutual goals.

Etiologies associated with *noncompliance* may include lack of knowledge, lack of necessary resources, denial of a health problem, information misinterpretation, or a belief that treatment measures are ineffective or unnecessary.

The following example illustrates some of the defining characteristics and etiologies of noncompliance:

Mr. Miller, age 65, is admitted to the hospital with an exacerbation of his emphysema. Within the past 12 months, Mr. Miller has entered the hospital three times with the same medical diagnosis. Each time, he received I.V. antibiotics, steroids, and oxygen.

During Mr. Miller's current admission, the nurse noted the following characteristics as part of the assessment: The patient is alert, exhibits circumoral cyanosis, has a respiratory rate of 32 breaths per minute with the use of accessory muscles, has breath sounds with scattered inspiratory and expiratory wheezes throughout and crackles in the posterior bases, has a cough productive of thick, yellow-green secretions, and states his shortness of breath has increased over the past 2 weeks, until he now needs assistance to perform his ADLs. The patient has a 50 pack-year history of smoking; he smokes one pack per day, which he refuses to decrease. He states that he quit taking his drugs 2 weeks before admission because they did not seem to make any difference in how he felt and were expensive. Upon further discussion, Mr. Miller could not state the effects of his drugs and treatments.

Mr. Miller lives with his wife, who also has several medical problems that require treatment. He is on a fixed income; he has insurance, the benefits of which are almost exhausted; Medicare; and Social Security. During the current admission, his respiratory status has improved. He performs his ADLs with minimal shortness of breath, although he needs oxygen at night. Upon discharge, he is to take prednisone 40 mg P.O., which should be tapered off over the next 2 weeks according to a set schedule, theophylline (Theo-Dur), furosemide (Lasix), potassium chloride (K-Lor), and cephalexin (Keflex) for 10 days, and use oxygen at night.

The defining characteristics for Mr. Miller include his repeated admissions for exacerbated emphysema, discontinued treatment, questionable understanding of the prescribed treatment, minimal resources to pay for treatment, and the nurse's assessment findings — including shortness of breath, wheezes and crackles, the use of accessory muscles for breathing, and an increased respiratory rate. The nurse needs to collect more information about Mr. Miller's disease knowledge and his beliefs about the effects of the treatment. The nurse may be dealing with *noncompliance related to a misunderstanding of the importance of the prescribed drug regimen* or *noncompliance related to a lack of financial resources.*

OTHER NURSING DIAGNOSES RELATED TO DRUG THERAPY

The nurse may formulate and use many other nursing diagnoses, depending on the potential or actual adverse effects of drug regimens. Some further nursing diagnoses include: *altered health maintenance related to cognitive inability to manage the prescribed drug regimen, potential for injury related to anticoagulant therapy, impaired skin integrity related to a reaction to the prescribed medication,* and *altered oral mucous membranes related to a superimposed infection,* which could be from steroids, chemotherapy, or antibiotic use. *Altered nutrition: less than body requirements, related to nausea, anorexia, and chemotherapy* and *sexual dysfunction related to prescribed medications,* such as propranolol (Inderal), represent still other diagnoses that the nurse might use.

With such nursing diagnoses, the defining characteristics will depend on the patient's specific reaction to the particular drug regimen. For example, with the diagnosis of *potential for injury related to anticoagulant therapy,* the defining characteristics may include petechiae, increased bruising, an elevated prothrombin time above therapeutic levels, or aspirin use. For the diagnosis of *altered nutrition,* the defining characteristics may include weight loss, eating less than 50% of meals, weakness, or a change in the way foods taste.

PLANNING RELATED TO DRUG THERAPY

Once the nursing diagnosis is formulated, the nurse can proceed to the planning step of the nursing process, determining the nursing plan of care for the patient. This consists of two major components: outcome criteria (patient goals) and nursing interventions.

OUTCOME CRITERIA

Outcome criteria, the first critical component of the nursing plan of care, represent patient goals and state the desired patient behaviors or responses that should result from the nursing care.

The nurse should ensure that outcome criteria exhibit certain characteristics. Each criterion should be measurable and objective, concise, realistic for the patient, and attainable by nursing management. Furthermore, for each criterion, the nurse should include only one behavior, express that behavior in terms of patient expectations, and indicate a time frame.

Typical outcome criteria are: *The patient verbalizes the major adverse effects related to his chemotherapy drugs before discharge* or *The patient demonstrates the proper administration of her antibiotic regimen before discharge.*

Components of an outcome criterion

The nurse must consider four major components in writing outcome criteria: the content area, an action verb, a time frame, and criterion modifiers.

The content area describes the subject that the patient will focus on or the physiologic or psychological response to be elicited. The focus of the content area may be the steps of I.V. administration of penicillin or the adverse effects of prednisone.

The action verb, the second component of the outcome criterion, describes how the patient will achieve the goal of the content area. Using action verbs with the two previously mentioned content areas could result in *Demonstrate the steps of the I.V. administration of penicillin* and *State the adverse effects of prednisone.*

The nurse should include a time frame—a target date for completion of the expected outcome criterion, which helps the nurse evaluate the patient's progress. For example, the statement *Demonstrate the steps of the I.V. administration of penicillin by the time of discharge* includes a specific time frame that tells the nurse when the patient should achieve the goals.

Criterion modifiers can add significant details to each outcome criterion. In some cases, criterion modifiers clarify what the patient should achieve by delineating specified limits for a specific action. For example, *The patient accurately demonstrates the steps of the I.V. administration of penicillin by the time of discharge* specifies that the patient must demonstrate the behaviors accurately.

When writing an outcome criterion, the nurse must include the content area, an action verb, and a time frame. Criterion modifiers are not essential, but are helpful. (For a summary of the components, see *Writing outcome criteria.*)

Writing outcome criteria

The essential components of outcome criteria and examples of those components follow.

CONTENT AREA

Describes the subject that the patient will focus on or the response to be elicited, such as
• action of digoxin
• pulse taking.

ACTION VERB

Describes how the patient will achieve the content area aim, such as
• *verbalize* the action of digoxin
• *demonstrate* pulse taking.

TIME FRAME

Gives a target date for completion of the outcome criteria, such as
• verbalize the action of digoxin *after the initial teaching session*
• demonstrate pulse taking *before discharge.*

CRITERION MODIFIERS

Add specificity to the subject, action, or time, such as
• *correctly* verbalize the major *action* of digoxin after the initial teaching session
• demonstrate pulse taking before discharge *with a degree of accuracy within 4 beats of the pulse the nurse takes.*

NURSING INTERVENTIONS

After developing the outcome criteria, the nurse determines the interventions needed to help the patient reach the desired behavior or response goals. Interventions are the actions that the nurse implements to help the patient meet the identified outcome criteria.

Nursing interventions are classified as independent, interdependent, or dependent. For example, altering the drug schedule to coincide with the patient's daily routine represents an independent intervention, whereas consulting with the physician and pharmacist to change a patient's medication because of adverse reactions represents an interdependent intervention. Administering an already-prescribed drug on time is a dependent intervention. The choice of which of the three types of nursing actions to use depends on the proposed outcome criteria for each stated nursing diagnosis. (For examples that illustrate the progression from diagnosis to outcome criteria to intervention, see *Three nursing care plans,* pages 80 and 81.)

When developing interventions for effective drug therapy, the nurse must include patient teaching to educate the patient about the prescribed drug regimen and enhance compliance.

Patient teaching

The patient must understand the prescribed drug regimen to achieve the maximum therapeutic effect from it. To promote patient learning, the nurse must understand basic learning principles and use basic teaching principles. (For more information, see *Basic learning and teaching principles,* page 81).

Development of an effective patient teaching program parallels the steps of the nursing process. The nurse uses the nursing process to assess patient learning needs, to develop a nursing diagnosis, to develop a teaching plan, to implement the plan, and to evaluate the teaching and learning that occurred. (For more information, see *Nursing process and patient teaching,* page 82.)

Developing a teaching plan also is an essential part of teaching the patient. Each teaching plan should include outcome criteria or behavioral objectives, teaching content, teaching methods, and evaluation. (For an example, see *Sample teaching plan,* page 83).

Outcome criteria. Outcome criteria are the desired patient behaviors or responses that result from the teaching. The nurse must focus the teaching on them and use them in formulating evaluation criteria.

Outcome criteria fall into three learning domains: cognitive, affective, and psychomotor. Within each domain, levels of behavior progress from simple to complex.

The cognitive domain addresses an individual's intellectual abilities and thinking processes. For example, the learner would be expected to know the actions and adverse effects of medications. The affective domain addresses an individual's feelings, beliefs, and values. In this domain, for example, the patient expresses feelings and beliefs about how medications affect daily routines and life-style. The psychomotor domain addresses an individual's ability to perform motor functions or skills, such as giving insulin injections. The level of the taxonomy helps determine the outcome criteria and the type of teaching strategies necessary.

Teaching content outline. The content outline identifies the specific information to teach in each session. Detail varies with the learner's needs and the teacher's knowledge of the topic. A more complete outline decreases the probability of omitting important ideas and information.

Teaching methods. The teaching methods selected, such as lecture, discussion, demonstration, or simulation, depend on the patient and the content. The learning domains can assist in determining the types of teaching method. The nurse may need to use more than one teaching method to enhance learning. For example, when instructing an individual about the importance of monitoring the pulse rate and blood pressure before administering propranolol, the nurse may use various teaching methods or strategies because the greater the number of senses (sight, hearing, touch) that the learner uses in the session, the greater the retention of information.

Media selection is another important component for the nurse to consider. When selecting different types of media, the nurse needs to remember the focus of the presentation. The selected media should support major concepts and highlight essential ideas.

When selecting learning materials for a patient, the nurse can go beyond prepackaged or published ones. The nurse's own informal materials, such as medication schedules, written lists, or drawings, also may be used. Whether the materials are prepackaged or handwritten, the nurse needs to verify that they are clear, concise, and written at the patient's level of understanding.

Evaluation. Evaluation is an important component of the teaching plan because it helps the nurse verify what the learner has accomplished. (For more information, see "Evaluating patient teaching" later in this chapter.)

Patient compliance

To achieve the optimal effects from drug therapy, the patient must comply with the prescribed regimen. Many factors, categorized as patient characteristics or clinical characteristics, can affect patient compliance.

Three nursing care plans

The first example gives the nursing care plan for Mrs. Kaminsky, for whom the nurse diagnosed *knowledge deficit related to the new drug regimen*. The second example gives Mr. Miller's nursing care plan for his diagnosis of *noncompliance related to a misunderstanding of the importance of the prescribed drug regimen*. The third nursing care plan is for a diagnosis of *potential for injury related to anticoagulant therapy*.

Knowledge deficit related to the new drug regimen

NURSING DIAGNOSIS
Knowledge deficit related to the new drug regimen (includes digoxin, furosemide [Lasix], and potassium chloride [K-Tab])

OUTCOME CRITERIA
Before discharge, Mrs. Kaminsky will:
• State the major action of each drug.
• Identify at least three adverse reactions that should be brought to the immediate attention of a health care professional.
• Describe the importance of monitoring daily weight.
• Demonstrate the ability to take her pulse accurately.

NURSING INTERVENTIONS
• Instruct Mrs. Kaminsky in the major actions of and possible adverse reactions to each drug.
• Instruct Mrs. Kaminsky about adverse reactions that need immediate medical attention, such as a sudden change in weight, nausea, loss of appetite, change in affect, palpitations, or lethargy.
• Provide Mrs. Kaminsky with a list of this information for home use.
• Discuss the importance of monitoring daily weight and noting more than a 2- to 3-pound (1- to 1.5-kg) increase.
• Provide Mrs. Kaminsky with written information on the major actions and adverse reactions of each drug as a guide for home use.
• Include Mrs. Kaminsky's son and daughter-in-law in the teaching, if possible.
• Instruct Mrs. Kaminsky on methods for taking her pulse, using demonstration and practice.

Noncompliance related to a misunderstanding of the importance of the prescribed drug regimen

NURSING DIAGNOSIS
Noncompliance related to a misunderstanding of the importance of the prescribed drug regimen (includes theophylline [Theo-Dur], metaproterenol [Alupent Inhaler], beclomethasone [Vancenase Inhaler], furosemide [Lasix], potassium chloride [K-Tab], and cephalexin [Keflex])

OUTCOME CRITERIA
By discharge, Mr. Miller will:
• State two reasons why he has exacerbated emphysema.
• Identify at least three signs or symptoms that may indicate exacerbated emphysema.
• Describe the major actions of the prescribed drugs.
• Describe the difference between adverse reactions to the drugs and the signs and symptoms of his emphysema.
• Describe the relationship between his drug regimen and his emphysema.
• Explain the importance of taking his prescribed drugs as ordered.

NURSING INTERVENTIONS
• Discuss emphysema with Mr. Miller, describing the disease process and why exacerbations occur—drug discontinuation, disease progression, or exposure to cold viruses.
• Review with Mr. Miller the signs and symptoms that indicated a need for medical attention before hospitalization and how to monitor them, including increased shortness of breath, increased use of oxygen, inability to perform activities of daily living, and changes in the color of secretions.
• Discuss and provide written information on the drug actions.
• Discuss the relationship of the prescribed drugs to his disease.
• Discuss the difference between the adverse reactions to the drugs and signs and symptoms that indicate an exacerbation of his emphysema or a change in his disease. Provide Mr. Miller with a list of the information.
• Contact the home health agency for follow-up care.
• Involve Mr. Miller's wife in the teaching sessions.
• Contact social services to assess the family finances, and refer Mr. Miller to hospital and community resources.

Potential for injury related to anticoagulant therapy

NURSING DIAGNOSIS
Potential for injury related to anticoagulant therapy

OUTCOME CRITERIA
The patient will:
• Describe the action of warfarin (Coumadin).
• State the importance of self-monitoring for signs of bleeding.
• List the signs of bleeding to report to the physician.
• Identify the reasons for carrying a medication alert identification card or wearing a bracelet.
• State the importance of the blood tests (prothrombin time) in monitoring the warfarin dosage.
• State the importance of not using products that contain aspirin.
• List at list three safety precautions to follow while on anticoagulant therapy.

NURSING INTERVENTIONS
• Teach the patient about the actions of warfarin.
• Discuss the signs of bleeding that the patient should be aware of, such as bleeding of the gums and increased bruising, and when to report these signs to the physician.
• Provide the patient with the medication alert information and discuss it.
• Discuss the need for follow-up blood tests (prothrombin time) to evaluate the warfarin dosage.
• Provide the patient with a booklet on anticoagulant therapy.
• Discuss the reasons for not using products that contain aspirin.
• Discuss the safety factors related to anticoagulant therapy, such as the use of a soft toothbrush and the careful use of razors.

Patient characteristics. Four kinds of factors reveal patient characteristics: demographic, physiologic, drug knowledge, and psychosocial factors.

Demographic factors include the patient's age, sex, culture or race, and educational level. The nurse should consider these factors when planning such interventions as patient teaching because they enable the nurse to present information at the appropriate level for each patient.

Physiologic factors include the duration and severity of the disease as well as the patient's knowledge about it. For example, a patient with chronic renal failure or chronic lung disease usually takes many drugs for extended periods, sometimes for life. In comparison, a patient with a bladder infection may take only a 7- or 10-day course of antibiotics. The patient requiring the longer treatment is less likely to maintain compliance and — lacking an adequate understanding of the prescribed therapy's desired outcome — may stop taking medications if the disease appears to improve.

Drug knowledge factors include the patient's understanding of the drug's therapeutic effects, adverse drug reactions, and drug interactions as well as a knowledge of the drug's administration (dose, dosage form, route, and

---

Basic learning and teaching principles

To develop and implement effective patient education, the nurse should apply learning principles, which provide information about factors that influence patient learning, and teaching principles, which influence teaching methods and strategies. The following list summarizes basic learning and teaching principles that the nurse can use when teaching about drug therapy.

LEARNING PRINCIPLES
• The patient needs to be motivated to learn.
• Physical and emotional readiness are essential for learning.
• Active participation by the patient can be critical to learning.
• Learning should be based on prior experiences and knowledge.
• Learning is more effective when knowledge can be applied immediately.
• Information presented to the patient must be congruent with the patient's expectations and goals.
• Repetition can reinforce learning.

TEACHING PRINCIPLES
• Establishing nurse-patient rapport aids patient teaching.
• Effective communication is essential.
• Environmental control can influence teaching effectiveness.
• Behavioral objectives can guide the teaching session and aid in evaluation.
• Cultural, ethnic, and religious beliefs must be considered in planning teaching sessions.
• Evaluation is an essential part of teaching.

Nursing process and patient teaching

This flow chart demonstrates the steps of the nursing process as they relate to patient teaching.

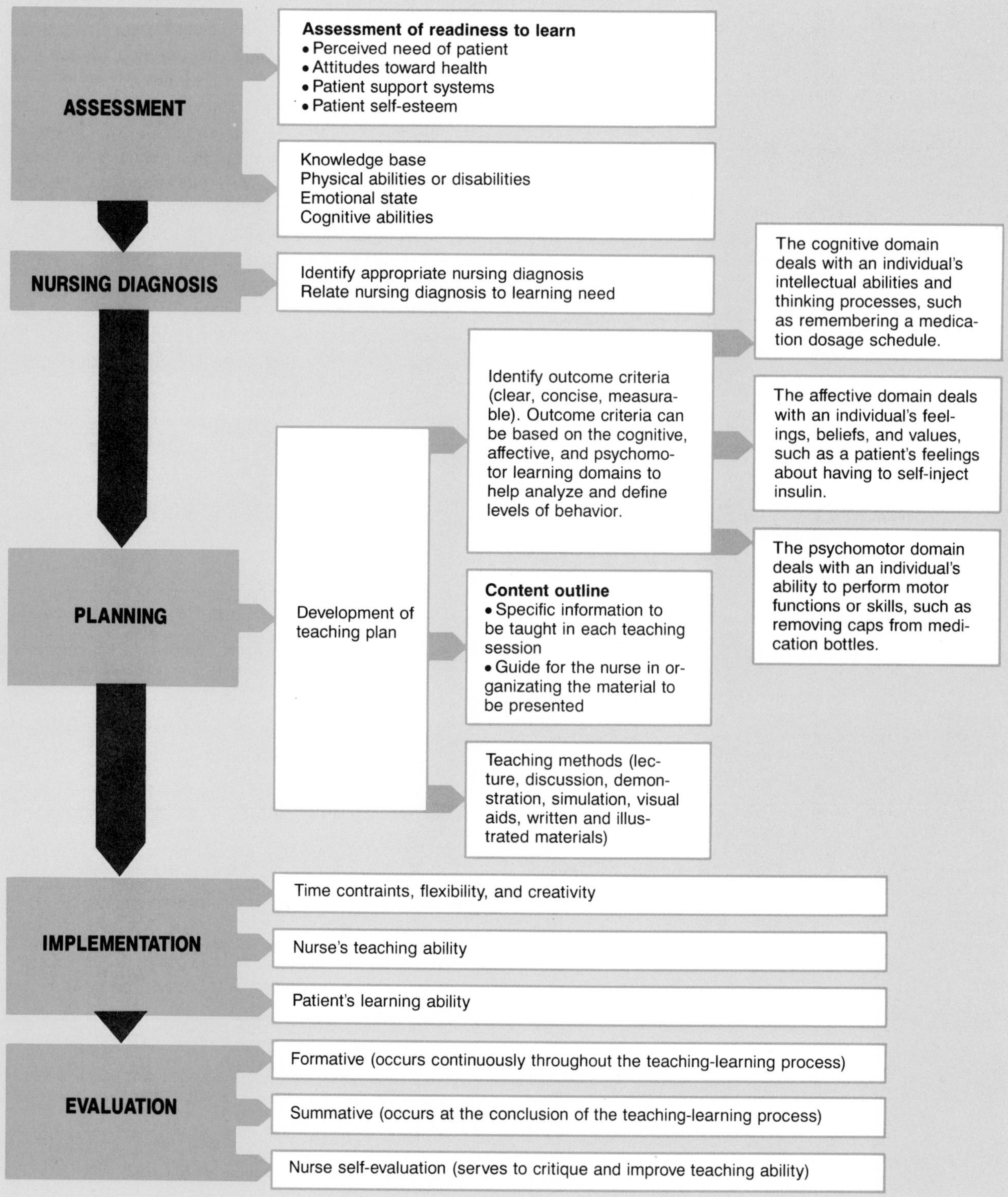

ASSESSMENT

Assessment of readiness to learn
- Perceived need of patient
- Attitudes toward health
- Patient support systems
- Patient self-esteem

Knowledge base
Physical abilities or disabilities
Emotional state
Cognitive abilities

NURSING DIAGNOSIS

Identify appropriate nursing diagnosis
Relate nursing diagnosis to learning need

The cognitive domain deals with an individual's intellectual abilities and thinking processes, such as remembering a medication dosage schedule.

PLANNING

Development of teaching plan

Identify outcome criteria (clear, concise, measurable). Outcome criteria can be based on the cognitive, affective, and psychomotor learning domains to help analyze and define levels of behavior.

The affective domain deals with an individual's feelings, beliefs, and values, such as a patient's feelings about having to self-inject insulin.

Content outline
- Specific information to be taught in each teaching session
- Guide for the nurse in organizating the material to be presented

The psychomotor domain deals with an individual's ability to perform motor functions or skills, such as removing caps from medication bottles.

Teaching methods (lecture, discussion, demonstration, simulation, visual aids, written and illustrated materials)

IMPLEMENTATION

Time contraints, flexibility, and creativity

Nurse's teaching ability

Patient's learning ability

EVALUATION

Formative (occurs continuously throughout the teaching-learning process)

Summative (occurs at the conclusion of the teaching-learning process)

Nurse self-evaluation (serves to critique and improve teaching ability)

timing). These factors are essential to compliance because the patient must understand the prescribed drug therapy before complying with it.

Psychosocial factors that affect compliance include support systems, patient attitudes and beliefs, and patient participation in treatment. A patient with a strong support system of family members or others usually maintains high self-esteem, which promotes compliance.

Positive attitudes and beliefs also strongly affect compliance. For example, a patient who believes that the benefits of a prescribed regimen outweigh its disadvantages, such as adverse effects and high cost, usually will be compliant. In addition, a patient who has a positive outlook for recovery and accepts responsibility for self-care will tend to be more compliant than one with a negative attitude.

Sample teaching plan

The following sample presents a teaching plan for Mrs. Davis, a patient with cancer who has the nursing diagnosis *knowledge deficit related to chemotherapy*. The nurse should include intended outcome criteria, content details to be covered, teaching methods, and standards for evaluation.

OUTCOME CRITERIA	CONTENT	TEACHING METHODS	EVALUATION
• Mrs. Davis will state the major actions of her chemotherapy drugs after the initial teaching session. • After the teaching session, Mrs. Davis will identify major adverse reactions to the chemotherapy drugs with 100% accuracy. • Before discharge, Mrs. Davis will list the adverse reactions that warrant contacting the physician. • Before discharge, Mrs. Davis will describe when she is at the greatest risk for infection.	Actions of fluorouracil and cisplatin: • attack and destroy the rapidly growing cancer cells • interfere with the ability of cancer cells to divide and grow. Adverse reactions to chemotherapy drugs: • occur mainly because chemotherapy drugs also affect other rapidly growing or dividing cells • most commonly involve hair loss (alopecia), mouth sores, nausea, vomiting, and diarrhea. Serious, unpredictable reactions: • include chills, fever, sore throat, unusual bleeding or bruising, swelling of feet or legs, and difficulty hearing • require the patient to contact the physician, if they occur at home. Other adverse reactions occur because of destruction of rapidly growing cells, including red blood cells, white blood cells, and platelets. • These reactions cause fatigue and weakness and increase the risk of infection. • The patient should avoid anyone who has an infection and must take care to avoid injury that could cause bleeding. • The peak effect of these actions is 7 to 14 days after chemotherapy administration.	Use lecture and discussion format. Plan two sessions, each 15 minutes. • The first session should cover the major actions and adverse reactions of chemotherapy. • The second session should cover all other information and review the first session's main points. Use a mix of media materials. • Give "Chemotherapy and You" slide-tape presentation. • Give the patient the "Chemotherapy and You" book; underline the two drugs she is receiving.	After the initial teaching session, Mrs. Davis: • stated the major actions of the chemotherapy drugs • selected the major adverse reactions when provided with a list. By discharge time, Mrs. Davis: • listed adverse reactions that warrant contacting the physician • described when she is at risk for an infection.

Compliance characteristics

This table lists patient and clinical characteristics that affect patient compliance. Understanding these characteristics helps the nurse develop and implement effective nursing interventions to promote patient compliance.

PATIENT CHARACTERISTICS

Demographic factors
• Age
• Sex
• Culture or race
• Educational level

Physiologic factors
• Disease duration and severity
• Knowledge about disease

Drug knowledge factors
• Understanding of therapeutic effects, adverse drug reactions, and drug interactions
• Understanding of the drug's administration (dose, dosage, dosage form, route, and timing)

Psychosocial factors
• Support systems
• Locus of control
• Attitudes and beliefs
• Participation in prescribed treatment

CLINICAL CHARACTERISTICS

Nurse-patient relationship
• Patient satisfaction
• Communication

Therapeutic regimen
• Complexity
• Cost
• Adverse reactions
• Effect on patient's life-style

Adapted with permission of Aspen Publishers, Inc., for McCord, M.A. (1986). Compliance: Self-care or compromise? *Topics in Clinical Nursing*, 7(4), 1-8.

Increased patient participation in the prescribed therapy and increased contact with the health care professional may affect compliance positively.

Clinical characteristics. Two major groups of clinical characteristics affect patient compliance: the nurse-patient relationship and the therapeutic regimen.

Factors in the nurse-patient relationship include patient satisfaction and communication. A nurse-patient relationship characterized by a trusting, informative interaction promotes patient satisfaction and compliance. The nurse who communicates a sense of concern for the patient's well-being instills confidence and trust in the patient—also a key to compliance.

The therapeutic regimen affects a patient's compliance through its complexity, cost, and adverse effects; the patient's life-style also affects compliance. A complex drug regimen may lead to patient noncompliance. The effects on patient compliance of a drug regimen's cost and adverse effects remain controversial. The same mixed results have occurred in studies of adverse reactions. If the patient views the adverse reactions as being unexpected or more traumatic than the disease, noncompliance may occur.

The patient whose personal routines are interrupted by the prescribed drug regimen also may become noncompliant. For example, suppose a telephone operator is scheduled to take digoxin at breakfast time, warfarin sodium at 2 p.m., isosorbide dinitrate four times a day (at 8 a.m., 1 p.m., 6 p.m., and 10 p.m.), and furosemide at 9 a.m. During work hours, 7 a.m. to 4 p.m., the patient must take four medications at different times. In addition, the patient will need to void frequently over several hours after taking furosemide. These interruptions may disturb the work schedule to such an extent that the patient may believe job performance is compromised and self-esteem is lost. Such conditions promote noncompliance. To avoid interfering with the patient's routine when establishing a drug regimen, the nurse or physician should discuss the times most convenient for the patient to take the medications. (For a summary, see *Compliance characteristics*.)

IMPLEMENTATION RELATED TO DRUG THERAPY

During the fourth step of the nursing process, implementation, the nurse puts interventions into action and provides care as described in the nursing care plan. By following the care plan and gearing actions toward the outcome criteria, the nurse can implement proposed interventions effectively.

In drug therapy, implementation includes all aspects of medication administration: working with the physician, administering drugs as prescribed, calculating dosages, preparing drugs, using appropriate administration techniques, and modifying techniques for patients with special needs, such as pediatric, geriatric, pregnant, and lactating patients. Other aspects of implementation include staying alert for medication errors, documenting drugs given, and teaching patients about drugs. Implementation also includes monitoring the patient to evaluate the effectiveness of drug therapy. (For more information about medication administration, see Chapters 7 through 12 of this unit.)

To increase effectiveness while implementing the care plan, the nurse must communicate—and collaborate—with the patient because any outcome that does not match the patient's perceived goals can decrease compliance. If necessary, the nurse may call on other health care professionals and resources to help implement the nursing care plan.

EVALUATION RELATED TO DRUG THERAPY

Integral to the nursing process, evaluation is a formal and systematic procedure for determining the effectiveness of nursing care. Evaluation provides descriptive data that enable the nurse to understand the patient's status and thereby make better-informed decisions about what to change and what to maintain.

EVALUATION CRITERIA

Typically considered the final step in the nursing process, evaluation helps the nurse review and, if necessary, modify each patient's care. Earlier in the process, the nurse has used the nursing diagnosis, or problem statement, to define the patient's current and potential problems and determine outcome criteria, or patient goals. The outcome criteria also suggest which nursing interventions may help the patient achieve these goals.

The nurse evaluates the care to determine whether the outcome criteria have been met. For example, the nurse might ask the patient if headache relief was achieved within 1 hour after administering a p.r.n. analgesic. If the headache was relieved, the outcome criterion was met. If the headache was better but not completely relieved, the outcome criterion was partially met. If the headache was the same or worse, the outcome criterion was not met.

Evaluation enables the nurse to design and implement a revised nursing care plan, reevaluating outcome criteria continually and replanning until each nursing diagnosis is resolved.

EVALUATING DRUG EFFECTS AND INTERACTIONS

The nurse can use evaluation to determine whether nursing interventions for drug administration have been effective. To do so, the nurse reassesses for therapeutic effects, adverse drug reactions, and drug interactions.

Therapeutic effects

The therapeutic effect is the body's response to a drug's pharmacologic action when that action produces a benefit for the patient. To understand how a drug produces its therapeutic effect, the nurse must understand the drug's mechanism of action. For example, some laxatives work by altering surface tension; others work through bowel lubrication or stimulation, saline catharsis, or bulk formation. The differences in their mechanisms of action could determine whether outcome criteria for a constipated patient are met or unmet—depending on the cause of constipation as well as on various other factors pertaining to the individual patient.

For example, most patients admitted to cardiac units receive a stool softener such as docusate sodium, an emollient laxative, to prevent constipation secondary to the inactivity of hospitalization. Docusate sodium works by reducing the surface tension of liquid bowel contents and promoting additional liquid absorption into the stool, resulting in a softer stool mass that the patient can pass without straining. Unless the patient is constipated initially, administration of docusate sodium helps meet these outcome criteria: *The patient will maintain usual bowel elimination pattern while hospitalized* and *The patient will not strain during bowel movements.*

If the patient had received a laxative with a different mechanism of action, the outcome criteria might not have been met. For example, a stimulant laxative such as bisacodyl would be inappropriate for the cardiac patient needing constipation prophylaxis because these laxatives work by increasing peristalsis of smooth muscle in the intestine to produce a stool within 6 to 8 hours and can cause abdominal cramping. Furthermore, frequent use can precipitate fluid and electrolyte imbalances that are undesirable for the cardiac patient. Finally, the cardiac patient needs a drug that prevents constipation, not one that treats the condition.

Evaluating a drug's effectiveness also requires that the nurse (1) know the time of the peak concentration, onset of action, and duration of action of the prescribed drug and (2) obtain a patient history covering any prior use of the drug and any allergic or adverse reactions that occurred. (For some standard questions the nurse can ask, see *Evaluation questions,* page 86.)

Adverse drug reactions

Adverse drug reactions are harmful, undesirable patient responses to a specific drug therapy. They may be dose related (predictable) or patient-sensitivity related (unpredictable). Dose-related adverse reactions result from the unknown pharmacologic effects of a drug. Patient-sensitivity-related adverse reactions are those that the physician or nurse cannot foresee, such as an allergic response. They are unrelated to dose.

Dose-related adverse drug reactions. Drowsiness, an adverse reaction to the antihistamine diphenhydramine, can be detrimental if the patient needs to remain alert. However,

Evaluation questions

To evaluate the effectiveness of a patient's drug therapy, the nurse must know the answers to these questions:

• What are the intended therapeutic effects of the drug therapy?
• What is the mechanism of action by which the drug produces its therapeutic effects?
• What are the adverse reactions associated with the drug?
• Which interactions between the drug and other drugs or foods could alter its therapeutic effect?
• Which adverse reactions to drugs, if any, has the patient experienced in the past?
• How is the drug administered?
• What should the patient know about the drug? Which factors might affect the patient's ability to follow the prescribed drug regimen?
• Which therapeutic effects has the drug produced on the patient? If none, or if the effects have been insufficient, which factors may be involved? (These may be related to the drug, the patient, or the health care professional.) Which nursing interventions are needed to remove the effects of these factors and achieve the original or revised outcome criteria?

diphenhydramine sometimes is administered specifically *for* the drowsiness it produces. For example, it may be given to a patient with insomnia. In this instance, the physician uses the drug's adverse reaction for therapeutic effect.

The nurse, however, usually works toward preventing or minimizing dose-related adverse drug reactions, such as the nausea and vomiting associated with many antineoplastic drugs.

Patient-sensitivity-related adverse drug reactions. These may occur as allergic reactions ranging from a mild rash or pruritus to severe anaphylaxis. The initial patient history compiled by the nurse can help avoid such reactions. If the patient had a previous allergic reaction, the nurse must determine its nature by asking the patient to describe it. The patient's description can help the nurse determine whether the reaction was an allergic response or a dose-related reaction.

Patient-sensitivity-related reactions (idiosyncratic responses) occur when a drug produces an effect opposite to its intended therapeutic effect. Suppose, for example, an elderly patient takes 15 mg of the hypnotic flurazepam approximately 30 minutes before bedtime to promote sleep. If, 1 hour later, the patient is awake, somewhat confused, and slightly combative, an idiosyncratic reaction is occurring. Very young and elderly patients are most likely to experience idiosyncratic reactions.

Drug interactions

A drug interaction occurs when one drug alters the pharmacokinetic or pharmacodynamic properties of another or when a drug interacts with food the patient has eaten. Most drug interactions of either type are minor and may go unnoticed by the patient and the nurse; however, a few drug interactions can produce serious consequences.

Some interactions between drugs can be beneficial. These may be initiated in various situations and include interactions that reduce toxicity or increase therapeutic effect. For example, the specific receptor-blocking agent naloxone is administered to counter the toxic effects of a narcotic overdose. Another beneficial interaction between drugs is the production of additive effects (effects that usually are equivalent to the sum of the effects of either drug administered alone in higher doses). For example, administering codeine with aspirin produces an additive effect, which allows pain relief with lower doses.

Beneficial and adverse interactions between drugs and food can occur. A beneficial interaction can occur in the patient taking supplemental doses of calcium to treat osteoporosis. If the patient eats foods rich in vitamins C and D, the vitamins assist in the absorption and use of calcium. The same patient may experience an adverse interaction, however, with high protein and fat intake because protein and fat inhibit calcium absorption.

EVALUATING PATIENT TEACHING

Evaluation, an essential component of the teaching plan, examines what the learner has accomplished. To evaluate the learner, the nurse uses outcome criteria or behavioral objectives. Behaviors specified in the outcome criteria determine how the evaluation should be conducted. For example, if the patient was to *state the action of digoxin at the end of the session,* the evaluation would be based on what the patient said. If the patient was to *demonstrate how to mix NPH and regular insulin in one syringe,* the evaluation would be based on what the patient did. Other forms of evaluation include paper and pencil tests, crossword puzzles, case studies, role-playing, and simulations or games.

Two other types of evaluation use outcome criteria. Formative (or concurrent) evaluation occurs continuously throughout the teaching and learning process. One benefit of this type of evaluation is that the nurse can adjust teaching strategies as necessary to enhance learning. Summative (or retrospective) evaluation occurs at the conclusion of the teaching and learning session. This evaluation, where feedback is given at the end of the session, does not allow for adjustment until after teaching and learning are finished.

EVALUATING PATIENT COMPLIANCE

Evaluation can help the nurse determine whether a patient is compliant with a prescribed drug regimen. If the patient is not responding to therapy, for example, the nurse's evaluation may reveal that the patient is socially isolated and is not receiving necessary support from family members. A patient who is confused or forgetful, who expresses doubt about the drug therapy, who fails to have a prescription filled, or who is involved in complex or expensive drug therapy also requires evaluation for compliance.

Current methods used to evaluate patient compliance do not always provide pure or true measurements, but they can help the nurse minimize factors that might lead to noncompliance. The methods include physiologic assessment, ratings by health care professionals, patient self-reporting, pill counts, and direct observation. Combining several methods provides more accurate measurement of compliance.

Physiologic assessment

Blood pressure measurements, serum or urine drug levels, and other assessments can provide objective evidence of whether the patient is complying with the prescribed drug therapy. However, some physiologic measurements, such as for blood pressure, may be inaccurate because of alteration by other factors. The blood pressure of a patient taking antihypertensive drugs, for example, can fluctuate according to the patient's anxiety level and ingestion of certain foods. As a result, the patient may be compliant with hypertensive drug therapy but still have high blood pressure. Serum or urine levels of a drug or its metabolites also may reflect compliance inaccurately if a noncompliant patient consumes the prescribed drug dose just before the test, producing a positive impression of compliance. Body weight and heart rate also provide objective measurements of compliance, but the nurse must interpret the information carefully and in relation to other assessment data.

Ratings by health care professionals

Physicians, nurses, pharmacists, and other professionals make judgments about a patient's compliance. These judgments may be arbitrary or based on experience that may not be applicable. Because they are subjective, such judgments should never be the only measurement used to determine patient compliance with drug therapy.

Patient self-reporting

Another subjective measurement of compliance, patient self-reporting sometimes requires the patient to recall complex behaviors over a long time. The patient is asked to recall whether the drug regimen was followed as prescribed, including verification that prescriptions were filled. Furthermore, the questions used to elicit the patient's information may call for objective as well as subjective responses. Researchers have shown that about half of noncompliant patients admit to noncompliance.

Pill counts

These counts objectively measure patient compliance. The nurse compares the number of doses in the patient's prescription container to the number that should be there if the patient has been compliant. Pill counts are not entirely reliable, however; if doses are missing, the patient may have spilled some of them or taken some at the wrong times. The nurse should consider the information derived from pill counts along with other compliance data.

Direct observation

Objective information about a patient's compliance can be obtained by the nurse through direct observation. Because the nurse must measure the drug dose and watch as the patient takes it, this method is practical mainly for hospital or clinical settings. It is impractical for measuring compliance when the patient takes drugs at home — unless a home health nurse visits regularly.

Combining two or more measurement methods produces more accurate evaluation of patient compliance. For example, for a patient who may have difficulty affording the prescribed drugs, the nurse may use self-reporting and pill counts to measure compliance. For an elderly patient with poor vision, the nurse may measure compliance using self-reporting, occasional direct observation by a home health nurse, and pill counts.

DOCUMENTATION RELATED TO DRUG THERAPY

Although documentation is not a step in the nursing process, the nurse legally is required to document activities related to drug therapy, including the time of administration, the quantity administered, and the patient's reaction to the drug. To deliver the best possible patient care, the nurse also should record evaluation data. Because other nurses must be able to read the evaluation and implement appropriate nursing care, documentation must be clear, concise, and complete. It should begin with an evaluation of outcome criteria and proceed to a reassessment of specific interventions.

The format used to document the evaluation step in the nursing process can vary. The nurse may combine progress notes with flow sheets or add an evaluation column to the nursing care plan.

The nurse also must document each teaching session in the patient's chart so that other nurses and members of the health care team know what was covered, what patient learning resulted, and which areas need refinement or further instruction. The nurse must remember that the patient's education is the concern of the entire health care team, each member having a different area of expertise. To provide optimal patient education, the nurse must work closely with all other team members.

The chart is one method of sharing information. Other methods include informal health care team meetings, educational rounds, family conferences with the health care team, and discharge planning rounds. Above all, the patient's medical record must include complete documentation of all teaching efforts.

CHAPTER SUMMARY

Chapter 6 presented the relationship between drug administration and the nursing process. The chapter focused on the assessment, nursing diagnosis, planning, implementation, and evaluation steps of the nursing process, detailing how each step relates to drug therapy. It also delineated the nurse's role in drug therapy. The nurse's responsibilities include obtaining a drug history, assessing pertinent body systems, identifying an appropriate nursing diagnosis, developing a plan that focuses on patient teaching and compliance, implementing the planned interventions, and evaluating the effectiveness of the care plan. Here are the highlights of Chapter 6.

• The nursing process involves assessment, nursing diagnosis, planning, implementation, and evaluation.

• The two major information categories used to compile a drug history are general information and prescription and OTC drugs. General information covers allergies, medical history, habits, socioeconomic status, life-style and beliefs, and sensory deficits. With prescription and OTC drugs, the nurse must assess the patient's knowledge of the reason for using the drug, frequency of use, dosage, drug efficacy, pattern of administration, and adverse reactions.

• In assessing the clinical behaviors of a patient before drug administration, the nurse determines the patient's cognitive abilities and body systems that may be affected by prescribed drugs. The nurse must know if the patient possesses the appropriate cognitive abilities to manage the prescribed drug regimen. The nurse's assessment of body systems, such as the cardiovascular or integumentary system, helps determine the potential effectiveness of a particular drug regimen.

• After performing the assessment step, the nurse formulates a nursing diagnosis by analyzing the essential data and identifying the specific signs or symptoms (defining characteristics) and the probable cause (etiology). *Knowledge deficit* and *noncompliance* are the two most common diagnostic labels used for patients receiving drug therapy.

• The planning step of the nursing process consists of two major components: outcome criteria and nursing interventions.

• An outcome criterion states a patient goal, or the desired patient behavior or response to be reached with nursing care. It should specify a content area and include an action verb, time frame, and, if needed, criterion modifiers.

• The implementation of independent, interdependent, or dependent nursing interventions helps the patient achieve the goals of the outcome criteria. During drug therapy, common nursing interventions include teaching the patient about the prescribed drug regimen and promoting patient compliance.

• To enhance patient learning, the nurse needs to understand basic learning principles, apply basic teaching principles, and develop a teaching plan. Components of a teaching plan include outcome criteria (patient goals or behavioral objectives), teaching content outline, teaching methods, and evaluation.

• Patient characteristics and clinical characteristics significantly influence patient compliance. Patient characteristics include demographic factors, physiologic factors, and psychosocial factors. Clinical characteristics include the nurse-patient relationship and the therapeutic regimen.

• The nurse evaluates a patient's drug therapy to determine if outcome criteria have been met. The outcome criteria serve as the basis for assessing the success (partial or total) or failure of a patient's drug therapy. If outcome criteria are not met, the nurse must reapply appropriate steps in the nursing process to implement effective interventions.

• For a client receiving drug therapy, the nurse evaluates therapeutic effects, adverse reactions, drug interactions, effectiveness of patient teaching, and patient compliance.

• The nurse should document all nursing actions and patient responses in the patient's chart. Documentation provides a legal record, acts as a reference for other health care professionals, and can help guide future drug therapy.

STUDY QUESTIONS

See Appendix 1 for answers.

1. Randall Jenkins, age 50, is admitted to the hospital with uncontrolled diabetes. He states that he takes 30 U of NPH

insulin "only when he feels his sugar is high." For Mr. Jenkins, which of the following is an appropriate nursing diagnosis?
(a) Noncompliance related to misunderstanding the importance of prescribed drug regimen
(b) Elevated glucose level related to uncontrolled diabetes
(c) Elevated glucose level related to patient noncompliance
(d) Inadequate insulin administration related to noncompliance

2. When preparing a care plan for Mr. Jenkins, the nurse writes several outcome criteria. Which of the following is written correctly?
(a) The patient adequately understands the need for insulin.
(b) The patient states the importance of taking insulin as prescribed.
(c) The patient knows he should take insulin as prescribed.
(d) The patient believes he should take insulin as prescribed.

3. At the shift change, the nurse on duty assesses Mr. Jenkins to determine if his medication was given at the proper time on the previous shift. This action demonstrates which type of nursing intervention?
(a) interdependent
(b) independent
(c) dependent
(d) intradependent

4. The nurse plans three patient-teaching sessions with Mr. Jenkins. Which of the following is *not* a component of the teaching plan?
(a) behavioral objectives
(b) evaluation methods
(c) assessment findings
(d) teaching methods

5. Before Mr. Jenkins is discharged, the nurse performs a thorough evaluation. What does the evaluation step of the nursing process determine?
(a) if the patient will recover
(b) if the outcome criteria have been met
(c) if the nurse has done a good job
(d) if the nursing diagnosis is correct

6. Alice Harding, age 31, will be taking an antihistamine to relieve her seasonal allergies. When teaching Ms. Harding, the nurse advises her to avoid tasks that require alertness, such as driving, because this drug may produce drowsiness. Which type of reaction is the nurse describing?
(a) dose-related reaction
(b) a patient-sensitivity-related reaction

(c) an idiosyncratic reaction
(d) a summation reaction

7. The nurse plans to evaluate Ms. Harding's compliance with the prescribed drug therapy. Which of the following methods allows objective evaluation of compliance?
(a) patient self-monitoring
(b) patient self-reporting
(c) rating by health care professionals
(d) direct observation

SELECTED REFERENCES

Gilmore, G., et al. (1988). *Needs assessment strategies for health education and health promotion.* Carmel, IN: Benchmark Press.

Gordon, M. (1976). Nursing diagnosis and the diagnostic process. *American Journal of Nursing, 76*(8), 1298.

Gordon, M. (1987). *Nursing diagnosis: Process and application.* New York: McGraw-Hill.

Lindberg, J., Hunter, M., and Kruzzewaki, A. (1990). *Introduction to nursing concepts, issues, and opportunities.* Philadelphia: Lippincott.

McCord, M. (1986). Compliance: Self-care or compromise? *Topics in clinical nursing, 7*(4), 1-8.

Morrison, E. (1989). Nursing assessment: What do nurses want to know? *Western Journal of Nursing Research,* 11(4), 469-476.

North American Nursing Diagnosis Association (NANDA). (1990). *Taxonomy I—Revised, with official diagnostic categories.* St. Louis: NANDA.

Redman, B. (1988). *The processes of patient education* (6th ed.). St. Louis: C.V. Mosby.

Tipton, J. (1989). A hospital-based approach to physical assessment. *Journal of Nursing Staff Development, 5*(2), 70-72.

Yura, H., and Walsh, M. (1988). *The nursing process* (5th ed.). East Norwalk, CT: Appleton & Lange.

RESPONSIBILITIES IN DRUG ADMINISTRATION

OBJECTIVES

After reading and studying this chapter, the student should be able to:

1. Identify the essential components of a properly written medication order.

2. Describe the purposes of the seven types of medication orders routinely used in the hospital.

3. Describe standard nursing practices that help the nurse achieve the five "rights" of drug administration.

4. Identify at least six other procedural safeguards against medication errors listed in the text.

5. Describe the nurse's responsibilities when using each of the four types of drug delivery systems.

6. Define malpractice and describe how it relates to the administration of medications.

7. Explain how the nurse applies the principles of autonomy, paternalism, truthfulness, beneficence, fidelity, and respect for property to professional practice.

INTRODUCTION

Chapter 7 discusses the nurse's role in drug administration. It presents essential background information about requirements for medication orders, the nurse's responsibilities in receiving and transcribing medication orders, and the proper procedures for preventing errors during drug administration. The chapter examines the advantages and disadvantages of various systems for delivering medications from the pharmacy to the nursing unit for administration. It also explores various legal expectations, such as what the nurse should know and do to administer medications safely. Chapter 7 explores the components that constitute malpractice and the special nursing responsibilities related to controlled drugs. It concludes with a discussion of some of the fundamental values and moral principles that guide nursing practice in medication administration.

MEDICATION ORDERS

Under the law, as outlined in the medical practice act of each state, licensed physicians as well as dentists, podiatrists, and in some states optometrists may prescribe, dispense, and administer drugs. In selected circumstances and within certain protocols, other health care professionals, such as nurses, pharmacists, or physicians' assistants, legally may prescribe and dispense drugs. Nevertheless, physicians write the vast majority of medication orders. Usually, pharmacists dispense the drugs, and nurses administer them to patients.

REQUIREMENTS FOR MEDICATION ORDERS

A medication order may take one of two forms, depending on whether the prescriber is treating a hospitalized patient or an outpatient. For the hospitalized patient, the prescriber can order medications, along with all other orders such as those for diet, X-rays, and laboratory work, on the order sheet in the patient's chart. The prescriber also can use a separate medication order sheet. For outpatients, the prescriber usually writes the medication order on a prescription pad sheet and gives it directly to the patient. The patient takes the medication order to a hospital or community pharmacy to be filled. (For a complete, properly written medication order for a hospitalized patient, see *Components of a medication order.*)

The prescriber's order sheet lists the patient's full name for identification purposes. The order sheet may be stamped with complete identifying information, including the patient's birth date, the hospital number, room number, and date of admission. Health care professionals must take extreme care in identifying patients, particularly if two or

Components of a medication order

The prescriber writes medication orders for hospitalized patients on the order sheet in the patient's chart. As shown in the sample below, the medication order should give the patient's full name, the name of the drug, the dosage form, the dose amount, the administration route, the time schedule, the prescriber's signature, and the date and time of the order. (*Note:* Prescriber's order sheets vary from one health care facility to another.)

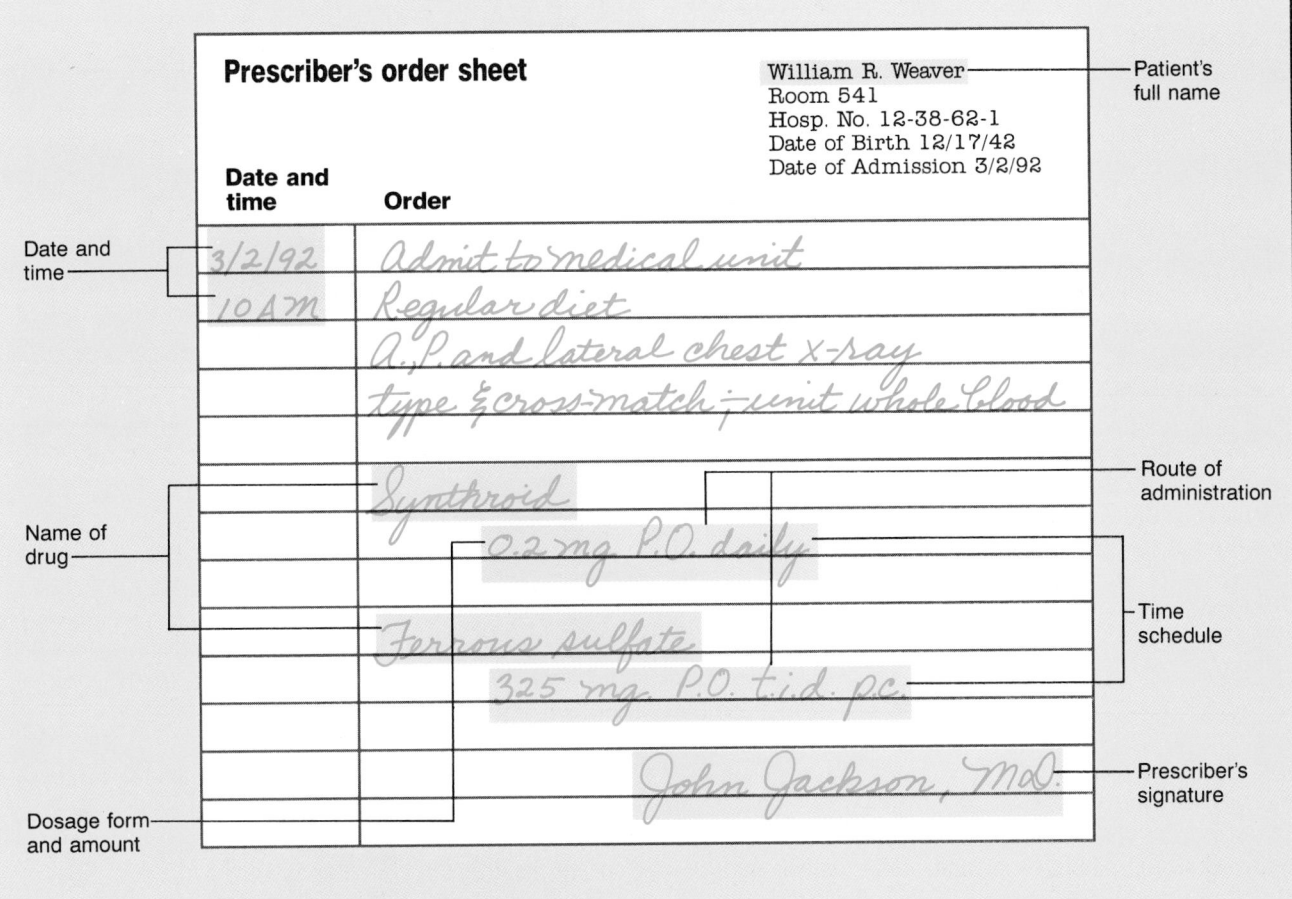

Prescriber's order sheet

William R. Weaver — Patient's full name
Room 541
Hosp. No. 12-38-62-1
Date of Birth 12/17/42
Date of Admission 3/2/92

Date and time — Date and time

Date and time	Order
3/2/92	Admit to medical unit
10 AM	Regular diet
	A.P. and lateral chest x-ray
	type & cross-match; unit whole blood

Name of drug — Synthroid

0.2 mg. P.O. daily — Route of administration / Time schedule

Ferrous sulfate
325 mg. P.O. t.i.d. p.c.

John Jackson, M.D. — Prescriber's signature

Dosage form and amount

---

more patients with the same or similar names appear on the unit.

The prescriber should give the generic or trade name of the drug and its dosage form, if more than one form of the drug is available. The prescriber should express the dose to be given at each administration in metric, apothecaries', or household measures and should state the administration route. The most common administration routes are oral, intramuscular, subcutaneous, and intravenous, although additional routes involving other body structures and cavities exist. Oral medications, representing the majority, tend to be the safest, least expensive, and most convenient for the patient to take.

The prescriber usually states the time schedule for administration as the number of times per day that the medication is to be administered. Upon noting the time schedule,

the nurse then schedules the specific hours according to how quickly a supply of the medication can be procured, the medication's characteristics, and institutional policies. The medication's characteristics, including its nature and onset and duration of action, primarily determine the schedule. For instance, if regular, intermittent peak blood concentration levels of antibiotics must be maintained to combat infections, the prescriber will schedule the drug administration at regular intervals around the clock.

To a lesser extent, institutional policy determines the schedule, such as a 10 a.m. administration for all drugs given only once a day. Sometimes, the specific responses of the patient to the illness and treatment determine the administration schedule. For example, the nurse may receive an order to administer 5 units of regular insulin to a diabetic patient whenever the blood glucose level exceeds 210 mg/dl.

The prescriber's signature, along with the date and time of day the order was written, also should appear. The date and time often are referred to when the order has an expiration date. For example, a narcotic order valid for 72 hours, written at noon on August 21, will expire at noon on August 24.

To implement a medication order properly, the nurse must understand dosage forms, measurement systems, administration routes, and accepted abbreviations. Prescribers should adhere strictly to the abbreviations approved by their specific institution. Adherence to approved abbreviations becomes particularly important in large institutions where health care professionals come from many different areas. Nonstandardized abbreviations lead to guesswork, which significantly increases the possibility of error. (For a list of many of the standardized, widely accepted abbreviations used today, see the appendix on Frequently Used Abbreviations in Drug Therapy.)

Outpatient medication orders usually are written as prescriptions. Before the patient leaves the outpatient setting, the nurse should clarify for the patient any abbreviations used in the prescription. By clarifying any doubtful abbreviations, the nurse can help avoid subsequent misinterpretation of the prescription by the patient. (For a list of abbreviations that patients often misunderstand, see the appendix on Frequently Misinterpreted Abbreviations in Drug Therapy.)

Like orders for hospitalized patients, prescriptions for outpatients identify the patient's name and address and the date the prescription was written. (For an illustration of how the prescriber writes a medication order for an outpatient, see *Outpatient medication order.*)

After *Rx*, which means "take thou," the prescriber writes the drug name, form, and dosage, along with instructions on the amount to be dispensed. Prescribing an adequate supply enables the health care professional to evaluate the patient's clinical response to the drug. After evaluating the patient's response, the health care professioanl may decide to change the medication. In such a case, by prescribing no more than an adequate supply, the health care professional saves the patient from incurring the unnecessary expense of the unused medication.

After the abbreviation *Sig.*, which means "let it be labeled," the prescriber writes directions to the patient for taking the medication. The directions are followed by the prescriber's signature, address, and telephone number. Finally, the prescriber indicates the number of times the prescription can be refilled. On some prescriptions, the physician's state medical license number also may appear. A prescription for any federally controlled drug also must include the prescriber's registration number with the Drug Enforcement Agency.

Outpatients must fill prescriptions for controlled substances within 6 months of the date written and cannot refill the prescription more than five times. Many prescriptions also will indicate whether the pharmacist should fill the prescription with generic or trade name products. If unspecified, most states allow the pharmacist to dispense the generic form of the drug, which may decrease the patient's expense. Patients should be aware that they have the right to ask the prescriber to write the prescription for the generic drug.

Besides the previously mentioned prescription requirements, all states now require the pharmacist to label each prescription container with the name, strength, and drug amount dispensed. These requirements contribute significantly to the patient's knowledge and understanding of the treatment regimen.

TYPES OF MEDICATION ORDERS

The following seven types of medication orders are routine in the hospital: standard written orders, single orders, stat orders, p.r.n. orders, standing orders, verbal (or oral) orders, and telephone orders.

Standard written orders

These orders apply indefinitely until the prescriber writes another order to alter or discontinue the first one. In some cases, the prescriber may specify on the standard written order a particular termination date. A standard written order with a termination date might read "Ergotrate (ergonovine) 0.2 mg P.O. q 4 hours × 3 days." In many cases, hospitals establish policies that indicate how long orders for certain classes of drugs remain valid. Examples of drugs with controlled termination dates include narcotic orders for 3 days and antibiotic orders for 7 days. If the patient still needs the drug after the expiration date, the prescriber must rewrite the order. The prescriber also must rewrite standard written orders postoperatively if the medications are to be continued.

Single orders

These orders are written for medications that are given only once. For example, a prescriber may order one tetanus toxoid injection for a patient with a laceration or puncture wound who received a primary tetanus toxoid series more than 10 years earlier.

Stat orders

Calls for medications that are to be administered immediately for an urgent patient problem are known as stat orders. For instance, a prescriber may order a single dose of an antianxiety drug to calm an acutely agitated patient.

Outpatient medication order

Community pharmacies usually fill outpatient medication orders. The following represents a typical prescription, showing its basic components.

HILLCREST MEDICAL ASSOCIATES

John Jackson, M.D. AJ 6051281
Richard Turner, M.D. AT 4051552

2813 Hillcrest Drive
Mayfield, PA 19682
Telephone: 814/613-5409

NAME: *Maria Fletcher*   AGE: *38*

ADDRESS: *206 Elmwood Drive*   DATE: *1/15/92*

Rx: *Penicillin VK 500 mg tablets orally*
Dispense #6

Sig.: *Take 4 tablets 1 hour before dental extraction then 2 tablets 6 hours later.*

_____*John Jackson*_____ M.D.

Generic equivalent permitted
Dispense as written

Refill: *2* times

P.R.N. orders

P.R.N. orders derive their name from a Latin phrase that means "as the occasion arises." Prescribers write p.r.n. orders for medications that are to be given when needed. The administration time results from the collaborative judgments of the nurse and the patient. Sometimes a p.r.n. order delineates the reason for giving the drug. For example, the prescriber may write "Tylenol 650 mg P.O. p.r.n. for a temperature above 101.3° F. (38.5° C.)." If an ordered drug, such as acetaminophen (Tylenol), serves multiple purposes, some hospital policies state that the nurse administer the drug only for the specific condition mentioned in the order. Under such a policy, the nurse would not give Tylenol ordered only for fever if the patient complained of a headache but had no fever. Other institutions allow the nurse to determine when to administer a p.r.n. drug. When administering a p.r.n. medication, the nurse should describe in the patient's record the reason for its use and its degree of subsequent effectiveness.

Standing orders

Also known as protocols, standing orders establish guidelines for treating a particular disease or set of symptoms. These orders require considerable judgment and expertise in assessing the patient's need for the medication and any dose-related adverse drug reactions that might occur.

Special care areas of the hospital, such as the coronary care unit, routinely establish standing orders that apply to such drug therapies as morphine sulfate for chest pain and anxiety, lidocaine (Xylocaine) for ventricular tachycardia, and furosemide (Lasix) for pulmonary congestion. Hospitals also may institute medication protocols that specifically designate drugs that a nurse may *not* give.

Verbal orders

Medication orders given orally rather than in writing are known as verbal orders. Health care professionals try to avoid using verbal orders because such orders can lead to miscommunication. In urgent situations, the nurse should write and sign the order dictated by the prescriber. Then the nurse should repeat the order aloud for the prescriber's verification and request the prescriber to spell the drug name if necessary. The prescriber should sign the verbal order that the nurse has written as soon as possible. The institution should have a policy that dictates the time period in which the prescriber must sign a verbal order. If a patient experiences hypoglycemic or insulin shock and the prescriber instructs the nurse to prepare immediately 50 ml of 50% glucose for I.V. administration, the nurse should show the prescriber the label on the empty glucose vial while simultaneously stating the drug's name and handing the syringe to the prescriber. Such actions allow the prescriber to confirm the accuracy of the drug and its dose.

Telephone orders

Verbal orders given to a nurse by a prescriber over the telephone may result in dangerous errors from mechanical problems involving the telephone and from the lack of nonverbal communication cues between the prescriber and nurse. Nurses should avoid telephone orders whenever possible. When a nurse must take a telephone order, the nurse should ask another nurse to monitor the call on an extension telephone. By monitoring the call, the second nurse can confirm the order. Unfortunately, nurses cannot always include such monitoring on the clinical unit. Besides verifying the drug name given during a telephone order, the nurse should repeat orally the individual digits of the dose. For instance, having understood the order to be 15 milligrams of meperidine (Demerol), the nurse might inquire, "You did say one-five milligrams of meperidine? Is that correct?" Repeating the order gives the prescriber the opportunity to confirm or correct the order, as in "No, that should be *fifty,* five-zero, milligrams of meperidine." The nurse then writes the order, indicating that it was a telephone order. Later, the prescriber must cosign the order within the time period established by institutional policy.

Unusual circumstances

The nurse will encounter situations related to the standard written order that require considerable nursing judgment in deciding whether and how to give the drug. On some occasions, the nurse may omit or at least delay a dose. This frequently occurs for patients prohibited from ingesting anything in preparation for certain diagnostic tests. In such cases, the nurse should confer with the prescriber. The nurse and prescriber may decide to omit the drug, give the drug orally with a very small amount of water, administer the drug by another route, or give the drug orally after completion of the test. Other circumstances may arise in which the nurse intentionally omits a dose of medication because the patient no longer needs it. For example, the nurse may omit a laxative dose if the patient has had a bowel movement since the medication order. The nurse sometimes omits medications because the patient refuses to take them.

Since the consumer movement of the 1960s, health care professionals and the public have placed considerable emphasis on the inclusion of the patient and family in making decisions about health care. Most health care professionals recognize a patient's right to know about specific drugs and to participate in making the decision to use the drugs. Before participating in such decisions, however, the patient should receive accurate information about the drug and its effects. Then the patient can make an informed decision. Health care professionals must assume the responsibility of supplying the necessary information and fully discussing the information with the patient.

Despite having the right to collaborate in the decision-making process, the patient still may refuse a drug, for various reasons. Patients may complain that the drug tastes bad and produces nausea, that injections hurt, that they do not understand the drug's purpose, or that they remain unconvinced that the drug will help. Patients also may believe that they are receiving the wrong medication. Some patients base their refusals on religious or cultural beliefs. In any case, the nurse should try to determine the patient's reason for refusing a medication.

The nurse may resolve problems by exploring the patient's feelings, listening to the patient's fears, and talking honestly to the patient about the need for the medication. Although the patient still may refuse the medication, the nurse should *never* give it by deceptive means, such as disguising it with food. In all instances in which patients do not receive an ordered medication, the nurse should indicate the omission on the medication administration record, describe the reason for the omission, and notify the patient's prescriber immediately if appropriate to do so.

PREVENTING MEDICATION ERRORS

The safe, accurate administration of medications demands that the nurse possess current, pertinent drug knowledge and follow safe procedures. From the beginning of a nursing student's professional preparation, educators make every effort to ensure the progressive accumulation of adequate knowledge about drug therapy.

Nursing educators encourage students to read pharmacology textbooks, examine brochures in medication packages, and consult clinical pharmacists. Because new medications constantly come into use, nurses must continue throughout their professional careers to seek drug information and develop the habit of pursuing continuing education offerings to maintain current drug knowledge.

Knowing about drugs as well as the factors to observe when preparing and administering each drug helps the nurse avoid medication errors. So does preparing medications in a quiet area, conducive to concentration.

After receiving a written order, the nurse transcribes it onto the appropriate working document approved by the hospital. The working document may be a medication administration record (MAR), a medication Kardex, medication cards or tickets, or a computer printout. Because the chance for error increases with the repeated copying of orders, the nurse must read each order carefully and prepare the medications directly from the approved document. The nurse must never rely on memory or personal worksheet notations. As a precaution against omitted orders, the established practices of many hospitals require the nurse to check periodically all MARs against the original order sheet. Also, the nurse preparing the change-of-shift report usually alerts the oncoming staff to any new medication orders.

THE FIVE "RIGHTS" OF MEDICATION ADMINISTRATION

Classic safeguards, known as the five "rights," exist to ensure accurate medication administration. Although the five "rights"—the right drug, dose, patient, time, and route—address various issues, health care professionals generally regard the safeguards as the minimum requirements for safety. Much additional forethought is required before any medication is administered.

Right drug

While working with the vast number of today's available drugs, the nurse must discriminate carefully among similar-sounding names. For example, digoxin (Lanoxin), digitoxin (Crystodigin), and Desoxyn (methamphetamine) all have similar-sounding names but are very different drugs. Digoxin and digitoxin represent different forms of the cardiac drug digitalis; Desoxyn is a drug used for weight reduction. The nurse always should compare the name of the drug on the container label to the medication order. For medications that are individually wrapped in single doses, the nurse should check the name when removing the drug from the drawer and again when unwrapping and giving the drug to the patient.

Before administering any drug, the nurse should tell the patient its name and action or use. Anytime a patient comments that the medication seems unusual, the nurse should recheck the drug name and strength. For example, a patient may say, "Nurse, this can't be my medication. I always take one pink pill, but you've given me two yellow pills." As a result, the nurse may discover a medication error or need to explain to the patient that the pink pill contains 10 mg of the drug whereas one yellow pill contains 5 mg of the same drug. Any patient comment mandates that the nurse explore the situation before administering the drug.

Right dose

The widespread use of unit-dose medications, individually wrapped and labeled single doses, has alleviated many problems related to drug dosage. Also, the many commercially prepared medications, available in various size tablets, decreases the number of calculations that the nurse must make to determine the dosage. The nurse should develop the standard practice of first mentally calculating the approximate dose, then calculating the actual dose in writing, using the correct formulas. For example, when giving 75 mg of a drug labeled 50 mg per ml, the nurse mentally can estimate the dosage to be 1.5 ml. Then the nurse can calculate the definitive dose by using the following formula:

$$50 : 1 :: 75 : X$$
$$50X = 75$$
$$X = 1.5 \text{ ml}$$

The nurse should recheck all calculations with another nurse or the pharmacist when possible. Many hospitals require double checks of dosage calculations for children's medications and for all drugs with narrow safety margins, such as heparin and insulin. Because more than one or two dosage units rarely are needed to prepare a prescribed dose, the nurse always should recheck the dosage if the calculations call for more than one tablet for a single dose or for a very small fraction of a dosage. The nurse also must be especially careful using decimal points because a misplaced or obscured decimal point can increase the dose many times or decrease it to a fraction of the intended dose. The nurse always should write a zero in front of a decimal point so that no one misreads a figure, such as 0.25 mg as 25 mg. Likewise, a zero should never follow a dosage that includes a decimal point because it easily could be misread and could increase the dosage tenfold. For example, the nurse should not write 0.250 for a dosage of 0.25 mg.

Occasionally, the nurse encounters unusual situations that cause difficulty in measuring the precise dose because of the supplied drug's form. The nurse should not break unscored tablets because the resulting doses will not be exact. The nurse should confer with the pharmacist to have an inconvenient form of a drug changed into a form that can be measured accurately.

To measure a dose of an oral liquid drug accurately, the nurse uses a medicine glass or cup. The nurse first sets the glass or cup at eye level when pouring, then reads the meniscus (a crescent shape on the liquid's surface) against the appropriate scale, that is, milliliters, drams, or ounces. By holding the bottle with the label toward the palm of the hand and pouring from the opposite side, the nurse avoids obliterating the label with dripping medication. The nurse should send bottles with illegible labels to the pharmacy and procure a new supply.

When measuring an injectable medication, the nurse must read carefully the correct scale on the syringe. Most syringes are marked in milliliters or cubic centimeters. Insulin syringes, marked according to the strength of insulin, may measure 40 or 100 units per cubic centimeter. The nurse must be sure to use the scale that correlates to the insulin concentration being used.

The nurse must never alter the dosage specified in the prescriber's order. For example, at the time of surgery, a physician orders 75 mg of meperidine (Demerol) for pain for the postoperative patient. The nurse later observes that the patient remains in excruciating pain and that the 75 mg of Demerol does not seem to be sufficient. The nurse may believe that 100 mg of Demerol would alleviate the patient's pain, but the nurse does *not* have the prerogative to change the dose. The nurse should consult with the physician and obtain a new written order. In many instances, prescribers now write medication orders with dosage ranges so that the nurse can decide the appropriate dose within the specified range.

Right patient

The nurse always should check the patient's identification bracelet carefully against the MAR before giving any medication. As a further check, the nurse should ask the patient to state his or her name. A nursing student may feel awkward about asking the patient's name, especially after working closely with a patient. However, the patient and nursing student can appreciate the reason for the precaution, and the feelings of awkwardness soon disappear when the patient sees that the procedure is standard practice. The nurse should not suggest the patient's name because a patient may

misunderstand the name or become confused and answer to the wrong name. Furthermore, the nurse should never assume that the patient in a correctly labeled bed is the right patient. A confused patient may get into the wrong bed.

Right time

Most hospitals establish routine times for drug administration. When administering a drug for which a consistent blood concentration level must be maintained to achieve therapeutic effects, the nurse observes equal time intervals around the clock. For example, the nurse may give the antiarrhythmic drug procainamide (Pronestyl) every 4 hours at 8 a.m., 12 noon, 4 p.m., 8 p.m., 12 midnight, and 4 a.m. The nurse also may have to measure certain patient responses to a therapy before administering another dose. For instance, the nurse should check the patient's apical pulse rate before giving a digitalis preparation and assess the patient's respiratory rate before administering a drug such as morphine.

For a drug with no dictating features, the nurse may space the divided doses over the patient's waking hours. For example, the nurse may give such a drug four times a day (q.i.d.) at 8 a.m., 12 noon, 4 p.m., and 8 p.m. Spacing the daily dosage serves to prevent adverse effects, which might be caused by a too-high concentration of the drug in the bloodstream at any given time. Bradycardia from propranolol (Inderal) use is an example of an adverse effect that the nurse can prevent by spacing daily doses. Sometimes, the nurse must consider other events, such as mealtime, when administering a drug. For example, a nurse giving a patient aspirin for a headache may administer the drug *before* meals to enhance absorption and speed pain relief. In another situation, the nurse deliberately may give a large dose of aspirin *after* meals to reduce drug-induced gastric irritation and to relieve pain more slowly but safely over a longer period.

By administering all drugs at evenly spaced intervals and at consistent times each day, the nurse can prevent errors and accommodate the patient's daily schedule. For example, quinidine gluconate (Quinaglute Dura-Tabs), used to treat certain cardiac arrhythmias, acts for 12 hours. Scheduling the drug for 8 a.m. and 8 p.m. administration maintains the necessary blood level without interfering with the patient's sleep. Routine administration schedules also help the patient develop the habit of taking the drug at a regular time. As a result, the patient is less likely to forget the drug after returning home.

To decrease further the risk of error in drug administration time, some institutions may require the nurse to use different ink colors when recording information about drugs. For example, the ink color may depend on whether the drug is to be given during the day, evening, or night shift. The nurse must pay attention to the hour of administration and the ink color. Errors can result even with the color-coding system. Other hospitals use the 24-hour system to decrease the number of medication errors related to timing. For example, the nurse would note a 10 p.m. medication time as 2200. By using the 24-hour system, the nurse cannot confuse 10 a.m. with 10 p.m.

The nurse should avoid scheduling medication administration at busy hours on the nursing unit, such as during a shift change. Instead of scheduling a twice-daily (b.i.d.) medication for 8 a.m. and 6 p.m., the nurse could schedule the administration for 9 a.m. and 7 p.m. to avoid the busy 8 a.m. hour after the shift change. Regardless of the exact schedule, the nurse should follow standard practice and allow a half hour before and after the designated time for medication administration. In many institutions, medications given beyond these time limits are considered errors.

Right route

The nurse must pay careful attention to the administration route specified in the medication order and on the product label. Some drugs must be given in certain manufactured forms to be appropriate for particular entry routes into the body. For example, the eye, with its delicate nature, requires special preparations. Also, the nurse should never inject a solution anywhere into the body unless the label clearly indicates that the solution is *for injection.*

The administration route also may affect the amount of the medication given. If given intramuscularly, 10 mg of morphine sulfate, a frequently used adult dose, relieves pain. If the drug is given I.V., the equivalent dose would decrease to 2 to 4 mg. If given orally, the morphine sulfate dose would need to be greater than 10 mg.

The procedure used to administer a drug also may affect the rate of drug absorption into the bloodstream. Some topical ointments, such as nitroglycerin paste, enter the bloodstream more rapidly and completely if spread over a large surface area and covered with plastic wrap or special paper supplied with the medication. On the other hand, crushing enteric-coated tablets or opening sustained-action capsules and dissolving the drug in liquid will result in improper absorption of the drug into the bloodstream and possibly unintended effects. (For more information about administering these types of drugs, see *Sustained-action drugs.* For details about proper techniques of medication administration, see Chapter 9, Routes and Techniques of Administration.)

PROCEDURAL SAFEGUARDS

Besides acknowledging the minimum requirements of the five "rights," the nurse practices other procedural safeguards to prevent errors. (For a summary, see *Nursing responsibilities associated with medication administration,* page 98.) This section discusses several special precautions,

---

Sustained-action drugs

Nurses increasingly encounter drugs designed to achieve an extended action over many hours. Prepared to dissolve at different rates, the drugs are released gradually but continuously into the bloodstream. Convenient for the patient, sustained-action drugs require fewer doses per day and provide more even control of symptoms.

Sustained-action drugs are supplied as plain tablets, coated tablets, and capsules filled with tiny granules. These drugs may be identified by "SA" after the drug name or by many prefixes used in the drug name to indicate prolonged effect. Common examples include Quinaglute *Dura-Tabs,* Dimetapp *Extentabs,* Chlor-Trimeton *Repetabs,* and Desoxyn *Gradumets.* Other names sometimes used include spansules, gyrocaps, and plateau caps.

The nurse must know that sustained-action tablets should never be split, crushed, or chewed, and that capsules should never be emptied into foods or beverages because doing so may alter the absorption rates, causing adverse reactions or a subtherapeutic level of activity. The nurse must be certain that the patient understands the importance of taking the sustained-action drug in its supplied form.

---

but the list is not all-inclusive. The nurse always should think of safety and analyze situations that could lead to medication errors.

• Health care professionals should handle and store drugs carefully to maintain the drugs' stability and strength. Because temperature, air, moisture, and light may affect a drug's stability, the nurse should follow drug-specific precautions. The nurse always should keep drugs in the containers in which the pharmacy dispensed them. Bottles should be capped tightly and stored away from sources of heat, light, and moisture. Some drugs are kept in brown bottles, and some I.V. medication bags are wrapped in aluminum foil to protect them from light during infusion. Some bottles of tablets contain small cylinders that absorb moisture and keep the product fresh. Ordinarily, drugs are stored at room temperature. Only those drugs that require cool temperatures are refrigerated because refrigeration causes moisture formation through condensation. Usually, the nurse allows refrigerated drugs to reach room temperature before administration.

• The law requires that narcotics and controlled substances be kept under double lock and key.

• The nurse always should note a drug's expiration date — the date after which the original potency of the drug is believed to change. The nurse should never administer an outdated drug or one that looks or smells unusual. If the manufacturer's drug package appears to have been tampered with, the nurse should not administer the drug but should return the package to the pharmacy for investigation. Drugs to be dispensed as powders may be reconstituted at

Nursing responsibilities associated with medication administration

When giving medication to any patient, the nurse must:
1. Assess the patient's physiologic and psychosocial status.
2. Form nursing diagnoses that identify actual or potential responses that require nursing intervention.
3. Administer the right drug in the right dose to the right patient at the right time by the right route.
4. Assess the patient's responses to drug therapy and determine if the drug is producing therapeutic or adverse effects.
5. Question medication orders that are not clear or that appear to be inappropriate for the patient.
6. Inform the prescriber of any necessary deviations in medication administration and of any adverse patient reactions to drug therapy.
7. Teach the patient about the safe, therapeutic self-administration of drugs.
8. Evaluate the effectiveness of nursing interventions.

administration time. Any unused medication should be labeled with the date, time, strength, and the nurse's initials or signature. The nurse should discard any drug that will remain stable for only a short time and will reach its expiration date before another dose is scheduled. The nurse should never administer a drug that has not been labeled properly after reconstitution. If the nurse finds an unlabeled syringe containing a medication, the nurse should discard it.

• When delivering drugs to a patient's room, the nurse should stay with the medication cart or tray. The nurse should never leave without locking the cart and taking it or the tray back to the medication room or to the usual storage place. The nurse should remain until the patient takes the medication to verify that it was taken as directed and should never leave medication doses at the patient's bedside unless a specific order to do so exists.

• The nurse should administer only medications prepared personally or by the pharmacist, unwrapping individual doses (unit doses) at the patient's bedside just before administration.

• Before administering a medication based on new orders, the nurse should review the patient's medication history to detect any known allergies or other idiosyncracies. The chart of any patient who has allergies should be labeled clearly.

• When administering an oral drug, the nurse should encourage the patient to drink a full glass of water, if appropriate. The water helps to move the medication through the esophagus and into the stomach and dilutes the drug, reducing the chance of gastric irritation.

• The prescriber must order drugs that are to be left at the patient's bedside for self-administration. Such drugs should be marked with the patient's name, the drug name and dose, and instructions. Drugs typically left at the patient's bedside include antacids, which the patient may take repeatedly, and nitroglycerin tablets, which the patient may need immediately for chest pain. The nurse remains responsible for supervising a patient whose drugs are left at the bedside. For example, the nurse must know how many nitroglycerin tablets the patient took, the exact times of self-administration, whether the patient obtained relief, and any unusual reactions to the drug. The nurse must record the information in the chart and report it to the prescriber.

• The nurse should chart drugs immediately after administering them. Delayed charting, especially of p.r.n. medications, can result in an error of repeated doses; early charting (charting before giving the medication) may result in omitted doses.

• The nurse should record observations of the patient's positive and negative responses to the medication. For instance, for a patient receiving an antibiotic for pneumonia, charted comments describing positive responses, such as a decreased amount of sputum, the absence of fever, and easier breathing, would confirm the drug's effectiveness. Negative reactions might include skin eruptions or gastric disturbances. Severe adverse reactions may prompt the prescriber to substitute another drug.

DRUG DELIVERY SYSTEMS

Several systems currently exist for procuring ordered drugs from the pharmacy. In each system, the nurse serves a vital coordinating function between the prescriber and the pharmacist.

Unit-dose system

When using the unit-dose system, the nurse transcribes the order on the patient's MAR and sends a carbon copy of the prescriber's order sheet directly to the pharmacy. The pharmacy may consist of a single, centralized department serving the entire hospital, or it may consist of several substations, or satellites, with a substation staffed by a pharmacist available on each nursing unit. The pharmacist transcribes the order and dispenses a supply of single doses, wrapped and labeled, of all forms of drugs—oral as well as injectable preparations, and I.V. solutions with additives. The pharmacist usually dispenses sufficient drugs and I.V. solutions to last 24 hours and also may prepare trays of medications for administration by the nurse at specified hours. The pharmacist may prepare unit doses or purchase them commercially. The pharmacist usually places drugs for each patient in individual drawers of a portable medication cart. The nurse keeps the drugs in their labeled wrappers until the actual administration time.

The nurse keeps the MAR in a Kardex or notebook on the medication cart and records all drugs immediately as they are administered to each patient. As a safeguard against errors from illegible longhand, the nurse prints the medication information on the MAR. The nurse should check the prescriber's order sheet and recopy the MAR anytime it becomes soiled or otherwise unreadable.

The unit-dose system reduces the chances for drug errors because (1) the prescriber and nurse collaborate with the pharmacist on the total drug regimen for the patient, (2) the prescriber, nurse, and pharmacist more readily can foresee and prevent therapeutic incompatibilities, possible adverse reactions, and incorrect dosages because the pharmacist keeps a detailed Kardex or record on each patient, (3) the system provides a double check for all medications, (4) health care professionals using the method waste fewer medications, and (5) nurses chart medications immediately. Furthermore, the unit-dose system reduces the risk of medication contamination because the pharmacist wraps medications as single doses and prepares I.V. medications under laminar airflow conditions in the pharmacy to assure sterility. The unit-dose system conveniently relieves the nurse of some of the preparation activities, thus allowing more time for other aspects of patient care. The system proves particularly useful in hospitals that do not have 24-hour pharmacy service because pharmacists may prepare drugs for later administration by the nurse.

For the unit-dose system to work properly, the number of pharmacy personnel may have to be increased, which some institutions may view as a disadvantage of the unit-dose system.

Automated systems

Automated systems essentially represent computerized versions of the unit-dose system. A mechanical medication-dispensing unit delivers individually wrapped and labeled medications upon command by the nurse. The pharmacist fills the unit and keeps it locked. A computer records all drug transactions on electronic tape and furnishes requested printouts. The automated system greatly simplifies the maintenance of accurate drug records because the system's computer can monitor and track drugs in every respect, from the original inventory to patient billing. The system's efficiency saves time and allows pharmacy personnel to expand their role to include more consultation and teaching. The system also relieves the nurse of the responsibilities of transcribing the medication order and procuring and storing the drug. The time saved frees the nurse to attend to other aspects of patient care.

Unfortunately, implementing an automated system can be expensive, and all mechanical systems are subject to failure. Because of possible computer downtime, hospitals using automated systems devise backup plans for administering and recording medications.

Although hospitals usually select and use one drug delivery system, some follow two systems. For example, an institution primarily using the unit-dose system may maintain small supplies of stock drugs in special care units for patients whose conditions may change rapidly, thus requiring that drugs be immediately available.

Individual prescriptions

When using the individual prescription system, the nurse transcribes the medication order and sends it to the pharmacy. The pharmacist fills the prescription using a container labeled for the particular patient. The nurse then administers the drug directly from the container. The nurse is less likely to commit the error of giving the drug to the wrong patient because the drug supply is designated for only one patient. Implementation, however, is slow in the individual prescription system because the medication order must travel from the nurse to the pharmacy and back to the nurse.

Floor stock system

The floor stock system, the oldest system in use, features the maintenance of a stock supply of medications on the nursing unit. Stock supplies usually are kept in a medication room and may be arranged alphabetically or in groups according to drug action. Upon receiving a medication order, the nurse immediately transcribes it onto the medication cards and a special medication Kardex. The medication cards or tickets give the patient's name, room, and bed number; the name, dose, and administration schedule of the medication; the name or initials of the nurse who noted the order; and the date of the order. The medication cards also may be color coded to call attention to the administration time schedule.

After transcribing the medication order, the nurse prepares the appropriate medication dose from the available stock supply, places the dose into an individual medication cup, and transports it to the patient on a tray or medication cart. The nurse who must dispense a large number of regularly scheduled medications should perform the charting in the nurses' station after administering all the medications for that hour.

The chief advantage of the floor stock system is that the nurse can implement medication orders quickly because the drug is immediately available on the unit. However, the system presents at least three distinct disadvantages: (1) the nurse must interpret the order and requisition of the medication alone, with no input from the pharmacist; (2) transcription errors easily can occur, particularly if many different nurses have transcribed the drug orders with no safeguard or check by the pharmacist; and (3) errors of omission also can occur if medication cards are misplaced.

Regardless of the drug delivery system used, the institution's nurses, physicians, and pharmacists must work collaboratively. Although many hospitals are instituting automated systems, nurses in most hospitals continue to note medication orders and to administer medications. The drug delivery system does not relieve the nurse of traditional responsibilities in administering medications, nor can the delivery system substitute for the nurse's judgment required in unusual patient circumstances where routine procedures do not apply.

LEGAL RESPONSIBILITIES

Chapter 1 discussed the sources and types of laws governing drug administration. This section covers specific nursing responsibilities imposed by the law. Practice acts passed by the legislature of each state govern the practice of each of the major health professions. Therefore, the nurse practice act, medical practice act, and pharmacy practice act of each state represent statutory laws and determine the scope of practice for those professionals. Essentially, practice acts allow physicians to prescribe, dispense, and administer drugs; pharmacists to prepare, dispense, and furnish drugs on the retail market; and nurses to administer medications and, if licensed to do so, prescribe. Also, the Controlled Substances Act, a federal legislation, regulates the manner in which narcotics and other controlled substances are dispensed and administered, thus directly affecting nursing practice.

EXPECTATIONS OF THE LAW

The law expects nurses who administer drugs to patients to know about those drugs. The nurse should know the goals of the drug therapy, the drug's mechanism of action, expected and unusual effects, dosage, proper administration methods, and any contraindications. The nurse also should assess the patient's medication responses and teach the patient about self-administration. The nurse practice acts in some states specifically include patient teaching as a legal expectation.

On receiving a medication order, the nurse should consider it carefully. If any part of the order seems unusual, the nurse should not implement it until clarifying the problem with the prescriber. Under no circumstances should the nurse *ignore* the medication order and fail to carry it out. The nurse has an obligation to seek clarification of

any questions concerning the order. Sometimes nurses are reluctant to approach a prescriber and question an order for fear of being rebuked. Questioning a medication order requires assertiveness and tact on the nurse's part. Frequently, nurses consult pharmacists or approved published drug references to confirm their knowledge of the drug before approaching a prescriber. When questioning an order, the nurse should discuss the matter with the prescriber privately, professionally, and with an attitude of objective scientific inquiry. If the prescriber's explanation is unacceptable, the nurse must notify the supervisor and withhold the medication until further clarification of the order is received.

MALPRACTICE

Malpractice refers to a professional's wrongful conduct, improper discharge of duties, or failure to meet standards of care that causes harm to another. Negligence is a form of malpractice. Negligence refers to the failure to do something that reasonably could be expected to be done by an individual in a given situation or the performance of an act that a reasonable and prudent person would not do (Creighton, 1987).

Under the law, nurses are judged to be responsible for their own actions. Thus, upon the implementation of an incorrect order, the nurse as well as the prescriber and the hospital may be held legally liable. Medication errors resulting in malpractice may take two forms: errors of omission and errors of commission. An error of omission occurs when the nurse omits an important part of care. For example, a nurse who overlooks a patient's 2 p.m. dose of cimetidine (Tagamet) makes an error of omission. An error of commission occurs when the nurse performs a procedure improperly. For example, a nurse administers 3 ml (0.15 mg) of digoxin (Lanoxin) to an infant I.M. rather than orally, and the infant suffers cardiac arrest. The nurse has made an error of commission.

Although malpractice may sound harsh, especially to the beginning nursing student, the student may feel reassured by learning that the law does not expect the nurse to be infallible. The law does expect sound knowledge, good judgment, and due care. Because medication errors, along with falls, rank at the top of the list of causes of malpractice suits, the nurse must safeguard against medication errors by carefully considering and following the five "rights" of medication administration.

Further legal expectations of the nurse arise when an error occurs. Upon discovery of the error, the nurse should (1) immediately notify the prescriber, the nursing supervisor, and the pharmacist, that is, *only* those personnel who can do something to rectify the error, (2) carefully assess the patient's condition and render care as necessary, and (3) complete a medication error incident report.

Medication error incident reports

Most hospitals include medication error incident reports among their unusual incident forms. The medication error incident report typically requires a clear description of the event, including the time and date of the error and what the nurse did about it. The prescriber completes a section describing the patient's condition and any medical action taken. The nurse should not neglect to fill out a medication error incident report for fear that the report will be used in disciplinary action. Administrative personnel can use medication error incident reports to help improve patient care by implementing policies or procedures to prevent similar errors from occurring in the future.

Circulation of a medication error incident report should be limited to administrative personnel who need to know the facts about a specific incident. The medication error incident report usually is not placed in the patient's chart, but the nurse's charting on the patient's record should explain what happened and what actions subsequently were taken.

CONFLICTS BETWEEN PRACTICE ACTS

A few special circumstances necessitate that the nurse must operate exactly within the provisions of the practice act and not infringe on the practice of one of the other professions. Nurse practice acts typically state that the nurse implements orders written by *licensed* physicians, podiatrists, and dentists. Medication orders written by physician's assistants do not meet the criterion. Therefore, a licensed physician must countersign any order written by a physician's assistant before the nurse implements the order.

Possible conflicts with pharmacy practice acts occasionally restrict nursing actions. For example, transferring medications from one bottle to another or relabeling bottles falls within the realm of pharmacy, not the realm of nursing. Also, nurse supervisors who need drugs from the pharmacy when it is closed may procure only enough medication for one dose. Pharmacy practice acts regard the taking of larger quantities as dispensing, a clear function of the pharmacist.

The emerging role of the nurse practitioner sometimes conflicts with medical practice acts. In 1981, the *Sermchief v. Gonzales* case in Missouri set a precedent. Under underprescribed protocols and the general guidance of staff physicians, two nurses employed as nurse practitioners in a family-planning clinic frequently diagnosed reproductive tract conditions and prescribed medications, such as antibiotic creams and contraceptive drugs and devices. A charge of practicing medicine without a license was brought against the two nurse practitioners. The state supreme court upheld the nurse practitioners' actions by ruling that they were operating within the provisions of the nurse practice act, which recently had been revised to allow for expanded nursing roles. All of the examples emphasize the need for the nurse to understand clearly the provisions of the nurse practice act established by the state in which the nurse is practicing.

CONTROLLED SUBSTANCES

The Controlled Substances Act of the federal government imposes a few special responsibilities on the nurse. Under its provisions, the nurse must account for the proper use of controlled drugs with specific patients. Thus, when administering a narcotic, a barbiturate, or another controlled drug, the nurse must sign for the drug on a special narcotics record. Every dose that the pharmacy dispenses must be accounted for, whether the dose was used for a particular patient or was discarded accidentally.

Most hospitals require change-of-shift controlled substance or narcotics counts to assure that the supply on hand correlates exactly with the records. A nurse going off duty and a nurse coming on duty cooperatively make the controlled substance or narcotics count, and both sign the form verifying the accuracy of the count. If the count indicates a discrepancy between the supply and the record, the reason for the discrepancy must be traced immediately. Someone simply may have forgotten to sign for a dose that was given to a patient, a dose may have been contaminated and wasted without an explanation on the narcotics record, or someone may have removed a dose from the supply without authorization.

The law also requires that controlled drugs be stored in locked cabinets. The nurse maintains the narcotics supply under double lock and key. The nurse always should carry the narcotics keys, never leaving them in a drawer or hung on a hook where unauthorized persons could have access to them.

ETHICAL OBLIGATIONS

Nursing ethics represent the application of moral principles and values to professional practice. Whereas legal affairs concern rights and correlated responsibilities, ethics deal with the duties and obligations that the nurse has to self, patients, and professional colleagues. Conflicts of value can occur when the nurse, patient, and physician express differences of opinion about what actions to take in a particular situation. Consider the following:

A nurse is caring for a patient with advanced cancer, and the patient's physician orders chemotherapy. The patient is reluctant to begin the chemotherapy and asks the nurse many questions about its efficacy and adverse effects. The nurse knows that the patient's disease is terminal and that the therapy may cause hair loss as well as severe nausea and vomiting. The nurse wants to be truthful and believes in the patient's right to refuse the therapy and live as desired. Yet the nurse also knows that the physician recommends the chemotherapy. Under the circumstances, the nurse's strong belief in the patient's right to self-determination, the role of the nurse as a patient advocate, and the nurse's sincere desire to be honest can produce ethical conflicts for the nurse.

Ethical conflicts always have existed in nursing but have become prominent today because of the quality-of-life issue. Rapidly advancing technology often prolongs life, resulting in conditions that some people may want to avoid.

Moral principles

The nurse applies six moral principles when considering all types of patient care, including medication administration. These principles are autonomy, paternalism, truthfulness, beneficence, fidelity, and respect for property. In analyzing ethical issues involving these principles, the nurse emphasizes:
• What is morally right and therefore ought to be done?
• What benefits and harms would result from this action?
• Who would be benefited or harmed?

Autonomy refers to the right of every person to make rational decisions about one's life. The nurse's belief in autonomy leads to a respect for the patient's decisions. The nurse actively helps the patient overcome fear, pain, and knowledge deficits that might interfere with the patient's rational thinking. The nurse must assess each patient and consider the patient's decision regarding medication administration.

Paternalism results when someone decides what is best for another person and acts without consulting the person. Anyone acting paternalistically toward a patient must consider whether the action is justifiable. Unjustified paternalism in no way supports the patient.

The nurse may practice justified paternalism when administering pain medication to a terminally ill patient who may refuse medication because the drug causes drowsiness. The nurse knows the positive and negative consequences of the medication and convinces the patient to take the medication by deemphasizing the drug's sedative effects. In such a situation, the nurse's justified paternalism benefits the patient.

Truthfulness refers to being honest. The nurse displays truthfulness by not withholding information. For example, if a patient's drug produced adverse reactions, such as severe nausea and vomiting, the nurse would disclose the full information about the drug's adverse effects while focusing on the positive benefits of the therapy and reassuring the patient that the nausea can be treated. The nurse must answer all questions honestly and provide or seek further information if necessary.

Beneficence refers to the concept that nursing actions always should cause beneficial effects, never harmful ones. All nursing procedures are based on the principle of beneficence. The nurse always should plan and implement actions that assure safe outcomes for the patient and avoid negative consequences, which might cause harm. Hence, the nurse reads drug labels repeatedly, double-checks dosage calculations, and compares the patient's identification band to the name on the medication order.

Fidelity requires the nurse to be faithful and truthful and to keep promises made to self, patients, families, coworkers, and employers. A nurse should not make a promise to a patient without absolute certainty that the promise can be kept.

Respect for property refers to the safekeeping of the patient's personal possessions. If a patient brings medications to the hospital, most hospitals require that the nurse take the medications from the patient upon admission and store them to prevent double dosing or undesirable drug interactions. The patient, however, must consent to the storage, and the nurse must return the medications to the patient upon discharge. Medications ordered from the pharmacy become the patient's personal property even though the nurse keeps the drugs in the medication cart and administers them. Therefore, the nurse would violate the patient's property rights by administering the drugs to another patient or by destroying the patient's drugs brought from home.

Placebos

Placebos (substances such as glucose pills and saline solution injections, used for nonspecific, psychological effects without the patient's immediate knowledge that a placebo is being given) create certain ethical quandaries. Placebo use requires the nurse to withhold information, which violates the moral principle of truthfulness. Traditionally, physicians and nurses have not told patients about placebos because doing so usually diminishes the chance of the placebo producing the desired effect. The success of placebo use seems to depend on a patient's susceptibility.

Health care professionals who administer placebos should acknowledge the extenuating circumstances and comply with the following guidelines:
• Use a placebo only after careful diagnosis.
• Use only an inert substance.
• Answer questions as truthfully as possible.

• Honor the patient's request if the patient specifically asks not to receive a placebo.
• Never give a placebo when other treatment is indicated or before exploring all treatment options.

CHAPTER SUMMARY

Chapter 7 presented the nurse's role in medication administration. Here are the chapter highlights.
• Medication orders usually originate with the physician or other prescriber and vary in form, depending on whether they apply to a hospitalized patient or to an outpatient. Prescribers write medication orders for hospitalized patients along with or in addition to all other medical orders.
• Requirements of the medication order include the patient's full name; the name, dose, and dosage form of the drug; the administration route; the schedule; the prescriber's signature; and the date and time.
• Prescribers write medication orders for outpatients as prescriptions. Prescriptions must include the patient's name and address; the date the prescription was written; the drug name, form, dose, and amount to be dispensed; directions for taking the drug; and the prescriber's signature, address, telephone number, and registration numbers.
• Seven types of medication orders are routine in the hospital: standard written, single, stat, p.r.n., standing, verbal, and telephone.
• Classic safeguards, known as the five "rights," exist to ensure accurate medication administration. Nurses ensure that they are giving the right drug and the right dose of the drug. Nurses also should check the patient's identification to ensure that they are giving the drug to the right patient. They also must establish and verify the right time for drug administration. Finally, nurses must be sure that they use the right administration route when giving a drug to a patient. The medication order and the drug product label specify the administration route.
• Other procedural safeguards, such as checking expiration dates, staying with the patient until the patient has taken the medication, and recording any observations of patient responses to the medication, can help the nurse prevent medication errors.
• Different systems are used for delivering medications from the pharmacy to the patient. When using the unit-dose system, the pharmacist dispenses medication supplies, storing the medications on trays or in a medication cart. The nurse then takes the medication cart or tray from room to room, administering the drugs. Automated systems essentially represent computerized versions of the unit-dose system. Hospitals using automated systems must establish a backup system for use during computer downtime. Using the individual prescription system, the pharmacist fills a single order, using a container labeled for the particular patient. The nurse then administers the drug directly from the container. With the floor stock system, each nursing unit maintains a stock supply of medications. By having the medications on hand, the nurse can implement medication orders quickly.
• The law expects the nurse administering medications to possess sound knowledge and good judgment and to exercise due care in executing procedures. The nurse is obligated to clarify any unusual or unclear medication orders with the prescriber before implementing them. The nurse cannot ignore a medication order, but can refuse to administer a medication if the prescriber cannot explain the order satisfactorily.
• Causes of malpractice include errors of omission, in which the nurse fails to give necessary care, and errors of commission, in which the nurse renders necessary care in an improper way. The nurse can be held liable for a patient's injury if the injury directly results from the nurse's action.
• The nurse must apply fundamental values and moral principles to professional nursing practice. Moral principles that the nurse applies when considering patient care include autonomy, paternalism, truthfulness, beneficence, fidelity, and respect for property.

STUDY QUESTIONS

See Appendix 1 for answers.

1. Salvatore Tandino, age 64, is admitted to the hospital, where his physician writes the following medication orders:
Regular insulin 5 U S.C. stat
NPH insulin 30 U S.C. daily before breakfast
Tylenol 650 mg P.O. q 4 hours p.r.n. headache
MOM 30 ml h.s. p.r.n.
Halcion 0.125 mg P.O. h.s. p.r.n.
Which of these orders is incomplete?
(a) NPH insulin 30 U S.C. daily before breakfast
(b) Halcion 0.125 mg P.O. h.s. p.r.n.
(c) MOM 30 ml h.s. p.r.n.
(d) Tylenol 650 mg P.O. q 4 hours p.r.n. headache

2. Mr. Tandino must receive regular insulin stat. When should the nurse administer this medication?
(a) when the patient requests it
(b) as the occasion arises
(c) immediately
(d) at bedtime

3. Mr. Tandino must receive several p.r.n. medications. When should the nurse administer these medications?
(a) at bedtime
(b) as needed
(c) only once
(d) immediately

4. The hospital pharmacy supplies individually wrapped single doses of Mr. Tandino's P.O. medications. To ensure administration of the right drug, how many times should the nurse check the drug?
(a) one
(b) two
(c) three
(d) four

5. Before administering medications to Mr. Tandino, the nurse must ensure that the drug is being given to the right patient. What is the best way to do this?
(a) Check the identification bracelet and ask the patient his name.
(b) Check the identification bracelet and call the patient by name.
(c) Check the identification bracelet against the name on the chart.
(d) Check the identification bracelet against the name on the bed.

6. At the women's health clinic, Carol Borden, age 23, seeks care for a vaginal infection. Her nurse practitioner prescribes miconazole (Monistat) based on a set of pre-established orders developed to treat particular diseases or sets of symptoms. Which type of orders are these?
(a) standard written orders
(b) single orders
(c) stat orders
(d) standing orders

7. The physician prescribes a sustained-action drug to treat Diane McKelvey's nasal congestion. When the nurse attempts to administer the drug, Ms. McKelvey states that the tablets are too large for her to swallow. What should the nurse do?
(a) Break the tablets into smaller pieces.
(b) Tell the patient to chew the tablets.
(c) Crush the tablets and mix them in her food.
(d) Consult with the physician about an alternative drug.

8. The physician recommends danazol (Danocrine) to treat Beth Minor's endometriosis. After discussing the drug's possible adverse effects, Ms. Minor, age 22, refuses to take it. By supporting Ms. Minor's decision to refuse medica-

tion, the nurse is demonstrating a belief in which moral principle?
(a) beneficence
(b) paternalism
(c) autonomy
(d) fidelity

SELECTED REFERENCES

Cohen, M. (1990). Better way to transcribe orders. *Nursing90, 20*(1), 9.

Creighton, H. (1987). Legal significance of charting. Part II. *Nursing Management, 18*(10), 14-15.

Donnelly, A. (1989). Multidisciplinary approach to improving documentation of medications used during surgical procedures. *American Journal of Hospital Pharmacy, 46*(4), 724-728.

Fuqua, R., and Stevens, K. (1988). What we know about medication errors: A literature review. *Journal of Nursing Quality Assurance, 3*(1), 1-17.

Kozier, B., and Erb, G. (1987). *Fundamentals of nursing: Concepts and procedures* (3rd ed.). Menlo Park, CA: Addison-Wesley.

Johnson, P., and Lloyd-Jones, J. (Eds.). (1988). *Drug delivery systems: Fundamentals and techniques.* New York: VCH Publications.

Lind, G. (1987). Sermchief v. Gonzales: The Missouri precedent...case to interpret a modern nurse practice act. *Missouri Nurse, 56*(1), 4.

Pawlak, R., and Herfert, L. (1989). *Administration in the NICU: A handbook for nurses* (2nd ed.). Petaluma, CA: Neonatal Network.

Scholz, D. (1990). Establishing an endemic medication error rate. *Journal of Nursing Quality Assurance, 21*(1), 11-17.

Stefos, K. (1989). Administering drugs safely, Part 1. *Nursing, 19*(5), 126-130.

DOSAGE MEASUREMENTS AND CALCULATIONS

OBJECTIVES

After reading and studying this chapter, the student should be able to:

1. Discuss factors that may influence drug dosages.
2. Explain the advantages of the metric system over the apothecaries' and household systems of measurement.
3. Give at least two clinical examples of how the metric, apothecaries', and household systems of measurement are used in medication administration.
4. Identify two drugs that use special systems of measurement developed by the manufacturers.
5. Use the fraction and ratio methods to calculate the dosage of a drug ordered in one system of measurement but available only in another system of measurement.
6. Perform the calculations for reconstituting a powdered drug for injection, an intravenous (I.V.) infusion rate, and a percentage solution, using the fraction and ratio methods.

INTRODUCTION

This chapter contains information related to administering safe, accurate dosages of drugs — a major responsibility for nurses. It begins by discussing factors that determine variations in drug dosages, followed by information about the major systems of drug weights and measures. The chapter includes the characteristics of each system of drug weights and measures, the units for liquid and solid measures in each system, and examples of physicians' orders for drugs measured in each system. It explains conversions between the systems of measurement and presents methods for calculating drug dosages within each system of drug weights and measures. Sample problems and their solutions appear throughout the chapter to assist in the step-by-step approach needed to calculate correct dosages. Practice computations and their answers also are presented. The chapter concludes

with a discussion of special considerations related to dosage calculations for pediatric and geriatric patients.

FACTORS INFLUENCING DRUG DOSAGES

Several major factors influence the amount of a drug that would prove most effective and safe for each patient.

Age
The first factor, the patient's age, predetermines to some extent body size and affects the functioning of the various body systems.

Health care professionals must give special consideration to infants and elderly patients. In an infant, immature body systems impede pharmacokinetics — the absorption, distribution, metabolism, and excretion of drugs. Elderly patients may experience age-related changes involving the degeneration of one or more of the major body systems. The degeneration of body systems increases the likelihood of chronic illnesses involving these systems. The resulting chronic illnesses subsequently may alter the absorption, distribution, metabolism, and excretion of drugs. The alterations in pharmacokinetics can produce adverse effects on the safety and effectiveness of an administered drug.

Size
A patient's size is determined by body weight and body-surface area. Both factors affect drug dosages. In most cases, a larger patient requires a larger dose of medication. For example, adult patients usually receive larger drug dosages than pediatric patients. In some instances, the patient's

weight determines the drug amount prescribed. In other cases, the patient's body-surface area affects drug dosage.

Integrity of body systems

The proper functioning of body systems is another important consideration when determining the drug dosage needed by a patient. Alterations in gastrointestinal functioning affect the time and amount of absorption of orally administered drugs. Alterations in cardiovascular functioning affect the absorption of injected medications. The integrity of the cardiovascular system also affects the transport of drugs from the absorption site to the action site. Because the liver metabolizes most drugs, any alteration in hepatic function disturbs the normal rate of such metabolism. Alterations in hepatic function and the resulting effects on drug metabolism lead to increasing blood concentration levels of a drug and the likelihood of a toxic effect, despite the administration of the drug within a safe dosage range.

Drug excretion occurs primarily through the renal system. Thus, alterations in renal function most significantly and adversely affect drug excretion. Patients with kidney disorders retain drugs and the end products of drug degradation. The retention causes increased blood concentration levels of the drug and end products and consequently increases the risk of toxicity.

Type and virulence of disease

The type and virulence of a patient's disease also affects the drug dosage. The same medication may be given for several purposes; however, the dosage varies according to the desired effect. For example, the antianxiety drug diazepam (Valium) may be given in a small dosage to control a patient's anxiety, but it also may be given in a larger dosage to produce an anesthetic effect. Similarly, the dosage of an antibiotic can vary, depending on the extent of infection evident.

Safe drug dosages

Drug companies and researchers extensively test each new drug before its approval for distribution to the general public. The research provides information about the drug's activities, effectiveness, adverse effects, and toxicity as well as about the drug's dosage ranges that yield desired outcomes. Drug manufacturers provide their research results to physicians for use in determining drug dosages.

The nurse's responsibilities include ensuring that all administered drugs fall within the safe ranges determined by manufacturers. To fulfill their responsibilities, nurses must be able to (1) determine equivalent measurements from among the metric, apothecaries', and household systems of measurement and (2) use appropriate mathematical formulas to calculate drug dosages, percentage solutions, and I.V. infusion rates. Mastery of the information presented in this chapter will provide an essential knowledge base for implementing these important nursing skills. (For additional information about the effects of patient characteristics on drug dosages and pharmacokinetics, see Chapter 2, Pharmacokinetics.)

SYSTEMS OF DRUG WEIGHTS AND MEASURES

Physicians use several systems of measurement when ordering drugs. The three systems of measurement most often used in clinical situations are the metric system, the apothecaries' system, and the household system. These systems are so widely used that the medication cup for liquid measurements may be calibrated in all three systems. A fourth system, the avoirdupois system, is used for ordering and purchasing pharmaceutical products and for weighing patients.

METRIC SYSTEM

The metric system, the most widely used and international system of measurement, is also the system used by the U.S. Pharmacopoeia. Among its many advantages, the metric system affords a way to achieve accuracy in calculating small drug dosages. Furthermore, the metric system uses Arabic numerals, which commonly are used by health care professionals throughout the world. Finally, most manufacturers calibrate newly developed drugs in the metric system.

Unfortunately, the general population in the United States has shown little eagerness to adopt the metric system. As a consequence, nurses and nursing students commonly view the metric system as a new and complicated concept. However, when they understand the general principles of this system, nurses easily can perform drug calculations and conversions within it. Nurses can use the metric system to measure liquids and solids. (For more information, see *Metric measures*.)

Liquid measures

The liter (L) of the metric system approximates 1 quart in volume. A milliliter (ml) equals one one-thousandth of a liter. Liters commonly are used when ordering and administering I.V. solutions. Milliliters are used in the administration of parenteral and some oral drugs.

Solid measures

In the metric system, the gram (g) serves as the basis for solid measures or units of weights. A milligram (mg) equals one one-thousandth of a gram. Many drugs are ordered in

Metric measures

This table shows the relationships among some commonly used measures. Several less commonly used measures, such as the hectogram, also appear.

LIQUIDS	
1 milliliter (ml)	= 1 cubic centimeter (cc)
1 deciliter (dl)	= 100 milliliters
1,000 milliliters	= 1 liter (L)
100 centiliters (cl)	= 1 liter
10 deciliters	= 1 liter
10 liters	= 1 dekaliter (dkl)
100 liters	= 1 hectoliter (hl)
1,000 liters	= 1 kiloliter (kl)

SOLIDS	
1,000 milligrams (mg)	= 1 gram (g)
1,000 grams	= 1 kilogram (kg)
100 centigrams (cg)	= 1 gram
10 decigrams (dg)	= 1 gram
10 grams	= 1 dekagram (dkg)
100 grams	= 1 hectogram (hg)

Apothecaries' measures

This table displays the relationships between measures, both liquid and solid, within the apothecaries' system.

LIQUIDS	
60 minims (℞)	= 1 fluidram (f℥)
8 fluidrams	= 1 fluidounce (f℥)
16 fluidounces	= 1 pint (pt)
2 pints	= 1 quart (qt)
4 quarts	= 1 gallon (gal)

SOLIDS	
20 grains (gr)	= 1 scruple (℈)
3 scruples	= 1 dram(℥)
8 drams	= 1 ounce (℥)
12 ounces	= 1 pound (lb)

milligrams. Body weight is recorded in kilograms (kg). A kilogram equals 1,000 grams.

The following examples represent possible orders using the metric system:
- 1 liter of 5% dextrose solution I.V. per 8 hours
- 30 ml (milliliters) Milk of Magnesia P.O. h.s.
- Ancef 1 g (gram) I.V.P.B. q6h
- Lanoxin 0.125 mg (milligram) P.O. daily
- Maintain 10 kg (kilogram) continuous traction

APOTHECARIES' SYSTEM

Though older than the metric system and still used to measure several medications, the apothecaries' system is being slowly phased out of use. The apothecaries' system possesses two unique features: the use of Roman numerals and the placement of the unit of measurement before the Roman numeral. For example, *5 grains* would be written as *grains v*. In the apothecaries' system, the equivalents among the various units of measure are close approximations. When using equivalents for calculations and conversions, keep in mind that the calculations, though not precise, will fall within acceptable standards. The apothecaries' system is the only system of measurement that uses symbols besides abbreviations to represent several of the units of measure. The nurse may use the apothecaries' system to measure liquids or solids. (For more information, see *Apothecaries' measures.*)

Liquid measures

Visualize the minim (℞), the smallest of the units, as the approximate size of a drop of water. Fifteen to sixteen minims comprise about 1 milliliter. (Note the approximation of the measure.)

Solid measures

The grain (gr) represents the solid measure or unit of weight in the apothecaries' system. Historians claim that the weight of an average grain of wheat originally determined the grain of the apothecaries' system.

The following examples represent possible orders using the apothecaries' system:
- multivitamin elixir ℞ (minims) xii P.O.
- Robitussin f℥ (fluidrams) iv P.O. q6h
- Mylanta f℥ (fluidounce) i P.O. 1 hour p.c.
- Tylenol gr (grains) x P.O. q4h p.r.n. headache

HOUSEHOLD SYSTEM

Most people in the United States are familiar with the household system of weights and measures. In most cases, food products, recipes, over-the-counter drugs, and home remedies use the household system. Although the units of measure in the household system may be the most familiar, discrepancies exist about quantities attributed to each measure and conversions between the measures. In the clinical setting, health care professionals seldom use the household system for drug administration; however, some household measures may prove useful.

Liquid measurement in the household system

To ensure the accuracy of dosages measured in teaspoons and tablespoons, the patient should receive information about obtaining a proper measuring device and the proper method of administration.

1. Obtain a spoon with hollow handle calibrated in teaspoons and tablespoons.

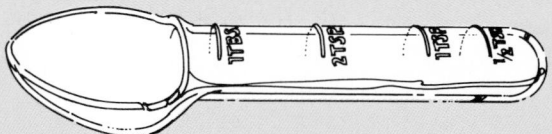

2. Check dose after filling. Hold spoon upright. Shaded area indicates dose of 2 tsp.

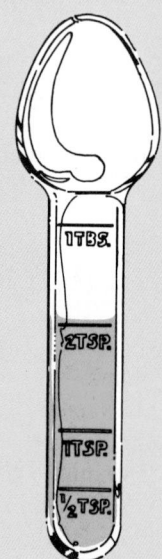

3. Administer by tilting the spoon so the medication (shaded area) fills the bowl of spoon. Then place the spoon in mouth.

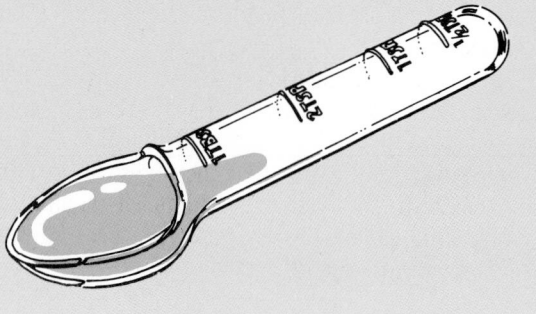

Liquid measures

Liquid measurements in the household system most often used in the clinical setting are teaspoons (tsp) and tablespoons (tbs). (For an illustration of a spoon that provides a more exact measure than the spoon used in the home for food preparation, see *Liquid measurement in the household system.*) The clinically used teaspoon and tablespoon have been standardized to equal 5 ml and 15 ml, respectively. Thus, 3 teaspoons equal 1 tablespoon, and 6 teaspoons equal 1 ounce (oz). Patients with prescribed medications to be taken in dosages of teaspoons or tablespoons should obtain clinical equipment calibrated in these measures to receive the exact prescribed dosage.

The following examples represent possible orders using the household system:
- 2 tsp (teaspoons) elixir of terpin hydrate P.O. b.i.d.
- Riopan 2 tbs (tablespoons) P.O. 1 hour a.c. and h.s.

AVOIRDUPOIS SYSTEM

The solid measures or units of weight in the avoirdupois system include the ounce (437.5 grains) and the pound (16 ounces or 7,000 grains). Note that the apothecaries' pound equals 12 ounces in contrast to the 16-ounce pound of the avoirdupois system.

MIXED SYSTEMS

Several units of measure may appear arbitrarily in the apothecaries', household, or avoirdupois systems. Two such units of measure, the drop and ounce, appear in the apothecaries' and household systems. The drop, traditionally considered equal to a drop of water, is an inexact measure that varies in size depending on the physical characteristics of the liquid being measured and the equipment used to form the drop. The drop is the unit of measure used when instilling liquid medication into such areas as the ear, nose, or conjunctival sac of the eye. When held vertically, a standard medication dropper usually is calibrated to deliver 20 drops of liquid per milliliter. Nurses also use the drop as the unit of measure when monitoring I.V. solutions. Standard I.V. administration sets usually deliver 10 to 20 drops per milliliter; microdrip sets deliver 60 drops per milliliter.

The pound and the ounce appear in the apothecaries' and avoirdupois systems. The determination of which system to place the pound and ounce within may vary from authority to authority, but the size and equivalents of the measures remain consistent within systems.

OTHER MEASURES

Some drugs require special systems developed by the manufacturers for measuring their quantities. The following discussion addresses special systems of measurement.

Units

Insulin, a drug used by many diabetic patients to assist in controlling blood sugar, is measured in units (U). Many types of insulin exist; however, all are measured in units. The international standard of U-100 insulin means that 1 milliliter of insulin solution contains 100 units of insulin regardless of type. Heparin, an anticoagulation drug, also is measured in units.

Several antibiotics, available in liquid, solid, and powder forms for oral or parenteral use, also have units as their basis of measure. Each drug manufacturer provides information about measurement of its drugs. For example, nystatin, an oral liquid preparation, contains 100,000 units per milliliter, but penicillin G benzathine suspension is available in two strengths (300,000 units per milliliter and 600,000 units per milliliter). The antibiotic penicillin also is manufactured in powdered form for later reconstitution for parenteral or oral administration, tablet form for oral use, and liquid form prepackaged in syringes for intramuscular (I.M.) injection.

The following examples represent possible orders using units:
- 14 U NPH insulin subcutaneous (S.C.) this a.m.
- heparin 5,000 U S.C. b.i.d.
- nystatin 200,000 U P.O. q6h
- 300,000 U procaine penicillin I.M. q4h

The nurse should keep in mind that the unit is not a standard measure. This means that drugs measured in units and produced by different manufacturers have no relationship to each other in quality or activity.

International units

International units (IU) represent the unit of measurement of biologicals, such as vitamins, enzymes, and hormones. For instance, the activity of calcitonin (Calcimar), a synthetic hormone used in calcium regulation, is expressed in international units.

Milliequivalents

Electrolytes may be measured in milliequivalents (mEq). The drug manufacturers provide information about the number of metric units required to provide the prescribed number of milliequivalents. The electrolyte potassium chloride usually is orderd in milliequivalents. Potassium preparations for I.V., oral, or other use come in liquid (elixir and parenteral) and solid (powder and tablet) forms.

The following examples represent possible orders using milliequivalents:
- 30 mEq (milliequivalents) KCl P.O. b.i.d.
- 1 liter of dextrose 5% in 0.9% saline solution with 40 mEq KCl to run at 125 ml per hour

CONVERSIONS BETWEEN SYSTEMS OF MEASUREMENT

Nurses sometimes must make conversions from one system of drug measurement to another. Conversions are necessary when a drug is ordered in one system of measurement but is available only in another system. To perform conversion calculations, the nurse must know the equivalents among the different systems of measurement. (For key equivalents, see *Units of exchange among systems of drug measurement,* page 110.)

Several methods can be used to convert a drug measurement from one unit to another. Use the method that feels most comfortable. Remember, dosage calculations may require converting measurements from one measure to another within the same system, or from one system to the equivalent measurement in another system. Making conversions associated with drug administration is a skill nurses use frequently.

Fraction method for conversions

The fraction method for conversions requires an equation consisting of two fractions. Set up the first fraction by placing the ordered dosage needed to convert over X units of the available dosage. For example, the physician orders 300 mg of aspirin. The bottle is labeled *aspirin gr v per tablet.* The milligram dosage represents the ordered dosage, and the grain dosage represents the available dosage. Because the amount of the available dosage is unknown, it is represented by an X. The first fraction of the equation appears as:

$$\frac{300 \text{ mg}}{X \text{ gr}}$$

Then set up the second fraction of the equation. The second fraction consists of the standard equivalents between the ordered and available measures. Because milligrams must be converted to grains, the second fraction appears as:

$$\frac{60 \text{ mg}}{1 \text{ gr}}$$

because 60 mg equal 1 gr. Remember, the same unit of measure appears in the numerator of both fractions. Like-

Units of exchange among systems of drug measurement

The following shows some approximate liquid equivalents among the household, apothecaries', and metric systems.

HOUSEHOLD	APOTHECARIES'	METRIC
1 teaspoonful (tsp)	1 fluidram (f℥)	5 ml
1 tablespoonful (tbs)	½ fluidounce (f℥)	15 ml
2 tbs	1 f℥	30 ml
1 measuring cupful	8 f℥	240 ml
1 pint (pt)	16 f℥	473 ml
1 quart (qt)	32 f℥	946 ml (1 liter)
1 gallon (gal)	128 f℥	3,785 ml

The following shows some approximate solid equivalents between the apothecaries' system and the metric system.

APOTHECARIES'	METRIC
15 grains (gr)	1 gram (g) (1,000 mg)
10 gr	0.6 g (600 mg)
7½ gr	0.5 g (500 mg)
5 gr	0.3 g (300 mg)
3 gr	0.2 g (200 mg)
1½ gr	0.1 g (100 mg)
1 gr	0.06 g (60 mg) or 0.065 g (65 mg)
¾ gr	0.05 g (50 mg)
½ gr	0.03 g (30 mg)
¼ gr	0.015 g (15 mg)
1/60 gr	0.001 g (1 mg)
1/100 gr	0.6 mg
1/120 gr	0.5 mg
1/150 gr	0.4 mg

The following lists some approximate solid equivalents among the avoirdupois, apothecaries', and metric systems.

AVOIRDUPOIS	APOTHECARIES'	METRIC
1 gr	1 gr	0.065 g
15.4 gr	15 gr	1 g
1 ounce (oz)	480 gr	28.35 g
437.5 gr	1 oz	31 g
1 pound (lb)	1.33 lb	454 g
0.75 lb	1 lb	373 g
2.2 lb	2.7 lb	1 kilogram (kg)

wise, the same unit of measure appears in both denominators. The entire equation should appear as:

$$\frac{300 \text{ mg}}{X \text{ gr}} = \frac{60 \text{ mg}}{1 \text{ gr}}$$

To solve for X, cross multiply:

$$300 \text{ mg} \times 1 \text{ gr} = 60 \text{ mg} \times X \text{ gr}$$
$$300 = 60X$$
$$\frac{300}{60} = \frac{60X}{60}$$
$$5 \text{ gr} = X$$

The patient should receive 5 gr (gr v) of aspirin, which in this case equal 1 tablet.

Ratio method for conversions

When using the ratio method to make conversions, first express the ordered dosage and available dosage as a ratio. For example, a physician's order calls for ASA (aspirin) gr x, but the aspirin is available in tablets measured in milligrams. As a result, the first ratio appears as 10 gr : X mg. The X represents the unknown dosage of milligrams. The second ratio represents the standard equivalents between the ordered and available measures. Because 60 mg equal 1 gr, the second ratio appears as 1 gr : 60 mg. Note that the same unit of measure (gr) appears in the first half of each ratio, and the same unit (mg) appears in the second half. The equation should appear as:

$$10 \text{ gr} : X \text{ mg} :: 1 \text{ gr} : 60 \text{ mg}$$

To solve for X, multiply the means of the ratio and the extremes (the outer portions of the ratio and the inner portions):

$$X \text{ mg} \times 1 \text{ gr} = 10 \text{ gr} \times 60 \text{ mg}$$
$$X = 600 \text{ mg}$$

Ten grains equal 600 milligrams.

Practice conversions with answers

1. The physician orders 15 gr of a drug. The drug label states that the tablets are measured in milligrams. Fifteen grains equal how many milligrams?
2. The physician orders 2 ml of a drug. The drug is available in minims. Two milliliters equal how many minims?
3. One-half ounce of a drug is ordered. The drug is dispensed in milliliters. How many milliliters should the patient receive?

The answers to the practice conversions are:

1.
$$\frac{15 \text{ gr}}{X \text{ mg}} = \frac{1 \text{ gr}}{60 \text{ mg}}$$
$$15 \text{ gr} \times 60 \text{ mg} = X \text{ mg} \times 1 \text{ gr}$$
$$900 \text{ mg} = X$$

Fifteen grains equal 900 mg.

2.
$$2 \text{ ml} : X \text{ M}_x :: 1 \text{ ml} : 15 \text{ M}_x$$
$$X \text{ M}_x \times 1 \text{ ml} = 2 \text{ ml} \times 15 \text{ M}_x$$
$$X = 30 \text{ M}_x$$

Two milliliters equal 30 M_x.

3.
$$\frac{0.5 \text{ oz}}{X \text{ ml}} = \frac{1 \text{ oz}}{30 \text{ ml}}$$
$$0.5 \text{ oz} \times 30 \text{ ml} = X \text{ ml} \times 1 \text{ oz}$$
$$15 \text{ m} = X$$

Fifteen milliliters equal ½ oz. Therefore, the patient should receive 15 ml.

COMPUTATION OF DRUG DOSAGES

Determining the drug dosage to be administered occurs after verification of the physician's order. Computing drug dosages is a two-step process. During the first step, ascertain if the drug ordered is available in units within the same system of measurement. If the ordered drug is available only in another system of measurement, perform the conversion between the two systems. Use the fraction method or the ratio method explained in the previous section. If the physician orders the drug in units that are available, proceed directly to the next step.

If the ordered units of measurement are available, calculate the quantity of a particular dosage form to be administered. For example, if the dose to be given calls for 250 mg, determine the quantity of tablets, powder, or liquid equal to 250 mg. To determine the quantity, use the fraction or ratio method, similar to the methods used for converting units of measure. Explanations of the fraction and ratio methods follow.

Fraction method

When using the fraction method to compute drug dosage, write an equation consisting of two fractions. First, set up a fraction showing the number of units to be given over X, which represents the quantity of the dosage form, or the number of tablets or milliliters. On the other side of the equation, form a fraction showing the number of units of drug in its dosage form over the quantity of dosage forms that contain the measure stated in the numerator. (Information provided on the drug label should supply the details needed to form the second fraction. The number of units and the quantity of dosage form are specific for each drug. In most cases the stated quantity equals 1 ml or 1 tablet.)

Here is an example of the fraction method for computation. If the number of units to be administered equals 250 mg, the first fraction in the equation is:

$$\frac{250 \text{ mg}}{X \text{ tab}}$$

The drug label states that each tablet contains 125 mg. The second fraction is:

$$\frac{125 \text{ mg}}{1 \text{ tab}}$$

The same units of measure must appear in the numerator of each fraction. Likewise, each denominator should show the same units of measure. The units of measure in the denominators will differ from the units in the numerators. The entire equation should appear as:

$$\frac{250 \text{ mg}}{X \text{ tab}} = \frac{125 \text{ mg}}{1 \text{ tab}}$$

Solving for *X* determines the quantity of the dosage form (number of tablets, in this example) to give to the patient. In this case, the patient should receive 2 tablets.

Ratio method

First, write the amount of the drug to be given and the quantity of the dosage (*X*) as a ratio. Using the example shown for the fraction method, in which the drug ordered equaled 250 mg, write the ratio as 250 mg : X tab. Next, complete the equation by forming a second ratio consisting of the number of units of the drug in the dosage form and the stated quantity of the dosage form. (Remember, the manufacturer's label provides information for the second ratio.) If, for example, each tablet contained 125 mg, write the second ratio as 125 mg : 1 tab. The entire equation is:

$$250 \text{ mg} : X \text{ tab} :: 125 \text{ mg} : 1 \text{ tab}$$

Solving for *X* determines the quantity of the dosage form.

The following example uses the ratio method for conversion between systems of measurement, then uses the fraction method to compute drug dosage. The physician orders 15 mg of phenobarbital for a patient. The drug is available in scored tablets containing gr $\overline{\text{ss}}$ (½ gr). How many tablets should the patient be given?

First, convert the milligrams of the metric system into grains of the apothecaries' system. The standard conversion is 60 mg = 1 gr. Using the ratio method, the equation is:

$$15 \text{ mg} : X \text{ gr} :: 60 \text{ mg} : 1 \text{ gr}$$

To solve for *X*, multiply the means and the extremes:

$$X \text{ gr} \times 60 \text{ mg} = 15 \text{ mg} \times 1 \text{ gr}$$
$$60X = 15$$
$$X = \frac{15}{60}$$

$$X = \frac{1}{4} = 0.25 \text{ gr}$$

Next, determine the drug dosage, in this case the number of tablets to administer. The drug label states that each tablet contains $\overline{\text{ss}}$ or ½ (0.5) gr of phenobarbital. The patient is to receive ¼ (0.25) gr or ½ tablet of phenobarbital. Using the fraction method, the equation is:

$$\frac{0.25 \text{ gr}}{X \text{ tab}} = \frac{0.5 \text{ gr}}{1 \text{ tab}}$$

To solve for X, cross multiply:

$$0.25 \text{ gr} \times 1 \text{ tab} = 0.5 \text{ gr} \times X \text{ tab}$$
$$0.25 = 0.5X$$
$$\frac{0.25}{0.5} = X$$
$$0.5 = X$$

The patient should receive ½ tablet of phenobarbital.

"Desired-available" method

The "desired (ordered)-available" method, also known as the dose over on-hand method (D/H), represents a third way to compute drug dosages. The desired-available method combines the conversion of ordered units into available units and the computation of drug dosage into one step. The equation for doing this is:

$$\text{ordered units} \times \text{conversion fraction} \times \frac{\text{quantity of dosage form}}{\text{stated quantity of drug within each dosage form}} = \text{X quantity to give}$$

The following situation shows how the equation works. The physician orders 10 gr of a drug. The drug is available only in 300-mg tablets. To determine the drug dosage, or the number of tablets to give to the patient, substitute 10 gr (the ordered number of units) for the first element of the equation. Then use the conversion fraction

$$\frac{60 \text{ mg}}{1 \text{ gr}}$$

as the second portion of the formula. The measure in the denominator of the conversion fraction must be the same as the measure in the ordered units. In this instance, the physician ordered 10 gr. As a result, grains appear in the denominator of the conversion fraction.

The third element of the equation shows the dosage form over the stated drug quantity within each dosage form. Because the drug is available in 300-mg tablets, the equation is:

$$\frac{1 \text{ tab}}{300 \text{ mg}}$$

The dosage form, in this case tablets, always should appear

in the numerator, and the quantity of drug in each dosage form always should appear in the denominator. The completed equation is:

$$10 \text{ gr} \times \frac{60 \text{ mg}}{1 \text{ gr}} \times \frac{1 \text{ tab}}{300 \text{ mg}} = X \text{ tab}$$

Solving for X shows that the patient should receive 2 tablets.

The desired-available method has the advantage of requiring only one equation. However, it requires memorizing an equation more elaborate than the one used in the fraction or ratio method. Having to memorize a more complicated equation may increase the chance of error. (For another example of a dosage calculation, see *Using the desired-available method*.)

SPECIAL COMPUTATIONS

The fraction, ratio, and desired-available methods can be used to compute drug dosage when the ordered drug and available form of the drug occur in the same units of measure. The three methods also can be used when the quantity of the particular dosage form differs from the units in which the dosage form will be administered. For example, if a patient is to receive 1,000 mg of a drug available in liquid form and measured in milligrams, with 100 mg contained in 6 ml, how many milliliters would the patient receive? Because the ordered and the available doses occur in milligrams, no initial conversion calculations need to be made. Simply use the ratio or fraction method to determine the number of milliliters of drug the patient should receive. The ratio method would be 1,000 mg : X ml :: 100 mg : 6 ml. Solving for X determines that 60 ml of the drug should be given.

Next, because the drug is to be administered in ounce form, determine the number of ounces needed, using a method of conversion. For the fraction method for conversion, the equation is:

$$\frac{60 \text{ ml}}{X \text{ oz}} = \frac{30 \text{ ml}}{1 \text{ oz}}$$

Solving for X indicates that the patient should receive 2 oz of the drug.

To use the desired-available method, simply change the order of the elements in the equation to correspond with the situation. The revised equation is:

$$\text{ordered units} \times \frac{\text{quantity of dosage form}}{\substack{\text{stated quantity} \\ \text{of drug within} \\ \text{each dosage form}}} \times \text{conversion fraction} = \text{X quantity to give}$$

Using the desired-available method

The physician orders 15 mg of phenobarbital. The drug is available only in tablets containing gr s̄s̄. Determine the drug dosage by solving for *X* as follows:

The ordered units would be 15 mg.

The conversion fraction is: $\dfrac{1 \text{ gr}}{60 \text{ mg}}$

$\dfrac{\text{The dosage form}}{\text{stated quantity}}$ is $\dfrac{1 \text{ tab}}{0.5 \text{ gr}}$

Use the information in the equation:

$$15 \text{ mg} \times \frac{1 \text{ gr}}{60 \text{ mg}} \times \frac{1 \text{ tab}}{0.5 \text{ gr}} = X \text{ tab}$$

Solve for *X*:

$$15 \times \frac{1}{60} \times \frac{1}{0.5} = X$$

$$\frac{15}{60 \times 0.5} = X$$

$$\frac{15}{30} = X$$

$$0.5 \text{ tab} = X$$

The patient should receive ½ tablet of phenobarbital.

Placing the given information into the equation results in:

$$1,000 \text{ mg} \times \frac{6 \text{ ml}}{100 \text{ mg}} \times \frac{1 \text{ oz}}{30 \text{ ml}} = X$$

Solving for X indicates that the patient should receive 2 oz of the drug.

Computing drug dosages in special systems

The three methods for drug dosage calculation may be used to calculate dosages of drugs measured in special systems. For example, the physician orders 3,000,000 U of penicillin for a patient. The penicillin is available in liquid form for I.M. use, with 5,000,000 U per milliliter; however, the dosage is to be administered in minims. When determining the number of minims to administer, first write the dosages as 5 m.U and 3 m.U instead of 5,000,000 and 3,000,000 U. The shorter notation eliminates the need for all the zeros in each dosage and makes the computation appear more manageable. The shorter notation also reduces the chance of error in miscopying the number of zeros during the calculation.

Using the fraction method, set up the initial equation as:

$$\frac{3 \text{ m.U}}{X \text{ ml}} = \frac{5 \text{ m.U}}{1 \text{ ml}}$$

Solving for X indicates that the patient should receive 0.6 ml of penicillin.

Using the ratio method to determine the number of minims to administer, set up the equation as:

$$0.6 \text{ ml} : X \text{ m} :: 1 \text{ ml} : 15 \text{ m}$$

Solving for X determines that the patient should receive 9 m of penicillin.

Using the desired-available method, the equation is:

$$3 \text{ m.U} \times \frac{1 \text{ ml}}{5 \text{ m.U}} \times \frac{15 \text{ m}}{1 \text{ ml}} = 9 \text{ m}$$

Solving the equation results in the same number of minims (9).

(For a problem using the fraction method to calculate the dosage of a drug measured in a special system, see *Computing dosages of heparin.*)

Inexact nature of conversions and computations

Converting drug measurements from one system to another and then determining the amount of a dosage form to give easily can produce inexact dosages. A rounding error during computation or discrepancies in the dosage to give may occur, depending on the conversion standard used in calculation. The nurse may determine a precise drug amount to be given, only to find that administering that amount is impossible. The nurse may determine, for example, that a patient should receive 0.97 tablet. Administering such an amount is impossible. The following general rule helps avoid calculation errors and discrepancies between theoretical and real dosages: *No more than 10% variation should exist between the dosage ordered and the dosage to be given.* Following the rule, a nurse who determined that the patient should receive 0.97 tablet could give 1 tablet permissibly.

The nurse often encounters such discrepancies when administering aspirin and acetaminophen (Tylenol). Physicians usually order aspirin and acetaminophen in grains (gr x being the usual adult dose); however, both drugs usually are available in 325-mg tablets. Converting gr x to milligrams indicates that 600 mg should be given, but 2 tablets would equal 650 mg, not 600 mg. To apply the rule concerning such discrepancies, first calculate 10% of 600 mg, which equals 60 mg. Adding 60 mg to 600 mg indicates that giving up to 660 mg is permissible. Because 2 tablets equal only 650 mg, the dosage would be safe to administer.

Practice computations with answers

1. The physician orders 30 mg of a drug available in tablets, each of which contains 1 gr. How many tablets should the patient receive?

2. The physician orders 200 mg of a drug available in an elixir that contains 100 mg/30 ml. How many ounces of the drug should be given?

3. The physician orders 5,000 U of a drug for a patient. The drug is available in a solution that contains 10,000 U per ml. How many minims should the patient receive?

The answers to the practice computations are:

1.
$$30 \text{ mg} : X \text{ gr} :: 60 \text{ mg} : 1 \text{ gr}$$
$$X \text{ gr} \times 60 \text{ mg} = 30 \text{ mg} \times 1 \text{ gr}$$
$$X = \frac{30}{60}$$
$$X = 0.5 \text{ gr}$$

Thirty milligrams equal 0.5 gr.

$$0.5 \text{ gr} : X \text{ tab} :: 1 \text{ gr} : 1 \text{ tab}$$
$$X \text{ tab} \times 1 \text{ gr} = 0.5 \text{ gr} \times 1 \text{ tab}$$
$$X = 0.5 \text{ tab}$$

The patient should receive ½ tablet.

2.
$$200 \text{ mg} \times \frac{30 \text{ ml}}{100 \text{ mg}} \times \frac{1 \text{ oz}}{30 \text{ ml}} = X \text{ oz}$$
$$200 \times \frac{30}{100} \times \frac{1}{3} = X$$
$$\frac{2}{1} = X$$
$$2 \text{ oz} = X$$

Two ounces of the drug should be given.

3.
$$\frac{5,000 \text{ U}}{X \text{ ml}} = \frac{10,000 \text{ U}}{1 \text{ ml}}$$

Computing dosages of heparin

The physician orders 5,000 U of heparin S.C. for a patient. On hand is heparin 10,000 U/ml. How many milliliters should the patient receive?

Using the fraction method, the equation is:

$$\frac{10,000 \text{ U}}{1 \text{ ml}} = \frac{5,000 \text{ U}}{X \text{ ml}}$$

After cross multiplying, the equation becomes:

$$10,000 \text{ X} = 5,000$$

Solving for X provides the answer:

$$X = \frac{5,000}{10,000} = 0.5 \text{ ml}$$

The patient should receive 0.5 or ½ ml of heparin.

$$5,000 \text{ U} \times 1 \text{ ml} = X \text{ ml} \times 10,000 \text{ U}$$

$$\frac{5,000}{10,000} = X$$

$$0.5 \text{ ml} = X$$

One-half of 1 ml contains 5,000 U.

$$\frac{0.5 \text{ ml}}{X \text{ ℳ}} = \frac{1 \text{ ml}}{15 \text{ (or 16)} \text{ ℳ}}$$

$$0.5 \text{ ml} \times 15 \text{ (or 16)} \text{ ℳ} = X \text{ ℳ} \times 1 \text{ ml}$$

$$7.5 \text{ or } 8 \text{ ℳ} = X$$

The patient should receive 7.5 or 8 ℳ.

COMPUTATION OF DRUGS FOR PARENTERAL ADMINISTRATION

The methods for computing drug dosages can be used for oral or parenteral routes. The following example shows how to determine drug dosages to be given via the parenteral route.

The physician orders 75 mg of Demerol. The package label reads: meperidine (Demerol), 100 mg/ml. Using the fraction method to determine the number of milliliters the patient should receive, the equation is:

$$\frac{75 \text{ mg}}{X \text{ml}} = \frac{100 \text{ mg}}{1 \text{ ml}}$$

To solve for *X,* cross multiply:

$$75 \text{ mg} \times 1 \text{ ml} = X \text{ ml} \times 100 \text{ mg}$$

$$75 = 100 \text{ X}$$

$$\frac{75}{100} = X$$

$$0.75 \text{ or } \tfrac{3}{4} \text{ ml} = X$$

The patient should receive 0.75 or ¾ ml.

The nurse might need to know the number of minims that would deliver the same dosage. The equation for the ratio method is:

$$0.75 \text{ ml.} : X \text{ ℳ} :: 1 \text{ ml} : 15 \text{ ℳ}$$

To solve for *X,* multiply the means and the extremes:

$$X \text{ ℳ} \ 1 \text{ ml} = 0.75 \text{ ml} \times 15 \text{ ℳ}$$

$$X = 12 \text{ ℳ}$$

Twelve minims equal 0.75 ml, which would contain the 75 mg of Demerol ordered by the physician.

RECONSTITUTION OF POWDERS FOR INJECTION

Although the pharmacist usually reconstitutes powders for parenteral use, nurses sometimes perform the function. The nurse also often computes I.V. fluid rates. The following

discussion addresses the reconstitution of powders for injection and the computation of I.V. drip rates.

When reconstituting powders for injection, consult the drug label for the needed information. The label gives the total quantity of drug in the vial or ampule, the amount and type of diluent to add to the powder, and the strength and shelf life (expiration date) of the resulting solution. When diluent is added to a powder, the powder increases the fluid volume. Therefore, the label calls for less diluent than the total volume of the prepared solution. For example, the nurse may have to add 1.7 ml of diluent to a vial of powdered drug to obtain a 2-ml total volume of prepared solution. Reconstituting a powdered drug simply requires following the directions on the drug label.

To determine the amount of solution to administer, use the manufacturer's information about the concentration of the solution. For example, if the nurse wants to administer 500 mg of a drug, and the concentration of the prepared

---

Reconstitution of a powder

The physician orders 500 mg of ampicillin for a patient. A 1-g vial of powdered ampicillin is available. The label states, "Add 4.5 ml sterile water to yield 1 g/5 ml." How many milliliters of reconstituted ampicillin should the patient be given?

The nurse first dilutes the powder according to the instructions on the label. The concentration listed on the label provides the first portion of the equation:

$$\frac{1 \text{ g}}{5 \text{ ml}}$$

The nurse then needs to assure that the same units of measure appear in both numerators of the equation. In this case, the units must be grams or milligrams; either choice is acceptable. If the nurse chooses to use milligrams and chooses the fraction method, the equation would be:

$$\frac{1,000 \text{ mg}}{5 \text{ ml}} = \frac{500 \text{ mg}}{X \text{ ml}}$$

The nurse then cross multiplies:

$$1,000 \text{ X} = 2,500$$

Then, to solve for *X,* the nurse divides:

$$X = \frac{2,500}{1,000}$$

$$X = 2.5 \text{ ml}$$

After computation, the nurse finds that 2.5 ml of reconstituted ampicillin provides 500 mg.

I.V. flow rates

The number of drops required to deliver 1 ml of I.V. solution varies with the type of administration set used and the manufacturer. To calculate the flow rate, the calibration of the drip rate for each manufacturer's product must be known. The chart below provides a quick reference guide.

MANUFACTURER	DROPS/ML	DROPS/MINUTE TO INFUSE					
		500 ml/ 24 hr	1,000 ml/ 24 hr	1,000 ml/ 20 hr	1,000 ml/ 10 hr	1,000 ml/ 8 hr	1,000 ml/ 6 hr
		21 ml/hr	42 ml/hr	50 ml/hr	100 ml/hr	125 ml/hr	166 ml/hr
Abbott	15	5 gtt	10 gtt	12 gtt	25 gtt	31 gtt	42 gtt
Baxter Healthcare	10	3 gtt	7 gtt	8 gtt	17 gtt	21 gtt	28 gtt
Cutter	20	7 gtt	14 gtt	17 gtt	34 gtt	42 gtt	56 gtt
IVAC	20	7 gtt	14 gtt	17 gtt	34 gtt	42 gtt	56 gtt
McGaw	15	5 gtt	10 gtt	12 gtt	25 gtt	31 gtt	42 gtt

solution is 1 g (1,000 mg) per 10 ml, the nurse can set up a fraction or ratio equation as follows:

Fraction method

$$\frac{500 \text{ mg}}{X \text{ ml}} = \frac{100 \text{ mg}}{10 \text{ ml}}$$

Ratio method

$$500 \text{ mg} : X \text{ ml} :: 1,000 \text{ mg} : 10 \text{ ml}$$

The patient should receive 5 ml of the prepared solution. (For another example of how the nurse might perform the required computations, see *Reconstitution of a powder,* page 115.)

I.V. drip rates and flow rates

For these special computations, first set up a fraction showing the volume of solution to be delivered over the number of minutes in which that volume is to be infused. For example, if a patient is to receive 100 ml of solution within 1 hour, the fraction would be written as

$$\frac{100 \text{ ml}}{60 \text{ min}}$$

Next, multiply the fraction by the drip factor (the number of drops contained in 1 ml) to determine the drip rate (the number of drops per minute to be infused). The drip factor varies among different I.V. sets and appears on the package containing the I.V. tubing administration set. Following the manufacturer's directions for drip factor is a crucial step. (For a discussion of the drip factors of several well-known I.V. administration sets, see *I.V. flow rates.*) Standard administration sets have drip factors of 10, 15, or 20 drops

per milliliter. A microdrip (minidrip) set has a drip factor of 60 drops per milliliter.

Use the following equation to determine the drip rate of an I.V. solution:

$$\frac{\text{Total no. of ml}}{\text{total no. of min.}} \times \text{drip factor} = \text{drops per minute}$$

The equation applies to I.V. solutions that infuse over many hours or to such small-volume infusions as those used for antibiotics, which are administered in less than 1 hour. (To see how the equation works in a specific situation, see *Calculating I.V. drip rate.*)

The nurse can modify the equation by first determining the number of milliliters to be infused over 1 hour (the flow rate). The nurse then divides the flow rate by 60 minutes. The resulting calculation is then multiplied by the drip factor to determine the number of drops per minute. The nurse also will use the flow rate when working with I.V. infusion pumps to set the number of milliliters to be delivered in 1 hour.

Quick methods for calculating drip rates

Besides the equation and its modified version, quicker methods exist for computing I.V. solution administration rates. To administer I.V. solutions via a microdrip set, adjust the flow rate (number of milliliters per hour) to equal the drip rate (number of drops per minute). Using the equation, divide the flow rate by 60 minutes and then multiply by the drip factor, which also equals 60. Because the flow rate and drip factor are equal, the two arithmetic operations "cancel out" each other. For example, if 125 ml of fluid

Calculating I.V. drip rate

The physician's order states: 1,000 ml dextrose 5% in 0.45% sodium chloride to infuse over 12 hours. The administration set delivers 15 drops per milliliter. What should the drip rate be?

Use the equation:

$$\frac{\text{Total no. of ml}}{\text{Total no. of min}} \times \text{drip factor} = \text{drip rate}$$

Set up the equation using the given data:

$$\frac{1,000 \text{ ml}}{12 \text{ hr} \times 60 \text{ min}} \times 15 \text{ gtt/ml} = \text{X gtt/min}$$

After multiplying the number of hours by 60 minutes in the denominator of the fraction, the equation is:

$$\frac{1,000 \text{ ml}}{720 \text{ min}} \times 5 \text{ gtt/ml} = \text{X gtt/min}$$

After dividing the fraction, the equation is:

$$1.39 \text{ ml/min} \times 15 \text{ gtt/ml} = \text{X gtt/min}$$

The final answer is 20.85 gtt/min, which can be rounded to 21 gtt/min. The drip rate is 21 drops per minute.

per hour represented the ordered flow rate, the equation would be:

$$\frac{125 \text{ ml}}{60 \text{ min}} \times 60 = \text{drip rate (125)}$$

Rather than spend the time calculating the equation, the nurse simply can use the number assigned to the flow rate as the drip rate.

For I.V. solution administration sets that deliver 15 drops per milliliter, the flow rate divided by 4 equals the drip rate. For sets with a drip factor of 10, the flow rate divided by 6 equals the drip rate.

Practice computations with answers
1. The patient is to receive 2 g of a drug available in powdered form. The drug label states: *Contains 3 g. Add 17 ml of sterile water to yield 1 g per 6 ml.* How many milliliters of solution should the patient receive?
2. The patient is to receive 3 liters of I.V. solution over 24 hours. The drip factor for the I.V. infusion set is 15 gtt (drops) per ml. How many milliliters should be infused each hour? What is the drip rate for the solution?
3. The physician orders 50 ml of a drug to be infused over 25 minutes. The I.V. infusion set has a drip factor of 10 gtt per ml. What is the drip rate for the solution?

The answers to the practice problems follow:

1.
$$2 \text{ g} : \text{X ml} :: 1 \text{ g} : 6 \text{ ml}$$
$$\text{X ml} \times 1 \text{ g} = 2 \text{ g} \times 6 \text{ ml}$$
$$\text{X} = 12 \text{ ml}$$

The patient should receive 12 ml of solution.

2.
$$\frac{3,000 \text{ ml}}{24 \text{ hr}} = \frac{\text{X ml}}{1 \text{ hr}}$$
$$3,000 \text{ ml} \times 1 \text{ hr} = 24 \text{ hr} \times \text{X ml}$$
$$\frac{3,000}{24} = \text{X}$$
$$125 \text{ ml} = \text{X}$$

The flow rate equals 125 ml per hour.

$$\frac{125 \text{ ml}}{60 \text{ min}} \times 15 \text{ gtt per ml} = \text{X gtt per min}$$
$$\frac{125}{60} \times 15 = \text{X}$$
$$31.25 = 31 \text{ gtt per min} = \text{X}$$

As an alternative, divide the flow rate by 4 (the quick method for sets with a drip factor of 15):

$$\frac{125}{4} = 31.25 = 31 \text{ gtt per min (drip rate)}$$

The drip rate equals 31 drops per minute.

3.
$$\frac{50 \text{ ml}}{25 \text{ min}} \times 10 \text{ gtt per ml} = \text{X gtt per min}$$
$$\frac{50}{25} \times 10 = \text{X}$$
$$2 \times 10 = \text{X}$$
$$20 \text{ gtt per min} = \text{X}$$

The drip rate equals 20 drops per minute.

PERCENTAGE SOLUTIONS

In most clinical settings, the pharmacy department or pharmaceutical companies prepare solutions containing drugs for topical use (for example, wound irrigation and the soaking of infected or inflamed body parts). Nurses, however, must prepare special percentage solutions for emergencies, such as resuscitation attempts after cardiac arrest. Furthermore, community health nurses working in home settings may need to prepare large-volume solutions if prepared solutions are not accessible to the patient.

Calculation of percentage solutions
An example of a percentage solution is 0.9% saline, which indicates that every 100 ml of solution contain 0.9 g of sodium chloride. Expressed as a fraction, the figures would appear as

$$\frac{0.9}{100}$$

The ratio form would appear as 0.9 : 100. A liter of 0.9% saline would contain 9 grams of sodium chloride. The figures for 1 liter would be

$$\frac{9}{1,000}$$

in fraction form, and 9 : 1,000 in ratio form.

The nurse may prepare percentage solutions by adding solutes (solid or liquid forms of drugs) to solvents (diluents). The solvents usually used include sterile water, normal saline solution, and dextrose 5% in water (D_5W). As a general rule when preparing solutions, the nurse should consider the solid form, whether crystals, powders, or tablets, to be 100% strength. The liquid form, also known as the stock solution, may vary in strength.

The nurse may use the following formulas to calculate the strength of percentage solutions. The fraction method offers two usable formulas:

$$\frac{\text{weaker solution}}{\text{stronger solution}} = \frac{\text{solute}}{\text{solvent}}$$

$$\frac{\text{small \% strength}}{\text{large \% strength}} = \frac{\text{small volume}}{\text{large volume}}$$

The ratio method also offers two formulas:

$$\text{weaker : stronger :: solute : solvent}$$

$$\text{small\%strength:large\%strength :: small volume:large volume}$$

Although a solid combined with a diluent will increase the total volume of the prepared solution, the increase usually is insignificant and may not need to be calculated. The increase, however, will prove significant and should be considered when adding a large amount of solid or a small amount of diluent. When adding a liquid, subtract the amount of the liquid from the total volume desired. This calculation tells the amount of diluent to add. For example, if the preparation of 1 liter of solution requires 50 ml of a liquid drug, add the 50 ml of liquid drug to 950 ml of diluent.

As an example, the nurse must prepare 500 ml of a 0.5% lidocaine (Xylocaine) solution and finds on hand a 2% Xylocaine solution and D_5W, which is the diluent. The nurse must determine the number of milliliters of Xylocaine solution to use, and the number of milliliters of dextrose solution to use. Using the ratio method, the nurse sets up the following equation:

$$0.5\% : 2\% :: X \text{ ml} : 500 \text{ ml}$$

Multiplying the means and the extremes gives $2X = 250$. The nurse then divides to solve for X:

$$X = \frac{250}{2}$$

$$X = 125 \text{ ml of 2\% Xylocaine solution}$$

Because the nurse wants a total volume of 500 ml and must use 125 ml of Xylocaine solution, the nurse next must determine the amount of dextrose solution to use as the diluent. Subtracting 125 from 500 yields the amount of dextrose solution to use:

$$500 \text{ ml} - 125 \text{ ml} = 375 \text{ ml of dextrose solution}$$

Practice computations with answers

1. An irrigation treatment scheduled for a patient requires the use of 500 milliliters of a 5% solution. The drug is available in solid form. How many grams of the drug are needed to prepare the solution for one treatment?

2. A nurse needs to prepare a liter of 4% solution. On hand is a 20% stock solution. How much of the stock solution should the nurse use? How many milliliters of water should the nurse add to the portion of the stock solution to obtain 1 liter of 4% solution?

3. A nurse is preparing 4 liters of 2% solution. The stock solution is 100% strength. How many milliliters of the stock solution does the nurse need? How many milliliters of water will the nurse add to prepare 4 liters of the desired solution?

The answers to the practice computations follow:

1.
$$5\% : 100\% :: X \text{ g} : 500 \text{ ml}$$
$$100 X = 5 \times 500$$
$$100 X = 2,500$$
$$X = 25 \text{ g}$$

The nurse needs 25 g of the drug to prepare enough solution for one treatment.

2.
$$\frac{4\%}{20\%} = \frac{X \text{ ml}}{1,000 \text{ ml}}$$
$$4 \times 1,000 = 20 \times X$$
$$4,000 = 20X$$
$$\frac{4,000}{20} = X$$
$$200 \text{ ml} = X$$

The nurse should use 200 ml of stock solution.

$$1,000 - 200 = X \text{ ml}$$
$$800 \text{ ml} = X$$

The nurse should add 800 ml of water to the stock solution.

3.
$$2\% : 100\% :: X \text{ ml} : 4,000 \text{ ml}$$
$$100 X = 2 \times 4,000$$
$$X = \frac{8,000}{100}$$
$$X = 80 \text{ ml}$$

The nurse needs 80 ml of stock solution.

$$4,000 \text{ ml} - 80 \text{ ml} = X \text{ ml}$$
$$3,920 \text{ ml} = X$$

The nurse will add 3,920 ml of water to the 80 ml of stock solution.

SPECIAL CONSIDERATIONS

Calculation of therapeutic drug dosages for pediatric and geriatric patients requires the use of special rules and considerations. Physicians and nurses use pediatric rules primarily to determine the safe pediatric dosage range when the safe adult range is known. The nurse should determine the safe dosage range to verify that the physician's order is appropriate for a particular child. The nurse's professional and legal responsibility requires such dosage verification in the administration of drugs.

One frequently used rule for calculating pediatric drug dosages involves the child's weight in kilograms; a second recommended method involves the child's body-surface area. Other methods of dosage calculations are not recommended.

Many institutions have adopted guidelines that determine the acceptable calculation method. Nurses in pediatric settings must familiarize themselves with the particular institution's policies regarding pediatric dosages. (For more information about special considerations regarding pediatric drug administration, see Chapter 10, The Pediatric Patient.)

Geriatric patients may require drug dosages that differ from the usual adult dosages because of chronic illnesses or the physiologic effects of aging, which may alter a drug's pharmacokinetics. As a result, the physician determines dosages for individual geriatric patients. No general rules exist. Because of the individual nature of the aging process and the unique medical history of each geriatric patient, the nurse in a gerontologic setting consistently must assess each patient's response to drugs. Although a patient may receive an average adult dosage, such a dosage does not account for individual differences. (For more information about special considerations regarding geriatric drug administration, see Chapter 11, The Geriatric Patient.)

CHAPTER SUMMARY

Chapter 8 explored the responsibilities of the nurse in administering safe and accurate doses of drugs. Information about the various ways to calculate drug dosages should assist the student nurse in reaching the goal of safe, accurate drug administration. Here are the chapter highlights.

• Factors that help determine the amount of a drug dosage include the patient's age, size, integrity of the body systems, and the type and virulence of the patient's disease. The purpose, action, and pharmacokinetic properties of a drug also affect the dosage ordered. Nurses must familiarize themselves with the recommended dosage ranges provided by pharmaceutical companies.

• The metric system is used internationally for ordering drugs, and most new drugs are measured in metric units. Use of the metric system is advantageous because it allows accurate calculation of small drug dosages. This system uses liquid measures based on the liter and solid measures based on the gram. Drugs measured in the metric system frequently are available in liters, milliliters, grams, and milligrams.

• The apothecaries' system, older and less precise than the metric system, is used less often. Equivalents in the apothecaries' system are approximate rather than exact. Liquids are measured in minims, fluidrams, fluidounces, pints, quarts, and gallons; solids are measured in grains, scruples, drams, ounces, and pounds.

• The household system, familiar because of its use in the measurement of foods, is the least used system of measurement in the clinical area. In many cases, over-the-counter medications are measured in the household system. Commonly used liquid measurements in the household system are teaspoons and tablespoons.

• Some drugs are measured in special systems developed by the manufacturer. Units and milliequivalents represent special drug measures. The labels of products manufactured in special measures give information on the size of the measures. Some drugs, such as insulin, require special equipment for measuring dosages.

• The nurse must make conversions from one system of drug measurement to another when a drug is ordered in one system but is available only in another system. The nurse must know the equivalents among the systems of measurement to make the conversion calculations.

• The fraction method for conversion uses an equation made up of two fractions. The first fraction shows the ordered dosage to be converted over X units of the available dosage. The second fraction consists of the standard equivalents between the ordered and available measures. The ratio method for conversion uses the same information; however, it is set up as ratios.

• If the physician orders the drug in available units, the nurse proceeds directly to computing the drug dosage. The nurse may use the fraction method, the ratio method, or the desired-available method to perform the calculation.

• When reconstituting powdered drugs before parenteral administration, the nurse should consult the drug label for needed information.

• The nurse calculates I.V. fluid rates regulated manually or by an I.V. fluid pump. The nurse must know how to calculate the hourly rate, or flow rate, as well as the drip rate, or number of drops per minute. Intravenous administration sets vary in the size of the drop produced. Therefore, the nurse must be familiar with the equipment in use and aware of the drip factor, or number of drops per milliliter that the equipment delivers.

• Sometimes the nurse must prepare special percentage solutions for emergencies. To prepare such solutions, the nurse adds solutes (solid or liquid forms of drugs) to solvents, such as normal saline solution. The nurse can use the fraction method or ratio method to calculate the amount of drug, or solute, and the volume of the solvent to use when preparing a solution of desired concentration.

• The nurse must be aware of special considerations related to pediatric and geriatric dosage determinations.

STUDY QUESTIONS

See Appendix 1 for answers.

1. Wesley Parker, age 80, is admitted to the hospital with congestive heart failure. How might Mr. Parker's age affect his treatment?
(a) It may affect the conversion calculations used for his drugs.
(b) It may determine the measurement system used for his drugs.
(c) It may alter the pharmacokinetics — and dosage — of his drugs.
(d) It may require special formulas for computing I.V. flow rates.

2. For Mr. Parker, the physician prescribes digoxin 0.25 mg I.V. daily. Which measurement system does this prescription represent?
(a) apothecaries' system
(b) metric system
(c) household system
(d) avoirdupois system

3. When preparing to administer I.V. digoxin to Mr. Parker, the nurse notes that the drug is contained in an ampule that contains 0.5 mg of digoxin per 2 ml. To administer a dose of 0.25 mg, how much should the nurse draw up?
(a) 4 ml
(b) 2 ml
(c) 1 ml
(d) 0.5 ml

4. Which equation would the nurse use to determine the I.V. drip rate?

(a) $\dfrac{\text{total no. of minutes} \times \text{drip factor}}{\text{total no. of ml}} = \text{drip rate}$

(b) $\dfrac{\text{total no. of minutes} \times \text{total no. of ml}}{\text{drip factor}} = \text{drip rate}$

(c) $\dfrac{\text{total no. of ml} \times \text{drip factor}}{\text{total no. of minutes}} = \text{drip rate}$

(d) $\dfrac{\text{total no. of minutes} \times \text{total no. of ml}}{\text{drip factor}} = \text{drip rate}$

5. Glen Richmond, age 44, seeks care for a peptic ulcer. His physician orders 1 fl. oz. of Mylanta P.O. 1 hour before and 3 hours after meals and h.s. In the metric system, what is the equivalent of each dose?
(a) 10 ml
(b) 20 ml
(c) 30 ml
(d) 40 ml

6. Carrie Pelham, age 68, takes 2.5 mg of nitroglycerin (Nitro-bid) P.O. b.i.d. to prevent angina. If converted to the apothecaries' system, how would this dosage be measured?
(a) grains
(b) grams
(c) drops
(d) milliliters

7. Alma White, age 62, tells the nurse she has been taking 2 teaspoons of Robitussin-DM daily for a persistent cough. When using the ratio method to determine the number of milliliters equal to 2 teaspoons, how should the nurse write the equation?
(a) 2 tsp : X ml :: 1 tsp : 5 ml
(b) 2 tsp : 1 tsp :: X ml : 15 ml
(c) X ml : 5 ml :: 1 tsp : 2 tsp
(d) X ml : 2 tsp :: 15 ml : 1 tsp

8. The physician prescribes Tylenol grains v. P.O. q4h p.r.n. for headaches for James Marshall. When calculating a conversion between the apothecaries' and metric systems, the nurse finds that the dosage is inexact. How much variation is allowed between dosage ordered and dosage delivered?
(a) no more than 5%
(b) no more than 10%
(c) no more than 15%
(d) no more than 20%

SELECTED REFERENCES

Deglin, J., and Mull, V. (1988). *Dosage calculations manual.* Springhouse, PA: Springhouse Corporation.

Deglin, J., and Mull, V. (1989). Dosage calculations. *Nursing89,* 19(9), 100-102.

Pickar, G. (1990). *Dosage calculations* (3rd ed.). Albany, NY: Delmar.

Medici, G. (1988). *Drug dosage calculations: A guide for clinical practice* (4th ed.). East Norwalk, CT: Appleton & Lange.

Olsen, J., Ablon, L., Giangrasso, A., and Siner-Weissman, H. (1987). *Medical dosage calculations* (4th ed.). Menlo Park, CA: Addison-Wesley.

Pauca, A. (1988). Constant-rate drug infusions: Two methods of preparation. *AANA Journal,* 56(6), 537-541.

ROUTES AND TECHNIQUES OF ADMINISTRATION

OBJECTIVES

After reading and studying this chapter, the student should be able to:

1. Differentiate among the following solid drug forms in terms of their disintegration and absorption sites: tablets, capsules, enteric-coated tablets, and wax matrix tablets.

2. Identify the composition of each of the following oral liquid drug forms: syrups, suspensions, tinctures, and elixirs.

3. Describe how suppository and inhalant drug forms are absorbed.

4. Identify the procedure for administering the following drug forms via the oral route: tablets, capsules, and liquids.

5. Explain how to administer a drug via a nasogastric tube or a gastrostomy tube.

6. Describe how to administer sublingual and buccal medications.

7. Explain the rationale for administering medications via the rectal route.

8. Describe how to insert a rectal suppository and administer a retention enema.

9. Describe how to reconstitute a powdered medication from a vial.

10. Differentiate among the techniques for administering medications via the following parenteral routes: intradermal, subcutaneous, intramuscular, and intravenous.

11. Explain the importance of rotating injection sites when administering parenteral medications.

12. Explain the rationales for using the intrathecal and epidural routes of drug administration.

13. Explain how to administer urethral and vaginal medications.

INTRODUCTION

The complexity and variety of available medications make proper administration a task requiring knowledge and skill. Before administering a medication, the nurse must know the pharmacokinetics, pharmacodynamics, pharmacotherapeutics, dosage range, drug interactions, adverse drug reactions, and nursing implications related to the specific drug. Also, the nurse must ensure that the five rights of medication administration are observed: the right patient, right drug, right route, right dose, and right time. (For further discussion of the five rights, see Chapter 7, Responsibilities in Drug Administration.)

Chapter 9 presents techniques as well as rationales for administering medications in the clinical setting. It begins by discussing drug packaging and forms, including solids, liquids, suppositories, inhalants, and others. Next, it describes techniques for oral, sublingual, buccal, and rectal administration. After exploring these gastrointestinal (GI) administration techniques, the chapter highlights parenteral administration techniques, such as intradermal, subcutaneous (S.C.), intramuscular (I.M.), and intravenous (I.V.) administration. It concludes with an overview of the following additional types of drug administration: intrathecal, epidural, intra-articular, dermal, ophthalmic, otic, nasal and sinus, respiratory, urethral, and vaginal administration.

DRUG PACKAGING AND FORMS

Drugs are packaged in numerous styles. When administering drugs, the nurse must consider packaging differences. Drugs may be packaged in unit-dose format, in which one dose of a drug comes in a labeled container or wrapper. They also can be packaged in bulk format, in which multiple doses of a drug are packaged in a container, bottle, or wrapper. The nurse always should remember to *read the label*. Valuable information appears on the label, and reading it helps the nurse administer medications properly. Other important information may appear in the package insert. For example, the insert may include information about changes in drug actions related to the consumption of food or alcohol with the drug.

The drug chlordiazepoxide serves as a good example of how reading package information can make a difference. When administering chlordiazepoxide intravenously, the nurse dilutes the drug with sterile water or saline solution. If, however, chlordiazepoxide is to be injected intramuscularly, the nurse must reconstitute the drug with the special diluent supplied by the manufacturer. If the nurse does not use the supplied diluent, the injection can result in severe pain.

Drugs are manufactured in many different forms, including solids, liquids, suppositories, inhalants, sprays, creams, lotions, patches, and lozenges. To administer drugs safely, the nurse must be knowledgeable about the different effects of the many drug forms. For example, nitroglycerin administered sublingually (allowing it to dissolve under the tongue) can relieve anginal pain in less than 1 minute. The same drug administered as an ointment applied to the chest wall may not relieve acute pain at all; however, it may be used prophylactically for anginal pain.

SOLIDS

The solid drug forms include tablets, capsules, enteric-coated tablets, and wax matrix tablets. A tablet is the result of compressing a drug, usually combined with inert ingredients, into one of many different shapes. Chewable tablets offer several advantages over other types of drug formulations: palatable taste, enhanced absorption, and easier ingestion for patients who have difficulty swallowing large tablets. Disintegration and some dissolution of chewed tablets take place in the mouth, and some absorption occurs in the stomach. Most of the absorption of the drug, however, occurs in the small intestine.

When swallowed, uncoated tablets disintegrate and dissolve in the stomach. They usually are absorbed in the small intestine. Sublingual tablets disintegrate in the mouth and are absorbed directly into the bloodstream by the blood vessels under the tongue; buccal tablets also disintegrate in the mouth, but are absorbed by blood vessels in the cheek.

A capsule is a hard or soft gelatin shell that contains a drug in a powder, in sustained-released beads, or in liquid form. Usually, solid drugs are contained in hard gelatin shells and liquid medications are contained in soft gelatin shells. Swallowed capsules disintegrate and dissolve in the stomach; absorption occurs in the small intestine. The precise degree of dissolution and absorption as well as the site of those activities depends on the specific drug.

Enteric-coated tablets have a thin coating that allows the tablet to pass through the stomach and disintegrate and dissolve in the small intestine, where the drug is absorbed. Because the enteric-coated drug form delivers a concentrated dose of drug to the intestinal mucosa, irritation or ulceration of the intestinal mucosa may result.

Unscored tablets, enteric-coated tablets, and capsules should *never* be divided. Each of these products may contain inert or other ingredients along with the drug, and dividing the drug form could result in incorrect dosage administration or damage to the stomach mucosa. Also, dividing an enteric-coated tablet destroys the enteric barrier, allowing stomach secretions to act on the medication and alter its absorption.

In the wax matrix form of an orally administered drug, the drug is deposited throughout a honeycomb-like structure made of a wax material. Many of these tablets are covered with an enteric-coated shell, allowing disintegration and absorption to occur in the small intestine. The wax matrix allows for the sustained release of a drug, which in turn provides a more constant blood level of the drug. The nurse should inform the patient taking a wax matrix preparation that the indigestible casing may be expelled in the feces.

LIQUIDS

Liquid medications usually are given parenterally or orally. The nurse also may administer liquid medications as irrigations, soaks, enemas, or gargles. Orally administered liquids, which contain the drug mixed with some type of fluid, are classified as syrups, suspensions, tinctures, or elixirs.

Syrups are drugs mixed in a sugar-water solution. Cough syrup frequently is given in this form.

Suspensions consist of finely divided drug particles suspended in a suitable liquid medium. The nurse or patient administering a suspension should shake the preparation thoroughly before using it. Shaking the suspension ensures that the drug particles are dispersed uniformly throughout the liquid. Antacids commonly are manufactured in suspension form.

Tinctures and elixirs are two types of alcoholic solution. Tinctures are hydroalcoholic drug solutions; elixirs are hydroalcoholic solutions plus glycerin, sorbitol, or another sweetener. The nurse or patient should consult a pharmacist before mixing an alcoholic solution with any liquid because some alcohol-soluble drugs may form a precipitate when mixed with any solution — even water. The nurse should never give an alcoholic solution to a patient who also takes the drug disulfiram (Antabuse) or any other drug that can cause disulfiram-like effects when taken with alcohol, such as metronidazole.

Liquids given parenterally are available in three packaging styles: vials, ampules, and self-contained systems or prefilled syringes.

Vials, which are bottles sealed with a rubber diaphragm, can contain a single dose or several doses. Multidose vials contain preservatives that enable them to be used for more than one dose, whereas single-dose vials do not contain such agents. The nurse must discard single-dose vials after one use or dose. The medication in vials may come in a liquid form or in a powder that the nurse must reconstitute before use.

An ampule contains a single dose of medication. The ampule is a glass container with a thin neck, which usually is scored so it can be snapped off. Ampules usually contain liquid medications.

Self-contained systems, or prefilled parenteral medications, contain a single dose of a drug in a plastic bag or in a prefilled syringe with an attached needle. Nurses and physicians use prefilled syringes for narcotics and other analgesics as well as for drugs used during cardiopulmonary resuscitation or advanced life-support activities. Prefilled syringes also are used in unit-dose drug administration systems.

SUPPOSITORIES

Administered rectally and vaginally, suppositories carry medications in a solid base that melts at body temperature. Suppositories produce local (analgesic, laxative, and anti-infective) and systemic (antiemetic, antipyretic, and analgesic) effects. Usually bullet-shaped, most suppositories are about 1 inch (2.5 cm) long and require lubrication for insertion. Because they melt at body temperature, suppositories usually require refrigeration until administration.

INHALANTS

Inhalants are powdered or liquid forms of a drug that are given via the respiratory route and are absorbed rapidly by the rich supply of capillaries in the lungs. Powdered forms must be broken into fine particles by means of a mechanical device before inhalation. Several frequently used methods of inhalation include ultrasonic nebulizers, metered-dose aerosol or turbo inhalers, and vaporizers.

OTHER DRUG FORMS

Other drug forms described in this chapter include sprays, which are used via several administration routes; creams, lotions, and patches, which are administered topically; and lozenges, which are used for local effects via the oral route.

GASTROINTESTINAL TRACT ADMINISTRATION TECHNIQUES

The GI tract provides a fairly safe but relatively slow-acting site for drug absorption. Oral, sublingual, buccal, and rectal preparations are given via the GI tract.

ORAL

Orally routed drug forms include tablets, capsules, liquids, and lozenges. As long as the patient is alert and able to swallow, oral administration is relatively simple and safe.

After checking the five rights of medication administration, the nurse must gather the necessary equipment. To administer tablets or capsules, the nurse needs a souffle cup (medicine cup), a glass of water or other suitable liquid, and the medication container. (If the facility uses the unit-dose system, the nurse should not need a souffle cup or separate medication container because the exact dose should be provided.) When using a bottle, the nurse should follow these instructions: (1) Shake the correct number of tablets or capsules comprising a dose into the lid, then transfer them to the souffle cup. Do not touch the medication directly, to avoid contamination of other tablets or capsules. (2) Take the souffle cup containing the appropriate number of tablets or capsules and the glass of water to the patient. If the tablets or capsules come in a unit-dose form, take the appropriate dose to the patient's bedside. (If the patient has difficulty handling the medication, the nurse may open the unit-dose packaging at the patient's bedside and place the dose in a souffle cup.) (3) Identify the patient by checking the armband and name tag and asking the patient to state his or her name. State the name of the drug and its action or use; then instruct the patient to place the tablets or capsules in the mouth and swallow them with the water. The patient may take the tablets or capsules one at a time or all at once. For the patient who has difficulty swallowing medications, suggest sitting in an upright position and drinking liquid before and while swallowing the capsules or tablets. The patient should drink at least 3 ounces (90 ml) of liquid after swallowing the medication to ensure that it travels down the esophagus and to decrease the risk of local irritation by the medication, particularly in an elderly patient. (4) Remain at the bedside until the patient swallows all of the medication, thus ensuring that the medication has not been aspirated and that it has entered the GI tract. Never leave the medication at the patient's bedside. This precaution ensures that the medication is not hoarded, lost, discarded, or ingested by someone other than the intended patient.

Some patients require special assistance or slightly altered techniques for oral administration. If the patient has difficulty swallowing medications, the nurse can encourage the patient to drink some liquid before and during swallowing of capsules or tablets. If the medication can be crushed, the nurse can place it in a small amount (usually a tablespoon) of applesauce, gelatin dessert, mashed potatoes, or other semisolid food. The nurse should use only small amounts of food because some medication may be lost if the patient does not ingest all of the food. This technique works well with toddlers and small children. It also is preferred for patients with dysphagia because they experience more difficulty swallowing liquids than semisolids.

A confused patient may refuse medication, but the nurse must distinguish between a patient who experiences confusion and one who makes an informed choice to refuse the medication. If the patient is confused, the nurse should return and offer the medication a few minutes later. The nurse may obtain the medication in a liquid form or may crush and mix it with a food or beverage. Under no circumstance should the nurse physically force the patient to swallow medication. Doing so is illegal and unprofessional and could lead to aspiration or other injuries.

All oral medications for infants are prescribed in liquid form. Infants can take medications through a bottle after the drug has been diluted with water or other liquid. Medications also may be given using a dropper, which is the preferred method. An infant taking medication through a bottle may receive an incomplete dose if all the liquid in the bottle is not ingested. When administering medications to an infant by the dropper method, the nurse first must identify the patient by checking the armband and name tag. Then the nurse follows these steps: (1) Place a bib on the infant to protect the clothing. (2) Hold the infant in one arm with the head at a 45-degree angle, taking care to restrain the infant's extremities. With the free hand, remove the correct dose of medicine from the bottle and hold the dropper to the infant's lips. (3) Instill the medication in the pocket between the infant's cheek and gum: instilling the drops in that location helps deter the infant from spitting out the medication. (4) Replace the dropper in the medication bottle if the bottle and medication are for an individual patient and the dropper is attached to the bottle cap. If the dropper is not attached to the bottle cap, rinse the dropper in warm water, dry it with a clean paper towel, and store it in a clean, airtight container for later use by the same patient.

Special techniques for oral administration

Giving medications through a gastric tube, such as a nasogastric (NG) tube or a gastrostomy tube, involves special techniques. Drugs administered through a gastric tube enter the stomach directly, thus bypassing the mouth and esophagus and the disintegration and dissolution processes that occur there. To administer a drug appropriately via an NG or gastrostomy tube, the nurse must reproduce the disintegration and dissolution processes by crushing a tablet and preparing a liquid form. When using an NG or gastrostomy tube, the nurse must know how the action of a medication changes when a tablet is crushed. A crushed tablet disintegrates immediately, and absorption from the GI tract occurs rapidly. These changes may not produce significant differences in blood levels and absorption rate if the tablet was designed for rapid disintegration and absorption. If, however, the tablet was designed for slow release and absorption, crushing can alter the drug's effect significantly. In some cases, the nurse may consult the physician about using a different form of the drug or a different route to achieve the intended effect.

The nurse must never place an intact tablet or capsule in a gastrostomy or NG tube. The small diameter of most tubes prevents tablets and capsules from passing through the lumen.

To determine which drugs can be crushed or should not be crushed, the nurse should read the label, consult a pharmacist, or check the package insert information. Uncoated tablets or those with sugar coatings designed only to camouflage a bitter taste usually can be crushed. Enteric-coated tablets should not be crushed because the coating is designed to protect the drug from stomach acids and ensure that it reaches and dissolves in the small intestine. When these tablets are crushed, gastric or esophageal irritation as well as altered drug action can result. Wax matrix tablets should not be crushed because the drug would dissolve faster, thereby increasing the serum level of the drug and causing it to be excreted more rapidly. The intended sustained-release action of the wax matrix tablet would become unpredictable.

The beads in sustained-release capsules should not be crushed because all of the drug would be released at once; the sustained-release action of the drug would be altered in much the same way as in crushing a wax matrix tablet. The nurse who must administer a sustained-release drug through a gastric tube should obtain and use a liquid form of the drug if possible. Otherwise, the patient may require more frequent doses, which may result in toxic effects. Capsules that contain a powder can be emptied for easy administration by gastric tube.

If crushing the tablet is necessary, the nurse should use a glass mortar and pestle or a special pill-crushing device. The hospital pharmacy may perform this service for patients who cannot take medications orally. Ideally, the tablet would be available in a unit-dose package and the nurse would crush it without opening the package. When a unit-dose package is not available, the nurse crushes the tablet using a clean, dry mortar and pestle or places the tablet in a souffle cup and uses the pill-crushing device. The nurse then removes the uniformly crushed powder from the unit-dose package, mortar, or souffle cup, mixes it with a liquid, and administers the dose to the patient through the NG or gastrostomy tube. Then the nurse washes the mortar and pestle with soap and water.

Powders can be dissolved in lukewarm water. For capsules containing a liquid, the nurse can prick the capsule in one end with a needle and squeeze the contents into the gastric tube. The nurse also can dissolve the whole capsule in a small amount of lukewarm water and then administer the dose. Dissolving the capsule ensures administration of the entire dose, but the dissolution process can take a long time.

Many medications that require administration via a gastric tube are available in liquid form, the use of which always is preferable to crushing tablets. Some of these medications also may be given parenterally. When using a gastric tube, the nurse should administer only room-temperature liquids. Liquids going through a gastric tube bypass the mouth and esophagus, which normally help warm or cool fluid entering the stomach. A burning or cramping sensation can occur in the patient's stomach if a liquid that is too hot or too cold is administered via a gastric tube. (For step-by-step procedures, see *Administering medication via an NG tube.*)

SUBLINGUAL AND BUCCAL

Uncoated tablets are used for sublingual and buccal routes, which differ from the oral route. Because the patient does not swallow the tablets, they do not enter the GI tract. Instead, the tablets disintegrate and dissolve in the mouth, under the tongue (sublingual) or between the cheek and gum (buccal). Furthermore, orally routed drugs are absorbed mainly in the small intestine. Sublingual and buccal drugs are absorbed directly into the bloodstream from the oral mucosa, thus bypassing the GI and hepatic systems.

When a drug bypasses the liver, first-pass metabolism cannot reduce significantly the percentage of drug that reaches the systemic circulation. (For more information about the first-pass effect, see Chapter 2, Pharmacokinetics.) The time required for a drug to begin therapeutic action also greatly diminishes when the drug bypasses the GI tract. The reduced time needed for therapeutic action can be advantageous in certain circumstances. For example, nitroglycerin given sublingually for acute anginal pain dissolves under the tongue, where it enters the bloodstream directly. The onset of action can occur in seconds. The same drug orally routed via a gastrostomy tube takes up to 30 minutes to produce effective action.

The time difference produced by sublingual and buccal routing also influences peak serum levels and the duration of action. For example, the duration of action of sublingual nitroglycerin for acute anginal pain is approximately 5 minutes. A patient experiencing acute anginal pain lasting longer than 5 minutes may need another dose of sublingual nitroglycerin.

Drugs given via the sublingual or buccal route include nitrates, such as nitroglycerin, isosorbide dinitrate, and ergotamine.

To administer drugs via the sublingual route, the nurse follows these steps: (1) Place the tablet in a souffle cup. (2) Identify the patient by checking the armband and name tag and asking the patient to state his or her name. (3) State the name of the drug and its action or use. (4) Ask the patient to open the mouth and touch the tip of the tongue to the roof of the mouth. (5) Place the tablet on the floor of the mouth and have the patient close the mouth. Instruct the patient not to swallow the tablet, but rather to hold it in place until it has been absorbed.

Another drug form used for sublingual administration is the spray. The nurse should identify the patient using the standard procedures and then administer the spray according to the manufacturer's instructions. For example, the nurse dispenses nitroglycerin spray by completely depressing the plunger on the pressurized aerosol container once. Doing so provides the patient with a metered dose of the drug. The nurse should deliver the dose while the patient maintains an open mouth with or without the tongue raised toward the roof of the mouth. The spray is deposited on the floor of the mouth, in the same location as a sublingual tablet. The patient then closes the mouth and resumes normal activity.

For drug administration via the buccal route, the nurse follows these steps: (1) Place the medication in a souffle cup. (2) Identify the patient using the standard procedure. (3) State the name of the drug and its action or use. (4) Have the patient open the mouth. (5) Place the tablet between the gum and cheek near the back of the mouth, and instruct the patient to close the mouth and keep the tablet against the cheek until it is absorbed.

Sublingual and buccal medications typically are kept at the patient's bedside for immediate use. In those instances, the medications are self-administered. Self-administration necessitates that the nurse provide adequate patient teaching and supervision and document it properly.

RECTAL

Nurses administer medications via the rectal route for various reasons. A postoperative patient may have an NG tube connected to continuous suction to keep the stomach de-

Administering medication via an NG tube

Before administering medication, the nurse identifies the patient by checking the armband and name tag and asking the patient to state his or her name, if appropriate. Then the nurse should state the name and action or use of the drug. To administer medication via an NG or gastrostomy tube, the nurse will need these supplies: a 50-ml syringe with a catheter tip that fits snugly into the gastric tube, a plastic medicine cup (containing the medication), a tissue or washcloth, a stethoscope, and a glass of tap water.

1 Check for NG tube displacement as shown below for the Salem Sump tube. To do this, connect the NG tube to the syringe and aspirate a small amount of stomach contents into the syringe. If stomach contents do not return upon aspiration, or if the diameter of the feeding tube is too small, insert a bolus of 10 cc of air into the tube while auscultating the abdomen midline, just below the xiphoid process. The stomach will emit a loud gurgle when the bolus of air enters. A patient with a gastrostomy tube will not require this procedure because the gastrostomy tube is placed directly into the stomach through a surgical incision.

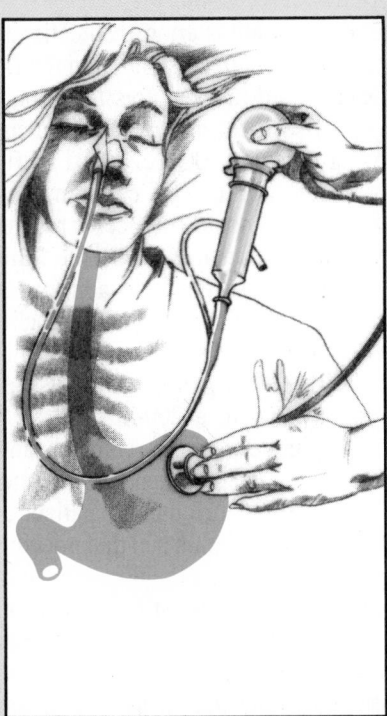

2 Remove the syringe from the tube. Then remove the plunger or bulb from the syringe and place the syringe back into the NG tube, making sure that it fits snugly.

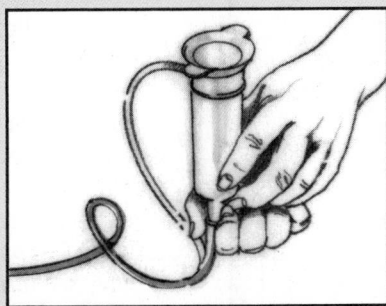

3 Slowly pour the medication into the syringe, which acts as a funnel.

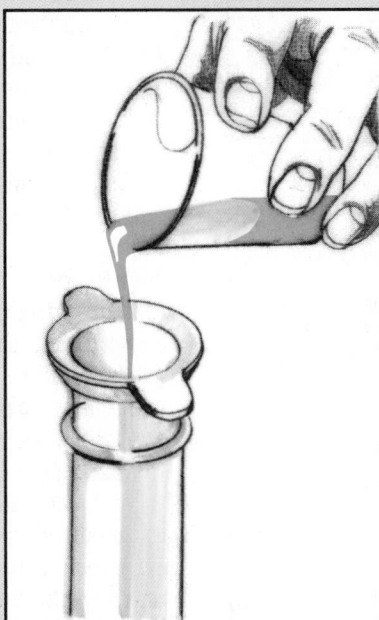

4 After the medication enters the gastric tube, measure 30 to 50 ml of room-temperature water in the medicine cup and pour it into the syringe. The amount of water needed depends on the length and diameter of the tube. Usually a large-bore tube requires 30 to 50 ml and a small-bore tube requires 15 to 25 ml. Flow into the gastric tube should occur by gravity. The water will help ensure that all medication is rinsed from the sides of the syringe, the gastric tube, and the medicine cup. This additional fluid also assists in maintaining tube patency. Any residue in the tube lumen may occlude the tube.

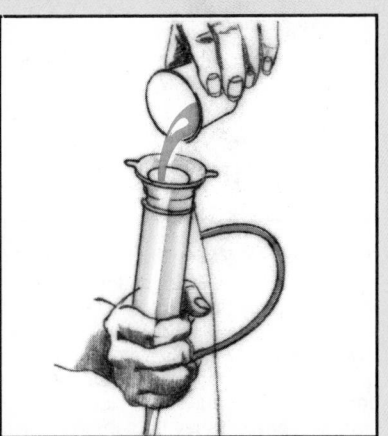

5 Remove the syringe from the tube while keeping a tissue or washcloth below the connection to catch any excess liquid. Then recap or clamp the gastric tube.

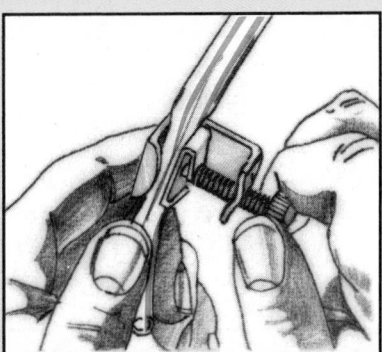

Inserting a rectal suppository

Before administering the medication, the nurse identifies the patient by checking the armband and name tag and asking the patient to state his or her name. Then the nurse states the name and action or use of the drug. To administer a suppository, the nurse will need these supplies: a finger cot or nonsterile disposable examination glove, a water-soluble lubricant, the foil-wrapped or unwrapped suppository, and a tissue or clean 4 × 4 gauze pad. The nurse should draw the curtains or close the door to ensure the patient's privacy.

1 After helping the patient into a comfortable position in which the anus is exposed, place the glove or finger cot on the index finger of the dominant hand. Then remove the foil wrapper, if present. Holding the suppository in the gloved hand, lubricate the tapered end of the suppository with approximately 1 teaspoon (5 ml) of lubricant.

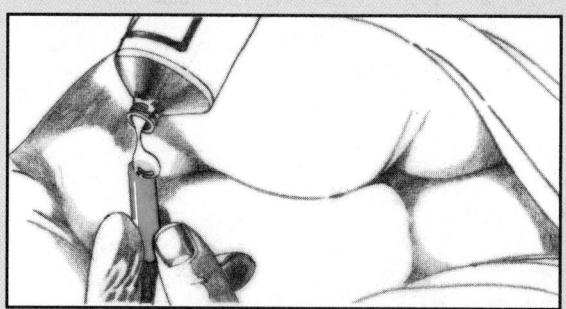

2 Spread the patient's buttocks and insert the suppository, tapered end first, into the anal opening, gently advancing the suppository past the anal sphincter. Use the index finger with the glove or the finger cot to advance the suppository far enough to pass the internal anal sphincter. In an adult, this distance is about 3 inches (7 cm); in a child, it may be considerably less depending on the child's size and age. Clean the excess lubricant from the anal area with the 4 × 4 gauze pad or tissue, and encourage the patient to retain the suppository for at least 20 minutes. If the suppository is not a cathartic, the patient may feel little or no urge to expel it. If, however, the suppository is intended to relieve constipation, the patient may want to expel it as soon as an urge to defecate occurs.

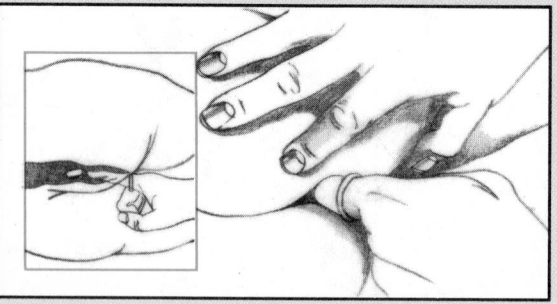

compressed, thus prohibiting the use of the oral route. In such circumstances, suppositories can provide a relatively convenient, painless route for some necessary drugs. Antiemetics given rectally to the nauseated patient usually are effective when the oral route cannot be used.

The rectal route also is the route of choice for circumstances in which certain local and systemic effects are desired. For example, bisacodyl suppositories are given to treat constipation. The nurse also can administer an enema such as sodium polystyrene sulfonate (Kayexalate) to decrease serum potassium levels. The rectal route also may represent the route of choice for unconscious patients because they cannot swallow.

Using the rectal route for administering medications poses several disadvantages. Receiving drugs rectally may embarrass the patient. Using the rectal route also can result in incomplete drug absorption if the patient cannot retain the medication or if the rectum contains feces. Also, pain can result if the patient has hemorrhoids or if the drug is irritating.

A drug may be administered via the rectal route in the form of a suppository or enema. (For an illustrated procedure, see *Inserting a rectal suppository*.)

The technique used for administering medications by enema depends on the time the patient must retain the fluid in the rectum. Medicated fluid that requires retention for at least 30 minutes is called a retention enema. In most cases, a retention enema contains 100 to 200 ml of fluid for adults and 75 to 150 ml of fluid for children ages 6 and over. Children under age 6 should not receive retention enemas because they cannot voluntarily retain the fluid.

The equipment that the nurse needs to administer a retention enema includes a rectal tube (14 or 20 French for adults and 12 to 14 French for children), water-soluble lubricant, a bedsaver pad, a 4 × 4 gauze pad or tissue, a rubber-tipped hemostat, a bedpan, a 200-ml catheter tip or bulb syringe with the plunger or bulb removed, and a paper towel. To administer the retention enema, the nurse follows these steps: (1) After identifying the patient and explaining the purpose of the medication and the procedure, ensure the patient's privacy by closing the door or drawing the curtains. (2) With the bed flat, assist the patient onto the left side with the right knee flexed. This position allows the medication to flow from the rectum into the colon. If the patient cannot assume this position, help the patient lie on the right side or the back. (3) Place the bedsaver pad well under the patient's buttocks to protect the bed linen. (4) Insert the tip of the syringe into the rectal tube. (The syringe will act as a funnel.) Purge the air from the rectal tube by first turning the tip of the tube upward and pinching it off with the fingers. (5) Pour a small amount of the medicated solution into the syringe, slowly lowering the tip of the tube until the solution flows out. Immediately turn the tip upward and attach the hemostat, or close the clamp, about 8 inches (20 cm) from the tip. *Do not* lay down the syringe and tube from this point until the medication is instilled and the tube removed from the patient. Laying these items down would allow the fluid to flow out, and the procedure would need to begin again. (6) After purging the air from the tube, lubricate the tip of the tube with the water-soluble lubricant. Place approximately 1 tablespoon (15 ml) of lubricant on the paper towel and roll the distal 2 inches (5 cm) of the tip of the tube in the lubricant. (7) Separate the patient's buttocks and insert the tube into the anus. Advance the tube about 4 inches (10 cm) in an adult and 2 to 3 inches (5 to 7 cm) in a child, directing it toward the umbilicus. This technique can be awkward because the tube must be inserted with the same hand that is holding the syringe. To help alleviate awkwardness, hold the tube and syringe in the dominant hand and spread the patient's buttocks with the nondominant hand. (8) Slowly pour the prescribed solution into the syringe, holding the tip of the syringe about 4 to 5 inches (10 to 13 cm) above the anus. Release the clamp and allow the fluid to flow into the patient by gravity. If the fluid level rises too far above the anus, the patient may experience cramping or a strong urge to defecate. Instruct the patient to take deep breaths during the insertion and instillation to aid relaxation and avoid the urge to defecate. After instilling all of the solution, clamp the tubing. Inform the patient that you are going to remove the tube. (9) Instruct the patient to take a deep breath. As the patient inhales, quickly remove the tube. Firmly apply pressure against the anus with the 4 × 4 gauze pad or tissue for 10 to 20 seconds or until the urge to defecate passes. (10) Clean the area of any solution or lubricant, and encourage the patient to wait the prescribed length of time (usually at least 30 minutes) before evacuating the enema. Leave the bedsaver pad in place and the bedpan near the patient until the patient has defecated.

For patients who require a retention enema but cannot retain the fluid, the nurse may need to use a catheter with an inflatable balloon for administration. The nurse inserts the catheter into the rectum, inflates the balloon with the appropriate amount of air or saline solution, and administers the medication. After administration, the nurse clamps the catheter, thereby helping the patient retain the fluid. After the retention period, the nurse unclamps and removes the catheter. Expulsion of the retained fluid usually occurs simultaneously with catheter removal.

Nonretention enemas, which may be medicated or unmedicated, are given to evacuate the lower bowel. Nonretention enemas contain 750 to 1,000 ml of fluid for adults and lesser amounts for children and infants. Ideally, the adult and older child retain the fluid for 10 minutes. To administer the nonretention enema, the nurse uses an enema bag.

PARENTERAL ADMINISTRATION TECHNIQUES

Administration via the parenteral route can involve all routes other than the GI tract. The discussion in this chapter, however, concentrates on those medications given by injection. Nurses use the parenteral route to provide a rapid onset of action and to ensure high blood levels of the drug. The parenteral route also is used when the GI route would inactivate the drug, in unconscious patients, and in unstable or seriously ill patients who require precise administration and monitoring.

PREPARATION

Medications can be injected into several body spaces, and the type of injection depends on the body space that is used. The techniques and equipment used for each injection type vary. All injections require a liquid form of the prescribed drug and some type of syringe and needle; the nurse must know and use the correct type of needle and syringe for the different kinds of injections. For example, an I.M. injection requires a long I.M. needle. A short S.C. needle would not reach the muscle, and pain or tissue damage could result. Using an incorrect needle also could alter the drug action and decrease the efficacy of the drug. (For illustrations and descriptions, see *Syringes and needles,* pages 130 and 131.)

Dead space
After selecting the correct needle and syringe, the nurse must prepare the syringe. Part of this preparation may include consideration of the dead space in the syringe. Dead space refers to the volume of fluid in a syringe and needle that remains after the plunger has been depressed completely. Although manufacturers calibrate syringes so that dead space compensation is not necessary, compensation for dead space sometimes is advantageous to parenteral administration. For example, the nurse may withdraw 0.2 cc of air after drawing the correct dose of a medication into the syringe. This air bubble not only compensates for dead space, but also keeps medication from tracking into the subcutaneous tissue when the drug is administered.

The package inserts of iron dextran and aluminum-adsorbed toxoids and vaccines recommend use of the air bubble. With iron dextran, an air bubble and the Z-track method of injection help prevent permanent staining of the

Syringes and needles

Because all injections require some type of needle and syringe, the nurse must know and use the correct type of needle and syringe for the different kinds of injections, as described below.

SYRINGES

Standard syringes are available in 3-, 5-, 10-, 20-, 25-, 30-, 35-, and 50-ml sizes. They are used to administer a wide variety of medications in numerous settings. Each one consists of a plunger, barrel, hub, needle, and dead space. The dead space in a syringe is the volume of fluid remaining in the syringe and needle when the plunger is depressed completely. Some syringes, such as insulin syringes, do not have dead space areas.

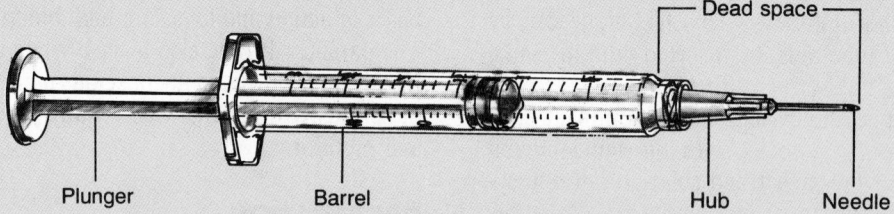

Dead space

Plunger   Barrel   Hub   Needle

The **insulin syringe** has an attached 25-gauge (25G) needle and no dead space. The syringe is divided into units rather than milliliters for measurement. This syringe should be used only for insulin administration.

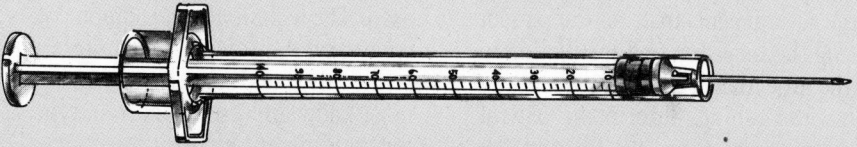

The **tuberculin syringe** holds up to 1 ml of medication. Used most commonly for intradermal injections, it also is used to administer small volumes of medication, such as might be required in pediatric and intensive care units.

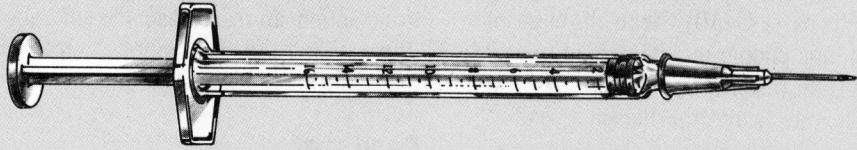

NEEDLES

When choosing a needle, the nurse must consider the needle gauge, bevel, and length. Gauge refers to the inside diameter of the needle. The smaller the gauge, the larger the diameter. Bevel refers to the angle at which the needle tip is opened, and length is the distance from the tip to the hub of the needle.

Needles usually used for **intradermal** injections are ⅜ to ⅝ inch (1 to 1.5 cm) long and are 25G. Such needles usually have short bevels.

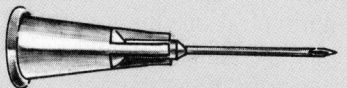

Needles for **subcutaneous** injections are ⅝ to ⅞ inch (1.5 to 2 cm) long, have medium bevels, and are 25G to 23G.

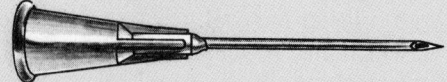

Needles for **intramuscular** use are 1 to 3 inches (2.5 to 7.5 cm) long, have medium bevels, and are 23G to 18G.

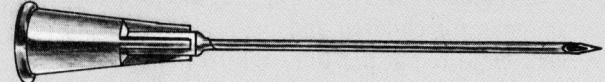

Syringes and needles (continued)

Needles for **intravenous** use are 1 to 3 inches long, have long bevels, and are 25G to 14G.

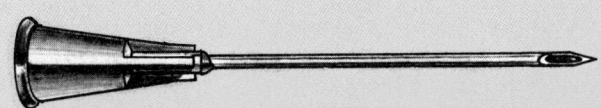

Microscopic pieces of rubber or glass may enter the solution when the nurse punctures the diaphragm of a vial with a needle or snaps open an ampule. The nurse can use a **filter needle** with a screening device contained within the hub to remove minute particles of foreign material from a liquid solution. Filter needles should not be used for injection. Filter needles are 1½ inches (4 cm) long, have medium bevels, and are 20G.

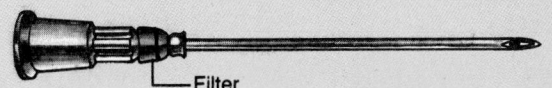
Filter

A **closed system device** comes with the needle in place. These devices come with the plunger attached (prefilled syringe) or as a cartridge to be inserted into a barrel with a plunger attached (cartridge-needle unit). Emergency drugs, such as atropine and lidocaine, are manufactured in prefilled syringes. Narcotic analgesics, heparin, and injectable vitamins are manufactured in cartridge-needle units.
    To prepare the prefilled syringe flip the protective caps off both ends. Remove the needle cap and expel any air in the system.
    To prepare the cartridge-needle unit, insert a cartridge into the reusable syringe. Twist the barrel until it is engaged. Then insert the plunger and twist until the barrel rotates in the reusable syringe. Remove the needle cap and purge the device of air and any extra medication.

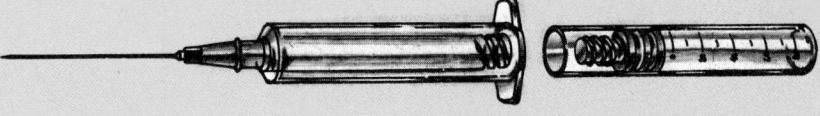

patient's skin should the solution leak into the subcutaneous tissue. (For more information, see *The Z-track method for I.M. injections,* page 132.) Tracking of aluminum toxoids can cause abscesses and tissue necrosis, and the sealing action of the air bubble technique helps prevent these problems.

However, the nurse should not use the air bubble method with other types of I.M. injections or with any S.C. injections. No scientific evidence supports the use of an air bubble to prevent bruising after S.C. heparin injections, nor does the air bubble decrease the pain associated with I.M. injections.

Reconstitution and withdrawal from a vial
Liquid and powdered medications for parenteral administration are packaged in sterile vials. The nurse can withdraw liquid medication into the syringe, but powdered forms must be reconstituted first. (For an illustrated procedure, see *Reconstituting and withdrawing medications,* page 133.) The nurse must use sterile technique during all medication preparation and injection procedures to decrease the risk of infection.

Small air bubbles may adhere to the interior surface of the syringe when medication is withdrawn from a vial. This small amount of air would not harm the patient if injected; however, it could change the dose of medication actually administered. Therefore, the nurse should remove the air bubbles. To do so, hold the syringe with the needle pointed upward, tap the side of the syringe until the bubbles accumulate at the hub, then slowly push the plunger until the air is expelled. If the amount of medication is not accurate after this procedure, withdraw more of the drug to complete the prescribed dose.

Withdrawal from an ampule
Liquid medications for parenteral administration also can be packaged in sterile ampules. Powdered ones rarely are packaged in ampules. Before administering medication from an ampule, the nurse must withdraw it carefully. (For an illustrated procedure, see *Withdrawing solution from an ampule,* page 134.)

Mixing drugs
The nurse frequently must mix drugs in one syringe. Probably the most commonly mixed drugs are insulin preparations. Because the onset of action, peak concentration level, and duration of action of insulin preparations vary, the nurse may have to combine a rapid-acting and a longer-

The Z-track method for I.M. injections

The Z-track method for I.M. injections involves pulling the skin in such a way that subcutaneous layers are staggered, causing the needle track to be sealed off after the injection, minimizing subcutaneous irritation and discoloration.

1 After withdrawing the appropriate amount of medication, draw 0.2 cc of air into the syringe. Then replace the needle with a sterile 3-inch (7.5-cm) needle.

Pull the skin laterally away from the intended injection site to ensure the needle's proper entry into the muscle tissue.

2 After cleaning the site, insert the needle, and inject the medication slowly.

When the injection is completed, wait 10 seconds before withdrawing the needle. Waiting prevents medication seepage from the site.

3 Withdraw the needle and syringe, and allow the retracted skin to resume its normal position, which effectively seals the needle track.

Never massage the site or allow the patient to wear tight-fitting clothing over the site immediately after an injection. Either action could force the medication into the subcutaneous tissue and cause irritation.

To increase the patient's absorption rate, encourage physical activity, such as walking. For subsequent injections, remember to rotate the sites.

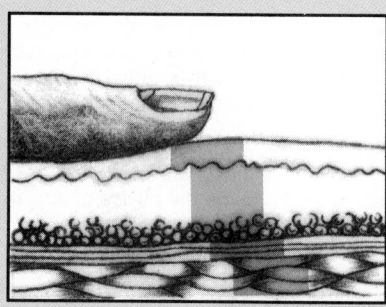
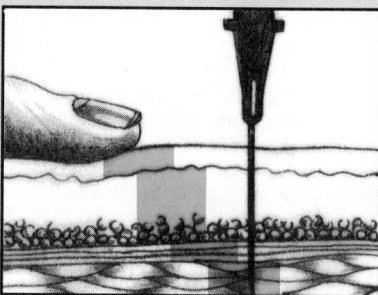
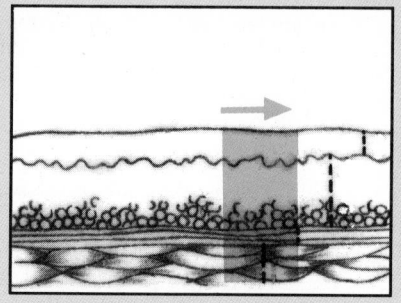

acting type to manage a patient's diabetes. (For a detailed discussion of insulin, see Chapter 49, Hypoglycemic Agents and Glucagon.) Rather than administer two injections, the nurse mixes the two insulins together and administers a single injection. For example, the nurse might mix 10 units of regular insulin with 33 units of NPH insulin.

Before mixing 10 units of regular insulin and 33 units of NPH insulin in one syringe, the nurse should gather these supplies: an insulin syringe calibrated in units equal to the insulin concentration, two alcohol swabs, a vial of NPH insulin, and a vial of regular insulin. To mix the drugs, the nurse may use the following technique: (1) Gently roll the NPH insulin vial between the hands to mix the particles into suspension. This action is not necessary for regular insulin. (2) Clean the tops of the vials with the alcohol swabs. (3) Remove the needle cap and withdraw the plunger until 43 units of air, which equals the total insulin dose, are in the syringe. (4) Carefully inject 33 units of air into the NPH insulin vial and then inject the remaining 10 units into the regular insulin vial. Do not inject air into the solution itself because doing so may produce air bubbles that can alter the dose. Without removing the needle, invert the vial of regular insulin and withdraw exactly 10 units

of regular insulin. (5) Insert the needle into the vial of NPH insulin. Invert the vial, and withdraw 33 units of NPH insulin. The plunger should be at the 43-unit calibration. The medications now are mixed in one syringe and ready for injection.

As in this example, regular insulin should be drawn up first to minimize the risk of contamination and potentially fatal adverse reactions. However, if accidental mixing is suspected in either vial, the nurse should discard it because the contents have been altered.

Skin preparation

After filling the syringe, the nurse must prepare the patient's skin for injection. Giving an injection disrupts the skin, the body's first line of defense, and provides an entry route for bacteria. In preparing the skin for injection, the nurse removes as many bacteria as possible; that is, disinfects the skin.

If the injection site is soiled, wash and dry the site thoroughly. Then use one of several antiseptic agents to disinfect the skin; ethyl alcohol and iodophor are two of the most commonly used. Use alcohol with intradermal injections because iodophor discolors the skin and can in-

Reconstituting and withdrawing medications

To reconstitute and withdraw medication from a vial, the nurse will need these supplies: the medication vial, a vial or ampule of an appropriate diluent, an iodophor or ethyl alcohol swab, a syringe, two needles of appropriate size, and a filter needle, if available, to screen particulate matter that may accumulate from reconstitution.

1 Place the medication vial on a counter top. Wipe the rubber diaphragm with the alcohol or iodophor swab. Do not rub the diaphragm vigorously because doing so can introduce bacteria from the nonsterile rim of the vial. Repeat the process with the vial of diluent.

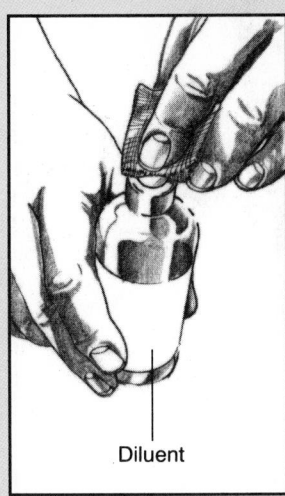

Diluent

2 Pick up the syringe, uncap the needle, and pull back on the plunger until the space inside the syringe equals the amount of diluent desired. Puncture the rubber diaphragm of the diluent vial with the needle, and inject the air. Injecting the air counters the fluid volume and creates a positive pressure. The positive pressure allows the fluid to be easily withdrawn from the vial and prevents a vacuum from forming after the contents are withdrawn. Invert the vial, and withdraw the desired amount of diluent.

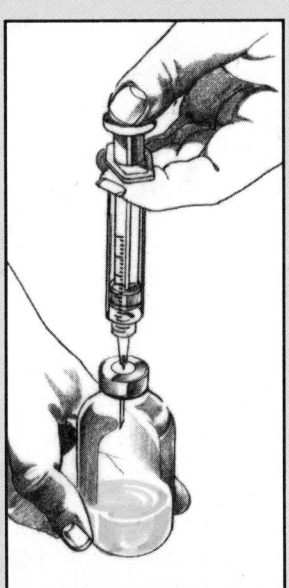

3 Inject the diluent into the medication vial, and withdraw the needle. Roll or shake the vial to mix the medication thoroughly. If a filter needle is available, remove the first needle, and attach the filter needle to the syringe and uncap it. If a filter needle is not available, leave the first needle attached to the syringe.

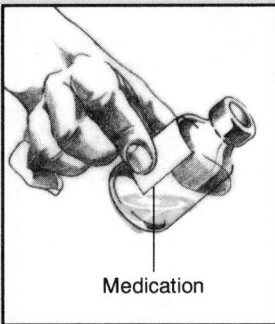

Medication

4 Pull back the plunger until the volume of air in the syringe equals the volume of medication to be given. Puncture the diaphragm of the medication vial, and inject the air. Invert the vial, and withdraw the correct amount of solution. Replace the original needle or the filter needle with a clean sterile needle because medication that may have adhered to the needle when the solution was withdrawn from the vial can irritate the patient's tissues. The syringe filled with medication is now ready to label and administer to the patient. If the medication is already in a liquid form, withdrawing it from a vial involves the same steps as previously described in handling a medication after reconstitution.

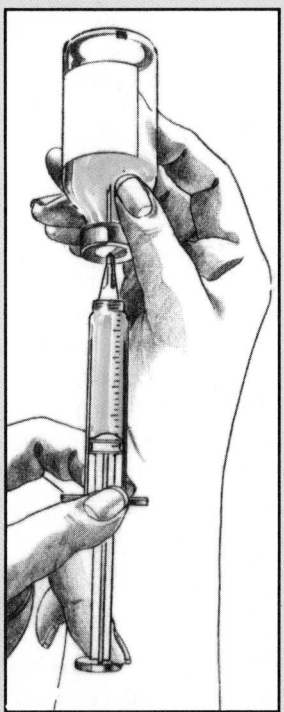

Withdrawing solution from an ampule

To withdraw medication from an ampule, the nurse will need these supplies: an ampule with the medication, a syringe, two needles of appropriate size, and a dry 2×2 gauze pad.

1 Make sure that all of the fluid is located in the base of the ampule; if any remains in the stem, or top portion, gently tap the stem to cause the liquid to flow through the thin neck to the base. If tapping the stem does not work, grasp the stem of the ampule, raise it to approximately eye level, and then quickly swing it down at arm's length.

Wrap the ampule stem with the 2 × 2 gauze pad to protect your fingers from cuts as the neck is snapped. Hold the body of the ampule in one hand and the tip between the thumb and finger of the other hand. While pointing the ampule away from you and others, snap off the top. Inspect the solution for small particles of glass. Discard the solution if any are present.

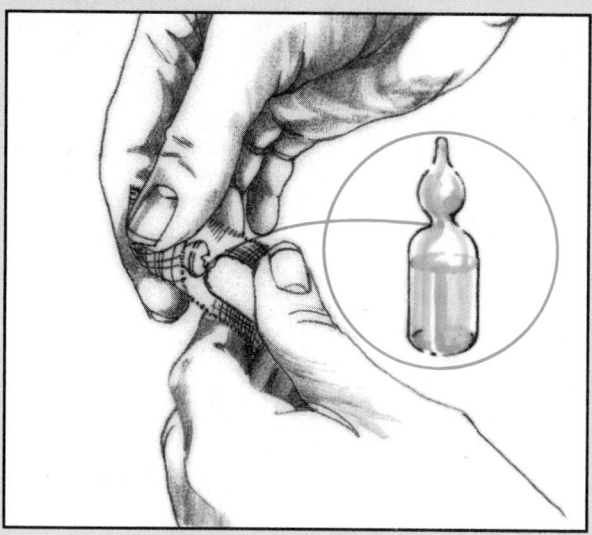

2 Place the first needle, such as a filter needle, on the syringe. Insert the needle into the fluid, and withdraw the appropriate amount of medication. Finally, replace this needle with the second needle for administering the medication. (By changing needles, the nurse prevents irritation that results from medication that remains on the outside of the first needle.) The medication is now ready for injection.

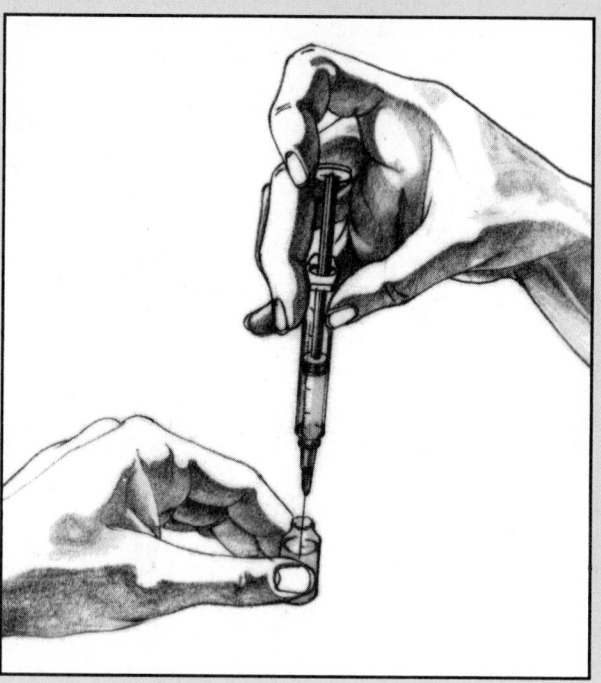

terfere with interpretation of skin test results. Also use alcohol with patients who are allergic to iodine.

Take care not to touch the patient's skin with anything except the sterile swab, cotton, or gauze impregnated with the disinfectant. When using a disinfectant, always begin at the point where the needle will be inserted and wipe in a spiral pattern from the center outward. Cleaning from the puncture site outward carries bacteria away from the site.

Before injecting the medication, allow the disinfected area to dry for about 1 minute. Do not blow on or fan the area to hasten the drying process because these activities increase the risk of contamination. Injecting while the skin is still moist introduces alcohol or iodophor into the tissues and causes irritation. Allowing the skin to dry before injection in many cases reduces injection pain.

ADMINISTRATION

Common administration techniques for parenteral drugs include intradermal, S.C., and I.M. injections as well as I.V. administration.

Intradermal

Intradermal injections are used for skin tests, such as the tuberculin or histoplasmin test. The results of the test usually are interpreted about 24 to 48 hours after the injection. Specific guidelines for each antigen determine whether a patient shows a positive or negative response. In most cases, an induration of 5 mm or greater indicates a positive response. However, the nurse should consult the package insert or drug reference manual for details on each test.

Most nurses seldom give intradermal injections. However, when they do, they should administer the injection

Giving an intradermal injection

Before giving an injection, the nurse must identify the patient according to standard procedure and must state the drug's name and action or use. To give the injection, the nurse will need a gauze pad, an alcohol swab, a syringe containing the drug, and a needle of appropriate size.

1 To identify the injection site on the ventral forearm, have the patient extend the forearm and rest it on a table with the palm up. Measure 2 to 3 finger-widths distal from the antecubital space. Then measure a hand-width proximal from the wrist. The space between these measures represents the area available for injection.
   Prepare the injection site with an alcohol swab. Expel any air in the syringe.

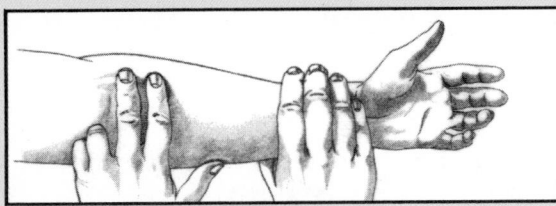

2 With the nondominant hand, retract the patient's skin proximal to the injection site until the skin over the site is taut. To prevent contamination, do not touch the injection site. With the other hand, place the syringe almost flat against the patient's skin (approximately at a 15-degree angle) with the bevel up. Insert the needle by pressing it slowly against the skin.

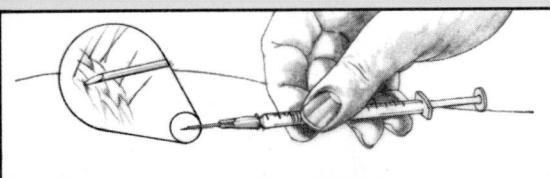

3 Inject the drug slowly and gently. During injection, the needle should be visible through the skin, and resistance should be felt. The area should display blanching and formation of a wheal about 6 mm in diameter.

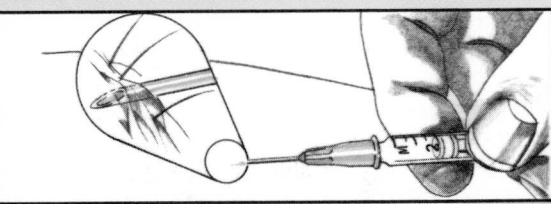

4 When the injection is completed, withdraw the needle and apply gentle pressure to the site. Do not massage the area because massage can irritate the site and interfere with results.

---

in the area of the scapula, upper chest, dorsal upper arm, or the ventral forearm. The ventral forearm is the site of choice. Any area with scars, blemishes, or abundant hair should not be used because it could hamper interpretation of the test results. Identify the patient by checking the armband and name tag. Then explain the medication and the procedure to the patient. (For an illustrated procedure, see *Giving an intradermal injection*.)

Subcutaneous

Subcutaneous injections provide a slow, sustained release of medication and a longer duration of action and are used when the total volume injected is no more than 1 ml of liquid. Many medications, including insulin, heparin, and epinephrine, are given by the S.C. route.

Subcutaneous injection sites, all areas relatively distant from bones and major blood vessels, include the area over the scapula, the lateral aspects of the upper arm and thigh, and the abdomen. At least a 1-inch (2.5-cm) pinched fold of skin and tissue is necessary for administering an S.C. injection. Burned, edematous, or scarred skin should not be used as an S.C. injection site, nor should the area 2 inches (5 cm) in diameter around the umbilicus or the belt line.

The nurse should ensure that injection sites are rotated and that a rotation pattern is established for patients who receive frequent S.C. injections. Site rotation helps promote adequate absorption of the medication and prevents the formation of hard nodules in the subcutaneous tissue. Because site rotation is especially critical for diabetic patients, the nurse must include it as part of the teaching plan for self-care.

The nurse should establish with the patient the convenient injection site areas, instruct the patient to use each site on a given area once before moving on to the next area, and encourage the patient to use the injection sites one after another in an orderly fashion. The nurse needs to stress the importance of establishing and using a systematic pattern.

One effective method of rotating sites is to use a diagram to represent the patient's pattern. (For a record-keeping diagram, see *Sites for S.C. injections,* page 136.)

When a patient does not self-administer injections, the rotation pattern being used must be communicated to other nurses. Most facilities have special flow sheets available to record the rotation patterns used for a specific patient. Notations also can be made on medication sheets.

In many cases, heparin and insulin are administered via the S.C. route using the abdominal sites. The administration technique for these sites resembles that used for the general S.C. injection, and the nurse or patient usually gives the injection holding the needle at a 90-degree angle. (For a step-by-step procedure, see *Giving an S.C. injection,* page 137.) Grasping a skin fold, however, is not always

Sites for S.C. injections

The nurse or patient can use a number of administration sites in several areas for S.C. injections. Systematic rotation of injections helps maintain those sites. In documenting a patient's site rotation pattern, the nurse frequently uses a diagram similar to this one.

In a typical patient, the nurse would administer the first injection in the site represented by a dot on the upper right quadrant and administer the next injection in the area represented by the second dot in that row. This continues until the sites represented by the top row of dots have been used once, then proceeds with the site represented by the dot on the figure's right side in the center row. When each of the sites on the abdomen have been used once, injections may begin in the right leg and follow a similar pattern. When all right leg sites have been used, injections can begin in another area.

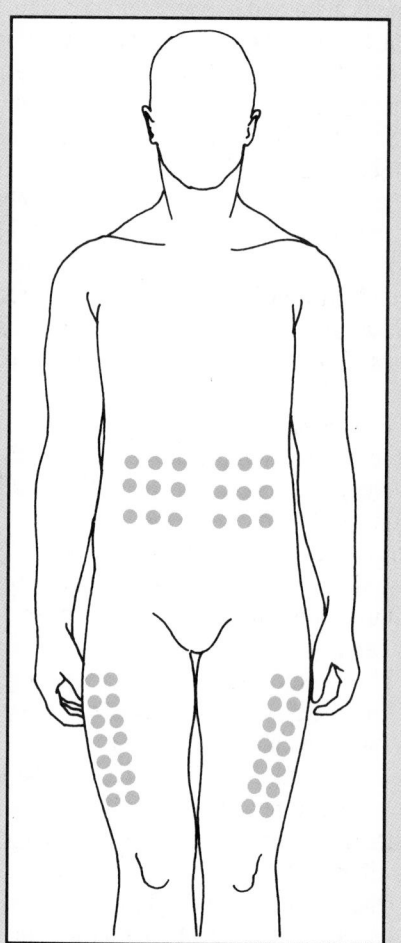
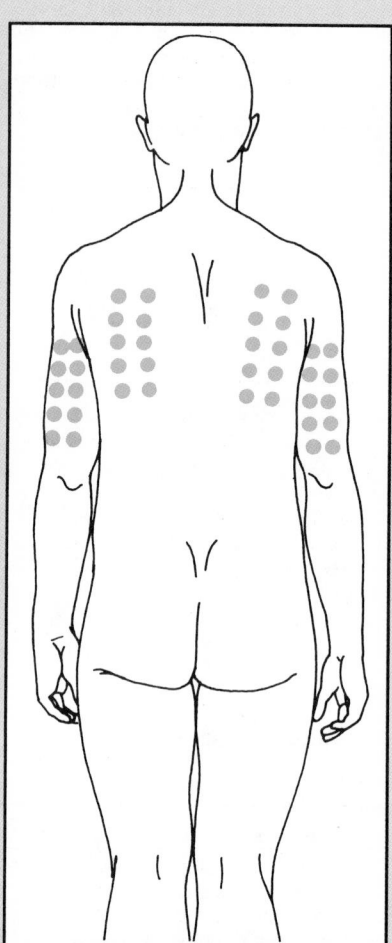

necessary at the abdominal site. Furthermore, if the patient is dehydrated, cachectic, or frail, the abdominal site may not provide adequate subcutaneous tissue for injections.

Aspiration is not necessary with S.C. injection because subcutaneous tissue usually contains only small blood vessels. Therefore, the danger of unintended I.V. injection is minimal. In fact, aspirating S.C. injections may cause tissue damage that could affect drug absorption adversely and in the case of insulin injection may lead to nodule formation in the subcutaneous tissue.

Insulin pumps. An insulin pump is a device that delivers a continuous infusion of insulin into a selected subcutaneous site, commonly the abdomen. The patient places the day's supply of insulin in a syringe and inserts the syringe into the pump. A length of special tubing is connected to the hub of the syringe, and a subcutaneous needle is attached to the distal end. The patient inserts the special needle into the abdomen at a 45-degree angle. Then the patient tapes the needle in place and begins the infusion.

Giving an S.C. injection

Before administering the medication, the nurse identifies the patient according to standard procedure and states the name and action or use of the drug. To administer an S.C. injection, the nurse will need a syringe with a 25G to 23G needle, the medication, and two alcohol or iodophor swabs.

1 Gather the necessary equipment. Then, identify and prepare the injection site using an alcohol swab.

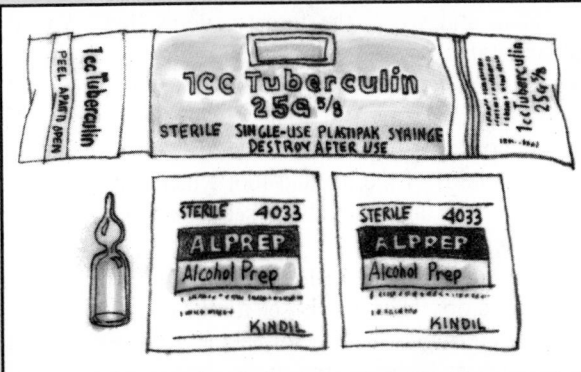

3 In the dominant hand, hold the syringe like a pencil with the bevel of the needle up. If the needle is ½ inch or shorter, hold it at a 90-degree angle to the skin fold. If the needle is ⅝ inch, as in the illustration, hold it at a 45-degree angle.

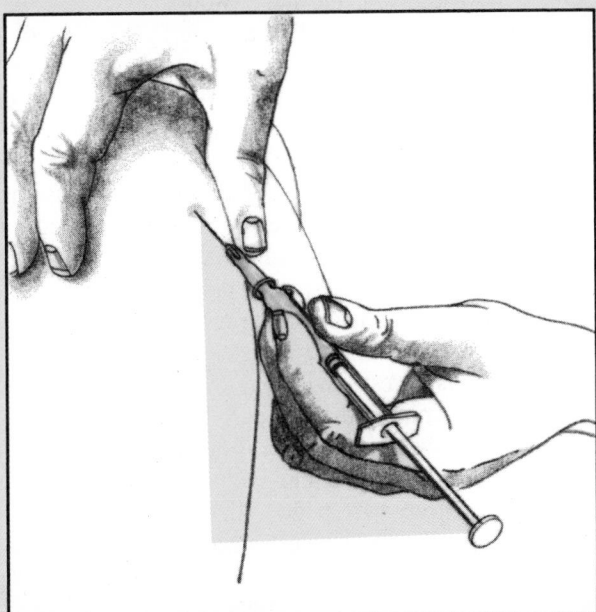

2 Open a second alcohol swab. To keep the swab accessible and maintain sterility of the portion that will contact the insertion site, remove the swab from the wrapper while touching only a corner. Place that same corner between the index and middle finger of the nondominant hand while administering the injection. Grasp at least a 1-inch (2.5-cm) skin fold of the prepared skin area between the thumb and first two fingers of the nondominant hand. Remember, the swab is also in this hand.

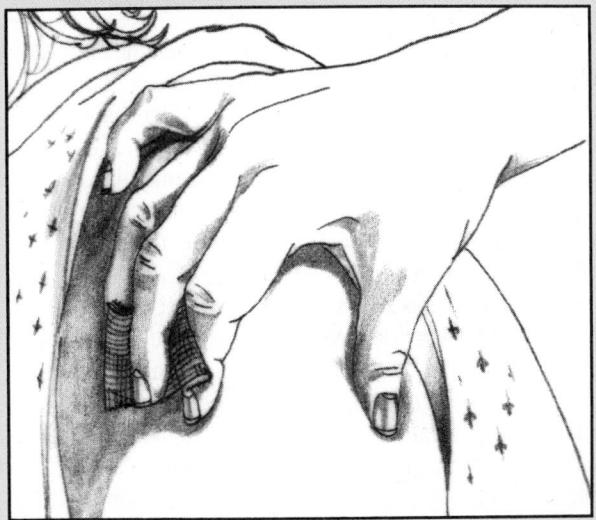

4 Insert the needle using a quick, dartlike motion. Then release the skin fold, and slowly inject the medication. When the plunger is completely depressed and all medication has been injected, place the sterile portion of the second alcohol swab over the insertion site. While gently applying downward pressure, quickly withdraw the needle and syringe. Continue to apply gentle pressure to the site for several seconds.

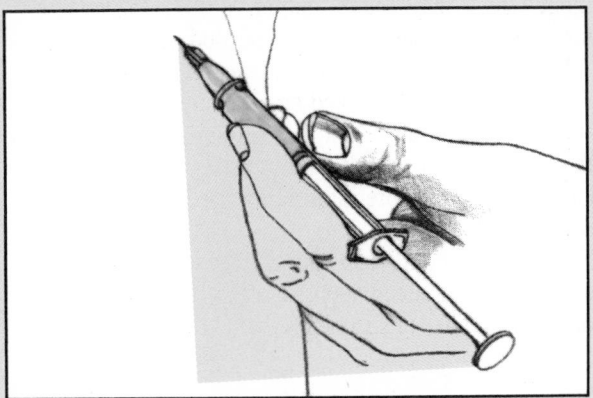

The nurse must instruct the patient to change the insertion site every 2 days and keep the site dry to prevent bacterial contamination. The nurse also must teach the patient how to operate the insulin pump and where to seek help if a problem arises at home.

Intramuscular

Intramuscular injections are given for various reasons, especially when the rapid absorption of medication is desired. The onset of action usually occurs within 10 to 15 minutes after an I.M. injection. However, the blood flow to the injection site affects the absorption rate. Intramuscular injections of drugs that irritate subcutaneous tissues cause less pain than S.C. injections. Also, a larger amount of fluid can be administered in an I.M. injection. The recommended maximum volume for a single I.M. injection for an adult is 5 ml.

Commonly used I.M. injection sites include the dorsogluteal, ventrogluteal, vastus lateralis, rectus femoris, and deltoid muscles. The nurse needs to identify I.M. injection sites accurately. Major blood vessels and nerves traverse the muscle groups used for I.M. injection. Therefore, using an inappropriate injection site could result in permanent damage to the patient. (For identification of the various injection sites, see *I.M. injection sites*.)

Damage to a muscle also can occur if the muscle group is overused for injections, which can be avoided by rotating sites. For example, if the nurse gives an injection in the left ventrogluteal muscle, the next injection might be in the left dorsogluteal or right ventrogluteal site, and a third injection might be given in the right dorsogluteal site. The nurse should record on the medication sheet each I.M. site used.

The injection technique for administering I.M. injections to an infant is the same as that for an adult. (For an illustrated procedure, see *Giving an I.M. injection,* page 140.) Positioning an infant requires special care so that the knees are flexed and arms restrained. This position provides easy access to the rectus femoris and vastus lateralis sites. Gentle restraint should be used to prevent the infant from jerking, which may cause trauma. Restraining and positioning an infant often requires a second adult. The nurse should use the rectus femoris and vastus lateralis sites for I.M. injections in infants and small children. The deltoid, ventrogluteal, and dorsogluteal sites are not used because of the immature muscle size at both sites and the increased risk of injury. (For more information, see Chapter 10, The Pediatric Patient.)

The nurse should use the Z-track method for I.M. injection when a medication, such as iron dextran (Imferon), can irritate or discolor subcutaneous tissue.

Intravenous

Medications are administered intravenously to obtain an immediate onset of action, to attain the highest possible blood concentration level of a drug, and to treat conditions that require the constant titration of medication. In many cases, life-threatening situations, such as shock, require such constant titration. Intravenous administration also is used when the medication is not available in another form and when the patient cannot tolerate the medication via other routes.

Sites used for I.V. administration include the veins on the hand and wrist, the forearm veins that traverse the antecubital fossa, the veins in the scalp and the umbilical vessels (for infants), the subclavian and internal and external jugular veins (for long-term administration or for medications that require rapid blood dilution), and the superficial veins of the leg and foot when other sites cannot be used. (For an illustration, see *Common sites for I.V. injection,* page 141.)

The equipment used for an I.V. injection depends on several factors. The vein chosen for the injection or infusion in part determines the type of needle used. For a one-time bolus of a medication, the nurse may use an antecubital vein because of the vein's accessibility and large size. For a bolus type of injection at an antecubital site, the nurse may use a syringe with a needle. For continuous or intermittent infusions lasting a few days, the nurse would select a vein of the hand, wrist, forearm, scalp, or umbilicus. For such an infusion, the nurse would use a cannula or scalp vein needle (also called a butterfly because of the winglike tabs used to hold the needle during insertion). If the solution is irritating, a smaller-gauge needle is recommended to create greater dilution by the blood flow.

Special catheters must be inserted into large veins for infusions that require rapid blood dilution and infusions or injections administered frequently over a prolonged time. Total parenteral nutrition is an example of this type of infusion. A physician inserts total parenteral nutrition catheters, commonly in the operating room, to reduce the risk of infection. The Hickman catheter is an example of this type of venous access device.

After determining the appropriate site and needle, the nurse performs a venipuncture. (For the procedure for inserting a butterfly needle into a dorsal hand vein, see *Performing a venipuncture,* pages 142 and 143.)

After completing the venipuncture, the nurse documents the date and time of the insertion, the type and gauge of needle inserted, and the initials of the person inserting the I.V. on the tape that secures the gauze pad. Once a venipuncture has been performed, I.V. administration of medication can begin.

Direct bolus. To administer medication by direct bolus, the nurse will need a syringe and a 20-gauge (20G) or

I.M. injection sites

The nurse must be familiar with the most commonly used I.M. injection sites: the ventrogluteal, dorsogluteal, deltoid, vastus lateralis, and rectus femoris muscles. To assist the nurse, the following illustrations identify each injection site and its anatomic landmarks.

Ventrogluteal

Used for all patients, this site is desirable because it is not only relatively free of large nerves and adipose tissue, but is also remote from the rectum (which minimizes the risk of contamination).

For this site, position the patient on the back or side.

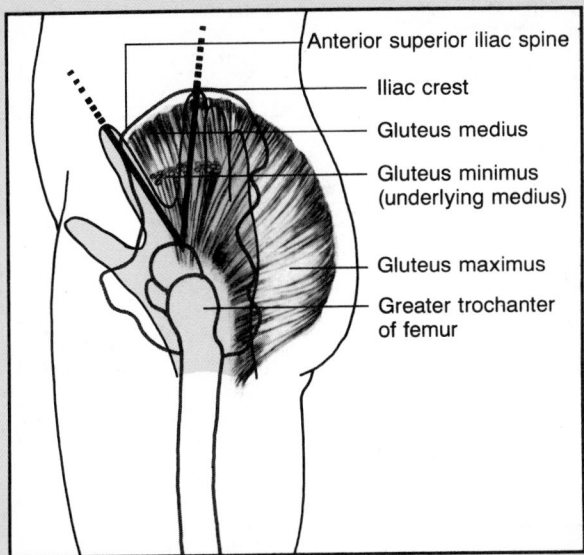

- Anterior superior iliac spine
- Iliac crest
- Gluteus medius
- Gluteus minimus (underlying medius)
- Gluteus maximus
- Greater trochanter of femur

Dorsogluteal

Commonly used for adults, the dorsogluteal site is not used for infants and children under age 3 because these muscles are not well developed.

Position the patient flat on the stomach with the toes pointed inward and the arms apart and flexed toward the head.

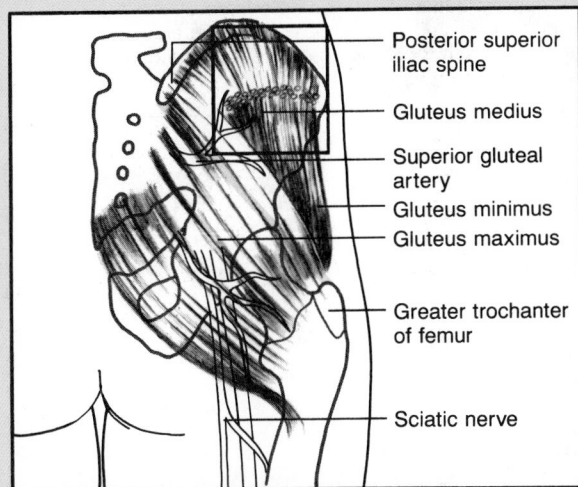

- Posterior superior iliac spine
- Gluteus medius
- Superior gluteal artery
- Gluteus minimus
- Gluteus maximus
- Greater trochanter of femur
- Sciatic nerve

Deltoid

Not usually used because the muscle is small and can accommodate only small doses of medications, the deltoid also is near the radial nerve.

For this site, seat the patient upright or have the patient lie flat with the arms apart.

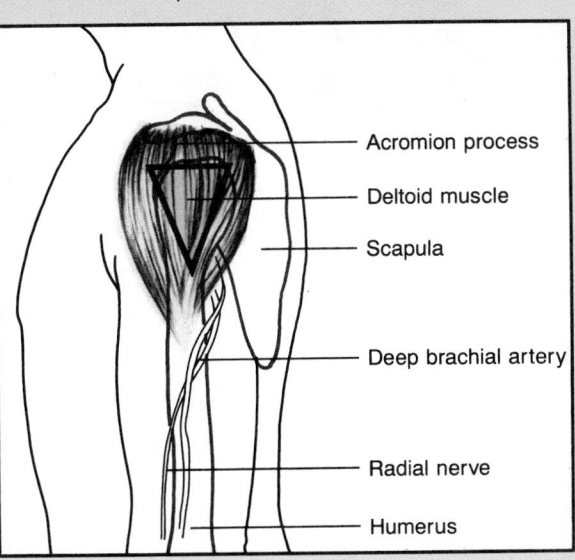

- Acromion process
- Deltoid muscle
- Scapula
- Deep brachial artery
- Radial nerve
- Humerus

Vastus lateralis and rectus femoris

The vastus lateralis is used for all patients, especially children. It is well developed and has few major blood vessels and nerves. The rectus femoris is used most commonly for self-injection because of its accessibility.

For this site, position the patient sitting up or lying flat.

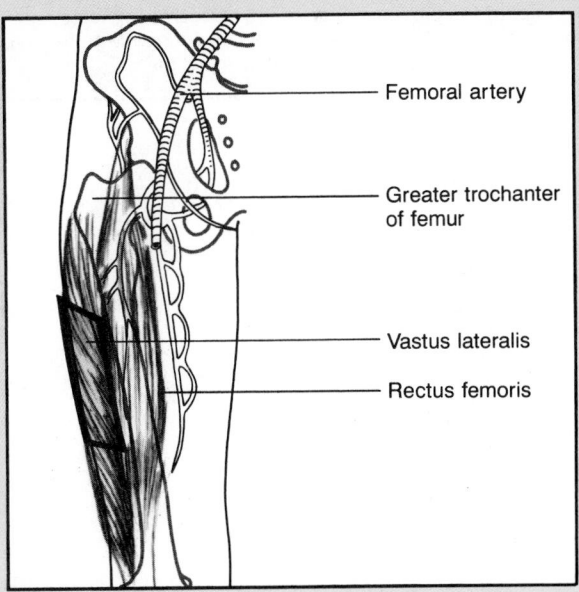

- Femoral artery
- Greater trochanter of femur
- Vastus lateralis
- Rectus femoris

Giving an I.M. injection

Before administering the medication, the nurse should identify the patient according to standard procedure and state the name and action or use of the drug. To administer a medication via an I.M. injection, the nurse will need two alcohol swabs, a syringe containing the medication to be injected, and a needle of appropriate size.

1 Expose the area where the injection will be administered. Remember to provide privacy for the patient if any site other than the deltoid muscle is being used. Palpate the appropriate anatomic landmarks, and identify the exact site for the injection. In this illustration, the vastus lateralis muscle is being used.

Prepare a 2-inch (5-cm) diameter area of skin around the injection site using an alcohol swab. Open a second alcohol swab and place it between the index and second finger of the nondominant hand.

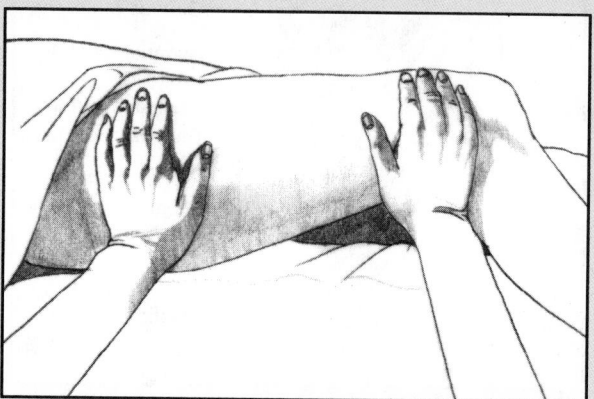

2 Grasp the syringe like a pencil in the dominant hand, and remove the needle cap. With the nondominant hand, spread the skin surrounding the injection site until it is taut. This action helps displace the subcutaneous tissue and brings the muscle closer to the surface.

With a quick, dartlike motion, insert the needle at a 90-degree angle into the muscle. Release the skin surrounding the injection site and use the nondominant hand to steady the syringe for aspiration.

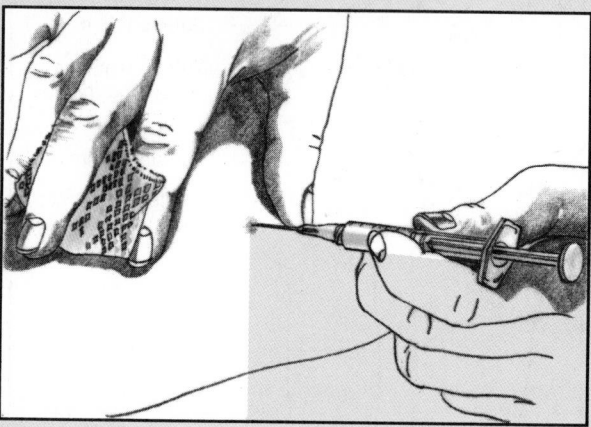

3 Gently aspirate; aspiration is used to determine if the inserted needle has entered a vessel. Pull back slightly on the plunger after inserting the needle into the injection site. If the needle has entered a vessel, blood will flow into the syringe. If blood is aspirated, remove and discard the syringe. Then start the procedure again. If no blood is aspirated, slowly inject the medication. Steady the syringe with the nondominant hand during aspiration and injection.

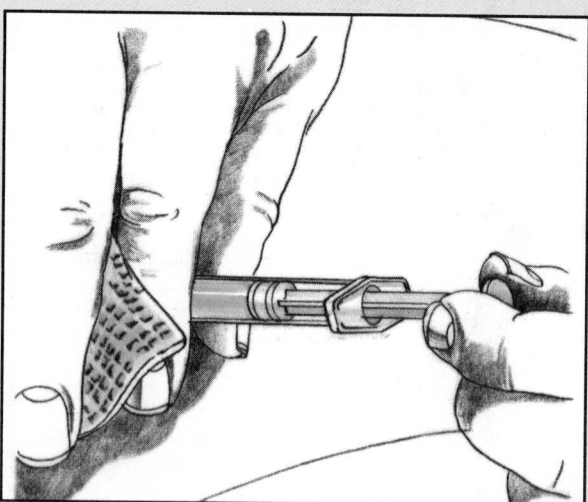

4 When the injection is completed, place the second alcohol swab over the insertion site and apply gentle downward pressure while quickly withdrawing the needle. Massage the site with the alcohol swab to help promote circulation to the area and decrease pain.

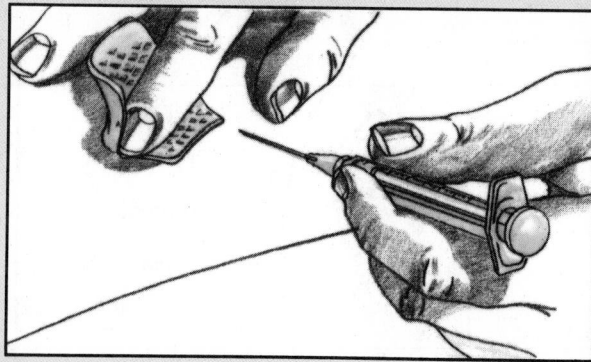

Common sites for I.V. injection

The primary sites for I.V. injection in the hand include the basilic, dorsal metacarpal, and cephalic veins. All of these vessels are relatively easy to locate. As the cephalic and basilic veins traverse the forearm, they branch into other vessels that also are easily accessible for I.V. injections.

smaller needle filled with 1 ml of 0.9% sodium chloride (normal saline) solution, a syringe and needle with the prescribed medication, a syringe and needle with 1 ml of heparin flush solution, and three iodophor or alcohol swabs.

The nurse follows these steps to administer the bolus: (1) Identify the patient and explain the medication and procedure. (2) Clean the intermittent infusion port with a swab. Puncture the center of the port with the syringe and needle containing the medication, and gently aspirate. A small amount of blood should return to ensure correct placement of the I.V. needle. Slowly inject the medication over the recommended time interval. (3) Withdraw the medication syringe, and clean the port with a second swab. Inject the saline-filled syringe to rinse all medication from the port and needle. (4) Remove the syringe and needle used to inject the saline solution. Swab the port a third time, and inject the heparin flush solution. Remove the needle and syringe.

Intermittent infusion. To administer medication using the intermittent infusion method, the nurse will need three alcohol or iodophor swabs, a syringe and needle with 1 ml of heparin flush solution, a syringe and needle with 1 ml of normal saline solution, I.V. administration tubing, a 20G or smaller needle, the I.V. bottle or bag of medication, and an I.V. pole.

The nurse follows these steps to administer the infusion: (1) Identify the patient and explain the procedure. Remove the I.V. administration tubing from the container and the protective cover from the medication bottle or bag. Close the roller clamp, which regulates fluid flow through the tubing. Remove the cap from the I.V. tubing spike, and insert it into the outlet port of the medication bag or bottle. Invert the bag or bottle and hang it from the I.V. pole. (2) Fill the drip chamber of the administration tubing. Remove the protective cap on the end of the tubing, and replace it with the 20G needle. Remove the needle cap, and slowly open the roller clamp, allowing the fluid to clear the tubing of air. Close the roller clamp when the liquid has reached the tip of the needle, and replace the needle cap. (3) Clean the intermittent infusion port. Remove the needle cap, and insert the needle into the port. Secure the needle with tape for the duration of the infusion. Open the roller clamp slightly, and lower the medication bag or bottle below the I.V. site. A backflow of blood confirms correct placement of the needle. Return the bottle or bag to the I.V. pole, and infuse the medication over the recommended time interval. (4) When the infusion is completed, remove and cap the infusion needle, clean the port with the second swab, and inject the saline solution. Use the third swab to clean the port, and inject the heparin flush solution.

(Text continues on page 144.)

Performing a venipuncture

Before beginning a venipuncture, the nurse identifies the patient according to standard protocol and explains the procedure. For a venipuncture into a dorsal hand vein, the nurse will need these supplies: a tourniquet, a butterfly needle (the gauge must be slightly smaller than the lumen of the vein), an iodophor swab, an alcohol swab, a sterile 2×2 gauze dressing, paper or silk tape, a package of antiseptic ointment, and a bedsaver pad.

1 Place the bedsaver pad under the patient's hand to be used for the venipuncture. Apply a tourniquet about 8 to 10 inches (20 to 25 cm) proximal to the needle insertion site.

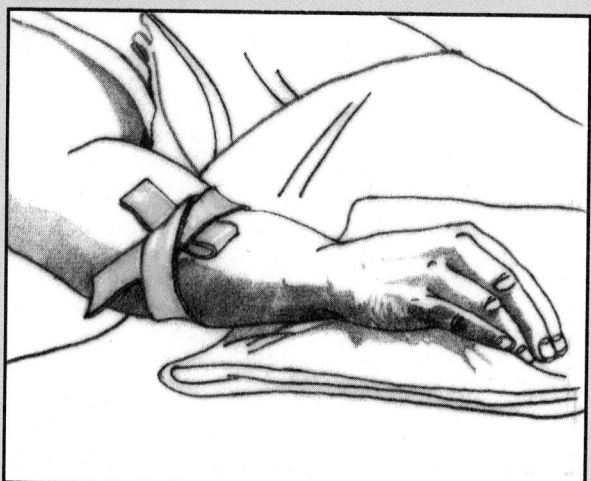

2 Prepare the injection site, using the iodophor swab first, then repeating the process with the alcohol swab. Using the alcohol swab removes some of the iodophor, allowing the vein to appear more clearly.

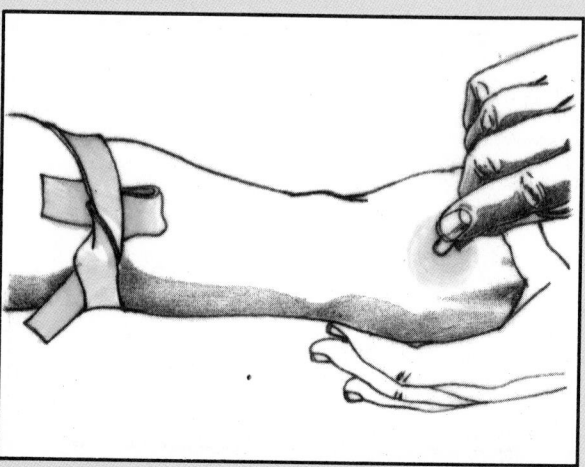

5 Direct the needle at a 30- to 45-degree angle to the skin and puncture the skin just to the side of the vein, using a slow, steady motion.

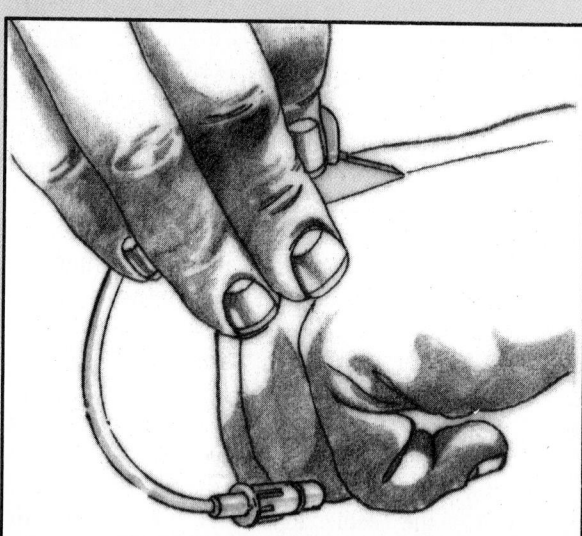

6 Once the entire bevel has penetrated the skin, reposition the needle slightly by directing it toward the vein and decreasing the angle until the needle is almost flat. Then puncture the vein wall. A backflow of blood confirms that the vein has been entered. Continue to insert the needle its full length.

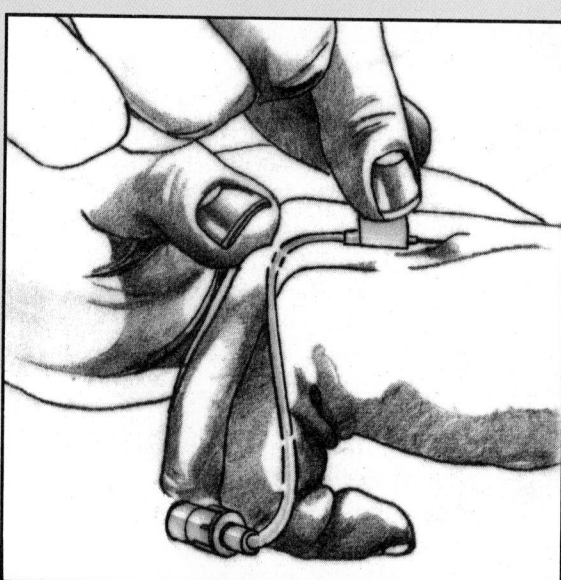

3 Remove the needle cover, and grasp the butterfly needle by its wings with the bevel up, using the thumb and forefinger of the dominant hand.

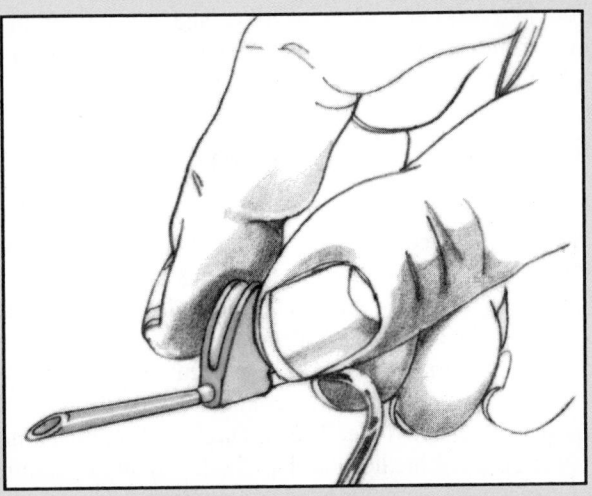

4 Stabilize the vein by gently retracting the skin just distal to the puncture site, using the thumb of the nondominant hand.

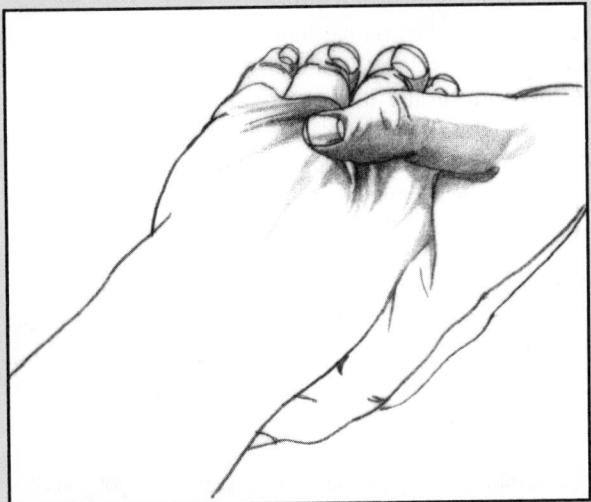

7 Secure the wings by placing a strip of tape over each side. Remove the protective cap on the end of the tubing, and attach an infusion set or intermittent infusion port.

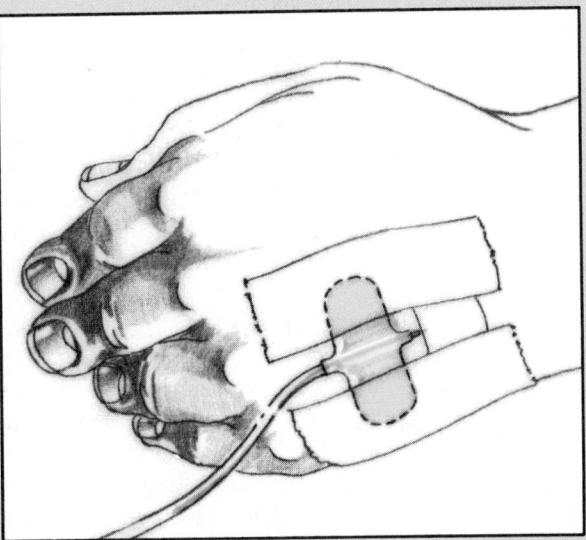

8 Do not cover the insertion site with the tape. Instead, place a small amount of iodophor or antibiotic ointment over the site and cover it with the gauze pad or another occlusive dressing. Apply a 2-inch-wide (5-cm) strip of tape over the gauze pad to hold it in place. Then loop the tubing and secure it with tape.

Leave the hub of the needle exposed so that it is easy to see and use. Remember to document the needle gauge, date and time of insertion, and your initials on the tape covering the site.

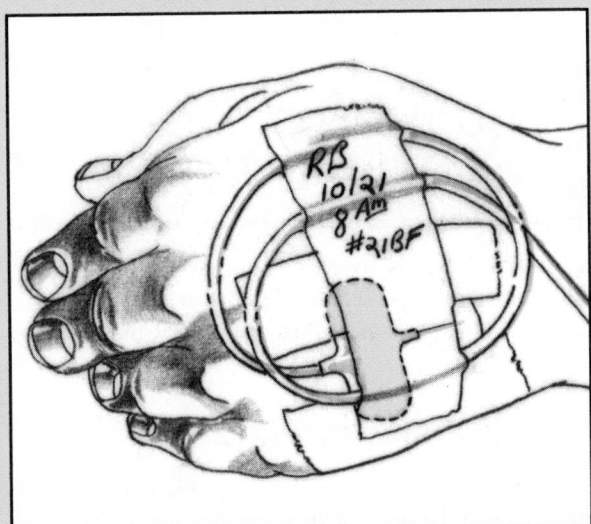

Continuous infusion. The procedure for administering a continuous I.V. infusion is similar to that used for the intermittent infusion, except for a longer duration of infusion. The I.V. administration tubing usually is used for a 24- to 48-hour period; however, the medication bottle or bag may need to be replaced during that period. To do so, the nurse clamps the tubing, inserts the sterile spike into the new bottle or bag of medication, unclamps the tubing, and continues the infusion.

Continuous I.V. medication administration often is facilitated by using an infusion pump. The nurse sets the electric or battery-powered infusion pump to deliver a constant amount of solution per minute or hour. To determine the pump settings, the nurse considers the total amount of fluid to be given and the interval over which it must be infused. Each of the different infusion pumps available comes with its own set of operating instructions. The nurse must follow the manufacturer's guidelines to ensure adequate functioning of the pump.

Hickman catheter administration. The Hickman catheter, one of the oldest and best-known venous access devices, is used when the patient requires frequent venous access over a sustained period. During such time, the nurse may obtain blood samples or administer medications or total parenteral nutrition.

The Hickman catheter and other similar venous access devices are implanted in a large vein, such as the cephalic or internal jugular vein. The tip of the catheter is introduced into the right atrium. The end of the catheter has an intermittent infusion port attached to it.

The procedures for injecting or infusing medication resemble those used for I.V. infusion or direct bolus. The volume of the heparin flush solution, however, is greater (3 ml).

OTHER ROUTES OF DRUG ADMINISTRATION

Other routes are used for medication administration, including the intrathecal, epidural, intra-articular, dermal, ophthalmic, otic, nasal and sinus, respiratory, urethral, and vaginal routes.

INTRATHECAL ADMINISTRATION

During intrathecal administration, an access device implanted beneath the scalp delivers medication to the brain. The access device, which consists of a dome-shaped reservoir and a ventricular catheter, is implanted surgically below the scalp on the top portion of the head. The catheter is threaded into a lateral ventricle. (For an illustration, see *Intrathecal access device.*)

Then a bolus of medication is injected into the pliable reservoir. When the filled reservoir is compressed, medication is ejected through the catheter into the brain. Intrathecal reservoir injections usually are not administered by nurses.

Intrathecal administration is used for patients requiring frequent chemotherapy treatments for lymphoma, leukemia, or meningeal metastases. The intrathecal device delivers chemotherapeutic agents at regular intervals and also provides greater patient mobility and freedom from repeated lumbar punctures. It also is used to administer antibiotics to patients with central nervous system infections.

EPIDURAL ADMINISTRATION

Using the epidural route requires that a catheter be placed into the spinal column via a lumbar puncture. The epidural route is used to administer anesthesia and narcotic analgesics, such as morphine. The route also is used postoperatively. In many cases, patients in intensive care units require epidural catheters. The procedure for injecting or infusing medication via the epidural catheter follows that used for the I.V. route. The epidural route requires much lower doses of medication than the I.V. route; in addition, the effects of the medication last longer.

INTRA-ARTICULAR ADMINISTRATION

Intra-articular injections seldom are given because of their high risk of infection. Furthermore, intra-articular injections may reduce the chances of success of future joint replacement surgery. Occasionally, patients with severe joint inflammation receive an intra-articular injection of corticosteroids, but these injections usually are not repeated. When giving an intra-articular injection, the physician uses a long needle to deposit the medication directly into the joint and observes strict aseptic technique.

DERMAL ADMINISTRATION

The dermal route also is known as the dermatomucosal route and, more commonly, the topical route. Dermal medications usually are used for their local rather than systemic effects. One of several exceptions, nitroglycerin is given via the dermal route for its systemic rather than local effect.

Medication forms given via the dermal route include creams, lotions, ointments, powders, and patches. The medication is absorbed through the epidermal layer into the dermis. The extent of absorption depends on the vascularity of and circulation in the region. To apply a cream, lotion, or ointment, the nurse begins at the midline and uses long,

Intrathecal access device

A catheter exits the dome-shaped reservoir on its inferior surface and projects into a lateral ventricle.

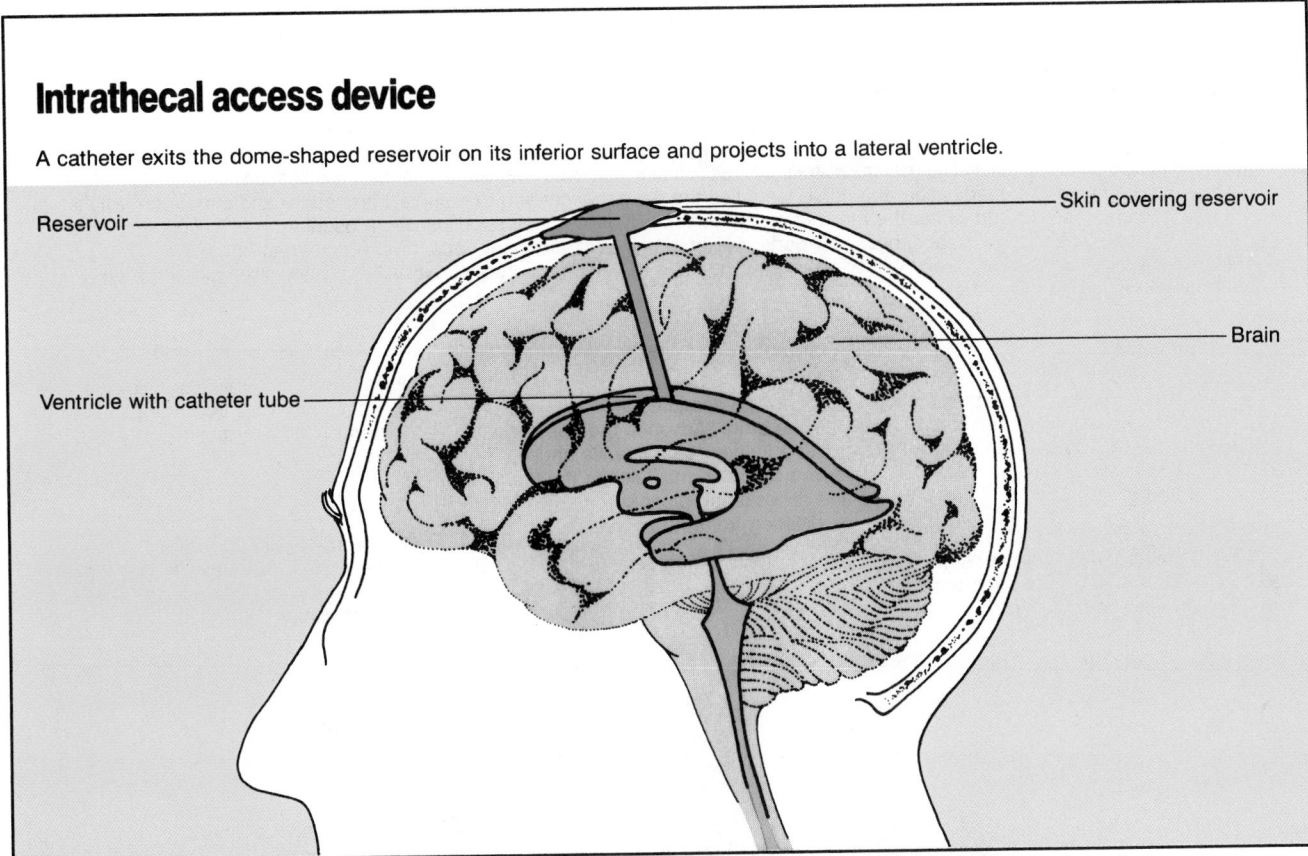

even strokes outward and downward, in the direction of hair growth. This application pattern reduces the risk of follicle irritation and skin inflammation. After applying a cream, lotion, or ointment, the nurse usually should rub the medication into the patient's skin; powders should not be rubbed into the skin.

Patches contain a measured dose of medication that is delivered over an extended time. Medications in patch form include nitroglycerin, scopolamine, clonidine, and estrogen. The nurse should apply the patch over clean, dry skin. Removal of excessive hair will ensure proper absorption. The drug is released through a thin membrane or from a gel base in the patch.

OPHTHALMIC ADMINISTRATION

Liquid and ointment medications are administered topically into the eye. The nurse usually instills liquid medications by the drop method. (For an illustrated procedure, see *Ophthalmic agent administration* in Chapter 71, Ophthalmic Agents.)

OTIC ADMINISTRATION

Liquid medications are administered topically into the ear. The nurse instills liquid medications by the drop method. (For an illustrated procedure, see *Using ear drops* in Chapter 72, Otic Agents.)

NASAL AND SINUS ADMINISTRATION

The nurse administers liquid and powdered forms of medications via the patient's nose and sinuses by instillation or by an atomizer or nasal aerosol device. Vasoconstrictors represent one kind of drug commonly administered by this route. (For instructions on instilling medication into the nose and sinuses, see Chapter 40, Decongestant Agents.)

The nasal aerosol device seldom is used. The technique for its use resembles that for the atomizer and drop instillation methods. The package insert provides specific information regarding the administration technique for this device.

RESPIRATORY ADMINISTRATION

Almost all drugs given via the respiratory route produce a systemic effect because of the rich blood supply in the lungs. The drug forms administered via this route include

Inserting a vaginal medication

The procedure is similar for administering all forms of vaginal medication, such as creams, suppositories, ointments, and gels. However, the nurse should follow the manufacturer's instructions for administering the prescribed medication.

Before inserting a vaginal medication, the nurse identifies the patient according to standard procedure and states the drug's name and action or use. To administer the medication, the nurse will need these supplies: the prescribed medication, applicator, gloves, water-soluble lubricant, tissues, bedsaver pad, several cotton balls, perineal pads, drape, and soap and water. The nurse should provide for the patient's privacy and explain the procedure to her. The nurse should ask the patient to void and then should use the following procedure.

1 Help the patient lie down with her knees flexed and legs spread apart. Place a bedsaver pad under her to protect the bed linen, and a drape over her legs, leaving only her perineum exposed. Put on gloves.

2 Using one cotton ball per stroke, clean the perineum with soap and water. Then spread the labia and clean this area.

3 Insert the medication into the applicator, and lubricate the applicator tip.

4 Spread the labia with one hand, and insert the applicator into the vagina with the other. Advance the applicator about 2 inches (5 cm), while angling it toward the sacrum. Release the labia and depress the plunger to expel the medication from the applicator.

5 Remove the applicator and wipe any excess lubricant from the perineum. Instruct the patient to remain supine for about 30 minutes to retain the medication.

6 Give the patient tissues to wipe away any medication that may drain when she stands. Instruct her to wear a perineal pad to prevent drainage stains on her clothes.

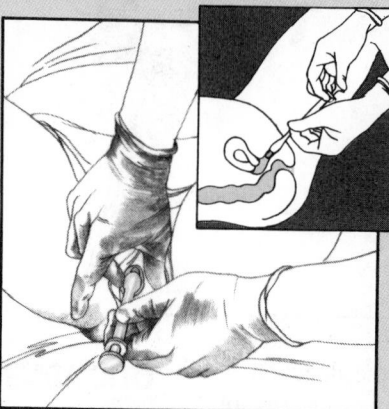

gas, such as oxygen; liquid, such as isoproterenol; and powder, such as cromolyn sodium.

Nebulization is a commonly used method for administering drugs via the respiratory route. The two major kinds of nebulizers are the ultrasonic nebulizer and the metered-dose aerosol or turbo inhaler. The ultrasonic nebulizer uses a small volume of medication (usually under 1 ml) combined with about 3 ml of normal saline solution. Air forced through the nebulizer delivers the medication in a fine mist, which the patient inhales by breathing deeply through a mouthpiece attached to the nebulizer.

Administering drugs via a metered-dose aerosol or turbo inhaler requires only the nebulizer, which is prefilled by the manufacturer with several doses of the drug. Each patient receives an individual nebulizer filled with the appropriate medication and dosage.

Powder is administered with a turbo inhaler. The nurse places a capsule of powdered drug inside the inhaler, and the patient inhales deeply through the mouth. As a result, the contents of the capsule are delivered in a fine powdered form to the lungs. (For detailed instructions on using the metered-dose aerosol and turbo inhaler, see *Cromolyn sodium* in the introduction to Unit Nine.)

URETHRAL ADMINISTRATION

Physicians and nurses use urethral administration for local antibiotic or antifungal therapy. After identifying the patient according to standard procedure and stating the drug's name and action or use, the nurse instills the liquid medication into the urethra through a small-diameter urinary catheter using sterile technique. The catheter then is removed or clamped so the medication can reach and bathe the bladder walls. How long the catheter remains clamped determines the duration of medication retention in the bladder. Occasionally, an intracath (the type used for I.V. administration), with the needle removed, is inserted into the urethra for the instillation of liquid medication. Severe cases of epididymitis may be treated in this manner.

Urethral administration may be repeated several times a day for about a week or only performed once. For repeated treatment, the nurse probably will use a special urinary catheter with an extra lumen for medication instillation.

The volume of medication can range from a few milliliters to almost a liter.

VAGINAL ADMINISTRATION

Vaginal administration is used for topical antibiotic or antifungal medications, in liquid, suppository, cream, ointment, tablet, or gel form. When administering drugs in liquid form, the nurse performs what commonly is called a douche or vaginal irrigation. The procedure resembles that used for a rectal retention enema except for the use of a special vaginal catheter. (See the section on rectal drugs for a description of the procedure for a retention enema.) When the nurse inserts the catheter tip into the vagina, the patient should be on a bedpan or toilet because no sphincter controls the vagina and the fluid will flow immediately out of the vaginal vault.

Other forms of vaginal medication are administered with the patient lying supine in bed. (For an illustrated procedure, see *Inserting a vaginal medication.*)

CHAPTER SUMMARY

Chapter 9 presented the different drug forms and routes of administration, including detailed descriptions of techniques used for the different routes. Here are the highlights of the chapter.

- Drugs are packaged in the unit-dose format (one dose in a labeled container) and bulk style (multiple doses in a labeled container).
- The major drug forms include solids, liquids, suppositories, and inhalants. The form of a drug affects the way the patient uses the drug.
- Solids include tablets, capsules, enteric-coated tablets, and wax matrix tablets. Solid drug forms are given orally and via the sublingual and buccal routes. Enteric-coated and wax matrix tablets should not be crushed because doing so alters the drug action and may irritate the esophageal and gastric mucosa. Buccal and sublingual medications are absorbed into the bloodstream without going through the GI tract.
- Liquids include syrups, suspensions, tinctures, and elixirs. Liquids usually are administered orally or parenterally via injection.
- Suppositories, which are administered rectally and vaginally, carry medications in a solid base that melts at body temperature.
- Inhalants are powdered or liquid forms of a drug that are administered via the respiratory route using an ultrasonic nebulizer, metered-dose aerosol or turbo inhaler, or vaporizer.
- Most medications are administered via the GI tract, which provides a fairly safe, but relatively slow-acting, site for drug absorption. Oral, sublingual, buccal, and rectal preparations are given via the GI tract.
- The technique for administering an enema depends on whether the drug requires retention.
- Parenteral liquids are packaged in vials, ampules, and self-contained or prefilled syringes. Parenteral medications in powdered form must be reconstituted before administration.
- Parenteral medications commonly are administered via the intradermal, S.C., I.M., and I.V. routes. Rotating injection sites improves absorption and minimizes patient discomfort.
- The nurse must match the type of syringe and appropriate needle size with the correct parenteral administration route. Alcohol most commonly is used to clean the skin before administration of parenteral medications.
- Intravenous medications may be administered as a bolus, intermittent infusion, or continuous infusion. An infusion pump may be used to deliver continuous I.V. medication.
- Other administration routes include intrathecal, epidural, intra-articular, dermal, ophthalmic, otic, nasal and sinus, respiratory, urethral, and vaginal.
- Intrathecal administration delivers medication to the brain through an access device implanted under the scalp.
- Epidural administration delivers medication to the spinal cord through a catheter.
- Intra-articular administration deposits medication directly into the joint.
- Medications administered via the dermal route include creams, lotions, ointments, powders, and patches.
- Ophthalmic medications are administered topically into the eyes; otic medications, into the ears.
- Liquid and powdered forms of medications may be administered to the patient's nose and sinuses by instillation, atomizer, or nasal aerosol device.
- Drug forms administered via the respiratory route include gas, such as oxygen; liquid, such as isoproterenol; and powder, such as cromolyn sodium.
- Urethral administration commonly is used for local antibiotic and antifungal therapy and involves instillation of liquid medication through a catheter.
- Vaginal administration is used for topical antibiotic or antifungal medications in liquid, suppository, cream, ointment, tablet, or gel form.

STUDY QUESTIONS

See Appendix 1 for answers.

1. To reduce GI distress for Hannah Selfridge, age 50, the physician prescribes enteric-coated aspirin. Where do enteric-coated tablets dissolve?
(a) in the mouth
(b) in the stomach
(c) in the intestine
(d) in the rectum

2. The nurse administers a cough elixir to 6-year-old Bobby Johnson, as prescribed. How does an elixir differ from a tincture?
(a) An elixir contains alcohol; a tincture does not.
(b) An elixir contains a sweetener; a tincture does not.
(c) A tincture contains alcohol; an elixir does not.
(d) A tincture contains water; an elixir does not.

3. Vera Danforth, age 63, has a history of coronary artery disease. Her physician has ordered nitroglycerine 1/150 gr. sublingual p.r.n. for chest pain. What should the nurse teach Ms. Danforth about taking this medication?
(a) Place the tablet between the cheek and gum.
(b) Chew the tablet thoroughly before swallowing.
(c) Place the tablet under the tongue.
(d) Swallow the tablet with at least 3 oz of water.

4. The nurse must administer a retention enema to Harlan Davies, age 69. To help ensure proper drug absorption from the enema, the nurse should encourage Mr. Davies to retain the medication for how long?
(a) at least 5 minutes
(b) at least 10 minutes
(c) at least 15 minutes
(d) at least 30 minutes

5. Later in the shift, the nurse must administer heparin subcutaneously to Mr. Davies. How many milliliters may be administered by the S.C. route?
(a) 1 ml
(b) 2 ml
(c) 3 ml
(d) 4 ml

6. Ellen Proctor, age 42, has an acute, painful musculoskeletal condition. Her physician orders orphenadrine (Norflex) 1 ampule (60 mg) I.M. q 12 hr. When should the nurse use the Z-track technique for I.M. injections?

(a) when a large dose is being administered
(b) when the drug is extremely irritating to tissue
(c) when the drug is extremely potent
(d) when the patient is uncooperative

7. Which administration route requires the nurse to aspirate for blood before injecting a medication?
(a) subcutaneous
(b) intradermal
(c) intramuscular
(d) intrathecal

8. The nurse administers a vaginal suppository, as prescribed, to Gwen Collins, age 35. To help Ms. Collins retain and absorb the medication, the nurse should advise her to remain supine for how long?
(a) 10 minutes
(b) 20 minutes
(c) 30 minutes
(d) 40 minutes

SELECTED REFERENCES

Davis, J. (1989). A practical system for narcotic control within the OR/PACU. *Journal of Post Anesthesia Nursing,* 4(1), 32-35.

Dick, L. (1989). Warning: Take only as directed. *RN,* 52(10), 83-88.

Drugs (2nd ed.). (1987). Nurse's Reference Library. Springhouse, PA: Springhouse Corporation.

Fuqua, R., and Stevens, K. (1988). What we know about medication errors: A literature review. *Journal of Nursing Quality Assurance,* 3(1), 1-17.

Kozier, B., and Erb, G. (1987). *Fundamentals of nursing: Concepts and procedures* (3rd ed.). Redwood City, CA: Addison-Wesley.

Ross, F. (1989). Doctor, nurse, and patient knowledge of prescribed medication in primary care. *Public Health,* 103(2), 131-137.

Smith, A., and Johnson, J. (1989). *Nurses guide to clinical procedures.* Philadelphia: Lippincott.

THE PEDIATRIC PATIENT

OBJECTIVES

After reading and studying this chapter, the student should be able to:

1. Explain how absorption, distribution, metabolism, and excretion of a drug differ between a child and an adult.

2. Describe how a drug's pharmacodynamics and pharmacotherapeutics are influenced by a child's age and individual response to the drug.

3. Calculate a correct pediatric dosage by weight and body-surface area.

4. Describe how to administer oral medications to children in different age-groups.

5. Select an appropriate intramuscular injection site and needle size for a pediatric patient.

6. Explain how to administer an intravenous medication safely to a pediatric patient.

7. Explain when and how to perform intraosseous medication administration.

8. Describe how absorption of a topical medication may differ in a neonate, infant, and small child.

9. Explain how to administer a drug rectally to a child.

10. Explain how to administer eye, ear, and nose drops to a child.

11. Develop a plan for teaching a pediatric patient and family members about the child's medications.

INTRODUCTION

Children are not small adults. Although the medication administration routes for children and adults are the same, pediatric injection sites, administration techniques, and especially dosages can differ greatly. Medication dosages for pediatric patients cannot be derived or scaled down from adult dosages, because the pharmacokinetics, pharmacodynamics, and pharmacotherapeutics of drugs in children vary substantially from those in adults. Physiologic differences and immature body systems exaggerate these variances and make medication effects less predictable—

sometimes even risky. The nurse must base all drug therapy on the child's physiologic and psychosocial development.

Chapter 8 begins by discussing factors that can influence the pharmacokinetic, pharmacodynamic, and pharmacotherapeutic processes in a pediatric patient. Next it describes the effects of drugs on growth and development. Then it explains pediatric dosage calculations, using body weight, body-surface area, and other rules for calculations. The chapter continues with techniques for oral, intramuscular (I.M.), subcutaneous (S.C.), intravenous (I.V.), topical, rectal, and other types of medication administration for pediatric patients. It concludes with information about patient and family education related to pediatric drug therapy.

PEDIATRIC PHARMACOLOGY

In a pediatric patient, many factors can influence the pharmacokinetic, pharmacodynamic, and pharmacotherapeutic processes that occur in the body. (For general information about these processes, see Chapter 2, Pharmacokinetics; Chapter 3, Pharmacodynamics; and Chapter 4, Pharmacotherapeutics.)

PHARMACOKINETICS

A child's age, physiologic state, body composition, immature organ function, and other factors can affect the absorption, distribution, metabolism, and excretion of a drug.

Absorption

After a drug is administered orally, its absorption depends on the child's age, the underlying disease, the dosage form, and the presence of other drugs or foods taken concurrently.

Differences in body composition

Total body water and extracellular fluid volume differ by age-group. These differences can affect significantly a drug's distribution. In a neonate, for example, the area for drug distribution and fluid volumes are proportionately greater than those in an adult. Because most drugs travel through extracellular fluid to reach their receptors, a drug is likely to become less concentrated and less effective in a neonate as it becomes more widely distributed.

AGE-GROUP	TOTAL BODY WATER (%)	EXTRACELLULAR FLUID VOLUME (%)
Premature neonate	94	50
Full-term neonate	85 to 90	35 to 40
Infant	75	35 to 40
Child	64	16 to 22
Adult	59	16

In a young child, the gastric pH is higher, or less acidic, than in an adult. In a premature infant, the pH differences are most dramatic because the immature gastrointestinal (GI) tract secretes a limited amount of acid. The gastric pH drops to an adult level sometime during the first year of life. Therefore, a child under age 1 will absorb more of those medications which react positively in a low-acid environment. For example, an infant would absorb more penicillin — a drug that is unstable in an acid environment — than an older child or an adult would. As the child develops, gastric pH decreases, acidity increases, and drug absorption is altered. Milk and formula also can affect gastric pH and may alter absorption. Therefore, most pediatric medications are administered when the child's stomach is empty.

Several other factors can influence drug absorption from the GI tract and make it less predictable and less efficient in a child under age 2. The shortness of the intestine and the presence of diarrhea can reduce the amount of time a drug is available for absorption. Decreased transit time through the GI tract also can decrease drug absorption.

Absorption of I.M. medications in infants may be unpredictable because of vasomotor instability and decreased muscle tone. Percutaneous absorption of S.C. medications in infants is increased because of an underdeveloped epidermal barrier and increased skin hydration.

A child will absorb a topical drug at about the same rate as an adult, but will absorb it more completely because of a greater body-surface area relative to total body mass. An occlusive dressing will enhance topical absorption further. Because young children absorb more medication topically, they are more likely than adults to experience adverse reactions to such topical drugs as steroid creams, salicylic acid, and silver sulfadiazine (when applied to burns that cover 20% or more of the body.)

Distribution

A drug's distribution is affected by its dilution in the body. In a neonate and an infant, total body water and extracellular fluid volume are higher than those of an older child or an adult. (For a comparison by age-group, see *Differences in body composition.*) The higher percentage of water in neonates and infants dilutes water-soluble drugs, reducing their blood concentration levels. That is why neonates and infants often require higher mg/kg dosages to achieve therapeutic drug concentration levels in the blood.

Body composition also affects the distribution of fat-soluble drugs, although to a lesser degree than water-soluble ones. As the percentage of fat increases with age, so does the distribution of fat-soluble drugs. Therefore, distribution of these drugs is more limited in children than in adults.

In a neonate, the immature liver also may affect drug distribution by decreasing formation of plasma proteins, which results in lower serum protein levels and higher fluid volume than in an adult. This reduces the number of plasma proteins for drugs to bind to. Because only unbound, or free, drugs produce a pharmacologic effect, the infant's decreased protein binding can intensify drug effects and possibly cause toxicity. Other adverse drug effects can occur when drugs, such as salicylates and sulfonamides, compete for the same protein-binding sites as endogenous substances, such as bilirubin and free fatty acids. Any medication that competes with bilirubin for protein-binding sites or inhibits the binding of bilirubin increases the risk of kernicterus (bilirubin accumulation in the central nervous system). The higher fluid volume in infants increases the volume of distribution and can dilute the drug.

Metabolism

In most people, the liver adequately metabolizes drugs. In an infant, however, the immature liver may metabolize drugs inefficiently. As the liver matures during the first year of life, drug metabolism improves.

Dosage and choice of therapeutic agent may be altered for an infant with immature liver function or liver disease. The immature liver function increases the risk of toxicity with some drugs, such as chloramphenicol. When the liver fails to inactivate this drug, toxic levels can accumulate in the blood and produce gray baby syndrome, characterized by rapid respirations, ashen gray cyanosis, vomiting, loose green stools, progressive abdominal distention, vasomotor collapse, and possibly death. Fortunately, drug discontinuation can reverse the syndrome if discontinuation occurs as soon as symptoms appear.

Children typically metabolize drugs that require oxidation, such as theophylline, caffeine, phenobarbital, and phenytoin, more rapidly than adults. The rate of metabolism for drugs such as aspirin and the sulfonamides that are catalyzed by microsomal or nonmicrosomal enzymes can vary among individuals and may be genetically determined.

In early infancy, drug metabolism and hepatic enzyme activity differ between the sexes and may be related to changes in diurnal rhythms. Before puberty, other sex-related differences in drug metabolism occur, especially in the microsomal enzymes that catalyze gonadal steroid metabolism.

Excretion

The rate of renal excretion of a drug depends on the rate of glomerular filtration, tubular reabsorption, and tubular secretion. Because most drug excretion occurs in the urine, the degree of renal development can affect drug excretion and, ultimately, dosage requirements for a pediatric patient.

At birth, the kidneys are immature, renal excretion is slow, and drug dosages must be adjusted carefully. As the kidneys mature during the first few months after birth, renal excretion of drugs increases, although the rate of increase is slow for a premature neonate. At about age 3 months, the kidneys can concentrate urine at the adult level. (For a summary of these developments, see *Physiologic characteristics of pediatric patients.*) Therefore, certain drugs, such as digoxin and most antibiotics, will need particularly careful dosage adjustments until the renal system matures completely.

Some drugs, such as nafcillin, are excreted by the biliary tree into the intestinal tract. In the first few days after birth, however, biliary blood flow is low, which can prolong the effects. Administering the drug in lower doses can prevent toxicity. Interactions with other drugs also may affect drug excretion. The nurse must be cognizant of these facts and familiar with possible drug interactions.

PHARMACODYNAMICS

Biochemically, a drug will display the same mechanism of action in all individuals. For example, if a drug normally inhibits the transfer of a substance into a cell, it will perform this action in anyone, child or adult. The response to a drug, however, can be affected by the maturity of the target organ and may require a dosage adjustment for a neonate, infant, or child. In addition, receptor sensitivity varies in infants and young children; it may be increased or decreased for certain drugs. Therefore, an infant or child may require a lower or higher dosage of a drug than expected.

Physiologic characteristics of pediatric patients

Body system immaturity and other physiologic characteristics of a pediatric patient can influence drug therapy.

AREA AFFECTED	CHARACTERISTIC
Renal system	• From birth until about age 3 months, the immature system has a decreased ability to concentrate urine. • Urinary excretion remains low until about age 2½, when the kidneys become functionally mature.
Gastrointestinal system	• Transit time through the GI tract increases until the toddler years, when it nears the adult rate. • Stomach acidity increases as the child becomes a toddler. • The immature liver interferes with the child's ability to metabolize drugs until about age 1. • The digestive processes mature by the preschool years.
Body-surface area	• The relationship between surface area and body weight changes as the child grows. The proportion of body-surface area to weight in an infant age 2 months may be 2½ times that of an adult, decreasing in a child ages 1 to 3 to roughly 2 times that of an adult. By age 12, the child's body-surface area to weight proportion is only slightly greater than an adult's.
Metabolism	• Metabolism is increased during infancy and childhood in relation to body weight.

PHARMACOTHERAPEUTICS

The goal of medication administration is to achieve and maintain a therapeutic drug level without producing toxicity. Achievement of a therapeutic level depends on the drug's absorption, distribution, metabolism, and excretion. For example, children between ages 2 and 6 clear the bronchodilator theophylline much faster than adults or neonates do, and male children clear and excrete the drug faster than female children. For this reason, the child may need higher doses more frequently or may need sustained-release preparations to achieve therapeutic drug levels.

To maintain therapeutic levels, the patient must receive repeated doses at intervals that may vary according to age. For example, a neonate probably would receive the antibiotic gentamicin every 12 hours initially because of an immature renal system that cannot excrete the drug as well as an older child's. An infant or child would be more likely to receive gentamicin every 8 hours initially because the more mature renal system can excrete the drug more efficiently. However, because the response to drugs is individual, the specific dosage for a pediatric patient is best determined by serum gentamicin levels.

The nurse must exercise extreme caution to achieve therapeutic effects without producing toxicity in a child. The nurse must calculate drug dosages and monitor the child's drug responses carefully.

Several drugs that commonly are used in pediatric patients have low therapeutic indexes (differences between therapeutic and toxic serum concentrations) and should be monitored by serum concentration levels. These drugs include aminoglycosides, digoxin, and phenytoin. Phenobarbital and other anticonvulsants can be monitored in the same way, although they have higher therapeutic indexes.

Dehydration and acid-base or electrolyte imbalances can alter the therapeutic and toxic effects of a medication. The nurse must monitor a child with these disorders closely for adverse drug reactions.

DRUG EFFECTS ON GROWTH AND DEVELOPMENT

Some drugs can have an adverse effect on a child's growth and development. Long-term treatment with glucocorticosteroids, which may be necessary for a child with an organ transplant or asthma, may stunt growth. In these cases, the benefits of drug therapy must be evaluated against the effects on growth. A jaundiced infant who receives drugs that compete with bilirubin-binding sites may develop kernicterus, which may result in mental retardation. The antibiotic tetracycline can produce tooth stains if given before the permanent teeth have formed. It also can bind calcium and phosphates and temporarily depress bone growth during the last half of gestation and during childhood from birth to age 8.

Drug excretion in breast milk
Many drugs are excreted in breast milk, and some can have an adverse effect on an infant. The nurse should advise a breast-feeding woman to avoid taking medications, if possible. (For more detailed information, see Chapter 12, The Pregnant or Lactating Patient.)

PEDIATRIC NURSING CONSIDERATIONS

When caring for a pediatric patient, the nurse must pay particular attention to dosage calculations, administration techniques, and education of patients and their families.

PEDIATRIC DOSAGE CALCULATIONS

To determine the correct pediatric dosage of a medication, physicians, pharmacists, and nurses usually use two computation methods. One is based on the child's weight in kilograms; the other uses the child's body-surface area. Other methods are less accurate and are not recommended.

Dosage range per kilogram of body weight
Currently, many pharmaceutical companies provide information on the safe dosage ranges for drugs given to children. The companies usually provide the dosage ranges in milligrams per kilogram of body weight and in many cases give similar information for adult dosage ranges. The following example and explanation indicate how to calculate the safe pediatric dosage range for a drug, using the company's suggested safe dosage range provided in milligrams per kilogram.

For a pediatric patient, a physician orders a drug with a suggested dosage range of 10 to 12 mg/kg of body weight per day. The child weighs 12 kg. What is the safe daily dosage range for the child?

The nurse must calculate the lower and upper limits of the dosage range provided by the manufacturer. The nurse first calculates the dosage based on 10 mg per kilogram of body weight, then calculates the dosage based on 12 mg per kilogram of body weight. The answers represent the lower and upper limits of the daily dosage range, expressed in milligrams per kilogram of the child's weight. (For a similar problem and its solution, see *Calculating pediatric dosages*.)

Body-surface area
A second method for calculating safe pediatric dosages uses the child's body-surface area as a factor. This method may provide a more accurate calculation because the child's body-surface area is thought to parallel the child's organ growth and maturation and metabolic rate.

The nurse determines the body-surface area of a child by using a three-columned chart called a nomogram. (For details on how to use a nomogram, see *Calculating pediatric dosages by body-surface area,* page 154.) The nurse marks the child's height in the first column and the child's weight in the third column, then draws a line between the two marks. The point at which the line intersects the vertical scale in the second column indicates the estimated body-surface area of the child in square meters. To calculate the child's approximate dose, the nurse uses the body-surface area measurement in the following equation:

$$\frac{\text{body-surface area of child}}{\text{average adult body-surface area (1.73 m}^2)} \times \frac{\text{average}}{\text{adult}} = \frac{\text{child's}}{\text{dose}}$$

The following example illustrates the use of the equation. Using a nomogram, the nurse finds that a 25-pound child 33 inches tall has a body-surface area of 0.52 square meters. The nurse needs to determine the child's dose of a drug with an average adult dose of 100 mg. The equation would appear as:

$$\frac{0.52 \text{ m}^2}{1.73 \text{ m}^2} \times 100 \text{ mg} = 30.06 \text{ mg (child's dose)}$$

The child should receive 30 mg of the drug.

Other rules

Because drug companies provide dosage ranges, nurses calculate pediatric dosages primarily to check and verify them. The importance of verifying dosages necessitates the nurse's understanding of the rules. Three other rules for calculating and verifying pediatric doses follow:

• Clark's rule (for children over age 2), based on *body weight* only:

$$\frac{\text{child's weight (1b)}}{150 \text{ lb (average adult weight)}} \times \frac{\text{average}}{\text{adult}} = \frac{\text{child's}}{\text{dose}}$$

• Fried's rule (for infants under age 1), based on child's *age* only:

$$\frac{\text{child's age (months)}}{\substack{150 \text{ months (age at which an} \\ \text{adult dose would be appropriate)}}} \times \frac{\text{average}}{\text{adult}} = \frac{\text{child's}}{\text{dose}}$$

• Young's rule (for children ages 2 to 12), based on child's *age* only:

$$\frac{\text{Child's age (yr)}}{\text{child's age (yr)} + 12} = \frac{\text{average}}{\text{adult}} = \frac{\text{child's}}{\text{dose}}$$

Clark's rule, Fried's rule, and Young's rule use an average adult dose as the standard from which to derive pediatric doses. The results are approximate. In practice, a safe adult dose of a particular drug usually falls within a range of doses, and depends on the individual. Therefore, the average adult dose used in the rules as a standard is imprecise.

Each rule also depends on an average developmental level of the child. For example, Fried's rule and Young's rule rely solely on the child's age. Fried's rule considers a child of 150 months (12.5 years) to be an adult, whereas

Calculating pediatric dosages

The physician orders 150 mg of a drug to be given q6h to an 18-kg child. (Remember that 1 kg equals 2.2 lb). The literature provided by the manufacturer indicates that the safe dosage range for the drug is 30 mg/kg to 35 mg/kg per day, to be given in divided doses. Can the nurse safely administer the ordered dosage?

Using the ratio method to determine the lower limit of the safe dosage range, the nurse sets up the following:

30 mg : X mg :: 1 kg : 18 kg

After cross multiplying the means and the extremes, the nurse finds that X = 540 mg; the 540 mg represents the low dosage.

Using the same method, the nurse then calculates the upper limit of the safe dosage range:

35 mg : X mg :: 1 kg : 18 kg

After cross multiplying the means and the extremes, the nurse finds that X = 630 mg, the high dosage.

The safe dosage range for the child is 540 to 630 mg per day. Because the physician ordered 150 mg to be given every 6 hours, the child would receive four doses per day, or a total daily dosage of 150 mg x four doses per day = 600 mg per day. This daily dosage falls within the safe range, so the nurse can safely administer 150 mg q6h.

Young's rule uses 12 years as the measure. Both rules assume that the child's body systems and functions achieve a particular level of maturity consistent with the child's chronological age. The assumption is somewhat unreliable because children at any age display a range of normal maturational levels. Furthermore, Fried's rule and Young's rule do not consider the child's weight and body size. The following example illustrates what can occur when using Fried's rule or Young's rule to calculate pediatric drug doses for a child of 15 months who does not fall within the age range for either of these rules.

A child of 15 months is to receive a drug usually given to adults in 100-milligram doses. If using Fried's rule, the nurse would calculate the following:

$$\frac{15 \text{ months}}{150 \text{ months}} \times 100 \text{ mg} = 10 \text{ mg (child's dose)}$$

With Young's rule, the calculations would be:

$$\frac{1.25 \text{ yr}}{1.25 \text{ yr} + 12 \text{ yr}} \times 100 \text{ mg} = 9.43 \text{ mg (child's dose)}$$

Using Fried's rule and Young's rule to calculate for the same situation results in a discrepancy of 0.57 mg.

Clark's rule considers the child's weight but not the child's age. By not considering the child's age, Clark's rule

Calculating pediatric dosages by body-surface area

The nurse can determine a correct pediatric drug dosage by estimating the child's body-surface area. If the child is average size, find the child's weight and corresponding surface area on the first, boxed scale. Otherwise, use the nomogram to the right. To do this, mark the child's height in the first column and weight in the third column; then draw a line between the two marks. Where the line intersects the scale in the second column indicates the estimated body-surface area of the child in square meters.

To calculate the child's dosage, complete this equation:

$$\frac{\text{body-surface area of child}}{\text{average adult body-surface area (1.73 m}^2\text{)}} \times \frac{\text{average adult dose}}{} = \frac{\text{child's dose}}{}$$

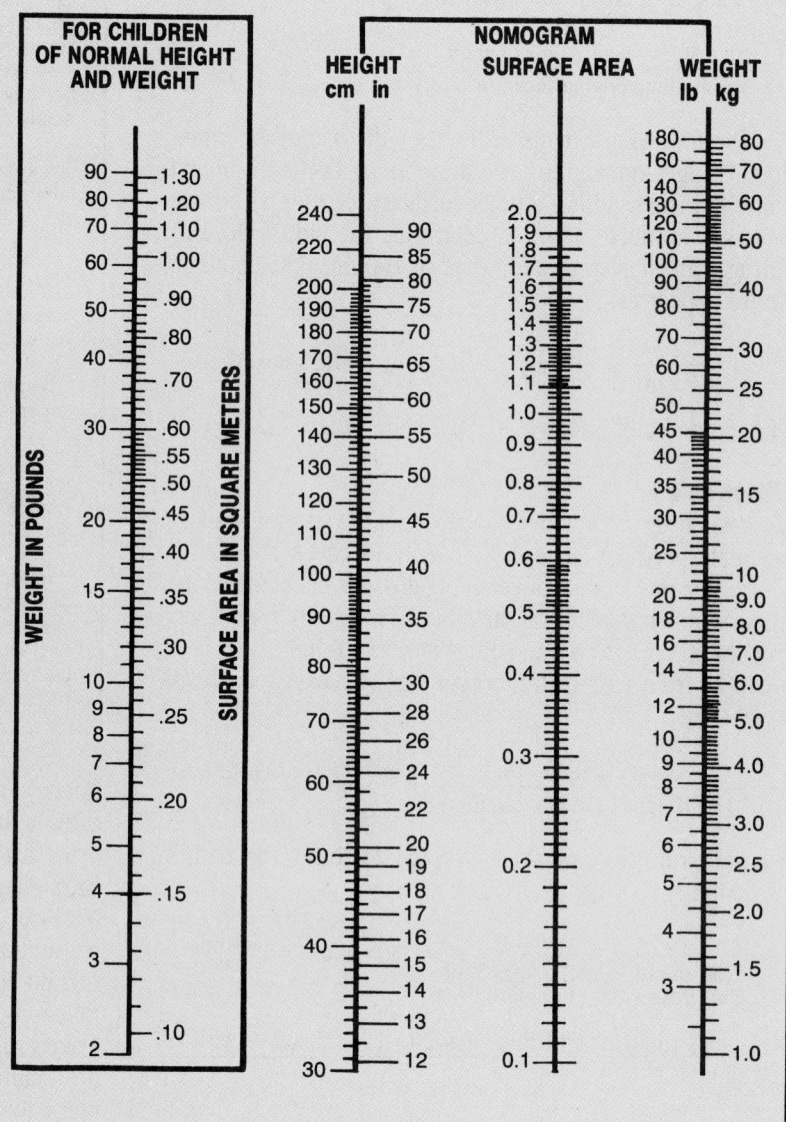

ignores individual differences in body system maturity. If the child of 15 months in the previous example weighed 27 pounds, calculating with Clark's rule would result in the following:

$$\frac{27 \text{ lb}}{150 \text{ lb}} \times 100 \text{ mg} = 18 \text{ mg (child's dose)}$$

Using Clark's rule results in a significantly larger dose than the doses calculated using Fried's rule or Young's rule. The child's dose could vary from 9.43 mg to 18 mg, almost twice the first amount. The discrepancies underscore that

pediatric doses calculated using specific equations represent, at best, approximations. Therefore, calculating with equations other than those involving dosage ranges per kilogram of body weight or body-surface area is *not* recommended for determining dosages.

PEDIATRIC ADMINISTRATION TECHNIQUES

Administering drugs safely to a child requires special attention to the five rights because any medication error can have a much greater impact on a child than on an adult.

The nurse must check for the right patient name by reading the child's identification band before giving each dose of medication. The nurse also must make sure that the medication is the right drug, in the right dose, for the right route, and at the right time and frequency.

Checking the drug's dosage is particularly important. The nurse can use the body weight or body-surface area method to check the dosage for accuracy. When preparing the medication, the nurse must calculate the dosage carefully and use the correct amount and type of diluent. When certain drugs, such as insulin, anticoagulants, or narcotics, are ordered, two nurses should calculate and check the dosage for accuracy. If an order seems incorrect, the nurse should check the drug's package insert or pediatric and pharmacologic references or call the pharmacist to verify the order. If the order is incorrect, the nurse should notify the physician so that the order can be corrected.

Administering medication to a child also requires careful attention to other details. Besides observing the five rights, the nurse also must be aware of adverse reactions and drug interactions. To ensure the pediatric patient's safety, the nurse should use this checklist for medication administration:
• Check the physician's order.
• Calculate the correct dosage.
• Have a second nurse calculate the dosage to verify accuracy.
• Prepare the right medication and dosage.
• Verify the patient's identity before administering the medication.
• Administer the medication as prescribed.
• Document the medication administration.
• Observe the patient for therapeutic effects and adverse drug reactions.

For each route of administration, the nurse must modify adult administration techniques for a pediatric patient. No matter which route is used, the nurse should try to elicit the child's cooperation to make medication administration as easy as possible. If the child is unable to cooperate, the nurse should enlist help to hold the child still during administration. (For further information, see *Administering pediatric medications,* page 156.)

Oral administration

Although absorption from the GI tract is less predictable than by other routes, oral administration frequently is prescribed because it is the least traumatic for the child. However, oral administration to a child can challenge a nurse's skills. Although a child willingly may swallow a medication at first, the child may begin to spit, drool, or choke after realizing that the medication tastes unpleasant. When this happens, the nurse must try to give the medication with as little distress as possible to the child. To do this, a nurse might hold a child in a bottle-feeding position, placing the child's inner arm behind the nurse's back, supporting the head in the crook of the nurse's elbow, and holding the child's free hand with the hand of the supporting arm. This position immobilizes the child's head in the crook of the nurse's arm and prevents the child from spilling the medication with either hand.

If an infant or small child must be restrained for medication administration, the nurse should use a syringe without a needle to administer small, controlled doses. To minimize the risk of choking or aspirating, the nurse should hold the child's head upright or to the side.

Then the nurse should slide the syringe into the child's mouth about halfway back between the gums and cheeks and squirt in a small amount of medication. This administration technique offers several advantages. Placement of the medication deep in the side of the mouth makes it difficult for the child to lose the medication by spitting or drooling. Although medication administration takes longer because the drug is given in small amounts, this technique reduces the risk of choking, coughing, and vomiting because it does not stimulate the gag reflex.

The nurse never should place medication in an infant's formula because it can lead to several problems. For example, the infant may not take the feeding if the medication alters its taste. If this happens, the nurse will not be able to determine how much medication the child actually took, and the child will not receive the drug's therapeutic effects or the formula's nutrition. Also, administration with formula can alter the absorption of some medications. For example, Osmolite can inhibit the absorption of phenytoin suspension.

During oral administration, the nurse can use certain techniques to enhance the pediatric patient's cooperation, depending on the child's development. An infant or small child may squirm less if the nurse talks soothingly and holds the child's head securely. Obviously, an explanation will not help an infant to cooperate, but it may reassure the child's caregiver. An explanation may help a toddler react better if it is given just before the nurse administers the medication. However, it will not help the toddler to cooperate. To promote cooperation, the nurse should praise the toddler's efforts. After receiving an explanation, preschoolers will attempt to cooperate. Young school-age children should be able to exercise more restraint and a greater degree of cooperation. The nurse should not shame preschool and young school-age children if they have difficulty cooperating but should help them gain some control by allowing choices when possible. For example, the nurse may ask if the child would like to take the medicine in a cup or a spoon.

Administering pediatric medications

To administer pediatric medications effectively, the nurse must understand how children of different ages think about and react to drugs and know how to intervene appropriately.

AGE-GROUP	PATIENT CHARACTERISTICS AND REACTIONS TO MEDICATION	NURSING INTERVENTIONS
Infant	• In a very young infant, lack of experience eliminates fear; the infant may take medication willingly. • Between ages 5 and 8 months, the infant begins to observe visual cues and anticipate unpleasant events. • By age 10 months, the infant will try to get away from anticipated unpleasantness and may spit, drool, or choke to avoid taking medication.	• Hold the infant still when giving an oral medication. • Make the medication palatable; if appropriate, mix it with syrup or applesauce. • Administer medication in a syringe placed in the side of the mouth or from a spoon placed far back on the tongue. • Allow the infant to suck medication from a nipple. • Give medication slowly to prevent choking and spitting. • Ask the parent or a coworker to hold the infant still during a painful administration. • Cuddle, rock, and speak soothingly to the infant after a painful procedure.
Toddler	• A toddler has a limited ability to express anger in words but will protest loudly. • A toddler may try to escape from the nurse or physician. • A toddler has a limited understanding of explanations and a poor concept of time. • The child may not be able to cooperate and may squirm because of a lack of self-control.	• Explain the procedure very simply just before performing it. • Mention that the child has no options about taking the medication. • Tell the child that you realize the procedure is unpleasant. Warn the child before a painful procedure. • Let the toddler exercise some control over the situation by allowing a choice of a spoon, straw, cup, or syringe to take an oral medication. • Try to improve the medication's taste by mixing it with a small amount of syrup or food, if appropriate. • Use the child's rituals to administer medication whenever possible. • Hold the child still, if necessary. Praise any attempts the child makes to hold still. • Encourage the child to express feelings, and offer reassurance that the child is not being punished. • Allow the parents to comfort the child after the procedure.
Preschooler	• A child in this age-group has a limited ability to understand a detailed explanation. • A preschooler will attempt to cooperate. • After an I.M. injection, a preschooler may think that body fluids will leak out of the injection site.	• Express faith in the child's ability to cooperate even with an unpleasant procedure. • Provide options, whenever possible, to give the child a sense of control over the situation. • Explain the procedure simply. • Warn the child before a painful procedure. • Praise the child for all attempts to cooperate. • Encourage the child to express feelings. • Offer the child an adhesive bandage after an I.M. injection. • Allow the parents or caregiver to comfort the child after the procedure. • Use therapeutic play before and after the procedure. Listen carefully to the child's play. Clear up any misconceptions, and provide further explanations as needed.
School-age child	• The older the school-age child, the greater the ability to exercise restraint and to cooperate.	• Explain the procedure in detail. • Allow the child to make choices, whenever possible. • Warn the child in advance when a painful procedure is scheduled. • Reassure the child that no one likes the procedure. • Praise the child for cooperating. • Listen to the child's concerns and feelings.
Adolescent	• An adolescent's reaction to medication is similar to an adult's. The ability to cooperate is highly developed.	• Include the adolescent in discussions and decisions about the procedure. • Allow the adolescent to make choices and to exercise as much control as possible. • Give support and encouragement, but do not treat the adolescent like a child.

I.M. injection sites

The nurse can use several landmarks to identify I.M. injection sites for pediatric patients. The vastus lateralis and rectus femoris muscles are the recommended sites for an infant or a toddler. The dorsogluteal and ventrogluteal sites can be used only after the toddler has been walking for about 1 year.

Dorsogluteal

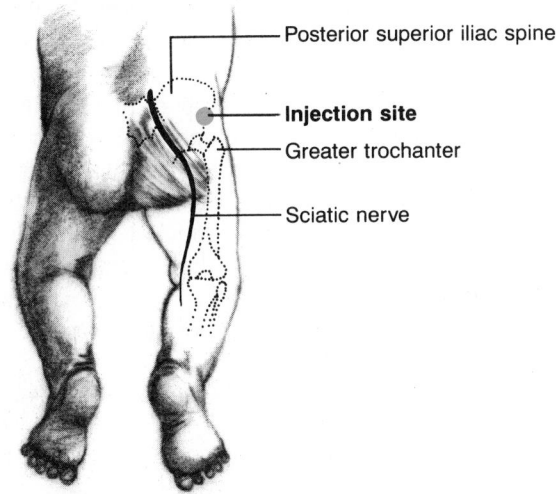

- Posterior superior iliac spine
- **Injection site**
- Greater trochanter
- Sciatic nerve

Ventrogluteal

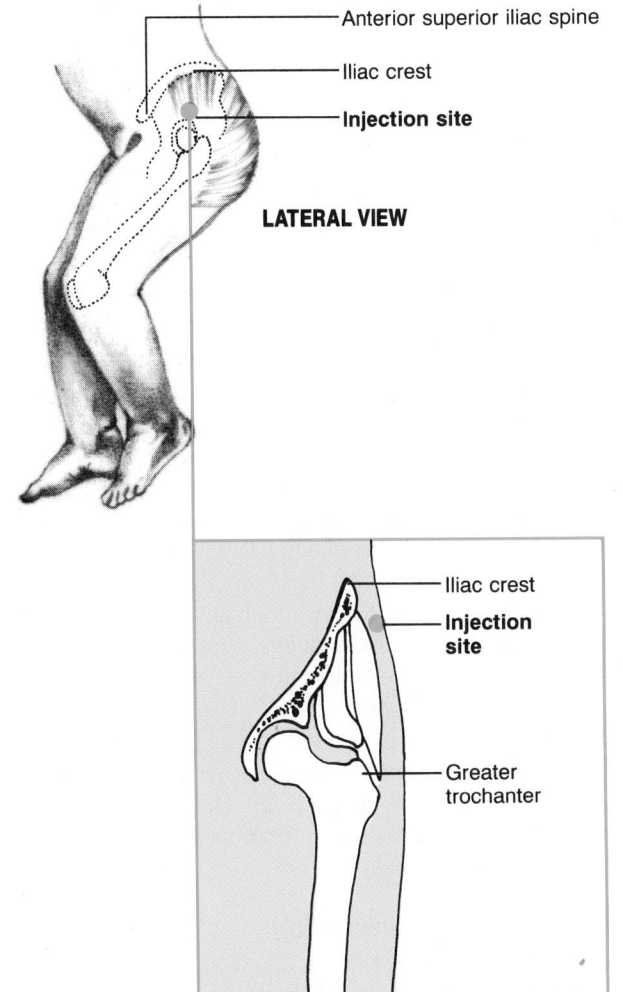

- Anterior superior iliac spine
- Iliac crest
- **Injection site**

LATERAL VIEW

- Iliac crest
- **Injection site**
- Greater trochanter

ANTERIOR VIEW

Vastus lateralis and rectus femoris

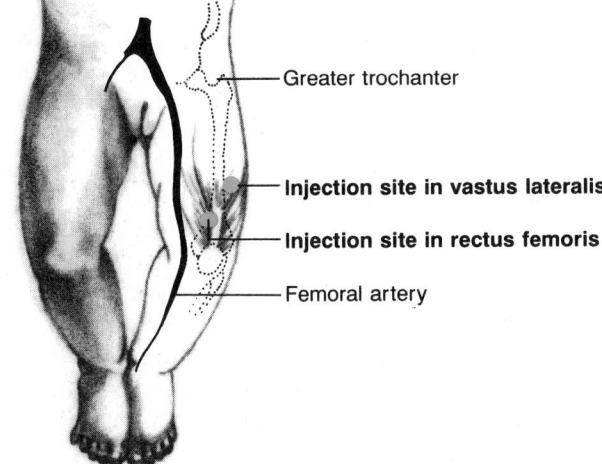

- Greater trochanter
- **Injection site in vastus lateralis**
- **Injection site in rectus femoris**
- Femoral artery

Intramuscular administration

For an I.M. injection, the nurse should use the smallest gauge needle appropriate for the medication. This usually is a needle that is 25G to 22G. The needle length should not exceed 1 inch (2.5 cm), except for an adult-size adolescent, who may require a 1½-inch (3.8-cm) needle.

The recommended injection sites vary with age. The vastus lateralis and rectus femoris muscles are the recommended sites for an infant or toddler. For a child who has been walking for about 1 year, the nurse can give an I.M. injection in the ventrogluteal or dorsogluteal area. Walking develops these muscles, thus reducing the risk of sciatic nerve damage during an I.M. injection. (For illustrations of these areas, see *I.M. injection sites.*) For an older child, the nurse may use an adult I.M. injection site, such as the deltoid, gluteus maximus, ventrogluteal, vastus lateralis, or rectus femoris muscle. The nurse uses the same I.M. injection technique for a child as for an adult. (For a description of this technique, see Chapter 9, Routes and Techniques of Administration.)

The air bubble technique, which uses an air bubble to clear the needle and hub after medication is drawn into the syringe, is not recommended for pediatric I.M. injections. Because the calibration on most syringes does include the amount in the hub and needle, an overdose can occur with the air bubble technique.

The nurse giving an I.M. injection can use certain techniques to help ensure a child's cooperation and safety. Before entering the child's room, the nurse should prepare the medication and syringe. The nurse should provide an explanation for all children regardless of age or ability to understand or cooperate. For the infant, the explanation will be helpful to the parent or primary caregiver. Although the toddler's understanding may be limited, the nurse should give a simple explanation immediately before the injection. Because the toddler will not be able to cooperate and may protest loudly, the nurse should make the explanation brief, perform the injection quickly, and allow the caregiver to comfort the child. If the child is alone, the nurse should hold and comfort the child after the injection. Before administering an injection to a preschooler, the nurse should explain the procedure simply and tell the child that the shot will hurt and that it is OK to cry. The nurse should emphasize that the child will need to hold still and that another nurse will help the child hold still, if necessary. Then the nurse should give the injection and praise the child for any cooperative efforts. A preschooler has a poor concept of body integrity and may think that body fluids will leak out of the injection site. To relieve this fear, the nurse should give the child an adhesive bandage. The school-age child should benefit from an explanation of the procedure and probably will be able to hold still. However, a young school-age child or one who is stressed might need help to hold still. The nurse must never shame the child, but should praise every attempt at cooperation. The adolescent generally has enough self-control to cooperate and benefits greatly from an explanation.

Subcutaneous administration

Subcutaneous administration is the same in a child as in an adult. (For a description of the technique, see Chapter 9, Routes and Techniques of Administration.) The needle should be 27G to 23G and $3/8$ to $5/8$ inch (1 to 1.5 cm) long. The nurse must remember to provide an age-appropriate explanation and to position the child properly, as described under "Intramuscular administration."

Intravenous administration

Pediatric I.V. administration poses several challenges for the nurse. For example, the nurse must assist with or perform the I.V. insertion, which can be traumatic for the child and parents. The nurse also must monitor the I.V. closely to maintain its patency.

The nurse should explain the procedure to the parents of a neonate or an infant, to prepare them for the necessity of the I.V. and the possibility that the infant's head will be shaved if the I.V. catheter is inserted in the scalp. The nurse also should tell the parents that the procedure may take some time so that they do not expect to see the infant again in a few minutes. For a toddler, the nurse should explain the procedure briefly just before taking the child to the treatment room, because the toddler's concept of time is not fully developed. A toddler probably will not be able to cooperate, so the nurse should plan to restrain the child carefully to ensure safe insertion of the I.V. catheter. For a preschooler, who has a better concept of time, the nurse may explain the procedure a short time before performing it. A preschooler especially needs to know that crying is permitted, but that he or she is expected to hold still. Although a young school-age child should be able to hold still without help for a painful procedure, the nurse should offer to help, by holding the child's hand, for instance. Generally, an older school-age child or an adolescent can hold still for this procedure.

For an infant or small child, the nurse uses a 24G to 22G I.V. catheter. For an older child, the nurse may use a 20G to 18G catheter. Silastic catheters are preferred because they are less irritating to the vein.

Before inserting the I.V. catheter, the nurse should proceed as follows: (1) tear off strips of tape and keep them ready to secure the inserted catheter; prime the I.V. tubing, removing all of the air bubbles, and cover the end with a sterile capped needle, a sterile capped T-connector, or the tubing's protective cover; and observe the I.V. fluids for contaminants and glass bottles for cracks or breaks. If irregularities are detected, the nurse should obtain a new container of I.V. fluid.

(2) Select a site for I.V. catheter insertion. Unlike in an adult, the antecubital fossa is not the first choice for a pediatric I.V. site; the child is likely to bend the arm with the inserted I.V. and dislodge the needle. Instead, start with the veins of the hand and lower arm to identify a site, and work from the distal to more proximal areas. That way, if an I.V. infiltrates in the lower hand, the nurse can use the veins of the wrist and forearm for other sites. The same rule applies to selecting an I.V. site in a lower extremity. Use the veins on the dorsum of the foot first and proceed upward to the ankle, if necessary.

(3) Insert the I.V. catheter as for an adult. (For a description of this technique, see Chapter 9, Routes and Techniques of Administration.)

(4) After inserting the I.V. catheter, secure it with the pretorn tape, restrain the extremity, and assess the circulation in the digits. At the end of the procedure, ensure that all tourniquets have been removed. A tourniquet inadvertently left in place can impair sensation and circulation in the affected extremity.

If a head vein is used for I.V. access in an infant, apply a "mummy" restraint, which holds the infant's head firmly in place and prevents body movement during the procedure, leaving the nurse's hands free to insert the catheter. Make sure that the infant can breathe adequately with this restraint in place.

If an extremity is used for I.V. access, use a padded board to secure the hand or foot. Some nurses prefer to secure the extremity to the board before starting the I.V., but others prefer to secure it afterward.

With either method, tape the I.V. so that the insertion site is visible for frequent monitoring. If the extremity must be immobilized by pinning the arm board to the sheet or using a sandbag, be careful to secure the I.V. so that hourly observation of the site can verify no signs of complications. Listen to the child to detect complications. If the child complains of pain at the I.V. site or if an infant or young child becomes unusually irritable, check closely for signs of infiltration or phlebitis, such as redness or swelling.

Infants, small children, and children with compromised cardiopulmonary status are particularly vulnerable to fluid overload with I.V. medication administration. To prevent this problem, the nurse should use a volume control set (a volume-control device in the I.V. tubing) and an infusion pump or syringe and place no more than 2 hours' worth of I.V. fluid in the volume control set at a time. These techniques help ensure that a limited amount of fluid is infused in a controlled manner.

Other factors can influence the amount and rapidity of medication administration. In tubing with a narrow lumen, the medication will reach the child faster than in tubing with a wide lumen because of increased pressure in the narrow tubing. If a child has a delicate fluid balance, an infusion (auto) syringe can deliver small amounts of fluid. With this technique, a syringe containing medication is secured in the cradle of an autoinfusion mechanism. The nurse can set the correct rate on the syringe to infuse the medication automatically.

Careful monitoring of intake and output can help prevent fluid overload and ensure that the child gets the amount of fluid ordered. Careful observation of the infusion will detect clot formation in the catheter, which is especially likely with a slow I.V. rate. Frequent assessment of the flow rate—particularly with gravity infusion—is important because position changes, crying, and restraints can impede the flow of fluids.

With all I.V. medications, the nurse must flush the volume control set and tubing before and after administration. Some medications are not compatible, and if they are mixed they may form a precipitate in the I.V. administration set. The nurse should check with the pharmacist if a question arises about medication compatibility. If a precipitate forms, the nurse must stop the infusion immediately and change all of the tubing.

Intraosseous administration

In an emergency, intraosseous drug administration may be used for a critically ill child under age 3. To administer medications by this route, the nurse inserts a bone marrow needle (or spinal needle with stylette, trephin, or standard 18G to 16G hypodermic needle) into the antero-medial surface of the proximal tibia 1 to 3 cm (1") below the tibial tuberosity. The nurse should direct the needle at a perpendicular or slightly inferior angle to avoid the epiphyseal plate.

When the needle is in the marrow cavity, the nurse will feel no resistance after the needle passes the bony cortex and will be able to aspirate bone marrow, the needle will remain upright without support, and the infusion will flow freely without subcutaneous infiltration. If bone or marrow obstructs the needle, the nurse should replace the needle by passing a second one through the cannula.

After ensuring that the needle is inserted properly, the nurse stabilizes and secures it with gauze dressing and tape. When the child is medically stable, the nurse should try to secure an intravenous route.

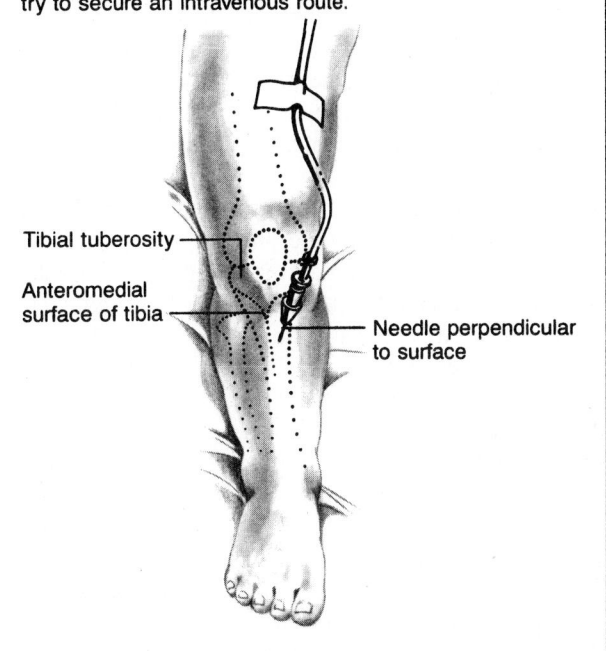

Tibial tuberosity

Anteromedial surface of tibia

Needle perpendicular to surface

Intraosseous administration

For a critically ill child under age 3, medications may be administered by the intraosseous route. This temporary administration route is used in emergencies, when I.V. access is unavailable. It allows drug infusion through a needle in the medullary cavity of a long bone. From there, marrow sinusoids allow the medication to drain into large medullary venous channels and then into the systemic circulation. This route may be used to administer fluids, blood, catechol-amines, calcium, digitalis, heparin, lidocaine, atropine, sodium bicarbonate, and antibiotics. (For more information, see *Intraosseous administration*.)

Topical administration

In a neonate, infant, or small child, thin epidermis and large body-surface area allow for increased drug absorption of topical medications and explain why a young pediatric patient is more likely to develop a toxic, systemic drug reaction than an older patient. Topical corticosteroids can produce particularly severe reactions. To decrease the risk of toxic effects, the nurse should wash a cleansing solution off an infant's skin, unless otherwise instructed, and apply a topical medication as thinly as possible and to as small a body-surface area as possible. When removing a topical medication from a jar, the nurse should use a tongue depressor to avoid contaminating the medication with the hand used to apply the medication.

Rectal administration

Drug absorption from the rectum may be unpredictable. The presence of stool in the rectum can delay, decrease, or block drug absorption. Nevertheless, medications often are administered rectally when oral administration is contraindicated or when they are designed for rectal administration. Children who are neutropenic or thrombocytopenic, however, should not receive rectal medications because of the increased risk of infection and bleeding caused by tissue trauma.

Before administering the rectal medication, the nurse should explain the procedure and the importance of retaining the suppository rather than expelling it. To administer the medication, the nurse uses a gloved hand to insert the unwrapped, lubricated suppository past the rectal sphincters. Then the nurse should hold the buttocks together so the child cannot expel the medication.

Some suppositories are scored and can be halved easily and accurately, if necessary. If an unscored suppository must be halved, the nurse should split it lengthwise to ensure even distribution of its medication.

Administration of eye, ear, and nose drops

To administer eyedrops, the nurse may need to have a coworker restrain an infant or toddler. For any pediatric patient, the nurse places the hand that holds the dropper on the child's forehead so that it will move as the child's head moves and decrease the risk of injury. With the other hand, the nurse can pull down the lower lid to expose the conjunctival sac. If the child is old enough to cooperate, the nurse should ask the child to look up and then instill the drops in the lower conjunctival sac. If the child will not cooperate, the nurse can place the eyedrops at the inner canthus while the child's eyes are closed. As the child's eyes open, the drops will be dispersed. After instillation, the nurse should encourage the child to blink or close the eyelids and rotate the eyes to distribute the medication.

Before administration, the nurse should warm ear drops almost to body temperature to prevent pain or vertigo when the drops come in contact with the child's tympanic membrane. The nurse should assist the child into a supine position with the head turned to the side and the affected ear up. For a child under age 3, the nurse will have to pull the pinna down and back to straighten the external auditory canal. For a child over age 3, the nurse should pull the pinna up and back. Then the nurse can administer the drops and massage the area in front of the tragus to promote their entry into the ear. If only one ear is affected, the child should lie on the unaffected side for several minutes after administration. If both ears are affected, the nurse should place a cotton ball in each external canal to prevent the medication from escaping.

To prevent nose drops from entering the throat rather than the nasal passages, the nurse should administer them to a child whose head is suspended over the edge of a pillow or bed or to an infant who is being held in the football position (tucked against the nurse's side with the infant on its back, its head at the nurse's head, and its feet against the nurse's waist). The nurse should keep the child in this position for 1 minute after medication administration to allow the drops to come in contact with as much of the nasal passages as possible.

PATIENT AND FAMILY TEACHING

Whether the child is treated in an outpatient or acute care setting, the nurse probably will be responsible for patient and family teaching to help increase medication compliance. Whenever patient or family teaching is required, the nurse should remember these teaching tips:

• Keep the instruction simple.
• Keep each session short.
• Repeat information.
• Allow time for questions.
• Provide written information.

(For further details, see *Steps for effective patient and family teaching.*)

Medication information should include the drug's name; its correct dosage, administration route, and frequency of administration; its therapeutic and adverse effects; and instructions for any required administration devices.

In this written information, the nurse should spell the name of the drug correctly and explain simply and clearly why the drug is being given. The nurse should instruct the family about the correct dosage and demonstrate how to prepare the correct amount for administration.

The nurse should describe the route of administration simply. For example, the nurse would use the phrase "by mouth" rather than "P.O." when talking to the parents and the patient. The nurse also should explain why the drug must be given in the exact way it is ordered. For example, the nurse might caution the parents to give a capsule without opening it because the capsule protects the medication from

---

Steps for effective patient and family teaching

To make patient and family teaching as effective as possible, the nurse should consider any psychosocial, physiologic, or cognitive deficits. Follow these steps:

- Decide who needs to be taught.
- Assess readiness to learn.
- Determine the necessary information to be taught.
- Present the information at a level that the learner can understand.
- Reinforce the teaching with printed materials.
- Assess the learner's ability to solve problems by asking "What if..." questions.
- Provide the necessary resources to meet the educational goals.
- Evaluate the learning and review information as needed.

---

destruction by stomach acids and allows it to be absorbed properly in the intestine. The frequency of administration requires careful discussion, too. If the timing of the doses presents a problem, the nurse should help the parents develop a schedule that will interfere as little as possible with their daily routine.

The parents and child also must learn what therapeutic and adverse effects to expect from the medication. For example, if theophylline is prescribed to treat a child's asthma, the nurse should explain that this drug should decrease or eliminate the wheezing; that the medication must be given at regular intervals to achieve the maximum effect; and that adverse reactions, such as irritability and nausea, may occur. Finally, the nurse should make sure that the family knows when to contact their physician about the drug therapy.

CHAPTER SUMMARY

Chapter 10 provided information on drug dosage calculations, routes and techniques of administration, and nursing techniques that are specific to the pediatric patient. Here are the chapter highlights.

- A child's age, physiologic state, body composition, immature organ function, and other factors can affect the absorption, distribution, metabolism, and excretion of a drug.
- Children may require wide variations of drug dosages to achieve therapeutic effects. Because of this, the nurse must monitor a pediatric patient closely to detect therapeutic

effects and adverse drug reactions. Pediatric patients are at particularly high risk for drug toxicity.

- The nurse should base accurate drug dosages on the child's weight or body-surface area.
- The nurse must administer medications carefully, delivering the right medication to the right patient at the right time by the right route and in the right amount.
- Although pediatric and adult routes of medication administration are the same, pediatric sites and techniques of administration vary considerably with age. The nurse must be familiar with the drug to be administered as well as the appropriate administration techniques for the child's age.
- Whenever possible, the nurse should explain the administration procedure to the patient and parents and try to elicit their cooperation in administering medications safely and effectively.
- Patient and family teaching is essential for compliance with a medication regimen at home. The nurse should provide oral and written instructions as a part of patient and family education.

STUDY QUESTIONS

See Appendix 1 for answers.

1. The physician prescribes an oral medication for Lynn Granger, age 1 month. Most oral medications should be administered in which manner?
(a) on an empty stomach
(b) on a full stomach
(c) with milk
(d) with juice

2. Lynn may need a higher mg/kg dosage to achieve therapeutic drug levels than an adult would. Which of the following accounts for this?
(a) her higher percentage of water
(b) her immature liver
(c) the longer GI tract
(d) her immature renal function

3. When administering an oral medication to Lynn, which technique should the nurse use?
(a) Use a syringe without a needle to give the medication.
(b) Mix the medication with the infant's food.
(c) Pour the medication into the infant's mouth.
(d) Place the medication in the infant's bottle.

4. Mark Shapiro, age 2 months, has been admitted to the hospital with epilepsy. The physician prescribes phenytoin (Dilantin) 5 mg/kg I.V. q8h. Which of Mark's organs may alter drug metabolism?
(a) heart
(b) lungs
(c) liver
(d) kidneys

5. Which of Mark's organs may interfere with drug elimination?
(a) heart
(b) lungs
(c) liver
(d) kidneys

6. Because Mark is receiving I.V. medication, the nurse should monitor him for which potential complication?
(a) fluid overload
(b) renal failure
(c) hyperglycemia
(d) hypoglycemia

7. During a regular checkup, Kate Mulligan, age 18 months, must receive I.M. immunization with diphtheria and tetanus toxoids and pertussis vaccine (DPT). Which of the following muscles is the most appropriate site for Kate's I.M. injection?
(a) deltoid
(b) vastus lateralis
(c) ventrogluteal
(d) gluteus maximus

8. During the checkup, Kate shows signs of otitis externa in her left ear. The physician prescribes neomycin sulfate 3 drops into the external auditory canal t.i.d. for 10 days. When administering ear drops to a toddler, how should the nurse straighten the ear canal?
(a) Pull the pinna up.
(b) Pull the pinna forward.
(c) Pull the pinna down and back.
(d) Pull the pinna down.

SELECTED REFERENCES

Behrman, R., and Vaughn, V., III. (1987). *Nelson's textbook of pediatrics* (13th ed.). Philadelphia: Saunders.

Chameides, L. (Ed.). (1988). *Textbook of pediatric advanced life support*. Dallas: American Heart Association and American Academy of Pediatrics.

Guyon, G. (1989). Pharmacokinetic considerations in neonatal drug therapy. *Neonatal Network*, 7(5), 9-30.

Handbook of pediatric drug therapy. (1990). Springhouse, PA: Springhouse Corporation.

Phillips, S. (1989). Monitoring vital sign changes in children. *Nursing89*, 19(10), 48-49.

Ragan, J., and Weinfield, A. (1989). VACNECCA: An eight-point check for neonatal assessment. *Journal of Practical Nursing*, 39(2), 39-43.

Shapiro, C. (1989). Pain in the neonate: Assessment and intervention. *Neonatal Network*, 8(1), 7-21.

CHAPTER

11

THE GERIATRIC PATIENT

OBJECTIVES

After reading and studying this chapter, the student should be able to:
1. Describe the general effects of aging on geriatric patients.
2. Explain how age can alter drug absorption, distribution, metabolism, and excretion.
3. Explain how a patient's age can alter a drug's action.
4. Discuss common drug-related problems in geriatric patients.
5. Describe the factors that may place a geriatric patient at risk for adverse drug reactions.
6. Describe safe and efficient systems to help the frail geriatric patient self-medicate at home.

INTRODUCTION

The geriatric population in the United States is growing faster than any other age-group. It may nearly double—from 12% to 21%—by the year 2030. Three factors account for this growth. First, improved medical care has reduced infant mortality, which has allowed more infants to survive and eventually reach old age. Second, medical advances and new treatments have decreased mortality from acute and chronic diseases—causing people to live longer. Third, while life expectancy has increased, the birth rate has decreased, amplifying the population shift.

Traditionally, the geriatric population has been defined as people age 65 and older. However, this definition is no longer useful because it encompasses at least two generations: those over age 85 and their children, who may be over age 65. Therefore, the geriatric population can be classified into three main subgroups: the young-old, ages 65 to 74; the middle-old, ages 75 to 84; and the old-old, ages 85 and older. The old-old group is the fastest growing and neediest and may have the greatest impact on the rest of society.

Within each of these three subgroups is another group, the frail elderly, which includes all individuals over age 65 who have one or more debilitating conditions. Members of this group are at especially high risk for adverse drug reactions. Some people under age 65 also may be considered part of the geriatric population because they have similar health care needs.

As the geriatric population grows, so will the need for nurses with advanced knowledge and skills in geriatric health care, especially in pharmacology. Traditionally, the nurse has been responsible for administering and monitoring prescribed medication regimens. This responsibility assumes even greater importance with geriatric patients, especially with frail elderly patients and those who live in long-term care facilities and routinely take several medications. The nurse must work closely with such patients to be aware of changes in their health and cognitive status, to detect subtle symptoms of an illness or adverse drug reaction, and to begin interventions.

To prepare the nurse for these responsibilities, Chapter 11 covers the effects of aging, age-related changes in pharmacokinetics and pharmacodynamics, significant drug-related problems that commonly affect geriatric patients, and nursing interventions for geriatric patients at high risk for adverse drug reactions.

EFFECTS OF AGING

Aging usually is accompanied by a decline in organ function, which can profoundly affect drug distribution and clearance, among other things. This physiologic decline is likely to be exacerbated by a disease or chronic disorder. This combination can significantly increase the geriatric patient's risk of drug toxicity and adverse reactions. (For an example, see *Geriatric case study,* page 164.)

Geriatric case study

This case study shows how a geriatric patient can develop adverse drug reactions when she uses over-the-counter (OTC) medications in conjunction with her prescription medications.

Rose Greenwald, age 78, lives alone on a fixed income and has been taking the same heart medications for years. When she developed a mild upper respiratory tract infection, Rose decided to purchase OTC remedies for symptomatic relief. She bought Nyquil, a cough suppressant that contains alcohol, to relieve her nighttime cough, and Dristan, an antihistamine, for her rhinorrhea and congestion. To relieve her fatigue, Rose opted for bed rest.

After Rose took the OTC medications and her usual medications as directed on the bottles, her appetite decreased, she felt too weak to prepare meals, and she ate and drank less. She also felt depressed but attributed this to the illness and continued to take the medications. She did not realize that the Nyquil decreased the cough reflex and appetite that were essential to her recovery. She did not know that the Dristan decreased her appetite, increased her feeling of lethargy, and produced urine retention. In fact, she was glad that she did not need to get up to urinate so often. After a few days, a neighbor noticed that Rose had not been outside lately. Upon investigation, the neighbor found her in bed, disoriented and incontinent.

Like many other elderly people, Rose Greenwald put herself at risk for adverse drug reactions in several ways. She diagnosed and treated herself, which could have been dangerous if her symptoms had been related to her history of congestive heart failure and not to a mild respiratory infection. She mixed OTC and prescription medications without consulting her physician or pharmacist about potential drug interactions or adverse reactions. Rose decreased her nutritional and fluid intake, which increased the concentration and effect of the medications. She also misjudged her reserve capacity to recover from this illness. Also, she did not keep track of the situation as it changed or alert her physician when her condition worsened.

Then Rose experienced disorientation and depression, two common symptoms of adverse drug reactions. If she had had anemia, low albumin levels, or a renal or hepatic dysfunction, or if her cardiovascular disease had worsened, the risk of a severe adverse reaction would have been high.

GENERAL EFFECTS

Multiple health problems and reduced reserve capacity commonly accompany aging and can lead to atypical signs and symptoms of disease. The nurse must be aware of these aging effects to assess the geriatric patient properly and to help distinguish between normal aging and disease.

Multiple health problems

The geriatric patient may experience multiple health problems and age-related changes and may take several medications. Because of the complex nature of geriatric health problems, the physician and the nurse must determine carefully which etiology or combination of etiologies is causing the signs and symptoms. They also must determine if the signs and symptoms are associated with normal aging or are the result of one drug or a combination of drugs. Basic knowledge of age-related changes and common pharmacotherapeutics helps the physician and the nurse to assess and treat the geriatric patient appropriately.

Reduced reserve capacity

Normal aging also can reduce normal body maintenance functions. For example, cardiac, kidney, liver, and endocrine functions all decline significantly with age. In many cases, elderly people—especially frail ones—cope poorly with illness or injury because they have a lowered reserve capacity (ability to compensate for disease) when challenged by adverse conditions. Their responses to illness or injury tend to be more catastrophic.

The reduced reserve capacity may be overlooked, however, because most geriatric patients maintain homeostasis fairly well when they are medically stable. However, the nurse must be alert to this deficit because a geriatric patient who seems well suddenly may become a high-risk patient when threatened by a condition as common as a urinary tract infection. One sign of reduced reserve capacity is orthostatic hypotension, a common condition in frail elderly people. The nurse's alertness to reduced reserve capacity and prompt intervention can avert a potentially fatal incident.

Atypical signs and symptoms

In geriatric patients, the effects of aging, multiple health problems, and reduced reserve capacity commonly lead to atypical signs and symptoms when compared to those exhibited by younger patients. For example, aging reduces the body's ability to regulate its temperature. This not only increases the geriatric patient's susceptibility to hyperthermia and heat stroke, but also decreases the ability to produce a fever in response to infection. Therefore, a low-grade or absent fever in a geriatric patient does not rule out severe infection. The nurse should assess this atypical sign further by checking for an increased white blood cell count. Otherwise, the geriatric patient may receive inadequate treatment and may develop serious complications.

A geriatric patient also may exhibit decreased pain perception. Such a patient may experience a bone fracture or "silent" myocardial infarction without feeling the pain that usually accompanies such an event. Because of this atypical symptom, the geriatric patient may not seek medical attention and may develop complications.

Adverse drug reactions also may produce subtle, nonspecific effects that may be mistaken for signs and symptoms of disease or dismissed as effects of aging. Many medications, such as anesthetic agents and analgesics, can cause confusion or depression in a geriatric patient, which the caregiver may attribute wrongly to aging or to the development of a new disorder.

Many people mistakenly consider forgetfulness to be a natural part of aging. The nurse must remember that the onset of confusion or memory loss is a common symptom of drug toxicity or altered health status in the geriatric patient. Any changes in a patient's health status require investigation to determine if they are related to illness or drug toxicity. For example, a fall that caused an injury may have resulted from confusion. The nurse's astute history taking, observation, and knowledge of adverse drug effects will help determine if the confusion is a symptom of an underlying health problem or a normal part of aging.

EFFECTS ON PHARMACOKINETICS

Many physiologic changes of aging affect drug absorption, distribution, metabolism, and excretion. The nurse must be especially aware of these changes when administering medications to a geriatric patient and when observing for adverse drug reactions.

Absorption

Several age-related changes in the gastrointestinal (GI) system can alter drug absorption patterns. Decreased gastric acidity may affect drug solubility and alter drug absorption. Reduced blood flow to the GI tract and the decreased number of cells available for absorption also can delay drug absorption. However, because the GI transit time is slowed, drugs remain in the system longer, which increases absorption. Overall, the effects of aging slow the absorption rate, but allow absorption to be as complete as in a younger patient.

The clinical effects of this altered absorption vary greatly. For example, an analgesic administered as a single dose for a headache may take longer to exert its effect because of delayed absorption. An anti-inflammatory agent administered regularly for arthritis will exhibit no difference in effect because the blood concentration remains fairly constant and so the absorption rate is not significant.

Distribution

Total body mass declines with age. Initially, this may be masked by an increase in the percentage of body fat. Eventually, however, total body fat decreases. Total body water also decreases with age. These changes in body composition lead to a relative increase in body fat and decrease in body water, which changes the distribution patterns for most drugs. A highly fat-soluble drug, such as diazepam, will have an increased volume of distribution and a prolonged distribution phase, leading to a prolonged half-life and duration of action. A highly water-soluble drug, such as gentamicin, will have a decreased volume of distribution.

Aging also reduces plasma levels of albumin, a blood protein that binds with and transports many drugs. As a result, more unbound drug may circulate, which typically increases the pharmacologic action of drugs that are extensively protein-bound. However, this effect is not always predictable because, as the amount of unbound drug increases, so does the amount of drug available for metabolism and excretion. For example, phenytoin—a highly protein-bound drug—undergoes increased metabolism and displays decreased serum concentrations, which reduces its therapeutic effect in geriatric patients. However, warfarin—another highly protein-bound drug—shows an increased effect in these patients. The nurse must account for such effects carefully, because some drugs may produce toxicity when administered at usual dosages to a geriatric patient.

Other factors that alter drug distribution in geriatric patients include declining cardiac output, poor nutrition, extremes of body weight, dehydration, electrolyte and mineral imbalances, inactivity, and prolonged bed rest. Perhaps the most significant factor is size: geriatric patients typically are smaller than younger patients. So if a geriatric patient receives the same drug dose as a younger patient, the geriatric patient's typically smaller volume can result in higher blood concentrations of the drug.

Metabolism

Aging reduces the liver's ability to metabolize drugs. A patient who lives to age 100 may have a liver weight decrease of almost 50%, with the greatest decrease occurring between age 60 and 70. Although the liver remains functional, its ability to metabolize drugs may change. Liver disease may compromise its functioning further. So may other diseases that reduce hepatic blood flow, such as congestive heart failure.

Drug metabolism by the liver depends primarily on two processes: hepatic blood flow and metabolic enzyme action. Because aging decreases blood flow to the liver, less drug is delivered for metabolism to inactive compounds, which can be especially significant for drugs, such as propranolol, that have metabolism rates dependent on hepatic blood flow.

The hepatic enzymes metabolize drugs in two major phases. Phase I metabolic reactions include oxidation, reduction, and hydrolysis of drug molecules. This metabolism leads to minor changes in drug molecules and usually produces an active metabolite. Phase II metabolic reactions couple the drug or its metabolite with acetic, glucuronic, sulfuric, or amino acid and lead to production of inactive compounds that are eliminated via the urine or feces. Aging reduces the efficiency of both phases, but Phase I reactions are affected more than Phase II reactions. Aging leads to different clinical effects, depending on whether a drug is metabolized in Phase I, Phase II, or both.

Some agents, such as cimetidine, may interfere with the liver's ability to metabolize other drugs. These agents, which inhibit some of the enzyme systems responsible for drug metabolism, may induce toxicity if dosage adjustments are not made for the other drugs.

Excretion

In any patient, renal function is an important factor in drug clearance and excretion. With aging, glomerular filtration and tubular secretion decline progressively. Also, dehydration and cardiovascular and renal diseases may impair renal function. Although serum creatinine levels typically remain unchanged in geriatric patients, creatinine production decreases because of decreased glomerular filtration. That means that a geriatric patient with renal dysfunction may not display increased creatinine levels until the dysfunction is severe. Therefore, the nurse should keep in mind that the geriatric patient has a smaller renal reserve than a younger patient, even if the blood urea nitrogen and serum creatinine levels appear normal.

The kidneys excrete many drugs. When the geriatric patient receives drugs that do not undergo metabolism, the nurse must monitor carefully for signs of toxicity because drug clearance and excretion may be delayed. Potentially nephrotoxic drugs, such as the aminoglycoside gentamicin, are of particular concern because they may cause more severe nephrotoxicity faster in a geriatric patient.

EFFECTS ON PHARMACODYNAMICS

Many changes in drug effect in geriatric patients do not result from pharmacokinetic factors. Instead, they may be caused by the aging organ system and its role in drug-receptor or drug-organ interactions.

Aging causes many receptors to function less efficiently and reduces the density of beta-adrenergic receptors. As a result, geriatric patients show diminished response to drugs such as isoproterenol and increased toxicity to beta-adrenergic blockers such as propranolol. Aging produces a decline in parasympathetic control, which enhances the effects of anticholinergic agents. It also reduces the number of neurotransmitters, particularly dopamine and acetylcho-

line. Reduced dopamine in the brain makes the geriatric patient more susceptible to the adverse extrapyramidal effects of neuroleptics, metoclopramide, and other drugs.

Changes in the central nervous system (CNS) include increased sensitivity to depressants and decreased blood flow. These changes increase susceptibility to sedation and to diminished cognitive function during drug therapy. Other CNS changes may include deterioration of the blood-brain barrier, which may allow a greater CNS concentration of some drugs and may account for the high incidence of drug-induced behavioral changes in geriatric patients. One such change, paradoxical excitement, commonly occurs with the use of sedatives and anxiolytics.

Age-related cardiovascular changes that may alter the response to a drug include decreased cardiac output, increased total peripheral resistance, increased circulating norepinephrine, and decreased sensitivity and function of baroreceptors. These changes may cause such common adverse drug reactions as orthostatic hypotension and heart failure.

Several endocrine changes may influence drug therapy. For example, the age-related decline in glucose tolerance may cause greater hyperglycemia in response to a thiazide diuretic. Reduced response to hypoglycemia may cause a geriatric patient to delay seeking treatment until the condition worsens. Reduced thyroid function may decrease body metabolism, which can slow drug metabolism.

COMMON DRUG-RELATED PROBLEMS

Drug-related problems in geriatric patients can affect the central nervous, cardiovascular, respiratory, GI, urinary, endocrine, and musculoskeletal systems. The drugs included in this section either are commonly prescribed or typically cause adverse drug reactions in geriatric patients. The nurse should keep in mind that some drugs are more likely to cause these problems than others. (For specific information, see the "Adverse drug reactions" sections in most chapters.)

CENTRAL NERVOUS SYSTEM

Several physiologic changes in the aging CNS may cause drug-related problems directly or indirectly. The decrease in the weight and water of the brain and the loss of neurons allow lipid-soluble drugs to accumulate in the CNS. Decreased brain activity and altered sleep patterns commonly cause insomnia. These factors make a geriatric patient much more sensitive to CNS depressants, such as barbiturates and general anesthetics.

Psychoactive drugs, such as sedatives and hypnotics, may produce adverse effects that can mimic the changes of aging, such as fatigue or depression. Because of these adverse effects, the patient may have difficulty dealing with a complex drug regimen, resulting in dosage errors. That, in turn, increases the risk of adverse drug reactions.

For a geriatric patient with peptic ulcer disease, cimetidine, a histamine$_2$ (H$_2$)-receptor antagonist, must be administered with extreme caution. Cimetidine inhibits the metabolism and excretion of several drugs, such as benzodiazepines and theophylline, and it causes several adverse CNS effects, including confusion and disorientation. In most geriatric patients with peptic ulcers, other H$_2$-receptor antagonists or sucralfate should be substituted.

Although the patient's intelligence may remain intact, aging slows learning speed, increasing the time needed to teach a geriatric patient about any drug. Insufficient patient instruction increases the likelihood of medication errors and adverse drug reactions.

CARDIOVASCULAR SYSTEM

Although aging produces few anatomic changes in the cardiovascular system, it may cause such functional changes as increased contraction time and decreased cardiac work load. Blood vessel elasticity decreases as a result of atherosclerosis, calcification, and increased collagen, decreasing blood flow to certain regions. Decreased cardiac output and blood flow redistribution may reduce hepatic and renal circulation, delaying metabolism and excretion of various drugs.

Although commonly used to treat cardiovascular disorders, diuretics can cause adverse cardiovascular effects. For example, they may produce extreme fluid volume deficit, causing decreased cardiac output and hypotension.

Aggressive use of antihypertensive agents also may lead to adverse cardiovascular effects, especially because a geriatric patient's cardiac output already is diminished. If the antihypertensive agent reduces the blood pressure too greatly, cardiac output may fall even further.

Anticholinergics, antihypertensives, diuretics, and many other drugs can produce orthostatic hypotension as an adverse reaction. In geriatric patients, this reaction is likely to be compounded by other disorders, such as neuropathy, organic brain disease, or dehydration.

RESPIRATORY SYSTEM

With age, the respiratory system shows a general decrease in function. This is reflected in most measures of lung function, such as vital capacity, flow rates, elastic recoil, and maximum breathing capacity. In geriatric patients, decreased respiratory function is a major factor in increased sensitivity to respiratory depressants, such as narcotics and barbiturates.

GASTROINTESTINAL SYSTEM

Aging causes decreased GI motility and activity and reduces the number of mucosal cells. These changes may result in constipation and greater sensitivity to the GI effects of anticholinergic agents. Constipation may lead to routine laxative use, which predisposes the patient to the adverse effects of laxatives, such as dehydration and electrolyte loss.

In the liver, albumin synthesis is reduced, which decreases the amount of protein-bound drug in circulation. That increases the level of unbound, or active, drug, which may lead to increased therapeutic and toxic effects or faster drug metabolism. Because most drugs are protein-bound to some degree, these are common drug-related problems.

URINARY SYSTEM

Renal function declines progressively with age, causing decreased renal blood flow, tubular secretion, and glomerular filtration. Therefore, drugs that are excreted primarily by the kidneys—especially by glomerular filtration (such as digoxin, aminoglycosides, and nitrofurantoin)—should be given in reduced dosages to prevent toxicity even if the geriatric patient shows no signs of renal disease. Because digoxin also has an extremely narrow therapeutic index, a geriatric patient receiving this drug is more likely to experience digitalis toxicity than a younger patient.

In a patient with renal disease, the kidneys produce vasodilating renal prostaglandins to help maintain renal perfusion. Nonsteroidal anti-inflammatory drugs (NSAIDs) significantly reduce production of these prostaglandins, which can lead to renal disease. Therefore, the nurse should monitor renal function carefully in a geriatric patient receiving an NSAID.

Because diuretics increase urinary frequency, they may precipitate incontinence in a geriatric patient, especially one who is predisposed to stress incontinence.

ENDOCRINE SYSTEM

With age, blood glucose normally rises slightly due to mild glucose intolerance. Therefore, the nurse must evaluate the patient's blood glucose level cautiously during therapy with a drug that causes hyperglycemia, such as propranolol.

Also, a geriatric patient may not display signs and symptoms of hypoglycemia as rapidly as a younger patient. So when a geriatric patient is taking a drug that causes hypoglycemia, such as insulin or an oral hypoglycemic agent, the nurse should check the blood glucose level regularly, and the patient must adhere to the therapeutic regimen closely to prevent severe hypoglycemia.

MUSCULOSKELETAL SYSTEM

Drugs such as beta carotene and cholecalciferol may cause changes in bone composition and other adverse musculoskeletal effects. Such drugs may increase the risk of fractures if the patient falls. Sedatives, hypnotics, and other drugs that cause muscle weakness or adverse CNS effects, such as drowsiness and dizziness, increase the risk of falls.

The diuretic furosemide should be used cautiously because it depletes serum calcium and, at high dosages, may contribute to osteoporosis — especially in women.

NURSING CONSIDERATIONS

Whenever a geriatric patient takes medications, the risk of medication errors and adverse reactions is high. Well-planned nursing interventions can help prevent drug-related problems.

HIGH-RISK FACTORS

Although elderly people constitute only about 12% of the population, they use about 30% of all prescription drugs sold annually. Also, they purchase up to 40% of nonprescription medications. Not only do elderly people use medications frequently, but they also experience adverse drug reactions two to seven times more frequently than younger people.

Geriatric patients tend to use more than one medication concurrently. In some studies of institutionalized geriatric patients, nearly 10% were taking 12 or more medications before admission. The average nursing home patient takes three to six prescription drugs a day. At this high rate of drug use, patients are likely to have adverse drug reactions.

Medication errors may increase further the risk of drug reactions. A quarter to a half of noninstitutionalized patients make medication errors, usually because of medication knowledge deficits. Geriatric patients are no exception. About 25% of all medication errors lead to a worsening of health problems and require medical care or hospital admission.

Several risk factors help identify geriatric patients who are prone to adverse drug reactions. Identification of high-risk geriatric patients can allow the nurse to protect them by monitoring closely, preventing medication errors, identifying drug-related problems promptly, and intervening as needed. The risk factors include advanced age, small physique, multiple illnesses, multiple medications, type of drugs prescribed (such as CNS depressants), previous adverse drug reactions, living alone, and malnutrition.

Many of the risk factors are interrelated. A geriatric patient who takes multiple medications is prone to medication errors and probably will have a history of adverse drug reactions. An elderly patient who lives alone is more likely to be malnourished and dehydrated than one who lives with family or in an institution. A patient who lives alone and has multiple illnesses also may lack support systems that assist with medication problems. Financial problems and lack of access to a pharmacy to obtain medications may compound these problems for such a patient.

NURSING INTERVENTIONS

To help a geriatric patient comply with the medication regimen and avoid adverse reactions, the nurse should simplify the medication schedule, educate the patient and family, review medications periodically, help the patient overcome cognitive and functional impairments, assess the patient's ability to obtain medications, plan for medical follow-up care, and assess the patient's risk level.

Simplify the medication schedule
Compliance drops sharply when more than three medications are prescribed. This drop may result from confusion about multiple schedules, concern about overmedicating or concern about the cost. Cost is especially important for patients who live on fixed incomes.

Devising the simplest possible medication schedule is the best way to increase compliance and reduce errors. The nurse should help the patient associate medications with meals, daily activities, or bedtime to aid memory and establish a routine.

If the patient has a memory or sensory deficit, the nurse may introduce a system to administer medications safely. For example, the nurse may suggest the use of prefilled insulin syringes for a diabetic patient with decreased vision. The syringes contain the correct amount of medication, can be stored in the refrigerator, and allow the patient to take the insulin safely every day. For another slightly impaired patient, the nurse may suggest individual prefilled envelopes or containers labeled with the medication, day of the week, and time of administration. The envelopes or containers, which can be refilled at scheduled intervals, allow the nurse to see how much medication has been taken. Medicine boxes based on this system are commercially available. They all provide compartments that hold medication doses, and the expensive models have programmable alarms that sound when medications are due. A labeled egg carton can serve the same compartmentalizing purpose at a much lower cost.

Another way to simplify the medication schedule is to give as few doses as possible. Although a simple schedule is best, high drug doses given at wider intervals may be dangerous to a geriatric patient because this schedule can produce a pattern of toxic blood concentrations followed by subtherapeutic ones. To avoid this toxic-subtherapeutic pattern and maintain even blood concentrations, the nurse may suggest using the drug in a sustained-release form or adjusting the dosage to twice a day, depending on the drug's half-life. A drug with a long half-life, such as digoxin, should be given once a day. A drug with a short half-life, such as acetaminophen, should be given several times a day, although perhaps not as frequently as a younger person might receive it.

Teach the patient and family

With many geriatric patients, nurses encounter a lack of knowledge about medications, including the reason for the prescription and the important therapeutic and adverse effects. These patients sometimes have difficulty learning about one drug, much less several. Hospitalized patients typically have little chance to learn about the medications that are administered to them or to make decisions about how to take them. All too often, insufficient patient education involves only a quick drug description during the intense activity that accompanies discharge. Because most individuals remember less than half of what they hear, and even less when under stress, many patients arrive home with little information about their medications. In a geriatric patient, who may be affected by sensory deficits, multisystem disease, and the stress of recent illness and hospitalization, retention of knowledge about medications is even less likely.

To avoid these pitfalls, the nurse must begin to teach the patient and the family about the prescribed medications well before discharge. To reinforce this teaching, the nurse can provide written information in large print and in simple terms geared to the patient's educational level and suitable for patient and family review at home. (For more information, see *Using a medication card.*)

Review medications periodically

The nursing care plan should include regular medication reviews even if the physician has prescribed no new medications. The nurse must determine which drugs the patient is taking, because a geriatric patient may stray from a regimen in several ways. The patient may:
• experiment with self-treatment by taking the medication of a friend who seems to have similar symptoms
• take a medication that was discontinued long ago if old symptoms reappear or discontinue a medication as symptoms diminish
• have drugs prescribed by a physician who may not know all the medications that the patient is taking

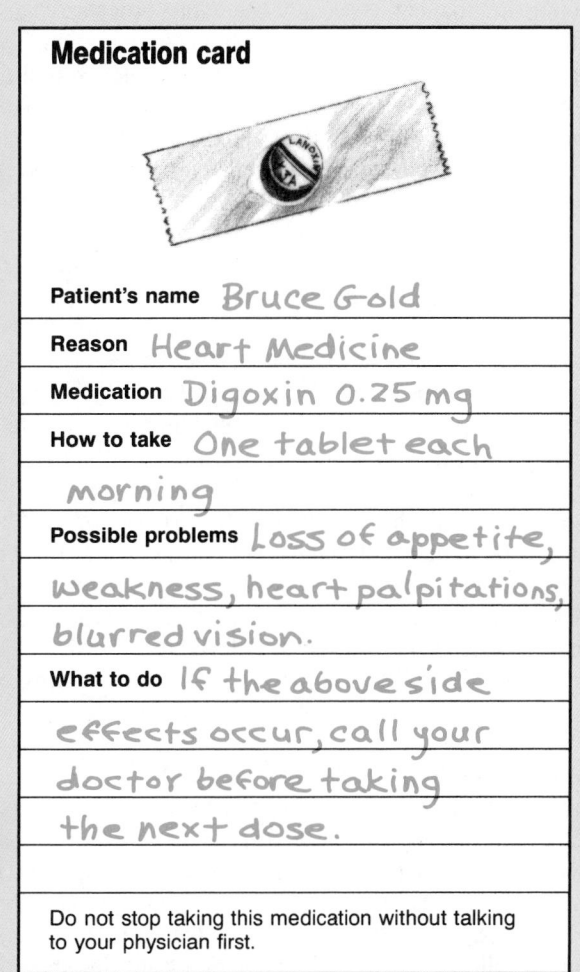

Using a medication card

As a follow-up to patient teaching, the nurse can compile drug information on a card, including the dose, the frequency of administration, and other information as shown on the sample card below. Taping a tablet or capsule onto the card also may be helpful in identifying the drug. The medication card can help the patient and family remember and comply with the drug regimen and serve as a guide to reordering the medication, if necessary. It also can help inform the physician about the patient's medications and be invaluable if an emergency arises or if the patient cannot communicate.

Medication card

Patient's name	Bruce Gold
Reason	Heart Medicine
Medication	Digoxin 0.25 mg
How to take	One tablet each morning
Possible problems	Loss of appetite, weakness, heart palpitations, blurred vision.
What to do	If the above side effects occur, call your doctor before taking the next dose.

Do not stop taking this medication without talking to your physician first.

• take one or more over-the-counter medications that may cause serious drug interactions or toxicity.

A periodic medication review allows the nurse to evaluate the total medication regimen, to report potential problems, and to coordinate the medication therapy safely. The potential for drug interactions requires special attention, and medications that follow the same metabolic pathways or that have long half-lives need careful consideration. The nurse should report any adverse reactions to the physician immediately.

The medication review is especially important for a home care nurse who may be the only health care professional to see which medications the patient is taking and to ensure that all prescribed drugs are current and appropriate. As part of the medication review, the home care nurse should inspect the medicine cabinet and other storage areas to remove out-of-date or dangerous drugs. (For more information about medication review, see *Drug use considerations.*)

Overcome cognitive and functional impairments

An impaired patient, especially one with a progressive disorder such as dementia, requires special consideration. The nurse must assure this patient's safety while promoting dignity and independence. The nurse can help a cognitively impaired patient by prepouring medications and putting away the excess. Strategies for overcoming a functional impairment depend on its nature, which may range from an inability to open containers to decreased vision or limited mobility. The nurse must question the patient carefully to form a workable plan for coping with the impairment.

Assess the ability to obtain medications

A geriatric patient usually is discharged from the hospital with various prescriptions. The hospital nurse can facilitate compliance by assessing the patient's ability to obtain medications. If the patient will be homebound, the nurse should develop a system that involves family, friends, or visiting nurses in obtaining medications. The nurse also may suggest the use of a pharmacy that delivers. Also, the nurse should assess the patient's financial status to ensure that the patient can pay for needed medications. Referral to a social worker may be necessary to obtain financial or other forms of assistance.

Plan for medical follow-up

Anyone who receives medications needs medical follow-up. A homebound, confused, or isolated geriatric patient is more likely to take a prescribed medication improperly, have adverse reactions, or combine prescription and OTC medications. The nurse should help the patient plan for medical follow-up before discharge by identifying the primary physician and discussing arrangements for physician contact.

Assess the patient's risk level

When assessing a geriatric patient, the nurse can use the high-risk factors described earlier as a guide for interventions. An isolated or malnourished patient may benefit from Meals On Wheels, meal programs at senior centers, or, possibly, nursing home placement. A patient who has experienced several adverse drug reactions may benefit from

---

Drug use considerations

When beginning or reviewing drug therapy for a geriatric patient, the nurse should consider the following basic questions, which frequently are overlooked.

Is drug therapy necessary?
Consider using nonpharmacologic treatments, especially for conditions that require only symptomatic treatment, such as anxiety and insomnia. Keep in mind that other disorders, such as hypertension and diabetes, also may respond to nonpharmacologic treatments, such as diet and exercise.

Is the appropriate drug or dosage form being prescribed? To evaluate the drug's appropriateness, carefully examine its adverse reaction profile to determine if it will cause problems for the geriatric patient. If the patient finds the regimen confusing or unpalatable, consult with the physician about substituting dosage forms that are visually distinctive or more palatable.

Is the drug dosage appropriate?
Expect to use the lowest possible dosage, as prescribed, especially for drugs excreted by the kidneys. Consider the significant adverse reactions for the dosage administered. For example, keep in mind that adverse central nervous system reactions are common in geriatric patients.

Has the patient been taught about the medications?
Ensure that the patient understands the name, purpose, dose, route, frequency, and adverse effects of each medication. Provide simple, concise instructions and reinforce them, when appropriate. Keep in mind that a geriatric patient may learn more slowly than a younger patient. To promote learning and retention, avoid distractions and plan to conduct shorter, more frequent teaching sessions.

---

prepoured medications, frequent nursing visits, reduced drug doses, or discontinuation of medications, as prescribed.

CHAPTER SUMMARY

Chapter 11 concentrated on the special medication needs of geriatric patients. Here are the chapter highlights.
• As the geriatric population grows, so does the need for skilled nursing care.
• General effects of aging include multiple health problems, reduced reserve capacity, and atypical signs and symptoms of diseases and drug toxicity. The nurse must be aware of these aging effects to assess the geriatric patient properly.
• Many physiologic changes of aging affect drug absorption, distribution, metabolism, and excretion. The nurse must be aware of these changes when administering medications

to a geriatric patient and when observing for adverse drug reactions.

• A geriatric patient may experience changes in a drug's effects that result from age-related changes in organ systems, such as alterations in drug receptors or in drug-organ interactions.

• Drug-related problems in geriatric patients commonly affect the central nervous, cardiovascular, respiratory, GI, urinary, endocrine, and musculoskeletal systems.

• Risk factors that make a geriatric patient prone to adverse drug reactions include advanced age, small physique, multiple illnesses, multiple medications, type of drugs prescribed, previous adverse drug reactions, living alone, and malnutrition.

• The nurse can further patient compliance with a self-medication regimen and reduce the likelihood of adverse reactions by simplifying the patient's medication schedule, educating the patient and family, reviewing medications periodically, helping the patient overcome cognitive and functional impairments, assessing the patient's ability to obtain medications, planning for follow-up care, and assessing the patient's risk level.

STUDY QUESTIONS

See Appendix 1 for answers.

1. Emma Leeds, age 75, is admitted to the critical care unit with a myocardial infarction that was discovered during a routine ECG. Ms. Leeds states that she experienced no chest pain. Which of the following most likely accounts for the absence of pain?
(a) reduced reserve capacity
(b) confusion or forgetfulness
(c) reduced severity of disorders
(d) decreased pain perception

2. Ms. Leeds suddenly displays confusion. Which of the following most likely explains this behavior change?
(a) drug toxicity
(b) effects of aging
(c) effects of the disease
(d) atypical signs and symptoms

3. The physician orders docusate calcium 240 mg P.O. daily for Ms. Leeds. In a geriatric patient, absorption of oral medication may be altered. What accounts for this alteration?
(a) decreased gastric acid secretion
(b) increased total body fat

(c) decreased total body mass
(d) decreased cardiac output

4. Laboratory results show that George Burford, age 72, has a staphylococcal infection. His physician prescribes gentamicin 1 mg/kg I.V. q 8 hours. In a geriatric patient, this water-soluble drug has a reduced volume of distribution. Which effect of aging accounts for this?
(a) decreased total body water
(b) increased total body mass
(c) increased lean body mass
(d) increased total body fat

5. Mr. Burford also is receiving the anticoagulant warfarin (Coumadin). A large proportion of this drug circulates bound to plasma proteins, placing Mr. Burford at risk for adverse drug reactions. Which effect of aging accounts for this risk?
(a) decreased albumin
(b) increased hemoglobin
(c) decreased fat
(d) increased water

6. Which of the following patients is at greatest risk for developing adverse drug reactions?
(a) Bill Johnson, age 80, is malnourished and has hypertension, diabetes, and coronary artery disease. He takes multiple medications and lives alone.
(b) Eloise Baines, age 76, has vascular disease and diabetes. She takes multiple medications and lives in a nursing home.
(c) Robert Cartwright, age 65, is well nourished although he lives alone. He has hypertension, which is controlled with one medication and diet.
(d) Hannah Egan, age 70, has diabetes, which she controls by adjusting her diet. Of average build, she lives with her family.

7. The nurse is preparing Margaret Walsh, age 81, for discharge. Which intervention can help increase her compliance with the prescribed drug regimen and reduce medication errors?
(a) Have a neighbor administer the medications at her convenience.
(b) Simplify the medication schedule according to her routine.
(c) Administer all the medications by the same route.
(d) Instruct her to follow the hospital schedule for medications.

SELECTED REFERENCES

American Association of Retired Persons. (1989). *A profile of older Americans.* Washington, DC: American Association of Retired Persons.

Atchley, R. (1990). *Social forces and aging: An introduction to social gerontology* (6th ed.). Belmont, CA: Wadsworth Publishing.

Bosker, G. (Ed.). (1987). Rapid detection of adverse drug reactions in the elderly. *Emergency Medicine Reports,* 8(20), 153-160.

Boynton, P. (1989). Health maintenance alteration: A nursing diagnosis of the elderly. *Clinical Nurse Specialist,* 3(1), 5-10.

Cooper, J. (1989). The aging of America: How to deal with the geriatric patient in a nursing home. *Journal of Geriatric Drug Therapy,* 4(1), 51-57.

Davis-Sharts, J. (1989). The elder and critical care: Sleep and mobility issues. *Nursing Clinics of North America,* 24(3), 755-767.

Fincham, J. (1989). The aging of America: How to deal with the geriatric patient in the community pharmacy. *Journal of Geriatric Drug Therapy,* 4(1), 33-49.

Freely, J., and Coakley, D. (1990). Altered pharmacodynamics in the elderly. *Clinics in Geriatric Medicine,* 6(2), 269-283.

Glen, L., and Anderson, J. (1989). Medications and the elderly: A review. *Journal of Geriatric Drug Therapy,* 4(1), 59-89.

Matteson, M., and McConnell, E. (1988). *Gerontological nursing: Concepts and practice.* Philadelphia: Saunders.

McEwan, R. (1989). Issues in evaluation: Evaluating assessments of elderly people using a combination of methods. *Journal of Advanced Nursing,* 14(2), 103-110.

Rietbrock, N., and Woodcock, B. (1987). *Clinical pharmacology in the aged.* Accord, MA: IPS.

Roberts, J., and Tumer, N. (1988). Pharmacodynamic basis for altered drug action in the elderly. *Clinics in Geriatric Medicine,* 4(1), 127-149.

Rossman, I. (Ed.). (1986). *Clinical geriatrics* (3rd ed.). Philadelphia: Lippincott.

Smith, M. (1989). Overview: The aging of America. *Journal of Geriatric Drug Therapy,* 4(1), 3-15.

Yuen, G. (1990). Altered pharmacokinetics in the elderly. *Clinics in Geriatric Medicine,* 6(2), 257-267.

THE PREGNANT OR LACTATING PATIENT

OBJECTIVES

After reading and studying this chapter, the student should be able to:

1. Identify factors that alter absorption, distribution, metabolism, and excretion of a drug ingested by a pregnant patient.

2. Describe the effects of drug exposure on the fetus at different times during gestation.

3. State clinical indications for using antacids, antiemetics, laxatives and stool softeners, and nonnarcotic analgesics during pregnancy.

4. Discuss the nurse's role when drugs are administered during labor and delivery.

5. Describe drug passage through breast milk.

6. Describe the components the nurse should include in the education of a pregnant or lactating patient.

INTRODUCTION

Pregnant and lactating patients require special consideration during drug therapy. Throughout gestation, especially during the first trimester, the fetus is sensitive to substances ingested by the mother. After birth, the breast-feeding infant also may be sensitive because of immature metabolism and excretion systems.

Although health care professionals recognize the potential adverse effects of drug use during pregnancy and lactation, women continue to take drugs. Many do so without medical supervision and without knowledge of the potential adverse effects on the fetus and infant.

Data about the precise effects of drugs on pregnant and lactating women remain incomplete. Consequently, most pharmaceutical compounds approved for use in the United States carry disclaimers that the safety of the drug has not been established for use in pregnant and lactating women. Thus, physicians and nurses are faced with the responsibility of counseling these patients without the benefit of well-documented, research-based information.

To prepare the nurse for these responsibilities, Chapter 12 explores drug use by pregnant and lactating patients. It begins by describing the effects of pregnancy on pharmacokinetic processes. After describing drug teratogenesis, it presents pharmacotherapeutics for common complaints of pregnancy and drug use during labor and delivery. The second part of the chapter is devoted to the lactating patient. It highlights breast anatomy and physiology, factors that influence drug passage through breast milk to the infant, and counseling guidelines about drug use for the breast-feeding patient.

THE PREGNANT PATIENT

Most drugs ingested by a pregnant patient cross the placenta to the fetus. In 1979, the Food and Drug Administration (FDA) established five categories (A, B, C, D, X) to indicate the level of risk to a fetus posed by drugs. Although these categories are helpful, they may not be entirely accurate. (For the FDA risk categories, see *Pregnancy drug risk categories,* page 174.)

A number of pregnancy-related changes and structures can alter the absorption, distribution, metabolism, and excretion of a drug ingested by the pregnant patient. The fetus also significantly influences drug distribution and disposition.

Pregnancy drug risk categories

The following summarizes the Food and Drug Administration (FDA) risk-factor categories for drugs used during pregnancy.

Category A: Controlled studies in women fail to demonstrate a risk to the fetus in the first trimester (no evidence of a risk in later trimesters); the possibility of fetal harm appears remote.

Category B: Either animal-reproduction studies have not demonstrated a fetal risk (no controlled studies in pregnant women), or animal-reproduction studies have shown an adverse effect other than decreased fertility that was not confirmed in controlled studies with women in the first trimester; no evidence of a risk in later trimesters.

Category C: Either animal studies have revealed teratogenic, embryocidal, or other adverse effects on the fetus (no controlled studies in women are available), or no studies in women or animals are available. Drugs should be administered only if the potential benefit justifies the potential risk to the fetus.

Category D: Positive evidence of human fetal risk exists, but the benefits from use in pregnant women may be acceptable despite the risk (for example, if the drug is needed in a life-threatening situation or for a serious disease for which safer drugs cannot be used or are ineffective).

Category X: Studies in animals or women have demonstrated fetal abnormalities, or evidence of fetal risk exists based on human experience, or both, and the risk in pregnant women clearly outweighs any possible benefit. The drug is contraindicated in women who are or may become pregnant.

Category NR: No rating available.

PHARMACOKINETICS

During pregnancy, the tone and motility of the gastrointestinal (GI) tract decrease, probably from increased progesterone production and decreased motilin levels (an intestinal hormone that causes increased intestinal motility and also stimulates pepsin secretion). These effects prolong the gastric emptying and intestinal transit times. The formation of hydrochloric acid in the stomach also decreases. All these factors delay absorption of drugs that require an acidic environment or that are absorbed in the small intestine.

Absorption of drugs administered parenterally also may be altered during pregnancy. Because of peripheral vasodilation, drugs administered subcutaneously, intramuscularly, or intradermally may be absorbed more rapidly.

The physiologic changes of pregnancy also alter drug distribution. Influencing factors include increased interstitial and cellular water and increased blood volume, elevated nearly 45% by the end of gestation. These increases change the ratios of blood constituents that affect drug distribution. For example, the ratio of albumin to water decreases during pregnancy, altering protein-binding capacity.

During pregnancy, estrogen and progesterone levels also rise, as do those of free fatty acids (triglycerides, cholesterol, and phospholipids) from increased fatty tissue metabolism. These effects are accompanied by increased competition for protein-binding sites. With fewer binding sites, a larger percentage of drug remains free to move to receptor sites or across the placenta.

Numerous changes in the urinary system occur during pregnancy and can affect drug excretion. The glomerular filtration rate and renal plasma flow increase early in pregnancy, and the former persists to delivery. Because of the increased renal plasma flow, drugs that normally are excreted easily may be eliminated even more rapidly.

The term "placental barrier" can be misleading because it implies that the placenta protects the fetus from drug effects. In fact, many drugs ingested by the pregnant patient will cross the placenta and reach the fetus. Although some drugs, such as insulin, do not cross the placenta, most do when administered at therapeutic levels.

Placental transport of substances to and from the fetus begins at approximately the fifth week of gestation. Substances of low molecular weight diffuse freely across the placenta, driven primarily by the concentration gradient, although active transport, facilitated diffusion, and other transport processes also are involved. Later in pregnancy when the placenta thins, drugs with high lipid solubility or low protein-binding ability pass more easily through the placenta.

Any condition that alters placental circulation, such as pregnancy-induced hypertension or diabetes mellitus, can affect drug transport. Differences in maternal and fetal pH also will increase the rate of drug transfer and reabsorption.

Because the placenta is metabolically active, it can affect drug disposition. The placenta appears to be capable of several enzymatic reactions, including reduction, hydrolysis, and conjugation, that can reduce the potency of a drug's metabolites. Conversely, these reactions may produce a more potent and toxic metabolite, thereby increasing fetal danger.

The fetus also significantly may affect drug distribution and disposition by fetal circulation, binding of plasma and tissue proteins, and excretory activity. Furthermore, enzyme systems that normally are deficient during fetal life can be stimulated by certain drugs. The fetus also has slower drug clearance than the adult, and drugs persist longer in the fetus's tissues and blood than in the mother's.

DRUG ADMINISTRATION

Drug effects on the fetus depend on the timing of drug administration in relation to gestational age. During the first week to the end of the second week of pregnancy, fertilization, implantation, and rudimentary placental formation occur. During the embryonic period, from the second through the eighth week, the major organ systems form (organogenesis). The fetal period, from the ninth week to the end of pregnancy, is one of rapid body growth. Some tissue differentiation also occurs. Functional maturation continues after birth.

The fetus is most susceptible to the adverse effects of drugs from the time of implantation to the embryonic period, with limb formation defects potentially occurring through the end of the first trimester. During conception and implantation, the ovum is bathed in fallopian tube fluid. At that time, any damage to the ovum from drug exposure usually is lethal; however, the ovum can recover completely from damage inflicted by a sublethal dose. During the embryonic period, major structural anomalies may occur after only a single exposure to a toxic drug. Teratogenic drug exposure (causing fetal anomalies) during the fetal period may slow cell growth and retard growth of the exposed part or of the entire fetus. Such an effect is called intrauterine growth retardation.

The care with which a drug is administered to the mother and fetus during the intrapartal period is critical to the safety of the fetus. Maternal-fetal equilibrium of drug levels usually is reached within 40 minutes after drug ingestion and more rapidly with parenteral or intravenous administration.

Drug teratogenesis

Drug exposure during pregnancy probably accounts for only about 1% of all congenital anomalies. Almost 60% of congenital anomalies have no known cause, and 20% are probably from hereditary tendencies and unknown environmental factors.

The mechanisms whereby drugs exert teratogenic effects are poorly understood. Drugs may alter maternal tissues with indirect effects on the fetus, or they may affect the embryonic cells directly, resulting in specific abnormalities. Drugs also may interfere with nutrient transport or alter placental metabolism, both of which may interfere with fetal nutrition.

Health care professionals increasingly are concerned with the adverse effects of drugs on the intellect and the social and functional behavior of the child. However, determining just how a drug produces such anomalies is difficult, especially given the number of intervening variables not related to drug use. Identifying causal relationship for drugs that may produce delayed effects after intrauterine exposure also is difficult. For example, researchers suspect that maternal ingestion of diethylstilbestrol leads to an increased risk of adenocarcinoma of the vagina in female offspring or abnormalities of the reproductive system in male offspring. However, an exact link has not been established. (For some other drugs that may cause adverse effects, see *Adverse effects of recreational drugs during pregnancy or lactation,* page 176.)

PHARMACOTHERAPEUTICS

When counseling the pregnant patient, the physician should evaluate each drug to determine whether equivalent benefits can be obtained through alternative measures. The patient should participate actively in these decisions. If a drug must be used, the physician should prescribe one that has been widely used during pregnancy for many years rather than a recently introduced drug with inadequately established effects.

The physician will substitute alternative measures, if possible, during the trimester when a drug may produce teratogenic effects. For example, a patient with diabetes mellitus that was controlled with oral hypoglycemic agents before pregnancy will receive insulin instead during pregnancy.

The physician and nurse should teach pregnant and nonpregnant patients of childbearing age about the use of drugs, including over-the-counter (OTC) medications. The nonpregnant patient should be instructed to be aware of her last menstrual period so that she can recognize a pregnancy at the earliest possible time; many women self-medicate without knowing they are pregnant. Those women attempting to conceive should discuss with their physician, nurse, nurse-midwife, or pharmacist any drug they are taking or considering. The pregnant patient should never self-medicate without consultating her physician.

Pregnancy usually produces some discomfort. The most common complaints involve the GI tract, including heartburn, nausea and vomiting, and constipation. The patient also may need a nonnarcotic analgesic throughout gestation to relieve headaches and minor muscle discomforts. The drugs frequently used to alleviate these symptoms include antacids, antiemetics, laxatives and stool softeners, and nonnarcotic analgesics. The nurse should be aware of these agents and the implications associated with their use.

Antacids. Antacids are used by approximately 50% of pregnant women for relief of heartburn and other reflux symptoms. Unfortunately, little data are available on the antacid effects on the fetus. Physicians currently consider most aluminum-, magnesium-, and calcium-containing antacids safe in therapeutic doses during the second and third trimesters. Sodium bicarbonate and magnesium trisilicate, however, should be avoided. The nurse counseling a pregnant patient about reflux symptoms should encourage the

Adverse effects of recreational drugs during pregnancy or lactation

The nurse should be aware that some socially used drugs can affect the fetus and breast-feeding neonate. This chart contains some drugs that may cause adverse effects during pregnancy, the postpartal period, and lactation.

DRUG	ADVERSE EFFECTS During pregnancy and postpartal period	During lactation
alcohol	Fetal alcohol syndrome	Large doses inhibit let-down reflex and may cause alcohol intoxication in neonate
caffeine	High intake (more than 6 to 8 cups daily) may be associated with complications, including infertility	Heavy maternal use produces irritability and poor sleeping patterns in infant
cocaine*	Depressed interactive abilities; impaired organizational abilities; increased rate of spontaneous abortion; with I.V. use, onset of labor with abruptio placentae	Neonate exhibits cocaine intoxication
heroin*	Intrauterine death may occur from meconium aspiration syndrome; potential increase in major fetal anomalies; low birth weight, underdevelopment for gestational age; impaired behavioral, perceptual, and organizational activities	Withdrawal of drug from mother induces withdrawal symptoms in infant; sufficient quantities can cause addiction in infant
marijuana (THC—active ingredient)	Not documented	May cause central nervous system suppression in infant
smoking (nicotine and carbon monoxide—active ingredients)	Reduced birth weight, increased perinatal mortality	May interfere with let-down reflex
phencyclidine (PCP)	Depressed neonate, craniofacial abnormalities, weakened muscular function of eyes and neck	May cause hallucinogenic effects in infant

*Effects of these drugs may be complicated by multiple drug use.

patient to avoid behaviors that aggravate heartburn (overeating, consuming fatty or fried foods, and lying down too soon after meals). Milk, hot tea, chewing gum, good posture, and small meals can prevent or minimize such symptoms.

Antiemetics. The antiemetic prochlorperazine maleate (Compazine) has been linked to an increased risk of cardiovascular and other malformations. Diphenhydramine hydrochloride (Benadryl) may cause cleft palate, and trimethobenzamide hydrochloride (Tigan) may produce other congenital anomalies. Phosphorated carbohydrate solution (Emetrol), an OTC liquid preparation used to treat morning sickness, has not been linked to toxicity.

The nurse counseling a pregnant patient about the nausea and vomiting associated with pregnancy can encourage nonpharmacologic practices to minimize the symptoms, including eating small, frequent meals; consuming liquid and dry foods separately; avoiding fried, odorous, spicy,

greasy, or gas-forming foods; and keeping crackers or other dry food at the bedside to be eaten in the morning before arising.

Laxatives and stool softeners. The pregnant patient may require a laxative or stool softener to treat the constipation and painful hemorrhoids that may accompany pregnancy. Certain laxatives are not safe during pregnancy. Castor oil may initiate premature uterine contractions; hyperosmotic saline cathartics, such as magnesium hydroxide, may promote sodium retention in the mother. Frequent use of lubricants, such as mineral oil, can lead to decreased absorption of fat-soluble vitamins, resulting in neonatal hypoprothrombinemia and hemorrhage.

Some stimulant laxatives, such as bisacodyl and senna, may be safe during pregnancy, as may stool softeners containing docusate sodium. Bulk-forming laxatives containing psyllium hydrophilic mucilloid also may be safe during pregnancy. As a component of patient teaching, the nurse should encourage nonpharmacologic measures to alleviate constipation or hemorrhoids, such as increasing fluid intake, walking as much as possible during the day, increasing dietary fiber, and avoiding straining while defecating.

Nonnarcotic analgesics. Headaches and minor muscle aches commonly occur during pregnancy. In therapeutic doses, acetaminophen is safe for short-term use during pregnancy for analgesic and antipyretic actions. High doses, especially during the first trimester, may result in severe liver damage in the fetus.

Aspirin, the drug most frequently ingested by pregnant women, has been associated with maternal anemia, antepartal and postpartal hemorrhage, and prolonged gestation and labor. The prolonged gestation and labor result from aspirin's inhibition of prostaglandin synthetase. Aspirin also may delay the induced-abortion time in nulliparous women and complicate delivery.

The adverse effects of aspirin on the fetus and neonate include increased perinatal mortality, intrauterine growth retardation, congenital salicylate intoxication, and depressed albumin-binding capacity. Aspirin given in low doses during the week before delivery may affect the neonate's clotting ability.

DRUGS DURING LABOR AND DELIVERY

The need to relieve pain during labor must be balanced with the delivery time and the drug dose to protect the fetus from a potentially toxic dose.

When administering an analgesic during labor and delivery, the nurse carefully monitors the maternal and fetal condition by frequent assessment of vital signs, careful observation, and assessment of internal or external monitor information. The nurse also assesses the progress of labor and prepares, if necessary, for a depressed neonate.

THE LACTATING PATIENT

Because most drugs and chemicals ingested by a mother appear in breast milk, physicians must evaluate drug effects on the lactating mother and the infant. Unfortunately, several factors complicate this evaluation: systematic, complete information on individual drugs is lacking; available information usually is questionable because of unscientific studies; measurements of drug concentration often are unrelated to dose timing; conclusions are based on studies of animals whose physiochemical milk properties differ from humans'; and reports on toxic effects do not include the quantity of the drug in breast milk.

Drugs that affect lactation

Certain drugs ingested by the mother may not affect the infant adversely but may interfere with the hormones controlling milk secretion and let-down (ejection), namely prolactin and oxytocin.

DRUG	EFFECT
anesthetics, sedatives alcohol	Decrease let-down reflex
diuretics (thiazides) bendroflumethiazide, chlorothiazide	May suppress lactation
hormones contraceptive pill with estrogen and progesterone	Decrease milk production and protein content
antipsychotics neuroleptics	Galactorrhea
stimulants nicotine	Decrease milk production
miscellaneous agents bromocriptine	Suppress lactation

Adapted with permission from American Academy of Pediatrics. (1983). *Pediatrics*, 72(3), 376-377.

Breast anatomy and physiology

A brief review of breast anatomy and physiology and of milk formation indicates how drugs pass through breast milk. However, the nurse should be aware that some drugs can affect lactation. (For a list of drugs and effects, see *Drugs that affect lactation.*) The breast is composed of approximately 15 to 20 lobes embedded in fatty stroma. The lobes are drained by the lactiferous ducts near the nipple. In the nipple, the ducts dilate slightly to form the lactiferous sinuses. Each lobe is separated by connective tissue septa through which blood vessels, lymphatic vessels, and nerves pass. This connective tissue further subdivides the lobes into lobules, each with its own excretory or interlobular duct.

The basic secretory units of the lobes are the alveoli, surrounded in a basketlike fashion by myoepithelial cells. With the proper stimulus, these cells contract and eject milk from the alveoli and alveolar ducts. Prolactin is the hormone responsible for milk secretion, and oxytocin regulates the let-down (milk-ejection) reflex. Both of these hormones are under neurohormonal control. (For a summary, see *Physiology of lactation,* page 178.)

Breast milk is an emulsion of fat in a protein-mineral-carbohydrate solution; lactose is the carbohydrate. The milk's curds and whey contain many proteins, including alpha-lactalbumin, lactoferrin, albumin, lysozyme, and im-

Pysiology of lactation

Before lactation can occur, hormones must prepare the breast as shown below.

Hormonal preparation of breast postpartum for lactation

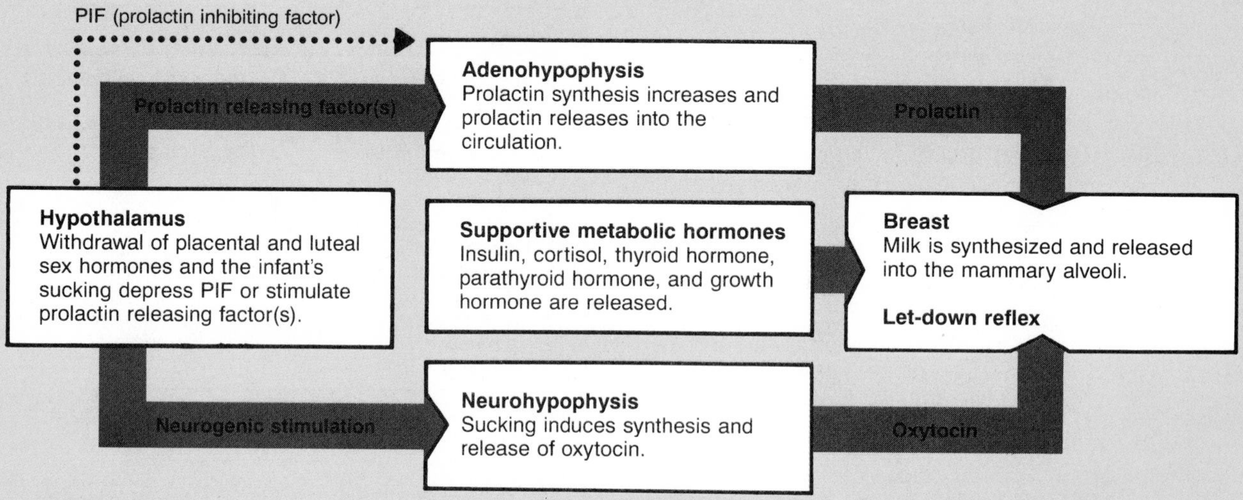

PIF (prolactin inhibiting factor)

Prolactin releasing factor(s)

Prolactin

Adenohypophysis
Prolactin synthesis increases and prolactin releases into the circulation.

Hypothalamus
Withdrawal of placental and luteal sex hormones and the infant's sucking depress PIF or stimulate prolactin releasing factor(s).

Supportive metabolic hormones
Insulin, cortisol, thyroid hormone, parathyroid hormone, and growth hormone are released.

Breast
Milk is synthesized and released into the mammary alveoli.

Let-down reflex

Neurogenic stimulation

Neurohypophysis
Sucking induces synthesis and release of oxytocin.

Oxytocin

Milk production takes place in the breast alveoli, tiny glands consisting of epithelial cells. A smooth-muscle layer of myoepithelial cells forms a dense meshwork of overlapping bands ensheathing the alveoli and lactiferous ducts—channels that convey milk to and through the nipples.

From the nutrient-rich blood in surrounding capillaries, alveoli draw the ingredients to make milk. Ten to one-hundred alveoli cluster to form lobules (as shown).

Although distributed throughout the breast, most lobules concentrate in the lower half and toward the axillae against the chest wall.

During pregnancy, the alveoli swell and their cells multiply rapidly. The start of lactation triggers fatty degeneration of cells in the lobule's center; these cells then are eliminated as colostrum corpuscles. Outer alveoli produce milk, which ejects into the cavity remaining in the middle of the lobule.

During pregnancy and lactation, myoepithelial cells multiply and expand. When exposed to oxytocin, a hormone released during breast-feeding, these cells contract, producing a squeezing effect on the lobule that forces milk down the ducts. When breast-feeding ends, myoepithelial cells decline in size and number.

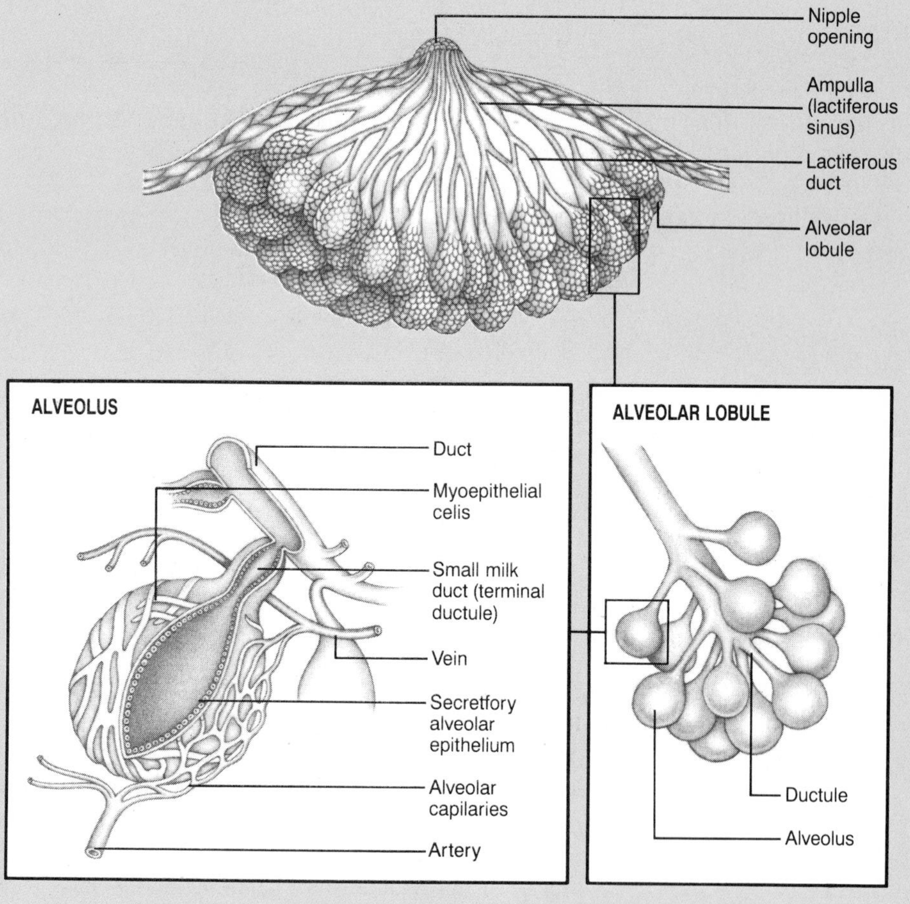

Nipple opening

Ampulla (lactiferous sinus)

Lactiferous duct

Alveolar lobule

ALVEOLUS

Duct

Myoepithelial celis

Small milk duct (terminal ductule)

Vein

Secretfory alveolar epithelium

Alveolar capilaries

Artery

ALVEOLAR LOBULE

Ductule

Alveolus

munoglobulin A, that may serve as molecules for drug binding and drug transport. The fat structure also may promote drug transport. In the protein-lactose-mineral aqueous component of milk, the lipid structure is suspended in fat globules that contain lipid surrounded by a lipoprotein membrane. Drugs may be transported by binding to the lipoprotein or be trapped within the milk-fat globule during fat formation.

Milk pH, another important variable affecting drug passage, ranges from 7.0 to 7.6, with an average of 7.2.

Drug characteristics

Before a drug can enter an alveolar cell from the maternal circulation, it must cross the capillary endothelium, extracellular water, cell basement membrane, and cell plasma membrane. Drugs usually are transported by passive diffusion and active transport.

Drug characteristics that affect the degree and rate of transport include molecular weight, solubility, maternal plasma protein binding, and ionization. A drug with a molecular weight greater than 200 has difficulty diffusing across cell membranes, and most drugs have a molecular weight of more than 200. Therefore, the passage of most drugs depends on the degree of lipid solubility and ionization. Highly lipid-soluble drugs cross the lipoprotein cell membrane more readily than more water-soluble drugs. Those bound to maternal plasma proteins are not readily transported; a nonprotein-bound (free) drug passes more easily into the milk.

Because most drugs are weak acids or bases, their crossing of a biological membrane is influenced greatly by ionization characteristics and pH differences. (For more information, see Chapter 2, Pharmacokinetics.) Because breast milk has a slightly lower pH than plasma, the milk's ions trap the basic drug compounds. The nonionized portion of a drug, however, can cross the lipid cell membrane.

Other factors that influence a drug's passage into breast milk include the route of administration, absorption rate, and drug half-life.

Maternal factors

Volume composition of breast milk may alter the amount of free drug available. Maternal factors, including nutrition, concurrent diseases, and infant intake, affect milk volume. Also, a high mammary blood flow during peak drug absorption could deliver a greater drug quantity to the milk. Milk fat content, which peaks between 6 a.m. and 10 a.m. and drops to its lowest level in the late evening, can affect drug availability, too. The composition of breast milk also varies depending on the infant's age. These changes in the milk may alter the amount of free (unbound) drug.

Drugs contraindicated during breast-feeding

Several drugs are contraindicated during breast-feeding. The nurse should be aware of these drugs to provide adequate patient teaching.

DRUG	SIGN OR SYMPTOM IN INFANT
methotrexate*	Possible immune suppression; unknown effect on growth or association with carcinogenesis
cimetidine†	May suppress gastric acidity in infant, inhibit drug metabolism, and produce central nervous system stimulation
cyclophosphamide*	Possible immune suppression; unknown effect on growth or association with carcinogenesis
ergotamine	Vomiting, diarrhea, seizures (doses used in migraine medications)
gold salts	Rash, inflammation of kidney and liver
methimazole	Potential for interfering with thyroid function
cyclosporine	Possible immune suppression; unknown effect on growth or association with carcinogenesis
doxorubicin	Possible immune suppression; unknown effect on growth or association with carcinogenesis
lithium	Produces 1/3 to 1/2 of the mother's therapeutic blood concentration in the infant

*Data unavailable for other cytotoxic agents.
†Drug is concentrated in breast milk.
Adapted with permission from American Academy of Pediatrics Committee on Drugs. (1983). Transfer of drugs and other chemicals into human breast milk. *Pediatrics*, 72(3), 375.

Infant characteristics

Unlike the fetus, the infant cannot depend on the placenta for the metabolism and excretion of maternally ingested drugs.

Infant sucking behavior, the amount consumed per feeding, and the frequency of breast-feeding affect the amount of drug the infant ingests. Low gastric acidity and slower absorption rates in the infant affect the amount of drug absorbed by the infant. Changes in plasma protein-binding in the infant may alter drug concentration levels at receptor sites. Further, drugs that are metabolized insufficiently and excreted by immature neonatal systems may accumulate, increasing the risk of toxicity.

Counseling guidelines

The nurse should inform the lactating patient that all drugs should be screened by a physician, nurse, or pharmacist for safety. The nurse should inform the patient about drugs that affect milk secretion.

The amount of drug that usually crosses to the milk is small, about 1% to 2% of the maternal dose. Nevertheless, the nurse should teach the mother to minimize the amount of a prescribed drug received by the infant. To do this, the mother should ingest the drug immediately after breast-feeding and postpone the next breast-feeding for 4 hours, if possible. Altering the administration schedule is another way to minimize the infant's drug exposure. For example, if the drug is to be administered once a day, the mother may take the dose before the infant's longest sleep period.

The nurse should teach the lactating patient the potential toxic effects of drugs on the infant. Easily recognizable effects include sedation, poor feeding, diarrhea, rash, and central nervous system stimulation. Some drugs may be contraindicated during breast-feeding. (For a list of drugs and their effects, see *Drugs contraindicated during breast-feeding,* page 179.) Others may require a temporary cessation of breast-feeding. The nurse also should discuss the effects of recreational drugs. (For a summary, see *Adverse effects of recreational drugs during pregnancy or lactation,* page 176.)

Should an infant become sick or fail to thrive for reasons that cannot be explained otherwise, the mother should discontinue the drug and temporarily discontinue breast-feeding. The mother may use a breast pump to maintain lactation while the infant's responses are monitored. The nurse should obtain samples of maternal plasma, breast milk, and infant plasma for drug assay.

CHAPTER SUMMARY

Chapter 12 covered the use of drugs during pregnancy and lactation. The fetus throughout gestation and the breast-feeding infant are sensitive to drugs ingested by the mother. Here are the chapter highlights.

• Maternal, placental, and fetal factors alter the absorption, distribution, metabolism, and excretion of a drug. Maternal factors include decreased tone and motility of the GI tract, increased blood volume, altered fat metabolism, increased glomerular filtration rate, and increased renal plasma flow. Placental factors include drug transport across the placenta and several enzymatic reactions, including reduction, hydrolysis, and conjugation. Fetal factors include fetal circulation, binding of plasma and tissue proteins, excretory activity, and the stimulation of normally deficient enzyme systems.

• The timing of drug administration during gestation determines the drug's effects on the fetus.

• When counseling a pregnant patient, the physician and nurse should discuss the benefits and risks of each drug. They should encourage her to use alternative nonpharmacologic measures and alternative drug treatments.

• The pregnant patient should use antacids, antiemetics, laxatives and stool softeners, and nonnarcotic analgesics with caution. She should consult the physician or nurse before using any OTC product.

• The need to relieve pain during labor must be balanced with the delivery time and the drug dose to protect the fetus from a potentially toxic dose.

• Most drugs and chemicals ingested by the mother appear in breast milk. When evaluating the use of drugs in a lactating patient, the physician considers drug characteristics, maternal factors, and infant characteristics.

• The nurse should inform the lactating patient about the signs and symptoms of drug toxicity that the infant may exhibit. If the mother must use a drug that is contraindicated during breast-feeding, she should discontinue breast-feeding temporarily.

STUDY QUESTIONS

See Appendix 1 for answers.

1. Ann Richards, a patient with diabetes mellitus controlled by glyburide (DiaBeta), is planning to become pregnant soon. She asks the nurse if she will be able to continue with her current drug regimen. The nurse checks the drug's risk-factor category for use during pregnancy. Drugs in which category should be used only if the potential benefit justifies the potential risk to the fetus?
(a) Category A
(b) Category B
(c) Category C
(d) Category X

2. The nurse teaches Ms. Richards that the physiologic changes of pregnancy may affect a drug's pharmacokinetics. Which physiologic change may alter drug distribution?
(a) decreased GI motility
(b) increased glomerular filtration
(c) decreased motilin levels
(d) increased blood volume

3. During pregnancy, how may physiologic changes in the urinary system affect drug excretion?
(a) They may slow excretion.
(b) They may speed excretion.
(c) They may cause variable excretion.
(d) They may produce unpredictable excretion.

4. The nurse advises Ms. Richards that ingestion of drugs during pregnancy may harm the fetus. During which trimester does drug use pose the greatest danger to fetal organ development?
(a) first
(b) second
(c) third
(d) all

5. After becoming pregnant, Ms. Richards complains of constipation during a prenatal visit. How should the nurse intervene?
(a) Advise her to take a prescription stool softener.
(b) Instruct her to use castor oil, as needed.
(c) Suggest that she take magnesium hydroxide.
(d) Tell her to increase her fluid and fiber intake.

6. After delivering a healthy, 9-pound boy, Janet Jones begins to breast-feed. How much of a drug usually passes through breast milk to the infant during breast-feeding?
(a) less than 1% of the maternal dose
(b) about 1% to 2% of the maternal dose
(c) from 10% to 20% of the maternal dose
(d) up to 50% of the maternal dose

7. One week after delivery, Ms. Jones develops a postpartal infection, for which the physician prescribes erythromycin. What should the nurse teach her about drug use during breast-feeding?
(a) Take the drug to meet her schedule.
(b) Take the drug immediately after a feeding.
(c) Take the drug 10 minutes before a feeding.
(d) Pump her breasts after taking the drug.

SELECTED REFERENCES

Atkinson, H., Begg, E., and Darlow, B. (1988). Drugs in human milk. *Clinical Pharmacokinetics,* 14(4), 217-240.

Bennett, P. (Ed.). (1988). *Drugs and human lactation.* New York: Elsevier.

Briggs, G., Freeman, R., and Yaffe, S. (1986). *Drugs in pregnancy and lactation* (2nd ed.). Baltimore: Williams & Wilkins.

Burrow, G., and Ferris, T. (1987). *Medical complications during pregnancy* (3rd ed.). Philadelphia: Saunders.

Dicke, J. (1989). Teratology: Principles and practice. *Medical Clinics of North America,* 73(3), 567-582.

Rivera-Calimlim, L. (1987). The significance of drugs in breast milk: Pharmacokinetic considerations. *Clinics in Perinatology,* 14(1), 51-70.

Zamula, E. (1989). Drugs and pregnancy: Often the two don't mix. *FDA Consumer,* 23(5), 7-10.

DRUGS AFFECTING THE AUTONOMIC NERVOUS SYSTEM

This unit focuses on drugs that influence one component of the nervous system: the efferent, or motor, limb of the peripheral nervous system. Yet the nurse must remember the interrelationship of all components of the nervous system when planning and monitoring drug therapy. The nurse can achieve clinical objectives for many autonomic nervous system disorders by understanding the system, how it communicates, and how it adapts to alterations in its environment.

The nervous system, which controls and coordinates functions throughout the body, has two major divisions: the central nervous system (CNS) containing the brain and spinal cord; and the peripheral nervous system containing afferent, or sensory, neurons (carrying information to the CNS) and efferent, or motor, neurons (carrying information from the CNS). The peripheral nervous system, which mediates between the CNS and the external and internal environments, is subdivided into the somatic nervous system and the autonomic nervous system.

The drugs discussed in Unit Three affect information transmittal by the motor neurons of the somatic and the autonomic divisions of the peripheral nervous system. To apply the nursing process when caring for a patient who is receiving such drug therapy, the nurse needs a working knowledge of this system.

ANATOMY AND PHYSIOLOGY

The somatic and autonomic nervous systems control and coordinate voluntary, involuntary, and reflex movements and visceral functions. However, these two systems have anatomic and physiologic differences that influence drug therapy and nursing assessment.

Somatic nervous system

Efferent neurons of the somatic nervous system travel to skeletal (striated) muscles and control reflex and voluntary movements. The cell bodies of these neurons lie within the CNS and send their axons directly to specialized synapses called neuromuscular junctions on the skeletal muscles that they innervate.

Autonomic nervous system

Efferent neurons of the autonomic nervous system innervate smooth and cardiac muscles, glands, and other viscera. Unlike the somatic nervous system, the autonomic nervous system is subdivided into the sympathetic nervous system (adrenergic) and the parasympathetic nervous system (cholinergic).

The sympathetic and parasympathetic nervous systems have two neurons (rather than one, as in the somatic nervous system) carrying information to the target sites. The cell bodies of the first neurons, like those of the somatic nervous system, originate in the CNS. The neurons of the sympathetic nervous system originate in the thoracic and lumbar regions of the spinal cord, and those of the parasympathetic nervous system originate in the brain stem or the sacral region of the spinal cord. The two systems are referred to, respectively, as the thoracolumbar and craniosacral divisions.

Axons from these first neurons leave the CNS and travel to ganglia where they synapse with a second neuron that travels to the target site. Because of the intervening ganglia, the axons of the first neurons are called preganglionic fibers; those of the second neurons, postganglionic fibers.

The preganglionic fibers of the sympathetic nervous system are short, terminating in ganglia that lie adjacent to the spinal cord (paravertebral chain) or a short distance from the cord (such as the celiac ganglion). The preganglionic fiber that innervates the adrenal medulla is an exception. It goes directly from the spinal cord to special cells in the adrenal medulla without synapsing. The adrenal medulla is analogous to a sympathetic postganglionic neuron (its secretory cells originate in nervous tissue) and releases norepinephrine and epinephrine directly into the circulation. Postganglionic fibers travel some distance to reach their target sites. (For an illustration of preganglionic

Glossary

Acetylcholine: choline acetic acid ester, present in many parts of the body, that facilitates impulse transmission from one nerve fiber to another or from a nerve to a muscle.

Acetylcholinesterase: enzyme that breaks down acetylcholine into acetic acid and choline.

Adrenergic: activated or transmitted by epinephrine, norepinephrine, or a similar substance.

Alpha-adrenergic receptor: adrenergic receptor of the sympathetic nervous system that responds to norepinephrine and various blocking agents.

Anticholinesterase: substance that inhibits the breakdown of acetylcholine by acetylcholinesterase.

Antimuscarinic: agent that inhibits stimulation of muscarinic receptors; also called anticholinergic or parasympatholytic.

Autonomic nervous system: portion of the nervous system that controls the involuntary visceral functions of the body.

Beta-adrenergic receptor: adrenergic receptor of the sympathetic nervous system that responds to epinephrine and various blocking agents.

Catecholamine: class of sympathomimetic neuroregulators that includes dobutamine, dopamine, isoproterenol, norepinephrine, and epinephrine.

Catechol-O-methyltransferase: enzyme diffusely present in all tissues that breaks down catecholamines.

Cholinergic: stimulated, activated, or transmitted by acetylcholine or a similar substance.

Ganglion: group of nerve cell bodies located outside the central nervous system.

Inotropic: altering the force of muscular contraction.

Monoamine oxidase: enzyme in the nerve endings that enhances deamination or breakdown of catecholamines.

Motor end plate: branching nerve terminals of a motor neuron of the voluntary muscles.

Muscarinic receptor: receptor located in effector cells that is stimulated by acetylcholine, muscarine, or a similar substance.

Neurohormone: hormone that stimulates the neural mechanism.

Neuromuscular junction: joining of a nerve ending and a muscle fiber.

Neuron: nerve cell; the structural unit of the nervous system.

Neurotransmitter: chemical substance secreted by the neuron at the synapse that acts on receptor proteins in the membrane of the adjacent neuron or muscle to stimulate, inhibit, or modify its activity.

Nicotinic receptor: receptor located in effector cells that is stimulated by acetylcholine and nicotine.

Parasympathetic nervous system: cholinergic division of the autonomic nervous system.

Parasympatholytic: agent that opposes the effects of impulses conveyed by the parasympathetic nervous system; also called anticholinergic or antimuscarinic.

Parasympathomimetic: agent that produces effects similar to those from stimulation of the parasympathetic nerves; also called cholinergic or muscarinic.

Sympathetic nervous system: adrenergic division of the autonomic nervous system.

Sympatholytic: agent that opposes the impulses conveyed by the adrenergic postganglionic fibers of the sympathetic nervous system.

Sympathomimetic: agent that produces effects similar to those of impulses conveyed by the adrenergic postganglionic fibers of the sympathetic nervous system.

Synapse: area surrounding the point of contact between the processes of two adjacent neurons or between a neuron and effector organ where an impulse is transmitted through the action of a neurotransmitter.

and postganglionic fibers and neurotransmission, see *Sympathetic division activity,* page 184.)

In contrast, most preganglionic fibers of the parasympathetic nervous system are long and travel to ganglia located close to or in the walls of their target sites. The postganglionic fibers of the parasympathetic nervous system are short. This dissimilarity in the distribution pattern of preganglionic and postganglionic fibers facilitates the contrasting effects of the two systems. The characteristics of the sympathetic nervous system permit a more generalized, widespread effect; those of the parasympathetic nervous system permit a more discrete, localized effect. (For an illustration of preganglionic and postganglionic fibers and neurotransmission, see *Parasympathetic division activity,* page 185.)

Usually, both systems send information to the same target sites. Exceptions include the adrenal medulla, sweat glands, spleen, and hair follicles, which are innervated by the sympathetic nervous system only. Because the physiologic functions of the two systems usually are opposite,

dual innervation balances physiologic effects. Drug therapy sometimes disrupts this critical balance, as when the parasympathetic nervous system is blocked and the activity of the sympathetic nervous system is unopposed. Knowing the physiologic effects of each system allows the nurse to predict what may happen when a particular drug is used therapeutically.

Stimulation of the somatic nervous system can be viewed as initiating a single activity, skeletal muscle contraction; however, the physiologic effects of the subdivisions of the autonomic nervous system are much more complex. In general, however, the sympathetic nervous system can be viewed as an activity-response system, and the parasympathetic nervous system as a vegetative-homeostatic system.

Stimulation of the sympathetic nervous system increases heart and respiratory rate, metabolic rate, and fat and glycogen breakdown; produces pupillary dilation, smooth muscle vasoconstriction, and skeletal muscle vasodilation; and decreases gastrointestinal (GI) activity. These effects

Sympathetic division activity

The sympathetic branch of the autonomic nervous system has two neurons that carry information to effector organs. Neurons originate from the thoracolumbar region within the central nervous system. Preganglionic and postganglionic fibers transmit nerve impulses. Preganglionic fibers are short, terminating in ganglia that lie adjacent to the spinal cord or a short distance from it. The preganglionic fiber that directly innervates the adrenal medulla without synapsing at a ganglion causes release of norepinephrine and epinephrine directly into the circulation. Postganglionic fibers are long and travel some distance through effector cells to reach effector organs. This transmittal is carried out by chemicals (neurotransmitters). Major neurotransmitters are norepinephrine, epinephrine, and to a lesser extent, dopamine and acetylcholine (ACh).

Major physiologic effects are alpha and beta adrenergic: vasoconstriction; vasodilation; heart rate, force of contraction, and conduction velocity increase; bronchial smooth muscle relaxation; gastrointestinal (GI) tract smooth muscle relaxation; GI sphincter contraction; urinary system smooth muscle relaxation; sphincter contraction; pupillary dilation and ciliary muscle relaxation; sweat gland secretion increase; pancreatic secretion decrease; and thick salivary secretions.

Drugs that influence these functions include adrenergic agonists and antagonists and ganglionic blocking agents.

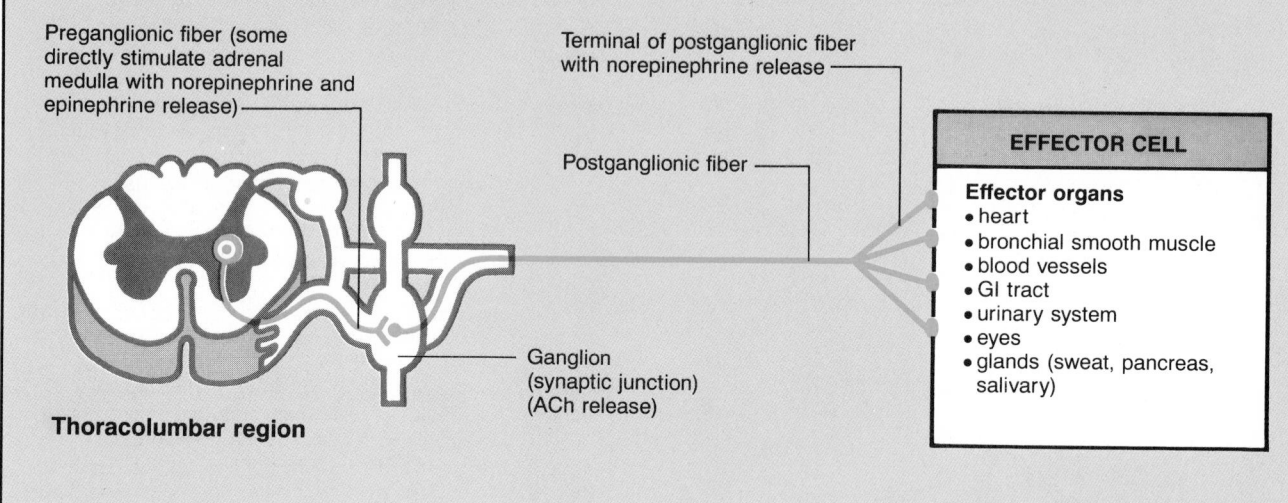

Preganglionic fiber (some directly stimulate adrenal medulla with norepinephrine and epinephrine release)

Terminal of postganglionic fiber with norepinephrine release

Postganglionic fiber

Ganglion (synaptic junction) (ACh release)

Thoracolumbar region

EFFECTOR CELL

Effector organs
- heart
- bronchial smooth muscle
- blood vessels
- GI tract
- urinary system
- eyes
- glands (sweat, pancreas, salivary)

sometimes are called the "fight or flight" response because they prepare the individual to face or run from something threatening.

Conversely, stimulation of the parasympathetic nervous system produces heart and respiratory rate decrease, pupil constriction and enhanced accommodation, digestion and elimination increase, GI tone enhancement, and sphincter tone relaxation. These activities are considered energy conserving and homeostatic.

Neuron communication

The nervous system communicates via chemicals called neuroregulators, or neurotransmitters, that transmit neuron information between adjacent cells. In the motor limb of the peripheral nervous system, the major neurotransmitters are acetylcholine, norepinephrine, epinephrine, and to a lesser extent, dopamine.

Acetylcholine is released from all preganglionic neurons of the autonomic nervous system, from all postganglionic neurons of the parasympathetic nervous system, from some postsynaptic neurons of the sympathetic nervous system,

and at neuromuscular junctions within the somatic nervous system. Acetylcholine's duration of action is short; it is degraded rapidly by the enzyme acetylcholinesterase.

Norepinephrine and epinephrine are released from the adrenal medulla. Norepinephrine also is released from the postganglionic adrenergic fibers of the sympathetic nervous system. The epinephrine and norepinephrine released from the adrenal medulla have effects similar to direct adrenergic neuronal stimulation but can reach and stimulate target sites that do not receive direct innervation from adrenergic fibers.

The duration of action of norepinephrine released at the synapse is extremely short because it rapidly re-enters the neuron from which it was released (reuptake), diffuses from the area, or is degraded by the enzymes monoamine oxidase or catechol-O-methyltransferase. The duration of action of the epinephrine and norepinephrine released from the adrenal medulla, however, may last 10 times longer because removal from the circulation is less rapid than from neuronal synapses. This slower removal from the circulation emphasizes the potential difference between the effects of

Parasympathetic division activity

The parasympathetic branch of the autonomic nervous system has two neurons that carry information to the cells of effector organs. Neurons originate in the craniosacral region of the central nervous system. Preganglionic and postganglionic fibers transmit nerve impulses. Most preganglionic fibers are long and travel to ganglia located close to or in the walls of the effector organs. In contrast, the postganglionic fibers are short. The major neurotransmitter is acetylcholine.

The physiologic effects include vasodilation of salivary glands; heart rate, force of contraction, and conduction velocity decrease; bronchial smooth muscle constriction; GI tract tone and peristalsis increase with sphincter relaxation; urinary system sphincter relaxation and bladder tone increase; pupillary constriction; and pancreatic, salivary, and lacrimal secretions increase.

Drugs that influence these functions include cholinergic agonists and antagonists and ganglionic blocking agents.

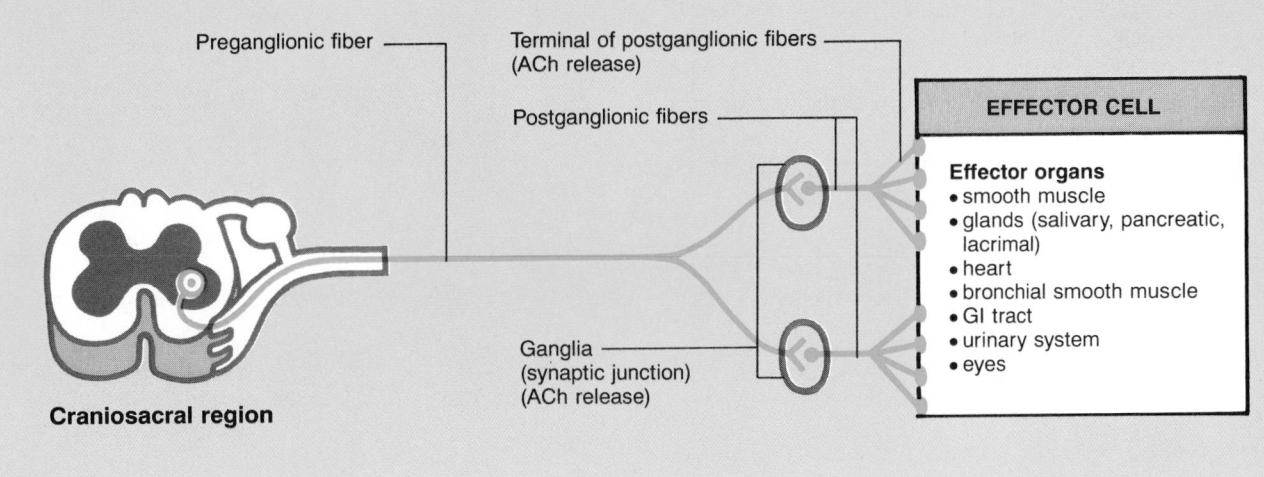

Preganglionic fiber

Terminal of postganglionic fibers (ACh release)

Postganglionic fibers

EFFECTOR CELL

Effector organs
- smooth muscle
- glands (salivary, pancreatic, lacrimal)
- heart
- bronchial smooth muscle
- GI tract
- urinary system
- eyes

Ganglia (synaptic junction) (ACh release)

Craniosacral region

administered drugs and endogenous substances released within the body.

Dopamine is a neurotransmitter and a precursor to norepinephrine. It can interact with dopaminergic, alpha- and beta-adrenergic receptors and can stimulate the release of norepinephrine from adrenergic fibers.

DRUG EFFECTS

Effects sometimes are achieved through a drug's interaction with specific receptors on a target cell. Receptors are dynamic cellular components that can be altered by many conditions. Knowledge of receptor physiology has improved drug specificity and the understanding of how the body adapts to exogenous drugs or an altered internal environment. The mechanisms of action for drugs discussed in this unit depend on receptor types, presynaptic receptors, receptor regulation, and nonspecific drug effects.

Types of receptors

The major classes of receptors currently identified in the motor limb of the peripheral nervous system include alpha-adrenergic receptors, beta-adrenergic receptors, dopamine receptors, muscarinic receptors, and nicotinic receptors.

Target tissues may have one or a combination of these receptors. A drug's effects are determined by the numbers of each receptor and the drug's specificity.

The catecholamines norepinephrine and epinephrine exert their effects by interacting with alpha- and beta-adrenergic receptors. Each has two subtypes: alpha$_1$ and alpha$_2$, and beta$_1$ and beta$_2$. Norepinephrine has a greater effect on alpha$_1$ and alpha$_2$, and beta$_1$ receptors than on beta$_2$ receptors; epinephrine has an equal effect on alpha and beta receptors. Thus epinephrine can exert greater metabolic, vasodilatory, and bronchodilatory effects than norepinephrine can.

Over the past decade, alpha-adrenergic receptors that regulate sympathetic transmission to the cardiovascular system also have been identifed in the CNS. Therefore, drugs that act on receptors in the CNS can influence the peripheral nervous system. Also, dopamine can interact with dopaminergic, alpha, and beta receptors, depending on its concentration.

Acetylcholine exerts its effect by interacting with nicotinic and muscarinic receptors. Nicotinic receptors are located in the autonomic ganglia (between pre- and postsynaptic fibers of the autonomic nervous system), in the motor end plates at the neuromuscular junction of the somatic nervous system, and in the CNS. The nicotinic receptors on skeletal muscle have different properties than those in the autonomic ganglia. Muscarinic receptors are found at the synapses of the postsynaptic fibers of the parasympathetic nervous system, on some postsynaptic fibers of the sympathetic nervous system, and in the CNS.

Presynaptic receptors

The amount of a neurotransmitter released from a neuron is modulated by neuroregulators and presynaptic receptors on the neuron. Presynaptic alpha-adrenergic receptors are alpha$_2$ receptors.

Presynaptic receptors have clinical importance. For example, an adrenergic blocking agent that nonselectively blocks alpha$_1$ and alpha$_2$ receptors will block the contraction of vascular smooth muscle (alpha$_1$) and the negative feedback to adrenergic fibers (alpha$_2$). The negative feedback block will release more norepinephrine that can stimulate the heart's beta-adrenergic receptors and cause tachycardia.

Receptor regulation

Altered environmental conditions can change receptor number or density (up or down regulation) or change the affinity of a receptor for an agonist or antagonist (uncoupling). Drug effects and withdrawal effects relate to receptor number or affinity. For instance, long-term administration of a beta agonist can decrease the density of beta receptors and reduce the drug's effect. In contrast, long-term administration of a beta antagonist, or blocker, can increase the density of receptors and the response to sudden withdrawal of a beta-blocking agent.

A number of clinical conditions, such as diabetes mellitus and hypothyroidism or hyperthyroidism, can affect receptor concentration or affinity. Thus the nurse must consider the patient's current clinical status when assessing drug therapy.

Nonspecificity

Drugs cannot be directed to a select body area or tissue site. Rather, they act on all receptors to which they have access and can bind. Because the CNS contains receptors for acetylcholine, norepinephrine, and epinephrine, drugs given to affect acetylcholine in the peripheral neurons can exert unwanted CNS effects if they cross the blood-brain barrier.

DRUG SELECTION AND USE

Drugs affect the neural transmission of information in several ways. For example, they may imitate a neurotransmitter's action, block its effect at a receptor site, or enhance or inhibit its synthesis, storage, release, or breakdown. Drugs also may alter the ability of postsynaptic target cells to recover from stimulation.

Drug selection is based on mechanism of action and clinical objectives. For example, if hypertension treatment is aimed at lowering norepinephrine levels to minimize vasoconstriction, a drug that inhibits norepinephrine's effects will be considered. Drug selection is based on specificity for a particular target tissue, efficacy, adverse effects and toxicity, and cost. The cost must be evaluated in dollars and effects on the patient's physical and psychological functioning (such as impotence from antihypertensive agents).

Drugs that influence the somatic or autonomic nervous systems can be categorized according to (1) location of their primary effect, (2) primary effect, such as facilitation or inhibition of sympathetic or parasympathetic effects, and (3) the receptor with which they interact. The drug categories discussed in this unit produce effects similar to acetylcholine, norepinephrine, or epinephrine, or inhibit the effects of those substances.

Drug categories that produce effects similar to acetylcholine include cholinergic agents, parasympathomimetic agents, cholinesterase inhibitors, muscarinic agents, and nicotinic agents. Drugs that inhibit the sympathetic nervous system also can permit acetylcholine's unopposed activity within the parasympathetic nervous system.

Drug categories that inhibit the effects of acetylcholine include cholinergic blocking agents, anticholinergic agents, parasympatholytic agents, antimuscarinic agents, ganglionic blocking agents, and neuromuscular blocking agents. Drugs that facilitate sympathetic nervous system activity also may antagonize acetylcholine's effects.

Drug categories that produce effects similar to norepinephrine and epinephrine include adrenergic agents (catecholamines or noncatecholamines that are alpha, beta, dopaminergic, or nonselective), sympathomimetic agents, and monoamine oxidase inhibitors. Drugs that inhibit the parasympathetic nervous system also may allow unopposed sympathetic nervous system activity.

Drug categories that inhibit the effects of norepinephrine and epinephrine include sympatholytic agents, adrenergic blocking agents, and ganglionic blocking agents — which block the sympathetic and parasympathetic nervous systems at the preganglionic level. Drugs that facilitate parasympathetic activity also indirectly may antagonize the effects of norepinephrine and epinephrine.

OVERVIEW OF CHAPTERS

The chapters in Unit Three explore the agents that affect the autonomic nervous system and the nurse's responsibilities when administering them. It addresses cholinergic, cholinergic blocking, adrenergic, adrenergic blocking, and neuromuscular blocking agents.

Chapter 13
Cholinergic Agents

Chapter 13 explores agents that mimic acetylcholine's effects and stimulate the parasympathetic nervous system. It highlights the three major clinical indications of cholinergic agents: to reduce intraocular pressure in patients with glaucoma or during ocular surgery; to treat atony of the GI tract or bladder; and to diagnose and treat myasthenia gravis. After discussing the two main classes of drugs used as cholinergic agents (cholinergic agonists and anticholinesterase agents), the chapter focuses on nursing care, especially management of the agents' effects.

Chapter 14
Cholinergic Blocking Agents

Chapter 14 focuses on agents that compete with acetylcholine at receptor sites in the CNS, autonomic ganglia, autonomic effector organs, and neuromuscular junctions. It reviews the uses of antimuscarinic agents, such as belladonna alkaloids, quaternary ammonium compounds, and tertiary amines, which include treatment of spastic conditions of the GI and urinary tracts, cardiac arrhythmias, motion sickness, parkinsonism, and chronic asthma. These agents also may be used as preanesthesia medications and as relaxants for the GI tract during diagnostic procedures and for the eye and pupil during ophthalmologic surgery. They serve as antidotes to cholinergic agents and organophosphate pesticides.

Chapter 15
Adrenergic Agents

Adrenergic agents, or catecholamines and noncatecholamines, are presented in Chapter 15. The discussion begins with a review of the physiologic actions of the adrenergic agents, similar to those produced by sympathetic nervous system stimulation. It differentiates among the effects of alpha, beta$_1$, and beta$_2$ receptor activity and the clinical uses of the adrenergic agents. Then the chapter describes the two drug classes of adrenergic agents: catecholamines and noncatecholamines. For each drug class, the chapter presents related nursing care.

Chapter 16
Adrenergic Blocking Agents

Chapter 16 explores alpha- and beta-adrenergic and ganglionic blocking agents used to inhibit sympathetic nervous system function. It discusses alpha-adrenergic blockers, which decrease blood pressure, and their adverse effects related to vasodilation. It investigates beta-adrenergic blocking agents, including their selective action on cardiospecific beta$_1$ receptors and their nonselective action on beta$_1$ and beta$_2$ receptors. The chapter details the clinical use of beta blockers in treating hypertension, cardiac ar-rhythmias, and angina. Then it discusses ganglionic blocking agents, which are nonselective in their blocking action, and their role in hypotension. Throughout, Chapter 16 emphasizes application of the nursing process during therapy with adrenergic blocking agents.

Chapter 17
Neuromuscular Blocking Agents

Chapter 17 examines the neuromuscular blocking agents as muscle relaxants that facilitate surgery. It explores the two types of neuromuscular blocking agents, nondepolarizing and depolarizing. A major emphasis of the chapter is the nursing care required for patient safety during the administration of these agents.

CHOLINERGIC AGENTS

OBJECTIVES

After reading and studying this chapter, the student should be able to:
1. Discuss the three major clinical indications for the cholinergic agents.
2. Describe the actions of acetylcholine and acetylcholinesterase in the parasympathetic nervous system.
3. Explain the pharmacokinetics of the cholinergic agonists.
4. Explain the pharmacokinetics of the anticholinesterase agents.
5. Contrast the mechanisms of action of the cholinergic agonists with those of the anticholinesterase agents.
6. Identify significant adverse effects of the cholinergic and anticholinesterase agents.
7. Describe how to apply the nursing process when caring for a patient who is receiving a cholinergic or anticholinesterase agent.

INTRODUCTION

Cholinergic agents are drugs that directly or indirectly promote the function of the neurotransmitter acetylcholine. The cholinergics also are called parasympathomimetics because they produce effects that imitate parasympathetic nerve stimulation.

Cholinergic agents have three major clinical indications. They are used to reduce intraocular pressure in patients with glaucoma or during ocular surgery, to treat atony of the gastrointestinal (GI) tract or bladder, and to diagnose and treat myasthenia gravis. Some of the cholinergic agents are important antidotes to neuromuscular blocking agents, tricyclic antidepressants, and belladonna alkaloids.

Cholinergic agents achieve their effects in one of two ways: They mimic the action of acetylcholine or inhibit its destruction at cholinergic receptor sites. Chapter 13 discusses the two main classes of drugs used as cholinergic agents: cholinergic agonists and anticholinesterase agents.

Physiology of the parasympathetic nervous system

Part of the autonomic nervous system, the parasympathetic nervous system controls the body's visceral functions: It conserves energy and maintains organ function.

The parasympathetic nervous system has two subdivisions: the cranial and the sacral. The cranial subdivision is made up of cranial nerves III (oculomotor), VII (facial), IX (glossopharyngeal), and X (vagus).

The oculomotor nerve innervates the pupillary sphincters and the ciliary muscles; the facial nerve innervates the lacrimal, sublingual, and submaxillary glands and mucous membranes of the nose and palate; and the glossopharyngeal nerve innervates the parotid gland. The vagus nerve carries about 75% of all parasympathetic fibers. The organs under vagal stimulation include the lungs, heart, stomach (including the pyloric valve), liver, small intestine, and the upper two-thirds of the colon and kidney. (For a depiction of the nerve-target organ relationships, see *Parasympathetic nervous system,* page 190.)

The cranial nerves give rise to preganglionic fibers that synapse with postganglionic fibers at ganglia near the target organs or, in the case of the vagus nerve, in the target organ itself. The postganglionic fibers innervate the target organs through autonomic effector cells, where acetylcholine is synthesized and secreted.

The sacral portion of the parasympathetic nervous system arises from the second, third, and fourth segments of the sacral spinal cord. The sacral parasympathetic fibers form the pelvic nerves, which distribute their fibers to the bladder, external genitalia, sex organs, distal colon, rectum, anal sphincter, and lower portion of the ureters.

The preganglionic and postganglionic fibers of the parasympathetic nervous system are cholinergic; that is, they synthesize and secrete the neurotransmitter acetylcholine. Acetylcholine's action lasts for a few seconds at most because most of it is quickly destroyed by the enzyme acetylcholinesterase.

Acetylcholine lasts long enough, however, to stimulate the target organ by combining with receptor sites on cell

SELECTED NURSING DIAGNOSES

Cholinergic agents

The following nursing diagnoses address representative problems and etiologies that a nurse may encounter when caring for a patient who is receiving a cholinergic agent. Some of these nursing diagnoses contain generalized etiologies, which the nurse must individualize based on the patient's needs. (For some common nursing diagnoses and related interventions for each drug class, see the "Nursing Process Application" sections of this chapter.)

- Activity intolerance related to skeletal muscle weakness caused by the anticholinesterase agent
- Altered health maintenance related to ineffectiveness of the cholinergic agent
- Altered urinary elimination related to urinary frequency caused by the cholinergic agonist
- Anxiety related to the adverse CNS effects of the cholinergic agent
- Decreased cardiac output related to the adverse cardiovascular effects of the cholinergic agonist
- Diarrhea related to increased GI motility caused by the cholinergic agent
- Fear related to the adverse CNS effects of the anticholinesterase agent
- Impaired physical mobility related to ineffectiveness of the anticholinesterase agent in a patient with myasthenia gravis taking a neuromuscular blocking agent or procainamide

- Ineffective breathing pattern related to bronchoconstriction caused by the cholinergic agent
- Knowledge deficit related to the prescribed cholinergic agent
- Potential fluid volume deficit related to the adverse GI effects of the cholinergic agent
- Potential for injury related to a preexisting condition that contraindicates the use of cholinergic agents
- Potential for injury related to a preexisting condition that requires cautious use of cholinergic agents
- Potential for injury related to adverse drug reactions
- Potential for injury related to drug interactions with the prescribed cholinergic agent
- Potential for trauma related to anticholinesterase-induced seizures
- Sensory-perceptual alteration (visual) related to the adverse CNS effects of the cholinergic agent

---

membranes. That allows calcium and sodium to enter the cells of the target organ, resulting in depolarization of the cell membrane and contraction of the target organ muscle.

Acetylcholine activates nicotinic and muscarinic receptors. Nicotinic receptors are present in the synapses between the preganglionic and postganglionic neurons of the sympathetic and parasympathetic nervous systems, in the motor end-plates of skeletal muscle at the neuromuscular function, and in the central nervous system (CNS). Muscarinic receptors are present in all the effector cells stimulated by postganglionic neurons of the parasympathetic nervous system, the postganglionic cholinergic neurons of the sympathetic nervous system, and in the CNS. Acetylcholine triggers representative responses in the eyes, salivary glands, bronchi, heart, GI tract, and urinary bladder. In these parasympathetic nervous system target organs, acetylcholine produces the following effects:
- Pupillary constriction
- Increased accommodation
- Increased salivation
- Bronchial constriction
- Increased bronchial secretion
- Decreased heart rate
- Decreased atrial contraction
- Increased GI secretions
- Increased GI peristalsis
- Relaxation of GI sphincter
- Voiding.

For a summary of representative drugs, see *Selected major drugs: Cholinergic agents,* page 197. For a listing of applicable nursing diagnoses that the nurse may formulate when caring for a patient receiving these agents, see *Selected nursing diagnoses: Cholinergic agents.* For detailed information on applying the nursing process, see Chapter 6, The Nursing Process and Drug Therapy.

CHOLINERGIC AGONISTS

Cholinergic agonists directly stimulate cholinergic receptors, thus mimicking the action of endogenous acetylcholine. They include synthetic acetylcholine; choline esters, such as bethanechol and carbachol; and naturally occurring cholinomimetic alkaloids such as pilocarpine.

Acetylcholine rarely is used clinically because it can act at nicotinic and muscarinic receptor sites, which can cause unpredictable effects, and because it is rapidly destroyed by acetylcholinesterase. Although the choline esters and cholinomimetic alkaloids resist breakdown by acetylcholinesterase, they too lack specificity of action. Clinically, they are used for their effects on the eye, the intestine, and the urinary bladder, but, because of their widespread parasympathomimetic actions, they have many adverse effects.

Parasympathetic nervous system

When parasympathetic nerves are stimulated, they release acetylcholine from the nerve endings. The acetylcholine binds with receptor sites on the target organs and stimulates muscle contraction. The nerves and their corresponding sites are shown below.

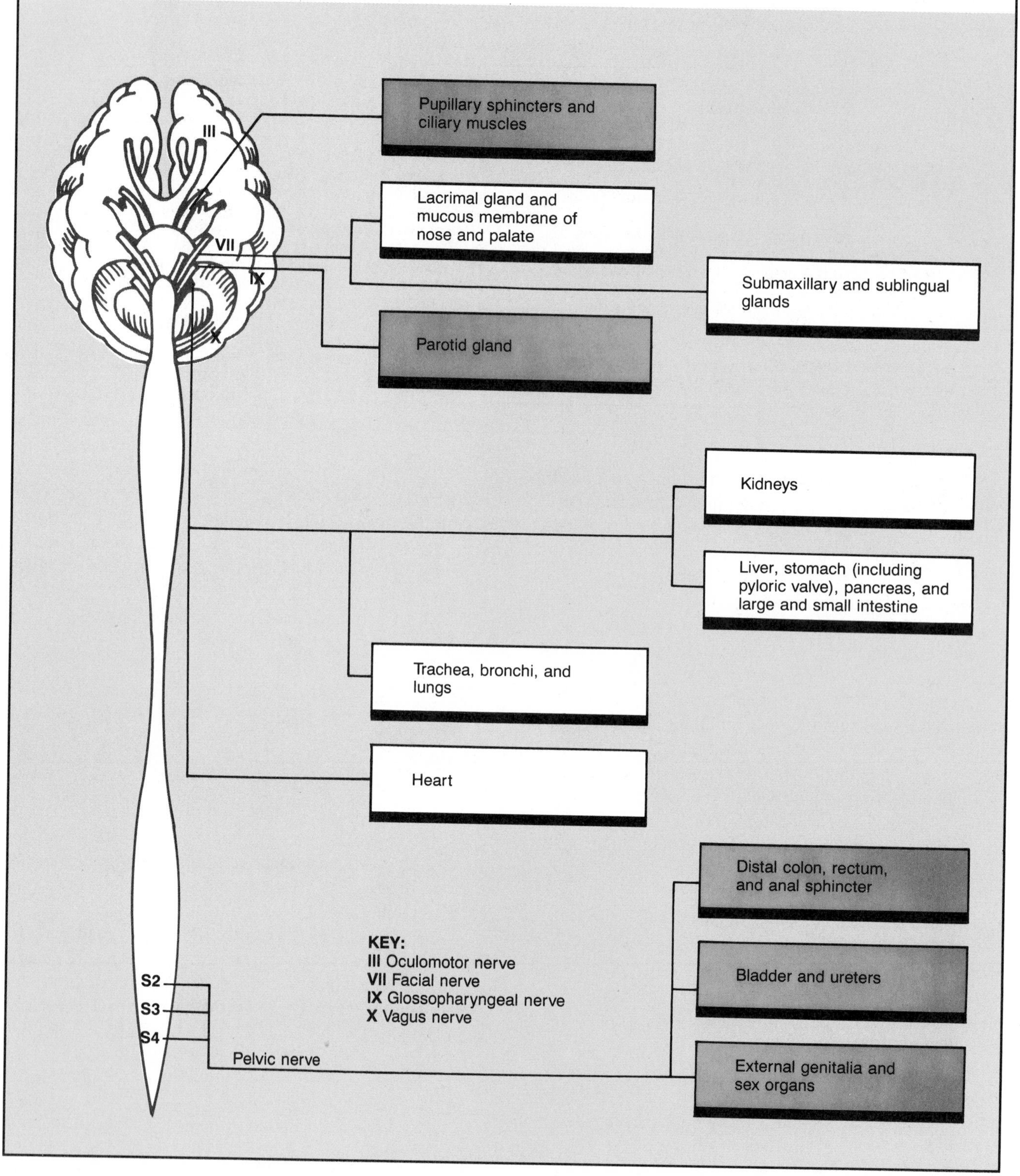

Pupillary sphincters and ciliary muscles

Lacrimal gland and mucous membrane of nose and palate

Submaxillary and sublingual glands

Parotid gland

Kidneys

Liver, stomach (including pyloric valve), pancreas, and large and small intestine

Trachea, bronchi, and lungs

Heart

Distal colon, rectum, and anal sphincter

Bladder and ureters

External genitalia and sex organs

III

VII

IX

X

S2

S3

S4

Pelvic nerve

KEY:
III Oculomotor nerve
VII Facial nerve
IX Glossopharyngeal nerve
X Vagus nerve

PHARMACOKINETICS

The action and metabolism of the cholinergic agonists vary widely, depending on their affinity for nicotinic or muscarinic receptors and on their susceptibility to inactivation by the enzyme acetylcholinesterase.

Absorption, distribution, metabolism, excretion

The cholinergic agonists rarely are administered I.M. or I.V. because they are subject to immediate breakdown by cholinesterases in the interstitial and intravascular spaces. In addition, cholinergic agonists administered I.M. and I.V. take effect rapidly and increase the likelihood of a cholinergic crisis.

Usually, the cholinergic agonists are administered intraocularly, orally, or subcutaneously. Because these routes limit drug absorption, the number of adverse effects is minimized. For example, when cholinergic agonists are administered in the eye, pressure applied on the inner canthus prevents their drainage through the lacrimal ducts and subsequent absorption through the nasal mucosa. This reduces systemic response to the medications. With oral administration, adverse effects seem to be reduced when the drugs are given on an empty stomach. Subcutaneous administration may result in a more rapid and effective response.

The most useful cholinergic agonists bind primarily with muscarinic receptors and are not susceptible to cholinesterases. For example, bethanechol has an affinity for muscarinic receptors in the bladder and GI tract and is resistant to cholinesterases. Drugs that bind with nicotinic and muscarinic receptors, such as carbachol, acetylcholine, and pilocarpine, are used intraocularly, where their absorption is limited.

All cholinergic agonists are metabolized by cholinesterases at the muscarinic and nicotinic receptor sites, in the plasma, and in the liver. However, some of the cholinergic agonists are more susceptible to the enzymes than others. Drugs such as acetylcholine, which are metabolized rapidly by cholinesterases, rarely are used clinically. Carbachol, bethanechol, and pilocarpine are more resistant to the action of these enzymes and therefore are more useful clinically. All drugs in this class are excreted by the kidneys.

Onset, peak, duration

When administered orally, bethanechol begins acting within 30 to 90 minutes, reaches a peak concentration level in 1 to 3 hours, and has a duration of action of 6 hours. Subcutaneously, bethanechol works much more rapidly, with an onset of action of 5 to 15 minutes, a peak concentration in 15 to 30 minutes, and a duration of 2 hours. (For a discussion of the ophthalmic cholinergic agonists carbachol and pilocarpine, see Chapter 71, Ophthalmic Agents.)

PHARMACODYNAMICS

The cholinergic agonists combine with cholinergic receptors at organs innervated by the parasympathetic nervous system, producing effects equivalent to those of postganglionic parasympathetic nerve impulses. (For a summary of the selective effects of these drugs on target organs, see *Pharmacologic actions of cholinergic agents,* page 192.)

Mechanism of action

Cholinergic agonists mimic the action of acetylcholine at the autonomic effector site. They bind with receptors on the cell membrane of smooth muscles, changing the permeability of the cell membrane and permitting calcium and sodium to flow into the cells. This depolarizes the cell membrane, causing muscle contraction.

PHARMACOTHERAPEUTICS

Clinical indications for the cholinergic agonists are twofold: to treat atonic bladder conditions and to reduce intraocular pressure in the anterior chamber of the eye. The latter indication is useful in patients with glaucoma and in those undergoing ocular surgery.

bethanechol chloride (Duvoid, Myotonachol, Urecholine). A choline ester that stimulates the smooth muscle of the GI tract and urinary bladder, bethanechol is used to treat urinary retention. Bethanechol also has been used to treat postoperative abdominal distention, GI atony, and other GI disorders, although its effectiveness in these indications has not been established.
Usual adult dosage: for urinary retention secondary to hypotonic or atonic bladder, up to 50 mg P.O. q.i.d.; for acute urine retention, 5 mg S.C.

carbachol (Carbacel, Isopto Carbachol, Miostat). A choline ester, intraocular carbachol is used to reduce intraocular pressure during ophthalmologic procedures; topical carbachol is used to treat open-angle and closed-angle glaucoma. (For a complete description, see Chapter 71, Ophthalmic Agents.)

pilocarpine hydrochloride (Adsorbocarpine, Akarpine, Isopto Carpine, Pilocar). A naturally occurring cholinomimetic alkaloid, pilocarpine reduces intraocular pressure in glaucoma. (For a complete description, see Chapter 71, Ophthalmic Agents.)

Drug interactions

The effect of the cholinergic agonists is intensified by the simultaneous presence of anticholinesterase agents, which inhibit the breakdown of acetylcholine at the receptor sites. The action of cholinergic agonists is limited by interaction

Pharmacologic actions of cholinergic agents

Cholinergic agents have a differential parasympathomimetic effect on the various body systems that are quantitative and selective for a body system. To provide quality patient care, the nurse should be aware of these differences.

DRUG	Bronchi	Cardiovascular system	Central nervous system	Eye	Gastrointestinal system	Myoneural junction	Salivary glands	Urinary bladder
Cholinergic agonists								
bethanechol	+ +	+ +	–	+ +	+ + +	–	+	+ + +
carbachol	+	+	–	+ + +	+ +	–	+	+ +
pilocarpine	+ +	+ + +	+ +	+ + +	+ +	–	+ + +	+ +
Anticholinesterase agents								
ambenonium	+	+	+	+	+	+ + +	+	+
edrophonium	+	+	–	+	+	+ +	+	+
neostigmine	+	+	+	+	+ +	+ + +	+	+ + +
physostigmine	+	+	+ + +	+	+	+ + +	+	+
pyridostigmine	+	+	+	+	+	+ + +	+	+

KEY + minor effect
+ + moderate effect
+ + + major effect
– no effect

with antimuscarinic drugs and sympathomimetics. Antimuscarinic drugs, such as atropine, block the action of the cholinergic agonists on the autonomic effector. Sympathomimetics produce a response opposite to that of the cholinergic agonists at muscarinic receptors. (For more information, see *Drug interactions: Cholinergic agonists.*)

ADVERSE DRUG REACTIONS

Adverse drug reactions to the cholinergic agonists usually result from their nonspecific effects throughout the parasympathetic nervous system. The cholinergic agonists typically bind with receptors in the parasympathetic nervous system, creating undesirable parasympathomimetic effects outside the target organ. For example, the use of bethanechol to reduce urinary retention also will increase GI motility, which may cause nausea, belching, vomiting, intestinal cramps, and diarrhea. Effects of the drug on the eye may include blurred vision and decreased accommodation. With high doses, cardiovascular responses may include vasodilation, decreased cardiac rate, and decreased force of cardiac contraction, which may cause hypotension. Salivation or sweating may increase greatly. The drug's

bronchoconstrictor effect may produce shortness of breath. Even the desired effect on the urinary bladder is problematic because urinary frequency may replace urinary retention. Usually, the greater the dose, the greater the generalized parasympathomimetic effect.

Cholinergic overstimulation can result from patient hypersensitivity, drug overdose, or, rarely, subcutaneous administration. This overstimulation may cause circulatory collapse, resulting in hypotension, shock, and cardiac arrest.

NURSING PROCESS APPLICATION

The following information assists the nurse in caring for a patient who is receiving a cholinergic agonist.

Assessment
• Review the patient's history for conditions that require cautious use of cholinergic agonists, such as asthma, coronary insufficiency, epilepsy, hypertension, hypotension, hyperthyroidism, GI tract inflammation, urinary tract obstruction, parkinsonism, or peptic ulcer.

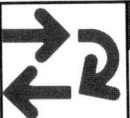

DRUG INTERACTIONS

Cholinergic agonists

Drug interactions involving the cholinergic agonists usually occur with drugs that also act at the autonomic effector cells.

DRUG	INTERACTING DRUGS	POSSIBLE EFFECTS	NURSING IMPLICATIONS
bethanechol, carbachol, pilocarpine	other cholinergic agents, particularly anticholinesterase agents (ambenonium, edrophonium, neostigmine, physostigmine, pyridostigmine)	Increase potential for cholinergic toxicity	• Observe the patient for signs of a toxic response, including generalized weakness, fasciculations, dysphagia, and respiratory weakness. • Observe the patient for signs of cardiovascular dysfunction, including bradycardia and hypotension. • Have atropine on hand as an antidote. • Have respiratory support equipment available: suction, oxygen, and mechanical ventilator.
	cholinergic blocking agents (atropine, belladonna, homatropine, methantheline, methscopolamine, propantheline, scopolamine)	Antagonize effect of acetylcholine at the muscarinic receptors	• Have atropine available as the antidote for cholinergic agonists. • Monitor the patient for decreased response to the prescribed cholinergic agonist.
	quinidine	Antagonizes effects of cholinergic agonists	• Monitor cardiovascular status in a patient with paroxysmal supraventricular tachycardia.

• Assess the patient for adverse reactions to the cholinergic agonist, such as increased GI motility, blurred vision, hypotension, shortness of breath, and increased salivation or sweating.
• Review the patient's medication history to identify use of drugs that may interact with cholinergic agonists, such as other cholinergic agents or cholinergic blocking agents.
• Assess the effectiveness of the cholinergic agonist regularly.
• Evaluate the patient's and family's knowledge about the prescribed cholinergic agonist.

Nursing diagnoses
The following examples represent appropriate nursing diagnoses for a patient receiving a cholinergic agonist.
• Potential for injury related to a preexisting condition that requires cautious use of cholinergic agonists
• Potential for injury related to adverse drug reactions
• Potential for injury related to drug interactions with the prescribed cholinergic agonist
• Altered health maintenance related to potential ineffectiveness of the cholinergic agonist
• Knowledge deficit related to the prescribed cholinergic agonist

Planning and implementation
• Administer a cholinergic agonist cautiously to a patient at risk because of a preexisting condition.
• Monitor the patient for adverse reactions when administering a cholinergic agonist.
• *Keep respiratory support equipment readily available.*
• *Observe the patient for 30 minutes to 1 hour after S.C. administration of bethanecol; have atropine (0.6 mg) available in a syringe to use as an antidote.*
• *Check vital signs and auscultate breath sounds when administering a cholinergic agonist.*
• Administer the cholinergic agonist when the patient's stomach is empty to minimize adverse reactions, unless the physician directs otherwise.
• Apply pressure on the inner canthus to prevent systemic absorption from ocular administration of a cholinergic agonist.
• Assist the patient with frequent oral hygiene, if increased salivation occurs.
• Change bed linens and clothing as needed to prevent skin breakdown in a patient with diaphoresis.
• Advise the physician if the patient has been taking another cholinergic agent or cholinergic blocking agent.
• *Monitor visual acuity closely if the patient received the cholinergic agonist to treat an ocular condition.*
• Notify the physician if the patient displays decreased effectiveness of the prescribed cholinergic agonist.

• *Monitor for urination in a patient who is receiving be-thanecol for acute urinary retention. Urination should occur within 1 hour. If not, notify the physician and expect to perform urinary catheterization.*

Patient teaching

• Teach the patient and family the name, dose, frequency, action, and adverse effects of the prescribed cholinergic agonist.

• *Instruct the patient to take the cholinergic agonist 1 hour before or 2 hours after meals to minimize adverse reactions.*

• Show the patient how and where to apply pressure when instilling a cholinergic agonist in the eye.

• *Advise the patient that vision may blur and accommodation may decrease.*

• Teach the patient to notify the physician if adverse reactions occur.

Evaluation

• The patient exhibits no signs of complications in the preexisting condition linked to the prescribed cholinergic agonist.

• The patient develops no adverse reactions to the prescribed cholinergic agonist.

• The patient uses no drugs that interact with the cholinergic agonist.

• The patient demonstrates reduced intraocular pressure.

• The patient urinates within one hour.

• The patient and family express an accurate understanding of the points taught about the prescribed cholinergic agonist.

• The patient names the prescribed cholinergic agonist and explains that it must be taken 1 hour before or 2 hours after meals.

ANTICHOLINESTERASE AGENTS

Anticholinesterase agents inhibit the enzyme acetylcholinesterase, thus slowing the destruction of acetylcholine. The subsequent buildup of acetylcholine produces continued stimulation of cholinergic receptors throughout the body. This action is short term in drugs that are used therapeutically, the so-called reversible anticholinesterase agents. The following reversible anticholinesterase agents are discussed here: ambenonium, edrophonium, neostigmine, physostigmine, and pyridostigmine.

Other anticholinesterase agents, the organophosphates, have a long-term or irreversible action. Used primarily as toxic insecticides and pesticides, they also have been used as nerve gases in chemical warfare. Only two of them, echothiophate and isoflurophate, have therapeutic usefulness. They are used to treat glaucoma and esotropia. (For more information about these drugs, see Chapter 71, Ophthalmic Agents.)

PHARMACOKINETICS

Reversible and *irreversible* refer to the duration of the anticholinesterase agents' blocking effect. With reversible anticholinesterase agents, the blocking effect lasts for minutes to hours; with the irreversible anticholinesterase agents, the effects are sustained for days or weeks. The major differences between these agents are their pharmacokinetics and adverse effects.

Absorption, distribution, metabolism, excretion

Many anticholinesterase agents are absorbed readily from the GI tract, subcutaneous tissue, and mucous membranes. The exceptions are neostigmine and related quaternary ammonium compounds, which are absorbed poorly from the GI tract and are given in larger doses when administered orally. If absorption from the GI tract is enhanced, overdose may occur.

Only physostigmine readily penetrates the blood-brain barrier. Most anticholinesterase agents are metabolized in the body by the plasma esterases and excreted in the urine.

Onset, peak, duration

Ambenonium begins acting in 20 to 30 minutes and continues for 3 to 8 hours. Edrophonium takes effect 2 to 10 minutes after I.M. administration and continues for 5 to 30 minutes. With I.V. administration, it has an onset of action of 30 to 60 seconds and a duration of action of 10 minutes. Oral neostigmine has a half-life of 40 to 60 minutes; its onset is 45 to 75 minutes, it reaches a peak concentration level in 1 to 2 hours, and its duration is 2 to 4 hours. Injectable neostigmine has a half-life of 50 to 90 minutes. When administered I.M., it takes effect in 20 minutes, reaches peak concentration in 30 minutes, and continues to act for 2 to 4 hours. With I.V. administration, onset is in 4 to 8 minutes and peak concentration is reached in 20 to 30 minutes; action continues for 2 to 4 hours. Physostigmine reaches peak concentration within 5 minutes of I.V. administration and has a duration of 30 minutes to 5 hours. When given I.M., pyridostigmine takes effect in less than 15 minutes and has a duration of 2 to 4 hours. With I.V. administration, it has an onset of 2 to 5 minutes and a duration of 2 to 4 hours.

PHARMACODYNAMICS

The anticholinesterase agents, like the cholinergic agonists, increase the effect of acetylcholine at receptor sites in the CNS, at autonomic ganglia, at autonomic effector cells on the viscera, and at the motor end-plate. Depending on the site and the drug's dose and duration of action, they can have stimulant and depressant effects on the cholinergic receptors.

Mechanism of action
Anticholinesterase agents act at the autonomic effector sites and at the neuromuscular junction to inhibit the action of the enzyme acetylcholinesterase. Ordinarily, this enzyme inactivates acetylcholine. Thus, the effect of the anticholinesterase agents is to increase the amount of acetylcholine available at the receptor sites and to prolong its effect.

PHARMACOTHERAPEUTICS

Anticholinesterase agents are important therapeutically because of their effects on the eye, the GI tract, and the skeletal neuromuscular junction. Their ability to reduce intraocular pressure makes them useful adjuncts to ocular surgery and glaucoma treatment. They stimulate tone and peristalsis in the GI tract in patients with gastroparesis. Probably their most important use is to promote muscle contraction in patients with myasthenia gravis. (Neostigmine and edrophonium also are used to diagnose myasthenia gravis.) Anticholinesterase agents also are antidotes to the competitive neuromuscular blocking agents, tricyclic antidepressants, belladonna alkaloids, and narcotics. They also are used to increase bladder tone.

ambenonium (Mytelase). A reversible anticholinesterase agent, ambenonium is used as an antimyasthenic. Its duration of action is longer than that of neostigmine or pyridostigmine, but its action is not as specific as that of the other agents and it produces many adverse reactions.
Usual adult dosage: 2.5 to 5 mg P.O. t.i.d. or q.i.d.; adjust as needed.

edrophonium chloride (Tensilon). A reversible anticholinesterase agent, edrophonium is a parenteral medication with multiple uses. Because of its short duration of action, it is the drug of choice for diagnosing myasthenia gravis; it also is used to differentiate myasthenia gravis from cholinergic toxicity. Edrophonium may be used as an antidote to the nondepolarizing blocking agents, such as metocurine iodide and pancuronium bromide, but it is not as effective as neostigmine or pyridostigmine. Rarely, it is used to terminate attacks of paroxysmal supraventricular tachycardia that are unresponsive to cardiac glycosides.

Usual adult dosage: for diagnosing myasthenia gravis, initially 10 mg I.M. or 1 to 2 mg I.V., followed by 8 mg I.V. if no response occurs in 45 seconds (keep respiratory support equipment and atropine at hand to counteract toxic effects); for differentiating myasthenia gravis from cholinergic toxicity, 1 mg I.V. followed by an additional 1 mg I.V. if the patient is not further impaired; for neuromuscular block, 10 mg I.V. given over 30 to 45 seconds, repeated to a maximum of 40 mg; for paroxysmal supraventricular tachycardia, 5 to 10 mg slow I.V. push, repeated in 10 minutes if necessary.

neostigmine (Prostigmin). A reversible anticholinesterase agent, neostigmine is available in oral and injectable forms. Oral neostigmine is an antimyasthenic agent. Parenteral neostigmine is widely used. Its clinical indications are the diagnosis and treatment of myasthenia gravis, the prevention and treatment of postoperative distention and urinary retention, and as an antidote to neuromuscular blocking agents.
Usual adult dosage: for myasthenia gravis, initially 15 mg P.O. every 3 to 4 hours or 0.5 to 2 mg I.M. or I.V. every 1 to 3 hours; for postoperative distention and urinary retention, 0.5 to 1 mg I.M. or S.C. every 4 to 6 hours; for neuromuscular blockade, 0.5 to 2 mg I.V., repeated as necessary.

physostigmine salicylate (Antilirium). A reversible anticholinesterase agent, physostigmine is used to treat tricyclic antidepressant overdose and to reverse the excessive anticholinergic effects of other drugs. However, because physostigmine may cause significant adverse reactions, it is used primarily as an adjunct in treating severe anticholinergic toxicity. Physostigmine also is used as an antiglaucoma agent and a miotic. (For additional information, see Chapter 71, Ophthalmic Agents.)
Usual adult dosage: 0.5 to 2 mg I.M. or I.V.; when given I.V., administer at a rate of not more than 1 mg/minute; repeat as necessary.

pyridostigmine (Mestinon, Regonol). A reversible anticholinesterase agent, pyridostigmine is used as an antimyasthenic agent and an antidote to the nondepolarizing neuromuscular blocking agents. It is available in oral and parenteral forms.
Usual adult dosage: for myasthenia gravis, 60 to 120 mg P.O. every 3 to 4 hours or 2 mg I.M. or I.V. every 2 to 3 hours, adjusted as needed; as an antidote, 10 to 20 mg I.V.

Drug interactions
Interacting drugs usually alter the actions of the anticholinesterase agents at the nicotinic or muscarinic receptor sites. Cholinergic agonists and other acetylcholinesterase inhibitors act at both sites. Therefore, combinations of the

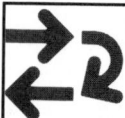

DRUG INTERACTIONS
Anticholinesterase agents

Drug interactions involving the anticholinesterase agents usually occur at nicotinic or muscarinic receptor sites.

DRUG	INTERACTING DRUGS	POSSIBLE EFFECTS	NURSING IMPLICATIONS
ambenonium, edrophonium, neostigmine, physostigmine, pyridostigmine	other cholinergic agents, particularly cholinergic agonists (bethanechol, carbachol, pilocarpine)	Increase the effect of acetylcholine at the neuromuscular junction	• Observe the patient for signs of a toxic response, including generalized weakness, fasciculations, dysphagia, and respiratory weakness. • Observe the patient for signs of cardiovascular dysfunction, including bradycardia and hypotension. • Have I.V. atropine on hand as an antidote. • Have respiratory support equipment on hand: suction, oxygen, and mechanical ventilator.
	cholinergic blocking agents (atropine, belladonna, homatropine, methantheline, methscopolamine, propantheline, scopolamine)	Antagonize effect of acetylcholine at muscarinic receptors; may mask early signs of cholinergic crisis	• Have I.V. atropine available as antidote. • Monitor the patient for adverse reactions.
	neuromuscular blocking agents (atracurium, gallamine, metocurine, pancuronium, tubocurarine, vecuronium)	Antagonize the effect of acetylcholine at the neuromuscular junction	• Monitor the patient for a decreased therapeutic response.
	ester anesthetics	Increase the risk of toxicity of anticholinesterase agents	• Monitor the patient for signs of toxicity, bradycardia, hypotension, shortness of breath, wheezing, diaphoresis, and diarrhea.
	procainamide	Antagnoizes neuromuscular blocking effect	• Monitor the patient for a decreased therapeutic response to the anticholinesterase agent.

drugs must be used with caution to avoid precipitating a toxic response. Drugs with neuromuscular blocking action antagonize the effect of the anticholinesterase agents at the muscarinic receptors in the skeletal muscle. These include selected antibiotics and anesthetics as well as neuromuscular blocking agents. Antimuscarinic agents such as atropine interfere with the anticholinesterase agents in the central and peripheral nervous systems. Therefore, they may be used as antidotes. Ganglionic blocking agents antagonize the effect of these drugs at the nicotinic receptor sites only. (For more details, see *Drug interactions: Anticholinesterase agents.*)

ADVERSE DRUG REACTIONS

Adverse reactions to the anticholinesterase agents almost invariably result from the increased action of acetylcholine at parasympathetic, motor, and CNS receptors. These reactions are difficult to control, particularly at high doses.

Parasympathomimetic effects are common. In the eye, they include blurred vision, decreased accommodation, and miosis; in the skin, increased sweating; in the GI system, increased salivation, belching, nausea, vomiting, intestinal cramps, and diarrhea. The bronchoconstrictor effect may occur as shortness of breath, wheezing, or tightness in the chest. Vasodilation, decreased cardiac rate, and decreased cardiac contraction can result in hypotension, although this effect is offset partially by decreased acetylcholine metabolism at the preganglionic receptor sites in the sympathetic nervous system. At the motor end-plate, hyperpolarization of the skeletal muscles reduces effective contractions. Adverse reactions in the CNS include irritability, anxiety or fear, and in some cases, seizures.

Reaction to the anticholinesterase agents is difficult to predict in a patient with myasthenia gravis. The therapeutic dose varies from day to day, and increased muscle weakness may result from underdosage, resistance to the drug, or overdosage. Differentiating between a toxic response and myasthenic crisis may be difficult. A physician who uses

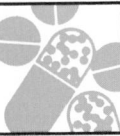

SELECTED MAJOR DRUGS

Cholinergic agents

This chart summarizes the major cholinergic agents in clinical use.

DRUG	MAJOR INDICATIONS	USUAL ADULT DOSAGES	CONTRAINDICATIONS AND PRECAUTIONS
Cholinergic agonists			
bethanechol	Urine retention	10 to 50 mg P.O. b.i.d. to q.i.d. or 5 mg S.C. t.i.d. or q.i.d.	• Administer with caution to a pregnant patient or one with asthma, coronary insufficiency, epilepsy, hypertension, hypotension, hyperthyroidism, GI tract inflammation, urinary tract obstruction, parkinsonism, or peptic ulcer.
Anticholinesterase agents			
edrophonium	Differential diagnosis of cholinergic toxicity and myasthenic crisis	1 mg I.V. followed by an additional 1 mg if patient is not impaired further	• Know that edrophonium is contraindicated in a patient with known sensitivity to the drug or a mechanical obstruction of the intestines or urinary tract. • Administer with caution to a pregnant patient or one with asthma, atelectasis, cardiac arrhythmias, intestinal or urinary tract obstruction, or pneumonia.
neostigmine	Myasthenia gravis	15 mg P.O. every 3 to 4 hours or 0.5 to 2 mg I.V. every 1 to 3 hours	• Know that neostigmine is contraindicated in a patient with known sensitivity to the drug, peritonitis, or a mechanical obstruction of the intestines or urinary tract. • Administer with caution to a pregnant patient or one with epilepsy, bronchial asthma, bradycardia, recent coronary occlusion, vagotonia, hyperthyroidism, cardiac arrhythmias, or peptic ulcer.
	Postoperative distention or urine retention	0.5 mg I.M. or S.C. every 4 to 6 hours	

edrophonium to distinguish between the two must have respiratory support equipment (a suction machine, oxygen, and a mechanical ventilator) and emergency drugs, such as atropine and pralidoxime, available to counteract cholinergic crisis.

NURSING PROCESS APPLICATION

The following information assists the nurse in caring for a patient who is receiving an anticholinesterase agent.

Assessment

• Review the patient's history for conditions that contraindicate the use of anticholinesterase agents, such as mechanical obstruction of the intestines or urinary tract, peritonitis, or known hypersensitivity to anticholinesterase agents.
• Review the patient's history for conditions that require cautious use of anticholinesterase agents, such as asthma, cardiac arrhythmias, epilepsy, recent coronary occlusion, hyperthyroidism, or peptic ulcer.

• Assess the patient for adverse reactions to the prescribed anticholinesterase agent, such as blurred vision; decreased accommodation; increased sweating, salivation, and GI motility; or hypotension.
• Assess the patient's emotional state, because anticholinesterase agents can produce anxiety and irritability.
• Review the patient's medication history to identify use of drugs that may interact with the prescribed anticholinesterase agent, such as other cholinergic agents, cholinergic blocking agents, neuromuscular blocking agents, ester anesthetics, and procainamide.
• Assess the effectiveness of anticholinesterase therapy regularly.
• Evaluate the patient's and family's knowledge about the prescribed anticholinesterase agent.

Nursing diagnoses

The following examples represent appropriate nursing diagnoses for a patient receiving an anticholinesterase agent.
• Potential for injury related to a preexisting condition that contraindicates the use of anticholinesterase agents

• Potential for injury related to a preexisting condition that requires cautious use of anticholinesterase agents
• Potential for injury related to adverse drug reactions
• Anxiety related to the adverse CNS effects of the anticholinesterase agent
• Impaired physical mobility related to ineffectiveness of the anticholinesterase agent in a patient with myasthenia gravis taking a neuromuscular blocking agent or procainamide
• Altered health maintenance related to potential ineffectiveness of anticholinesterase therapy
• Knowledge deficit related to the prescribed anticholinesterase agent

Planning and implementation

• Do not administer an anticholinesterase agent to a patient with a condition that contraindicates its use.
• Administer an anticholinesterase agent cautiously to a patient at risk because of a preexisting condition.
• *Have respiratory support equipment available. Keep suction equipment, oxygen, and a mechanical ventilator on hand if edrophonium is used.*
• Observe the patient periodically for adverse reactions to the anticholinesterase agent.
• *Monitor vital signs and auscultate breath sounds at least once every 4 hours.*
• Monitor the patient closely for signs of a toxic response, such as generalized weakness, fasciculations, dysphagia, and respiratory weakness.
• *Keep atropine (0.6 mg) readily available in a syringe as an antidote.*
• Take safety precautions if the patient develops visual disturbances. For example, move the call bell close to the patient and supervise ambulation.
• *Take seizure precautions.*
• Notify the physician if adverse reactions occur.
• Monitor the patient's emotional state periodically.
• Maintain a calm environment.
• Encourage the patient to verbalize feelings of anxiety.
• Notify the physician if anxiety occurs. Also reassure the patient and family that anxiety is an adverse reaction to the anticholinesterase agent.
• Monitor the patient for signs of decreased therapeutic response.
• *Monitor and record changes in muscle strength daily when administering an anticholinesterase agent.*
• Expect to administer a higher dosage of the anticholinesterase agent if the patient demonstrates decreased muscle strength.

Patient teaching

• Teach the patient and family the name, dose, frequency, action, and adverse effects of the prescribed anticholinesterase agent.

• *Help the patient develop a system for keeping track of each dose and its effect.*
• Describe ways to manage common adverse reactions. For example, tell the patient to take the drug with food or milk if nausea occurs after oral administration.
• *Show the patient how to assess and record changes in muscle strength and help the patient practice this assessment.*
• Advise the patient to report adverse reactions to the physician.

Evaluation

The following examples represent appropriate evaluation statements for a patient receiving an anticholinesterase agent.
• The patient has no conditions that contraindicate anticholinesterase agent therapy.
• The patient exhibits no signs of complications in the preexisting condition linked to the prescribed anticholinesterase agent.
• The patient reports no adverse reactions to the prescribed anticholinesterase agent.
• The patient reports no feelings of anxiety.
• The patient uses no drugs that interact with anticholinesterase agents.
• The patient maintains muscle strength.
• The patient and family express an accurate understanding of the points taught about the prescribed anticholinesterase agent.
• The patient demonstrates how to record changes in muscle strength.
• The patient develops a system that tracks each dose and its effect.

CHAPTER SUMMARY

Chapter 13 presented cholinergic agonists and anticholinesterase agents and explained their actions on the parasympathetic nervous system. Here are the chapter highlights.
• Cholinergic agents directly or indirectly mimic the effects of acetylcholine in the body. Because these effects usually are similar to the effects of the parasympathetic nervous system, the cholinergic agents also are called parasympathomimetic drugs.
• Cholinergic agonists replicate the action of acetylcholine at the autonomic effector site. They bind with receptors on the cell membrane of smooth muscles, changing cell membrane permeability and permitting calcium and sodium to flow into the cells. This depolarizes the cell membrane, causing muscle contraction. Therapeutically, they are used

for their actions on the eye, the GI tract, and the urinary bladder.

• The anticholinesterase agents facilitate the action of acetylcholine by inhibiting its destruction by the acetylcholinesterase enzyme at the autonomic effector sites and at the neuromuscular junction. Their primary therapeutic use is to diagnose and treat myasthenia gravis and to counteract neuromuscular blocking agents. Occasionally, they are used to treat glaucoma, to treat hypotonia of the GI tract or urinary bladder, and in ocular surgery.

• The adverse effects of the cholinergic agents result primarily from their nonspecific effects on the parasympathetic nervous system; those of the anticholinesterase agents almost invariably result from the increased action of acetylcholine at parasympathetic, motor, and CNS receptors.

• Nursing care for a patient receiving a cholinergic agent should include managing and teaching about adverse drug reactions. For a patient who takes an anticholinesterase agent for long-term treatment of myasthenia gravis, the nurse should supply detailed instructions.

STUDY QUESTIONS

See Appendix 1 for answers.

1. Ann White, age 36, comes to the emergency department (ED) because she has been unable to void for the past 12 hours. She has multiple sclerosis, which began 6 years ago, and now worries that this symptom signals exacerbation of the disease. The physician orders bethanechol (Duvoid), 5 mg S.C., to relieve acute urinary retention. When bethanechol is administered S.C., what is its onset of action?
(a) 5 to 15 minutes
(b) 15 to 30 minutes
(c) 30 to 90 minutes
(d) 1 to 3 hours

2. If the nurse had to administer bethanechol I.V., which nursing action would be appropriate?
(a) Have atropine readily available.
(b) Administer the medication slowly.
(c) Divide the dose in half.
(d) Assess for adverse reactions.

3. The nurse should assess Ms. White for which common adverse reactions to bethanechol?
(a) dry mouth, flushed face, and constipation
(b) skin rash, shortness of breath, and nasal congestion
(c) nausea, vomiting, diarrhea, and abdominal cramps
(d) fasciculations, dysphagia, and respiratory distress

4. The ambulance brings Bill Koster, age 29, to the ED in extreme respiratory distress. He has myasthenia gravis, for which he takes neostigmine (Prostigmin) to promote muscle contraction. What is this drug's mechanism of action?
(a) It increases available receptor sites for acetylcholine.
(b) It stimulates the release of acetylcholine at the neuromuscular junction.
(c) It mimics the action of acetylcholine at the neuromuscular junction.
(d) It inhibits the action of acetylcholinesterase, which usually inactivates acetylcholine.

5. The physician is most likely to use which of the following drugs to help distinguish between myasthenic crisis and cholinergic toxicity?
(a) atropine
(b) edrophonium
(c) ambenonium
(d) physostigmine

6. In addition to monitoring Mr. Koster for any change in muscle strength, the nurse should assess for which other adverse drug reaction?
(a) dry skin
(b) constipation
(c) hypertension
(d) blurred vision

7. When Mr. Koster develops a respiratory infection, the physician prescribes an antibiotic that antagonizes the effects of acetylcholine at the neuromuscular junction. As a result of this drug interaction, the nurse may need to take which action to produce a therapeutic response?
(a) Decrease the neostigmine dosage.
(b) Increase the neostigmine dosage.
(c) Administer atropine with the antibiotic.
(d) Administer the antibiotic I.V.

SELECTED REFERENCES

AHFS drug information 90. (1990). Bethesda, MD: American Society of Hospital Pharmacists.

Bell, J. (1989). Understanding and managing myasthenia gravis. *Focus on Critical Care,* 16(1), 57-65.

Glass, P. (1989). Reversal of muscle relaxants. *Journal of Post Anesthesia Nursing,* 4(2), 112-115.

Gravenstein, J. (1988). Another look at anticholinergic drugs. *Current Reviews for Nurse Anesthetists,* 11(10), 74-80.

Hansten, P., and Horn, J. (1989). *Drug interactions* (6th ed.). Philadelphia: Lea & Febiger.

USPDI. (1991). *Drug information for the health care professional* (Vol. I, 11th ed.). Rockville, MD: United States Pharmacopeial Convention.

USPDI. (1991). *Advice for the patient* (Vol. II, 11th ed.). Rockville, MD: United States Pharmacopeial Convention.

Youngbluth, J., Henry J., and McAnallen, K. (1988). Recovery characteristics following antagonism of vecuronium with edrophonium, neostigmine, or pyridostigmine. *AANA Journal,* 56(2), 127-133.

CHAPTER

14

CHOLINERGIC BLOCKING AGENTS

OBJECTIVES

After reading and studying this chapter, the student should be able to:

1. Describe the mechanism of action of the cholinergic blocking agents.

2. Identify the effect that cholinergic blocking agents have on target organs innervated by the parasympathetic nervous system.

3. Differentiate among the types of antimuscarinic cholinergic blocking agents.

4. Describe the pharmacokinetics of the cholinergic blocking agents.

5. List the major clinical indications for the cholinergic blocking agents.

6. Describe the major adverse reactions to these drugs.

7. Teach the patient the safe administration of a drug having a narrow margin of safety between therapeutic and toxic dosages.

8. Describe how to apply the nursing process when caring for a patient who is receiving a cholinergic blocking agent.

INTRODUCTION

Cholinergic blocking agents interrupt parasympathetic nerve impulses in the central and autonomic nervous systems. Their primary clinical indications include spastic conditions of the gastrointestinal (GI) and urinary tracts, cardiac arrhythmias, motion sickness, parkinsonism, and chronic asthma. They also are used as preanesthesia medications and as relaxants for the GI tract during diagnostic procedures and for the eye and pupil during ophthalmologic surgery. They serve as antidotes to cholinergic agents and certain organophosphate pesticides.

As a group, cholinergic blocking agents have various names. Because they oppose the effects of parasympathetic nerve impulses, they are called parasympatholytic drugs. Because they block the action of acetylcholine (which transmits parasympathetic nerve impulses), they are known as anticholinergic drugs. Because their sites of activity are muscarinic receptors, they also are called antimuscarinic drugs.

Cholinergic blocking agents constitute two classes: ganglionic blocking agents and antimuscarinic drugs. Although ganglionic blocking agents block the transmission of adrenergic and cholinergic stimuli, their clinical use is limited to their adrenergic effects. Therefore, they are discussed in Chapter 16, Adrenergic Blocking Agents.

The antimuscarinic drugs, of which atropine sulfate is the prototype, exert their blockade effect at postganglionic cholinergic nerve endings at the muscarinic receptor sites. They are the focus of this chapter.

Physiology of the muscarinic receptor

Understanding the cholinergic blocking agents depends on understanding the physiology of the parasympathetic nervous system and the pharmacology of the cholinergic agents. (For a detailed discussion, see Chapter 13, Cholinergic Agents.)

Cholinergic blocking agents compete in a dose-dependent manner with acetylcholine at muscarinic receptor sites in the central nervous system (CNS), the autonomic ganglia, smooth muscle innervated by parasympathetic nerves, and at the neuromuscular junction. This means that the higher the drug dose, the greater the competition with acetylcholine. (For a further discussion, see Chapter 17, Neuromuscular Blocking Agents.)

The cholinergic blocking agents usually block the effects of the parasympathetic nerves, allowing the effects of the sympathetic adrenergic nervous system to predominate. These agents affect the brain, eyes, salivary glands, bronchi, heart, GI tract, and urinary bladder. In these target agents, cholinergic blocking agents produce the following effects:

- Excitation followed by depression
- Pupillary dilation
- Decreased accommodation
- Decreased salivation
- Bronchial dilation
- Decreased bronchial secretion

Cholinergic blocking agents

The following nursing diagnoses address representative problems and etiologies that a nurse may encounter when caring for a patient who is receiving a cholinergic blocking agent. Some of these nursing diagnoses contain generalized etiologies, which the nurse must individualize based on the patient's needs. (For some common nursing diagnoses and related interventions for each drug class, see the "Nursing Process Application" section of this chapter.)

- Altered health maintenance related to ineffectiveness of the prescribed cholinergic blocker
- Altered role performance related to CNS excitation caused by cholinergic blocker toxicity
- Altered thought processes related to cholinergic blocker toxicity
- Decreased cardiac output related to cholinergic blocker-induced cardiac arrhythmias
- Impaired physical mobility related to CNS depression caused by cholinergic blocker toxicity
- Knowledge deficit related to the prescribed cholinergic blocker
- Potential altered body temperature related to risk of heatstroke caused by cholinergic blockers
- Potential for injury related to a preexisting condition that contraindicates the use of cholinergic blockers
- Potential for injury related to a preexisting condition that requires cautious use of cholinergic blockers
- Potential for injury related to adverse drug reactions
- Potential for injury related to use of a drug that interacts with the prescribed cholinergic blocker
- Sensory-perceptual alteration (visual) related to the adverse effects of a cholinergic blocker in a patient with undiagnosed glaucoma
- Urine retention related to urinary obstruction in a patient with benign prostatic hypertrophy

- Increased heart rate
- Increased cardiac contractility
- Decreased GI secretions
- Decreased GI peristalsis
- Urine retention.

Some cholinergic blocking agents that can cross the blood-brain barrier have a further effect on the CNS. The brain contains two kinds of muscarinic receptors, M_1 and M_2. M_1 receptors predominate in the cerebral cortex and the gray matter of the corpus striatum and the hippocampus. M_2 receptors are most common in the cerebellum. When cholinergic blocking agents in low to moderate doses combine with these receptors, the CNS is stimulated; if the dosage level increases, the CNS is depressed.

Muscarinic receptors also are present in the medulla oblongata, which controls the heart. Vagal stimulation of the heart results from muscarinic action in the CNS and in the heart muscle. The resulting cholinergic blockade can reverse sinus bradycardia and some other arrhythmias.

For a summary of representative drugs, see *Selected major drugs: Cholinergic blocking agents,* page 208. For a listing of applicable nursing diagnoses that the nurse may formulate when caring for a patient receiving these agents, see *Selected nursing diagnoses: Cholinergic blocking agents.* For detailed information on applying the nursing process, see Chapter 6, The Nursing Process and Drug Therapy.

CHOLINERGIC BLOCKERS

The cholinergic blocking agents block the action of acetylcholine at muscarinic receptors in the parasympathetic nervous system. The major drugs in this class are the belladonna alkaloids (atropine sulfate, homatropine hydrobromide, hyoscyamine sulfate, and scopolamine hydrobromide), their synthetic derivatives (the quaternary ammonium agents clidinium bromide, glycopyrrolate, and propantheline bromide), and the tertiary amines (benztropine mesylate, dicyclomine hydrochloride, oxybutynin chloride, ethopropazine hydrochloride, and trihexyphenidyl hydrochloride). Because benztropine, ethopropazine, and trihexyphenidyl are almost exclusively treatments for parkinsonism, they are discussed fully in Chapter 19, Antiparkinsonian Agents.

PHARMACOKINETICS

The belladonna alkaloids are absorbed more readily and distributed more widely in the body than are their derivatives. Onset of action depends more on how the drug is administered than on the drug used.

Absorption, distribution, metabolism, excretion
The belladonna alkaloids are absorbed from the GI tract, the mucous membranes, the skin, and the eyes. The quaternary ammonium derivatives and tertiary amines are absorbed primarily through the GI tract, although much less readily than the alkaloids.

The belladonna alkaloids are distributed more widely than the quaternary ammonium derivatives or dicyclomine. The alkaloids readily cross the blood-brain barrier; the other drugs in this class do not. Scopolamine has a greater effect on the CNS than does atropine. Scopolamine also strongly affects the eye and its secretory glands. Atropine has a greater effect on the heart, the intestine, the urinary tract, and the bronchi. The quaternary ammonium derivatives have an affinity for the GI tract and, to a lesser degree, for the urinary bladder. They also have an effect on the nicotinic receptors, which affect the cardiovascular system and the neuromuscular junctions.

The belladonna alkaloids have low to moderate binding with serum proteins, are metabolized in the liver by hydrolysis (splitting by the addition of water), and are excreted by the kidneys as unchanged drug and metabolites. The metabolism of the quaternary ammonium derivatives is more complicated. Hydrolysis occurs in the GI tract and the liver; excretion is in feces and urine. Dicyclomine's metabolism is unknown, but it is excreted approximately 50% in urine and 50% in feces.

Onset, peak, duration

For the most part, the route chosen to administer the cholinergic blocking agents determines how quickly they take effect. Administered I.V., most have an onset of action of 1 minute; I.M. or S.C., onset takes about 30 minutes; orally, about 30 to 60 minutes. Belladonna is administered orally only, and its onset takes 1 to 2 hours. The duration of action of the belladonna alkaloids lasts up to 6 hours, depending on the drug chosen; the elimination half-life ranges from 3½ to 24 hours, depending on the drug. The quaternary ammonium derivatives and tertiary amines have a similar duration but shorter half-lives.

PHARMACODYNAMICS

The cholinergic blocking agents compete with acetylcholine and cholinergic agonists at muscarinic receptor sites in the CNS and at the junction between the postganglionic parasympathetic nerve and the smooth muscle (neuromuscular junction). The resulting blockade of the nerve stimulus may be overcome by increasing acetylcholine concentrations at the receptor sites, accomplished by administering the anticholinesterase agent physostigmine (the antidote for cholinergic blocking agents), which blocks the enzyme that destroys acetylcholine.

Mechanism of action

The action of the cholinergic blocking agents is stimulating or depressing, depending on the target organ. In the brain, they seem to do both — low drug levels stimulate, and high levels depress. Drug effects also are determined by the condition being treated. Parkinsonism, for example, is characterized by a dopamine deficiency that intensifies the stimulating effects of acetylcholine. Antimuscarinic agents blunt or depress this effect. In other cases, the effects of these on the CNS seem to be stimulatory.

PHARMACOTHERAPEUTICS

All the cholinergic blocking agents are used to treat spastic conditions of the GI and urinary tracts because they relax muscles and decrease GI secretions. The quaternary ammonium compounds, such as propantheline, are the drugs of choice for these conditions because they cause fewer adverse reactions than the belladonna alkaloids. However, the alkaloids are used with morphine to treat biliary colic. Parenteral doses of cholinergic blocking agents are used before such diagnostic procedures as endoscopy or sigmoidoscopy to relax the GI smooth muscle.

Because cholinergic blocking agents counteract bronchospasm and reduce respiratory secretions, they are used to treat chronic asthma. As preanesthesia medications, they reduce salivation and gastric secretions and depress the respiratory system. They also block cardiac vagal inhibition during anesthesia.

The belladonna alkaloids have several therapeutic CNS effects. Scopolamine, given with morphine or meperidine, reduces excitement and produces amnesia in the preanesthesia patient. It is also the drug of choice in treating motion sickness. Although other drugs are more effective for other dyskinesias, the cholinergic blocking agents play an important role in treating extrapyramidal symptoms from drugs and in treating parkinsonism.

The belladonna alkaloids also have important therapeutic effects on the heart. Parenteral atropine is the drug of choice to treat sinus bradycardia. It blocks the vagal effects of the SA (sinoatrial) nodal pacemaker and is particularly useful when arrhythmia results from anesthetics, choline esters, or succinylcholine.

Cholinergic blocking agents also are used as cycloplegics to paralyze the ciliary muscles of the eye, altering the shape of the lens, and as mydriatics to dilate the pupils. They make it easier to measure refractive errors during an ophthalmic examination or to perform ophthalmologic surgery. Occasionally, they are used as adjuncts to antibiotics in treating eye infections.

The belladonna alkaloids, particularly atropine and hyoscyamine, are effective antidotes to cholinergic and anticholinesterase agents. Atropine is the drug of choice to treat poisoning from organophosphate pesticides. Atropine and hyoscyamine also counteract the effects of the neuromuscular blocking agents by competing for the same receptor sites.

atropine sulfate (Arco-Lase Plus, Atropine Sulfate Injection). The prototype of the cholinergic blocking agents, atropine sulfate is a belladonna alkaloid that has the broadest clinical application of any drug in this class. Atropine stimulates or depresses the CNS, depending on the dose. It has a more potent action on the heart, intestine, and bronchial muscle than the other belladonna alkaloids and is used to treat bradycardia, spastic conditions of the GI tract, and occasionally, asthma. As a preanesthesia medication, atropine reduces secretions and minimizes vagal reflexes. It also is used as an antidote to cholinergic agents and neuromuscular blocking agents. (For more information about atropine's role as an antiarrhythmic, see Chapter 30, Antiarrhythmic Agents.) Atropine is available in oral and parenteral forms.

Usual adult dosage: to reverse arrhythmias, bradycardia, or sinus arrest, 0.4 to 1 mg I.V. every 2 hours, as needed, up to a maximum of 2 mg; as a preanesthesia medication to reduce secretions, 0.2 to 0.6 mg I.M. given 30 to 60 minutes before surgery; and to reverse neuromuscular blockade, 0.6 to 1.2 mg I.V. before or concurrently with 0.5 to 2.5 mg of neostigmine in a separate syringe.

belladonna. A crude botanical preparation, belladonna contains atropine, hyoscyamine, scopolamine, and minor alkaloids. It is used primarily to decrease GI motility and inhibit gastric secretions in peptic ulcer, irritable bowel syndrome, and other GI disorders. Although belladonna once was used to treat vertigo and dyskinesia, more effective agents now are available. Belladonna is available as tablets and tincture.

Usual adult dosage: 15-mg tablet P.O. t.i.d. or q.i.d., 30 minutes before meals and h.s.; 0.6 to 1 ml of tincture P.O. t.i.d. or q.i.d., 30 minutes before meals and h.s.

benztropine mesylate (Cogentin). A tertiary amine, benztropine is used primarily to treat parkinsonism. (For more information, see Chapter 19, Antiparkinsonian Agents.)

clidinium bromide (Quarzan). A quaternary ammonium derivative of the belladonna alkaloids, clidinium is used to treat peptic ulcer disease. Although available as a single agent, it usually is used in a fixed combination with chlordiazepoxide (Librax).

Usual adult dosage: 2.5 to 5 mg P.O. t.i.d. or q.i.d. before meals and h.s.

dicyclomine hydrochloride (Antispas, Bentyl, Viscerol). A tertiary amine derivative, dicyclomine is used to treat irritable bowel syndrome. It is absorbed rapidly after oral or I.M. administration, but effects occur only with large doses.

Usual adult dosage: 20 mg P.O. q.i.d. initially; can be increased up to a total of 160 mg/day; 20 mg I.M. daily in 4 divided doses.

ethopropazine hydrochloride (Parsidol). A phenothiazine derivative that has antimuscarinic properties, ethopropazine is used as a cholinergic blocking agent for its antidyskinetic properties in treating parkinsonism. (For more information, see Chapter 19, Antiparkinsonian Agents.)

glycopyrrolate (Robinul, Robinul Forte). A quaternary ammonium derivative, glycopyrrolate is the synthetic cholinergic blocking agent that most closely approximates the action of atropine. Even so, its action on the CNS is minimal, and GI absorption is poor. Glycopyrrolate is used to treat peptic ulcer. As a preanesthesia medication, it reduces secretions, helps prevent aspiration of gastric contents, and reduces arrhythmias. Glycopyrrolate is administered concurrently with anticholinesterase agents in reversing neuromuscular blockade. It is available in oral and parenteral forms.

Usual adult dosage: for peptic ulcer, 1 to 2 mg P.O. b.i.d. or t.i.d., or 0.1 to 0.2 mg I.M. or I.V. t.i.d. to q.i.d.; as preanesthesia medication, 0.004 mg/kg of body weight I.M. given 30 to 60 minutes before the anesthetic is to be administered; as a cholinergic adjunct in reversing neuromuscular blockade, 0.2 mg I.V. for each mg of neostigmine, in the same syringe.

homatropine hydrobromide (Homatrocel Ophthalmic, Isopto Homatropine). A quaternary ammonium derivative, homatropine is an ophthalmic solution used as a cycloplegic and a mydriatic. (For further information, see Chapter 71, Ophthalmic Agents.)

hyoscyamine sulfate (Anaspaz, Cystospaz-M, Levsin). A belladonna alkaloid, hyoscyamine's actions are similar to those of atropine, but with more potent central and peripheral effects. It is effective at half the dosage of atropine. The drug is available in oral and parenteral forms.

Usual adult dosage: for spastic GI disorders, 0.125 to 0.25 mg P.O. t.i.d. or q.i.d., 30 to 60 minutes before meals and h.s., or 0.25 to 0.5 mg I.M., I.V., or S.C. every 6 to 8 hours; as a cholinergic adjunct in reversing neuromuscular blockade, 0.3 to 0.6 mg I.V. for each 0.5 to 2 mg of neostigmine, in a separate syringe.

oxybutynin chloride (Ditropan). A tertiary amine, this agent produces a direct spasmolytic effect on the urinary bladder and provides some local anesthesia and mild analgesia.

Usual adult dosage: for neurogenic bladder, 5 mg P.O. b.i.d. or t.i.d., up to a maximum of 5 mg P.O. q.i.d.

propantheline bromide (Pro-Banthine). A quaternary ammonium derivative, propantheline is used mainly to reduce secretions and spasms in the GI tract. It provides symptomatic relief in patients with peptic ulcer, pancreatitis, gastritis, irritable bowel syndrome, diverticulitis, and colitis and also acts as a spasmolytic for the ureters and urinary bladder.

Usual adult dosage: 15 mg P.O. q.i.d. 30 minutes before meals and h.s.

scopolamine hydrobromide (Transderm Scop, Triptone). A belladonna alkaloid, scopolamine has a greater effect on the CNS than any other drug in this class, making it the

drug of choice for motion sickness. Scopolamine also is useful as a preanesthesia medication. It not only reduces excessive salivation and respiratory tract secretions during anesthesia, but also produces a sense of euphoria and amnesia. Scopolamine is absorbed readily from the GI tract and the mucous membranes. In treating motion sickness, scopolamine usually is administered topically via a skin patch behind the ear. One transdermal system delivers 0.5 mg of medication over a period of 3 days. The drug also is available in oral and parenteral dosage forms.
Usual adult dosage: for motion sickness, a 0.5-mg transdermal patch or 0.25 to 0.75 mg P.O. 1 hour before the effect is desired; as a preanesthesia medication, 0.3 to 0.6 mg I.M., I.V., or S.C. 30 to 60 minutes before surgery.

trihexyphenidyl hydrochloride (Artane, Trihexane, Trihexidyl). A synthetic drug structurally similar to the belladonna alkaloids, trihexyphenidyl is used primarily as an antidyskinetic in treating parkinsonism. (For more information, see Chapter 19, Antiparkinsonian Agents.)

Drug interactions

Because cholinergic blocking agents decrease gastric motility and delay gastric emptying, they may increase the absorption of other medications. Additionally, the delayed gastric emptying keeps the drugs in prolonged contact with the GI mucosa, which can increase their adverse effects. Cholinergic blocking agents can be affected adversely by antacids and antidiarrheals, which may reduce drug absorption.

Some interactions change the action of the cholinergic blocking agents. Most common is a general enhancement of the whole range of anticholinergic effects. Drugs that do this include antiarrhythmics, antidepressants, antidyskinetics, antiemetics, antihistamines, antipsychotics, antivertigo agents, CNS stimulants, and skeletal muscle relaxants. (For more details, see *Drug interactions: Cholinergic blocking agents,* page 206.)

ADVERSE DRUG REACTIONS

The widespread action of the cholinergic blocking agents commonly produces therapeutic benefits that are accompanied by undesirable effects. The use of drugs that interact with cholinergic blocking agents further increases the possibility of adverse reactions.

Adverse reactions are a function of the affinity of the muscarinic receptors for specific drugs and of the drug dosage. Dosage is particularly crucial: the difference between a therapeutic and a toxic dosage is small with the cholinergic blocking agents. Also, some people are much more susceptible than others to the effects of these drugs. These include infants, elderly patients, fair-skinned children with Down's syndrome, and children with spastic paralysis or brain damage.

Adverse reactions increase in severity as the dosage increases. Small doses are accompanied by decreases in salivation, bronchial secretions, and sweating—reducing the patient's ability to cope with heat. As the dosage increases, the pupils dilate, visual accommodation decreases, and heart rate increases. Still larger doses inhibit urination and intestinal motility, followed by a decrease in gastric secretions and motility.

With drug overdose, all these effects are exaggerated. Patients who experience cholinergic blocking agent toxicity are described in the mnemonic "Hot as a hare, blind as a bat, dry as a bone, and mad as a hatter." CNS excitation is prominent at toxic levels. The patient becomes restless, irritable, and disoriented, even hallucinatory or delirious. (Scopolamine may cause this reaction even in therapeutic doses, although the reaction is more likely if the patient has severe pain.) If the process is not reversed (physostigmine is the usual antidote), the excitatory phase is followed by CNS depression, unconsciousness, medullary paralysis, and death.

Cholinergic blocking agents may precipitate problems in patients with some underlying diseases. The drugs sometimes cause a dangerous rise in intraocular pressure in those with unrecognized narrow-angle glaucoma. Because aqueous humor cannot drain from the anterior chamber of the eye, severe pain and blindness result. These drugs should be administered cautiously to a patient over age 40 because of the chance of undiagnosed glaucoma. The incidence of temporary drug-induced blindness has increased as the use of topical scopolamine has increased.

In a patient with coronary artery disease, tachycardia secondary to the administration of cholinergic blocking agents can lead to circulatory failure. This may be compounded by the atrial and ventricular arrhythmias that sometimes occur with the cholinergic blocking agents.

In a patient with benign prostatic hypertrophy, cholinergic blocking agents may cause urine retention. The agents therefore should be used cautiously in elderly male patients.

Heatstroke is another potential complication with these drugs because they inhibit such heat-regulating mechanisms as sweating. It produces extreme elevation in body temperature, dehydration, flushing, and mental changes. (The flush associated with toxic doses of the belladonna alkaloids may be the body's attempt to compensate for this effect by peripheral vasodilation.) Heatstroke occurs more commonly with strenuous activity and high environmental temperatures. Elderly patients with cardiovascular disease are most susceptible to heatstroke.

DRUG INTERACTIONS
Cholinergic blocking agents

The nurse must be aware of the many commonly administered medications that interact with the cholinergic blocking agents.

DRUG	INTERACTING DRUGS	POSSIBLE EFFECTS	NURSING IMPLICATIONS
atropine, belladonna, clidinium, dicyclomine, glycopyrrolate, hyoscyamine, oxybutynin, propantheline, scopolamine	disopyramide, tricyclic and tetracyclic antidepressants, antidyskinetics (including amantadine), antiemetics and antivertigo agents (including buclizine, cyclizine, meclizine, and diphenhydramine), antipsychotics (including haloperidol, phenothiazines, thioxanthenes, cyclobenzaprine, and orphenadrine)	Enhance anticholinergic effect	• Monitor the patient for signs of adverse reactions to cholinergic blockers. • Monitor for constipation, which may become severe or result in paralytic ileus.
	cholinergic agonists (bethanechol), anticholinesterase agents (neostigmine, pyridostigmine)	Antagonize antimuscarinic effect	• Monitor the patient for therapeutic effects of the cholinergic blocking agents.
	digoxin	Increase serum concentration levels of digoxin by decreasing gastrointestinal (GI) motility	• Monitor the patient's apical pulse frequently. • Observe the patient for signs of digitalis toxicity, such as GI, cardiac, and neurologic effects.
	opiate-like analgesics	Decrease GI motility	• Monitor the patient for constipation, which may become severe or result in paralytic ileus. • Monitor the patient's bowel sounds frequently.
	nitroglycerin	Delay sublingual absorption of nitroglycerin because of dry mouth	• Offer the patient sips of water before administering nitroglycerin.

NURSING PROCESS APPLICATION

The following information assists the nurse in caring for a patient who is receiving a cholinergic blocking agent.

Assessment
• Review the patient's history for conditions that contraindicate the use of cholinergic blockers, such as known hypersensitivity to the drug, narrow-angle glaucoma, renal or GI obstructive disease, reflux esophagitis, or myasthenia gravis.
• Review the patient's history for conditions that require cautious use of cholinergic blockers, such as coronary heart disease, GI infection, open-angle glaucoma, prostatic hypertrophy, hypertension, hyperthyroidism, ulcerative colitis, autonomic neuropathy, or hiatal hernia associated with reflux esophagitis.
• Assess the patient for adverse reactions to the prescribed cholinergic blocker, such as decreased salivation, bronchial secretions, sweating, visual accommodation, gastric secretions, and gastric motility; restlessness; and disorientation.
• Assess the patient for signs of heatstroke, such as extreme elevation in body temperature, dehydration, and mental changes.
• Assess the patient for urine retention.
• Assess the effectiveness of the prescribed cholinergic blocker regularly.
• Evaluate the patient's and family's knowledge about the prescribed cholinergic blocker.

Nursing diagnoses
The following examples represent appropriate nursing diagnoses for a patient receiving a cholinergic blocking agent.
• Potential for injury related to a preexisting condition that contraindicates the use of cholinergic blockers
• Potential for injury related to a preexisting condition that requires cautious use of cholinergic blockers
• Potential for injury related to adverse drug reactions

• Potential altered body temperature related to risk of heatstroke caused by cholinergic blockers

• Urinary retention related to urinary obstruction in a patient with benign prostatic hypertrophy

• Altered health maintenance related to ineffectiveness of the prescribed cholinergic blocker

• Knowledge deficit related to the prescribed cholinergic blocker

Planning and implementation

• Do not administer a cholinergic blocker to a patient with a condition that contraindicates its use.

• Administer a cholinergic blocker cautiously to a patient at risk because of a preexisting condition.

• *Monitor the patient regularly for adverse drug reactions. Closely monitor an infant, elderly patient, fair-skinned child with Down's syndrome, or child with spastic paralysis or brain damage because such a patient is at increased risk for developing adverse reactions to a cholinergic blocker. Keep in mind that adverse reactions increase in severity as the dosage increases.*

• Monitor the patient's vital signs at least every 4 hours.

• Administer an analgesic, as prescribed, to a patient who is in pain and is receiving a cholinergic blocker. This helps reduce the risk of CNS excitation.

• *Administer a cholinergic blocker 30 minutes before meals and at bedtime when used to reduce GI motility.*

• Notify the physician if adverse reactions occur.

• *Monitor the patient for signs of heatstroke, such as dehydration, flushing, and altered level of consciousness. Be aware that heatstroke induced by a cholinergic blocker occurs is more common during strenuous activity, in hot weather, and in elderly patients with cardiovascular disease.*

• Keep the patient's room temperature cool.

• Encourage the patient to drink additional fluids (if not contraindicated) when engaging in a strenuous activity or when the weather is hot.

• Be prepared to perform emergency interventions if heatstroke occurs.

• Record fluid intake and output for a patient with benign prostatic hypertrophy who is taking a cholinergic blocker.

• *Monitor the patient for signs and symptoms of urine retention, such as urinary frequency with voiding of small amounts.*

• Notify the physician if urine retention occurs.

• Monitor the patient for increased GI or urinary tract spasticity, which may be exhibited by a change in bowel or bladder function.

• Notify the physician if spasticity occurs or increases.

Patient teaching

• Teach the patient and family the name, dose, frequency, action, and adverse reactions of the prescribed cholinergic blocker.

• *Teach the patient to avoid drug toxicity by taking only the amount of medicine ordered. Advise the patient who misses a dose to take it as soon as possible; if it is almost time for the next dose, the patient should wait until then and take a single dose only. Stress that the patient should not double the dose without consulting the physician.*

• Teach the patient to reduce the risk of heatstroke by moving slowly and staying in the shade in hot weather, avoiding strenuous exercise, and using fans or air conditioners.

• *Advise the patient to limit milk and bedtime snacks because they increase gastric secretions.*

• Teach the patient to consume a high-fiber diet and plenty of fluids to help prevent constipation.

• Teach the patient how to stroke the abdomen or use Credé's maneuver (bladder massage) if voiding becomes difficult.

• Recommend that the patient wear dark glasses and avoid driving if drug therapy produces mydriasis and cycloplegia.

• *Teach the patient about the need for scrupulous oral hygiene to decrease the likelihood of caries and periodontal disease caused by decreased salivation.*

• Recommend sugarless gum, hard sugarless candies, or ice to reduce dry mouth.

Evaluation

The following examples represent appropriate evaluation statements for a patient receiving a cholinergic blocking agent.

• The patient has no conditions that contraindicate the use of cholinergic blockers.

• The patient exhibits no signs of complications in the preexisting condition linked to the prescribed cholinergic blocker.

• The patient displays no adverse reactions to the prescribed cholinergic blocker.

• The patient maintains normal body temperature.

• The patient maintains normal voiding patterns.

• The patient exhibits no signs of increased GI spasticity, such as cramping abdominal pain or diarrhea.

• The patient exhibits no signs of increased urinary tract spasticity, such as bladder spasms or urinary urgency or frequency.

• The patient and family express an accurate understanding of the points taught about the prescribed cholinergic blocker.

• The patient demonstrates the proper technique for Credé's maneuver.

• The patient correctly lists precautions to take to prevent heatstroke.

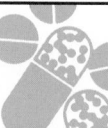

SELECTED MAJOR DRUGS

Cholinergic blocking agents

This chart summarizes the cholinergic blocking agents in clinical use.

DRUG	MAJOR INDICATIONS	USUAL ADULT DOSAGES	CONTRAINDICATIONS AND PRECAUTIONS
atropine	Reversal of arrhythmias, brady-cardia, and sinus arrest Preanesthesia medication Cholinergic adjunct to reverse neuromuscular blockade Dyskinesia in parkinsonism	0.4 to 1 mg I.V. every 2 hours, as needed, up to a maximum of 2 mg 0.2 to 0.6 mg I.M. 30 to 60 minutes before surgery 0.6 to 1.2 mg I.V. before or concurrently with 2 to 2.5 mg of neostigmine in a separate syringe 0.1 to 0.2 mg P.O. q.i.d.	• Know that atropine is contraindicated in a patient with known hypersensitivity to the drug or narrow-angle glaucoma. • Administer with caution to a pediatric or geriatric patient or one with open-angle glaucoma. • Administer with caution to a patient with coronary heart disease or a gastrointestinal (GI) infection or obstructive disease.
dicyclomine	Irritable bowel syndrome	20 mg P.O. t.i.d. or q.i.d., up to a maximum of 160 mg/day, or 20 mg I.M. daily in 4 divided doses	• Know that dicyclomine is contraindicated in a patient with known hypersensitivity to the drug, obstructive uropathy, obstructive disease of the GI tract, reflux esophagitis, narrow-angle glaucoma, or myasthenia gravis. • Administer with caution to a patient with prostatic hypertrophy, coronary heart disease, hypertension, hyperthyroidism, ulcerative colitis, open-angle glaucoma, hepatic or renal disease, and autonomic neuropathy.
propantheline	Peptic ulcer and spastic bladder	15 mg q.i.d., 30 minutes before meals and h.s.	• Know that propantheline is contraindicated in a patient with known hypersensitivity to the drug, narrow-angle glaucoma, renal or GI obstructive disease, or myasthenia gravis. • Administer with caution to a pregnant patient, a patient over age 40 (because of the chance of undiagnosed glaucoma), or one with autonomic neuropathy, hepatic or renal disease, open-angle glaucoma, hyperthyroidism, coronary artery disease, or hiatal hernia associated with reflux esophagitis.
scopolamine	Preanesthesia medication Motion sickness	0.3 to 0.6 mg I.M., I.V., or S.C. 30 to 60 minutes before surgery 0.5 mg topically to postauricular skin (lasts for 3 days) or 0.25 to 0.75 mg P.O. 1 hour before effect is desired	• Know that scopolamine is contraindicated in a patient with known hypersensitivity to the drug or narrow-angle glaucoma. • Administer with caution to a patient with pyloric, intestinal, or urinary bladder neck obstruction; open-angle glaucoma; or impaired metabolic, liver, or kidney function. • Administer with caution to an elderly, pregnant, or lactating patient.

CHAPTER SUMMARY

Chapter 14 focused on the antimuscarinic cholinergic blocking agents, which exert a blockade effect at postganglionic cholinergic nerve endings. Here are the chapter highlights.

• Cholinergic blocking agents interrupt parasympathetic nerve impulses in the central and autonomic nervous systems by competing with the neurotransmitter acetylcholine at muscarinic receptor sites.

• The antimuscarinic drugs, of which atropine is the prototype, include the belladonna alkaloids, their quaternary ammonium derivatives, and the tertiary amines.

• Clinical indications for the cholinergic blocking agents include cardiac arrhythmias, motion sickness, parkinsonism, chronic asthma, spastic conditions of the GI and urinary tracts, poisoning by organophosphate pesticides, and toxicity from cholinergic agents or neuromuscular blocking agents. They also are used to decrease salivary and respiratory secretions during anesthesia, relax the GI tract during diagnostic procedures, and relax eye muscles and dilate the pupil during ophthalmologic examinations and surgery.

• Because of the drugs' lack of selectivity, even therapeutic doses of the cholinergic blocking agents may cause multiple adverse reactions, usually extensions of the anticholinergic actions. Adverse drug reactions increase in severity as the dosage increases: The margin of safety between therapeutic and toxic doses is extremely small.

• Cholinergic blocking agents may precipitate a dangerous rise in intraocular pressure in a patient with unrecognized narrow-angle glaucoma, tachycardia leading to circulatory failure in a patient with coronary artery disease, urine retention in a patient with benign prostatic hypertrophy, and heatstroke, particularly in an elderly patient with cardiovascular disease.

• The nurse must teach the patient about the prescribed cholinergic blocking agent, including its adverse effects and how to prevent, recognize, and obtain treatment for toxicity.

STUDY QUESTIONS

See Appendix 1 for answers.

1. Mark Kane, age 50, is scheduled for repair of an inguinal hernia. The physician prescribes preoperative sedation with meperidine (Demerol) 50 mg I.M. and the cholinergic blocker atropine (Arco-Lase Plus) 0.4 mg I.M. Before administering a cholinergic blocker, the nurse should assess for which contraindication?
(a) constipation
(b) narrow-angle glaucoma
(c) asthma
(d) Parkinson's disease

2. A belladonna alkaloid, atropine is absorbed from the GI tract, mucous membranes, skin, and eyes. Through which site are the quaternary ammonium agents primarily absorbed?
(a) GI tract
(b) skin
(c) eyes
(d) blood

3. Emma Jackson, age 66, has been invited to tour British Columbia by automobile with her sister and brother-in-law.

However, she is hesitant to go because she suffers from motion sickness. Her physician prescribes the cholinergic blocking agent scopolamine (Triptone) 0.75 mg P.O. 1 hour before traveling to prevent motion sickness. How does a cholinergic blocking agent, such as scopolamine, produce its therapeutic effects?
(a) It mimics the action of acetylcholine at the muscarinic receptor sites.
(b) It competes with acetylcholine at the muscarinic receptor sites.
(c) It metabolizes acetylcholine at the postjunctional membrane.
(d) It blocks the action of acetylcholine at the nicotinic receptor sites.

4. Which of the following effects explains why scopolamine is the drug of choice in the belladonna alkaloid class for treating motion sickness?
(a) It has a greater effect on the CNS than any other drug in this class.
(b) It produces a sense of euphoria and amnesia.
(c) It heightens activity in the sympathetic nervous system.
(d) It heightens activity in the parasympathetic nervous system.

5. During the trip, Ms. Jackson experienced motion sickness, so she tripled her intake of scopolamine. Shortly thereafter, she became restless, irritable, and disoriented. Her husband took her to the emergency department (ED). The physician determined that Ms. Jackson was experiencing toxic effects caused by scopolamine. Which drug should be administered to reverse these effects?
(a) atracurium
(b) bethanechol
(c) trimethaphan
(d) physostigmine

6. Albert Emlen, age 70, has GI tract spasms, for which his physician prescribes propanthelene (Pro-Banthine) 15 mg P.O. q.i.d. During propanthelene therapy, Mr. Emlen is likely to display which of the following adverse reactions?
(a) skin rash and nasal congestion
(b) vomiting and diarrhea
(c) dry mouth and pupillary dilation
(d) decreased level of consciousness and ataxia

7. Mr. Emlen reports constipation during propanthelene therapy. How should the nurse intervene?
(a) Reduce the propanthelene dosage.
(b) Increase the patient's fluid and fiber intake.
(c) Advise the patient to increase milk intake.
(d) Tell the patient to take the drug with meals.

SELECTED REFERENCES

AHFS drug information 90. (1990). Bethesda, MD: American Society of Hospital Pharmacists.

Beta-blockers and aerobic exercise. (1989). *Nurses Drug Alert,* 13(1), 2-3.

Crowe, D. (1986). The beta and calcium channel blockers. *Topics in Emergency Medicine,* 8(1), 26-33.

Hansten, P., and Horn, J. (1989). *Drug interactions.* Philadelphia: Lea & Febiger.

Manzo, M. (1988). Atropine: A versatile drug. *Nursing88.* 18(11), 24.

Miracle, V. (1987). The effect of nursing intervention on serum lipid level of patients taking beta blockers. *Kentucky Nurse,* 35(6), 22-23.

Teplitz, L. (1989). LEAD drugs for cardiac emergencies: Clinical close-up on atropine. *Nursing89,* 19(11), 44-47.

ADRENERGIC AGENTS

OBJECTIVES

After reading and studying this chapter, the student should be able to:

1. Differentiate between catecholamines and noncatecholamines.

2. Compare the methods of action of adrenergic agents: direct, indirect, or dual.

3. Differentiate among the effects of alpha-, beta₁-, and beta₂-receptor stimulation.

4. Explain the relationship between an agent's therapeutic use and its receptor activity.

5. Describe clinical situations that require catecholamine use.

6. Describe clinical situations in which the noncatecholamines are useful.

7. Discuss the adverse effects of the catecholamines and the noncatecholamines.

8. Describe how to apply the nursing process when caring for a patient who is receiving a catecholamine or noncatecholamine agent.

INTRODUCTION

Pharmacologically, adrenergic agents are compounds that cause biological responses similar to those produced by activation of the sympathetic nervous system (SNS). The SNS is a large part of the autonomic nervous system (ANS), which is the part of the nervous system concerned with control of involuntary bodily functions. The SNS consists of ganglia, nerves, and plexuses that supply the involuntary muscles. Most of the nerves of the SNS are motor, but some are sensory.

Adrenergic agents, which also are called sympathomimetics, include a large number of endogenous substances and synthetic drugs that have a wide range of therapeutic uses. Classifying adrenergic agents is thus difficult. The classification system used in this chapter divides adrenergic agents into two groups: catecholamines (including endogenous and synthetic agents) and noncatecholamines.

Adrenergic agents may be divided further by their method of action. They may be direct-acting (acting directly on the sympathetically innervated organ or tissue), indirect-acting (triggering the release of a neurotransmitter, usually norepinephrine), or dual-acting (combining direct and indirect actions).

For a summary of representative drugs, see *Selected major drugs: Adrenergic agents,* pages 228 and 229. For a listing of applicable nursing diagnoses that the nurse may formulate when caring for a patient receiving these agents, see *Selected nursing diagnoses: Adrenergic agents,* page 212. For detailed informaton on applying the nursing process, see Chapter 6, The Nursing Process and Drug Therapy.

Endogenous catecholamines (such as epinephrine, norepinephrine, and dopamine hydrochloride) and synthetic catecholamines (such as isoproterenol hydrochloride, isoproterenol sulfate, and dobutamine hydrochloride) are direct-acting. Noncatecholamines may be direct-acting (such as albuterol, isoetharine hydrochloride, isoetharine mesylate, metaproterenol sulfate, methoxamine hydrochloride, nylidrin hydrochloride, phenylephrine hydrochloride, ritodrine hydrochloride, and terbutaline sulfate), indirect-acting (such as amphetamines), or dual-acting (such as ephedrine sulfate, mephentermine sulfate, and metaraminol bitartrate). These agents can activate the SNS alpha and beta receptors selectively, nonselectively, or in combination.

The therapeutic use of adrenergic agents depends on the receptor activity of the particular agent. (For location and effect of the receptor sites, see *Adrenergic receptor sites,* page 213. Most adrenergic agents stimulate alpha or beta receptors to produce their pharmacologic effects, thus mimicking the action of norepinephrine or epinephrine. Other adrenergic agents, called dopaminergic agents, act primarily on the SNS receptors stimulated by dopamine. Individual drugs differ in receptor activity, although in some the differences may be only quantitative.

Agents that act on alpha receptors are called alphamimetics or alpha agonists. Their most important effects therapeutically involve vasoconstriction of arterioles in the skin, kidneys, mesentery, and splanchnic area. The local

SELECTED NURSING DIAGNOSES

Adrenergic agents

The following nursing diagnoses address representative problems and etiologies that a nurse may encounter when caring for a patient who is receiving an adrenergic agent. Some of these nursing diagnoses contain generalized etiologies, which the nurse must individualize based on the patient's needs. (For some common nursing diagnoses and related interventions for each drug class, see the "Nursing Process Application" sections of this chapter.)

- Activity intolerance related to skeletal muscle weakness caused by the adrenergic agent
- Altered peripheral tissue perfusion related to the adverse cardiovascular effects of the noncatecholamine agent
- Altered thought processes related to noncatecholamine-induced incoherence
- Altered tissue perfusion related to the adverse effects of the adrenergic agent
- Altered health maintenance related to ineffectiveness of the prescribed adrenergic agent
- Anxiety related to the adverse CNS effects of the prescribed adrenergic agent
- Decreased cardiac output related to the adverse cardiovascular effects of the adrenergic agent
- Diarrhea related to the adverse GI effects of the catecholamine agent
- Fear related to the adverse CNS effects of a catecholamine
- Fluid volume deficit related to catecholamine-induced nausea and severe vomiting
- Impaired gas exchange related to paradoxical bronchospasm caused by the noncatecholamine agent
- Impaired tissue integrity related to tissue necrosis from extravasation of the parenteral catecholamine
- Knowledge deficit related to the prescribed adrenergic agent
- Pain related to adrenergic-induced anginal pain
- Pain related to severe headache caused by the adrenergic agent
- Potential for injury related to a preexisting condition that contraindicates the use of adrenergic agents
- Potential for injury related to a preexisting condition that requires cautious use of adrenergic agents
- Potential for injury related to adverse drug reactions
- Potential for trauma related to noncatecholamine-induced seizures
- Potential for trauma related to the adverse CNS effects of the prescribed adrenergic agent
- Sensory-perceptual alteration (visual or gustatory) related to the adverse effects of the noncatecholamine agent
- Sleep pattern disturbance related to insomnia caused by the adrenergic agent
- Total incontinence related to the adverse genitourinary effects of the noncatecholamine agent

---

effects of alpha$_1$-receptor stimulation are used for hemostasis, pupil dilation, nasal and ophthalmic decongestion, and hypotension associated with allergic reactions. The vasopressor effects of alpha$_1$-receptor stimulation are useful in clinical conditions involving hypotension, shock, and decreased cardiac and cerebral circulation. The therapeutic potential of alpha$_2$-receptor stimulants has not been researched fully, although some antihypertensive agents are known to have alpha$_2$-receptor activity in the central nervous system (CNS).

Agents that act on beta receptors are called betamimetics or beta agonists. Their most important effects therapeutically are cardiac stimulation, smooth muscle relaxation, and vasodilation of blood vessels in the brain, heart, and skeletal muscle. The cardiac stimulant effects of beta$_1$-receptor activation are used only under certain restricted conditions. The beta$_2$-receptor effects of smooth muscle relaxation have important therapeutic uses, including bronchial relaxation in asthma or chronic obstructive pulmonary disease. The beta$_2$-receptor effects of vasodilation are therapeutically used in conditions requiring increased blood flow to these organs. When administering catecholamines, the nurse must remember that the pharmacologic actions of these nonselective drugs may overlap, producing undesirable adverse reactions.

Agents that act on dopamine receptors are called dopaminergic agents or agonists. Dopamine receptors are found primarily in the CNS; dopaminergic agonists are used most often to treat parkinsonism. (For more information, see Chapter 19, Antiparkinsonian Agents.) Dopamine, however, also stimulates beta$_1$ receptors in the heart where it increases the force of myocardial contraction (produces a positive inotropic effect). Dopamine also possesses indirect activity, stimulating the release of norepinephrine.

CATECHOLAMINES

Catecholamines include dobutamine hydrochloride, dopamine hydrochloride, epinephrine, epinephrine hydrochloride, epinephrine bitartrate, isoproterenol hydrochloride, isoproterenol sulfate, and norepinephrine (levarterenol). These drugs may be endogenous or synthetic. Endogenous catecholamines share a complex pathway of synthesis: Tyrosine is acted upon by tyrosine hydroxylase to become dopa; dopa is then acted upon by dopa decarboxylase to become dopamine. Dopamine, in turn, is acted upon by

Adrenergic receptor sites

This chart lists specific receptor types and locations and identifies the effect of an adrenergic or dopaminergic drug on the receptor.

RECEPTOR TYPE	LOCATION	EFFECT
Adrenergic agents		
alpha₁	Blood vessels • arterioles	Constriction
	Sphincters • urinary bladder	Contraction
	Muscles • eye (radial) • skin (pilomotor)	Contraction Contraction
	Glands • salivary • pancreas	Secretion Decreased insulin secretion
alpha₂	Adipose tissue	Inhibition of lipolysis
	Skeletal blood vessels	Constriction
beta₁	Heart	Increased rate, conduction, and contractility
	Adipose tissue	Lipolysis
	Kidneys	Renin release
beta₂	Smooth muscle • bronchial • GI tract • urinary bladder	Relaxation Relaxation Relaxation
	Skeletal blood vessels	Dilation
	Uterus	Relaxation
	Liver	Glycogenolysis
Dopaminergic agents		
	Coronary arteries	Dilation
	Renal blood vessels	Dilation
	Mesenteric or visceral blood vessels	Dilation

dopamine beta-hydroxylase to become norepinephrine, which, in the adrenal medulla, then may be acted upon by methyltransferase to become epinephrine.

Because of their common basic chemical structure, catecholamines share certain properties. Although they may produce some CNS effects, such as anxiety, headache, or tremors, they penetrate the blood-brain barrier poorly or not at all. They are ineffective when ingested orally because they are inactivated rapidly in the gastrointestinal (GI) tract and liver. Compared to noncatecholamines, they have a short duration of action. They are relatively unstable, especially in solution, and readily decompose.

Before administering a catecholamine, the nurse must assess the patient carefully for a history of conditions, such as hypertension, diabetes mellitus, and hyperthyroidism, or medications (including over-the-counter medications) that might contraindicate the use of these drugs. The physical examination and interview are important in determining the probability of therapeutic drug effects, adverse drug reactions, and possible drug interactions.

PHARMACOKINETICS

Catecholamines are inactivated rapidly by monoamine oxidase (MAO) and catechol-O-methyltransferase (COMT) in the GI tract and liver, so they must be administered parenterally or via mucous membranes.

Absorption, distribution, metabolism, excretion

Catecholamines are destroyed by digestive enzymes, but rapidly absorbed from mucous membranes. When given sublingually, a catecholamine must be absorbed completely to prevent its rapid metabolism by swallowed saliva. Subcutaneous absorption is slowed by local vasoconstriction secondary to the drug's administration. Intramuscular absorption is more rapid because this route results in less local vasoconstriction.

These drugs are distributed widely in the body, with norepinephrine found primarily in the SNS nerve terminals. They do not cross the blood-brain barrier (such as dopamine and dobutamine) or cross it poorly (such as epinephrine, isoproterenol, and norepinephrine); epinephrine and norepinephrine can cross the placenta.

Metabolism with inactivation of the drugs occurs in the GI tract, lungs, kidneys, plasma, and other tissues, but most occurs in the liver through the action of MAO and COMT. Interference with these enzymes will prolong the drug's duration of action.

Metabolites and some unchanged drugs are excreted primarily in the urine; a small amount of isoproterenol is excreted in the feces, and some epinephrine is excreted in breast milk.

Onset, peak, duration

The route of administration largely determines the onset of action, peak concentration levels, and duration of action. (For comparative information, see *Catecholamines: Summary of pharmacokinetics,* page 214.) Onset usually is rapid with all catecholamines. I.V. administration is the

Catecholamines: Summary of pharmacokinetics

The pharmacokinetics of the catecholamines directly affect their therapeutic uses. Data are available for all properties except half-life of epinephrine, isoproterenol, and norepinephrine. Half-life of dobutamine and dopamine is 2 minutes.

DRUG	ROUTE	ONSET	PEAK	DURATION
dobutamine	I.V. infusion	1 to 3 min	10 min or less	Short
dopamine	I.V. infusion	2 to 5 min	Immediate	5 to 10 min
epinephrine	S.C. injection	3 to 5 min	20 min	Unknown
	Parenteral suspension	5 to 10 min	Immediate upon absorption	8 to 10 hr
	Oral inhalation	1 min	Immediate upon absorption	Unknown
	Topical	1 to 60 min	4 to 8 hr	1 to 24 hr
isoproterenol	I.V.	Immediate	Immediate	Less than 1 hr
	Parenteral	Rapid	Immediate upon absorption	1 to 2 hr
	Oral inhalation	Rapid	Immediate upon absorption	1 to 2 hr
	Sublingual	Rapid	Immediate upon absorption	1 to 2 hr
	Rectal	Rapid	Immediate upon absorption	2 to 4 hr
norepinephrine	I.V. infusion	Immediate	Immediate	1 to 2 min

most rapid route; topical administration is the slowest. Subcutaneous administration involves a delay in onset from vasoconstriction, an effect that is lessened with I.M. injection. Concentrations peak early with most catecholamines, but depend largely on the drug itself and its administration route. The duration also depends on the route, with drugs administered by parenteral suspension lasting longer than those administered by I.V. infusion. The half-life of catecholamines usually is short.

PHARMACODYNAMICS

Catecholamines function as adrenergic neurotransmitters. The endogenous catecholamine epinephrine also is classified as a neurohormone and functions not only as a neural activator but also as an endocrine regulator. The effects of exogenous epinephrine may be different from the endogenous chemical because circulating levels are much higher than endogenous epinephrine levels.

Physiologic release of epinephrine, which is about 10 to 30 mcg/minute, increases heart rate and cardiac output and shunts blood from the peritoneal cavity to the skeletal muscles, myocardium, and liver. Epinephrine amounts in excess of this, as might be given exogenously, can produce a generalized alpha-type effect on blood vessels with resulting widespread vasoconstriction.

Mechanism of action

When catecholamines combine with alpha or beta receptors, chemical or electrical events occur that produce excitatory or inhibitory effects. In most cases, alpha-receptor activation generates an excitatory response (except for intestinal relaxation). Beta-receptor activation is mostly inhibitory (except in the myocardial cells, where norepinephrine elicits excitatory effects). (For more information, see *Adrenergic agents: Receptor activity, drug action, and use.*)

Catecholamines are inactivated quickly by uptake into nerve terminals, enzymatic transformation, or diffusion. The reuptake process involves active transport and is the most important mechanism for inactivation. This mechanism also results in conservation and recycling of the drug,

Adrenergic agents: Receptor activity, drug action, and use

This chart summarizes the receptor activity of the major catecholamines and noncatecholamines, the physical effects they produce, and their clinical use. This information forms an important knowledge base for the nurse administering these drugs.

DRUG	RECEPTOR ACTIVITY	ACTION	USE
Catecholamines			
Direct-acting			
dobutamine	Beta$_1$	Cardiac stimulation	Inotropic drug
dopamine	Dopaminergic, alpha (only at high doses), beta$_1$	Vasoconstriction at high doses Renal vessel dilation at low doses	Shock, hypotension, inotropic drug
epinephrine	Alpha, beta$_1$, beta$_2$	Cardiac stimulation Vasoconstriction Bronchodilation	Anaphylaxis, acute hypotension, cardiac arrest, topical vasoconstriction, glaucoma
isoproterenol	Beta$_1$, beta$_2$	Cardiac stimulation Bronchodilation	Shock, digitalis toxicity, asthma
norepinephrine or levarterenol	Alpha, beta$_1$	Vasoconstriction	Shock, hypotension
Noncatecholamines			
Direct-acting			
albuterol	Beta$_1$ < beta$_2$	Bronchodilation	Asthma, bronchitis, emphysema
isoetharine	Beta$_1$ < beta$_2$	Bronchodilation	Inhalation therapy
metaproterenol	Beta$_1$ < beta$_2$	Bronchodilation	Inhalation therapy
methoxamine	Alpha	Vasoconstriction	Hypotension, termination of paroxysmal atrial tachycardia
nylidrin	Beta$_1$, beta$_2$	Vasodilation	Peripheral vascular disorders
phenylephrine	Alpha, beta (weak)	Vasoconstriction	Shock, hypotension, nasal congestion, termination of paroxysmal atrial tachycardia
ritodrine	Beta$_1$ < beta$_2$	Smooth muscle relaxation	Preterm labor for uterine relaxation
terbutaline	Beta$_1$ < beta$_2$	Bronchodilation Uterine relaxation	Emphysema, asthma, preterm labor
Dual-acting			
ephedrine	Alpha, beta, CNS	Bronchodilation Vasoconstriction	Nasal congestion, hypotension, narcolepsy
mephentermine	Alpha < beta	Vasoconstriction Appetite depression	Hypotension, appetite depression
metaraminol	Alpha > beta	Vasoconstriction	Shock, hypotension

which is not destroyed. Enzymatically, endogenous catecholamines are inactivated primarily by MAO; exogenous catecholamines are inactivated primarily by COMT. The diffusion process, whereby catecholamines are absorbed into the circulation and metabolized elsewhere in the body, accounts for only a small portion of catecholamine inactivation.

Norepinephrine, dobutamine, and epinephrine are less potent than isoproterenol in stimulating beta receptors. Dopamine has a weak, indirect action on alpha receptors, stimulating release of norepinephrine. Norepinephrine and epinephrine are equal in their $alpha_1$-stimulating abilities. This $alpha_1$ activation usually stimulates smooth muscle contraction.

Because $alpha_1$ receptors control blood vessels in the internal organs, mucosal surface, and skin, a systemic increase in blood pressure results from $alpha_1$ activation. However, $alpha_2$ receptors serve as a negative feedback system to limit norepinephrine release from the neuron. Norepinephrine also activates $alpha_2$ receptors on the nerve terminal, inhibiting further endogenous norepinephrine release.

Isoproterenol, which stimulates $beta_1$ and $beta_2$ receptors, is a more potent $beta_1$-receptor stimulant than epinephrine or norepinephrine. Dobutamine also is a $beta_1$ stimulant, exerting a weak, indirect effect. $Beta_1$ receptors in the conduction tissue of the heart speed cell repolarization when stimulated, leading to positive chronotropic (rate) and inotropic (force) effects. $Beta_1$ stimulation in fat tissue produces fat breakdown, releasing fatty acids for heart and liver energy sources. However, this effect has no therapeutic application.

Norepinephrine, dopamine, and dobutamine are weak $beta_2$-adrenergic receptor stimulants; epinephrine and isoproterenol are equally strong in activating $beta_2$ sites. $Beta_2$ stimulants cause bronchodilation by relaxing bronchial smooth muscle via $beta_2$ activation. Additional $beta_2$ effects include vasodilation and shunting of blood to the skeletal muscles, brain, and heart. An effect of $beta_2$ stimulation not used therapeutically is liver glycogenolysis (also an $alpha_1$ effect).

The combination of $alpha_1$, $beta_1$, and $beta_2$ actions is valuable in the fight or flight response. $Beta_1$ stimulation by norepinephrine is reinforced by epinephrine, producing an increased heart rate and cardiac output, with blood shunted to muscles, brain, and heart by $beta_2$ vasodilation action. $Alpha_1$ receptors control calcium entry into cells, which leads to enzyme changes and produces $alpha_1$ effects (including vasoconstriction of the skin and abdominal organs), and epinephrine provides energy by producing glycogenolysis in the liver and lipolysis in fat cells. $Alpha_2$ receptors oppose beta-receptor action by inhibiting adenylate cyclase, an enzyme necessary for this reaction.

The clinical effects of catecholamines depend on the dosage and the route of administration. In the cardiovascular system, these effects also may depend on the vascular bed. The positive inotropic action (marked increase in strength of contraction) results from the influx of calcium into cardiac fibers, producing more complete emptying of the ventricles and increasing cardiac work load and oxygen consumption. Also, the positive inotropic action may occur with catecholamine agents as well as a positive chronotropic effect from the increased rate of membrane depolarization in the pacemaker cells of the sinus node. This produces a more rapid attainment of the action potential threshold, so the pacemaker cells fire more often. Reflex bradycardia may occur from increased vasoconstriction and blood pressure. Catecholamines may precipitate spontaneous firing in the Purkinje fibers, producing pacemaker activity and possibly producing premature ventricular contractions and fibrillation. Epinephrine is likelier than norepinephrine to produce this spontaneous firing.

Although the catecholamines cross the blood-brain barrier poorly, their use produces various CNS effects. Epinephrine and isoproterenol produce alertness, tremulousness, respiratory stimulation, and anxiety; less anxiety and tremulousness are noted with norepinephrine. Epinephrine and norepinephrine improve cerebral blood flow through their effect on peripheral circulation, resulting in increased systemic blood flow.

Catecholamines produce general relaxation of nonvascular smooth muscles. One effect of this is bronchodilation. Isoproterenol exerts greater effects than epinephrine, and epinephrine exerts greater effects than norepinephrine. Epinephrine also may act to decrease bronchial secretions by constricting bronchial vessels.

Catecholamines reduce peristalsis in the GI tract. Epinephrine causes the urinary bladder sphincter to contract and the detrusor muscle to relax. The physiologic effects of dopamine primarily are dose-related. With low doses of dopamine, only dopaminergic receptors are activated, with the resultant vasodilation of the renal arteries leading to increased renal blood flow and, usually, increased urine output. With high doses of dopamine, alpha and beta effects are noted.

Epinephrine inhibits insulin secretion. Also, catecholamines stimulate glycogenolysis in liver and skeletal muscle and lipolysis in adipose tissue. This results in increased circulating blood glucose and free fatty acids. Norepinephrine, epinephrine, and isoproterenol also increase oxygen consumption.

Although catecholamines usually produce decreased glandular secretions, causing such an effect as a dry mouth, epinephrine may increase saliva. Also, local sweating of the palms, axillae, and genital area may occur with some catecholamines.

PHARMACOTHERAPEUTICS

The particular receptor activity that exists alone or predominates if more than one receptor type is activated determines how the drug is used therapeutically. Of the catecholamines, norepinephrine has the most nearly pure alpha activity. Drugs with only beta-related therapeutic uses include dobutamine and isoproterenol, and epinephrine stimulates alpha and beta receptors. Dopamine primarily exhibits dopaminergic activity.

The therapeutic uses of catecholamines are related not only to their systemic effects, but also to their local effects. The local vasoconstrictive actions of the drugs make them useful as nasal decongestants to treat inflammatory and allergic conditions; as ophthalmic decongestants to treat conjunctivitis and ocular congestion; as an adjunct to topical miotics, beta-adrenergic blockers, osmotic agents, or systemic carbonic anhydrase inhibitors to treat simple open-angle glaucoma; as topical hemostatics to control superficial bleeding; as local anesthetic adjuncts to prolong action by retarding absorption; and as antiallergens to treat hypersensitivity and anaphylaxis. Local application of various drugs dilates pupils without concurrent cycloplegia (paralysis of ciliary muscles) or increased intraocular pressure. These effects are beneficial primarily in ophthalmic examinations and glaucoma treatment.

The alpha stimulators can be used systemically to relieve hypotension. Hypotension may be caused by numerous conditions, including sympathectomy, pheochromocytomectomy, spinal anesthesia, myocardial infarction, transfusion reaction, septicemia, drug reactions, or shock. As a rule, the pressor effects are used for conditions related to loss of vasomotor tone or loss of adequate circulating blood volume.

$Beta_1$-active drugs are used to treat bradycardia and heart block (as seen in Stokes-Adams syndrome and carotid sinus syndrome) and insufficient cardiac output. They also may be used to terminate paroxysmal atrial or nodal tachycardia. Because they are believed to make the heart more responsive to defibrillation, they are used in cases of ventricular fibrillation, asystole, or cardiac arrest.

Catecholamines that exert $beta_2$ activity are used to treat acute and chronic bronchial asthma, emphysema, bronchitis, and acute hypersensitivity reactions to drugs.

The effects of drugs that are exogenously administered differ somewhat from the natural effects of endogenous catecholamines. Thus the patient's response also will differ somewhat from the normal physiologic response to endogenous catecholamines. The effects of catecholamines administered exogenously will be of short duration, which may limit their therapeutic usefulness.

Isoproterenol is longer-acting and less toxic than epinephrine. Epinephrine, dopamine, dobutamine, and isoproterenol increase cardiac output; norepinephrine may have no effect or may lower it slightly. (The potent vasoconstricting action may cause a reflex bradycardia). Epinephrine increases atrioventricular conduction and may produce more severe tachycardia than norepinephrine because epinephrine is a more potent beta stimulant. Isoproterenol usually produces tachycardia but improves cardiac output because of the drug's positive inotropic and chronotropic actions. Decreased blood pressure may result from low-dose epinephrine because of decreased total peripheral vascular resistance, or from isoproterenol because of a pure vasodilator action. Increased blood pressure may result from high-dose epinephrine, high-dose dopamine, or norepinephrine because of the increased total peripheral vascular resistance with activation of alpha receptors. Norepinephrine and dopamine decrease blood flow in skeletal muscle; epinephrine increases perfusion to skeletal muscle by $beta_2$-induced vasodilation.

In most cases, epinephrine is useful therapeutically for its alpha activities in allergic reactions. It is the drug of choice for anaphylactic shock because it counteracts the hypotensive effects of histamine. The pressor effects are also beneficial for local vasoconstriction when prolongation of locally administered drugs is desired. Epinephrine also is used clinically for its beta effects of bronchodilation in acute asthma attacks and for its cardiac effects.

Norepinephrine, with its alpha vasopressor effects, counteracts hypotension from septicemic shock and spinal anesthesia.

Dopamine's therapeutic value is based on its dopaminergic, $beta_1$, and alpha-agonist activity. The drug is used in low doses to dilate renal arteries, preventing renal shutdown in cardiogenic or bacteremic shock. Dopamine also may be helpful in treating chronic refractory congestive heart failure because of its positive inotropic activity.

The beta effects of dobutamine are valuable clinically to increase cardiac contractility and output without an undue increase in heart rate or conductivity in patients with congestive heart failure.

Isoproterenol is useful therapeutically for its beta actions on the heart in shock or heart block.

dobutamine hydrochloride (Dobutrex). A synthetic direct-acting beta-active agent, dobutamine is administered only intravenously, with actions similar to those of isoproterenol and low doses of dopamine. This drug is used to increase cardiac output for patients with acute congestive heart failure and those undergoing cardiopulmonary bypass surgery.

Usual adult dosage: I.V. infusion only; 2.5 to 10 mcg/kg/minute. The drug is reconstituted in 10 to 20 ml of sterile water or D_5W and then further diluted in D_5W, normal saline, or ⅙M sodium lactate solution. Infusion rates up to 40 mcg/kg/minute may be required.

dopamine hydrochloride (Intropin, Dopastat). A naturally occurring neurotransmitter, dopamine is a precursor of epinephrine and norepinephrine. Its actions are dose-dependent, with dopaminergic activity only at approximately 2 to 5 mcg/kg/minute, mixed dopaminergic and beta activity at 5 to 10 mcg/kg/minute, and predominantly alpha activity at greater than 10 mcg/kg/minute. It acts directly and indirectly (releases norepinephrine stores) on alpha and beta$_1$ receptors. It is used to treat shock with related renal shutdown and chronic refractory congestive heart failure. Discontinue the drug gradually.

Usual adult dosage: I.V. infusion only, usually by an electronic infusion pump; initially, 1 to 5 mcg/kg/minute diluted in appropriate sterile solution as recommended by manufacturer. For severely ill patients, increase by 5 to 10 mcg/kg/minute increments to a total of 20 to 50 mcg/kg/minute.

epinephrine hydrochloride and **epinephrine bitartrate** (Parenteral: Adrenalin, Sus-Phrine), (Inhalation: AsthmaHaler, Medihaler-Epi), **epinephrine** (Inhalation: Bronkaid Mist, Primatene Mist). Epinephrine is the prototype sympathomimetic agent. Available in many forms, it is used widely for bronchodilation, pulmonary decongestion, potentiation and prolongation of anesthetic action, and topical hemostasis. It also is used to treat acute asthmatic attacks; anaphylactic, allergic, and hypersensitivity reactions; acute hypotension; and cardiac arrest. (For use in glaucoma and ocular congestion, see Chapter 71, Ophthalmic Agents.)

Usual adult dosage: for cardiac arrest, 1 to 10 ml I.V. of a 1:10,000 concentration repeated at 5-minute intervals as required. If no I.V. site is available, 10 ml of 1:10,000 solution via endotracheal tube. Dosage for bronchospasm, hypersensitivity reactions, and anaphylaxis is 0.1 to 0.5 ml of 1:1,000 solution I.M. or S.C. For acute asthmatic attacks, the dosage is one inhalation of a 1:100 solution, repeated once if needed after at least 1 minute. As adjunct to local anesthesia, a concentration of 1:200,000 to 1:20,000 is used. For nasal congestion, 0.1% solution applied topically; as a hemostatic, topically applied 1:50,000 or 1:1,000 solution; for spinal anesthesia, 0.2 to 0.4 ml 1:1,000 added to anesthetic solution and administered intraspinally.

Usual pediatric dosage: for bronchospasm, 0.005 to 0.01 mg/kg of a 1:200 suspension administered S.C., used only in emergency situations.

isoproterenol hydrochloride (Oral: Isuprel. Inhalation: Vaso-Iso), **isoproterenol sulfate** (Inhalation: Medihaler-Iso). A powerful, direct-acting beta-receptor stimulator, isoproterenol may have longer action and be less toxic than epinephrine. Uses include treatment of asthma; bronchospasm associated with respiratory disorders and general anesthesia; and adjunct management of shock, cardiac ar-

rest, Stokes-Adams syndrome, atrioventricular block, and carotid sinus hypersensitivity.

Usual adult dosage: for bronchospasm during anesthesia, 0.01 to 0.02 mg of a 1:50,000 solution in normal saline or D$_5$W I.V. For shock, 0.25 to 2.5 ml/minute (0.5 to 5 mcg/minute) of a 1:500,000 solution in D$_5$W I.V. In cardiac arrest, I.V. injection of 1 to 3 ml (0.02 to 0.06 mg) of a 1:50,000 dilution, or I.V. infusion of 1.25 ml/minute (5 mcg/minute) of a 1:250,000 solution, or 1 ml (0.2 mg) undiluted I.M. or S.C. For intracardiac administration, 0.1 ml (0.02 mg) of 1:5,000 solution. For heart block, initially 10 mg sublingually, with range of 5 to 50 mg, or initially 5 mg rectal administration, with 5 to 15 mg for maintenance. For bronchospasm, sublingual or rectal administration of 10 to 20 mg t.i.d. or q.i.d., to a maximum of 60 mg/day; or inhalation of solution, 120 to 262 mcg (one to two inhalations) 4 to 6 times a day; or aerosol, 80 to 160 mcg (one to two inhalations) 4 to 6 times a day.

norepinephrine formerly **levarterenol** (Levophed, Noradrenaline). Norepinephrine is a direct-acting sympathomimetic amine with predominantly alpha-adrenergic activity and minor beta$_1$ activity in the heart. It is used for acute hypotension and shock, adjunct treatment of cardiac arrest, myocardial infarction, and anaphylaxis.

Usual adult dosage: I.V. infusion only; initially 2 to 3 ml/minute (8 to 12 mcg/minute) of a 4-mg norepinephrine:1,000 ml D$_5$W solution (4 mcg/ml dilution). Maintenance dosage is 0.5 to 1 ml/minute (2 to 4 mcg/minute).

Drug interactions

Knowledge of the interactions between catecholamines and other agents is essential because of the potential for additive effects, which might lead to a hypertensive crisis or cardiac arrhythmias. (For interacting drugs, possible effects, and nursing implications, see *Drug interactions: Catecholamines.*)

ADVERSE DRUG REACTIONS

Because of the widespread actions of the catecholamines, adverse reactions affect the CNS, cardiovascular system, GI tract, skeletal and smooth muscles, and all other body systems. Although the reactions vary from drug to drug, the nurse must be aware of their possibility and must monitor and assess patients carefully when they are receiving catecholamine therapy.

Many CNS manifestations may be noted, including restlessness, nervousness, anxiety, fear, dizziness, vertigo, headache (throbbing to severe), and insomnia. Adverse cardiovascular reactions include pallor or flushing, palpitations, cardiac arrhythmias, tachycardia or slow and forceful heartbeat, hypotension or hypertension, cerebrovascular accident, and angina. Skeletal muscle adverse reactions may

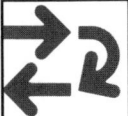

DRUG INTERACTIONS

Catecholamines

Drug interactions involving catecholamines can be among the most serious, causing hypotension, hypertension, cardiac arrhythmias, seizures, and hyperglycemia in diabetics. If catecholamines must be administered with other drugs, the patient must be monitored frequently. Note that all interactions may not occur between all catecholamines and drugs listed.

DRUG	INTERACTING DRUGS	POSSIBLE EFFECTS	NURSING IMPLICATIONS
dobutamine, dopamine, epinephrine, isoproterenol, norepinephrine	alpha blockers (phentolamine)	Antagonize catecholamines with alpha activity, causing hypotension	• Administer with caution. • Monitor the patient's blood pressure.
	oral hypoglycemic agents	Inhibit insulin, inducing hyperglycemia	• Monitor the patient's blood glucose level.
	beta blockers (propranolol)	Mutually antagonize effects; may allow the domination of alpha effects of the adrenergic, causing hypertension; inhibit adrenergic stimulation of heart, bronchial tree (bronchial constriction, asthma)	• Monitor the patient's blood pressure.
	sympathomimetics	Produce additive effects (hypertension, cardiac arrhythmias), enhance adverse effect	• Alternate drugs as prescribed, or monitor closely. • Monitor the patient's pulse rate and blood pressure.

include weakness or mild tremors. The most common GI adverse reactions include nausea, vomiting (which may be severe), and diarrhea.

With extravasation of I.V. catecholamines, necrosis can occur from local vasoconstriction. Tissue sloughing may follow.

NURSING PROCESS APPLICATION

The following information assists the nurse in caring for a patient who is receiving a catecholamine.

Assessment
• Review the patient's history for conditions that contraindicate the use of catecholamines, such as cardiovascular disease, pheochromocytoma, or diabetes.
• Review the patient's history for conditions that require cautious use of catecholamines, such as advanced age, hypertension, hyperthyroidism, diabetes, psychoneurosis, or pregnancy.
• Assess the patient for adverse reactions to the prescribed catecholamine, such as headache, restlessness, flushing, palpitations, cardiac arrhythmias, hypotension or hypertension, weakness, nausea, and vomiting.
• Evaluate the patient's and family's knowledge about the prescribed catecholamine.

Nursing diagnoses
The following examples represent appropriate nursing diagnoses for a patient receiving a catecholamine.
• Potential for injury related to a preexisting condition that contraindicates the use of catecholamines
• Potential for injury related to a preexisting condition that requires cautious use of catecholamines
• Potential for injury related to adverse drug reactions
• Knowledge deficit related to the prescribed catecholamine

Planning and implementation
• Do not administer a catecholamine to a patient with a condition that contraindicates its use.
• Administer a catecholamine cautiously to a patient at risk because of a preexisting condition.
• *Have oxygen and emergency respiratory equipment readily available.*
• Correct hypovolemia, as prescribed, before catecholamine therapy begins.
• *Check the prescription closely, particularly noting the solution concentration, dosage, and rate.*
• *Do not administer isoproterenol and inhaled epinephrine concurrently; space 4 hours apart.*
• Monitor the patient closely for adverse reactions to catecholamines.
• Obtain blood glucose levels, as needed, for the diabetic patient.

Proper preparation and administration of catecholamines

Besides observing other important implications, the nurse should remember these points before administering any catechol-amines.

Preparation

- Do not expose solutions to heat, light, or air; they may deteriorate rapidly.
- Do not use any solution that is yellow or amber-colored or that contains a precipitate.
- In patients dependent on catecholamines for blood pressure support, keep an additional bag of the solution available.

- Use a syringe with calibrations small enough to ensure accurate dosage measurement.
- Always have antidotal drug (phentolamine) on hand when administering I.V. drugs.

Administration

- Always aspirate with the syringe before S.C. or I.M. injection to avoid systemic effects.
- For I.V. infusion, use a large vein (preferably a central line) when possible and rotate peripheral I.V. insertion sites to minimize the risk of necrosis from infiltration.
- Never administer catecholamines for hypotension through the proximal port of a pulmonary artery catheter being used for cardiac output measurement; the patient inadvertently might receive a bolus of the drug.
- Use an infusion control device to ensure accurate drug delivery and prevent overdose.
- With I.V. administration, gradually titrate up dose and monitor blood pressure and pulse rate every 3 to 5 minutes until they stabilize, then every 15 minutes.
- With all catecholamines, gradually decrease the infusion rate when weaning off the drug. Continue monitoring vital signs every 15 minutes to ensure circulatory stability.
- With I.V. administration, observe closely for cyanosis or pallor (signs of shock or excessive peripheral vasoconstriction).
- During drug infusion, continually monitor electrocardiogram, blood pressure, cardiac rate, cardiac rhythm, and, when possible, cardiac output and pulmonary wedge pressure.
- Monitor for bradycardia; the rate of the infusion of alpha stimulants should be decreased as prescribed to return the

heart rate to normal; atropine, isoproterenol, dopamine, or dobutamine may be ordered if necessary.
- With I.V. drugs, decrease or discontinue the drug as prescribed if the heart rate exceeds 120 beats/minute.
- Note that duration of I.V. drug action is brief, and the effects terminate shortly after discontinuation of I.V. infusion.
- Massage S.C. and I.M. injection sites to hasten absorption.
- Always dilute dopamine, dobutamine, isoproterenol, and norepinephrine as prescribed before I.V. administration.
- Do not give I.V. infusion of vasoconstrictors into leg veins, especially in elderly patients, because of the possibility of occlusive vascular disease.
- With inhalant drugs, allow 1 to 2 minutes between inhalations to prevent systemic effects.
- Monitor urine output regularly to assess for renal perfusion and urine retention.
- To prevent systemic effects with inhalation drugs, use the minimum number of inhalations to relieve the symptoms.
- If I.V. norepinephrine extravasates, stop the infusion immediately and infiltrate with 10 to 15 ml of normal saline solution containing 5 to 10 mg phentolamine as prescribed.
- Do not infuse concurrently in I.V. lines being used to administer blood products or heparin because of incompatibility.

- *Monitor the patient's respiratory rate when administering isoproterenol to detect rebound bronchospasm.*
- Prepare and administer the catecholamine carefully. (For details, see *Proper preparation and administration of catecholamines.*)
- Notify the physician if adverse reactions occur.

Patient teaching
- Teach the patient and family the name, dose, frequency, action, and adverse effects of the prescribed catecholamine.
- *Teach the patient and family how to take a pulse rate.*
- *Show the patient and family how to use inhalant devices correctly. Emphasize using the lowest number of inhalations possible.*
- Teach the patient using an inhaler to rinse the mouth with water after administration to prevent dry mouth.

- Advise the patient using an intranasal drug that rebound congestion and hyperemia commonly occur with too frequent use of epinephrine.
- Advise the patient using an intranasal drug that it will sting, but that the discomfort will be temporary.
- *Teach the diabetic patient to notify the physician if glucose test results change or if signs and symptoms of hyperglycemia occur.*
- Tell the patient to notify the physician if adverse reactions occur.

Evaluation
The following examples represent appropriate evaluation statements for a patient receiving a catecholamine.
- The patient has no conditions that contraindicate catecholamine therapy.

• The patient exhibits no signs of complications in the preexisting condition linked to the prescribed catecholamine.

• The patient exhibits no adverse reactions to the prescribed catecholamine.

• The patient and family express an accurate understanding of the points taught about the prescribed catecholamine.

• The patient correctly uses the inhalant device.

• The patient demonstrates an appropriate technique for pulse rate measurement.

NONCATECHOLAMINES

Noncatecholamine adrenergic drugs have a wide variety of therapeutic uses. This wide use is related to the many physiologic effects of these drugs, including local or systemic vasoconstriction (mephentermine, metaraminol, methoxamine, phenylephrine), nasal and ophthalmic decongestion and bronchodilation (albuterol, ephedrine, isoetharine, metaproterenol, terbutaline), and smooth muscle relaxation (nylidrin, terbutaline, ritodrine).

In this chapter, drugs are discussed in relation to their direct- or dual-acting mechanism of action and their adrenergic receptor activity (alpha, beta$_1$, or beta$_2$).

Before administering noncatecholamine adrenergic drugs, the nurse must assess the patient carefully for a history of conditions or medications that might contraindicate such therapy. The physical examination and interview are essential to assess the efficacy of the drug therapy and to detect signs or symptoms of adverse reactions.

PHARMACOKINETICS

Unlike catecholamines, most noncatecholamine adrenergic drugs are effective orally (isoetharine, however, is degraded if swallowed). These drugs usually have a longer duration of action than catecholamines and may act directly or indirectly on the adrenergic receptors or may exert a combination of the two actions.

Absorption, distribution, metabolism, excretion

The absorption of noncatecholamine adrenergic drugs depends on the route of administration. Drugs administered by inhalation, such as albuterol, are absorbed gradually from the bronchi, causing lower systemic drug levels after the patient inhales recommended doses. Oral drugs are absorbed well from the GI tract and are distributed widely in the body fluids and tissues. Some drugs cross the blood-brain barrier (for example, ephedrine) and may be found in high concentrations in the brain and cerebrospinal fluid.

Albuterol is one drug that does not cross the blood-brain barrier. Albuterol, terbutaline, ritodrine, and possibly ephedrine cross the placenta, and ephedrine and terbutaline are excreted in breast milk.

Metabolism and inactivation of the noncatecholamines occur primarily in the liver, where large concentrations of MAO are found, but also occur in the lungs, GI tract, and other tissues.

These drugs and their metabolites are excreted primarily in the urine. Some, such as inhaled albuterol, are excreted within 24 hours; others, such as oral albuterol, within 3 days. Of minor clinical importance, acidic urine increases excretion of many noncatecholamine drugs; alkaline urine slows excretion.

Onset, peak, and duration

Variations in the onset of action, peak concentration levels, and duration of action of noncatecholamine drugs are primarily functions of the route of administration. (For comparative information, see *Noncatecholamines: Summary of pharmacokinetics,* page 222.) The onset generally is rapid after most routes of administration, occurring between 1 and 30 minutes after inhalation, between 10 and 120 minutes after oral ingestion, between 1 and 60 minutes after I.V. infusion, and between 5 and 60 minutes after I.M., S.C., or topical application.

The peak action usually is between 5 and 15 minutes for inhalation, between 1 and 8 hours for oral administration, and between 30 and 60 minutes after parenteral administration.

The duration ranges from 15 minutes after I.M. administration of metaraminol to 6 hours after inhalation or oral administration of albuterol. The specific half-life of many of these drugs is unknown but ranges between 3 and 5 hours. Nasal decongestants usually have a fairly long duration and therefore should be used only two to three times a day.

PHARMACODYNAMICS

Noncatecholamine adrenergic drugs may be direct-acting, indirect-acting, or dual-acting (unlike catecholamines, which are primarily direct-acting). Direct-acting noncatecholamine drugs achieve their effects by occupying receptor sites on organs and structures innervated by the SNS. Drugs that exhibit primarily alpha activity include methoxamine and phenylephrine; those that selectively exert beta$_2$ activity include albuterol, isoetharine, metaproterenol, nylidrin, ritodrine, and terbutaline.

Indirect-acting noncatecholamines exert their effects by stimulating norepinephrine release from its storage sites. Dual-acting noncatecholamine adrenergic drugs combine both actions; they include ephedrine, mephentermine, and metaraminol. Nylidrin also acts directly on smooth muscle

Noncatecholamines: Summary of pharmacokinetics

The nurse administering noncatecholamines must be aware of their pharmacokinetic properties to assess the patient's therapeutic response.

DRUG	ROUTE	ONSET	PEAK	DURATION	HALF-LIFE
albuterol	Inhalation	5 to 15 min	0.5 to 2 hr	3 to 4 hr	4 to 6 hr
	Oral	30 min	2 to 3 min	4 to 6 hr	4 to 6 hr
ephedrine	Oral, nasal	15 to 60 min	*	2 to 4 hr	3 to 6 hr
	I.V., I.M., S.C.	Rapid	Rapid	1 hr	3 to 6 hr
isoetharine	Inhalation	1 min	5 to 15 min	1 to 4 hr	*
mephentermine	I.M.	5 to 15 min	*	1 to 4 hr	*
	I.V.	Immediate	*	30 to 45 min	*
	S.C.	5 to 15 min	*	30 to 60 min	*
metaproterenol	Oral	15 min	1 hr	3 to 4 hr	*
	Inhalation	1 to 5 min	30 min to 1 hr	1 to 5 hr	*
metaraminol	I.M.	10 min	*	20 to 60 min	*
	I.V.	1 to 2 min	*	20 to 60 min	*
	S.C.	5 to 20 min	*	20 to 60 min	*
methoxamine	I.M.	15 to 20 min	15 to 20 min	60 to 90 min	*
	I.V.	Immediate	0.5 to 2 min	10 to 15 min	*
nylidrin	Oral	10 min	30 to 90 min	2 hr	*
phenylephrine	I.V.	Immediate	Rapid	15 to 20 min	*
	S.C., I.M.	1 to 15 min	*	30 to 50 min	*
	Intranasal	10 to 15 min	*	3 to 4 hr	*
ritodrine	Oral	10 to 120 min	2 to 3 hr	4 to 6 hr	10 hr
	I.V.	Immediate	Rapid	1.5 to 2 hr	10 hr
terbutaline	Oral	30 min	1 to 2 hr	4 to 8 hr	13 to 18 hr
	Inhalation	5 to 30 min	30 to 60 min	3 to 6 hr	13 to 18 hr
	S.C.	6 to 15 min	30 to 60 min	1.5 to 4 hr	13 to 18 hr

*Information unknown or unavailable

to cause relaxation. (For more information, see *Noncatecholamines: Summary of receptor activity.*)

Mechanism of action

All of the noncatecholamine adrenergic drugs share a similar chemical structure with the catecholamines. In contrast to the catecholamines, most noncatecholamines are effective when given orally and may act longer. This is partly because of their resistance to the inactivating enzymes of the liver and other tissues and partly because of relatively large doses. They are, however, largely inactivated by MAO, as are catecholamines, and therefore are potentiated by MAO inhibitors. Methoxamine and metaraminol, used pri-

Noncatecholamines: Summary of receptor activity

This table summarizes the pharmacologic activity of the noncatecholamines.

DRUG	RECEPTORS ACTIVATED
Direct-acting agents	
albuterol	Beta$_2$ effects greater than beta$_1$
isoetharine	Beta$_2$ effects greater than beta$_1$
metaproterenol	Beta$_2$ effects greater than beta$_1$
methoxamine	Alpha
nylidrin	Beta$_1$, beta$_2$
phenylephrine	Alpha, beta$_1$ (weak)
ritodrine	Beta$_2$ effects greater than beta$_1$
terbutaline	Beta$_2$ effects greater than beta$_1$
Dual-acting agents	
ephedrine	Alpha, beta
mephentermine	Beta effects greater than alpha
metaraminol	Alpha effects greater than beta

marily as vasopressors, act directly and indirectly to produce generalized vasoconstriction.

Bronchodilating drugs may be direct- or dual-acting and nonselectively may activate alpha and beta receptors or selectively activate primarily beta$_2$ receptors. Nonspecific receptor effects include tachycardia, increased blood pressure, and increased cardiac output; beta$_2$-selective receptor effects include relaxation of bronchial, uterine, and vascular smooth muscle.

Drugs used to relax smooth muscles (nylidrin, ritodrine, terbutaline, and albuterol) exert a direct, predominantly beta-specific activity. Nylidrin also exerts a direct effect on vascular smooth muscle, not affected by beta blockade.

PHARMACOTHERAPEUTICS

Because noncatecholamines stimulate the SNS and produce varied physiologic effects, they are used widely. The bronchodilatory effects of such drugs as albuterol, metaproterenol, and terbutaline are used to treat acute and chronic bronchial asthma, emphysema, pulmonary fibrosis, and chronic bronchitis.

Ephedrine, methoxamine, phenylephrine, mephentermine, and metaraminol may be used for their pressor effects with spinal anesthesia, for treating hypotension, for vasoconstriction during regional anesthesia, and for nosebleeds.

Metaraminol may be used (rarely) to treat hypotension in patients with septicemia, or after barbiturate overdose, myocardial infarction, or trauma.

Ephedrine is used primarily to treat nasal congestion, ophthalmic conditions, allergic disorders, bronchospasm associated with asthma, or as a CNS stimulant in narcolepsy.

Various noncatecholamines may be used for migraine headache, certain dermatoses, low cardiac output, allergic reactions, anaphylactic reactions, paroxysmal supraventricular tachycardia (phenylephrine or methoxamine), and wide-angle glaucoma. They also may be given to produce mydriasis (pupil dilatation) with ocular examination or uveitis (phenylephrine), to reduce spasms associated with ureteral and biliary colic, for dysmenorrhea, or to delay delivery in preterm labor (terbutaline or ritodrine).

Many differences exist among the drugs, making general statements difficult. The various drugs are more or less effective depending on the route of administration, the dose, and the desired therapeutic effect and patient tolerance. For example, when bronchodilation is desired, metaproterenol might be chosen over the catecholamine isoproterenol. Although the two drugs are similar chemically and pharmacologically, patients are less likely to develop a tolerance to metaproterenol. Metaproterenol is a more effective bronchodilator orally than ephedrine and is longer-acting than isoproterenol. Albuterol is only one-half to one-quarter as active as isoproterenol in producing increased heart rate in some patients and might be chosen as a bronchodilator for a patient who also has cardiac disease or hypertension. Ephedrine is pharmacologically similar to epinephrine, but is longer-acting, less potent, and has a slower onset of action. Metaraminol is similar in overall effects to norepinephrine but is less potent and has a slower onset and a longer duration of action. Methoxamine and phenylephrine have similar pharmacologic effects.

albuterol (Proventil, Ventolin). This direct-acting drug is comparatively long-acting and relatively selective for beta$_2$ receptors, particularly in bronchial, uterine, and vascular smooth muscle, and in mast cells. Albuterol is used primarily for bronchospasm associated with reversible obstructive airway disease. It also may be used to treat several conditions, including prevention of exercise-induced bronchospasm and preterm labor.
Usual adult dosage: as an inhalation (metered spray), one to two inhalations of 90 to 180 mcg every 4 to 6 hours; the initial oral dose is 2 to 4 mg t.i.d. or q.i.d.; maximum daily dosage is 32 mg.
Usual pediatric dosage: for ages 6 to 12, 2 mg P.O. q.i.d.

ephedrine sulfate (Efedron, Vatronol). Ephedrine is a dual-acting drug that activates alpha and beta receptors. Although pharmacologically similar to epinephrine, it is longer-acting, less potent, and has a slower onset of action. It is used for its nasal decongestant effects with hay fever, allergic rhinitis, and sinusitis; for its bronchodilator effects with acute and chronic asthma; and occasionally for its CNS stimulant actions for narcolepsy. Rarely, it also is used for hypotension, enuresis, myasthenia gravis, Stokes-Adams syndrome, and to produce mydriasis. Ephedrine is not recommended for elderly patients because of its CNS effects.

Usual adult dosage: 25 to 50 mg P.O., S.C., I.M., or slow I.V., as necessary, to maximum daily dosage of 150 mg; as an intranasal drug, two to three drops of a 0.5% solution or a small amount of 0.6% jelly in each nostril four or fewer times a day for 3 to 4 consecutive days; do not repeat before 2 hours.

Usual pediatric dosage: for ages 6 to 12, 6.25 to 12.5 mg every 4 to 6 hours; for ages 2 to 6, 0.3 to 0.5 mg/kg every 4 to 6 hours.

isoetharine hydrochloride (Arm-A-Med, Beta-2, Bronkosol, Dey-Lute, Dispos-a-Med), **isoetharine mesylate** (Bronkometer). Isoetharine is a direct-acting, beta$_2$-selective agent with a particular affinity for bronchial and selected arteriolar muscle receptors that produces few cardiac symptoms. It is used for its bronchodilatory effects with bronchial asthma, bronchitis, and emphysema.

Usual adult dosage: three to seven undiluted inhalations by hand-held nebulizer; one to two inhalations by aerosol nebulizer every 4 to 6 hours to a total of 12 per day; wait after the initial inhalation to see if a second is necessary. With intermittent positive-pressure breathing, 0.25 to 1 ml, diluted with normal saline solution (1:3) or other diluent; or use 2 to 8 ml of a unit-dose vial.

mephentermine sulfate (Wyamine). Mephentermine is a dual-acting agent with predominately beta$_1$, but also alpha receptor activity. CNS effects are prominent only with large doses. It is used for its pressor effects to treat hypotension related to ganglionic blockade, spinal anesthesia, hemorrhage, and cardiogenic shock.

Usual adult dosage: 15 to 45 mg single dose as I.M. or I.V. injection, 30 mg supplements as needed; 1 mg/minute of 0.1% solution in D$_5$W by I.V. infusion.

metaproterenol sulfate (Alupent, Metaprel). A direct-acting beta$_2$-selective agent, metaproterenol is used for its bronchodilatory effects to treat asthma, bronchitis, and emphysema. This drug also is under investigation for treatment and prophylaxis of heart block and for management of premature labor.

Usual adult dosage: 20 mg P.O. t.i.d. or q.i.d.; 10 inhalations of 5% solution by hand-held nebulizer; two to three (0.65-mg) sprays by aerosol nebulizer every 3 to 4 hours to a maximum of 12 per day; or two inhalations from a metered-dose inhaler t.i.d.

Usual pediatric dosage: for ages 6 to 9, or less than 60 pounds (27 kg), 10 mg t.i.d. or q.i.d. Not recommended for children under age 6.

metaraminol bitartrate (Aramine). A potent dual-acting synthetic agent that acts predominantly on alpha receptors, but also acts on beta$_1$ receptors, metaraminol is used for its vasopressor effects to treat shock caused by hemorrhage, medication reactions, surgical complications, cardiogenic shock, and septicemia.

Usual adult dosage: 2 to 10 mg S.C. or I.M., with at least 10 minutes before an additional dose is given, to prevent cumulative effects; for severe shock, I.V. injection of 0.5 to 5 mg, followed by I.V. infusion of 15 to 100 mg/500 ml of D$_5$W or normal saline solution (adjust infusion rate to maintain blood pressure at desired level).

Usual pediatric dosage: 0.1 mg/kg S.C. or I.M.; I.V. injection of 0.01 mg/kg; 0.4 mg/kg I.V. infusion.

methoxamine hydrochloride (Vasoxyl). A direct-acting agent that acts on alpha receptors, methoxamine is related pharmacologically to phenylephrine. It has no direct effect on the heart, but tends to slow heart rate as a reflex action from increased peripheral vasoconstriction. It is used for its pressor effects during anesthesia and for paroxysmal atrial tachycardia.

Usual adult dosage: for vasopressor effects in emergencies, 3 to 5 mg slow I.V. or 10 to 15 mg I.M.; for tachycardia, 10 mg slow I.V., or 10 to 20 mg I.M., repeated if necessary, only after 15 minutes.

nylidrin hydrochloride (Arlidin). A direct-acting agent that acts predominantly on beta receptors, nylidrin also acts directly on muscle, producing relaxation that is not blocked by beta blockers. It is used for its direct smooth muscle and arteriolar smooth muscle relaxant effects for symptomatic relief to treat such peripheral vascular disorders as diabetic vascular disease, Raynaud's disease, acrocyanosis, frostbite, night leg cramps, thromboangiitis obliterans, ischemic ulcer, thrombophlebitis, Ménière's disease, and circulatory disturbances of the inner ear.

Usual adult dosage: 3 to 12 mg P.O. t.i.d. or q.i.d.

phenylephrine hydrochloride (Neo-Synephrine). A potent, direct-acting agent with strong alpha-receptor and weak beta-receptor actions, phenylephrine produces little or no CNS activity. It is used for its systemic and topical vasopressor effects with anesthesia and for treating shock, paroxysmal supraventricular tachycardia, rhinitis, allergies, uveitis, and to produce mydriasis.

Usual adult dosage: for its pressor effects, 2 to 5 mg I.M. or S.C. initial dose, not to exceed 5 mg every 10 to 15 minutes; by I.V. injection, 0.1 to 0.5 mg, subsequent doses no more often than 10 to 15 minutes in increments no larger

than 0.2 mg; I.V. infusion of 100 to 200 drops/minute of a 1:50,000 solution of D_5W or normal saline solution until stable, then 40 to 60 drops/minute. As an intranasal drug, two to three drops, one to two sprays (0.25% to 0.5%), or a small amount of nasal jelly placed into each nostril every 3 to 4 hours. (For use as an ophthalmic decongestant and mydriatic, see Chapter 71, Ophthalmic Agents.)
Usual pediatric dosage: 0.1 mg/kg S.C. or I.M.

ritodrine hydrochloride (Yutopar). Ritodrine is a direct-acting agent that preferentially stimulates $beta_2$ receptors in uterine smooth muscle, causing reduced intensity and frequency of contractions. Other effects include bronchial relaxation and some vascular smooth muscle relaxation. This drug is used for preterm labor in selected patients, but its safety and effectiveness during advanced labor have not been established.
Usual adult dosage: initially 0.1 mg/minute by I.V. infusion, increased by 50 mcg/minute every 10 minutes to a maximum of 350 mcg/minute. Continue for 12 hours after labor has ceased. Oral therapy of 10 mg is begun 30 minutes before terminating I.V. infusion, then 10 mg every 2 hours for 24 hours, then 10 to 20 mg every 4 to 6 hours as long as necessary. The total dosage should not exceed 120 mg/day.

terbutaline sulfate (Brethaire, Brethine, Bricanyl). A direct-acting synthetic agent with selective $beta_2$ activity, terbutaline is used for its bronchodilation effects to treat bronchial asthma, bronchitis, and emphysema. It also may be used to delay delivery in preterm labor.
Usual adult dosage: 10 mcg/minute by I.V. infusion with maximum dose of 80 mcg/minute for 4 hours, then oral therapy until term. Oral therapy of 2.5 to 5 mg t.i.d.; 0.25 mg S.C., repeat in 15 to 30 minutes if needed; two inhalations separated by 1 minute no more than every 6 hours.
Usual pediatric dosage: over age 12, 2.5 mg t.i.d. or q.i.d.

Drug interactions

Drugs known to interact with various noncatecholamines include MAO inhibitors, furazolidone, beta blockers (for example, propranolol), other sympathomimetics, acetazolamide, sodium bicarbonate, ammonium chloride, ascorbic acid, barbiturates, guanethidine, phenothiazines, anesthetics (especially cyclopropane and halogenated hydrocarbons), corticosteroids, digitalis, methyldopa, rauwolfia alkaloids, oxytocics, tricyclic antidepressants, lithium, ergot alkaloids, and reserpine. All interactions vary from drug to drug, but the nurse must be aware of their potential for causing interactions. Many of these drugs also are contraindicated with catecholamines. (For details, see *Drug interactions: Noncatecholamines,* page 226.)

ADVERSE DRUG REACTIONS

Adverse reactions to noncatecholamine adrenergic drugs primarily affect the CNS, cardiovascular system, GI and genitourinary tracts, skeletal and smooth muscles, and all other body systems. The adverse effects of any noncatecholamine drug depend on its receptor activity. Other considerations include the intended therapeutic effect of the drug and whether the drug crosses the blood-brain barrier. For example, if ephedrine given for its bronchodilation effects interferes with sleep, the insomnia is considered an adverse reaction; however, if the drug is given to treat narcolepsy, the insomnia is the desired therapeutic effect. Although adverse reactions vary from drug to drug, the nurse must know their potential and must monitor the patient closely.

In the CNS, adverse reactions to the noncatecholamines include headache, restlessness, nervousness, anxiety or euphoria, irritability, trembling, drowsiness or insomnia, lethargy, dizziness, light-headedness, incoherence, and seizures. Possible adverse cardiovascular reactions include hypertension or hypotension, palpitations, bradycardia or tachycardia, arrhythmias, cardiac arrest, cerebral hemorrhage, tingling or coldness in the extremities, pallor or flushing, anginal pain, and alterations in maternal and fetal heart rates and blood pressures. Elderly patients are particularly susceptible to CNS reactions, such as confusion and anxiety, and to cardiovascular reactions, such as increased systolic blood pressure, coldness in the extremities, and anginal pain.

Skeletal muscle reactions may include weakness, mild tremors, or muscle cramps. Other possible adverse reactions include sweating, urinary urgency or incontinence, pilomotor stimulation, stinging and burning of the nasal mucosa or eyes, blurred vision, sneezing, dryness of the orpharynx, nausea, vomiting, unusual taste, erythema, and transient elevations in blood glucose level and increased insulin requirements in diabetic patients. These drugs should not be used in diabetic patients because the vasoconstriction induced may aggravate the already compromised microcirculation.

Prolonged use of certain noncatecholamine drugs, such as metaraminol, may result in shock because continued vasoconstriction prevents volume expansion. Hypotension can occur after discontinuation of these drugs because of depletion of the intrinsic catecholamines in the storage granules of the nerve endings.

Although rare, overdose of nasal decongestants can cause marked somnolence, sedation, hypotension, bradycardia, and even coma. Methoxamine and other drugs can cause severe headache and sustained, severe hypertension. In rare instances, ephedrine and other agents may cause respiratory depression.

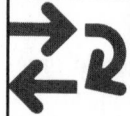

DRUG INTERACTIONS

Noncatecholamines

Noncatecholamines can produce significant reactions, including hypotension, hypertension, cardiac arrhythmias, seizures, and hyperglycemia in diabetics. If noncatecholamines must be administered with other drugs, the patient must be monitored frequently. Note that all interactions may not occur between all noncatecholamines and the drugs listed.

DRUG	INTERACTING DRUGS	POSSIBLE EFFECTS	NURSING IMPLICATIONS
albuterol, ephedrine, isoetharine, mephentermine, metaproterenol, metaraminol, methoxamine, nylidrin, phenylephrine, ritodrine, terbutaline	anesthetics (general), cyclopropane, and halogenated hydrocarbons	Sensitize the heart to adrenergic agents, cause cardiac arrhythmias from increased cardiac irritability, increase hypotension if used with agents having predominant beta₂ activity (ritodrine, terbutaline)	• Avoid, or administer with extreme caution to patients scheduled for surgery if general anesthesia is to be used. • Monitor the patient's blood pressure.
	MAO inhibitors	Cause severe hypertension from potentiation of pressor effects of both drugs	• Avoid concurrent administration. • Monitor the patient's blood pressure.
	oxytocics	Counteract oxytocic effects (terbutaline and ritodrine), cause hypertensive crisis from potentiation of effects of both drugs, produce cerebrovascular accident	• Avoid concurrent use; maintain blood pressure under 130/80 mm Hg.
	tricyclic antidepressants	Increase pressor effects, increase hypertension from potentiation of pressor effects of both drugs, cause cardiac arrhythmias	• If administered concurrently, reduce adrenergic dosage as prescribed. • Monitor the patient's pulse rate and blood pressure.
	urine alkalinizers (acetazolamide, sodium bicarbonate)	Cause decreased excretion, prolong action	• Monitor the patient for increased adverse reactions.

Confusion, delirium, or even hallucinations, as well as tremors, may follow large doses of ephedrine. This drug also may produce paradoxical bronchospasm or aggravate ketoacidosis. Parotid gland enlargement is a rare result of metaproterenol administration. Care must be exercised with I.V. ritodrine and terbutaline because hypokalemia, lactic acidosis, chest pain, arrhythmias, dyspnea, bloating, chills, or anaphylactic shock may occur.

NURSING PROCESS APPLICATION

The following information assists the nurse in caring for a patient who is receiving a noncatecholamine.

Assessment

• Review the patient's history for conditions that contraindicate the use of noncatecholamines, such as known hypersensitivity, arrhythmias associated with tachycardia, or hypovolemia.

• Review the patient's history for conditions that require cautious use of noncatecholamines, such as diabetes, hyperthyroidism, or cardiovascular disorders.

• Assess the patient for adverse reactions to the prescribed noncatecholamine, such as headache, dizziness, incoherence, hypotension or hypertension, palpitations, cardiac arrhythmias, flushing, or weakness.

• Evaluate the patient's and family's knowledge about the prescribed noncatecholamine.

Nursing diagnoses

The following examples represent appropriate nursing diagnoses for a patient receiving a noncatecholamine.

• Potential for injury related to a preexisting condition that contraindicates the use of noncatecholamines

• Potential for injury related to a preexisting condition that requires cautious use of noncatecholamines

• Potential for injury related to adverse drug reactions

• Knowledge deficit related to the prescribed noncatecholamine

Planning and implementation
• Do not administer a noncatecholamine to a patient with a condition that contraindicates its use.
• Administer a noncatecholamine cautiously to a patient at risk because of a preexisting condition.
• *Monitor vital signs, mental status, and muscle strength at least every 4 hours.*
• Obtain electrolyte levels in all patients who are beginning therapy; obtain blood pH, PCO_2, and bicarbonate levels in patients who are receiving prolonged drug therapy, as prescribed.
• *Monitor the serum potassium level closely to detect hypokalemia in a patient receiving prolonged infusion of ritrodrine or terbutaline.*
• *Obtain the diabetic patient's serum glucose level, as prescribed, and observe closely for signs and symptoms of hyperglycemia.*
• Monitor the patient's fluid intake and output and voiding pattern to assess renal response; initially, it may decrease, then increase as blood pressure rises, then decrease again if the dosage is excessive.
• *Monitor the patient for 12 hours after terbutaline is discontinued because cardiovascular symptoms may recur.*
• Administer an oral noncatecholamine with food to reduce GI symptoms unless otherwise indicated.
• Administer S.C. terbutaline in the lateral deltoid area.
• *Place the patient in a left lateral recumbent position to prevent hypotension during I.V. infusion of ritrodrine or terbutaline.*
• Monitor blood pressure and maternal and fetal heart rate when administering ritodrine or terbutaline for preterm labor.
• *Infuse I.V. ritodine and terbutaline into a large vein to avoid extravasation. If extravasation occurs, inject the area within 12 hours with 10 to 15 ml of normal saline solution containing phentolamine (regitine), as prescribed.*
• *Discontinue ephedrine and notify the physician if wheezing or bronchospasm occurs after therapy.*
• Be aware that a patient may greatly exceed the prescribed dose because tolerance and extreme psychological dependence are likely to develop.
• Notify the physician if adverse reactions occur.

Patient teaching
• Teach the patient and family the name, dose, frequency, action, and adverse effects of the prescribed noncatecholamine.
• Instruct the patient to initiate inhalation therapy before meals to improve lung ventilation and to reduce fatigue caused by eating.

• Teach the patient self-assessment techniques to determine the need for administration or repeat administration of the drug. For example, instruct the patient to assess for dyspnea, wheezing, and chest discomfort.
• *Teach the patient the proper inhalation technique.*
• Teach the patient to blow the nose gently, with both nostrils open to clear nasal passages before administering a nasal medication.
• Teach the patient to avoid contact between the inhaled drug and the eyes.
• Teach the patient to rinse the mouth after inhalation to minimize dryness and irritation.
• *Teach the patient to use no other aerosol bronchodilator during terbutaline inhalation therapy.*
• Advise the patient of the prescribed interval between albuterol inhalations, which may vary from 1 to 10 minutes.
• Teach the patient to take the drug only as prescribed because of possible adverse reactions.
• Teach the patient to protect these drugs from light, excessive heat or cold, and moisture, and not to use discolored drugs.
• Teach the patient to notify the physician if symptoms are not relieved or if adverse reactions occur.

Evaluation
The following examples represent appropriate evaluation statements for a patient receiving a noncatecholamine.
• The patient has no conditions that contraindicate the use of a noncatecholamine.
• The patient exhibits no signs of complications in the preexisting condition linked to the prescribed noncatecholamine.
• The patient displays no adverse reactions to the prescribed noncatecholamine.
• The patient and family express an accurate understanding of the points taught about the prescribed noncatecholamine.
• The patient correctly demonstrates inhalation technique.
• The patient describes self-assessment for drug administration.

OTHER ADRENERGIC AGENTS

This section contains information about cerebral stimulating agents, such as CNS stimulants and appetite suppressants. These drugs share many noncatecholamine characteristics.

(Text continues on page 230.)

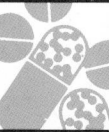

Adrenergic agents

This chart summarizes the indications, dosages, and precautions for the major adrenergic agents currently in clinical use.

DRUG	MAJOR INDICATIONS	USUAL ADULT DOSAGES	CONTRAINDICATIONS AND PRECAUTIONS
Catecholamines			
dobutamine	Acute congestive heart failure, cardiopulmonary bypass surgery	I.V. infusion: 2.5 to 10 mcg/kg/min of a 250-mcg/ml, 500-mcg/ml, or 1,000-mcg/ml solution in D_5W or normal saline solution; rates up to 40 mcg/kg/min may be required	• Know that dobutamine is contraindicated in a patient with known hypersensitivity to the drug or idiopathic hypertrophic subaortic stenosis. • Administer with caution to a pregnant patient.
dopamine	Shock, decreased renal function	I.V. infusion: initially 1 to 5 mcg/kg/min diluted as recommended; may increase by 5- to 10-mcg/kg/min increments to 20 to 50 mcg/kg/min in critically ill patients	• Know that dopamine is contraindicated in a patient with known hypersensitivity to the drug or pheochromocytoma. • Administer with caution to a pregnant patient or one with hypovolemia or occlusive vascular disease.
epinephrine	Bronchospasm, asthma, nasal and ophthalmic congestion, simple open-angle glaucoma, allergic conditions, hypotension, cardiac arrest, superficial bleeding control	Cardiac arrest: 1 to 10 ml of a 1:10,000 solution I.V., repeated at 5 minute intervals; 10 ml of 1:10,000 solution via endotracheal tube Bronchospasm: 0.1 to 0.5 ml of a 1:1,000 solution S.C. or I.M., or 0.1 to 0.3 ml of 1:200 S.C.; one inhalation, repeat once after at least 1 minute, if needed Hemostasis: 1:50,000 to 1:1,000 topically applied Local anesthetic adjunct: 1:200,000 to 1:20,000 mixed with local anesthetic Bronchospasm in children: 0.005 to 0.01 mg/kg of a 1:200 solution S.C.	• Know that epinephrine is contraindicated in a patient with narrow-angle glaucoma, shock, or organic brain damage. It also is contraindicated during general anesthesia with halogenated hydrocarbons or cyclopropane. • Administer with caution to an elderly or pregnant patient or one with cardiovascular disease, hypertension, diabetes, hyperthyroidism, bronchial asthma, emphysema, or psychoneurosis.
isoproterenol	Asthma, bronchospasm, shock, cardiac arrest, selected arrhythmias	Bronchospasm: 10 to 20 mg sublingually or rectally t.i.d. or q.i.d. to a maximum of 60 mg/day; 120 to 262 mcg 4 to 6 times/day by hand-held nebulizer; 80 to 160 mcg 4 to 6 times/day by aerosol nebulizer	• Know that isoproterenol is contraindicated in a patient with arrhythmias caused by digitalis toxicity, ventricular arrhythmias, or angina pectoris. • Administer with caution to a pregnant or lactating patient or one with coronary artery disease, coronary insufficiency, diabetes, hyperthyroidism, or sensitivity to sympathomimetic amines.
norepinephrine	Acute hypotension, shock, cardiac arrest, myocardial infarction, anaphylaxis	I.V. infusion: 2 to 3 ml/min of a 4-mg norepinephrine:1,000 ml 5% dextrose solution initially; maintenance dosage is 0.5 to 1 ml/min	• Know that norepinephrine is contraindicated in a patient with mesenteric or peripheral vascular thrombosis.

SELECTED MAJOR DRUGS

Adrenergic agents *(continued)*

DRUG	MAJOR INDICATIONS	USUAL ADULT DOSAGES	CONTRAINDICATIONS AND PRECAUTIONS
Noncatecholamines			
albuterol	Bronchospasm	One to two inhalations every 4 to 6 hours 2 to 4 mg P.O. t.i.d. to q.i.d., to a maximum of 32 mg/day	• Know that albuterol is contraindicated in a patient with known hypersensitivity to the drug. • Administer with caution to a pregnant or lactating patient; one with a cardiovascular or convulsive disorder, hyperthyroidism, or diabetes; or one who is unusually responsive to sympathomimetic amines.
metaproterenol	Bronchodilation	Oral: 20 mg t.i.d. to q.i.d., initially Hand-held nebulizer: 10 inhalations of a 5% solution; aerosol nebulizer: 2 to 3 sprays every 3 to 4 hours to a maximum of 12/day Children: age 6 to 9 or less than 60 lb (27 kg), 10 mg t.i.d. to q.i.d.	• Know that metaproterenol is contraindicated in a patient with known hypersensitivity to the drug or cardiac arrhythmias associated with tachycardia. • Administer with caution to a pregnant or lactating patient; one with a cardiovascular or convulsive disorder, hyperthyroidism, or diabetes; or one who is unusually responsive to sympathomimetic amines.
ritodrine	Preterm labor	Initially, 0.1 mg/min, by I.V. infusion; increase by 50 mcg/min every 10 minutes to a maximum of 350 mcg/min; continue for 12 hours after labor has ceased 10 mg P.O. begun 30 minutes before terminating I.V. infusion, then 10 mg every 2 hours for 24 hours; then 10 to 20 mg every 4 to 6 hours as long as necessary	• Know that ritodrine is contraindicated in a pregnant patient (before 20 weeks) and in one with known hypersensitivity to the drug, hypovolemia, cardiac arrhythmias associated with tachycardia or digitalis toxicity, uncontrolled hypertension, pheochromocytoma, or bronchial asthma that is treated with a betamimetic or steroid agent.
terbutaline	Bronchodilation, preterm labor	10 mcg/min I.V. infusion with maximum dose of 80 mcg/min for 4 hours, then oral therapy until term 2.5 to 5 mg P.O. t.i.d.; 0.25 mg S.C., repeat in 15 to 30 minutes if needed Inhalation: two inhalations separated by 1 minute no more often than every 6 hours	• Know that terbutaline is contraindicated in a patient with known hypersensitivity to the drug. • Administer with caution to a patient with a cardiovascular disorder, hyperthyroidism, or diabetes or one who is unusually responsive to sympathomimetic amines.

amphetamine sulfate (Benzedrine). A Schedule II drug, amphetamine may be used to treat narcolepsy, attention deficit disorder (ADD), or exogenous obesity.

bitolterol mesylate (Tornalate). This substance is hydrolyzed to colterol, which is a long-acting bronchodilator similar to albuterol. It is selective for beta$_2$ receptors and is used primarily to treat bronchial asthma.

dextroamphetamine sulfate (Dexampex, Dexedrine, Spancap). A Schedule II drug, dextroamphetamine is used to treat narcolepsy, exogenous obesity, and ADD. Its CNS-stimulating effect is about twice that of amphetamine, and it sometimes is given with amphetamine in the combination product Biphetamine.

fenfluramine hydrochloride (Pondimin). A Schedule IV drug, fenfluramine commonly is used to treat exogenous obesity. It also may be helpful in treating autistic children with elevated serotonin levels, although it has not received Food and Drug Administration approval for this use yet.

mazindol (Mazanor, Sanorex). A Schedule IV drug, mazindol is used only as a short-term adjunct in treating exogenous obesity.

methylphenidate hydrochloride (Ritalin). A Schedule II drug, methylphenidate is used to treat narcolepsy in adults and ADD in children.

pirbuterol acetate (Maxair). Pirbuterol is indicated for the prevention and reversal of bronchospasm in patients with reversible bronchospasm, including asthma. It may be used with or without concurrent theophylline or steroid therapy.

phenylpropranolamine hydrochloride (Acutrim, Dexatrim, Prolamine). Phenylpropanolamine directly stimulates alpha and beta receptors. It is used primarily in nasal decongestant products and sold over the counter in appetite-suppressing products as well as many cold and influenza preparations.

CHAPTER SUMMARY

Chapter 15 covered the catecholamine and noncatecholamine adrenergic drugs. Drugs in each class were described in relation to their pharmacokinetics, pharmacodynamics, pharmacotherapeutics, adverse drug reactions, and nursing care. Here are the highlights of the chapter.

• Adrenergic drugs produce biological responses similar to those produced by the SNS.
• The therapeutic use of a drug depends on its receptor activity.
• Alpha activation produces primarily vasoconstrictive and smooth muscle contraction effects; beta$_1$ activation produces primarily cardiac stimulant effects; and beta$_2$ activation produces primarily smooth muscle relaxation as well as bronchodilatory and vasodilatory effects.
• Catecholamines may be endogenous or synthetic.
• Catecholamines are ineffective when administered orally.
• Catecholamines function as adrenergic neurotransmitters, causing direct action at alpha, beta$_1$, or beta$_2$ adrenergic receptor sites.
• Alpha-active drugs are used primarily to relieve hypotension.
• Beta-active drugs are used primarily to treat respiratory disorders, such as bronchial asthma, emphysema, and bronchitis, and acute hypersensitivity reactions to drugs. They also are used for cardiac stimulation.
• Noncatecholamine drugs are active orally and generally have a longer duration of action than catecholamines.
• Noncatecholamine adrenergic drugs exert effects on sympathetic receptor sites through direct, indirect, or dual action.
• Noncatecholamine drugs primarily produce bronchodilation, vasopression, smooth muscle relaxation, and cardiac stimulation.
• Adverse reactions to adrenergic agents can involve all body systems.
• Other drugs that share noncatecholamine characteristics include cerebral stimulating agents, such as CNS stimulants and appetite suppressants.
• When caring for a client who is receiving an adrenergic agent, the nurse should apply the nursing process. Care typically includes monitoring the patient for therapeutic and adverse effects based on the drug's indications, preparing and administering the drugs properly, and teaching the patient how to self-administer the drugs correctly.

STUDY QUESTIONS

See Appendix 1 for answers.

1. Olga Johansen, age 27, is undergoing I.V. pyelography to determine the cause of acute pain in her left flank. Five minutes after the radiographic dye is injected, she begins to wheeze, and her eyes, lips, and tongue begin to swell. Her blood pressure drops to 80/60 mm Hg, her pulse increases to 120 beats/minute, and her respirations are 30

breaths/minute. The radiologist administers epinephrine 0.5 ml of 1:1,000 solution S.C. What is the action of this adrenergic agent?
(a) It metabolizes neurotransmitters at the receptor sites.
(b) It acts directly on sympathetically innervated organs and tissue.
(c) It competes directly with the neurotransmitter for receptor sites.
(d) It triggers the release of a neurotransmitter, usually norepinephrine.

2. Because epinephrine acts on alpha and beta receptors, it is used to treat anaphylactic shock. Which of the following result from epinephrine's action on these receptors?
(a) vasoconstriction, cardiac stimulation, and bronchodilation
(b) vasodilation, cardiac stimulation, and bronchodilation
(c) vasoconstriction, coronary artery dilation, and bronchoconstriction
(d) vasodilation, cardiac stimulation, and bronchodilation

3. Ms. Johansen received epinephrine subcutaneously. Which of the following explains why catecholamines are not administered orally?
(a) They are inactivated in the GI tract and liver.
(b) They produce toxic effects when administered orally.
(c) Absorption after oral administration is delayed and unpredictable.
(d) Normal intestinal flora destroy the drug by phagocytosis.

4. To maintain Ms. Johansen's blood pressure, the physician prescribes a dopamine drip 1 to 5 mcg/kg/minute. While receiving dopamine, she develops a headache. What may this symptom indicate?
(a) catecholamine toxicity
(b) inadequate catecholamine dosage
(c) catecholamine hypersensitivity
(d) adverse reaction to catecholamine

5. Rita Miller, age 49, takes the noncatecholamine metaproterenol (Alupent), 20 mg P.O. q.i.d. as prescribed, for asthma. How do catecholamines differ from noncatecholamines?
(a) Catecholamines cross the blood-brain barrier; noncatecholamines do not.
(b) Catecholamines stimulate alpha receptors; noncatecholamines stimulate beta receptors.
(c) Catecholamines are not effective when given orally; most noncatecholamines are.
(d) Catecholamines do not affect the heart; noncatecholamines affect the heart in many ways.

6. What makes metaproterenol (Alupent) effective in treating Ms. Miller's asthma?
(a) It is a direct-acting alpha$_1$-selective agent.
(b) It is a direct-acting beta$_2$-selective agent.
(c) It is an indirect-acting alpha$_1$-selective agent.
(d) It is an indirect-acting beta$_1$-selective agent.

7. The nurse obtains a drug history from Ms. Miller because many drugs interact with adrenergic agents. Which of the following drugs can potentiate the effects of noncatecholamines?
(a) MAO inhibitors
(b) alpha and beta blockers
(c) anticholinesterase agents
(d) neuromuscular blocking agents

SELECTED REFERENCES

AHFS drug information 90. (1990). Bethesda, MD: American Society of Hospital Pharmacists.

Anderson, M. (1989). The pharmacology of intervention for respiratory emergencies. *Emergency Care Quarterly,* 5(1), 23-36.

Carter, R. (1988). The relevance of adrenergic receptor reactions. *Journal of the American Academy of Physician Assistants,* 1(4), 324-328.

Hansten, P., and Horn, J. (1989). *Drug interactions.* Philadelphia: Lea & Febiger.

Morley, T., Marozsan, E., and Zappasodi, S. (1988). Comparison of beta-adrenergic agents delivered by nebulizer vs. metered dose inhaler with InspirEase in hospitalized asthmatic patients. *Chest: The Cardiopulmonary Journal,* 94(6), 1205-1210.

ADRENERGIC BLOCKING AGENTS

OBJECTIVES

After reading and studying this chapter, the student should be able to:

1. Distinguish among alpha-adrenergic, beta-adrenergic, and autonomic ganglionic blocking agents.

2. Identify the major drugs in each class of adrenergic blocking agents.

3. Describe the major physiologic effects and mechanisms of action of each class of adrenergic blocking agents.

4. Discuss therapeutic uses for each class of adrenergic blocking agents.

5. Explain why arteriosclerosis, bronchospastic disease, congestive heart failure, hypertension, diabetes mellitus, and thyrotoxicosis require cautious administration of beta-adrenergic blocking agents.

6. Identify the major drug interactions and adverse reactions for each class of adrenergic blocking agents.

7. Describe how to apply the nursing process when caring for a patient who is receiving an adrenergic blocking agent.

INTRODUCTION

Adrenergic blocking agents, or sympatholytics, are used therapeutically to disrupt sympathetic nervous system (SNS) function. These agents may block impulse transmission (and thus SNS stimulation) at adrenergic neurons or adrenergic receptor sites. This action at these sites may be exerted by interrupting the action of sympathomimetic (adrenergic) agents (see Chapter 15, Adrenergic Agents), by reducing available norepinephrine or by preventing the action of cholinergic agents (see Chapter 13, Cholinergic Agents). Adrenergic blocking agents are classified according to their site of action as, respectively, alpha blockers, beta blockers, or autonomic ganglionic blockers. For a summary of representative drugs, see *Selected major drugs: Adrenergic blocking agents,* pages 248 and 249. For a listing of applicable nursing diagnoses that the nurse may formulate when caring for a patient receiving these agents, see *Selected nursing diagnoses: Adrenergic blocking agents.* For detailed

SELECTED NURSING DIAGNOSES

Adrenergic blocking agents

The following nursing diagnoses address representative problems and etiologies that a nurse may encounter when caring for a patient who is receiving an adrenergic blocking agent. Some of these nursing diagnoses contain generalized etiologies, which the nurse must individualize based on the patient's needs. (For some common nursing diagnoses and related interventions for each drug class, see the "Nursing Process Application" sectons of this chapter.)

- Activity intolerance related to muscle weakness caused by the adrenergic blocker
- Altered nutrition: less than body requirements, related to the adverse GI effects of an adrenergic blocker
- Altered protection related to the adverse hematologic effects of an adrenergic blocker
- Altered tissue perfusion: cardiopulmonary, related to drug interaction between the beta-adrenergic blocker and another prescribed drug
- Altered urinary elimination related to the adverse genitourinary effects of the alpha-adrenergic blocker
- Diarrhea related to the adverse GI effects of the adrenergic blocker
- Ineffective breathing pattern related to respiratory depression caused by the ganglionic blocker
- Knowledge deficit related to the prescribed adrenergic blocking agent
- Pain related to ineffectiveness of ergotamine
- Pain (headache or abdominal pain) related to the adverse effects of the alpha-adrenergic blocker
- Potential for injury related to a preexisting condition that contraindicates the use of an adrenergic blocking agent
- Potential for injury related to a preexisting condition that requires cautious use of an adrenergic blocking agent
- Potential for injury related to adverse drug reactions
- Potential for trauma related to the adverse CNS effects of the alpha-adrenergic blocker
- Sexual dysfunction related to impotence caused by the adrenergic blocker

information on applying the nursing process, see Chapter 6, The Nursing Process and Drug Therapy.

ALPHA-ADRENERGIC BLOCKERS

Alpha-adrenergic blocking agents interrupt the actions of sympathomimetic agents at alpha-adrenergic receptor sites, relaxing vascular smooth muscle, increasing peripheral vasodilation, and decreasing blood pressure. Drugs in this class include ergoloid mesylates, ergotamine tartrate, phenoxybenzamine hydrochloride, phentolamine mesylate, and prazosin hydrochloride. (For information on prazosin, see Chapter 32, Antihypertensive Agents.)

PHARMACOKINETICS

The action of alpha-adrenergic blocking agents in the body is not well understood. Most of these agents are absorbed erratically when administered orally and more rapidly and completely when administered sublingually or by inhalation.

Absorption, distribution, metabolism, excretion

For the most part, ergoloid mesylates are inactivated by the first-pass effect; only about one-third of the drug reaches the systemic circulation. Ergotamine is distributed throughout the body and sequestered in tissues (explaining its long duration of action), then excreted in the bile after hepatic metabolism. Absorption of phenoxybenzamine is erratic, with only 20% to 30% of the drug reaching the systemic circulation. Little is known about phenoxybenzamine's distribution, metabolism, and excretion. The pharmacokinetics of phentolamine are unknown.

Onset, peak, duration

The various alpha adrenergic blocking agents vary considerably in their onset of action, peak concentration levels, and duration of action. The onset varies widely: that of ergoloid mesylates is unknown; that of ergotamine is erratic or rapid (when administered by inhalation). Phentolamine has an onset within 2 to 20 minutes, whereas phenoxybenzamine takes 2 hours.

Peak concentrations occur in 1 to 2 hours with ergoloid mesylates, 1 to 3 hours with ergotamine, and 4 to 6 hours with phenoxybenzamine. The peak concentration of phentolamine is 2 to 20 minutes. The duration of phentolamine is short — 15 to 45 minutes, depending on administration route; ergotamine's duration is 24 hours, and phenoxyben-

zamine's is 3 to 4 days. Ergoloid mesylate's duration is unknown.

PHARMACODYNAMICS

Alpha-adrenergic blockers exert two main pharmacologic actions: they interfere with or block the synthesis, storage, release, and reuptake of norepinephrine by neurons; and they competitively or noncompetitively antagonize epinephrine, norepinephrine, or sympathomimetic agents at alpha-receptor sites.

Alpha-receptor sites are categorized as alpha$_1$ or alpha$_2$. Alpha$_1$ receptors are located postsynaptically; alpha$_2$ receptors, primarily presynaptically, where they mediate a feedback system that controls norepinephrine release.

Pharmacologic classification does not recognize the specificity of alpha-receptor activity; the category of alpha-adrenergic blockers includes drugs that block the stimulation of alpha$_1$ receptors and that also may or may not block alpha$_2$ stimulation.

Mechanism of action

Alpha-adrenergic blockers occupy alpha-receptor sites on the vascular smooth muscle. (For a description of this process, see *How alpha-adrenergic blockers affect peripheral blood vessels,* page 234.) This action prevents the excitatory response to sympathetic stimulation or sympathomimetic agents. In most patients, this action produces vasodilation, which increases local blood flow to the skin and other organs. The decreased peripheral vascular resistance decreases blood pressure.

The degree of therapeutic effect depends on the sympathetic tone before drug administration. Only a small change in blood pressure is produced with the patient in a supine position; however, orthostatic hypotension develops when the patient shifts to a standing position because the ability of the SNS to prevent peripheral blood pooling is blocked.

In most cases, alpha-adrenergic blockers, such as phenoxybenzamine and phentolamine, cause tachycardia in addition to lowering blood pressure. This is because the decrease in systemic blood pressure, particularly when the patient is standing, activates baroreceptor reflexes that increase impulse activity in sympathetic cardiac nerves, producing a reflex tachycardia. If severe, this tachycardia may precipitate coronary insufficiency, angina, or even heart failure.

Ergotamine not only acts on receptors but also stimulates smooth muscle directly, producing vasoconstriction primarily in the uterus and blood vessels. This action reduces extracranial blood flow, which produces decreased cerebral blood flow and a decline in arterial pressure.

Phenoxybenzamine acts by forming a stable bond with the alpha-receptor site. Phentolamine competes for alpha-

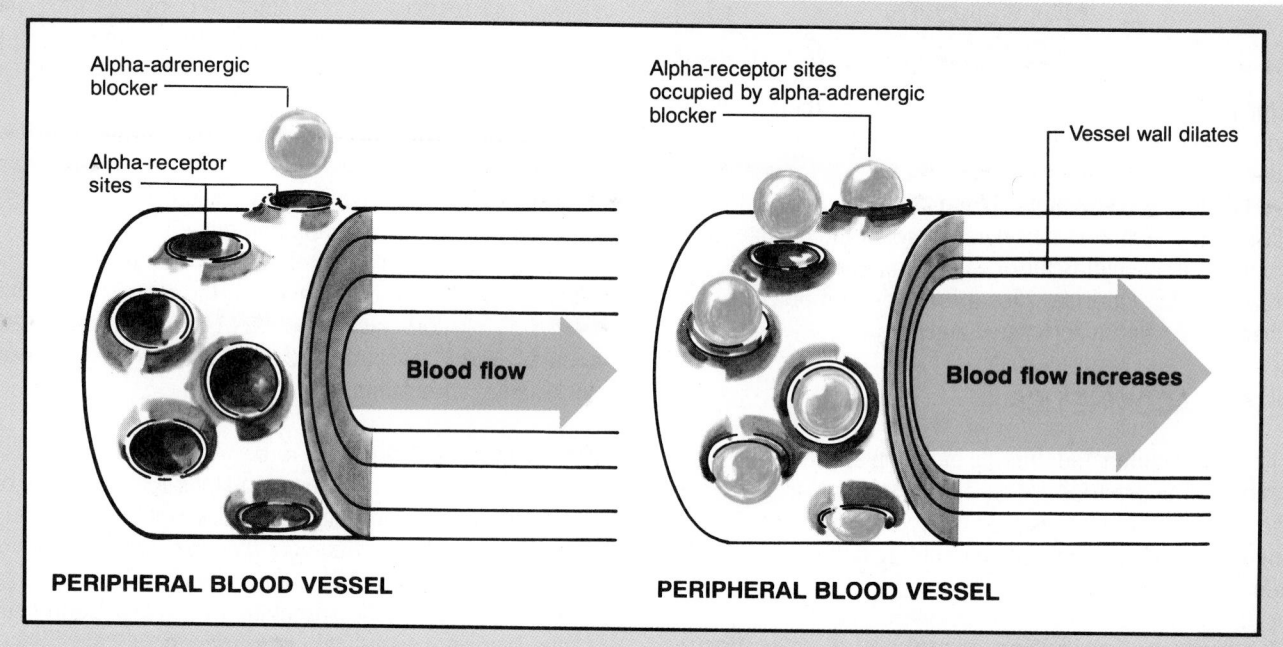

How alpha-adrenergic blockers affect peripheral blood vessels

By occupying alpha-receptor sites, the alpha-adrenergic blockers cause vessel muscle-wall relaxation, vasodilation, and reduced peripheral vascular resistance. These effects can cause orthostatic hypotension when the patient changes position from supine to standing because of altered blood flow redistribution.

Alpha-adrenergic blocker

Alpha-receptor sites

Blood flow

PERIPHERAL BLOOD VESSEL

Alpha-receptor sites occupied by alpha-adrenergic blocker

Vessel wall dilates

Blood flow increases

PERIPHERAL BLOOD VESSEL

receptor sites, but this blockade is short-acting, persisting only for a few hours.

PHARMACOTHERAPEUTICS

Therapeutic use of alpha-adrenergic blockers is based on their smooth muscle relaxation and vasodilation and the resultant increased local blood flow to skin and other organs and decreased blood pressure from decreased peripheral vascular resistance. Conditions in which these effects prove beneficial include hypertension and peripheral vascular disorders.

Because of the risk of rebound tachycardia in a patient receiving the alpha-adrenergic blockers phenoxybenzamine and phentolamine, these drugs rarely (if ever) are used to treat primary (essential) hypertension. However, they are important in treating the secondary hypertension caused by pheochromocytoma, a chromaffin-cell tumor of the adrenal gland that secretes excessive epinephrine and norepinephrine.

Certain peripheral vascular disorders—mainly those with a vasospastic component causing poor local blood flow, such as Raynaud's disease (intermittent pallor, cyanosis, or redness of fingers), acrocyanosis (symmetrical mottled cy-

anosis of the hands and feet), and aftereffects of frostbite—respond well to alpha-adrenergic therapy.

ergoloid mesylates (Deapril-ST, Hydergine). This combination of three hydrogenated ergot alkaloid derivatives may increase cerebral vasodilation, may decrease blood pressure slightly, and may increase metabolic activity in the brain and improve cerebral circulation. As a result, it is used to treat symptoms attributed to cerebral arteriosclerosis—decreased or impaired mental capacity and function, depression, and anxiety—especially in elderly patients. *Usual adult dosage:* 1 mg P.O. or sublingually t.i.d.; dosage is adjusted gradually for optimal individual effect. Alleviation of symptoms usually is gradual; 3 or 4 weeks may be needed for full therapeutic effect.

ergotamine tartrate (Ergomar, Ergostat, Medihaler Ergotamine). This natural amino acid alkaloid of ergot is used to relieve the pain of vascular headaches, such as migraines. Its mechanism of action is complex because ergotamine has alpha agonist and alpha antagonist properties and because it prevents the reuptake of norepinephrine into adrenergic nerve terminals. In vascular headache, ergotamine's agonist properties allow constriction of the dilated cerebral arterial vessels. Its ability to prevent norepinephrine reuptake may add to this effect. The net result is decreased pulsatile blood flow through the cerebral vessels and symptom relief.

Combining ergotamine with caffeine (in such products as Cafergot, Cafetrate, Ercatab, and Cafergot suppositories) potentiates the cranial vasconstricting action of both substances; caffeine enhances the vasoconstrictor effects and enhances ergotamine absorption. Belladonna alkaloids also are combined with ergotamine; their anticholinergic and antiemetic effects combat the excessive nausea and vomiting some patients experience during migraine attacks. Phenobarbital is added in some products (Cafergot P-B tablets and suppositories) for sedation. Another combination containing ergotamine, caffeine, and tartaric acid (Wigraine suppositories) is used when belladonna is not required. *Usual adult dosage:* 2 mg P.O. or sublingually at onset of attack, then 2 mg every 30 minutes until resolution occurs, or maximum dosage (6 mg per attack or 10 mg per week) is reached; inhalations (0.36 mg) 5 minutes apart until pain is relieved (maximum of 6 inhalations a day or 15 inhalations a week); for combination therapy, one or two tablets or suppositories every 15 minutes to 1 hour. Do not exceed six tablets or two suppositories per attack, or ten tablets or five suppositories per week.

phenoxybenzamine hydrochloride (Dibenzyline). This long-acting, noncompetitive alpha-adrenergic blocking agent can produce and maintain a state called chemical sympathectomy. It acts on alpha$_1$- and alpha$_2$-receptor sites (although about 100 times more potently on alpha$_1$-receptor sites) to increase blood flow to the skin, mucosa, and viscera and to lower blood pressure whether the patient is supine or erect. It has no parasympathetic activity and produces no increase in cardiac output or liver or kidney perfusion. Although rarely used today, phenoxybenzamine has been used to treat Raynaud's disease, post-frostbite syndrome, acrocyanosis, arteriosclerosis obliterans, and other peripheral vascular disorders. It also is used sometimes to control the hypertension and diaphoresis associated with pheochromocytoma.

Usual adult dosage: initially, 10 mg P.O. b.i.d., increasing by 10 mg every 2 to 4 days to achieve maximum effect with minimal adverse reactions (may take several weeks to reach maximal effects); usual range is 20 to 60 mg/day.

phentolamine mesylate (Regitine). An alpha-adrenergic blocker with transient and incomplete action, phentolamine exerts alpha-adrenergic blocking as well as direct smooth muscle, parasympathomimetic, and some sympathomimetic and histamine-like actions. It is used to diagnose pheochromocytoma (using the Regitine-blocking test) and to control hypertension in patients with pheochromocytoma during surgical excision of the tumor. It also is used to prevent tissue necrosis and sloughing related to extrava-

sation of I.V. vasopressor drugs, such as norepinephrine or dopamine.

Usual adult dosage: for hypertension associated with pheochromocytoma, 5 mg I.M. or I.V. before surgery, 5 mg I.V., if needed, during surgery; for necrosis prevention, 5 to 10 mg in 10 ml normal saline solution injected into the area of extravasation.

Drug interactions

Many agents interact synergistically with alpha-adrenergic blocking agents and can potentiate or cause mutually additive effects, often with serious sequelae. The most serious include severe hypotension or vascular collapse; blockage of therapeutic blood pressure decreases, possibly leading to hypertensive crisis, cerebrovascular accident, or any of the many other complications of hypertension; and increased cardiac stimulation, causing arrhythmias or angina. (For detailed information, see *Drug interactions: Alpha-adrenergic blockers,* page 236.)

ADVERSE DRUG REACTIONS

Adverse reactions caused by blockage of alpha receptors are related primarily to the vasodilation effect of the drugs. However, because of the varied mechanisms of action of the alpha-adrenergic blocking agents, many adverse reactions are possible with these drugs.

Reactions may include such cardiovascular manifestations as orthostatic hypotension or severe hypertensive episodes, bradycardia or tachycardia, edema, dyspnea, lightheadedness, flushing, arrhythmias, angina, myocardial infarction (MI), cerebrovascular spasm, or a shocklike state. With long-acting noncompetitive alpha-adrenergic blockers, such as phenoxybenzamine, the beta-adrenergic receptors are left unopposed, possibly leading to an exaggerated hypotensive response and tachycardia.

Central nervous system (CNS) manifestations may include paresthesias, tingling of extremities, muscle weakness, fatigue, nervousness, depression, insomnia, drowsiness, lethargy, sedation, vertigo, syncope, confusion, headache, or CNS stimulation.

The nurse also may note eye, ear, nose, and throat manifestations, such as nasal stuffiness, blurred vision, increased nasopharyngeal secretions, epistaxis, miosis (pinpoint pupils), conjunctival infection, ptosis (drooping of the eyelids), tinnitus, reddened sclera, or dry mouth.

Gastrointestinal (GI) manifestations are common and may consist of sublingual irritation, nausea, vomiting, heartburn, diarrhea, abdominal pain, or exacerbation of peptic ulcer.

Genitourinary reactions may include urinary frequency, impotence, incontinence, or priapism.

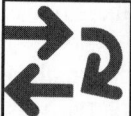

DRUG INTERACTIONS
Alpha-adrenergic blockers

Drug interactions involving alpha-adrenergic blocking agents primarily affect the cardiovascular system and may include profound hypotension or vascular collapse, hypertension, and cardiac arrhythmias.

DRUG	INTERACTING DRUGS	POSSIBLE EFFECTS	NURSING IMPLICATIONS
ergoloid mesylates, ergotamine	alcohol	May cause hypotension	• Monitor the patient's blood pressure frequently.
	caffeine	Increases ergotamine effect	• Monitor the patient for an increased therapeutic effect.
	dopamine	Increase pressor effects	• Monitor the patient's blood pressure frequently.
	nitroglycerin	May cause hypotension by excessive vasodilation	• Monitor the patient's blood pressure frequently.
	sympathomimetics, including many over-the-counter medications	Enhance cardiac stimulation; may cause hypotension with rebound hypertension	• Monitor the patient's blood pressure and heart rate frequently.

Hematologic manifestations are rare; however, granulocytopenia, leukopenia, thrombocytopenia, and pancytopenia have been reported with some agents.

Various dermatologic manifestations may occur, including rash, allergic dermatitis, pruritus, alopecia, or lichen planus.

Other adverse reactions reported are allergic phenomena, including shock, diaphoresis, and arthralgia. Increased serum uric acid and blood urea nitrogen levels also may occur. Overuse of ergotamine may produce ergotism. (For more information, see *Ergotism.*)

NURSING PROCESS APPLICATION

The following information assists the nurse in caring for a patient who is receiving an alpha-adrenergic blocker.

Assessment
• Review the patient's history for conditions that contraindicate the use of an alpha-adrenergic blocker, such as MI, coronary insufficiency, or angina.
• Review the patient's history for conditions that require cautious use of an alpha-adrenergic blocker, such as pregnancy or lactation.
• Assess the patient for adverse reactions to the prescribed alpha-adrenergic blocker, such as orthostatic hypotension, arrhythmias, light-headedness, tingling of extremities, muscle weakness, lethargy, GI distress, and urinary frequency.

• Assess the effectiveness of the prescribed alpha-adrenergic blocker periodically.
• Assess for impotence in a male patient who is taking an alpha-adrenergic blocker.
• Evaluate the patient's and family's knowledge about the prescribed alpha-adrenergic blocker.

Nursing diagnoses
The following examples represent appropriate nursing diagnoses for a patient receiving an alpha-adrenergic blocker.
• Potential for injury related to a preexisting condition that contraindicates the use of an alpha-adrenergic blocker
• Potential for injury related to a preexisting condition that requires cautious use of an alpha-adrenergic blocker
• Potential for injury related to adverse drug reactions
• Pain related to ineffectiveness of ergotamine
• Sexual dysfunction related to impotence caused by the alpha-adrenergic blocker
• Knowledge deficit related to the prescribed alpha-adrenergic blocker

Planning and implementation
• Do not administer an alpha-adrenergic blocker to a patient with a condition that contraindicates its use.
• Administer an alpha-adrenergic blocker cautiously to a patient at risk because of a preexisting condition.
• Monitor the patient for adverse reactions to the alpha-adrenergic blocker.

Ergotism

Prolonged ergotamine use, overdose, or chronic poisoning related to diseases that increase sensitivity to the drug may induce a condition known as ergotism. In this condition, prolonged constriction of blood vessels causes the extremities to become cold, pale, and numb. Arterial peripheral pulses diminish and eventually disappear. Muscle pain may occur even at rest, and the patient also may experience confusion, vomiting, seizures, or vision loss. Untreated, vasoconstriction can cause a severe lack of blood flow that could lead to tissue damage, even gangrene. Treatment includes immediate discontinuation of the drug and symptomatic therapy.

• *Measure the patient's vital signs frequently, noting any change in blood pressure from the supine to standing position. Auscultate breath sounds frequently during therapy with an alpha-adrenergic blocker.*

• *Take safety measures if the patient develops light-headedness, weakness, or changes in mental status. For example, elevate the side rails and assist with mobility, as appropriate.*

• *Notify the physician immediately if the patient develops chest pain.* Obtain an electrocardiogram and treat the patient as prescribed.

• *Place the patient in the Trendelenburg position if a shocklike state occurs (and if not contraindicated). Also, notify the physician immediately and begin emergency interventions according to health care facility guidelines.*

• *Monitor for signs of vascular insufficiency (numbness, coldness, and tingling or weakness in the extremities) in a patient receiving ergotamine.*

• *Administer oral drugs with milk to reduce GI distress.*

• Notify the physician if the patient displays any adverse reactions to an alpha-adrenergic blocker.

• *Administer ergotamine in the early stage of a migraine attack to maximize effectiveness.*

• *Have the patient lie quietly in a darkened room after taking ergotamine to increase its effectiveness.*

• Monitor pain relief after ergotamine administration.

• Notify the physician if ergotamine does not relieve the patient's migraine.

• Encourage the patient to report impotence; notify the physician if it occurs.

• Offer to arrange for sexual counseling for the patient and partner if the alpha-adrenergic agent cannot be replaced with another agent that does not cause impotence.

Patient teaching

• Teach the patient and family the name, dose, frequency, action, and adverse effects of the prescribed alpha-adrenergic blocker.

• *Teach the patient to minimize orthostatic hypotension by arising slowly from a supine position and by dangling the feet for a few minutes before standing.*

• *Instruct the patient to assume a head-low position or to lie down if light-headedness, faintness, or weakness occurs.*

• Advise the patient not to exceed the prescribed dosage. Explain that adverse reactions can result from higher dosages.

• Teach the patient to avoid alcohol consumption. Explain that alcohol used with an alpha-adrenergic blocking agents may cause hypotension.

• *Instruct the patient to avoid over-the-counter cough, cold, allergy, or weight-loss medications that contain alcohol or caffeine unless they have been approved by the physician.*

• Instruct the patient to store medications in a light-resistant, airtight container.

• Instruct the patient to notify the physician if adverse reactions occur.

Evaluation

The following examples represent appropriate evaluation statements for a patient receiving an alpha-adrenergic blocker.

• The patient has no conditions that contraindicate the use of an alpha-adrenergic blocker.

• The patient exhibits no signs of complications in the preexisting condition linked to the prescribed alpha-adrenergic blocker.

• The patient develops no adverse reactions to the prescribed alpha-adrenergic blocker.

• The patient reports migraine headache relief.

• The patient verifies that the drug has not caused impotence.

• The patient and family express an accurate understanding of the points taught about the prescribed alpha-adrenergic blocker.

• The patient correctly demonstrates how to manage orthostatic hypotension.

BETA-ADRENERGIC BLOCKERS

Beta-adrenergic blocking agents, the most widely used adrenergic blockers, prevent SNS stimulation by inhibiting the action of catecholamines and other sympathomimetic agents at beta-adrenergic receptor sites. (For more information about this group of drugs, see Chapter 31, Antianginal Agents, and Chapter 32, Antihypertensive Agents.)

Many beta-adrenergic blocking agents (including carteolol, labetalol hydrochloride, nadolol, propranolol hydrochloride, and timolol maleate) are nonselective in their blocking action, affecting beta₁-receptor sites (located mainly in the heart) and beta₂-receptor sites (located in bronchi, blood vessels, and the uterus). (For information about carteolol, see Chapter 32, Antihypertensive Agents.) The newer beta-adrenergic blocking agents acebutolol hydrochloride, atenolol, betaxolol hydrochloride, esmolol hydrochloride, and metoprolol tartrate are selective: they primarily affect beta₁-receptor sites. (For information about betaxolol hydrochloride, see Chapter 71, Ophthalmic Agents. For a discussion of esmolol hydrochloride, see Chapter 30, Antiarrhythmic Agents.) Some beta-adrenergic blockers also exhibit a pharmacologic property known as intrinsic sympathetic activity (ISA). Drugs that exhibit ISA, such as pindolol and acebutolol, sometimes are classified as partial agonists.

Beta-adrenergic blockers are used extensively to treat hypertension, cardiac arrhythmias, and angina pectoris as well as hyperthyroidism and other related disorders of SNS overstimulation.

PHARMACOKINETICS

Beta-adrenergic blockers usually are absorbed rapidly and well from the GI tract and are protein bound to some extent.

Absorption, distribution, metabolism, excretion

Food does not inhibit their absorption and may enhance absorption of some agents. Some beta-adrenergic blockers are absorbed more completely than others; for instance, only 50% of oral atenolol is absorbed, whereas 75% or more of oral propranolol is absorbed. Most agents are protein bound to some extent. Acebutolol, atenolol, metoprolol, and timolol are weakly protein bound; pindolol, nadolol, and labetalol, moderately protein bound; and propranolol, highly protein bound (up to 90%).

Beta-adrenergic blockers are distributed widely in body tissues, with the highest concentrations found in the heart, liver, lungs, and saliva. Some agents (such as metoprolol and timolol) cross the blood-brain barrier; timolol crosses the placental barrier.

With the exception of nadolol and atenolol, beta-adrenergic blockers are metabolized to some extent in the liver. Acebutolol, labetalol, metoprolol, propranolol, and timolol undergo extensive first-pass metabolism in the liver; 60% to 65% of pindolol is metabolized in the liver. As a result of this extensive first-pass metabolism, only a small percentage of the drug reaches the circulation. Excretion is primarily in the urine, as metabolites or in unchanged form, with some excretion also occurring in feces and bile, and some secretion in breast milk. Nadolol is not metabolized, is excreted unchanged in the urine (about 70%) and

feces, and is secreted in breast milk. Atenolol is excreted primarily unchanged in urine.

Onset, peak, duration

The onset of action of beta-adrenergic blockers is primarily dose- and drug-dependent; peak concentration levels are route-dependent. Duration of action varies according to dose and usually ranges from 4 hours for oral timolol to 24 hours for oral atenolol. Half-life varies from a low of 3 to 4 hours for timolol and pindolol to a high of 10 to 24 hours for nadolol. (For more information, see *Beta-adrenergic blockers: Summary of pharmacokinetics.*)

PHARMACODYNAMICS

Beta-adrenergic blocking agents act primarily as competitive adrenergic antagonists, preventing beta-adrenergic receptors from responding to sympathetic impulses, catecholamines, or other adrenergic agents. Physiologically, these drugs compete for the available beta-receptor sites located on the membrane of cardiac muscle (primarily beta₁ receptors) and smooth muscle of bronchi and blood vessels (beta₂ receptors). Some agents, in addition to their beta activity, also exhibit other cardiac effects; acebutolol and pindolol demonstrate ISA, occupying a receptor site to exert a weak activation in preference to occupation of the site by a stronger stimulating agent. The minimal decrease in cardiac output and pulse rate is evidence of pindolol's ISA. This makes it a useful agent for patients with bradycardia and reduced cardiac reserve.

Mechanism of action

Beta-adrenergic blocking agents produce a competitive blocking action not only at adrenergic nerve endings but also in the adrenal medulla; that accounts for their widespread effects. Some researchers speculate that certain beta-adrenergic blockers, such as metoprolol and propranolol, produce CNS activity, with effects exerted at the vasomotor center in the brain stem to reduce tonic sympathetic nerve impulse transmission. These agents can reduce or block myocardial stimulation, vasodilation, bronchodilation, glycogenolysis (production of glucose from glycogen), and lipolysis (fat hydrolysis). The effects of this blockade include increased peripheral vascular resistance, decreased systemic blood pressure, decreased contractile force, decreased myocardial oxygen consumption, slowed atrioventricular (AV) conduction, and decreased cardiac output. Pulmonary manifestations include increased bronchial smooth muscle tone; metabolic manifestations include inhibition of the sympathetic response to hypoglycemia. CNS manifestations include weakness, lethargy, and fatigue. Other manifestations include decreased plasma renin activity (particularly in patients with high levels before beta-adrenergic blocker therapy) and decreased production of

Beta-adrenergic blockers: Summary of pharmacokinetics

This chart provides a quick reference for administration routes and pharmacokinetic processes of the beta-adrenergic blocking agents. The nurse who administers these agents should be familiar with the variations.

DRUG	ROUTE	ONSET	PEAK	DURATION	HALF-LIFE
acebutolol	Oral	Unknown	2½ to 3½ hours	Unknown	3 to 4 hours
atenolol	Oral	1 hour	2 to 4 hours	24 hours	6 to 9 hours
labetalol	Oral	Rapid	1 to 2 hours	8 to 10 hours	6 to 8 hours
	I.V.	Immediate	5 minutes	Unknown	5 to 8 hours
metoprolol	Oral	10 minutes	1½ hours	Up to 6 hours	3 to 4 hours
	I.V.	Rapid	20 minutes	5 to 8 hours	3 to 4 hours
nadolol	Oral	Unknown	2 to 4 hours	24 hours	10 to 24 hours
pindolol	Oral	Rapid	1 to 2 hours	24 hours	3 to 4 hours
propranolol	Oral	30 minutes	1 to 1½ hours	6 hours	3 to 6 hours
	I.V.	2 minutes	15 minutes	3 to 6 hours	3 to 6 hours
timolol	Oral	30 minutes	1 to 2 hours	4 to 6 hours	3 to 4 hours
	Ophthalmic	15 to 30 minutes	1 to 2 hours	24 hours	Unknown

aqueous humor in the eye, not accompanied by miosis or hyperemia (increased blood).

The ophthalmic actions of beta-adrenergic blockers are of great importance; agents such as betaxolol rapidly are becoming the drugs of choice in treating glaucoma. (For more information, see Chapter 71, Ophthalmic Agents.) The cardiovascular actions also are of great clinical significance, as is the decreased renin activity. Currently, the bronchial and CNS actions primarily are viewed as causes of adverse effects, although investigations eventually may demonstrate that the CNS effects have some psychiatric or neurologic value.

Some physiologic manifestations of the various beta-adrenergic blocking agents are related to the drugs' classification as selective or nonselective. Selective beta-adrenergic blockers, which preferentially block beta$_1$-receptor sites, produce effects primarily related to prevention of cardiac excitation. Nonselective beta-adrenergic blockers, which block beta$_1$- and beta$_2$-receptor sites, prevent not only cardiac excitement but also bronchiolar dilation. For instance, nonselective beta-adrenergic blockers can cause bronchospasm in patients with chronic obstructive lung disorders, but this adverse effect largely is eliminated with the use of selective drugs, which have minimal beta$_2$ activity.

PHARMACOTHERAPEUTICS

Beta-adrenergic blockers are used to treat many conditions and are under investigation for use in many more. As mentioned earlier, their clinical usefulness is based largely (but not exclusively) on their cardiovascular effects. (For more information, see *Major effects of beta-adrenergic blockers,* page 240.) Cardiovascular indications for beta-adrenergic blockers include hypertension, angina pectoris, prevention of reinfarction after MI, supraventricular arrhythmias, and hypertrophic cardiomyopathy. Other uses include the treatment of migraine headaches, anxiety, wide-angle glaucoma, pheochromocytoma, and the cardiovascular symptoms associated with thyrotoxicosis.

acebutolol hydrochloride (Sectral). This selective beta$_1$-adrenergic blocking agent exerts mild intrinsic sympathomimetic activity. It acts to lower heart rate, blood pressure, and cardiac output, making it useful in treating hypertension and ventricular arrhythmias.

Usual adult dosage: initially, 200 mg P.O. b.i.d. or 400 mg P.O. daily, with the dosage gradually increased to achieve optimal response (for hypertension, the range is 400 to 800 mg/day; for ventricular arrhythmia, 600 to 1,200 mg/day). A lower maintenance dosage is required for an elderly patient; avoid giving more than 800 mg/day.

Major effects of beta-adrenergic blockers

By blocking the action of endogenous catecholamines and other sympathomimetic agents at beta-receptor sites, beta-adrenergic blockers counteract the stimulating effects of these agents. The diagram below shows the effects of beta-adrenergic blockers on the pulmonary and cardiovascular systems.

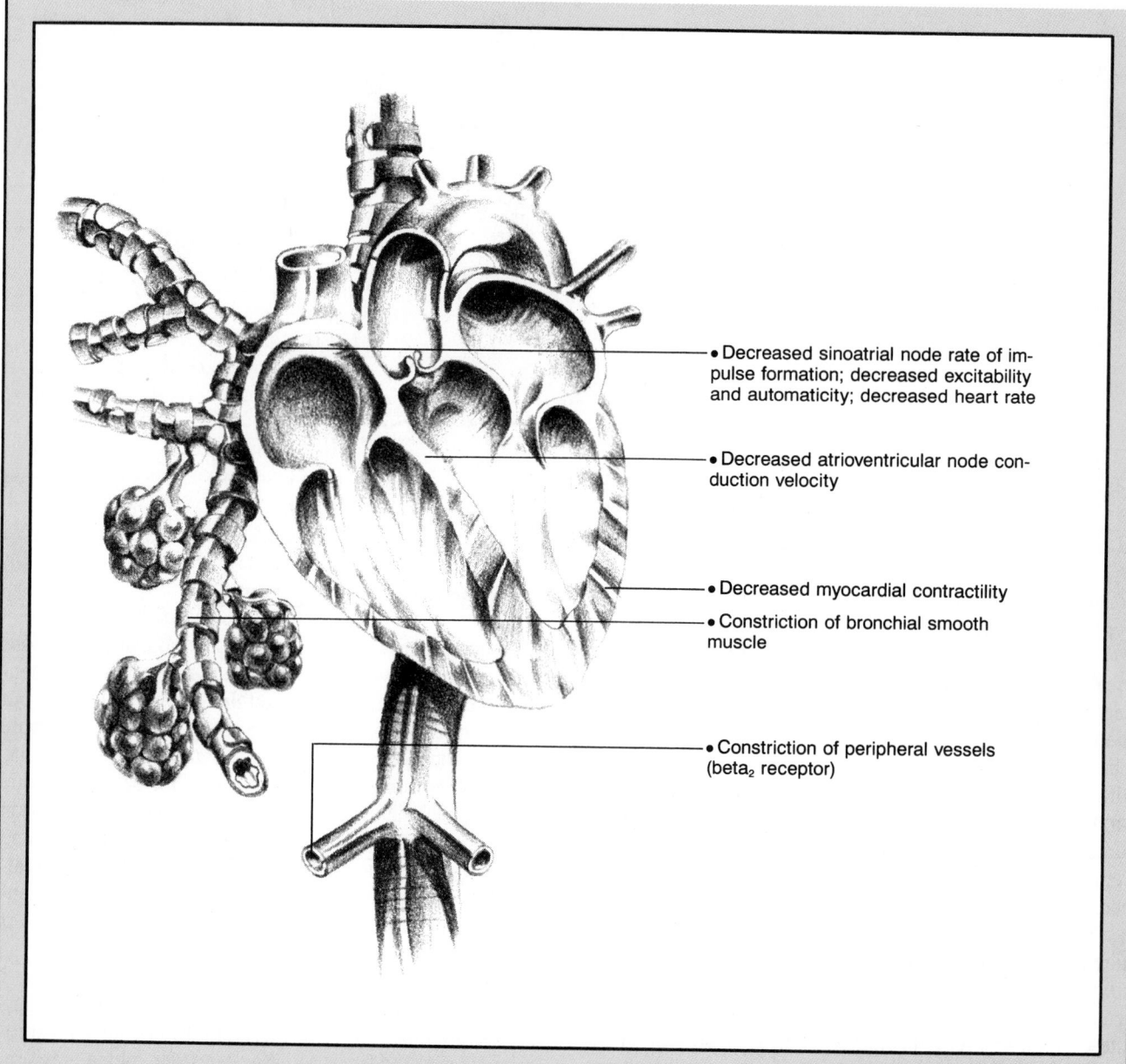

• Decreased sinoatrial node rate of impulse formation; decreased excitability and automaticity; decreased heart rate

• Decreased atrioventricular node conduction velocity

• Decreased myocardial contractility
• Constriction of bronchial smooth muscle

• Constriction of peripheral vessels (beta₂ receptor)

atenolol (Tenormin). This long-acting, selective beta₁ blocker exhibits minimal protein binding. It decreases cardiac output and systolic and diastolic blood pressure; however, like other beta-adrenergic blocking agents, it increases peripheral vascular resistance at rest and with exercise. Atenolol is used as a first-step agent in treating hypertension, alone or with other agents, and also has been used for prophylactic management of stable angina pectoris.
Usual adult dosage: initially, 50 mg P.O. once a day; increase to 100 mg once a day, if necessary, after 1 to 2 weeks; reduce to 50 mg on alternate days for patients with renal failure.

labetalol hydrochloride (Trandate, Normodyne). This selective alpha$_1$- and nonselective beta-adrenergic blocking agent decreases blood pressure without reflex tachycardia or a marked decrease in heart rate; it is used to control blood pressure in severe hypertension.

Usual adult dosage: initially 100 mg P.O. b.i.d., alone or with diuretic therapy. After 2 or 3 days, increase by 100 mg b.i.d. to achieve the desired therapeutic effect; maintenance dosage is individualized, with a usual range of 200 to 400 mg b.i.d. (Severe hypertension may require 1,200 to 2,400 mg/day.) For I.V. injection, 20 mg by slow injection over 2 minutes, repeat every 10 minutes to a maximum of 300 mg; I.V. infusion, 40 ml (two 100-mg ampules) in 160 ml of I.V. fluid (approximately 1 mg:1 ml) administered at 2 ml/minute (2 mg/minute), or 40 ml (two 100-mg ampules) in 250 ml I.V. fluid (approximately 2 mg:3 ml) administered at a rate of 3 ml/minute to deliver 2 mg/minute. Rate is adjusted according to blood pressure response. When a satisfactory response is reached (usually after infusion of 50 to 200 mg), oral therapy is begun at a 200-mg initial dose, followed in 6 to 12 hours by a 200- to 400-mg dose and adjusted according to the individual's response.

metoprolol tartrate (Lopressor, Betaloc). This selective beta$_1$ blocker produces few unwanted beta$_2$ effects except at high doses. It has some CNS activity and is used alone or in combination as a second-step antihypertensive agent or for MI.

Usual adult dosage: for hypertension, initially, 100 mg/day P.O. in single or divided doses, increased weekly until optimal effects are obtained (usual range is 100 to 450 mg/day); for MI, 5 mg I.V., 2 minutes apart, for three doses; then 50 mg P.O. every 6 hours for 48 hours, then 100 mg P.O. every 12 hours.

nadolol (Corgard). This nonselective beta-adrenergic blocker, which does not cross the blood-brain barrier, decreases standing and supine blood pressures as well as plasma renin activity. It is used to treat hypertension and may be combined with a diuretic for enhanced effects. It also is used for long-term prophylactic management of stable angina pectoris. The drug is administered orally, in a single daily dosage. Because it is excreted unchanged in the urine, the dosage must be reduced in patients with impaired renal function.

Usual adult dosage: for hypertension, initially, 40 mg/day P.O., increased gradually in 40 to 80 mg doses to a maximum of 640 mg/day (usual range, 80 to 320 mg); for angina, initially, 40 mg P.O. once a day, increased every 3 to 7 days to achieve optimal effects (usual range is 80 to 240 mg once a day). For a patient with renal failure, dosing intervals are based on creatinine clearance levels.

pindolol (Visken). This nonselective beta-adrenergic blocking agent has significant partial beta-agonist activity and some intrinsic sympathomimetic activity. As a result, it causes less reduction in cardiac contractility and heart rate and slows conduction less markedly than do other beta-adrenergic blockers. This drug is used in the first-step management of hypertension, alone or with other agents.

Usual adult dosage: initially, 5 mg P.O. b.i.d., increased by 10 mg every 3 to 4 weeks (to a maximum of 60 mg) until optimal effects are achieved.

propranolol hydrochloride (Inderal). This nonselective beta-adrenergic blocking agent produces some centrally mediated peripheral vasodilation and also decreases the heart rate by slowing conduction through the atria and the AV node. Propranolol increases exercise tolerance by blocking the sympathetic effects of exertion (such as increased heart rate and blood pressure) and decreases myocardial oxygen requirements in patients with angina. This drug is used to manage many conditions, including first-step management of hypertension, cardiac arrhythmias, MI, prophylactic management of angina pectoris, hypertrophic subaortic stenosis, and migraine. It undergoes extensive first-pass metabolism in the liver—the reason for the significant difference between oral and I.V. dosages.

Usual adult dosage: for hypertension, initially, 40 mg P.O. b.i.d., increased until optimal effects are reached (usual range is 120 to 240 mg in two or three divided doses or 120 to 160 mg of sustained-release capsules once a day) to a maximum of 640 mg/day; for angina, initially, 10 to 20 mg P.O. t.i.d. or q.i.d., increased every 3 to 7 days until optimal effects are obtained (usual dosage is 160 mg/day in divided doses) to a maximum of 320 mg/day; for arrhythmias, 10 to 30 mg P.O. t.i.d. or q.i.d.; for hypertrophic subaortic stenosis, 20 to 40 mg P.O. t.i.d. or q.i.d., or 80 to 160 mg of sustained-release capsules once a day; for MI, 180 to 240 mg P.O. daily in three or four divided doses to a maximum of 240 mg/day; for migraine, 80 mg P.O. daily in divided doses, increased as necessary (usual range, 160 to 240 mg/day); for parenteral administration in an emergency, 1 to 3 mg I.V. at an infusion rate of 1 mg/minute; a second dose may be given within 2 to 3 minutes.

timolol maleate (Blocadren, Timoptic). This nonselective beta-adrenergic blocking agent, although structurally similar to propranolol, is approximately 5 to 10 times more potent than propranolol and does not cross the blood-brain barrier. This drug is a valuable agent in treating chronic open-angle glaucoma, aphakic glaucoma, secondary glaucoma, and ocular hypertension. (For a summary of the drug's ophthalmic uses, see Chapter 71, Ophthalmic Agents.) The oral form is used as a first-step agent, alone or with other agents, to manage hypertension as well as to prevent reinfarction after MI.

Usual adult dosage: initially, 10 mg P.O. b.i.d.; maintenance dosage, 20 to 40 mg/day in two divided doses; maximum 60 mg/day in two divided doses.

Drug interactions

Many agents can interact synergistically with beta-adrenergic blocking agents to cause potentially dangerous effects, by potentiating or creating additive effects of one or both drugs or by inhibiting the desired effects of the drugs. Some of the most serious potential effects include cardiac depression, arrhythmias, respiratory depression, severe bronchospasm, and severe hypotension that could lead to vascular collapse. (For details, see *Drug interactions: Beta-adrenergic blockers.*)

ADVERSE DRUG REACTIONS

Generally, beta-adrenergic blockers cause few adverse reactions. Most that do occur are drug- or dose-dependent. Adverse reactions occur most often from I.V. rather than oral administration and in elderly patients and those with impaired renal or hepatic function.

Beta-adrenergic blocker toxicity is marked primarily by arrhythmias, orthostatic hypotension, CNS disturbances, and GI or respiratory distress. Cardiovascular reactions include hypotension, bradycardia, peripheral vascular insufficiency (Raynaud's disease), AV block, and congestive heart failure. Elderly patients are especially likely to experience peripheral vascular insufficiency and congestive heart failure.

The most common respiratory reaction is bronchospasm. Although selective agents are less likely than nonselective agents to cause bronchospasm, caution is nevertheless advisable when administering all beta-adrenergic blockers, particularly to patients with bronchial asthma, bronchitis, or emphysema. GI manifestations commonly include diarrhea, nausea, vomiting, constipation, abdominal discomfort, anorexia, and flatulence. CNS effects may include dizziness, insomnia, fatigue, weakness, lethargy, disorientation, memory loss, visual disturbances, sedation, hallucinations, or behavioral changes. Elderly patients, in particular, are at increased risk for CNS effects, such as cognitive impairment and depression. Hematologic adverse reactions, also rare, include decreased platelet agglutination, granulocytopenia, and thrombocytopenic purpura. Other reported adverse reactions include headache, impotence or decreased libido; nasal stuffiness; diaphoresis; tinnitus; and dry mouth, eyes, and skin.

Adverse reactions indicating an allergic response include rash, fever with sore throat, laryngospasm, and possibly respiratory distress. Although most patients tolerate beta-adrenergic blockers fairly well, patients with various preexisting chronic conditions are at special risk for adverse reactions to beta-adrenergic blocker therapy. (For a list of these conditions and associated adverse drug reactions, see *Adverse beta-adrenergic blocker reactions in chronic disease,* page 244.)

NURSING PROCESS APPLICATION

The following information assists the nurse in caring for a patient who is receiving a beta-adrenergic blocker.

Assessment

• Review the patient's history for conditions that contraindicate the use of a beta-adrenergic blocker, such as congestive heart failure, sinus bradycardia, heart block greater than first degree, cardiogenic shock, or bronchospastic disease.
• Review the patient's history for conditions that require cautious use of a beta-adrenergic blocker, such as diabetes, hypoglycemia, or impaired hepatic or renal function.
• Assess the patient for adverse reactions to the beta-adrenergic blocker, such as arrhythmias, orthostatic hypotension, bronchospasm, dizziness, disorientation, memory loss, visual disturbances, diarrhea, vomiting, or anorexia.
• Review the patient's medication history to identify use of drugs that may interact with the beta-adrenergic blocker, such as antacids, cardiac glycosides, or calcium channel blockers.
• Evaluate the patient's and family's knowledge about the prescribed beta-adrenergic blocker.

Nursing diagnoses

The following examples represent appropriate nursing diagnoses for a patient receiving a beta-adrenergic blocker.
• Potential for injury related to a preexisting condition that contraindicates the use of a beta-adrenergic blocker.
• Potential for injury related to a preexisting condition that requires cautious use of a beta-adrenergic blocker
• Potential for injury related to adverse drug reactions
• Altered tissue perfusion: cardiopulmonary, related to drug interaction between the beta-adrenergic blocker and another prescribed drug
• Knowledge deficit related to the prescribed beta-adrenergic blocker

Planning and implementation

• Do not administer a beta-adrenergic blocker to a patient with a condition that contraindicates its use.
• Administer a beta-adrenergic blocker cautiously to a patient at risk because of a preexisting condition.
• *Monitor the patient periodically for adverse reactions to the beta-adrenergic blocker. For example, closely monitor the patient's vital signs, fluid intake and output, daily weight, breath sounds, and peripheral circulation before*

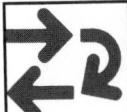

DRUG INTERACTIONS

Beta-adrenergic blockers

Drug interactions involving beta-adrenergic blockers primarily affect the cardiovascular and respiratory systems.

DRUG	INTERACTING DRUGS	POSSIBLE EFFECTS	NURSING IMPLICATIONS
acebutolol, atenolol, labetalol, metoprolol, nadolol, pindolol, propranolol, timolol	antacids	Delay absorption of drug from GI tract	• Administer several hours apart. • Monitor the patient for a decreased therapeutic effect.
	lidocaine	Increase plasma levels of lidocaine (potential toxicity); may cause additive cardiac depressant effects	• Monitor the patient for signs of lidocaine toxicity, such as confusion, restlessness, and tremors.
	insulin and oral hypoglycemic agents	May cause hypoglycemia or hyperglycemia; may mask tachycardia as a sign of hypoglycemia (diaphoresis and agitation still present)	• Administer these drugs cautiously. • Monitor the patient's blood glucose levels frequently.
	anti-inflammatories (indomethacin, salicylates)	Decrease hypotensive effects of beta-adrenergic blockers by inhibiting prostaglandin synthesis	• Monitor the patient for altered beta-adrenergic blocker effects.
	barbiturates	Stimulate metabolism of beta-adrenergic blockers that are metabolized extensively	• Monitor the patient for altered response to beta-adrenergic blockers that are metabolized by the liver (propranolol, metoprolol).
	cardiac glycosides	May cause additive bradycardia and depression of atrioventricular conduction	• Monitor the patient's blood pressure and heart rate frequently.
	calcium channel blockers (primarily verapamil)	Increase pharmacologic and toxicologic effects of both agents	• Monitor the patient for adverse reactions.
	sympathomimetics (epinephrine, dobutamine, dopamine, isoproterenol, terbutaline, metaproterenol, albuterol, ritodrine)	May cause hypertension and reflex bradycardia from unopposed alpha effects (vasoconstriction) and increased vagal tone	• Monitor the patient's blood pressure and heart rate frequently.
	cimetidine	Reduces metabolism of beta-adrenergic blockers; enhances ability of beta-adrenergic blockers to reduce pulse rate	• Monitor the patient for altered response to beta-adrenergic blockers.
	rifampin	Inhibits therapeutic response to metoprolol and propranolol	• Monitor the patient for altered response to the beta-adrenergic blocker.
	theophyllines	Impair bronchodilating effects of theophyllines by nonselective beta-adrenergic blockers	• Monitor the patient's therapeutic response.
	clonidine	Causes unopposed alpha effects when clonidine is discontinued, leading to a life-threatening increase in blood pressure	• Monitor the patient's blood pressure closely.
labetalol	halothane anesthetics	Increase hypotension	• Monitor the patient's blood pressure closely.

Adverse beta-adrenergic blocker reactions in chronic disease

This table lists common chronic disorders that place affected patients at increased risk for adverse reactions to beta-adrenergic blockers, along with the potential effects and etiologic mechanisms.

DISORDERS	POSSIBLE REACTIONS	CAUSES
Arteriosclerosis	Reflex tachycardia, acute angina pectoris, cardiac failure	Lowered blood pressure from direct cardiac action of some beta-adrenergic blocking agents
Bronchospastic disease	Severe respiratory distress	Inhibition of beta$_2$ effect, resulting in bronchospasm
Congestive heart failure, hypertension	Further cardiac failure	Increased myocardial depression
Diabetes mellitus	Masking of hypoglycemic signs and symptoms	Suppression of hypoglycemic response
Thyrotoxicosis	Masking of clinical signs	Suppression of tachycardia
	Thyroid storm	Abrupt beta-adrenergic blocker withdrawal

and during administration of the beta-adrenergic blocker. Be aware that adverse reactions most commonly occur from I.V. rather than oral administration and in elderly patients and those with impaired renal or hepatic function.
• *Obtain blood glucose levels frequently for the diabetic patient because beta-adrenergic blockers can potentiate hypoglycemia and masks its signs and symptoms.*
• Use safety precautions, such as elevating side rails and assisting with mobility, if the patient develops mental changes, such as disorientation or memory loss.
• *Keep the following emergency drugs on hand when administering an I.V. beta-adrenergic blocker: atropine for possible bradycardia, epinephrine (or another vasopressor) for possible hypotension, and isoproterenol and aminophylline for possible bronchospasm.*
• Administer oral beta-adrenergic blockers before meals or at bedtime to facilitate absorption. Avoid late-evening doses if insomnia occurs.
• *Check the patient's apical pulse rate before drug administration (especially if the patient is taking digitalis). Withhold the drug if the patient has a pulse rate below 60 or exhibits adverse reactions to the beta-adrenergic blocker.*
• *Notify the physician immediately if the patient experiences cardiac or respiratory depression, arrhythmias, severe bronchospasm, or severe hypotension. Institute emergency care according to the health care facility's guidelines.*
• *Administer antacids several hours before or after the oral beta-adrenergic blocker.*

• Help prevent drug interactions by alerting all consulting physicians that the patient is receiving a beta-adrenergic blocker.
• Monitor closely for increased effects of the prescribed beta-adrenergic blocker if the patient is receiving other agents known to potentiate or create additive effects, such as cardiac glycosides or calcium channel blockers.

Patient teaching
• Teach the patient and family the name, dose, frequency, action, and adverse effects of the prescribed beta-adrenergic blocker.
• *Advise the patient not to stop taking the drug abruptly or alter the prescribed dosage, unless ordered. Explain that abrupt withdrawal can cause MI, arrhythmias, or other serious complications.*
• *Teach the patient to measure the pulse rate and report slowing or irregularity to the physician.*
• Teach the patient to minimize the effects of orthostatic hypotension by changing position slowly, especially supine to upright, and by dangling the legs over the bedside for a few minutes before standing.
• *Instruct the patient to sit or lie down immediately if dizziness or faintness occurs.*
• *Advise the patient not to drive or operate machinery until after adjusting to the drug's CNS effects.*
• Advise the patient receiving metoprolol that the drug may take up to 1 week to produce optimal effects; if the drug produces insomnia, the patient should avoid late-evening doses.

• *Teach the patient with impaired renal function to report a weight gain of 3 to 4 pounds (1.4 to 1.8 kg) per day, cough, orthopnea, fatigue, tachycardia, dyspnea on exertion, edema, or anxiety.*

• Teach the patient to store the beta-adrenergic blocker at room temperature and to protect it from moisture, light, and air.

• Tell the patient and family to notify the physician of any adverse drug reactions.

Evaluation

The following examples represent appropriate evaluation statements for a patient receiving a beta-adrenergic blocker.

• The patient has no conditions that contraindicate the use of beta-adrenergic blockers.

• The patient exhibits no signs of complications in the preexisting condition linked to the prescribed beta-adrenergic blocker.

• The patient develops no adverse drug reactions to the prescribed beta-adrenergic blocker.

• The patient displays adequate cardiopulmonary tissue perfusion.

• The patient and family express an accurate understanding of the points taught about the prescribed beta-adrenergic blocking agent.

• The patient correctly demonstrates how to measure the pulse rate.

• The patient states that the drug will be stored in a kitchen cabinet.

AUTONOMIC GANGLIONIC BLOCKERS

All nerve impulse transmission from preganglionic to postganglionic fibers in the autonomic nervous system (the parasympathetic and the sympathetic branches) is mediated by the neurotransmitter acetylcholine. By inhibiting the action of acetylcholine, ganglionic blocking agents reduce or prevent impulse transmission in the autonomic nervous system. These drugs are classified according to their type of action as depolarizing or nondepolarizing agents. Depolarizing agents initially stimulate postganglionic fibers, then block further activity by continuing to occupy the receptor sites, thereby preventing postganglionic repolarization. Nondepolarizing agents function as competitive antagonists of acetylcholine at postganglionic receptor sites and exert no initial stimulatory action. The clinically useful ganglionic blockers, such as trimethaphan camsylate and mecamylamine hydrochloride, belong to the nondepolarizing category and cause primarily sympatholytic effects: vasodilation and decreased blood pressure.

Because of their broad and somewhat unpredictable effects and because other, more specific agents are available, ganglionic blocking agents have limited clinical uses. Like alpha- and beta-adrenergic blocking agents, they exert potent hypotensive effects, but they also produce such problematic parasympatholytic effects as constipation, paralytic ileus, and decreased urinary bladder tone with urine retention.

PHARMACOKINETICS

The two ganglionic blocking agents in use today, trimethaphan and mecamylamine, have similar pharmacokinetic actions, differing primarily in route of administration.

Absorption, distribution, metabolism, excretion

Administered orally, ganglionic blocking agents are absorbed well from the GI tract, but at erratic rates. Higher doses usually are required at night; lower doses in warm weather. The drugs are distributed widely throughout the body. Trimethaphan and mecamylamine cross the placenta; mecamylamine also crosses the blood-brain barrier. Possibly metabolized by pseudocholinesterase, the drugs are excreted by the kidneys, largely in unchanged form. Excretion of mecamylamine is enhanced by acidic urine and slowed by alkaline urine. A small amount is excreted in the feces.

Onset, peak, duration

The onset of action of ganglionic blockers is route-dependent, beginning immediately after I.V. administration and within 30 minutes to 2 hours after oral administration. With oral therapy, peak concentration levels are reached 3 to 5 hours after administration; duration of action is 6 to 12 hours. Note, however, that full therapeutic effects may not be achieved for 2 to 3 days with oral medication. With I.V. therapy, the duration is 10 to 30 minutes, with rebound hypertension occurring shortly after discontinuation.

PHARMACODYNAMICS

Ganglionic blocking agents prevent nerve transmission by competing with acetylcholine at the postganglionic synapses of the autonomic nervous system. They work not only at the ganglia of the autonomic nervous system but also in the adrenal medulla, where the drugs prevent the cells from secreting epinephrine and norepinephrine into the circulation, thereby blocking sympathetic impulses to cells. Administration of ganglionic blocking agents causes vasodilation, which may be accompanied by a loss of the baroreceptor reflex action that serves to normalize blood pressure.

Mechanism of action

Besides blocking sympathetic stimulation of the adrenal medulla to prevent the secretion of epinephrine and norepinephrine into the systemic circulation, ganglionic blocking agents block acetylcholine at postganglionic cells by competitive inhibition. This blockage of impulse transmission and reduction of circulating catecholamines diminish vasoconstrictor tone, leading to vascular dilation and decreased arterial pressure. When the patient stands, the compensatory vasoconstrictor reflexes that respond to position changes by regulating blood pressure are suppressed. As a result, blood collects in the leg veins, causing decreased venous return and decreased cardiac output. Trimethaphan also may have a direct vasodilation effect on blood vessels. Along with the desired decrease in arterial pressure, decreased venous return and decreased cardiac output can lead to such undesirable effects as orthostatic hypotension and syncope. Other undesirable effects include inhibited diaphoresis, loss of body heat, and lowered body temperature from vasodilation in the skin.

PHARMACOTHERAPEUTICS

Clinical use of ganglionic blocking agents is limited by the drugs' many potential adverse effects, including significant orthostatic hypotension, paralytic ileus, and urine retention. The drugs are used selectively, however, to treat hypertensive emergencies, pulmonary edema resulting from pulmonary hypertension, and uncomplicated malignant hypertension; to provide controlled hypotension during surgery, such as for brain tumors, cerebral aneurysms, AV fistulas, aortic grafts and transplants, and coarctations; and to predict the effects of a sympathectomy.

mecamylamine hydrochloride (Inversine). This competitive antagonist of acetylcholine is a potent, long-acting agent that decreases blood pressure in normotensive and hypertensive patients. Tolerance to mecamylamine rarely develops, and its effects are most pronounced while the patient is standing or sitting. Rarely, the drug is used to control moderate to severe essential hypertension and uncomplicated malignant hypertension.
Usual adult dosage: initially, 2.5 mg P.O. b.i.d., increased by 2.5-mg increments every 2 days until the optimum effects are obtained; average total daily dosage, 25 mg, usually given in three divided doses.

trimethaphan camsylate (Arfonad). This potent, short-acting, competitive ganglionic blocking agent directly relaxes vascular smooth muscle. It also can stimulate histamine release. Tolerance to this agent can develop in 48 hours after therapy is begun. Trimethaphan is administered by continuous I.V. infusion for controlled hypotension during neurologic, ophthalmic, and cosmetic surgery proce-

dures, for short-term control of blood pressure during hypertensive emergencies, and for emergency treatment of pulmonary hypertension causing pulmonary edema. It is under investigation for use in managing dissecting aortic aneurysm and ischemic heart disease when other agents cannot be used.
Usual adult dosage: initially, 3 to 4 ml/minute I.V. of a 1-mg/ml solution (500 mg, or 10 ml of drug in 500 ml of D$_5$W); adjust to individual need within range of 0.3 to 6 mg/minute.

Drug interactions

Many agents can interact with ganglionic blocking agents to cause potentially dangerous effects, by potentiating or creating additive effects of either or both drugs or by inhibiting the desired effects of the drugs. Perhaps the most dangerous effect is severe hypotension, which can progress to vascular collapse. (For more details, see *Drug interactions: Autonomic ganglionic blockers.*)

ADVERSE DRUG REACTIONS

Adverse reactions to ganglionic blocking agents are related to their broad, nonspecific blocking effects on the parasympathetic and sympathetic nervous systems.

Mild adverse reactions commonly are associated with ganglionic blocking agents and can involve many body systems. Possible cardiovascular manifestations include tachycardia or bradycardia and orthostatic hypotension. CNS effects may include restlessness, weakness, fatigue, sedation, cycloplegia, or mydriasis. GI and genitourinary signs and symptoms may include glossitis, nausea, vomiting, or anorexia as well as parasympathetic manifestations — dry mouth, constipation (sometimes preceded by small, frequent, liquid stools), decreased bowel sounds, loss of GI tract tone, and decreased bladder tone with urinary hesitancy. Other reactions may include suppression of diaphoresis and respiratory depression.

Severe adverse reactions — often dose-related — can include extreme hypotension, rapid pulse, cyanosis, angina-like pain, vascular collapse, abdominal distention, paralytic ileus, urine retention, dizziness, syncope, tremors, mental disturbance, paresthesias, and impaired sexual function.

Patients who have undergone sympathectomy, have hypertensive encephalopathy, or are on low-sodium diets are particularly sensitive to these agents.

Allergic manifestations may include urticaria, pruritus, and a histamine-like reaction of the vein when the I.V. agent is administered.

NURSING PROCESS APPLICATION

The following information assists the nurse in caring for a patient who is receiving an autonomic ganglionic blocker.

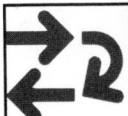

DRUG INTERACTIONS
Autonomic ganglionic blockers

Combining certain drugs with ganglionic blocking agents can cause significant adverse reactions, including hypotension and respiratory depression. This table summarizes the interactions that can cause these and other reactions and their nursing implications.

DRUG	INTERACTING DRUGS	POSSIBLE EFFECTS	NURSING IMPLICATIONS
trimethaphan, mecamylamine	anesthetics	Increase hypotensive effects	• Monitor the patient's blood pressure.
	depolarizing muscle relaxants	Increase neuromuscular blocking effects with prolonged respiratory depression	• Monitor the patient's respiratory rate and provide mechanical ventilatory support, as needed.
	nondepolarizing muscle relaxants	Increase neuromuscular blocking effects with prolonged respiratory depression	• Monitor the patient's respiratory rate and provide mechanical ventilatory support, as needed.

Assessment
• Review the patient's history for conditions that contraindicate the use of an autonomic ganglionic blocker, such as uncorrected anemia, hypovolemia, shock, asphyxia, or uncorrected respiratory insufficiency.
• Review the patient's history for conditions that require cautious use of an autonomic ganglionic blocker, such as allergies, advanced age, or debilitation.
• Assess the patient for adverse reactions to the autonomic ganglionic blocker, such as tachycardia, bradycardia, orthostatic hypotension, restlessness, weakness, constipation, decreased GI tract tone, and decreased bladder tone with urinary hesitancy.
• Assess the patient's nutritional intake during autonomic ganglionic blocker therapy.
• Evaluate the patient's and family's knowledge about the prescribed autonomic ganglionic blocker.

Nursing diagnoses
The following examples represent appropriate nursing diagnoses for a patient receiving an autonomic ganglionic blocker.
• Potential for injury related to a preexisting condition that contraindicates the use of an autonomic ganglionic blocker
• Potential for injury related to a preexisting condition that requires cautious use of an autonomic ganglionic blocker
• Potential for injury related to adverse drug reactions
• Altered nutrition: less than body requirements, related to the adverse GI effects of autonomic ganglionic blocker therapy
• Knowledge deficit related to the prescribed autonomic ganglionic blocker

Planning and implementation
• Do not administer an autonomic ganglionic blocker to a patient with a condition that contraindicates its use.
• Administer an autonomic ganglionic blocker cautiously to a patient at risk because of a preexisting condition.
• Monitor the patient periodically for adverse reactions to the autonomic ganglionic blocker. Be aware that a patient who has undergone sympathectomy, has hypertensive encephalopathy, or is on a low-sodium diet is particularly sensitive to such an agent.
• *Have the following equipment and supplies available to treat a hypotensive reaction: oxygen, resuscitation and ventilation equipment, and vasopressor medication.*
• *Administer an autonomic ganglionic blocker carefully to a patient with a history of allergies because they may cause histamine release.*
• Monitor the patient's vital signs periodically during and after administration of an autonomic ganglionic blocker.
• *Dilute trimethaphan (1 mg/1 ml of D_5W) before administration and do not mix it with any other drug for I.V. administration.*
• Administer I.V. trimethaphan via continuous infusion, titrating the dose in response to the patient's blood pressure. Use microdrip tubing or an infusion pump to facilitate accurate administration.
• *Minimize the risk of severe hypotension by administering trimethapan with the patient in a supine or head-down position. Be aware that the drug's action is enhanced by the reverse Trendelenburg position.*
• *Discontinue an I.V. infusion of trimethaphan gradually.*
• *Give smaller doses of an autonomic ganglionic blocker in the morning, when the patient's response usually is greater.*

SELECTED MAJOR DRUGS

Adrenergic blocking agents

This chart summarizes the major adrenergic blockers currently in clinical use.

DRUG	MAJOR INDICATIONS	USUAL ADULT DOSAGES	CONTRAINDICATIONS AND PRECAUTIONS
Apha-adrenergic blockers			
phentolamine	Hypertension associated with pheochromocytoma	5 mg I.M. or I.V. before surgery; 5 mg I.V. if needed, during surgery	• Know that phentolamine is contraindicated in a patient with known hypersensitivity to the drug, myocardial infarction, coronary insufficiency, or angina.
	Prevention of necrosis related to extravasation	5 to 10 mg in 10 ml normal saline solution injected into the area of extravasation	• Administer with caution to a pregnant or lactating patient.
Beta-adrenergic blockers			
atenolol	Hypertension, angina	50 mg P.O. once/day; increase to 100 mg/day after 1 to 2 weeks if necessary; reduce to 50 mg every other day for patients with renal failure	• Know that atenolol is contraindicated in a patient with sinus bradycardia, heart block greater than first degree, cardiogenic shock, or overt cardiac failure. • Administer with extreme caution to a patient with respiratory conditions, such as asthma, hay fever, bronchitis, emphysema, or allergic rhinitis. Severe bronchospasm may occur. • Administer with caution to a pregnant or lactating patient or one with impaired renal function.
metoprolol	Hypertension	100 mg/day P.O. with weekly increase to achieve desired effects. Maintenance dosage: 100 to 450 mg/day	• Know that metaprolol is contraindicated in a patient with sinus bradycardia, heart block greater than first degree, cardiogenic shock, overt cardiac failure, or bronchospastic disease.
	Myocardial infarction	5 mg I.V. every 2 minutes for three doses; then 50 mg P.O. every 6 hours for 48 hours; then 100 mg every 12 hours	• Administer with caution to a pregnant or lactating patient or one with diabetes, hypoglycemia, or impaired hepatic function.
nadolol	Hypertension	40 mg P.O. once a day; increased gradually in 40- to 80-mg doses to a maximum of 640 mg/day (usual range, 80 to 320 mg). For a patient with renal failure, dosing intervals are based on creatinine clearance levels.	• Know that nadolol is contraindicated in a lactating patient or one with bronchial asthma, sinus bradycardia, heart block greater than first degree, cardiogenic shock, bronchospastic disease, or overt cardiac failure. • Administer with caution to a pregnant patient or one with impaired respiratory or renal function.
	Angina	40 mg P.O. once a day; increased every 3 to 7 days to desired effect (range, 80 to 240 mg/day). For a patient with renal failure, dosing intervals are based on creatinine clearance levels.	

SELECTED MAJOR DRUGS

Adrenergic blocking agents (continued)

DRUG	MAJOR INDICATIONS	USUAL ADULT DOSAGES	CONTRAINDICATIONS AND PRECAUTIONS
Beta-adrenergic blockers (continued)			
propranolol	Hypertension	40 mg P.O. b.i.d. to desired effect (usual range, 120 to 240 mg in two or three divided doses, or 120 to 160 mg of sustained-release capsules once a day)	• Know that propranolol is contraindicated in a patient with cardiogenic shock, sinus bradycardia, heart block greater than first degree, bronchial asthma, or congestive heart failure.
	Angina	10 to 20 mg P.O. t.i.d. or q.i.d. increased every 3 to 7 days to achieve desired effects (usual dosage, 160 mg/day in divided doses)	• Administer with caution to a pregnant or lactating patient or one with impaired renal or hepatic function.
	Arrhythmias	10 to 30 mg P.O. t.i.d. or q.i.d. Emergencies: 1 to 3 mg I.V. push (1 mg/minute) repeated in 2 to 3 minutes	
	Hypertrophic subaortic stenosis	20 to 40 mg P.O. t.i.d. or q.i.d. or 80 to 160 mg of sustained-release capsules once a day	
	Myocardial infarction	180 to 240 mg P.O. daily in 3 or 4 divided doses	
	Migraine	80 mg P.O. daily in divided doses, increased as necessary (usual range, 160 to 240 mg/day)	
Autonomic ganglionic blocker			
trimethaphan	Hypertension, controlled hypotension in surgery	3 to 4 ml/minute I.V. of a 1 mg/ml solution (500 mg or 10 ml of drug in 500 ml D$_5$W); adjust individually (within a 0.3 to 6 mg/minute range)	• Know that trimethaphan is contraindicated in a lactating patient or one with a condition that increases the risk of hypotension, such as uncorrected anemia, hypovolemia, shock, asphyxia, or uncorrected respiratory insufficiency. • Administer with extreme caution to a pregnant patient. • Administer with caution to an elderly or debilitated patient or one with allergies.

• *Monitor the patient for rebound hypertension, which can lead to hypertensive crisis, during withdrawal of the autonomic ganglionic blocker.*
• Notify the physician if adverse drug reactions occur.
• Observe the patient for nutritional deficits and weight loss.
• Encourage the patient to eat nutritious foods for snacks.
• Provide small, frequent meals throughout the day.
• Provide nutritional, vitamin, or mineral supplements, if prescribed.

• Notify the physician if the patient develops nutritional deficits or loses more than 2 pounds per week.

Patient teaching
• Teach the patient and family the name, dose, frequency, action, and adverse effects of the prescribed autonomic ganglionic blocker.
• *Teach the patient to minimize orthostatic hypotension by arising slowly from the supine position and dangling the legs over the bedside for a short time before standing.*

• Teach the patient how to prevent constipation by increasing the intake of fluids and high-fiber foods.
• Instruct the patient and family to inform the physician of any adverse drug reactions.

Evaluation

The following examples represent appropriate evaluation statements for a patient receiving an autonomic ganglionic blocker.
• The patient has no conditions that contraindicate the use of an autonomic ganglionic blocker.
• The patient exhibits no signs of complications in the preexisting condition linked to the prescribed autonomic ganglionic blocker.
• The patient develops no adverse reactions to the prescribed autonomic ganglionic blocker.
• The patient maintains body weight and obtains adequate nutrition.
• The patient and family express an accurate understanding of the points taught about the prescribed autonomic ganglionic blocker.
• The patient lists appropriate techniques to minimize orthostatic hypotension and constipation.

ergic blockers block beta$_1$- and beta$_2$-receptor sites. Both types prevent cardiac excitation.
• Because of their cardiovascular effects, beta-adrenergic blockers are used extensively to treat hypertension, cardiac arrhythmias, and angina pectoris. They also are used to treat hyperthyroidism and related disorders of sympathetic nervous system overstimulation.
• Beta-adrenergic blockers are absorbed rapidly and well, somewhat protein bound, distributed widely in the body, and excreted primarily in the urine.
• Autonomic ganglionic blocking agents, like alpha- and beta-adrenergic blockers, exert potent hypotensive effects. They work at the postganglionic fibers of the autonomic nervous system and the adrenal medulla to prevent epinephrine and norepinephrine secretion.
• The use of ganglionic blocking agents is limited by the drugs' many potential adverse effects, including significant orthostatic hypotension, paralytic ileus, and urine retention.
• When caring for a patient who receives an adrenergic blocking agent, the nurse should apply the nursing process, providing care that includes careful monitoring for adverse reactions, screening for drug interactions, and providing patient teaching.

CHAPTER SUMMARY

Chapter 16 discussed adrenergic blockers as they are used therapeutically to disrupt sympathetic nervous system function. Here are the highlights of the chapter.
• Adrenergic blocking agents, also called sympatholytics, are used therapeutically to block sympathetic nervous system function. This drug class includes alpha-adrenergic blockers, beta-adrenergic blockers, and autonomic ganglionic blockers.
• Blockage of alpha-adrenergic receptor sites decreases blood pressure by relaxing the smooth muscles surrounding the arterioles. As a result, alpha-adrenergic blockers provide some therapeutic benefit in treating certain types of hypertension.
• The pharmacokinetics of alpha-adrenergic blocking agents are not well understood. Most of these agents are absorbed erratically when administered orally and more rapidly and completely when administered sublingually or by inhalation.
• Adverse reactions to alpha-adrenergic blockers primarily are related to the vasodilation effect of the drugs and mainly involve the cardiovascular system.
• Beta-adrenergic blockers are classified as selective or nonselective. Selective beta-adrenergic blockers preferentially block beta$_1$-receptor sites; nonselective beta-adren-

STUDY QUESTIONS

See Appendix 1 for answers.

1. Alan Brown, age 30, has hypertension. To determine whether the hypertension is primary or secondary, the physician orders the Regitine-blocking test. Phentolamine (Regitine) is an alpha-adrenergic blocking agent. What is its primary use?
(a) reduction of peripheral vascular resistance
(b) coronary artery dilation
(c) constriction of bronchi
(d) skeletal muscle relaxation

2. Administration of an alpha-adrenergic blocker typically lowers the blood pressure. It also may cause which of the following effects?
(a) bradycardia
(b) reflex tachycardia
(c) bronchodilation
(d) constipation

3. Elva Kelly, age 62, is admitted to the hospital for treatment of uncontrolled hypertension. The physician prescribes the nonselective beta-adrenergic blocker propranolol

(Inderal) 40 mg P.O. b.i.d. How do beta-adrenergic blocking agents produce their therapeutic effects?
(a) They act as competitive adrenergic antagonists at beta-receptor sites.
(b) They stimulate metabolism of neurotransmitters.
(c) They inhibit neurotransmitter production.
(d) They chemically inactivate neurotransmitters at receptor sites.

4. Before administering propranolol to Ms. Kelly, the nurse assesses for a history of bronchial asthma. Why?
(a) Propranolol may cause bronchospasms.
(b) Propranolol may cause bronchodilation.
(c) Propranolol may increase respiratory secretions.
(d) Propranolol may decrease the respiratory rate.

5. When teaching Ms. Kelly about propranolol, the nurse should include which of the following instructions?
(a) Stop taking the medication if insomnia develops.
(b) Take the medication with meals or snacks.
(c) Store the medication in the refrigerator.
(d) Do not discontinue the medication abruptly.

6. Rita Fisher, age 48, has moderate essential hypertension. Her physician orders the autonomic ganglionic blocker mecamylamine (Inversine) 2.5 mg P.O. b.i.d. Clinical use of autonomic ganglionic blockers is limited. Which factor may help account for this?
(a) erratic rate of absorption
(b) extremely short duration of action
(c) narrow range of therapeutic effects
(d) broad, somewhat unpredictable effects

7. What is the mechanism of action of the autonomic ganglionic blockers?
(a) They compete with catecholamine at receptor sites in the sympathetic nervous system.
(b) They compete with acetylcholine at receptor sites in the parasympathetic nervous system.
(c) They compete with catecholamines at receptor sites in the autonomic nervous system.
(d) They compete with acetylcholine at postganglionic synapses in the autonomic nervous system.

SELECTED REFERENCES

AHFS drug information 90. (1990). Bethesda, MD: American Society of Hospital Pharmacists.

Dix-Sheldon, D. (1989). Pharmacologic management of myocardial ischemia. *Journal of Cardiovascular Nursing,* 3(4), 17-30.

Hansten, P., and Horn, J. (1989). *Drug interactions.* Philadelphia: Lea & Febiger.

Miller, C. (1988). Medication in angina. *Focus on Critical Care,* 15(4), 23-29.

Streedback, N. (1988). Beta-adrenoceptor blockade and anesthesia. *AANA Journal,* 56(4), 334-337.

Williams, J. (1989). Update on beta blockers. *AANA Journal,* 57(1), 29-36.

Withdrawal syndrome following beta-blocker taper. (1988). *Nurses Drug Alert,* 12(10), 73-4.

NEUROMUSCULAR BLOCKING AGENTS

OBJECTIVES

After reading and studying this chapter, the student should be able to:

1. List the major clinical indications for the neuromuscular blocking agents.

2. Describe the physiology of the motor end plate where neuromuscular blocking agents exert their effect.

3. Describe the pharmacokinetics of the neuromuscular blocking agents.

4. Differentiate between the actions of nondepolarizing and depolarizing neuromuscular blocking agents.

5. Explain the additive effects that result when drugs interact with the neuromuscular blocking agents.

6. Identify the antidotes to the neuromuscular blocking agents.

7. Describe how to apply the nursing process when caring for a patient who is receiving a neuromuscular blocking agent.

INTRODUCTION

Neuromuscular blocking agents are drugs that act to relax the skeletal muscles by disrupting the transmission of nerve impulses. Because the drugs do not cross the blood-brain barrier, the patient remains conscious and aware of pain.

Neuromuscular blocking agents have three major clinical indications: to relax skeletal muscles during surgery, to reduce the intensity of muscle spasms in drug or electrically induced convulsions, or to manage patients who are fighting mechanical ventilation. Chapter 17 discusses the two main classes of natural and synthetic drugs used as neuromuscular blocking agents: nondepolarizing and depolarizing blocking agents.

For a summary of representative drugs, see *Selected major drugs: Neuromuscular blocking agents,* page 259. For a listing of applicable nursing diagnoses that the nurse

---

SELECTED NURSING DIAGNOSES

Neuromuscular blocking agents

The following nursing diagnoses address representative problems and etiologies that a nurse may encounter when caring for a patient who is receiving a neuromuscular blocking agent. Some of these nursing diagnoses contain generalized etiologies, which the nurse must individualize based on the patient's needs. (For some common nursing diagnoses and related interventions for each drug class, see the "Nursing Process Application" sections of this chapter.)

- Altered protection related to tachyphylaxis from repeated doses of succinylcholine
- Anxiety related to immobility and inability to communicate
- Decreased tissue perfusion: renal, related to hypotension caused by the nondepolarizing blocking agent
- Impaired gas exchange related to bronchospasm caused by the nondepolarizing blocking agent
- Impaired physical mobility related to the muscle relaxing effects of the neuromuscular blocking agent
- Impaired verbal communication related to the muscle relaxing effects of the neuromuscular blocking agent
- Ineffective airway clearance related to excessive bronchial secretions caused by the nondepolarizing blocking agent
- Ineffective breathing pattern related to respiratory muscle paralysis
- Knowledge deficit related to the prescribed neuromuscular blocking agent
- Pain related to muscle fasciculation during Phase I of succinylcholine's action
- Potential for injury related to a preexisting condition that contraindicates the use of a neuromuscular blocking agent
- Potential for injury related to a preexisting condition that requires cautious the use of a neuromuscular blocking agent
- Potential for injury related to adverse drug reactions

Motor end plate

The motor nerve axon divides to form branching terminals called motor end plates. These are enfolded in muscle fibers but are separated from the fibers by the synaptic cleft.

A stimulus to the nerve causes the release of acetylcholine into the synaptic cleft. There, acetylcholine occupies receptor sites on the muscle cell membrane, depolarizing the membrane and causing muscle contraction. Neuromuscular blocking agents act at the motor end plate by competing with acetylcholine for the receptor sites or by blocking depolarization.

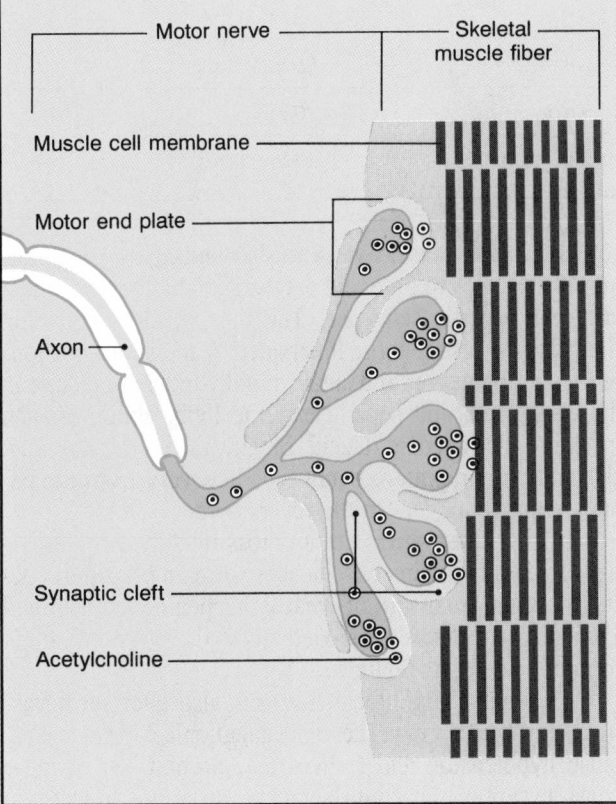

may formulate when caring for a patient receiving these agents, see *Selected nursing diagnoses: Neuromuscular blocking agents.* For detailed information on applying the nursing process, see Chapter 6, The Nursing Process and Drug Therapy.

Physiology of the motor end plate

Neuromuscular blocking agents act at the motor end plate of the motor unit. The motor end plate is the junction between the motor nerve and the skeletal muscle. (For an illustration and a description of the events that lead to muscle contraction, see *Motor end plate.*)

Motor nerves arise from anterior horn cells in the spinal cord; at the neuromuscular junction, the nerve axon divides

to form branching terminals called the motor end plate. These terminals are insulated from surrounding fluid by Schwann's cells. The terminals are enfolded into the muscle fiber but are separated from it by a space called the synaptic cleft.

The sequence of events that triggers muscle contraction begins with a stimulus to the nerve. When the impulse reaches the neuromuscular junction, depolarization occurs, resulting in an influx of calcium ions from the extracellular fluid into the terminals, which then release acetylcholine into the synaptic cleft. The acetylcholine combines with receptor sites on the postjunctional muscle cell membrane, depolarizing it and facilitating the entry of sodium (and, to a lesser extent, calcium). The result is a muscle contraction. Almost immediately after the muscle fibers are stimulated, acetylcholine is inactivated by the enzyme acetylcholinesterase.

NONDEPOLARIZING BLOCKING AGENTS

The nondepolarizing blocking agents, also called competitive or stabilizing agents, are derived curare alkaloids and their synthetic analogues. They include atracurium besylate, gallamine triethiodide, metocurine iodide, pancuronium bromide, pipecuronium bromide, tubocurarine chloride, and vecuronium bromide. These agents produce intermediate to prolonged muscle relaxation, such as that required for intubation and ventilation during surgery.

PHARMACOKINETICS

Because plasma levels of the nondepolarizing blocking agents are difficult to predict, nerve stimulators are used to assess drug effects on the patient.

Absorption, distribution, metabolism, excretion

Because nondepolarizing blocking agents are absorbed poorly from the gastrointestinal (GI) tract, they are administered parenterally. The I.V. route is preferred because the action is more predictable. The drugs, which are distributed rapidly throughout the body, act on the motor end plates and, to a lesser degree, on the autonomic ganglia. A variable but large proportion of the nondepolarizing agents is excreted unchanged in the urine. Some of the newer drugs, such as atracurium, pancuronium, pipecuronium, and vecuronium, are metabolized partially in the liver.

Pharmacokinetics of the nondepolarizing agents

This chart compares the onset of action, peak concentration level, and duration of action of the nondepolarizing blocking agents. Note that all have rapid onset and reach peak concentration in 3 to 5 minutes. Their durations vary greatly.

DRUG	ONSET OF ACTION	PEAK CONCENTRATION LEVEL	DURATION OF ACTION
atracurium	2 min	3 to 5 min	20 to 70 min
gallamine	1 to 2 min	3 to 5 min	15 to 30 min
metocurine	1 to 4 min	3 to 5 min	25 to 90 min
pancuronium	less than 1 min	3 to 5 min	12 to 60 min
pipecuronium	1 to 3 min	3 to 5 min	60 to 120 min
tubocurarine	1 to 2 min	3 to 5 min	60 min
vecuronium	1 to 2 min	3 to 5 min	20 to 30 min

Onset, peak, duration

Nondepolarizing blocking agents have a rapid onset of action after I.V. administration. Their half-lives vary from 20 minutes to 4 hours. For atracurium, pancuronium, and vecuronium, the onset, clinical effect, and rate of recovery depend on dosage as well as numerous other factors. Acidosis, inhalation anesthetics, renal or hepatic dysfunction, and hypothermia may prolong the action of these agents. The duration of action of metocurine and tubocurarine is related directly to the total dosage and the depth of anesthesia produced by the accompanying anesthetic agent. Repeated doses of metocurine and tubocurarine result in a cumulative effect. The duration of paralysis associated with gallamine is related to total dosage, the type of anesthetic, and the depth of anesthesia. (For more information, see *Pharmacokinetics of the nondepolarizing agents*.)

PHARMACODYNAMICS

The therapeutic action of the nondepolarizing blocking agents is based on the relaxation or paralysis of the skeletal muscles.

Mechanism of action

The nondepolarizing blocking agents compete with acetylcholine at the cholinergic receptor sites of the skeletal muscle membrane. This blocks acetycholine's transmitter action, preventing the muscle membrane from depolarizing. The effect can be counteracted clinically by anticholinesterase drugs, such as neostigmine or pyridostigmine, which inhibit the action of acetylcholinesterase, the enzyme that destroys acetylcholine.

The initial muscle weakness produced by the drugs quickly changes to a flaccid paralysis that affects the muscles in a specific sequence. The first muscles to exhibit flaccid paralysis are those innervated by the motor portions of the cranial nerves and small, rapidly moving muscles in the eyes, face, and neck. Next, the limb, abdomen, and trunk muscles become flaccid. Finally, the intercostal muscles and diaphragm are paralyzed. Recovery from the paralysis usually occurs in the reverse order.

Because these drugs do not cross the blood-brain barrier, no alterations in consciousness or pain perception occur. Patients are aware of what is happening to them and may experience extreme anxiety and pain, but they cannot communicate their feelings.

Nondepolarizing blocking agents also alter cardiovascular dynamics. First, the mild ganglionic blockade may cause hypotension and tachycardia. Second, all of these drugs except vecuronium increase histamine release to varying degrees, which may accentuate the hypotension. Pancuronium causes minimal histamine release and no ganglionic blockade. Histamine release also produces bronchial spasm and excessive bronchial or salivary secretions. These manifestations are accentuated further by decreased venous return and diminished respiratory excursion from loss of skeletal muscle tone.

PHARMACOTHERAPEUTICS

Nondepolarizing blocking agents are used for intermediate or prolonged muscle relaxation. They facilitate endotracheal intubation and are used during surgery to decrease the amount of anesthetic required and to facilitate manipulations. They also are used to paralyze patients who need ventilatory support but who fight the endotracheal tube and ventilator. Some nondepolarizing blocking agents also prevent muscle injury during electroconvulsive therapy (ECT) by reducing the intensity of muscle spasms.

atracurium besylate (Tracrium). Atracurium is used primarily as an adjunct to anesthesia. Unlike the other drugs in this class, atracurium does not appear to have a cumulative effect on the duration of blockade if recovery is allowed to begin before each maintenance dose is given. Doses thus may be administered at relatively regular intervals with predictable blocking effects.
Usual adult dosage: initially, 0.4 to 0.5 mg/kg of body weight I.V.; maintenance dosage, usually 0.08 to 0.1 mg/kg every 20 to 45 minutes, depending on duration of action.

gallamine triethiodide (Flaxedil). Gallamine is used to manage patients undergoing mechanical ventilation. It sometimes is replaced by pancuronium for long-term ventilation and by succinylcholine for short intubation procedures.
Usual adult dosage: initially, 1 mg/kg of body weight I.V.; then 0.5 to 1.0 mg/kg every 30 to 40 minutes, not to exceed 100 mg per dose.

metocurine iodide (Metubine). Metocurine is used to reduce trauma during ECT and to manage patients undergoing mechanical ventilation.
Usual adult dosage: for endotracheal intubation, 0.2 to 0.4 mg/kg I.V. given over 30 to 60 seconds; supplemental dosage during anesthesia, 0.5 to 1 mg I.V. For ECT, 1.75 to 5.5 mg I.V. given slowly.

pancuronium bromide (Pavulon). Used to manage patients undergoing intubation and mechanical ventilation, pancuronium has minimal histamine-releasing effects, does not block sympathetic ganglia, and therefore does not produce hypotension and bronchospasm. However, it affects the vagus nerve, resulting in an increased pulse rate as well as increased systolic blood pressure and cardiac output.
Usual adult dosage: for endotracheal intubation and ventilation, 0.06 to 0.1 mg/kg of body weight I.V. bolus. For anesthesia, 0.04 to 0.1 mg/kg of body weight I.V.; repeated doses of 0.01 to 0.02 mg/kg administered every 20 to 60 minutes.

pipecuronium bromide (Arduan). This drug is used as an adjunct to general anesthesia for skeletal muscle relaxation during surgery.
Usual adult dosage: Dosage is highly individualized. A representative dosage for endotracheal intubation is 70 to 85 mcg/kg I.V.; for maintenance during anesthesia, 10 to 15 mcg/kg I.V., which provides relaxation for about 50 minutes.

tubocurarine chloride (Tubarine). Used as an adjunct in anesthesia and to manage patients undergoing endotracheal intubation and mechanical ventilation, tubocurarine also may be used to reduce the intensity of muscle spasms in drug-induced or electrically induced convulsions.
Usual adult dosage: for anesthesia, intubation, and ventilation, initially 6 to 9 mg I.V. slowly over 60 to 90 seconds, then 3 to 4.5 mg I.V. in 3 to 5 minutes; for ECT, 0.165 mg/kg I.V. slowly.

vecuronium bromide (Norcuron). Vecuronium is used for intermediate and long-term neuromuscular blockade in patients with heart disease or asthma because it does not cause histamine release, which results in hypotension and bronchospasm.
Usual adult dosage: 0.08 to 0.1 mg/kg of body weight I.V.; maintenance dosage, 0.01 to 0.015 mg/kg I.V. every 12 to 15 minutes.

Drug interactions

Most drugs that interact with the nondepolarizing blocking agents have an additive effect. For example, some antibiotics and anesthetics potentiate the neuromuscular blockade. Drugs that alter the serum levels of calcium, magnesium, or potassium also alter the effects of the nondepolarizing blocking agents. The anticholinesterases (neostigmine, pyridostigmine, and edrophonium) are antagonistic to nondepolarizing blocking agents and are used as antidotes to the nondepolarizing blocking agents. (For more information, see *Drug interactions: Nondepolarizing blocking agents,* page 256.)

ADVERSE DRUG REACTIONS

Nondepolarizing blocking agents most commonly produce adverse reactions when given to patients who are debilitated, have fluid and electrolyte imbalances, or have respiratory, hepatic, neuromuscular, or renal disorders.

The prolonged pharmacologic effects of these drugs are responsible for most adverse reactions. The most serious adverse reaction is apnea. Ganglionic blockade and histamine release may cause a cardiovascular reaction, usually hypotension. Histamine release also may produce skin reactions, bronchospasm, and excessive bronchial and salivary secretions. Antidotes used to restore breathing may accentuate the hypotension and bronchospasms. Allergic reactions to nondepolarizing blocking agents are rare.

Pancuronium and gallamine selectively block the vagus nerve and may result in tachycardia, cardiac arrhythmias, and hypertension.

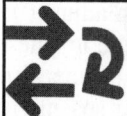

DRUG INTERACTIONS

Nondepolarizing blocking agents

Most interacting drugs enhance the blocking action of the neuromuscular blocking agents and require that the patient be observed closely to prevent fatal complications.

DRUG	INTERACTING DRUGS	POSSIBLE EFFECTS	NURSING IMPLICATIONS
atracurium, gallamine, metocurine, pancuronium, pipecuronium, tubocurarine, vecuronium	inhalation anesthetics	Potentiate neuromuscular blockade by stabilizing the postjunctional membrane Potentiate neuromuscular blockade by inhibiting acetylcholine release at the preganglionic terminal and by stabilizing the postjunctional membrane	• Anticipate possible prolonged apnea. • Keep equipment available to provide mechanical ventilation. • Monitor the patient's heart rate and rhythm and blood pressure for signs of cardiovascular collapse. • Be prepared to replace fluids and electrolytes, as necessary. • Keep the antidotes neostigmine and pyridostigmine available.
	aminoglycosides	Potentiate neuromuscular blockade by inhibiting acetylcholine release at the preganglionic terminal and by stabilizing the postjunctional membrane	• Anticipate possible prolonged apnea. • Keep equipment available to provide mechanical ventilation. • Monitor the patient's heart rate and rhythm and blood pressure for signs of cardiovascular collapse. • Be prepared to replace fluids and electrolytes, as necessary. • Keep the antidotes neostigmine and pyridostigmine available.
	clindamycin, polymyxin, calcium channel blockers, magnesium salts	Potentiate neuromuscular blockade	• Monitor the patient for adverse drug reactions and consult the physician regarding a dosage decrease.
	cholinesterase inhibitors	Antagonize neuromuscular blockade	• Be aware that these agents may be used as antidotes for the nondepolarizing agents.
	potassium-depleting medications	Potentiate neuromuscular blockade	• Assess potassium level before administration. • Closely monitor patients with decreased renal function.

NURSING PROCESS APPLICATION

The following information assists the nurse in caring for a patient who is receiving a nondepolarizing blocking agent.

Assessment
• Review the patient's history for conditions that contraindicate the use of a nondepolarizing blocking agent, such as bromide hypersensitivity.
• Review the patient's history for conditions that require cautious use of a nondepolarizing blocking agent, such as renal, hepatic, cardiac, or pulmonary impairment; fluid and electrolyte imbalance; or myasthenia gravis.
• Assess the patient for adverse reactions to the nondepolarizing blocking agent, such as apnea, hypotension, cardiac arrhythmias, skin reactions, bronchospasm, and excessive bronchial and salivary secretions.

• Assess the patient's emotional response to nondepolarizing blocking agent therapy.
• Assess the patient's respiratory rate and pattern, particularly noting decreased respirations. Auscultate breath sounds to detect wheezing or crackles.
• Evaluate the patient's and family's knowledge about the prescribed nondepolarizing blocking agent.

Nursing diagnoses
The following examples represent appropriate nursing diagnoses for a patient receiving a nondepolarizing blocking agent.
• Potential for injury related to a preexisting condition that contraindicates the use of a nondepolarizing blocking agent
• Potential for injury related to a preexisting condition that requires cautious use of a nondepolarizing blocking agent
• Potential for injury related to adverse drug reactions

• Anxiety related to immobility and inability to communicate
• Ineffective breathing pattern related to respiratory muscle paralysis
• Knowledge deficit related to the nondepolarizing blocking agent

Planning and implementation

• Do not administer a nondepolarizing blocking agent to a patient with a condition that contraindicates its use.
• Administer a nondepolarizing blocking agent cautiously to a patient at risk because of a preexisting condition.
• *Keep antidotes to the nondepolarizing blocking agent readily available.*
• *Keep endotracheal equipment, oxygen, suction equipment, and a mechanical ventilator available for respiratory support.*
• Monitor the patient closely for signs of adverse reactions to the nondepolarizing blocking agent. Keep in mind that a patient who is debilitated or has a fluid or electrolyte imbalance or a respiratory, hepatic, or neuromuscular disorder has increased susceptibility to adverse drug reactions.
• *Monitor the patient's vital signs frequently during administration of a nondepolarizing blocking agent to detect cardiovascular reactions.*
• Monitor fluid intake and output and obtain electrolyte levels, as prescribed, for a patient with renal disease.
• Provide total care for the immobilized patient to prevent complications, such as pneumonia or skin breakdown.
• Notify the physician if adverse drug reactions occur or if the patient's condition deteriorates.
• *Reduce anxiety for the patient who is completely paralyzed and cannot communicate. Maintain a calm environment, provide reassurance regularly, and explain all procedures and outcomes to the patient.*
• *Monitor respirations closely until the patient is fully recovered from neuromuscular blockage, as evidenced by tests of muscle strength (hand grip, head lift, and ability to cough).*
• Check mechanical ventilator settings and functions frequently to ensure that it is operating properly. *Never turn off the ventilator alarm.*
• Turn the patient every 2 hours and provide chest physiotherapy, as prescribed.
• Suction the patient, as needed, because the nondepolarizing blocking agent suppresses the cough reflex and may increase respiratory secretions.
• *Reassure the patient that breathing will return to normal after the nondepolarizing blocking agent is discontinued.*
• Notify the physician of any changes in the patient's respiratory status during administration of a nondepolarizing blocking agent.

Patient teaching

• Teach the patient and family about the prescribed nondepolarizing blocking agent.
• Encourage the patient and family to ask questions about nondepolarizing agents before administration, if possible.
• Inform the patient fully of all procedures in advance. Provide reassurance that the nurse will monitor the patient continually during administration of the nondepolarizing blocking agent.

Evaluation

The following examples represent appropriate evaluation statements for a patient receiving a nondepolarizing blocking agent.
• The patient has no conditions that contraindicate nondepolarizing blocking agent therapy.
• The patient exhibits no signs of complications in the preexisting condition linked to the prescribed cholinergic agonist.
• The patient displays no adverse reactions to the nondepolarizing blocking agent.
• The patient acts more relaxed and less anxious.
• The patient maintains adequate ventilation.
• The patient and family express an accurate understanding of the points taught about the prescribed nondepolarizing blocking agent.
• The patient asks appropriate questions during the teaching session before drug administration.

DEPOLARIZING BLOCKING AGENTS

Succinylcholine is the only therapeutic depolarizing blocking agent. Although it is similar to the nondepolarizing blocking agents in its therapeutic effect, its mechanism of action differs.

PHARMACOKINETICS

Because succinylcholine is absorbed poorly from the GI tract, the preferred administration route is I.V., but the I.M. route may be used if necessary. When given I.V., succinylcholine has an onset of action of 30 seconds. The drug reaches a peak concentration level in 1 minute; its duration of action is 4 to 10 minutes. It is hydrolyzed in the liver and plasma by pseudocholinesterase, and a resulting metabolite, succinylmonocholine, produces a nondepolarizing blocking action. Succinylcholine is excreted via the kidneys; approximately 10% is excreted unchanged.

PHARMACODYNAMICS

Succinylcholine produces a biphasic effect. In Phase I blockade, it acts like acetylcholine and depolarizes the postsynaptic membrane of the muscle. However, succinylcholine is not inactivated by cholinesterase, so the depolarization persists. This results in brief periods of repetitive excitation — manifested by muscle fasciculations (uncoordinated contractions of muscle fibers) — followed by muscle paralysis and flaccidity. Phase II blockade normally is not seen except with a high drug concentration or repeated doses. In this phase, the muscle gradually repolarizes toward normal, although the drug persists in the synaptic cleft. It remains unresponsive to nerve stimulation, causing prolonged blockade. This action may result from desensitization of acetylcholine receptors and other factors.

PHARMACOTHERAPEUTICS

Succinylcholine is the drug of choice for short-term muscle relaxation, such as during intubation and ECT.

succinylcholine (Anectine, Quelicin, Sucostrin). Succinylcholine is used primarily to induce short-term muscle relaxation.
Usual adult dosage: for short procedures or treatments, 0.3 to 1.1 mg/kg of body weight; for longer procedures or treatments, continuous I.V. infusion of 0.1% to 0.2% solution at a rate of 0.5 to 10.0 mg/minute for up to 1 hour, then 0.04 to 0.07 mg/kg of body weight.

Drug interactions
The action of succinylcholine is potentiated by a number of anesthetics and antibiotics. However, succinylcholine does not interact with most drugs that alter serum electrolyte levels. In contrast to their interaction with nondepolarizing blockers, anticholinesterases increase succinylcholine blockade.

ADVERSE DRUG REACTIONS

The primary adverse drug reactions to succinylcholine are the same as those to the nondepolarizing blocking agents: prolonged apnea and cardiovascular alterations.

Patients commonly experience muscle pain from the fasciculations that occur in Phase I. These also may cause myoglobinemia and myoglobinuria, especially in children. The concomitant rise in the serum potassium level can be dangerous to patients with renal or neuromuscular disorders. The transient elevation of intraocular pressure that occurs during Phase I may be harmful to patients with previously elevated intraocular pressure.

Neuromuscular blockade may be potentiated by certain genetic predispositions, such as a low pseudocholinesterase level and the tendency to develop malignant hyperthermia. A low pseudocholinesterase level also is present in liver disorders because pseudocholinesterase is synthesized in the liver. To determine the patient's sensitivity to succinylcholine, an initial test dose of 10 mg may be administered.

Phase II blockade may occur with repeated doses of succinylcholine.

NURSING PROCESS APPLICATION

The following information illustrates general application of the nursing process for a patient who is receiving succinylcholine.

Assessment
• Review the patient's history for conditions that contraindicate the use of succinylcholine, such as malignant hyperthermia, known sensitivity, acute narrow-angle glaucoma, or penetrating eye injuries.
• Review the patient's history for conditions that require cautious use of succinylcholine, such as a renal, pulmonary, or neuromuscular disorder; fluid and electrolyte imbalance; or increased intraocular pressure.
• Assess the patient for adverse reactions to succinylcholine, such as apnea, cardiovascular alterations, and tachyphylaxis.
• Assess the patient for muscle fasciculations.
• Assess the patient's respiratory rate and pattern and auscultate breath sounds.
• Evaluate the patient's and family's knowledge about succinylcholine.

Nursing diagnoses
The following examples represent appropriate nursing diagnoses for a patient receiving succinylcholine.
• Potential for injury related to a preexisting condition that contraindicates the use of succinylcholine
• Potential for injury related to a preexisting condition that requires cautious use of succinylcholine
• Potential for injury related to adverse drug reactions
• Pain related to muscle fasciculation during Phase I of succinylcholine's action
• Ineffective breathing pattern related to succinylcholine's effect on respiratory muscles
• Knowledge deficit related to succinylcholine

Planning and implementation
• Do not administer succinylcholine to a patient with a condition that contraindicates its use.
• Administer succinylcholine cautiously to a patient at risk because of a preexisting condition.
• Monitor the patient for adverse reactions periodically. Keep in mind that genetic factors, such as a low pseudo-

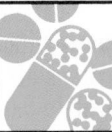

SELECTED MAJOR DRUGS

Neuromuscular blocking agents

Physicians prescribe neuromuscular blocking agents to induce short- and long-term muscle relaxation. Patients receiving these agents must be monitored closely because of drug effects. Patients may require ventilatory support.

DRUG	MAJOR INDICATIONS	USUAL ADULT DOSAGES	CONTRAINDICATIONS AND PRECAUTIONS
Nondepolarizing blocking agents			
pancuronium	Adjunct to anesthesia	0.04 to 0.1 mg/kg of body weight I.V.; repeat doses of 0.01 to 0.02 mg/kg every 20 to 60 minutes as needed.	• Know that pancuronium is contraindicated in a patient with bromide hypersensitivity. • Administer with caution to a patient with renal, hepatic, cardiac, or pulmonary impairment; fluid and electrolyte imbalance; or myasthenia gravis.
	Assistance in intubation and mechanical ventilation	0.06 to 0.1 mg/kg of body weight I.V. bolus	
tubocurarine	Adjunct to anesthesia Assistance in intubation and mechanical ventilation Prevention of trauma during electroconvulsive therapy (ECT)	For anesthesia, intubation, and ventilation, 6 to 9 mg I.V. slowly over 60 to 90 seconds initially, then 3 to 4.5 mg in 3 to 5 minutes; for electroshock therapy, 0.165 mg/kg of body weight I.V. slowly	• Administer with caution to a patient with renal, hepatic, cardiac, or pulmonary impairment; fluid and electrolyte imbalance; or myasthenia gravis. Also use caution in a patient undergoing cesarean delivery.
Depolarizing blocking agents			
succinylcholine	Procedures that facilitate intubation or orthopedic manipulation Prevention of trauma during ECT	For short procedures or treatments, 0.3 to 1.1 mg/kg of body weight I.V.; then 0.04 to 0.07 mg/kg of body weight as needed; for longer procedures or treatments, continuous I.V. infusion of 0.1% to 0.2% solution at a rate of 0.5 to 10 mg/min for up to 1 hour.	• Know that succinylcholine is contraindicated in a patient with malignant hyperthermia, known hypersensitivity to the drug, acute narrow-angle glaucoma, penetrating eye injury, myopathy (with elevated creatinine phosphokinase) and genetic plasma pseudocholinesterase. • Administer with caution to a patient with a renal, pulmonary, or neuromuscular disorder; fluid and electrolyte imbalance; increased intraocular pressure; or a family history of malignant hyperthermia or low serum pseudocholinesterase levels.

cholinesterase level and a tendency to develop malignant hyperthermia, may potentiate neuromuscular blockade.
• Monitor the patient's vital signs frequently throughout succinylcholine infusion.
• Monitor the serum potassium level closely during succinylcholine infusion, particularly in a patient with a renal or neuromuscular disorder.
• *Notify the physician immediately if adverse reactions occur. Be prepared to give emergency care according to health care facility guidelines.*
• *Reassure the patient that pain from Phase I of succinylcholine's action is transient.*
• *Maintain a patent airway for the patient.*

• *Keep endotracheal equipment, oxygen, suction equipment, and a mechanical ventilator available for respiratory support.*
• *Check the patient's respiratory rate and pattern every 5 to 10 minutes during infusion.*
• *Monitor the patient closely until recovery from neuromuscular blockade is complete. Signs of complete recovery include a renewed ability to cough and a return to previous levels of muscle strength on hand-grip and head-lift tests.*
• Notify the physician of any change in the patient's respiratory status.

Patient teaching
• Teach the patient and family about succinylcholine.
• Encourage the patient and family to ask questions about succinylcholine before administration, if possible.

• Inform the patient and family fully of all procedures in advance. Provide reassurance that the nurse will monitor the patient continually during succinylcholine administration.

Evaluation

The following examples represent appropriate evaluation statements for a patient receiving succinylcholine.

• The patient has no conditions that contraindicate succinylcholine administration.

• The patient exhibits no signs of complications in the preexisting condition linked to succinylcholine.

• The patient displays no adverse reactions to succinylcholine.

• The patient reports transient pain during succinylcholine administration.

• The patient maintains adequate ventilation.

• The patient and family express an accurate understanding of the points taught about succinylcholine.

• The patient and family ask appropriate questions about succinylcholine before its administration.

CHAPTER SUMMARY

Chapter 17 discussed nondepolarizing and depolarizing neuromuscular blocking agents, which are used to relax the skeletal muscles by disrupting the transmission of nerve impulses. Here are the chapter highlights.

• Neuromuscular blocking agents relax skeletal muscles by disrupting nerve impulse transmission. They have three major uses: to relax skeletal muscles during surgery, to reduce the intensity of muscle spasms in drug-induced or electrically induced convulsions, or to manage patients who are fighting mechanical ventilation.

• The two classes of neuromuscular blocking agents are nondepolarizing and depolarizing blocking agents.

• The nondepolarizing blocking agents are used when intermediate or prolonged duration of action is required. They compete with acetylcholine at the cholinergic receptor sites of the skeletal muscle membrane, blocking the depolarization required for muscle contraction. This class is composed of curare alkaloids and their synthetic derivatives.

• Initially, the depolarizing blocking agent acts like acetylcholine and results in depolarization of the postsynaptic membrane. However, unlike acetylcholine, the depolarizing agent is not inactivated by cholinesterase. Therefore, the depolarization lasts longer. With continued drug use, the depolarizing blocking action changes to a nondepolarizing blocking action. Succinylcholine is the drug of choice for short-term muscle relaxation.

• The nurse must monitor the vital functions of any patient receiving these drugs. The maintenance of respiratory function is the top priority. However, because these drugs also alter cardiovascular function and fluid and electrolyte balance, careful monitoring is required.

STUDY QUESTIONS

See Appendix 1 for answers.

1. Evelyn Thomas, age 35, is admitted to the intensive care unit after a craniotomy for a subarachnoid hemorrhage. When placed on a mechanical ventilator, she fights it, which raises her PCO_2 level and intracranial pressure. To help maintain adequate ventilation, the physician orders the neuromuscular blocking agent pancuronium (Pavulon) 0.1 mg/kg of body weight. What is the mechanism of action of pancuronium?
(a) It competes with acetylcholine at cholinergic receptor sites in the skeletal muscle.
(b) It stimulates muscarinic receptors at effector organs.
(c) It inhibits the action of cholinesterase at the motor end plate.
(d) It enhances the muscle's ability to respond to the neurotransmitter.

2. After administering pancuronium to Ms. Thomas, the nurse can expect paralysis to occur in which sequence?
(a) diaphragm, arms, and legs
(b) neck, diaphragm, and legs
(c) diaphragm, eyes, and legs
(d) face, arms, and diaphragm

3. Throughout pancuronium therapy, Ms. Thomas will be able to perceive pain. What accounts for this?
(a) Pancuronium reduces the production of endogenous endorphins.
(b) Pancuronium does not cross the blood-brain barrier.
(c) Pancuronium stimulates the reticular-activating system.
(d) Pancuronium increases the amount of serotonin in the sustantia gelantinosa.

4. The nurse should give which problem top priority when Ms. Thomas is receiving pancuronium?
(a) pain
(b) fluid volume excess
(c) ineffective breathing pattern
(d) altered tissue perfusion

5. Alice Brown, age 40, has depression, for which her psychiatrist prescribes ECT. Before therapy, Ms. Brown receives succinylcholine. Why is succinylcholine administered before ECT?
(a) to sedate the patient
(b) to provide short-term muscle relaxation
(c) to relieve pain
(d) to increase muscle contractions

6. After ECT, Ms. Brown complains of muscle pain. What is the most likely cause of this reaction?
(a) action of succinylcholine in Phase I
(b) action of succinylcholine in Phase II
(c) succinylcholine toxicity
(d) adverse effects of ECT

SELECTED REFERENCES

AHFS drug information 90. (1990). Bethesda, MD: American Society of Hospital Pharmacists.

Bruton-Maree, N. (1989). Neuromuscular blocking drugs. *Journal of Neuroscience Nursing,* 21(3), 198-200.

Clinton, J., and Ruiz, E. (1988). Emergency airway management: Methods to meet the challenge. *Topics in Emergency Medicine,* 10(1), 31-41.

Hansten, P., and Horn, J. (1989). *Drug interactions.* Philadelphia: Lea & Febiger.

Loper, K., Butler, S., Nessly, M., and Wild, L. (1989). Paralyzed with pain: The need for education. *Pain,* 37(3), 315-316.

Miyagawa, C. (1987). Sedation of the mechanically ventilated patient in the intensive care unit. *Respiratory Care,* 32(9), 792-800.

DRUGS TO TREAT NEUROLOGIC AND NEUROMUSCULAR SYSTEM DISORDERS

Unit Four discusses pharmacologic agents used to treat neurologic and neuromuscular system disorders, such as musculoskeletal spasms, Parkinson's disease, and seizure disorders. These agents include skeletal muscle relaxing, antiparkinsonian, and anticonvulsant agents. Although their pharmacokinetics, pharmacodynamics, and pharmacotherapeutics vary greatly, they all affect the neurologic or neuromuscular system.

To help the nurse understand the actions and uses of these agents, this introduction provides an overview of the anatomy and physiology of the nervous system.

ANATOMY OF THE NERVOUS SYSTEM

The nervous system is composed of the central and peripheral divisions. The central nervous system (CNS) consists of the brain and spinal cord. (For an illustration of the components, see *Structures of the central nervous system,* page 264.)

The brain is composed of the cerebrum, diencephalon, cerebellum, and brain stem. Two structurally matched hemispheres make up the cerebrum, the largest portion of the brain. Each hemisphere contains four lobes — frontal, parietal, temporal, and occipital. The surface of the cerebrum (cortex) is composed of gray matter made of neuron cell bodies, axon terminals, and dendrites. The interior of the cerebrum is composed of white matter made of basal ganglia. The corpus callosum facilitates communication between corresponding areas in the two hemispheres.

The diencephalon, located anterior to the brain stem, includes the hypothalamus and thalamus. The cerebellum lies at the base of the brain below the occipital lobes of the cerebrum. The brain stem, composed of the midbrain, pons, and medulla oblongata, relays all messages between the upper and lower levels of the nervous system; cranial nerves III through XII originate there.

The spinal cord serves as a communication pathway between the brain and the peripheral nervous system, and its gray matter functions as a reflex center for spinal reflexes. It joins the brain stem at the level of the foramen magnum and terminates near the second lumbar vertebra. The spinal cord comprises a central H-shaped mass of gray matter divided into dorsal (or posterior) and ventral (or anterior) horns. Cell bodies in the dorsal horn relay sensory (afferent) impulses, and those in the ventral horn relay motor (efferent) impulses. White matter surrounding these horns consists of myelinated axons of sensory and motor nerves grouped in ascending and descending tracts. (For a depiction of these structures, see *Cross section of the spinal cord,* page 265.)

The peripheral nervous system is composed of the cranial and spinal nerves, which carry sensory messages from organs and tissues to the brain and motor instructions from the brain to target organs.

The 12 pairs of cranial nerves provide for the sensory and motor needs primarily of the head but also of the neck, chest, and abdomen. Cranial nerves I and II originate in the frontal lobe; III through XII originate in the brain stem.

The 31 pairs of spinal nerves originate in the spinal cord. These paired nerves include 8 cervical, 12 thoracic, 5 lumbar, 5 sacral, and 1 coccygeal. Cervical 3 to thoracic 2 supply the upper extremities; thoracic 9 through 12 supply the lower extremities.

PHYSIOLOGY OF THE NERVOUS SYSTEM

The nervous system governs all movement, sensation, thought, and emotion. Two types of cells constitute the nervous system: neuroglial cells and neurons. Neuroglial cells perform specialized support functions, such as supplying nutrients to the neurons, assisting in the production of cerebrospinal fluid, and providing electrical insulation for the axons of the CNS neurons.

The neuron consists of a cell body and two types of appendages — a long one (an axon) and one or more shorter ones (dendrites). Cell bodies form the gray matter in the brain, brain stem, and spinal cord. The axon transmits impulses from the cell body to other neurons, whereas

Glossary

Absence seizure: generalized seizure characterized by an abrupt loss of consciousness or unawareness with staring; also called petit mal seizure.

Actin: protein in muscle filaments that acts with myosin to contract and relax muscle.

Agonist: drug that has an affinity for a receptor and enhances or stimulates the receptor's functional properties.

Akinesia: abnormal absence of movement.

Ataxia: impaired ability to coordinate movement.

Atonic seizure: generalized seizure accompanied by akinesia and usually loss of consciousness.

Axon: cylindrical extension of a nerve cell that carries impulses away from the neuron cell body.

Clonic seizure: generalized seizure characterized by rhythmic contraction and relaxation of muscles, loss of consciousness, and marked autonomic signs and symptoms.

Dendrite: branching process that extends from the nerve cell and carries impulses to the cell body.

Dopamine: neurotransmitter produced by the decarboxylation of dopa, an intermediate product in norepinephrine synthesis.

Dopaminergic: stimulated, activated, or transmitted by dopamine.

Dyskinesia: impaired power of voluntary movement resulting in fragmentary or incomplete movements.

Dystonia: disordered muscle tone.

Electroencephalogram: graphic recording of electrical currents produced in the brain.

Epilepsy: disorder characterized by one or more of the following signs and symptoms: paroxysmally recurring impairment or loss of consciousness, involuntary excess or cessation of muscle movements, psychic or sensory disturbances, and derangement of the autonomic nervous system.

Ganglion: group of nerve cell bodies located outside the central nervous system.

Generalized seizure: bilaterally symmetrical, violent, involuntary contractions of voluntary muscles involving loss of consciousness; more specifically classified as absence, myoclonic, clonic, tonic, tonic-clonic, or atonic seizure.

Hyperkinesia: abnormally increased motor function or activity.

Hyperpyrexia: highly elevated body temperature.

Hypotonia: abnormally decreased muscle tone, tension, or activity.

Interneuron: any neuron in a chain of neurons that is situated between the primary afferent neuron and the final motor neuron.

Monoamine oxidase (MAO) inhibitor: substance that opposes the action of monoamine oxidase, an enzyme in the nerve endings that deaminates, or breaks down, catecholamines.

Myoclonic seizure: generalized seizure characterized by bilaterally symmetrical, involuntary lightning jerks of voluntary muscles lasting from seconds to minutes; consciousness is maintained.

Myofibril: slender, threadlike contractile element that parallels the long axis of a muscle fiber.

Myosin: abundant muscle protein that acts with actin to produce muscle contraction and relaxation.

Neuromuscular junction: joining of a nerve ending and a muscle fiber at the fiber's midpoint so that action potential in the fiber travels bidirectionally.

Neurotransmitter: chemical substance secreted by the neuron at the synapse that acts on receptor proteins in the membrane of the adjacent neuron to stimulate, inhibit, or modify the neuron's activity.

Parkinson's disease: disorder characterized by muscular rigidity, immobile facies, tremors that disappear upon volitional movement, and loss of associated autonomic movement and salivation.

Partial seizure: focal or local violent, involuntary contractions of voluntary muscles; more specifically classified as simple or complex.

Relaxant: agent that reduces or lessens muscle tension.

Rigidity: abnormal muscle stiffness or inflexibility.

Sarcolemma: delicate elastic sheath that surrounds a striated muscle fiber.

Sarcoplasmic reticulum: network of tubular and flat vesicular structures that conduct electrical impulses and coordinate the contraction of myofibrils.

Spasm: sudden, violent, involuntary contraction of a muscle or group of muscles, accompanied by pain, dysfunction, involuntary movement, and distortion.

Spasticity: increased muscle tension resulting in continually increased resistance to stretching.

Status epilepticus: series of rapidly repeated epileptic seizures without periods of consciousness separating them.

Synapse: area of contact between the processes of two adjacent neurons where an impulse is transmitted.

Synaptic cleft: space between a nerve fiber terminal and the fiber membrane.

Tonic-clonic seizure: generalized seizure characterized by contraction of all skeletal muscles in rhythmic alternating tonic and clonic patterns, followed by depression of all central functions; also known as grand mal seizure.

Tonic seizure: generalized seizure characterized by an abrupt increase in muscle tone, resulting in contraction, loss of consciousness, and marked autonomic signs and symptoms.

Tremor: involuntary trembling or quivering.

---

dendrites receive impulses from nearby cells and conduct them toward the cell body.

Neurons perform one of three roles in transmitting impulses: reception of sensory stimuli, transmission of motor responses, or integration of activities and coordination of communication between body parts. Sensory neurons carry stimuli from the peripheral sensory organs, such as the skin, to the spinal cord and brain. Motor neurons carry impulses from the brain and spinal cord to tissues and organs. Interneurons relay impulses within the CNS.

All human functions rely on the electrical and chemical transmission of impulses from neuron to neuron. This trans-

Structures of the central nervous system

The brain, brain stem, and spinal cord function synergistically to control movement, sensation, thought, and emotion. Major structures and their functions are shown below.

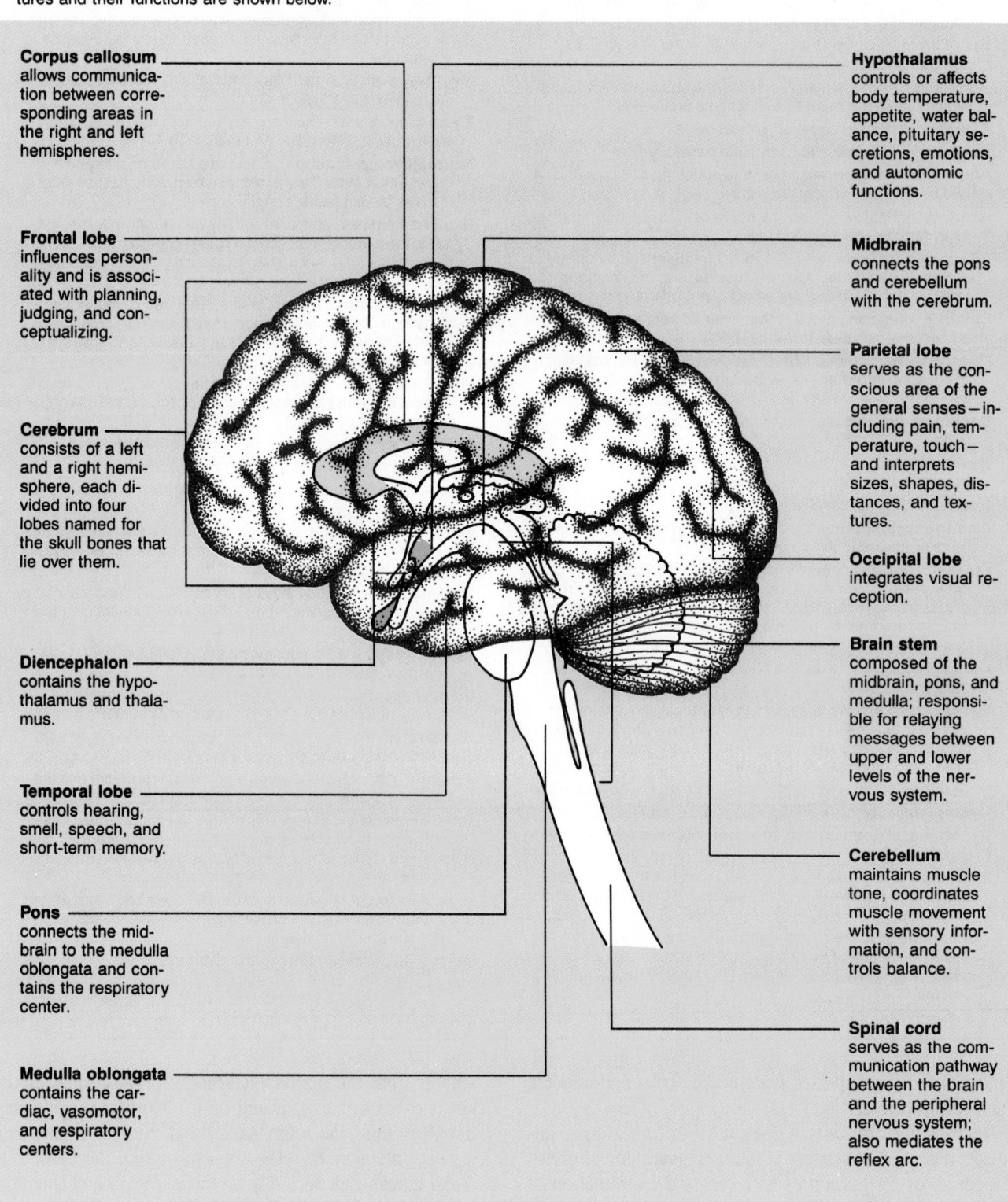

Corpus callosum allows communication between corresponding areas in the right and left hemispheres.

Frontal lobe influences personality and is associated with planning, judging, and conceptualizing.

Cerebrum consists of a left and a right hemisphere, each divided into four lobes named for the skull bones that lie over them.

Diencephalon contains the hypothalamus and thalamus.

Temporal lobe controls hearing, smell, speech, and short-term memory.

Pons connects the midbrain to the medulla oblongata and contains the respiratory center.

Medulla oblongata contains the cardiac, vasomotor, and respiratory centers.

Hypothalamus controls or affects body temperature, appetite, water balance, pituitary secretions, emotions, and autonomic functions.

Midbrain connects the pons and cerebellum with the cerebrum.

Parietal lobe serves as the conscious area of the general senses—including pain, temperature, touch—and interprets sizes, shapes, distances, and textures.

Occipital lobe integrates visual reception.

Brain stem composed of the midbrain, pons, and medulla; responsible for relaying messages between upper and lower levels of the nervous system.

Cerebellum maintains muscle tone, coordinates muscle movement with sensory information, and controls balance.

Spinal cord serves as the communication pathway between the brain and the peripheral nervous system; also mediates the reflex arc.

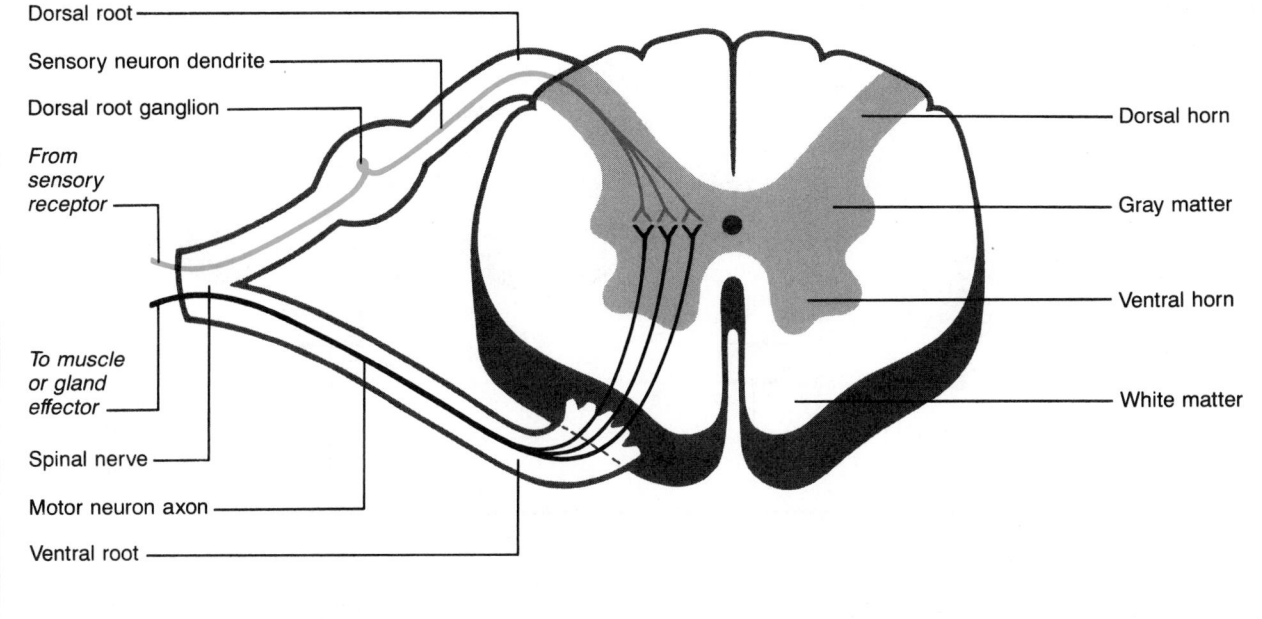

Cross section of the spinal cord

The spinal cord consists of gray matter, including the ventral and dorsal horn, surrounded by white matter. White matter contains many nerve fiber tracts that relay messages to and from the brain. When a peripheral nerve is stimulated, the impulse travels to the dorsal root ganglion through the sensory neuron dendrite to the dorsal horn. The impulse travels to the brain via the nerve fiber tracts. Then the brain's responses travel down the spinal cord and out the ventral root to the motor neuron axon. A motor response results.

Dorsal root

Sensory neuron dendrite

Dorsal root ganglion

From sensory receptor

To muscle or gland effector

Spinal nerve

Motor neuron axon

Ventral root

Dorsal horn

Gray matter

Ventral horn

White matter

---

mission occurs across a synapse, or the contact point between two neurons. Neurotransmission is facilitated by neurotransmitters, such as acetylcholine and dopamine. (For an illustration of this process, see *Neurotransmission,* page 266.)

OVERVIEW OF CHAPTERS

The chapters in Unit Four focus on drugs used to treat neurologic and neuromuscular system disorders. These drugs include skeletal muscle relaxing, antiparkinsonian, and anticonvulsant agents.

Chapter 18
Skeletal Muscle Relaxing Agents

Chapter 18 discusses centrally and peripherally acting agents used to treat musculoskeletal spasms and spasticity. Beginning with an overview of normal muscle physiology, the chapter provides a clinical delineation of musculoskeletal spasms and spasticity. Next it details the mechanisms of action of the two types of muscle relaxing agents. Then it presents pharmacotherapeutic uses of the various agents, followed by related nursing care, including patient teaching.

Chapter 19
Antiparkinsonian Agents

Chapter 19 describes Parkinson's disease and the drugs in the two major classes used to treat it: the synthetic anticholinergic agents and the dopaminergic agents. It emphasizes the clinical benefits for the patient and potential adverse reactions. It also explores associated nursing implications and specific nursing interventions, including patient teaching.

Chapter 20
Anticonvulsant Agents

The chapter introduction discusses the four factors used to select an anticonvulsant. Then it presents the international classification system for seizure disorders, including clinical characteristics. The remainder of Chapter 20 discusses the classes of anticonvulsants: hydantoins, barbiturates, iminostilbenes, benzodiazepines, succinimides, and valproic acid. For each drug, it delineates the specific clinical uses and other pharmacologic properties. It also highlights application of the nursing process when caring for a patient receiving these drugs.

Neurotransmission

Neurotransmission is the conduction of impulses across the synapse. It involves the presynaptic terminal of the transmitter neuron, the target receptor neuron (postsynaptic receptor), and the synaptic cleft between the two neurons. Numerous presynaptic terminals branch from the tips of axons. These terminals contain synaptic vesicles, which, when stimulated, release neurotransmitter substances into the synaptic cleft to excite or inhibit the target receptor neuron. On a larger scale, the interneuron transmits impulses to the sensory neuron and the motor neuron, as shown below.

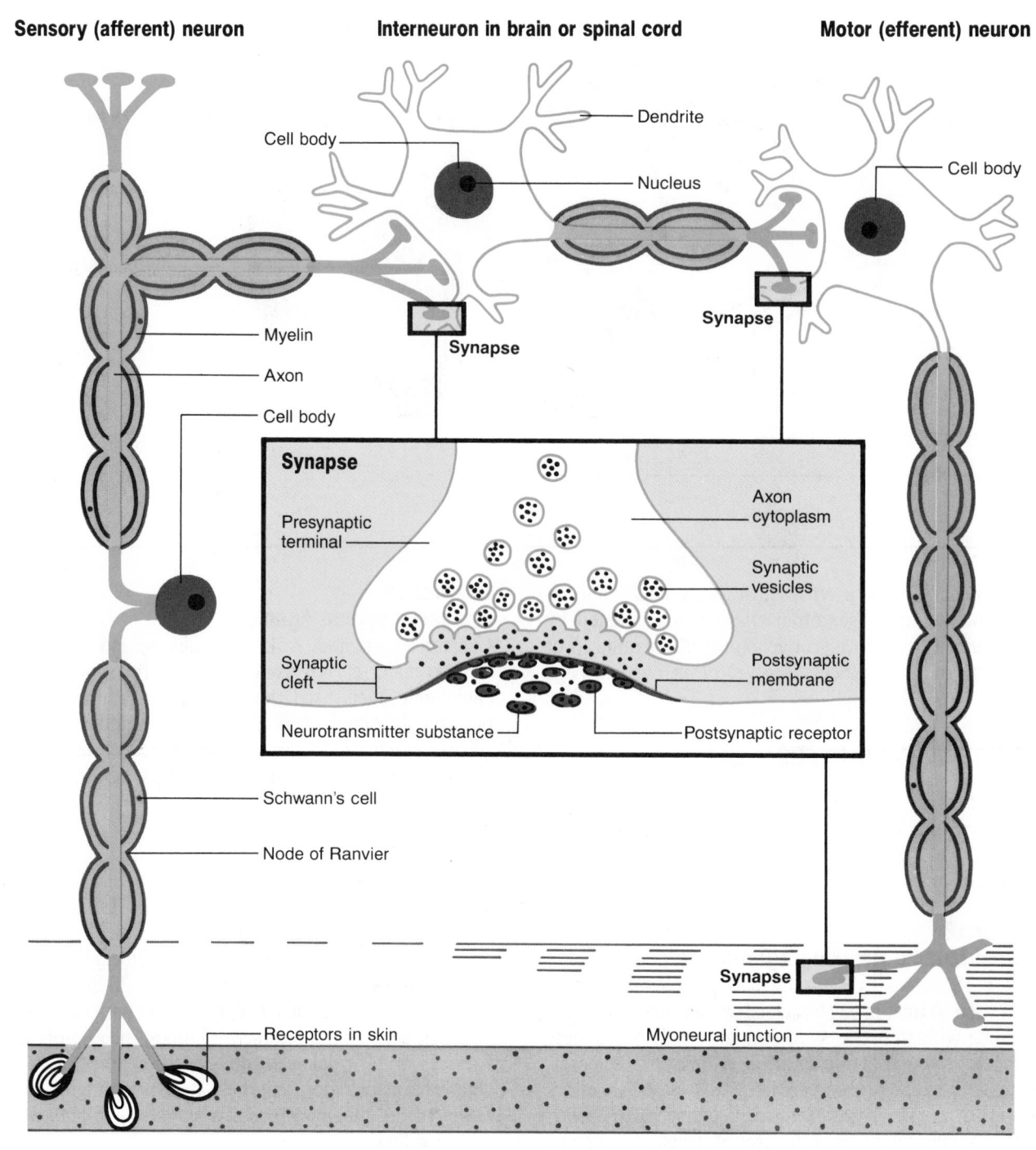

Sensory (afferent) neuron

Interneuron in brain or spinal cord

Motor (efferent) neuron

Cell body

Dendrite

Nucleus

Cell body

Myelin

Axon

Cell body

Synapse

Synapse

Synapse

Presynaptic terminal

Axon cytoplasm

Synaptic vesicles

Synaptic cleft

Postsynaptic membrane

Neurotransmitter substance

Postsynaptic receptor

Schwann's cell

Node of Ranvier

Synapse

Receptors in skin

Myoneural junction

SKELETAL MUSCLE RELAXING AGENTS

OBJECTIVES

After reading and studying this chapter, the student should be able to:

1. Discuss the physiology of skeletal muscle contraction.
2. Define spasm and spasticity.
3. Differentiate among the skeletal muscle relaxing agents that act centrally and those that act peripherally.
4. Describe the mechanism of action of the centrally and peripherally acting skeletal muscle relaxing agents.
5. List the therapeutic uses for the various groups of skeletal muscle relaxing agents.
6. Describe the adverse reactions that occur when these agents are given with central nervous system (CNS) depressants.
7. Describe how to apply the nursing process when caring for a patient who is receiving a skeletal muscle relaxing agent.

INTRODUCTION

Skeletal muscle relaxing agents relieve musculoskeletal pain or spasm and severe musculoskeletal spasticity. They are used to treat acute, painful musculoskeletal conditions and the muscle spasticity associated with multiple sclerosis, cerebral palsy, cerebrovascular accident, and spinal cord injuries. Chapter 18 discusses the two main classes of skeletal muscle relaxing agents — centrally acting and peripherally acting — and baclofen and diazepam, two other drugs that are used to manage musculoskeletal disorders.

Physiology of skeletal muscle contraction

Skeletal muscles are innervated by large nerve fibers containing motor neurons that originate in the anterior horns of the spinal cord, but the neurotransmitters that relay excitatory or inhibitory signals to the spinal motor neurons are not understood completely. Five have been identi-

fied — acetylcholine, norepinephrine, serotonin, glycine, and gamma-aminobutyric acid (GABA); of them, acetylcholine is an excitatory neurotransmitter, and glycine and GABA are inhibitory.

Nerve endings join muscle fibers at the neuromuscular junction. Skeletal muscles themselves are made up of muscle fibers composed of actin and myosin filaments — protein molecule compounds that are responsible for muscle contraction. These filaments are embedded in the sarcoplasm, which also holds a network of tubules, the sarcoplasmic reticulum. Skeletal muscle contraction apparently is triggered by high concentrations of sodium, which trigger the release of calcium ions from the sarcoplasmic reticulum. (For an illustration of this process, see Chapter 17, Neuromuscular Blocking Agents.)

Some drugs that relieve skeletal muscle spasticity are believed to act in the spinal cord to alter neurotransmitter function; others act peripherally on the skeletal muscle itself. The centrally acting skeletal muscle relaxants probably inhibit interneuron activity in the spinal cord and the brain.

Acute musculoskeletal spasms and spasticity

Severe cold, lack of blood flow to a muscle, or overexertion can elicit pain or other sensory impulses that are transmitted by the posterior sensory nerve fibers to the spinal cord and the higher levels of the CNS. These sensory impulses may cause a reflex (involuntary) muscle contraction, or spasm. The muscle contraction further stimulates the sensory receptors to a more intense contraction, establishing a cycle. The centrally acting muscle relaxants are believed to break this cycle by acting as CNS depressants.

Spasticity is a motor disorder characterized by an increase in muscle tone from hyperexcitability of the anterior motor neurons. This hyperexcitability may arise from a lack of inhibition or from excess stimulation produced by signals transmitted from the brain through the interneurons

SELECTED NURSING DIAGNOSES

Skeletal muscle relaxing agents

The following nursing diagnoses address representative problems and etiologies that a nurse may encounter when caring for a patient who is receiving a skeletal muscle relaxing agent. Some of these nursing diagnoses contain generalized etiologies, which the nurse must individualize based on the patient's needs. (For some nursing diagnoses and related interventions for each drug class, see the "Nursing Process Application" sections of the chapter.)

- Altered thought processes related to psychiatric disturbances caused by a skeletal muscle relaxing agent
- Constipation related to the adverse GI effects of a skeletal muscle relaxing agent
- Diarrhea related to the adverse GI effects of a skeletal muscle relaxing agent
- Fluid volume deficit related to nausea, vomiting, or diarrhea caused by a skeletal muscle relaxant
- Impaired adjustment related to physical and psychological dependence on a centrally acting skeletal muscle relaxant
- Impaired gas exchange related to respiratory depression caused by a skeletal muscle relaxant
- Impaired physical mobility related to flaccid paralysis caused by a centrally acting skeletal muscle relaxing agent
- Impaired physical mobility related to ineffectiveness of dantrolene
- Knowledge deficit related to the prescribed skeletal muscle relaxing agent
- Pain related to ineffectiveness of a centrally acting skeletal muscle relaxant
- Potential activity intolerance related to possible ineffectiveness of baclofen or another skeletal muscle relaxing agent
- Potential for injury related to a preexisting condition that contraindicates the use of a skeletal muscle relaxing agent
- Potential for injury related to a preexisting condition that requires cautious use of a skeletal muscle relaxing agent
- Potential for injury related to adverse drug reactions
- Potential for injury related to drug interactions with the prescribed skeletal muscle relaxing agent
- Potential for trauma related to drowsiness or dizziness caused by a skeletal muscle relaxing agent
- Sensory-perceptual alteration (visual, gustatory, or auditory) related to the adverse effects of a skeletal muscle relaxing agent
- Urinary retention related to the anticholinergic effects of a skeletal muscle relaxing agent

in the spinal cord to the anterior motor neurons. Spasticity is associated with various clinical conditions, called upper motor neuron disorders, including multiple sclerosis, cerebral palsy, cerebrovascular accident (stroke), and spinal cord injuries. The skeletal muscle relaxants vary in their efficacy; they apparently reduce spasticity by reducing hyperexcitability.

For a summary of representative drugs, see *Selected major drugs: Skeletal muscle relaxing agents,* page 277. For a listing of applicable nursing diagnoses that the nurse may formulate when caring for a patient receiving these agents, see *Selected nursing diagnoses: Skeletal muscle relaxing agents.* For detailed information on applying the nursing process, see Chapter 6, The Nursing Process and Drug Therapy.

CENTRALLY ACTING SKELETAL MUSCLE RELAXANTS

Such conditions as trauma, inflammation, anxiety, and pain can be associated with acute muscle spasms. The following drugs may relieve such spasms: carisoprodol, chlorphenesin carbamate, chlorzoxazone, cyclobenzaprine hydrochloride, metaxalone, methocarbamol, and orphenadrine citrate. However, they are ineffective in treating spasticity associated with chronic neurologic disease. Lack of controlled clinical trials makes assessing these agents difficult.

PHARMACOKINETICS

Currently, the pharmacokinetic properties of the centrally acting skeletal muscle relaxants are not well defined. In general, these drugs are absorbed from the gastrointestinal (GI) tract, widely distributed in the body, metabolized in the liver, and excreted by the kidneys. The centrally acting muscle relaxants have an onset of action between 30 and 60 minutes; their duration of action varies from 3 to 24 hours. (For detailed information, see *Pharmacokinetics of the centrally acting skeletal muscle relaxants.*)

PHARMACODYNAMICS

The precise mechanism of action of these drugs is unknown. However, they are known to be CNS depressants.

Mechanism of action
The skeletal muscle relaxant effects of the centrally acting agents are minimal and may be related to their sedative effects. The drugs do not relax skeletal muscle directly or depress neuronal conduction, neuromuscular transmission, or muscle excitability.

Carisoprodol is related structurally to meprobamate, a CNS depressant. Chlorphenesin and methocarbamol are related chemically to each other, and both have sedative effects. Chlorzoxazone is a benzoxazole derivative unre-

Pharmacokinetics of the centrally acting skeletal muscle relaxants

As this chart shows, the onset of action of the centrally acting skeletal muscle relaxants is 30 minutes to 1 hour. Cyclobenzaprine has the longest duration of action at 12 to 24 hours.

DRUG	ONSET OF ACTION	TIME TO PEAK CONCENTRATION	DURATION OF ACTION
carisoprodol	30 minutes	4 hours	4 to 6 hours
chlorphenesin	Not available	1 to 3 hours	4 to 6 hours
chlorzoxazone	1 hour	3 to 4 hours	3 to 4 hours
cyclobenzaprine	1 hour	4 to 8 hours	12 to 24 hours
metaxalone	1 hour	2 hours	4 to 6 hours
methocarbamol	30 minutes	1 to 2 hours	Not available
orphenadrine	1 hour	2 hours	4 to 6 hours

lated to the other centrally acting skeletal muscle relaxants, but with similar activity. Cyclobenzaprine is related structurally to the tricyclic antidepressants, and, like them, it enhances the effects of norepinephrine and has anticholinergic effects. Metaxalone is an oxazolidinone derivative. Oxazolidinone is a cyclic carbamate of methocarbamol.

Orphenadrine is an anticholinergic agent that may reduce skeletal muscle spasm through an atropine-like central action. It also blocks the effects of the excitatory neurotransmitter acetylcholine. Although orphenadrine does not relax skeletal muscle directly, it may produce analgesic effects. Orphenadrine also produces antihistaminic effects, but it stimulates rather than depresses the CNS.

PHARMACOTHERAPEUTICS

The centrally acting skeletal muscle relaxants are used as adjuncts to rest and physical therapy in treating acute, painful musculoskeletal conditions. Their beneficial effects probably derive from their sedative properties, and they do not appear to be as effective as diazepam for treating musculoskeletal pain. They are ineffective in treating skeletal muscle hyperactivity secondary to such chronic neurologic disorders as cerebral palsy.

carisoprodol (Soma). Carisoprodol is used to treat acute, painful musculoskeletal conditions.
Usual adult dosage: 350 mg P.O. t.i.d. and h.s.

chlorphenesin carbamate (Maolate). Used for short-term treatment of acute, painful musculoskeletal conditions, chlorphenesin should not be given for more than 8 weeks.

Usual adult dosage: 800 mg P.O. t.i.d. until a beneficial response is obtained; then the dosage should be reduced to the lowest effective level, with maintenance at 400 mg P.O. q.i.d.

chlorzoxazone (Paraflex). Used to treat acute, painful musculoskeletal conditions or severe muscle spasm, chlorzoxazone should be taken with food to avoid gastric distress.
Usual adult dosage: for musculoskeletal conditions, 250 mg P.O. t.i.d. or q.i.d.; for spasm, 500 mg t.i.d. or q.i.d. initially, then increased up to 750 mg P.O. t.i.d. or q.i.d. until a beneficial response is obtained, then reduced to the lowest effective level.

cyclobenzaprine hydrochloride (Flexeril). Used for short-term treatment of muscle spasm, cyclobenzaprine should not be given for more than 3 weeks.
Usual adult dosage: 10 mg P.O. b.i.d. to q.i.d.; increased to a maximum of 60 mg daily, if needed.

metaxalone (Skelaxin). Metaxalone is used to treat acute, painful musculoskeletal conditions.
Usual adult dosage: 800 mg P.O. t.i.d. or q.i.d.

methocarbamol (Robaxin). Used to treat acute, painful musculoskeletal conditions, methocarbamol also is used as supportive therapy in tetanus management.
Usual adult dosage: for musculoskeletal conditions, initially 1.5 to 2 g P.O. q.i.d. for 48 to 72 hours, with maintenance at 4 to 4.5 g P.O. daily in three to six divided doses, or not more than 500 mg (5 ml) I.M. into each buttock every 8 hours, or 1 to 3 g (10 to 30 ml) I.V. daily directly into I.V. tubing at 3 ml/minute, or 1 g in 250 ml of D₅W or

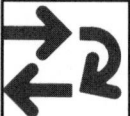

DRUG INTERACTIONS

Centrally acting skeletal muscle relaxants

Drug interactions involving the centrally acting skeletal muscle relaxants are infrequent; they usually result from simultaneous administration of central nervous system (CNS) depressant drugs, including alcohol.

DRUG	INTERACTING DRUGS	POSSIBLE EFFECTS	NURSING IMPLICATIONS
carisoprodol, chlorphenesin, chlorzoxazone, cyclobenzaprine, metaxalone, methocarbamol, orphenadrine	CNS depressants (alcohol, narcotics, barbiturates, anticonvulsants, tricyclic antidepressants, antianxiety agents)	Increase sedative and other CNS effects, including motor skill impairment and respiratory depression	• Monitor the patient for changes in level of consciousness. • Monitor the patient for signs of respiratory depression. • Advise the patient of possible additive effects, especially with alcohol.
cyclobenzaprine	Monoamine oxidase (MAO) inhibitors	May cause hyperpyrexia, excitation, and seizures	• Expect 14 days to elapse between the administration of the last dose of an MAO inhibitor and the first dose of cyclobenzaprine. • Monitor the patient's CNS status and body temperature frequently.
	Cholinergic blocking agents	Increase anticholinergic effects, including confusion and hallucinations	• Monitor the patient for signs and symptoms of an adverse reaction; be prepared to administer a reduced dosage of the cholinergic blocking agent as prescribed.
orphenadrine	Cholinergic blocking agents	Increase anticholinergic effects, including confusion and hallucinations	• Monitor the patient for signs and symptoms of an adverse reaction; be prepared to administer a reduced dosage of the cholinergic blocking agent as prescribed.

normal saline solution—maximum dosage 3 g daily; I.M. and I.V. dosages should not exceed 3 g daily for 3 consecutive days. For tetanus, 1 to 2 g into the tubing of an infusing I.V. line at a rate of 300 mg/minute or 1 to 3 g as an infusion every 6 hours.
Usual pediatric dosage: for tetanus, 15 mg/kg of body weight I.V. every 6 hours.

orphenadrine citrate (Norflex, Norgesic). Used to treat acute, painful musculoskeletal conditions, orphenadrine is highly toxic at even slight overdoses.
Usual adult dosage: 100-mg extended-release tablet P.O. every 12 hours, or 25- to 50-mg compound (with aspirin and caffeine) P.O. t.i.d. or q.i.d., or 60 mg I.M. or I.V. every 12 hours p.r.n. injected over 5 minutes with the patient in the supine position; switch to oral form for maintenance.

Drug interactions
The centrally acting skeletal muscle relaxants interact with few drugs, but all interact with other CNS depressants (including alcohol), causing additive depression of the CNS. Cyclobenzaprine interacts with monoamine oxidase (MAO) inhibitors: 14 days must elapse between the last dose of an MAO inhibitor and the first dose of cyclobenzaprine. Cyclobenzaprine may decrease the effects of the antihy-

pertensive agents guanethidine and clonidine. Orphenadrine and cyclobenzaprine sometimes enhance the effects of cholinergic blocking agents. Methocarbamol may antagonize the cholinergic effects of the anticholinesterase agents used to treat myasthenia gravis. (For more information, see *Drug interactions: Centrally acting skeletal muscle relaxants.*)

The centrally acting skeletal muscle relaxants also interfere with some laboratory tests. Metaxalone may produce false-positive results for glucose with the copper reduction method. (It does not interfere with the glucose oxidase method.) Methocarbamol may cause false-positive results for urine 5-hydroxyindoleacetic acid and for urine vanillylmandelic acid.

ADVERSE DRUG REACTIONS

The most common adverse reactions to the centrally acting skeletal muscle relaxants are extensions of their therapeutic effects on the CNS.

Drowsiness and dizziness are the most common adverse reactions to drugs in this class. Occasionally, nausea, vomiting, diarrhea, constipation, heartburn, abdominal distress, or ataxia occurs. Areflexia, flaccid paralysis, respiratory depression, and hypotension are seen occasionally after oral administration of any of these drugs except methocarbamol. With parenteral administration, reactions may include syncope, hypotension, flushing, blurred vision, asthenia, lethargy, vertigo, lack of coordination, and bradycardia.

Because orphenadrine has an anticholinergic effect, adverse reactions may include dry mouth, urine retention, urinary hesitancy, blurred vision, and tachycardia. Orphenadrine overdose may cause seizures, shock, respiratory arrest, coma, or death. At high doses, cyclobenzaprine, which is structurally similar to the tricyclic antidepressants, shares their toxic potential; reactions include tachycardia and orthostatic hypotension. Physical and psychological dependence is a possibility after long-term use of these agents; abrupt cessation of the drug may cause severe withdrawal symptoms.

Rarely, parenteral orphenadrine causes an anaphylactic reaction. Chlorphenesin contains tartrazine dye, which may cause an allergic reaction.

NURSING PROCESS APPLICATION

The following information assists the nurse in caring for a patient who is receiving a centrally acting skeletal muscle relaxant.

Assessment
• Review the patient's history for conditions that contraindicate the use of centrally acting skeletal muscle relaxants, such as known hypersensitivity to these drugs and pregnancy.
• Review the patient's history for conditions that require cautious use of centrally acting skeletal muscle relaxants, such as impaired liver or kidney function.
• Assess the patient for adverse reactions to a centrally acting skeletal muscle relaxant, such as drowsiness, dizziness, GI distress, ataxia, hypotension, blurred vision, bradycardia, and urine retention.
• Review the patient's medication history to identify use of drugs that may interact with the prescribed centrally acting skeletal muscle relaxant, such as CNS depressants, MAO inhibitors, or cholinergic blocking agents.
• Assess the effectiveness of the prescribed centrally acting skeletal muscle relaxant periodically.
• Assess the patient for signs of physical or psychological dependence on the prescribed centrally acting skeletal muscle relaxant.
• Evaluate the patient's and family's knowledge about the prescribed centrally acting skeletal muscle relaxant.

Nursing diagnoses
The following examples represent appropriate nursing diagnoses for a patient receiving a centrally acting skeletal muscle relaxant.

• Potential for injury related to a preexisting condition that contraindicates the use of a centrally acting skeletal muscle relaxant
• Potential for injury related to a preexisting condition that requires cautious use of a centrally acting skeletal muscle relaxant
• Potential for injury related to selected adverse drug reactions
• Potential for injury related to drug interactions with the prescribed centrally acting skeletal muscle relaxant
• Pain related to ineffectiveness of the centrally acting skeletal muscle relaxant
• Impaired adjustment related to physical and psychological dependence on the centrally acting skeletal muscle relaxant
• Knowledge deficit related to the prescribed centrally acting skeletal muscle relaxant

Planning and implementation
• Do not administer a centrally acting skeletal muscle relaxant to a patient with a condition that contraindicates its use.
• Administer a centrally acting skeletal muscle relaxant cautiously to a patient at risk because of a preexisting condition.
• Monitor the patient periodically for adverse reactions during therapy with a centrally acting skeletal muscle relaxant.
• Document the patient's fluid intake and output and ensure that the patient voids regularly during orphenadrine therapy.
• *Avoid abrupt discontinuation of a centrally acting skeletal muscle relaxant.*
• *Give parenteral orphenadrine over 5 minutes with the patient in the supine position; keep the patient supine for 5 to 10 more minutes. Then help the patient to a sitting position and supervise ambulation.*
• *Monitor the I.V. site in a patient who receives parenteral methocarbamol. Watch for extravasation because thrombophlebitis, sloughing, and pain may result.*
• *Administer I.V. methocarbamol slowly at a maximum rate of 3 ml/min. Inject I.M. methocarbamol deeply and slowly, only in the upper outer quadrant of the buttocks, with a maximum of 5 ml in each buttock.*
• Keep epinephrine, antihistamines, and corticosteroids on hand during methocarbamol therapy to correct syncope that does not resolve with supportive therapy.
• *Avoid administering methocarbamol subcutaneously.*
• *Monitor respiratory status for a patient receiving a CNS depressant along with a centrally acting skeletal muscle relaxant. Keep emergency equipment available.*
• *Monitor the level of consciousness and mental status for a patient receiving a CNS depressant or cholinergic blocking agent along with a centrally acting skeletal muscle relaxant. Take safety precautions if drug interactions produce effects such as sedation, confusion, or motor skill impairment.*

• Monitor for hyperpyrexia, excitation, and seizures in a patient receiving an MAO inhibitor along with a centrally acting skeletal muscle relaxant. Take seizure precautions, if indicated.

• Notify the physician if drug interactions occur.

• Determine the degree of pain relief produced by the centrally acting skeletal muscle relaxant.

• Monitor the patient's activity level.

• Notify the physician if the centrally acting skeletal muscle relaxant does not relieve pain or muscle spasm.

• Verify the patient's need for continued use of the centrally acting skeletal muscle relaxant.

• Reduce the dosage gradually for a centrally acting skeletal muscle relaxant, as prescribed.

• Provide a referral for psychological evaluation if the patient refuses to reduce drug use when the drug no longer is needed.

Patient teaching

• Teach the patient and family the name, dose, frequency, action, and adverse effects of the prescribed centrally acting skeletal muscle relaxant.

• Inform the patient that a centrally acting skeletal muscle relaxant may impair mental alertness or physical coordination, increasing the risk of operating machinery or driving a motor vehicle.

• *Instruct the patient to take an oral centrally acting agent with meals or milk to prevent GI distress.*

• Advise the patient taking orphenadrine to relieve dry mouth with sugarless candy or gum and cool beverages, if permitted. Also, advise the patient to contact the physician if urine retention occurs.

• *Inform the patient that chlorzoxazone may harmlessly discolor urine an orange or purple-red; methocarbamol, green, black, or brown.*

• Teach the diabetic patient that metaxalone may cause false-positive results for glucose with the copper reduction method.

• Teach the patient to notify the physician if adverse reactions occur.

Evaluation

The following examples represent appropriate evaluation statements for a patient receiving a centrally acting skeletal muscle relaxant.

• The patient's history reveals no conditions that contraindicate the use of a centrally acting skeletal muscle relaxant.

• The patient exhibits no signs of complications in the preexisting condition linked to the prescribed centrally acting skeletal muscle relaxant.

• The patient exhibits no adverse reactions to the prescribed centrally acting skeletal muscle relaxant.

• The patient uses no drugs that interact with centrally acting skeletal muscle relaxants.

• The patient reports relief of muscle pain.

• The patient reports discontinuation of the centrally acting skeletal muscle relaxant.

• The patient and family express an accurate understanding of the points taught about the prescribed centrally acting skeletal muscle relaxant.

• The patient reports taking the centrally acting skeletal muscle relaxant with breakfast, lunch, and dinner.

PERIPHERALLY ACTING SKELETAL MUSCLE RELAXANTS

Dantrolene sodium is the only peripherally acting skeletal muscle relaxant. Similar to the centrally acting agents in its therapeutic effect, dantrolene differs in its mechanism of action. Because its major effect is on the muscle, dantrolene has a lower incidence of adverse CNS effects, but high therapeutic doses are hepatotoxic. Clinically, dantrolene seems most effective for spasticity of cerebral origin. Because it produces muscle weakness, dantrolene is of questionable benefit in patients with borderline strength.

PHARMACOKINETICS

Dantrolene is absorbed poorly from the GI tract. It is highly plasma protein bound, metabolized by the liver, and excreted in the urine.

Absorption, distribution, metabolism, excretion

Only about 35% of an oral dose of dantrolene is absorbed from the GI tract, and blood concentrations vary widely among patients after oral administration — partly because dantrolene has a strong affinity for plasma protein binding, particularly with albumin. Dantrolene undergoes significant liver metabolism to compounds that are much less active than the parent molecule; these metabolites are excreted primarily in the urine.

Onset, peak, duration

Although the peak concentration level of a single dose of dantrolene occurs about 5 hours after it is ingested, the drug's therapeutic benefit may not be evident for a week or more. Dosage increases should not exceed two per week. Dantrolene's elimination half-life in healthy adults is about 9 hours. Because dantrolene undergoes significant hepatic metabolism, however, its half-life may be prolonged in patients with impaired liver function.

PHARMACODYNAMICS

Dantrolene is chemically and pharmacologically unrelated to the other skeletal muscle relaxants. It probably acts directly on the muscle contractile mechanism, as opposed to affecting reflex pathways in the CNS.

Mechanism of action

Dantrolene may act by inhibiting calcium release from the sarcoplasmic reticulum in muscle cells. The sarcoplasmic reticulum stores calcium until the muscle is activated electrically by an action potential; then it releases calcium, which triggers muscle contraction.

Although dantrolene appears to affect the CNS as well, any central effect remains unproven. CNS effects, such as drowsiness, possibly result indirectly from decreased skeletal muscle activity. At therapeutic concentrations, dantrolene has little effect on cardiac or intestinal smooth muscle.

PHARMACOTHERAPEUTICS

Dantrolene helps manage all types of spasticity, regardless of lesion location, but is most effective when the lesion is cerebral. Patients with multiple sclerosis, cerebral palsy, spinal cord injury, or cerebrovascular accident may benefit from dantrolene. It is particularly useful for reducing spasticity in patients whose nursing care is impeded by severe muscle contractions. It also benefits patients whose rehabilitation program has been slowed by spasticity. If these patients have reversible spasticity, its relief should speed restoration of residual function. The patient's gait or ability to stand or sit also may improve.

Dantrolene also is used to treat and prevent malignant hyperthermic crisis. (For more information, see *Malignant hyperthermic crisis.*)

dantrolene sodium (Dantrium). Dosages must be titrated to the individual patient's response, always using the lowest dosage possible. Maintain each dosage level for 4 to 7 days to determine the patient's response. If benefits are not evident in 45 days, discontinue therapy to avoid liver damage. *Usual adult dosage:* for spasticity, 25 mg P.O. daily, increased to 25 mg b.i.d., t.i.d., or q.i.d., and then by increments of 25 mg to a maximum of 100 mg q.i.d.; for preventing malignant hyperthermic crisis, 4 to 8 mg/kg of body weight daily P.O. in four divided doses for 1 to 2 days before surgery with the last dose 3 to 4 hours before surgery; for managing malignant hyperthermic crisis, 1 mg/kg of body weight by rapid I.V. infusion, which may be repeated up to a cumulative total of 10 mg/kg; for preventing recurrence of malignant hyperthermic crisis, 4 to

---

Malignant hyperthermic crisis

This hereditary and fatal defect is triggered by inhalation anesthetics, depolarizing muscle relaxants, and curare-like neuromuscular blocking agents. The drugs prolong an increase in the release of calcium from the sarcoplasmic reticulum, producing intense muscle contraction, body heat, and metabolic acidosis. Dantrolene is the drug of choice to prevent or treat malignant hyperthermic crisis because it reduces the release of calcium by the sarcoplasmic reticulum.

---

8 mg/kg of body weight daily P.O. in four divided doses for 3 days after the crisis.

Drug interactions

CNS depressants combined with dantrolene increase CNS depression, which may lead to sedation, motor skill impairment, and respiratory depression. No other interactions are reported.

ADVERSE DRUG REACTIONS

The most common adverse reaction to dantrolene is muscle weakness. The drug also may depress liver function or cause idiosyncratic hepatitis.

Dose-related adverse reactions to dantrolene usually are transient, lasting up to 4 days after therapy begins. The most common is muscle weakness, rarely severe enough to cause slurring of speech, drooling, and enuresis. Other common reactions include drowsiness, dizziness, lightheadedness, diarrhea, nausea, malaise, and fatigue. If weakness or diarrhea is severe, the dosage may be decreased or the drug discontinued. Other adverse GI reactions that may respond to a dosage decrease include anorexia, vomiting, gastric irritation, abdominal cramps, constipation, difficulty swallowing, and GI bleeding. Constipation sometimes is severe enough to resemble bowel obstruction.

Neurologic adverse reactions include visual and speech disturbances, headache, taste alteration, depression, confusion, hallucinations, nervousness, insomnia, and seizures.

Urogenital reactions include urinary frequency, incontinence, nocturia, difficult urination, urine retention, hematuria, crystalluria, and difficult erection.

Cardiovascular reactions include tachycardia, erratic blood pressure, phlebitis, and pleural effusion with pericarditis.

Fatal and nonfatal hepatitis from dantrolene appear to be idiosyncratic reactions. In most cases, nausea, anorexia, vomiting, and abdominal discomfort precede hepatitis, which occurs most commonly in patients receiving more than 300 mg daily for longer than 2 months. The risk of dantrolene hepatotoxicity is greatest in women over age 35 who simultaneously take estrogens and in patients with baseline liver function test abnormalities. The abnormal liver function test results induced by dantrolene may return to normal when the drug is discontinued. Other reactions include acneiform rash, erratic blood pressure, pruritus, urticaria, excessive tearing, chills and fever, and a feeling of suffocation.

NURSING PROCESS APPLICATION

The following information assists the nurse in caring for a patient who is receiving dantrolene.

Assessment
• Review the patient's history for conditions that contra-indicate the use of dantrolene, such as pregnancy, lactation, or hepatic disease.
• Review the patient's history for conditions that require cautious use of dantrolene, such as impaired cardiac or pulmonary function.
• Assess the patient for adverse reactions to dantrolene, such as muscle weakness, depressed liver function, drowsiness, dizziness, GI irritation, headache, confusion, or urine retention.
• Review the patient's medication history to identify use of drugs that may interact with dantrolene, such as CNS depressants.
• Assess the effectiveness of dantrolene regularly.
• Assess the patient for constipation during dantrolene therapy.
• Evaluate the patient's and family's knowledge about dantrolene.

Nursing diagnoses
The following examples represent appropriate nursing diagnoses for a patient receiving dantrolene.
• Potential for injury related to a preexisting condition that contraindicates the use of dantrolene
• Potential for injury related to a preexisting condition that requires cautious use of dantrolene
• Potential for injury related to adverse drug reactions
• Potential for injury related to drug interactions with dantrolene
• Impaired physical mobility related to ineffectiveness of dantrolene
• Constipation related to the adverse GI effects of dantrolene
• Knowledge deficit related to dantrolene

Planning and implementation
• Do not administer dantrolene to a patient with a condition that contraindicates its use.
• Administer dantrolene cautiously to a patient at risk because of a preexisting condition.
• Monitor closely any patient with severe cardiac or pulmonary disease who receives dantrolene.
• *Monitor the patient's liver function before and during dantrolene therapy with the ALT (formerly SGPT), AST (formerly SGOT), alkaline phosphatase, and total bilirubin tests, as prescribed.*
• Observe closely for adverse drug reactions.
• Document the patient's fluid intake and output at least once daily.
• Take safety precautions if the patient exhibits neurologic reactions; for example, take seizure precautions and supervise all activities.
• *Empty dantrolene capsules into fruit juice or another liquid immediately before administration to a patient who has difficulty swallowing.*
• *Reconstitute dantrolene with 60 ml of sterile, not bacteriostatic, water for I.V. administration.*
• Notify the physician if adverse reactions occur.
• *Monitor for sedation, motor skill impairment, and respiratory depression in a patient receiving dantrolene and a CNS depressant.*
• Take safety precautions if the patient develops sedation or motor skill impairment.
• *Keep emergency equipment nearby to treat respiratory depression.*
• Notify the physician if drug interactions occur.
• Monitor the patient's level of spasticity during dantrolene therapy.
• Notify the physician if physical mobility does not improve while the patient is taking dantrolene.
• *Encourage the patient to increase fluid and high-fiber food intake during dantrolene therapy.*
• Auscultate the patient's bowel sounds at least every 8 hours.
• Consult the physician about additional measures, such as laxative or enema administration, if constipation persists.

Patient teaching
• Teach the patient and family about dantrolene, including its name, dose, frequency, action, and adverse effects.
• Teach the patient about dantrolene's possible effects, such as weakness, drowsiness, and dizziness. Reassure the patient that these effects usually subside in a few days.
• *Instruct the patient to take dantrolene with meals or milk to prevent gastric irritation.*
• Advise the patient to expect frequent blood testing of liver function.
• Teach the patient and family to notify the physician if adverse reactions occur.

Evaluation

The following examples represent appropriate evaluation statements for a patient receiving dantrolene.

• The patient's history reveals no conditions that contraindicate the use of dantrolene.

• The patient exhibits no signs of complications in the preexisting condition linked to dantrolene.

• The patient displays no adverse reactions to dantrolene.

• The patient uses no drugs that interact with dantrolene.

• The patient reports greatly reduced spasticity.

• The patient engages in significantly more activities than before dantrolene therapy.

• The patient reports a return to normal bowel pattern.

• The patient and family express an accurate understanding of the points taught about dantrolene.

• The patient schedules follow-up visits for blood testing.

OTHER SKELETAL MUSCLE RELAXANTS

Two other drugs, diazepam and baclofen, are used as skeletal muscle relaxants. Diazepam is primarily an antianxiety agent and is discussed more fully in Chapter 27, Antianxiety Agents. Its use as a skeletal muscle relaxant is summarized in *Diazepam as a skeletal muscle relaxing agent.*

Baclofen is an analogue of the neurotransmitter GABA and probably acts in the spinal cord. Because baclofen produces less sedation than diazepam and less peripheral muscle weakness than dantrolene, it is the drug of choice to treat spasticity.

PHARMACOKINETICS

Baclofen is absorbed rapidly from the GI tract. It is distributed widely, undergoes minimal liver metabolism, and is excreted primarily unchanged in the urine.

Absorption, distribution, metabolism, excretion

Baclofen is absorbed in varying amounts from the GI tract. The amount varies widely from patient to patient and is reduced as the dosage is increased.

Baclofen is distributed widely throughout the body, but only small amounts cross the blood-brain barrier. Although concentrations of baclofen therefore are considerably lower in the brain and nerve tissue than in the blood, they decline more slowly there. At therapeutic blood concentrations, baclofen is about 30% bound to serum proteins. The drug crosses the placenta, but its distribution into breast milk is uncertain.

Diazepam as a skeletal muscle relaxing agent

Diazepam (Valium) is a benzodiazepine with antispastic effects besides its antianxiety, hypnotic, and anticonvulsant ones. Useful in various chronic disorders in which spasticity is a component, diazepam is one of the most effective agents available for treating acute muscle spasms. It seems to work by enhancing the inhibitory effect on muscle contraction of the neurotransmitter gamma-aminobutyric acid.

In treating spasticity, diazepam is useful alone or with other drugs, especially in patients with spinal cord lesions and occasionally in patients with cerebral palsy. It is useful in patients who have painful continuous muscle spasms and are not too susceptible to the drug's sedative effect. However, its tranquilizing properties may be helpful in anxious patients. Diazepam's use is limited by its central nervous system effects and the tolerance that develops with prolonged use.

Diazepam therapy is initiated with 2 mg P.O. twice daily; the dosage is increased slowly every few days until adverse reactions develop or until it reaches 10 mg t.i.d. A slow upward titration will minimize the sedation associated with diazepam. In the elderly patient, the initial dosage should not exceed 2 mg daily. For more information on diazepam, see Chapter 27, Antianxiety Agents.

Baclofen undergoes limited liver metabolism and is excreted almost completely within 72 hours after oral administration; 70% to 80% is excreted in the urine unchanged or as metabolites, and the remainder is excreted in the feces.

Onset, peak, duration

The beneficial effects of baclofen may or may not occur immediately—the onset of therapeutic effect ranges from hours to weeks. Peak blood concentration levels of the drug are attained in 2 to 3 hours and are sustained for 8 hours. The elimination half-life of baclofen is 2.5 to 4 hours. Abrupt withdrawal of the drug may precipitate hallucinations, seizures, and acute exacerbations of spasticity.

PHARMACODYNAMICS

The exact mechanism of action of baclofen has not been established. It is believed to work in the spinal cord. Biochemically, baclofen resembles an inhibitory neurotransmitter.

Mechanism of action

Animal studies have helped to identify baclofen's site of action as the spinal cord. However, some of its adverse effects, such as respiratory depression at higher doses, enhanced electroencephalogram activity, and sedation, suggest an additional supraspinal site of action.

Baclofen seems to depress neuron activity, decreasing the degree and frequency of muscle spasms and reducing muscle tone. Researchers question whether baclofen produces these effects by suppressing excitatory neurotransmitter release, by directly inhibiting spinal pathways, or both. Baclofen resembles the inhibitory neurotransmitter GABA. Although baclofen does not displace GABA from its receptor-binding sites, it may compete with GABA at presynaptic GABA receptors. Its overall effect reduces the frequency and severity of painful flexor or extensor muscle spasms. Baclofen also reduces protracted muscle spasms of the lower extremities in patients with spinal spasticity.

PHARMACOTHERAPEUTICS

Baclofen's principal clinical indication is for the paraplegic or quadriplegic patient with spinal cord lesions, most commonly caused by multiple sclerosis or trauma. For these patients, baclofen significantly reduces the number and severity of painful flexor spasms. Aside from waking patients at night, these spasms are painful and unpleasant in the day and may cause sudden falls in ambulatory patients. Baclofen also improves bladder and bowel control, and it may make the patient's hygiene and nursing care more comfortable by relaxing tightly flexed legs. Aside from these benefits, however, baclofen does not improve stiff gait, increase manual dexterity, or improve residual muscle function.

Baclofen and diazepam have comparable antispastic effects in patients with multiple sclerosis; however, baclofen usually is preferred because it produces a lower incidence of sedation.

Baclofen has been used experimentally to treat a number of other conditions, with limited success.

baclofen (Lioresal). Because the dosage must be individualized to produce the best response without adverse effects, baclofen should be started at low doses and titrated slowly. Full clinical benefit may require 1 to 2 months of treatment.

Usual adult dosage: initially, 5 mg P.O. t.i.d., increased by 15 mg daily at 3-day intervals until an optimal response is achieved, usually at 40 to 80 mg daily in three or four divided doses not to exceed 80 mg/day.

Drug interactions

Few drug interactions are reported with baclofen; the most significant is an increase in CNS depression when baclofen is administered with other CNS depressants, including alcohol. Other drug interactions include prolonged analgesia when fentanyl and baclofen are administered concomitantly, aggravation of hyperkinesis when lithium carbonate and baclofen are administered concomitantly, and increased muscle relaxation when tricyclic antidepressants and baclofen are administered concomitantly.

ADVERSE DRUG REACTIONS

Baclofen causes few major adverse reactions when administered appropriately to patients with spinal lesions. General CNS depression produces the most problems.

The most common adverse reaction to baclofen is transient drowsiness. Other, less frequent adverse reactions include nausea, fatigue, vertigo, hypotonia, muscle weakness, depression, and headache. These can be avoided by a slow titration of the dose.

Elderly patients or patients with cerebrovascular accidents and brain disorders may experience psychiatric disturbances, such as hallucinations, euphoria, depression, confusion, and anxiety. Dosage increases should be made even more slowly in these patients.

Other rare neuropsychiatric disturbances include insomnia, muscle pain, paresthesia, tinnitus, slurred speech, tremor, rigidity, ataxia, seizures, blurred vision, strabismus, nystagmus, diplopia, and dysarthria. Baclofen rarely causes adverse genitourinary reactions. Cardiovascular reactions include hypotension and, rarely, dyspnea, chest pain, and syncope. Adverse GI reactions include nausea, vomiting, constipation, and, rarely, dry mouth, anorexia, taste disorders, and diarrhea.

Rash, allergic skin disorders, and pruritus have occurred with baclofen, as have ankle edema, weight gain, and excessive diaphoresis.

NURSING PROCESS APPLICATION

The following information assists the nurse in caring for a patient who is receiving baclofen or another skeletal muscle relaxant.

Assessment
• Review the patient's history for conditions that contraindicate the use of baclofen or another skeletal muscle relaxant, such as pregnancy or known hypersensitivity to the drug.
• Review the patient's history for conditions that require cautious use of baclofen or another skeletal muscle relaxant, such as brain disorders.
• Assess the patient for adverse drug reactions to baclofen, such as drowsiness, fatigue, nausea, muscle weakness, headache, confusion, anxiety, and rash.
• Assess the effectiveness of baclofen or another skeletal muscle relaxant periodically.
• Evaluate the patient's and family's knowledge about the prescribed skeletal muscle relaxant.

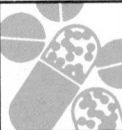

SELECTED MAJOR DRUGS

Skeletal muscle relaxing agents

This table summarizes the major skeletal muscle relaxing agents currently in clinical use. Diazepam is discussed in detail in Chapter 27, Antianxiety Agents.

DRUG	MAJOR INDICATIONS	USUAL ADULT DOSAGES	CONTRAINDICATIONS AND PRECAUTIONS
Centrally acting agents			
carisoprodol	Acute muscle spasms	350 mg P.O. t.i.d. and h.s.	• Know that carisoprodol is contraindicated in a pregnant patient or one with known hypersensitivity to this drug. • Administer with caution to a patient with impaired liver or kidney function.
Peripherally acting agents			
dantrolene	Spasticity	25 mg daily to 100 mg P.O. q.i.d.	• Know that dantrolene is contraindicated in a pregnant or lactating patient or one with hepatic disease. • Administer with caution to a patient with impaired pulmonary function, as in obstructive pulmonary disease, or with severely impaired cardiac function, as in myocardial disease.
	Prevention of malignant hyperthermic crisis	4 to 8 mg/kg P.O. daily for 1 to 2 days before surgery or for 3 days after crisis	
	Treatment of malignant hyperthermic crisis	1 mg/kg I.V. to a cumulative total of 10 mg/kg	
Other agents			
baclofen	Spasticity	40 to 80 mg P.O. daily	• Know that baclofen is contraindicated in a pregnant patient or one with known hypersensitivity to this drug. • Administer with caution to an elderly patient or one with a cerebrovascular accident or other brain disorder.

Nursing diagnoses

The following examples represent appropriate nursing diagnoses for a patient receiving baclofen or another skeletal muscle relaxant.

• Potential for injury related to a preexisting condition that contraindicates the use of baclofen or another skeletal muscle relaxant

• Potential for injury related to a preexisting condition that requires cautious use of baclofen or another skeletal muscle relaxant

• Potential for injury related to adverse drug reactions

• Potential activity intolerance related to possible ineffectiveness of baclofen or another skeletal muscle relaxant

• Knowledge deficit related to baclofen

Planning and implementation

• Do not administer baclofen or another skeletal muscle relaxant to a patient with a condition that contraindicates its use.

• Administer baclofen or another skeletal muscle relaxant cautiously to a patient at risk because of a preexisting condition.

• Monitor the patient for adverse reactions periodically.

• *Monitor for impaired renal function by documenting the patient's fluid intake and output and body weight daily. Impaired renal function may require dosage reduction because baclofen is excreted primarily in the urine.*

• Take seizure precautions for a patient with a seizure disorder or one who develops seizures during baclofen therapy.

• Manage overdose, as indicated. Induce emesis if the patient is conscious or use gastric lavage if the patient is comatose, as prescribed. If necessary, assist with endotracheal intubation to maintain respiratory function, but do not administer respiratory stimulants.

• Notify the physician if adverse reactions occur.

• Monitor the number and severity of painful flexor spasms.

• Assess the patient's degree of bowel and bladder control.

• *Notify the physician if the skeletal muscle relaxant does not improve the patient's spasticity or bowel and bladder control.*

Patient teaching

• Teach the patient and family the name, dose, frequency, action, and adverse effects of the prescribed skeletal muscle relaxant.
• Inform the patient that baclofen may impair mental alertness or physical coordination, increasing the risks associated with operating machinery or driving a motor vehicle.
• *Advise the patient to avoid alcohol while taking baclofen.*
• *Instruct the patient to take baclofen with meals or milk to prevent GI distress.*

Evaluation

The following examples represent appropriate evaluation statements for a patient receiving baclofen or another skeletal muscle relaxant.
• The patient's history reveals no conditions that contraindicate use of the prescribed skeletal muscle relaxant.
• The patient exhibits no signs of complications in the preexisting condition linked to the prescribed skeletal muscle relaxant.
• The patient exhibits no adverse drug reactions.
• The patient reports decreased flexor spasms and increased activity level.
• The patient and family express an accurate understanding of the points taught about the prescribed skeletal muscle relaxant.
• The patient reports taking baclofen with breakfast, lunch, and dinner.

CHAPTER SUMMARY

Chapter 18 investigated the skeletal muscle relaxing agents, which act to relieve musculoskeletal pain or spasm and severe musculoskeletal spasticity. Here are the chapter highlights.
• Some skeletal muscle relaxing drugs act in the spinal cord to alter neurotransmitter function; these are centrally acting drugs. Others act on the skeletal muscle itself; these are peripherally acting drugs.
• Two other drugs—baclofen, which may act on the spinal cord, and diazepam, an antianxiety agent—have valuable antispastic effects.
• The centrally acting skeletal muscle relaxants probably relieve acute musculoskeletal spasms as a result of their CNS depressant activity. Drugs in this class are carisoprodol, chlorphenesin, chlorzoxazone, cyclobenzaprine, metaxalone, methocarbamol, and orphenadrine.
• Patients with multiple sclerosis, cerebral palsy, spinal cord injury, or cerebrovascular accident may benefit from the peripherally acting agent dantrolene, although some patients may not respond to the drug. If a patient does not benefit from dantrolene, it should be discontinued because of its hepatotoxic potential.
• Diazepam may be the most effective skeletal muscle relaxant available for the relief of acute muscle spasms. It also is effective for the relief of spasticity associated with chronic neurologic disorders. Diazepam is as effective as baclofen or dantrolene for relieving spasticity, but it has a higher incidence of adverse CNS effects.
• Baclofen's principal indication is for the paraplegic or quadriplegic patient with spinal cord lesions, most commonly caused by multiple sclerosis or trauma.

STUDY QUESTIONS

See Appendix 1 for answers.

1. Ken Baker, age 35, is admitted to the hospital with low back strain. His physician prescribes orphenadrine (Norflex) 50 mg P.O. t.i.d. What is orphenadrine's mechanism of action?
(a) It produces an atropine-like central action.
(b) It enhances the action of norepinephrine.
(c) It acts directly on the skeletal muscle.
(d) It depresses neuromuscular transmission.

2. The nurse is extremely careful when administering orphenadrine to Mr. Baker. What may occur with even a slight overdose?
(a) drug ineffectiveness
(b) drug toxicity
(c) hypertension
(d) tachycardia

3. Evelyn Carver, age 55, develops malignant hyperthermic crisis after surgery. Her physician prescribes the peripherally acting skeletal muscle relaxant dantrolene (Dantrium) 1 mg/kg of body weight I.V. How does dantrolene exert its therapeutic effects?
(a) It depresses the central nervous system.
(b) It promotes calcium release from the sarcoplasmic reticulum.
(c) It inhibits calcium release from the sacroplasmic reticulum.
(d) It affects reflex pathways in the central nervous system.

4. When receiving dantrolene, Ms. Carver is most likely to develop which adverse reaction?
(a) muscle weakness
(b) hypotension
(c) hepatitis
(d) seizures

5. Ellen Crane, age 30, has multiple sclerosis. To relieve her muscle spasms, the physician orders baclofen (Lioresal). The nurse instructs Ms. Crane not to discontinue baclofen abruptly. What might happen with abrupt discontinuation?
(a) hypotension
(b) muscle weakness
(c) respiratory distress
(d) exacerbation of spasticity

6. What is the most likely reason for the physician's prescription of baclofen rather than diazepam to reduce Ms. Crane's muscle spasms?
(a) Baclofen is more effective than diazepam.
(b) Baclofen produces less sedation than diazepam.
(c) Baclofen can be used safely in patients with impaired renal function; diazepam cannot.
(d) Baclofen does not require dosage titration; diazepam does.

7. Elvin Dee, age 30, seeks care for a sprained ankle and muscle spasms, which he incurred while playing basketball. His physician prescribes diazepam (Valium). This drug is not indicated for prolonged use because it may cause which of the following problems?
(a) hepatotoxicity
(b) constipation
(c) hypotension
(d) tolerance

SELECTED REFERENCES

AHFS drug information 90. (1990). Bethesda, MD: American Society of Hospital Pharmacists.

Biddle, C. (1988). Adverse reactions to drugs used in anesthesia. *Current Reviews for Nurse Anesthetists,* 10(25), 195-200.

Goodman and Gilman's the pharmacological basis of therapeutics (8th ed.; 1990). Elmsford, NY: Pergamon Press.

Hansten, P., and Horn, J. (1989). *Drug interactions* (6th ed.). Philadelphia: Lea & Febiger.

Hildebrand, R. (1988). Muscle relaxants: A review. *Journal of Post Anesthesia Nursing,* 3(3), 165-167.

Drug facts and comparisons. (1991). St. Louis: Facts and Comparisons Division, Lippincott.

Mediphor Editorial Group. (1987). *Drug interaction facts 1987.* St. Louis: Lippincott.

CHAPTER

19

ANTIPARKINSONIAN AGENTS

OBJECTIVES

After reading and studying this chapter, the student should be able to:

1. Describe the signs, symptoms, and effects of Parkinson's disease.

2. Describe the pharmacokinetics of the antiparkinsonian agents.

3. Explain the mechanisms of action of the antiparkinsonian agents.

4. Identify the major adverse effects of the antiparkinsonian agents.

5. Compare the uses of anticholinergic and dopaminergic agents in treating parkinsonism.

6. Describe how to apply the nursing process when caring for a patient who is receiving an antiparkinsonian agents.

INTRODUCTION

Drug therapy is an important part of the treatment for Parkinson's disease, also known as paralysis agitans. Parkinson's disease is a progressive, idiopathic neurologic disorder caused by depletion, degeneration, or destruction of dopamine in the neurons of the brain's basal ganglia. It produces parkinsonism, an involuntary movement disorder characterized by four cardinal features: tremor at rest, akinesia (complete or partial loss of muscle movement), rigidity (increased muscle tone), and disturbances of posture and equilibrium. Parkinsonism also can result from drugs, encephalitis, neurotoxins, trauma, arteriosclerosis, or other neurologic disorders. Only 15% of all cases of parkinsonism result from these causes. The remaining 85% are idiopathic and result from Parkinson's disease.

This chapter includes synthetic anticholinergic and dopaminergic agents used to treat parkinsonism.

For a summary of representative drugs, see *Selected major drugs: Antiparkinsonian agents*, page 291. For a listing of applicable nursing diagnoses that the nurse may formulate when caring for a patient receiving these agents, see *Selected nursing diagnoses: Antiparkinsonian agents.*

SELECTED NURSING DIAGNOSES

Antiparkinsonian agents

The following nursing diagnoses address representative problems and etiologies that a nurse may encounter when caring for a patient who is receiving an antiparkinsonian agent. Some of these nursing diagnoses contain generalized etiologies, which the nurse must individualize based on the patient's needs. (For some common nursing diagnoses and related interventions for each drug class, see the "Nursing Process Application" sections of this chapter.)

- Altered health maintenance related to ineffectiveness of the prescribed antiparkinsonian agent
- Altered protection related to adverse hematologic effects of the antiparkinsonian agent
- Altered thought processes related to the adverse CNS effects of an antiparkinsonian agent
- Altered urinary elimination related to the adverse genitourinary effects of a dopaminergic agent
- Decreased cardiac output related to bromocriptine-induced arrhythmias
- Diarrhea related to the adverse GI effects of selegiline
- Hyperthermia related to levodopa withdrawal
- Impaired physical mobility related to ineffectiveness of dopaminergic agents, particularly levodopa
- Impaired skin integrity related to a dermatologic hypersensitivity reaction to an anticholinergic agent
- Knowledge deficit related to the prescribed antiparkinsonian agent
- Noncompliance related to long-term use of an antiparkinsonian agent
- Potential for injury related to a preexisting condition that contraindicates the use of an antiparkinsonian agent
- Potential for injury related to a preexisting condition that requires cautious use of an antiparkinsonian agent
- Potential for injury related to adverse drug reactions
- Potential for injury related to an interaction between levodopa and foods
- Urinary retention related to use of an antiparkinsonian agent

For detailed information on applying the nursing process, see Chapter 6, The Nursing Process and Drug Therapy.

ANTICHOLINERGIC AGENTS

Anticholinergic agents sometimes are called parasympatholytics because they antagonize functions that are controlled primarily by the parasympathetic nervous system.

Anticholinergics that are used to treat parkinsonism are classified in three chemical categories: synthetic tertiary amines, phenothiazine derivatives, and antihistamines. The synthetic tertiary amines constitute the largest group, including benztropine mesylate, biperiden hydrochloride, biperiden lactate, procyclidine hydrochloride, and trihexyphenidyl hydrochloride. Ethopropazine (a phenothiazine derivative) and diphenhydramine hydrochloride and orphenadrine citrate (antihistamines) constitute the remainder of these anticholinergics.

PHARMACOKINETICS

In general, the anticholinergic agents are well absorbed from the gastrointestinal (GI) tract and cross the blood-brain barrier to their action site in the brain. Most of them undergo hepatic metabolism and renal excretion.

Absorption, distribution, metabolism, excretion

Although detailed information on the pharmacokinetics of specific anticholinergic agents is unknown, their pharmacokinetic processes follow a general pattern.

After oral administration, nearly complete absorption occurs readily in the GI tract. (Food does not significantly reduce absorption of anticholinergic agents.) A large amount of diphenhydramine undergoes first-pass metabolism after oral administration: Only 40% to 50% of a dose reaches the circulation unchanged.

The exact distribution of most of these agents is undetermined. However, most researchers believe that anticholinergics cross the blood-brain barrier and penetrate brain tissue because they affect the central nervous system (CNS).

The liver metabolizes most anticholinergic agents at least partially. Diphenhydramine is metabolized almost completely. So is orphenadrine, which is metabolized to at least eight compounds.

Anticholinergics usually are excreted in urine as metabolites and unchanged drug. Trihexyphenidyl also may be excreted by the kidneys, but principally as an unchanged drug.

Onset, peak, duration

For most of the anticholinergic agents, onset of action occurs within 1 hour, peak concentration is reached in 2 to 4 hours, and duration of action is up to 6 hours.

Benztropine is a long-acting drug with a duration of action up to 24 hours in some patients. For most anticholinergic agents, the half-life is undetermined.

PHARMACODYNAMICS

In the brain, anticholinergic agents counteract the cholinergic activity that is believed to be present in Parkinson's disease.

Mechanism of action

Parkinson's disease results from the degeneration of dopaminergic neurons in the basal ganglia. Because dopamine helps control motor activity, a lack of it will cause problems in coordinating smooth motor movements. At the same time, an excess of acetylcholine activity develops, producing an excitatory effect on the CNS, which may cause the parkinsonian tremor.

The mechanism of action of the anticholinergic agents is not known, but these drugs may inhibit cerebral motor centers. They also suppress central cholinergic activity and the characteristic tremor of parkinsonism.

PHARMACOTHERAPEUTICS

Anticholinergic agents are used to treat all forms of parkinsonism, but are most commonly used in the early stages of Parkinson's disease when symptoms are mild and do not have a major impact on the patient's life-style. These agents effectively control sialorrhea (excessive flow of saliva) and are about 20% effective in reducing the incidence and severity of akinesia and rigidity.

Anticholinergics may be used alone or with amantadine in the early stages of Parkinson's disease. They may be given with levodopa during the later stages to relieve symptoms further. No single anticholinergic is consistently superior, but a patient may respond more favorably to one agent than to another. Trihexyphenidyl is the most widely used drug of the group. Benztropine and diphenhydramine also are used commonly.

Most anticholinergics maintain their effectiveness with long-term administration and rarely require dosage adjustment after the proper dosage is reached. However, as the disease advances, anticholinergics alone are not effective enough. If any antiparkinsonian agent must be discontinued and replaced with another drug, dosage should be reduced gradually. Abrupt withdrawal of anticholinergics can produce confusion, exhaustion, and exacerbation of parkinsonian symptoms.

The adverse effects of the anticholinergics usually are dose-limiting; that is, they increase with the dosage and may limit the amount the patient can take. Ethopropazine has a high incidence of adverse effects that are intolerable to some patients. Because the anticholinergics are more likely to cause adverse CNS effects in elderly patients, these drugs may be more successful in younger patients.

Diphenhydramine, benztropine, and biperiden may be administered I.V. or I.M. to treat parkinsonism. But these parenteral routes usually are reserved for use when the disease is acute or when oral administration is not feasible. In most cases of parkinsonism, I.V. administration usually is not needed to achieve a rapid response.

benztropine mesylate (Cogentin). Used alone or with other antiparkinsonian agents to treat all forms of parkinsonism, benztropine may be especially useful in treating elderly patients who cannot tolerate the CNS-stimulating properties of other anticholinergics, such as orphenadrine and trihexyphenidyl. Because the drug's effects are cumulative, benztropine may take 2 to 3 days to become fully effective. Therefore, dosage increases should be slow, allowing time for the drug to take effect.
Usual adult dosage: 0.5 to 1 mg P.O. daily, preferably as a single dose h.s. for the first few days, increased by 0.5 mg every few days, until the most effective dosage (maximum of 6 mg/day) is reached; maintenance dosage, 1 to 2 mg P.O., I.V., or I.M. daily. Some patients will achieve 24-hour symptom control with a single bedtime dose of 2 mg or more.

biperiden hydrochloride (Akineton) and **biperiden lactate** (Akineton Lactate). This anticholinergic agent is useful for initial or adjunct treatment of all forms of parkinsonism.
Usual adult dosage: for idiopathic Parkinson's disease, 2 mg P.O. t.i.d. or q.i.d.; for acute drug-induced parkinsonism, 2 mg I.M. or I.V. repeated every 30 minutes up to a maximum parenteral dosage of 8 mg in 24 hours. The oral dosage should be adjusted according to the patient's requirements and tolerance for adverse reactions. With prolonged therapy, drug tolerance may develop, requiring a dosage increase.

procyclidine hydrochloride (Kemadrin). Indications for this agent include initial or adjunct treatment of all forms of parkinsonism. Procyclidine may relieve muscle rigidity more than tremor. Its dosage should be individualized according to the patient's age, therapeutic response, and form of parkinsonism. For instance, younger patients usually tolerate and require larger doses than elderly patients, and drug-induced parkinsonism may require a larger dosage than idiopathic Parkinson's disease.

Usual adult dosage: initially, 2.5 mg P.O. b.i.d. or t.i.d. after meals; if tolerated, dosage is gradually increased up to 5 mg t.i.d. or q.i.d; maintenance dosage ranges from 10 to 20 mg P.O. daily, but may reach 60 mg/day in severe cases.

trihexyphenidyl hydrochloride (Artane, Hexaphen, Trihexane). This agent is used for initial or adjunct treatment of all forms of parkinsonism, including idiopathic, postencephalitic, and drug-induced. Although 50% to 75% of patients will respond to trihexyphenidyl, maximum response commonly requires combining this drug with others. Trihexyphenidyl is available in regular tablets, in sustained-release capsules, and as an elixir. Dosages of trihexyphenidyl should be adjusted carefully to the patient's requirements and response.
Usual adult dosage: initially, 1 mg P.O. daily, increased by 2 mg every 3 to 5 days until a desirable response is achieved, intolerable adverse reactions occur, or a daily dosage of 10 mg is reached; the dosage usually ranges from 3 to 15 mg P.O. t.i.d. Patients with postencephalitic parkinsonism may require 12 to 15 mg daily. Concurrent administration of levodopa and trihexyphenidyl may require a dosage reduction, adjusted to individual response and tolerance. If trihexyphenidyl is replacing another anticholinergic agent, the trihexyphenidyl dosage should be increased gradually while the other agent is withdrawn gradually. Tolerance to trihexyphenidyl may develop with prolonged use.

ethopropazine (Parsidol). A phenothiazine derivative, ethopropazine is distinct from other drugs in its class and can be used as an adjunct treatment for all forms of parkinsonism.
Usual adult dosage: initially, 50 mg P.O. once or twice daily, increased gradually to the lowest possible effective dosage: 100 to 400 mg P.O. daily for mild to moderate symptoms, 500 to 600 mg P.O. daily for severe symptoms. Adverse effects limit ethopropazine's usefulness.

diphenhydramine hydrochloride (Benadryl). This antihistamine's anticholinergic properties are responsible for its effectiveness in treating all forms of parkinsonism. Also a sleep aid, diphenhydramine may be useful for elderly patients who cannot tolerate more potent CNS-stimulating agents and for those with insomnia. For patients with mild cases of parkinsonism, diphenhydramine may be used alone or with other anticholinergics. Diphenhydramine may be administered orally, I.V., or I.M.; it also is available as an oral syrup and an elixir, containing 5% and 14% alcohol, respectively.
Usual adult dosage: initially, 25 mg P.O. t.i.d., increased gradually to 25 to 50 mg P.O. t.i.d. or q.i.d. at 4- to 6-hour intervals, according to the patient's response and tolerance; 10 to 100 mg I.M. or I.V. The maximum adult

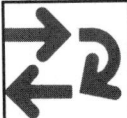

DRUG INTERACTIONS

Anticholinergic agents

The most common interactions occur between anticholinergic agents and drugs that have anticholinergic properties. Other interactions involving antipsychotic drugs may produce serious problems.

DRUG	INTERACTING DRUGS	POSSIBLE EFFECTS	NURSING IMPLICATIONS
benztropine, biperiden, procyclidine, trihexyphenidyl, ethopropazine, diphenhydramine, or-phenadrine	amantadine	Increases anticholinergic adverse effects	• Monitor the patient for changes in mental status and other adverse reactions, such as urine retention, dry mouth, blurred vision, and constipation. • Expect to reduce the dose of either agent, as prescribed, if intolerable anticholinergic adverse reactions occur.
	levodopa	Decrease levodopa absorption, which could lead to worsening parkinsonian signs and symptoms	• Monitor the patient for increased rigidity, bradykinesia, and tremor. Instruct the patient to report any of these problems to the physician. • Expect to increase the levodopa dosage, as prescribed.
	antipsychotics (phenothiazines, thiothixene, haloperidol, loxapine)	Decrease effectiveness of anticholinergics; decrease effectiveness of antipsychotics; increase incidence of anticholinergic adverse reactions	• Avoid concomitant use of anticholinergics and antipsychotics. • Observe the patient for an increase in parkinsonian signs or deterioration in mental status. Instruct the patient and family to report either of these problems to the physician. • Monitor the patient for increased anticholinergic adverse reactions.
	over-the-counter cough or cold preparations, diet aids, or analeptics (agents used to stay awake)	Increase anticholinergic effects	• Advise the patient not to take these drugs without consulting the physician because they may contain ingredients that have anticholinergic properties.
	alcohol	Increases depression of the central nervous system	• Teach the patient that alcohol may increase the drowsiness produced by the anticholinergic agent.

daily dosage is 300 mg orally or 400 mg parenterally. (For more information on diphenhydramine, see Chapter 56, Antihistaminic Agents.)

orphenadrine citrate (Norflex). This antihistamine is used in the adjunct treatment of all forms of parkinsonism and for pain relief in musculoskeletal disorders. Orphenadrine produces slight CNS stimulation and may cause mild euphoria. The oral sustained-release preparation is used to treat Parkinson's disease.
Usual adult dosage: initially, 50 mg P.O. t.i.d., increased gradually up to 250 mg P.O. daily, according to the patient's tolerance and response. (For more information, see Chapter 56, Antihistaminic Agents.)

Drug interactions
A few drugs, such as amantadine, levodopa, and the antipsychotics, produce clinically significant interactions when used with anticholinergics. (For details, see *Drug interactions: Anticholinergic agents.*)

ADVERSE DRUG REACTIONS

Most of the adverse effects of the anticholinergics are an extension of their pharmacologic effects. Mild, dose-related adverse reactions are seen in 30% to 50% of patients. Typically, reactions decrease as treatment continues, but they limit the dosage that the patient can tolerate. One way to review the various dose-related adverse reactions is to start at the head of the body and move down. (For details, see *Dose-related adverse reactions to the anticholinergics,* page 284.)

Dose-related adverse reactions to the anticholinergics

Common dose-related adverse reactions to anticholinergic agents are described below. Use this illustration as a head-to-toe guide when assessing a patient.

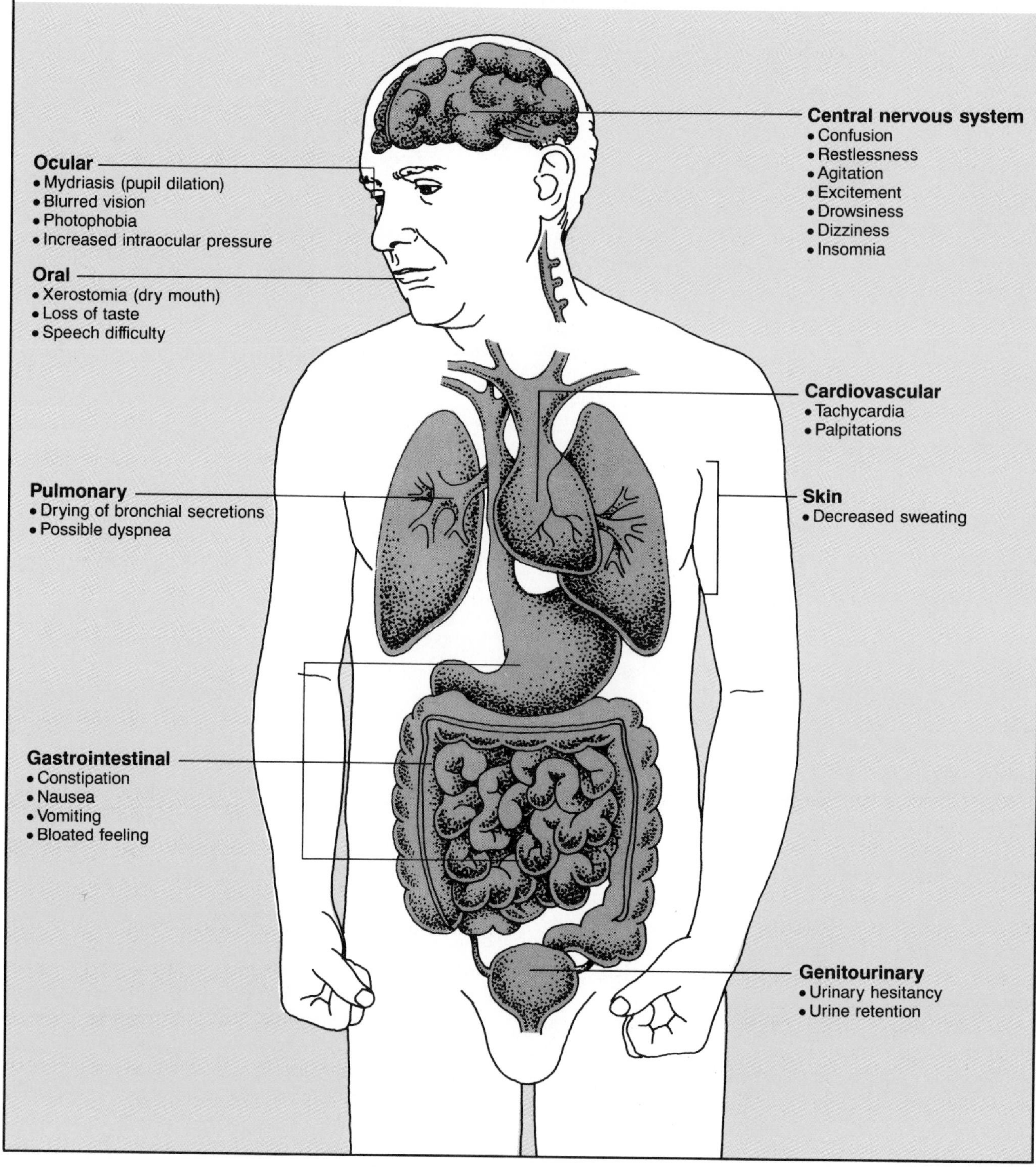

Ocular
- Mydriasis (pupil dilation)
- Blurred vision
- Photophobia
- Increased intraocular pressure

Oral
- Xerostomia (dry mouth)
- Loss of taste
- Speech difficulty

Pulmonary
- Drying of bronchial secretions
- Possible dyspnea

Gastrointestinal
- Constipation
- Nausea
- Vomiting
- Bloated feeling

Central nervous system
- Confusion
- Restlessness
- Agitation
- Excitement
- Drowsiness
- Dizziness
- Insomnia

Cardiovascular
- Tachycardia
- Palpitations

Skin
- Decreased sweating

Genitourinary
- Urinary hesitancy
- Urine retention

Anticholinergic agents also can produce various patient-sensitivity-related adverse reactions, including urticaria and allergic skin rashes that may lead to exfoliation. Diphenhydramine also can produce a photosensitivity reaction (abnormal reaction of the skin to sunlight), causing burning and redness with minimal exposure.

Rare adverse effects include blood dyscrasias. Prolonged therapy with some antihistamines may precipitate narrow-angle glaucoma and psychiatric disturbances that differ from the confusion usually associated with anticholinergic therapy.

NURSING PROCESS APPLICATION

The following information assists the nurse in caring for a patient who is receiving an anticholinergic agent.

Assessment
• Review the patient's history for conditions that contraindicate the use of an anticholinergic agent, such as narrow-angle glaucoma.
• Review the patient's history for conditions that require cautious use of an anticholinergic agent, such as gastric ulcer, prostatic hypertrophy, esophageal reflux, chronic pulmonary disease, and cardiovascular disease.
• Assess the patient for adverse reactions to the prescribed anticholinergic agent, such as constipation, nausea, xerostomia (dry mouth), confusion, tachycardia, dyspnea, or allergic skin rashes.
• Assess the effectiveness of anticholinergic therapy regularly.
• Assess for urine retention in a patient with prostatic hypertrophy who is taking an anticholinergic agent.
• Evaluate the patient's and family's knowledge about the prescribed anticholinergic agent.

Nursing diagnoses
The following examples represent appropriate nursing diagnoses for a patient receiving an anticholinergic agent.
• Potential for injury related to a preexisting condition that contraindicates the use of an anticholinergic agent
• Potential for injury related to a preexisting condition that requires cautious use of an anticholinergic agent
• Potential for injury related to adverse drug reactions
• Altered health maintenance related to ineffectiveness of the anticholinergic agent
• Urine retention related to use of an anticholinergic agent in a patient with prostatic hypertrophy
• Knowledge deficit related to the prescribed anticholinergic agent

Planning and implementation
• Do not administer an anticholinergic agent to a patient with a condition that contraindicates its use.
• Administer an anticholinergic agent cautiously to a patient at risk because of a preexisting condition.
• *Auscultate breath sounds at least every 8 hours in a patient with chronic pulmonary disease because secretions may thicken and cause dyspnea during anticholinergic therapy.*
• *Monitor the patient's heart rate for tachycardia.*
• Monitor for confusion when administering an anticholinergic agent to an elderly patient or one with dementia.
• Monitor for signs of an allergic reaction, such as skin rash.
• *Administer an anticholinergic agent during or shortly after meals to prevent adverse GI reactions.*
• Encourage a patient with constipation to ambulate and to increase fluid and dietary fiber intake, if possible. Administer a bulk-forming laxative or stool softener, as prescribed. Auscultate the patient's bowel sounds at least every 8 hours to detect signs of GI obstruction.
• Notify the physician if the patient experiences adverse reactions.
• Monitor the patient's degree of salivation, akinesia, and rigidity.
• Review the patient's medication history periodically to identify new use of a drug that decreases the anticholinergic agent's effectiveness, especially if parkinsonian signs and symptoms increase.
• Report to the physician any change in the patient's parkinsonian signs and symptoms.
• *Record fluid intake and output for a patient taking an anticholinergic agent. Observe for decreased output.*
• Notify the physician if the patient experiences urine retention.

Patient teaching
• Teach the patient and family the name, dose, frequency, action, and adverse effects of the prescribed anticholinergic agent.
• Encourage the patient and family to ask questions about the prescribed anticholinergic agent.
• *Teach the patient to relieve xerostomia by drinking cold beverages, sucking on hard candy, or using a nonprescription saliva substitute. Encourage proper oral hygiene.*
• *Instruct the patient to use caution when performing tasks that require alertness because of the risk from adverse reactions such as drowsiness or blurred vision.*
• *Advise the patient to avoid prolonged exposure to high temperatures because an anticholinergic increases the risk of heat stroke by reducing sweating.*
• Teach the patient not to discontinue long-term anticholinergic therapy before consulting the physician.

• Instruct the patient not to take over-the-counter cough or cold preparations, diet aids, or analeptics (agents used to stay awake) without consulting the physician because of potential interactions with the prescribed anticholinergic agent.

• Teach the patient that alcohol may increase the drowsiness produced by the anticholinergic agent.

• Advise the patient and family to inform the physician of improving or worsening of parkinsonian signs and symptoms.

• Advise the patient to notify the physician of adverse drug reactions.

• *Instruct family members to inform the physician of any signs of confusion or mental changes in the patient, especially in an elderly patient.*

• Give the patient written instructions about the prescribed anticholinergic agent.

Evaluation

The following examples represent appropriate evaluation statements for a patient receiving an anticholinergic agent.

• The patient has no conditions that contraindicate anticholinergic therapy.

• The patient exhibits no signs of complications in the preexisting condition linked to the prescribed anticholinergic agent.

• The patient demonstrates no adverse reactions to the prescribed anticholinergic agent.

• The patient states that signs and symptoms (tremors, akinesia, rigidity, and disturbance of posture and equilibrium) are under control.

• The patient maintains normal fluid balance.

• The patient and family express an accurate understanding of the points taught about the prescribed anticholinergic agent.

• The patient correctly describes how to relieve xerostomia.

DOPAMINERGIC AGENTS

Dopaminergics include six chemically unrelated drugs: levodopa, the metabolic precursor to dopamine; carbidopa-levodopa, a combination drug composed of the substance carbidopa, along with levodopa; amantadine hydrochloride, an antiviral agent; bromocriptine mesylate, a semisynthetic ergot alkaloid; pergolide mesylate, a dopamine agonist; and selegiline, a type B monoamine oxidase (MAO) inhibitor.

PHARMACOKINETICS

Like anticholinergics, dopaminergic agents are absorbed from the GI tract into the bloodstream and are delivered to their action site in the brain. They are metabolized extensively in various areas of the body and eliminated by the liver, kidneys, or both.

Absorption, distribution, metabolism, excretion

Levodopa competes with dietary amino acids for absorption from the small intestine and is absorbed by active transport. Consequently, absorption is slowed when the drug is ingested with food. The body absorbs most of a levodopa, carbidopa-levodopa, or an amantadine dose from the GI tract after oral administration, but it absorbs only about 28% of a bromocriptine dose. The body may absorb a significant amount of pergolide, although its absorption percentage is not fully known. It absorbs about 73% of an oral dose of selegiline.

Levodopa is widely distributed into most body tissues, including the GI tract, liver, pancreas, kidneys, salivary glands, and skin. Carbidopa-levodopa also is widely distributed. Amantadine is distributed in saliva, nasal secretions, and breast milk. Bromocriptine is 90% to 96% bound to serum albumin. Pergolide is approximately 90% protein bound. The distribution of selegiline is unknown.

Large amounts of levodopa are metabolized in the lumen of the stomach and during the first pass through the liver. After absorption, more than 95% is converted into dopamine peripherally (outside the CNS). But peripherally produced dopamine is ineffective because it cannot penetrate the CNS, where it is needed. To work, levodopa must undergo conversion to dopamine in the brain.

Carbidopa alone has no antiparkinsonian activity. When combined with levodopa, however, it blocks the peripheral conversion of levodopa to dopamine and allows levodopa to cross the blood-brain barrier. The levodopa then is converted to dopamine in the brain. Carbidopa also increases plasma levodopa concentrations, which may make smaller levodopa doses effective. When used with carbidopa, the levodopa dosage may be reduced by 70% to 75%. This in turn reduces the number of adverse reactions from levodopa alone.

Carbidopa is not metabolized extensively. The kidneys excrete approximately one-third of it as unchanged drug within 24 hours. Levodopa is metabolized extensively to various compounds that are excreted by the kidneys.

The pharmacokinetic processes of amantadine and bromocriptine are not understood completely. Amantadine is excreted mostly unchanged by the kidneys. Therefore, an elderly patient or a patient with renal insufficiency will require a lower dosage of amantadine based on the degree of renal impairment. In contrast, bromocriptine undergoes substantial first-pass metabolism in the liver; almost all of it is metabolized hepatically to pharmacologically inactive compounds. Elimination of bromocriptine and its metabolites occurs primarily in the feces; only 2.5% to 5.5% is excreted in the urine.

After pergolide is metabolized, it is excreted by the kidneys. Selegiline is metabolized to amphetamine, methamphetamine, and n-desmethyldeprenyl (the major metabolite), which are eliminated in the urine.

Onset, peak, duration

The onset of action, peak concentration levels, and duration of action of levodopa—with or without carbidopa—vary widely in patients. Levodopa's onset usually occurs in 30 to 45 minutes, its peak concentration is reached in about 1 hour, and its duration ranges from 2 to 5 hours. Administration of levodopa with food may delay its onset. Levodopa produces a short-term improvement that subsides 5 hours after a dose and a long-term improvement with prolonged therapy. The half-life of carbidopa-levodopa is approximately 2 hours, or about double that of levodopa alone.

Amantadine's peak concentration is reached approximately 1 to 4 hours after administration. Its half-life varies greatly but averages 24 hours. If the patient does not respond to amantadine in 2 weeks, the drug should be discontinued.

Bromocriptine's onset varies somewhat; improvement in parkinsonian signs may occur 30 to 90 minutes after a single dose. Peak concentration occurs in approximately 2 hours, and the duration of action is 3 to 5 hours. Bromocriptine has a half-life of 6 hours.

Pergolide's onset ranges from 15 to 20 minutes. It reaches peak concentration in 1 to 3 hours. Its duration of action and half-life are unknown.

After oral administration, selegiline attains peak concentration in 2 hours. Its onset, duration, and half-life have not been identified.

PHARMACODYNAMICS

The dopaminergic agents act in the brain by increasing the dopamine concentration or by enhancing neurotransmission of dopamine. These two mechanisms help improve motor function.

Mechanism of action

Levodopa is pharmacologically inactive until it crosses the blood-brain barrier and is converted to dopamine by enzymes in the brain. After this conversion, levodopa acts primarily by increasing dopamine concentrations in the basal ganglia. Carbidopa enhances levodopa's effectiveness.

Amantadine's mechanism of action is less clear. It may increase the amount of dopamine in the brain by increasing dopamine release or by blocking dopamine reuptake from presynaptic neurons.

Bromocriptine stimulates dopamine receptors in the brain, producing effects that are similar to dopamine's.

Pergolide directly stimulates postsynaptic dopamine receptors in the CNS.

Selegiline may increase dopaminergic activity by inhibiting type B MAO activity or by other mechanisms.

PHARMACOTHERAPEUTICS

Usually, dopaminergic agents are used to treat patients with severe parkinsonism or those who do not respond to anticholinergics alone.

levodopa (Dopar, Larodopa, Levopa). The most effective drug for parkinsonism, levodopa is used to treat the idiopathic and postencephalitic forms, especially in moderate to severe cases in advanced stages. Levodopa can be administered alone or with other drugs.
Usual adult dosage: initially, 0.5 to 1 gram P.O. b.i.d., t.i.d., or q.i.d., increased by 100 to 750 mg every 3 to 7 days until an optimum response is achieved or the maximum dosage of 8 grams is reached. The usual optimum dosage ranges from 3 to 6 grams P.O. in three or more divided doses. The typical patient reaches this level in 6 to 8 weeks.

carbidopa-levodopa (Sinemet). In this combination drug, carbidopa allows more levodopa to be converted to dopamine in the brain by inhibiting peripheral conversion. Physicians prescribe carbidopa-levodopa to treat idiopathic, postencephalitic, and symptomatic parkinsonism. Carbidopa-levodopa is available as combination tablets of 10 mg carbidopa/100 mg levodopa, 25 mg carbidopa/100 mg levodopa, or 25 mg carbidopa/250 mg levodopa. Carbidopa (Lodosyn) also is available alone in a 25-mg tablet.
Usual adult dosage: initially, 25 mg carbidopa/250 mg levodopa P.O. t.i.d.; if the patient is not receiving levodopa currently, initiate dosage with 25 mg carbidopa/100 mg levodopa t.i.d. Increase by one tablet daily or every other day to a dosage of 6 tablets per day. The usual dosage of carbidopa-levodopa ranges from 75/300 to 200/2,000 mg P.O. daily.

In a patient switching from levodopa alone to carbidopa-levodopa, discontinue levodopa at least 8 hours before initiating combination therapy. Then start carbidopa-levodopa with a daily dosage of no more than 25% of the previous levodopa dosage. Patients on combination therapy require close monitoring because therapeutic and adverse effects develop more rapidly.

amantadine hydrochloride (Symmetrel). This drug may be used alone in the early stages of parkinsonism or with other drugs in the advanced stages. Available as a capsule or as syrup, amantadine is especially effective against rigidity and bradykinesia, but less effective against tremor.

Usual adult dosage: 100 mg P.O. b.i.d.; adjust dosage as prescribed in patients with renal insufficiency; in patients with other serious illnesses or active seizure disorders and in those already receiving other antiparkinsonian agents, 100 mg P.O. daily for at least 1 week, then 100 mg b.i.d. If amantadine must be withdrawn, do so gradually to avoid precipitating parkinsonian crisis and possible life-threatening complications.

bromocriptine mesylate (Parlodel). This drug is used primarily as an adjunct to levodopa in the later stages of idiopathic or postencephalitic parkinsonism. When used with levodopa, bromocriptine may reduce levodopa's long-term adverse effects.
Usual adult dosage: initially, 1.25 mg P.O. once or twice daily with meals, increased by 1.25 to 2.5 mg every 2 to 3 days. The safety of bromocriptine in dosages greater than 100 mg P.O. daily has not been established. The usual adult maintenance dosage ranges from 10 to 40 mg P.O. daily. The patient's therapeutic response needs to be assessed every 2 weeks to ensure that the lowest effective dosage is being used. To prevent levodopa's adverse effects, the levodopa dose may need to be reduced as the bromocriptine dose is increased. If necessary, bromocriptine should be withdrawn gradually.

pergolide mesylate (Permax). This drug is used as an adjunct to carbidopa-levodopa in managing the signs and symptoms of Parkinson's disease.
Usual adult dosage: initially, 0.05 mg P.O. daily for 2 days; then increased gradually by 0.1 to 0.15 mg daily every third day over the next 12 days; then increased by 0.25 mg daily every third day until a therapeutic dosage is reached. The mean daily dosage is 3 mg P.O. Efficacy of dosages greater than 5 mg daily has not been established. During the pergolide dosage titration, the dosage of concurrent levodopa-carbidopa may be decreased slowly.

selegiline (Eldepryl). This drug is used as an adjunct in managing Parkinson's disease in patients receiving levodopa or carbidopa-levodopa who exhibit a reduced response to therapy.
Usual adult dosage: 5 to 10 mg P.O. daily. When administered with levodopa, the levodopa dosage may be reduced by 20% to 50%.

Drug interactions

The most serious interactions between the dopaminergics and other drugs occur when levodopa is combined with a type A MAO inhibitor, which can cause hypertensive crisis, or with meperidine, which can lead to death. Other interactions between dopaminergics and other drugs usually decrease the effectiveness of the dopaminergic agents. (For a summary, see *Drug interactions: Dopaminergic agents.*)

In some patients, levodopa may produce a significant interaction with foods. Dietary amino acids can decrease levodopa's effectiveness by competing with it for absorption from the intestine and slowing its transport to the brain. Therefore, if a patient's response deteriorates regularly after meals, the patient may need to reduce protein intake and avoid taking levodopa with meals to minimize this interaction.

ADVERSE DRUG REACTIONS

Among the dopaminergics, amantadine produces the fewest adverse reactions. Adverse reactions to bromocriptine, pergolide, and levodopa are mainly dose-related and can occur peripherally or in the CNS. With daily recommended dosages, selegiline produces few adverse reactions.

Adverse reactions to levodopa or carbidopa-levodopa usually are dose-related and reversible. Carbidopa decreases levodopa's peripheral effects but not its CNS effects. Levodopa commonly produces adverse GI reactions, such as nausea, vomiting, and anorexia. It also can cause orthostatic (postural) hypotension as well as other, less common adverse cardiovascular reactions, such as palpitations, tachycardia, arrhythmias, flushing, and hypertension. Additional adverse reactions include dark-colored urine and sweat, urinary frequency or urine retention, CNS disturbances (irritability, confusion, and hallucinations), and visual difficulties.

After withdrawal of levodopa, some patients experience hyperpyrexia (extreme elevation of body temperature) and neuroleptic malignant syndrome (characterized by hyperthermia, akinesia, altered consciousness, muscular rigidity, and profuse sweating). Both of these reactions can be fatal. Hematologic effects—such as leukopenia, granulocytopenia, thrombocytopenia, hemolytic anemia, and decreased hemoglobin and hematocrit levels—also may occur. When used alone, levodopa can cause transient elevations of liver enzymes, bilirubin, and blood urea nitrogen (BUN). When combined with carbidopa, levodopa may produce lower BUN, serum creatinine, and uric acid laboratory test values.

The most distressing problem with levodopa is the drug's loss of effectiveness after 3 to 5 years. The problem takes one of two forms: the on-off phenomenon, characterized by sharp fluctuations between mobility and immobility, or the end-of-dose deterioration (also known as the wearing-off effect), a progressive decrease in the duration of beneficial effects from each levodopa dose. The use of smaller, more frequent doses of levodopa and the addition of bromocriptine to the regimen can reduce both problems.

Amantadine produces relatively few adverse reactions at usual dosages. However, long-term therapy may produce livedo reticularis (diffuse, mottled reddening of the skin usually confined to the lower extremities), which commonly is accompanied by mild ankle edema. Other relatively com-

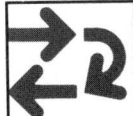

DRUG INTERACTIONS

Dopaminergic agents

Among the dopaminergic agents, levodopa causes most of the significant interactions with other drugs and with foods. Levodopa and monoamine oxidase (MAO) inhibitors can produce a hypertensive crisis when given concomitantly. Selegiline and meperidine may cause a fatal reaction. Less serious drug interactions also can occur with other dopaminergics, producing additive toxicities or decreasing the effectiveness of the dopaminergic agent.

DRUG	INTERACTING DRUGS	POSSIBLE EFFECTS	NURSING IMPLICATIONS
levodopa	pyridoxine (vitamin B$_6$)	Decreases effectiveness of levodopa caused by increased peripheral conversion of levodopa to dopamine by vitamin B$_6$	• Instruct the patient taking levodopa without carbidopa to avoid vitamin B$_6$ supplements or multiple vitamins containing vitamin B$_6$. • Be aware that this drug interaction may not occur in a patient taking carbidopa-levodopa.
	type A MAO inhibitors and furazolidone	Cause hypertensive crisis; increase toxic effects of levodopa	• Monitor the patient for hypertension if this combination is given. • Document and inform the physician if the patient starting levodopa has taken an MAO inhibitor in the past 2 weeks.
	phenytoin	Decreases effectiveness of levodopa	• Observe the patient for increased parkinsonian signs, such as bradykinesia, rigidity, and tremor. • Tell the patient to report any worsening of parkinsonian symptoms to the physician. • Expect to increase the levodopa dosage or administer an alternative anticonvulsant as prescribed.
	benzodiazepines	Inhibit effectiveness of levodopa	• Avoid concomitant administration of these drugs, if possible. • Observe the patient for increased parkinsonian signs, such as bradykinesia, rigidity, and tremor, if this combination is given.
	papaverine	Decreases effectiveness of levodopa	• Avoid concomitant administration, if possible.
levodopa, pergolide	antipsychotics (phenothiazines, thiothixene, haloperidol, loxapine)	Decrease effectiveness of levodopa and pergolide	• Avoid concomitant use of antipsychotics. If an antipsychotic medication is required, thioridazine usually is preferred. • Observe the patient for increased parkinsonian signs, such as bradykinesia, rigidity, and tremor, if this combination is given.
	reserpine	Decreases therapeutic response to levodopa by depleting dopamine stores in the brain	• Avoid administering reserpine to a patient receiving levodopa. • Observe the patient for increased parkinsonian signs, such as bradykinesia, rigidity, and tremor, if this combination is given.
levodopa, amantadine	anticholinergics	Increase anticholinergic adverse effects with amantadine, including adverse effects on mental function; decrease levodopa absorption, possibly leading to worsening of parkinsonian signs and symptoms or exacerbation of abnormal involuntary movements	• Monitor the patient taking amantadine for changes in mental status and other adverse reactions, such as urine retention, dry mouth, blurred vision, and constipation. • Expect to reduce the dosage of either agent, as prescribed, if intolerable anticholinergic adverse reactions occur. • Monitor the patient taking levodopa for increased rigidity, bradykinesia, and tremor or for exacerbation of abnormal involuntary movements.
selegiline	meperidine	May cause fatal reactions by an unknown mechanism of action	• Avoid concomitant administration.

mon adverse reactions include urine retention, orthostatic hypotension, anorexia, nausea, and constipation. Adverse CNS reactions may include inability to concentrate, confusion, light-headedness, anxiety, insomnia, irritability, dizziness, and hallucinations. Rare reactions include skin rash, leukopenia, eczematoid dermatitis, seizures, oculogyric episodes, and lingual and facial dyskinesias (movement impairments).

Besides cost, adverse reactions are the most important factor limiting the use of bromocriptine. Adverse reactions are more common at the start of therapy and when dosage exceeds 20 mg/day. Adverse GI reactions, such as nausea, occur commonly. Other common initial adverse reactions include orthostatic hypotension, vomiting, acute anxiety, dizziness, and sedation. Erythromelalgia (intermittent reddening and burning and throbbing sensations in the extremities) also may occur. Bromocriptine can cause adverse reactions in the cardiovascular system by producing persistent orthostatic hypotension (which may result in syncope), edema in the ankles and feet, palpitations, ventricular tachycardia, bradycardia, and exacerbation of angina. Confusion, hallucinations, delusions, nightmares, and erythromelalgia are notable especially during long-term or high-dosage (100 mg or more daily) bromocriptine therapy, but they usually are reversible. The presence of adverse CNS reactions usually limits the dosage and is the main reason for discontinuation of bromocriptine therapy.

Bromocriptine therapy has been associated with pleuropulmonary reactions, such as pulmonary infiltrates, pleural effusions, and thickening of the pleura. Bladder dysfunction with incontinence, urinary frequency, and urine retention also have been reported. Signs and symptoms of ergotism, including numbness and tingling of the extremities, cold feet, and muscle cramps in the legs and feet, also may occur.

The most common adverse reactions to pergolide include confusion, dyskinesia, hallucinations, nausea, and constipation. Hypertension is less common. Other adverse reactions may include abdominal pain, dizziness, drowsiness, flulike symptoms, orthostatic hypotension, lower back pain, rhinitis, and weakness; they may require medical attention if they continue or are bothersome. Rarely, pergolide has been associated with cerebrovascular hemorrhage, myocardial infarction, chills, diarrhea, xerostomia, facial edema, appetite loss, and vomiting.

Selegiline usually does not cause serious adverse reactions. However, it may produce nausea, dry mouth, dizziness, light-headedness, fainting, confusion, and hallucinations. Additional adverse reactions include vivid dreams, dyskinesia, headache, generalized achiness, anxiety, tension, diarrhea, insomnia, lethargy, leg pain, low back pain, palpitations, urine retention, and weight loss.

NURSING PROCESS APPLICATION

The following information assists the nurse in caring for a patient who is receiving dopaminergic agents.

Assessment
• Review the patient's history for conditions that contraindicate the use of dopaminergic agents, such as narrow-angle glaucoma or known hypersensitivity to these drugs.
• Review the patient's history for conditions that require cautious use of dopaminergic agents, such as cardiopulmonary, renal, hepatic, or endocrine disease; seizure disorders; and psychosis.
• Assess the patient for adverse reactions to the prescribed dopaminergic agent, such as nausea, orthostatic hypotension, peripheral edema, insomnia, hallucinations, and confusion.
• Assess the patient's diet for consumption of foods that may interact with levodopa.
• Assess the effectiveness of the dopaminergic agent periodically.
• Evaluate the patient's and family's knowledge about the prescribed dopaminergic agent.

Nursing diagnoses
The following examples represent appropriate nursing diagnoses for a patient receiving dopaminergic agents.
• Potential for injury related to a preexisting condition that contraindicates the use of dopaminergic agents
• Potential for injury related to a preexisting condition that requires cautious use of dopaminergic agents
• Potential for injury related to adverse drug reactions
• Potential for injury related to an interaction between levodopa and foods
• Impaired physical mobility related to ineffectiveness of dopaminergic agents, particularly levodopa
• Knowledge deficit related to the prescribed dopaminergic agent

Planning and implementation
• Do not administer a dopaminergic agent to a patient with a condition that contraindicates its use.
• Administer a dopaminergic agent cautiously to a patient at risk because of a preexisting condition.
• *Monitor the patient's blood pressure for orthostatic hypotension or, if the patient is taking an MAO inhibitor, hypertension.*
• Observe for adverse CNS reactions.
• Be aware that levodopa or carbidopa-levodopa may produce false-positive or false-negative results on urine glucose test strips (Testape, Diastix).
• Expect to reduce the bromocriptine dosage for a patient with hepatic dysfunction.

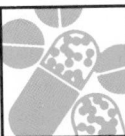

SELECTED MAJOR DRUGS

Antiparkinsonian agents

This chart summarizes the most commonly used agents for treating all forms of parkinsonism.

DRUG	MAJOR INDICATIONS	USUAL ADULT DOSAGES	CONTRAINDICATIONS AND PRECAUTIONS
Anticholinergic agents			
trihexyphenidyl benztropine diphenhydramine	Parkinsonism, especially control of symptoms in the early stages of Parkinson's disease (administered alone or with amantadine) and in the advanced stages (administered with levodopa)	3 to 15 mg P.O. t.i.d. 1 to 2 mg P.O., I.V., or I.M. daily 25 to 50 mg P.O. t.i.d. or q.i.d., or 10 to 100 mg I.M. or I.V. t.i.d. or q.i.d.	• Know that anticholinergics are contraindicated in a patient with known hypersensitivity to these drugs or one with narrow-angle glaucoma. • Administer with caution to a patient with gastric ulcer, esophageal reflux, hiatal hernia associated with reflux esophagitis, tachycardia, cardiac arrhythmias, hypotension, hypertension, hyperthyriodism, coronary artery disease, congestive heart failure, chronic pulmonary disease, or prostatic hypertrophy.
Dopaminergic agents			
levodopa carbidopa-levodopa	Parkinsonism, especially control of moderate to severe symptoms in Parkinson's disease (timing of initiation of levodopa therapy is controversial) Parkinsonism, especially control of moderate to severe symptoms in Parkinson's disease	3 to 6 grams P.O. daily in three or more divided doses 75/300 to 200/2,000 mg P.O. daily in divided doses	• Know that dopaminergic agents are contraindicated in a patient with known hypersensitivity to these drugs. • Know that levodopa is contraindicated in a patient with narrow-angle glaucoma. • Administer dopaminergic agents with caution to a patient with residual arrhythmias after myocardial infarction; one with a history of peptic ulcer disease, psychosis, or seizure disorders; or one experiencing hallucinations, confusion, or dyskinesia. • Administer levodopa with caution to a patient with bronchial asthma; emphysema; severe cardiovascular, pulmonary, renal, hepatic, or endocrine disease; or a need for a sympathomimetic agent such as epinephrine. • Advise a female patient to notify the physician if she is pregnant or lactating.
pergolide	Adjunct therapy with levodopa and carbidopa-levodopa to treat Parkinson's disease	0.05 mg P.O. daily initially for 2 days, increased by 0.1 to 0.15 mg daily every third day for 12 days, then increased by 0.25 mg daily every third day until a therapeutic dosage is reached	• Know that dopaminergic agents are contraindicated in a patient with known hypersensitivity to these drugs. • Administer dopaminergic agents with caution to a patient with residual arrhythmias after myocardial infarction; one with a history of peptic ulcer disease, psychosis, or seizure disorders; or one experiencing hallucinations, confusion, or dyskinesia. • Advise a female patient to notify the physician if she is pregnant or lactating.
selegiline	Adjunct therapy with levodopa and carbidopa-levodopa to treat Parkinson's disease	5 to 10 mg P.O. daily	• Know that dopaminergic agents are contraindicated in a patient with known hypersensitivity to these drugs. • Know that selegiline is contraindicated in a patient who is taking meperidine. • Administer dopaminergic agents with caution to a patient with residual arrhythmias after myocardial infarction; one with a history of peptic ulcer disease, psychosis, or seizure disorders; or one experiencing hallucinations, confusion, or dyskinesia. • Advise a female patient to notify the physician if she is pregnant or lactating.

• *Avoid administering levodopa with meals to prevent a drug-food interaction that may result in a decrease in the rate of drug absorption.*
• Expect to start pergolide therapy in small doses and titrate slowly to minimize hypotensive effects.
• Give the second daily dose of amantadine earlier in the evening if the patient experiences insomnia.
• *Elevate the patient's legs to help relieve drug-induced edema.*
• Monitor the patient's degree of physical mobility.
• Report decreased mobility to the physician.

Patient teaching

• Teach the patient and family the name, dose, frequency, action, and adverse effects of the prescribed dopaminergic agent.
• Advise the patient not to exceed the prescribed daily dosage because serious adverse reactions could result.
• Explain the importance of frequent blood pressure measurements, and teach the patient to recognize the symptoms of hypotension (such as dizziness and light-headedness) as well as hypertension (such as headache and vision changes).
• Instruct the family how to maintain a safe environment to prevent patient injury during periods of confusion.
• *Inform the patient that levodopa may cause harmless discoloration of urine and sweat.*
• Teach the patient who is taking levodopa about the on-off phenomenon.
• Instruct the female patient to notify her physician if she becomes pregnant or is lactating during dopaminergic therapy.
• Inform the patient that the levodopa-carbidopa dosage may be decreased after adjunct therapy begins with another dopaminergic agent.
• *Instruct the patient who is beginning levodopa therapy that the drug may take several weeks or months to reach its maximum effectiveness.*
• *Teach the patient not to discontinue long-term levodopa, amantadine, or bromocriptine therapy before consulting the physician.*
• Teach the diabetic patient how to monitor glucose levels using a blood glucose test.
• Instruct the patient to notify the physician if adverse reactions occur.
• Instruct family members to inform the physician if the patient experiences confusion or mental changes.
• Give the patient written instructions about the prescribed dopaminergic agent.

Evaluation

The following examples represent appropriate evaluation statements for a patient receiving a dopaminergic agent.
• The patient has no conditions that contraindicate dopaminergic agent therapy.

• The patient exhibits no signs of complications in the preexisting condition linked to the prescribed dopaminergic agent.
• The patient demonstrates no adverse reactions to the prescribed dopaminergic agent.
• The patient states that physical mobility has not decreased.
• The patient and family express an accurate understanding of the points taught about the prescribed dopaminergic agent.
• The patient schedules regular follow-up visits for blood pressure measurement.

CHAPTER SUMMARY

Chapter 19 concentrated on drugs for Parkinson's disease. Here are the highlights.
• Two major drug classes, the anticholinergics and the dopaminergics, are used to treat parkinsonism, which may result from idiopathic Parkinson's disease or other causes.
• Anticholinergic agents may be used alone or with amantadine in the early stages of Parkinson's disease and with levodopa in the more advanced stages. Although trihexyphenidyl, benztropine, and diphenhydramine are used most commonly, no single anticholinergic agent is clinically superior to the others. Effectiveness depends on the patient.
• Most adverse reactions to anticholinergics are an extension of their pharmacologic effects. Typically, they decrease as treatment continues, but limit the dosage that the patient can take.
• Levodopa, a dopaminergic agent, is the most effective drug used to treat Parkinson's disease. Levodopa therapy usually begins during advanced stages, either alone or with other drugs. Carbidopa given with levodopa is preferred because it reduces the levodopa dosage, decreasing GI and cardiovascular adverse effects.
• Levodopa presents two major therapeutic problems after 3 to 5 years of treatment: sharp fluctuations between mobility and immobility in the patient and a progressive decrease in beneficial effects. Although smaller, more frequent doses help, both problems become increasingly difficult to manage as the disease progresses.
• Amantadine may be used by itself in the early stages of Parkinson's disease or with other drugs, such as levodopa, in the advanced stages. Patients taking amantadine commonly develop a tolerance to it shortly after therapy begins. Tolerance does not develop, however, when the drug is used with levodopa or bromocriptine. Amantadine produces relatively benign adverse effects, but can produce more severe

ones if its dosage is not reduced for elderly patients or patients with renal insufficiency or seizure disorders.

• Bromocriptine, another dopaminergic agent, serves primarily as an adjunct to levodopa in advanced stages of Parkinson's disease. Bromocriptine's major drawbacks are its high cost and its adverse effects.

• When given with carbidopa-levodopa, pergolide and selegiline may decrease the required levodopa dosage, improve the duration of response, and decrease on-off fluctuations.

STUDY QUESTIONS

See Appendix 1 for answers.

1. Edna Miller, age 60, has just received a diagnosis of early-stage Parkinson's disease. The physician prescribes the anticholinergic agent benztropine mesylate (Cogentin) for her. Before administering this drug to Ms. Miller, the nurse assesses her history. Which of the following history findings contraindicates use of benztropine?
(a) nystagmus
(b) narrow-angle glaucoma
(c) cataracts
(d) blurred vision

2. Which of the following best describes benztropine's mechanism of action?
(a) It inhibits cerebral motor centers.
(b) It blocks the action of dopamine.
(c) It replaces depleted stores of dopamine.
(d) It triggers central cholinergic activity.

3. When Ms. Miller's disease progresses, benztropine no longer is effective in managing her signs and symptoms. How should the nurse expect to proceed with benztropine therapy?
(a) Discontinue benztropine immediately, then begin the new agent.
(b) Administer equal doses of each antiparkinsonian agent.
(c) Substitute the new agent and gradually discontinue benztropine.
(d) Provide a loading dose of the new agent, then stop the benztropine.

4. Which anticholinergic agent is most likely to be prescribed if Ms. Miller cannot tolerate a potent CNS-stimulating agent or if she experiences insomnia?
(a) orphenadrine
(b) diphenhydramine
(c) trihexyphenidyl
(d) benztropine

5. Rita Cunningham, age 65, takes levodopa, as prescribed, for moderate Parkinson's disease. Where does levodopa exert its action?
(a) in the brain
(b) in the stomach
(c) in the small intestine
(d) in the circulatory system

6. Which drug might the physician prescribe for Ms. Cunningham to enhance the effects of levodopa by inhibiting its peripheral conversion?
(a) carbidopa
(b) amantadine
(c) bromocriptine
(d) diphenhydramine

7. Before administering levodopa, the nurse obtains Ms. Cunningham's drug history. Which of the following interactions may occur if she takes a type A MAO inhibitor?
(a) hypotension
(b) hypertensive crisis
(c) nausea and vomiting
(d) tachycardia

SELECTED REFERENCES

AHFS drug information 90. (1990). Bethesda, MD: American Society of Hospital Pharmacists.

Berg, M., et al. (1987). Parkinsonism: Drug treatment, part I. *Drug Intelligence and Clinical Pharmacy,* 21(1), 10-21.

Calne, S. (1988). Parkinson's disease problems in nursing management related to medications. *Axon,* 9(4), 55-58.

Diet modification may improve response to levodopa. (1988). *Nurses Drug Alert,* 12(12), 95-96.

Hansten, P., and Horn, J. (1989). *Drug interactions* (6th ed.). Philadelphia: Lea & Febiger.

Pergolide and selegiline for Parkinson's disease. (1989). *The Medical Letter on Drugs and Therapeutics,* 31(800), 81-83.

CHAPTER 20

ANTICONVULSANT AGENTS

OBJECTIVES

After reading and studying this chapter, the student should be able to:
1. Describe the clinical characteristics of the major types of seizures identified by the international classification of epileptic seizures.
2. Identify the four factors that physicians consider when choosing a specific anticonvulsant agent for a patient.
3. Describe the mechanisms of action and the types of seizures treated by hydantoins, barbiturates, iminostilbenes, benzodiazepines, succinimides, and valproic acid.
4. Describe the important adverse reactions associated with each of the six major classes of anticonvulsants.
5. Describe how to apply the nursing process when caring for patients who are receiving drugs from each class of anticonvulsants.

INTRODUCTION

Anticonvulsant drugs are prescribed for long-term management of chronic epilepsy (recurrent seizures) and for short-term management of acute isolated seizures not caused by epilepsy. The short-term use of anticonvulsants also provides prophylaxis after trauma or a craniotomy. Selected anticonvulsants are indicated in the emergency treatment of status epilepticus, which is characterized by a series of rapidly repeating seizures without intervening periods of consciousness.

Seizures can be classified in various ways, but health care professionals usually use the international classification of epileptic seizures as the standard system. (For more information, see *International Classification of Epileptic Seizures,* page 296.)

The accurate diagnosis of a seizure requires a reliable patient history, careful patient observations, and an electroencephalogram. It also may require a computerized tomography scan or magnetic resonance imaging. The pharmacologic therapy used to treat seizures differs de-

pending on the type of seizure. The goal of anticonvulsant therapy is to control or prevent seizures. For many patients, anticonvulsant therapy is lifelong. Some patients, however, may have their drug therapy tapered off and eventually discontinued if they do not experience any seizures for a year.

Anticonvulsants fall into six major classes: hydantoins, barbiturates, iminostilbenes, benzodiazepines, succinimides, and valproic acid. The physician determines the specific anticonvulsant drug for a patient by considering four factors:
• the accurate diagnosis of the seizure type
• the ability of the drug to control seizures while producing only minimal adverse reactions
• the use of a single anticonvulsant when possible
• the appropriateness of the anticonvulsant for the patient's age and health.

The nurse must be aware of several nursing implications concerning administration, adverse reactions, and patient teaching.

For a summary of representative drugs, see *Selected major drugs: Anticonvulsant agents,* page 318. For a listing of applicable nursing diagnoses that the nurse may formulate when caring for a patient receiving these agents, see *Selected nursing diagnoses: Anticonvulsant agents.* For detailed information on applying the nursing process, see Chapter 6, The Nursing Process and Drug Therapy.

HYDANTOINS

Phenytoin, the most commonly prescribed anticonvulsant agent, belongs to the hydantoin class of drugs. Mephenytoin and ethotoin are also hydantoin anticonvulsants.

SELECTED NURSING DIAGNOSES

Anticonvulsant agents

The following nursing diagnoses address representative problems and etiologies that a nurse may encounter when caring for a patient who is receiving an anticonvulsant agent. Some of these nursing diagnoses contain generalized etiologies, which the nurse must individualize based on the patient's needs. (For some nursing diagnoses and related interventions for each drug class, see the "Nursing Process Application" sections of this chapter.)

- Activity intolerance related to anticonvulsant-induced weakness
- Altered health maintenance related to hydantoin-induced hyperglycemia
- Altered health maintenance related to ineffectiveness of the prescribed anticonvulsant agent
- Altered nutrition: less than body requirements, related to weight loss from succinimide therapy
- Altered oral mucous membrane related to succinimide-induced gum hypertrophy
- Altered protection related to drowsiness, dizziness, and other adverse CNS effects of an anticonvulsant agent
- Altered protection related to anticonvulsant-induced hematologic dysfunction
- Altered thought processes related to the adverse CNS effects of an anticonvulsant agent
- Altered urinary elimination related to the adverse genitourinary effects of a succinimide
- Body image disturbance related to cosmetic toxicity from hydantoin use
- Constipation related to the GI effects of an anticonvulsant agent
- Decreased cardiac output related to anticonvulsant-induced arrhythmias
- Diarrhea related to the adverse GI effects of a succinimide

- Fluid volume deficit related to the adverse GI effects of an anticonvulsant agent
- Fluid volume excess related to water intoxication with long-term use of carbamazepine
- Health-seeking behaviors related to possible interaction between carbamazepine and an oral contraceptive
- Impaired gas exchange related to barbiturate-induced respiratory depression or laryngospasm
- Impaired physical mobility related to the sedative effects of a barbiturate or valproic acid
- Knowledge deficit related to the prescribed anticonvulsant agent
- Noncompliance related to long-term use of the prescribed anticonvulsant agent
- Potential for injury related to a preexisting condition that contraindicates the use of an anticonvulsant agent
- Potential for injury related to a preexisting condition that requires cautious use of an anticonvulsant agent
- Potential for injury related to adverse drug reactions
- Potential for injury related to valproic acid therapy during pregnancy
- Sensory-perceptual alteration (visual) related to the adverse CNS effects of an anticonvulsant agent
- Sexual dysfunction related to primidone-induced impotence
- Urinary retention related to the adverse genitourinary effects of carbamazepine

PHARMACOKINETICS

Usually the hydantoin anticonvulsants are absorbed slowly, rapidly distributed, and extensively protein bound. These drugs usually are metabolized by hepatic microsomal enzymes and excreted as metabolites in the urine.

Absorption, distribution, metabolism, excretion

Phenytoin is absorbed slowly after oral administration and absorbed poorly after I.M. administration. Absorption rates, however, may vary with different phenytoin preparations. For example, Dilantin Kapseals are designed to provide extended therapy and therefore are absorbed more slowly; they also reach peak concentrations more slowly than other preparations. Clinically, the physician must differentiate among the various preparations and their administration routes to determine which preparation meets the therapeutic needs of a specific patient.

Phenytoin is distributed rapidly to all tissues; it also is bound extensively (90%) to plasma proteins, primarily albumin. Decreased protein binding occurs in neonates and in patients who are hypoalbuminemic or uremic. This de-

creased protein binding causes a higher free phenytoin serum concentration that can cause toxicity, even with normal measured serum concentrations.

Phenytoin is metabolized in the liver by the hepatic microsomal enzymes. Between 60% and 70% of a single dose of phenytoin is metabolized to an inactive metabolite, a parahydroxyphenyl derivative excreted as a glucuronide in the urine. Metabolism of phenytoin also produces other inactive metabolites.

Phenytoin metabolism is dose dependent, demonstrating saturation kinetics; that is, at a certain drug concentration the hepatic enzymes that metabolize phenytoin become saturated. When saturation occurs, further increase in drug concentration does not result in a direct linear increment but instead demonstrates a disproportionate increase in plasma concentration. Therefore, incremental increases in phenytoin dosage must be made cautiously. (For more information and an illustration, see *Phenytoin saturation kinetics,* page 297.)

The inactive metabolites of phenytoin are excreted in bile and then reabsorbed from the gastrointestinal (GI) tract. Eventually, however, they are excreted in the urine,

International Classification of Epileptic Seizures

Rational anticonvulsant therapy depends primarily on the accurate diagnosis of the seizure type. The following two classifications conform with the international classification scheme and reflect the current practice related to seizure types and their clinical characteristics. A third category of epileptic seizures remains unclassified because of inadequate or incomplete data. Earlier terminology appears in parentheses.

SEIZURE CLASSIFICATION	CLINICAL CHARACTERISTICS
Partial seizures—focal or local seizures	
Simple partial seizures (focal; jacksonian) • sensory • motor • autonomic • psychic	Most common in older children and adults. Consciousness not impaired; an aura is a simple partial seizure.
Complex partial seizures (psychomotor epilepsy) or **temporal lobe seizures**	Most common in older children and adults; brief impairment of consciousness; characterized by loss of contact with reality, automatisms (automatic behaviors such as chewing, lip smacking), and confusion that may last 1 to 2 minutes after seizure subsides.
Partial seizures evolving to secondarily generalized seizures	Partial seizures may spread, or "march," and ultimately involve all other parts of the brain with subsequent loss of consciousness. A tonic-clonic seizure follows.
Generalized seizures—convulsive or nonconvulsive	
Absence seizures (petit mal) • typical	Onset between ages 4 and 8; abrupt loss of consciousness, amnesia, or unawareness characterized by staring and a 3-cycle/second spike and waveform on electroencephalogram; attack lasts 10 to 30 seconds; may occur as frequently as 50 to 100 times/day. No postictal or confused state follows the attack.
• atypical	Slower onset and cessation of attacks than usually is seen with absence seizures.
Myoclonic seizures	Occur in older children and adults; myoclonic, lightning jerks (flexor or extensor) without loss of consciousness; last from seconds to minutes or longer and may occur daily.
Clonic seizures	Rhythmic clonic contraction and relaxation of muscles, loss of consciousness, and marked autonomic signs and symptoms.
Tonic seizures	Abrupt increase in muscle tone (contraction), loss of consciousness, and marked autonomic signs and symptoms.
Tonic-clonic seizures (grand mal)	Can occur at any age. May be preceded by an aura or an outcry. Contraction of all skeletal muscle masses occurs in rhythmic, alternating clonic and tonic patterns, followed by depression of all central functions, a state called the postictal period. Urinary and fecal incontinence may occur. Usually lasts 2 to 5 minutes but may last much longer. The frequency of attacks varies.
Atonic seizures	Seen in older children and adults. Consciousness usually lost, accompanied by loss of postural tone or akinesia. Lasts a few seconds to minutes and may occur daily.

with an alkaline urine enhancing urinary excretion. Less than 5% of the phenytoin is excreted unchanged in the urine. Phenytoin also is excreted via lacrimation and lactation.

Mephenytoin is absorbed rapidly after oral administration. The drug then exhibits moderate protein binding (60%) in the plasma. Metabolism of mephenytoin by the liver results in 5,5-ethylphenylhydantoin, an active metabolite believed to possess the therapeutic and toxic effects attributed to mephenytoin. Excretion occurs via the urine.

Ethotoin is metabolized by the hepatic microsomal enzyme system. Extensively protein bound, ethotoin is excreted in the urine, primarily as metabolites.

Phenytoin saturation kinetics

Phenytoin demonstrates saturation kinetics at varying serum concentrations. When saturation kinetics occur, the liver enzymes become saturated and unable to degrade more of the drug, and the serum concentration rises disproportionately. The daily drug dosages necessary to reach the serum concentration consistent with saturation vary for each individual. As illustrated on the following graph, patient A would receive 100 mg daily, whereas patient E would receive 500 mg to reach a therapeutic concentration. Beyond that level, saturation and rapid disproportionate increase in serum concentration occur.

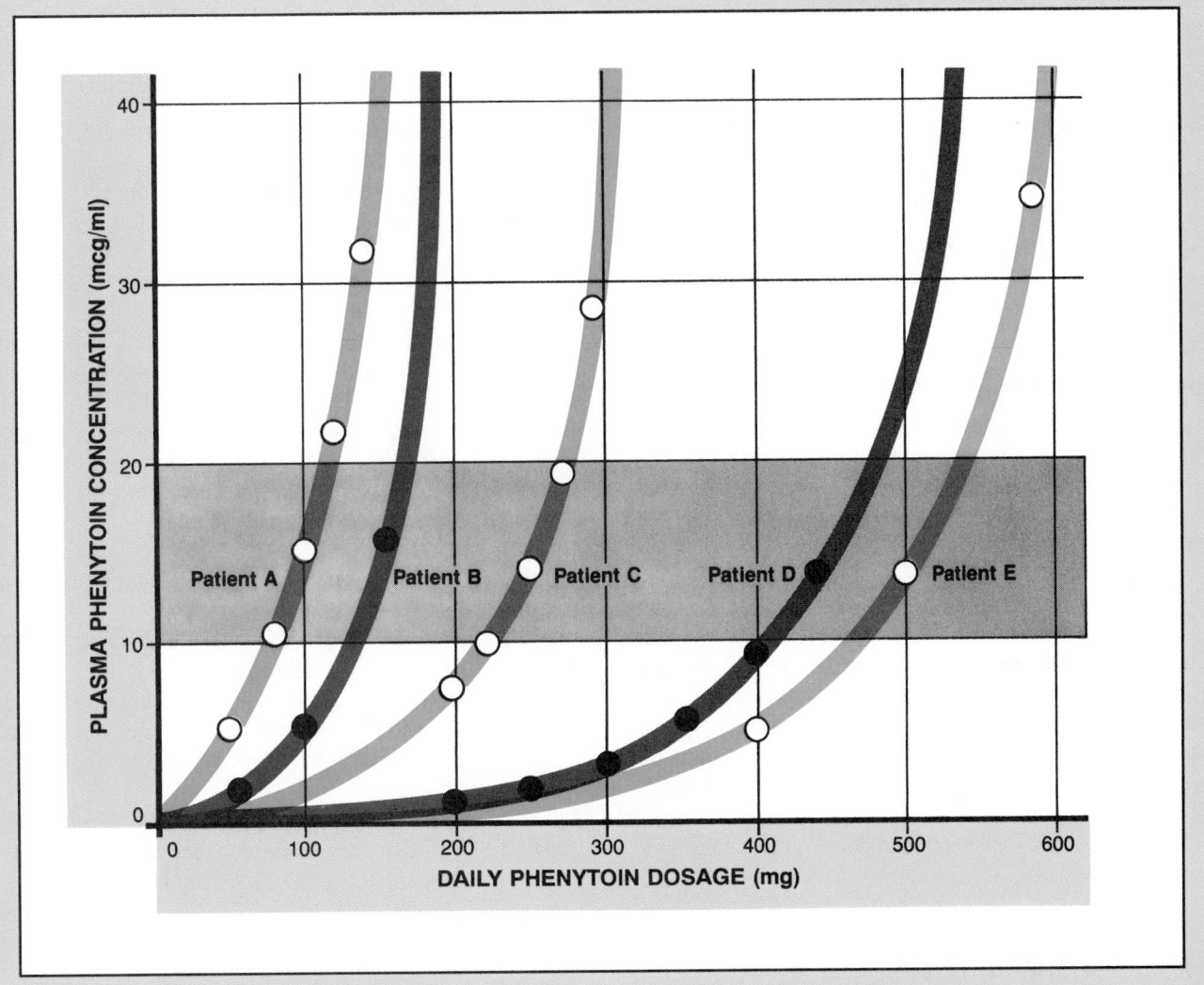

Reprinted with permission from Winter, M. (1980). *Basic clinical pharmacokinetics* (2nd ed.). Spokane, Wash.: Applied Therapeutics, Inc.

Onset, peak, duration

When administered orally, phenytoin demonstrates a variable onset of action from 30 minutes to 2 hours. When phenytoin is administered I.V., the onset occurs within 3 to 5 minutes.

The peak plasma concentration level for prompt-acting phenytoin preparations occurs in 1.5 to 3 hours, although the sustained-release preparations produce peak serum concentrations in 4 to 12 hours.

The duration of action for phenytoin depends on the time the drug remains in the therapeutic range. The plasma half-life after oral administration averages 22 hours, with a range of 7 to 42 hours. The range is so large because half-life changes with changes in serum concentration. (For an illustration of the significance of varying phenytoin serum levels, see *Phenytoin saturation kinetics.*) Steady-state serum phenytoin concentrations usually are achieved 7 to 10 days after initiating therapy. The clinically effective serum concentration range is between 10 and 20 mcg/ml in patients with normal serum albumin levels and normal renal function. For a more immediate clinical effect, loading doses administered over 8 to 12 hours produce a therapeutic serum concentration within 24 hours in most patients.

Mephenytoin exhibits a rapid onset of action, achieving peak serum concentrations in 2 to 4 hours. The duration of action of mephenytoin and its major metabolite, 5,5-ethylphenylhydantoin, is longer than that of phenytoin: 24 to 48 hours. Half-lives of 32 to 144 hours have been reported with mephenytoin because half-life changes with changes in serum concentration.

Ethotoin demonstrates a rapid onset of action, achieving peak serum concentrations in 2 to 4 hours. Ethotoin appears to undergo saturation kinetics, as does phenytoin, and its half-life ranges from 3 to 9 hours.

PHARMACODYNAMICS

In most cases, the hydantoin anticonvulsants can stabilize nerve cells against hyperexcitability.

Mechanism of action

The primary site of action appears to be the motor cortex, where the drugs inhibit the spread of seizure activity. Specifically, phenytoin alters ion movement across cell membranes. The pharmacodynamics of mephenytoin and ethotoin are thought to mimic those of phenytoin.

Because of its general effect of stabilizing excitable cells, phenytoin also exerts significant effects on excitable tissues outside the central nervous system (CNS). Phenytoin exhibits antiarrhythmic properties similar to those of quinidine or procainamide. It decreases the force of myocardial contractions, suppresses ectopic pacemaker activity, improves atrioventricular conduction depressed by digitalis glycosides, and increases the effective refractory period. (For a discussion of these effects, see Chapter 30, Antiarrhythmic Agents.) Phenytoin also exerts a membrane-stabilizing effect on the pancreas and may inhibit effective insulin release.

PHARMACOTHERAPEUTICS

Because of its clinical efficacy and relatively low toxicity, phenytoin is the most commonly prescribed anticonvulsant. Phenytoin represents one of the drugs of choice to treat complex partial (also called psychomotor or temporal lobe) and tonic-clonic seizures. Physicians sometimes prescribe mephenytoin and ethotoin as adjunct therapy for partial and tonic-clonic seizures in patients who are refractory to, or intolerant of, other anticonvulsants.

phenytoin and **phenytoin sodium** (Dilantin). Phenytoin is the drug of choice to treat complex partial (psychomotor)

and tonic-clonic seizures. Individualized dosage is required to achieve a therapeutic blood concentration of 10 to 20 mcg/ml.

Usual adult dosage: 300 mg P.O. of a prompt-acting preparation in three divided doses daily, or sustained-release preparations in a single daily dose; maintenance dosage, usually 300 to 400 mg or 3 to 5 mg/kg/day with a maximum dosage of 600 mg; in the acute treatment of status epilepticus, usually 15 mg/kg I.V. push at a rate not to exceed 50 mg/minute with an additional 5 mg/kg 12 hours later if required. In a geriatric patient with heart disease, the rate should not exceed 50 mg over 2 to 3 minutes.

Usual pediatric dosage: 5 mg/kg/day administered in two to three equally divided doses; suggested maintenance dosage, 4 to 8 mg/kg/day with a maximum of 300 mg/day (children over age 6 may require the minimum adult dosage of 300 mg/day); in the acute treatment of status epilepticus, 10 to 15 mg/kg administered I.V., usually at a rate not to exceed 1 to 2 mg/kg/minute in patients whose seizures are refractory to less toxic anticonvulsants.

The pediatric forms of phenytoin, tablets and suspension, are the free acid form rather than the sodium salt used in the adult, sustained-release, and I.V. forms. The free acid form supplies about 8% more phenytoin than the sodium salt form. Therefore, the nurse must monitor serum concentration carefully when using different forms of preparations to manage the same patient.

mephenytoin (Mesantoin). This drug is used primarily to treat partial and tonic-clonic seizures.

Usual adult dosage: 50 to 100 mg P.O. daily during the first week of treatment. Subsequent weekly increases of the same amount are administered until the maintenance dosage is achieved. For maintenance therapy, 200 to 600 mg P.O. daily in three equal doses, up to 800 mg or more P.O. daily.

Usual pediatric dosage: 50 to 100 mg P.O. daily during the first week of treatment. Subsequent weekly increases of the same amount are administered until the maintenance dosage, 100 to 400 mg P.O. daily in three equal doses, is achieved.

ethotoin (Peganone). This drug is used for complex partial (psychomotor) and tonic-clonic seizures.

Usual adult dosage: 1 gram or less P.O. daily, in four to six divided doses after meals. Subsequent dosages are increased gradually over several days. Maintenance therapy, 2 to 3 grams P.O. daily in four to six divided doses.

Usual pediatric dosage: initially, less than 750 mg P.O. daily in four to six divided doses; maintenance dosage, usually 500 mg to 1 gram P.O. daily. Occasionally, children may require larger dosages for maintenance therapy.

Drug interactions

Hydantoins interact with a number of other drugs. As a result, the activities of phenytoin, the other drug, or both are altered. (For detailed information, see *Drug interactions: Hydantoins,* pages 300 to 302.)

ADVERSE DRUG REACTIONS

The adverse effects of hydantoin anticonvulsants involve the central nervous, cardiovascular, GI, and hematopoietic systems, as well as cosmetic effects. The adverse reactions presented here relate directly to phenytoin. Ethotoin produces similar reactions; mephenytoin may produce more serious blood dyscrasias, including aplastic anemia.

In the CNS, adverse reactions to hydantoins include drowsiness, ataxia, irritability, headache, restlessness, nystagmus, dizziness, vertigo, and dysarthria. Adverse CNS reactions to phenytoin reflect the drug's blood concentration. For example, nystagmus and diplopia occur at 25 to 30 mcg/ml; ataxia, lethargy, and asterixis, at 30 to 40 mcg/ml; and decreased consciousness and coma, at 40 to 50 mcg/ml. Phenytoin also may cause toxic amblyopia and mental dullness.

The major adverse GI reactions include nausea, vomiting, epigastric pain, and anorexia. The adverse cardiovascular reactions are depressed atrial and ventricular conduction and, in toxic states, ventricular fibrillation. With I.V. administration, the adverse cardiovascular reactions include bradycardia, hypotension, and potential cardiac arrest. The primary adverse reaction of the hematopoietic system is a folic acid deficiency that can cause macrocytic anemia.

Cosmetic toxicity includes gingival hyperplasia, hirsutism, and facial coarsening. Other adverse reactions include hyperglycemia, glycosuria, and osteomalacia. Toxic doses of phenytoin paradoxically may induce seizures.

Hypersensitivity reactions to hydantoins typically are manifested as pruritus, fever, arthralgia, and a measleslike rash; exfoliative, purpuric, or bullous dermatitis; Stevens-Johnson syndrome; lymphadenopathy; acute renal failure; hepatitis; and liver necrosis. Several adverse reactions also relate to the hematopoietic system, including thrombocytopenia, leukopenia, leukocytosis, agranulocytosis, pancytopenia, eosinophilia, macrocytosis, and various anemias.

NURSING PROCESS APPLICATION

The following information assists the nurse in caring for a patient who is receiving a hydantoin.

Assessment

• Review the patient's history for conditions that contraindicate the use of a hydantoin, such as known hypersensitivity to the drug.
• Review the patient's history for conditions that require cautious use of a hydantoin, such as pregnancy.
• Assess the patient for adverse reactions to the prescribed hydantoin, such as drowsiness, ataxia, irritability, headache, restlessness, nystagmus, GI distress, depressed atrial and ventricular conduction, bradycardia, hypotension, folic acid deficiency, gingival hyperplasia, and hyperglycemia.
• Assess the effectiveness of the prescribed hydantoin periodically.
• Assess the patient regularly for signs and symptoms of hyperglycemia.
• Assess for perceived changes in body image if the patient develops cosmetic adverse reactions.
• Evaluate the patient's and family's knowledge about the prescribed hydantoin.

Nursing diagnoses

The following examples represent appropriate nursing diagnoses for a patient receiving a hydantoin.
• Potential for injury related to a preexisting condition that contraindicates the use of hydantoins
• Potential for injury related to a preexisting condition that requires cautious use of hydantoins
• Potential for injury related to adverse drug reactions
• Altered health maintenance related to ineffectiveness of the prescribed hydantoin
• Altered health maintenance related to hydantoin-induced hyperglycemia
• Body image disturbance related to cosmetic toxicity from hydantoin use
• Knowledge deficit related to the prescribed hydantoin

Planning and implementation

• Do not administer a hydantoin to a patient with a condition that contraindicates its use.
• Administer a hydantoin cautiously to a patient at risk because of a preexisting condition. Be aware that safe use of an anticonvulsant in a woman of childbearing age as well as a pregnant or lactating woman has not been established.
• Monitor the patient's serum phenytoin concentration because many adverse reactions are dose-related.
• *Keep oxygen, suction, and resuscitation equipment available when administering phenytoin I.V.*
• Monitor the patient regularly for signs of adverse reactions to the prescribed hydantoin.
• *Administer I.V. phenytoin at a rate not to exceed 50 mg/minute (or 50 mg/3 minutes in a geriatric patient with heart disease) because of its cardiotoxicity. Also monitor*

(Text continues on page 302.)

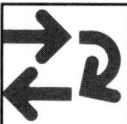

DRUG INTERACTIONS

Hydantoins

The following drug interactions may occur with the use of phenytoin or any other hydantoin anticonvulsant. Because phenytoin interacts with many drugs, this chart has been limited to interactions that have major to moderate clinical significance. Drug interactions of lesser clinical significance, involving such drugs as acetaminophen, allopurinol, antacids, and dopamine, have not been included.

DRUG	INTERACTING DRUGS	POSSIBLE EFFECTS	NURSING IMPLICATIONS
phenytoin, mephen-ytoin, ethotoin	cimetidine, disulfiram, iso-niazid, sulfonamides	Inhibit phenytoin metabo-lism, resulting in increased toxic adverse effects of phenytoin	• Monitor serum phenytoin concentration; phe-nytoin dosage may need to be decreased. • Advise the patient to report adverse reactions. • Carefully monitor complete blood count (CBC), platelet and reticulocyte counts, and liver function tests.
	oral anticoagulants	Increase serum phenytoin concentrations when phe-nytoin therapy begins first; produce a transient in-crease in anticoagulant ef-fect, followed by a de-crease in anticoagulant effect when oral anticoag-ulant therapy begins first	• Monitor serum phenytoin concentration; phe-nytoin dosage may need to be decreased. • Advise the patient to report adverse reac-tions. • Carefully monitor CBC, platelet and reticulo-cyte counts, and liver function tests.
	phenobarbital	Produces variable interac-tion mechanism, usually resulting in decreased phenytoin concentration; occasionally, may cause increased phenytoin con-centration	• Monitor phenytoin and phenobarbital serum concentrations. • Monitor CBC, platelet and reticulocyte counts, and liver function tests. • Advise the patient to report any change in adverse reactions or seizure frequency.
	diazoxide	Increases induction of phenytoin metabolism, re-sulting in decreased effi-cacy of phenytoin	• Monitor serum phenytoin concentration.
	levodopa	Cause unknown interac-tion mechanism, resulting in decreased efficacy of levodopa	• Observe for increased signs or symptoms of Parkinson's disease. • Advise the patient to report any change in parkinsonian signs or symptoms. • Be aware that the levodopa dosage may need to be increased because of decreased effect.
	chloramphenicol	Inhibits phenytoin metabo-lism, resulting in increased toxic adverse effects of phenytoin; unknown inter-action mechanism, result-ing in decreased efficacy of chloramphenicol	• Monitor serum phenytoin concentration; ad-vise the patient to report adverse reactions. • Monitor CBC, platelet and reticulocyte counts, and liver function tests. • Monitor serum chloramphenicol concentra-tion. • Be aware that the chloramphenicol dosage may need to be increased because of de-creased effect.
	amiodarone	Inhibits phenytoin metabo-lism, resulting in twofold to threefold increase in phe-nytoin concentration;	• Monitor serum phenytoin concentration. • Observe the patient for signs of phenytoin toxicity. • Expect to decrease the phenytoin dosage.

DRUG INTERACTIONS

Hydantoins *(continued)*

DRUG	INTERACTING DRUGS	POSSIBLE EFFECTS	NURSING IMPLICATIONS
phenytoin, mephenytoin, ethotoin *(continued)*		cause induction of amiodarone metabolism, resulting in decreased amiodarone efficacy	• Be aware that the amiodarone dosage may need to be increased because of decreased effect. • Advise the patient to see the physician frequently for monitoring of cardiac status. • Alert the patient to report signs or symptoms of arrhythmias, such as palpitations and irregular pulse.
	corticosteroids	Cause induction of corticosteroid metabolism, resulting in decreased efficacy of corticosteroids	• Be aware that the corticosteroid dosage may need to be increased because of decreased effect. • Monitor the patient's blood pressure and weight. • Monitor serum electrolyte levels.
	doxycycline	Cause induction of doxycycline metabolism, resulting in decreased efficacy of doxycycline	• Monitor the patient closely because of decreased effect. Be aware that the doxycycline dosage may need to be increased.
	methadone	Cause induction of methadone metabolism, resulting in decreased efficacy of methadone	• Be aware that the methadone dosage may need to be increased because of decreased effect. • Alert the patient to watch for signs of withdrawal.
	metyrapone	Cause induction of metyrapone metabolism, resulting in decreased efficacy of metyrapone	• Monitor the patient closely. Be aware that the metyrapone dosage may need to be increased because of decreased effect.
	quinidine, mexiletine	Cause induction of metabolism, resulting in decreased efficacy of these drugs	• Be aware that the dosage of these drugs may need to be increased because of decreased effect. • Advise the patient to see the physician frequently for monitoring of cardiac status. • Alert the patient to report signs or symptoms of arrhythmias, such as palpitations and irregular pulse.
	theophylline	Produces unknown interaction mechanism, resulting in decreased efficacy of phenytoin; cause induction of metabolism, resulting in decreased efficacy of theophylline	• Be aware that the phenytoin and theophylline dosages may need to be increased because of their decreased effects. • Monitor serum concentrations of both drugs. • Advise the patient to report increased shortness of breath to the physician. • Monitor CBC, platelet and reticulocyte counts, and liver function tests.
	thyroid hormone	Increase metabolism of thyroid hormone	• Monitor the patient closely because of increased thyroid hormone metabolism. • Be aware that the thyroid hormone dosage may need to be increased.
	oral contraceptives	Cause induction of contraceptive metabolism, resulting in decreased efficacy of contraceptives	• Be aware that the patient may need an alternative contraceptive method because of decreased efficacy.

(continued)

DRUG INTERACTIONS

Hydantoins *(continued)*

DRUG	INTERACTING DRUGS	POSSIBLE EFFECTS	NURSING IMPLICATIONS
phenytoin, mephen-ytoin, ethotoin *(continued)*	valproic acid	Produces unpredictable effects; may cause displacement of phenytoin protein binding, resulting in a transient decrease in phenytoin concentrations; may inhibit phenytoin metabolism, causing increased phenytoin concentrations	• Monitor phenytoin concentration carefully. • Be aware that breakthrough seizures may occur with use of valproic acid-phenytoin combination.
	cyclosporine	Decrease cyclosporine absorption, resulting in decreased serum concentrations	• Monitor cyclosporine concentration.
	digitoxin	Decrease digitoxin effect	• Monitor the patient closely. • Be aware that the digitoxin dosage may need to be increased because of decreased effect.

the patient's blood pressure, pulse, and respirations every 5 minutes during administration and every 15 minutes thereafter until the patient becomes stable. If blood pressure decreases during drug administration, reduce the infusion rate.

• Minimize vein irritation by infusing normal saline solution after I.V. phenytoin administration, as prescribed.

• *Do not mix I.V. phenytoin with any other drug to avoid phenytoin precipitation.*

• *Avoid I.M. injections because phenytoin precipitates in muscle tissue, which decreases drug bioavailability.*

• *Administer an oral hydantoin with meals to minimize GI distress.*

• Use only sustained-release capsules (Dilantin Kapseals) for once-a-day dosing of phenytoin. The chewable tablets are not intended for once-a-day dosing. Furthermore, the chewable tablets are not dose-exchangeable with the capsules, because the free acid tablet and the sodium capsule provide different strengths of phenytoin.

• Shake suspension preparations vigorously before pouring to ensure uniform distribution and exact measurement of the drug.

• *Discontinue phenytoin immediately and notify the physician if the patient develops a skin rash.*

• Expect to administer vitamin K to treat hypoprothrombinemia in a neonate whose mother received a hydantoin during pregnancy.

• *Monitor the patient's liver and kidney function tests and blood count periodically.*

• Notify the physician if the patient displays adverse drug reactions.

• Monitor the patient's frequency of seizure activity.

• Notify the physician if the patient displays continued seizure activity.

• *Monitor the patient regularly for signs and symptoms of hyperglycemia, such as polyuria, polyphagia, polydipsia, and weight loss.*

• *Obtain blood glucose levels at least once daily.*

• Expect to alter the diabetic patient's treatment for diabetes if hyperglycemia occurs with hydantoin administration.

• Encourage the patient to express feelings about body image if cosmetic adverse reactions occur.

• Explore ways to mask undesired cosmetic changes, such as by using makeup and hair removal preparations for the female patient.

• Consult with the physician about switching to a different anticonvulsant agent if the patient is disturbed greatly by cosmetic adverse reactions.

Patient teaching

• Provide basic information about hydantoin therapy. (For specifics, see *General patient-teaching tips.*)

• Teach the patient and family the name, dose, frequency, action, and adverse effects of the prescribed hydantoin agent.

• *Recommend that the female patient who is taking an oral contraceptive and a hydantoin use an additional or different contraceptive method.*

General patient-teaching tips

Regardless of the anticonvulsant prescribed, the following patient-teaching tips apply.
• Instruct the patient not to alter the prescribed drug regimen.
• Instruct the patient to notify the physician if seizure control deteriorates.
• Alert the patient that abrupt discontinuation of the prescribed drug could precipitate seizures or status epilepticus.
• Remind the patient to check all prescription refills to ensure that the drug preparation is the same as the previous preparation.
• Advise the patient to avoid hazardous activities until the dosage and adverse reactions become stabilized.
• Teach the patient's family how to care for the patient during a seizure.
• Advise the patient not to self-medicate with over-the-counter drugs.
• Advise the patient to refrain from ingesting alcohol because of its possible interactive effects with some anticonvulsants.
• Emphasize the importance of frequent follow-up care for the patient, and provide information about voluntary community organizations that provide information and support.

• Encourage the patient with gingival hyperplasia to brush the teeth meticulously and floss daily.
• *Remind the patient to notify the dentist about hydantoin therapy.*
• *Inform the patient that phenytoin may cause harmless pink, red, or red-brown discoloration of urine.*
• Advise the patient to report adverse drug reactions to the physician.
• *Advise the diabetic patient to monitor blood glucose levels because the hydantoin may increase blood glucose levels.*

Evaluation
The following examples represent appropriate evaluation statements for a patient receiving a hydantoin agent.
• The patient has no conditions that contraindicate hydantoin therapy.
• The patient exhibits no signs of complications in the preexisting condition linked to the prescribed hydantoin.
• The patient experiences no adverse reactions to the prescribed hydantoin.
• The patient displays no seizure activity.
• The patient's blood glucose level remains normal.
• The patient expresses acceptance of cosmetic changes and demonstrates a willingness to address these changes appropriately.
• The patient and family express an accurate understanding of the points taught about the prescribed hydantoin.

• The patient correctly lists adverse reactions to the prescribed hydantoin and describes what to do if they occur.

BARBITURATES

The long-acting barbiturate phenobarbital is also one of the most widely employed anticonvulsants. Phenobarbital is used in long-term treatment of epilepsy and is prescribed selectively for acute treatment of status epilepticus. Mephobarbital, also a long-acting barbiturate, is used less commonly as an anticonvulsant. Primidone, a deoxybarbiturate that is closely related chemically to the barbiturates, also is used in the chronic treatment of epilepsy. (For a discussion of barbiturates as sedatives and hypnotics, see Chapter 25, Sedative and Hypnotic Agents.)

PHARMACOKINETICS

The barbiturate anticonvulsants are metabolized in the liver. Metabolites and unchanged drug are excreted in the urine.

Absorption, distribution, metabolism, excretion
Phenobarbital is absorbed slowly but well (about 70% to 90%) from the GI tract. Peak plasma concentration levels occur 8 to 12 hours after a single dose. The drug is 20% to 45% bound to serum proteins and to a similar extent to other tissues, including the brain.

About 75% of a phenobarbital dose is metabolized by hepatic microsomal enzymes, and 25% is excreted unchanged in the urine. Renal excretion can be increased by alkalinizing the urine or increasing the urinary flow rate. Phenobarbital also is excreted in breast milk.

Almost 50% of a mephobarbital dose is absorbed from the GI tract and well distributed in body tissues. The drug is bound to tissue and plasma proteins. Mephobarbital undergoes extensive metabolism by hepatic microsomal enzymes. This metabolism converts approximately 75% of a single mephobarbital dose to the major metabolite phenobarbital within 24 hours. Only 1% to 2% of a dose is excreted unchanged in the urine.

From 60% to 80% of a primidone dose is absorbed from the GI tract and distributed evenly among body tissues. The drug is protein bound to a small extent in the plasma, as is one of its active metabolites, phenylethylmalonamide (PEMA). Primidone is metabolized by hepatic microsomal enzymes to two active metabolites, phenobarbital and PEMA, which share in the anticonvulsant activity of primidone. From 15% to 25% of primidone is excreted unchanged in the urine, 15% to 25% is metabolized to phenobarbital, and 50% to 70% is excreted in the urine as PEMA. Primidone also is excreted in breast milk.

Onset, peak, duration

Phenobarbital provides an onset of action within 30 minutes after oral administration. Peak anticonvulsant effect occurs in 8 to 12 hours. The onset after I.V. administration occurs within 5 minutes, with peak anticonvulsant effect within 30 minutes. Phenobarbital has an extremely long half-life of 50 to 170 hours and thus requires 10 to 35 days to reach a steady state.

Mephobarbital demonstrates a rapid onset, with peak anticonvulsant effect in 6 to 8 hours. The half-life of mephobarbital is 11 to 67 hours, with a steady state in 6 to 15 days.

Primidone displays a rapid onset, with peak anticonvulsant effect in 4 hours. The half-life of primidone varies from 10 to 21 hours. The time needed for the drug and its metabolites to reach steady-state levels varies as follows: primidone, 2 days; PEMA, 1 week; and phenobarbital, 10 to 35 days.

PHARMACODYNAMICS

The barbiturates exhibit anticonvulsant action at subhypnotic dosages. For this reason, the barbiturates usually do not produce addiction when used to treat epilepsy.

Mechanism of action

The barbiturate anticonvulsants limit seizure activity by increasing the threshold for motor cortex stimuli. This increase may be due, at least in part, to reduction of monosynaptic and polysynaptic transmission.

PHARMACOTHERAPEUTICS

The barbiturate anticonvulsants are effective in treating partial, tonic-clonic, and febrile seizures when used alone or with other anticonvulsants. I.V. phenobarbital also is used to treat status epilepticus. The major disadvantage of using phenobarbital for status epilepticus is delayed onset of action. Barbiturate anticonvulsants are ineffective in treating absence seizures.

Mephobarbital offers no advantage over phenobarbital; it is used when the patient cannot tolerate the adverse effects of phenobarbital. Primidone is used primarily with other anticonvulsants. Some clinicians, however, consider it the drug of choice for complex partial seizures.

phenobarbital, phenobarbital sodium (Luminal). A Schedule IV drug, phenobarbital is used for long-term treatment of partial and tonic-clonic seizures and for the acute management of status epilepticus and febrile seizures. The

therapeutic plasma concentration range for adults and children is 15 to 40 mcg/ml.
Usual adult dosage: for partial and tonic-clonic seizures, 100 to 300 mg, or 1 to 5 mg/kg P.O. daily; for status epilepticus, 5 to 10 mg/kg I.V. at a rate not to exceed 60 mg/minute.
Usual pediatric dosage: for partial and tonic-clonic seizures, 3 to 5 mg/kg P.O. daily in two equal doses.

mephobarbital (Mebaral). A Schedule IV drug, mephobarbital is used to treat the same types of seizures as phenobarbital, with the exception of status epilepticus. The therapeutic serum concentration of phenobarbital determines the dosage adjustments of mephobarbital, because mephobarbital is metabolized to phenobarbital.
Usual adult dosage: 400 to 600 mg P.O. daily.
Usual pediatric dosage: 16 to 32 mg P.O. t.i.d. to q.i.d. as ordered for children under age 5; for children over age 5, 32 to 64 mg P.O. t.i.d. to q.i.d.

primidone (Mysoline). A deoxybarbiturate, primidone is used for long-term treatment of partial seizures and tonic-clonic seizures. Primidone is ineffective in treating status epilepticus and absence seizures. When measuring serum concentrations of primidone, phenobarbital also must be measured because it is an active metabolite.
Usual adult dosage: initially, 125 mg P.O. daily in divided doses, gradually increased by 125 mg every 3 days to 250 mg P.O. t.i.d. to q.i.d. up to a maximum dosage of 2 grams per day. The therapeutic plasma concentrations of primidone are phenobarbital, 15 to 40 mcg/ml, and primidone, 5 to 12 mcg/ml. (PEMA concentrations are not measured in clinical practice.) The maximum dosage is 2 grams.
Usual pediatric dosage: initially, 50 mg P.O. daily for the first 3 days, then 50 mg b.i.d. for days 4 through 6, and 100 mg b.i.d for days 7 through 9; for maintenance, 125 to 250 mg P.O. t.i.d., or 10 to 25 mg/kg/day in divided doses.

Drug interactions

Phenobarbital interacts with many drugs, usually altering their metabolic rate. For example, such drugs as the hydantoins and chloramphenicol inhibit phenobarbital metabolism, increasing the drug's toxic effects. Mephobarbital and primidone interact with the same drugs and in the same way as phenobarbital because both drugs are metabolized to phenobarbital. (For more information, see *Drug interactions: Barbiturates.*)

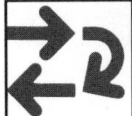

DRUG INTERACTIONS

Barbiturates

Most of the clinically significant interactions involving barbiturates occur with phenobarbital. Mephobarbital and primidone interact with the same drugs as phenobarbital. Because primidone is converted to phenobarbital in the body, concurrent administration of primidone and phenobarbital may result in an elevated serum phenobarbital concentration.

DRUG	INTERACTING DRUGS	POSSIBLE EFFECTS	NURSING IMPLICATIONS
phenobarbital, mephobarbital, primidone	hydantoins	Inhibit phenobarbital metabolism, resulting in increased toxic effects	• Monitor serum concentrations; phenobarbital dosage may need to be decreased. • Advise the patient to report adverse reactions. • Alert the patient not to drive or operate heavy machinery until the effect of the drug combination in the patient is known. • Advise the patient to avoid alcohol consumption.
	beta blockers (metoprolol, propranolol)	Cause induction of beta blocker metabolism, resulting in decreased effectiveness of beta blockers	• Monitor desired effect in the patient (antianginal, antihypertensive, and antiarrhythmic); beta blocker dosage may need to be increased. • Instruct the patient to report changes in desired effect in drug therapy. • Advise the patient to report periodically for blood pressure and pulse checks.
	chloramphenicol	Cause induction of chloramphenicol metabolism, resulting in decreased effectiveness of chloramphenicol; inhibits phenobarbital metabolism	• Monitor desired effect in the patient (anti-infective); chloramphenicol dosage may need to be increased. • Monitor serum chloramphenicol and phenobarbital concentrations.
	corticosteroids	Cause induction of corticosteroid metabolism, resulting in decreased effectiveness of corticosteroids	• Be aware that the corticosteroid dosage may need to be increased because of decreased effect. • Monitor the patient's weight and blood pressure. • Monitor serum electrolyte levels.
	doxycycline	Cause induction of doxycycline metabolism, resulting in decreased effectiveness of doxycycline	• Be aware that the doxycycline dosage may need to be increased or that tetracycline may be substituted because of decreased effect.
	oral anticoagulants	Produce induction of oral anticoagulant metabolism, resulting in decreased effectiveness of oral anticoagulants	• Monitor prothrombin level; anticoagulant dosage may need to be increased. • Advise the patient to be alert for signs and symptoms of thrombus formation, such as pain, tenderness, and edema in the calf.
	oral contraceptives	Produce induction of oral contraceptive metabolism, resulting in decreased effectiveness of oral contraceptives	• Alert the patient that contraceptive effect may be impaired; breakthrough bleeding may occur. • Suggest alternative or additional contraceptive method.
	quinidine	Cause induction of quinidine metabolism, resulting in decreased effectiveness of quinidine	• Be aware the the quinidine dosage may need to be increased because of decreased effect. • Advise the patient to see the physician frequently for monitoring of cardiac status. • Alert the patient to report any signs and symptoms of arrhythmias, such as palpitations and irregular pulse.

(continued)

DRUG INTERACTIONS

Barbiturates *(continued)*

DRUG	INTERACTING DRUGS	POSSIBLE EFFECTS	NURSING IMPLICATIONS
phenobarbital, mephobarbital, primidone *(continued)*	methoxyflurane	Causes possible induction of hepatic microsomal enzymes by barbiturates that may stimulate metabolism of methoxyflurane to nephrotoxic metabolites	• Avoid concurrent administration of phenobarbital and methoxyflurane.
	phenothiazines	Cause induction of phenothiazine metabolism, resulting in decreased effectiveness of phenothiazine	• Be aware that the phenothiazine dosage may need to be increased because of decreased effect. • Monitor the patient's behavior closely. • Advise the patient and family members to report promptly to the physician any changes in behavior.
	tricyclic antidepressants	Cause induction of tricyclic antidepressant metabolism, resulting in decreased effectiveness of tricyclic antidepressant	• Be aware that the tricyclic antidepressant dosage may need to be increased because of decreased effect. • Monitor the serum concentration of the tricyclic antidepressant. • Advise the patient to report any change in therapeutic effect, such as lack of mood elevation.
	CNS depressants (antianxiety agents, sedative-hypnotics, most narcotic analgesics, and alcohol)	Produce additive effects, resulting in increased sedative toxicity	• Assess frequently for changes in level of consciousness and respirations. • Supervise ambulation; raise side rails, especially with elderly patients. • Alert the patient not to drive or use heavy machinery until the effects of the drug combination in the patient is known. • Advise the patient not to drink alcohol while taking these medications.
	valproic acid	Inhibits the hepatic metabolism of phenobarbital	• Monitor for excessive phenobarbital effect, such as drowsiness. • Be aware that the phenobarbital dosage may need to be decreased because of increased serum phenobarbital concentration.
	metronidazole	Increase metronidazole metabolism	• Be aware that the metronidazole dosage may need to be increased.
	digitoxin	Decrease digitoxin effectiveness	• Monitor the patient for signs of digitoxin's effectiveness. • Be aware that the digitoxin dosage may need to be increased.
	theophylline	Increase rate of theophylline metabolism, resulting in decreased serum theophylline concentration	• Monitor theophylline concentration, as prescribed. • Be aware that the theophylline dosage may need to be increased.
	cyclosporine	May decrease plasma cyclosporine concentration	• Monitor cyclosporine concentration regularly; the cyclosporine dosage may need to be increased.

ADVERSE DRUG REACTIONS

The toxicity of the barbiturate anticonvulsants results primarily in adverse reactions in the CNS. Significant GI reactions, blood dyscrasias, and emotional or psychiatric reactions also occur.

The most common dose-related CNS effects of phenobarbital include drowsiness, lethargy, and dizziness; nystagmus; confusion; and ataxia with large doses.

The adverse GI reactions include nausea and vomiting. These adverse reactions are most common when primidone therapy begins, which explains why the primidone dosage is increased gradually.

Folate deficiencies and osteomalacia secondary to the induced metabolism of vitamin D also may occur. When administered I.V., phenobarbital can cause laryngospasm, respiratory depression, and hypotension secondary to decreased cardiac output. Signs of overdose include respiratory depression, pupillary constriction, oliguria, hypothermia, circulatory collapse, and pulmonary edema.

Mephobarbital produces adverse reactions similar to phenobarbital. Primidone evokes the same CNS and GI adverse reactions as phenobarbital. Primidone also has been implicated in the development of acute psychoses in patients with complex partial seizures. It also may cause alopecia, impotence, and osteomalacia.

Rare hematologic adverse effects of the barbiturates include agranulocytosis, thrombocytopenia, leukopenia, eosinophilia, decreased serum folate levels, and megaloblastic anemia. All three barbiturate anticonvulsants can produce a hypersensitivity rash. These drugs also may produce a morbilliform rash, lupus erythematosus-like syndrome, and lymphadenopathy. Paradoxical excitement in elderly patients and children and hyperkinetic behavior in children may occur.

NURSING PROCESS APPLICATION

The following information assists the nurse in caring for a patient who is receiving a barbiturate anticonvulsant.

Assessment

• Review the patient's history for conditions that contraindicate the use of a barbiturate, such as known hypersensitivity to the drug, bronchopneumonia, or other severe pulmonary insufficiency.
• Review the patient's history for conditions that require cautious use of a parenteral barbiturate, such as hypertension, hypotension, or pulmonary or cardiovascular disease.
• Assess the patient for adverse reactions to the barbiturate, such as drowsiness, lethargy, nystagmus, ataxia, nausea, vomiting, folate deficiency, hypotension, respiratory depression, and hypothermia.

• Assess the patient's physical mobility during barbiturate therapy and compare it to baseline levels.
• Evaluate the patient's and family's knowledge about the prescribed barbiturate.

Nursing diagnoses

The following examples represent appropriate nursing diagnoses for a patient receiving a barbiturate.
• Potential for injury related to a preexisting condition that contraindicates the use of a barbiturate
• Potential for injury related to a preexisting condition that requires cautious use of a barbiturate
• Potential for injury related to adverse drug reactions
• Impaired physical mobility related to the sedative effects of a barbiturate
• Knowledge deficit related to the prescribed barbiturate

Planning and implementation

• Do not administer a barbiturate to a patient with a condition that contraindicates its use.
• Administer a barbiturate cautiously to a patient at risk because of a preexisting condition.
• *Keep resuscitative drugs and equipment nearby when administering an I.V. barbiturate.*
• *Do not exceed a rate of 60 mg/minute when giving an I.V. barbiturate.*
• *Do not use a cloudy solution when giving an I.V. barbiturate. Administer a reconstituted solution within 30 minutes of preparation.*
• *Monitor vital signs frequently—especially respirations and blood pressure—when administering an I.V. barbiturate.*
• Be sure that the patient actually swallows the drug when administering an oral barbiturate.
• Monitor the patient's phenobarbital blood concentrations and serum folate levels during prolonged therapy.
• *Raise the side rails for a child or an elderly patient because barbiturate therapy may precipitate paradoxical excitement or CNS depression.*
• *Monitor the patient's physical mobility during barbiturate therapy.*
• Notify the physician if the barbiturate's sedative effects interfere with the patient's physical mobility.

Patient teaching

• Provide basic information about anticonvulsant therapy. (For specifics, see *General patient-teaching tips,* page 303.)
• Teach the patient and family the name, dose, frequency, action, and adverse effects of the prescribed barbiturate.
• *Reassure the patient that the prescribed barbiturate is not addictive when used in subhypnotic doses for seizures.*
• Advise the patient to keep the prescribed barbiturate in a secure place to prevent others, including children, from taking the drug.

• *Inform the male patient that impotence may occur.*
• *Inform the patient that a barbiturate can impair mental alertness, which may require avoidance of activities that require alertness.*
• Instruct the patient to report adverse reactions to the physician.

Evaluation

The following examples represent appropriate evaluation statements for a patient receiving a barbiturate.
• The patient has no conditions that contraindicate barbiturate therapy.
• The patient exhibits no signs of complications in the preexisting condition linked to the prescribed barbiturate.
• The patient demonstrates no adverse reactions to the prescribed barbiturate.
• The patient reports normal physical activity.
• The patient and family express an accurate understanding of the points taught about the prescribed barbiturate.
• The patient states that the barbiturate will be stored in a locked desk at home.

IMINOSTILBENES

Carbamazepine, an iminostilbene derivative, acts as an effective anticonvulsant for partial and generalized tonic-clonic seizures, and mixed seizure types. Carbamazepine also produces sedative, anticholinergic, antidepressant, muscle-relaxant, antiarrhythmic, antidiuretic, and neuromuscular transmission-inhibiting actions. Also, carbamazepine is the only anticonvulsant compound that has a chemical structure similar to the tricyclic antidepressant drugs, such as imipramine. This similarity helps explain the drug's effects on behavior and emotions.

PHARMACOKINETICS

Carbamazepine is absorbed slowly and erratically from the GI tract. The drug is distributed rapidly to all tissues, and 75% to 90% is bound to plasma proteins. Metabolism occurs in the liver, and carbamazepine is excreted as glucuronides in the urine.

Absorption, distribution, metabolism, excretion

The GI tract absorption of carbamazepine is slow, erratic, and possibly incomplete. After carbamazepine is distributed widely in body tissues, 75% to 90% of the drug becomes protein bound. Carbamazepine is metabolized in the liver by oxidative enzyme induction to an active metabolite, 10,11-epoxide, and five other metabolites. From 1% to 3%

is excreted unchanged in the urine. The active metabolite 10,11-epoxide is metabolized to inactive compounds, which are excreted in urine and bile. A small amount crosses the placenta and some is secreted in breast milk.

Onset, peak, duration

The onset of action varies, with the peak serum concentration level occurring after 2 to 8 hours. The half-life also varies greatly, as a result of the autoinduction of drug-metabolizing hepatic enzymes and a change in the metabolism rate caused by other drugs.

PHARMACODYNAMICS

Carbamazepine exerts an anticonvulsant effect similar to that of phenytoin. The drug's anticonvulsant action may occur because of its ability to inhibit the spread of seizure activity or neuromuscular transmission in general. Carbamazepine also increases the discharge of noradrenergic neurons—an action that may contribute to its antiepileptic effects.

PHARMACOTHERAPEUTICS

Carbamazepine is used to treat generalized tonic-clonic seizures as well as simple and complex partial seizures in adults and children. The efficacy of carbamazepine makes it a drug of choice for treating these seizures. Use of the drug also relieves pain when used to treat trigeminal neuralgia (tic douloureux).

carbamazepine (Tegretol). This drug is used to treat adults and children.
Usual adult dosage: initially, 200 mg P.O. b.i.d.; gradually increased in small increments up to 400 mg P.O. t.i.d. until desired response is obtained; for maintenance, 1,200 mg P.O. daily in adults and children over age 15. Some patients require 1,600 to 2,400 mg/day.
Usual pediatric dosage: for children ages 6 to 12, 20 to 30 mg/kg, beginning with 100 mg P.O. b.i.d.; increased by 100 mg P.O. daily using at least a t.i.d. regimen. Generally, the dosage should not exceed 1 gram P.O. daily. The maintenance dosage is 400 to 800 mg P.O. daily in three divided doses for children under age 12; 800 to 1,200 mg P.O. daily in children ages 12 to 15. Therapeutic serum concentration is 4 to 12 mcg/ml.

Drug interactions

Carbamazepine possesses enzyme-inducing properties and generally decreases the steady-state levels of other drugs. Some anticonvulsant drugs, however, decrease the steady-state levels of carbamazepine. (For more information, see *Drug interactions: Iminostilbenes.*)

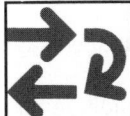

DRUG INTERACTIONS

Iminostilbenes

The following chart lists the drug interactions between carbamazepine, an iminostilbene derivative, and other drugs.

DRUG	INTERACTING DRUGS	POSSIBLE EFFECTS	NURSING IMPLICATIONS
carbamazepine	erythromycin, isoniazid, propoxyphene, troleando-mycin, cimetidine	Inhibit carbamazepine metabolism, resulting in increased toxic adverse reactions	• Monitor serum carbamazepine concentrations carefully; decreased carbamazepine dosage may be needed. • Monitor complete blood count and platelet and reticulocyte counts; hematopoietic toxicity warrants immediate withdrawal. • Advise the patient and family to notify the physician immediately if the following signs or symptoms occur: fever, sore throat or mouth, malaise, unusual fatigue, or tendency to bruise or bleed. • Monitor the pulse and cardiac function frequently in a patient with heart disease because toxic doses may precipitate cardiac arrhythmias. • Advise the patient to avoid hazardous tasks that require mental alertness and physical coordination, such as operating a motor vehicle or using heavy machinery because dizziness, drowsiness, and ataxia may occur.
	doxycycline	Decreases efficacy of doxycycline because of increased breakdown by the liver, resulting in decreased therapeutic effect of doxycycline	• Be aware that the doxycycline dosage may need to be increased because of decreased effect.
	theophylline	Decreases efficacy of theophylline because of increased breakdown by the liver, resulting in decreased therapeutic effect of theophylline	• Be aware that the theophylline dosage may need to be increased because of decreased effect.
	warfarin	Decreases efficacy of warfarin because of increased breakdown by the liver, resulting in decreased therapeutic effect of warfarin	• Monitor prothrombin time frequently; the warfarin dosage may need to be increased. • Observe for signs of thrombus formation, such as Homans' sign, tenderness, or edema.
	lithium	Causes unknown interaction mechanism, resulting in neurotoxicity	• Assess for changes in level of consciousness. • Instruct the patient to report dizziness, headache, fatigue, or slurred speech immediately. • Advise the patient not to operate a motor vehicle or heavy machinery until the drug combination effects on the patient are known.
	oral contraceptives	Increases metabolism of oral contraceptives, resulting in decreased efficacy of contraceptives	• Advise the patient to use an alternative contraceptive method during carbamazepine therapy.

ADVERSE DRUG REACTIONS

Most adverse reactions produced by carbamazepine are tolerable and relatively minor, if the drug therapy begins slowly at a low dosage and advances gradually to tolerance. Occasionally, however, serious hematologic toxicity occurs. Furthermore, because carbamazepine is related structurally to the tricyclic antidepressants, it can cause similar toxicities.

Dose-related adverse reactions include drowsiness, diplopia, ataxia, vertigo, nystagmus, headaches, tremor, and dry mouth. Because carbamazepine is related to the tricyclic antidepressants, it can produce many of the same adverse reactions, including heart failure, hypertension or hypotension, syncope, arrhythmias, and myocardial infarction. Carbamazepine's action as a mild anticholinergic may result in urine retention, constipation, and increased intraocular pressure. With long-term use, the drug also can cause syndrome of inappropriate antidiuretic hormone secretion (SIADH) and water intoxication.

Urticaria and Stevens-Johnson syndrome have been reported with carbamazepine use. The occasional but significant hematologic reactions include aplastic anemia (rare), agranulocytosis, thrombocytopenia, and leukopenia. Rare instances of cholestatic and hepatocellular jaundice also have been noted. Rare psychiatric reactions have been noted, including activation of latent psychosis, mental depression with agitation, and talkativeness.

NURSING PROCESS APPLICATION

The following information assists the nurse in caring for a patient who is receiving the iminostilbene carbamazepine.

Assessment
• Review the patient's history for conditions that contraindicate the use of carbamazepine, such as known hypersensitivity to the drug or bone marrow depression.
• Review the patient's history for conditions that require cautious use of carbamazepine, such as cardiac, hepatic, or renal damage.
• Assess the patient for adverse reactions to carbamazepine, such as drowsiness, ataxia, headaches, dry mouth, arrhythmias, hypertension or hypotension, urine retention, constipation, and increased intraocular pressure.
• Assess the female patient for concurrent use of an oral contraceptive and carbamazepine.
• Assess for fluid overload in a patient who is receiving long-term therapy with carbamazepine.
• Evaluate the patient's and family's knowledge about carbamazepine.

Nursing diagnoses
The following examples represent appropriate nursing diagnoses for a patient receiving carbamazepine.
• Potential for injury related to a preexisting condition that contraindicates the use of carbamazepine
• Potential for injury related to a preexisting condition that requires cautious use of carbamazepine
• Potential for injury related to adverse drug reactions
• Health-seeking behaviors related to possible interaction between carbamazepine and an oral contraceptive
• Fluid volume excess related to water intoxication with long-term use of carbamazepine
• Knowledge deficit related to carbamazepine

Planning and implementation
• Do not administer carbamazepine to a patient with a condition that contraindicates its use.
• Administer carbamazepine cautiously to a patient at risk because of a preexisting condition.
• Monitor the patient for adverse drug reactions.
• Monitor the patient's vital signs during carbamazepine therapy.
• Obtain complete blood cell counts with differential, as prescribed.
• *Take bleeding and infection precautions, if the patient develops thrombocytopenia or leukopenia.*
• *Take safety precautions if the patient exhibits drowsiness, diplopia, ataxia, vertigo, or syncope.*
• *Check for early signs of urine retention by documenting fluid intake and output carefully and palpating the bladder after the patient voids.*
• Notify the physician if the patient develops any adverse reactions to carbamazepine.
• *Recommend that the female patient who uses an oral contraceptive use an additional or different contraceptive method.*
• Discuss the advantages and disadvantages of various contraceptive methods, if requested.
• *Auscultate breath sounds at least every 4 hours to detect crackles.*
• *Assess the patient for dependent edema, especially in the ankles.*
• *Weigh the patient daily.*
• Document fluid intake and output and note changes in vital signs, such as increased blood pressure, pulse, and respirations, at least daily.
• *Limit the patient's fluid and salt intake.*
• Notify the physician if the patient develops signs of fluid excess, such as shortness of breath.

Patient teaching

• Provide basic information about anticonvulsant therapy. (For specifics, see *General patient-teaching tips,* page 303.)
• Teach the patient and family about carbamazepine's name, dose, frequency, action, and adverse effects.
• *Advise the patient to take carbamazepine with meals to decrease GI distress and enhance absorption.*
• *Instruct the patient and family to notify the physician immediately if the patient displays early signs of hematologic problems, such as fever, sore throat, malaise, unusual fatigue, or a tendency to bruise or bleed.*

Evaluation

The following examples represent appropriate evaluation statements for a patient receiving carbamazepine.
• The patient has no conditions that contraindicate carbamazepine therapy.
• The patient exhibits no signs of complications in the preexisting condition linked to carbamazepine use.
• The patient displays no adverse reactions to carbamazepine.
• The patient selects an additional contraceptive method to use during carbamazepine therapy.
• The patient maintains a normal fluid balance.
• The patient and family demonstrate an accurate understanding of the points taught about carbamazepine therapy.
• The patient correctly lists early signs of hematologic problems and describes what to do if they occur.

BENZODIAZEPINES

The three drugs from the benzodiazepine class that provide anticonvulsant effects are diazepam (parenteral), clonazepam, and clorazepate dipotassium. Only clonazepam is recommended for long-term treatment of epilepsy; diazepam is restricted to acute treatment of status epilepticus. Clorazepate is prescribed as an adjunct in treating partial seizures. (For the major discussion of benzodiazepines, see Chapter 27, Antianxiety Agents.)

PHARMACOKINETICS

The benzodiazepines are metabolized in the liver to multiple metabolites, which subsequently are excreted in the urine.

Absorption, distribution, metabolism, excretion

The benzodiazepines are absorbed rapidly and almost completely from the GI tract, but are distributed at different rates. Protein binding of benzodiazepines ranges from 85%

to 90%. Based on the rate of excretion or elimination, benzodiazepines are classified as long-acting, intermediate-acting, or short-acting. Metabolism of the long-acting compounds results in the formation of the major plasma metabolite N-desmethyldiazepam, which has a long half-life. The long half-life of the metabolite probably accounts for some of the pharmacologic action. The metabolites of the benzodiazepines eventually are excreted in urine. The benzodiazepines are distributed readily across the placenta and are excreted in breast milk.

Onset, peak, duration

The onset of action for the benzodiazepines is 5 to 10 minutes, with peak concentration levels reached within 60 to 90 minutes. Diazepam and clorazepate have half-lives of 1 to 2 days, but their active metabolite N-desmethyldiazepam has a half-life of 30 to 200 hours. Clonazepam's half-life is about 1 day. The half-lives of the benzodiazepines correlate poorly with their anticonvulsant duration of action.

PHARMACODYNAMICS

The benzodiazepines provide anticonvulsant, antianxiety, sedative-hypnotic, and muscle-relaxant effects.

Mechanism of action

Although not clearly understood, benzodiazepine anticonvulsant action may increase availability of the inhibitory neurotransmitter gamma-aminobutyric acid (GABA) to brain neurons.

PHARMACOTHERAPEUTICS

Clonazepam is used to treat absence (petit mal), atypical absence (Lennox-Gastaut syndrome), atonic, and myoclonic seizures. Diazepam is not recommended for long-term treatment because of the high serum concentrations required to control seizures and its addictive potential. Intravenously, it is used routinely as the initial control for status epilepticus. Because it is distributed so rapidly, diazepam provides only short-term effects of less than 1 hour. Consequently, a long-acting anticonvulsant, such as phenytoin or phenobarbital, also must be given during diazepam therapy. Clorazepate is used with other drugs to treat partial seizures. The therapeutic serum concentrations for the benzodiazepines have not been well established.

clonazepam (Klonopin). A Schedule IV drug, clonazepam is used to treat absence, atypical absence, atonic, and myoclonic seizures. The dosage required for seizure control is highly individualized.
Usual adult dosage: initially, 1.5 mg P.O. daily in three divided doses; increased by increments of 0.5 to 1 mg every

3 days until the seizures become controlled or until adverse reactions preclude further increases. The maximum recommended dosage is 20 mg P.O. daily.

Usual pediatric dosage: for children up to age 10 or weighing up to 30 kg, initially, 0.01 to 0.03 mg/kg P.O. daily in three divided doses, not to exceed 0.05 mg/kg/day; gradual increments of 0.25 to 0.5 mg P.O. may be added every 3 days; for maintenance, 0.1 to 0.2 mg/kg P.O. daily in three divided doses.

diazepam (Valium). A Schedule IV drug, diazepam is indicated to treat status epilepticus only.

Usual adult dosage: 5 to 10 mg I.V. at a rate not to exceed 5 mg/minute; may be repeated at 10- to 15-minute intervals up to a maximum dosage of 30 mg. The regimen can be repeated in 2 to 4 hours if necessary, but the total dosage should not exceed 100 mg in 24 hours.

Usual pediatric dosage: for children over age 5, 1 mg I.V. over at least 3 minutes initially, followed by repeated doses every 2 to 5 minutes until a maximum dosage of 10 mg has been given. This regimen can be repeated in 2 to 4 hours if necessary.

clorazepate dipotassium (Tranxene). A Schedule IV drug, clorazepate is recommended for adjunctive treatment of partial seizures only.

Usual adult dosage: 22.5 mg P.O. daily in three divided doses. Daily dosages should be increased by not more than 7.5 mg per week. The maximum dosage is 90 mg P.O. daily.

Usual pediatric dosage: initially, 15 mg P.O. daily in two divided doses. Daily dosages should be increased by not more than 7.5 mg per week. The maximum dosage for children is 60 mg/day. Clorazepate is not recommended for use in children under age 9.

Drug interactions
Drug interactions between benzodiazepines and other CNS depressant drugs can occur. (For detailed information, see *Drug interactions: Benzodiazepines.*)

ADVERSE DRUG REACTIONS

The dose-related adverse reactions to the benzodiazepines are primarily neurologic and include drowsiness, confusion, ataxia, weakness, dizziness, nystagmus, vertigo, syncope, dysarthria, headache, tremor, and a glassy-eyed appearance. These dose-related reactions diminish as therapy continues. Cardiorespiratory depression may occur with high doses and with I.V. diazepam. Elderly patients are particularly susceptible to confusion, ataxia, and paradoxical excitement.

Idiosyncratic reactions to the benzodiazepines include a rash and acute hypersensitivity reactions. Hepatomegaly, leukopenia, thrombocytopenia, and eosinophilia have been reported rarely.

NURSING PROCESS APPLICATION

The following information assists the nurse in caring for a patient who is receiving a benzodiazepine anticonvulsant.

Assessment
• Review the patient's history for conditions that contraindicate the use of a benzodiazepine, such as known hypersensitivity to the drug, liver disease, acute narrow-angle glaucoma, pregnancy, and lactation.
• Review the patient's history for conditions that require cautious use of a benzodiazepine, such as impaired renal function or chronic respiratory disease.
• Assess the patient for adverse reactions to a benzodiazepine, such as drowsiness, ataxia, weakness, vertigo, syncope, tremor, or cardiorespiratory depression.
• Evaluate the patient's and family's knowledge about the prescribed benzodiazepine.

Nursing diagnoses
The following examples represent appropriate nursing diagnoses for a patient receiving a benzodiazepine.
• Potential for injury related to a preexisting condition that contraindicates the use of a benzodiazepine
• Potential for injury related to a preexisting condition that requires cautious use of a benzodiazepine
• Potential for injury related to adverse drug reactions
• Knowledge deficit related to the prescribed benzodiazepine

Planning and implementation
• Do not administer a benzodiazepine to a patient with a condition that contradicts its use.
• Administer a benzodiazepine cautiously to a patient at risk because of a preexisting condition.
• Monitor the patient for adverse drug reactions. Monitor the elderly patient closely for confusion, ataxia, and excitability.
• Monitor vital signs during I.V. administration of diazepam, and keep resuscitation equipment readily available.
• *Administer I.V. diazepam no faster than 5 mg/minute in adults and over at least 3 minutes in children. Avoid starting an I.V. line in small veins. Use care to prevent extravasation.*
• *Do not mix I.V. diazepam with other drugs in the same syringe. Give direct I.V. push only. Do not give the drug as an infusion.*
• Verify patient compliance with oral doses of a benzodiazepine to detect hoarding.

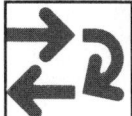

DRUG INTERACTIONS

Benzodiazepines

Drug interactions involving the benzodiazepines discussed in this chapter occur infrequently. However, when interactions occur, they usually involve concurrent use of other central nervous system (CNS) depressant drugs, including alcohol. The additive effects of CNS drugs with benzodiazepines can be lethal.

DRUG	INTERACTING DRUGS	POSSIBLE EFFECTS	NURSING IMPLICATIONS
clonazepam, clorazepate, diazepam	CNS depressants	Enhance sedative and other CNS depressant effects. Effects may be supra-additive, causing motor skill impairment and respiratory depression. Possible lethal effect, especially with high doses. Combination with anticonvulsant drugs can cause changes in seizures, especially in frequency or severity.	• Monitor for changes in level of consciousness and muscle coordination. • Monitor for signs of respiratory depression. • Advise about possible additive effects of other CNS depressant drugs. • Warn patient that alcohol increases the effect of the drug and can cause serious CNS depression. • Supervise ambulation; raise side rails, especially with elderly patients. • Advise against operating a motor vehicle or heavy machinery because of possibly impaired motor skills. • Observe for changes in frequency and severity of seizures when these drugs are used with anticonvulsant drugs.
	cimetidine	Inhibits hepatic metabolism, resulting in excessive sedation and increasing CNS depression	• Monitor for signs of increasing CNS depressant effects; notify the physician if any changes are noted. • Advise against operating a motor vehicle or heavy machinery because increased sedation is possible. • Supervise ambulation; raise side rails, especially with elderly patients.
	oral contraceptives	Decrease oxidative metabolism of these benzodiazepines	• Monitor for signs of excessive sedation. • Be aware that the benzodiazepine dosage may need to be decreased.

• Store an oral benzodiazepine in a light-resistant container at room temperature, unless otherwise specified by the manufacturer.
• Notify the physician if the patient develops adverse reactions to the prescribed benzodiazepine.
• *Monitor the patient for signs and symptoms of overdose, such as somnolence, confusion, diminished reflexes, and coma.*
• *Perform emergency interventions if a patient overdoses on a benzodiazepine. Maintain an open airway, ventilate if necessary, monitor vital signs, and administer fluids; perform gastric lavage, and administer a vasopressor as prescribed.*

Patient teaching
• Provide basic information about anticonvulsant therapy. (For specifics, see *General patient-teaching tips,* page 303.)
• Teach the patient and family the name, dose, frequency, action, and adverse effects of the prescribed benzodiazepine.

• Instruct the patient to contact the physician if adverse reactions occur.
• Instruct the patient to notify the physician if seizure control deteriorates.
• *Instruct the patient to take the benzodiazepine exactly as prescribed to prevent drug dependence. Teach the patient and family to recognize and report to the physician signs of drug dependence, such as nervousness, insomnia, or diarrhea.*

Evaluation
The following examples represent appropriate evaluation statements for a patient receiving a benzodiazepine.
• The patient has no conditions that contraindicate benzodiazepine therapy.
• The patient exhibits no signs of complications in the preexisting condition linked to the prescribed benzodiazepine.
• The patient experiences no adverse drug reactions.

• The patient and family express an accurate understanding of the points taught about the prescribed benzodiazepine.
• The patient and family correctly list signs of drug dependence and steps to take if these signs appear.

SUCCINIMIDES

Three drugs from the succinimide class are used to treat absence (petit mal) seizures: ethosuximide, methsuximide, and phensuximide.

PHARMACOKINETICS

The succinimides are absorbed well from the GI tract and distributed widely throughout body tissues. Plasma protein binding of the drugs is negligible. The succinimides are metabolized in the liver by microsomal enzymes. Almost 50% of ethosuximide is metabolized to its primary metabolite, the inactive hydroxyethyl derivative. This metabolite, as well as those of the other succinimides, is excreted as a glucuronide in the urine. Approximately 20% of ethosuximide is excreted unchanged in the urine.

The onset of action for the succinimides occurs rapidly. Peak serum concentration levels are reached at the following rates: methsuximide, 2 hours; phensuximide, 1 to 4 hours; ethosuximide, about 4 hours. The half-life varies from 4 to 12 hours for phensuximide, 23 to 57 hours for methsuximide and its active metabolite, and 60 hours for ethosuximide.

PHARMACODYNAMICS

The succinimides reduce frequency of absence seizures in children and adults, apparently by depressing nerve transmission in the motor cortex and increasing the seizure threshold for stimulus.

PHARMACOTHERAPEUTICS

Ethosuximide is the drug of choice for treating absence seizures. Methsuximide is prescribed less frequently because of the high incidence of toxicity associated with it. Methsuximide is indicated, however, for absence seizures and with other anticonvulsants to treat complex partial seizures. Phensuximide rarely is used because it is less effective. If used alone for mixed types of seizures, succinimides may increase the frequency of tonic-clonic seizures. However, methsuximide is least likely to precipitate tonic-clonic seizures.

ethosuximide (Zarontin). This drug is used to treat absence seizures. The dosage needed to control the seizures is highly individualized.
Usual adult dosage: initially, 250 mg P.O. b.i.d., with dosage increases in increments of 250 mg every 4 to 7 days until seizure control is achieved with minimal adverse reactions; for maintenance, 20 to 40 mg/kg P.O.; maximum dosage usually should not exceed 1.5 grams daily. The therapeutic serum concentration required to control seizures is 40 to 100 mcg/ml.
Usual pediatric dosage: initially, for children over age 6, 250 mg P.O. b.i.d.; for children ages 3 to 6, 250 mg P.O. daily; recommended dosage increment is 250 mg P.O. every 4 to 7 days until seizure control is achieved with minimal adverse reactions; for maintenance, 20 mg/kg, with a maximum dosage of 1 gram for children up to age 6.

methsuximide (Celontin). This drug is used to treat absence seizures refractory to other drugs.
Usual adult and pediatric dosage: initially, 300 mg P.O. daily for the first week, increased by 300 mg/day at weekly intervals if required; for maintenance, 600 to 1,200 mg; maximum dosage is 1.2 grams daily in divided doses.

phensuximide (Milontin). This drug is used to treat absence seizures. Highly individualized dosages are required to maintain seizure control.
Usual adult and pediatric dosage: initially, 0.5 to 1 gram P.O. b.i.d. to t.i.d.; maximum total dosage may vary between 1 to 3 grams P.O. daily.

Drug interactions

The succinimides may inhibit the metabolism of hydantoin anticonvulsants. Carbamazepine may decrease the concentration of a succinimide by induction.

ADVERSE DRUG REACTIONS

The succinimides produce GI, neurologic, hematologic, and genitourinary adverse reactions. In the GI tract, adverse reactions include nausea, vomiting, weight loss, abdominal pain, constipation, and diarrhea. The neurologic complaints are ataxia, dizziness, drowsiness, headache, euphoria, restlessness, irritability, lethargy, and confusion. Psychosis and suicidal ideation have occurred, but rarely. The hematologic adverse reactions include eosinophilia, leukopenia, thrombocytopenia, agranulocytosis, and aplastic anemia. The genitourinary adverse reactions are urinary frequency, hematuria, and albuminuria.

Methsuximide also can produce renal and hepatic damage. Other toxic reactions include increased libido, hirsutism, alopecia, and gum hypertrophy. The following hypersensitivity reactions to succinimides can occur: Stevens-Johnson syndrome, pruritic skin eruptions, exfoliative dermatitis, and systemic lupus erythematosus.

NURSING PROCESS APPLICATION

The following information assists the nurse in caring for a patient who is receiving a succinimide.

Assessment
• Review the patient's history for conditions that contraindicate use of a succinimide, such as known hypersensitivity to the drug.
• Review the patient's history for conditions that require cautious use of a succinimide, such as pregnancy or hepatic or renal disease.
• Assess the patient for adverse reactions to a succinimide, such as GI distress, weight loss, ataxia, dizziness, restlessness, irritability, lethargy, and confusion.
• Assess the effectiveness of the prescribed succinimide periodically.
• Assess the patient for signs and symptoms of nutritional deficiencies.
• Assess the patient's mental status at least every 4 hours.
• Evaluate the patient's and family's knowledge about the prescribed succinimide.

Nursing diagnoses
The following examples represent appropriate nursing diagnoses for a patient receiving a succinimide.
• Potential for injury related to a preexisting condition that contraindicates the use of a succinimide
• Potential for injury related to a preexisting condition that requires cautious use of a succinimide
• Potential for injury related to adverse drug reactions
• Altered health maintenance related to ineffectiveness of the prescribed succinimide
• Altered nutrition: less than body requirements, related to weight loss from succinimide therapy
• Altered thought processes related to the adverse CNS effects of a succinimide
• Knowledge deficit related to the prescribed succinimide

Planning and implementation
• Do not administer a succinimide to a patient with a condition that contraindicates its use.
• Administer a succinimide cautiously to a patient at risk because of a preexisting condition.
• Observe the patient for adverse drug reactions. Adjust the dosage, as prescribed.
• Monitor the patient for signs of toxicity when adjusting the dosage or when adding or eliminating any other medication.
• *Note that methsuximide contains FD&C Yellow Dye No. 5, which can cause allergic reactions in a patient with* *asthma or allergies to aspirin or other nonsteroidal anti-inflammatory drugs.*
• *Administer a succinimide with meals if adverse GI reactions occur.*
• Store the succinimide away from heat. Shake all suspensions well before administration.
• Monitor the serum drug concentration.
• Take bleeding precautions if thrombocytopenia occurs and infection precautions if leukopenia occurs.
• Report evidence of adverse drug reactions to the physician.
• Monitor the patient for signs of efficacy when adjusting the dosage or when adding or eliminating any other medication.
• Monitor seizure activity.
• Weigh the patient daily.
• *Monitor the patient for nutritional deficiencies during succinimide therapy.*
• Encourage the patient to eat a well-balanced diet.
• Administer nutritional supplements as prescribed, if weight loss becomes significant.
• *Notify the physician if weight loss exceeds 5 pounds during succinimide therapy.*
• Monitor the patient's mental status frequently.
• *Take safety precautions if mental status alters. For example, keep the side rails up at all times, keep the bed in a low position, and supervise ambulation.*
• Reorient the confused patient, as needed.
• Notify the physician if the patient displays mental status changes.

Patient teaching
• Provide basic information about anticonvulsant therapy. (For specifics, see *General patient-teaching tips,* page 303.)
• Teach the patient and family the name, dose, frequency, action, and adverse effects of the prescribed succinimide.
• *Instruct the patient with GI distress to take the prescribed succinimide with meals.*
• *Inform the patient that phensuximide may cause harmless pink, red, or red-brown discoloration of urine.*
• Instruct the patient to contact the physician if adverse reactions occur.

Evaluation
The following examples represent appropriate evaluation statements for a patient receiving a succinimide.
• The patient has no conditions that contraindicate succinimide therapy.
• The patient exhibits no signs of complications in the preexisting condition linked to the prescribed succinimide.
• The patient displays no adverse reactions to the prescribed succinimide.
• The patient demonstrates no seizure activity.
• The patient maintains adequate nutrition and body weight.

• The patient remains alert and oriented.
• The patient and family express an accurate understanding of the points taught about the prescribed succinimide.
• The patient reports taking the succinimide with breakfast and dinner, as prescribed.

VALPROIC ACID

Valproic acid, a carboxylic acid with anticonvulsant activity, is unrelated structurally to the other anticonvulsants. The two major drugs in the valproic acid class are valproate sodium and divalproex sodium.

PHARMACOKINETICS

Valproate sodium is converted rapidly to valproic acid in the stomach. Divalproex is a pro-drug (precursor) of valproic acid and becomes dissociated (separated into molecular fragments) to valproic acid in the GI tract. Valproic acid is absorbed well when administered as valproate or divalproex. Once absorbed, it is strongly protein bound and is metabolized in the liver. Metabolites and unchanged drug are excreted in urine.

Absorption, distribution, metabolism, excretion
The absorption rate of valproic acid depends on the dosage form. Valproic acid is 90% bound to plasma proteins, but that percentage decreases as the total serum concentration increases throughout the therapeutic range.

Valproic acid is metabolized in the liver to the conjugate ester of glucuronic acid. Other metabolites result from the beta oxidation by the mitochondria. The major active metabolites having anticonvulsant activity are 2-propyl-2-pentenoic acid and 2-propyl-3-oxopentanoic acid. These active metabolites, along with 3% of the unchanged drug, are excreted in urine. Valproic acid readily crosses the placental barrier and also appears in breast milk.

Onset, peak, duration
The onset of action of valproic acid occurs in 20 to 30 minutes. The peak serum concentration level of valproate sodium occurs in 1 to 4 hours. Serum concentration of divalproex sodium peaks in 3 to 5 hours. The time needed to reach peak concentration is longer if the patient has a full stomach or receives enteric-coated tablets. In patients not taking other drugs, the half-life is 13 to 16 hours. For patients taking other anticonvulsants, the half-life drops to 6 to 10 hours, probably as a result of hepatic enzyme induction.

PHARMACODYNAMICS

The mechanism of action for valproic acid remains unknown, but it may be related to the increased availability of the inhibitory neurotransmitter GABA to brain neurons. Valproic acid may inhibit GABA transaminase or succinic semialdehyde dehydrogenase, which would account for the increased GABA.

PHARMACOTHERAPEUTICS

Valproic acid is prescribed for long-term treatment of absence, myoclonic, and tonic-clonic seizures. It also is administered rectally for status epilepticus refractory to other anticonvulsants. Valproic acid must be used cautiously in a young child or a patient receiving multiple anticonvulsants because of possible fatal hepatotoxicity. This risk limits the use of valproic acid as a drug of choice for seizure disorders.

valproate sodium (Depakene) and **divalproex sodium** (Depakote). A steady-state concentration of valproate sodium is reached 1 to 4 days after initiation. The effective serum concentration for adults and children is 50 to 100 mcg/ml. With divalproex, a twice-daily dosing regimen is recommended.
Usual adult and pediatric dosage: initially, 15 mg/kg P.O. daily, increased at weekly intervals by 5 to 10 mg/kg until seizures are under control or unacceptable adverse reactions develop; maximum dosage is 60 mg/kg/day, and divided doses are recommended when the total daily dosage exceeds 250 mg.

Drug interactions
The most clinically significant drug interactions associated with valproic acid are inhibition of platelet aggregation, which may cause prolonged bleeding times in patients who also are receiving anticoagulants, and inhibition of the hepatic metabolism of phenobarbital. Valproic acid also can produce a false-positive result on urine ketone tests.

ADVERSE DRUG REACTIONS

Most adverse reactions associated with valproic acid are tolerable and dose related; however, rare fatal hepatotoxicity has occurred. The drug is not prescribed routinely because of the possibility of hepatotoxicity.

The dose-related adverse reactions affect the GI and CNS. The adverse GI reactions include nausea, vomiting, appetite changes, diarrhea, and constipation. Divalproex produces fewer adverse GI reactions than valproate. The adverse CNS reactions include sedation, drowsiness, dizziness, ataxia, headache, decreased alertness, and muscle weakness.

Adverse hematologic reactions include inhibited platelet aggregation and prolonged bleeding time. Rare adverse psychiatric reactions include depression, hallucinations, and behavioral disorders in children.

The rare, fatal hepatotoxicity that has been reported usually is preceded by nonspecific symptoms, such as loss of seizure control, malaise, jaundice, weakness, lethargy, facial edema, anorexia, and vomiting. The reaction may develop at any time from 3 days to 6 months after initiation of therapy. At the greatest risk are children and patients who receive other anticonvulsants along with valproic acid.

A drug rash may occur, as may hyperammonemia with normal liver function. The use of valproic acid also may produce blood dyscrasias, such as anemia, leukopenia, and thrombocytopenia.

NURSING PROCESS APPLICATION

The following information assists the nurse in caring for a patient who is receiving valproic acid.

Assessment
• Review the patient's history for conditions that contraindicate the use of valproic acid, such as hepatic dysfunction and known hypersensitivity to the drug.
• Assess the female patient for pregnancy, which requires cautious use of valproic acid.
• Assess the patient for adverse reactions to valproic acid, such as hepatotoxicity, GI distress, sedation, drowsiness, ataxia, headache, decreased alertness, muscle weakness, inhibited platelet aggregation, and prolonged bleeding time.
• Assess the effectiveness of valproic acid regularly.
• Evaluate the patient's and family's knowledge about valproic acid.

Nursing diagnoses
The following examples represent appropriate nursing diagnoses for a patient receiving valproic acid
• Potential for injury related to a preexisting condition that contraindicates the use of valproic acid
• Potential for injury related to valproic acid therapy during pregnancy
• Potential for injury related to adverse drug reactions
• Altered health maintenance related to ineffectiveness of valproic acid
• Knowledge deficit related to valproic acid

Planning and implementation
• Do not administer valproic acid to a patient with a condition that contraindicates its use.
• *Administer valproic acid cautiously to a pregnant patient.*
• *Monitor the patient for adverse reactions to valproic acid.*

• *Monitor liver function and coagulation studies periodically.*
• *Take bleeding precautions, such as avoiding I.M. and S.C. injections if possible and having the patient use a soft-bristle toothbrush and an electric razor.*
• *Take safety measures, if decreased mental alertness occurs. For example, keep the bed side rails up at all times, maintain the bed in a low position, and supervise all patient activity.*
• Do not administer treatment for ketonemia based solely on urine ketone results because valproic acid can produce a false-positive result on urine ketone tests.
• *Administer valproic acid with meals to decrease adverse GI reactions. Keep the flavorful red syrup out of the reach of children.*
• Notify the physician if adverse drug reactions occur.
• Monitor the serum concentration of valproic acid regularly.
• Monitor seizure activity.
• Notify the physician of any change in seizure activity and serum drug concentrations.

Patient teaching
• Provide basic information about anticonvulsant therapy. (For specifics, see *General patient-teaching tips,* page 303.)
• Teach the patient and family the name, dose, frequency, action, and adverse effects of valproic acid.
• *Instruct the patient to swallow each capsule whole because the free drug can irritate the GI mucosa.*
• *Alert the diabetic patient that the drug may produce a false-positive result on a urine ketone test.*
• Teach the patient to recognize the signs and symptoms of hepatotoxicity and to contact the physician immediately if any occur.
• *Remind the patient to report immediately any signs of bleeding so that platelet function can be assessed.*
• Instruct the patient to inform the physician of valproic acid therapy before any surgery, including dental surgery.

Evaluation
The following examples represent appropriate evaluation statements for a patient receiving valproic acid.
• The patient has no conditions that contraindicate valproic acid therapy.
• The neonate exhibits no signs of complications, such as birth defects, linked to valproic acid administered during the mother's pregnancy.
• The patient exhibits no adverse reactions to valproic acid.
• The patient's seizure activity is under control and serum drug concentration is within a therapeutic range.
• The patient and family express an accurate understanding of the points taught about valproic acid.
• The patient correctly identifies the signs and symptoms of hepatotoxicity.

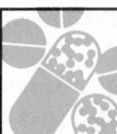

Anticonvulsant agents

This chart summarizes the major anticonvulsant agents currently in clinical use.

DRUG	MAJOR INDICATIONS	USUAL ADULT DOSAGES	CONTRAINDICATIONS AND PRECAUTIONS
Hydantoin			
phenytoin	Complex partial seizures, tonic-clonic seizures	300 to 400 mg P.O. daily in divided doses if a prompt-acting preparation is used; sustained-release preparations are administered as single doses	• Know that phenytoin is contraindicated in a patient with known hypersensitivity to the drug. • Administer with caution to a pregnant patient.
Barbiturate			
phenobarbital	Partial seizures, tonic-clonic seizures	60 to 300 mg P.O. daily in divided doses	• Know that phenobarbital is contraindicated in a patient with known hypersensitivity to the drug, bronchopneumonia, or other severe pulmonary insufficiency. • Administer the parenteral form with caution to a patient with hypertension, hypotension, or pulmonary or cardiovascular disease.
Iminostilbene			
carbamazepine	Partial seizures, tonic-clonic seizures	200 mg P.O. b.i.d. initially; gradually increased in small increments up to 400 mg P.O. t.i.d. until desired response is obtained	• Know that carbamazepine is contraindicated in a patient with known hypersensitivity to the drug or bone marrow depression. • Administer with caution to a pregnant patient or one with cardiac, hepatic, or renal damage; a mixed seizure disorder with atypical absence seizures; adverse hematologic reactions to other drugs; or interrupted courses of therapy with carbamazepine.
Benzodiazepine			
clonazepam	Absence seizures (petit mal); atypical absence, atonic, and myoclonic seizures	1.5 mg P.O. daily in three divided doses; highly individualized	• Know that clonazepam is contraindicated in a pregnant or lactating patient or one with known hypersensitivity to the drug, significant liver disease, or acute narrow-angle glaucoma. • Administer with caution to a patient with impaired renal function or chronic respiratory disease.
Succinimide			
ethosuximide	Absence seizures (petit mal)	250 mg P.O. b.i.d.; 20 to 40 mg/kg P.O. daily as maintenance dosage; highly individualized	• Know that ethosuximide is contraindicated in a patient with known hypersensitivity to the drug. • Administer with caution to a pregnant patient or one with hepatic or renal disease.
Valproic acid			
valproate sodium, divalproex sodium	Absence seizures (petit mal); myoclonic and tonic-clonic seizures	15 mg/kg P.O. daily; maximum dosage is 60 mg/kg P.O. daily; dosages are highly individualized and should be divided if they exceed 250 mg/day	• Know that valproic acid is contraindicated in a patient with hepatic disease or known hypersensitivity to the drug. • Administer with caution to a pregnant patient.

OTHER ANTICONVULSANTS

This section contains information about other drugs used less frequently to treat seizure disorders.

acetazolamide (Diamox). A carbonic anhydrase inhibitor and a sulfonamide derivative, acetazolamide is used primarily as a diuretic, but also possesses anticonvulsant properties. Acetazolamide sometimes is used as adjunctive or intermittent therapy in absence, partial, and generalized tonic-clonic seizures.

The mechanism of action remains unknown, but acetazolamide may suppress the spread of paroxysmal discharges. Hypokalemia and metabolic acidosis represent potentially serious effects associated with the use of acetazolamide. The nurse should caution patients treated with this drug to visit their physician frequently for electrolyte studies. (For a further discussion of acetazolamide, see Chapter 33, Diuretic Agents.)

trimethadione (Tridione) and **paramethadione** (Paradione). These drugs are oxazolidinediones. Since the introduction of the succinimides, trimethadione and paramethadione are used only occasionally as sole or adjunctive treatment for refractory absence seizures.

Both drugs are metabolized to an active metabolite, dimethadione, with a prolonged half-life of 10 days to 2 weeks. Trimethadione and paramethadione cause significant GI and CNS toxicity and are less effective than the succinimides.

magnesium sulfate. This drug prevents or controls seizures by blocking neuromuscular transmission. Magnesium sulfate is used primarily as an anticonvulsant in preeclampsia or eclampsia. Magnesium sulfate also is used to treat hypomagnesemic seizures.

CHAPTER SUMMARY

Chapter 20 centered on anticonvulsant drugs. Here are the highlights of the chapter.
• Anticonvulsants are prescribed for long-term treatment of epilepsy and for short-term control of acute isolated seizures not caused by epilepsy. Drug choice depends on an accurate diagnosis of the seizure type, the ability of the drug to control seizures with minimal adverse effects, the use of a single drug whenever possible, and the appropriateness of the drug for the patient's age and health.
• The major classes of drugs used to treat patients with seizure disorders include hydantoins, barbiturates, iminostilbenes, benzodiazepines, succinimides, and valproic acid.
• The drugs of choice for complex partial seizures are phenytoin and carbamazepine, and possibly primidone. Phenobarbital is one of the most widely used anticonvulsants in long-term treatment of epilepsy. It also may be used for acute treatment of status epilepticus. Ethosuximide is the drug of choice for absence seizures.
• Most anticonvulsants demonstrate linear kinetics; however, phenytoin exhibits saturation kinetics. Dosage increases of phenytoin must be made carefully in small increments to avoid toxicity.
• Anticonvulsants commonly interact with other drugs, sometimes producing drug toxicity. To help prevent drug interactions, the nurse should maintain an up-to-date drug history.
• Some anticonvulsants are an increased risk factor when administered to women of childbearing age or to pregnant or lactating women. Teratogenic effects have occurred in patients using anticonvulsants.
• The nurse should monitor serum concentrations of anticonvulsants frequently. Additional laboratory studies are recommended depending on the potential for toxicity.

STUDY QUESTIONS

See Appendix 1 for answers.

1. Larry Stokes, age 18, is admitted to the hospital after experiencing his first seizure. His mother states that Larry fell to the floor without warning, became rigid for a few seconds, thrashed around for a couple of minutes, and then was unconscious for 5 to 10 minutes. Larry arrives at the hospital groggy and confused. His physician orders phenytoin (Dilantin) 300 mg P.O. h.s. daily. Which of the following best describes the absorption rate of oral phenytoin?
(a) rapid
(b) slow
(c) erratic
(d) poor

2. By which mechanism does phenytoin prevent seizure activity?
(a) by altering ion movement
(b) by increasing the threshold for motor cortex stimuli
(c) by inhibiting neurotransmission
(d) by increasing the availability of GABA to brain neurons

3. For about 8 years, Elaine Coggins, age 27, has been taking phenobarbital 60 mg P.O. daily for long-term treatment of partial seizures. Which of the following accurately characterizes the use of this Schedule IV drug as an anticonvulsant?
(a) Addiction can occur with small doses.
(b) Addiction is unlikely because the dosage is at subhypnotic levels.
(c) Addiction occurs after long-term use.
(d) Addiction is likely when phenobarbital alone is used to control seizures.

4. Kenny Borden, age 7, suffers from tonic-clonic seizures. His physician prescribes the iminostilbene carbamazepine (Tegretol) 100 mg P.O. b.i.d. Carbamazepine is related structurally to which drugs?
(a) phenothiazines
(b) tricyclic antidepressants
(c) benzodiazepines
(d) barbiturates

5. The nurse should include which of the following in the teaching of Kenny's parents?
(a) Administer the drug on an empty stomach to improve absorption.
(b) Be alert for hyperkinetic effects.
(c) Be alert for signs of hematologic problems, such as fever and bleeding.
(d) Be alert for sedation.

6. Ben Gordon, age 35, is brought to the emergency department with seizures. The physician orders diazepam (Valium) 5 mg I.V. initially. For which type of seizure is diazepam used?
(a) partial seizure
(b) tonic-clonic seizure
(c) status epilepticus
(d) absence seizure

7. Judy Green, age 34, has a seizure disorder, which her physician decides to treat with ethosuximide (Zarontin). This anticonvulsant is the drug of choice for which type of seizure?
(a) partial seizure
(b) tonic-clonic seizure
(c) status epilepticus
(d) absence seizure

8. As an alternative, the physician could have prescribed valproate sodium (Depakene) for Ms. Green. However, this drug is not administered routinely. Which adverse reaction limits the use of valproate?
(a) sedation
(b) hepatotoxicity
(c) nausea
(d) muscle weakness

SELECTED REFERENCES

AHFS drug information 90. (1990). Bethesda, MD: American Society of Hospital Pharmacists.

Conley, N., and Olshanky, E. (1987). Current controversies in pregnancy and epilepsy: A unique challenge to nursing. *JOGNN,* 16(5), 321-328.

Friedman, D. (1988). Taking the scare out of caring for seizure patients. *Nursing88,* 18(2), 52-60.

Goodman and Gilman's the pharmacological basis of therapeutics (8th ed., 1990). Elmsford, NY: Pergamon Press.

Hansten, P., and Horn, J. (1989). *Drug interactions* (6th ed.). Philadelphia: Lea & Febiger.

Parks, B., Jr. (1988). Febrile seizures. *Pediatric Nursing,* 14(6), 518.

DRUGS TO PREVENT AND TREAT PAIN

Pain, a basic protective mechanism, is a symptom of an underlying physiologic or psychological problem. Pain usually indicates that something is wrong and that health care is desirable.

Because pain is subjective, only the patient can describe it. Pain is whatever sensation the patient perceives it to be; one person's pain perceptions may vary widely from another's. Emotional states and ethnic, cultural, and religious factors all contribute to the patient's pain perception.

PAIN DETECTION AND TRANSMISSION

Pain sensation begins in the nociceptors, which are part of an afferent neuron. Nociceptors are free nerve endings located primarily in the skin, periosteum, joint surfaces, and arterial walls. They may be activated by mechanical, chemical, or thermal stimuli. They also are activated by chemical mediators that are released or synthesized in response to tissue damage. Regardless of the etiology, even if only minor tissue damage occurs, the chemical mediators are synthesized and stimulate the nociceptors.

Prostaglandins, histamine, bradykinin, and serotonin are chemical mediators that activate the nociceptors. Acetylsalicylic acid and other nonsteroidal anti-inflammatory drugs (NSAIDs) decrease pain by inhibiting these mediators.

Once the pain process is initiated, the impulse is communicated from the peripheral terminals of the nociceptors to the spinal cord. (For an illustration, see *Pain pathways,* page 323.) Two types of nociceptors exist: the myelinated A-delta fibers and the smaller, unmyelinated, more numerous C fibers. The faster-conducting A-delta fibers signal sharp, well-localized pain; the slower-conducting C fibers signal dull, poorly localized pain.

All nociceptors terminate in the dorsal horn of the spinal cord. The dorsal horn is the control center for incoming information from the afferent neurons, for local modulation (pain impulse regulation), and for descending influences from higher centers in the central nervous system (CNS), such as emotion, attention, and memory.

PAIN THEORY

Several theories have been suggested to define pain transmission; however, much still is unknown.

The Melzack-Wall gate control theory, the most widely accepted pain theory, states that neural mechanisms in the dorsal horn act as a regulator between the peripheral fibers and the higher processing centers in the CNS. The dorsal horn receives pain- and non-pain-related signals from the various peripheral nerves; pain messages depend on the total information. This process, or gating effect, modulates, or regulates, afferent input before an impulse is sent to the CNS and pain is perceived. Therefore, pain perception may be inhibited by the simultaneous activation of sensory neurons carrying non-pain information.

At least two major and several minor ascending pathways in the spinal cord transmit messages to the brain when pain-related signals activate pain-transmission neurons in the dorsal root. The two major pathways are the spinothalamic tract and the spinoreticulothalamic tract; the former probably is the more important. Both pathways travel up the spinal cord and terminate in two separate areas of the thalamus. The two thalamic regions project to different sites in the cerebral cortex.

The thalamus is a relay station for all incoming sensory stimuli, including pain. A primitive awareness of pain occurs in the thalamus, but the sensation is not well localized or specific. From the thalamus, pain messages are directed to the cerebral cortex, where more specific localization and characterization of the pain sensation occur. The emotional aspect of pain is related partially to thalamic and limbic stimulation when incoming sensory data are relayed to the cortex.

The brain contains opiate receptors and opiate peptides (endorphins, enkephalins, and dynorphins). The endogenous peptides have a high affinity for the opiate receptors and may modulate pain sensation. These peptides, however, are not the only pain neurotransmitters. Other peptides, amino acids, and biogenic amines also are active.

Glossary

Analgesia: absence of sensitivity to pain.

Anesthesia: loss of feeling or sensation.

Balanced anesthesia: combination of drugs that produces a loss of feeling or sensation, with maximum beneficial drug effects and minimum adverse drug reactions.

Competitive inhibition: displacement of an agent from an opiate receptor site by an antagonist.

Endorphin: endogenous opiate in the hypothalamus and pituitary.

Enkephalin: endogenous opiate throughout the central and peripheral nervous systems.

Epidural block: loss of feeling or sensation produced by injecting an anesthetic agent between the vertebrae and beneath the ligaments into the space surrounding the dura.

Equianalgesic dose: amount of an analgesic drug that will produce the same level of pain relief as a standard agent used for comparison.

Field block: regional loss of feeling or sensation produced by using several injections of an anesthetic agent to create a pain-free area around an operative site.

Inflammation: tissue reaction to injury characterized by pain, heat, redness, edema, and sometimes loss of function.

Local infiltration: loss of feeling or sensation in a confined area produced by injecting an anesthetic agent.

Narcotic: drug derived from opium or synthetically produced that alters pain perception, induces mental changes, promotes deep sleep, depresses respirations, constricts pupils, and decreases gastrointestinal motility.

Nerve block: regional loss of feeling or sensation produced by injecting an anesthetic agent around or near a nerve to interrupt its conductivity.

Neuralgia: paroxysmal pain extending along one or more nerves.

Neuroleptanesthesia: loss of feeling or sensation produced by using a narcotic, a neuroleptic, and nitrous oxide.

Neurolysis: destruction or dissolution of nerve tissue.

Peripheral nerve block: loss of feeling or sensation produced by injecting an anesthetic agent near or around nerve fibers outside the central nervous system.

Prostaglandins: naturally occurring fatty acids abundant in cells that affect many different cellular functions.

Regional anesthesia: loss of feeling or sensation produced by interrupting the sensory nerve conductivity from a specific body area.

Salicylism: toxic effects of excessive salicylic acid ingestion.

Spinal block: loss of feeling or sensation produced by injecting an anesthetic agent into the cerebrospinal fluid in the subarachnoid space around the spinal cord.

Sympathetic block: loss of feeling or sensation produced by the paravertebral injection of an anesthetic agent to block the sympathetic trunk.

Topical anesthesia: loss of feeling or sensation produced by direct application of a local anesthetic agent to a specified area.

Most biological systems have an autoregulation mechanism, and the pain system is no exception. This internal regulation occurs in a descending pathway of the CNS and is responsible for maintaining the normal pain-free state.

MECHANISMS OF INFLAMMATION

Pain may occur alone or with inflammation. Both are reactions to tissue irritation. Inflammation is an immune-mediated process characterized by redness, heat, swelling, loss of function, and pain at the site. Some of the chemical mediators of pain, including prostaglandins, bradykinin, and histamine, also mediate the inflammatory response. (For more information about inflammation, see Unit Thirteen, Drugs to Control Inflammation, Allergy, and Organ Rejection.)

TEMPERATURE REGULATION

The hypothalamus regulates body temperature by balancing heat production and loss. Pyrogens, secreted by toxic bacteria or released from protein breakdown as in degenerating body tissue, can cause the hypothalamic thermostat to rise. This in turn increases body temperature. Recent research also indicates that pyrogens may increase body temperature by causing production of prostaglandin E_1 in the hypothalamus. Some of the drugs used to control pain inhibit prostaglandins and produce an antipyretic effect.

OVERVIEW OF CHAPTERS

The chapters in this unit discuss the pharmacologic management of pain. They present drugs that range from mild, over-the-counter preparations, such as acetaminophen, to potent general anesthetics, which are administered only by highly trained professionals in a controlled environment.

Chapter 21
Nonnarcotic Analgesic, Antipyretic, and Nonsteroidal Anti-Inflammatory Agents

Chapter 21 discusses the three subclasses of nonnarcotic agents (salicylates, para-aminophenol derivatives, and NSAIDs), describing their mechanisms of action, clinical uses, and adverse effects, such as salicylism. The chapter also explores nursing activities related to the administration of these agents.

Pain pathways

When stimulated, the A-delta fiber and C fiber nociceptors transmit an afferent impulse through the dorsal root ganglia to the dorsal horn. Peripheral nerves also transmit information to the dorsal horn. The dorsal horn then modulates all of this information and may transmit an impulse via the spinothalamic tract to the cerebral cortex. Descending pathways carry inhibitory information from the brain to the dorsal horn to be used for further modulation.

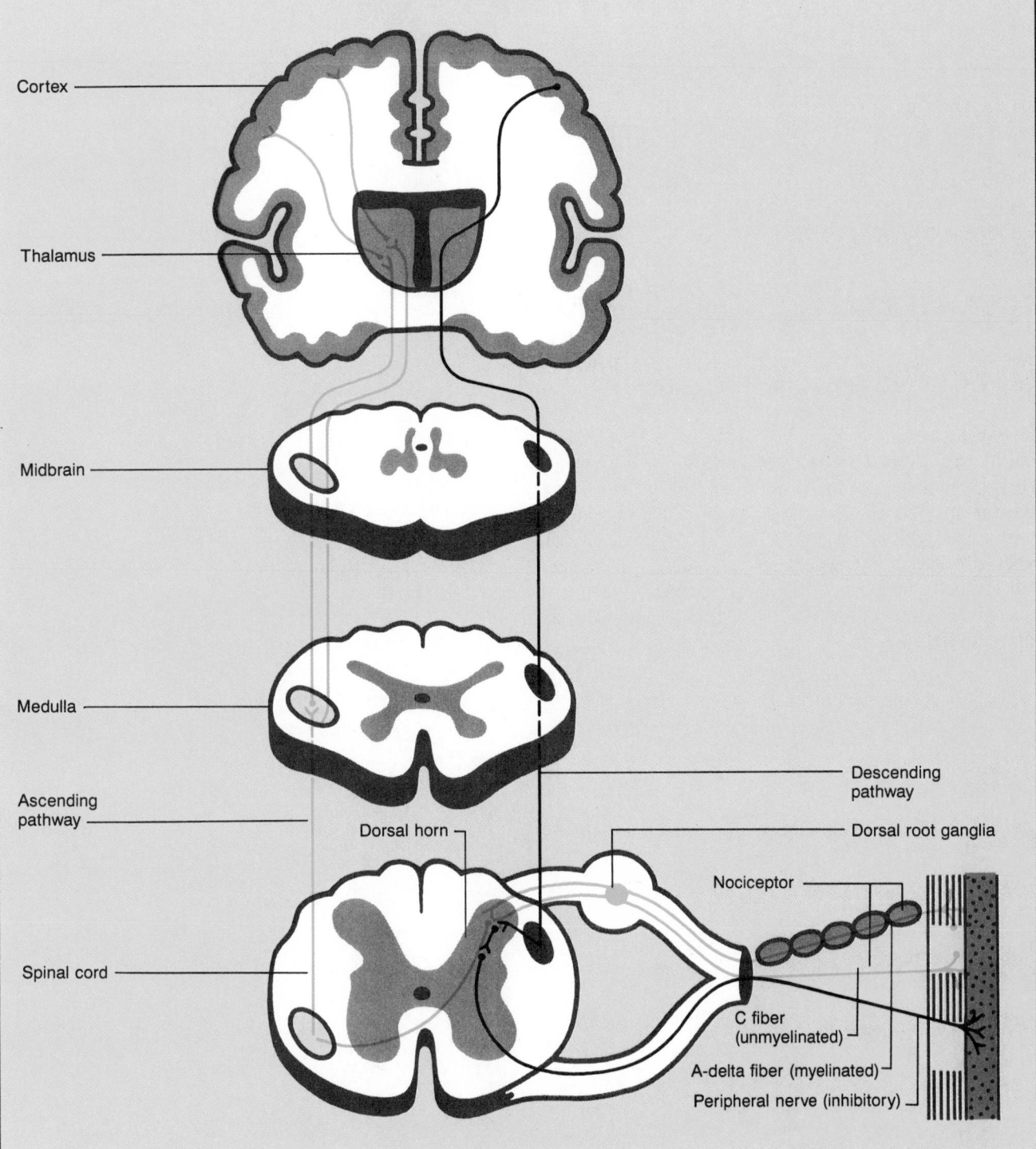

Cortex

Thalamus

Midbrain

Medulla

Ascending pathway

Dorsal horn

Spinal cord

Descending pathway

Dorsal root ganglia

Nociceptor

C fiber (unmyelinated)

A-delta fiber (myelinated)

Peripheral nerve (inhibitory)

Chapter 22
Narcotic Agonist and Antagonist Agents

Chapter 22 discusses three types of narcotic agents: narcotic agonists, mixed narcotic agonist-antagonists, and narcotic antagonists. Narcotic agonists include opium derivatives and synthetic agents with similar pharmacologic properties. The chapter discusses their uses in inhibiting pain impulse transmission, suppressing the cough mechanism, and decreasing gastrointestinal (GI) motility. Mixed narcotic agonist-antagonists offer pain relief similar to that of morphine but have little or no antitussive or GI effect. Chapter 22 concludes by describing narcotic antagonists that are used to treat narcotic-related problems, such as narcotic overdose and dependence. For each type of narcotic agent, the chapter highlights related nursing care.

Chapter 23
General Anesthetic Agents

Chapter 23 reviews general anesthesia and associated pharmacologic agents. It discusses various types of anesthesia, including balanced and neuroleptic, and the four stages and their clinical characteristics. The chapter presents inhalation and injection anesthetic agents, addressing their systemic effects and associated nursing responsibilities.

Chapter 24
Local and Topical Anesthetic Agents

This chapter discusses the local and topical agents used to interrupt pain impulse transmission from the peripheral nerves of a specific, limited body area. It describes several types of blocks, including field, spinal, epidural, peripheral, and sympathetic. It also details the pharmacodynamics, clinical uses, application, and nursing implications of the topical anesthetics.

NONNARCOTIC ANALGESIC, ANTIPYRETIC, AND NONSTEROIDAL ANTI-INFLAMMATORY AGENTS

OBJECTIVES

After reading and studying this chapter, the student should be able to:

1. Describe the pharmacodynamics of the salicylates, acetaminophen, and nonsteroidal anti-inflammatory drugs (NSAIDs).

2. Compare the therapeutic uses of the salicylates, acetaminophen, and the NSAIDs.

3. Contrast the drug interactions associated with the salicylates, acetaminophen, and the NSAIDs.

4. Compare the adverse drug reactions to salicylates, acetaminophen, and the NSAIDs.

5. Explain the inflammatory process.

6. Identify the signs and symptoms of salicylate toxicity.

7. Discuss the signs, symptoms, and treatment of acetaminophen overdose.

8. Describe how to apply the nursing process when caring for a patient who is receiving salicylates, acetaminophen, or NSAIDs.

INTRODUCTION

The drugs discussed in this chapter form a heterogenous collection that produce analgesic, antipyretic, and anti-inflammatory effects. Among these drugs, salicylates — especially aspirin — are the most widely used. This chapter discusses the salicylates, the para-aminophenol derivative acetaminophen, NSAIDs, and the urinary tract analgesic phenazopyridine hydrochloride.

For a summary of representative drugs, see *Selected major drugs: Nonnarcotic analgesics, antipyretic agents, and NSAIDs*, pages 342 and 343. For a listing of applicable nursing diagnoses that the nurse may formulate when caring

---

SELECTED NURSING DIAGNOSES

Nonnarcotic analgesics, antipyretic agents, and NSAIDs

The following nursing diagnoses address representative problems and etiologies that a nurse may encounter when caring for a patient who is receiving a nonnarcotic analgesic, antipyretic agent, or nonsteroidal anti-inflammatory drug (NSAID). Some of these nursing diagnoses contain generalized etiologies, which the nurse must individualize based on the patient's needs. (For some common nursing diagnoses and related interventions for each drug class, see the "Nursing Process Application" sections of this chapter.)

- Altered protection related to hemorrhagic tendencies associated with salicylate use
- Diarrhea related to the adverse gastrointestinal (GI) effects of the prescribed NSAID
- Fluid volume excess related to sodium and water retention caused by an NSAID
- Impaired tissue integrity related to gastric ulceration caused by salicylate or NSAID use
- Knowledge deficit related to the prescribed nonnarcotic analgesic, antipyretic agent, or NSAID
- Pain related to ineffectiveness of the prescribed nonnarcotic analgesic, antipyretic agent, or NSAID
- Potential fluid volume deficit related to the diaphoresis and adverse GI reactions to the salicylate
- Potential for injury related to a preexisting condition that contraindicates the use of a nonnarcotic analgesic, antipyretic agent, or NSAID
- Potential for injury related to a preexisting condition that requires cautious use of a nonnarcotic analgesic, antipyretic agent, or NSAID
- Potential for injury related to adverse drug reactions
- Sensory-perceptual alteration (auditory) related to salicylate-induced hearing problems

for a patient receiving these agents, see *Selected nursing diagnoses: Nonnarcotic analgesics, antipyretic agents, and NSAIDs,* page 325. For detailed information on applying the nursing process, see Chapter 6, The Nursing Process and Drug Therapy.

SALICYLATES

These agents possess analgesic, antipyretic, and anti-inflammatory properties. They usually cost less than other analgesics and most are readily available without a prescription. In fact, many over-the-counter (OTC) medications for pain, colds, and influenza contain salicylates along with other agents.

This section discusses the following salicylates: aspirin, choline magnesium trisalicylate, choline salicylate, diflunisal, salsalate, and sodium salicylate. Despite the recent development of new products, however, aspirin remains the cornerstone of anti-inflammatory drug therapy.

PHARMACOKINETICS

Salicylates are absorbed readily and distributed widely throughout the body. They are metabolized in the liver at dose-dependent rates and excreted by the kidneys.

Absorption, distribution, metabolism, excretion

After oral administration, salicylate absorption occurs partly in the stomach but mainly in the upper part of the small intestine through passive diffusion. Although absorption usually occurs within 30 minutes, the rate depends on the dosage form, the gastric and intestinal pH, the presence of food or antacids in the stomach, and the gastric-emptying time. The pure and buffered forms of aspirin are absorbed readily, but sustained-release and enteric-coated salicylate preparations or food or antacids in the stomach delay absorption.

Salicylates are distributed widely throughout the body tissues and fluids, including breast milk. They cross the placenta easily and are highly protein bound.

The liver metabolizes salicylates extensively into several metabolites. This pharmacokinetic process is dose-dependent. As the salicylate dose and serum concentration levels increase, some metabolic pathways become saturated and cannot metabolize the drug completely. When this happens, metabolism shifts to alternate pathways, resulting in increased formation of toxic metabolites. Therapeutic salicylate concentrations range from 30 to 300 mcg/ml. Blood levels that exceed this amount may be toxic. Decreasing the salicylate dose even slightly usually decreases toxic metabolite formation. Blood levels of a salicylate can determine whether a dose has produced an adequate anti-inflammatory effect or has caused toxicity.

The kidneys excrete the salicylate metabolites and some unchanged drug. The amount of unchanged drug excreted is pH-dependent, with about 2% being excreted in acidic urine and 30% in alkaline urine.

Onset, peak, duration

The onset of action of salicylates begins about 30 to 60 minutes after administration. When the drugs reach peak plasma concentrations in 2 hours, they are 50% to 90% serum protein bound. The amount of protein binding, however, depends on the serum salicylate concentration. At a low serum concentration, such as 100 mcg/ml, protein binding nears 90%; at a higher concentration, such as 400 mcg/ml, protein binding drops to 76%. The half-life of salicylates ranges from 3 hours for a low dose to 30 hours for a high dose.

PHARMACODYNAMICS

The salicylates produce analgesia primarily by inhibiting prostaglandin synthesis; reduce fever through hypothalamic stimulation leading to vasodilation and increased diaphoresis; and reduce inflammation through a poorly understood process that may involve their ability to inhibit prostaglandin synthesis and release during inflammation.

Mechanism of action

Prostaglandins play an important role in the inflammatory process, and pain impulse transmission from the periphery to the spinal cord requires prostaglandin E. Salicylates produce anti-inflammatory and analgesic effects primarily by inhibiting prostaglandin synthesis through inactivation of cyclooxygenase (prostaglandin synthetase). (For more details, see *The inflammatory process*.) Salicylates also may stabilize membranes, preventing the release of substances that cause inflammation.

The antipyretic effects of these drugs, caused by prostaglandin inhibition in the brain, seem to stimulate the heat-regulating center in the hypothalamus, increasing heat elimination. The hypothalamic center then stimulates peripheral vasodilation and increases perspiration.

Aspirin inhibits platelet aggregation through irreversible pathways by interfering with thromboxane A_2 production, which is necessary for platelet clumping. (For more information on the use of aspirin as an antiplatelet agent, see Chapter 36, Anticoagulant Agents.)

The inflammatory process

Anti-inflammatory drugs act by interrupting the inflammatory process. This process usually begins when tissue injury causes the release of bradykinin and histamine, which in turn cause increased capillary permeability and vasodilation. The change in capillary permeability leads to swelling and pain, and the vasodilation leads to redness and heat. Bradykinin plays a role in the formation and release of prostaglandins, which cause pain. Salicylates and nonsteroidal anti-inflammatory drugs act primarily as antiprostaglandin agents, disrupting the inflammatory process and relieving pain and inflammation.

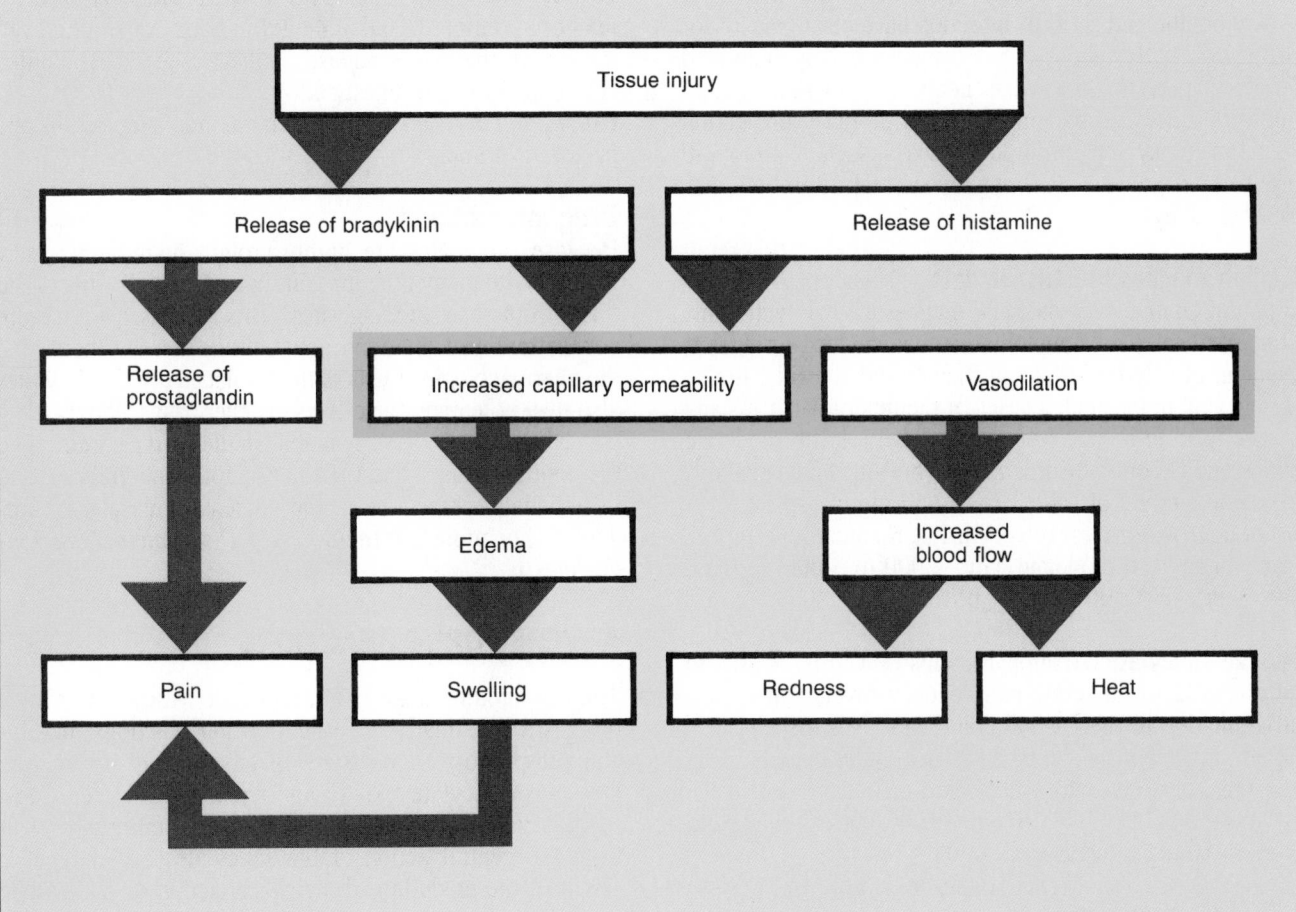

PHARMACOTHERAPEUTICS

Salicylates are used primarily to relieve pain and reduce fever. However, they cannot effectively relieve visceral pain or severe pain from trauma.

Salicylates have little or no effect on normal body temperature but cause a marked fall if body temperature is elevated. This is especially true of aspirin. Salicylates are often the drugs of choice for relief of fever associated with common colds or influenza because they can relieve headache and muscle ache as well.

Salicylates suppress inflammation, probably by inhibiting prostaglandin synthesis. Used to reduce inflammation in rheumatic fever and rheumatoid arthritis, they can provide considerable relief in 24 hours. No matter what the clinical indication, the main guideline of salicylate therapy is to use the lowest dose that provides relief.

aspirin (A.S.A., Bayer Timed-Release, Empirin). Aspirin is the most widely used salicylate and effectively relieves headache, neuritis, neuralgia, myalgia, rheumatoid arthritis, and dysmenorrhea.

Aspirin appears in many preparations, even in analgesic combinations with narcotics, such as oxycodone and codeine. Unlike aspirin alone, medications that contain aspirin and a narcotic require a prescription.

No pediatric dosages are listed because aspirin is contraindicated in a child with varicella or influenza. Many health care professionals discourage aspirin use in anyone under age 18, except for rheumatic fever.

Usual adult dosage: for fever or mild to moderate pain such as headache or musculoskeletal pain, 325 to 650 mg P.O. every 3 to 4 hours p.r.n.; for dysmenorrhea, 650 mg P.O. every 4 to 6 hours, beginning 1 or 2 days before the onset of menses and continuing until the second or third day of menses, taken monthly for maximum effect; for rheumatic fever, 975 to 1,300 mg P.O. four to six times daily, individualized to the patient's needs, until fever and inflammation subside (about 1 week) or until the patient is asymptomatic and signs of infection have disappeared; for rheumatoid arthritis, 3.6 to 5.4 grams P.O. daily in divided doses; to prevent transient ischemic attacks (TIAs), 325 mg P.O. q.i.d. or 650 mg P.O. b.i.d. (TIA prevention sometimes may occur with lower doses, such as 40 to 150 mg/day); to prevent recurrent myocardial infarction, 325 mg P.O. daily.

choline magnesium trisalicylate (Trilisate). A combination of choline salicylate and magnesium salicylate, this drug is indicated for symptomatic relief and long-term management of osteoarthritis and rheumatoid arthritis. It also is indicated in the acute phases of rheumatoid arthritis and can be used to reduce fever and relieve mild to moderate pain related to other disorders. Each 500-mg tablet contains the same amount of salicylate as 650 mg of aspirin.
Usual adult dosage: for osteoarthritis, rheumatoid arthritis, fever, or mild to moderate pain, 2,000 to 3,000 mg P.O. once a day or 1,500 mg P.O. b.i.d.

choline salicylate (Arthropan). This OTC drug is used to relieve mild to moderate pain, reduce fever, and reduce inflammation in rheumatoid conditions. It is dispensed in liquid form and may be mixed with fruit juice, a carbonated beverage, or water before administration. One teaspoon (5 ml) of the liquid contains 870 mg of choline salicylate and equals 650 mg of aspirin.
Usual adult dosage: for pain or fever, 2.5 to 5 ml (435 to 870 mg) P.O. every 4 hours up to a maximum of six doses daily; for inflammation, 5 to 10 ml (870 to 1740 mg) P.O. t.i.d. or q.i.d.

diflunisal (Dolobid). A salicylic acid derivative, diflunisal has analgesic, anti-inflammatory, and antipyretic actions, although it is not indicated for antipyretic therapy. It may be used for acute or long-term relief of mild to moderate pain caused by musculoskeletal problems or osteoarthritis. Diflunisal requires a prescription. Because metabolism of this drug depends on its blood concentration, small dosage changes may cause large changes in the blood concentration, leading to toxicity.
Usual adult dosage: for mild to moderate pain, initially 500 to 1,000 mg P.O., followed by 250 to 500 mg every 8 to 12 hours; for osteoarthritis, 500 to 1,000 mg/day P.O. in two divided doses; not to exceed 1,500 mg/day.

salsalate (Disalcid, Mono-Gesic). Salsalate is used for temporary relief of the symptoms of osteoarthritis, rheumatoid arthritis, and related rheumatic conditions. It is available in 750- and 1,500-mg tablets.
Usual adult dosage: for osteoarthritis, rheumatoid arthritis, or rheumatic conditions, 1,500 mg P.O. b.i.d. or 750 mg P.O. q.i.d., not to exceed 4,000 mg/day.

sodium salicylate (Pabalate). This salicylate is used for temporary relief of mild to moderate pain. An enteric coating delays the drug's release until it reaches the alkaline environment of the intestine.
Usual adult dosage: for mild to moderate pain, 325 to 650 mg every 4 hours.

Drug interactions

Because salicylates are highly protein bound, they may interact with many other protein-bound drugs by displacing them from their binding sites. This increases the serum concentration of unbound active drug, thereby increasing the pharmacologic effects of the displaced drug. Salicylates also may potentiate the effects of other drugs. Rarely, they can cause false-positive reactions in diabetic patients using the copper reduction test (Clinitest) for urine glucose, and false-negative reactions to the glucose oxidase test (Tes-Tape). (For more information, see *Drug interactions: Salicylates.*)

ADVERSE DRUG REACTIONS

The most common adverse reactions to salicylates involve the gastrointestinal (GI) system. Other reactions may include respiratory alkalosis and metabolic acidosis, hearing problems, salicylate toxicity, and hypersensitivity reactions.

Gastric distress, nausea, and vomiting commonly result from the central action of the salicylates on the emetic center of the medulla and their local action on the gastric mucosa secretions that protect the stomach from gastric acid. Although sodium bicarbonate may help prevent GI irritation, it also promotes salicylate excretion by the kidneys.

Large or toxic salicylate doses can cause respiratory alkalosis and increase the rate and depth of respiration. If the respiratory problem is not corrected, metabolic acidosis can occur as the body attempts to compensate for the respiratory alkalosis.

Prolonged use of salicylates sometimes causes bilateral hearing loss of 30 to 40 decibels that usually resolves within 2 weeks after therapy is discontinued. Tinnitus may occur with dosage levels used to treat arthritis, requiring a small dosage reduction. An elderly patient or a patient with impaired hearing, who may not notice the ringing sound until it is severe, should be monitored closely.

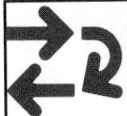

DRUG INTERACTIONS

Salicylates

Drug interactions involving salicylates are common and sometimes severe. They typically occur with concurrent use of other highly protein-bound or ulcerogenic agents. Because salicylates are so widely used, the nurse must obtain a thorough drug history and be alert for possible drug interactions.

DRUG	INTERACTING DRUGS	POSSIBLE EFFECTS	NURSING IMPLICATIONS
aspirin, choline magnesium trisalicylate, choline salicylate, diflunisal, salsalate, sodium salicylate	alcohol	Increases the ulcerogenic effect, leading to gastrointestinal (GI) bleeding	• Monitor the patient for signs of GI bleeding, such as epigastric pain, abdominal pain or cramps, or black or tarry stools.
	oral anticoagulants and heparin	Increase the anticoagulant effect, increasing risk of bleeding	• Monitor the patient for signs of increased anticoagulant effect, such as gingival bleeding, black or tarry stools, blood in the urine, petechiae, bruises, and prolonged bleeding from cuts.
	corticosteroids	Decrease the plasma salicylate concentrations and increase the ulcerogenic effect	• Assess the patient for the salicylate's effectiveness. If it does not provide relief, obtain a prescription for a different analgesic. • Monitor the patient for epigastric pain, especially 1 to 2 hours after meals. Also assess the patient for other signs of GI bleeding, such as abdominal pain or cramps or black or tarry stools.
	methotrexate	Increase the methotrexate effect and toxicity, causing pancytopenia	• Question any prescription for salicylates for a patient receiving methotrexate. Avoid concurrent use, if possible. • Monitor the patient for signs of methotrexate toxicity, such as diarrhea and stomatitis. • Monitor the patient for signs of severe bone marrow depression, such as fatigue, pallor, and fever.
	probenecid, sulfinpyrazone	Decrease the uricosuric effect	• Be aware that even small doses of salicylates can decrease the uricosuric effects of probenecid or sulfinpyrazone. • Instruct the patient not to take aspirin or other over-the-counter drugs containing salicylates unless specifically directed by the physician.
	antacids	Alkalinize urine, leading to reduced renal tubular reabsorption	• Observe the patient for signs and symptoms of reduced salicylate response, such as increased pain and inflammation. • Expect serum salicylate concentrations to decrease, requiring a dosage adjustment.
	oral hypoglycemics (sulfonylureas)	Increase the hypoglycemic effect	• Monitor the patient for signs and symptoms of hypoglycemia, such as fatigue, tremors, hunger, drowsiness, headache, diaphoresis, anxiety, numb mouth or tongue, or incoherent speech.
	zidovudine	Inhibit zidovudine metabolism, possible causing toxicity	• Avoid concurrent use of these drugs.

(continued)

DRUG INTERACTIONS

Salicylates *(continued)*

DRUG	INTERACTING DRUGS	POSSIBLE EFFECTS	NURSING IMPLICATIONS
aspirin, choline magnesium trisalicylate, choline salicylate, diflunisal, salsalate, sodium salicylate *(continued)*	alkalinizing agents	Increase salicylate excretion, if salicylate dosage exceeds 50 mg/kg/day	• Monitor the patient for decreased salicylate effectiveness.
	spironolactone	Reduce spironolactone effectiveness	• Monitor the patient's fluid intake and output. • Monitor the patient's serum potassium level.
	acetazolamide	May cause acetazolamide intoxication	• Monitor the patient for signs and symptoms of central nervous system toxicity, such as lethargy, confusion, or anorexia.

Mild salicylate toxicity, or salicylism, characteristically causes nausea, vomiting, diarrhea, thirst, diaphoresis, tinnitus, confusion, dizziness, impaired vision, and hyperventilation. When these signs and symptoms appear with doses used to treat rheumatic conditions, a reduction of 325 mg/day usually reduces them to a tolerable level. Indications of severe toxicity include metabolic acidosis and related acid-base imbalances, hemorrhagic tendencies, hypoglycemia, restlessness, incoherent speech, apprehension, delirium, hallucinations, and seizures.

In a child with a varicella infection or flulike symptoms, salicylates may lead to Reye's syndrome, a potentially fatal disorder that causes encephalopathy and fatty infiltration of the internal organs. Although a direct causal relationship has not been established, the U.S. Food and Drug Administration discourages the use of salicylates in children and teenagers who have varicella or influenza infections.

Common hypersensitivity reactions to salicylates include rash and, in asthmatics with nasal polyps, bronchospasm and asthma. Anaphylaxis rarely occurs.

NURSING PROCESS APPLICATION

The following information assists the nurse in caring for a patient who is receiving a salicylate.

Assessment
• Review the patient's history for conditions that contraindicate the use of a salicylate, such as known hypersensitivity to the drug, bleeding disorder, the last trimester of pregnancy, or a history of acute asthmatic attacks, urticaria, or rhinitis precipitated by aspirin.
• Review the patient's history for conditions that require cautious use of a salicylate, such as GI lesions or impaired renal function.
• Assess the patient for adverse reactions to the salicylate, such as GI distress, signs of respiratory alkalosis and metabolic acidosis, hearing problems, hypersensitivity reac-

tions, or salicylate toxicity. (For more information about toxicity, see *Signs and symptoms of salicylate toxicity*.)
• Review the patient's medication history to identify use of drugs that may interact with the salicylate, such as alcohol, oral anticoagulants, heparin, corticosteroids, or antacids.
• Assess the effectiveness of the salicylate.
• Assess the patient for dehydration if nausea, vomiting, diarrhea, or excessive diaphoresis occurs.
• Evaluate the patient's and family's knowledge about the salicylate.

Nursing diagnoses
The following examples represent appropriate nursing diagnoses for a patient receiving a salicylate.
• Potential for injury related to a preexisting condition that contraindicates the use of the salicylate
• Potential for injury related to a preexisting condition that requires cautious use of the salicylate
• Potential for injury related to adverse drug reactions
• Potential fluid volume deficit related to the excessive diaphoresis and adverse GI reactions to the salicylate
• Sensory-perceptual alteration (auditory) related to salicylate-induced hearing problems
• Pain related to salicylate ineffectiveness
• Knowledge deficit related to the salicylate

Planning and implementation
• Do not administer a salicylate to a patient with a condition that contraindicates its use. Keep in mind that an asthmatic patient with nasal polyps is particularly vulnerable to acute asthmatic attack and bronchospasm, usually 15 to 30 minutes after salicylate ingestion.
• *Do not administer aspirin to a patient in the third trimester of pregnancy.* If she ingests aspirin or an aspirin-containing product up to 2 weeks before delivery, observe the neonate closely for bleeding.
• Do not administer diflunisal for antipyretic therapy.

Signs and symptoms of salicylate toxicity

Whether mild or severe, salicylate toxicity requires early detection and appropriate action to prevent more serious problems.

Mild toxicity

Mild toxicity typically affects patients taking high doses of salicylates for rheumatoid arthritis and related conditions. Its signs and symptoms may indicate that the maximum tolerable dosage has been reached and that a slight reduction is required. Signs and symptoms include:
- hearing loss
- dizziness
- drowsiness
- headache
- hyperventilation
- confusion
- nausea and vomiting
- reduced visual acuity
- diaphoresis
- thirst
- tinnitus
- diarrhea.

Severe toxicity

Severe toxicity, which occurs most commonly in infants and young children who have ingested large amounts of aspirin, requires immediate medical attention. Signs and symptoms include:
- electroencephalogram changes
- hypoglycemia
- skin eruptions
- marked changes in acid-base balance; respiratory alkalosis leading to metabolic acidosis
- central nervous system depression, seizures, coma
- hemorrhagic tendencies.

• Administer a salicylate cautiously to a patient at risk because of a preexisting condition.

• Question any prescription of sodium salicylate for a patient with hypertension or on a sodium-restricted diet. Advise such a patient not to use effervescent aspirin products, which have a high sodium content.

• Observe the patient frequently for adverse reactions to the salicylate.

• Take the patient's vital signs at least every 4 hours. If respirations increase in rate and depth, notify the physician; the patient may be compensating for or developing an acid-base imbalance.

• Check the diflunisal dose carefully before administration. Small dosage changes may cause large changes in the blood concentration, leading to toxicity.

• *Administer the salicylate with at least 8 ounces of liquid.*

• Do not check the diabetic patient's urine for glucose with the copper reduction test (Clinitest) or glucose oxidase test (Tes-Tape). These tests may provide incorrect results during salicylate use.

• Monitor the diabetic patient who takes a salicylate and sulfonylurea for hypoglycemia.

• Expect to discontinue aspirin 1 week before major surgery to reduce the risk of bleeding.

• *Observe for early signs and symptoms of salicylate toxicity.* Take safety precautions if confusion, dizziness, or impaired vision occur. Keep the bed in a low position, change the patient's position slowly, and supervise ambulation. Expect to reduce the salicylate dosage.

• Observe for these signs of bleeding if the patient receives concurrent anticoagulant therapy: gingival bleeding, black or tarry stools, blood in the urine, petechiae, bruises, or prolonged bleeding from a cut. Report these signs to the physician.

• Notify the physician of any other adverse reactions or evidence of salicylate toxicity.

• Document the patient's fluid intake and output if nausea, vomiting, diarrhea, or excessive diaphoresis occurs.

• Encourage the nauseated patient to take 1 to 2 ounces of an iced beverage every hour to combat dehydration.

• Keep the patient cool and dry; prevent shivering if diaphoresis occurs.

• Weigh the patient daily. Notify the physician if the patient loses more than 2 pounds within 24 hours or exhibits signs of dehydration.

• *Encourage the patient to report hearing changes because bilateral hearing loss of 30 to 40 decibels can occur with prolonged use of a salicylate.* Reassure the patient that hearing usually returns to normal within 2 weeks after discontinuation of salicylate therapy.

• Monitor for tinnitus in the arthritic patient who is receiving high-dosage salicylate therapy. If tinnitus occurs, notify the physician and expect a small dosage reduction.

• Monitor an elderly patient or one with tinnitus for other signs of salicylate toxicity, such as nausea, vomiting, diarrhea, thrush, impaired vision, and hyperventilation. Such a patient may not notice tinnitus until it is severe.

• Monitor the patient for pain relief during salicylate therapy. If pain relief does not occur, obtain a prescription for a different analgesic. Be aware that concomitant use of certain drugs, such as corticosteroids and antacids, may decrease the analgesic effect of salicylates.

Patient teaching

• Teach the patient and family the name, dose, frequency, action, and adverse effects of the prescribed salicylate.

• Discourage the use of salicylates—even "children's aspirin"—in a patient under age 18.

• Advise an aspirin-sensitive patient to read labels carefully on OTC drugs because many contain aspirin or another salicylate.

• Teach the patient to recognize such signs as gingival bleeding, prolonged bleeding from a cut, black or tarry stools, dark urine (which may indicate blood in the urine), petechiae, and bruises. Advise the patient to report any of these signs to the physician immediately.

• Inform the patient to keep the salicylate in a cool, dry place because exposure to heat and moisture will weaken its potency.

• Advise the patient to discard tablets with a vinegarlike odor—a sign of salicylate deterioration.

• Inform the patient that buffered aspirin contains too little antacid to reduce gastric irritation. Suggest that the patient take plain aspirin with food, milk, or 1 to 2 teaspoons of antacid to prevent GI distress more effectively at less expense. (If aspirin is taken with an antacid, the patient may require an increased aspirin dosage.)

• Advise the patient taking sodium salicylate tablets not to crush or chew them or take them within 1 hour of ingesting milk or antacids, which may disrupt the enteric coating.

• Advise the patient taking diflunisal tablets not to crush or chew them. Expect to administer a decreased diflunisal dosage to a patient with renal failure.

• Encourage the patient to use the salicylate as prescribed. Because many salicylates have been available for years and can be purchased OTC, some patients question their therapeutic effectiveness.

• Inform the patient that concurrent use of alcohol and a salicylate increases the risk of bleeding.

• Tell the diabetic patient who must test urine for glucose to use products other than Clinitest or Tes-Tape and to be alert for signs of hypoglycemia.

• Caution the pregnant patient not to take salicylates during the last trimester.

• Advise the asthmatic patient with nasal polyps to avoid using salicylates when self-medicating for minor aches and pains because these drugs may induce an acute asthma attack.

• Instruct the patient to notify the physician of any adverse reactions to the salicylate.

Evaluation

The following examples represent appropriate evaluation statements for a patient receiving a salicylate.

• The patient has no conditions that contraindicate salicylate therapy.

• The patient exhibits no signs of complications in the preexisting condition linked to the prescribed salicylate.

• The patient demonstrates no adverse reactions to the prescribed salicylate.

• The patient remains hydrated during salicylate therapy.

• The patient reports no hearing problems during salicylate therapy.

• The patient reports pain relief during salicylate therapy.

• The patient and family express an accurate understanding of the points taughts about the prescribed salicylate.

• The patient correctly identifies signs of bleeding and describes what to do if they occur.

PARA-AMINOPHENOL DERIVATIVES

Although this subclass contains two substances—phenacetin and acetaminophen—only acetaminophen is available in the United States. Phenacetin was removed from all preparations in the United States because it was associated with anemia, acidosis, kidney damage, and methemoglobinemia. Acetaminophen, an analgesic and antipyretic, appears in many products to relieve pain, colds, and influenza. It has no anti-inflammatory properties. Physicians frequently choose acetaminophen over a salicylate for a patient with a history of GI bleeding, ulcers, or salicylate hypersensitivity.

PHARMACOKINETICS

Acetaminophen is absorbed rapidly and completely from the GI tract and is absorbed well from the rectal mucosa. It is distributed widely in body fluids and readily crosses the placenta. After acetaminophen undergoes metabolism by hepatic enzymes, it is excreted by the kidneys and, in small amounts, in breast milk.

The drug's plasma concentration level peaks in 10 to 60 minutes, and its duration of action ranges from 3 to 5 hours. Acetaminophen's plasma protein binding is about 25%, and its half-life ranges from 1 to 3 hours.

PHARMACODYNAMICS

Acetaminophen offers significant analgesic and antipyretic actions, but unlike salicylates, does not act on inflammation or platelet function.

Although acetaminophen's mechanism of analgesic action is not understood fully, the drug may act centrally by inhibiting prostaglandin synthesis and peripherally in some unknown way. The drug's antipyretic effect results from its direct action on the heat-regulating center in the hypothalamus.

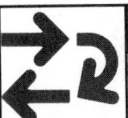

DRUG INTERACTIONS
Para-aminophenol derivatives

When acetaminophen is given with certain drugs, its absorption may decrease. This interaction requires the nurse to time the doses properly. Other interactions require different nursing interventions.

DRUG	INTERACTING DRUGS	POSSIBLE EFFECTS	NURSING IMPLICATIONS
acetaminophen	alcohol (chronic use)	Increases risk of hepato-toxicity	• Inform a patient with known or suspected chronic alcoholism of the increased risk of liver damage. Because acetaminophen is available over the counter, patient teaching is the only way to prevent this problem.
	charcoal	Reduces GI absorption of acetaminophen	• Administer the charcoal and acetaminophen doses several hours apart unless charcoal is being administered for acetaminophen over-dose.
	cholestyramine, colestipol	Reduce GI absorption of acetaminophen	• Administer acetaminophen 1 hour before or 6 hours after cholestyramine or colestipol administration.

PHARMACOTHERAPEUTICS

Acetaminophen offers an alternative to patients who cannot tolerate aspirin and who do not need an analgesic with anti-inflammatory properties. An OTC drug, acetaminophen reduces fever and relieves headache, muscle ache, and pain in general but cannot relieve intense or visceral pain. It is the drug of choice to treat fever and flulike symptoms in children.

A patient with osteoarthritis may benefit from acetaminophen because this common form of arthritis does not result from an inflammatory process. Some physicians consider acetaminophen the drug of choice for osteoarthritis.

Besides its presence in many OTC preparations, acetaminophen is included in several combination prescription drugs, such as oxycodone hydrochloride and some codeine compounds.

acetaminophen (Datril, Panadol, Tylenol). This drug commonly is administered to relieve headache, alleviate mild to moderate pain, and reduce fever. It is available in regular tablets, chewable tablets, caplets, elixirs, solutions, and rectal suppositories.
Usual adult dosage: for headache, mild to moderate pain, fever, or osteoarthritis, 325 to 650 mg P.O. or rectally every 3 to 4 hours p.r.n., not to exceed 4 grams daily.
Usual pediatric dosage: for headache, mild to moderate pain, or fever, 5 to 10 mg/kg P.O. every 4 to 6 hours.

Drug interactions
Few significant interactions occur between acetaminophen and other drugs. (For more information, see *Drug interactions: Para-aminophenol derivatives*.) Acetaminophen may increase slightly the effects of oral anticoagulants. Antacids, anticholinergics, and narcotics may reduce acetaminophen's absorption by slowing intestinal motility; however, these interactions are not clinically significant.

ADVERSE DRUG REACTIONS

Most patients tolerate acetaminophen well. Unlike the salicylates, acetaminophen rarely causes gastric irritation or hemorrhagic tendencies.

Similar to an overdose, chronic use of high doses of acetaminophen can cause hypoglycemia, methemoglobinemia, leukopenia, kidney damage, renal failure, hepatotoxicity leading to coagulation defects, cyanosis, and vascular collapse. (For detailed information, see *Detection and treatment of acetaminophen-induced hepatotoxicity*, page 334.)

Hypersensitivity reactions to acetaminophen usually take the form of skin rashes but rarely may include fever and angioedema. Such reactions are much less common with acetaminophen than with aspirin.

NURSING PROCESS APPLICATION

The following information assists the nurse in caring for a patient who is receiving acetaminophen.

Detection and treatment of acetaminophen-induced hepatotoxicity

Ingestion of 10 grams or more of acetaminophen may cause a severe adverse reaction: hepatotoxicity. Although hepatotoxicity signs and symptoms appear within 24 hours, they mimic common illnesses in many cases and permit the real problem to go undetected. Specific clinical and laboratory signs may not appear for 48 to 72 hours.

DETECTION
The nurse can detect hepatotoxicity by monitoring the patient for the following signs and symptoms of acetaminophen overdose:

1 to 24 hours after ingestion
- nausea
- vomiting
- diaphoresis
- malaise
- pallor

24 to 48 hours after ingestion
- decreased urine output
- abdominal pain in the right upper quadrant

2 to 6 days after ingestion
- bruises, petechiae, and bleeding caused by coagulation defects
- jaundice
- hypoglycemia
- renal failure
- encephalopathy
- cardiomyopathy
- elevated bilirubin and liver enzymes
- prolonged prothrombin and partial thromboplastin times.

TREATMENT
A patient with signs and symptoms of acetaminophen-induced hepatotoxicity requires hospitalization for close monitoring and prompt treatment. To treat acetaminophen overdose and prevent hepatic injury, the nurse can expect to perform gastric lavage immediately or induce emesis with ipecac syrup, followed by the oral administration of activated charcoal. Then the nurse should obtain blood for liver function tests and blood acetaminophen concentrations. (Blood should not be obtained for acetaminophen concentrations until at least 4 hours after ingestion.) If less than 24 hours have elapsed since ingestion, the nurse can expect to administer oral acetylcysteine (Mucomyst), an antidote that crosses liver cell membranes and inactivates acetaminophen metabolites. Because its odor and taste are unpleasant, acetylcysteine should be chilled and added to cola or to orange or grapefruit juice before administration.

Assessment

- Review the patient's history for conditions that contraindicate the use of acetaminophen, such as known hypersensitivity to the drug, or contraindicate repeated administration, such as anemia or cardiac, pulmonary, renal, or hepatic disease.
- Review the patient's history for conditions that require cautious use of acetaminophen, such as asthma.
- Assess the patient who receives long-term high doses of acetaminophen for adverse reactions, such as hypoglycemia, renal failure, hepatotoxicity, coagulation defects, cyanosis, or vascular collapse.
- Review the patient's medication history to identify use of drugs that may interact with acetaminophen, such as alcohol, charcoal, cholestyramine, or colestipol.
- Assess the effectiveness of acetaminophen.
- Evaluate the patient's and family's knowledge about acetaminophen.

Nursing diagnoses

The following examples represent appropriate nursing diagnoses for a patient receiving acetaminophen.
- Potential for injury related to a preexisting condition that contraindicates the use of acetaminophen
- Potential for injury related to a preexisting condition that requires cautious use of acetaminophen
- Potential for injury related to adverse drug reactions
- Pain related to ineffectiveness of acetaminophen
- Knowledge deficit related to acetaminophen

Planning and implementation

- Do not administer acetaminophen to a patient with a condition that contraindicates its use.
- Administer acetaminophen cautiously to a patient at risk because of a preexisting condition.
- Obtain a baseline liver function test before beginning acetaminophen therapy and monitor liver function test results periodically during therapy, as prescribed.
- Monitor the patient for adverse reactions throughout acetaminophen therapy.
- Obtain blood glucose levels frequently for a diabetic patient to identify hypoglycemia, particularly if the patient must take sustained high doses of acetaminophen.
- Document the patient's fluid intake and output and daily weight to help detect renal failure during long-term, high-dose acetaminophen therapy.
- Monitor the patient's vital signs at least every 8 hours. Decreased blood pressure and increased pulse rate and respirations may be early signs of impending vascular collapse.
- Observe for signs of bleeding and monitor coagulation studies for a patient receiving long-term, high-dose acetaminophen therapy.
- *Withhold acetaminophen and notify the physician if the patient develops a rash, unexplained fever, or angioedema.* Also notify the physician of any other adverse reactions.
- Monitor the patient for pain relief after administering acetaminophen. If pain does not subside, obtain a prescription for a different analgesic.

Patient teaching

• Teach the patient and family the name, dose, frequency, action, and adverse effects of acetaminophen.

• Inform the patient that high doses or unsupervised long-term use of this drug can cause liver damage and that excessive alcohol ingestion may increase this risk.

• Teach the patient that acetaminophen is safe and effective only when used as directed on the label. Because this drug is readily available OTC and is advertised widely, many patients assume that it is nontoxic. This assumption can lead to accidental overdose when a patient attempts to relieve severe or persistent headache, fever, or pain.

• Advise the asthmatic or hypersensitive patient to read all drug labels carefully. Acetaminophen is an ingredient in many OTC drugs with brand names that do not signal its presence.

• Explain that if fever or pain lasts more than 3 days, the patient should obtain medical advice.

• Teach the patient to store the drug in a light-resistant container, because transfer to a clear glass or plastic container eventually may affect the drug's potency.

• Advise the diabetic patient on long-term, high-dose acetaminophen therapy to monitor blood glucose levels at least daily for hypoglycemia.

• Instruct the patient to notify the physician if adverse drug reactions occur.

Evaluation

The following examples represent appropriate evaluation statements for a patient receiving acetaminophen.

• The patient has no conditions that contraindicate acetaminophen therapy.

• The patient exhibits no signs of complications in the preexisting condition linked to acetaminophen.

• The patient demonstrates no adverse reactions to acetaminophen.

• The patient reports pain relief.

• The patient and family express an accurate understanding of the points taught about acetaminophen.

• The patient stores acetaminophen in a white plastic container away from light.

NONSTEROIDAL ANTI-INFLAMMATORY DRUGS

With chemical structures that differ from those of corticosteroids, NSAIDs have anti-inflammatory, analgesic, and antipyretic properties, although they are seldom prescribed for fever. Their anti-inflammatory action equals that of aspirin.

The NSAIDs are derived from many different chemical sources. Fenoprofen calcium, flurbiprofen, ibuprofen, ketoprofen, naproxen, and naproxen sodium are propionic acid derivatives (fenamates). Meclofenamate and mefenamic acid are anthranilic acid derivatives. Phenylbutazone is a pyrazolon derivative. Piroxicam is an oxicam derivative. Indomethacin and ketorolac tromethamine are indoleacetic acid derivatives. Tolmetin sodium is a pyrrole acetic acid derivative. Sulindac is an indeneacetic acid derivative. Diclofenac is a phenylacetic acid derivative.

NSAIDs can relieve mild to moderate pain from dental extractions and such conditions as soft-tissue athletic injuries and dysmenorrhea. They also can relieve the pain and inflammation of arthritis and related conditions.

PHARMACOKINETICS

All NSAIDs, except ketorolac tromethamine, are absorbed in the GI tract and, for the most part, metabolized in the liver and excreted primarily by the kidneys. They differ widely, however, in their onset of action, duration of action, and half-life.

Absorption, distribution, metabolism, excretion

After oral administration, all NSAIDs, except ketorolac, are absorbed rapidly in the GI tract. (The presence of food in the stomach can delay absorption significantly but will not affect the total amount of drug absorbed.) Ketorolac is absorbed rapidly from muscle tissue. NSAIDs are distributed widely in the body. Most are metabolized in the liver and excreted primarily in the urine. Sulindac must be metabolized to a clinically active metabolite to be effective.

Onset, peak, duration

Onset of action varies considerably among the NSAIDs, although their analgesic effects always precede their antirheumatic effects—which may take 1 to 3 weeks to appear. Naproxen sodium and ketorolac, the fastest-acting NSAIDs, relieve pain effectively in 1 hour. Indomethacin and similar drugs reach peak plasma concentrations in 1 to 2 hours if the stomach is empty. Their duration of action varies widely, from 2 to 85 hours, affecting the dosage frequency. Their plasma protein binding, which ranges from 90% to 99%, may contribute to potential drug interactions. Ketorolac has a half-life of 5 hours. Phenylbutazone has the longest half-life—78 to 85 hours—and a long duration. Naproxen has a relatively long half-life (10 to 20 hours) and duration of action, allowing twice-a-day administration. Piroxicam's half-life is 50 hours, which allows once-a-day administration; sulindac's is 7.8 hours, which allows twice-a-day administration.

PHARMACODYNAMICS

Unlike the corticosteroids, the NSAIDs do not reduce inflammation by stimulating the pituitary-adrenal system. Instead they decrease inflammation and pain by inhibiting prostaglandin activity.

Mechanism of action

Researchers believe the NSAIDs inhibit prostaglandin synthetase, retard polymorphonuclear leukocyte motility, and affect the release and activity of lysosomal enzymes. Their ability to decrease prostaglandin concentrations in peripheral tissues may account for their anti-inflammatory effects. Fenamates may act in another way because studies have shown that they compete with prostaglandins at receptor-binding sites.

PHARMACOTHERAPEUTICS

NSAIDs are used primarily to decrease inflammation and secondarily to relieve pain. Although the NSAIDs share similar indications and mechanisms of action, individual responses vary greatly: A patient may respond poorly to one drug and very well to another. Therefore, the choice of an NSAID must be made empirically. Usually, a patient receives an NSAID for a trial period of 2 to 4 weeks. If this NSAID does not produce a therapeutic response, it usually is discontinued and replaced with a second drug for another trial period. This procedure may be repeated until relief is obtained.

Indications for NSAIDs include ankylosing spondylitis; moderate to severe rheumatoid arthritis; osteoarthritis in the hip, shoulder, or other large joints; osteoarthritis accompanied by inflammation; and acute gouty arthritis. The nurse may see these drugs prescribed interchangeably. For example, tolmetin is the only NSAID specifically indicated for juvenile arthritis, although naproxen, indomethacin, and ibuprofen are effective and are used in many cases. Because of their toxicity, indomethacin and phenylbutazone should be used only after other drugs have proven ineffective.

diclofenac (Voltaren). This phenylacetic acid derivative is used to relieve acute or chronic pain from rheumatoid arthritis, osteoarthritis, and ankylosing spondylitis.
Usual adult dosage: for rheumatoid arthritis, 150 to 200 mg P.O. daily in two to four divided doses; for osteoarthritis, 100 to 150 mg P.O. daily in two or three divided doses; for ankylosing spondylitis, 100 to 125 mg P.O. daily in 25 mg doses q.i.d. with an additional 25 mg at bedtime, as needed.

fenoprofen calcium (Nalfon). Fenoprofen, a propionic acid derivative, is used primarily for symptomatic relief of acute

and chronic osteoarthritis and rheumatoid arthritis; it also may be used to relieve mild to moderate pain.
Usual adult dosage: for osteoarthritis and rheumatoid arthritis, 300 to 600 mg P.O. t.i.d. or q.i.d. up to a maximum of 3,200 mg/day; for mild to moderate pain, 200 mg P.O. every 4 to 6 hours.

flurbiprofen (Ansaid). This propionic acid derivative is used for acute or long-term symptomatic treatment of rheumatoid arthritis and osteoarthritis.
Usual adult dosage: for rheumatoid arthritis and osteoarthritis, 200 to 300 mg P.O. daily in two to four divided doses. The largest recommended single dose in a multiple-dose regimen is 100 mg.

ibuprofen (Advil, Motrin, Nuprin). The only OTC NSAID, ibuprofen is used to relieve the signs and symptoms of osteoarthritis and rheumatoid arthritis, to relieve mild to moderate pain, and to treat dysmenorrhea. It is available in 200-mg tablets. Higher dosage forms require a prescription.
Usual adult dosage: for mild to moderate pain, 200 to 400 mg P.O. every 4 to 6 hours; for dysmenorrhea, 400 mg P.O. every 4 hours, p.r.n., given as soon as pain begins; for arthritis, 400 to 800 mg P.O. t.i.d. or q.i.d. A patient with rheumatoid arthritis usually requires a higher dosage than a patient with osteoarthritis.

indomethacin (Indocin). This NSAID, an indoleacetic acid derivative, usually is reserved for adults with rheumatoid arthritis or osteoarthritis who do not respond to salicylates or other treatments. It controls the pain and inflammation associated with the active stages of moderate to severe rheumatoid arthritis; with acute flare-ups of chronic rheumatoid arthritis; and with ankylosing spondylitis, bursitis, and acute gouty arthritis. For oral administration, indomethacin is available in 25- and 50-mg capsules and in a sustained-release 75-mg capsule. For rectal administration, it is available in 50-mg suppositories.
Usual adult dosage: for moderate to severe rheumatoid arthritis or osteoarthritis, acute flare-ups of chronic rheumatoid arthritis, and ankylosing spondylitis, 25 to 50 mg P.O. t.i.d. of regular indomethacin with food, increased to a maximum of 200 mg/day. For night pain and morning stiffness associated with osteoarthritis, 100 mg of the total daily dosage may be given P.O. or rectally at bedtime. For bursitis or tendinitis, 75 to 150 mg P.O. may be given in three or four divided doses. For gouty arthritis, 50 mg P.O. t.i.d. may be given. The 75-mg sustained-release preparation can be given for all indications except gouty arthritis.

ketoprofen (Orudis). This NSAID, a propionic acid derivative, is used to treat the signs and symptoms of osteoarthritis and rheumatoid arthritis.

Usual adult dosage: for osteoarthritis and rheumatoid arthritis, 75 mg P.O. t.i.d. or 50 mg P.O. q.i.d. initially, given with milk or food, increased to a maximum of 300 mg/day, if needed.

ketorolac tromethamine (Toradol). Ketorolac, an indoleacetic acid derivative, is the only injected NSAID for short-term pain management.
Usual adult dosage: 30 or 60 mg I.M. initially, followed by half the loading dose (15 or 30 mg) every 6 hours as needed for pain control. The recommended maximum daily dosage is 150 mg for the first day, then 120 mg daily. Lower dosages are recommended for patients who weigh less than 50 kg (110 lb), are over age 65, or have decreased renal function.

meclofenamate (Meclomen). Meclofenamate, an anthranilic acid derivative, can relieve the signs and symptoms of acute and chronic rheumatoid arthritis and osteoarthritis. However, it should not be used as a first-line drug because it can cause severe adverse reactions.
Usual adult dosage: for acute and chronic rheumatoid arthritis and osteoarthritis, 200 to 400 mg P.O. daily, given in three or four equal doses of 50 to 100 mg each. Therapy should begin at a low dose and increase based on the patient's response.

mefenamic acid (Ponstel). This NSAID, an anthranilic acid derivative, may be prescribed for short-term management of dysmenorrhea or acute moderate pain of less than 1 week's duration such as that associated with insertion of an intrauterine device or postoperative pain.
Usual adult dosage: for dysmenorrhea and acute moderate pain of short duration, 500 mg P.O. initially, followed by 250 mg every 6 hours p.r.n., for no more than 7 days.

naproxen (Naprosyn). Naproxen, a propionic acid derivative, is used to relieve mild to moderate pain and to treat osteoarthritis, rheumatoid arthritis, ankylosing spondylitis, tendinitis, bursitis, acute gout, and dysmenorrhea. Its 13-hour half-life allows twice-a-day administration.
Usual adult dosage: for acute tendinitis and bursitis, dysmenorrhea, and mild to moderate pain, 500 mg P.O. initially, followed by 250 mg P.O. every 6 to 8 hours p.r.n.; for osteoarthritis, rheumatoid arthritis, and ankylosing spondylitis, 250 to 375 mg P.O. in the morning and evening separated by about 12 hours, increased to a maximum of 1,000 mg/day, if needed. A patient who awakens with morning pain should take unequal doses, with the larger one in the evening.

naproxen sodium (Anaprox). Naproxen sodium is a propionic acid derivative used for the same indications as naproxen, with one major advantage: more rapid absorption.
Usual adult dosage: for dysmenorrhea, acute tendinitis and bursitis, and mild to moderate pain, two 275-mg tablets P.O. initially, followed by 275 mg every 6 to 8 hours p.r.n., up to a maximum of 1,375 mg/day; for rheumatoid arthritis, osteoarthritis, and ankylosing spondylitis, two 275-mg tablets P.O. initially, morning and evening, or 275 mg in the morning and 550 mg in the evening, increased to a maximum of 1,100 mg/day.

phenylbutazone (Butazolidin). Phenylbutazone, a pyrazolon derivative, is reserved for use when other NSAIDs have proven unsatisfactory because it can cause severe adverse reactions. It is used mainly for symptomatic relief of severe rheumatoid arthritis, ankylosing spondylitis, and osteoarthritis of the hips and knees.
Usual adult dosage: for rheumatoid arthritis, ankylosing spondylitis, and osteoarthritis, 300 to 600 mg P.O. daily given in three or four divided doses until condition improves, then decreased to the minimum dosage needed to produce a satisfactory response—usually 100 to 200 mg, but less than 400 mg/day. If a favorable response does not occur within 7 days of therapy, the patient should receive a different drug.

piroxicam (Feldene). Piroxicam, an oxicam derivative, is indicated for symptomatic relief of acute and chronic osteoarthritis and rheumatoid arthritis. Piroxicam has a long half-life (50 hours), making a single daily dose possible. However, it does not produce maximum effects for about 2 weeks.
Usual adult dosage: for acute and chronic osteoarthritis and rheumatoid arthritis, 20 mg P.O. once daily or 10 mg every 12 hours.

sulindac (Clinoril). Sulindac, an indeneacetic acid derivative, is indicated for acute or long-term use. Sulindac provides symptomatic relief of osteoarthritis, rheumatoid arthritis, ankylosing spondylitis, bursitis, and acute gouty arthritis.
Usual adult dosage: for osteoarthritis, rheumatoid arthritis, ankylosing spondylitis, bursitis, and acute gouty arthritis, 150 to 200 mg P.O. b.i.d. with food, not to exceed 400 mg/day.

tolmetin sodium (Tolectin). Tolmetin, a pyrrole acetic acid derivative, is used to relieve the signs and symptoms of osteoarthritis, rheumatoid arthritis, and juvenile rheumatoid arthritis.
Usual adult dosage: for osteoarthritis and rheumatoid arthritis, initially 400 mg P.O. t.i.d., including one dose upon arising and one at bedtime; increase as needed up to a maximum of 1,800 mg/day in four divided doses.

Usual pediatric dosage: for juvenile rheumatoid arthritis, initially 20 mg/kg/day for children over age 2; then 15 to 30 mg/kg/day.

Drug interactions

A wide variety of drugs can interact with NSAIDs, especially with indomethacin, mefenamic acid, phenylbutazone, piroxicam, and sulindac. Because they are highly protein bound, NSAIDs are likely to interact with other protein-bound drugs, such as oral anticoagulants. They also may interfere with antihypertensive drugs, such as beta-adrenergic blockers and thiazides, decreasing their antihypertensive effects. This interaction is not documented fully, however, and may not occur with all NSAIDs. (For further information about significant interactions, see *Drug interactions: Nonsteroidal anti-inflammatory drugs*.)

ADVERSE DRUG REACTIONS

All NSAIDs produce similar adverse reactions that rarely require discontinuation of therapy. In general, the NSAIDs are better tolerated than salicylates or corticosteroids.

GI tract disturbances are the most common adverse reactions to NSAIDs. Other reactions affect the central nervous system (CNS), the renal system, and the eyes. Adverse CNS and renal reactions are particularly common in geriatric patients. (For detailed information, see *Nonsteroidal anti-inflammatory drugs: Summary of adverse reactions*, page 341.)

Phenylbutazone has an unusually high incidence of adverse reactions, commonly causing nausea, vomiting, abdominal discomfort, dyspepsia, diarrhea, and skin rashes. Other reactions include gastric ulceration and hemorrhage, vertigo, insomnia, and the combination of sodium and water retention, increased plasma volume, and decreased urine volume—which may lead to peripheral edema, acute pulmonary edema, and cardiac symptoms. Phenylbutazone sometimes causes thrombocytopenia, aplastic anemia, granulocytopenia, and other blood dyscrasias. At highest risk for adverse reactions are elderly patients, especially women, and patients receiving high doses or long-term therapy. Adverse reactions limit phenylbutazone's use to short-term therapy—1 week or less for a patient over age 60.

NSAIDs can cause hypersensitivity reactions, evidenced by skin rashes, urticaria, angioedema, hypotension, dyspnea, and an asthmalike syndrome. With phenylbutazone, hypersensitivity reactions include pruritus, fever, arthralgia, polyarthritis, Stevens-Johnson syndrome, and anaphylaxis. With piroxicam, skin rashes and photosensitivity occur more commonly than with the other NSAIDs. With any NSAID, therapy should be discontinued at the first sign of a hypersensitivity reaction.

NURSING PROCESS APPLICATION

The following information assists the nurse in caring for a patient who is receiving an NSAID.

Assessment
• Review the patient's history for conditions that contraindicate the use of an NSAID, such as GI lesions or known hypersensitivity to the drug.
• Review the patient's history for conditions that require cautious use of an NSAID, such as cardiac decompensation, hypertension, fluid retention, or coagulation defects.
• Assess the patient for adverse reactions to the NSAID, such as GI distress or CNS, renal, or ophthalmic dysfunction.
• Review the patient's medication history to identify use of drugs that may interact with an NSAID, such as corticosteroids, captopril, loop diuretics, oral anticoagulants, or lithium.
• Assess the effectiveness of the prescribed NSAID.
• Assess the patient for signs of fluid volume excess, such as unexplained weight gain, peripheral edema, crackles on lung auscultation, and shortness of breath.
• Monitor the patient for signs of gastric ulceration, such as gastric discomfort, nausea, vomiting, and black, tarry stools.
• Evaluate the patient's and family's knowledge about the prescribed NSAID.

Nursing diagnoses
The following examples represent appropriate nursing diagnoses for a patient receiving an NSAID.
• Potential for injury related to a preexisting condition that contraindicates the use of an NSAID
• Potential for injury related to a preexisting condition that requires cautious use of an NSAID
• Potential for injury related to adverse drug reactions
• Pain related to ineffectiveness of an NSAID
• Fluid volume excess related to sodium and water retention caused by an NSAID
• Knowledge deficit related to the prescribed NSAID

Planning and implementation
• Do not administer an NSAID to a patient with a condition that contraindicates its use. Keep in mind that a patient with aspirin hypersensitivity also may be hypersensitive to NSAIDs.
• Administer an NSAID cautiously to a patient at risk because of a preexisting condition.
• Observe the patient for adverse reactions during NSAID therapy.
• Monitor the results of the patient's liver and kidney function tests, hemoglobin counts, and ophthalmic examinations during long-term NSAID therapy.

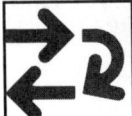

DRUG INTERACTIONS

Nonsteroidal anti-inflammatory drugs

Drug interactions with the nonsteroidal anti-inflammatory drugs (NSAIDs) are common and can be severe. They typically require dosage adjustment, drug discontinuation, or drug substitution.

DRUG	INTERACTING DRUGS	POSSIBLE EFFECTS	NURSING IMPLICATIONS
diclofenac, fenopro-fen, flurbiprofen, ibuprofen, indo-methacin, ketopro-fen, meclofena-mate, mefenamic acid, naproxen, na-proxen sodium, pir-oxicam, tolmetin	corticosteroids	Increase the ulcerogenic effect	• Monitor the patient for epigastric and abdom-inal pain, abdominal cramps—especially 1 to 2 hours after eating, and signs of gastrointesti-nal bleeding, such as bloody or tarry stools.
	captopril, enalapril, lisino-pril	Decrease the antihyper-tensive effect of these agents	• Monitor the patient for increased blood pres-sure. • Expect to adjust the antihypertensive agent dosage as prescribed.
	loop diuretics	Decrease the antihyper-tensive and diuretic effects of loop diuretics	• Monitor the patient's blood pressure and fluid intake and output to detect decreased effects. • Anticipate substitution of a different NSAID, such as sulindac, for indomethacin.
	oral anticoagulants	Increase the anticoagulant effect	• Monitor the patient for gingival bleeding, black or tarry stools, blood in the urine, pete-chiae, bruises, or prolonged bleeding from a cut. • Monitor the patient's prothrombin time and partial thromboplastin time, and adjust the an-ticoagulant dosage as prescribed.
	lithium	Increase lithium concen-tration	• Monitor the patient's lithium concentration.
	beta-adrenergic blockers	May inhibit synthesis of renal prostaglandins, pos-sibly causing hypertension	• Monitor the patient's blood pressure fre-quently.
	methotrexate	May increase methotrex-ate toxicity by decreasing tubular secretion	• Avoid concurrent use. If this is unavoidable, monitor for increased adverse reactions to methotrexate, such as fatigue, bone marrow suppression, and stomatitis.
	zidovudine	Inhibit zidovudine metabo-lism, which may lead to toxicity	• Avoid concomitant use of these agents.
sulindac	oral anticoagulants	Increases hypoprothrom-binemic activity, causing bleeding	• Avoid concurrent use. If this is unavoidable, monitor the patient for signs of bleeding, such as blood-tinged urine, black or tarry stools, or easy bruising. • Expect to substitute ibuprofen, naproxen, or tolmetin for sulindac as prescribed; these drugs are less likely to interact with anticoagu-lants.
phenylbutazone	oral anticoagulants	Inhibits anticoagulant me-tabolism	• Expect to substitute ibuprofen, naproxen, or tolmetin for phenylbutazone as prescribed; these drugs are less likely to interact with an-ticoagulants.

(continued)

DRUG INTERACTIONS

Nonsteroidal anti-inflammatory drugs (continued)

DRUG	INTERACTING DRUGS	POSSIBLE EFFECTS	NURSING IMPLICATIONS
phenylbutazone (continued)	oral hypoglycemics (sulfonylureas)	Increases the hypoglycemic effect	• Observe the patient for signs and symptoms of hypoglycemia, such as tremors, light-headedness, and diaphoresis. • Expect to adjust the oral hypoglycemic dosage as ordered.
	methotrexate	Displaces methotrexate from plasma protein-binding sites, causing methotrexate toxicity	• Avoid concurrent use. If this is unavoidable, monitor the patient for signs and symptoms of methotrexate toxicity, such as thrombocytopenia, ulcerated stomatitis, enteritis, and alopecia.
	phenytoin	Extends the half-life of phenytoin, leading to toxicity	• Monitor the patient for signs and symptoms of phenytoin toxicity, such as confusion, hypotension, and arrhythmias.
indomethacin	nonamphetamine anorexigenic agents	May cause hypertension	• Avoid concurrent use. • Monitor the patient's blood pressure when concurrent use is unavoidable.
ketorolac	salicylates	Increase plasma concentrations of unbound ketorolac	• Avoid concurrent use.

• Administer phenylbutazone cautiously because it commonly causes adverse reactions, particularly in elderly patients—especially women—and patients receiving high-dose or long-term therapy.

• Do not administer phenylbutazone to a patient over age 60 for more than 1 week because of the high incidence of adverse reactions.

• Discontinue NSAID therapy and notify the physician at the first sign of a hypersensitivity reaction to the drug.

• Withhold meclofenamate or mefenamic acid and consult the physician if diarrhea occurs.

• Monitor the patient's vision. If an alteration or problem develops, expect to discontinue the NSAID until an ophthalmic examination rules out drug therapy as the cause.

• Monitor the patient's blood pressure frequently during concurrent therapy with an NSAID and captopril, enalapril, lisinopril, or a loop diuretic. Expect to adjust the antihypertensive dosage or substitute sulindac for the interacting NSAID.

• *Administer the prescribed NSAID with food or milk to decrease GI irritation, unless directed otherwise.*

• Question any prescription for medications that contain alcohol, aspirin, or other drugs that may cause GI irritation and bleeding during concomitant NSAID therapy.

• Monitor the patient with a history of peptic ulcer for ulcer reactivation and gastric bleeding during NSAID therapy.

• Monitor the patient for signs of GI irritation, such as nausea, vomiting, abdominal pain, or black, tarry stools.

Notify the physician immediately if the patient displays any signs of GI irritation.

• *Monitor the patient for bleeding during concurrent therapy with an NSAID and an oral anticoagulant.* Expect to monitor the patient's prothrombin time and partial thromboplastin time and adjust the anticoagulant dosage, as prescribed. Also expect to substitute ibuprofen, naproxen, or tolmetin for the prescribed NSAID; these drugs are less likely to interact with anticoagulants.

• Obtain regular blood glucose measurements during concurrent therapy with phenylbutazone and an oral hypoglycemic in a diabetic patient. Also monitor the diabetic patient for signs and symptoms of hypoglycemia, such as tremors, light-headedness, and diaphoresis. Expect to adjust the oral hypoglycemic dosage, if hypoglycemia occurs.

• Monitor the patient for signs of phenytoin toxicity, such as confusion, hypotension, and arrhythmias, during concurrent therapy with phenylbutazone and phenytoin.

• Do not administer indomethacin and nonamphetamine anorexigenic agents concurrently because hypertension may occur.

• Do not administer salicylates and ketorolac concurrently; salicylates increase unbound ketorolac plasma concentrations.

• Monitor the patient for signs of infection. Keep in mind that indomethacin may mask some signs.

• Notify the physician of any adverse reactions to the prescribed NSAID.

Nonsteroidal anti-inflammatory drugs: Summary of adverse reactions

NSAIDs can produce numerous adverse reactions in four major body systems: the central nervous system, the gastrointestinal system (most common site), the renal system, and the eyes.

Central nervous system

- Drowsiness
- Headache
- Dizziness
- Confusion
- Tinnitus
- Vertigo
- Depression

Gastrointestinal system

- Abdominal pain
- Bleeding
- Anemia
- Diarrhea
- Nausea
- Ulcerations
- Perforation
- Hepatotoxicity

Renal system

- Cystitis
- Hematuria
- Kidney necrosis
- Nephrotic syndrome (rare)

Eyes

- Blurred vision
- Decreased acuity
- Corneal deposits

- Evaluate the degree of pain relief during NSAID therapy. Note that 2 to 4 weeks may elapse before the prescribed NSAID provides relief.
- Expect to administer a different NSAID if pain is not relieved within 4 weeks of NSAID therapy.
- Expect to administer a larger dose of naproxen in the evening to a patient who awakens with morning pain.
- Monitor the patient's vital signs at least every 8 hours. Note any significant increase in blood pressure, which may indicate increased plasma volume.
- Weigh the patient daily and report any sudden, unexplained weight gain. Be aware that fluid retention and edema may occur during NSAID therapy.

- Monitor the patient regularly for signs of fluid retention, such as ankle edema, crackles, and shortness of breath.
- Limit the patient's sodium and fluid intake, unless prescribed by the physician.
- Document the patient's intake and output daily to detect a fluid imbalance.
- *Alert the physician if the patient displays signs of fluid retention.*

Patient teaching
- Teach the patient and family the name, dose, frequency, action, and adverse effects of the prescribed NSAID.
- Stress the importance of returning for periodic blood tests as prescribed.
- Advise the patient receiving indomethacin to avoid driving or operating machinery until the drug's effects are evaluated, because drowsiness and dizziness commonly occur at the beginning of therapy.
- Advise the patient that some NSAIDs, such as naproxen, ibuprofen, and fenoprofen, may take several weeks to produce the maximum therapeutic effect.
- Instruct the patient to take the prescribed NSAID with milk or food to decrease gastric irritation, unless directed otherwise.
- Advise the patient with aspirin hypersensitivity to avoid ibuprofen.
- Instruct the patient who self-medicates with an NSAID to discontinue the drug and consult a physician if pain lasts longer than 72 hours.
- Advise the patient to avoid alcohol, aspirin, and other drugs that may cause GI irritation and bleeding.
- Instruct the patient taking an oral anticoagulant along with the prescribed NSAID to be alert for bleeding tendencies, such as easy bruising, nosebleeds, and black, tarry stools. Also advise the patient to institute bleeding precautions, such as using an electric razor when shaving and avoiding forceful nose blowing and bumps and trauma to the skin.
- Teach the diabetic patient taking an oral hypoglycemic and phenylbutazone to monitor blood glucose levels frequently and watch for signs of hypoglycemia, such as tremors, light-headedness, and diaphoresis.
- Instruct the patient taking indomethacin to avoid nonamphetamine anorexigenic agents to prevent hypertension.
- Advise the patient taking ketorolac not to take a salicylate concurrently.
- Teach the patient to avoid high-sodium foods and to limit fluid, unless directed by the physician, because fluid retention can occur.
- Instruct the patient to notify the physician if adverse drug reactions occur.

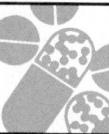

SELECTED MAJOR DRUGS

Nonnarcotic analgesics, antipyretic agents, and NSAIDs

The following chart features the most frequently used salicylates, para-aminophenol derivatives, and nonsteroidal anti-inflammatory drugs.

DRUG	MAJOR INDICATIONS	USUAL ADULT DOSAGES	CONTRAINDICATIONS AND PRECAUTIONS
Salicylates			
aspirin	Mild to moderate pain, fever	325 to 650 mg P.O. every 3 to 4 hours p.r.n.	• Know that aspirin is contraindicated in a child or adolescent with varicella or influenza (unless directed by a physician), in a woman during the last 3 months of pregnancy, and in any patient with a bleeding disorder or known hypersensitivity to the drug, or one in whom acute asthmatic attacks, urticaria, or rhinitis are precipitated by aspirin.
	Dysmenorrhea	650 mg P.O. every 4 to 6 hours, beginning 1 or 2 days before the onset of menses and continuing until the second or third day of menses	• Administer with extreme caution to a patient receiving an anticoagulant or to one with advanced chronic renal insufficiency, hypoprothrombinemia, vitamin K deficiency, thrombocytopenia, thrombotic thrombocytopenic purpura, or severe hepatic impairment.
	Rheumatic fever	975 to 1,300 mg P.O. four to six times daily until fever and inflammation subside	• Administer highly buffered aspirin solutions with extreme caution to a patient with congestive heart failure or other condition in which a high sodium intake would be harmful.
	Rheumatoid arthritis	3.6 to 5.4 grams P.O. daily in divided doses	• Administer with caution to a lactating patient or one with gastrointestinal (GI) lesions or impaired renal function.
	Transient ischemic attacks	325 mg P.O. q.i.d. or 650 mg P.O. b.i.d.	
diflunisal	Mild to moderate musculoskeletal pain	500 to 1,000 mg P.O. initially, followed by 250 to 500 mg every 8 to 12 hours; not to exceed 1,500 mg/day	• Know that diflunisal is contraindicated in a patient with known hypersensitivity to the drug or diflunisal-induced acute asthmatic attacks, urticaria, or rhinitis.
	Osteoarthritis	500 to 1,000 mg P.O. daily in two divided doses	• Administer with caution to a pregnant or lactating patient or one with compromised cardiac function; hypertension or other condition that predisposes to fluid retention; reduced renal reserve, or upper or lower GI disease.
Para-aminophenol derivatives			
acetaminophen	Headache, mild to moderate pain, fever, osteoarthritis	325 to 650 mg P.O. or rectally every 3 to 4 hours p.r.n., not to exceed 4 grams/day	• Know that acetaminophen is contraindicated in a patient with known hypersensitivity to the drug and that repeated acetaminophen administration is contraindicated in a patient with anemia or cardiac, pulmonary, renal, or hepatic disease. • Administer with caution to an asthmatic patient.
Nonsteroidal anti-inflammatory drugs (NSAIDs)			
diclofenac	Ankylosing spondylitis	100 to 125 mg P.O. daily in 25-mg doses q.i.d. with an additional 25 mg h.s. as needed	• Know that diclofenac is contraindicated in a lactating patient or one with known hypersensitivity to the drug, hepatic porphyria, or aspirin- or NSAID-induced asthma, urticaria, or other allergic-type reactions.
	Osteoarthritis	100 to 150 mg P.O. daily in two or three divided doses	• Administer with caution to a patient with cardiac decompensation, hypertension, or other condition that predisposes to fluid retention.
	Rheumatoid arthritis	150 to 200 mg P.O. daily in two to four divided doses	

SELECTED MAJOR DRUGS

Nonnarcotic analgesics, antipyretic agents, and NSAIDs *(continued)*

DRUG	MAJOR INDICATIONS	USUAL ADULT DOSAGES	CONTRAINDICATIONS AND PRECAUTIONS
Nonsteroidal anti-inflammatory drugs (NSAIDs) *(continued)*			
ibuprofen	Mild to moderate pain	200 to 400 mg P.O. every 4 to 6 hours	• Know that ibuprofen is contraindicated in a pregnant or lactating patient or one with known hypersensitivity to the drug or with nasal polyps, angioedema, and bronchospastic reactivity to aspirin or other NSAIDs. • Administer with caution to a patient who is receiving anticoagulant therapy or one with cardiac decompensation, hypertension, or intrinsic coagulation defects.
	Dysmenorrhea	400 mg P.O. every 4 hours p.r.n. as soon as pain begins	
	Osteoarthritis, rheumatoid arthritis	400 to 800 mg P.O. t.i.d. or q.i.d.	
indomethacin	Rheumatoid arthritis, osteoarthritis, ankylosing spondylitis	25 to 50 mg P.O. t.i.d., increased to a maximum of 200 mg/day	• Know that indomethacin is contraindicated in a pregnant or lactating patient or one with known hypersensitivity to the drug, active or recurrent GI lesions, or aspirin- or NSAID-induced acute asthmatic attacks, urticaria, or rhinitis. Suppositories are contraindicated in a patient with proctitis or recent rectal bleeding. • Administer with caution to a patient with reduced renal reserve, cardiac dysfunction, hypertension, or a condition that predisposes the patient to fluid retention or coagulation defects.
	Acute gouty arthritis	50 mg P.O. t.i.d.	
	Bursitis and tendinitis	75 to 150 mg P.O. in three or four divided doses	
naproxen	Osteoarthritis, rheumatoid arthritis, ankylosing spondylitis	250 to 375 mg P.O. morning and evening, increased to a maximum of 1,000 mg/day, if needed	• Know that naproxen is contraindicated in a lactating patient or pregnant patient in the third trimester or one with known hypersensitivity to the drug or in whom aspirin, other NSAIDs, or analgesic drugs induce asthma, rhinitis, and nasal polyps. • Administer with caution to a patient with significantly impaired renal function, chronic alcoholic liver disease, other forms of cirrhosis, fluid retention, hypertension, or heart failure.
	Tendinitis, bursitis, dysmenorrhea, mild to moderate pain	500 mg P.O. initially, then 250 mg every 6 to 8 hours p.r.n.	
tolmetin	Osteoarthritis, rheumatoid arthritis	400 mg P.O. t.i.d. initially, including a dose upon arising and at bedtime, increased as needed to a maximum of 1,800 mg/day given in four divided doses	• Know that tolmetin is contraindicated in a lactating patient or one with a known hypersensitivity to the drug or aspirin- or NSAID-induced asthma, rhinitis, urticaria, or other symptoms of allergic or anaphylactic reactions. • Administer with caution to a pregnant patient or one with compromised cardiac function, hypertension, or other condition predisposing the patient to fluid retention.

Evaluation

The following examples represent appropriate evaluation statements for a patient receiving an NSAID.

• The patient has no conditions that contraindicate NSAID therapy.

• The patient exhibits no signs of complications in the preexisting condition linked to the prescribed NSAID.

• The patient demonstrates no adverse reactions to the prescribed NSAID.

• The patient reports pain relief.

• The patient maintains normal fluid balance.

• The patient experiences no GI irritation.

• The patient and family express an accurate understanding of the points taught about the prescribed NSAID.

• The patient schedules follow-up visits for blood tests.

URINARY TRACT ANALGESIC

Phenazopyridine hydrochloride (Azodine, Pyridium), an azo dye, produces a local analgesic effect on the urinary tract, usually within 24 to 48 hours after therapy begins. It relieves the pain, burning, urgency, and frequency that occur with urinary tract infections.

The usual dosage ranges from 100 to 200 mg P.O. t.i.d. after meals for 2 days only. After oral administration, phenazopyridine is 35% metabolized in the liver, with the remainder excreted unchanged in the urine. The drug colors the urine orange or red, which permanently may stain fabrics it contacts. A yellow tinge to the skin or sclera may indicate drug accumulation and the need to discontinue phenazopyridine therapy. Because this drug can alter the results of some urine glucose tests, such as Tes-Tape and Clinistix, the nurse should use Clinitest for a more accurate urine glucose determination.

CHAPTER SUMMARY

Chapter 21 covered nonnarcotic analgesic, antipyretic, and nonsteroidal anti-inflammatory drugs. Here are the highlights of the chapter.
• The three subclasses of nonnarcotic analgesics include salicylates, para-aminophenol derivatives, and NSAIDs.
• Aspirin, a salicylate and the most widely used analgesic, is available alone or with other ingredients in OTC remedies for pain, colds, and influenza.
• Salicylates produce analgesia by inhibiting prostaglandin synthesis. They also can act as antipyretics. The anti-inflammatory action of salicylates is understood poorly. Salicylates are used to treat headache, neuralgia, myalgia, dysmenorrhea, and arthritis. The major adverse reactions involve the GI system. Other reactions may include respiratory alkalosis and metabolic acidosis, hearing problems, salicylate toxicity, and hypersensitivity reactions.
• Acetaminophen is currently the only para-aminophenol derivative used in the United States. Its effects are antipyretic and analgesic but not anti-inflammatory. A common ingredient in many OTC analgesics, acetaminophen causes few adverse reactions when taken in recommended doses.
• The NSAID category includes many drugs that may act by inhibiting prostaglandin synthetase, retarding polymorphonuclear leukocyte motility, and affecting the release and activity of lysosomal enzymes. These drugs are used primarily to relieve the symptoms of arthritis and related conditions as well as mild to moderate pain in such conditions as dysmenorrhea. Most NSAIDs are highly protein bound, accounting for many of their drug interactions. They commonly cause adverse reactions in the GI system. Other adverse reactions affect the CNS, renal system, and eyes.
• The only urinary tract analgesic, phenazopyridine, acts locally. It is used to relieve the pain, burning, and urinary urgency and frequency associated with urinary tract infections.
• When caring for a patient receiving a nonnarcotic analgesic, antipyretic, or NSAID, the nurse should monitor the patient closely for adverse reactions. Because many of these drugs are used commonly and are available without a prescription, the nurse also should teach the patient about the drug and its effects whenever possible.

STUDY QUESTIONS

See Appendix 1 for answers.

1. Arlene Hummel, age 30, takes 4 grams of aspirin a day for rheumatoid arthritis. The nurse might expect to see which common adverse drug reactions in Ms. Hummel?
(a) increased rate and depth of respirations
(b) dizziness and vision changes
(c) nausea, vomiting, and GI distress
(d) tinnitus and hearing loss

2. The nurse assesses Ms. Hummel's drug history closely for anticoagulant use. A drug interaction between aspirin and an anticoagulant may cause which problem?
(a) bleeding
(b) clot formation
(c) aspirin inactivation
(d) salicylate toxicity

3. Eleanor Dean brings her daughter Katie, age 8, to the pediatrician after 2 days of fever, aches, and flulike symptoms. The nurse tells Ms. Dean *not* to give Katie aspirin to treat the flulike symptoms. Why?
(a) Salicylates may cause Reye's syndrome.
(b) Salicylates are not as effective in children as in adults.
(c) Salicylates are too irritating to a child's GI mucosa.
(d) Salicylates may lead to excessive bleeding.

4. Ruth Brown, age 72, takes acetaminophen, as prescribed, for arthritis. Which of the following types of arthritis responds best to acetaminophen?
(a) gouty arthritis
(b) rheumatoid arthritis
(c) juvenile arthritis
(d) osteoarthritis

5. Long-term use of high doses of acetaminophen can increase Ms. Brown's risk for which of the following adverse reactions?
(a) hypertension
(b) hepatotoxicity
(c) peptic ulcer
(d) hemorrhage

6. Frank Harmon, age 60, has gouty arthritis. His physician prescribes the NSAID indomethacin (Indocin) 50 mg P.O. t.i.d. The nurse reviews Mr. Harmon's drug history carefully to anticipate drug interactions. Which statement may account for the high potential for drug interactions with NSAID use?
(a) Most NSAIDs are highly protein bound.
(b) Most NSAIDs circulate unbound.
(c) Most NSAIDs have a long half-life.
(d) Most NSAIDs have a short half-life.

7. During NSAID therapy, the nurse monitors Mr. Harmon for adverse drug reactions. Which of the following adverse reactions most commonly occurs with NSAID use?
(a) pruritus
(b) hypotension
(c) dyspnea
(d) GI disturbances

8. What should the nurse teach Mr. Harmon about his medication schedule to minimize adverse reactions?
(a) Take the drug on an empty stomach.
(b) Take the drug with milk or food.
(c) Take the drug before meals.
(d) Take the drug with water.

SELECTED REFERENCES

AHFS drug information 90. (1990). Bethesda, MD: American Society of Hospital Pharmacists.

Burton, S. (1989). Drugs to treat rheumatic disorders. *Nursing,* 3(34), 27-29.

Drug facts and comparisons. (1991). St. Louis: Facts and Comparisons Division, J.B. Lippincott.

Hansten, P., and Horn, J. (1989). *Drug interactions: Clinical significance of drug-drug interactions* (6th ed.). Philadelphia: Lea & Febiger.

Hord, A., et al. (1989). Postoperative pain: A review of management methods. *Hospital Formulary,* 24(1), 28-40.

Moulds, R. (1988). Analgesic guidelines, part 1. *Australian Nurses Journal,* 18(4), 28-29.

Pain control in the hospital, part 1. (1989). *Harvard Medical School Health Letter,* 14(8), 1-4.

Stephany, T. (1989). Oral medication for pain relief. *Home Health Care Nurse,* 7(2), 44-45.

USPDI. (1991). *Drug information for the health care professional* (Vol. I, 11th ed.). Rockville, MD: United States Pharmacopeial Convention.

NARCOTIC AGONIST AND ANTAGONIST AGENTS

OBJECTIVES

After reading and studying this chapter, the student should be able to:

1. Discuss how narcotic agonists act to relieve pain.
2. Distinguish between narcotic agonists and narcotic antagonists.
3. Discuss the clinical indications for the various narcotic agents.
4. Describe the common adverse reactions to narcotic drugs.
5. Describe the pain-relieving action of the mixed narcotic agonist-antagonists.
6. Describe the action of naloxone hydrochloride and its use in treating narcotic overdose.
7. Describe how to apply the nursing process when caring for a patient who is receiving narcotic agonists, mixed narcotic agonist-antagonists, or narcotic antagonists.

INTRODUCTION

Narcotic agonists (analgesics), which include opium derivatives and synthetic drugs with similar pharmacologic properties, can relieve or decrease pain without causing loss of consciousness. Most narcotic agonists also possess antitussive and antidiarrheal actions. Morphine sulfate is the narcotic agonist against which all others are compared.

Narcotic agonists can alter the patient's perception of pain and emotional response to it. These drugs alter pain perception by (1) inhibiting the transmission of pain impulses in sensory pathways in the spinal cord, (2) reducing cortical responses to painful stimuli in the brain stem, thalamus, and limbic system, and (3) altering behavioral responses to pain as they are mediated in the frontal lobe. As a result of this threefold action, pain decreases, and the patient may become less tense and more tranquil. The patient even may become euphoric, probably as a result of the narcotic's effects on the limbic system. This euphoria,

however, may lead to repeated drug use, even in the absence of pain, possibly resulting in drug dependence. (For more information about drug dependence, see the appendix on Substance Abuse.)

With continuous use, the patient may develop tolerance to many of the effects of narcotic agonists. Tolerance can occur even in the absence of psychological or physical dependence and usually is manifested by a decreased duration of analgesia. Thus the patient requires larger doses to produce the analgesic effects. Another kind of tolerance occurs with continuous narcotic use, as the body adapts to such physiologic effects as respiratory depression and sedation. Tolerance to the smooth muscle effects of narcotic drugs develop more slowly, causing constipation with regular use of narcotic agonists.

Narcotic agonists act as analgesics to relieve pain by attaching to opiate receptor sites. Narcotic antagonists block the effects of narcotic agonists, including pain relief and adverse drug reactions, most notably respiratory depression. Some narcotic analgesics, called mixed narcotic agonist-antagonists, display agonist and antagonist properties: The agonist component relieves pain; the antagonist component decreases the risk of toxicity and drug dependence. These mixed narcotic agonist-antagonists are less likely than pure agonists to result in respiratory depression and drug abuse.

Researchers have isolated endogenous morphinelike compounds, endorphins and enkephalins, from subcortical brain areas. Beta-endorphin, found in largest amounts in the pituitary gland, is the principal endorphin and one of the most potent. Methionine enkephalin and leucine enkephalin are the principal enkephalins. Occurring primarily in the basal ganglia, brain stem, and spinal cord, enkephalins seem to modify pain impulse transmission in the same way as the narcotic agonists, by attaching to opiate receptor sites. Whether released in the presence of a narcotic agonist or in response to other stimuli, enkephalins

SELECTED NURSING DIAGNOSES

Narcotic agonist and antagonist agents

The following nursing diagnoses address representative problems and etiologies that a nurse may encounter when caring for a patient who is receiving a narcotic agonist or antagonist agent. Some of these nursing diagnoses contain generalized etiologies, which the nurse must individualize based on the patient's needs. (For some common nursing diagnoses and related interventions for each drug class, see the "Nursing Process Application" sections of this chapter.)

- Altered thought processes related to the adverse central nervous system (CNS) effects of a narcotic agonist or antagonist agent
- Altered urinary elimination related to naltrexone-induced urinary frequency
- Anxiety related to the adverse effects of naltrexone
- Body image disturbance related to the adverse dermatologic effects of naltrexone
- Constipation related to the anticholinergic effects of a narcotic agonist or antagonist agent
- Diarrhea related to the adverse gastrointestinal effects of naltrexone
- Fluid volume excess related to naltrexone-induced edema
- Impaired adjustment related to dependence on a narcotic agonist
- Ineffective breathing pattern related to the adverse respiratory effects of a narcotic agonist
- Knowledge deficit related to the prescribed narcotic agonist or antagonist agent
- Pain related to ineffectiveness of a narcotic agonist or antagonist agent

- Potential fluid volume deficit related to nausea or vomiting caused by a narcotic agonist or antagonist agent
- Potential for injury related to a preexisting condition that contraindicates the use of a narcotic agonist or antagonist agent
- Potential for injury related to a preexisting condition that requires cautious use of a narcotic agonist or antagonist agent
- Potential for injury related to adverse drug reactions
- Potential for trauma related to narcotic agonist-induced seizures
- Sensory-perceptual alterations (visual or auditory) related to the adverse CNS effects of a mixed narcotic agonist-antagonist or naltrexone
- Sexual dysfunction related to the genitourinary effects of naltrexone
- Sleep pattern disturbance related to insomnia caused by a mixed narcotic agonist-antagonist
- Urinary retention related to the adverse genitourinary effects of a narcotic agonist or antagonist agent

also may decrease the patient's perception of pain and emotional response to it.

Neither endorphins nor enkephalins are absorbed orally, and both are degraded rapidly by enzymes. As a result, they are of little clinical value at present. However, endorphins and enkephalins may facilitate placebo-induced analgesia, which occurs in about one-third of patients with anginal, arthritic, dental, or postoperative pain who receive placebos. The narcotic antagonist naloxone blocks attachment of narcotic analgesics to opiate receptor sites and placebo-induced analgesia—leading researchers to conclude that endorphins and enkephalins act via receptor combination.

This chapter discusses the narcotic agonist, mixed narcotic agonist-antagonist, and narcotic antagonist agents. For a summary of representative drugs, see *Selected major drugs: Narcotic agonist and antagonist agents,* pages 362 and 363. For a listing of applicable nursing diagnoses that the nurse may formulate when caring for a patient receiving these agents, see *Selected nursing diagnoses: Narcotic agonist and antagonist agents.* For detailed information on applying the nursing process, see Chapter 6, The Nursing Process and Drug Therapy.

NARCOTIC AGONISTS

The term *narcotic* refers to any analgesic derived from active opium poppy alkaloids as well as to compounds chemically similar to the alkaloids. Because the Harrison Narcotic Act of 1914 established a legal definition of narcotics based on their habit-forming nature, however, the term *narcotic* commonly is used inaccurately to refer to any drug that can produce dependence or is restricted by the Controlled Substance Act.

This chapter presents the following narcotic agonists: codeine, fentanyl citrate, hydrocodone bitartrate and acetaminophen, hydrocodone and phenyltoloxamine, hydromorphone hydrochloride, levorphanol tartrate, meperidine hydrochloride, methadone hydrochloride, morphine sulfate (including morphine sulfate sustained-release tablets and intensified oral solution), oxycodone hydrochloride (alone or with acetaminophen or aspirin), oxymorphone hydrochloride, propoxyphene hydrochloride, and propoxyphene napsylate.

Morphine sulfate serves as a standard against which the effectiveness and adverse reactions of other narcotic drugs as well as nonnarcotic analgesics are measured.

Pharmacokinetics of selected narcotic agonists

All narcotic agonists have a rapid onset of action when administered I.V. and reach peak concentration levels in 20 to 40 minutes; duration of action varies primarily according to the drug administered. This chart outlines the pharmacokinetics of narcotic agonists administered I.M.

DRUG	ONSET OF ACTION (MINUTES)	PEAK CONCENTRATION LEVEL (MINUTES)	DURATION OF ACTION (HOURS)
codeine	15 to 30	60 to 90	4 to 6
morphine	5 to 20	30 to 90	4 to 6
hydromorphone hydrochloride	15 to 30	30 to 90	3 to 5
levorphanol tartrate	15 to 45	60 to 90	6 to 8
meperidine	15 to 30	30 to 60	2 to 4
methadone hydrochloride	10 to 15	60 to 120	4 to 6; 12 to 15 with long-term therapy
oxymorphone hydrochloride	5 to 10	30 to 60	3 to 6

PHARMACOKINETICS

Narcotic agonists are absorbed well from the gastrointestinal (GI) tract and the rectal mucosa and are distributed to most body tissues. Parenteral administration produces the most rapid onset of action. The duration of action varies, depending on the drug and the route of administration used.

Absorption, distribution, metabolism, excretion

The narcotic agonists are administered by the oral, intravenous (I.V.), subcutaneous (S.C.), intramuscular (I.M.), epidural, intrathecal, sublingual, and rectal routes. Opium derivatives are absorbed well from the nasal mucosa and lung surface; oral doses are absorbed readily from the GI tract. I.V. administration produces the most rapid (almost immediate) and reliable analgesic effects. Absorption from S.C. and I.M. injections depends on the lipid solubility of the narcotic drug administered and the amount of the patient's fatty tissue. The S.C. and I.M. routes may result in delayed absorption and peak concentration of the drug, especially in patients with impaired tissue perfusion.

In the past, parenteral routes were preferred for morphine administration, because the first-pass effect causes rapid metabolism and inactivation of oral doses. However, a concentrated oral solution and a sustained-release tablet now are available for use in cancer patients and others with severe chronic pain. Although these relatively new dosage forms do not avoid the first-pass effect, they enable the patient to receive morphine in smaller solution volumes or in sustained-release tablets, thereby avoiding the need for injections or I.V. lines. The oral form allows the patient and the patient's family more mobility.

Narcotic agonists are distributed widely throughout body tissues, displaying relatively low plasma protein-binding capacity (30% to 35%). The drugs are metabolized extensively in the liver, and the metabolites are excreted by the kidneys. A minor amount, 7% to 10% of the dose, is excreted in feces via the biliary tract.

Meperidine is metabolized to normeperidine, a toxic metabolite with a longer half-life than meperidine. With long-term administration or high doses of meperidine (especially by the oral route), normeperidine may accumulate and cause seizures. Normeperidine accumulation also occurs commonly in patients with renal failure or sickle-cell disease. Normeperidine also is excreted by the kidneys.

Onset, peak, duration

After parenteral administration of a narcotic agonist, onset of action usually occurs within 30 minutes. Duration of action varies, depending on the drug administered. The peak drug concentration is reached within 20 to 40 minutes after I.V. administration and 60 to 120 minutes after S.C. or I.M. injection, depending on the drug administered. Narcotic agonist half-life varies, depending on the drug administered and the route of administration. (For a comparison of the drugs in this class, see *Pharmacokinetics of selected narcotic agonists.*)

PHARMACODYNAMICS

Narcotic agonists act primarily at opiate receptor sites, binding to the receptors centrally and peripherally and activating the endogenous pain relief system. This receptor-site binding produces the therapeutic effects of analgesia and cough suppression along with narcotic adverse reactions, including respiratory depression and constipation.

Mechanism of action

The opiate receptors that narcotic agonists occupy in the central and peripheral nervous systems are most numerous in the hypothalamus, limbic system, midbrain, thalamus, and substantia gelatinosa of the spinal cord. In sensory neurons, pure narcotic analgesics alter the release of neurotransmitters, including acetylcholine, dopamine, norepinephrine, and substance P.

The existence of five types of opiate receptors (mu, kappa, sigma, delta, and epsilon) has been postulated but not proved; pure narcotic agonists appear to act primarily at the mu receptors. Researchers have observed that when a narcotic occupies the presumed mu, kappa, and sigma receptors, identifiable clinical effects occur. This is not the case with the delta and epsilon receptors (which may be related to enkephalins or beta-endorphin): their narcotic-related clinical effects have not been determined yet. (For information about the physiologic effects of these receptors, see *Opiate receptors and their effects.*)

The mechanism of action and therapeutic uses of the synthetic narcotic agonists are similar to those of the opium derivatives. A notable exception is the antitussive effect of the opium derivatives, which is lacking in some of the synthetic narcotic agonists.

Narcotic agonists, especially morphine, affect the smooth muscle of the GI and genitourinary tracts, causing bladder and ureter contraction and decreased intestinal peristalsis. The narcotic agonists also cause blood vessel dilation, especially in the face, head, and neck. Narcotic agonists also depress the cough center in the brain, thereby producing antitussive effects and causing constriction of the bronchial musculature. Any of these effects can become adverse reactions. (For an illustration of the various sites and effects of narcotic agonists, see *Narcotic sites of action,* page 350.)

PHARMACOTHERAPEUTICS

Narcotic agonists are used to relieve severe pain in acute, chronic, and terminal illnesses and to reduce preanesthesia patient anxiety. They also have antidiarrheal and antitussive effects. Morphine reduces the dyspnea of pulmonary edema and left ventricular failure by reducing anxiety and by producing peripheral vasodilation, which decreases cardiac work load. Rarely, opium derivatives are used in obstetric

---

Opiate receptors and their effects

Narcotic agonists stimulate five types of opiate receptors: mu, kappa, sigma, delta, and epsilon. The following chart lists three receptors and the physiologic effects that can occur when a narcotic agonist binds to each. Clinical effects for delta and epsilon are unknown.

TYPE OF OPIATE RECEPTOR	CLINICAL EFFECT
mu	• Euphoria • Physical dependence • Respiratory depression • Supraspinal analgesia
kappa	• Miosis • Sedation • Spinal analgesia • Respiratory depression
sigma	• Dysphoria • Hallucinations • Respiratory stimulation • Vasomotor stimulation

---

analgesia, and only with extreme caution because these drugs cross the placenta and can compromise neonatal respirations.

An equianalgesic dose of a narcotic drug is a dose that produces the same level of analgesia as an agent and dose selected as a standard, usually 10 mg of morphine I.M. Occasionally, a patient must be changed from one narcotic drug to another (for example, when the postoperative patient is allowed to take drugs orally). When this is necessary, referring to the equianalgesic dose decreases the risk of toxicity and inadequate pain relief. (For the various narcotic agonist doses equianalgesic to 10 mg of morphine I.M., see *Narcotic agonists: Equianalgesic doses,* page 351.)

codeine. A Schedule II drug, codeine is used for relief of mild to moderate pain and as an antitussive. Codeine, which possesses good oral potency, commonly is combined with 650 mg of aspirin or acetaminophen for an additive analgesic effect. Such a combination places the medication in Schedule III because the potential for abuse is diminished. However, the combination increases the potential for adverse drug reactions and drug interactions, because aspirin and acetaminophen are potent medications. Codeine usually is not used for chronic severe pain because it exhibits an analgesic ceiling effect — as the oral or parenteral codeine dose is increased, the level of analgesia increases only slightly after a dose of 60 to 120 mg (P.O.) is reached, but adverse drug reactions (most notably GI upset and constipation) become more pronounced. As a result, the patient cannot tolerate the codeine. For cough suppression

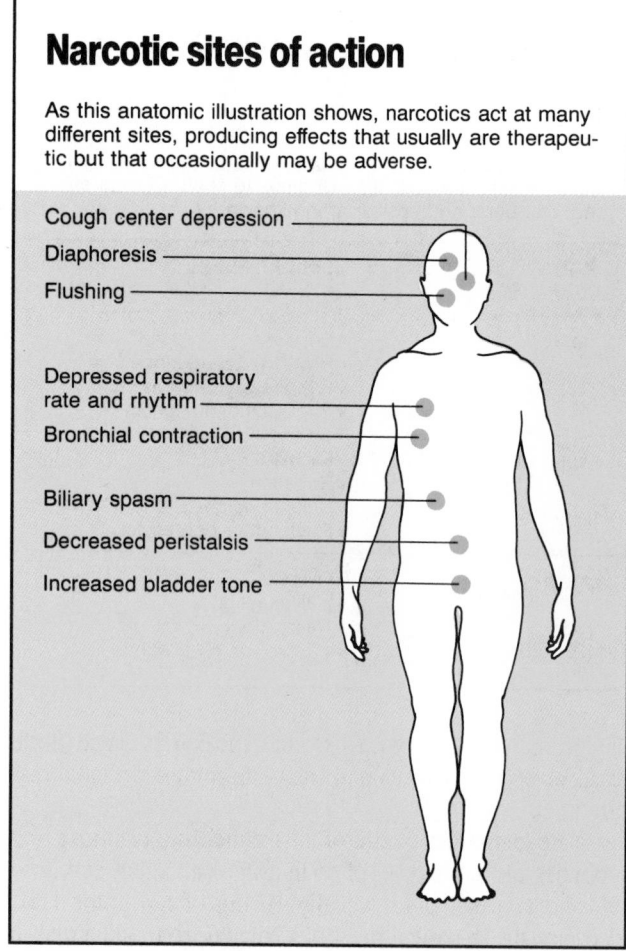

Narcotic sites of action

As this anatomic illustration shows, narcotics act at many different sites, producing effects that usually are therapeutic but that occasionally may be adverse.

Cough center depression

Diaphoresis

Flushing

Depressed respiratory rate and rhythm

Bronchial contraction

Biliary spasm

Decreased peristalsis

Increased bladder tone

in adult patients, the low potential for abuse, good oral potency, and relatively low dose required to suppress the cough make codeine a preferred agent.
Usual adult dosage: for analgesia, 15 to 60 mg P.O., S.C., or I.M. every 4 to 6 hours; for cough suppression, 10 to 20 mg P.O. every 4 to 6 hours, usually in liquid form.

fentanyl citrate (Sublimaze). A Schedule II drug, fentanyl is a potent synthetic narcotic agonist available for parenteral use. Fentanyl is administered I.V. before, during, and immediately after surgery. The drug also is used as an anesthetic agent with oxygen in selected high-risk surgical patients and as an obstetric analgesic—a use not approved by the Food and Drug Administration (FDA). Fentanyl can be given by continuous infusion and via the epidural route.
Usual adult dosage: except for anesthesia maintenance during surgery, 0.05 to 0.1 mg I.M. or I.V.; for anesthesia maintenance during surgery, 0.025 to 0.05 mg I.V.; 100 mcg (0.1 mg) is equianalgesic to 10 mg of morphine I.M. or 75 mg of meperidine I.M.

hydrocodone bitartrate and acetaminophen (Vicodin). This combination product is used to relieve mild to moderate pain. Each tablet contains 5 mg hydrocodone and 500 mg acetaminophen.
Usual adult dosage: one to two tablets every 4 to 6 hours for pain relief.

hydrocodone and phenyltoloxamine (Tussionex). A long-acting antitussive combination, hydrocodone and phenyltoloxamine is available in capsule, liquid, and tablet form. The usual dose contains 5 mg of hydrocodone and 10 mg of phenyltoloxamine. Children over age 5 can receive the drug at 12-hour intervals; however, the antitussive agent of choice for children is dextromethorphan. Because hydrocodone and phenyltoloxamine has a high potential for abuse, it should be prescribed only when dextromethorphan or codeine is undesirable or ineffective.
Usual adult dosage: one capsule or tablet or 1 teaspoonful (5 ml) every 8 to 12 hours.

hydromorphone hydrochloride (Dilaudid). A Schedule II drug, hydromorphone is a potent synthetic narcotic agonist that is related to morphine. Used to relieve moderate to severe pain, hydromorphone can be administered orally, rectally, or parenterally. Continuous I.V. infusions of hydromorphone are used to relieve severe pain.

Unlike codeine, hydromorphone does not exhibit a ceiling effect: As the dose of hydromorphone increases, so does the level of analgesia. Therefore, hydromorphone is useful in treating chronic severe pain. Hydromorphone is highly soluble in water, and a highly concentrated solution for parenteral use is available for patients requiring high doses. Hydromorphone powder also can be used to make highly concentrated parenteral solutions, if needed.
Usual adult dosage: for parenteral use, a starting dose of 1 to 2 mg S.C., I.V., or I.M. every 4 to 6 hours to control pain; for oral administration, a starting dose of 2 mg every 4 to 6 hours, which may be increased to 12 to 15 mg every 4 hours in patients with severe pain; for rectal administration, one 3-mg suppository every 6 to 8 hours.

levorphanol tartrate (Levo-Dromoran). A Schedule II drug, levorphanol is a synthetic narcotic agonist possessing good oral potency. It is used to relieve moderate or severe pain; pain from myocardial infarction (MI), severe trauma, or renal or biliary colic; postoperative pain; and intractable pain from cancer or other causes. It also is used for preoperative analgesia. Levorphanol is available in oral tablets and in parenteral solution.
Usual adult dosage: for relief of moderate to severe pain, 2 mg P.O. or S.C., which may be increased to 3 mg, if necessary.

Narcotic agonists: Equianalgesic doses

The so-called standard narcotic agonist dose, 10 mg of morphine sulfate I.M., is used to calculate equally effective (equianalgesic) doses of the various narcotic agonists. This method is particularly useful when a patient must be switched from one narcotic agonist to another with no change in dose effectiveness. In this chart, which lists equianalgesic doses of selected narcotic agonists, all doses are I.M. except for codeine, which is administered orally.

NARCOTIC AGONIST	EQUIANALGESIC DOSE
codeine	120 mg
morphine	10 mg
hydromorphone	1.5 mg
levorphanol	2 mg
meperidine	75 to 100 mg
methadone	8 to 10 mg
fentanyl	0.1 to 0.2 mg
oxymorphone	1.0 to 1.5 mg

meperidine hydrochloride (Demerol). A Schedule II drug, meperidine is a synthetic narcotic agonist most commonly prescribed for postoperative pain. Meperidine can be administered P.O., I.M., S.C., or I.V. It is available as a tablet, parenteral liquid, or oral syrup. Parenteral meperidine is effective for the relief of moderate to severe visceral pain, for obstetric analgesia, and as a preoperative medication.
Usual adult dosage: for moderate to severe pain, 50 to 150 mg parenterally or P.O. every 3 to 4 hours; for preoperative analgesia, 50 to 100 mg I.M. or S.C. 30 to 90 minutes before surgery; for obstetric analgesia, 50 to 100 mg I.M. or S.C. (sometimes combined with scopolamine), possibly repeated at 1- to 3-hour intervals.

methadone hydrochloride (Dolophine). A Schedule II drug, methadone is a synthetic narcotic agonist indicated for relief of severe pain, detoxification treatment of narcotic addiction, and management of narcotic dependence—although the drug produces tolerance and physical and psychological dependence. Methadone is used for analgesia in terminal illness on a scheduled basis (every 6 to 12 hours around the clock). Methadone has good oral potency; 20 mg P.O. are equianalgesic to 10 mg of morphine sulfate I.M. The drug can accumulate in patients with impaired hepatic or renal function and in elderly patients, sometimes causing respiratory depression. Methadone should be administered I.V. only with extreme caution.

Methadone is dispensed daily only by hospitals, pharmacies, FDA-approved community agencies, and designated state authorities with maintenance or detoxification programs. Detoxification programs administer smaller and smaller doses until the physical dependence is reduced and the drug can be stopped. Maintenance programs provide enough methadone to replace the amount of illegal narcotic taken. Some physicians feel that methadone maintenance therapy administered once daily allows psychosocial rehabilitation of the participant. Symptoms of anxiety or stress do not necessarily reflect withdrawal and should not form the basis for dosage increase.
Usual adult dosage: for pain relief, 2.5 to 10 mg I.M., S.C., or P.O. every 3 to 4 hours, as needed; for detoxification, 15 to 20 mg P.O. daily in liquid form initially, with additional doses if withdrawal symptoms do not subside or if symptoms recur; for stabilization after initial detoxification, 40 mg P.O. daily in a single dose or divided doses. After stabilization, maintenance dosages vary depending on the amount of narcotic taken.

morphine sulfate (Duramorph). A Schedule II drug, naturally occurring morphine is considered the best narcotic agonist for relief of severe pain. Among its many indications, morphine is used to relieve pain from surgery, MI, and terminal cancer. Morphine sulfate is available in oral tablets, solutions, rectal suppositories, sustained-release tablets, and parenteral forms. It can be administered by many routes—oral, rectal, sublingual, S.C., I.M., I.V., epidural, and intrathecal—and by implantable pumps. Because morphine does not exhibit a ceiling effect, the level of analgesia increases as the dose is increased. Morphine commonly is used as a continuous infusion in patients with severe pain.
Usual adult dosage: initially, 10 mg/70 kg of body weight when given parenterally (a 60-mg oral dose of morphine is equianalgesic to a 10-mg parenteral dose). Reportedly, some patients can tolerate doses of 8 grams or more per day.

morphine sulfate sustained-release tablets (MS Contin, Roxanol SR). These Schedule II products contain morphine sulfate in a sustained-release formula that allows morphine to be released slowly and continuously as the tablet travels through the GI tract. This helps the patient remain pain-free for a longer time (6 to 12 hours) than with rapid-release tablets, which provide pain relief for 3 to 4 hours. Morphine sulfate sustained-release tablets are indicated for prolonged relief of chronic, severe pain. They should not be administered as needed because the release of medication is slowed and the products are not indicated for mild or intermittent pain. Because dosage titration is difficult with sustained-release tablets, regular tablets or liquid should be used initially.

Usual adult dosage: variable (titrated to the patient's individual needs); a starting dose of 30 mg every 8 to 12 hours may be used when the narcotic need is not known. Some patients may need to take the drug at 8-hour intervals.

morphine sulfate intensified oral solution (Roxanol). A Schedule II drug dispensed in bottles of 30 and 120 ml containing 20 mg/ml, morphine sulfate intensified solution is used to relieve severe acute pain and chronic pain in patients unable to swallow tablets. These solutions also are indicated for patients with high narcotic requirements who cannot tolerate the large volume of solution required with regular morphine sulfate solution (5 mg/5 ml). Intensified oral solutions and sustained-release tablets usually are used for terminally ill patients who require medication on a regularly scheduled basis to achieve effective relief. Once pain is relieved, the patient may sleep for a number of hours after each dose. The nurse should be careful not to interpret this reaction as indicating a need for a dosage decrease. Such patients may be experiencing rebound sleep because the previously uncontrolled pain had deprived them of sleep. The dosage should be maintained for at least 2 days before reduction, as long as the patient's respiratory and cardiovascular status remains adequate.

Usual adult dosage: initially, 10 to 30 mg every 4 hours. However, dosage is variable, depending on patient response, and should be titrated to pain relief.

oxycodone hydrochloride (Roxicodone). A Schedule II drug, oxycodone is a semisynthetic oral narcotic analgesic structurally similar to codeine. Oxycodone is available in 5-mg tablets and in a 5 mg/5 ml suspension and is prescribed most commonly with aspirin or acetaminophen.

Usual adult dosage: for pain relief, a starting dose of 5 mg P.O. every 3 to 6 hours.

oxycodone hydrochloride and acetaminophen (Percocet, Tylox). Each Schedule II Percocet tablet contains 5 mg of oxycodone and 325 mg of acetaminophen; each Tylox capsule contains 5 mg of oxycodone and 500 mg of acetaminophen. These combination products are used to relieve moderate to moderately severe pain. Nurses should be aware of the antipyretic effect of acetaminophen when assessing the vital signs of a patient taking this combination drug.

Usual adult dosage: one tablet or capsule P.O. every 6 hours for pain relief; dosage increases for patients with severe pain are limited by the amount of acetaminophen contained in the tablets. The maximum recommended daily dosage of acetaminophen is 4 grams.

oxycodone hydrochloride and aspirin (Percodan). Each Schedule II Percodan tablet contains 4.8 mg of oxycodone and 325 mg of aspirin. Percodan is indicated for moderate to moderately severe pain. The nurse should be aware of the antipyretic effect of this combination product because it contains aspirin.

Usual adult dosage: one tablet P.O. every 6 hours for pain relief.

oxymorphone hydrochloride (Numorphan). A Schedule II drug, oxymorphone is a potent synthetic narcotic analgesic effective for moderate to severe pain. Clinical indications for oxymorphone include preoperative and obstetric analgesia and relief of pain caused by pulmonary edema or left ventricular failure. One milligram of oxymorphone administered parenterally is equianalgesic to 10 mg I.M. of morphine sulfate.

Usual adult dosage: for obstetric analgesia, 0.5 to 1 mg I.M.; for other indications, 1 to 1.5 mg S.C. or I.M. every 4 to 6 hours, 0.5 mg I.V. initially followed by cautious increases until satisfactory effects are obtained, or 5-mg rectal suppository every 4 to 6 hours.

propoxyphene hydrochloride (Darvon). A Schedule IV drug, propoxyphene is a weak synthetic narcotic agonist used to relieve mild pain. In many cases, the drug is combined with aspirin (Darvon Compound). Propoxyphene is available as 32- or 65-mg capsules. Darvon Compound contains 389 mg of aspirin and 32 mg of caffeine in addition to propoxyphene.

Usual adult dosage: one 65-mg capsule P.O. every 4 hours, as needed.

propoxyphene napsylate (Darvon-N). A Schedule IV drug, propoxyphene napsylate is a more stable salt of propoxyphene than propoxyphene hydrochloride and is available in liquid and tablet form. A 100-mg dose of the napsylate salt is equianalgesic to 65 mg of the hydrochloride, the difference being molecular weight. Darvon-N contains 100 mg of propoxyphene napsylate. Doses of 50 and 100 mg are combined with 325 and 650 mg of acetaminophen, respectively, in Darvocet-N 50 and Darvocet-N 100. Darvon-N with A.S.A. contains 100 mg of propoxyphene napsylate and 325 mg of aspirin.

Usual adult dosage: one tablet or capsule every 4 hours, as needed.

Drug interactions

The use of narcotic agonists with any other drugs known to decrease respiration, including alcohol, sedatives, hypnotics, and anesthetics, increases the patient's risk of severe respiratory depression. Concomitant therapy with tricyclic antidepressants, phenothiazines, or anticholinergics may

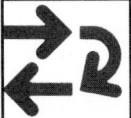

DRUG INTERACTIONS
Narcotic agonists

Drug interactions involving the narcotic agonists commonly lead to increased (and possibly lethal) respiratory and central nervous system (CNS) depression.

DRUG	INTERACTING DRUGS	POSSIBLE EFFECTS	NURSING IMPLICATIONS
codeine, fentanyl, hydromorphone, levorphanol, meperidine, methadone, morphine, oxymorphone	alcohol	Increases CNS depression, especially respiratory depression	• Advise the patient to avoid concomitant alcohol ingestion. Teach the patient to read labels on all over-the-counter cough syrups and cold remedies for possible alcohol content. • Monitor the patient's respirations every 30 minutes for 2 hours if alcohol ingestion occurs, and report any change to the physician.
	barbiturates	Cause additive CNS effects; increase sedation	• Administer doses at least 2 hours apart, as prescribed, to avoid extreme patient drowsiness or deep sleep. • Monitor the patient for signs of respiratory depression every 20 to 30 minutes for 2 hours after concomitant administration.
	cimetidine	May inhibit narcotic metabolism, leading to increased respiratory and CNS depression	• Monitor the patient for increased sedation. • Monitor the patient's respiratory rate every 20 to 30 minutes for 2 hours after concomitant administration.
meperidine	monoamine oxidase (MAO) inhibitors	Increase effects of meperidine; cause rigidity, hypotension, excitation	• Avoid administering meperidine to a patient within 10 days after administration of an MAO inhibitor.
methadone	hydantoins	Induce methadone metabolism	• Monitor the patient for signs of withdrawal. • Expect to increase the methadone dosage.

cause severe constipation and urine retention. (For detailed information, see *Drug interactions: Narcotic agonists*.)

ADVERSE DRUG REACTIONS

Narcotic agonists produce numerous adverse reactions that affect most body systems. Central nervous system (CNS) reactions, the most common, usually affect the respiratory and GI tracts.

One of the most common adverse reactions to the opium derivatives is decreased rate and depth of respiration that worsens as the dosage is increased. This may cause periodic, irregular breathing or precipitate asthmatic attacks in susceptible patients. The cough-suppressant effect of narcotic agonists usually is considered therapeutic; however, as these adverse reactions indicate, it sometimes may be undesirable.

Dilation of peripheral arteries and veins from narcotic agonists leads to flushing and orthostatic hypotension; the patient may feel drowsy or light-headed, and the extremities may feel warm and heavy. (Little change in blood pressure or pulse rate occurs when the patient is recumbent.) In-

creased respirations may be from a medullary effect of the drug.

Adverse GI reactions include nausea, vomiting, biliary colic, and constipation. Nausea and vomiting are more likely to occur in ambulatory patients; however, this reaction differs with specific narcotic agonists, even in the same patient. Biliary colic is most likely to occur with morphine; meperidine is least likely to produce or exacerbate this condition. Narcotic agonists may cause constipation through sedation that reduces response to the defecation impulse, through significant reduction in peristalsis, and through increased water absorption from intestinal contents.

Some patients receiving these drugs, especially males with prostatic hypertrophy, experience urine retention. Narcotic agonists also may prolong labor and produce respiratory depression in the neonate.

Pupil constriction (miosis) also occurs with narcotic agonists and persists throughout long-term therapy.

Narcotic agonists are contraindicated in patients with head injury or increased intracranial pressure because the drugs may mask changes in level of consciousness. These changes, which may be subtle, are early signs that the patient is developing CNS problems.

The incidence and severity of adverse reactions to narcotic agonists may increase as the dosage increases. For example, euphoria and mood elevation may become heightened, and depressed respirations may become slower and more shallow. When toxic concentrations are reached, blood pressure and pulse decline, and bronchoconstriction may develop. The patient also may experience seizures. Death from narcotic overdose usually results from respiratory failure.

Health care professionals always must be alert for the development of patient tolerance to the effects of narcotic drugs. When a patient who has become tolerant to a narcotic drug suddenly stops receiving it, withdrawal symptoms may occur, including increased sensory perceptions (especially those of pain and touch), tactile hallucinations, increased GI secretions, nasopharyngeal secretions, diarrhea, dilated pupils, and photophobia.

Responses to a narcotic agonist vary from patient to patient and even in the same patient over the course of the therapy. Although pain increases the patient's tolerance to the narcotic agonist, the severity of adverse reactions usually does not increase. Patients with hypothyroidism, multiple sclerosis, or myasthenia gravis are particularly sensitive to opiates. Renal or hepatic dysfunction interferes with the elimination of these drugs, prolongs their duration of action, and may increase the risk of accumulation—and CNS stimulation and seizures—especially with meperidine and methadone. An accumulation of normeperidine may cause CNS stimulation and seizures. Infants and patients with compromised respiratory function (for example, cor pulmonale or obstructive lung disease) can be particularly sensitive to the respiratory effects of opiates. Elderly patients may have increased respiratory depression and may become restless after narcotic administration.

Meperidine frequently produces tremors, palpitations, tachycardia, and delirium.

Severe hypersensitivity reactions to narcotic agonists are rare and usually occur as urticaria or a skin rash; even I.V. administration rarely causes anaphylaxis. Some patients may experience itching or wheal formation at the injection site, but this is usually a local, histamine-mediated response.

NURSING PROCESS APPLICATION

The following information assists the nurse in caring for a patient who is receiving a narcotic agonist.

Assessment
- Review the patient's history for conditions that contraindicate the use of a narcotic agonist, such as known hypersensitivity to the drug or recent use of monoamine oxidase inhibitors.
- Review the patient's history for conditions that require cautious use of a narcotic agonist, such as head injury, increased intracranial or intraocular pressure, hepatic or renal dysfunction, or pregnancy.
- Assess the patient for adverse reactions to the prescribed narcotic agonist, such as respiratory depression, asthmatic attacks, orthostatic hypotension, nausea, vomiting, constipation, urine retention, and miosis.
- Assess the effectiveness of the narcotic agonist.
- Review the patient's medication history to identify use of drugs that may interact with the narcotic agonist.
- Observe the patient for signs of dependence on the narcotic agonist.
- Assess the patient's respiratory status at least every 4 hours.
- Assess the patient's pain level.
- Evaluate the patient's and family's knowledge about the prescribed narcotic agonist.

Nursing diagnoses
The following examples represent appropriate nursing diagnoses for a patient receiving a narcotic agonist.
- Potential for injury related to a preexisting condition that contraindicates the use of a narcotic agonist
- Potential for injury related to a preexisting condition that requires cautious use of a narcotic agonist
- Potential for injury related to adverse drug reactions
- Impaired adjustment related to dependence on a narcotic agonist
- Ineffective breathing pattern related to the adverse respiratory effects of a narcotic agonist
- Pain related to ineffectiveness of a narcotic agonist
- Knowledge deficit related to the prescribed narcotic agonist

Planning and implementation
- Do not administer a narcotic agonist to a patient with a condition that contraindicates its use.
- Administer a narcotic agonist cautiously to a patient at risk because of a preexisting condition.
- Observe the patient periodically for adverse reactions to narcotic agonists. Keep in mind that the incidence and severity of adverse reactions to narcotic agonists may increase as the dosage increases and that vomiting and orthostatic hypotension are more likely to occur in ambulatory than in recumbent patients. Also keep in mind that patients with hypothyroidism, multiple sclerosis, or myasthenia gravis are particularly sensitive to narcotic agonists.

• Obtain the patient's baseline blood pressure, pulse, and respirations before administering the initial dose of a narcotic agonist. Continue to monitor these vital signs throughout narcotic agonist therapy.

• *Note the patient's respiratory rate, depth, and rhythm before administering each narcotic agonist dose. Withhold the dose and consult the physician if the patient's respiratory rate is 8 to 10 breaths/minute or less. Keep in mind that an infant or a patient with compromised respiratory function may be particularly sensitive to the respiratory effects of a narcotic agonist.*

• Do not allow the patient to walk without assistance immediately after a dose or until the patient's response to the narcotic is determined.

• *Keep the bed rails up and place the bed in the low position for an elderly patient who may become restless.*

• Measure and record the patient's fluid intake and output to assess for urine retention.

• Monitor the patient for decreased peristalsis, abdominal distention, and constipation. If constipation develops, consult with the physician about a prescription for a laxative or stool softener.

• Encourage regular deep breathing, coughing, and turning in a postoperative patient.

• Notify the physician of any adverse reactions to the narcotic agonist.

• Observe for signs of patient tolerance to the effects of the narcotic agonist, such as inadequate pain relief and requests for increased drug administration.

• *Do not discontinue the narcotic agonist suddenly in a drug-dependent patient.* This may cause withdrawal symptoms, such as increased sensory perceptions, tactile hallucinations, increased GI or nasopharyngeal secretions, diarrhea, dilated pupils, and photophobia.

• Encourage the patient to seek help in combating drug dependence.

• Assess the patient's pain before and after each dose of narcotic agonist; determine and record the onset, duration, location, intensity, and quality of the pain as well as the degree of pain relief obtained after each dose. Keep in mind that narcotic agonists are most effective when administered before pain becomes severe.

• *Do not crush or break morphine sulfate sustained-release tablets; this will negate the sustained-release effect.*

• Discuss with the physician the addition of a nonnarcotic analgesic agent to improve pain control, if needed.

Patient teaching

• Teach the patient and family the name, dose, frequency, action, and adverse effects of the prescribed narcotic agonist.

• Instruct the patient not to smoke or walk immediately after receiving a narcotic agonist because of its sedative effects. Also caution the patient against operating a motor vehicle or performing any other activity that requires alertness.

• Advise the patient to avoid alcohol or other CNS depressants, which may cause excessive sedation and respiratory depression.

• Instruct the patient to lie down if drowsiness, nausea, or light-headedness occurs.

• Teach the patient ways to prevent constipation, such as increasing fluid and fiber intake.

• Advise the patient to note any change in voiding patterns because urine retention may occur.

• Caution the patient to take the narcotic agonist exactly as prescribed because misuse can lead to dependence.

• Teach the patient pain management techniques, such as guided imagery, distraction, and meditation, to minimize the need for prolonged use or large doses of the narcotic agonist.

• Instruct the patient to take the prescribed narcotic agonist before the pain becomes severe for greatest effectiveness.

• Instruct the patient taking morphine sulfate sustained-release tablets not to crush or break them because this will negate the sustained-release effect.

• Instruct the patient and family to notify the physician if adverse reactions occur.

• Provide written instructions about the prescribed narcotic agonist.

Evaluation

The following examples represent appropriate evaluation statements for a patient receiving a narcotic agonist.

• The patient has no conditions that contraindicate narcotic agonist therapy.

• The patient exhibits no signs of complications in the preexisting condition linked to the prescribed narcotic agonist.

• The patient demonstrates no adverse reactions to the prescribed narcotic agonist.

• The patient shows no signs of narcotic agonist dependence.

• The patient's respirations are 15 breaths/minute with normal depth and regularity.

• The patient reports decreased pain during narcotic agonist therapy.

• The patient and family express an accurate understanding of the points taught about the prescribed narcotic agonist.

• The patient increases consumption of fluids, fruits, vegetables, and grain products.

MIXED NARCOTIC AGONIST-ANTAGONISTS

The mixed narcotic agonist-antagonists—buprenorphine hydrochloride, butorphanol tartrate, dezocine, nalbuphine hydrochloride, and pentazocine—originally appeared to have less abuse potential than the pure narcotic agonists. However, butorphanol and pentazocine reportedly have caused dependence.

PHARMACOKINETICS

The pharmacokinetics of the mixed narcotic agonist-antagonists closely resemble those of morphine, with some differences in onset and duration of action.

Absorption, distribution, metabolism, excretion

The mixed narcotic agonist-antagonists can be administered orally or by the S.C., I.M., or I.V. route, but pentazocine is the only drug in this category available in oral form. Absorption occurs rapidly from parenteral sites. These drugs are distributed to most body tissues and also cross the placenta. They are metabolized in the liver and excreted primarily by the kidneys, although more than 10% of a butorphanol dose and a small amount of dezocine and pentazocine doses are excreted in the feces.

Mixed narcotic agonist-antagonists: Equianalgesic doses

This chart lists the equianalgesic I.M. doses (based on the standard dose of 10 mg of morphine sulfate I.M.) for the mixed narcotic agonist-antagonist agents.

MIXED NARCOTIC AGONIST-ANTAGONIST	EQUIANALGESIC DOSE
buprenorphine (Buprenex)	0.3 mg
butorphanol (Stadol)	2 mg
dezocine (Dalgan)	10 mg
nalbuphine (Nubain)	10 mg
pentazocine (Talwin)	30 mg

Onset, peak, duration

Slight variations exist among the onset of action, peak concentration, and duration of action of parenterally administered mixed narcotic agonist-antagonists. The onset of buprenorphine is 15 minutes, the drug's peak concentration is reached in 60 minutes, and its duration is 5 to 6 hours. The onset of butorphanol occurs within 10 to 30 minutes, peak concentration occurs within 30 to 60 minutes, and the drug's duration is 3 to 4 hours. Dezocine begins to act in 15 to 30 minutes, peaks at 60 minutes, and lasts 4 to 6 hours. Nalbuphine has an onset of less than 15 minutes, reaches peak concentration in 20 to 45 minutes, and has a duration of 3 to 6 hours. Orally administered pentazocine has an onset of 15 to 30 minutes, reaches peak concentration in less than an hour, and has a duration of 3 to 4 hours.

The plasma half-life of buprenorphine is about 2 hours after I.V. injection. The plasma half-life of butorphanol after I.V. administration is 3 to 4 hours. The half-life of nalbuphine is 5 hours. The half-life of pentazocine is 2 to 3 hours.

PHARMACODYNAMICS

Although the mixed narcotic agonist-antagonists occupy the same opiate receptor sites as the narcotic agonists, they have few or no antitussive effects and produce fewer GI effects than the pure agonists.

Mechanism of action

The exact mechanism of action of the mixed narcotic agonist-antagonists has not been established. Buprenorphine seems to dissociate slowly from binding sites and therefore has a longer duration of action than the other drugs in this class. The site of action of butorphanol may be opiate receptors in the limbic system. Like pentazocine, butorphanol also acts on pulmonary circulation, increasing pulmonary artery and pulmonary capillary wedge pressures and pulmonary vascular resistance. Both drugs also increase systemic arterial pressure and the overall cardiac work load. Dezocine reportedly increases cardiac index, stroke volume, and pulmonary vascular resistance.

PHARMACOTHERAPEUTICS

Mixed narcotic agonist-antagonists are prescribed primarily for the relief of moderate to severe pain, for obstetric analgesia in selected cases, and for preoperative medication to reduce anxiety and pain perception. (For equianalgesic doses comparable to 10 mg of morphine sulfate I.M., see *Mixed narcotic agonist-antagonists: Equianalgesic doses*.)

Mixed narcotic agonist-antagonists sometimes are preferred because the risk of drug dependence is lower with them than with the narcotic agonists. Mixed narcotic agonist-antagonists also are less likely to cause respiratory depression.

buprenorphine hydrochloride (Buprenex). A Schedule IV drug and a semisynthetic opioid, buprenorphine has an analgesic effect approximately 30 times as potent as that of morphine sulfate. Buprenorphine is used to relieve moderate to severe pain.
Usual adult dosage: for adults and children over age 13, 0.3 mg I.M. or by slow I.V. injection at intervals of 6 or more hours, as needed. Doses may be increased to 0.6 mg or intervals shortened to 4 hours, depending on patient response and pain severity.

butorphanol tartrate (Stadol). A potent analgesic, butorphanol is indicated for moderate to severe pain, for obstetric analgesia during labor, and for preoperative medication.
Usual adult dosage: 2 mg I.M. every 3 to 4 hours, with a dosage range of 1 to 4 mg (higher doses are not recommended); or 1 mg I.V. every 3 to 4 hours, with a dosage range of 0.5 to 2 mg.

dezocine (Dalgan). Dezocine is indicated for postoperative and other types of analgesia.
Usual adult dosage: 5 to 15 mg I.M., S.C., or I.V.

nalbuphine hydrochloride (Nubain). Equianalgesic to morphine sulfate on a milligram-to-milligram basis, nalbuphine is indicated for relief of moderate to severe pain and for preoperative and obstetric analgesia.
Usual adult dosage: 10 mg per 70 kg of body weight I.V., I.M., or S.C. every 3 to 6 hours, as necessary; not to exceed 160 mg/day.

pentazocine hydrochloride and pentazocine lactate (Talwin). A Schedule IV drug, pentazocine is used for the relief of moderate pain, as a preoperative medication, and as a supplement to surgical anesthesia. For the lactate form, the S.C. route should be used only when necessary, because severe tissue damage can result. Pentazocine may cause psychotomimetic effects, such as dysphoria, especially with long-term administration; this limits its usefulness in patients with chronic or severe pain.
Usual adult dosage: for pain relief, 50 to 100 mg of pentazocine hydrochloride P.O. every 3 to 4 hours, or 30 mg of pentazocine lactate I.M., I.V., or S.C., repeated every 3 to 4 hours. Doses should not exceed 30 mg I.V. or 60 mg I.M. or S.C.

pentazocine hydrochloride and naloxone hydrochloride (Talwin-Nx). In this product, 50 mg of oral pentazocine is combined with 0.5 mg of naloxone. The naloxone was added after reports that narcotic addicts were injecting themselves with a solution made from crushing the tablets.

Usual adult dosage: 50 to 100 mg P.O. every 3 to 4 hours.

pentazocine hydrochloride and aspirin (Talwin Compound). Each tablet contains 12.5 mg of pentazocine and 325 mg of aspirin. Two tablets produce an additive analgesic effect of pentazocine and aspirin as well as the anti-inflammatory and antipyretic action of aspirin. This compound is used to relieve moderate pain.
Usual adult dosage: two tablets P.O. t.i.d. or q.i.d.

pentazocine hydrochloride and acetaminophen (Talacen). Each caplet contains 25 mg of pentazocine and 650 mg of acetaminophen. This drug is used to relieve moderate pain.
Usual adult dosage: one caplet P.O. every 3 to 4 hours.

Drug interactions

Patients who have become dependent on narcotic agonists almost always will experience withdrawal symptoms if they are given mixed narcotic agonist-antagonists. The exception is nalbuphine, which can be administered just before, together with, or just after an injection of a narcotic agonist without antagonizing it. Patients with a known or suspected history of narcotic abuse should not receive any of the mixed narcotic agonist-antagonists. Supportive measures should be readily available in the event that one of these drugs is administered inadvertently to a narcotic-dependent patient.

Increased CNS depression and an additive decrease in respiratory rate and depth may result if mixed narcotic agonist-antagonists are administered to patients taking or using other CNS depressants, such as barbiturates or alcohol. If concomitant administration is necessary, the dosage of one of the drugs should be reduced.

ADVERSE DRUG REACTIONS

Adverse reactions to the mixed narcotic agonist-antagonists are less common than reactions to narcotic agonists and usually affect the CNS and the GI tract.

The most common adverse reactions to these drugs include nausea, vomiting, light-headedness, sedation, and euphoria. Dysphoria, visual hallucinations, confusion, and disorientation also may occur (especially in elderly patients). These effects limit the long-term use of these agents in patients with severe pain. Respiration may be depressed with initial doses but does not worsen with increased dosage. Insomnia and disturbed dreams may occur, especially with pentazocine and nalbuphine, and anticholinergic effects (dry mouth, blurred vision, constipation, and urine retention) are common. The patient may experience blood pressure changes, primarily hypertension, especially with nalbuphine. The mixed narcotic agonist-antagonists also can cause hypersensitivity reactions.

NURSING PROCESS APPLICATION

The following information assists the nurse in caring for a patient who is receiving a mixed narcotic agonist-antagonist.

Assessment
• Review the patient's history for conditions that contra-indicate the use of a mixed narcotic agonist-antagonist, such as known hypersensitivity to the drug.
• Review the patient's history for conditions that require cautious use of a mixed narcotic agonist-antagonist, such as head injury, increased intracranial pressure, cardiac or pulmonary dysfunction, renal or hepatic impairment, pregnancy, lactation, or known prior drug abuse.
• Assess the patient for adverse reactions to the mixed narcotic agonist-antagonist, such as CNS and GI problems.
• Review the patient's medication history to identify the use of drugs that may interact with the mixed narcotic agonist-antagonist.
• Assess the patient daily for constipation.
• Assess the effectiveness of the mixed narcotic agonist-antagonist periodically.
• Evaluate the patient's and family's knowledge about the prescribed mixed narcotic agonist-antagonist.

Nursing diagnoses
The following examples represent appropriate nursing diagnoses for a patient receiving a mixed narcotic agonist-antagonist.
• Potential for injury related to a preexisting condition that contraindicates the use of a mixed narcotic agonist-antagonist
• Potential for injury related to a preexisting condition that requires cautious use of a mixed narcotic agonist-antagonist
• Potential for injury related to adverse drug reactions
• Constipation related to the anticholinergic effects of a mixed narcotic agonist-antagonist
• Pain related to ineffectiveness of the prescribed mixed narcotic agonist-antagonist
• Knowledge deficit related to the prescribed narcotic agonist-antagonist

Planning and implementation
• Do not administer a mixed narcotic agonist-antagonist to a patient with a condition that contraindicates its use.
• Administer a mixed narcotic agonist-antagonist cautiously to a patient at risk because of a preexisting condition.
• Monitor the patient for adverse reactions throughout drug therapy. Be aware that a mixed narcotic agonist-antagonist may obscure signs of increasing intracranial pressure, such as confusion or changes in level of consciousness. *Monitor at least every 4 hours for a patient with a head injury or other condition that could cause increased intracranial pressure.*
• Monitor respiratory status during therapy. Have emergency equipment readily available.
• Expect to decrease the dosage of the mixed narcotic agonist-antagonist or of a CNS depressant, if concomitant administration is necessary, to prevent additive CNS or respiratory effects.
• *Do not administer a mixed narcotic agonist-antagonist to a narcotic-dependent patient; it may precipitate withdrawal symptoms.*
• Take safety precautions and provide psychological support if a mixed narcotic agonist-antagonist is administered inadvertently to a narcotic-dependent patient. Observe the patient frequently and take necessary safety precautions if the patient develops mental status changes. For example, keep the bed rails up and place the bed in the low position.
• Evaluate the patient for urine retention—for example, by recording fluid intake and output at least every 8 hours.
• *Do not mix pentazocine in the same syringe as a barbiturate.*
• *Question any prescription for S.C. pentazocine because it may cause severe tissue damage when administered by S.C. injection.* If the patient must receive the drug S.C., record, inspect, and rotate injection sites.
• *Provide emergency care if an overdose occurs; use mechanical ventilation, as prescribed.* Keep in mind that naloxone can reverse the effects of pentazocine and nalbuphine, but will not reverse totally the effects of buprenorphine.
• Notify the physician if adverse drug reactions occur.
• Provide high-fiber foods and 2 to 3 liters of fluid daily, unless contraindicated, to prevent constipation.
• Consult with the physician about the need for a laxative or stool softener if the patient becomes constipated.
• Rate the patient's pain before and after each dose of a mixed narcotic agonist-antagonist agent; determine and record the onset, duration, location, intensity, and quality of the pain as well as the degree of pain relief obtained after drug administration.
• Notify the physician if the prescribed mixed narcotic agonist-antagonist does not relieve the patient's pain.

Patient teaching
• Teach the patient and family the name, dose, frequency, action, and adverse effects of the prescribed mixed narcotic agonist-antagonist.
• Advise the patient to avoid activities that require alertness until response to the drug has been determined.
• Inform the narcotic-dependent patient that administration of a mixed narcotic agonist-antagonist may precipitate withdrawal symptoms; encourage honesty in reporting all drug use.

• Advise the patient not to take alcohol or any over-the-counter medication containing alcohol without consulting the physician because of the increased risk of CNS and respiratory depression.

• Instruct the patient to drink 2 to 3 liters of fluid daily and increase fiber in diet to prevent constipation.

• Alert the patient and family that dysphoria, blurred vision, visual hallucinations, confusion, and disorientation may occur. Instruct the family to handle these adverse reactions by taking safety measures, such as constant supervision, until the effects of the drug wear off.

• Instruct the patient to relieve dry mouth by drinking cold beverages, sucking on hard candy, or using a nonprescription saliva substitute. Also encourage frequent oral hygiene.

• Instruct the patient and family to notify the physician if adverse reactions occur or if pain is not relieved.

Evaluation

The following examples represent appropriate evaluation statements for a patient receiving a mixed narcotic agonist-antagonist.

• The patient has no conditions that contraindicate therapy with a mixed narcotic agonist-antagonist.

• The patient exhibits no signs of complications in the preexisting condition linked to the prescribed mixed narcotic agonist-antagonist.

• The patient demonstrates no adverse reactions to the prescribed mixed narcotic agonist-antagonist.

• The patient maintains normal bowel patterns.

• The patient reports adequate pain relief.

• The patient and family express an accurate understanding of the points taught about the prescribed mixed narcotic agonist-antagonist.

• The patient brushes the teeth and uses a mouthwash four times a day.

NARCOTIC ANTAGONISTS

The pure narcotic antagonists naloxone hydrochloride and naltrexone hydrochloride have an affinity for the opiate receptors but do not stimulate them. Instead, these drugs attach to the receptors and prevent narcotic drugs, enkephalins, and endorphins from producing their effects. Naloxone is used to treat narcotic overdose. Naltrexone is used as an adjunct therapy to keep detoxified patients drug-free, similar to the use of disulfiram (Antabuse) to prevent resumption of alcohol abuse.

PHARMACOKINETICS

Naloxone is administered I.M. or I.V.; naltrexone is administered orally in tablet or liquid form. Both drugs are metabolized by the liver and excreted by the kidneys.

Absorption, distribution, metabolism, excretion

Naloxone usually is administered I.V. even though it is absorbed readily from I.M. injection sites. Because it is deactivated rapidly after oral administration, naloxone is not administered by this route. Naltrexone is administered orally because it is absorbed rapidly and almost completely from the GI tract after oral administration. Both drugs occupy opiate receptor sites without initiating any response (in the absence of narcotic drugs); both also are deactivated rapidly by first-pass metabolism in the liver and are excreted by the kidneys. A small portion of a naltrexone dose is excreted in the feces.

Onset, peak, duration

Naloxone has an immediate onset of action, but its duration of action depends on the dose and administration route. For example, I.M. administration produces a more prolonged effect than I.V. administration. The nurse must monitor the patient carefully because the effects of the narcotic overdose in many cases last longer than the effects of the antagonist, and repeated doses may be necessary. Onset of naltrexone occurs within 20 to 30 minutes; peak concentration occurs in 1 hour. The plasma half-life of naloxone is 60 to 90 minutes. The half-life of naltrexone is 13 hours.

PHARMACODYNAMICS

Narcotic antagonists block the effects of narcotics by occupying the opiate receptor sites, displacing any narcotic molecules already present, and blocking further narcotic binding at these sites. This is known as competitive inhibition. Naloxone and naltrexone seem to have the highest affinity for the mu opiate receptors.

PHARMACOTHERAPEUTICS

Naloxone is the drug of choice for managing a narcotic overdose because it reverses the respiratory depression and sedation and helps stabilize the patient's vital signs within seconds after administration. Naloxone administration also reverses the analgesic effects of narcotic drugs, so a patient who was given a narcotic drug for pain relief may complain of pain or even experience withdrawal symptoms. The severity of these symptoms depends on the narcotic used and the amount.

If repeated injections of naloxone are needed but the patient does not improve after receiving three doses or 10 mg, supportive methods such as mechanical ventilation should be instituted; lingering depressant effects may be from nonnarcotic drugs or a mixed overdose.

Naltrexone is used only as an adjunct to psychotherapy or counseling for patients who have been detoxified from narcotic drugs and wish to remain so. Before naltrexone treatment is initiated, a naloxone challenge test may be given after the patient has been without narcotics for 7 to 10 days. (For more information, see *Naloxone challenge test*.)

naloxone hydrochloride (Narcan). A narcotic antagonist related to oxymorphone, naloxone is the drug of choice for complete or partial reversal of respiratory depression caused by narcotic overdose. Naloxone also is used to diagnose suspected narcotic overdose.
Usual adult dosage: initially, 0.4 to 2 mg I.V., I.M., or S.C., repeated every 2 to 3 minutes as needed, depending on the degree of counteraction achieved. The I.V. route is preferred in emergencies. If the patient does not respond after 10 mg have been administered, the diagnosis of narcotic overdose should be reevaluated.
Usual pediatric dosage: initially, for opiate-induced asphyxia neonatorum, 0.01 mg/kg I.V. via the umbilical vein, if no response, give 0.1 mg/kg, as prescribed. If an I.V. route is unavailable, the drug may be given I.M., S.C., or by endotrachael tube.

naltrexone hydrochloride (Trexan). Naltrexone is used as an adjunct to psychotherapy or counseling for detoxified addicts who have been narcotic-free for 7 to 10 days, as verified by urinalysis. The patient also should be free of withdrawal symptoms before starting naltrexone treatment. A naloxone challenge test may be obtained before naltrexone treatment is initiated.
Usual adult dosage: 50 mg P.O. every 24 hours; other dosage schedules include 50 mg on weekdays, 100 mg on Saturday, and nothing on Sunday; 100 mg every 48 hours; or 150 mg every 72 hours. The total weekly dosage should be 350 mg given in at least three doses.

Drug interactions

Naloxone produces no significant drug interactions. Naltrexone will cause withdrawal symptoms if given to a patient receiving a narcotic agonist or to a narcotic addict.

ADVERSE DRUG REACTIONS

Naloxone may cause nausea, vomiting, and, occasionally, hypertension and tachycardia. An unconscious patient returned to consciousness abruptly after naloxone administration may hyperventilate and experience tremors.

Naltrexone produces numerous adverse reactions affecting various body systems. (For details, see *Naltrexone:*

Naloxone challenge test

Planned use of naltrexone commonly requires that a negative naloxone challenge test be obtained before administration of the first naltrexone dose.

For an I.V. naloxone challenge, 0.8 mg is drawn up into a sterile syringe and 0.2 mg is injected. While the needle is still in place, observe the patient for 30 seconds for signs and symptoms of withdrawal. If no evidence of withdrawal appears, inject the remaining 0.6 mg and observe the patient for an additional 20 minutes.

For an S.C. naloxone challenge, 0.8 mg is administered S.C., and the patient is observed for 45 minutes for withdrawal symptoms.

With either test, occurrence of withdrawal symptoms indicates a potential risk to the patient, and naltrexone therapy should *not* be initiated. The naloxone challenge test can be repeated in 24 hours. If no withdrawal symptoms occur, naltrexone therapy may begin.

Summary of adverse reactions.) The variety and number of adverse reactions to this drug have delayed its full acceptance in maintaining narcotic abstinence. Patients should be monitored frequently, even if they receive the drug on an outpatient basis.

NURSING PROCESS APPLICATION

The following information assists the nurse in caring for a patient who is receiving a narcotic antagonist.

Assessment
• Review the patient's history for conditions that contraindicate the use of a narcotic antagonist, such as known hypersensitivity to the drug.
• Review the patient's history for conditions that require cautious use of a narcotic antagonist, such as cardiac disease, pregnancy, lactation, or the use of cardiotoxic drugs.
• Assess the patient for adverse reactions to the narcotic antagonist, such as nausea, vomiting, hypertension, tachycardia, anxiety, disorientation, itching, nasal congestion, and urinary frequency.
• Review the patient's medication history to identify use of drugs that may interact with the narcotic antagonist.
• Assess the effectiveness of the narcotic antagonist.
• Question the patient receiving naltrexone about changes in libido or delayed ejaculation.
• Evaluate the patient's and family's knowledge about the prescribed narcotic antagonist.

Naltrexone: Summary of adverse reactions

Adverse reactions to naltrexone can take many forms, as this chart demonstrates. (Hepatotoxicity may occur in a small number of patients.)

Cardiopulmonary

- Edema
- Hypertension
- Palpitations
- Phlebitis
- Shortness of breath

Central nervous system

- Anxiety
- Depression
- Disorientation
- Dizziness
- Headache
- Nervousness

Eye, ear, nose, and throat

- Blurred vision
- Cough
- Epistaxis
- Nasal congestion
- Tinnitus

Gastrointestinal

- Anorexia
- Diarrhea or constipation
- Nausea
- Thirst
- Vomiting

Genitourinary

- Changes in libido
- Delayed ejaculation
- Urinary frequency

Skin

- Acne
- Alopecia
- Itching
- Rash

Nursing diagnoses

The following examples represent appropriate nursing diagnoses for a patient receiving a narcotic antagonist.

- Potential for injury related to a preexisting condition that contraindicates the use of a narcotic antagonist
- Potential for injury related to a preexisting condition that requires cautious use of a narcotic antagonist
- Potential for injury related to adverse drug reactions
- Sexual dysfunction related to the genitourinary effects of naltrexone
- Knowledge deficit related to the prescribed narcotic antagonist

Planning and implementation

- Do not administer a narcotic antagonist to a patient with a condition that contraindicates its use.
- Do not administer naltrexone until a negative naloxone challenge test is obtained. Also, do not administer naltrexone to a patient who is receiving narcotic drugs, is addicted to narcotic drugs, or is in the acute phase of narcotic withdrawal because acute withdrawal may occur or worsen.
- Administer a narcotic antagonist cautiously to a patient at risk because of a preexisting condition.
- Observe the patient for adverse reactions throughout narcotic antagonist therapy.
- *Be prepared to administer another dose of naloxone, as prescribed, if respiratory depression occurs.* Also monitor the patient's respiratory rate and depth, and be prepared to provide oxygen, ventilation, and other resuscitation measures, as needed. Keep in mind that the duration of action of a narcotic may exceed naloxone's duration of action, and that naloxone does not reverse respiratory depression produced by diazepam.
- Encourage the patient taking naltrexone to report signs and symptoms of sexual dysfunction, such as changes in libido and delayed ejaculation. Reassure the patient that these effects will disappear when naltrexone is discontinued.

Patient teaching

- Teach the family about the use and purpose of naloxone to treat narcotic overdose in the patient.
- Inform the family that naloxone cannot reverse the effects of all drugs and that other emergency care may be required, such as mechanical ventilation.
- Advise the family that an unconscious patient returned to consciousness abruptly after naloxone administration may hyperventilate and experience tremors.
- Encourage the family to ask questions about naloxone use.
- Teach the patient and family the name, dose, frequency, action, and adverse effects of naltrexone.
- Inform the patient that naltrexone blocks the action of narcotics and may precipitate narcotic withdrawal. Advise the patient to be honest with the physician about narcotic use.
- Instruct the patient about the naloxone challenge test.
- Teach the patient how to manage a nosebleed, which may occur during naltrexone therapy.

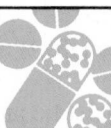

Narcotic agonist and antagonist agents

This chart summarizes the narcotic agonists, mixed narcotic agonist-antagonists, and narcotic antagonists in clinical use.

DRUG	MAJOR INDICATIONS	USUAL ADULT DOSAGES	CONTRAINDICATIONS AND PRECAUTIONS
Narcotic agonists			
meperidine	Moderate to severe visceral pain	50 to 150 mg parenterally or P.O. every 3 to 4 hours, as needed	• Know that meperidine is contraindicated in a patient with known hypersensitivity to the drug or one who is receiving an MAO inhibitor.
	Preoperative medication, obstetric analgesia	50 to 100 mg I.M. or S.C.	• Administer with extreme caution to a pregnant or lactating patient; a patient with head injury or increased intracranial pressure, asthma or other respiratory conditions; or a patient with susceptibility to hypotension, which may result from surgery or volume depletion. Also administer with extreme caution to a patient who is receiving other central nervous system depressants, phenothiazines, or certain anesthetics.
			• Administer with caution to a patient with hepatic or renal impairment because of the increased risk for normeperidine accumulation.
morphine	Severe pain from myocardial infarction, cancer, major surgery, pulmonary edema	10 mg/70 kg of body weight parenterally, titrated to pain relief	• Know that morphine is contraindicated in a patient with known hypersensitivity to the drug. I.V. administration is contraindicated in a patient with acute bronchial asthma or upper airway obstruction.
morphine, sustained-release	Terminal cancer pain or other conditions in which prolonged pain relief is desirable	30 mg P.O. every 8 to 12 hours, titrated to pain relief	• Administer with extreme caution to an elderly or debilitated patient or one with head injury or increased intracranial or intraocular pressure.
morphine, intensified oral solution	Severe acute pain, chronic pain	10 to 30 mg P.O. every 4 hours; dosage varies with patient response	• Administer with caution to a pregnant or lactating patient or one with hepatic or renal dysfunction.
propoxyphene	Mild to moderate pain	65 mg P.O. every 4 hours, as needed	• Know that propoxyphene is contraindicated in a patient with known hypersensitivity to the drug.
			• Administer with extreme caution to a patient with peptic ulcer disease or coagulation abnormalities.
			• Administer with caution to a pregnant patient or one with hepatic or renal impairment.
Mixed narcotic agonist-antagonists			
butorphanol	Moderate to severe pain, obstetric analgesia, preoperative medication	2 mg I.M. every 3 to 4 hours or 1 mg I.V. every 3 to 4 hours	• Know that butorphanol is contraindicated in a patient with known hypersensitivity to the drug.
			• Administer with extreme caution to a patient with head injury, increased intracranial pressure, acute myocardial infarction, ventricular dysfunction, or coronary insufficiency.
			• Administer with caution to a pregnant or lactating patient, one under age 18, or one with impaired renal or hepatic function, hypertension, known prior drug abuse, a respiratory disorder such as bronchial asthma, or an obstructive respiratory disorder.

SELECTED MAJOR DRUGS

Narcotic agonist and antagonist agents (continued)

DRUG	MAJOR INDICATIONS	USUAL ADULT DOSAGES	CONTRAINDICATIONS AND PRECAUTIONS
nalbuphine	Moderate to severe pain, obstetric analgesia, preoperative medication	10 mg/70 kg of body weight I.V., I.M., or S.C. every 3 to 6 hours; not to exceed 160 mg/day	• Know that nalbuphine is contraindicated in a patient with known hypersensitivity to the drug. • Administer with extreme caution to a patient with head injury or increased intracranial pressure. • Administer with caution to a pregnant patient or one with impaired respirations, myocardial infarction, biliary tract surgery, hepatic or renal dysfunction, or known prior drug abuse.
Narcotic antagonist			
naloxone	Narcotic overdose	0.4 to 2 mg I.V. every 2 to 3 minutes depending on patient response; also may be given I.M. or S.C.	• Know that naloxone is contraindicated in a patient with known hypersensitivity to the drug. • Administer with caution to a neonate of an opioid-dependent mother, a pregnant or lactating patient, one with cardiac disease, or one who is receiving potentially cardiotoxic drugs.

• Advise the patient to change positions slowly and not to engage in activities that require concentration if naltrexone produces dizziness, blurred vision, or mental status changes.
• Instruct the patient to eat small, frequent meals if naltrexone produces anorexia. Also advise the patient to consume 2 to 3 liters of fluid a day and adequate fiber to prevent naltrexone-induced constipation.
• Inform the patient about naltrexone's genitourinary effects, such as change in libido and delayed ejaculation.
• Instruct the patient to notify the physician if adverse reactions to naltrexone occur.

Evaluation

The following examples represent appropriate evaluation statements for a patient receiving a narcotic antagonist.
• The patient has no conditions that contraindicate narcotic antagonist therapy.
• The patient exhibits no signs of complications in the preexisting condition linked to the prescribed narcotic antagonist.
• The patient displays no adverse reactions to the prescribed narcotic antagonist.
• The patient reports normal sexual activity.
• The patient and family express an accurate understanding of the points taught about the prescribed narcotic antagonist
• The patient reports eating six small meals daily.

CHAPTER SUMMARY

Chapter 22 explored narcotic agonists, mixed narcotic agonist-antagonists, and narcotic antagonists. Here are the highlights of the chapter.
• Narcotic agonists modify the sensation of pain by inhibiting the transmission of pain impulses in sensory pathways in the spinal cord, reducing cortical responses to painful stimuli, and altering behavioral responses to pain.
• Narcotic agonists include the opium derivatives and the synthetic narcotics used to relieve pain. Oral, rectal, and parenteral forms are available.
• Morphine is considered the narcotic standard; all narcotic drugs are compared with it.
• Oxycodone with acetaminophen or aspirin (Percocet or Percodan) is a combination drug that exemplifies the additive effect of nonnarcotic-narcotic combination analgesics. Concentrated oral solutions of morphine and a sustained-release tablet may be used to treat cancer pain and chronic intractable pain. Among the synthetic narcotic agonists, meperidine (Demerol) is the most commonly used for postoperative pain.
• Adverse reactions to narcotic agonists include respiratory depression, orthostatic hypotension, and constipation. Tolerance as well as psychological and physical dependence may occur with long-term narcotic use.

• Mixed narcotic agonist-antagonists produce analgesic effects similar to those of morphine. They have few or no antitussive effects.

• Pentazocine, a mixed narcotic agonist-antagonist, is an effective analgesic for moderate pain. An oral dosage form (Talwin Compound) combines pentazocine with aspirin, providing an additive analgesic effect and anti-inflammatory and antipyretic actions.

• Buprenorphine and nalbuphine, also mixed narcotic agonist-antagonists, have a longer duration of action than pentazocine — up to 6 hours. Both effectively relieve moderate to severe pain.

• The respiratory depression caused by mixed narcotic agonist-antagonists does not worsen with higher doses.

• The narcotic antagonists naloxone and naltrexone work by competitive inhibition at the opiate receptor sites, displacing narcotic molecules and preventing them from exerting their effects.

• Naloxone is used to treat narcotic overdose. Naltrexone is used as an adjunct treatment with detoxified addicts who are highly motivated to remain drug-free.

• Naltrexone produces numerous adverse reactions in many body systems.

STUDY QUESTIONS

See Appendix 1 for answers.

1. George Richards, age 46, is recovering from a cholecystectomy. For postoperative pain, the physician prescribes the narcotic agonist meperidine (Demerol), 100 mg I.M. every 4 hours p.r.n. Which of the following statements best describes the action of a narcotic agonist?
(a) It inhibits prostaglandin synthesis.
(b) It inhibits binding to opiate receptors.
(c) It inactivates the pain impulse.
(d) It alters the perception of, and response to, pain.

2. Robert Potamkin, age 52, seeks care for a severe cough. His physician orders a narcotic agonist. Which narcotic agonist commonly is used for cough suppression?
(a) paregoric
(b) morphine
(c) oxycodone
(d) codeine

3. The nurse teaches Mr. Potamkin to avoid alcohol while taking the narcotic agonist to avoid which drug interaction?
(a) severe respiratory depression
(b) severe constipation
(c) urine retention
(d) tachycardia

4. The ambulance squad brings Kevin Bolton, age 21, to the emergency department (ED) with a head injury. Although Mr. Bolton is in pain, the physician does not order a narcotic agonist. Why?
(a) The risk of drug dependence is highest in patients with head injuries.
(b) Narcotic agonists mask changes in the level of consciousness.
(c) In such a patient, narcotic agonists may have a paradoxical effect.
(d) The level of consciousness is likely to increase suddenly.

5. Shelley Johnson, age 25, is in labor. To ease her pain, her physician prescribes butorphanol (Stadol), a mixed narcotic agonist-antagonist. What is the difference between a narcotic agonist and a mixed narcotic agonist-antagonist?
(a) Less of a mixed narcotic agonist-antagonist is needed to relieve pain.
(b) More of a mixed narcotic agonist-antagonist is needed to relieve pain.
(c) A mixed narcotic agonist-antagonist is more likely to cause drug dependence.
(d) A mixed narcotic agonist-antagonist is less likely to cause respiratory depression.

6. Before administering butorphanol, the nurse assesses Ms. Johnson for use of narcotic agonists. Administering a mixed narcotic agonist-antagonist to a patient who is dependent on narcotic agonists may cause which of the following reactions?
(a) hypersensitivity reaction
(b) hepatotoxicity
(c) urinary incontinence
(d) withdrawal symptoms

7. Coretta Smith, age 58, takes morphine for chronic pain caused by metastatic bone cancer. To relieve increasingly severe pain, she increases her morphine dosage. When her husband finds her unresponsive with shallow respirations, he brings her to the ED. Which drug is most likely to be prescribed to treat morphine overdose?
(a) naloxone
(b) naltrexone
(c) pentazocine
(d) butorphanol

8. The physician prescribes a narcotic antagonist to treat Ms. Smith. When administering this drug, the nurse should consider which fact?

(a) Narcotic antagonists have a rapid onset and are long-lasting.

(b) Narcotic antagonists have a slow onset but a long duration of action.

(c) Narcotic antagonist effects seldom last as long as the overdose effects.

(d) Narcotic antagonists require only a single dose to be effective.

SELECTED REFERENCES

AHFS drug information 90. (1990). Bethesda, MD: American Society of Hospital Pharmacists.

Compendium of pharmaceuticals and specialties: The Canadian reference for health professionals. (1990). Toronto: CK Productions.

Hansten, P., and Horn, J. (1989). *Drug interactions* (6th ed.). Philadelphia: Lea & Febiger.

McCaffrey M., and Beebe, A. (1989). Giving narcotics for pain: The secrets to giving equianalgesic doses. *Nursing89,* 19(10), 161-165.

McCaffrey, M., and Beebe, A. (1989). Managing your patients' adverse reactions to narcotics. *Nursing89,* 19(10), 166-168.

Molitor, R., Jr., Lain, D., and Dupen, S. (1988). Home epidural infusions of opiate agonists and bupivacaine-epinephrine. *American Journal of Hospital Pharmacy,* 45(9), 1861-1862.

Peplin, N. (1989). Intractable pain management with intravenous narcotic administration at home. *Journal of Intravenous Nursing,* 12(4), 228-232.

Portenoy, R. (1988). Practical aspects of pain control in the patient with cancer. *CA: A Cancer Journal for Clinicians,* 38(6), 327-352.

Speight, T. (1987). *Avery's drug treatment: Principles and practice of clinical pharmacology and therapeutics* (3rd ed.). Baltimore: Williams & Wilkins.

Three opioids compared for postsurgical pain. (1989). *Nurses Drug Alert,* 13(9), 71-72.

CHAPTER

23

GENERAL ANESTHETIC AGENTS

OBJECTIVES

After reading and studying this chapter, the student should be able to:

1. Explain the differences between balanced anesthesia and neuroleptanesthesia.

2. Describe the stages of anesthesia.

3. Define and distinguish between inhalation and injection anesthetic agents.

4. Discuss the pharmacokinetics and mechanism of action of inhalation anesthetic agents.

5. Describe the adverse effects of inhalation anesthetic agents.

6. Discuss the pharmacokinetics and mechanism of action of injection anesthetics.

7. Describe the adverse effects of injection anesthetics.

8. Describe how to apply the nursing process when caring for a patient who is receiving a general anesthetic agent.

INTRODUCTION

General anesthetic agents depress the central nervous system (CNS) to produce loss of consciousness, loss of responsiveness to sensory stimulation including pain, and muscle relaxation. General anesthesia may result from one or a combination of drugs.

These drugs are volatile liquids or gases vaporized in oxygen and administered by inhalation or nonvolatile solutions administered by injection.

In many cases, drug combinations are used to produce anesthesia. One kind of anesthesia, neuroleptanesthesia, is produced by administering a neuroleptic drug (a tranquilizer or an antipsychotic) with an opiate analgesic and nitrous oxide. The patient can be aroused almost immediately from this anesthesia if necessary. Another kind of anesthesia, balanced anesthesia, is produced by administering a barbiturate, an opiate analgesic, and a cholinergic blocking agent, then inducing anesthesia with another barbiturate and maintaining it with inhalation and injection anesthetics plus a neuromuscular blocking agent. When properly ad-

ministered, balanced anesthesia minimizes cardiovascular effects, allows an early return to consciousness, and reduces postoperative nausea, vomiting, and excitement.

The practice of anesthesia includes more than proper administration of anesthetic agents. Monitoring and maintaining vital signs, fluids, electrolytes, acid-base balance, body temperature, and positioning, and assuring the patient's well-being from before surgery through recovery are vital components of anesthesia practice.

The choice of a particular anesthetic agent for a patient involves several considerations, including the patient's physiologic state and medical history, the type of surgical procedure, and the anticipated postoperative course.

Chapter 23 discusses the two main classes of general anesthetics — inhalation and injection — and their use singly and in combination.

Anesthesia administration

Anesthesia administration is divided into three parts: induction, maintenance, and emergence.

Induction is the initiation of anesthesia and usually is accomplished with an intravenous (I.V.) agent that has a rapid onset of action and a short duration of action. Its purpose is to produce a rapid, pleasant, and stressless transition from consciousness to sleep. Induction agents include the ultra-short-acting barbiturates (thiopental sodium, thiamylal sodium, and methohexital sodium); the benzodiazepine sedatives (diazepam, lorazepam, and midazolam); or the rapid-acting hypnotic agents (etomidate and propofol).

Administration of the primary anesthetic — the maintenance stage — begins during induction. The transition to maintenance anesthesia is completed as the induction stage effects diminish. Maintenance levels of anesthesia can be continued for many hours if necessary, until surgery is completed.

Emergence follows the withdrawal of anesthetic agents. Drugs are administered to reverse the effects, and the patient exhales or otherwise excretes the anesthetic agents. The anesthesia process is completed after the postoperative

SELECTED NURSING DIAGNOSES

General anesthetic agents

The following nursing diagnoses address representative problems and etiologies that a nurse may encounter when caring for a patient who is receiving a general anesthetic agent. Some of these nursing diagnoses contain generalized etiologies, which the nurse must individualize based on the patient's needs. (For some common nursing diagnoses and related interventions for each drug class, see the "Nursing Process Application" sections of this chapter.)

- Altered thought processes related to prolonged recovery from the general anesthetic agent
- Altered urinary elimination related to nephrotoxicity from methoxyflurane
- Hypothermia related to a postoperative reaction to the inhalation anesthetic
- Impaired tissue integrity related to phlebitis caused by parenteral diazepam administration
- Ineffective breathing pattern related to the adverse respiratory effects of the general anesthetic agent
- Knowledge deficit related to the general anesthetic agent
- Pain related to muscle rigidity and spasms caused by injection anesthetic administration
- Potential altered body temperature related to possible development of hypothermia or hyperthermia during inhalation anesthetic administration
- Potential for fluid volume deficit related to nausea, vomiting, or excess salivation and tearing caused by the general anesthetic agent
- Potential for injury related to a preexisting condition that contraindicates the use of the general anesthetic agent
- Potential for injury related to a preexisting condition that requires cautious use of the general anesthetic agent
- Potential for injury related to adverse drug reactions
- Potential for injury related to drug interactions with the general anesthetic agent
- Potential for injury related to increased cerebrospinal fluid and intraocular pressure caused by ketamine administration
- Potential for trauma related to halothane-induced liver necrosis

patient recovers from the effects of the administered anesthetic.

During surgery, the anesthesiologist or nurse anesthetist continuously monitors and adjusts the depth of anesthesia—the degree of CNS depression.

Stages of anesthesia

The depth of anesthesia is gauged in four stages, originally described for ether anesthesia in the 1920s.

Stage 1 – analgesia. This stage begins with onset of anesthesia and ends with loss of consciousness. Smell and pain sensations are lost before unconsciousness ensues. The patient may experience hallucinations and dreams. Inhalation anesthetics may cause coughing or choking at this stage if other anesthetic agents are not used.

Stage 2 – excitement. This stage begins with loss of consciousness. Reflexes become more prominent and respirations irregular; autonomic activity increases. Complications of anesthesia occur most commonly in this stage. Stages 1 and 2 correspond to induction of anesthesia.

Stage 3 – surgical anesthesia. This stage reaches the degree of anesthesia under which the procedure may be performed safely. Respirations normalize. Surgical anesthesia extends across four planes that represent increasing depth of anesthesia and diminution of reflexes and muscle tone. Precise maintenance of anesthesia depth is necessary for successful completion of a surgical procedure.

Stage 4 – medullary paralysis. Also referred to as the toxic stage, stage 4 signifies the loss of respirations and collapse of the circulatory system, requiring mechanical ventilation and perfusion. This stage, which represents anesthetic overdose, easily is avoided in clinical practice.

Anesthesia-related drugs

Apart from the general anesthesic agents, other drugs are used before, during, and after anesthesia to help manage the patient. Before surgery, the nurse anesthetist has two concerns: to allay the patient's anxiety over the procedure and to control secretions that could complicate the anesthesia. Other preoperative needs include producing amnesia for the period of the operation and combating postoperative nausea. Various drugs are used as preoperative medications, including antihistamines, opiates, sedatives, neuroleptics, and anticholinergics. (For more information about these medications, see *Selected preoperative medications*, page 368.)

Drugs used during surgery include neuromuscular blocking agents, which permit mechanical ventilation or allow access to areas guarded by large muscle groups, such as the abdomen. Other seemingly unrelated drugs, such as vasodilators, alpha-adrenergic blocking agents, ganglionic blocking agents, corticosteroids, vasopressors, and cardiac agents, are used during surgery to prevent or rectify various problems as well as to compensate for the effects of coexisting medical conditions.

Postoperative drugs are given to reverse the effects of drugs given before or during surgery. For example, atropine,

Selected preoperative medications

The nurse typically administers preoperative medications. Many drug combinations are used, but the most common is a narcotic combined with an antianxiety agent and a cholinergic blocking agent. The following are commonly administered preoperative drugs, their dosages, and actions. Before administration, the nurse should explain the drug effects to the patient, provide privacy by closing the curtains, and ensure safety by pulling up the bed side rails.

DRUG	DOSAGE	ACTION
Narcotics		
meperidine	50 to 100 mg I.M. or S.C. 30 to 90 minutes before surgery	Alters perception of, and emotional response to, pain
morphine	8 to 12 mg I.M. 30 to 90 minutes before surgery	Alters perception of, and emotional response to, pain
Barbiturates		
pentobarbital sodium	150 to 200 mg I.M. 40 to 60 minutes before surgery	Sedates the patient
secobarbital	200 to 300 mg P.O. 1 to 2 hours before surgery	Sedates the patient
Cholinergic blocking agents		
atropine	0.4 to 0.6 mg I.M. 45 to 60 minutes before surgery	Reduces secretions, vomiting, and laryngospasm
scopolamine	0.4 to 0.6 mg S.C. 45 to 60 minutes before surgery	Reduces secretions, vomiting, and laryngospasm
Antianxiety agents		
diazepam	5 to 10 mg I.V. immediately before surgery	Sedates the patient and reduces anxiety
hydroxyzine	25 to 100 mg I.M. 30 to 60 minutes before surgery	Reduces anxiety
midazolam	0.07 to 0.08 mg/kg I.M. 60 minutes before surgery	Sedates the patient and reduces anxiety

neostigmine, or pyridostigmine antagonizes neuromuscular blocking agents; naloxone reverses the effects of opiates; antiemetic antihistamines and major tranquilizers counteract the nausea from potent inhalation anesthetic agents; and opiates and other analgesics combat pain.

For a summary of representative drugs, see *Selected major drugs: General anesthetic agents,* page 377. For a listing of applicable nursing diagnoses that the nurse may formulate when caring for a patient receiving these agents, see *Selected nursing diagnoses: General anesthetic agents,* page 367. For detailed information on applying the nursing process, see Chapter 6, The Nursing Process and Drug Therapy.

INHALATION ANESTHETICS

Commonly used inhalation anesthetics include enflurane, halothane, isoflurane, and nitrous oxide. Another inhalation anesthetic, methoxyflurane, has limited use because it produces renal toxicity at high doses.

PHARMACOKINETICS

Inhalation anesthetics are absorbed at varying rates, distributed most rapidly to organs with high blood flow, metabolized, and excreted by the lungs and liver.

Absorption, distribution, metabolism, excretion

The absorption and elimination rates of an anesthetic are governed by the anesthetic's solubility in blood. Basically, the lower the solubility, the faster the absorption and elimination. Nitrous oxide, with the lowest solubility, is absorbed and eliminated the fastest, followed by isoflurane, enflurane, halothane, and methoxyflurane.

Absorption also is affected by alveolar ventilation—the provision of air or gas to the alveoli—and perfusion—the amount of blood passing through the alveoli. Such diseases as emphysema or congestive heart failure can increase or decrease the absorption of inhalation anesthetics by changing ventilation or perfusion.

Inhalation anesthetics enter the blood from the lungs and are distributed to other tissues. Distribution is most rapid to organs with high blood flow: the brain, liver, kidneys, and heart. All inhalation anesthetics cross the blood-brain barrier, some at greater concentrations than others. This characteristic determines the potency of the agent. Methoxyflurane is the most potent inhalation anesthetic. Halothane, isoflurane, enflurane, and nitrous oxide follow in order of decreasing potency.

The inhalation anesthetics are eliminated primarily by the lungs, but also by the liver in the case of enflurane, halothane, and methoxyflurane. Metabolites are excreted in the urine.

Onset, peak, duration

Onset of action and peak concentration levels of the inhalation anesthetics vary greatly, depending on therapeutic and patient factors. Therapeutic variables include the anesthetic concentration and the presence of other CNS-depressant drugs in the blood. Patient variables include age, pregnancy, respiratory and circulatory status, hypotension, and hypothermia.

The duration of action for each inhalation anesthetic is determined by the rate at which it leaves the brain.

PHARMACODYNAMICS

Inhalation anesthetics are general depressants of the CNS, although they affect other organ systems.

Mechanism of action

The ability of an inhalation anesthetic to enter the brain depends on its degree of lipid solubility. Movement of the inhalation anesthetics throughout the brain and spinal cord is rapid and efficient, but little more is known about their mechanism of action.

Usually, inhalation anesthetics depress the CNS, but paradoxically some seem to increase the potential for seizure activity. Outside the CNS, the halogenated anesthetics affect other organ systems. They interfere with nerve impulse transmission, relax skeletal and uterine smooth mus-

cles, reduce arterial blood pressure and redirect blood flow (which may endanger circulation in the brain and kidneys), decrease respirations, increase the fraction of carbon dioxide in the blood, depress the exchange of oxygen and carbon dioxide in the lungs, and decrease renal and hepatic blood flow and hepatic enzyme activity.

Nitrous oxide counteracts the cardiovascular effects of the halogenated anesthetics while increasing their anesthetic effects. It appears to have little effect on respiratory function alone but adds to respiratory depression when used with a halogenated agent. It has no effect on the musculature, liver, or gastrointestinal (GI) tract; long-term use may cause changes in red and white blood cell and vitamin production.

PHARMACOTHERAPEUTICS

Inhalation anesthetics are used for surgery because they offer more precise and rapid control of depth of anesthesia than injection anesthetics. Enflurane, halothane, isoflurane, and methoxyflurane are halogenated anesthetics, which are simple compounds. Their molecular structure consists of a hydrocarbon chain (usually an ether derivative, except for halothane). These anesthetics, which are liquids at room temperature, require a vaporizer and special delivery system for safe use. They may be administered only by skilled practitioners.

Of the inhalation anesthetics available, enflurane and isoflurane are the most commonly used, usually with nitrous oxide. Which anesthetic is used depends on a careful evaluation of the patient's physical condition, medical history, and medication profile; the type of surgical procedure; and an assessment of anticipated postoperative needs.

Inhalation anesthetics are administered as gases, so dosages are not expressed in weight, as with other drugs. Because the amount of anesthetic in the lungs is known to be proportional to the amount in the brain at equilibrium, the quantity of anesthetic agent needed can be determined by a measurement called the minimum alveolar concentration (MAC). MAC is the alveolar anesthetic concentration at which 50% of patients do not move during a surgical incision.

enflurane (Ethrane). During induction, enflurane causes marked CNS excitation, and seizures resembling generalized tonic-clonic seizures have been reported when high concentrations were administered to hypocapnic patients. *Usual adult dosage:* dosages are individualized and continuously monitored and altered throughout surgery.

halothane (Fluothane). Halothane relaxes the bronchial smooth muscle, making it useful for anesthesia during surgery on patients with asthma. Because halothane sensitizes the heart to the action of catecholamines, which may lead

to cardiac arrhythmias, catecholamine dosages should be reduced in patients receiving halothane. This inhalation anesthetic rarely is used for adults because of the risk of hepatotoxicity. However, it remains the primary anesthetic for children because they rarely exhibit halothane-related liver dysfunction.
Usual adult dosage: dosages are individualized and continuously monitored and altered throughout surgery.

isoflurane (Forane). Isoflurane produces the greatest degree of skeletal muscle relaxation of all the inhalation anesthetics. Because of its lack of serious toxicity, this agent currently is the most widely used inhalation anesthetic.
Usual adult dosage: dosages are individualized and continuously monitored and altered throughout surgery.

methoxyflurane (Penthrane). Because methoxyflurane can produce renal toxicity at high doses, it is used only occasionally for analgesia during obstetric procedures.
Usual adult dosage: dosages are individualized and continuously monitored and altered throughout labor.

nitrous oxide. A rapidly acting anesthetic agent, nitrous oxide produces little or no toxicity in clinically useful concentrations. Much less potent than the halogenated anesthetics, it is used primarily as an adjunct to them or to the injection anesthetics.
Usual adult dosage: dosages are individualized and continuously monitored and altered throughout surgery.

Drug interactions
The most important drug interactions involving inhalation anesthetics are with other CNS, cardiac, or respiratory depressant drugs. The potent anesthetics greatly enhance the depressant effects of normally safe concentrations of these drugs. (For details, see *Drug interactions: Inhalation anesthetics*.)

ADVERSE DRUG REACTIONS

Many adverse reactions can be planned for when the anesthesiologist or nurse anesthetist collects data preoperatively.

The most common adverse reaction associated with inhalation anesthetics is an exaggerated patient response to a normal dose. A surgical patient who is debilitated is predisposed to an exaggerated response, and even smaller-than-normal doses may result in hypotension, prolonged respiratory depression, and prolonged recovery. These effects can be avoided by using a detailed medical history before surgery to plan anesthesia. In elderly patients, confusion, agitation, and memory loss may accompany a prolonged recovery from the anesthesia and may be mistaken for signs of dementia.

The postoperative reactions are much the same as those seen with other CNS depressant drugs: cardiopulmonary depression, confusion, sedation, nausea, vomiting, ataxia, and hypothermia.

Methoxyflurane sometimes causes dose-related nephrotoxicity. Called high-output renal failure, the syndrome begins 2 to 4 days postoperatively as the patient suddenly produces massive amounts of dilute urine. Treatment involves aggressive maintenance of fluid and electrolyte balance; mortality has been reported as high as 50%, which accounts for the limited use of this drug.

Malignant hyperthermia, characterized by a sudden and often lethal increase in body temperature, is a serious and unexpected reaction to inhalation anesthetic agents. It occurs in genetically susceptible patients only and may result from a failure in calcium uptake by muscle cells. The skeletal muscle relaxant dantrolene is used to treat this condition.

In approximately 1 in 35,000 cases, liver necrosis develops several days after halothane use. Although it is not infective in origin, the necrosis resembles hepatitis clinically, so it is called halothane hepatitis. Symptoms include rash, fever, jaundice, nausea, vomiting, eosinophilia, and alterations in liver function. This often fatal syndrome occurs most commonly with multiple exposures to the drug. An immunologic or chemical response to a toxic metabolite may explain this phenomenon. Treatment is symptomatic.

NURSING PROCESS APPLICATION

The following information assists the nurse in caring for a patient who is receiving an inhalation anesthetic.

Assessment
• Review the patient's history for conditions that contraindicate the use of an inhalation anesthetic, such as known hypersensitivity to the anesthetic, hepatic disorders, or malignant hyperthermia.
• Assess the patient's history for conditions that require cautious use of an inhalation anesthetic, such as pregnancy or lactation.
• Assess the patient for adverse reactions to the inhalation anesthetic, such as an exaggerated response, hypotension, prolonged respiratory depression, confusion, ataxia, or nausea and vomiting.
• Assess the effectiveness of the inhalation anesthetic continuously throughout the procedure.
• Review the patient's medication history to identify use of drugs that may interact with the inhalation anesthetic, such as alcohol, labetalol, CNS depressants, xanthines, and neuromuscular blocking agents.
• Monitor the patient for temperature changes.
• Monitor the patient's fluid intake and output.

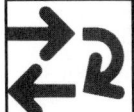

DRUG INTERACTIONS

Inhalation anesthetics

The most significant drug interactions involving inhalation anesthetics are caused by other central nervous system (CNS) depressants.

DRUG	INTERACTING DRUGS	POSSIBLE EFFECTS	NURSING IMPLICATIONS
enflurane, halothane, isoflurane, methoxyflurane, nitrous oxide	alcohol	Increases anesthetic requirement	• Monitor the patient's respirations, blood pressure, pulse rate, and level of consciousness.
	labetalol	Increases hypotensive effects	• Monitor the patient's blood pressure frequently.
	CNS depressants	Increase CNS and respiratory depression and cause hypotension	• Monitor the patient's rate and rhythm of respirations, level of consciousness, and blood pressure.
	xanthines (caffeine, theophylline)	Increase risk of arrhythmias	• Monitor the patient's pulse rate and characteristics, blood pressure, and respirations.
enflurane, halothane, isoflurane, methoxyflurane	neuromuscular blocking agents	Increase neuromuscular blockage	• Monitor the patient's respirations. • Monitor the patient's ability to move limbs as anesthesia diminishes.
	catecholamines (dopamine, epinephrine, norepinephrine), doxapram, ephedrine, metaraminol, methoxamine; other sympathomimetics	Increase risk of arrhythmias	• Monitor the patient's pulse rate and characteristics and blood pressure.
	ketamine	Increases risk of hypotension	• Monitor the patient's blood pressure and level of consciousness. • Provide supportive therapy, such as drugs, fluids, and volume expanders, as prescribed.
	ritodrine	Increases risk of hypotension and arrhythmias	• Monitor the patient's vital signs frequently.
	succinylcholine	Increases risk of malignant hyperthermia and neuromuscular blockade; repeated use increases risk of bradycardia	• Monitor the patient's temperature and other vital signs frequently. • Monitor the patient's airway and ability to move limbs.
	nondepolarizing blocking agents	Potentiate neuromuscular blockade	• Monitor the patient for signs of cardiovascular collapse, such as decreased heart rate and blood pressure.
enflurane	isoniazid	Increases release of nephrotoxic fluorine from enflurane	• Monitor the patient's urine output and blood urea nitrogen (BUN) and serum creatinine levels.
methoxyflurane	aminoglycosides, tetracyclines, barbiturates	Increase risk of nephrotoxicity	• Monitor the patient's urine output and BUN and serum creatinine levels.

• Evaluate the patient's and family's knowledge about the inhalation anesthetic to be used.

Nursing diagnoses
The following examples represent appropriate nursing diagnoses for a patient receiving an inhalation anesthetic.
• Potential for injury related to a preexisting condition that contraindicates the use of an inhalation anesthetic

• Potential for injury related to a preexisting condition that requires cautious use of an inhalation anesthetic
• Potential for injury related to adverse drug reactions
• Potential altered body temperature related to possible development of hypothermia or malignant hyperthermia during inhalation anesthetic administration
• Altered patterns of urinary elimination related to nephrotoxicity from methoxyflurane
• Knowledge deficit related to the inhalation anesthetic

Planning and implementation
• Know that an inhalation anesthetic must not be administered to a patient with a condition that contraindicates its use.
• Know that an inhalation anesthetic must be administered cautiously to a patient at risk because of a preexisting condition.
• Observe the patient for adverse reactions to the inhalation anesthetic throughout administration and recovery.
• Monitor the patient's vital signs frequently to detect potential problems. Assess the adequacy, rate, and depth of the patient's respirations. Maintain a patent airway. Assess the patient's level of consciousness, arousal, and orientation.
• Provide symptomatic care for a patient with adverse reactions, such as cardiovascular and respiratory depression, prolonged sedation, and nausea and vomiting; these reactions usually are reversible. Inform the anesthesiologist of severe adverse reactions.
• *Keep atropine available to reverse bradycardia, if prescribed.*
• Exercise extreme caution when giving additional analgesics before recovery from anesthesia is complete. The analgesic dose will vary, depending on the residual analgesic effect of the inhalation anesthetic. Monitor closely for signs of respiratory depression if the patient receives narcotic analgesics for pain control within 8 hours of surgery.
• *Take safety precautions, such as helping the patient with ambulation and keeping the bed in a low position.*
• Assess for confusion, agitation, and memory loss in an elderly patient; these may signal prolonged recovery from the anesthesia, rather than dementia.
• Monitor the patient's temperature frequently. Be aware that hypothermia is a common effect of inhalation anesthesia and that shivering is normal during recovery. If the patient is shivering, administer oxygen, as prescribed, to compensate for the increased oxygen demand.
• Keep the patient warm if hypothermia occurs.
• *Notify the anesthesiologist immediately if the patient's temperature increases suddenly. This may signal malignant hyperthermia, a sudden, potentially lethal reaction to the inhalation anesthetic.*

• *Keep dantrolene readily available to treat malignant hyperthermia.*
• *Record the patient's fluid intake and output until discharge. Be aware that high-output renal failure may occur 2 to 4 days after the use of methoxyflurane.*
• *Notify the physician immediately if massive diuresis occurs.*

Patient teaching
• Teach the patient and family the name, action, and adverse effects of the inhalation anesthetic to be used.
• Advise the patient not to eat for at least 8 hours before surgery to prevent aspiration of stomach contents into the lungs during anesthesia.
• Inform the patient that psychomotor functions may be impaired for 24 hours or more after inhalation anesthesia.
• Advise the patient not to drink alcohol or use any other CNS depressants for at least 24 hours after anesthesia.
• Instruct the patient to report any adverse reactions or unusual symptoms to the physician immediately.

Evaluation
The following examples represent appropriate evaluation statements for a patient receiving an inhalation anesthetic.
• The patient has no conditions that contraindicate the use of an inhalation anesthetic.
• The patient exhibits no signs of complications in the preexisting condition linked to the inhalation anesthetic.
• The patient demonstrates no adverse reactions to the inhalation anesthetic.
• The patient maintains a normal body temperature.
• The patient maintains normal renal function after receiving methoxyflurane.
• The patient and family express an appropriate understanding of the points taughts about the inhalation anesthetic.
• The patient reports that the last meal was eaten 10 hours before surgery.

INJECTION ANESTHETICS

Injection anesthetics usually are used in situations requiring a short duration of anesthesia, such as outpatient surgery. The injection anesthetics also are used to promote rapid induction of anesthesia or to supplement inhalation anesthetics.

This section discusses the following injection anesthetics: alfentanil, diazepam, droperidol, etomidate, fentanyl citrate, ketamine hydrochloride, lorazepam, meperidine hydrochloride, methohexital sodium, midazolam hydrochloride, morphine sulfate, propofol, sufentanil citrate, thiamylal sodium, and thiopental sodium.

Four agents in this class — droperidol, etomidate, propofol, and ketamine hydrochloride — are used solely as injected general anesthetics. The rest are drawn from other chemical categories, such as barbiturates and benzodiazepines, and are used secondarily as anesthetics. Detailed considerations of primary uses of barbiturates and benzodiazepines appear in Chapter 25, Sedative and Hypnotic Agents, and Chapter 27, Antianxiety Agents.

PHARMACOKINETICS

All injection anesthetics bypass the mechanisms that reduce bioavailability, distributing rapidly into the CNS.

Absorption, distribution, metabolism, excretion
Effects of the injection anesthetics appear quickly, beginning 15 seconds to a few minutes after administration. Intramuscular (I.M.) injection of the opiates may delay absorption and decrease peak effect when compared to I.V. administration.

The barbiturates depend on hepatic transformation for elimination, as do the benzodiazepine and opiate agents and the hypnotic etomidate.

Onset, peak, duration
All the injection anesthetics have a rapid onset of action and are short-acting, except for diazepam, which is long-acting. Etomidate, the opiates, propofol, and the barbiturates begin to act within 60 seconds; the benzodiazepines act within 1 to 15 minutes. The opiates reach peak concentration levels in 3 to 20 minutes. Rapid redistribution of barbiturates, propofol, etomidate, and ketamine from the brain to other tissues ends anesthetic action; therefore, their duration of action is much shorter than would be anticipated from their half-lives.

PHARMACODYNAMICS

Because the injection anesthetics come from different chemical classes, their mechanisms of action differ.

Mechanism of action
Barbiturates seem to enhance responses to the CNS neurotransmitter gamma-aminobutyric acid (GABA) and to depress the excitability of CNS neurons. The benzodiazepines also stimulate responses to GABA, thus inhibiting the brain's response to stimulation of the reticular activating system (RAS), the area of the brain stem that controls alertness. Etomidate, too, may have GABA-like effects, including direct inhibition of the RAS. Droperidol induces neurolepsis by blocking postsynaptic dopamine receptors

in sections of the brain. The opiates occupy sites on specialized receptors scattered throughout the CNS and modify the release of neurotransmitters from sensory nerves entering the CNS. Ketamine appears to interact with N-methyl-D-aspartate receptors, which may account for its inhibitory anesthetic action.

PHARMACOTHERAPEUTICS

The short duration of action of these agents is an advantage in shorter surgical procedures — including outpatient surgery. However, only skilled practitioners may administer these agents for anesthesia.

The subcategories of injection anesthetics have various pharmacologic characteristics. The barbiturates are used alone in surgery that is not expected to be painful and as adjuncts to other agents in more extensive procedures. The benzodiazepines produce sedation and amnesia, but not analgesia. Etomidate is used to induce anesthesia and to supplement low-potency inhalation anesthetics such as nitrous oxide. The opiates provide analgesia and supplement other anesthetic agents. Droperidol is used with analgesics, but rarely alone.

alfentanil (Alfenta). An ultra-short-acting drug, alfentanil may be used with nitrous oxide, with a barbiturate and nitrous oxide, or as the primary anesthetic in surgery in which ventilatory assistance is maintained.
Usual adult dosage: for induction of anesthesia, 130 to 245 mcg/kg of body weight I.V., followed by an infusion of 0.5 to 1.5 mcg/kg/minute; for analgesia, 8 to 20 mcg/kg of body weight I.V., followed by 3 to 5 mcg/kg or a continuous infusion of 0.5 to 1 mcg/kg/minute in patients who will breathe unassisted; dose in ventilator patients is 20 to 50 mcg/kg I.V., followed by incremental doses of 5 to 15 mcg/kg.

diazepam (Valium). A widely used benzodiazepine, diazepam is used to increase the sedative and amnesic effects of other anesthetic agents.
Usual adult dosage: 10 to 20 mg I.M. or I.V. before surgery.

droperidol (Inapsine). Droperidol is the only neuroleptic agent used for general anesthesia.
Usual adult dosage: for induction, 2.5 mg/9 to 11 kg of body weight I.V. with an analgesic or a general anesthetic; for maintenance, 1.25 to 2.5 mg I.V.

etomidate (Amidate). Etomidate is used to induce anesthesia rapidly or to augment another anesthetic agent during maintenance anesthesia.
Usual adult dosage: for induction, 0.2 to 0.6 mg/kg of body weight I.V., administered over 30 to 60 seconds; for main-

tenance, smaller individual I.V. doses or a continuous I.V. infusion.

fentanyl citrate (Sublimaze). A narcotic analgesic, fentanyl is one of a series of compounds with potent but brief opiate-like activity. Fentanyl is used as an adjunct to general anesthesia, in balanced anesthesia, as a primary drug for induction of anesthesia, and as a preoperative and postoperative analgesic.
Usual adult dosage: for induction, 0.05 to 0.1 mg/kg of body weight by slow I.V.; as an adjunct to general anesthesia, 0.002 to 0.05 mg/kg of body weight I.V., depending on the procedure and on other agents used. In balanced anesthesia, 0.05 to 0.1 mg/kg of body weight I.V. For preoperative analgesia, 0.05 to 0.1 mg I.M. 30 to 60 minutes before surgery. For postoperative analgesia, 0.05 to 0.1 mg I.M., repeated in 1 to 2 hours if necessary.

ketamine hydrochloride (Ketalar). Used as an anesthetic in minor surgical or diagnostic procedures, ketamine also is used for induction or as the sole anesthetic agent in high-risk patients for whom cardiac or respiratory depressant drugs are contraindicated.
Usual adult dosage: for induction, 1 to 2 mg/kg of body weight I.V. or 5 to 10 mg/kg of body weight I.M.; for maintenance, 0.1 to 0.5 mg/minute by slow I.V. microdrip infusion, adjusted according to the patient's vital signs and response.

lorazepam (Ativan). A benzodiazepine, lorazepam is used mainly to induce anterograde amnesia.
Usual adult dosage: 0.05 mg/kg of body weight (to a maximum of 4 mg) I.M. at least 2 hours before surgery or 0.044 mg/kg of body weight (to a maximum of 2 mg) I.V. at least 15 minutes before anesthesia.

meperidine hydrochloride (Demerol). An opiate, meperidine is used as an adjunct to general anesthesia, as an obstetric anesthetic, and as a preoperative analgesic.
Usual adult dosage: as an adjunct, dose is dependent on patient response, delivered I.V. by repeated slow injection or continuous infusion; for obstetric anesthesia, 50 to 100 mg I.M. or S.C. at 1- to 3-hour intervals when contractions are regular; as a preoperative analgesic, 50 to 100 mg I.M. 30 to 90 minutes before surgery.

methohexital sodium (Brevital). Methohexital is a barbiturate used where a short duration of action is tolerable or desirable, as in anesthesia for electroshock therapy.
Usual adult dosage: for induction, 5 to 12 ml (50 to 120 mg) I.V. as a 1% solution (some sources recommend a 2-ml test dose before the induction dose); for maintenance, 2 to 4 ml (20 to 40 mg) I.V. as a 1% solution for 5 to 7 minutes of anesthesia. Some anesthesiologists prefer a con-

tinuous infusion of a 0.2% solution with the rate modulated to the patient's response.

midazolam hydrochloride (Versed). Midazolam is a benzodiazepine used for preoperative sedation, induction of anesthesia, or maintenance of anesthesia in short procedures.
Usual adult dosage: for preoperative sedation, 0.07 to 0.08 mg/kg I.M. 1 hour before surgery; for induction in premedicated patients, 150 to 350 mcg/kg I.V.; for induction in nonpremedicated patients, 200 to 350 mcg/kg I.V. Dosage is titrated according to the patient's age and clinical status.

morphine sulfate. Like meperidine, the opiate morphine is used as an adjunct to general anesthesia, as an obstetric anesthetic, and as a preoperative analgesic.
Usual adult dosage: as an adjunct, dose is dependent on patient response, delivered I.V. by continuous infusion; for obstetric anesthesia, 10 mg I.M. or S.C.; as a preoperative analgesic, 5 to 12 mg I.M. or S.C.

propofol (Diprivan). Propofol is a short-acting anesthetic used for induction and maintenance in balanced anesthesia.
Usual adult dosage: for induction, 2 to 2.5 mg/kg of body weight I.V.; for maintenance, 0.1 to 0.2 mg/kg/minute by I.V. infusion or 25 to 50 mg by intermittent bolus injection.

sufentanil citrate (Sufenta). A derivative of fentanyl, sufentanil is approximately eight times as potent as its parent drug, but somewhat shorter-acting. Sufentanil is used as an adjunct to other anesthetics and in balanced anesthesia.
Usual adult dosage: as an adjunct, initially 1 to 2 mcg/kg of body weight I.V., depending on the procedure and other agents used, with supplemental doses of 10 to 25 mcg/kg of body weight I.V., as necessary; in balanced anesthesia, initially 8 to 30 mcg/kg of body weight I.V., with supplemental doses of 25 to 50 mcg/kg of body weight I.V., as necessary.

thiamylal sodium (Surital). Thiamylal is an ultra-short-acting barbiturate used where a short duration of action is tolerable or desirable, as in anesthesia for electroshock therapy.
Usual adult dosage: for induction of anesthesia, 3 to 5 mg/kg of body weight I.V. as a 2.5% solution (a 2-ml test dose sometimes is recommended). For maintenance, 50 to 100 mg I.V. as a 2.5% solution every 30 to 40 seconds until the desired effect is obtained.

thiopental sodium (Pentothal Sodium). Thiopental is an ultra-short-acting barbiturate used where a short duration of action is tolerable or desirable, as in anesthesia for electroshock therapy.

Usual adult dosage: for induction, 3 to 4 mg/kg of body weight I.V. or 2 to 3 ml (50 to 75 mg) every 30 to 40 seconds until the desired effect is obtained, as a 2.5% solution (a 1- to 3-ml test dose sometimes is given). For maintenance, 2 to 4 ml (50 to 100 mg), as required. Some anesthesiologists use continuous infusions of 0.2% to 0.4% solutions; the dose is adjusted by altering the infusion rate.

Drug interactions

Injection anesthetics interact with many other drugs. As with the inhalation anesthetics, most of these interactions require the nurse to monitor the patient's vital signs, airway, and level of consciousness. The opiates, barbiturates, and benzodiazepines and their interactions are covered in Chapter 22, Narcotic Agonist and Antagonist Agents; Chapter 25, Sedative and Hypnotic Agents; and Chapter 27, Antianxiety Agents. (For more information on drugs that interact with droperidol, etomidate, ketamine, and propofol, see *Drug interactions: Injection anesthetics,* page 376.)

ADVERSE DRUG REACTIONS

Adverse reactions to the injection anesthetics frequently are extensions of their therapeutic effects.

Adverse CNS reactions are most common after ketamine anesthesia; they include prolonged recovery, unpleasant dreams, irrational behavior, excitement, disorientation, delirium, and hallucinations. The barbiturates and propofol cause respiratory depression. Thiopental, etomidate, and propofol can produce airway reflex hyperactivity with hiccoughs, coughing, and muscle twitching and jerking. Thiopental also depresses cardiac function and causes peripheral vasodilation, whereas ketamine increases heart rate, cardiac output, and blood pressure in patients who are not severely ill. The opiates sometimes cause changes in heart rate, including arrhythmias. The rare circulatory failure and respiratory arrest seen with the benzodiazepines appear to be associated with too-rapid drug administration or concomitant narcotic administration. Phlebitis has been reported with diazepam administration.

Muscle rigidity and spasms follow administration of several of the injection anesthetics, including ketamine and the opiates; the reaction seems to be directly proportional to the infusion rate. Fentanyl and ketamine may cause seizures. Extrapyramidal manifestations are the most prominent adverse reactions to droperidol.

Etomidate, ketamine, and propofol can cause nausea and vomiting. Ketamine also may produce excess salivation, tearing, shivering, and increased cerebrospinal fluid and intraccular pressure. In a patient under stress, etomidate may cause reduced cortisol levels. The only other major adverse reaction to etomidate is pain on administration, which can be avoided by rapid administration into a large vein or with use of a preoperative analgesic.

Rash and hypersensitivity reactions are uncommon with etomidate, the opiates, and the barbiturates; anaphylaxis has been reported with the barbiturates only. Extravasation of the barbiturates may cause neuritis and vasospasm.

NURSING PROCESS APPLICATION

The following information assists the nurse in caring for a patient who is receiving an injection anesthetic.

Assessment

• Review the patient's history for conditions that contraindicate the use of an injection anesthetic, such as known hypersensitivity to the drug or acute intermittent porphyria.
• Review the patient's history for conditions that require cautious use of an injection anesthetic, such as cardiovascular disease, increased intracranial pressure, or pregnancy.
• Assess the patient for adverse reactions to the injection anesthetic, such as excitement, disorientation, respiratory depression, altered cardiac function, decreased cortisol levels, muscle rigidity, and spasms.
• Review the patient's medication history to identify use of drugs that may interact with the injection anesthetic, such as CNS depressants, hypotensive agents, antidepressants, or inhalation anesthetics..
• Assess the effectiveness of the injection anesthetic throughout the procedure.
• Assess the patient's respiratory status continuously.
• Assess the patient for discomfort.
• Evaluate the patient's and family's knowledge about the injection anesthetic to be used.

Nursing diagnoses

The following examples represent appropriate nursing diagnoses for a patient receiving an injection anesthetic.
• Potential for injury related to a preexisting condition that contraindicates the use of an injection anesthetic
• Potential for injury related to a preexisting condition that requires cautious use of an injection anesthetic
• Potential for injury related to adverse drug reactions
• Ineffective breathing pattern related to the adverse respiratory effects of the injection anesthetic
• Pain related to administration of the injection anesthetic
• Knowledge deficit related to the injection anesthetic

Planning and implementation

• Know that an injection anesthetic must not be administered to a patient with a condition that contraindicates its use.
• Be aware that an injection anesthetic must be administered cautiously to a patient at risk because of a preexisting condition.
• Monitor the patient for adverse reactions throughout injection anesthetic administration and recovery.

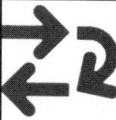

DRUG INTERACTIONS

Injection anesthetics

Because drug interactions involving the injection anesthetics can cause increased central nervous system (CNS) depression and hypotension, the nurse must assess the patient's vital signs and level of consciousness frequently.

DRUG	INTERACTING DRUGS	POSSIBLE EFFECTS	NURSING IMPLICATIONS
droperidol	CNS depressants	Increase CNS depressant effects	• Monitor the patient's vital signs, level of consciousness, and ability to move limbs.
	hypotensive agents	Increase hypotensive effects	• Monitor the patient's blood pressure frequently.
	neuroleptics, metoclopramide	Increase risk of extrapyramidal effects	• Monitor the patient for tremors. • Monitor the patient's vital signs.
etomidate	antidepressants, antihypertensives with CNS depressant effects, magnesium sulfate, monoamine oxidase inhibitors	Increase CNS depressant effects	• Monitor the patient's vital signs, level of consciousness, and ability to move limbs.
	hypotensive agents	Increase hypotensive effects	• Monitor the patient's blood pressure frequently.
ketamine	inhalation anesthetics	Increase risk of hypotension, decrease cardiac output	• Monitor the patient's vital signs, level of consciousness, and ability to move limbs.
	antihypertensives with CNS depressant effects (reserpine, clonidine, and methyldopa)	Increase risk of hypotension and respiratory depression	• Monitor the patient's blood pressure and respirations frequently.
propofol	benzodiazepines, opiates, barbiturates, chloral hydrate, droperidol	Increase effects of propofol	• Expect the propofol dosage to be reduced. • Monitor the patient's blood pressure and cardiac output carefully.

• Observe for extrapyramidal reactions in a patient receiving droperidol.

• Monitor the patient's vital signs before, during, and after injection anesthetic administration.

• *Keep resuscitative equipment and emergency drugs readily available.*

• *Keep I.V. fluids and vasopressors readily available to treat hypotension, as prescribed, for a patient receiving thiopental.*

• *Be aware that barbiturates and ketamine should not be mixed in the same syringe; they are chemically incompatible.*

• *Expect to see methohexital used with dextrose 5% in water (D_5W) or normal saline solution because it is incompatible with lactated Ringer's solution or acid drug solutions, such as atropine.*

• *Know that ampules of propofol must be shaken well before use to distribute the emulsion evenly.*

• *Expect propofol to be prepared using sterile technique because it is dissolved in an I.V. fat emulsion, which gives it a high potential for bacterial infection.*

• Use glass containers for propofol solutions because plastic containers hasten the drug's loss of potency.

• Provide physical support for the patient during injection anesthetic administration because the onset of action is rapid.

• Keep environmental stimulation to a minimum to prevent emergence reactions, such as excitement and restlessness.

• Prepare to administer an exogenous corticosteroid replacement, if prescribed.

• *Notify the physician immediately if adverse reactions occur.*

• *Observe for respiratory depression in a patient receiving a barbiturate or propofol; and for airway reflex hyperactivity with hiccoughs, coughing, and muscle twitching in a patient receiving thiopental, etomidate, or propofol.*

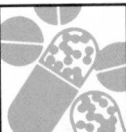

SELECTED MAJOR DRUGS

General anesthetic agents

This chart summarizes the major inhalation and injection anesthetics currently in clinical use.

DRUG	MAJOR INDICATIONS	USUAL ADULT DOSAGES	CONTRAINDICATIONS AND PRECAUTIONS
Inhalation anesthetics			
isoflurane	General anesthesia	Individualized and continuously monitored and altered throughout surgery	• Know that isoflurane is contraindicated in a patient with known hypersensitivity to this drug or other halogenated anesthetics or with known or suspected genetic susceptibility to malignant hyperthermia. • Administer with caution to a pregnant or lactating patient.
nitrous oxide	General anesthesia	Individualized and continuously monitored and altered throughout surgery	• Know that nitrous oxide is contraindicated in a patient with known hypersensitivity to this drug. • Administer with caution to a pregnant or lactating patient.
Injection anesthetics			
etomidate	General anesthesia induction and maintenance	For induction, 0.2 to 0.6 mg/kg of body weight I.V. over 30 to 60 seconds; for maintenance, smaller individual I.V. doses or a continuous I.V. infusion	• Know that etomidate is contraindicated during labor and delivery, including cesarean deliveries.
fentanyl	Preoperative analgesia Adjunct to general anesthesia	0.05 to 0.1 mg I.M. 30 to 60 minutes before surgery 0.002 to 0.05 mg/kg of body weight I.V.	• Know that fentanyl is contraindicated in a patient with known intolerance to the drug. • Administer with caution to a pregnant or lactating patient or one with head injury, brain tumor, chronic obstructive pulmonary disease, decreased respiratory reserve, potentially compromised respirations, impaired hepatic or renal function, or bradyarrhythmias.
ketamine	General anesthesia induction and maintenance	For induction, 1 to 2 mg/kg of body weight I.V. or 5 to 10 mg/kg of body weight I.M.; for maintenance, adjusted according to the patient's vital signs and response	• Know that ketamine is contraindicated in a patient with a history of stroke; with significant hypertension or severe cardiac decompensation; in one who would be endangered by a significant rise in blood pressure; and in surgery of the pharynx, larynx, or bronchial tree (unless used with muscle relaxants). • Administer with caution to a pregnant or lactating patient, chronic alcoholic patient, alcohol-intoxicated patient, or a patient with elevated cerebrospinal fluid pressure.
thiopental sodium	General anesthesia induction and maintenance	For induction, 3 to 4 mg/kg of body weight I.V. as a 2.5% solution; for maintenance, 50 to 100 mg I.V., as required	• Know that thiopental sodium is contraindicated in a patient with known hypersensitivity to barbiturates or one with variegate or acute intermittent porphyria. • Administer with extreme caution to a patient with severe cardiovascular disease, hypotension, shock, a condition in which the hypnotic effect may be prolonged or potentiated, or status asthmaticus. • Administer with caution to a pregnant patient or one with cardiac disease, increased intracranial pressure, ophthalmoplegia, asthma, myasthenia gravis, or endocrine insufficiency.

• *Monitor the patient's respiratory status throughout the administration of, and recovery from, an injection anesthetic.*

• *Know that a benzodiazepine should not be administered too rapidly or concurrently with a narcotic agent; respiratory arrest can result.*

• *Notify the physician of changes in the patient's respiratory status.*

• Watch for muscle rigidity and spasms after administration of ketamine and an opiate; these signs are directly proportional to the infusion rate.

• *Expect to see etomidate administered rapidly into a large vein or with a preoperative analgesic to prevent pain during administration.*

• Monitor the patient's I.V. site closely; barbiturate extravasation may cause neuritis and vasospasm, resulting in pain.

• Notify the physician if pain occurs with injection anesthetic administration.

Patient teaching

• Teach the patient and family the name, action, and adverse effects of the injection anesthetic to be used.

• Advise the patient not to eat for at least 8 hours before surgery.

• Instruct the patient not to drink alcohol or use any other CNS depressants for at least 24 hours after receiving an injection anesthetic.

• Stress the importance of notifying the nurse or physician of any unusual symptoms up to 24 hours after receiving an injection anesthetic.

Evaluation

The following examples represent appropriate evaluation statements for a patient receiving an injection anesthetic.

• The patient has no conditions that contraindicate the use of the injection anesthetic.

• The patient exhibits no signs of complications in the preexisting condition linked to the injection anesthetic.

• The patient displays no adverse reactions to the injection anesthetic.

• The patient maintains adequate ventilation throughout injection anesthetic administration.

• The patient shows no signs of pain.

• The patient and family express an accurate understanding of the points taught about the injection anesthetic to be used.

• The patient reports that the last meal was eaten 12 hours before surgery.

COMBINATION ANESTHETICS

Two or more anesthetics used together to produce a desired anesthesia state constitute a combination anesthetic. The two types of combination anesthetics are neuroleptanesthesia and balanced anesthesia.

Neuroleptanalgesia is a state of altered consciousness free of pain from administration of an opiate analgesic and a neuroleptic drug (an antipsychotic drug without hypnotic effects, such as a tranquilizer). When nitrous oxide is added, neuroleptanesthesia results: the patient is unconscious but can be roused easily if necessary. Neuroleptanesthesia is valuable when the patient's cooperation is necessary during surgery.

The drugs most commonly used in neuroleptanesthesia are droperidol and fentanyl, although diazepam and ketamine also have been combined with other opiates, such as meperidine, morphine, and pentazocine.

Balanced anesthesia combines nitrous oxide with a more potent general anesthetic, such as a barbiturate, and with an opiate analgesic and a neuromuscular blocking agent. The opiate is given as premedication; the barbiturate and nitrous oxide induce anesthesia. The opiate is given again in small doses after induction to provide the desired level of analgesia. The neuromuscular blocking agent makes surgical manipulation easier, but it requires assisted ventilation.

A common balanced anesthesia combination includes fentanyl (opiate) and thiopental (barbiturate) with atropine (cholinergic blocking agent), nitrous oxide, and a neuromuscular blocking agent such as succinylcholine. Morphine may be used instead of fentanyl in patients for whom minimal cardiovascular effects are desired.

Naloxone, which reverses the effects of opiates, commonly is used at the end of surgery to reduce postoperative analgesia. The patient must be observed frequently until the analgesic is eliminated from the body.

When properly administered, balanced anesthesia minimizes cardiovascular effects, allows an early return of consciousness, and prevents postoperative nausea, vomiting, excitement, and pain.

Balanced anesthesia is contraindicated in patients who cannot tolerate FIO_2 of 25% to 40% or whose anemia limits the ability of the blood to carry oxygen.

CHAPTER SUMMARY

Chapter 23 explained the types of anesthesia and presented the inhalation and injection general anesthetics that produce them. Here are the chapter highlights.

• General anesthesia may be induced with one or combined agents. These drugs are volatile liquids or gases vaporized in oxygen and administered by inhalation or nonvolatile solutions administered by injection.

• Anesthesia administration is divided into three parts: induction, maintenance, and emergence.

• The four stages of anesthesia include stage 1, analgesia; stage 2, excitement; stage 3, surgical anesthesia; and stage 4, medullary paralysis. Depth of anesthesia must be controlled precisely to permit successful surgery.

• Medications may be administered before surgery to sedate the patient, cause amnesia, or prevent undesirable conditions during surgery. Preoperative medications may include antihistamines, opiates, sedatives, neuroleptics, and anticholinergics.

• Enflurane, halothane, isoflurane, methoxyflurane, and nitrous oxide are the inhalation anesthetics in current use.

• Four agents—droperidol, etomidate, ketamine, and propofol—are used solely as injection anesthetics. Drugs from other categories, such as barbiturates and benzodiazepines, are used secondarily as injection anesthetics.

• Many drugs interact with inhalation and injection anesthetics; thus, caution is needed when medicating a patient after anesthesia.

• Anesthetics can be combined to produce neuroleptanesthesia or balanced anesthesia. Neuroleptanesthesia produces an unconscious patient who can be roused easily. Balanced anesthesia minimizes cardiovascular effects, allows an early return to consciousness, and prevents certain postoperative adverse reactions.

• Although an anesthesiologist or nurse anesthetist typically administers general anesthetics, the nurse uses the nursing process to provide patient care. For all general anesthetics, the nurse must monitor the patient's vital signs closely, maintain airway patency, and observe the return to consciousness.

STUDY QUESTIONS

See Appendix 1 for answers.

1. Richard Deglin, age 35, is scheduled to receive the inhalation anesthetics halothane and nitrous oxide before surgery to repair a torn Achilles tendon. During which stage of anesthesia do complications occur most commonly?
(a) stage 1
(b) stage 2
(c) stage 3
(d) stage 4

2. Absorption and elimination of inhalation anesthetics depend primarily on which factor?
(a) the patient's renal function
(b) the patient's liver function
(c) previous exposure to anesthesia
(d) the drug's solubility in blood

3. What determines the potency of the inhalation anesthetic agent Mr. Deglin will receive?
(a) the rate of drug absorption
(b) the drug concentration that crosses the blood-brain barrier
(c) the elimination route of the drug and any metabolites
(d) the amount of alveolar ventilation and perfusion

4. What is the advantage of using an inhalation over an injection anesthetic?
(a) Inhalation anesthetics produce a longer stage 2 than injection anesthetics.
(b) Inhalation anesthetics produce more precise and rapid control of anesthesia depth.
(c) Inhalation anesthetics are absorbed more quickly than injection anesthetics.
(d) Inhalation anesthetics are distributed more evenly than injection anesthetics.

5. The nurse monitors Mr. Deglin for adverse reactions. What is the most common adverse reaction to inhalation anesthetics?
(a) nausea and vomiting
(b) respiratory distress
(c) hypersensitivity reaction
(d) exaggerated response to a normal dose

6. Linda Dean, age 49, is about to undergo outpatient surgery to repair a broken finger. Which type of anesthesia is most likely to be used for this type of surgery?
(a) injection anesthesia
(b) balanced anesthesia
(c) neuroleptanesthesia
(d) inhalation anesthesia

7. Ms. Dean receives ketamine. During ketamine administration, the nurse should assess carefully for which adverse reaction?
(a) high blood pressure
(b) low blood pressure
(c) increased respiratory rate
(d) severe bradycardia

8. Amy Chen, 28, is scheduled for a cesarean delivery. During this procedure, she will receive neuroleptanesthesia. What are the major advantages of this type of anesthesia?
(a) It minimizes cardiovascular effects.
(b) It reduces postoperative nausea and vomiting.
(c) It allows easy arousal of the patient.
(d) It reduces postoperative excitement.

SELECTED REFERENCES

AHFS drug information 90. (1990). Bethesda, MD: American Society of Hospital Pharmacists.

Civetta, J. (1988, July 14). Perioperative effects of anesthesia. *Current Review for Nurse Anesthetists,* 11(3), 18-24.

General vs. spinal anesthesia in the elderly. (1988, February). *Nurses Drug Alert,* 12(2), 9-10.

Gravenstein, J. (1988, January 30). The induction of general anesthesia. *Current Review for Nurse Anesthetists,* 11(2), 11-16.

Hansten, P., and Horn, J. (1989). *Drug interactions* (6th ed.). Philadelphia: Lea & Febiger.

Marshall, B., and Long-Necker, D. (1990). General anesthetics. In A. Gilman, et al. (Eds.), *Goodman and Gilman's the pharmacological basis of therapeutics* (8th ed.; pp. 285-310). Elmsford, NY: Pergamon Press.

Marshall, M. (1989, March/April). Demystifying general anesthesia. *Canadian Critical Care Nursing Journal,* 6(1), 13-19.

Drug facts and comparisons. (1991). St. Louis: Facts and Comparisons Division. J.B. Lippincott.

Miller, R. (1990). *Anesthesia* (3rd ed.). New York: Churchill Livingstone.

Smith, N., Miller, R., and Corbascio, A. (1981). *Drug interactions in anesthesia.* Philadelphia: Lea & Febiger.

USPDI. (1991). *Drug information for the health care professional* (Vol. I). Rockville, MD: United States Pharmacopeial Convention.

LOCAL AND TOPICAL ANESTHETIC AGENTS

OBJECTIVES

After reading and studying this chapter, the student should be able to:

1. Differentiate between local and topical anesthetics.

2. Describe how pain impulses are conducted in the body.

3. Explain how a nerve block works.

4. Identify the major drug interactions and adverse reactions for local and topical anesthetics.

5. Explain why vasoconstrictors sometimes are used with local anesthetics.

6. Explain why local anesthetics without preservatives must be used in certain nerve block procedures.

7. Describe how to apply the nursing process when caring for a patient who is receiving a local or topical anesthetic agent.

INTRODUCTION

Local and topical anesthetics are used to interrupt the transmission of pain impulses from peripheral nerves by causing a temporary loss of sensation in a limited area of the body. Local anesthetics must be injected to produce anesthesia; topical anesthetics are applied directly to the skin or mucous membranes. Some local anesthetics can be used topically.

Physiology of pain

Pain is one of the brain's interpretations of signals sent from nerve endings in the skin and other tissues. These signals are transmitted by the peripheral and central nervous systems. Researchers are unclear about the characteristics of the stimuli that produce the cerebral interpretation of pain.

Nerve cells transmit an electrical impulse that results from differences in the intracellular and extracellular fluids and the semipermeable cell membrane that separates them. The exterior surface of the cell membrane normally carries a positive electrical charge produced by extracellular sodium concentrations. The charge of the interior surface is more negative than that of the exterior. This relative negative charge results mainly from the lower concentration of positive charges—mostly potassium—found in the interior. When a painful stimulus activates the free nerve endings, the permeability of the membrane temporarily changes, allowing sodium to enter the cell and potassium to leave. This shift in the content of intracellular and extracellular fluids, called depolarization, changes the electrical charge of the membrane, allowing an electrical impulse to be transmitted.

The electrical current from one stimulated nerve cell is transmitted to adjoining cells, causing similar shifts in fluid content and electrical charge. These shifts continue toward the spinal cord, travel through the cord, and enter the brain.

After a nerve cell transmits the current, it pumps sodium out through the membrane and returns to its original condition, ready to send another impulse; this is repolarization.

Different types of nerves exist in different parts of the body. Large nerves, coated with a protein called myelin, relay pain messages in the spinal nerves of the central nervous system (CNS) and proximal parts of the autonomic nervous system (ANS). These myelinated nerves transmit information much faster than the smaller, uncoated nerves found in the ANS. Both types of nerves may relay pain messages at the same time, but the patient will feel the two types of pain at slightly different times. The first sensation—a sharp, penetrating pain—occurs immediately after the stimulus and comes from the large, myelinated fibers. The second sensation—a burning pain—appears shortly after the first and probably is transmitted by small, nonmyelinated nerves.

Local and topical anesthetics

The following nursing diagnoses address representative problems and etiologies that a nurse may encounter when caring for a patient who is receiving a local or topical anesthetic agent. Some of these nursing diagnoses contain generalized etiologies, which the nurse must individualize based on the patient's needs. (For some common nursing diagnoses and related interventions for each drug class, see the "Nursing Process Application" sections of this chapter.)

- Anxiety related to high plasma concentration of a local anesthetic
- Altered thought processes related to the adverse central nervous system (CNS) effects of a local or topical anesthetic
- Decreased cardiac output related to myocardial depression from use of a local or topical anesthetic
- Impaired gas exchange related to local anesthetic-induced methemoglobinemia
- Impaired tissue integrity related to tissue necrosis and sloughing at the injection site of a local anesthetic
- Ineffective breathing pattern related to CNS depression caused by a local or topical anesthetic
- Knowledge deficit related to the prescribed local or topical anesthetic
- Pain related to use of a local anesthetic with a vasoconstrictor
- Potential for injury related to a preexisting condition that contraindicates the use of a local or topical anesthetic
- Potential for injury related to a preexisting condition that requires cautious use of a local or topical anesthetic
- Potential for injury related to adverse drug reactions
- Potential for suffocation related to throat swelling caused by a hypersensitivity reaction to a topical anesthetic
- Potential for trauma related to frostbite caused by a topical anesthetic with a refrigerant
- Potential for trauma related to the adverse CNS effects of a local or topical anesthetic
- Sensory-perceptual alterations (visual or auditory) related to blurred vision or tinnitus caused by a local or topical anesthetic

Pain control

Some pain, such as that from a surgical or dental procedure, may be prevented. Other pain, such as that from a disease or injury, can be relieved only after it occurs. In either case, physicians can use local and topical anesthetics to manage the pain.

Local—and some topical—agents cause anesthesia by blocking a nerve, causing a temporary interruption in the transmission of impulses through nerves that come in contact with the anesthetic. When local anesthetics block large nerves that carry impulses from large areas of skin and tissue, they produce a wide field of anesthesia. This makes

possible diagnostic procedures or treatments that otherwise would be intolerable.

For a summary of representative drugs, see *Selected major drugs: Local and topical anesthetic agents,* pages 392 and 393. For a listing of applicable nursing diagnoses that the nurse may formulate when caring for a patient receiving these agents, see *Selected nursing diagnoses: Local and topical anesthetics.* For detailed information on applying the nursing process, see Chapter 6, The Nursing Process and Drug Therapy.

LOCAL ANESTHETICS

Many clinical situations require local anesthetics to prevent or relieve pain. These agents also offer a safe alternative to general anesthesia for elderly or debilitated patients. Local anesthetics may be amide agents (ones with nitrogen in the molecular chain) or ester agents (ones with oxygen in the molecular chain). Amide anesthetics include bupivacaine hydrochloride, etidocaine hydrochloride, lidocaine hydrochloride, mepivacaine hydrochloride, and prilocaine hydrochloride. Ester anesthetics include chloroprocaine hydrochloride, procaine hydrochloride, propoxycaine hydrochloride, and tetracaine hydrochloride.

The physician can administer local anesthetics in various places to block different groups of nerves. Local anesthetics can be used for local effects as well as central, peripheral, intravenous (I.V.), regional, retrobulbar, or transtracheal nerve blocks. (For an illustration of some of these areas, see *Blocking the pain pathway*.)

Local infiltration involves injecting a local anesthetic into an area that has been injured or that will undergo surgery. One particularly useful type of local infiltration is the field block, which uses several injections to produce a wall of anesthetic around a lesion or an incision. (For an illustration of this technique, see *Field block,* page 384.)

A *central nerve block* can be given in the spinal, perineal, epidural, caudal, or lumbar area to produce anesthesia in the CNS. A *spinal* (or subarachnoid) *block* requires penetrating the second layer of the spinal cord (the arachnoid membrane at the base of the spine) and injecting a local anesthetic into the cerebrospinal fluid (CSF). In a *saddle block,* the anesthetic is administered near the lower end of the spinal column, where it is confined to the perineal or saddle area. An *epidural block* places the local anesthetic next to the outermost covering of the spinal cord, the dura mater. A *caudal block,* a special type of epidural block, is administered near the sacrum. A *lumbar block* is a type of epidural block administered low in the spinal column, near the lumbar vertebrae.

Blocking the pain pathway

Nerve endings transmit pain signals through the peripheral and central nervous systems to the brain. Administering an anesthetic at any point on this pain pathway can block the signal transmission and relieve pain. The illustration below shows several points where an anesthetic may be administered.

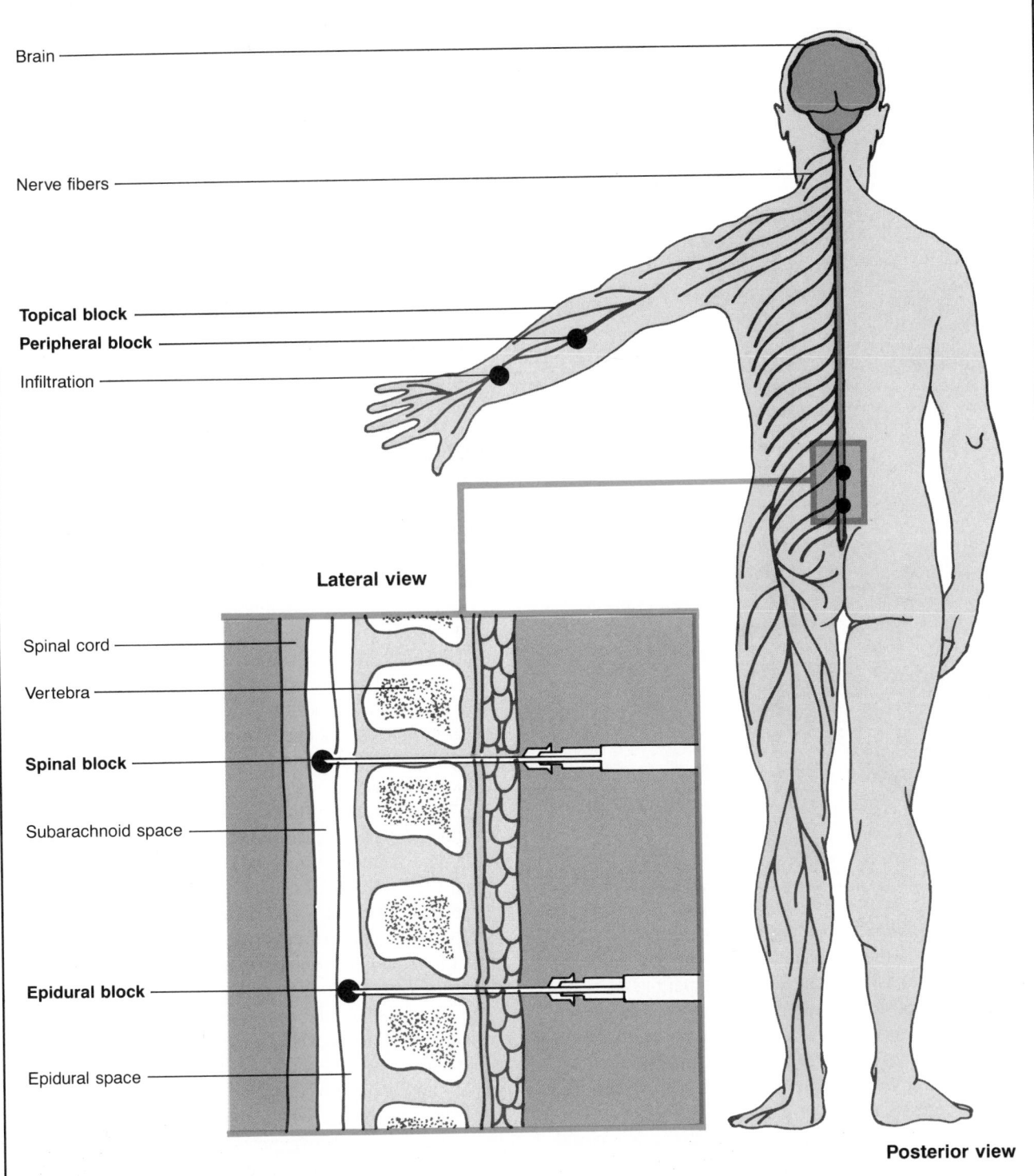

Brain

Nerve fibers

Topical block

Peripheral block

Infiltration

Lateral view

Spinal cord

Vertebra

Spinal block

Subarachnoid space

Epidural block

Epidural space

Posterior view

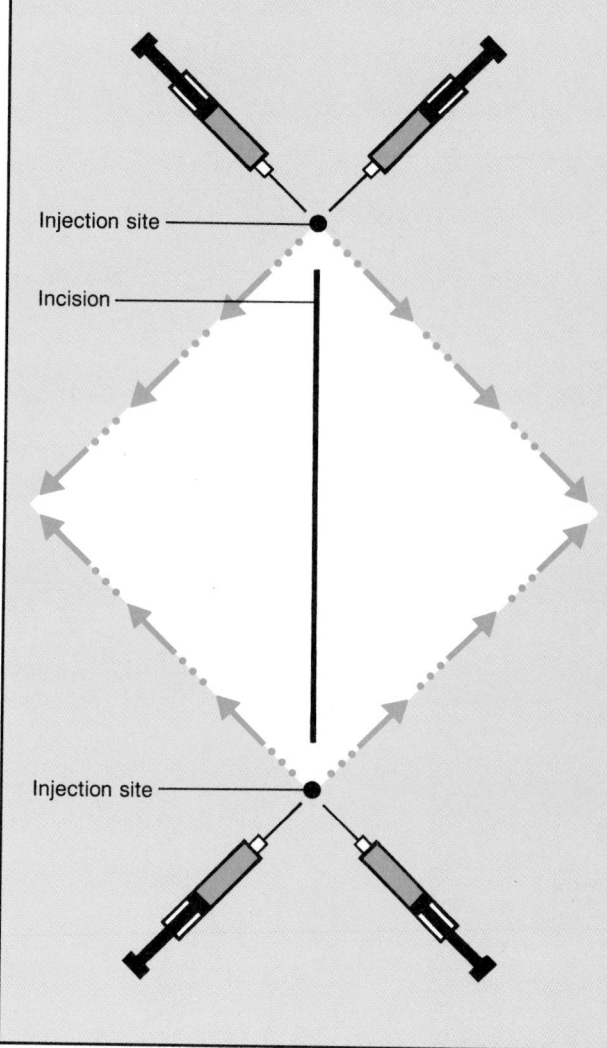

Field block

To produce a wall of anesthesia around a lesion or an incision, the physician can use a field block. Injections must be given to delineate the anesthetized area, or field. In the field block illustrated below, the arrows show the direction of the injections.

Injection site

Incision

Injection site

A *peripheral nerve block* places a local anesthetic next to nerve fibers in the peripheral nervous system. Paracervical and pudendal blocks are types of peripheral nerve blocks used in obstetric procedures. A *sympathetic block* is a peripheral nerve block of sympathetic nerve trunks that is used to relieve pain resulting from injury to the arms or legs and injury or disease of the internal organs. An *intercostal block* is a type of peripheral nerve block produced by injection of an anesthetic near the intercostal nerves.

An *I.V. regional nerve block* is reserved for specific surgical procedures, such as hand or foot surgery. To prepare the patient for this type of anesthesia, the physician applies a tourniquet to the proximal end of the patient's arm or leg and then applies a pressure bandage to force blood away from the area to be anesthetized. A local anesthetic solution is infused into the limb to provide anesthesia during the procedure.

A *retrobulbar nerve block* involves injecting a local anesthetic into nerves behind the eyeball in preparation for ocular surgery.

A *transtracheal nerve block* eliminates reflex activity that occurs from contact with mucous membranes during upper airway surgery. It requires inserting a needle through the cricoid cartilage into the larynx so that an anesthetic solution can be sprayed on the laryngeal mucosa.

PHARMACOKINETICS

Absorption of local anesthetics varies widely, yet distribution occurs throughout the body. Esters and amides undergo different types of metabolism, but both yield metabolites that are excreted in the urine.

Absorption, distribution, metabolism, excretion

The rate and extent of absorption varies with the dose, the drug's characteristics, and the administration site. For example, injection in a highly vascular area will produce faster absorption by more tissues than will injection in a less vascular area.

Local anesthetics are distributed throughout the body, including the CNS. They also can cross the placenta in inverse proportion to the extent that they are bound to plasma proteins. In other words, a highly protein-bound local anesthetic reaches the fetus in smaller quantities than a less protein-bound one. Bupivacaine is highly bound to plasma proteins, making its placental transfer the lowest of the local anesthetics.

When a local anesthetic is administered in the spine, several factors influence its distribution. The type of solution injected helps direct the anesthesia to the part of the spinal cord where it is needed. Hypobaric solutions—less dense than the CSF—rise above the point of injection. Isobaric solutions—of equal density as the CSF—remain near the injection site. Hyperbaric solutions—more dense than the CSF—tend to fall with gravity below the injection site. The direction the drug travels also depends on the patient's position, movement, spine curvature, amount of subarachnoid space, and the drug dose and the specific gravity and volume of the drug solution.

Ester anesthetics, which contain oxygen, are metabolized readily into inactive components by esterase enzymes in the plasma. They also undergo some metabolism in the liver. Amide anesthetics, which contain nitrogen, are metabolized by microsomal enzymes in the liver. The inactive metabolites of ester and amide anesthetics are excreted in the urine along with small amounts of unchanged drug.

Onset, peak, duration

The onset of action varies with the drug used, administration site, and technique. For example, a local lidocaine injection can cause anesthesia in 30 seconds, whereas a local chloroprocaine hydrochloride injection may require 10 minutes to take effect. Although lidocaine works quickly as a local injection, it requires at least 5 minutes to produce anesthesia with epidural administration. (For more information, see *Local anesthetics: Onset and duration.*)

PHARMACODYNAMICS

Researchers believe that local anesthetics block the transmission of impulses across the nerve cell membranes.

Mechanism of action

Local anesthetics block nerve impulses at the point of contact in all kinds of nerves. They apparently accumulate and cause the nerve cell membrane to expand. As the membrane expands, the cell loses its ability to depolarize, which is necessary for impulse transmission. Small nerves and nerves without myelin sheaths exhibit anesthetic effects before large, myelinated nerves.

PHARMACOTHERAPEUTICS

Clinical indications for local anesthetics include preventing and relieving pain from a medical procedure, disease, or injury. Local anesthetics are used for severe pain that topical anesthetics or analgesics cannot relieve. Also, they usually are preferred to general anesthetics for surgery in an elderly or debilitated patient or a patient with a disorder that affects respiratory function, such as chronic obstructive pulmonary disease or myasthenia gravis.

For some procedures, a local anesthetic is combined with a vasoconstrictor, primarily epinephrine, to produce local vasoconstriction that controls local bleeding and reduces anesthetic absorption. Reduced absorption prolongs the anesthetic's action at the site and limits its distribution and CNS effects. However, the use of epinephrine with a local anesthetic is contraindicated in a patient with cardiovascular disease and in an elderly patient because systemic absorption of this vasoconstrictor can cause tachycardia, palpitations, and chest pain. Epinephrine also should be avoided when anesthetizing an area with small vessels, such as the fingers, toes, nose, and ears, because ischemia and necrosis could result.

In other procedures, an anesthetic that contains a preservative (for example, mepivacaine multidose container) may be used. However, this type of anesthetic would not

Local anesthetics: Onset and duration

The onset and duration of action of a local anesthetic vary with the drug used. The nurse can use the data below to predict when a drug's effect will wear off and to anticipate the patient's need for more medication.

DRUG	ONSET OF ACTION	DURATION OF ACTION
bupivacaine for dental anesthesia	2 to 10 minutes	up 7 hours
bupivacaine for epidural anesthesia	4 to 17 minutes	3 to 9 hours
bupivacaine for spinal anesthesia	1 minute	2 hours
chloroprocaine	6 to 12 minutes	30 to 60 minutes
etidocaine	2 to 8 minutes	4.5 to 13 hours
lidocaine	30 seconds to 5 minutes	75 to 140 minutes
mepivacaine	7 to 15 minutes	115 to 150 minutes
prilocaine	less than 2 minutes	1 to 2 hours
procaine	2 to 5 minutes	1 hour
propoxycaine	2 to 5 minutes	2 to 3 hours
tetracaine	15 minutes	1.5 to 3 hours

be used for subarachnoid or epidural anesthesia because it can cause chronic inflammation of the arachnoid membrane.

To guard against adverse reactions during an epidural block, a test dose of the anesthetic should be given before the full dose is administered.

For all local anesthetics, the dosage varies greatly, depending on the procedure to be performed, the depth and duration of anesthesia required, the degree of muscle relaxation needed, tissue vascularity, and the patient's physical condition. Therefore, only skilled practitioners may administer these agents. Local anesthetics typically produce their effects in a predictable pattern. (For details, see *Typical reactions to local anesthetics,* page 386.)

Because the patient typically receives the smallest dose and concentration that will produce the desired effect, this section provides this information for the local anesthetics. (For usual adult dosages used for specific anesthetic pro-

Typical reactions to local anesthetics

After a local anesthetic is administered, a patient's sensory reactions typically diminish in the order shown in this chart. Sensory functions usually return in reverse order. After epidural or spinal anesthesia, sympathetic activity does not necessarily return simultaneously with sensation.

Skin veins dilate because of vasomotor paralysis.	Fast pain sensation disappears.	Sense of touch is dulled.
Temperature perception usually undergoes the following changes:	Slow pain sensation disappears.	Fibers carrying motor impulses are blocked.
The sensation of cold disappears.	Pain sensation is blocked.	Muscle, tendon, and joint sense decrease.
A sense of warmth occurs briefly.	Then, neither warmth nor cold is felt.	Deep pressure sense weakens but may not disappear completely.

cedures, see *Selected major drugs: Local and topical anesthetic agents,* pages 392 and 393.)

bupivacaine hydrochloride (Marcaine). An amide anesthetic, bupivacaine is used in infiltration, spinal, and epidural (caudal and lumbar) anesthesia, and peripheral and sympathetic nerve blocks.
Usual adult dosage: a single bupivacaine dose should not exceed 175 mg when administered alone or 225 mg when administered with epinephrine (1:200,000); daily dosage should not exceed 400 mg of solution without preservatives. Doses usually should not be repeated more than once every

3 hours. With long-acting bupivacaine, the dose should not need to be repeated for 12 hours when it is given with epinephrine.

chloroprocaine hydrochloride (Nesacaine, Nesacaine-CE). An ester anesthetic, chloroprocaine is used for infiltration anesthesia as well as for peripheral, sympathetic, and epidural blocks.
Usual adult dosage: a chloroprocaine dose should not exceed 800 mg when administered alone or 1 gram when administered with epinephrine.

etidocaine hydrochloride (Duranest). An amide anesthetic, etidocaine is used for peripheral, sympathetic, and epidural anesthesia. Other uses include I.V. regional anesthesia, paracervical block in obstetrics, and intercostal nerve block. Highly protein bound, etidocaine is less likely to cross the placenta than other agents. It is long-acting and potent with a high risk of toxicity.
Usual adult dosage: a dose of etidocaine should not exceed 300 mg when administered alone or 400 mg when administered with epinephrine.

lidocaine hydrochloride [lignocaine] (Xylocaine Hydrochloride). An amide anesthetic, lidocaine may be used for infiltration anesthesia or for peripheral, sympathetic, epidural, or spinal blocks. It also has been used intraperitoneally to anesthetize the peritoneum and pelvic organs. A rapid-acting agent, lidocaine is somewhat toxic. In addition to its use as a local anesthetic, lidocaine also is effective as a topical anesthetic (see the section of topical anesthetics later in this chapter) and as an antiarrhythmic (see Chapter 30, Antiarrhythmic Agents).
Usual adult dosage: a single adult dose of lidocaine should not exceed 4 to 5 mg/kg or 300 mg—whichever is lower. When given with epinephrine, lidocaine should not exceed 7 mg/kg or 300 mg.

mepivacaine hydrochloride (Carbocaine, Isocaine). An amide anesthetic, mepivacaine is used for infiltration and epidural anesthesia and for peripheral and sympathetic nerve blocks. Its toxicity resembles that of lidocaine. Because it is effective without a vasoconstrictor, mepivacaine is useful for elderly patients or those with cardiovascular disease.
Usual adult dosage: a single dose or a series of doses used for one procedure should not exceed 400 mg. The total 24-hour dosage should not exceed 1 gram.

prilocaine hydrochloride (Citanest). An amide anesthetic, prilocaine is used for infiltration and nerve block anesthesia in dental procedures. Its use as a spinal anesthetic is declining because it can produce methemoglobinemia.
Usual adult dosage: the total amount given over 2 hours should not exceed 400 mg.

procaine hydrochloride (Novocain). An ester anesthetic, procaine can produce infiltration and spinal anesthesia and peripheral and sympathetic nerve block. In dental procedures, this drug is used for infiltration and anesthesia nerve block. In other settings, it is administered I.V. to manage intractable pain. It is the least toxic local anesthetic.
Usual adult dosage: the initial dose of procaine should not exceed 1 gram.

propoxycaine hydrochloride (Ravocaine). An ester anesthetic, propoxycaine is used with procaine and levonordefrin, a vasoconstrictor. Its primary uses include infiltration and nerve block in dental procedures.
Usual adult dosage: during a procedure, the total dosage should not exceed 0.275 ml/kg of body weight.

tetracaine hydrochloride (Pontocaine). An ester anesthetic, tetracaine is the most widely used spinal anesthetic. Its high lipid solubility allows it to be rapidly absorbed throughout the body.
Usual adult dosage: the tetracaine dose should not exceed 15 mg, except in rare cases.

Drug interactions

Local anesthetics produce few significant interactions with other drugs. Severe interactions can occur, however, when anesthetics with vasoconstrictors are given concurrently with certain other drugs. (For details, see *Drug interactions: Local anesthetic agents,* page 388.) No interactions between local anesthetics and food occur.

ADVERSE DRUG REACTIONS

Adverse reactions to local anesthetics usually result from three main causes: overdose, hypersensitivity, and improper injection technique.

High plasma concentrations of local anesthetics can cause CNS and cardiovascular reactions. The dose-related CNS reactions to stimulation include anxiety, apprehension, restlessness, nervousness, disorientation, confusion, dizziness, blurred vision, tremor, twitching, shivering, and seizures. CNS depression follows, with drowsiness, unconsciousness, and respiratory arrest. The stimulatory phase may not occur, however, if the patient has received lidocaine or another amide anesthetic. Other CNS reactions may include nausea, vomiting, chills, miosis, and tinnitus. Cardiovascular reactions usually are dose-related and typically occur with high plasma concentrations of local anesthetics. These effects may include myocardial depression, bradycardia, cardiac arrhythmias, hypotension, cardiovascular collapse, and cardiac arrest.

Local anesthetic solutions that contain vasoconstrictors such as epinephrine also can produce CNS and cardiovascular reactions, including anxiety, dizziness, headache, restlessness, tremor, palpitations, tachycardia, anginal pain, and hypertension. Extreme reactions include pulmonary edema and ventricular fibrillation. Norepinephrine may be less likely to cause cardiac arrhythmias, but it may cause reflex bradycardia. A burning sensation at the injection site also occurs commonly with these drugs. In rare cases, this reaction may be severe, producing pain, skin discoloration, tissue irritation, swelling, neuritis, neurolysis, and tissue necrosis and sloughing.

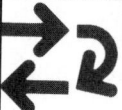

DRUG INTERACTIONS
Local anesthetic agents

Anesthetics with vasoconstrictors can interact with other drugs to produce serious adverse reactions. The nursing implications for these and other local anesthetics are detailed below.

DRUG	INTERACTING DRUGS	POSSIBLE EFFECTS	NURSING IMPLICATIONS
bupivacaine, chloroprocaine, etidocaine, lidocaine, mepivacaine, prilocaine, procaine, propoxycaine, tetracaine	central nervous system (CNS) depressants	Cause additive CNS depression	• Monitor the patient's vital signs and level of consciousness.
lidocaine	beta-adrenergic blocking agents, cimetidine	Increase risk of lidocaine toxicity	• Monitor for signs of lidocaine toxicity, such as confusion, restlessness, and tremor.
anesthetics with vasoconstrictors	inhalation anesthetics	Cause arrhythmias	• If concurrent use is unavoidable, monitor the electrocardiogram continuously while the patient is receiving an inhalation anesthetic.
	tricyclic antidepressants, monoamine oxidase inhibitors, ergot oxytocics	Cause severe hypertension	• Monitor the patient's blood pressure, and alert the physician to any changes.

Ester anesthetics and preservatives in amide anesthetics can cause hypersensitivity reactions, with dermatologic symptoms, edema, status asthmaticus, or anaphylaxis. A patient who is hypersensitive to an ester anesthetic probably will not be sensitive to an amide agent, although the patient may be sensitive to other ester anesthetics. A local anesthetic solution with a preservative such as paraben, phenol, or bisulfite may produce chronic inflammation of the arachnoid membrane if it is used for subarachnoid or epidural anesthesia.

Local anesthetics may produce methemoglobinemia (the presence in the blood of oxidized hemoglobin that cannot combine irreversibly with oxygen). Although this reaction is rare, it occurs most commonly with prilocaine. Cyanosis may be the only symptom, but if it is severe, oxygen and methylene blue may be needed.

Because local anesthetics rapidly cross the placenta, they may produce adverse reactions in the fetus, such as bradycardia and acidosis.

NURSING PROCESS APPLICATION

The following information assists the nurse in caring for a patient who is receiving a local anesthetic.

Assessment
• Review the patient's history for a preexisting condition that contraindicates the use of a local anesthetic, such as known hypersensitivity to the drug.

• Review the patient's history for conditions that require cautious use of a local anesthetic, such as hepatic disease, hypotension, or heart block.
• Assess the patient for adverse reactions to the local anesthetic, such as CNS, cardiovascular, or hypersensitivity reactions.
• Monitor the effectiveness of the local anesthetic used.
• Review the patient's medication history to identify use of drugs that may interact with the local anesthetic, such as CNS depressants, beta-adrenergic blocking agents, inhalation anesthetics, or tricyclic antidepressants.
• Assess the patient receiving a local anesthetic with a vasoconstrictor for anginal pain or discomfort at the injection site.
• Evaluate the patient's and family's knowledge about the local anesthetic.

Nursing diagnoses
The following examples represent appropriate nursing diagnoses for a patient receiving a local anesthesia.
• Potential for injury related to a preexisting condition that contraindicates the use of a local anesthetic
• Potential for injury related to a preexisting condition that requires cautious use of a local anesthetic
• Potential for injury related to adverse drug reactions
• Pain related to use of a local anesthetic with a vasoconstrictor
• Knowledge deficit related to the local anesthetic used.

Planning and implementation

• Do not administer a local anesthetic to a patient with a condition that contraindicates its use, such as known hypersensitivity to the drug.

• Administer a local anesthetic cautiously to a patient at risk because of a preexisting condition. For example, an amide anesthetic, which is metabolized in the liver, must be used with caution in a patient with hepatic dysfunction.

• Observe the patient for adverse reactions to the local anesthetic. Keep in mind that the higher the dose of a local anesthetic, the higher the incidence of adverse reactions.

• *Keep emergency drugs and resuscitation equipment on hand when the patient must receive a parenteral local anesthetic.*

• Position the patient as directed for a subarachnoid block to prevent CSF leakage and headache and to ensure proper anesthetic distribution. Afterward, ensure that the patient stays flat in bed with the bed rails up for the time instructed by the physician.

• *Do not administer a local anesthetic with a vasoconstrictor if a halogenated inhalation anesthetic may be used later.*

• Expect to see a test dose given before the full dose is administered for an epidural block with a local anesthetic agent.

• Expect to monitor the fetus, especially during paracervical block, to detect any fetal bradycardia and acidosis.

• Expect that anesthesia for an obstetric procedure will not be injected during a contraction or when the patient is bearing down, because excess absorption could result.

• Monitor vital signs, contractions, and labor progress. An anesthetic that contains a vasoconstrictor may decrease the intensity of uterine contractions, prolong labor, and cause severe hypertension by interacting with an ergot-type oxytocic agent. Keep in mind that peripheral anesthesia may alter the dynamics of childbirth, increasing the need for forceps-assisted delivery.

• Help prevent maternal hypotension by elevating the patient's legs and positioning her on her left side after peripheral or epidural anesthesia.

• Observe the extremity that has undergone regional anesthesia. Check its peripheral pulse, color, and temperature, and compare it to the unaffected extremity.

• *Ensure that the gag reflex has returned before feeding a patient whose throat has been anesthetized.*

• *Discard partially used vials of local anesthetics that do not contain preservatives.*

• Take safety measures, such as constant patient supervision and seizure precautions, if the patient develops CNS reactions to the local anesthetic, including dizziness, disorientation, blurred vision, drowsiness, or seizures. If CNS depression occurs, alert the physician immediately because unconsciousness and respiratory arrest can occur. *Be prepared to take emergency measures for respiratory arrest.*

• *Monitor the patient for signs of methemoglobinemia, such as cyanosis, and keep oxygen and methylene blue readily available.*

• Notify the physician if adverse reactions occur.

• Monitor the patient with angina for anginal pain when administering a local anesthetic that contains a vasoconstrictor. Ensure that the patient's nitroglycerin is nearby.

• Alert the physician to the occurrence, frequency, and severity of anginal attacks. Be prepared to take emergency measures if anginal pain is not relieved.

• Reassure the patient that a burning sensation at the injection site is normal with use of a local anesthetic that contains a vasoconstrictor.

Patient teaching

• Teach the patient and family the name, action, and adverse effects of the prescribed local anesthetic.

• Stress the importance of remaining supine after receiving a spinal anesthetic.

• Teach the patient to protect numb areas until sensation returns.

• Instruct the patient to alert the nurse or physician immediately if adverse reactions occur.

Evaluation

The following examples represent appropriate evaluation statements for a patient receiving a local anesthetic.

• The patient has no conditions that contraindicate the use of a local anesthetic.

• The patient exhibits no signs of complications in the preexisting condition linked to the prescribed local anesthetic.

• The patient demonstrates no adverse reactions to the local anesthetic.

• The patient reports a transient burning sensation — but no anginal pain — from a local anesthetic that contains a vasoconstrictor.

• The patient and family express an accurate understanding of the points taught about the prescribed local anesthetic.

• The patient protects numb areas until sensation returns.

TOPICAL ANESTHETICS

Applied directly to the skin or mucous membranes, topical anesthetics include benzocaine, benzyl alcohol, butacaine sulfate, butamben picrate, clove oil, cocaine hydrochloride, dibucaine hydrochloride, dyclonine hydrochloride, ethyl chloride, lidocaine, menthol, pramoxine hydrochloride, and tetracaine. Some injectable local anesthetics, such as lidocaine and tetracaine, also are effective topically. All these agents may be used to prevent or relieve minor pain.

Some of these agents also are used in combination products for topical anesthesia. For example, the combination drug tetracaine-adrenaline-cocaine (TAC) is used instead of lidocaine infiltration to achieve local anesthesia without injection for scalp and facial wounds. Most TAC preparations contain tetracaine 0.5%, epinephrine 1:2,000, and cocaine 11.8%. In pediatric patients, TAC produces anesthesia with less anxiety and allows faster, superior wound closure. However, the drug's high cocaine concentration has caused seizures and deaths after application to mucous membranes. To prevent excessive cocaine absorption, TAC should not be used for large wounds or mucous membrane wounds.

Another combination product, eutectic mixture of local anesthetics (EMLA) contains equal amounts of lidocaine and prilocaine. It is used for topical anesthesia in minor invasive procesures, such as venipuncture, I.V. cannula placement, and lumbar puncture. Widely used in Europe, EMLA is pending approval by the Food and Drug Administration in the United States. Several clinical trials have demonstrated the effectiveness of EMLA in adults and children. EMLA reportedly causes no serious adverse reactions, but may produce mild ones, such as erythema and skin blanching.

Tetracaine also is used as a topical ophthalmic anesthetic. (For information about its uses in ophthalmology, see Chapter 71, Ophthalmic Agents.) Benzocaine is used with other agents in several otic preparations. (For more information, see Chapter 72, Otic Agents.)

PHARMACOKINETICS

Topical application of these anesthetics does not produce significant systemic absorption, except for mucosal application of cocaine. However, systemic absorption may occur with frequent or high-dose application to the eye or large areas of burned or injured skin. Tetracaine and other esters are metabolized extensively in the blood and to a lesser extent in the liver. Dibucaine, lidocaine, and other amides are metabolized primarily in the liver. Both types of topical anesthetics are excreted in the urine.

Topical anesthetics have a rapid onset of action, producing anesthesia in a few minutes. However, the peak concentration level and duration of action vary with the drug used. For example, cocaine reaches peak concentration in 2 to 5 minutes, and its effects last for 30 minutes. Dyclonine reaches peak effectiveness in less than 10 minutes and has a duration of less than 1 hour. With lidocaine administration, peak effects occur in 2 to 5 minutes, and the anesthetic action lasts for 30 minutes to 1 hour. Pramoxine's activity peaks in 3 to 5 minutes. Tetracaine's activity peaks in 3 to 8 minutes and lasts for 30 minutes to 1 hour.

PHARMACODYNAMICS

Benzocaine, butacaine, butamben, cocaine, dyclonine, and pramoxine produce topical anesthesia by blocking transmission of nerve impulses. They accumulate in the nerve cell membrane, causing it to expand and lose its ability to depolarize, thus blocking transmission of impulses.

The aromatic compounds, such as benzyl alcohol and clove oil, appear to stimulate the nerve endings. Clove oil may stimulate the nerve endings by counterirritation that interferes with pain perception.

Ethyl chloride superficially freezes the tissue, stimulating the cold sensation receptors and blocking the nerve endings in the frozen area. Dibucaine, lidocaine, and tetracaine may block impulse transmission across the nerve cell membranes. Menthol selectively stimulates the sensory nerve endings for cold, causing a cool sensation and some local analgesic effects.

PHARMACOTHERAPEUTICS

Topical anesthetics relieve or prevent pain—especially minor burn pain—as well as itching and irritation. They also are used to anesthetize an area before an injection is given and to numb mucosal surfaces before a tube, such as an indwelling (Foley) catheter, is inserted. In a spray or solution, a topical anesthetic also is used to alleviate sore throat or mouth pain.

benzocaine (Americaine, Anbesol, Ora-Jel, Solarcaine). An ester anesthetic, benzocaine is active topically only. Available in ointments, creams, and sprays in concentrations of 0.5% to 20%, it is used to treat sunburn pain, pruritus, and hemorrhoidal itching and pain. Benzocaine also is available as a jelly, syrup, or lozenge for toothache or mouth sores.
Usual adult dosage: apply locally b.i.d. or t.i.d.

benzyl alcohol. This clear, colorless, oily liquid is the base of ester local anesthetics. It is used topically to relieve itching.
Usual adult dosage: 5% gel apply locally t.i.d. or q.i.d.

butacaine sulfate. An ester anesthetic, butacaine is used topically as a 4% ointment to relieve pain associated with dental appliances, such as braces.
Usual adult dosage: apply as needed for temporary relief of dental pain.

butamben picrate (Butesin Picrate). Butamben is available as a 1% anesthetic ointment for skin irritations and minor burns.
Usual adult dosage: apply thinly on painful or denuded lesions.

clove oil. An aromatic oil distilled from the dried buds of the clove tree, clove oil's major active ingredient is eugenol. It is used in dentistry to decrease the sensation of pain.
Usual adult dosage: apply as needed for temporary relief of dental pain.

cocaine hydrochloride. This controlled substance, Schedule II drug, the original ester anesthetic, may be applied to the mucosa to provide topical anesthesia during head and throat surgery. It also acts as a vasoconstrictor.
Usual adult dosage: a typical concentration is the 4% solution applied locally.

dibucaine hydrochloride (Nupercainal). This topical anesthetic may be used to treat painful skin and mucosal conditions, such as sunburn, abrasions, and hemorrhoids.
Usual adult dosage: 0.5% to 1% lotion, cream, or ointment applied locally several times a day for up to 7 days.

dyclonine hydrochloride (Dyclone). A ketone anesthetic, dyclonine may be useful for a patient who is hypersensitive to ester or amide anesthetics. This topical anesthetic may be used to relieve surface pain and itching and to anesthetize mucous membranes in endoscopic or cystoscopic procedures. It is contraindicated in cystoscopy after an I.V. pyelogram because it will produce a precipitate with the iodine in the contrast material.
Usual adult dosage: 0.5% or 1% solution applied locally as needed.

ethyl chloride. Ethyl chloride freezes the skin to produce anesthesia. It can reduce skin irritation, produce local anesthesia for minor operative procedures, and relieve the pain of insect stings, burns, and myofascial and visceral pain syndromes.
Usual adult dosage: for skin irritation, spray affected area once or twice from a distance of 24 inches (61 cm) and repeat as needed; for local anesthesia, apply a fine spray from a distance of 12 inches (30 cm); for other indications, apply the smallest dosage possible to produce the desired effect.

lidocaine (Xylocaine). Available as lidocaine or lidocaine hydrochloride, this anesthetic usually is used on mucous membranes as a gel or viscous liquid to ease the discomfort caused by instruments used during urethral catheterization or gastroscopy. It also is used in cancer patients to relieve stomatitis, although it decreases the gag reflex and the sense of taste.
Usual adult dosage: apply 2% to 5% gel or ointment or 15 ml of viscous liquid as needed.

menthol. A benzyl alcohol derivative, menthol's anesthetic action is used to relieve pruritus. It is available in creams and lotions in varying concentrations.
Usual adult dosage: apply 0.25% or 2% lotion or cream as needed for a total of 750 mg/day for pain relief or 600 mg in 6 hours for procedural preparation.

pramoxine hydrochloride (Tronothane). This topically administered local anesthetic contains hydrocortisone and is used as a 1% cream or lotion to ease minor irritations of the skin and mucous membranes.
Usual adult dosage: apply 1% cream or jelly every 3 to 4 hours as needed.

tetracaine (Pontocaine). This ester anesthetic is available as tetracaine or tetracaine hydrochloride in ointment (0.5%) and cream (1%) forms. It usually is used to relieve minor skin and mucous membrane irritation.
Usual adult dosage: apply 0.5% ointment or 1% cream as needed up to a maximum of 28 grams/day.

Drug interactions

Few interactions with other drugs occur with topical anesthetics because they are not absorbed well systemically. When used topically, lidocaine can interact with beta-adrenergic blocking agents and cimetidine, increasing the risk of lidocaine toxicity. When these medications must be given concurrently, the nurse must monitor the patient for signs of toxicity, such as confusion, restlessness, and tremors.

No interactions between the topical anesthetics and food have been described.

ADVERSE DRUG REACTIONS

Adverse reactions to topical anesthetics vary with the chemical class. Agents that are used as local anesthetics may produce CNS and cardiovascular reactions. (See the section on adverse drug reactions under local anesthetics earlier in this chapter.) Benzyl alcohol can cause topical reactions, such as skin irritation. Refrigerants such as ethyl chloride may produce frostbite in the application area.

Any topical anesthetic can cause a hypersensitivity reaction that may include a rash, pruritus, urticaria, swelling of the mouth and throat, and breathing difficulty.

NURSING PROCESS APPLICATION

The following information assists the nurse in caring for a patient who is receiving a topical anesthetic.

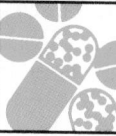

SELECTED MAJOR DRUGS

Local and topical anesthetic agents

This chart summarizes the major local and topical anesthetics currently in clinical use.

DRUG	MAJOR INDICATIONS	USUAL ADULT DOSAGES	CONTRAINDICATIONS AND PRECAUTIONS
Local anesthetics			
bupivacaine	Caudal anesthesia	37.5 to 150 mg	• Know that bupivacaine is contraindicated in a patient with known hypersensitivity to this drug, any amide local anesthetic, or other components of Marcaine solutions; and in obstetric paracervical block. • Administer with caution to a patient with hepatic disease, hypotension, or heart block.
	Infiltration anesthesia	Up to 175 mg	
	Peripheral anesthesia	12.5 to 25 mg	
	Retrobulbar anesthesia	5 to 30 mg	
	Spinal anesthesia	6 to 12 mg	
chloroprocaine	Caudal anesthesia	300 to 750 mg	• Know that chloroprocaine is contraindicated in a patient with known hypersensitivity to any ester anesthetic. • Administer with extreme caution to a patient receiving lumbar or caudal epidural anesthesia who has a neurologic disease, spinal deformity, septicemia, or severe hypertension. • Administer with caution to a patient with hypotension, heart block, other cardiovascular dysfunction, or hepatic disease.
	Epidural anesthesia	40 to 75 mg/segment	
	Infiltration anesthesia	Variable	
	Peripheral anesthesia	10 to 800 mg	
lidocaine	Caudal anesthesia	200 to 300 mg	• Know that lidocaine is contraindicated in a patient with known hypersensitivity to amide local anesthetics. • Administer with extreme caution to a patient with a neurologic disease, spinal deformity, septicemia, or severe hypertension who is receiving lumbar or caudal epidural anesthesia. • Administer with caution to a patient with severe shock, heart block, other cardiovascular dysfunction, or hepatic disease.
	Infiltration anesthesia	5 to 300 mg	
	Peripheral anesthesia	20 to 300 mg	
	Spinal anesthesia	9 to 120 mg	
procaine	Infiltration anesthesia	350 to 600 mg	• Know that spinal anesthesia with procaine is contraindicated in a patient with generalized septicemia; sepsis at the proposed injection site; certain cerebrospinal diseases, such as meningitis and syphilis; or known hypersensitivity to this drug, other ester anesthetics, drugs of a similar chemical configuration, or aminobenzoic acid or its derivatives. • Administer with caution to a patient with known drug allergies and sensitivities, severe disturbances of cardiac rhythm, shock, or heart block.
	Peripheral anesthesia	500 mg	
	Spinal anesthesia	50 to 200 mg	
Topical anesthetics			
benzocaine	Dermal anesthesia, mucosal anesthesia	Apply locally b.i.d. or t.i.d.	• Know that benzocaine is contraindicated in a patient who is allergic to procaine or para-aminobenzoic acid (PABA), an ingredient in many sunscreens.

SELECTED MAJOR DRUGS

Local and topical anesthetic agents *(continued)*

DRUG	MAJOR INDICATIONS	USUAL ADULT DOSAGES	CONTRAINDICATIONS AND PRECAUTIONS
Topical anesthetics *(continued)*			
cocaine	Mucosal anesthesia	4% solution applied locally	• Know that cocaine is contraindicated in a patient with known hypersensitivity to any ester anesthetic. • Administer with caution to a patient with hypertension, cardiovascular disease, or hyperthyroidism.
dibucaine	Dermal anesthesia, mucosal anesthesia	Apply 0.5% to 1% lotion, cream, or ointment locally several times a day for up to 7 days	• Know that dibucaine is contraindicated in a patient with known hypersensitivity to this drug or any amide-type anesthetic. It should not be used in large quantities, especially over denuded or blistered areas.
ethyl chloride	Dermal anesthesia	Spray affected area once or twice from a distance of 12 to 24 inches (30 to 61 cm)	• Know that ethyl chloride is contraindicated in a patient with known hypersensitivity to this drug.
lidocaine	Dermal anesthesia, mucosal anesthesia	Apply as 2% to 5% gel or ointment, or 15 ml viscous liquid as needed	• Know that lidocaine is contraindicated in a patient with known hypersensitivity to amide local anesthetics. • Administer with caution to an elderly patient or one with large areas of broken skin or mucous membranes.
tetracaine	Dermal anesthesia, mucosal anesthesia	Apply 0.5% ointment or 1% cream, as needed, up to maximum of 28 grams/day	• Know that tetracaine is contraindicated in a patient with an allergy to procaine or PABA, or known hypersensitivity to any ester anesthetic.

Assessment
• Review the patient's history for a preexisting condition that contraindicates the use of a topical anesthetic, such as known hypersensitivity to the drug.
• Review the patient's history for a preexisting condition that requires cautious use of a topical anesthetic, such as hypertension or cardiovascular disease.
• Assess the patient for adverse reactions to the topical anesthetic, such as CNS and cardiovascular reactions.
• Monitor the effectiveness of the topical anesthetic used.
• Review the patient's medication history to identify the use of drugs that may interact with the topical anesthetic, such as beta-adrenergic blocking agents and cimetidine.
• Evaluate the patient's and family's knowledge about the prescribed topical anesthetic.

Nursing diagnoses
The following examples represent appropriate nursing diagnoses for a patient receiving a topical anesthetic.
• Potential for injury related to a preexisting condition that contraindicates the use of a topical anesthetic

• Potential for injury related to a preexisting condition that requires cautious use of a topical anesthetic
• Potential for injury related to adverse drug reactions
• Knowledge deficit related to the prescribed topical anesthetic

Planning and implementation
• Do not administer a topical anesthetic to a patient with a condition that contraindicates its use.
• Administer a topical anesthetic cautiously to a patient at risk because of a preexisting condition.
• Observe the patient regularly for adverse reactions to the topical anesthetic.
• *Administer topical lidocaine with caution in an elderly patient or a patient with large areas of broken skin or mucous membranes.*
• Monitor for signs of localized frostbite in a patient receiving a refrigerant, such as ethyl chloride, and for skin irritation and other topical reactions in a patient receiving benzyl alcohol.
• *Do not apply a refrigerant to broken skin or mucous membranes.*

• Expect to administer a smaller dose of the topical anesthetic to a child or elderly patient.
• *Use the lowest dose necessary for relief of symptoms.*
• Clean and dry the area thoroughly before applying an anesthetic rectally.
• *Avoid contact with eyes.*
• Discontinue use if a rash develops.
• Notify the physician if adverse reactions occur.

Patient teaching
• Teach the patient and family the name, action, frequency, and adverse effects of the prescribed topical anesthetic.
• Show the patient and family how to apply a topical anesthetic if prescribed for home use. Tell them to use it only as directed.
• Discourage prolonged use of a topical anesthetic without medical supervision.
• Advise the patient to keep dibucaine out of the reach of children to prevent ingestion and accidental poisoning.
• Advise the patient whose oropharyngeal mucosa has been anesthetized to delay eating until sensation returns.
• Instruct the patient to alert the nurse or physician if any adverse reactions occur.

Evaluation
The following examples represent appropriate evaluation statements for a patient receiving a topical anesthetic.
• The patient has no conditions that contraindicate the use of topical anesthetics.
• The patient exhibits no signs of complications in the preexisting condition linked to the prescribed topical anesthetic.
• The patient demonstrates no adverse reactions to the prescribed topical anesthetic.
• The patient and family express an accurate understanding of the points taught about the prescribed topical anesthetic.
• The patient correctly demonstrates application of the topical anesthetic.

CHAPTER SUMMARY

Local and topical anesthetics can interrupt pain impulses at their point of contact with nerves. Local anesthetics usually are injected, but some are applied topically; topical anesthetics are applied directly to skin or mucous membranes. Here are the chapter highlights.
• Local anesthetics produce their effect in a limited body area, but they are distributed throughout the body.

• When injected near nerves, local anesthetics can produce nerve block anesthesia for pain relief or surgery.
• When applied to the skin or mucous membranes, topical anesthetics can relieve minor irritation or prevent discomfort during diagnostic testing or other procedures.
• Most topical anesthetics are applied to the surface of the skin or mucous membranes. In special formulations, they also may be used in the eyes and ears. Some topical anesthetics appear in combination products, such as TAC and EMLA, and are used for specific purposes.
• Hypersensitivity reactions may occur with local and topical anesthetic agents, especially with ester anesthetics.
• The nurse uses the nursing process when caring for a patient receiving a local or topical anesthetic. Nursing care commonly includes screening for potential drug interactions, monitoring for adverse drug reactions, and patient teaching.

STUDY QUESTIONS

See Appendix 1 for answers.

1. Cindy Williams, age 30, has been in labor for 12 hours. Her physician orders a saddle block with bupivacaine. Where is a saddle block administered?
(a) into the subarachnoid space
(b) next to the dura mater
(c) into the peripheral nerve
(d) into the epidural space

2. Bupivacaine is an amide anesthetic. What is the difference between amide and ester anesthetics?
(a) Amide anesthetics have a longer duration of action and produce fewer hypersensitivity reactions.
(b) Amide anesthetics are metabolized in the liver; ester anesthetics are metabolized in the plasma and liver.
(c) Amide anesthetics are less stable and require larger doses.
(d) Amide anesthetics are excreted in urine; ester anesthetics are excreted in urine and feces.

3. Besides the drug's specific gravity, what other factors affect distribution of spinal anesthesia?
(a) patient's age
(b) patient's position
(c) pain's severity
(d) drug's absorption rate

4. By which mechanism of action does the local anesthetic bupivacaine produce its effect?
(a) It inhibits nerve cell depolarization.
(b) It transforms myelinated into demyelinated nerve cells.
(c) It inhibits pain impulse transmission in the CNS.
(d) It blocks nerve impulses in the spinal cord.

5. Joey Birnbaum, age 9, has a sunburn. His mother applies the topical anesthetic benzocaine (Solarcaine) to relieve his pain. How do topical anesthetics differ from local anesthetics?
(a) Topical anesthetics are longer acting than local anesthetics.
(b) Topical anesthetics are better absorbed than local anesthetics.
(c) Topical anesthetics are more toxic than local anesthetics.
(d) Topical anesthetics are applied to the skin or mucous membranes; local anesthetics are injected.

6. How does benzocaine relieve Joey's sunburn pain?
(a) It numbs the skin surface, decreasing the perception of pain.
(b) It causes vasoconstriction to the area, minimizing the sense of pain.
(c) It blocks nerve impulse transmission by preventing nerve cell depolarization.
(d) It freezes the skin, which prevents nerve impulse transmission.

7. After receiving chemotherapy for metastatic breast cancer, Lynn Schubert, age 42, develops stomatitis, which is treated with topical lidocaine (Xylocaine). Which problem may result from topical lidocaine use?
(a) diarrhea
(b) poor nutrient absorption
(c) GI distress
(d) decreased gag reflex

SELECTED REFERENCES

AHFS drug information 90. (1990). Bethesda, MD: American Society of Hospital Pharmacists.

Collins, V. (1989). *Principles of anesthesiology* (3rd ed.). Philadelphia: Lea & Febiger.

Drug facts and comparisons. (1991). St. Louis: Facts and Comparisons Division, J.B. Lippincott.

Hansten, P., and Horn, J. (1988). *Drug interactions: Clinical significance of drug-drug interactions* (6th ed.). Philadelphia: Lea & Febiger.

Houghton, K. (1988). Local anaesthesia. *Nursing Times,* 84(41), 63-66.

Luczun, M. (Ed.). (1987). *Handbook of postanesthesia nursing.* Rockville, MD: Aspen Publishers.

Miller, R. (1990). *Anesthesia* (3rd ed.). New York: Churchill Livingstone.

Recommended practices: Monitoring the patient receiving local anesthesia. (1989). *AORN Journal,* 50(3), 624-625.

USPDI. (1991). *Drug information for the health care professional* (Vol. I, 11th ed.). Rockville, MD: United States Pharmacopeial Convention.

U N I T

6

DRUGS TO ALTER PSYCHOGENIC BEHAVIOR AND PROMOTE SLEEP

The pharmacologic treatment of psychiatric disorders is relatively new. The discovery of chlorpromazine and its value in treating schizophrenia did not occur until the 1950s. Before this, the psychiatric hospital stay was lengthy, with little to offer the patient but custodial care. With the discovery of phenothiazines, the prognosis for schizophrenia improved dramatically. Patients were able to leave hospitals sooner, live in the community, and take part in other therapies previously unavailable to them. The role of the nurse as patient custodian was redefined; emphasis was placed instead on the therapeutic nurse-patient relationship.

In the past 35 years, newer drugs have become available for various psychiatric disorders. Antianxiety agents, such as diazepam, and antidepressant agents, such as amitriptyline, are prescribed commonly. Although these medications sometimes are used alone, psychiatric drugs usually are intended to be used with other therapeutic modalities, such as psychotherapy.

When caring for a patient who is receiving a drug to alter psychogenic behavior or promote sleep, the nurse should keep in mind that such a drug is likely to be prescribed for long-term therapy. Because of this and because the drug may cause intolerable adverse reactions, the nurse should monitor the patient closely for adverse reactions, check the blood level of the drug as instructed, and watch for signs of noncompliance, such as a return of the original symptoms. Because some of these drugs are addictive, the nurse also should be alert for signs of dependence and, when the drug is discontinued, withdrawal symptoms.

OVERVIEW OF CHAPTERS

Unit Six presents drugs that are used to treat various sleep and psychogenic disorders, such as insomnia, agitation, depression, mania, bipolar disorders, anxiety, and schizophrenia.

Chapter 25
Sedative and Hypnotic Agents

Chapter 25 explores three main classes of sedative and hypnotic agents. It begins with an overview of the physiology of sleep, the four major categories of sleep disorders, and the process for assessing sleep and rest habits. Then it describes the clinical uses of these agents. The chapter also presents the nursing activities associated with sedative and hypnotic administration. It concludes with a discussion of other drugs used as sedative and hypnotic agents, such as alcohol and over-the-counter preparations.

Chapter 26
Antidepressant and Antimanic Agents

Chapter 26 presents the characteristics and pathophysiology of such affective disorders as depression and mania. It then discusses the major classes of agents used to treat those disorders, including monamine oxidase inhibitors, tricyclic antidepressants, second-generation antidepressants, and lithium. The chapter also discusses the rationales for selecting one drug over another and related nursing care, including patient teaching.

Chapter 27
Antianxiety Agents

The introduction to Chapter 27 discusses the huge degree to which the population experiences anxiety and describes the symptoms and classifications of anxiety. Then the chapter presents the major drug classes used to treat anxiety, including benzodiazepines, buspirone, and barbiturates, as well as drugs that are used rarely to treat anxiety, such as meprobamate, antihistamines, and beta blockers. For each drug, the chapter details the rationales for selection and major adverse reactions. It also demonstrates how to use the nursing process when caring for a patient who receives an antianxiety agent.

Glossary

Affective disorder: mood disturbance in the presence of an elated or depressive state.

Akathisia: continuous restlessness or inability to sit or stand still; a common adverse reaction to antipsychotic agents.

Antidepressant: agent that prevents or relieves depression.

Antimanic: agent that prevents or diminishes mania.

Antipsychotic: agent that prevents or diminishes psychosis.

Anxiety: feeling of apprehension, uncertainty, and fear.

Anxiety disorder: primary medical condition or disorder secondary to another medical or social problem. An anxiety disorder may be nonphobic, such as a generalized anxiety, obsessive-compulsive, or panic disorder; or it may be phobic, such as a fear of crowds or heights.

Anxiolytic: agent that prevents or diminishes anxiety.

Ataxia: impaired ability to coordinate movement.

Bipolar disorder: mood disorder in which manic and depressive episodes occur.

Dementia: progressive mental or intellectual decline.

Depression: emotional dejection characterized by an absence of cheerfulness and hope disproportionate to circumstances.

Drug holiday: discontinuation of an antipsychotic agent for 4 or more weeks to detect tardive dyskinesia, which may be masked by the drug's effects.

Dystonia: disordered muscle tone; a common adverse reaction to antipsychotic agents.

Euphoria: exaggerated sense of well-being.

Gamma-aminobutyric acid (GABA): inhibitory neurotransmitter secreted by nerve terminals in the spinal cord, the cerebellum, the basal ganglia, and many areas of the cerebral cortex.

Gilles de la Tourette's syndrome: disease characterized by motor incoordination, the meaningless repetition of words, and the use of obscene language.

Huntington's chorea: hereditary disease characterized by chronic, progressive motor disturbances and mental deterioration.

Hypersomnia: disorder of excessive somnolence, such as narcolepsy (sleep attacks).

Hypnotic: agent that induces sleep.

Insomnia: inability to sleep; abnormal wakefulness.

Mania: mood disorder characterized by an expansive emotional state, elation, hyperirritability, over-talkativeness, a flight of ideas, and increased motor activity.

Manic-depressive disorder: bipolar mental disorder characterized by fluctuations between mania and depression.

Monoamine oxidase (MAO): enzyme in the nerve endings that breaks down catecholamines.

Narcosis: reversible condition characterized by stupor or insensibility produced by drugs.

Neuroleptic: drug with an action that resembles a nervous system disorder; an antipsychotic agent.

Non-rapid eye movement (NREM) sleep: first four stages of sleep, which progress from light to deep sleep and are characterized by non-rapid eye movement.

Obsessive-compulsive disorder: mental disorder characterized by the need to perform certain acts repetitively or to carry out certain rituals.

Panic: extreme, unreasoned anxiety or fear.

Parasomnia: dysfunction associated with sleep, sleep stages, or partial arousals.

Phobia: persistent, abnormal dread or fear.

Pseudoparkinsonism: state resembling Parkinson's disease and characterized by muscle rigidity, tremors, shuffling gait, drooling, and decreased arm swing and associative movements when walking; a common adverse reaction to antipsychotic agents.

Psychosis: mental disorder characterized by loss of contact with reality and derangement of personality.

Rapid eye movement (REM) sleep: fifth and last stage of sleep characterized by rapid eye movements. REM sleep is essential for physiologic and mental restoration.

Schizophrenia: group of severe emotional disorders characterized by delusions, hallucinations, loss of contact with reality, and bizarre or regressive behavior.

Sedative: agent that allays excitement and produces drowsiness.

Serotonin: neurotransmitter secreted by the raphe nuclei that inhibits pain pathways and helps control an individual's mood; it may induce sleep.

Tardive dyskinesia: neurologic syndrome characterized by abnormal muscle movement, particularly around the mouth (such as lip smacking, rhythmic darting of the tongue, and constant chewing movements), and slow, aimless involuntary movements of the arms and legs; a common adverse reaction to antipsychotic agents.

Chapter 28
Antipsychotic Agents

Chapter 28 discusses antipsychotic, or neuroleptic, agents and their clinical uses. It begins with a brief review of the anatomy and physiology of some areas of the central nervous system, including the pyramidal and extrapyramidal tracts and the limbic system. Then the chapter discusses the pharmacokinetic, pharmacodynamic, and pharmacotherapeutic properties of the two major classes of neuroleptic drugs, phenothiazines and nonphenothiazines. For both classes, it emphasizes early recognition of neurologic adverse reactions, such as extrapyramidal symptoms and tardive dyskinesia, that may accompany their use. The chapter also highlights nursing activities related to the administration of antipsychotic agents.

SEDATIVE AND HYPNOTIC AGENTS

OBJECTIVES

After reading and studying this chapter, the student should be able to:

1. Differentiate between a sedative and a hypnotic.

2. Describe a typical sleep cycle from stage 1 through stage 5 sleep.

3. Describe the four major categories of sleep disorders.

4. Describe the pharmacokinetic properties of the benzodiazepines, barbiturates, and the nonbenzodiazepines-nonbarbiturates.

5. Discuss the clinical indications for each of the three major groups of sedative and hypnotic agents.

6. Describe significant adverse reactions associated with each of the three major classes of sedative and hypnotic agents.

7. Describe how alcohol and over-the-counter (OTC) products function as sleep aids.

8. Describe how to use the nursing process when caring for a patient who is receiving a sedative or hypnotic agent.

INTRODUCTION

Sedatives are drugs that act to reduce activity or excitement, calming a patient. Some degree of drowsiness commonly accompanies sedative use. When administered in large doses, sedatives are considered hypnotics, which induce a state resembling natural sleep. Chapter 25 discusses three main classes of synthetic drugs used as sedatives and hypnotics: the benzodiazepines, the barbiturates, and the nonbenzodiazepine-nonbarbiturate drugs. The chapter also discusses other sedatives, including alcohol and OTC sleep aids.

Physiology of sleep

Sleep represents an active state of unconsciousness from which a person can be awakened with an appropriate stimulus. A naturally occurring state, sleep occupies about one-third of an adult's life. Although researchers know that a lack of sleep causes physical and psychological symptoms and generally believe that the body requires sleep for restoration, they have not yet identified the precise relationship between sleep and cellular renewal.

While sleeping, a person passes through several cycles, each cycle involving five stages. The first four stages, characterized by non-rapid eye movement (NREM), account for 75% to 80% of a typical period of sleep. The stages progress from light sleep, stages 1 and 2, to deep sleep, stages 3 and 4. NREM, especially stage 4, helps maintain physical health and well-being and represents what some people refer to as obligatory sleep. After completing stage 4, the sleeper regresses through stages 3 and 2 to reach the fifth and last stage, called rapid eye movement (REM) sleep. REM sleep accounts for the remaining 20% to 25% of a normal period of sleep. A physiologically active period characterized by rapid eye movements, REM sleep is essential for physiologic and mental restoration. During REM sleep, the person integrates new learning and experiences into the memory.

After REM sleep, the sleeper begins a second cycle, proceeding through stages 2 to 4, then back through stages 3 and 2, and finally into a longer period of REM sleep. Changes in body position usually mark the transition from one stage of sleep to another. A typical cycle averages 90 minutes, with the duration of stage 4 decreasing and the REM stage lengthening with each cycle. Each time a person awakens, a new cycle begins. (For more information, see *NREM and REM sleep,* page 400.)

SELECTED NURSING DIAGNOSES

Sedative and hypnotic agents

The following nursing diagnoses address representative problems and etiologies that a nurse may encounter when caring for a patient who is receiving a sedative or hypnotic agent. Some of these nursing diagnoses contain generalized etiologies, which the nurse must individualize based on the patient's needs. (For some common nursing diagnoses and related interventions for each drug class, see the "Nursing Process Application" sections of this chapter.)

- Altered health maintenance related to ineffectiveness of the prescribed sedative or hypnotic agent
- Altered protection related to barbiturate-induced blood dyscrasias
- Altered role performance related to dependence on a sedative or hypnotic agent
- Anxiety related to a paradoxical reaction to the barbiturate
- Diarrhea related to the adverse gastrointestinal effects of the barbiturate
- Fatigue related to the adverse effects or a benzodiazepine
- Impaired gas exchange related to the adverse respiratory effects of the sedative or hypnotic agent
- Impaired home maintenance management related to the sedative effects of the prescribed sedative or hypnotic agent
- Ineffective breathing pattern related to respiratory depression cause by a sedative or hypnotic agent
- Knowledge deficit related to the prescribed sedative or hypnotic agent

- Pain related to barbiturate-induced headache
- Potential activity intolerance related to benzodiazepine-induced muscle weakness
- Potential fluid volume deficit related to nausea and vomiting caused by a hypnotic or sedative agent
- Potential for injury related to a preexisting condition that contraindicates the use of a sedative or hypnotic agent
- Potential for injury related to a preexisting condition that requires cautious use of a sedative or hypnotic agent
- Potential for injury related to adverse drug reactions
- Potential for injury related to drug interactions with the prescribed sedative or hypnotic agent
- Potential for injury related to impaired judgment and motor skills caused by the hangover effects of a barbiturate
- Potential for trauma related to dizziness, drowsiness, and other adverse central nervous system effects of the sedative or hypnotic agent
- Sensory-perceptual alterations (visual) related to photosensitivity caused by a sedative or hypnotic agent
- Sleep pattern disturbance related to rebound insomnia caused by a sedative or hypnotic agent

Sleep disorders

The four major categories of sleep disorders are (1) insomnias, or disorders of initiating and maintaining sleep, (2) hypersomnias, or disorders of excessive somnolence, (3) parasomnias, or dysfunctions associated with sleep, sleep stages, or partial arousals, and (4) disorders of the sleep-awake schedule.

Insomnias represent the most common sleep problems in our society. Hypersomnias may occur as difficulties in arousing from sleep, excessive daytime sleeping and napping, and actual "sleep attacks" (narcolepsy) such as falling asleep while driving or eating. Narcolepsy accounts for about 60% of all hypersomnias; sleep apnea accounts for another 20% to 25%. Sleep apnea, a condition characterized by the cessation of respirations, occurs intermittently during the sleep cycle and may last anywhere from a few seconds to more than a minute. Parasomnias, which occur during normal sleep periods, include sleepwalking (somnambulism), night terrors, nocturnal enuresis (bed-wetting), and nightmares. Disorders of the sleep-awake schedule typically accompany sudden time changes. Workers changing shifts at their jobs and travelers flying across several time zones typically experience disorders of the sleep-awake schedule.

Assessment of sleep and rest habits

Because sedatives and hypnotics commonly are prescribed p.r.n., a comprehensive nursing assessment of the need for the drugs is especially important. The nurse must assess the patient's sleep and rest habits before identifying any present or potential sleep and rest problems. Assessing the sleep and rest habits of hospitalized patients also helps the nurse develop a plan to minimize any disruption of established patterns. A sleep history documents the patient's usual pattern of sleep and rest. When obtaining a sleep history, the nurse should focus questions on the patient's usual sleep habits to determine if they have changed over the past month. The nurse should address the following topics.

- History (personal history of allergies; past and present medical conditions; complete drug history including all prescription and over-the-counter sleep aids; caffeine intake including coffee, tea, and soda; family history; general emotional state and affect)
- Number of hours of sleep per day
- Sleep pattern (usual time of retiring and arising)
- Usual length of time to fall asleep; any difficulties associated with falling asleep
- Usual number of awakenings during the sleep period; reasons for awakenings (bladder tension, dreams, anxiety

NREM and REM sleep

Non-rapid eye movement (NREM) sleep and rapid eye movement (REM) sleep differ from each other significantly in terms of the following characteristics: brain activity, eye movements, muscle activity, physiologic activity, and dreams.

CHARACTERISTICS	NREM	REM
Brain activity (electroencephalogram)	Progressive from relatively fast alpha waves (stage 1) to large, slow delta waves (stage 4)	Irregular, rapid brain waves (resemble waking state)
Eye movements (electrooculogram)	Slow and rolling (stages 1 and 2) or no eye movement (stages 3 and 4)	Rapid, darting movements
Muscle activity (electromyelogram)	Decreased muscle tone (stage 1) progressing to complete muscle relaxation (stage 4)	Muscle tone at lowest level; complete relaxation of skeletal muscles
Physiologic activity	Steady decrease in vital signs and slowing of bodily functions—for example, decreased metabolic rate and decreased GI tract activity	Pulse and blood pressure increased and erratic; respirations variable with some periods of apnea possible; increased bodily functions, such as increased metabolic rate and increased GI tract activity
Dreams	Stage 1—sense of floating with drifting thoughts; stage 2—fragmented thoughts; stage 3—low intensity dreams; stage 4—realistic dreams, resembling normal thought processes, rarely recalled	Vivid, detailed, emotionally charged, more likely to be recalled than NREM dreams; account for 80% to 85% of REM

or depression); difficulty falling back to sleep after awakening
• Feeling upon awakening (rested, groggy, tired, disoriented)
• Usual sleep environment (type of bed, number of pillows, blankets, amount of light, noise, ventilation)
• Prebedtime routines (exercise habits, use of such beverages as warm milk or tea, warm bath or shower, reading, watching TV, other relaxation measures)
• Number, time of day, and length of daytime naps.

For example, if a patient identifies insomnia as a problem, the nurse must obtain a thorough sleep history and assess the signs and symptoms that indicate a lack of sleep. The nurse also should identify the amount of sleep that the patient considers necessary in 24 hours for optimal functioning. Considering all the factors as well as the patient's perception of the quality of sleep in the past month helps the nurse identify the potential or actual sleep problem. Once the sleep problem has been identified, the nurse can determine the appropriate nursing interventions.

For a summary of the drugs discussed in this chapter, see *Selected major drugs: Sedative and hypnotic agents,* pages 416 to 418. For a listing of applicable nursing diagnoses that the nurse may formulate when caring for a patient receiving these agents, see *Selected nursing diagnoses: Sedative and hypnotic agents,* page 399. For detailed information on applying the nursing process, see Chapter 6, The Nursing Process and Drug Therapy.

BENZODIAZEPINES

Benzodiazepines produce many actions, including daytime and preanesthetic sedation, sleep induction, relief of anxiety and tension, skeletal muscle relaxation, and anticonvulsant activity. The benzodiazepines discussed here are used mainly for their sedative or hypnotic effects. Such benzodiazepines include flurazepam hydrochloride, lorazepam, quazepam, temazepam, and triazolam. When other benzodiazepines are used clinically, they secondarily exert a sedative or hypnotic effect. Discussions of the other benzodiazepines appear in the appropriate chapters related to their primary clinical use.

PHARMACOKINETICS

Benzodiazepines are absorbed well and distributed widely in the body. All benzodiazepines are metabolized in the liver and excreted primarily in the urine.

Absorption, distribution, metabolism, excretion

When taken orally, benzodiazepines are absorbed from the gastrointestinal (GI) tract, with peak concentration levels occurring at any time between 30 minutes and 8 hours, but usually within 1 to 3 hours. An intramuscular (I.M.) injection of a benzodiazepine results in erratic absorption, with the exception of lorazepam, which is absorbed readily to peak concentration in 60 to 90 minutes.

These drugs are distributed widely into body tissues; they also cross the blood-brain barrier and placenta. The lipid solubility of benzodiazepines increases their distribution and potential for redistribution; the redistribution of the drugs enhances their duration of action. Conversely, protein binding decreases the distribution of benzodiazepines. Most benzodiazepines and their active metabolites bind to plasma proteins.

The benzodiazepines are metabolized extensively in the liver by various microsomal enzyme systems. For example, metabolism of flurazepam occurs via hydroxylation, which produces active metabolites with long half-lives; metabolism of lorazepam and temazepam occurs via glucuronic acid conjugation. Metabolized benzodiazepines are excreted in the urine.

Onset, peak, duration

Most benzodiazepines register a relatively rapid onset of action: under 30 minutes. However, flurazepam and lorazepam have a slower onset, from 1 to 2 hours in some patients, because of slow absorption. The peak concentration and duration of action vary among patients as well as among the specific drugs. For example, triazolam reaches a peak concentration in just over 1 hour but has a short duration and an elimination half-life of 2 to 3 hours. By comparison, flurazepam takes 1 to 3 hours to reach a peak concentration but has a duration of up to 18 hours, including a half-life of 47 to 100 hours. Flurazepam becomes more effective after two consecutive uses because the active metabolite accumulates in the body. Because of age-related factors, flurazepam used by elderly patients exhibits a significantly prolonged half-life, with a mean half-life of 120 hours in females and 160 hours in males. In patients with severe liver dysfunction, the half-life of flurazepam also is prolonged because the liver, which metabolizes the drug, cannot work efficiently. Other sedatives and hypnotics do not form long-acting active metabolites, and, as a result, their actions are not as prolonged in elderly patients and in patients with significant liver dysfunction.

PHARMACODYNAMICS

Researchers have not established the locations of drug action or the mechanisms of action for the benzodiazepines. Although the drug action sites remain unknown, researchers believe the principal sites are the cerebral cortex and the limbic, thalamic, and hypothalamic levels of the central nervous system (CNS).

Mechanism of action

Researchers believe that benzodiazepines act at several sites in the CNS. One theory suggests that the drugs enhance the effects of the inhibitory neurotransmitter gamma-aminobutyric acid (GABA). Because GABA is inhibitory, receptor stimulation increases inhibition and blocks limbic and cortical arousal. Another theory suggests that because benzodiazepine receptors are found in various structures of the CNS, but not outside it, the drugs have little effect on other body systems.

When administered at low therapeutic doses, benzodiazepines decrease anxiety by acting on the limbic system and related brain areas that help regulate emotional activity. The drugs usually can calm or sedate the patient without causing drowsiness. (For a detailed discussion of benzodiazepines used to treat anxiety, see Chapter 27, Antianxiety Agents.) At higher doses, benzodiazepines exhibit sleep-producing properties, probably because the drugs depress the activating system located in the reticular formation of the midbrain.

The clinical use of benzodiazepines results in a net increase in total sleep time and produces a deep, refreshing sleep. Many experts hypothesize that the benzodiazepines improve the quality of sleep because of their effect on REM sleep. In most cases, benzodiazepines decrease the frequency of eyeball movement and the time spent in REM sleep. Flurazepam (in low doses) and temazepam, however, shorten stages 3 and 4 of NREM sleep and do not diminish REM sleep significantly. If temazepam has any effect on REM sleep, the effect resembles that of triazolam, which decreases REM sleep in the early hours but allows the sleeper to make up the lost REM time later in the sleep period. Benzodiazepines that do decrease total REM sleep time also allow for more frequent REM cycles later in the sleep period.

PHARMACOTHERAPEUTICS

Clinical indications for the benzodiazepines include relaxing and calming the patient during the day or before surgery and treating insomnia characterized by difficulty falling or staying asleep or early-morning awakenings. Other clinical indications include producing intravenous (I.V.) anesthesia, treating alcohol withdrawal, treating anxiety and seizure disorders, and producing skeletal muscle relaxation. More information about these clinical indications for the benzodiazepines appears in the appropriate chapters of this book.

In most cases, benzodiazepines are preferred to barbiturates because of their effectiveness and safety. Benzodiazepines offer many advantages, including fewer adverse effects and less abuse, few drug interactions, a wide margin of safety between therapeutic and toxic doses that makes overdose less likely, and a rare incidence of physical and psychological dependence with therapeutic doses.

Despite their many advantages, benzodiazepines do have disadvantages. Abuse of the drugs can cause overdose, but with much less frequency than barbiturates. The potential for physical and psychological dependence exists with high doses and long-term use. Also, benzodiazepines can produce a synergistic action with other CNS depressants, further enhancing the depressant effects of the other drugs. If combined, such drugs can be lethal.

flurazepam hydrochloride (Dalmane). A Schedule IV drug, flurazepam is used as a hypnotic in patients with insomnia, such as those with poor sleep habits, and in acute or chronic medical situations requiring restful sleep. It is only for short-term and intermittent use.
Usual adult dosage: 15 to 30 mg P.O. at bedtime. Elderly and debilitated patients receive 15 mg P.O. at bedtime.

lorazepam (Ativan). A Schedule IV drug, lorazepam is used for sedation before surgery, insomnia from anxiety or transient situational stress, anxiety disorders, short-term relief of anxiety, or anxiety associated with depressive symptoms. This drug is for short-term and intermittent use only.
Usual adult dosage: for preoperative sedation, 0.05 mg/kg up to 4 mg I.M. 2 hours before the procedure; for hypnotic effects, 2 to 4 mg P.O. at bedtime. Elderly and debilitated patients receive 1 to 2 mg at bedtime for sleep.

quazepam (Doral). A Schedule IV drug, quazepam is used only as a hypnotic to relieve insomnia associated with difficulty falling asleep or early morning awakenings.
Usual adult dosage: for hypnotic effects, 15 mg P.O. at bedtime until the patient's response is determined; then decreased to 7.5 mg, if possible. Elderly and debilitated patients should receive 7.5 mg P.O. at bedtime.

temazepam (Restoril). A Schedule IV drug, temazepam is used only as a hypnotic to relieve insomnia associated with complaints of difficulty falling asleep, frequent nocturnal awakenings, or early-morning awakenings.
Usual adult dosage: for hypnotic effects, 15 to 30 mg P.O. at bedtime. Elderly and debilitated patients receive 15 mg P.O. initially.

triazolam (Halcion). A Schedule IV drug, triazolam is used to treat insomnia from various physical or psychological states. It is short-acting and therefore has less tendency to cause morning drowsiness (hangover effect). This drug should not be used for longer than 1 month for managing insomnia.

Usual adult dosage: 0.125 to 0.25 mg P.O. at bedtime. Elderly and debilitated patients may receive 0.125 mg P.O. at bedtime.

Drug interactions

Except for other CNS depressants, few drugs interact with benzodiazepines. (For details, see *Drug interactions: Benzodiazepines.*) No interactions between drugs and food involving benzodiazepines have been documented.

ADVERSE DRUG REACTIONS

Benzodiazepines cause few adverse reactions. Some mild allergic reactions and idiosyncratic effects have been reported.

Common adverse reactions, such as daytime sedation and hangover effect, can occur with clinically effective doses of benzodiazepines, but these occur less commonly than those accompanying barbiturates. Dose-related dizziness and ataxia also may occur. Rebound insomnia may occur, especially with short-acting drugs such as triazolam. Some benzodiazepines may cause amnesia. Elderly patients, debilitated patients, and patients with liver disease are more likely to experience dose-related adverse reactions to benzodiazepines.

Fatigue, muscle weakness, mouth dryness, nausea, and vomiting result occasionally from benzodiazepine use. Respiratory depression more commonly occurs with elderly or debilitated patients, patients with limited ventilatory reserve, and patients receiving other CNS depressants. Signs and symptoms of psychological and physical dependence occur with prolonged use and high doses, but rarely with usual doses. If a patient becomes physically dependent, sudden withdrawal may cause weakness, delirium, and tonic-clonic seizures.

Rare and usually mild allergic reactions to benzodiazepines include skin rash, pruritus, urticaria, burning eyes, and photosensitivity. Rare idiosyncratic reactions, which occur primarily in elderly patients, include nervousness, restlessness, talkativeness, apprehension, euphoria, and excitement.

NURSING PROCESS APPLICATION

The following information assists the nurse in caring for a patient who is receiving a benzodiazepine as a sedative or hypnotic.

Assessment
• Review the patient's history for a condition that contraindicates the use of a benzodiazepine, such as pregnancy or known hypersensitivity to the drug.
• Review the patient's history for a condition that requires cautious use of a benzodiazepine, such as depression, im-

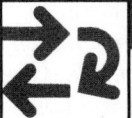

DRUG INTERACTIONS

Benzodiazepines

Few drug interactions involving the benzodiazepines discussed in this chapter occur. However, when interactions occur, they are seen more commonly with the concurrent use of other central nervous system (CNS) depressants, including alcohol. The additive effects of CNS drugs and benzodiazepines can be lethal.

DRUG	INTERACTING DRUGS	POSSIBLE EFFECTS	NURSING IMPLICATIONS
flurazepam, lorazepam, quazepam, temazepam, triazolam	CNS depressants	Enhance sedative and other CNS depressant effects. Effects may be supra-additive, causing motor skill impairment and respiratory depression. Possible lethal effect especially with high doses. Combination with anticonvulsant drugs, which also are CNS depressants, can cause changes in seizures, especially in frequency or severity.	• Monitor for changes in level of consciousness and muscle coordination. • Monitor for signs of respiratory depression. • Advise the patient about possible additive effects of other CNS depressant drugs. • Warn the patient that alcohol increases the effect of the drug and can cause serious CNS depression. • Supervise ambulation; raise bed rails, especially with elderly patients. • Advise against operating a motor vehicle or heavy machinery because of possible impaired motor skills. • Observe for changes in frequency and severity of seizures when these drugs are used with anticonvulsant drugs.
flurazepam, quazepam, triazolam	cimetidine	Inhibits hepatic metabolism, causing excessive sedation and increasing CNS depression	• Monitor for signs of increasing CNS depressant effects; notify the physician of any changes. • Advise against operating a motor vehicle or heavy machinery because increased sedation is possible. • Supervise ambulation; raise bed rails, especially with elderly patients.
flurazepam	oral contraceptives	Decrease oxidative metabolism	• Monitor the patient for excessive sedation. • Expect to decrease the benzodiazepine dosage.
lorazepam, temazepam	oral contraceptives	Increase glucuronide conjugation	• Expect to increase the benzodiazepine dosage to produce the desired effect.

paired renal or hepatic function, chronic pulmonary insufficiency, or lactation.

• Assess the patient for adverse reactions to the benzodiazepine, such as daytime sedation, hangover effect, dizziness, ataxia, fatigue, dry mouth, nausea, vomiting, and respiratory depression.

• Review the patient's medication history to identify the use of drugs that may interact with the benzodiazepine, such as CNS depressants, cimetidine, or oral contraceptives.

• Assess the patient for signs of benzodiazepine dependence, such as drug ineffectiveness or repeated requests for additional doses or an increased dosage.

• Evaluate the patient's and family's knowledge about the prescribed benzodiazepine.

Nursing diagnoses

The following examples represent appropriate nursing diagnoses for a patient receiving a benzodiazepine as a sedative or hypnotic.

• Potential for injury related to a preexisting condition that contraindicates the use of a benzodiazepine as a sedative or hypnotic

• Potential for injury related to a preexisting condition that requires cautious use of a benzodiazepine as a sedative or hypnotic

• Potential for injury related to adverse drug reactions

• Ineffective breathing pattern related to the respiratory depression caused by a benzodiazepine

• Altered role performance related to benzodiazepine dependence

• Knowledge deficit related to the prescribed benzodiazepine

Patient-teaching tips for sedative and hypnotic agents

Regardless of the sedative or hypnotic prescribed, the following patient-teaching tips apply. The nurse should give oral instructions first, then written ones to take home.
• Teach the patient to take the drug exactly as prescribed and not to change the dosage without consulting the physician.
• Advise the patient not to discontinue the drug suddenly without consulting the physician because withdrawal symptoms may occur.
• Instruct the patient not to operate a motor vehicle or heavy machinery, at least until the patient knows the drug's effects on mental alertness.
• Instruct the patient not to drink alcohol during drug therapy because respiratory depression can occur.
• Instruct the patient to read drug labels and avoid over-the-counter drugs that contain central nervous system depressants, such as alcohol or antihistamines.
• Advise the patient to consult the physician before taking any tranquilizers, narcotics, or other prescription pain relievers.
• Instruct the patient to notify the nurse or physician when beginning or discontinuing any other drug during sedative or hypnotic therapy.
• Counsel the patient not to give any prescribed drugs to family members or friends.
• Advise the patient to keep the drug and all other medications out of the reach of children.

Planning and implementation

• Do not administer a benzodiazepine to a patient with a condition that contraindicates its use.
• Administer a benzodiazepine cautiously to a patient at risk because of a preexisting condition.
• Monitor the patient regularly for adverse reactions to the prescribed benzodiazepine, especially in an elderly or debilitated patient or one with liver disease.
• *Consult with the physician if other CNS depressants also are prescribed during benzodiazepine therapy; this drug combination may cause lethal depressant effects.*
• Expect to discontinue benzodiazepine therapy in a patient who hallucinates or behaves violently.
• Assist with gastric lavage, respiratory support, and other support measures, such as I.V. fluid or drug administration, if overdose occurs. Frequently monitor vital signs and fluid intake and output.
• *Keep epinephrine and corticosteroids readily available for emergency care of a patient with a hypersensitivity reaction to the prescribed benzodiazepine.*
• Plan care and administer drugs based on the hospitalized patient's daily routines and bedtime rituals. Do not awaken a patient to administer a benzodiazepine.
• Watch the patient take the benzodiazepine to prevent drug hoarding for later use.

• *Take safety measures after administering the drug, such as raising the bed rails and assisting with ambulation, because the patient may become dizzy and weak. Give special assistance to an elderly patient during ambulation.*
• Do not apply restraints if a patient awakens confused and excited. Instead, attempt to calm the patient, orient the patient to the surroundings, and talk quietly until the patient relaxes.
• Do not awaken the patient during the night, unless necessary. Allow the patient at least 90 minutes of uninterrupted rest or sleep whenever possible and use times when the patient awakens spontaneously to make necessary checks or to administer required treatments. Question the rationale for routines that require waking the patient, especially during the night.
• Use nursing judgment when considering administration of a second p.r.n. dose of a benzodiazepine during the night. Try to find out why the patient cannot sleep. If pain is causing insomnia, use comfort measures, such as back rubs, and administer analgesics. Remember, the hangover effect can result from injudicious use of a benzodiazepine during the night.
• Notify the physician if adverse reactions occur.
• Monitor the patient's vital signs frequently, particularly noting signs of respiratory depression, such as decreased respirations or respiratory pattern changes.
• *Perform a respiratory assessment before and after giving each dose of the prescribed benzodiazepine.*
• *Withhold the benzodiazepine dose and notify the physician if respiratory depression occurs.*
• Expect to reduce the benzodiazepine dosage for a patient who is receiving another CNS depressant because of the risk of increased respiratory depression.
• Position the debilitated patient to maximize respiratory function. For example, help the patient into a semi-Fowler's or high Fowler's position.
• Encourage the patient to be honest about use of the prescribed benzodiazepine because dependence can occur with long-term or high-dose use of benzodiazepines.
• *Do not discontinue benzodiazepine therapy abruptly. The patient may develop withdrawal symptoms, such as weakness, delirium, and tonic-clonic seizures.*
• Alert the physician to suspected benzodiazepine dependence.

Patient teaching

• Provide general instructions about benzodiazepine use. (For details, see *Patient-teaching tips for sedative and hypnotic agents*.)
• Teach the patient and family the name, dose, frequency, action, and adverse effects of the prescribed benzodiazepine.
• Instruct the patient with insomnia or a similar sleep disorder to try other measures before taking the prescribed

benzodiazepine. Suggest a warm bath or shower or a glass of warm milk before the patient retires, encourage moderate daily exercise several hours before sleeping, advise the patient to eliminate daytime naps, and encourage reading and the use of other relaxation techniques.
• Instruct the family to take safety measures, such as assisting with ambulation, during the patient's benzodiazepine therapy.
• Teach the family what to do if the patient awakens confused and excited after taking a benzodiazepine. Tell them not to awaken the patient during the night unless necessary.
• Instruct the patient and family to alert the physician if adverse reactions occur.

Evaluation

The following examples represent appropriate evaluation statements for a patient receiving a benzodiazepine.
• The patient has no conditions that contraindicate benzodiazepine therapy.
• The patient exhibits no signs of complications in the preexisting condition linked to the prescribed benzodiazepine.
• The patient experiences no adverse reactions to the prescribed benzodiazepine.
• The patient maintains a normal respiratory rate and pattern.
• The patient shows no signs of benzodiazepine dependence.
• The patient and family express an accurate understanding of the points taught about the prescribed benzodiazepine.
• The patient reads and uses other relaxation techniques at bedtime.

BARBITURATES

The major pharmacologic action of the barbiturates reduces overall CNS alertness. The uses of barbiturates include daytime and preoperative sedation, hypnotic effects for patients complaining of insomnia, anesthesia, relief of anxiety, and anticonvulsant activity. This section discusses the barbiturates used primarily as sedatives and hypnotics, including amobarbital, aprobarbital, butabarbital, mephobarbital, pentobarbital, phenobarbital, and secobarbital.

PHARMACOKINETICS

Barbiturates are absorbed well, distributed rapidly, metabolized by the liver, and excreted via the metabolic processes as well as in the urine.

Absorption, distribution, metabolism, excretion

Barbiturates are absorbed well after oral and I.M. administration. The I.M. route usually is avoided, however, because the alkalinity of the soluble preparations causes pain and necrosis at the injection site.

Barbiturates, which are weak acids, are distributed rapidly to all body tissues and fluids. The highest concentrations go to the brain, liver, and kidneys. Barbiturates also cross the placental barrier and can depress neonatal respirations and the CNS. Lipid solubility is the dominant factor in the distribution of barbiturates within the body. The more lipid-soluble the barbiturate, the more rapidly the drug penetrates all body tissues. Secobarbital displays the highest lipid solubility; phenobarbital, the lowest.

Barbiturates are metabolized primarily by the microsomal enzymes in the liver. Longer-acting barbiturates metabolize more slowly than shorter-acting ones.

Barbiturates are excreted primarily by the kidneys. Some, such as mephobarbital, undergo metabolic changes in the liver before they are excreted. Others, such as aprobarbital and phenobarbital, are excreted partly in an altered form and partly in their unchanged forms. Still others, such as butabarbital, pentobarbital, and secobarbital, are excreted in a completely altered form. The more slowly the system metabolizes or excretes a barbiturate, the more prolonged the drug's action.

Onset, peak, duration

The duration of action represents the main difference among barbiturates. The duration may be ultrashort-acting, short-acting, intermediate-acting, or long-acting. Peak concentration levels also vary, depending on the onset of action. (For information about onset, peak, and duration, see *Comparing the onset, peak, and duration of barbiturates,* page 406.)

The duration of a barbiturate depends in part on the rate of drug metabolism and the rate of drug redistribution throughout the body. The duration varies among patients and even in the same patient from time to time. The half-lives of barbiturates vary from drug to drug. For example, secobarbital has a half-life of 15 to 40 hours, mephobarbital 11 to 67 hours, and phenobarbital 50 to 170 hours. Note, however, that because of the rapid distribution of some barbiturates, no correlation exists between duration and half-life. When used over an extended time, all barbiturates will accumulate.

PHARMACODYNAMICS

Researchers do not know the primary sites of drug action and the mechanisms of action of barbiturates. They believe the primary action sites to be the neuronal fibers and synapses that integrate the sleep-awake centers of the brain,

Comparing the onset, peak, and duration of barbiturates

The onset of action, peak concentration level, and duration of action vary significantly depending on the specific barbiturate. The following graph illustrates the comparison of short-acting, intermediate-acting, and long-acting barbiturates.

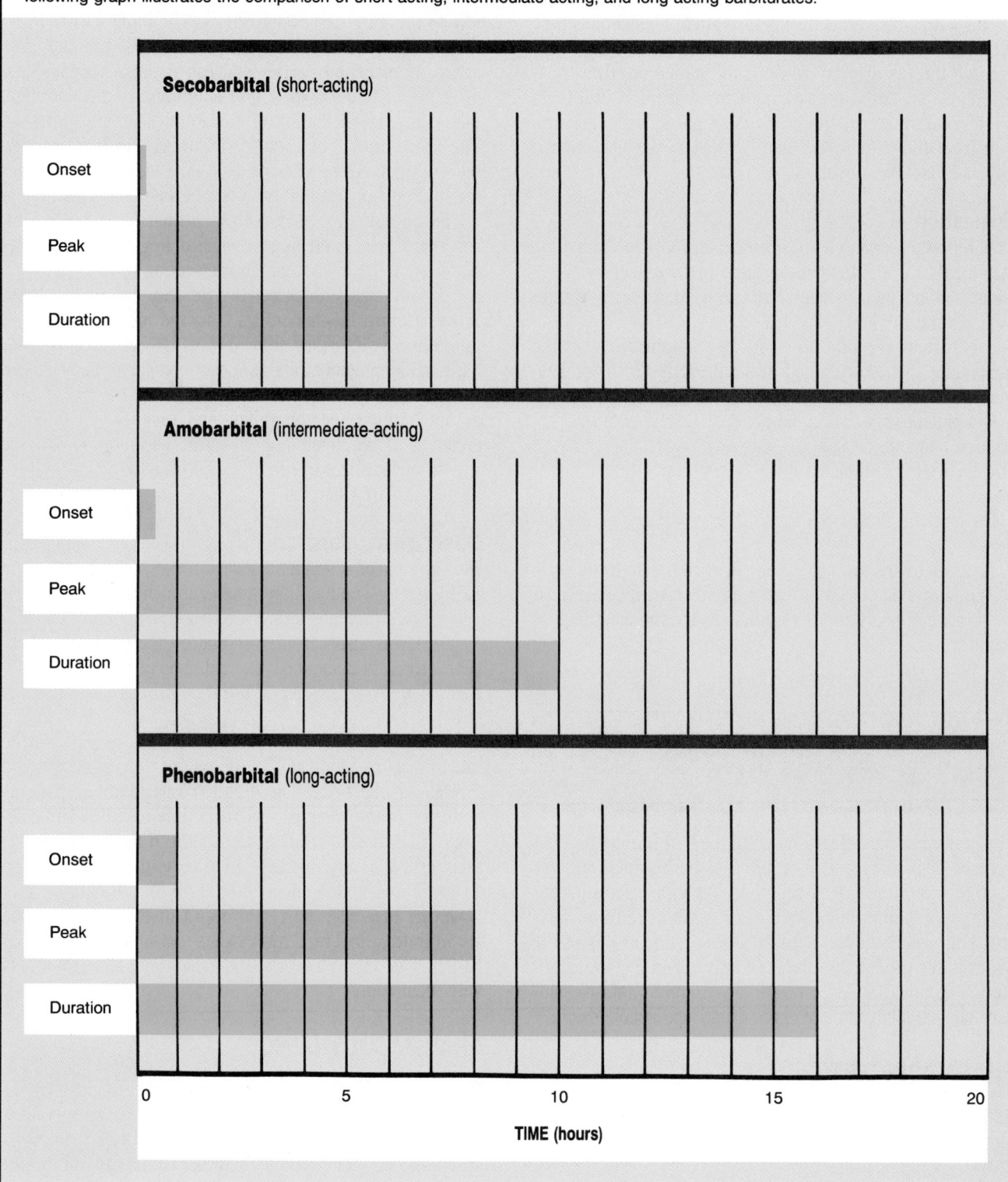

primarily at the level of the thalamus and the ascending reticular formation.

Mechanism of action

Barbiturates are considered to be nonspecific CNS depressants. The sites of barbiturate action appear to be less selective than the sites of benzodiazepine action. As sedative-hypnotics, barbiturates depress the sensory cortex, decrease motor activity, alter cerebral function, and produce drowsiness, sedation, and hypnosis. These drugs appear to act at the level of the thalamus, where they inhibit the ascending conduction in the reticular formation, thus interfering with impulse transmission to the cortex.

Barbiturates produce a sequence of CNS depressant effects, ranging from mild sedation and relief of anxiety to anesthesia and coma. (For more information, see *Effects of barbiturates,* page 408.) The degree of CNS depression depends on the drug dose and administration route as well as the patient's age and emotional state.

Barbiturates decrease stages 3 and 4 of NREM sleep. They also reduce the amount of time a person spends in REM sleep or dream sleep. If barbiturates are prescribed for long periods and then abruptly withdrawn, the patient may experience REM sleep rebound, with a marked increase in dreaming, nightmares, or insomnia.

Patients also can develop a tolerance for barbiturates, which decreases the sedative, hypnotic, and mood-altering effects of the drugs. Also, as tolerance increases, the therapeutic index decreases and the drugs become less safe. Tolerance can occur after only weeks or after a few months of therapy.

PHARMACOTHERAPEUTICS

Barbiturates have many clinical indications including daytime sedation, hypnotic effects, anesthesia, and anticonvulsant effects. (For details about the use of barbiturates as anticonvulsants, see Chapter 20, Anticonvulsant Agents.) Barbiturates usually are not used for daytime sedation. When used, they are given for short periods, typically less than 2 weeks. The use of barbiturates as sedatives and hypnotics is declining because benzodiazepines now are regarded as the sedatives and hypnotics of choice.

Barbiturates offer no real advantages over the benzodiazepines as sedatives and hypnotics. In fact, they present many disadvantages, including a greater probability of causing drug tolerance, a high potential for physical and psychological dependence, a high liability for abuse, severe withdrawal symptoms when drug use is discontinued suddenly after long-term use, life-threatening toxicity resulting from overdose, potentially lethal CNS depressant effects if used concurrently with alcohol or other CNS depressants, and respiratory center depression after large doses. More toxic than the benzodiazepines, barbiturates, especially

long-acting forms, are more prone to accumulate in the system.

Elderly or debilitated patients should receive a lower dosage than other adults.

amobarbital, amobarbital sodium (Amytal). A Schedule II drug, amobarbital is used for conditions that require degrees of sedation. Minimal doses are used to relieve anxiety and tension, hypnotic doses to treat insomnia and acute agitated episodes in psychotic disorders.
Usual adult dosage: for sedation, 30 to 50 mg P.O. or I.M. b.i.d. or t.i.d.; for hypnotic effect, 65 to 200 mg P.O. or I.M. at bedtime.

aprobarbital (Alurate). A Schedule III drug, aprobarbital is used for daytime sedation and the induction of sleep on a short-term basis.
Usual adult dosage: for sedation, 40 mg P.O. t.i.d.; for hypnotic effect, 40 to 160 mg P.O. at bedtime.

butabarbital sodium (Butisol, Buticaps). A Schedule III drug, butabarbital is used as a daytime mild sedative for anxiety, as a preoperative sedative, and for insomnia for use up to 2 weeks.
Usual adult dosage: for sedation, 15 to 30 mg P.O. t.i.d. or q.i.d.; for preoperative sedation, 50 to 100 mg P.O. 60 to 90 minutes before surgery; for hypnotic effect, 50 to 100 mg P.O. at bedtime.

mephobarbital (Mebaral). A Schedule IV drug, mephobarbital is used for daytime sedation to relieve anxiety, tension, and apprehension, and as adjunct therapy for generalized tonic-clonic and absence seizures.
Usual adult dosage: for daytime sedation, 32 to 100 mg P.O. t.i.d. or q.i.d.

pentobarbital sodium (Nembutal). A Schedule II drug, pentobarbital is used as a daytime sedative to reduce nervous tension in patients with various medical and psychiatric conditions; as a preoperative sedative for minor diagnostic or surgical procedures; for short-term treatment of insomnia for up to 2 weeks; and for the emergency control of seizures.
Usual adult dosage: for daytime sedation, 20 to 40 mg P.O. b.i.d. to q.i.d.; for preoperative sedation, 150 to 200 mg P.O. or I.M.; for hypnotic effect, 100 mg P.O., 120 to 200 mg rectal, or 100 to 200 mg I.M.

phenobarbital, phenobarbital sodium (Luminal). A Schedule IV drug, phenobarbital is used as a sedative to relieve mild to moderate anxiety or tension, as a preoperative sedative, as treatment for insomnia, and as an anticonvulsant.

Effects of barbiturates

Barbiturates produce a wide range of sequential effects depending on the size of the dose. The same effects would occur with benzodiazepines and the nonbenzodiazepine-nonbarbiturate drugs, but would require much higher doses than barbiturates to produce such effects.

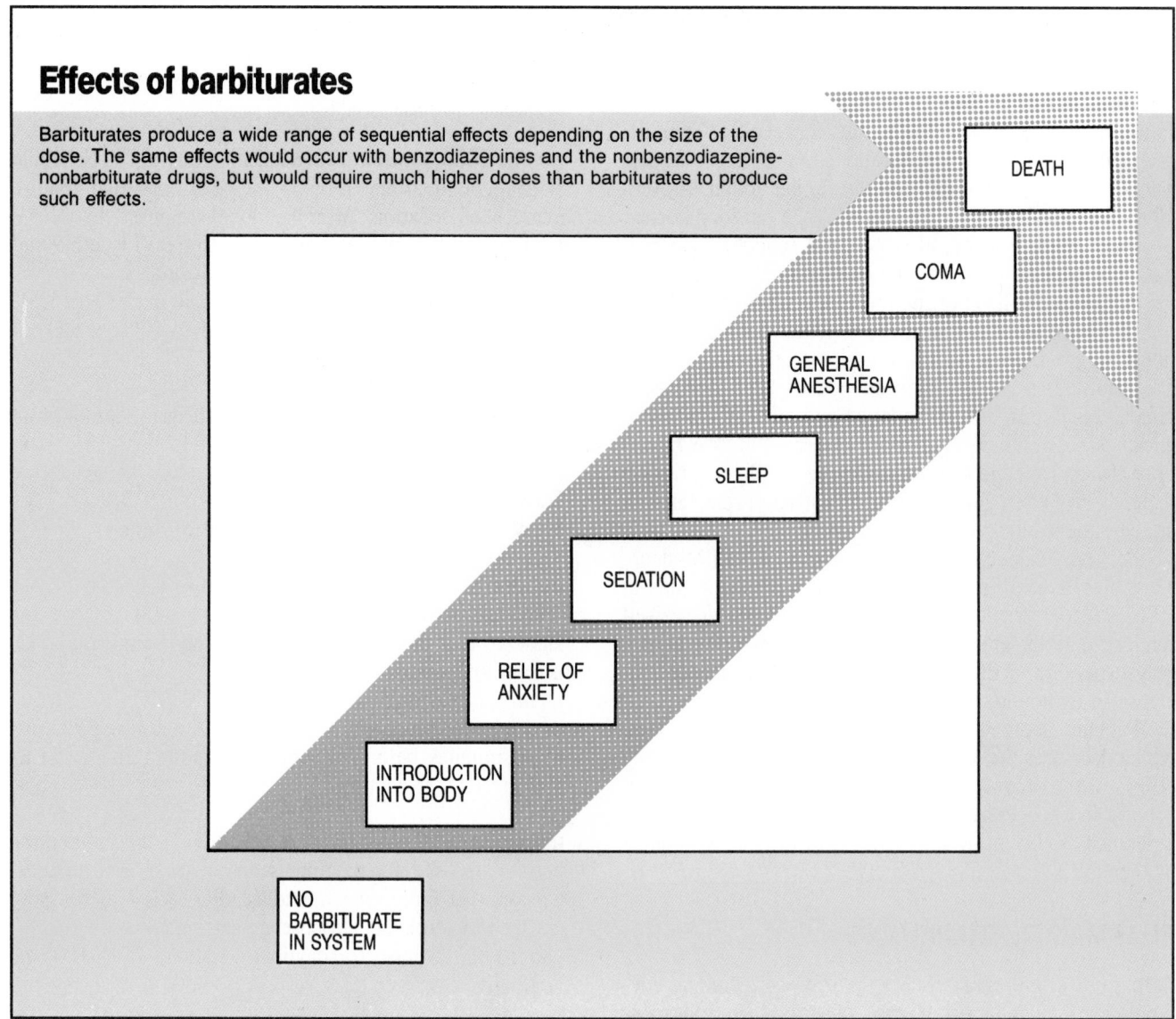

DEATH

COMA

GENERAL ANESTHESIA

SLEEP

SEDATION

RELIEF OF ANXIETY

INTRODUCTION INTO BODY

NO BARBITURATE IN SYSTEM

Usual adult dosage: for daytime sedation, 15 to 30 mg P.O. b.i.d. to q.i.d.; for preoperative sedation, 100 to 200 mg I.M. 60 to 90 minutes before surgery; for hypnotic effect, 100 to 320 mg P.O. or I.M. at bedtime.

secobarbital sodium (Seconal). A Schedule II drug, secobarbital is used as a mild sedative; as a short-acting hypnotic for insomnia, especially in patients with difficulty falling asleep; and as treatment for acute convulsive disorders, such as local anesthetic reactions, tetanus, and status epilepticus.

Usual adult dosage: for daytime sedation, 30 to 50 mg P.O. t.i.d. to q.i.d. or 120 to 200 mg rectal suppository; for preoperative sedation, 200 to 300 mg P.O. 1 to 2 hours before surgery; for hypnotic effect, 100 to 200 mg P.O., 120 to 200 mg rectally, or 100 to 200 mg I.M. at bedtime.

Drug interactions

Barbiturates interact with many other drugs. (For details, see *Drug interactions: Barbiturates.*)

ADVERSE DRUG REACTIONS

Barbiturates cause many adverse drug reactions, some of which are minor. Other more serious drug reactions include severe CNS and respiratory depression.

The most frequently reported adverse reactions relate to the CNS and include drowsiness, lethargy, headache, depression, and vertigo. After hypnotic doses, the hangover effect commonly occurs, accompanied by impairment of judgment and motor skills that can last for many hours and may lead to falls in elderly patients. When hypnotic doses are discontinued, the patient may experience REM sleep rebound as well as a decrease in stage 2 NREM sleep.

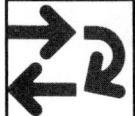

DRUG INTERACTIONS

Barbiturates

Drug interactions involving barbiturates are common and can be serious. Interactions typically occur with concurrent use of other central nervous system (CNS) depressants, including alcohol. The additive effects can be lethal. Most of the clinically significant interactions from barbiturates occur with phenobarbital, and some of the barbiturates are converted to phenobarbital in the body.

DRUG	INTERACTING DRUGS	POSSIBLE EFFECTS	NURSING IMPLICATIONS
amobarbital, aprobarbital, butabarbital, mephobarbital, pentobarbital, phenobarbital, secobarbital	hydantoins	Inhibit phenobarbital metabolism, resulting in increased toxic effects	• Monitor serum concentration levels; phenobarbital dosage may need to be decreased. • Advise the patient to report adverse reactions. • Assess for change in level of consciousness. • Alert the patient not to operate a motor vehicle or heavy machinery until the effect of the drug combination is known. • Advise the patient to avoid alcohol consumption.
	beta blockers (metoprolol, propranolol)	Cause induction of beta-blocker metabolism, resulting in decreased effectiveness of beta blockers	• Monitor desired effect in the patient (antianginal, antihypertensive, or antiarrhythmic); beta-blocker dosage may need to be increased. • Instruct the patient to report changes in desired effect in drug therapy. • Advise the patient to report periodically for blood pressure and pulse check.
	chloramphenicol	Cause induction of chloramphenicol metabolism, resulting in decreased effectiveness of chloramphenicol; inhibits phenobarbital metabolism	• Monitor desired effect in the patient (anti-infective); chloramphenicol dosage may need to be increased. • Monitor serum chloramphenicol and phenobarbital levels.
	corticosteroids	Induce corticosteroid metabolism, resulting in decreased effectiveness of corticosteroids	• Expect to increase the corticosteroid dosage because of the drug's decreased effectiveness. • Monitor the patient's weight and blood pressure. • Monitor serum electrolyte levels.
	doxycycline	Induce doxycycline metabolism, resulting in decreased effectiveness of doxycycline	• Expect to substitute tetracycline for doxycycline or increase the doxycycline dosage because of the drug's decreased effectiveness.
	oral anticoagulants	Induce oral anticoagulant metabolism, resulting in decreased effectiveness of oral anticoagulants	• Monitor prothrombin levels; anticoagulant dosage may need to be increased. • Advise the patient to be alert for signs and symptoms of thrombus formation: pain, tenderness, edema in the calf.
	oral contraceptives	Induce oral contraceptive metabolism, resulting in decreased effectiveness of oral contraceptives	• Alert the patient that contraceptive effect may be impaired; breakthrough bleeding may occur. • Suggest alternative or additional contraceptive method.
	quinidine	Induce quinidine metabolism, resulting in decreased effectiveness of quinidine	• Expect to increase the quinidine dosage, if needed. • Advise the patient to see the physician frequently for monitoring of cardiac status. • Alert the patient to report signs and symptoms of arrhythmias, such as palpitations and irregular pulse.
	methoxyflurane	May induce hepatic microsomal enzymes that may stimulate metabolism of methoxyflurane to nephrotoxic metabolites	• Avoid concurrent administration of phenobarbital and methoxyflurane.

(continued)

DRUG INTERACTIONS

Barbiturates (continued)

DRUG	INTERACTING DRUGS	POSSIBLE EFFECTS	NURSING IMPLICATIONS
amobarbital, aprobarbital, butabarbital, mephobarbital, pentobarbital, phenobarbital, secobarbital (continued)	tricyclic antidepressants	Induce tricyclic antidepressant metabolism, resulting in decreased effectiveness of tricyclic antidepressants	• Expect to increase the tricyclic antidepressant dosage, if needed. • Monitor serum levels of tricyclic antidepressants. • Advise the patient to report any change in therapeutic effect, such as lack of mood elevation.
	CNS depressants (antianxiety agents, sedatives, hypnotics, most narcotic analgesics, and alcohol)	Produce additive CNS effects, resulting in increased sedative toxicity	• Assess frequently for changes in level of consciousness and respirations. • Supervise ambulation; raise bed rails, especially for elderly patients. • Alert the patient not to operate a motor vehicle or heavy machinery until the effects of the drug combination are known. • Advise the patient not to drink alcohol while taking these medications.
	valproic acid	Inhibits the hepatic metabolism of phenobarbital	• Monitor for excessive phenobarbital effect, such as drowsiness. • Expect to reduce the phenobarbital dosage because of increased phenobarbital serum levels.
	metronidazole	Increase metronidazole metabolism	• Expect to increase the metronidazole dosage, if needed.
	digitoxin	Decrease digitoxin effect	• Monitor the patient for the desired effect of digitoxin related to arrhythmias and cardiac function. • Expect to increase the digitoxin dosage, if needed.
	theophylline	Increase the rate of theophylline metabolism, which decreases serum theophylline concentration level	• Monitor the patient's serum theophylline level. • Adjust the theophylline dosage, as prescribed.
	cyclosporine	May decrease plasma cyclosporine level	• Monitor the patient's cyclosporine level. • Expect to increase the cyclosporine dosage, if needed.

Patients, especially elderly ones, may exhibit excitement and confusion, particularly when taking short-acting compounds such as secobarbital.

The patient can experience serious adverse respiratory reactions, including hypoventilation, laryngospasm, bronchospasm, and severe respiratory depression, specifically when large doses are administered I.V. and too rapidly. Large doses of barbiturates suppress the hypoxic and chemoreceptor drive of the respiratory system, resulting in decreased respiratory rate and rhythm.

The patient also can sustain adverse cardiovascular reactions such as mild bradycardia and hypotension. Less commonly, adverse reactions to barbiturates affect the GI tract, resulting in nausea, vomiting, diarrhea, and epigastric pain.

Acute barbiturate toxicity causes overdose symptoms, which can be severe. The symptoms are characterized by CNS and respiratory depression, and death can result from respiratory failure followed by cardiac arrest.

With prolonged use, the patient can develop drug tolerance as well as psychological and physical dependence on the barbiturate. Withdrawal symptoms resemble those associated with chronic alcoholism and occur with sudden discontinuation after long-term use.

Allergic reactions mainly involve the skin and mucous membranes and occur more commonly in patients with past allergies or asthma. Allergic reactions include these signs and symptoms: skin rashes of various kinds, urticaria, angioedema, and fever. Rare occurrences of photosensitivity also have been reported. Other signs and symptoms of allergic reactions to barbiturates include rare blood dyscrasias, such as pancytopenia, leukopenia, granulocytopenia, thrombocytopenia, and megaloblastic anemia secondary to folic acid depletion.

Idiosyncratic reactions include paradoxical anxiety, agitation, restlessness, and rage or paradoxical excitement (delirium rather than sedation). The idiosyncratic reactions occur most commonly among elderly patients and those with severe uncontrolled pain.

NURSING PROCESS APPLICATION

The following information assists the nurse in caring for a patient who is receiving a barbiturate as a sedative or hypnotic.

Assessment
• Review the patient's history for a condition that contraindicates the use of a barbiturate, such as known hypersensitivity to the drug, porphyria, pregnancy, nephritis, renal insufficiency, or premonitory signs of hepatic coma.
• Review the patient's history for a condition that requires cautious use of a barbiturate, such as lactation, depression, suicidal tendencies, hepatic damage, or a history of drug abuse.
• Assess the patient for adverse reactions to the prescribed barbiturate, such as CNS or respiratory depression, mild bradycardia, hypotension, or GI distress.
• Review the patient's medication history to identify the use of drugs that may interact with the prescribed barbiturate, such as CNS depressants, oral anticoagulants, hydantoins, and beta blockers.
• Assess the patient for signs of barbiturate dependence, such as drug ineffectiveness or repeated requests for additional doses or dosage increases.
• Evaluate the patient's and family's knowledge about the prescribed barbiturate.

Nursing diagnoses
The following examples represent appropriate nursing diagnoses for a patient receiving a barbiturate as a sedative or hypnotic.
• Potential for injury related to a preexisting condition that contraindicates the use of a barbiturate as a sedative or hypnotic
• Potential for injury related to a preexisting condition that requires cautious use of a barbiturate as a sedative or hypnotic
• Potential for injury related to adverse drug reactions
• Ineffective breathing pattern related to barbiturate-induced respiratory depression
• Altered role performance related to barbiturate dependence
• Knowledge deficit related to the prescribed barbiturate

Planning and implementation
• Do not administer a barbiturate to a patient with a condition that contraindicates its use.
• Administer a barbiturate cautiously to a patient at risk because of a preexisting condition.
• Monitor the patient periodically for adverse reactions to the prescribed barbiturate. Be alert for idiosyncratic reactions, such as paradoxical anxiety or excitement, in an elderly patient or one with severe uncontrolled pain.
• Expect to administer a reduced dosage, as needed, to an elderly or debilitated patient.
• Discontinue the drug slowly after long-term therapy, as prescribed, to prevent REM sleep rebound.
• Monitor prothrombin time, as directed, for a patient who is receiving an anticoagulant. Keep in mind that abrupt withdrawal of barbiturates may cause serious bleeding. Adjust the anticoagulant dosage as prescribed.
• *Take safety measures when administering the prescribed barbiturate, especially to an elderly patient. For example, place the bed in a low position, keep the bed rails up, and assist with ambulation.*
• *Rotate the amobarbital ampule (do not shake); mix the solution with sterile water only;* discard solutions that do not clear within 5 minutes; use the solution within 30 minutes after opening to minimize deterioration; and inject the solution slowly and deeply into a large muscle mass when using the I.M. route of administration.
• *Do not use a cloudy pentobarbital, phenobarbital, or secobarbital solution or mix the solution with other medications;* use the solution within 30 minutes after opening to minimize deterioration; and inject the solution into a large muscle mass when administering I.M.
• Remember, the I.M. route is a poor route for administering barbiturates.
• Notify the physician if adverse reactions occur.
• Monitor the patient's vital signs frequently, particularly noting such signs of respiratory depression as decreased respirations or respiratory pattern changes.
• *Perform a respiratory assessment before and after administering each dose of the prescribed barbiturate.*
• *Withhold the barbiturate dose and notify the physician if respiratory depression occurs.*
• Position the debilitated patient to maximize respiratory function. For example, place the patient in a semi-Fowler's or high Fowler's position.
• Encourage the patient to be honest about barbiturate use because dependence can occur with long-term use.
• *Do not discontinue barbiturate therapy abruptly.* Otherwise, the patient receiving long-term therapy may develop withdrawal symptoms similar to those associated with alcoholism.
• Alert the physician to suspected barbiturate dependence.

Patient teaching
• Provide general instructions about barbiturate use. (For details, see *Patient-teaching tips for sedative and hypnotic agents,* page 404.)
• Teach the patient and family the name, dose, frequency, action, and adverse effects of the prescribed barbiturate.

Evaluation
The following examples represent appropriate evaluation statements for a patient receiving a barbiturate as a sedative or hypnotic.
• The patient has no conditions that contraindicate barbiturate therapy.
• The patient exhibits no signs of complications in the preexisting condition linked to the prescribed barbiturate.
• The patient displays no adverse reactions to the prescribed barbiturate.
• The patient maintains a normal respiratory rate and pattern.
• The patient exhibits no signs of barbiturate dependence.
• The patient and family express an accurate understanding of the points taught about the prescribed barbiturate.
• The patient reviews all prescriptions with the physician before taking any other drugs during barbiturate therapy.

NONBENZODIAZEPINES-NONBARBITURATES

Like the barbiturates, the nonbenzodiazepine-nonbarbiturate drugs act as hypnotics for short-term treatment of simple insomnia, but lose their effectiveness by the end of the second week. These drugs also provide preoperative sedation and sedation before electroencephalogram studies. This section discusses nonbenzodiazepine-nonbarbiturate drugs, including chloral hydrate, ethchlorvynol, glutethimide, methyprylon, and paraldehyde.

PHARMACOKINETICS

Nonbenzodiazepine-nonbarbiturate drugs are absorbed rapidly from the GI tract, metabolized in the liver, and excreted in the urine.

Absorption, distribution, metabolism, excretion
Rapid absorption from the GI tract occurs after oral administration, with the exception of glutethimide, which is absorbed erratically. The drugs generally are distributed to the cerebrospinal fluid, breast milk, and fetal circulation.
    The nonbenzodiazepine-nonbarbiturate drugs are metabolized primarily in the endoplasmic reticulum of the liver. Glutethimide and ethchlorvynol undergo extensive enterohepatic recirculation, with the liver destroying 80% to 90% of the drugs. Excretion occurs primarily through the urine via the kidneys and to a small degree in the feces via bile. Following therapeutic doses, clinically insignificant amounts are excreted in breast milk.

Onset, peak, duration
The onset of action for nonbenzodiazepine-nonbarbiturate drugs is rapid in most cases, with chloral hydrate displaying an onset within 10 to 15 minutes. The other drugs have an onset of 15 to 45 minutes. Drug action usually reaches a peak concentration level at 1 to 2 hours, with the exception of glutethimide, which reaches peak concentration at 1 to 6 hours from erratic absorption from the GI tract.
    The duration of action, including half-life, varies among the drugs. Generally, however, the duration is 4 to 8 hours. Ethchlorvynol has a duration and half-life of 10 to 25 hours, the longest among the nonbenzodiazepine-nonbarbiturate drugs.

PHARMACODYNAMICS

The mechanisms of action for the nonbenzodiazepine-nonbarbiturate drugs are not fully known, but the drugs produce depressant effects similar to the barbiturates. At high doses, the drugs can produce CNS depression of the respiratory center, causing respiratory failure and death.

PHARMACOTHERAPEUTICS

Nonbenzodiazepine-nonbarbiturate drugs typically are used for short-term treatment of simple insomnia and to sedate the patient before surgery. The drugs offer no special advantages over other sedatives and hypnotics and, in fact, are similar to the barbiturates. Many physicians believe that chloral hydrate produces less excitement in elderly patients than the barbiturates, but this has not been confirmed. The disadvantages of the drugs include being habit-forming, causing physical dependence, and being subject to abuse.

chloral hydrate (Noctec, SK-Chloral Hydrate). A Schedule IV drug, chloral hydrate is used as a daytime sedative and as a hypnotic to relieve insomnia.
Usual adult dosage: for sedation, 250 mg P.O. or 325 mg rectally t.i.d. after meals; for hypnotic effect, 0.5 to 1 gram P.O. or rectally 15 to 30 minutes before bedtime. The chloral hydrate dosage should not exceed 2 grams daily.

ethchlorvynol (Placidyl). A Schedule IV drug, ethchlorvynol is used for daytime sedation and short-term hypnotic therapy of insomnia (not to exceed 1 week).

Usual adult dosage: for sedation, 200 mg P.O. b.i.d. or t.i.d.; for hypnotic effect, 0.5 to 1 gram P.O. at bedtime. The dose should be adjusted carefully in elderly and debilitated patients.

glutethimide (Doriden). A Schedule III drug, glutethimide is used as a daytime and preoperative sedative and for the short-term treatment of insomnia (not to exceed 1 week). *Usual adult dosage:* for hypnotic effect, 250 to 500 mg P.O. at bedtime.

methyprylon (Noludar). A Schedule III drug, methyprylon is used as a hypnotic for transient or intermittent insomnia. *Usual adult dosage:* 200 to 400 mg P.O. at bedtime.

paraldehyde (Paral). A Schedule IV drug, paraldehyde is used infrequently to produce sedation, provide hypnotic therapy for insomnia, treat alcohol withdrawal syndrome, and control seizures caused by tetanus. Its most common use is for alcohol withdrawal.
Usual adult dosage: for sedation, 5 to 10 ml P.O. or rectally; for hypnotic effect, 10 to 30 ml P.O. or rectally at bedtime; for anticonvulsant effect, 5 to 10 ml I.M. or 5 ml I.V. diluted in normal saline solution; for alcohol withdrawal, 5 to 10 ml P.O. or 5 ml I.M. every 4 to 6 hours up to a maximum of 60 ml P.O. or 30 ml I.M. during the first 24 hours, then 5 to 10 ml P.O. or 5 ml I.M. every 6 hours to a maximum of 40 ml/day P.O. or 30 ml I.M. until desired response is achieved. I.V. dosages rarely are administered and are reserved for emergencies.

Drug interactions

The main interaction between nonbenzodiazepine-nonbarbiturate drugs occurs when they are used with other CNS depressants, causing additive CNS depression. (For details, see *Drug interactions: Nonbenzodiazepines-nonbarbiturates,* page 414.) No interactions occur between the drugs and food.

ADVERSE DRUG REACTIONS

The most common dose-related adverse reactions involving nonbenzodiazepine-nonbarbiturate drugs include GI symptoms and some hangover effects. Adverse GI reactions include nausea, vomiting, and some gastric irritation. The affected CNS, which occurs especially with hypnotic doses, can produce the hangover effect. Compared to the hangover produced by barbiturates and benzodiazepines, the nonbenzodiazepine-nonbarbiturate hangover occurs less commonly, especially in elderly patients.

At high doses, the drugs can produce CNS depression of the respiratory center, causing respiratory depression, respiratory failure, and death, especially in elderly patients. Habitual use can cause tolerance and dependence. Chronic and acute toxicity can occur, and abrupt withdrawal from large doses may cause dangerous withdrawal symptoms similar to those seen with barbiturate withdrawal.

Rare and mild hypersensitivity reactions to these drugs include skin rashes and urticaria. Also rare, idiosyncratic reactions can include marked excitement, hysteria, prolonged hypnosis, profound muscle weakness, and syncope without marked hypotension.

NURSING PROCESS APPLICATION

The following information assists the nurse in caring for a patient who is receiving a nonbenzodiazepine-nonbarbiturate agent.

Assessment
• Review the patient's history for a condition that contraindicates the use of a nonbenzodiazepine-nonbarbiturate, such as known hypersensitivity to the drug, severe renal impairment, gastroenteritis, ulcers, or porphyria.
• Review the patient's history for a condition that requires cautious use of a nonbenzodiazepine-nonbarbiturate, such as depression, suicidal tendencies, renal or hepatic impairment, or a history of drug abuse.
• Assess the patient for adverse reactions to the prescribed nonbenzodiazepine-nonbarbiturate, such as nausea, vomiting, gastric irritation, hangover effect, or respiratory depression.
• Review the patient's medication history to identify the use of drugs that may interact with the nonbenzodiazepine-nonbarbiturate, such as CNS depressants, oral anticoagulants, or disulfiram.
• Assess the patient for nonbenzodiazepine-nonbarbiturate dependence.
• Evaluate the patient's and family's knowledge about the prescribed nonbenzodiazepine-nonbarbiturate agent.

Nursing diagnoses
The following examples represent appropriate nursing diagnoses for a patient receiving a nonbenzodiazepine-nonbarbiturate.
• Potential for injury related to a preexisting condition that contraindicates the use of a nonbenzodiazepine-nonbarbiturate
• Potential for injury related to a preexisting condition that requires cautious use of a nonbenzodiazepine-nonbarbiturate
• Potential for injury related to adverse drug reactions
• Ineffective breathing pattern related to the respiratory depressant effects of the prescribed nonbenzodiazepine-nonbarbiturate
• Altered role performance related to nonbenzodiazepine-nonbarbiturate dependence

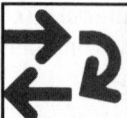

DRUG INTERACTIONS

Nonbenzodiazepines-nonbarbiturates

Drug interactions that occur with this class of drug are mainly from nonbenzodiazepines-nonbarbiturates used with other central nervous system (CNS) depressants.

DRUG	INTERACTING DRUGS	POSSIBLE EFFECTS	NURSING IMPLICATIONS
chloral hydrate, ethchlorvynol, glutethimide, methyprylon, paraldehyde	CNS depressant drugs	Cause drowsiness, respiratory depression, stupor, coma, or death	• Assess for CNS and respiratory changes. • Advise the patient to prohibit or sharply curtail alcohol use during administration. (Combination of alcohol with chloral hydrate is called a "Mickey Finn.") • Supervise ambulation; use bed rails, especially with elderly patients. • Caution the patient not to operate a motor vehicle or heavy machinery until the drug effects are known.
chloral hydrate	oral anticoagulants	Increases bleeding	• Monitor the patient's prothrombin time (PT); adjust the anticoagulant dosage, as prescribed. • Assess the patient for signs of bleeding, such as epistaxis, bleeding gums, hematuria, or bruising.
paraldehyde	disulfiram	Increases paraldehyde blood levels, causing increased CNS depression; possibly toxic disulfiram reaction (respiratory depression, cardiac arrhythmias, seizures, unconsciousness)	• Monitor for increased signs of CNS and respiratory depression. • Warn the patient not to consume alcohol because doing so can be lethal.
glutethimide, ethchlorvynol	oral anticoagulants	Increase risk of clotting	• Monitor the patient's PT carefully; anticoagulant dosage may need to be adjusted. • Assess the patient for signs of thromboembolism, such as pain, swelling, and redness in calf, and for signs of pulmonary embolism, such as shortness of breath, chest pain, and fever.

• Knowledge deficit related to the prescribed nonbenzodiazepine-nonbarbiturate agent

Planning and implementation

• Do not administer a nonbenzodiazepine-nonbarbiturate to a patient with a condition that contraindicates its use.
• Administer a nonbenzodiazepine-nonbarbiturate cautiously to a patient at risk because of a preexisting condition.
• Monitor the patient regularly for adverse drug reactions.
• Expect to administer a lower dosage to an elderly or debilitated patient than to other adults.
• *Take safety precautions after administering the nonbenzodiazepine-nonbarbiturate, such as placing the bed in a low position, keeping the bed rails up, and supervising ambulation.*
• To minimize gastric irritation from chloral hydrate liquid or capsules, give the drug after meals. Dilute liquid chloral hydrate with a fluid that minimizes its upleasant taste, such as juice or soda. Store chloral hydrate in a dark container and refrigerate suppositories.
• Store ethchlorvynol and glutethimide in tight, light-resistant containers to avoid possible deterioration; a slight darkening of the liquid from exposure to light and air will not affect safety or potency.
• Use paraldehyde from containers that have been opened for less than 24 hours because the drug decomposes upon exposure to light; do not give the drug if it is brown or has an acetic acid odor. Dilute the oral liquid form in iced milk, syrup, or fruit juice to disguise the taste and odor and reduce gastric distress.
• Use glass syringes and metal needles with paraldehyde because the drug reacts with some plastics. When administering I.M., inject deep into a large muscle mass and massage the site. For rectal administration, minimize ir-

ritation by diluting the drug with vegetable oil (one part drug to two parts diluent); then administer as a retention enema.

• Notify the physician if adverse reactions occur.

• *Monitor the patient's vital signs frequently, particularly noting such signs of respiratory depression as decreased respirations or respiratory pattern changes.*

• *Perform a respiratory assessment before and after giving each dose of the prescribed nonbenzodiazepine-nonbarbiturate.*

• *Withhold the prescribed dose and notify the physician if respiratory depression occurs.*

• Position the debilitated patient to maximize respiratory function. For example, help the patient into a semi-Fowler's or high Fowler's position.

• Encourage the patient to be honest about use of nonbenzodiazepines-nonbarbiturates because dependence can occur.

• *Do not discontinue large doses abruptly.* Otherwise, the patient may develop withdrawal symptoms similar to those associated with alcoholism.

• Alert the physician to suspected nonbenzodiazepine-nonbarbiturate dependence.

Patient teaching

• Provide general instructions about nonbenzodiazepine-nonbarbiturate use. (For details, see *Patient-teaching tips for sedative and hypnotic agents,* page 404.)

• Teach the patient and family the name, dose, frequency, action, and adverse effects of the prescribed nonbenzodiazepine-nonbarbiturate.

• Advise the patient and family to take safety precautions during nonbenzodiazepine-nonbarbiturate therapy.

• Describe clearly the risk of drug dependence.

• Teach the patient how to self-administer and store chloral hydrate.

• Teach the patient how to dilute and self-administer oral paraldehyde.

• Instruct the patient to inform the physician of any adverse reactions.

Evaluation

The following examples represent appropriate evaluation statements for a patient receiving a nonbenzodiazepine-nonbarbiturate agent.

• The patient has no conditions that contraindicate nonbenzodiazepine-nonbarbiturate therapy.

• The patient exhibits no signs of complications in the preexisting condition linked to the prescribed nonbenzodiazepine-nonbarbiturate.

• The patient develops no adverse drug reactions.

• The patient maintains a normal respiratory rate and pattern.

• The patient shows no signs of nonbenzodiazepine-nonbarbiturate dependence.

• The patient and family express an accurate understanding of the points taught about the prescribed nonbenzodiazepine-nonbarbiturate agent.

• The patient correctly demonstrates how to dilute and self-administer oral paraldehyde.

OTHER SEDATIVES

Alcohol and many OTC products, especially those containing antihistamines, often are used as sedatives.

Alcohol is the most widely used and abused drug in the United States. Alcohol is a CNS depressant and can be considered a sleep aid, a purpose it has served since ancient times. After rapid absorption from an empty stomach, alcohol enters the bloodstream and quickly travels to the CNS, where it diffuses past the blood-brain barrier. Metabolism occurs primarily in the liver, where most of the absorbed alcohol is broken down for the production of energy, with the unchanged remainder leaving the body in the urine and respirations. Small amounts of alcohol have been used to improve appetite and digestion and, in elderly patients, to promote sleep. Alcohol causes many adverse reactions in the body, and continual consumption of large amounts can have serious effects on gastric and hepatic function. Alcohol use with other CNS depressants can be lethal. Nurses need to be prepared to teach patients about alcohol and its effects on the body.

OTC sleep aids are readily available for purchase in the United States. These drugs usually contain an antihistamine (diphenhydramine, doxylamine, or pyrilamine), which has some sedative properties. The common antihistamines pyrilamine maleate and diphenhydramine are found in Nevine, Nytol, Sleep-eze, and Sominex. The antihistamines, being CNS depressants, affect sleep; however, researchers have not studied the effect extensively. (For more information about antihistamines, see Chapter 56, Antihistaminic Agents.) Minor atropine-like adverse reactions, such as dry mouth, can result from use of OTC sleep aids. Confusion and disorientation also can occur, especially in elderly patients.

(Text continues on page 418.)

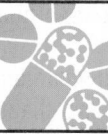

SELECTED MAJOR DRUGS

Sedative and hypnotic agents

This chart summarizes the major sedative and hypnotic drugs currently in clinical use.

DRUG	MAJOR INDICATIONS	USUAL ADULT DOSAGES	CONTRAINDICATIONS AND PRECAUTIONS
Benzodiazepines			
flurazepam	Hypnotic for insomnia	15 to 30 mg P.O. h.s.	• Know that flurazepam is contraindicated in a pregnant patient or one with known hypersensitivity to the drug. • Administer with caution to a patient with severe or latent depression, impaired renal or hepatic function, or chronic pulmonary insufficiency.
lorazepam	Sedative before surgery Hypnotic for insomnia from anxiety or transient situational stress, anxiety disorders	0.05 mg/kg up to 4 mg I.M. 2 hours before operative procedure 2 to 4 mg P.O. h.s.	• Know that lorazepam is contraindicated in a pregnant patient or one with known hypersensitivity to the drug, acute narrow-angle glaucoma, a primary depressive disorder, or psychosis. • Administer with caution to a lactating or elderly patient, one with impaired renal or hepatic function, or any patient over a prolonged time.
quazepam	Hypnotic for insomnia	15 mg P.O. h.s. until the response is measured; then decreased to 7.5 mg, if possible	• Know that quazepam is contraindicated in a pregnant patient or one with known hypersensitivity to the drug. • Administer with caution to a patient with impaired renal or hepatic function.
temazepam	Hypnotic for insomnia	15 to 30 mg P.O. h.s.	• Know that temazepam is contraindicated in a pregnant patient or one with known hypersensitivity to the drug. • Administer with caution to a lactating patient or one with severe or latent depression, impaired renal or hepatic function, or chronic pulmonary insufficiency.
triazolam	Hypnotic for insomnia	0.125 to 0.25 mg P.O. h.s.	• Know that triazolam is contraindicated in a pregnant or lactating patient or one with known hypersensitivity to the drug. • Administer with caution to a patient with depression, impaired renal or hepatic function, or chronic pulmonary insufficiency.
Barbiturates			
amobarbital	Sedative for anxiety and tension Hypnotic for insomnia	30 to 50 mg P.O. or I.M. b.i.d. or t.i.d. 65 to 200 mg P.O. or I.M. h.s.	• Know that amobarbital is contraindicated in a pregnant patient or one with porphyria or known hypersensitivity to the drug.
aprobarbital	Daytime sedative Hypnotic for insomnia	40 mg P.O. t.i.d. 40 to 160 mg P.O. h.s.	• Know that aprobarbital is contraindicated in a pregnant or lactating patient or one with known hypersensitivity to the drug, porphyria, nephritis, renal insufficiency, or premonitory signs of hepatic coma. • Administer with caution to a patient with depression, suicidal tendencies, hepatic damage, or a history of drug abuse.

SELECTED MAJOR DRUGS

Sedative and hypnotic agents *(continued)*

DRUG	MAJOR INDICATIONS	USUAL ADULT DOSAGES	CONTRAINDICATIONS AND PRECAUTIONS
Barbiturates *(continued)*			
mephobarbital	Daytime sedative	32 to 100 mg P.O. t.i.d. or q.i.d.	• Know that mephobarbital is contraindicated in a pregnant patient or one with known hypersensitivity to the drug, porphyria, nephritis, renal insufficiency, or premonitory signs of hepatic coma. • Administer with caution to a lactating patient or one with depression, suicidal tendencies, myasthenia gravis, myxedema, a history of drug abuse, or impaired hepatic, cardiac, or respiratory function.
pentobarbital	Daytime sedative	20 to 40 mg P.O. b.i.d. to q.i.d.	• Know that pentobarbital is contraindicated in a pregnant patient or one with porphyria or known hypersensitivity to the drug. • Administer with caution to a lactating patient or one with depression, suicidal tendencies, hepatic damage, or a history of drug abuse.
	Sedative before surgery	150 to 200 mg P.O. or I.M.	
	Hypnotic for insomnia	100 mg P.O., 120 to 200 mg rectal, 100 to 200 mg I.M.	
phenobarbital	Daytime sedative	15 to 30 mg P.O. b.i.d. to q.i.d.	• Know that phenobarbital is contraindicated in a pregnant patient or one with porphyria, nephritis, renal insufficiency, or known hypersensitivity to the drug. • Administer with caution to a lactating patient or one with depression, suicidal tendencies, hepatic damage, or a history of drug abuse.
	Sedative before surgery	100 to 200 mg I.M. 60 to 90 minutes before surgery	
	Hypnotic for insomnia	100 to 320 mg P.O. or I.M. h.s.	
secobarbital	Daytime sedative	30 to 50 mg P.O. t.i.d. to q.i.d., 120 to 200 mg rectal	• Know that secobarbital is contraindicated in a pregnant patient or one with porphyria or known hypersensitivity to the drug. • Administer with caution to a lactating patient or one with depression, suicidal tendencies, hepatic damage, or a history of drug abuse.
	Sedative before surgery	200 to 300 mg P.O. 1 to 2 hours before surgery	
	Hypnotic for insomnia	100 to 200 mg P.O., 120 to 200 mg rectal, 100 to 200 mg I.M. h.s.	
Nonbenzodiazepines-nonbarbiturates			
chloral hydrate	Daytime sedative	250 mg P.O. or 325 mg rectal t.i.d. after meals	• Know that chloral hydrate is contraindicated in a patient with known hypersensitivity to the drug, gastroenteritis, or ulcers. • Administer with caution to a pregnant or lactating patient or one with depression, suicidal tendencies, or severe hepatic, renal, or cardiac disease.
	Hypnotic for insomnia	0.5 to 1 g P.O. or rectal 15 to 30 minutes before bedtime	
ethchlorvynol	Daytime sedative	200 mg P.O. b.i.d. or t.i.d.	• Know that ethchlorvynol is contraindicated in a patient with porphyria or known hypersensitivity to the drug. • Administer with caution to a pregnant or lactating patient or one with suicidal tendencies, impaired renal or hepatic function, or a history of drug abuse.
	Hypnotic for insomnia	0.5 to 1 g P.O. h.s.	

(continued)

SELECTED MAJOR DRUGS

Sedative and hypnotic agents (continued)

DRUG	MAJOR INDICATIONS	USUAL ADULT DOSAGES	CONTRAINDICATIONS AND PRECAUTIONS
Nonbenzodiazepines-nonbarbiturates (continued)			
glutethimide	Hypnotic for insomnia	250 to 500 mg P.O. h.s.	• Know that glutethimide is contraindicated in a patient with porphyria, severe renal impairment, or known hypersensitivity to the drug. • Administer with caution to a pregnant or lactating patient or one with depression, suicidal tendencies, or a history of drug abuse.
methyprylon	Hypnotic for insomnia	200 to 400 mg P.O. h.s.	• Know that methyprylon is contraindicated in a patient with known hypersensitivity to the drug. • Administer with caution to a lactating patient or one with porphyria or renal or hepatic impairment.
paraldehyde	Sedative Hypnotic for insomnia	5 to 10 ml P.O. or rectal 10 to 30 ml P.O. or rectal h.s.	• Know that paraldehyde is contraindicated in a patient with ulcerative gastroenteritis or known hypersensitivity to the drug. • Administer with caution to a patient with impaired hepatic function or a pulmonary disease, such as asthma.

CHAPTER SUMMARY

Chapter 25 presented sedatives, which act to reduce activity or excitement and calm a patient, and hypnotics, which are sedatives given in large doses to induce a state resembling natural sleep. Here are the chapter highlights.

• The three main classes of sedative and hypnotic drugs are benzodiazepines, barbiturates, and nonbenzodiazepine-nonbarbiturate agents. Alcohol and OTC drugs also are used to promote sleep.

• Sleep is an active state of unconsciousness from which a person can be awakened with appropriate stimulus. During a sleep period, a person passes through several cycles. Each cycle consists of four stages of NREM sleep and one stage of REM sleep.

• The four major sleep disorders include insomnia, hypersomnia, parasomnia, and disorders of the sleep-awake schedule.

• The benzodiazepines include five primary sedative and hypnotic drugs: flurazepam, lorazepam, quazepam, temazepam, and triazolam. The benzodiazepines usually are preferred because of their effectiveness and safety.

• Drug interactions with the benzodiazepines are rare and mainly occur with the use of other CNS depressant drugs, causing an additive effect that can be lethal.

• Benzodiazepines produce few adverse reactions.

• Barbiturates include amobarbital, aprobarbital, butabarbital, mephobarbital, pentobarbital, phenobarbital, and secobarbital. Like benzodiazepines, barbiturates are CNS depressants capable of producing a wide range of effects, from sedation to hypnosis to anesthesia to coma.

• Barbiturates exhibit a high potential for physical and psychological dependence, high abuse level, and life-threatening toxicity with overdose, causing severe CNS and respiratory depression. Several drug interactions involving barbiturates can occur, including the additive effects when combined with other CNS depressants, including alcohol. Adverse reactions are common and include CNS and respiratory depression.

• Nonbenzodiazepine-nonbarbiturate drugs include chloral hydrate, ethchlorvynol, glutethimide, methyprylon, and paraldehyde. The most common adverse reactions to these drugs are GI distress and some hangover effects. Respiratory depression also can occur. Hypersensitivity and idiosyncratic reactions to these drugs are rare.

• Other sources of sedative and hypnotic effects include alcohol and OTC drugs. OTC sleep aids contain antihistamines, primarily diphenhydramine, doxylamine, and pyrilamine.

• When caring for a patient who is receiving a sedative or hypnotic agent, the nurse applies the nursing process, paying particular attention to prevention of respiratory depression, detection of drug dependence, and safety measures.

STUDY QUESTIONS

See Appendix 1 for answers.

1. Joan Moffet, age 44, is scheduled for a cholecystectomy. Her physician prescribes the benzodiazepine triazolam (Halcion) 0.125 mg P.O. h.s. as a hypnotic the night before surgery. What is the difference between a sedative and a hypnotic?
(a) Sedatives reduce activity or excitement; hypnotics induce sleep.
(b) Sedatives require larger doses than hypnotics to obtain desired effects.
(c) Sedatives are Schedule II drugs; hypnotics are Schedule IV drugs.
(d) Sedatives produce more adverse reactions than hypnotics do.

2. Ms. Moffet will receive triazolam orally. Why isn't the I.M. route used for most benzodiazepines?
(a) I.M. injections irritate the tissue.
(b) I.M. injections produce more adverse reactions.
(c) I.M. injections are absorbed erratically.
(d) I.M. injections reduce the duration of action.

3. The physician prescribes 50 mg P.O. h.s. of the barbiturate butabarbital for Philip Ambrose, age 58, for sedation the night before surgery. Barbiturates are not used as commonly as benzodiazepines. Which characteristic of barbiturates may account for this?
(a) high potential for drug dependence
(b) unpredictable therapeutic effects
(c) high incidence of hepatotoxicity
(d) paradoxical effects with prolonged use

4. When Mr. Ambrose awakens in the morning, he says he feels like he has a hangover. What is probably responsible for this reaction?
(a) anxiety related to impending surgery
(b) unusually large dose of barbiturate
(c) hypersensitivity to barbiturates
(d) adverse reaction to barbiturates

5. Grace Brown, age 61, has been having difficulty sleeping. Her physician prescribes the nonbenzodiazepine-nonbarbiturate chloral hydrate 0.5 gram P.O. h.s. Which statement accurately characterizes nonbenzodiazepines-nonbarbiturates?
(a) They produce the most adverse reactions of all sedatives and hypnotics.
(b) They are the most potent of all sedatives and hypnotics.

(c) They lose their effectiveness by the end of the second week.
(d) They are the safest of all sedatives and hypnotics.

6. Ms. Brown is *most* likely to experience which of the following adverse reactions?
(a) severe CNS and respiratory depression
(b) severe withdrawal symptoms
(c) hypersensitivity reactions
(d) GI symptoms and hangover effects

7. John Madara, age 48, receives the nonbenzodiazepine-nonbarbiturate paraldehyde to treat alcohol withdrawal syndrome. How should the nurse administer oral paraldehyde to Mr. Madara?
(a) on an empty stomach to speed absorption
(b) with meals to prolong absorption
(c) with juice to disguise the taste and odor
(d) with milk to delay absorption

SELECTED REFERENCES

AHFS drug information 90. (1990). Bethesda, MD: American Society of Hospital Pharmacists.

Davies, D. (Ed.). (1987). *Textbook of adverse drug reactions* (3rd ed.). New York: Oxford Press.

Drug facts and comparisons. (1991). St. Louis: Facts and Comparisons Division, J.B. Lippincott.

Goodman and Gilman's the pharmacological basis of therapeutics (8th ed.; 1990). Elmsford, NY: Pergamon Press.

Hansten, P., and Horn, J. (1989). *Drug interactions: Clinical significance of drug-drug interactions* (6th ed.). Philadelphia: Lea & Febiger.

North American Nursing Diagnosis Association. (1990). *Taxonomy I-Revised, with official categories.* St. Louis: NANDA.

Rabel, R. (Ed.). (1989). *Conn's current therapy 1989.* Philadelphia: Saunders.

USPDI. (1991). *Drug information for the health care professional* (Vol. I, 11th ed.). Rockville, MD: United States Pharmacopeial Convention.

USPDI. (1991). *Advice for the patient* (Vol. II, 11th ed.). Rockville, MD: United States Pharmacopeial Convention.

ANTIDEPRESSANT AND ANTIMANIC AGENTS

OBJECTIVES

After reading and studying this chapter, the student should be able to:

1. Discuss the clinical indications for antidepressant and antimanic agents.

2. Explain the mechanism of action of the monoamine oxidase (MAO) inhibitors.

3. Teach the patient which drugs and foods to avoid during MAO inhibitor therapy.

4. Describe the major adverse effects of MAO inhibitors.

5. Describe the major adverse effects of tricyclic antidepressants.

6. Compare the pharmacokinetic, pharmacodynamic, and pharmacotherapeutic properties of the tricyclic antidepressants with those of the second-generation antidepressants.

7. Identify the major drugs that interact with lithium.

8. Describe the major adverse effects of lithium.

9. Describe how to apply the nursing process when caring for a patient who is receiving an antidepressant or antimanic agent.

INTRODUCTION

Antidepressant and antimanic agents are used to treat affective disorders. MAO inhibitors, tricyclic antidepressants, and second-generation antidepressants are used to treat unipolar disorders, characterized by periods of clinical depression. Lithium is used to treat bipolar disorders, characterized by alternating periods of manic behavior and clinical depression.

Affective disorders

Depression and mania are the most common affective disorders – or syndromes – producing mood disturbances not related to any other physical or psychiatric conditions. These disorders affect twice as many women as men, with unipolar depressions accounting for 90% of the cases. This type of depression typically has a gradual onset of vague complaints, making it difficult to diagnose.

Diagnosis requires a prominent and persistent mood disturbance and the presence of several of the following signs and symptoms for at least 2 weeks: poor appetite, weight loss, sleep disturbances, agitation, loss of interest in activities, fatigue, feelings of worthlessness, slowed thinking or the inability to concentrate, and thoughts of death.

For 30% to 50% of these patients, depression occurs as a single episode; for the remainder, depression recurs. All these patients may require treatment with such drugs as MAO inhibitors, tricyclic antidepressants, second-generation antidepressants, or (occasionally) lithium.

Unlike depression, mania produces periods of euphoria, rapid speech, flight of ideas, lack of need for sleep, and overactivity. Mania may occur alone or it may alternate with depression, resulting in manic-depressive illness, a bipolar disorder. Manic-depressive illness is much less common than depression. Lithium is the drug of choice to treat mania and manic-depressive illness.

Because diminished concentration levels of one or both of the neurotransmitters norepinephrine and serotonin occur in depression, and because excessive neurotransmitter concentration levels occur in mania, many theorists believed that depletion of norepinephrine or serotonin was the biological cause of depression. This belief led to the discovery of agents to treat depression that could increase neurotransmitter availability in the brain.

Researchers were puzzled when antidepressant and antimanic drugs took weeks to produce a therapeutic response. Later, the receptor-sensitivity theory explained this phenomenon: in depression, the receptor site for norepinephrine and serotonin is hyposensitive to stimulation of the alpha-adrenergic receptor that releases the neurotrans-

SELECTED NURSING DIAGNOSES

Antidepressant and antimanic agents

The following nursing diagnoses address representative problems and etiologies that a nurse may encounter when caring for a patient who is receiving an antidepressant or antimanic agent. Some of these nursing diagnoses contain generalized etiologies, which the nurse must individualize based on the patient's needs. (For some common nursing diagnoses and related interventions for each drug class, see the "Nursing Process Application" sections of this chapter.)

- Altered health maintenance related to ineffectiveness of the prescribed antidepressant or antimanic agent
- Altered protection related to the adverse hematologic effects of an antidepressant or antimanic agent
- Constipation related to the anticholinergic effects of the prescribed antidepressant agent
- Diarrhea related to the adverse gastrointestinal (GI) effects of fluoxetine
- Fluid volume excess related to exacerbation of congestive heart failure caused by a tricyclic antidepressant
- Knowledge deficit related to the prescribed antidepressant or antimanic agent
- Noncompliance related to long-term use of an antidepressant or antimanic agent
- Pain related to headache caused by an MAO inhibitor or fluoxetine
- Potential fluid volume deficit related to possible lithium-induced diabetes insipidus syndrome
- Potential fluid volume deficit related to possible adverse GI effects and excessive diaphoresis associated with fluoxetine
- Potential for injury related to a preexisting condition that contraindicates the use of an antidepressant or antimanic agent

- Potential for injury related to a preexisting condition that requires cautious use of an antidepressant or antimanic agent
- Potential for injury related to adverse drug reactions
- Potential for injury related to drug interactions
- Potential for injury related to hypertensive crisis induced by an MAO inhibitor
- Potential for trauma related to syncope caused by an MAO inhibitor
- Potential for trauma related to seizures caused by antidepressant or antimanic agent
- Sensory-perceptual alterations (tactile) related to paresthesias caused by an MAO inhibitor
- Sensory-perceptual alterations (visual) related to blurred vision or photosensitivity caused by an MAO inhibitor or tricyclic antidepressant
- Sexual dysfunction related to the adverse genitourinary effects of an antidepressant agent
- Sleep pattern disturbance related to insomnia caused by bupropion
- Urinary retention related to the adverse genitourinary effects of an antidepressant agent

---

mitters norepinephrine and serotonin; in mania, the receptor site is hypersensitive. Antidepressant agents produce adaptive changes over several weeks that return the receptor to normal sensitivity.

For a summary of representative drugs, see *Selected major drugs: Antidepressant and antimanic agents,* pages 434 and 435. For a listing of applicable nursing diagnoses that the nurse may formulate when caring for a patient receiving these agents, see *Selected nursing diagnoses: Antidepressant and antimanic agents*. For detailed information on applying the nursing process, see Chapter 6, The Nursing Process and Drug Therapy.

M.A.O. INHIBITORS

MAO inhibitors are divided into two classifications based on chemical structure: the hydrazines, which include isocarboxazid and phenelzine sulfate, and the single nonhy-

drazine tranylcypromine sulfate. All of these drugs nonselectively inhibit the enzyme monoamine oxidase, which metabolizes neurotransmitters at receptor sites. Researchers have subdivided this enzyme into type A, which can produce hypertensive crisis in a patient who eats food containing tyramine, and type B, which is sensitive to different amines and not associated with hypertensive reactions. Currently available MAO inhibitors affect type A and type B enzymes; however, research continues for agents that selectively will affect type A and type B enzymes. In the future, administering a type B MAO inhibitor may allow the patient to eat tyramine-rich foods without fear of hypertensive crisis, a severe interaction between a drug and a food. Selegiline is an MAO inhibitor with some type B selectivity, but its effects in depression vary.

PHARMACOKINETICS

Little information exists regarding the pharmacokinetics of these agents.

Absorption, distribution, metabolism, excretion

MAO inhibitors are absorbed rapidly and completely from the gastrointestinal (GI) tract and are metabolized in the liver to inactive metabolites. These metabolites are excreted mainly by the GI tract and to a lesser degree by the kidneys.

Onset, peak, duration

The onset of action of an MAO inhibitor ranges from 1 to 2 weeks, and a full clinical response may be delayed for 3 to 4 weeks. The therapeutic effects may continue for 1 to 2 weeks after discontinuation. Several factors account for the delayed onset of these drugs. The MAO inhibitors have relatively short half-lives (measured in hours), but the half-life of the enzyme they inhibit is about 12 days. The drugs inhibit enzyme production within a short time but have no effect on the circulating enzyme. Thus, the effects of the existing enzyme may take 1 to 2 weeks to dissipate.

No correlation exists between plasma MAO inhibition and plasma levels of MAO inhibitors. However, a direct correlation has been demonstrated between platelet MAO inhibition and therapeutic response.

PHARMACODYNAMICS

Administering these agents inhibits monoamine oxidase synthesis and action, thus increasing the concentration of the neurotransmitters norepinephrine and serotonin.

Mechanism of action

Although their exact mechanism of action is unclear, MAO inhibitors appear to work by inhibiting monoamine oxidase (the enzyme that normally metabolizes the neurotransmitters norepinephrine and serotonin) because they inhibit neurotransmitter intracellular metabolism. This action makes more norepinephrine and serotonin available to the receptors, relieving the symptoms of depression.

PHARMACOTHERAPEUTICS

MAO inhibitors are used to treat psychiatric conditions, especially atypical depression. This disorder produces the signs opposite to those of typical depression. For example, the patient gains weight, lacks suicidal tendencies, and has an increased libido. In treating atypical depression, MAO inhibitors are more effective than tricyclic antidepressants and have a shorter onset of action than usual—approximately 3 to 5 days.

MAO inhibitors may be used to treat typical depression when it is resistant to other therapies or when other therapies are contraindicated.

Other clinical uses include depression accompanied by anxiety, phobic anxieties, neurodermatitis, hypochondriasis, and refractory narcoleptic states. The safety and ef-

fectiveness of MAO inhibitors in patients under age 16 have not been established.

isocarboxazid (Marplan). This MAO inhibitor exerts its effects within 1 week in patients who are depressed and have symptoms, such as weight gain or overeating. Its therapeutic use is declining, however, because of its lack of consistent effectiveness.
Usual adult dosage: 30 mg P.O. daily as a single dose or in divided doses, decreased to 10 to 20 mg/day when a therapeutic response occurs. Dosages that exceed 30 mg/day can increase adverse reactions and are not recommended.

phenelzine sulfate (Nardil). Phenelzine is less potent than other MAO inhibitors, less likely to produce hypertensive crisis, and produces fewer adverse reactions than tranylcypromine. It may be most effective in treating panic or phobic disorders.
Usual adult dosage: 15 mg P.O. t.i.d. or approximately 1 mg/kg/day, increased rapidly to 60 to 90 mg depending on the patient's tolerance and therapeutic response. In 2 to 6 weeks after the maximum response occurs, the dosage is decreased slowly to a maintenance level as low as 15 mg/day.

tranylcypromine sulfate (Parnate). This nonhydrazine compound acts more rapidly than phenelzine but has more adverse effects. Its mild central nervous system (CNS) stimulant effects preclude administering an evening dose.
Usual adult dosage: 10 mg P.O. b.i.d., increased to 20 mg in the morning and 10 mg in the afternoon if the response is inadequate after 2 to 3 weeks. If a therapeutic response does not appear after 1 week at this dosage, it is unlikely to occur. Dosages in excess of 30 mg/day are more likely to have adverse effects.

Drug interactions

Certain foods and drugs can interact with MAO inhibitors and may produce severe reactions. The most serious reactions involve tyramine-rich foods and sympathomimetic agents. (For more information about these interactions, see *Drug interactions: MAO inhibitors,* and *Foods that may interact with MAO inhibitors,* page 424.)

ADVERSE DRUG REACTIONS

Although MAO inhibitors can produce a significant number of adverse reactions, they may produce fewer adverse reactions than tricyclic antidepressants do. The most serious adverse reaction is hypertensive crisis, which can lead to death. Hypertensive crisis is characterized by increased blood pressure, severe headache, palpitations, nausea, vomiting, neck stiffness or soreness, fever, clammy skin, my-

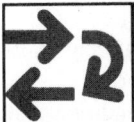

DRUG INTERACTIONS

MAO inhibitors

MAO inhibitors can interact with several commonly used drugs, causing potentially severe effects.

DRUG	INTERACTING DRUGS	POSSIBLE EFFECTS	NURSING IMPLICATIONS
isocarboxazid, phenelzine, tranylcypromine	amphetamines	Increase catecholamine release and hypertension	• Do not administer amphetamines with an MAO inhibitor.
	fluoxetine, tricyclic antidepressants, cyclobenzaprine	Cause hyperpyrexia, excitation, seizures	• Monitor the patient's temperature and level of consciousness.
	doxapram	Cause hypertension and arrhythmias; potentiate the adverse effects of doxapram	• Monitor the patient's vital signs frequently.
	sympathomimetics, non-amphetamine anorexigenic agents	Increase catecholamine release and hypertension	• Avoid giving sympathomimetics or nonamphetamine anorexigenic agents to a patient receiving an MAO inhibitor.
	levodopa	Increase storage and release of dopamine, norepinephrine, or both, leading to hypertension	• Avoid giving levodopa to a patient receiving an MAO inhibitor.
	hypoglycemic agents	Cause hypoglycemia	• Monitor the patient closely for signs of hypoglycemia, such as hunger, diaphoresis, weakness, tremor, dizziness, and tachycardia.
	meperidine	Causes excitation, hypertension or hypotension, hyperpyrexia, and coma	• Avoid concurrent use of meperidine as well as use within 10 days of last MAO inhibitor dose.

driasis, or photophobia or other visual disturbances. It also may be associated with tachycardia or bradycardia, constricting chest pain, or intracranial hemorrhage.

The most common adverse reactions are restlessness, drowsiness, dizziness, headache, insomnia, constipation, anorexia, nausea, vomiting, weakness, arthralgia, dry mouth, blurred vision, peripheral edema, urine retention, transient impotence, rash, and purpura. Orthostatic hypotension also is common and may lead to syncope with high doses. Orthostatic hypotension usually occurs in patients with preexisting hypertension, although it also may occur in patients with normal blood pressure.

Other adverse reactions to MAO inhibitors include urinary frequency, increased appetite, weight gain, increased perspiration, flushing, numbness, paresthesia, muscle spasms, tremor, myoclonic jerks, and hyperreflexia. With high dosages, these drugs may cause hyperexcitability, agitation, activation of latent schizophrenic disorder, mania, and hypomania. Such reactions require a dosage reduction or concomitant use of a phenothiazine.

Rare reactions include amblyopia, aggravation of glaucoma, other visual disturbances, impaired water excretion,

leukopenia, granulocytopenia, thrombocytopenia, and normocytic, normochromic anemia.

With high dosages of tranylcypromine, dependence and addiction can occur. When this drug is discontinued, the patient may display anxiety, depression, confusion, hallucinations, diarrhea, and other withdrawal symptoms.

NURSING PROCESS APPLICATION

The following information assists the nurse in caring for a patient who is receiving an MAO inhibitor.

Assessment

• Review the patient's history for a condition that contraindicates the use of an MAO inhibitor, such as cardiovascular disease, pheochromocytoma, known hypersensitivity to the drug, or concomitant use of high-tryptophan foods, high-tyramine foods, excessive amounts of caffeine, CNS depressants, or sympathomimetic drugs.

• Review the patient's history for a condition that requires cautious use of an MAO inhibitor, such as diabetes, epilepsy, pregnancy, or lactation.

Foods that may interact with MAO inhibitors

Foods that contain tyramine can produce a hypertensive crisis in a patient receiving an MAO inhibitor. Hypertensive crisis is signaled by a sudden severe increase in blood pressure, severe headache, sudden visual changes, and dizziness. To avoid this severe drug-food interaction, teach the patient which foods to avoid during treatment. Foods with a high tyramine content should be avoided completely, those with a moderate content may be eaten occasionally, and those with low tyramine levels are allowable in limited quantities.

Foods with a high tyramine content

- Red wines, such as Chianti and burgundy
- Beer
- Aged cheeses, such as bleu, Swiss, and cheddar
- Aged or smoked meats, such as herring, sausage, and corned beef
- Liver, such as chicken or beef liver
- Yeast extracts, such as brewer's yeast
- Fava or broad beans, such as Italian green beans

Foods with a moderate tyramine content

- Sour cream
- Ripe avocados
- Yogurt
- Ripe bananas
- Meat extracts, such as bouillon

Foods with a low tyramine content

- Chocolate
- Figs
- American, mozzarella, cottage, and cream cheeses
- Distilled spirits, such as gin, vodka, and Scotch
- White wines

- Assess the patient for adverse reactions to the prescribed MAO inhibitor, such as hypertensive crisis, orthostatic hypotension, impotence, edema, drowsiness, insomnia, urine retention, dry mouth, or paresthesias.
- Review the patient's medication history to identify the use of drugs that may interact with the prescribed MAO inhibitor, such as amphetamines, tricyclic antidepressants, sympathomimetic agents, levodopa, and hypoglycemic agents.
- Ask the male patient about impotence during MAO inhibitor therapy.
- Evaluate the patient's and family's knowledge about the prescribed MAO inhibitor.

Nursing diagnoses

The following examples represent appropriate nursing diagnoses for a patient receiving an MAO inhibitor.
- Potential for injury related to a preexisting condition that contraindicates the use of an MAO inhibitor
- Potential for injury related to a preexisting condition that requires cautious use of an MAO inhibitor
- Potential for injury related to adverse drug reactions
- Urinary retention related to the adverse genitourinary effects of the prescribed MAO inhibitor
- Sexual dysfunction related to impotence from MAO inhibitor use
- Knowledge deficit related to the prescribed MAO inhibitor

Planning and implementation

- Do not administer an MAO inhibitor to a patient with a condition that contraindicates its use.
- Administer an MAO inhibitor cautiously to a patient at risk because of a preexisting condition.
- Monitor the patient regularly for adverse reactions to the prescribed MAO inhibitor.
- *Monitor the patient closely for signs of hypertensive crisis, such as increased blood pressure, severe headache, palpitations, neck stiffness or soreness, nausea, or vomiting.*
- *Prepare for emergency interventions if hypertensive crisis occurs. For example, expect to discontinue the MAO inhibitor immediately and administer 5 to 10 mg of phentolamine by I.V. injection to reduce the blood pressure, as prescribed.*
- Expect to change the patient to a different MAO inhibitor if adverse reactions do not diminish with time or a dosage adjustment.
- Expect to change the administration time to the early evening or the morning if drowsiness or insomnia occurs.
- *Do not discontinue tranylcypromine therapy abruptly.* If discontinuation is necessary, expect to taper off the drug dosage over 2 weeks to prevent withdrawal reactions, such as anxiety, depression, confusion, and hallucinations.
- *Withhold the prescribed MAO inhibitor and notify the physician if the patient develops signs or symptoms of an intentional overdose, such as palpitations, frequent headaches, or severe hypertension, which typically result from a suicide attempt.*
- *Have the patient sit up for 1 minute before getting out of bed to reduce the effects of orthostatic hypotension. Supervise the patient's ambulation.*
- Continue patient monitoring for 7 to 10 days after discontinuation of the prescribed MAO inhibitor because of its long-lasting effects.
- Notify the physician if adverse reactions occur.

• Record the patient's fluid intake and output to help detect urine retention. Also, palpate and percuss the bladder after the patient voids.

• Ask the patient to report symptoms of urine retention, such as urinary hesitancy, frequent voiding of small amounts, and a sensation of fullness in the lower abdomen.

• Notify the physician if urine retention occurs and prepare to catheterize the patient, as directed.

• Reassure the patient that drug-induced impotence should resolve when the MAO inhibitor is discontinued.

• Discuss alternative ways for the impotent patient and sexual partner to achieve sexual satisfaction.

Patient teaching

• Teach the patient and family the name, dose, frequency, action, and adverse effects of the prescribed MAO inhibitor.

• Teach the patient which drugs and foods to avoid during MAO inhibitor therapy; provide a written list.

• Teach the patient and family to recognize the signs of a hypertensive crisis, such as severe headache, sudden visual changes, and dizziness.

• Instruct the patient to inform other physicians about the MAO inhibitor therapy because, for example, the drug should be discontinued 10 to 14 days before surgery.

• Caution the patient not to stop taking the MAO inhibitor abruptly and explain that the therapy should be tapered off as prescribed by the physician.

• Instruct the patient to take the drug at bedtime if it produces drowsiness or to take the last daily dose in the afternoon if it causes insomnia.

• Inform the male patient that impotence may occur during MAO inhibitor therapy but should subside when the drug is discontinued.

• Teach the patient to recognize — and report to the physician — signs of urine retention.

• Instruct the patient to notify the physician of any other adverse reactions.

Evaluation

The following examples represent appropriate evaluation statements for a patient receiving an MAO inhibitor.

• The patient has no conditions that contraindicate MAO inhibitor therapy.

• The patient exhibits no complications in the preexisting condition linked to the prescribed MAO inhibitor.

• The patient experiences no adverse reactions to the prescribed MAO inhibitor.

• The patient maintains a normal fluid balance.

• The patient reports satisfactory sexual activity.

• The patient and family express an accurate understanding of the points taught about the prescribed MAO inhibitor.

• The patient correctly identifies signs of urine retention.

TRICYCLIC ANTIDEPRESSANTS

Most tricyclic antidepressants produce similar effects in treating depression, but differ in their abilities to increase neurotransmitter concentration levels. This section discusses the following tricyclic antidepressants: amitriptyline hydrochloride, desipramine hydrochloride, doxepin hydrochloride, imipramine hydrochloride, nortriptyline hydrochloride, protriptyline hydrochloride, and trimipramine maleate. It also discusses the tricyclic antidepressant clomipramine, which is the first agent approved by the Food and Drug Administration (FDA) to treat obsessive-compulsive disorder.

PHARMACOKINETICS

After oral administration, the tricyclic antidepressants undergo extensive hepatic metabolism that varies considerably among individuals.

Absorption, distribution, metabolism, excretion

Tricyclic antidepressants are absorbed completely after oral administration, but their bioavailability ranges from 30% to 70% because of the first-pass effect. The extreme fat solubility of these drugs accounts for their wide distribution throughout the body (the highest concentrations appear in the brain and heart), slow excretion, and long half-life.

The tricyclic antidepressants are metabolized extensively in the liver. All of the tricyclic antidepressants are active pharmacologically, and some of their metabolites also are active. Eventually, the metabolites are hydroxylated and then conjugated to form inactive compounds that are excreted in the urine. Only small amounts of active drug are excreted.

Onset, peak, duration

The half-lives of the tricyclic antidepressants vary from 8 to 120 hours and average 24 hours, except for that of protriptyline hydrochloride, which is 3 to 4 days. Because the tricyclic antidepressants have long half-lives, a noticeable response may not occur for 10 to 14 days; a full response, for up to 30 days.

Plasma tricyclic antidepressant levels vary widely because of individual differences in metabolism. Subtherapeutic or toxic concentration levels may reflect a patient's metabolic status.

PHARMACODYNAMICS

Tricyclic antidepressant administration increases neurotransmitter concentrations, reducing the signs and symptoms of depression.

Mechanism of action

Researchers hypothesize that tricyclic antidepressants increase the amount of norepinephrine, serotonin, or both, normalizing the hyposensitive receptor site associated with depression. Normalization takes up to several weeks, slowing the onset of antidepressant action.

PHARMACOTHERAPEUTICS

Tricyclic antidepressants are the drugs of choice for episodes of major depression. They are especially effective in treating depression of insidious onset accompanied by weight loss, anorexia, or insomnia. Physical signs and symptoms may respond after 1 to 2 weeks of therapy; psychological symptoms, after 2 to 4 weeks. Tricyclic antidepressants are much less effective in patients with hypochondriasis, atypical depression, or depression accompanied by delusions. However, they may be helpful in treating acute episodes of depression, producing a response in about two-thirds of these patients. After a patient's acute depressive episode, the dosage is reduced to the lowest level that will relieve symptoms. This maintenance therapy is continued for 6 to 12 months, and then the dosage is decreased every 3 to 7 days until the drug is discontinued. A patient who experiences two acute episodic relapses in 2 years may require long-term tricyclic antidepressant therapy, which may last for several years.

Currently, clomipramine is the only tricyclic antidepressant used to treat obsessive-compulsive disorder. However, tricyclic antidepressants also are being investigated for use in preventing migraine headaches and in treating phobias, enuresis, attention deficit disorders, duodenal or peptic ulcer disease, and diabetic neuropathies.

The relative effectiveness of the tricyclic antidepressants has not been established; therefore, a patient who fails to respond to one tricyclic antidepressant may respond to a different one, to a combination of lithium and a tricyclic antidepressant, or to a combination of an MAO inhibitor and a tricyclic antidepressant (if special precautions are taken). Although a once-daily dosage is possible because of the tricyclic antidepressants' long half-life, the dosage is divided to decrease the risk of adverse effects or to allow the patient to adjust to them before changing to a once-daily dosage. Dosages should be reduced for elderly patients.

amitriptyline hydrochloride (Elavil, Emitrip, Endep). This tricyclic antidepressant is used primarily to treat depression. It is as potent as desipramine, doxepin hydrochloride, imipramine, and trimipramine maleate, but produces greater sedative and anticholinergic effects.
Usual adult dosage: initially, 50 to 75 mg P.O. increased by 25 to 50 mg every 1 to 2 days as tolerated, to 200 mg; if no response occurs after 1 week, the dosage is increased by 25 mg daily, as tolerated, to a maximum of 300 mg daily. Amitriptyline may be given I.M. at 20 to 30 mg q.i.d. or as a single dose h.s. Elderly or adolescent patients may require an initial dosage of 30 mg P.O. daily in divided doses, increased to 100 mg as tolerated.

clomipramine (Anafranil). Structurally related to imipramine, clomipramine is the first drug approved by the FDA to treat obsessive-compulsive disorder.
Usual adult dosage: initially, 25 mg P.O. h.s., increased in 25-mg increments to 100 mg during the first 2 weeks; then increased by 25 mg every week, as needed, to a maximum of 250 mg daily. Elderly patients usually require lower dosages.

desipramine hydrochloride (Norpramin, Pertofrane). Used to treat depression, desipramine is a metabolite of imipramine but produces fewer sedative and anticholinergic effects.
Usual adult dosage: initially, 50 to 75 mg P.O., increased to a maximum of 300 mg daily; for an elderly patient, 25 to 50 mg P.O. daily, increased to 100 mg. Higher dosages may be prescribed with caution.

doxepin hydrochloride (Adapin, Sinequan). Doxepin is used to treat depression.
Usual adult dosage: initially, 25 to 50 mg P.O. daily in divided doses or as a single dose h.s., gradually increased to 150 mg with a maximum of 300 mg daily, if needed; for an elderly patient, initially 25 to 50 mg P.O. daily, gradually increased to a maximum of 100 mg, if needed.

imipramine hydrochloride (Janimine, SK-Pramine, Tofranil). Imipramine shares amitriptyline's dosage schedule for treating depression. It also is used to treat enuresis in children ages 6 and over.
Usual adult dosage: initially, 50 to 75 mg P.O. daily increased to a maximum of 300 mg, or 30 to 40 mg daily increased to 100 mg in an elderly or debilitated patient.
Usual pediatric dosage: for enuresis in children ages 6 and over, 25 mg 1 hour before bedtime, up to a maximum of 50 mg daily in children under age 12 and 75 mg daily in children ages 12 and older. Imipramine also is available in injectable form for administration using the same dosage schedule up to a maximum of 100 mg/day.

nortriptyline hydrochloride (Aventyl, Pamelor). This drug is twice as potent as most of the other tricyclic antide-

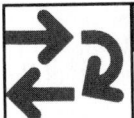

DRUG INTERACTIONS
Tricyclic antidepressants

Tricyclic antidepressants can interact with several commonly used drugs, causing potentially severe effects.

DRUG	INTERACTING DRUGS	POSSIBLE EFFECTS	NURSING IMPLICATIONS
amitriptyline, clomipramine, desipramine, doxepin, imipramine, nortriptyline, protriptyline, trimipramine	amphetamines	Increase catecholamine effects, leading to hypertension	• Administer amphetamines cautiously to a patient receiving tricyclic antidepressants. • Monitor the patient's blood pressure frequently.
	barbiturates	Increase metabolism and decrease blood levels of tricyclic antidepressants	• Monitor the patient for a decreased therapeutic effect.
	cimetidine	Impairs hepatic metabolism of tricyclic antidepressants, leading to toxicity	• Monitor the patient for signs of toxicity, such as dry mouth, blurred vision, orthostatic hypotension, urine retention, and tachycardia, if these drugs must be given together.
	MAO inhibitors	Cause hyperpyrexia, excitation, seizures	• Monitor the patient's body temperature and level of consciousness.
	sympathomimetics	Increase catecholamine effects, leading to hypertension	• Monitor the patient's blood pressure and heart rate frequently, if these drugs must be given together.
	anticholinergic agents	Enhance anticholinergic effect	• Monitor the patient for signs of anticholinergic effects, such as dry mouth, urine retention, and constipation.
	clonidine, guanethidine	Inhibit antihypertensive effects	• Avoid concomitant administration, if possible. • Monitor the patient's blood pressure frequently.

pressants. As a result, the dosages are much lower for treating depression.

Usual adult dosage: initially, 25 mg P.O. t.i.d. or q.i.d., increased every 1 to 2 days by 10 to 25 mg, as tolerated. If the response is inadequate after 1 week, the dosage can be increased by 10 mg daily to a maximum of 150 mg. The dosage for elderly patients should not exceed 100 mg daily.

protriptyline hydrochloride (Vivactil). The most potent tricyclic antidepressant, protriptyline is about five times more potent than amitriptyline. Usually, this agent is used to treat depression; it produces the mildest sedative effects of all the tricyclic antidepressants.

Usual adult dosage: initially, 10 to 15 mg P.O. daily increased by 5 mg every 1 to 2 days, as tolerated, to 30 mg daily. If the response is inadequate after 1 week, the dosage can be increased by 5 mg daily, as tolerated, to a maximum of 60 mg daily. Elderly patients usually receive lower dosages.

trimipramine maleate (Surmontil). Trimipramine is used to treat depression and is under investigation for treating duodenal ulcers.

Usual adult dosage: for depression, initially, 50 to 75 mg P.O. daily, increased to a maximum of 300 mg daily; for duodenal ulcers, 50 mg P.O. daily. A patient receiving more than 200 mg daily will require close observation because of the increased incidence of adverse reactions. Elderly patients rarely receive more than 100 mg daily.

Drug interactions

Tricyclic antidepressants can interact with many drugs, especially MAO inhibitors and sympathomimetics. (For detailed information, see *Drug interactions: Tricyclic antidepressants.*)

ADVERSE DRUG REACTIONS

Reactions to tricyclic antidepressants commonly include orthostatic hypotension, cardiovascular effects, anticholinergic effects, and sedation. Because adverse reactions can differ markedly among agents and because no one agent is more effective than the others, the patient's therapy can be changed from one tricyclic antidepressant to another to eliminate intolerable adverse reactions.

Orthostatic hypotension commonly occurs with tricyclic antidepressant therapy. In these cases, the dosage may be reduced or nortriptyline may be prescribed—especially for elderly patients—because it is less likely to cause this adverse reaction.

A conduction delay, demonstrated by a widening QT interval, also may occur with tricyclic antidepressant therapy. This adverse reaction can exacerbate congestive heart failure or an existing bundle branch block. A patient taking a tricyclic antidepressant will need to be monitored for palpitations, tachycardia, and electrocardiogram (ECG) changes. In therapeutic concentrations, these agents can act as antiarrhythmics, but in toxic concentrations, they can induce arrhythmias.

Anticholinergic adverse reactions commonly occur with tricyclic antidepressant therapy, but may diminish or disappear as treatment continues. Reactions include blurred vision, urine retention, dry mouth, and constipation.

At high dosages, tricyclic antidepressants can cause seizures. Other adverse reactions include sedation, jaundice, a fine resting tremor, decreased libido, inhibited ejaculation, transient eosinophilia and leukopenia, and, rarely, granulocytopenia (agranulocytosis).

Rashes may occur during the first 2 months of therapy, particularly with amitriptyline and imipramine. They usually are mild and do not require discontinuation of therapy. Photosensitivity reactions also may occur.

NURSING PROCESS APPLICATION

The following information assists the nurse in caring for a patient who is receiving a tricyclic antidepressant.

Assessment

• Review the patient's history for a condition that contraindicates the use of a tricyclic antidepressant, such as a known hypersensitivity to the drug, urine retention, or narrow-angle glaucoma.
• Review the patient's history for a condition that requires cautious use of a tricyclic antidepressant, such as pregnancy, lactation, suicidal tendencies, cardiovascular disease, or impaired hepatic function.
• Assess the patient for adverse reactions to the prescribed tricyclic antidepressant, such as orthostatic hypotension, cardiovascular effects, anticholinergic effects, seizures, sedation, and urine retention.
• Review the patient's medication history to identify the use of drugs that may interact with the tricyclic antidepressant, such as amphetamines, MAO inhibitors, sympathomimetics, and anticholinergic agents.
• Monitor the patient for signs of urine retention.

• Assess the patient daily for constipation.
• Question the male patient about sexual dysfunction.
• Evaluate the patient's and family's knowledge about the prescribed tricyclic antidepressant.

Nursing diagnoses

The following examples represent appropriate nursing diagnoses for a patient receiving a tricyclic antidepressant.
• Potential for injury related to a preexisting condition that contraindicates the use of a tricyclic antidepressant
• Potential for injury related to a preexisting condition that requires cautious use of a tricyclic antidepressant
• Potential for injury related to adverse drug reactions
• Urinary retention related to the adverse genitourinary effects of the prescribed tricyclic antidepressant
• Constipation related to the anticholinergic effects of the prescribed tricyclic antidepressant
• Sexual dysfunction related to the adverse genitourinary effects of the tricyclic antidepressant
• Knowledge deficit related to the prescribed tricyclic antidepressant

Planning and implementation

• Do not administer a tricyclic antidepressant to a patient with a condition that contraindicates its use.
• Administer a tricyclic antidepressant cautiously to a patient at risk because of a preexisting condition.
• Monitor the patient frequently for adverse reactions to the prescribed tricyclic antidepressant. Closely observe any patient who receives more than 200 mg daily of trimipramine maleate because of the increased incidence of adverse reactions with high doses.
• Expect to change the patient to a different tricyclic antidepressant if intolerable adverse reactions occur because adverse reactions can differ markedly among these agents.
• Consult with the physician about dividing a once-daily dosage if adverse reactions occur because smaller doses given more frequently decrease the risk of adverse reactions.
• Expect to use a lower dosage of tricyclic antidepressant for an elderly patient, as prescribed, to minimize adverse reactions.
• Monitor the patient's blood pressure and heart rate frequently to detect adverse cardiovascular effects. Also monitor the patient for palpitations, tachycardia, and ECG changes. Be aware that an elderly patient should have an ECG before beginning tricyclic antidepressant therapy.
• *Notify the physician if the QT interval widens on the ECG.*
• *Have the patient sit up for 1 minute before getting out of bed to reduce the effects of orthostatic hypotension. Supervise the patient's ambulation.*

• *Take safety precautions if blurred vision or sedation occurs. For example, place the bed in a low position and keep the bed rails up.*

• *Take seizure precautions, such as padding the bed rails when the patient must receive a high dosage of tricyclic antidepressants.*

• *Monitor a suicidal patient closely until the drug takes full effect.*

• Reassure the patient that anticholinergic adverse reactions may diminish or disappear as therapy continues.

• Notify the physician if adverse reactions occur.

• Record the patient's fluid intake and output to detect signs of urine retention. Also palpate and percuss the bladder after the patient voids.

• Ask the patient to report symptoms of urine retention, such as urinary hesitancy, frequent voiding of small amounts, or a sensation of fullness in the lower abdomen.

• Notify the physician if urine retention occurs. Be prepared to catheterize the patient, as prescribed.

• Provide a high-fiber diet and plenty of fluids (unless contraindicated) to help prevent or correct constipation.

• Consult with the physician for a prescription for a stool softener to relieve the patient's constipation, if needed.

• Reassure the patient that drug-induced decreased libido and inhibited ejaculation should resolve when the tricyclic antidepressant is discontinued.

Patient teaching

• Teach the patient and family the name, dose, frequency, action, and adverse effects of the prescribed tricyclic antidepressant.

• Caution the patient not to stop taking a tricyclic antidepressant abruptly after long-term use; abrupt withdrawal can produce nausea, headache, and malaise.

• Advise the patient not to operate a motor vehicle or dangerous machinery if blurred vision or sedation occurs.

• Inform the patient that urine retention can occur.

• Teach the patient to identify high-fiber foods and include them in the diet to prevent constipation.

• Teach the patient how to manage orthostatic hypotension.

• Inform the patient that decreased libido may occur. Tell the male patient that inhibited ejaculation also may occur.

• Alert the patient that a full therapeutic response may take up to 30 days.

• Instruct the patient to take the entire drug dosage at bedtime to avoid sedation and anticholinergic effects, unless otherwise prescribed.

• Warn the patient that the use of alcohol or other CNS depressants may increase sedation.

• Warn the patient to keep tricyclic antidepressants out of the reach of children.

• Instruct the patient to notify the physician if adverse reactions occur.

Evaluation

The following examples represent appropriate evaluation statements for a patient receiving a tricyclic antidepressant.

• The patient has no conditions that contraindicate tricyclic antidepressant therapy.

• The patient exhibits no signs of complications in the preexisting condition linked to the prescribed tricyclic antidepressant.

• The patient displays no adverse reactions to the prescribed tricyclic antidepressant.

• The patient maintains normal fluid balance.

• The patient maintains normal bowel patterns.

• The patient states that sexual activity remains satisfactory.

• The patient and family express an accurate understanding of the points taught about the prescribed tricyclic antidepressant.

• The patient correctly identifies high-fiber foods and plans to include some at each meal.

SECOND-GENERATION ANTIDEPRESSANTS

Developed to treat depression with fewer adverse reactions, these antidepressants are chemically different from each other and from tricyclic antidepressants and MAO inhibitors. Five second-generation antidepressants currently are available: amoxapine, bupropion hydrochloride, fluoxetine hydrochloride, maprotiline hydrochloride, and trazodone hydrochloride.

PHARMACOKINETICS

The second-generation antidepressants are chemically distinct from one another and differ somewhat in their pharmacokinetic properties.

Absorption, distribution, metabolism, excretion

All of these agents are absorbed completely after oral administration and distributed widely throughout the body, except for cardiac tissue.

Amoxapine undergoes extensive metabolism in the liver, producing some active metabolites. Only 3% of it is excreted unchanged by the kidneys; the rest is excreted as glucuronides.

Bupropion is metabolized extensively to several active metabolites. Insignificant amounts are excreted in the urine as unchanged drug.

Fluoxetine is metabolized by the liver to several metabolites. The primary route of elimination appears to be hepatic metabolism with inactive metabolites excreted in the urine.

Maprotiline also is metabolized in the liver, producing some active metabolites. Most of the drug is excreted in the urine, but 30% leaves the body in the feces.

Although trazodone is metabolized extensively in the liver, the therapeutic activity of its metabolites is unknown. The kidneys excrete most of this drug.

Onset, peak, duration

Some of these drugs have shorter half-lives than other antidepressants. Amoxapine achieves a peak concentration level in 1 to 2 hours and has a half-life of 8 hours. Some of its active metabolites have half-lives of up to 30 hours. Steady-state concentration can be attained in 2 to 7 days.

Bupropion reaches peak concentration within 2 hours. Its half-life ranges from 8 to 24 hours and averages 14 hours.

Fluoxetine achieves peak plasma concentrations 6 to 8 hours after administration. The half-life of fluoxetine is 2 to 3 days; of its one known active metabolite, 7 to 9 days. Because of these long half-lives, fluoxetine does not attain a steady-state concentration until week 4 or 5 of therapy.

Maprotiline reaches peak concentration in 8 to 24 hours. Its half-life is about 43 hours, and a steady-state concentration is attained in 8 to 10 days.

The trazodone concentration peaks in 1 to 2 hours. This drug has a relatively short half-life of 4 to 12 hours and can achieve a steady-state concentration in 2 days.

PHARMACODYNAMICS

The biochemical activity of second-generation antidepressants resembles that of the tricyclic antidepressants.

Mechanism of action

Like the tricyclic antidepressants, second-generation antidepressants inhibit reuptake of the neurotransmitters norepinephrine or serotonin, or both, thus restoring hyposensitive receptor sites to normal so that increased neurotransmitter concentrations can exert a therapeutic effect. Amoxapine and maprotiline primarily inhibit the reuptake of norepinephrine, inhibiting serotonin reuptake to a lesser extent. Trazodone inhibits reuptake of serotonin only. Bupropion weakly blocks reuptake of serotonin and norepinephrine. Fluoxetine strongly inhibits serotonin reuptake and has some inhibiting effect on norepinephrine reuptake.

PHARMACOTHERAPEUTICS

Second-generation antidepressants are used to treat the same major depressive episodes as the tricyclic antidepressants and have the same degree of effectiveness.

amoxapine (Asendin). A loxapine derivative, amoxapine possesses some antipsychotic effects besides its antidepressant effects.
Usual adult dosage: initially, 50 mg P.O. t.i.d., increased to 300 mg/day after 3 days, if tolerated; after 2 weeks, increased to a maximum of 400 mg/day, if necessary. For an elderly patient, the initial dose is 25 mg P.O. t.i.d.

bupropion hydrochloride (Wellbutrin). This drug is used to treat depression in patients who fail to respond to or cannot tolerate other antidepressants.
Usual adult dosage: initially, 100 mg P.O. b.i.d; may be increased to 100 mg t.i.d. after 3 days based on clinical response. Dosages above 300 mg/day are not recommended unless the patient fails to show improvement after several weeks of therapy. In such a patient, the maximum recommended dosage is 450 mg/day. After depression resolves, the dosage should be decreased to the lowest possible maintenance therapy. Elderly patients usually receive lower dosages.

fluoxetine hydrochloride (Prozac). Fluoxetine is chemically unrelated to tricyclic and other antidepressant compounds. It is used to treat major depressive disorders.
Usual adult dosage: initially, 20 mg P.O. daily in the morning; increased slowly to a maximum of 80 mg/day, if no improvement occurs after 2 to 4 weeks. Dosages above 20 mg/day should be administered in two divided doses—in the morning and at noon. Elderly patients should receive lower dosages, usually 20 mg.

maprotiline hydrochloride (Ludiomil). Maprotiline has significant sedative properties and is used to treat depression.
Usual adult dosage: initially, 50 to 100 mg P.O. daily, given in two divided doses or as a single dose; increased after 2 weeks, as needed and tolerated, by 25-mg increments to 150 to 200 mg daily, up to a maximum of 300 mg, if necessary. An elderly patient may require an initial dosage of 25 mg P.O. daily.

trazodone hydrochloride (Desyrel). This second-generation agent is used to treat depression. It has the least anticholinergic activity of the second-generation antidepressants and may be somewhat less effective.
Usual adult dosage: initially, 150 mg P.O. daily in divided doses, increased by 50 mg every 3 to 4 days up to a maximum of 400 mg/day (600 mg/day for a severely ill hospitalized patient). For an elderly patient, the initial dosage is 50 mg P.O. daily.

Drug interactions

Few interactions have been documented between amoxapine or maprotiline and other drugs. Patients receiving drugs that interact with tricyclic antidepressants, however, should be observed for similar interactions with the second-generation antidepressants.

Bupropion may stimulate hepatic enzymes needed for drug metabolism. Caution should be used with concomitant administration of other drugs that may affect drug metabolism, such as carbamazepine, cimetidine, phenobarbital, and phenytoin. Bupropion may increase levodopa's adverse effects when used concurrently. Therefore, bupropion therapy should begin with small doses and increase gradually in a patient receiving levodopa.

Fluoxetine increases the half-life of diazepam and displaces highly protein-bound drugs, which can lead to drug toxicity. Fluoxetine also may produce a potentially fatal interaction when used with MAO inhibitors; this drug combination should be avoided. This second-generation antidepressant also may increase serum levels of other antidepressants during concomitant therapy.

Trazodone may produce additive effects when combined with other drugs. For instance, it can increase sedation when combined with a CNS depressant and may produce an additive hypotensive effect when used with a hypotensive agent. It also can increase phenytoin levels during concomitant therapy.

ADVERSE DRUG REACTIONS

Second-generation antidepressants produce fewer adverse reactions than tricyclic antidepressants do. Seizures may occur with all of these antidepressants, particularly high dosages of protiline and bupropion. To prevent seizures, dosages should be prescribed below the maximum. Amoxapine and maprotiline also may cause anticholinergic effects, orthostatic hypotension, and tachycardia.

Because it is structurally similar to the anorexigenic agent diethylpropion, bupropion causes dose-related CNS stimulation, including restlessness, hallucinations, seizures, insomnia, and psychotic episodes. This distinguishes bupropion from the other tricyclic antidepressants, which commonly produce sedation. Bupropion produces fewer cardiovascular and anticholinergic symptoms than other antidepressants.

The most common adverse reactions to fluoxetine are headache, nervousness, anxiety, insomnia, nausea, anorexia, diarrhea, and diaphoresis. A rash also may occur.

Trazodone sometimes produces sedation and dizziness, but rarely produces anticholinergic effects; to minimize these adverse reactions, give the drug before bedtime or with food. It also can produce priapism.

NURSING PROCESS APPLICATION

The following information assists the nurse incaring for a patient who is receiving a second-generation antidepressant.

Assessment

• Review the patient's history for a condition that contraindicates the use of a second-generation antidepressant, such as a known hypersensitivity to the drug.
• Review the patient's history for a condition that requires cautious use of a second-generation antidepressant, such as cardiac disease, pregnancy, or lactation.
• Assess the patient for adverse reactions to the prescribed second-generation antidepressant, such as seizures or anticholinergic, cardiovascular, or CNS effects.
• Review the patient's medication history to identify the use of drugs that may interact with the prescribed second-generation antidepressant, such as CNS depressants, levodopa, MAO inhibitors, sympathomimetics, or anticholinergics.
• Evaluate the patient's and family's knowledge about the prescribed second-generation antidepressant.

Nursing diagnoses

The following examples represent appropriate nursing diagnoses for a patient receiving a second-generation antidepressant.
• Potential for injury related to a preexisting condition that contraindicates the use of a second-generation antidepressant
• Potential for injury related to a preexisting condition that requires cautious use of a second-generation antidepressant
• Potential for injury related to adverse drug reactions
• Knowledge deficit related to the prescribed second-generation antidepressant

Planning and implementation

• Do not administer a second-generation antidepressant to a patient with a condition that contraindicates its use.
• Administer a second-generation antidepressant cautiously to a patient at risk because of a preexisting condition.
• Monitor the patient periodically for adverse drug reactions.
• *Take seizure precautions, such as padding the bed rails, during therapy with these agents.* Also, expect to administer less-than-maximum dosages of maprotiline and bupropion to prevent seizures.
• *Take safety precautions if sedation or dizziness occurs. For example, place the bed in a low position, keep the bed rails up, and supervise patient ambulation.*
• Give the drug before bedtime or with food to minimize anticholinergic effects.

• *Have the patient sit up for 1 minute before getting out of bed to reduce the effects of orthostatic hypotension.*
• Expect to administer a fluoxetine dosage that exceeds 20 mg/day in two divided doses — in the morning and at noon.
• Expect to begin bupropion therapy with small doses and increase them gradually in a patient who also is receiving levodopa.
• *Withhold fluoxetine and notify the physician if the patient develops a rash.* Also notify the physician if other adverse reactions occur.
• Notify the physician if GI upset occurs. Obtain an order for an antiemetic or antidiarrheal agent, as needed.

Patient teaching
• Teach the patient and family the name, dose, frequency, action, and adverse effects of the prescribed second-generation antidepressant.
• Advise the patient to avoid operating a motor vehible or dangerous machinery, because sedation can occur.
• Teach the patient to take most of the dosage at bedtime if sedation is a problem.
• Instruct the patient to take the drug with meals or a snack to enhance absorption and decrease dizziness.
• Instruct the female patient to notify her physician if she becomes pregnant or intends to become pregnant.
• Advise the patient to notify the physician if adverse reactions occur.

Evaluation
The following examples represent appropriate evaluation statements for a patient receiving a second-generation antidepressant.
• The patient has no conditions that contraindicate the use of a second-generation antidepressant.
• The patient exhibit no signs of complications in the pre-existing condition linked to the prescribed second-generation antidepressant.
• The patient demonstrates no adverse reactions to the prescribed second-generation antidepressant.
• The patient and family express an accurate understanding of the points taught abou the prescribed second-generation antidepressant.
• The patient plans to take the second-generation antidepressant with meals to reduce dizziness.

LITHIUM

Lithium is the drug of choice to prevent or treat mania. Its discovery was a milestone in treating mania and bipolar disorders.

PHARMACOKINETICS

An active drug, lithium is not metabolized and is excreted from the body unchanged.

Absorption, distribution, metabolism, excretion
After oral administration, lithium is absorbed rapidly and completely and is distributed to body tissues, with highest concentrations occurring in the kidneys, thyroid gland, and bone. The kidneys excrete lithium unchanged at a rate that parallels the glomerular filtration rate (GFR). Because 80% of the lithium is reabsorbed in the renal tubules, the renal clearance rate is 20% of the GFR.

Lithium crosses the placenta and is detectable in the fetus. It also is excreted in breast milk.

Onset, peak, duration
The serum concentration level of lithium peaks 2 to 3 hours after administration. Initially, the half-life is 2 hours, but it increases to 20 hours as therapy continues. Steady-state concentration is reached in 6 days with fixed-dose administration.

PHARMACODYNAMICS

Although the exact mechanism of action is unknown, lithium reduces the excessive catecholamine response in mania.

Mechanism of action
In mania, the patient experiences excessive catecholamine stimulation. In a bipolar disorder, the patient is affected by swings between the excessive catecholamine stimulation of mania and the diminished catecholamine stimulation of depression. Lithium may normalize the catecholamine receptors by increasing norepinephrine and serotonin uptake, reducing the release of norepinephrine from the synaptic vesicles, and inhibiting norepinephrine's postsynaptic action.

PHARMACOTHERAPEUTICS

Lithium is used primarily to treat acute episodes of mania and to prevent relapses of bipolar disorders. It can produce 70% to 80% improvement in manic patients within 1 to 2 weeks and can reduce the 2-year relapse incidence to 50%. After an acute manic episode, lithium therapy typically is continued for 3 to 6 months and then tapered off. A patient who experiences a relapse every 1 to 2 years, however, may require long-term prophylactic therapy.

Other uses of lithium under investigation include preventing unipolar depression and migraine headaches and treating resistant depression, alcohol dependence, anorexia nervosa, inappropriate secretion of antidiuretic hormone, and neutropenia.

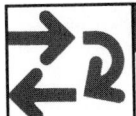

DRUG INTERACTIONS

Lithium

Lithium can interact with several drugs; most interactions affect lithium excretion and can be managed with dosage adjustments.

DRUG	INTERACTING DRUGS	POSSIBLE EFFECTS	NURSING IMPLICATIONS
lithium	thiazide diuretics, loop diuretics	Increase lithium reabsorption in the kidneys	• Monitor the patient's serum lithium level and renal function.
	nonsteroidal anti-inflammatory drugs (NSAIDs)	Inhibit lithium excretion	• Monitor the patient's serum lithium level. • Expect to substitute sulindac for the interacting NSAID.
	potassium iodide	Increases hypothyroid activity	• Avoid concomitant use. If these drugs must be given together, observe the patient for signs and symptoms of hypothyroidism, such as fatigue, cold sensitivity, and a decreased pulse rate.
	sodium bicarbonate	Increases lithium excretion	• Monitor the patient's serum lithium level.
	sodium chloride	Alters lithium excretion in proportion to sodium chloride intake	• Be aware that a patient on a severe salt-restricted diet is susceptible to lithium toxicity. • Advise the patient that increased salt intake will decrease lithium's therapeutic effects.
	carbamazepine	May cause neurotoxicity	• Assess the patient's level of consciousness. • Instruct the patient to report dizziness, headache, fatigue, or slurred speech.
	phenothiazines	May cause neurotoxicity and seizures	• Assess the patient's level of consciousness. • Instruct the patient to report dizziness, headache, fatigue, or slurred speech. • Take seizure precautions, such as padding the patient's bed rails.
	theophylline	Increases renal clearance of lithium	• Monitor the patient's serum lithium level.

lithium carbonate and **lithium citrate** (Eskalith, Lithane, Lithobid). Lithium's two salts have identical effects and dosage schedules, but lithium citrate is more soluble. Because lithium's therapeutic dosage range is narrow, dosages require regular adjustment. Blood levels monitored 12 hours after the last daily dose serve as an adjustment guide. *Usual adult dosage:* to treat acute mania, 300 to 600 mg P.O. up to q.i.d., adjusted to achieve a blood level of 1 to 1.5 mEq/liter; to prevent a relapse of a bipolar disorder, a drug dosage adjusted to achieve a blood level of 0.6 to 1.2 mEq/liter or a maximum of 2 mEq/liter.

Drug interactions
Serious interactions with other drugs can occur because of lithium's narrow therapeutic range. They may occur in the kidneys, where the clearance can increase or decrease, or at the receptor site, where potentiation takes place. (For more information, see *Drug interactions: Lithium*.)

ADVERSE DRUG REACTIONS

Adverse reactions to lithium affect various body systems and may occur in any phase of therapy; most are dose-related. Because GI complaints are associated with increasing blood levels of lithium, they are most frequent during the initial phase of therapy and after dosage adjustments. About 50% of patients experience a fine tremor that may diminish with dosage reduction and worsen with dosage increase. Polyuria of 2 to 3 liters/day may appear, accompanied by polydipsia. When blood levels exceed 1.5 mEq/liter, toxicity may occur, producing confusion, lethargy, slurred speech, hyperreflexia, and seizures.

Long-term lithium therapy may result in distal tubule atrophy and decreased GFR. A diabetes insipidus syndrome can occur, producing a daily urine output exceeding 3 liters and a low urine specific gravity. Hypothyroidism and nontoxic goiters may affect about 4% of patients. Other adverse

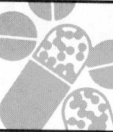

SELECTED MAJOR DRUGS

Antidepressant and antimanic agents

This chart summarizes the major antidepressant and antimanic drugs currently in clinical use.

DRUG	MAJOR INDICATIONS	USUAL ADULT DOSAGES	CONTRAINDICATIONS AND PRECAUTIONS
MAO inhibitors			
isocarboxazid	Atypical depression	30 mg P.O. daily in a single dose or divided doses, reduced to 10 to 20 mg/day when condition improves	• Know that isocarboxazid is contraindicated in an elderly or debilitated patient and in a patient with severe hepatic or renal impairment; congestive heart failure; pheochromocytoma; hypertensive, cardiovascular, or cerebrovascular disease; severe or frequent headaches; or known hypersensitivity to the drug. It also is contraindicated within 10 days of elective surgery requiring general anesthesia, cocaine, or a local anesthetic containing sympathomimetic vasoconstrictors; and with concurrent use of other MAO inhibitors, dibenzazepines, buspirone, clomipramine, central nervous system depressants, sympathomimetic drugs, high-tryptophan foods, high-tyramine foods, or excessive amounts of caffeine. • Administer with caution to a hyperactive, agitated, schizophrenic, or suicidal patient and to a patient with diabetes or epilepsy or one taking antihypertensive drugs including thiazide diuretics. Also administer with caution to a pregnant or lactating patient.
tranylcypromine	Atypical depression	10 mg P.O. b.i.d., increased to a maximum of 30 mg/day after 2 to 3 weeks, if necessary	• Know that tranylcypromine is contraindicated in a patient with cerebrovascular defects, cardiovascular disorders, pheochromocytoma, liver disease, known hypersensitivity to the drug, or with concurrent use of MAO inhibitors, dibenzazepines, fluoxetine, buspirone, sympathomimetics, meperidine, dextromethorphan, or high-tyramine foods. It also is contraindicated in a patient undergoing elective surgery or one who uses narcotics, alcohol, hypotensive agents, or excessive amounts of caffeine. • Administer with caution to a pregnant or lactating patient; one with impaired renal function, epilepsy, diabetes, or hyperthydroidism; or one who is receiving antiparkinsonian agents or disulfiram (Antabuse).
Tricyclic antidepressants			
amitriptyline	Depression	50 to 75 mg P.O. increased to 200 mg/day, then to a maximum of 300 mg daily, if needed; or 20 to 30 mg I.M. q.i.d. or as a single dose h.s.	• Know that amitriptyline is contraindicated in a patient with a known hypersensitivity to the drug or during the acute recovery phase of myocardial infarction. • Administer with caution to a pregnant or lactating patient, a patient receiving electroconvulsive therapy or undergoing elective surgery, or one with seizures, suicidal tendencies, urine retention, narrow-angle glaucoma, increased intraocular pressure, cardiovascular disease, hyperthyroidism, or impaired hepatic function.

SELECTED MAJOR DRUGS

Antidepressant and antimanic agents (continued)

DRUG	MAJOR INDICATIONS	USUAL ADULT DOSAGES	CONTRAINDICATIONS AND PRECAUTIONS
Tricyclic antidepressants (continued)			
doxepin	Depression	25 to 50 mg P.O. daily initially, increased to a maximum of 300 mg daily, if necessary	• Know that doxepin is contraindicated in a patient with urine retention, narrow-angle glaucoma, or known hypersensitivity to the drug . • Administer with caution to a pregnant or lactating patient or one with suicidal tendencies.
Second-generation antidepressants			
trazodone	Depression	150 mg P.O. daily in divided doses, increased by 50 mg/day every 3 to 4 days up to a maximum of 400 mg/day; (600 mg/day for a severely ill patient)	• Know that trazodone is contraindicated in a patient with known hypersensitivity to the drug. • Administer with caution to a pregnant or lactating patient or one with cardiac disease.
Lithium			
lithium	Mania and bipolar disorder relapse	300 to 600 mg P.O. up to q.i.d., adjusted to achieve lithium blood level of 1 to 1.5 mEq/liter for acute mania, 0.6 to 1.2 mEq/liter to prevent bipolar disorder relapses, and 2 mEq/liter as a maximum dose	• Know that lithium is contraindicated in a pregnant, lactating, elderly, or debilitated patient; a patient who cannot be monitored closely; or one with epilepsy, renal or cardiovascular disease, brain damage, severe dehydration, or sodium depletion. • Administer with caution to a patient with a thyroid disorder.

reactions include weight gain, skin eruptions, alopecia, and leukocytosis.

NURSING PROCESS APPLICATION

The following information assists the nurse in caring for a patient who is receiving lithium.

Assessment
• Review the patient's history for a condition that contraindicates the use of lithium, such as epilepsy, renal or cardiovascular disease, brain damage, severe dehydration, sodium depletion, pregnancy, or lactation.
• Review the patient's history for a condition that requires cautious use of lithium, such as a thyroid disorder.
• Assess the patient for adverse reactions to lithium, such as GI upset, tremor, polyuria, polydipsia, thyroid problems, weight gain, skin eruptions, alopecia, or leukocytosis.
• Review the patient's medication history to identify the use of drugs that may interact with lithium, such as thiazide diuretics, loop diuretics, nonsteroidal anti-inflammatory drugs, sodium bicarbonate, or sodium chloride.
• Monitor the patient with diabetes insipidus syndrome for signs of dehydration, such as a weight loss that exceeds 2 pounds/day, dry mucous membranes, and poor skin turgor.

• Evaluate the patient's and family's knowledge about lithium.

Nursing diagnoses
The following examples represent appropriate nursing diagnoses for a patient receiving lithium.
• Potential for injury related to a preexisting condition that contraindicates the use of lithium
• Potential for injury related to a preexisting condition that requires cautious use of lithium
• Potential for injury related to adverse drug reactions
• Potential fluid volume deficit related to possible lithium-induced diabetes insipidus syndrome
• Knowledge deficit related to lithium

Planning and implementation
• Do not administer lithium to a patient with a condition that contraindicates its use.
• Administer lithium cautiously to a patient at risk because of a preexisting condition.
• Observe the patient frequently for adverse drug reactions. Be aware that most adverse reactions to lithium are dose-related.
• Obtain baseline tests of the patient's thyroid and renal functions and an ECG reading, as prescribed.

- Monitor the patient's lithium concentration periodically during therapy and after dosage adjustments. Expect to draw blood and evaluate lithium concentration 12 hours after the last daily dose. Particularly note a concentration that exceeds 1.5 mEq/liter, which may cause toxicity.
- Monitor the patient's white blood cell (WBC) count.
- Monitor the patient closely for drug interactions.
- Monitor the patient closely for GI complaints, especially during the initial phase of lithium therapy.
- Administer lithium with food to reduce GI distress.
- Notify the physician if adverse reactions occur.
- Record the patient's fluid intake and output; polyuria of 2 to 3 liters/day may occur with diabetes insipidus syndrome.
- *Monitor the patient with polyuria for signs of dehydration, such as dry mucous membranes, polydipsia, and poor skin turgor.*
- Note the patient's urine specific gravity and color. With diabetes insipidus syndrome, the specific gravity is low and the urine is light yellow (diluted) rather than dark yellow (concentrated), which usually occurs in dehydration.
- *Notify the physician if the urine output significantly exceeds fluid intake.*
- Administer fluids to replace fluid loss, as needed.

Patient teaching
- Teach the patient and family the name, dose, frequency, action, and adverse effects of lithium.
- Advise the patient that lithium may take 1 to 2 weeks to produce a therapeutic response.
- Instruct the patient to take lithium with food to reduce GI distress.
- Stress the importance of having blood drawn for lithium level and WBC count, as prescribed.
- Teach the patient and family to recognize signs of toxicity (confusion, lethargy, slurred speech, hyperreflexia, and seizures) and to notify the physician if toxicity occurs before administering the next dose.
- Instruct the patient to notify other physicians about lithium therapy to avoid serious drug interactions.
- Advise the patient to measure fluid intake and output and to notify the physician if output exceeds 3 quarts a day.
- Advise the patient who develops a fine tremor that it may diminish with a dosage reduction and worsen with a dosage increase. Reassure the patient that the tremor will cease when lithium is discontinued.
- Reassure the patient that weight gain, skin eruptions, and alopecia will disappear when lithium is discontinued.
- Instruct the female patient to notify the physician if she becomes pregnant or intends to become pregnant.

- Instruct the patient to notify the physician if adverse drug reactions occur.

Evaluation
The following examples represent appropriate evaluation statements for a patient receiving lithium.
- The patient has no conditions that contraindicate lithium therapy.
- The patient exhibits no signs of complications in the preexisting condition linked to lithium.
- The patient experiences no adverse reactions to lithium.
- The patient maintains normal hydration.
- The patient and family express an accurate understanding of the points taught about lithium.
- The patient schedules follow-up appointments for blood tests for lithium level and WBC count.

CHAPTER SUMMARY

Chapter 26 discussed the antimanic and antidepressant agents. Here are the highlights of the chapter.
- Various agents are used to treat depression, mania, and bipolar disorders, such as manic-depressive illness.
- Although MAO inhibitors can interact with many drugs and foods, they remain the treatment of choice for atypical depression. They also may be used to treat other types of depression when it is resistant to other therapies or when other therapies are contraindicated.
- The tricyclic antidepressants are preferred for treating major depressive episodes. However, they can interact with numerous drugs.
- The second-generation antidepressants are used to treat depression. They have fewer adverse effects than tricyclic antidepressants and MAO inhibitors. No second-generation antidepressant is more effective than the tricyclic antidepressants.
- Lithium effectively treats manic episodes and prevents relapses of bipolar disorders. This drug has a narrow therapeutic range and a high incidence of adverse effects, however, so lithium therapy requires close patient monitoring.
- For a patient who is receiving an antidepressant or antimanic agent, the nurse applies the nursing process and emphasizes monitoring for CNS effects, taking safety precautions, and ensuring compliance with the drug regimen.

STUDY QUESTIONS

See Appendix 1 for answers.

1. Carla Blakely, age 43, seeks care because she feels depressed and has been gaining weight. She is diagnosed as having atypical depression. Which type of antidepressant is the physician most likely to prescribe for Ms. Blakely?
(a) lithium
(b) an MAO inhibitor
(c) a tricyclic antidepressant
(d) a second-generation antidepressant

2. Ms. Blakely's physician prescribes isocarboxazid (Marplan) 30 mg P.O. daily. During the patient-teaching session, the nurse should advise her to avoid which food completely?
(a) aged cheese
(b) fresh pork
(c) chocolate
(d) cream cheese

3. The nurse teaches Ms. Blakely to avoid high-tyramine foods. What may occur if the patient's MAO inhibitor interacts with these foods?
(a) MAO inhibitor inactivation
(b) MAO inhibitor hypersensitivity
(c) paradoxical drug effects
(d) hypertensive crisis

4. Patricia Potts, age 51, has depression associated with weight loss, anorexia, and insomnia. Her physician prescribes the tricyclic antidepressant amitriptyline (Elavil) 75 mg P.O. daily. How does amitriptyline reverse depression?
(a) It increases neurotransmitter concentration levels.
(b) It stimulates hyposensitive receptor sites.
(c) It stimulates the reuptake of neurotransmitters.
(d) It stimulates GABA activity at receptor sites.

5. Ms. Potts reports that she feels dizzy when she stands. To decrease the effects of orthostatic hypotension, what should the nurse tell Ms. Potts?
(a) Decrease the amitriptyline dosage.
(b) Arise gradually from a supine position.
(c) Drink more fluids, especially juices.
(d) Take the drug in the morning, not at bedtime.

6. The physician changes Ms. Potts's medication to the second-generation antidepressant fluoxetine 20 mg P.O. daily. How do second-generation antidepressants differ from tricyclic antidepressants?

(a) They have longer half-lives.
(b) They are more effective.
(c) They cause fewer adverse reactions.
(d) They are metabolized in the intestines; tricyclic antidepressants, in the liver.

7. Leo Hart, age 38, has manic-depression. His physician prescribes lithium citrate 300 mg P.O. t.i.d. Because lithium's therapeutic index is narrow, the nurse should take which action to help prevent toxicity?
(a) Assess Mr. Hart's behavior during treatment.
(b) Assess for exophthalmos and tinnitus.
(c) Monitor the lithium concentration regularly.
(d) Maintain the lithium concentration under 0.5 mEq/liter.

SELECTED REFERENCES

AHFS drug information 90. (1990). Bethesda, MD: American Society of Hospital Pharmacists.

American Psychiatric Association. (1987). *Diagnostic and statistical manual of mental disorders: DSM-III-R* (3rd ed. rev.). Washington, DC: American Psychiatric Association.

Bupropion for depression. (1989). *Medical Letter on Drugs and Therapeutics,* 31(804), 97-98.

Clomipramine for obsessive-compulsive disorder. (1988). *Medical Letter on Drugs and Therapeutics,* 30(778), 102-104.

Davies, D. (Ed.). (1987). *Textbook of adverse drug reactions* (3rd ed.). New York: Oxford Press.

Dreyfus, J. (1988). The treatment of depression in an ambulatory care setting. *Nurse Practitioner,* 13(7), 14-25.

Goodman and Gilman's the pharmacological basis of therapeutics (8th ed.; 1990). Elmsford, NY: Pergamon Press.

Hansten, P., and Horn, J. (1989). *Drug interactions* (6th ed.). Philadelphia: Lea & Febiger.

Harris, E. (1988). Psych drugs: The antidepressants. *AJN,* 88(11), 1512-1518.

North American Nursing Diagnosis Association. (1990). *Taxonomy I-Revised, with official diagnostic categories.* St. Louis: NANDA.

Perry, P., et al. (1989). *Psychotropic drug handbook* (5th ed.). Cincinnati: Harvey Whitney Books.

USPDI. (1991). *Drug information for the health care professional* (Vol. I, 11th ed.). Rockville, MD: United States Pharmacopeial Convention.

USPDI. (1991). *Advice for the patient* (Vol. II, 11th ed.). Rockville, MD: United States Pharmacopeial Convention.

CHAPTER

27

ANTIANXIETY AGENTS

OBJECTIVES

After reading and studying this chapter, the student should be able to:
1. Describe the three major types of antianxiety agents.
2. Explain why the benzodiazepines are the drugs of choice for treating anxiety.
3. Compare the mechanism of action of the benzodiazepines with that of the barbiturates, and describe how each type of drug produces different adverse reactions.
4. Explain why the benzodiazepines tend to be prescribed as antianxiety agents more often than the barbiturates.
5. Describe the pharmacokinetic, pharmacodynamic, and pharmacotherapeutic properties of buspirone.
6. Describe how to apply the nursing process when caring for a patient who is receiving an antianxiety agent.

INTRODUCTION

Antianxiety agents, also called anxiolytics, include some of the most commonly prescribed drugs in the United States. They are used primarily to treat anxiety disorders, which affect 7% to 18% of Americans.

This chapter presents the three main types of drugs used to treat anxiety disorders: the commonly prescribed benzodiazepines; buspirone; and the former drugs of choice, the barbiturates. It also will discuss briefly meprobamate and several other drugs that are used (rarely) to treat anxiety.

Anxiety disorders

The American Psychiatric Association divides anxiety disorders into two main types: nonphobic and phobic. Nonphobic anxieties can be subdivided into generalized anxiety disorders (the most common), obsessive-compulsive disorder, and panic disorders. Phobic anxieties can take many forms, such as phobias of crowds or heights. An anxiety disorder may be a primary medical condition or may occur secondary to another medical or social problem.

SELECTED NURSING DIAGNOSES

Antianxiety agents

The following nursing diagnoses address representative problems and etiologies that a nurse may encounter when caring for a patient who is receiving an antianxiety agent. Some of these nursing diagnoses contain generalized etiologies, which the nurse must individualize based on the patient's needs. (For some common nursing diagnoses and related interventions for each drug class, see the "Nursing Process Application" sections of this chapter.)

- Altered health maintenance related to ineffectiveness of the prescribed antianxiety agent
- Altered protection related to barbiturate-induced blood dyscrasias
- Altered role performance related to benzodiazepine or barbiturate dependence
- Altered thought processes related to the adverse central nervous system (CNS) effects of the antianxiety agent
- Impaired physical mobility related to barbiturate-induced impairment of motor coordination
- Impaired skin integrity related to dermatologic allergic reactions to the prescribed benzodiazepine or barbiturate
- Ineffective breathing pattern related to the adverse respiratory effects of the prescribed barbiturate
- Knowledge deficit related to the prescribed antianxiety agent
- Noncompliance related to long-term use of an antianxiety agent
- Pain related to headache caused by buspirone or a barbiturate
- Potential for injury related to a preexisting condition that contraindicates the use of an antianxiety agent
- Potential for injury related to a preexisting condition that requires cautious use of an antianxiety agent
- Potential for injury related to adverse drug reactions
- Potential for injury related to drug interactions
- Potential for trauma related to the adverse CNS effects of the antianxiety agent
- Sleep pattern disturbance related to buspirone-induced insomnia

Whatever its type, anxiety disorder symptoms include nervousness and tension as well as tremors, tachycardia, bowel and urinary complaints, diaphoresis, and palpitations.

Neither the etiologies of anxiety disorders nor the actions of the drugs used to treat them are understood fully. However, researchers have discovered that antianxiety agents relieve the symptoms of anxiety by mediating neurotransmitters in the midbrain. Today, medical specialists in many different fields (only one-fourth of them psychiatrists) treat these common disorders with antianxiety agents.

For a summary of representative drugs, see *Selected major drugs: Antianxiety agents,* page 446. For a listing of applicable nursing diagnoses that the nurse may formulate when caring for a patient receiving these agents, see *Selected nursing diagnoses: Antianxiety agents.* For detailed information on applying the nursing process, see Chapter 6, The Nursing Process and Drug Therapy.

BENZODIAZEPINES

Currently, the benzodiazepines are the drugs of choice to treat anxiety disorders. Although 12 benzodiazepines are marketed in the United States, one is used solely as an anticonvulsant, and three others as hypnotics. The remaining benzodiazepines are used as antianxiety agents. They include alprazolam, chlordiazepoxide hydrochloride, clorazepate dipotassium, diazepam, halazepam, lorazepam, oxazepam, and prazepam. Diazepam also is used as a muscle relaxant. However, with dosage adjustment, almost any benzodiazepine can be used as an antianxiety, hypnotic, or anticonvulsant agent.

PHARMACOKINETICS

Benzodiazepines are absorbed well and distributed widely in the body. In the liver, long-acting agents are broken down into active metabolites that may have even longer half-lives than the parent compounds. Short-acting agents are metabolized to inactive metabolites. (However, alprazolam is a short- to intermediate-acting agent that is metabolized to an active compound.) All benzodiazepines are excreted primarily in the urine.

Absorption, distribution, metabolism, excretion

After oral administration, benzodiazepines are absorbed rapidly and completely from the gastrointestinal (GI) tract. Even clorazepate dipotassium, an inactive compound, is absorbed rapidly after decarboxylation (splitting off of car-

bon dioxide molecules) in the GI tract. Its active metabolite desmethyldiazepam also is absorbed rapidly. Prazepam and oxazepam undergo much slower absorption. After intramuscular (I.M.) injection, chlordiazepoxide and diazepam are absorbed slowly and erratically, but lorazepam is absorbed rapidly and completely.

Benzodiazepines and their metabolites are distributed well throughout the body. Because long-acting agents are more lipophilic (have a greater affinity for fat) than short-acting agents, they can accumulate in fatty tissue with continued therapy. All benzodiazepines and their metabolites cross the placenta, and fetal concentrations of diazepam may equal those of the mother.

Metabolism occurs in one of two ways. For lorazepam, oxazepam, and certain other benzodiazepines, metabolism involves hepatic conjugation with glucuronic acid. This produces water-soluble inactive compounds that are excreted in the urine. For alprazolam, chlordiazepoxide, clorazepate, diazepam, halazepam, and prazepam, metabolism involves hepatic oxidation to active compounds with half-lives that may be longer than those of the parent compounds. Then these metabolites are conjugated to inactive compounds that are excreted in the urine.

Onset, peak, duration

After oral administration, most benzodiazepines reach peak concentration levels in 1 to 2 hours. Prazepam and oxazepam typically peak later, however. Peak concentration of prazepam's active metabolite occurs about 6 hours after administration; oxazepam concentration peaks between 2½ and 8 hours after administration.

Benzodiazepines produce antianxiety, muscle relaxant, and anticonvulsant effects after the first dose. These effects increase until steady-state concentrations are reached. Long-acting agents accumulate with repeated doses to reach steady-state concentrations and produce a full therapeutic response in 5 to 10 days. After steady-state concentrations are attained, these agents can be given once or twice daily; the therapeutic response will persist for days after discontinuation.

Prolonged half-lives of the long-acting agents, such as diazepam, may occur in elderly patients and in patients with liver disease because these patients have an increased percentage of fatty tissue in their bodies. Short-acting benzodiazepines with no active metabolites will accumulate more rapidly and reach steady-state concentrations in 2 to 4 days. These agents require multiple doses every day. If the patient misses 1 day of therapy, the blood level—and the therapeutic response—will decline rapidly.

PHARMACODYNAMICS

Although researchers have not established the exact mechanism of action of benzodiazepines, most believe that these drugs inhibit excitation. The principal sites are the cerebral cortex and the limbic, thalamic, and hypothalamic levels of the central nervous system (CNS).

Mechanism of action

Current theories suggest that the benzodiazepines enhance the effects of gamma-aminobutyric acid (GABA). A natural inhibitor of excitatory stimulation, GABA affects the limbic system and helps control emotions. Enhancement of GABA activity is responsible for the action of benzodiazepines.

Unlike barbiturates, which can depress the CNS directly, benzodiazepines work indirectly by enhancing GABA activity. This synergistic action may explain the safer adverse reaction profile of the benzodiazepines, especially in overdoses.

PHARMACOTHERAPEUTICS

Benzodiazepines are used for short-term treatment of generalized anxiety. Other clinical uses include producing sedative and hypnotic effects, treating seizure disorders, producing skeletal muscle relaxation, treating insomnia, providing light anesthesia, and managing alcohol withdrawal. Alprazolam also is used to treat panic attacks. (More information about these clinical indications appears in the appropriate chapters of this book.)

Currently, the benzodiazepines are the drugs of choice for treating anxiety. They have replaced the barbiturates because they produce fewer adverse reactions, less respiratory depression, and fewer drug interactions, and because they have a relatively low abuse potential and produce milder withdrawal symptoms. They are, however, more expensive than barbiturates.

alprazolam (Xanax). A Schedule IV drug, alprazolam is not as effective as the tricyclic antidepressants, but is useful in treating panic attacks and anxiety associated with depression.
Usual adult dosage: for anxiety, initially, 0.25 to 0.5 mg P.O. t.i.d., increased as tolerated to a maximum of 4 mg/day in divided doses; for elderly or debilitated patients, initially, 0.25 mg P.O. b.i.d. or t.i.d., increased gradually; for panic attacks, 0.5 mg P.O. t.i.d., increased by up to 1 mg daily every 3 to 4 days to a maximum of 10 mg/day.

chlordiazepoxide hydrochloride (A-poxide, Librium). A Schedule IV drug, chlordiazepoxide can be used to treat anxiety and alcohol withdrawal. This drug is available in oral or injectable form. I.M. injections, not recommended for children under age 12, must be prepared with the diluent provided and must be administered deep I.M.
Usual adult dosage: for anxiety, 5 to 10 mg P.O. t.i.d., increased to 25 mg t.i.d. or q.i.d. as needed; for anxiety in an elderly patient, 5 mg P.O. b.i.d. to q.i.d. increased as needed; for alcohol withdrawal, 50 to 100 mg P.O., I.M., or I.V. to a maximum of 300 mg/day.

clorazepate dipotassium (Tranxene). A Schedule IV drug, clorazepate is used to treat anxiety and alcohol withdrawal and can be used as an adjunct in managing partial seizures. (For seizure dosage information, see Chapter 20, Anticonvulsant Agents.)
Usual adult dosage: for anxiety, 7.5 mg P.O. t.i.d., or 15 mg P.O. h.s., increased as tolerated and as needed, to a maximum of 60 mg/day; for anxiety in an elderly patient, 7.5 to 15 mg P.O. daily, increased as needed. For acute alcohol withdrawal: day 1–30 mg P.O. initially, followed by 30 to 60 mg P.O. in divided doses; day 2–45 to 90 mg P.O. in divided doses; day 3–22.5 to 45 mg P.O. in divided doses; day 4–15 to 30 mg P.O. in divided doses; gradually reduce daily dosage to 7.5 to 15 mg P.O.

diazepam (Valium, Valrelease). A Schedule IV drug, diazepam is used to treat anxiety, alcohol withdrawal, skeletal muscle spasms, and status epilepticus. Besides the standard oral form, diazepam is available in I.V., I.M., and sustained-release oral forms.
Usual adult dosage: for anxiety, 2 to 10 mg P.O. b.i.d. to q.i.d. (initially, 1 to 2 mg P.O. b.i.d. for an elderly patient) or 15 to 30 mg P.O. of sustained-release capsule once daily; for alcohol withdrawal, 10 mg P.O. t.i.d. or q.i.d. for the first 24 hours, decreased to 5 mg t.i.d. or q.i.d. as needed; for skeletal muscle spasms, 2 to 10 mg P.O. t.i.d. or q.i.d.; for status epilepticus, 5 to 10 mg slow I.V. push at no more than 5 mg/minute, repeated as needed every 10 to 15 minutes to a maximum of 30 mg.

halazepam (Paxipam). A Schedule IV drug, halazepam is used to treat anxiety.
Usual adult dosage: for anxiety, 20 to 40 mg P.O. t.i.d. or q.i.d.; for anxiety in an elderly patient, 20 mg P.O. once a day or b.i.d. The optimal daily dosage ranges from 80 to 160 mg.

lorazepam (Ativan). A Schedule IV drug, lorazepam is used to treat anxiety and to provide preoperative sedation.
Usual adult dosage: for anxiety, 2 to 3 mg P.O. b.i.d. or t.i.d., increased to a maximum of 6 mg/day; for anxiety in an elderly patient, 1 to 2 mg P.O. b.i.d. or t.i.d., increased as needed; for preoperative sedation, 2 to 4 mg I.M. or I.V.

oxazepam (Serax). A Schedule IV drug, oxazepam is used to treat anxiety, especially in patients with hepatic disease. It is safe for these patients because it does not accumulate the way long-acting benzodiazepines with active metabolites do.
Usual adult dosage: for anxiety, 10 to 15 mg P.O. t.i.d. or q.i.d., increased as needed to 15 to 30 mg t.i.d. or q.i.d.; for anxiety in an elderly patient, 10 mg P.O. t.i.d., increased to 15 mg t.i.d. or q.i.d. as needed.

prazepam (Centrax). A Schedule IV drug, prazepam also is used to treat anxiety disorders.
Usual adult dosage: for anxiety, 10 mg P.O. t.i.d., increased to a maximum of 60 mg/day as needed; for anxiety in an elderly patient, 10 to 15 mg P.O. daily, in divided doses increased as needed.

Drug interactions

Fewer, less severe drug interactions occur with the benzodiazepines than with the barbiturates. The major interactions relate to the use of benzodiazepines with other CNS depressants, producing additive effects. (For detailed information, see *Drug interactions: Benzodiazepines* in Chapter 20, Anticonvulsant Agents.)

ADVERSE DRUG REACTIONS

Most adverse reactions to the benzodiazepines affect the CNS; less than 1% affect other body systems. Sedation is the most common adverse reaction, affecting 4% to 12% of all patients taking chlordiazepoxide or diazepam. A dosage reduction may eliminate this reaction. Benzodiazepines also can impair motor coordination, reaction time, and cognitive reasoning, especially in elderly patients. Although these reactions usually affect driving skills, some anxious patients actually drive better because their anxieties are relieved. Benzodiazepines — particularly alprazolam, diazepam, and lorazepam — also can cause dosage-related amnesia.

The benzodiazepines have a potential for abuse, tolerance, and physical dependence. As a result, abrupt discontinuation of long-term, high-dosage therapy can cause a withdrawal reaction with such symptoms as weakness, delirium, and tonic-clonic seizures. Because some benzodiazepines have long half-lives, withdrawal symptoms may take a week to appear. This reaction may occur less commonly with benzodiazepines than with other antianxiety agents, although its true incidence is unknown. Aprazolam is most likely to cause withdrawal symptoms because it is used in high dosages, usually for long periods, to treat panic attacks. Therefore, the drug must be tapered off when therapy is discontinued to prevent withdrawal symptoms.

Rarely, benzodiazepines may cause mild allergic reactions, such as skin rash, pruritus, and urticaria. They also may cause paradoxical excitation in elderly patients.

NURSING PROCESS APPLICATION

The following information assists the nurse in caring for a patient who is receiving a benzodiazepine as an antianxiety agent.

Assessment
• Review the patient's history for a condition that contraindicates the use of a benzodiazepine, such as acute narrow-angle glaucoma, depressive neuroses, psychotic reactions, pregnancy, or known hypersensitivity to the drug.
• Review the patient's history for a condition that requires cautious use of a benzodiazepine, such as impaired renal or hepatic function or drug dependence.
• Assess the patient for adverse reactions to the prescribed benzodiazepine, such as sedation; impaired motor coordination, reaction time, or cognitive reasoning; or amnesia.
• Review the patient's medication history to identify the use of drugs that may interact with the prescribed benzodiazepine, such as CNS depressants, cimetidine, or oral contraceptives.
• Assess the patient for benzodiazepine dependence.
• Evaluate the patient's and family's knowledge about the prescribed benzodiazepine.

Nursing diagnoses
The following examples represent appropriate nursing diagnoses for a patient receiving a benzodiazepine as an antianxiety agent.
• Potential for injury related to a preexisting condition that contraindicates the use of a benzodiazepine as an antianxiety agent
• Potential for injury related to a preexisting condition that requires cautious use of a benzodiazepine as an antianxiety agent
• Potential for injury related to adverse drug reactions
• Altered thought processes related to the adverse CNS effects of the prescribed benzodiazepine
• Altered role performance related to benzodiazepine dependence
• Knowledge deficit related to the prescribed benzodiazepine

Planning and implementation
• Do not administer a benzodiazepine to a patient with a condition that contraindicates its use.
• Administer a benzodiazepine cautiously to a patient at risk because of a preexisting condition.

• Monitor the patient periodically for adverse reactions to the prescribed benzodiazepine, especially in an elderly or debilitated patient or one with liver disease.

• *Consult with the physician if other CNS depressants also are prescribed during benzodiazepine therapy; this drug combination may cause lethal depressant effects.*

• Monitor the patient for a therapeutic response to a long-acting benzodiazepine. Keep in mind that, after steady-state levels are reached, the therapeutic response may persist for days after discontinuation.

• *Avoid I.M. administration, if possible because absorption after I.M. injection is slow and erratic.*

• Prepare I.M. chlordiazepoxide with the diluent provided and administer it deep I.M.

• *Administer I.V. preparations slowly to reduce the risk of phlebitis and cardiovascular collapse.* Administer I.V. diazepam at no more than 5 mg/minute and repeat, as needed, every 10 to 15 minutes to a maximum of 30 mg as prescribed.

• Notify the physician if adverse reactions occur.

• *Take safety precautions if the patient develops adverse CNS reactions, such as sedation or amnesia. For example, place the bed in a low position, keep the bed rails up, and supervise patient ambulation.*

• Expect to decrease the benzodiazepine dosage, as prescribed, if CNS reactions occur.

• Help with decisions about such things as menu selections and discharge arrangements, if the patient's cognitive reasoning becomes impaired.

• Encourage the patient to be honest about benzodiazepine use because dependence can occur.

• *Do not discontinue benzodiazepine therapy abruptly.* Otherwise, the patient may develop withdrawal symptoms, such as weakness, delirium, and tonic-clonic seizures.

• Notify the physician of suspected drug dependence.

Patient teaching

• Provide general instructions about benzodiazepine use. (For details, see *Patient-teaching tips for sedative and hypnotic agents* in Chapter 25.)

• Teach the patient and family the name, dose, frequency, action, and adverse effects of the prescribed benzodiazepine.

• Instruct the female patient to notify her physician if she becomes pregnant or intends to become pregnant.

• Advise the family to provide close supervision and take safety measures, such as assisting with ambulation, if the patient experiences adverse CNS reactions.

• Instruct the patient and family to notify the physician if adverse reactions occur.

Evaluation

The following examples represent appropriate evaluation statements for a patient receiving a benzodiazepine as an antianxiety agent.

• The patient has no conditions that contraindicate benzodiazepine therapy.

• The patient exhibits no signs of complications in the preexisting condition linked to the prescribed benzodiazepine.

• The patient demonstrates no adverse reactions to the prescribed benzodiazepine.

• The patient maintains usual patterns of thought.

• The patient shows no signs of benzodiazepine dependence.

• The patient and family express an accurate understanding of the points taught about the prescribed benzodiazepine.

• The patient correctly identifies possible adverse reactions to the prescribed benzodiazepine and describes how to manage them.

BUSPIRONE

The first anxiolytic in a new class of agents, buspirone hydrochloride's structure and mechanism of action differ from those of other antianxiety agents.

PHARMACOKINETICS

Buspirone is absorbed rapidly and metabolized by the liver. Few other details about its metabolism are known.

Absorption, distribution, metabolism, excretion

After oral administration, buspirone is absorbed rapidly. Its bioavailability is decreased, however, because of a large first-pass effect. Although buspirone's distribution has not been explained fully, researchers have found that some of its metabolites accumulate in the brain at higher levels than the parent compound does. Buspirone's metabolism also remains largely unknown. After administration, 40% of a dose appears in the urine as metabolites, less than 1% is excreted unchanged, and nearly 60% is unaccounted for.

Onset, peak, duration

The plasma concentration level peaks 1 hour after oral administration. The half-life averages 2.5 hours and ranges from 0.9 to 9.4 hours. However, buspirone's onset of action ranges from 1 to 2 weeks.

PHARMACODYNAMICS

Researchers have not yet identified buspirone's site and mechanism of action, but they know that, in contrast to theories about the benzodiazepines, buspirone does not affect GABA receptors. Rather, it seems to produce various effects in the midbrain and acts as a midbrain modulator.

PHARMACOTHERAPEUTICS

Currently, buspirone is indicated to treat generalized anxiety states. Few clinical trials have compared buspirone to other agents, but patients who have not been exposed previously to benzodiazepines seem to respond better to buspirone. This drug's slow onset of action, however, makes it ineffective for p.r.n. use.

buspirone hydrochloride (Buspar). So far, five clinical trials have demonstrated that buspirone is as effective as diazepam or clorazepate in relieving anxiety. Milligram for milligram, buspirone equals diazepam in potency.
Usual adult dosage: 5 mg P.O. t.i.d., increased by 5 mg daily every 2 to 3 days, as needed, to a maximum dosage of 60 mg/day. For most patients, the maintenance dosage is 20 to 30 mg/day.

Drug interactions
When buspirone is given concomitantly with monoamine oxidase (MAO) inhibitors, hypertensive reactions may occur. Therefore, these drugs should not be used together. Unlike other antianxiety agents, buspirone does not interact with alcohol or other CNS depressants.

ADVERSE DRUG REACTIONS

Buspirone produces far fewer adverse reactions than the benzodiazepines. The most common reactions include dizziness, light-headedness, insomnia, and headache. At this time, no data exist regarding buspirone overdose, and the drug does not appear to have an abuse potential.

NURSING PROCESS APPLICATION

The following information assists the nurse in caring for a patient who is receiving buspirone.

Assessment
• Review the patient's history for a condition that contraindicates the use of buspirone, such as impaired renal or hepatic function, lactation, concomitant use of MAO inhibitors, or known hypersensitivity to the drug.
• Review the patient's history for a condition that requires cautious use of buspirone, such as pregnancy.

• Assess the patient for adverse reactions to buspirone, such as dizziness, light-headedness, insomnia, or headache.
• Evaluate the patient's and family's knowledge about buspirone.

Nursing diagnoses
The following examples represent appropriate nursing diagnoses for a patient receiving buspirone.
• Potential for injury related to a preexisting condition that contraindicates the use of buspirone
• Potential for injury related to a preexisting condition that requires cautious use of buspirone
• Potential for injury related to adverse drug reactions
• Sleep pattern disturbance related to buspirone-induced insomnia
• Knowledge deficit related to buspirone

Planning and implementation
• Do not administer buspirone to a patient with a condition that contraindicates its use.
• Administer buspirone cautiously to a patient at risk because of a preexisting condition.
• Monitor the patient regularly for adverse reactions to buspirone.
• Expect to change a patient from long-term benzodiazepine therapy to buspirone by tapering off the benzodiazepine dosage as prescribed to avoid a benzodiazepine withdrawal reaction.
• *Take safety measures if the patient develops dizziness or light-headedness. For example, place the bed in a low position, keep the bed rails up, and supervise ambulation.*
• Request an order for an analgesic if headache results from buspirone use.
• Notify the physician if adverse reactions occur.
• Prevent insomnia by administering the last daily dose of buspirone several hours before bedtime, if permissible.
• Help the patient explore alternative methods for inducing sleep if insomnia occurs, such as a warm bath or quiet meditation. If appropriate, obtain an order for a hypnotic agent.

Patient teaching
• Teach the patient and family the name, dose, frequency, action, and adverse effects of buspirone.
• Instruct the patient to use safety precautions at home if dizziness or light-headedness occurs. Tell family members to supervise the patient's ambulation.
• Instruct the patient to take the last daily dose of buspirone several hours before bedtime to prevent insomnia. Also suggest alternative methods for inducing sleep if insomnia occurs.
• Advise the patient to ask the physician to recommend an analgesic if headaches occur.

• Instruct the female patient to notify her physician if she becomes pregnant or plans to breast-feed.
• Instruct the patient to notify the physician if adverse reactions occur.

Evaluation

The following examples represent appropriate evaluation statements for a patient receiving buspirone.
• The patient has no conditions that contraindicate buspirone therapy.
• The patient exhibit no complications in the preexisting condition linked to buspirone.
• The patient experiences no adverse reactions to buspirone.
• The patient reports satisfactory sleeping patterns.
• The patient and family express an accurate understanding of the points taught about buspirone.
• The patient successfully uses alternative methods for inducing sleep.

BARBITURATES

Until the benzodiazepines were introduced about 30 years ago, the barbiturates were the most commonly prescribed antianxiety agents. Although no longer the drugs of choice, barbiturates still are used for their antianxiety, anticonvulsant, preanesthetic, sedative, and hypnotic effects.

This section presents two representative barbiturates: phenobarbital sodium, a long-acting agent commonly used for its anticonvulsant and sedative effects; and pentobarbital sodium, a short- to intermediate-acting agent principally used for its hypnotic and sedative properties. (For more information about barbiturates, see Chapter 25, Sedative and Hypnotic Agents.)

PHARMACOKINETICS

Barbiturates are absorbed well, distributed rapidly, metabolized in the liver, and excreted in the urine. They fall into four classifications based on duration of action: long-acting agents, intermediate-acting agents, short-acting agents, and ultrashort-acting agents. The ultrashort-acting agents are used to induce and maintain anesthesia.

Absorption, distribution, metabolism, excretion

The barbiturates are absorbed well after oral administration. For oral administration, the sodium salt form is absorbed more rapidly than the acid form.

Because barbiturates are lipophilic, they are distributed throughout the body and highly concentrated in the fatty tissue of the liver and brain. Phenobarbital, which has a reduced lipophilic effect, enters and exits the brain more slowly, so it has an extended duration of action. Barbiturates also cross the placenta.

Slowly metabolized by microsomal enzymes in the liver, barbiturates produce inactive metabolites. The kidneys eliminate most barbiturates as metabolites, except for phenobarbital: 25% to 50% of phenobarbital is excreted unchanged in the urine.

Onset, peak, duration

After oral administration, phenobarbital reaches a peak plasma concentration level in 8 to 12 hours and a steady-state concentration in 3 to 4 weeks if a loading dose is not given. Its half-life ranges from 50 to 170 hours.

Pentobarbital demonstrates onset of action in 15 to 60 minutes after oral administration and achieves a peak concentration in 30 to 60 minutes. The half-life of pentobarbital ranges from 15 to 48 hours.

PHARMACODYNAMICS

The mechanism of action of the barbiturates for treating anxiety is not completely understood. However, these agents may cause an imbalance in the central inhibitory and facilitatory mechanisms, which affects the cerebral cortext and reticular formation.

PHARMACOTHERAPEUTICS

In treating anxiety, barbiturates are more effective than meprobamate and equally as effective as the benzodiazepines. Because barbiturates cause many adverse reactions, including severe respiratory depression, they largely have been replaced by the benzodiazepines as antianxiety agents. Barbiturates most commonly are prescribed as anticonvulsant, anesthetic, sedative, and hypnotic agents. (For more information about these uses, see Chapter 20, Anticonvulsant Agents; Chapter 23, General Anesthetic Agents; and Chapter 25, Sedative and Hypnotic Agents.) Phenobarbital also is used to manage barbiturate or nonbarbiturate withdrawal in dependent patients and is under investigation for use in treating congenital biliary defects and hyperbilirubinemia in neonates.

pentobarbital sodium (Nembutal Sodium). A Schedule II drug, pentobarbital usually is used as a hypnotic but can be used as a sedative or antianxiety agent.
Usual adult dosage: for sedation or to relieve anxiety, 20 mg P.O. t.i.d. or q.i.d. The dosage must be individualized for each patient and reduced for an elderly patient.

phenobarbital sodium (Luminal Sodium). A Schedule IV drug, phenobarbital can be used as an antianxiety agent.

Usual adult dosage: 30 to 120 mg P.O. daily in two or three divided doses. The dosage must be individualized for each patient and reduced for an elderly patient.

Drug interactions

When administered with other CNS depressants, the barbiturates can produce additive depressant effects. Other drug interactions also are likely to occur because barbiturates can stimulate the enzymes that degrade other drugs, decreasing their duration of action. (For more information, see *Drug interactions: Barbiturates* in Chapter 25, Sedative and Hypnotic Agents.)

ADVERSE DRUG REACTIONS

The most serious adverse reactions involve the CNS and the respiratory system. Other, less serious, reactions can occur, including allergic reactions and GI complaints.

The most common dose-related adverse reactions involve the CNS and include sedation, lethargy, ataxia, headache, depression, and impaired motor coordination and reaction time. When used as hypnotics, barbiturates can produce a hangover effect or confused state the next day, especially in elderly patients.

In an otherwise healthy person, barbiturates produce respiratory depression equal to that produced by sleep. In a patient with a pulmonary disease, respiratory depressant effects are more pronounced. Even low doses of phenobarbital can produce severe changes in the blood oxygen saturation and blood pH levels. Respiratory effects are more drastic in a patient who has taken an overdose.

Long-term use can lead to tolerance and physical or psychological dependence on the barbiturate. If therapy is discontinued abruptly, a withdrawal reaction can occur in 8 to 12 hours. Withdrawal symptoms include anxiety, insomnia, nausea, vomiting, hallucinations, muscle twitches, and seizures. To avoid a potentially fatal withdrawal reaction, long-term therapy should be tapered off over 1 to 2 weeks.

Other reactions include dermatologic and allergic manifestations, paradoxical excitation, and blood dyscrasias.

NURSING PROCESS APPLICATION

The following information assists the nurse in caring for a patient who is receiving a barbiturate as an antianxiety agent.

Assessment
• Review the patient's history for a condition that contraindicates the use of a barbiturate, such as porphyria, nephritis, renal insufficiency, pregnancy, or known hypersensitivity to the drug.

• Review the patient's history for a condition that requires cautious use of a barbiturate, such as depression, suicidal tendencies, hepatic dysfunction, or a history of drug abuse.
• Assess the patient for adverse reactions to the prescribed barbiturate, such as CNS and respiratory depression.
• Review the patient's medication history to identify the use of drugs that may interact with the prescribed barbiturate, such as hydantoins, beta blockers, oral anticoagulants, or CNS depressants.
• Assess the patient for barbiturate dependence.
• Evaluate the patient's and family's knowledge about the prescribed barbiturate.

Nursing diagnoses
The following examples represent appropriate nursing diagnoses for a patient receiving a barbiturate as an antianxiety agent.
• Potential for injury related to a preexisting condition that contraindicates the use of a barbiturate
• Potential for injury related to a preexisting condition that requires cautious use of a barbiturate
• Potential for injury related to adverse drug reactions
• Ineffective breathing pattern related to the adverse respiratory effects of the prescribed barbiturate
• Altered role performance related to barbiturate dependence
• Knowledge deficit related to the prescribed barbiturate

Planning and implementation
• Do not administer a barbiturate to a patient with a condition that contraindicates its use.
• Administer a barbiturate cautiously to a patient at risk because of a preexisting condition.
• Monitor the patient frequently for adverse reactions to the prescribed barbiturate.
• Expect to administer a lower barbiturate dosage to an elderly patient as prescribed.
• Monitor the patient's prothrombin time, if the patient is receiving an anticoagulant. Adjust the anticoagulant dosage, as prescribed. Remember that abrupt withdrawal of barbiturates may cause bleeding.
• *Take safety measures when administering the barbiturate. For example, place the bed in a low position, keep the bed rails up, and assist with ambulation.*
• Notify the physician if adverse reactions occur.
• Monitor the patient's vital signs frequently, particularly noting such signs of respiratory depression as decreased respirations or respiratory pattern changes.
• *Perform a respiratory assessment before and after giving each dose of the prescribed barbiturate.*
• *Delay the prescribed barbiturate dose until the physician is notified, if respiratory depression occurs.*

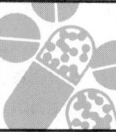

SELECTED MAJOR DRUGS

Antianxiety agents

This chart summarizes the most common antianxiety agents currently in clinical use.

DRUG	MAJOR INDICATIONS	USUAL ADULT DOSAGES	CONTRAINDICATIONS AND PRECAUTIONS
Benzodiazepines			
alprazolam	Anxiety associated with depression	0.025 to 0.5 mg P.O. t.i.d. increased as tolerated to a maximum of 4 mg/day in divided doses	• Know that alprazolam is contraindicated in a pregnant or lactating patient or one with acute narrow-angle glaucoma or known hypersensitivity to the drug. • Administer with caution to an elderly or debilitated patient, a patient receiving another psychotropic agent, or one with impaired renal or hepatic function or a history of drug dependence.
diazepam	Anxiety	2 to 10 mg P.O. b.i.d. to q.i.d.	• Know that diazepam is contraindicated in a child under age 6 months, a pregnant patient, or one with acute narrow-angle glaucoma or known hypersensitivity to the drug. • Administer with caution to a patient with severe or latent depression, impaired renal or hepatic function, or a history of drug dependence.
	Alcohol withdrawal	10 mg P.O. t.i.d. or q.i.d. for 24 hours, decreased to 5 mg t.i.d. or q.i.d.	
	Skeletal muscle spasms	2 to 10 mg P.O. t.i.d. or q.i.d.	
	Status epilepticus	5 to 10 mg slow I.V. push repeated every 10 to 15 minutes to a maximum of 30 mg	
Buspirone			
buspirone	Anxiety	5 mg P.O. t.i.d., increased by 5 mg q 2 to 3 days, as needed, to a maximum of 60 mg/day	• Know that buspirone is contraindicated in a lactating patient, one with impaired renal or hepatic function or known hypersensitivity to the drug, or one who uses monoamine oxidase inhibitors concomitantly. • Administer with caution to a pregnant patient.
Barbiturates			
pentobarbital	Anxiety, sedation	20 mg P.O. t.i.d. or q.i.d.	• Know that pentobarbital is contraindicated in a pregnant patient or one with porphyria or known hypersensitivity to the drug. • Administer with caution to a lactating patient or one with depression, suicidal tendencies, hepatic damage, or a history of drug abuse.
phenobarbital	Anxiety	30 to 120 mg P.O. daily in two or three divided doses	• Know that phenobarbital is contraindicated in a pregnant patient or one with porphyria, nephritis, renal insufficiency, or known hypersensitivity to the drug. • Administer with caution to a lactating patient or one with depression, suicidal tendencies, hepatic damage, or a history of drug abuse.

CHAPTER 27 • ANTIANXIETY AGENTS: CHAPTER SUMMARY 447

• Position the debilitated patient to maximize respiratory function. For example, help the patient into the semi-Fowler's or high Fowler's position.
• Encourage the patient to be honest about barbiturate use because dependence can occur.
• *Do not discontinue the prescribed barbiturate abruptly.* Otherwise, the patient may develop withdrawal symptoms, such as anxiety, insomnia, nausea, vomiting, hallucinations, muscle twitches, and seizures.
• Notify the physician of suspected drug dependence.

Patient teaching
• Provide general instructions about barbiturate use. (For details, see *Patient-teaching tips for sedative and hypnotic agents* in Chapter 25.)
• Teach the patient and family the name, dose, frequency, action, and adverse effects of the prescribed barbiturate.

Evaluation
The following examples represent appropriate evaluation statements for a patient receiving a barbiturate as an antianxiety agent.
• The patient has no conditions that contraindicate barbiturate therapy.
• The patient exhibits no signs of complications in the preexisting condition linked to the prescribed barbiturate.
• The patient reports no adverse reactions to the prescribed barbiturate.
• The patient maintains a normal respiratory rate and pattern.
• The patient shows no signs of barbiturate dependence.
• The patient and family express an accurate understanding of the points taught about the prescribed barbiturate.
• The patient correctly identifies adverse reactions to the prescribed barbiturate.

OTHER ANTIANXIETY AGENTS

Although benzodiazepines, buspirone, and barbiturates commonly are used to treat anxiety disorders, meprobamate, beta blockers, and antihistamines also may be used as antianxiety agents.

meprobamate (Equanil, Meprocon, Miltown, SK-Bamate). This drug was used widely in the past to treat anxiety. It rarely is used today, however, because of its low degree of effectiveness, the severity of its adverse effects, and the advent of safer, more effective agents. A carbamate derivative, meprobamate is the only drug of its class to be used as an antianxiety agent rather than a muscle relaxant. After oral administration, meprobamate is absorbed well from the intestines and distributed uniformly throughout the body. It is metabolized partially in the liver to inactive metabolites and is excreted by the kidneys. Although meprobamate is a CNS depressant, its exact site and mechanism of action in anxiety relief is unknown.

When administered with other CNS depressant drugs, meprobamate usually causes additive depressant effects. Meprobamate's CNS depressant action accounts for its adverse effects, which commonly include sedation, ataxia, and hypotension. Dependence can develop, and severe withdrawal reactions have occurred after abrupt discontinuation of high dosages administered for several weeks. Other reactions also may occur, including allergic reactions, paradoxical excitement, and congenital heart defects, if given during the first 6 weeks of pregnancy. Although meprobamate use is rare, the nurse must be prepared to instruct the patient about this drug's adverse effects and interactions with CNS depressant drugs.

beta blockers. These drugs can relieve the somatic symptoms associated with anxiety. Although most studies show that benzodiazepines are more effective in treating anxiety disorders, beta blockers are useful in treating acute situational anxiety that causes somatic symptoms.

antihistamines. These drugs, particularly hydroxyzine hydrochloride and diphenhydramine hydrochloride, may be used to treat anxiety. This use of antihistamines is rare, however, and most studies indicate that they are not effective antianxiety agents.

CHAPTER SUMMARY

Chapter 27 explored drugs used to treat anxiety disorders. These antianxiety agents include some of the most commonly prescribed drugs in the United States. Here are the chapter highlights.
• Benzodiazepines have replaced barbiturates as the drugs of choice to treat anxiety. They interact with fewer drugs and offer a safer adverse reaction profile. The major drug interaction is with other CNS depressants, causing additive effects. The most common adverse reactions affect the CNS, producing drowsiness, motor incoordination, and decreased reaction time. Other adverse reactions are less common.
• Buspirone is the newest antianxiety agent. Preliminary data indicate it interacts only with MAO inhibitors. Buspirone appears to have no abuse potential, causes almost no sedation, and produces only minor adverse reactions,

such as dizziness and headache. Nevertheless, a patient receiving buspirone must be monitored closely until researchers discover more about its long-term effects.

• Although barbiturates are effective in treating anxiety, they largely have been replaced by the benzodiazepines for several reasons. Barbiturates interact with many drugs because they can stimulate the enzymes that degrade those drugs and decrease their duration of action. They also cause many adverse reactions, including respiratory depression, which is especially dangerous in a patient who has a pulmonary disease or an overdose. They also are associated with dermatologic and allergic reactions.

• Meprobamate seems less effective than other antianxiety agents and rarely is used today to treat anxiety disorders. Other drugs that are used rarely to treat anxiety include beta blockers and antihistamines.

• When caring for a patient receiving an antianxiety agent, the nurse uses the nursing process. Key aspects of nursing care include monitoring the drug's effectiveness, observing for signs of drug tolerance, assessing for adverse reactions, and ensuring patient safety.

STUDY QUESTIONS

See Appendix 1 for answers.

1. Ruth Cowelton, age 75, is admitted to the medical-surgical unit for a biopsy and possible mastectomy of her right breast. Nervous about the impending surgery, she shows signs of anxiety, including tachycardia, tremors, and sweating. Her physician prescribes the benzodiazepine diazepam (Valium). For an elderly patient like Ms. Cowelton, the nurse should expect to administer a reduced dosage of diazepam. Why?
(a) Elderly patients have increased GABA activity, which inhibits excitatory stimulation.
(b) Elderly patients have a higher percentage of fatty tissue, which prolongs the drug's half-life.
(c) Elderly patients have decreased cardiac output, which affects drug distribution.
(d) Elderly patient have decreased GI motility, which delays drug absorption.

2. Which diazepam dosage would be most appropriate for treating Ms. Cowelton's anxiety?
(a) 1 to 2 mg P.O. b.i.d.
(b) 2 to 10 mg P.O. b.i.d. to q.i.d.
(c) 10 to 15 mg P.O. t.i.d. to q.i.d.
(d) 15 to 30 mg P.O. t.i.d. to q.i.d.

3. Benzodiazepines effectively reduce anxiety by which of the following mechanisms of action?
(a) midbrain modulation
(b) direct depression of the CNS
(c) enhancement of GABA activity
(d) inhibition of neurotransmitter release

4. Ms. Cowelton is *most* likely to experience which adverse reaction to diazepam?
(a) tachycardia
(b) skin rash
(c) hypertension
(d) sedation

5. Louise Harper, age 42, has had generalized anxiety since her daughter left for college. Her physician prescribes buspirone (Buspar) 5 mg P.O. t.i.d. How do the pharmacodynamics of buspirone differ from that of the benzodiazepines and barbiturates?
(a) Buspirone does not affect the CNS.
(b) Buspirone does not affect the cerebral cortex.
(c) Buspirone does not affect GABA receptors.
(d) Buspirone does not affect the midbrain.

6. Which of the following statements accurately characterizes buspirone?
(a) Buspirone has a rapid onset of action.
(b) Buspirone has a high potential for abuse.
(c) Buspirone does not interact with alcohol or other CNS depressants.
(d) Buspirone produces more adverse reactions than benzodiazepines.

7. Edgar Manning, age 70, has been admitted to the hospital for surgery. Because Mr. Manning is anxious, the surgeon prescribes the barbiturate pentobarbital (Nembutal) 20 mg P.O. t.i.d. Where are the highest concentrations of barbiturates found?
(a) in the bones
(b) in fatty tissue
(c) in cerebrospinal fluid
(d) in the thyroid gland

8. Barbiturates should be used with caution in patients with certain diseases. Before administering pentobarbital, the nurse should assess Mr. Manning for which of the following diseases?
(a) epilepsy
(b) narrow-angle glaucoma
(c) anorexia nervosa
(d) pulmonary disease

SELECTED REFERENCES

AHFS drug information 90. (1990). Bethesda, MD: American Society of Hospital Pharmacists.

Derogatis, L., and Wise, T. (Eds.). (1988). *Anxiety and depressive disorders in the medical patient.* Washington, DC: American Psychiatric Press.

Drug facts and comparisons. (1991). St. Louis: Facts and Comparisons Division, J.B. Lippincott.

Goldman, H. (1988). *Review of general psychiatry* (2nd ed.). Norwalk, CT: Appleton & Lange.

Goodman and Gilman's the pharmacological basis of therapeutics (8th ed.; 1990). Elmsford, NY: Pergamon Press.

Hansten, P., and Horn, J. (1989). *Drug interactions: Clinical significance of drug-drug interactions* (6th ed.). Philadelphia: Lea & Febiger.

Levy, D. (1988). Benzodiazepine review. *Emergency, 20*(3), 18-21.

Menza, M., Murray, G., Holmes, V., and Rafuls, W. (1988). Controlled study of extrapydramidal reactions in the management of delirious, medically ill patients: Intravenous haloperidol versus intravenous haloperidol plus benzodiazepines. *Heart & Lung, 17*(3), 238-241.

North American Nursing Diagnosis Association. (1990). *Taxonomy I-Revised, with official categories.* St. Louis: NANDA.

Perry, P., et al. (1989). *Psychotropic drug handbook* (5th ed.). Cincinnati: Harvey Whitney Books.

Tyrer, P. (Ed.). (1989). *Psychopharmacology of anxiety.* New York: Oxford University Press.

USPDI. (1991). *Drug information for the health care professional* (Vol. I, 11th ed). Rockville, MD: United States Pharmacopeial Convention.

USPDI. (1991). *Advice for the patient* (Vol. II, 11th ed.). Rockville, MD: United States Pharmacopeial Convention.

ANTIPSYCHOTIC AGENTS

OBJECTIVES

After reading and studying this chapter, the student should be able to:
1. Identify medications that commonly are prescribed as antipsychotic agents.
2. Discuss the clinical indications for the antipsychotic agents.
3. Describe the mechanism of action of the antipsychotic agents.
4. Identify common adverse reactions to the antipsychotic agents.
5. Explain the importance of early detection of symptoms of tardive dyskinesia.
6. Explain the drug regimen and adverse effects of an antipsychotic agent to the patient.
7. Describe how to apply the nursing process when caring for a patient receiving an antipsychotic agent.

INTRODUCTION

Widely used in psychiatric hospitals as well as nonpsychiatric settings, antipsychotic agents can control psychotic symptoms, such as delusions, hallucinations, and thought disorders, that can occur with schizophrenia, mania, and other psychoses. They can help treat organic psychiatric disorders, such as dementia, delirium, and stimulant-induced psychoses, and can sedate agitated patients. They also are used to treat the movement disorders of Gilles de la Tourette's syndrome and Huntington's chorea; to augment the effects of analgesics and anesthetics preoperatively to control pain; and to treat nausea, vomiting, intractable hiccups, and pruritus.

Antipsychotic agents also are called major tranquilizers or neuroleptics: *antipsychotic* because they can eliminate signs and symptoms of psychoses; *major tranquilizer* because they can calm an agitated patient; *neuroleptic* because they have a neurobiological adverse effect that causes abnormal body movements. Many people prefer *neuroleptic*

because it accurately describes the drugs' broader use in nonpsychiatric settings.

Regardless of what they are called, all antipsychotic agents belong to one of two major groups: phenothiazines and nonphenothiazines. This chapter discusses both groups.

An understanding of the effects of antipsychotic drugs requires a knowledge of the anatomy and physiology of the central nervous system (CNS), including the functions of the pyramidal and extrapyramidal tracts, the limbic system, and related structures in the brain.

An area of the brain's cerebral cortex known as the primary motor, or pyramidal, area controls voluntary motor functions. Motor signals are transmitted from this area to the anterior motor neurons through the pyramidal tract. The extrapyramidal tracts primarily control involuntary motor functions by transmitting motor signals from the cortex and spinal cord to the brain. Some extrapyramidal pathways pass through the substantia nigra, one of the lower basal ganglia composed of neurons that connect with other associated areas of the extrapyramidal system. The limbic system of the brain includes all of the basal ganglia and controls emotional behavior and drive. The basal ganglia work with the motor cortex and cerebellum to provide motor control in the body. Although stimulation of certain parts of the basal ganglia can produce muscle contractions or complex movements, the ganglia usually inhibit excessive muscle tone and prevent rigidity or spasticity. This action requires dopamine at synaptic receptor sites. Dopamine, a neurotransmitter substance, is released by the substantia nigra.

One theory suggests that schizophrenia results from excess dopamine in the limbic system. This theory is based on evidence that dissociated thought patterns and drives, hallucinations, and delusions tend to disappear when psychotic patients receive antipsychotic drugs inhibiting dopamine action.

For a summary of representative drugs, see *Selected major drugs: Antipsychotic agents,* page 462. For a listing of applicable nursing diagnoses that the nurse may formulate when caring for a patient receiving these agents,

SELECTED NURSING DIAGNOSES

Antipsychotic agents

The following nursing diagnoses address representative problems and etiologies that a nurse may encounter when caring for a patient who is receiving an antipsychotic agent. Some of these nursing diagnoses contain generalized etiologies, which the nurse must individualize based on the patient's needs. (For some common nursing diagnoses and related interventions for each drug class, see the "Nursing Process Application" sections of this chapter.)

- Altered health maintenance related to ineffectiveness of the antipsychotic agent
- Altered protection related to antipsychotic-induced blood dyscrasias
- Altered thought processes related to the sedative effects of the antipsychotic agent
- Altered tissue perfusion: cerebral, related to the hypotensive effects of the antipsychotic agent
- Constipation related to the anticholinergic effects of the antipsychotic agent
- Hyperthermia related to neuroleptic malignant syndrome caused by the eantipsychotic agent
- Impaired physical mobility related to the extrapyramidal effects of the antipsychotic agent
- Knowledge deficit related to the prescribed antipsychotic agent
- Noncompliance related to long-term use of the prescribed antipsychotic agent
- Potential for injury related to a preexisting condition that contraindicates the use of an antipsychotic agent
- Potential for injury related to a preexisting condition that requires cautious use of an antipsychotic agent
- Potential for injury related to adverse drug reactions
- Potential for injury related to drug interactions
- Sensory-perceptual alterations (tactile) related to antipsychotic-induced photosensitivity reaction
- Urinary retention related to the anticholinergic effects of the antipsychotic agent

see *Selected nursing diagnoses: Antipsychotic agents.* For detailed information on applying the nursing process, see Chapter 6, The Nursing Process and Drug Therapy.

PHENOTHIAZINES

Antipsychotics can be classified on the basis of chemical structure. Many clinicians believe that one of these groups, the phenothiazines, should be treated as three distinct drug classes because of their differences in adverse effects. The three classes include aliphatics (which primarily cause se-

dation and anticholinergic effects), piperazines (which primarily cause extrapyramidal reactions), and piperidines (which primarily cause sedation).

The phenothiazines include chlorpromazine hydrochloride and promazine hydrochloride of the aliphatic subgroup; acetophenazine maleate, fluphenazine decanoate, fluphenazine enanthate, fluphenazine hydrochloride, perphenazine, and trifluoperazine hydrochloride of the piperazine subgroup; and mesoridazine besylate and thioridazine hydrochloride of the piperidine subgroup. Prochlorperazine, also a phenothiazine, is used almost exclusively for nausea and vomiting control. (For a discussion of this drug, see Chapter 43, Emetic and Antiemetic Agents.)

Because their chemical structures vary, each subgroup produces slightly different actions and adverse reactions, but all are equally effective in treating the symptoms of psychoses. The choice of a drug must be based on its therapeutic and adverse effects in a particular patient.

PHARMACOKINETICS

Although the phenothiazines are absorbed erratically, they are distributed to many tissues and are highly concentrated in the brain. All phenothiazines are metabolized in the liver and excreted in urine and bile.

Absorption, distribution, metabolism, excretion

After oral administration, phenothiazines are absorbed erratically, although liquid preparations tend to be better absorbed than tablets or capsules. After intramuscular (I.M.) administration, the drugs are absorbed more completely.

The drugs are distributed to most body tissues and are highly concentrated in the CNS. They are 91% to 99% bound to plasma proteins and are highly lipophilic (having a high affinity for fatty tissue). The unchanged drug and its metabolites are stored in tissues with a good blood supply, such as the brain and lungs. Phenothiazines also can enter fetal circulation.

The phenothiazines are metabolized extensively in the liver by hepatic enzymes. Active metabolites accumulate in fatty tissues and prolong drug activity up to 3 months after discontinuation.

Metabolized phenothiazines are excreted by the kidneys in urine and to a lesser degree in the bile, although elderly patients exhibit a decreased capacity to eliminate them. Metabolites may appear in the urine up to 3 months after the last dose.

Onset, peak, duration

The onset of action varies with the type of preparation. A liquid preparation will produce effects in 2 to 4 hours. The onset with tablets is unpredictable. An I.M. injection usually produces effects in 15 to 30 minutes. Although the onset of action and tranquilizing effects usually occur in a few hours, the antipsychotic effects (the normalizing of thoughts, moods, and actions) may take several weeks to appear.

The duration of action for a single dose is up to 24 hours. This long action permits once-daily dosing after the optimum therapeutic dosage has been determined. The half-life ranges from 10 to 30 hours for an oral phenothiazine and up to 9 days for some long-acting preparations. Because fatty tissues slowly release accumulated phenothiazine metabolites into the plasma, the phenothiazines may produce effects up to 3 months after their discontinuation.

PHARMACODYNAMICS

Although the mechanism of action of phenothiazines is not understood fully, researchers believe that these drugs depress the reticular activating system, the hypothalamus, the chemoreceptor trigger zone (CTZ), and to some extent, the vomiting center. Phenothiazines also stimulate the extrapyramidal system.

Mechanism of action

Researchers believe that the phenothiazines cause a reduction of stimuli to the brain stem reticular activating system, which produces a sedative action. They further postulate that these drugs block postsynaptic dopamine receptors in the limbic system and hypothalamus to produce an antipsychotic action. At the same time, the phenothiazines may interfere with the transmitter function of dopamine in the extrapyramidal tract, causing extrapyramidal symptoms (abnormal body movements).

Researchers also theorize that phenothiazines inhibit the medullary CTZ, thereby producing an antiemetic effect on chemically induced nausea and vomiting, as after surgery. (The drugs, however, cannot reduce nausea and vomiting related to gastric irritants or vestibular disorders, such as motion sickness.) Additional actions include alpha-adrenergic blocking effects and anticholinergic effects, which account for some of the adverse drug reactions.

PHARMACOTHERAPEUTICS

Phenothiazines are used primarily to treat schizophrenia, calm anxious or agitated patients, improve thought processes, and alleviate delusions and hallucinations. These agents may be used to treat other psychiatric disorders, such as brief reactive psychosis, atypical psychosis, schizoaffective psychosis, pervasive development disorder (autism), bipolar affective disorder (manic-depressive disorder), and major depression with psychosis. In manic-depressive patients, the phenothiazines are administered with lithium until the slower-acting lithium becomes effective. The phenothiazines can be used to quiet mentally

retarded children and agitated elderly patients, particularly those with organic brain syndrome. However, they may cause extrapyramidal symptoms, especially in elderly women.

Shortly after phenothiazine administration, a quieting and calming effect occurs, but this sedation differs from that produced by CNS depressants. With the phenothiazines, the patient is easily aroused, alert, responsive, and has good motor coordination. After several days of phenothiazine therapy, affective changes occur. Formerly fearful schizophrenic patients no longer are bothered by delusions and hallucinations, and autistic and withdrawn patients become more responsive and open to communication. After several weeks of therapy, the patient becomes more coherent, and hallucinations and delusions commonly disappear. Unfortunately, symptoms usually return when medication is discontinued.

The phenothiazines also are used to augment the preoperative effects of analgesics and to manage pain, anxiety, and nausea in cancer patients. Additional indications vary with the specific phenothiazine. Chlorpromazine is used to treat intractable hiccups and shivering associated with CNS damage. It also serves as an effective antiemetic, as does prochlorperazine. (For more information about these uses, see Chapter 43, Emetic and Antiemetic Agents.) These drugs do not cause physical dependence, but they can cause psychological dependence.

Initial dosing with phenothiazines can be rapid or slow, depending on the severity of symptoms and the patient's age and physical condition. In acute psychosis, the patient receives a loading dose; a patient receiving a high dosage must be hospitalized so that the drug's effectiveness and adverse reactions can be monitored. When the symptoms are under control, the patient receives a low maintenance dosage. Because phenothiazines have long half-lives, the maintenance dosage may consist of a single bedtime dose. If severe orthostatic hypotension occurs in the morning, the patient may require divided doses.

Unlike other adults, an elderly or debilitated patient will receive a small initial dosage that is increased gradually until a favorable response is achieved. After the patient has taken that dosage for about 2 weeks, it is reduced gradually to the lowest effective maintenance dosage.

This section describes the typical dosages for the phenothiazines. Higher dosages may be used, however, particularly in institutional settings.

chlorpromazine hydrochloride (Thorazine). An aliphatic phenothiazine, chlorpromazine was the pharmacologic prototype for all the phenothiazines and was the first antipsychotic agent marketed. It is used to treat schizophrenia and other psychoses, intractable hiccups, and nausea or vomiting. Most patients develop a tolerance to its sedative effects. Patients over age 40 who do not tolerate chlorpromazine well will have an increased incidence of dizziness, hypotension, ocular changes, and dyskinesia.

Usual adult dosage: for psychosis, 200 to 600 mg P.O. in divided doses initially, increased to a maintenance dosage of 500 to 1,000 mg P.O. daily in divided doses, although some adults may receive up to 2 grams/day, or 25 mg I.M. initially, repeated with an additional 25 to 50 mg in 1 hour if needed and tolerated, then in 3 to 12 hours p.r.n. For nausea and vomiting, 50 to 100 mg rectally every 6 to 8 hours p.r.n., 10 to 25 mg P.O. every 4 to 6 hours p.r.n., or 25 to 50 mg I.M. every 3 to 4 hours p.r.n; for intractable hiccups, 25 to 50 mg P.O. or I.M. t.i.d. or q.i.d.

promazine hydrochloride (Sparine). An aliphatic phenothiazine, promazine is used as a sedative because it lacks antipsychotic properties.

Usual adult dosage: for sedation in mild to moderate agitation, 10 to 200 mg P.O. or I.M. every 4 to 6 hours; for sedation in severe agitation, 50 to 150 mg I.M., repeated in 30 minutes if needed, up to a maximum of 300 mg.

acetophenazine maleate (Tindal). A piperazine phenothiazine, this drug is used solely to treat psychotic disorders.

Usual adult dosage: initially, 20 mg P.O. t.i.d. or q.i.d. adjusted to 40 to 80 mg/day for nonhospitalized patients or 80 to 120 mg/day for hospitalized patients. Hospitalized patients with severe schizophrenia may receive doses from 400 to 600 mg/day.

fluphenazine decanoate (Prolixin), **fluphenazine enanthate** (Prolixin Enanthate), and **fluphenazine hydrochloride** (Permitil Hydrochloride). A piperazine phenothiazine, fluphenazine is available in several forms to treat psychotic symptoms. The decanoate and enanthate salts are depot forms of injection. They are stored in the fat and released slowly into the blood to provide extended action. Because their effects last for up to 6 weeks, they are used commonly with chronically ill patients when compliance is a problem. After the maintenance dosage has been established, these drugs can be given on an outpatient basis. The decanoate form usually is preferred because it has a longer duration of action than the enanthate form. The hydrochloride salt is available in two forms: a nondepot injection and an oral preparation.

Usual adult dosage: with fluphenazine decanoate or enanthate injection, 12.5 to 25 mg I.M. or S.C. every 1 to 6 weeks initially, then 25 to 100 mg p.r.n. for maintenance; with fluphenazine hydrochloride injection, 1.25 to 2.5 mg I.M. every 6 to 8 hours; with fluphenazine hydrochloride oral preparations, 0.5 to 10 mg daily in divided doses every 6 to 8 hours, increased up to 20 mg/day. To determine response, the shorter-acting fluphenazine hydrocloride usually is prescribed for the patient who never has taken phenothiazines.

perphenazine (Trilafon). A piperazine phenothiazine, perphenazine is used to treat psychoses.

Usual adult dosage: for control of psychotic symptoms in hospitalized patients, 8 to 16 mg P.O. b.i.d., t.i.d., or q.i.d. initially, increased to 64 mg/day; in nonhospitalized patients, 4 to 8 mg P.O. t.i.d.

trifluoperazine hydrochloride (Stelazine). A piperazine phenothiazine, this agent is used to control the manifestations of psychoses.

Usual adult dosage: 1 to 5 mg P.O. b.i.d., possibly increased gradually up to 40 mg/day, or 1 to 2 mg I.M. every 4 to 6 hours p.r.n. Even if the I.M. dosage exceeds 10 mg/24 hours, the injections should be administered at intervals of at least 4 hours.

mesoridazine besylate (Serentil). A piperidine phenothiazine, this antipsychotic is also an effective sedative.

Usual adult dosage: for antipsychotic effects, 10 to 50 mg P.O. b.i.d. or t.i.d., or 25 mg I.M. repeated in 30 to 60 minutes p.r.n.; for schizophrenia, up to 400 mg P.O. daily; for anxiety, 10 mg P.O. t.i.d. up to 150 mg/day.

thioridazine hydrochloride (Mellaril). A piperidine phenothiazine, thioridazine is used to treat the symptoms of psychoses. It also is an effective sedative and is used for dementia (in elderly patients) and depressive neurosis as well as for alcohol withdrawal — although it cannot correct the nausea and vomiting associated with it.

Usual adult dosage: to control psychotic symptoms, 50 to 100 mg P.O. t.i.d., gradually increased up to 800 mg/day in divided doses, if needed. Usual maintenance dosage is 200 to 800 mg/day. Dosage must not exceed 800 mg/day because retinal pigmentation may result. For dementia, 10 to 25 mg b.i.d. or at bedtime. For nonpsychotic uses, 25 mg P.O. t.i.d., increased to 200 mg/day in divided doses.

Drug interactions

The use of phenothiazines with alcohol and CNS depressants, such as barbiturates and narcotics, may enhance depressant effects, causing hypotension, respiratory depression, or coma. Phenothiazines also may enhance the effects of antihypertensives by increasing the alpha-adrenergic blocking action, and they may increase such adverse reactions as dry mouth or blurred vision when taken with anticholinergics, such as atropine. They can interact with other drugs as well. (For other possible effects, see *Drug interactions: Phenothiazines,* page 454.)

ADVERSE DRUG REACTIONS

Phenothiazines produce various adverse reactions ranging from mild, such as dry mouth, to severe, such as tardive dyskinesia. A suitable drug produces minimal adverse re-

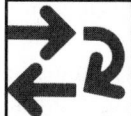

DRUG INTERACTIONS
Phenothiazines

Drug interactions involving phenothiazines can be serious. Interactions occur commonly with concurrent use of alcohol or other central nervous system (CNS) depressants.

DRUG	INTERACTING DRUGS	POSSIBLE EFFECTS	NURSING IMPLICATIONS
chlorpromazine, fluphenazine, mesoridazine, perphenazine, promazine, thioridazine, trifluoperazine	guanethidine	Inhibit uptake of guanethidine	• Monitor the patient's blood pressure frequently. • Expect to increase the guanethidine dose or replace guanethidine with another antihypertensive agent, as prescribed.
	amphetamines, nonamphetamine anorexigenic agents	Inhibit effects of both drugs	• Do not administer these drugs concurrently.
	anticholinergics	Increase anticholinergic effects; decrease antipsychotic effects	• Do not administer together routinely. If the drugs must be given concurrently, assess the patient for signs of reduced phenothiazine effects, such as increased psychotic behavior or agitation. • Perform abdominal assessments to monitor the patient for diminished or absent bowel sounds, abdominal pain, constipation, and other abdominal problems.
	CNS depressants (barbiturates, narcotic analgesics, general anesthetics, alcohol)	Increase CNS depressant effects; increase phenothiazine metabolism	• Observe the patient for erratic therapeutic effects by behavior changes, such as increased psychotic behavior or agitation; for hypotension and CNS and respiratory depression; and for increased depressant effect, such as stupor.
	levodopa	Reduce antiparkinsonian effects of levodopa when phenothiazines block dopamine receptors in the CNS	• Avoid concurrent administration, if possible. • Monitor the patient for an increase in parkinsonian symptoms.
	lithium	Increase chance of neurotoxicity, seizures, delirium, and encephalopathy in manic patients; can produce respiratory depression and hypotension	• Monitor the patient for reduced phenothiazine response and changes in neurologic status. • Monitor the patient's vital signs frequently.
	droperidol	Increase risk of extrapyramidal effects	• Monitor the patient for tremors. • Monitor the patient's vital signs frequently.
	anticonvulsants	May lower the seizure threshold	• Monitor the patient for seizures. • Be aware that the anticonvulsant dosage may be increased.
	tricyclic antidepressants, beta blockers	Increase serum levels of either agent	• Monitor the patient for adverse reactions to either agent.

actions, but a physician cannot always predict a specific agent's effects on a given patient and may not obtain reliable information from a mentally ill patient. To monitor phenothiazine therapy accurately, the nurse must have a thorough knowledge of the potential adverse reactions to these drugs.

Neurologic reactions are the most common and serious. They include extrapyramidal effects, which may appear any time after the first few days of therapy, and tardive dyskinesia, which usually occurs after several years of treatment. Phenothiazines also may lower the seizure threshold. (For details about these adverse reactions, see *Common neurologic effects of antipsychotic agents*.)

Phenothiazines can cause severe—possibly irreversible—tardive dyskinesia, especially in elderly and debilitated patients. However, their actions sometimes mask

Common neurologic effects of antipsychotic agents

Phenothiazines and other antipsychotic drugs commonly produce adverse neurologic reactions ranging from extrapyramidal effects, such as dystonia, akathisia, and pseudoparkinsonism, to tardive dyskinesia.

Dystonia

In the first week of antipsychotic therapy, the patient may exhibit an acute dystonic reaction, an extrapyramidal effect manifested by spasms in the tongue, face, neck, back, and sometimes legs that may resemble a seizure. Spasms sometimes affect certain groups of muscles only. Contracted cervical muscles can result in torticollis, an unnatural or twisted position of the neck. Opisthotonos, grimacing, perioral spasms, or pharyngeal or laryngeal spasms with dysphagia or dyspnea also can occur. Eye muscle spasms can cause oculogyrations—abnormal eye movements. Frequently accompanied by excessive salivation, these dystonic spasms typically occur when a patient receives large doses of an antipsychotic agent that is likely to produce extrapyramidal symptoms. They usually disappear with a dosage reduction or administration of 25 to 50 mg I.M. of diphenhydramine (Benadryl) or 1 to 2 mg I.M. or I.V. of benztropine (Cogentin).

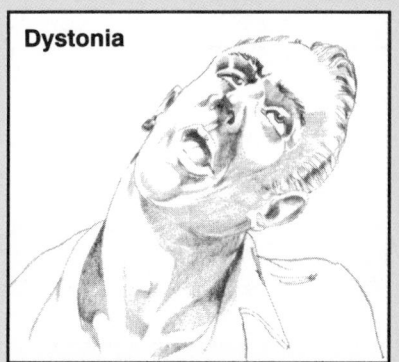

Dystonia

Pseudoparkinsonism

Later in the course of treatment, pseudoparkinsonism may occur. This extrapyramidal effect produces muscle tremors, cogwheel rigidity (muscle rigidity that gives way in little jerks when the muscle is stretched passively), shuffling gait, drooling, and a decrease in arm swing and associative movements when walking. Bradykinesia (slow movement) and akinesia (immobility) also may occur. Pseudoparkinsonism results from a direct blockade of dopamine receptors by antipsychotic agents. This reaction may be controlled with the use of antiparkinsonian agents, such as amantadine.

Pseudoparkinsonism

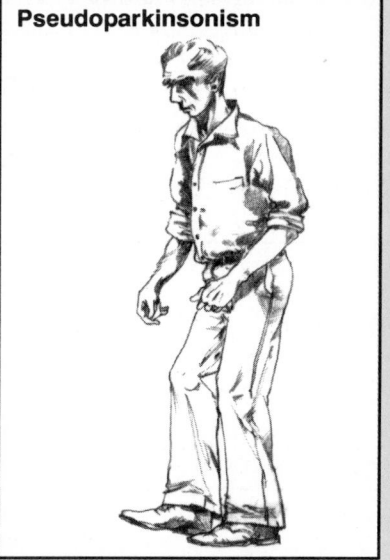

Tardive dyskinesia

Tardive dyskinesia may appear after several months or years of treatment with antipsychotic drugs. It is characterized by abnormal muscle movement, primarily around the mouth, such as lip smacking, rhythmic darting of the tongue, and constant chewing movements. Slow, aimless involuntary movements of the arms or legs also may occur. Although the exact mechanism of tardive dyskinesia is not clear, researchers believe that it may differ from that of the other extrapyramidal symptoms. Tardive dyskinesia usually affects elderly women, but can occur in younger patients as well, even after short-term antipsychotic therapy. If the medication is discontinued when first signs, such as fine wormlike tongue movements, are detected, tardive dyskinesia sometimes can be prevented.

Prevention of this adverse reaction is vital because no effective treatment is available and the reaction usually is irreversible.

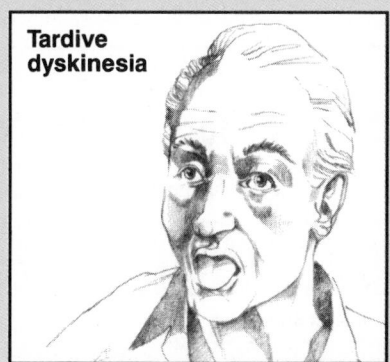

Tardive dyskinesia

Akathisia

Another extrapyramidal effect, akathisia (a continuous restlessness or inability to sit or stand still) may occur in the first 90 days of therapy. The patient attempts to relieve the discomfort of remaining quiet by tapping a foot, moving about in a chair, or pacing constantly. This symptom easily can be mistaken for agitation, which requires treatment with a higher dose of antipsychotic. However, akathisia should be managed by decreasing the antipsychotic dose or by giving an antiparkinsonian agent, such as benztropine.

Akathisia

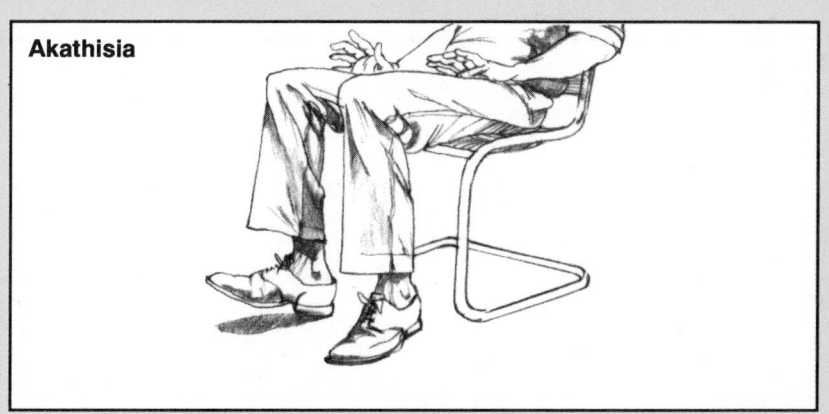

tardive dyskinesia. A "drug holiday" may be prescribed for a long-term phenothiazine patient to unmask this adverse reaction. The patient receives no antipsychotic drugs for 4 or more weeks and is observed for adverse reactions. A drug holiday also is used to delay the appearance of tardive dyskinesia, which is related to the total accumulated phenothiazine dosage.

Phenothiazines are not associated with psychological dependence, tolerance, or addiction. Upon abrupt withdrawal, however, they produce symptoms that resemble physical dependence, such as nausea, vomiting, gastritis, dizziness, tremors, sweating, tachycardiac, headache, and insomia.

Phenothiazines also may produce adverse reactions in the autonomic nervous and endocrine systems, including sedation, hypotension, orthostatic hypotension, and anticholinergic effects. (For more information, see *Relative effects of phenothiazines*.)

Hypersensitivity to phenothiazines can cause additional reactions. For example, photosensitive skin reactions commonly occur and can be serious enough to warrant instructing all patients to stay out of the sun or use a sunscreen with a skin protection factor of 15 or more. Other skin reactions, such as urticaria and dermatitis, are less common.

Although they are less common, more serious adverse reactions can occur, including blood dyscrasias, jaundice, and neuroleptic malignant syndrome (NMS), which pro-

duces muscle rigidity, hyperpyrexia, and cardiovascular collapse. When these reactions occur, the phenothiazine should be discontinued or, if the patient is psychiatrically unstable, the dosage should be reduced.

NURSING PROCESS APPLICATION

The following information assists the nurse in caring for a patient who is receiving a phenothiazine.

Assessment
• Review the patient's history for a condition that contraindicates the use of a phenothiazine, such as coma, pregnancy, lactation, blood dyscrasia, liver damage, or known hypersensitivity to the drug.
• Review the patient's history for a condition that requires cautious use of a phenothiazine, such as cardiovascular, liver, or chronic respiratory disease.
• Assess the patient for adverse reactions to the prescribed phenothiazine, such as sedation, extrapyramidal symptoms, tardive dyskinesia, hypotension, or anticholinergic effects.
• Review the patient's medication history to identify the use of drugs that may interact with the prescribed phenothiazine, such as CNS depressants, antihypertensives, anticonvulsants, or anticholinergics.
• Evaluate the patient's and family's knowledge about the prescribed phenothiazine, if possible.

Relative effects of phenothiazines

The chart below indicates the relative ability of phenothiazines to produce specific adverse effects.

PHENOTHIAZINES	SEDATION	EXTRAPYRAMIDAL SYMPTOMS	HYPOTENSION	ANTICHOLINERGIC EFFECTS
Aliphatic subgroup				
chlorpromazine	High	Moderate	High	High
promazine	Moderate	Moderate	High	High
Piperazine subgroup				
acetophenazine	Moderate	Moderate	Low	Moderate
fluphenazine	Low	High	Low	Low
perphenazine	Moderate	Moderate	Low	Low
trifluoperazine	Low	High	Low	Low
Piperidine subgroup				
mesoridazine	High	Low	Moderate	Moderate
thioridazine	High	Low	Moderate	Very high

Nursing diagnoses

The following examples represent appropriate nursing diagnoses for a patient receiving a phenothiazine.

• Potential for injury related to a preexisting condition that contraindicates the use of a phenothiazine

• Potential for injury related to a preexisting condition that requires cautious use of a phenothiazine

• Potential for injury related to adverse drug reactions

• Altered tissue perfusion: cerebral, related to the hypotensive effects of the phenothiazine

• Urinary retention related to the anticholinergic effects of the phenothiazine

• Knowledge deficit related to the prescribed phenothiazine

Planning and implementation

• Do not administer a phenothiazine to a patient with a condition that contraindicates its use.

• Administer a phenothiazine cautiously to a patient at risk because of a preexisting condition.

• Observe for neurologic and other common adverse reactions regularly throughout phenothiazine therapy.

• *Monitor for signs of less common, more serious adverse reactions, including blood dyscrasias, jaundice, and NMS. Notify the physician if the patient develops signs and symptoms of these reactions; expect to discontinue the phenothiazine or, if the patient is psychiatrically unstable, to decrease the dosage.*

• Review the results of laboratory and diagnostic tests, such as complete blood count (CBC) and liver studies, to detect adverse hematologic and hepatic reactions.

• *Observe for extrapyramidal symptoms. Notify the physician immediately if the patient exhibits acute dystonic reactions, particularly if face or neck spasms interfere with swallowing or breathing.*

• Watch for other signs of an underlying disease because phenothiazines may mask nausea and suppress vomiting.

• Assess the patient for early signs of tardive dyskinesia, such as wormlike movements of the tongue. If these signs appear, suggest a change in the drug regimen.

• Expect a drug holiday to be prescribed to check for tardive dyskinesia in a patient receiving long-term phenothiazine therapy. When beginning the drug holiday, remember not to discontinue the drug abruptly to prevent withdrawal symptoms. During the 4 or more weeks of the drug holiday, observe the patient closely for tardive dyskinesia, exhibited by abnormal muscle movement primarily around the mouth (such as lip smacking, rhythmic darting of the tongue, and constant chewing movements) and by slow, aimless, involuntary movements.

• *Continue to take safety precautions, such as close supervision of the patient and removal of harmful objects from the patient's environment, during the first several weeks of phenothiazine therapy.* Antipsychotic effects may take several weeks to appear.

• Expect to administer a small initial dose of the prescribed phenothiazine, and gradually increase it until a favorable response is achieved in an elderly or debilitated patient.

• Do not give I.M. trifluoperazine injections more frequently than every 4 hours if the dosage exceeds 10 mg/24 hours because of the drug's cumulative effects.

• Do not administer more than 800 mg/day of thioridazine because retinal pigmentation may occur.

• *Watch for respiratory depression and decreased level of consciousness in a patient who receives phenothiazines and CNS depressants;* for increased seizure activity in one who also receives anticonvulsants or has a history of seizures; for increased blood pressure in one who also receives antihypertensives; and for increased anticholinergic effects, such as dry mouth, urine retention, or blurred vision, in one who also receives anticholinergics.

• Relieve anticholinergeric effects—for example, by offering the patient sugarless gum or chipped ice to relieve dry mouth and increasing the patient's fluid and fiber intake to prevent constipation.

• Observe and report patient behavior carefully because the response to treatment can vary widely among individuals.

• Document the effects of therapy so that the patient may receive the lowest effective dosage. Note, in particular, whether the patient is sedated, stimulated, agitated, or overactive, and describe any changes in thought patterns and speech that might indicate hallucinations or delusions.

• Notify the physician if adverse reactions occur.

• Monitor the patient's blood pressure regularly to detect hypotension.

• *Use caution when administering phenothiazines with narcotics or other CNS depressants because they can induce hypotension.*

• Expect to administer the prescribed phenothiazine in divided doses if severe orthostatic hypotension occurs in the morning.

• Have the patient sit up for 1 to 2 minutes before standing to minimize the effects of orthostatic hypotension.

• *Monitor the patient closely for signs of altered cerebral perfusion, such as decreased blood pressure or changes in level of consciousness or behavior. If these signs occur, take safety precautions and notify the physician.*

• Monitor the patient closely for signs of urine retention, such as frequent trips to the bathroom, complaints of a sense of fullness in the lower abdomen, dullness on percussion of the lower abdomen, and palpation of a distended bladder.

• Notify the physician and prepare to catheterize the patient if assessment findings suggest urine retention. Expect to decrease the phenothiazine dosage or change the patient to a different drug.

Patient teaching

• Teach the patient (if appropriate) and family the name, dose, frequency, action, and adverse effects of the prescribed phenothiazine.

• Alert the family that psychological dependence can occur with phenothiazine use.

• Inform the family that they can expect to see normalization of thoughts, moods, and actions in the patient after several weeks or months of phenothiazine therapy.

• Stress the importance of taking the phenothiazine exactly as prescribed and not discontinuing it without physician approval because psychotic symptoms may return.

• Ask the family to tell the physician if the patient does not comply with the drug regiman. The physician may change the drug to fluphenazine decanoate or enanthate because their effects last for up to 6 weeks.

• Advise the patient to obtain physician approval before ingesting other CNS depressants.

• Teach the patient how to manage troublesome anticholinergic effects.

• Instruct the patient to return regularly for follow-up care that includes periodic dosage adjustments.

• Instruct the family to notify the physician at the first sign of tardive dyskinesia to prevent permanent damage.

• Prepare the patient receiving long-term phenothiazine therapy for a drug holiday, as instructed. During the 4 or more weeks of the drug holiday, the patient and family should watch for—and report to the physician—signs of tardive dyskinesia.

• Advise the patient not to discontinue the drug abruptly.

• Teach the patient how to manage orthostatic hypotension.

• Instruct the family to use safety precautions, such as supervising ambulation, if mild sedation occurs and to alert the physician if sedation worsens or seizures occur.

• Teach the patient to recognize and report the signs of urine retention.

• Instruct the patient and family to notify the physician of any other adverse reactions or changes in psychotic symptoms.

Evaluation

The following examples represent appropriate evaluation statements for a patient receiving a phenothiazine.

• The patient has no conditions that contraindicate phenothiazine therapy.

• The patient exhibits no complications in the preexisting condition linked to the prescribed phenothiazine.

• The patient displays no adverse reactions to the prescribed phenothiazine.

• The patient maintains normal cerebral tissue perfusion.

• The patient maintains a normal voiding pattern during phenothiazine therapy.

• The patient and family express an accurate understanding of the points taught about the prescribed phenothiazine.

• The patient and family correctly identify signs of tardive dyskinesia and describe what to do if they occur.

NONPHENOTHIAZINES

Based on their chemical structures, nonphenothiazine antipsychotics can be divided into several drug classes, including the butyrophenones, such as haloperidol and haloperidol decanoate; dibenzodiazepines, such as clozapine; dibenzoxazepines, such as loxapine succinate; dihydroindolones, such as molindone hydrochloride; diphenylbutylpiperidines, such as pimozide; and thioxanthenes, such as chlorprothixene and thiothixene.

Although chemically different from the phenothiazines, the nonphenothiazines are used to treat psychotic symptoms with equal effectiveness and produce similar actions and adverse reactions. Individual reactions to nonphenothiazines can vary. Therefore, a physician usually prescribes the nonphenothiazine that produces the greatest therapeutic action and fewest adverse reactions for each patient.

PHARMACOKINETICS

Nonphenothiazines are absorbed, distributed, metabolized, and excreted in the same manner as the phenothiazines. Their onset of action, peak concentration levels, and duration of action are similar to those of the phenothiazines.

PHARMACODYNAMICS

Except for clozapine, the mechanism of action of the nonphenothiazines resembles that of the phenothiazines. Clozapine's structure differs from that of the other nonphenothiazines. Unlike the other drugs in this category, which block dopamine receptors, clozapine is a weak blocker of dopamine receptors but a potent blocker of serotonin activity.

PHARMACOTHERAPEUTICS

As a group, nonphenothiazines are used to treat psychotic disorders. Specific drugs in this group may serve additional functions. For example, thiothixene also is used to control acute agitation. Haloperidol and pimozide may be used to treat Gilles de la Tourette's syndrome. Because of its adverse effects, clozapine is reserved for patients who have not responded to therapy with other antipsychotic agents or who have developed tardive dyskinesia.

haloperidol (Haldol) and **haloperidol decanoate** (Haldol Decanoate). A butyrophenone nonphenothiazine, this antipsychotic agent is available in short-acting and long-acting (decanoate) forms. Both are used to treat dyskinesia in Gilles de la Tourette's syndrome and symptoms of psychoses. In elderly patients, they may be used to treat the symptoms of dementia.

Usual adult dosage: 0.5 to 5 mg P.O. b.i.d. or t.i.d. of the short-acting form, increased p.r.n. up to 100 mg/day for a limited period in a hospital setting; 2 to 5 mg I.M. of the short-acting form repeated every hour p.r.n. until symptoms are controlled and then repeated at 4- to 8-hour intervals; up to 100 mg I.M. initially of the long-acting form repeated at monthly intervals in doses of up to 300 mg. Elderly patients usually receive 0.5 to 2 mg P.O. h.s. or b.i.d. of the short-acting form. Haloperidol decanoate is not to be administered I.V. As an unlabeled use, the short-acting form (not the decanoate form) may be administered I.V. for some acute psychiatric conditions.

clozapine (Clozaril). This tricyclic dibenzodiazepine is reserved for treating patients who do not respond to standard schizophrenia treatments and for those with tardive dyskinesia.

Usual adult dosage: initially, 25 mg P.O. once or twice daily for 2 weeks, increased by 25 to 50 mg/day, as needed and tolerated, up to a dosage of 300 to 450 mg/day. Subsequent dosage adjustments should not exceed 100 mg and should be made no more than once or twice a week. Most patients respond to dosages of 300 to 600 mg/day, but some have required higher amounts. The maximum dosage is 900 mg/day.

loxapine succinate (Loxitane). A dibenzoxazepine nonphenothiazine, loxapine is used to treat the manifestations of psychoses.

Usual adult dosage: 10 mg P.O. b.i.d. to q.i.d., increased to 60 to 100 mg/day; for severe agitation, 12.5 to 50 mg I.M. every 4 to 6 hours.

molindone hydrochloride (Moban). A dihydroindolone nonphenothiazine, molindone is used to control psychotic symptoms.

Usual adult dosage: 50 to 75 mg P.O. daily, increased to 225 mg P.O. daily in 3 or 4 divided doses.

pimozide (Orap). This diphenyl-butylpiperidine nonphenothiazine suppresses severe motor and phonic tics in patients with Gilles de la Tourette's syndrome when these symptoms do not respond to other treatments.

Usual adult dosage: 1 to 2 mg P.O. daily in divided doses, increased to a maintenance dosage from 7 to 16 mg P.O. daily, not to exceed 0.3 mg/kg/day.

chlorprothixene (Taractan). A thioxanthene nonphenothiazine, this antipsychotic agent also is effective as a sedative for agitation in patients with severe neurosis and depression.

Usual adult dosage: for psychotic disorders, 25 to 50 mg P.O. t.i.d. or q.i.d., increased gradually up to 600 mg/day; for sedation of an agitated patient, 25 to 50 mg I.M. t.i.d. or q.i.d., increased as needed up to 600 mg/day. Transfer to oral doses may be accomplished by alternating I.M. and P.O. routes of administration as prescribed.

thiothixene (Navane). A thioxanthene nonphenothiazine, this agent is used to treat acute psychosis.

Usual adult dosage: initially, 4 mg I.M. b.i.d. to q.i.d., increased gradually until symptoms are controlled; then 6 to 10 mg/day P.O. in divided doses; may be increased gradually to optimal dosage of 20 to 30 mg/day or, if indicated, up to a dosage of 60 mg/day until symptoms are controlled, then decreased gradually. For elderly patients, one-half to one-third of the I.M. or oral dosage is prescribed.

Drug interactions

Nonphenothiazines interact with fewer drugs than the phenothiazines do. However, their dopamine-blocking activity can inhibit levodopa and may cause disorientation in patients receiving both medications.

Haloperidol also may augment the effects of lithium, producing encephalopathy. When given concurrently with lithium, haloperidol should be used initially to control acute symptoms and then decreased as lithium is added to the regimen.

Concomitant administration of clozapine with anticholinergic agents may have added anticholinergic effects. The hypotensive effects of antihypertensive agents may be potentiated by clozapine administration; blood pressure should be monitored closely in this patients receiving both medications. Additive CNS effects may result when clozapine is administered with other agents that affect the CNS. Clozapine may cause agranulocytosis and should not be administered with other agents known to suppress bone marrow. Because clozapine is highly protein bound, it may cause protein-binding displacement when administered with such other highly bound drugs as warfarin or phenytoin. Closely monitor the patient for drug toxicity during concomitant administration.

ADVERSE DRUG REACTIONS

Most nonphenothiazines cause the same adverse reactions as the phenothiazines. (For details, see *Relative effects of nonphenothiazines,* page 460.)

Compared to the other nonphenothiazines, clozapine produces fewer extrapyramidal reactions and no tardive dyskinesia. Divided doses and cautious titration of cloza-

Relative effects of nonphenothiazines

The chart below indicates the relative ability of nonphenothiazines to produce specific adverse effects.

NONPHENOTHIAZINES	SEDATION	EXTRAPYRAMIDAL SYMPTOMS	HYPOTENSION	ANTICHOLINERGIC EFFECTS
Butyrophenone subgroup				
haloperidol	Low	Very high	Low	Very low
Dibenzoxazepine subgroup				
clozapine	High	Very low	Moderate	Very high
loxapine	Low	Moderate	Low	Low
Dihydroindolone subgroup				
molindone	Moderate	Moderate	Low	Low
Thioxanthene subgroup				
chlorprothixene	High	Moderate	Moderate	Moderate
thiothixene	Low	Moderate	Moderate	Low
Diphenyl-butylpiperidine subgroup				
pimozide	Low	Very high	Low	Moderate

pine help to minimize the risk of hypotension, sedation, and seizures. Its major adverse reaction is the development of life-threatening neutropenia or agranulocytosis, which typically occurs within the first 6 months of therapy. To detect this reaction, a white blood cell (WBC) count should be performed weekly during clozapine therapy.

NURSING PROCESS APPLICATION

The following information assists the nurse in caring for a patient who is receiving a nonphenothiazine.

Assessment
• Review the patient's history for a condition that contraindicates the use of a nonphenothiazine, such as CNS depression, coma, Parkinson's disease, pregnancy, lactation, or known hypersensitivity to the drug.
• Review the patient's history for a condition that requires cautious use of a nonphenothiazine, such as cardiovascular disease or drug allergies.
• Assess the patient for adverse reactions to the prescribed nonphenothiazine, such as sedation, extrapryamidal symptoms, tardive dyskinesia, hypotension, and anticholinergic effects.
• Review the patient's medication history to identify the use of drugs that may interact with the prescribed non-

phenothiazine, such as levodopa, lithium, anticholinergics, or antihypertensive agents.
• Evaluate the patient's and family's knowledge about the prescribed nonphenothiazine, if appropriate.

Nursing diagnoses
The following examples represent appropriate nursing diagnoses for a patient receiving a nonphenothiazine.
• Potential for injury related to a preexisting condition that contraindicates the use of a nonphenothiazine
• Potential for injury related to a preexisting condition that requires cautious use of a nonphenothiazine
• Potential for injury related to adverse drug reactions
• Altered tissue perfusion: cerebral, related to the hypotensive effects of the nonphenothiazine
• Urinary retention related to the anticholinergic effects of the nonphenothiazine
• Knowledge deficit related to the prescribed nonphenothiazine

Planning and implementation
• Do not administer a nonphenothiazine to a patient with a condition that contraindicates its use.
• Administer a nonphenothiazine cautiously to a patient at risk because of a preexisting condition.

• Observe for neurologic and other common adverse reactions regularly throughout nonphenothiazine therapy.
• *Monitor for signs of serious adverse reactions, such as blood dyscrasias, jaundice, and NMS. Notify the physician if the patient develops signs of these reactions; expect to discontinue the nonphenothiazine, or if the patient is psychiatrically unstable, to decrease the dosage.*
• Review the results of laboratory and diagnostic tests, such as regular CBCs, liver studies, or (for a patient receiving clozapine) weekly WBC counts, to detect adverse hematologic and hepatic reactions.
• *Observe for extrapyramidal symptoms. Notify the physician immediately if the patient exhibits acute dystonic reactions, particularly if face or neck spasms interfere with swallowing or breathing.*
• Assess the patient for early signs of tardive dyskinesia, such as wormlike movements of the tongue. If these signs appear, suggest a change in the drug regimen.
• Expect a drug-holiday to be prescribed to check for tardive dyskinesia in a patient receiving long-term nonphenothiazine therapy. During the 4 or more weeks of the drug holiday, observe the patient closely for tardive dyskinesia, exhibited by abnormal muscle movement primarily around the mouth (such as lip smacking, rhythmic darting of the tongue, and constant chewing movements) and by slow, aimless, involuntary movements of the arms or legs.
• Expect the patient to be changed to clozapine if tardive dyskinesia occurs or if the patient does not respond to standard drug therapy.
• Administer clozapine in divided doses and titrate it cautiously to minimize the risk of hypotension, sedation, and seizures, as prescribed.
• Monitor the patient taking chlorprothixene for an allergic reaction because it contains tartrazine.
• *Continue to take safety precautions, such as close patient supervision and removal of harmful objects from the patient's environment, during the first several weeks of nonphenothiazine therapy.* Antipsychotic effects may take several weeks to appear.
• Expect to administer a small initial dosage of the prescribed nonphenothiazine and gradually increase it until a favorable response is achieved in an elderly or debilitated patient. With thiothixene, an elderly patient should receive only one-half to one-third of the normal I.M. or P.O. dosage.
• *Do not administer haloperidol decanoate I.V.*
• Protect haloperidol from exposure to light. Haloperidol may be administered if it becomes slightly yellow, but it must be discarded if the solution is markedly discolored because its potency will have decreased.
• *Avoid abrupt discontinuation of the prescribed nonphenothiazine unless severe adverse reactions make this necessary.*

• *Monitor for disorientation in a patient who is receiving a nonphenothiazine and levodopa.*
• Expect concurrent use of haloperidol and lithium to proceed as follows to prevent encephalopathy: Administer haloperidol initially to control acute symptoms and then decrease it when lithium is added to the regimen.
• Relieve anticholinergic effects, for example, by offering the patient sugarless gum or chipped ice to relieve dry mouth and increasing the patient's fluid and fiber intake to prevent constipation, unless otherwise contraindicated.
• Observe and report patient behavior carefully because the response to treatment can vary widely among individuals.
• Document the effects of therapy so that the patient may receive the lowest effective dosage. Note, in particular, whether the patient is stimulated, agitated, or overactive, and describe any changes in thought patterns and speech that might indicate hallucinations or delusions.
• Notify the physician if adverse reactions occur.
• Monitor the patient's blood pressure regularly to detect hypotension.
• Have the patient sit up for 1 to 2 minutes before standing to minimize the effects of orthostatic hypotension.
• *Monitor the patient closely for signs of altered cerebral perfusion, such as decreased blood pressure or a change in level of consciousness or behavior. If these signs occur, take safety precautions and notify the physician.*
• Monitor the patient closely for signs of urine retention, such as frequent trips to the bathroom, complaints of a sense of fullness in the lower abdomen, dullness on percussion of the lower abdomen, and palpation of a distended bladder.
• Notify the physician and prepare to catheterize the patient if assessment findings suggest urine retention. Expect to decrease the nonphenothiazine dosage or change the patient to another drug.

Patient teaching
• Teach the patient (if appropriate) and family the name, dose, frequency, action, and adverse reactions of the prescribed nonphenothiazine.
• Inform the family that they can expect to see normalization of thoughts, moods, and actions in the patient after several weeks or months of nonphenothiazine therapy.
• Stress the importance of taking the nonphenothiazine exactly as prescribed and not discontinuing it without physician approval because psychotic symptoms may return.
• Teach the patient how to manage troublesome anticholinergic effects.
• Encourage the patient to return regularly for follow-up care that includes periodic dosage adjustments and laboratory studies.
• Instruct the family to notify the physician at the first sign of tardive dyskinesia to prevent permanent damage.

SELECTED MAJOR DRUGS

Antipsychotic agents

This chart summarizes the major antipsychotic agents currently in clinical use.

DRUG	MAJOR INDICATIONS	USUAL ADULT DOSAGES	CONTRAINDICATIONS AND PRECAUTIONS
Phenothiazines			
chlorpromazine	Symptomatic relief of psychoses	200 to 600 mg P.O. daily in divided doses initially, increased to a maintenance dosage of 500 to 1,000 mg P.O. daily in divided doses	• Know that chlorpromazine is contraindicated in a pregnant or lactating patient; a patient with bone marrow depression or known hypersensitivity to the drug; a comatose patient; a patient receiving a high dosage of central nervous system (CNS) depressants; or a child or adolescent with signs and symptoms of Reye's syndrome. • Administer with caution to an elderly or debilitated patient or to one with cardiovascular or liver disease; a history of seizures; a chronic respiratory disorder, such as severe asthma or emphysema; acute respiratory infections (especially a child); glaucoma; exposure to extreme heat or organophosphorus insecticides; or to a patient receiving atropine or a related drug.
fluphenazine decanoate	Symptomatic relief of psychoses when compliance is a problem	12.5 to 25 mg I.M. or S.C. every 1 to 6 weeks initially, then 25 to 100 mg p.r.n. for maintenance	• Know that fluphenazine decanoate is contraindicated in a child under age 12, a comatose or severely depressed patient, or one with known hypersensitivity to the drug, suspected or proven subcortical brain damage, blood dyscrasia, or liver damage. • Administer with caution to an elderly, debilitated, or pregnant patient; a patient undergoing surgery who takes large doses of fluphenazine; or one with cholestatic jaundice, dermatoses or other allergic reactions to phenothiazine derivatives, a seizure disorder, cardiovascular disease such as mitral insufficiency, pheochromocytoma, or exposure to extreme heat or organophosphorus insecticides.
Nonphenothiazines			
haloperidol, haloperidol decanoate	Symptomatic relief of psychoses, relief of dyskinesia in Gilles de la Tourette's syndrome	0.5 to 5 mg P.O. b.i.d. or t.i.d., increased p.r.n. up to 100 mg/day	• Know that haloperidol and haloperidol decanoate are contraindicated in a pregnant or lactating patient or one with toxic CNS depression, coma, Parkinson's disease, or known hypersensitivity. • Administer with caution to a patient with severe cardiovascular disease or known allergies, or to a patient who also receives an anticonvulsant or anticoagulant.

• Prepare the patient receiving long-term nonphenothiazine therapy for a drug holiday, as instructed. During the 4 or more weeks of the drug holiday, the patient and family should watch for—and report to the physician—signs of tardive dyskinesia.

• Advise the patient to use a sunscreen and wear protective clothing otudoors to prevent a photosensitivity reaction.

• Teach the patient how to manage orthostatic hypotension.

• Teach the patient to recognize and report the signs of urine retention.

• Instruct the patient and family to notify the physician of any other adverse reactions or changes in psychotic symptoms.

Evaluation

The following examples represent appropriate evaluation statements for a patient receiving a nonphenothiazine.

• The patient has no conditions that contraindicate nonphenothiazine therapy.

• The patient exhibits no signs of complications in the preexisting condition linked to the prescribed nonphenothiazine.

• The patient experiences no adverse reactions to the prescribed nonphenothiazine.

• The patient maintains normal cerebral tissue perfusion.

• The patient maintains a normal voiding pattern during nonphenothiazine therapy.

• The patient and family express an accurate understanding of the points taught about the prescribed nonphenothiazine.

• The patient schedules follow-up visits for periodic dosage adjustments and laboratory studies.

CHAPTER SUMMARY

Chapter 28 presented antipsychotic agents, or neuroleptics, used to control the symptoms of psychoses, especially schizophrenia. Although they cannot cure mental illness, they can improve the quality of life for many mentally ill patients and their families. They allow patients who might otherwise be institutionalized for life to function independently in the community. Here are the highlights of this chapter.

• All antipsychotic agents belong to one of two major groups: phenothiazines and nonphenothiazines. Phenothiazines include chlorpromazine, promazine, acetophenazine, fluphenazine, perphenazine, trifluoperazine, mesoridazine, and thioridazine. Nonphenothiazines include haloperidol, clozapine, loxapine, molindone, pimozide, chlorprothixene, and thiothixene.

• Antipsychotic agents also are used to calm or sedate agitated or disturbed patients with psychotic symptoms, alleviate nausea and vomiting, and enhance the effects of analgesics and anesthetics preoperatively to control pain.

• Neurologic reactions are the most common and serious adverse reactions to antipsychotic agents and include sedation, extrapyramidal symptoms, and tardive dyskinesia. Other reactions include hypotension, seizures, anticholinergic effects, photosensitivity, blood dyscrasias, jaundice, and NMS.

• The newest nonphenothiazine, clozapine can cause severe neutropenia and agranulocytosis. Because of these adverse reactions, clozapine is reserved for patients who do not respond to therapy with standard antipsychotic agents or who have tardive dyskinesia.

• Except for clozapine, phenothiazines and nonphenothiazines produce similar actions and adverse reactions, but the response to these drugs varies widely from patient to patient. Therefore, effective antipsychotic therapy requires the nurse to observe accurately and report the patient's behavior and the drug's effects.

• During antipsychotic therapy, the nurse uses the nursing process to guide patient care. Nursing activities typically include monitoring the patient and promoting compliance. The nurse also should teach the patient about the drug, its regimen, its therapeutic and adverse effects, and other considerations.

STUDY QUESTIONS

See Appendix 1 for answers.

1. Gordon Wills, age 26, is admitted to the psychiatric unit for treatment of acute schizophrenia. His physician prescribes the phenothiazine chlorpromazine (Thorazine) 125 mg P.O. q.i.d. When can the nurse expect to see the antipsychotic effects of this drug?
(a) 15 to 30 minutes after administration
(b) 2 to 4 hours after administration
(c) 24 to 48 hours after administration
(d) several weeks after administration

2. How does sedation caused by phenothiazines differ from that produced by many CNS depressants?
(a) Phenothiazines produce greater sedation than other CNS depressants.
(b) Phenothiazines produce deeper sleep than other CNS depressants.
(c) Phenothiazines produce a calming effect from which the patient is easily aroused.
(d) Phenothiazines produce more prolonged sedative effects, making the patient difficult to arouse.

3. After receiving chlorpromazine for a week, Mr. Wills develops urine retention. Which drug effect is responsible for this adverse reaction?
(a) antiadrenergic
(b) anticholinergic
(c) extrapyramidal
(d) adrenergic

4. During the patient-teaching session, which instructions should the nurse provide about chlorpromazine therapy?
(a) Stop taking the drug as soon as he begins to feel better.
(b) Take the drug exactly as prescribed, even if symptoms disappear.
(c) Take the drug with an antacid if gastric distress occurs.
(d) Increase or decrease the dosage, depending on how he feels.

5. Hannah Atkins, age 75, has dementia and is agitated. Her physician prescribes the nonphenothiazine haloperidol (Haldol) 0.5 mg I.M. b.i.d until symptoms are controlled. When preparing a haloperidol injection for Ms. Atkins, the nurse notices that the medication is slightly yellow. What should the nurse do?

(a) Administer the medication; a slightly yellow color is acceptable.

(b) Administer the medication; the normal color is light yellow.

(c) Discard the medication; its potency will have decreased.

(d) Double the dosage to offset light deterioration of the drug.

6. After taking haloperidol for a few months, Ms. Atkins develops wormlike movements of the tongue and slow, aimless, involuntary movements of her arms. What is the most likely cause of these signs?

(a) development of Parkinson's disease

(b) neurologic effects of haloperidol

(c) hypersensitivity to haloperidol

(d) preexisting dementia

7. After 16 months of loxapine therapy, Tony Carson, age 37, develops tardive dyskinesia. However, he still needs an antipsychotic agent to control the symptoms of psychosis. Which drug is most likely to be prescribed?

(a) thioridazine hydrochloride

(b) trifluoperazine hydrochloride

(c) clozapine

(d) thiothixene

SELECTED REFERENCES

Alper, J. (1988). Tranquilizers: A user's guide. *Health,* 20(11), 35-86.

Ashton, H. (Ed.). (1987). *Brain systems, disorders, and psychotropic drugs.* New York: Oxford University Press.

Bickal, T. (1987). A protocol for the diagnosis and treatment of extrapyramidal symptoms of neuroleptic drugs. *Nurse Practitioner,* 12(1), 25-38.

Bostrum, A. (1988). Assessment scales for tardive dyskinesia. *Journal of Psychosocial Nursing,* 26(6), 9-12.

Dahl, S. (1986). *Clinical pharmacology in psychology.* New York: Springer-Verlag.

Davies, D. (Ed.). (1987). *Textbook of adverse drug reactions* (3rd ed.). New York: Oxford University Press.

Drug facts and comparisons. (1991). St. Louis: Facts and Comparisons Division, J.B. Lippincott.

Gelenberg, A. (1987). Treating extrapyramidal reactions: Some current issues. *Journal of Clinical Psychiatry,* 8(9)(Suppl.), 24-27.

Goodman and Gilman's the pharmacological basis of therapeutics (8th ed; 1990). Elmsford, NY: Pergamon Press.

Hansten, P., and Horn, J. (1989). *Drug interactions: Clinical significance of drug-drug interactions* (6th ed.). Philadelphia: Lea & Febiger.

Marder, S., and Van Putten, T. (1988). Who should receive clozapine? *Archives of General Psychiatry,* 45(9), 865-867.

Middlemiss, M., and Beeber, L. (1989). Update on psychopharmacology: Issues in the use of depot antipsychotics. *Journal of Psychosocial Nursing and Mental Health Services,* 27(6), 36-37.

North American Nursing Diagnosis Association. (1990). *Taxonomy I-Revised, with official categories.* St. Louis: NANDA.

Patients' and nurses' reports of neuroleptic side effects. (1989). *Nurses Drug Alert,* 13(9), 70.

Perry, P., et al. (1989). *Psychotropic drug handbook* (5th ed.). Cincinnati: Harvey Whitney.

Singh, H., and Simpson, G. (1988). Tardive dyskinesia: Clinical features. In M. Wolf and A. Mosnaim (Eds.), *Tardive dyskinesia: Biological mechanisms and clinical aspects* (pp. 69-86). Washington, DC: American Psychiatric Press.

USPDI. (1991). *Drug information for the health care professional* (Vol. I, 11th ed.). Rockville, MD: United States Pharmacopeial Convention.

USPDI. (1991). *Advice for the patient* (Vol. II, 11th ed.). Rockville, MD: United States Pharmacopeial Convention.

Weiden, P., Shaw, E., and Mann, J. (1987). Causes of neuroleptic noncompliance. *Psychiatric Annals,* 16(10), 567-568.

Weintraub, M., and Evans, P. (1989). Clozapine: A neuroleptic agent for selected schizophrenics and patients with tardive dyskinesia. *Hospital Formulary,* 24, 16-27.

7

DRUGS TO IMPROVE CARDIOVASCULAR FUNCTION

The circulatory system includes the heart and blood vessels. In this system, arteries generally carry oxygen and nutrients to the cells, and veins carry away the unoxygenated blood and the waste products of cellular metabolism. Because this system represents a vital function, a dysfunction in the heart or kidneys seriously can affect an individual's health.

CIRCULATION

Blood flow results from pressure differences in the circulatory system, which are caused by the force of the blood flow through the vessels and the force or resistance to that blood flow.

Blood pressure refers to the force exerted by the blood against the vessel walls. Arterial blood pressure is determined by cardiac output and peripheral resistance. Usually, an increase or decrease in cardiac output or peripheral resistance will increase or decrease blood pressure correspondingly. Similarly, increases or decreases in blood flow and tissue perfusion will accompany blood pressure changes. Cardiac output is a function of the heart rate and stroke volume.

Peripheral circulation refers to blood ejected from the left side of the heart. Pulmonary circulation refers to blood ejected from the right side.

In peripheral circulation, the heart pumps blood to all body tissues and organs except the lungs. Arteries and arterioles carry the blood away from the heart; capillaries allow the exchange of nutrients for cellular waste products; then the venules and veins return the blood to the right side of the heart.

In pulmonary circulation, the heart pumps blood to the lungs via the pulmonary arteries, and the pulmonary veins return the blood to the left side of the heart. Unlike peripheral circulation, pulmonary circulation uses the veins to carry oxygen-rich blood and the arteries to carry unoxygenated blood and waste products.

HEART

Coronary arteries supply blood to the myocardium; coronary veins carry away the waste products of metabolism. (For an illustration, see *Coronary circulation,* page 467.) The coronary arteries arise from the aorta and fill during diastole.

Cardiac function depends on conduction of electrical impulses throughout the myocardium. When recorded by an electrocardiogram (ECG), the electrical activity of the heart appears as deflection points designated by the letters P, Q, R, S, T, and U. This electrical activity results in contraction of the heart and ejection of blood. (For an illustration of this activity, see *Electrical activity and the ECG,* page 468.)

KIDNEYS

The kidneys regulate the body's fluid and electrolyte balance and dispose of waste products. Blood enters the kidneys through the renal arteries and is filtered at the glomerulus. The filtrate enters the renal tubular system, where it is altered and concentrated or diluted. Then the concentrated or diluted urine leaves the kidneys through the renal pelvis and ureters to the bladder for excretion. Blood leaves the kidneys through the renal veins.

The kidneys also help regulate blood pressure through the renin-angiotensin system. They release the hormone renin in response to a decrease in renal blood flow or, more specifically, to a decrease in the glomerular filtration rate. Renin acts on angiotensinogen (a plasma protein) to form angiotensin I. Angiotensin I is converted to angiotensin II as it circulates through the lungs. Angiotensin II, a potent vasoconstrictor, increases peripheral resistance and sodium and water resorption, contributing to an increase in blood pressure.

Glossary

Afterload: pressure in the arteries leading from the ventricle that must be overcome for ejection to occur.

Arrhythmia: abnormal variation in cardiac conduction, rhythm, or rate.

Atrioventricular (AV) block: obstructed transmission of electrical impulses from the atria to the ventricles caused by AV node damage or depression.

Automaticity: ability to generate an electrical impulse independently.

Bathmotropic: increasing or decreasing the excitability of muscle tissue, especially cardiac tissue.

Cardiac output: amount of blood pumped by the heart per unit of time, normally about 5 liters/minute.

Chronotropic: altering the rate of cardiac muscle contraction; a drug with a negative chronotropic effect slows the heart rate.

Conductivity: capacity of cells to conduct current.

Contractility: capacity for shortening or contracting in response to a stimulus.

Depolarization: neutralization of electrical polarity in cardiac cells caused by an influx of sodium ions.

Diastole: period of ventricular dilation that occurs between the second and first heart sounds.

Diastolic blood pressure: pressure exerted in the vessels when the ventricles are at rest.

Dromotropic: influencing conduction; a drug with a negative dromotropic effect slows conduction through the AV node.

Ectopy: generation of electrical impulses by cardiac cells outside the normal conduction pathways.

Excitability: readiness of a cell to respond to a stimulus.

Fibrillation: twitching movements of cardiac muscle resulting from so rapid a transmission of independent impulses that coordinated contractions cannot occur.

Frank-Starling law of the heart: principle which states that the force of ventricular contraction is related to the length of cardiac muscle fibers; within limits, the greater the length of stretched fibers, the stronger the contraction.

Hyperlipoproteinemia: excess lipids in the blood.

Hypertension: systolic blood pressure of 160 mm Hg or higher and diastolic blood pressure of 95 mm Hg or higher on two or more occasions.

Infarction: formation of a localized area of tissue necrosis caused by hypoxia resulting from inadequate blood flow to the area.

Inotropic: affecting the force of cardiac muscle contraction; a drug with a positive inotropic effect increases the strength of the muscle contraction.

Ischemia: decreased blood supply to an area caused by vascular constriction or obstruction.

Lipid: fatty substance in the blood.

Lipoprotein: combination of different lipids with proteins.

Mean arterial pressure: average blood pressure throughout each cardiac cycle, usually about 96 mm Hg.

Orthostatic hypotension: decrease in blood pressure that occurs when a person stands erect; also called postural hypotension.

Peripheral vascular resistance: pressure that blood must overcome as it flows in a vessel.

Phospholipid: phosphoric acid ester of lipid substances.

Preload: blood volume in the ventricle at the end of diastole.

Proarrhythmia: arrythmia that occurs when another already is present.

Pulse pressure: difference between systolic and diastolic blood pressures, usually about 40 mm Hg.

Reentry or **circus movement:** abnormal transmission of an electrical impulse around and around in cardiac muscle without stopping.

Refractory period: period of depolarization after excitation, during which cardiac muscle cannot respond to another normal cardiac impulse.

Repolarization: restoration of electrical polarity in cardiac cells caused by an outflow of potassium ions from the cells.

Stroke volume: blood output from the ventricle during systole, usually about 70 ml.

Systole: period of ventricular contraction that occurs between the first and second heart sounds.

Systolic blood pressure: pressure exerted in the vessels when the ventricles contract.

OVERVIEW OF CHAPTERS

Unit Seven investigates various agents that are used to treat cardiovascular disorders, such as congestive heart failure, arrhythmias, angina, hypertension, and hyperlipoproteinemia.

Chapter 29
Cardiac Glycoside Agents and Bipyridines

Chapter 29 explores inotropic agents used to treat congestive heart failure and supraventricular arrhythmias by decreasing contractility. It discusses the cardiac glycosides digoxin and digitoxin as well as the bipyridine amrinone,

highlighting their pharmacokinetics, pharmacodynamics, pharmacotherapeutics, and adverse effects. The chapter concludes with nursing care related to these agents.

Chapter 30
Antiarrhythmic Agents

After providing an overview of the conduction system of the heart, Chapter 30 examines the seven classes of antiarrhythmic agents (drugs used to treat abnormalities of cardiac electrical activity). It describes the mechanisms of action of these agents, which primarily block three cardiac mechanisms: the fast sodium channel, the slow calcium channel, and the autonomic innervation of myocardial cells.

Coronary circulation

Coronary arteries arise from the aorta and supply blood to the myocardium. The coronary veins carry blood from the myocardium via the coronary sinus. The illustration below shows the location of the major structures of the coronary circulation.

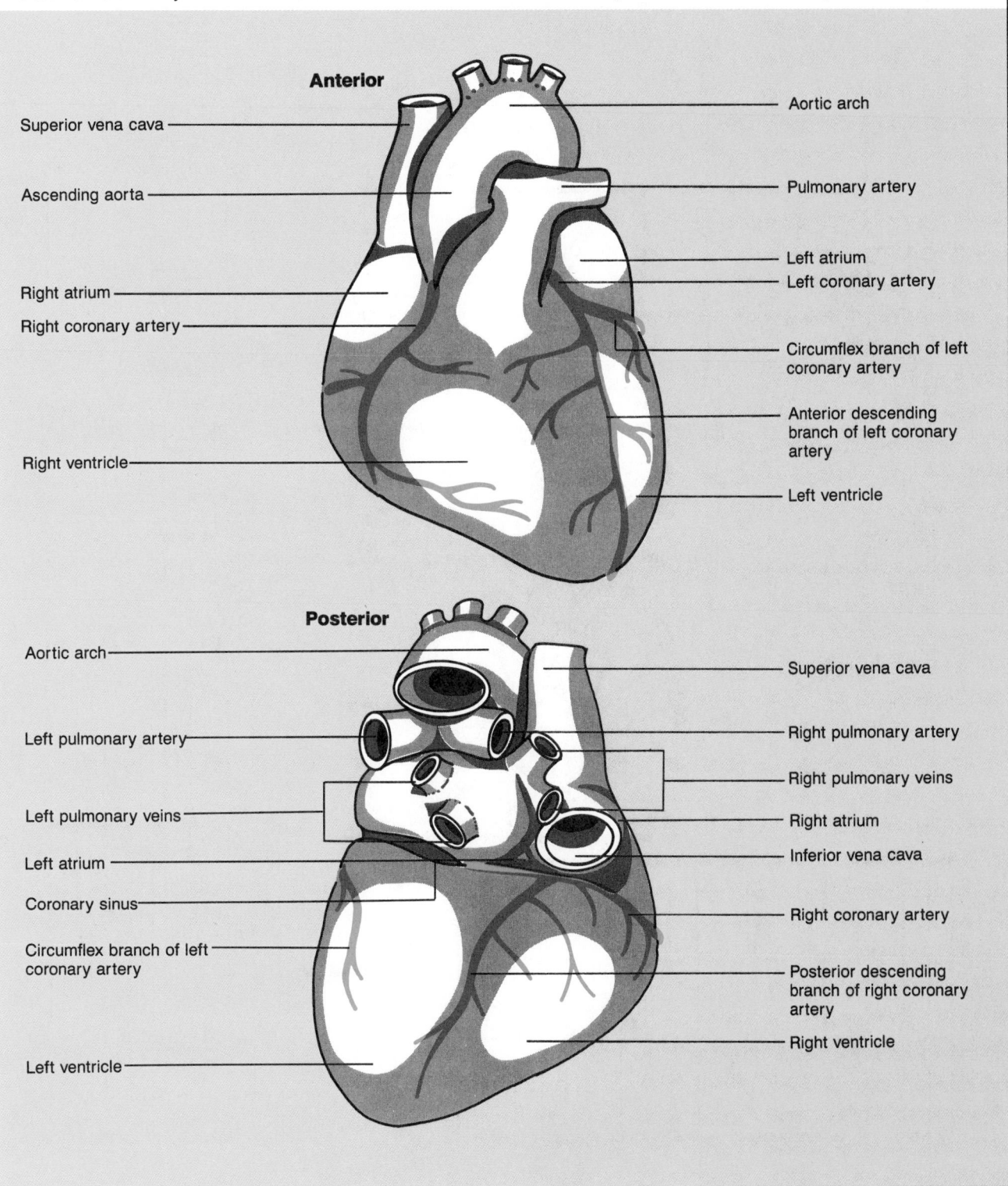

Anterior

Superior vena cava

Ascending aorta

Right atrium

Right coronary artery

Right ventricle

Aortic arch

Pulmonary artery

Left atrium

Left coronary artery

Circumflex branch of left coronary artery

Anterior descending branch of left coronary artery

Left ventricle

Posterior

Aortic arch

Left pulmonary artery

Left pulmonary veins

Left atrium

Coronary sinus

Circumflex branch of left coronary artery

Left ventricle

Superior vena cava

Right pulmonary artery

Right pulmonary veins

Right atrium

Inferior vena cava

Right coronary artery

Posterior descending branch of right coronary artery

Right ventricle

Electrical activity and the ECG

On an ECG tracing, electrical activity in the myocardium appears as a series of deflection points. Each deflection point—P, Q, R, S, T—corresponds to a specific area where electrical activity occurs. (Note: A U wave also may occur.)

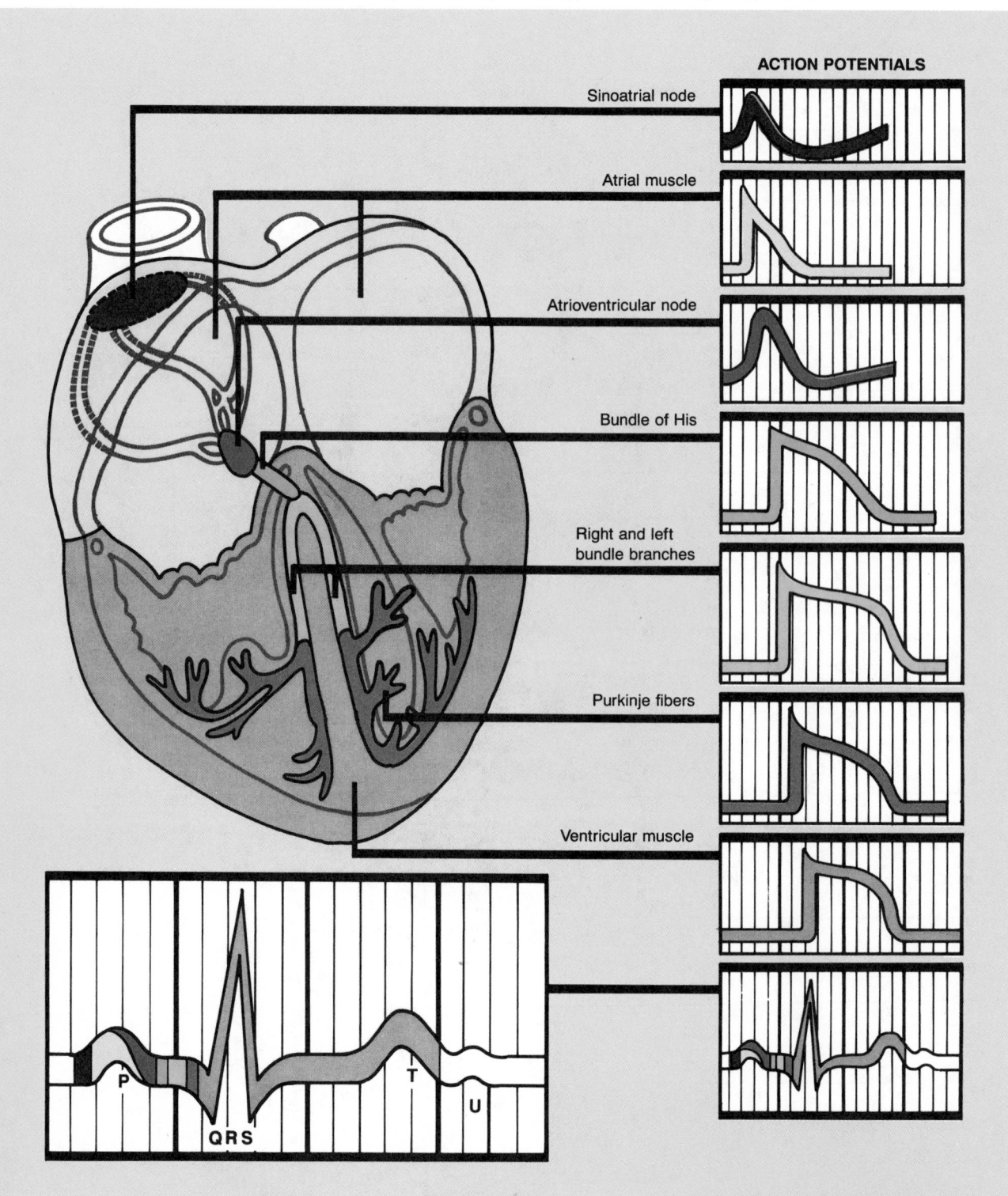

For each class, the chapter defines the uses, dosages, and adverse effects of the drugs as well as appropriate nursing care.

Chapter 31
Antianginal Agents

Chapter 31 presents the drugs used to treat angina: nitrates, beta blockers, and calcium channel blockers. To provide a framework for understanding these drugs, the chapter presents an overview of coronary blood flow and oxygen consumption and a survey of abnormalities that produce angina. Then it differentiates among the pharmacologic properties of the various classes of antianginal agents. The chapter also demonstrates how to apply the nursing process when caring for a patient receiving an antianginal agent.

Chapter 32
Antihypertensive Agents

Chapter 32 focuses on the agents used to treat hypertension, a disease that affects millions of Americans. Beginning with a brief review of the physiology of blood pressure, the chapter next defines the various types of hypertension. Then it discusses clinical assessments, nondrug therapies, and the stepped-care approach to hypertension management. The chapter presents the many types of sympatholytic agents, vasodilating agents, and angiotensin-converting enzyme (ACE) inhibitors. For each drug class, it shows how to use the nursing process to provide appropriate care.

Chapter 33
Diuretic Agents

Drugs that increase the renal excretion of water and electrolytes are the topic of Chapter 33. These diuretic agents are presented according to their classification: thiazide and thiazide-like diuretics, loop diuretics, potassium-sparing diuretics, osmotic diuretics, and other agents, such as carbonic anhydrase inhibitor and mercurial diuretics. After investigating the adverse effects of these agents, the chapter highlights related nursing care using the nursing process.

Chapter 34
Antilipemic Agents

Chapter 34 examines the antilipemic agents, which are used to lower abnormally high blood lipid levels. It begins with an overview of the composition and role of lipids in the body. Then it describes the clinical conditions managed with bile sequestering agents, fibric acid derivatives, and cholesterol synthesis inhibitors. It concludes with a discussion of nursing care as it relates to antilipemic agent therapy.

CARDIAC GLYCOSIDE AGENTS AND BIPYRIDINES

OBJECTIVES

After reading and studying this chapter, the student should be able to:

1. Describe the clinical indications of the cardiac glycosides, digoxin and digitoxin, and the bipyridine amrinone lactate.

2. Identify conditions that contraindicate or require cautious use of cardiac glycosides and bipyridines.

3. Differentiate between the pharmacokinetic properties of digoxin and digitoxin.

4. Describe the actions of cardiac glycosides and bipyridines in treating congestive heart failure.

5. Explain why digitalis toxicity commonly occurs, and describe its signs and symptoms.

6. Describe how to apply the nursing process when caring for a patient receiving a cardiac glycoside or bipyridine.

INTRODUCTION

Cardiac glycosides (digitalis compounds) and bipyridines increase the force of cardiac contraction; that is, they exert a positive inotropic effect. For this reason, they also are called inotropic agents. Cardiac glycosides also slow the heart rate (a negative chronotropic effect) and slow electrical impulse conduction through the atrioventricular (AV) node (a negative dromotropic effect). These actions make cardiac glycosides and bipyridines useful in treating congestive heart failure and make cardiac glycosides useful in treating certain supraventricular arrhythmias.

To understand how these agents improve congestive heart failure, the nurse must comprehend several key concepts in cardiovascular physiology. Cardiac output (the amount of blood pumped from the heart in 1 minute) is determined by multiplying the stroke volume (the amount of blood ejected by the left ventricle with each contraction) by the heart rate (the number of beats per minute). Stroke volume is affected by myocardial contractility, preload, and afterload. Heart rate is affected by the autonomic nervous system, the ability of the heart to function, and various drugs. The amount of blood returned to the right atrium is called the venous return. Usually, the venous return equals the cardiac output. At times, however, they differ because of blood storage in areas of circulation. This blood volume determines the length of ventricular fibers in the left ventricule at the end of diastole, which is known as the preload. Afterload refers to the impedance of the forward flow of blood against which the left ventricle must contract. The tone of the arterial tree (systemic vascular resistance) contributes significantly to afterload. Preload helps determine the force of ventricular contractions. This principle forms the basis of Starling's law of the heart: Within the limits of the heart, the greater the length of the stretched fibers, the stronger the contraction.

Congestive heart failure results from a decrease in cardiac output. It typically produces decreased myocardial contractility and increased preload and afterload. To try to maintain vital organ perfusion, the body uses compensatory mechanisms: It increases sympathetic tone, causes ventricular hypertrophy (increased cardiac muscle size), and increases renin-angiotensin-aldosterone system activity. Although these mechanisms help maintain adequate perfusion, they increase myocardial work. Eventually, the patient's condition worsens and drug treatment becomes necessary.

When this occurs, the physician may prescribe cardiac glycosides or bipyridines to improve myocardial contractility or diuretics or vasodilators to improve preload and afterload. However, the usefulness of cardiac glycosides and bipyridines to treat congestive heart failure is controversial, compared to the usefulness of diuretics and angiotensin-converting enzyme (ACE) inhibitors. The ideal positive inotropic agent should (1) be effective when given orally, (2) increase the force of contraction without pro-

---

SELECTED NURSING DIAGNOSES

Cardiac glycoside agents and bipyridines

The following nursing diagnoses address representative problems and etiologies that a nurse may encounter when caring for a patient who is receiving a cardiac glycoside agent or bipyridine. Some of these nursing diagnoses contain generalized etiologies, which the nurse must individualize based on the patient's needs. (For some common nursing diagnoses and related interventions for each drug class, see the "Nursing Process Application" sections of this chapter.)

- Altered health maintenance related to ineffectiveness of the prescribed cardiac glycoside or bipyridine
- Altered protection related to eosinophilia caused by the cardiac glycoside
- Altered protection related to amrinone-induced thrombocytopenia
- Altered thought processes related to confusion caused by a cardiac glycoside
- Decreased cardiac output related to the adverse effects of a cardiac glycoside
- Diarrhea related to the adverse GI effects of the cardiac glycoside
- Hyperthermia related to a hypersensitivity reaction to the cardiac glycoside or bipyridine
- Knowledge deficit related to the prescribed cardiac glycoside or bipyridine
- Noncompliance related to adverse drug reactions

- Pain related to abdominal or chest pain caused by a cardiac glycoside or bipyridine
- Potential activity intolerance related to weakness caused by a cardiac glycoside
- Potential fluid volume deficit related to the adverse GI effects of a cardiac glycoside or bipyridine
- Potential for injury related to a preexisting condition that contraindicates the use of a cardiac glycoside or bipyridine
- Potential for injury related to a preexisting condition that requires cautious use of a cardiac glycoside or bipyridine
- Potential for injury related to adverse drug reactions
- Potential for injury related to drug interactions
- Sensory-perceptual alterations (visual) related to the central nervous system effects of a cardiac glycoside
- Sleep pattern disturbance related to insomnia caused by digitalis toxicity

---

ducing adverse electrophysiologic effects, (3) decrease peripheral vascular resistance and myocardial oxygen consumption, (4) produce improvement without drug tolerance, (5) improve patient symptoms and life expectancy, and (6) cause no serious adverse drug reactions. Although cardiac glycosides and bipyridines meet some of these criteria, they do not meet all of them.

In supraventricular arrhythmias (such as atrial fibrillation or atrial flutter), cardiac glycosides are used to slow electrical impulse conduction through the AV node. By doing so, they slow the ventricular rate. Cardiac glycosides commonly are used with quinidine in these disorders. They are used to slow the ventricular response while quinidine is used to convert the abnormal rhythm to a normal sinus rhythm.

For a summary of representative drugs, see *Selected major drugs: Cardiac glycoside agents and bipyridines,* page 481. For a listing of applicable nursing diagnoses that the nurse may formulate when caring for a patient receiving these agents, see *Selected nursing diagnoses: Cardiac glycoside agents and bipyridines.* For detailed information on applying the nursing process, see Chapter 6, The Nursing Process and Drug Therapy.

CARDIAC GLYCOSIDES

Cardiac glycosides are a group of drugs composed of digitalis, a substance that occurs naturally in the foxglove plant, certain toads, and squill (a marine plant). Also called digitalis compounds, these drugs are structurally similar. They each have a ring (aglycone), which produces pharmacologic activity, and different sugar molecules, which modify the drug's properties. Digoxin and digitoxin are the two most frequently used cardiac glycosides. Others, such as deslanoside, oubain, and digitalis leaf, rarely are used.

The therapeutic range for cardiac glycosides is relatively narrow; therapeutic dosages are close to toxic ones. Fortunately, reliable assays are now available to measure the serum concentrations of digoxin and digitoxin, which has contributed to safer use of these drugs. Despite widespread use of cardiac glycosides for more than 200 years, controversy still exists about their efficacy and safety.

PHARMACOKINETICS

Although the pharmacotherapeutic properties of digoxin and digitoxin are the same, the pharmacokinetic properties differ significantly.

Absorption, distribution, metabolism, excretion

The intestinal absorption of digoxin varies greatly, especially among products from different manufacturers. Digoxin absorption ranges from 60% to 80% in tablet form, from 70% to 85% in elixir form, and from 90% to 100% in capsule form. When taken with meals, the absorption rate may slow, but the extent of absorption rarely is affected, except when the drug is consumed with a high-bran meal, which decreases the amount of drug absorbed.

Once absorbed or given by intravenous (I.V.) injection, digoxin takes about 8 hours to reach equilibrium at the tissue-binding sites. This is known as the distribution phase of the drug. Digoxin is distributed widely throughout the body, is bound extensively to skeletal muscles, and does not penetrate well into body fat. About 20% to 30% of digoxin in the plasma binds to albumin. This distribution volume can be affected by factors that may alter tissue- or plasma- binding sites, such as renal failure, heart failure, hypoalbuminemia, or age extremes. A patient affected by these factors may require a modification of the usual loading dose. (For more information on loading doses, see the "Drug excretion" section of Chapter 2, Pharmacokinetics.)

A small percentage of digoxin is metabolized by the liver and by gastrointestinal (GI) flora. Several metabolites have been identified, some of which have pharmacologic activity.

The remaining digoxin is eliminated by the kidneys as unchanged drug. In a patient with normal renal function, digoxin's half-life is 36 hours. A patient with renal dysfunction will require a decreased digoxin dosage.

Because it is more lipid soluble than digoxin, oral digitoxin is absorbed more completely (90% to 100%). It is distributed to most body tissues. With therapeutic plasma concentrations, 90% of digitoxin in the blood is bound to plasma proteins, primarily albumin. Digitoxin is metabolized extensively in the liver to inactive metabolites. About 8% of the drug is converted to digoxin. The inactive and active metabolites are eliminated by the kidneys. The half-life of digitoxin is about 7 days.

Onset, peak, duration

After an oral dose, the onset of action ranges from 30 minutes to 2 hours for digoxin, and from 1 to 6 hours for digitoxin. With an I.V. dose, the onset may occur within 5 to 30 minutes for digoxin, and within 30 minutes to 2 hours for digitoxin, depending on the infusion rate.

The peak effect of digoxin occurs 2 to 6 hours after an oral dose and 1 to 4 hours after an I.V. dose. The peak effect of digitoxin occurs 6 to 12 hours after an oral dose and 4 to 8 hours after an I.V. dose. The effects of cardiac glycosides correspond to the concentration of unbound drug at receptor sites in the tissue. Therefore, the peak serum concentration level may be misleading, especially if the serum sample is taken before the drug has had sufficient time to distribute adequately to the tissues.

The duration of action varies with the patient's ability to eliminate the drug. The average duration for digoxin is 2 to 6 days with a half-life of 36 hours. For digitoxin, the average duration is 2 to 3 weeks with a half-life of 5 to 7 days.

Because cadiac glycosides have long half-lives, a patient would need several days of drug therapy before achieving a therapeutic blood level. (For more information, see *Steady-state dosing* in Chapter 2, Pharmacokinetics.) To achieve a therapeutic blood level more rapidly, the patient may receive a loading, or digitalizing, dose. (For details, see *Adult dosage considerations for cardiac glycosides*, and *Pediatric dosage considerations for cardiac glycosides*, page 474.)

The use of assays to measure digoxin and digitoxin serum concentrations has reduced the incidence of digitalis toxicity. To interpret them correctly, however, serum samples must be taken after the drug has distributed to the tissues. If the serum is taken during the distribution phase of the drug, the assay will show a falsely elevated serum concentration. Serum samples should be taken at least 6 hours after an I.V. dose and 8 hours after an oral dose. In most cases, a serum sample is taken immediately before the daily maintenance dosage is given, about 24 hours after the last dose.

The therapeutic serum concentration for digoxin usually is 0.5 to 2 ng/ml (nanogram per milliliter); for digitoxin, 14 to 26 ng/ml. However, the serum concentration must be interpreted with caution. Several conditions may lead to digoxin-like immunoreactive substances (DLIS) in the blood, such as renal dysfunction, pregnancy, hepatic failure, preeclampsia, and young age (neonates and infants). In a patient with one of these conditions, endogenous DLIS may interfere with accurate determination of serum digoxin concentrations.

PHARMACODYNAMICS

Digoxin and digitoxin produce positive inotropic effects and negative chronotropic and dromotropic effects.

Mechanism of action

Cardiac glycosides are used to treat congestive heart failure because of their positive inotropic action, which may result from three mechanisms. First, they may bind to and inhibit the sodium-potassium-adenosine triphosphatase (ATPase) pump, which normally maintains the sodium and potassium concentration differences across the cell membrane. Pump inhibition may increase intracellular sodium, which then is exchanged for calcium. This makes increased intracellular calcium available to the contractile elements of the myocardium, leading to enhanced force of contraction.

Adult dosage considerations for cardiac glycosides

Because the half-lives of digoxin (36 hours) and digitoxin (7 days) are relatively long, a loading dose (or digitalizing dose) must be given to reach the therapeutic steady state concentration rapidly, followed by regular maintenance dosages. Specific dosage considerations vary, depending on whether the patient must receive a loading dose or a maintenance dosage.

Loading (digitalizing) dose

- Expect to administer a digoxin loading dose that is 10 to 15 mcg/kg of the patient's ideal or lean body weight.
- Administer the drug I.V. or P.O. in divided doses.
- Give one-half of the loading dose initially, followed by one-quarter of the dose 3 to 6 hours later, and then by the remainder of the dose if the patient does not respond 3 to 6 hours after the second dose.
- Expect to reduce the loading dose of digoxin if the patient has a condition that affects drug distribution to the receptor site, such as renal dysfunction or use of quinidine.
- Give the digitoxin loading dose as prescribed. The usual loading dose is 0.6 mg initially, followed by 0.4 mg, then 0.2 mg every 4 to 6 hours.

Maintenance dosage

- Know that the maintenance dosage of a cardiac glycoside is determined by its half-life. The most common maintenance dosage of digoxin is 0.25 mg P.O. daily; of digitoxin, 0.15 mg P.O. daily.
- Expect to use a lower maintenance dosage of digoxin in a patient with renal dysfunction to avoid toxicity.
- Administer a lower maintenance dosage to an elderly patient because of reduced renal function and increased drug sensitivity.
- Continue to monitor the patient after the maintenance dosage is discontinued because the cardiac glycoside's half-life determines the amount of time needed before the drug effect is diminished. In a patient with normal renal function, digoxin requires 6 to 8 days before the drug effect is eliminated completely; digitoxin, 3 to 5 weeks.

Some evidence suggests that cardiac glycosides may enhance the movement of calcium into the myocardial cell. Other evidence points to a third mechanism for the inotropic effect: Cardiac glycosides may stimulate the release, or block the reuptake, of norepinephrine at the adrenergic nerve terminal.

Cardiac glycosides also have electrophysiologic properties that make them useful in managing specific supraventricular arrhythmias. They affect the autonomic nervous system by stimulating the parasympathetic division, which increases vagal tone. This vagal effect slows the heart rate, increases the refractory period, and slows conduction through the AV node and junctional tissue.

Because of this action, cardiac glycosides must be used with caution in patients with atrial fibrillation or flutter and an anomalous conduction pathway, such as in Wolff-Parkinson-White syndrome. By slowing conduction through the normal pathway, cardiac glycosides allow more impulses to be conducted through the anomalous (abnormal) pathway, leading to a rapid ventricular response and an unstable hemodynamic situation in these patients.

The effects of cardiac glycosides are antagonized by conditions that reduce vagal tone or enhance sympathetic activity, such as atropine use, exercise, fever, thyrotoxicosis, or decompensated heart failure.

PHARMACOTHERAPEUTICS

Cardiac glycosides are prescribed to treat congestive heart failure, atrial fibrillation and flutter, and paroxysmal atrial tachycardia. These agents are beneficial in patients with dilated failing hearts, impaired systolic function, or a third heart sound (S_3). They also are helpful in patients with heart failure complicated by supraventricular tachyarrhythmias, such as atrial fibrillation. In patients with heart failure caused by diastolic dysfunction, cardiac glycosides are beneficial only if a supraventricular arrhythmia also is present.

Cardiac glycosides also may improve cardiac hemodynamics when used with diuretics or vasodilators in managing mild to moderate heart failure. In patients with acute myocardial infarction (MI), cardiac glycosides must be used with caution. The risk of adverse effects on cardiac rhythm and increasing myocardial oxygen consumption may outweigh the potential benefits in a patient who does not have supraventricular arrhythmias. However, these agents clearly are indicated in a patient with an MI who has atrial fibrillation and a rapid ventricular response.

Although cardiac glycosides may cause arrhythmias, they have a role as antiarrhythmic agents. These drugs slow conduction and increase the refractory period in the specialized conducting tissue in the heart, which decreases the heart rate. Therefore, cardiac glycosides are useful in controlling the rapid ventricular rates associated with atrial fibrillation or atrial flutter. Supraventricular arrhythmias of the reentrant type, such as paroxysmal supraventricular tachycardia, usually are treated with verapamil. However, cardiac glycosides may be used if the patient has a ventricular dysfunction that could worsen with administration of verapamil or a beta blocker.

Because the cardiac glycosides have long half-lives, a loading dose must be given to a patient who requires immediate drug effects, as in superventricular arrhythmia. Without a loading dose, the drug takes three half-lives to reach 88% of its steady state concentration. For example,

Pediatric dosage considerations for cardiac glycosides

For a pediatric patient, loading and maintenance dosage considerations depend on the cardiac glycoside to be administered and the patient's age.

DIGOXIN

- Know that an I.V. loading dose is 80% of an oral loading dose.
- Divide the loading dose and give half the total followed by one-quarter after 4 hours and one-quarter after 8 hours.
- Be aware that loading and maintenance dosages for children are based on age and weight as shown in the chart below.

Age	Loading dose (oral)	Daily maintenance dosage
Under age 1 month (premature neonate)	20 to 30 mcg/kg	20% to 30% of loading dose
Under age 1 month (full-term neonate)	25 to 35 mcg/kg	25% to 35% of loading dose
Ages 1 to 24 months	35 to 60 mcg/kg	25% to 35% of loading dose
Ages 2 to 5	30 to 40 mcg/kg	25% to 35% of loading dose
Ages 5 to 10	20 to 35 mcg/kg	25% to 35% of loading dose
Over age 10	10 to 15 mcg/kg	25% to 35% of loading dose

DIGITOXIN

- Divide the loading dose into three or four portions, and give each portion at 6- to 8-hour intervals.
- Be aware that loading and maintenance dosages for children are based on age and weight as shown in the chart below.

Age	Loading dose (oral)	Daily maintenance dosage
Under age 1	45 mcg/kg	10% of loading dose
Ages 1 to 2	40 mcg/kg	10% of loading dose
Over age 2	30 mcg/kg or 750 mcg/m²	10% of loading dose

for a patient receiving a usual daily maintenance dosage of digoxin, steady state concentration would be reached in 7 days; for one receiving digitoxin, in nearly 1 month. If the maintenance dosage of either drug is changed, the patient requires five half-lives before reaching a new steady state concentration.

digoxin (Lanoxin, Lanoxicaps). This drug is the most commonly used cardiac glycoside. Its bioavailability in capsules and elixirs is slightly higher than in tablets, so dosages for these forms are slightly lower. Digoxin is used to treat heart failure, atrial fibrillation, atrial flutter, and paroxysmal atrial tachycardia.
Usual adult dosage: 0.75 to 1.25 mg P.O. or 0.5 to 1 mg I.V. as a loading dose; 0.125 mg to 0.5 mg P.O. as a daily maintenance dosage. For patients with supraventricular arrhythmias, the dosage should be titrated to control the ventricular rate and usually is higher than that used to treat heart failure. I.M. injection of digoxin is not recommended because it causes severe pain at the injection site and increased serum creatine phosphokinase (CPK), which complicates interpretation of enzyme levels.
Usual pediatric dosage: 15 to 60 mcg/kg P.O. or I.V. as a loading dose; 25% to 35% of the loading dose as a daily maintenance dosage, given in two divided doses to avoid abnormally high serum concentrations.

digitoxin (Crystodigin). This cardiac glycoside is used to treat heart failure, atrial fibrillation, atrial flutter, and supraventricular tachycardia. It rarely is used because it has a long half-life, which prolongs the duration of adverse effects. However, it may be prescribed when digoxin is contraindicated because of renal failure. It is available in 0.05-, 0.1-, 0.15-, and 0.2-mg tablets.
Usual adult dosage: for slow digitalization, a loading dose of 0.2 mg P.O. b.i.d. for 4 days, followed by a maintenance dosage of 0.05 to 0.3 mg P.O. daily; for rapid digitalization, a loading dose of 0.6 mg P.O. initially, followed by 0.4 mg and then 0.2 mg at 4- to 6-hour intervals, followed by a maintenance dosage of 0.05 to 0.3 mg P.O. daily. The most common maintenance dosage is 0.15 mg P.O. daily.
Usual pediatric dosage: 0.03 to 0.045 mcg/kg P.O. as a loading dose, depending on the patient's age; 10% of the loading dose as a daily maintenance dosage.

Drug interactions
Many drugs can interact with cardiac glycosides. Some drugs reduce their absorption, which can reduce their therapeutic effect; others enhance their absorption or pharmacologic effects, which can lead to toxicity.

For example, quinidine may double a patient's serum digoxin concentration because quinidine decreases the digoxin distribution volume and elimination rate. Therefore,

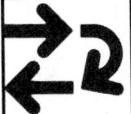

DRUG INTERACTIONS

Cardiac glycosides

Digoxin and digitoxin interact with several drugs. The interactions may result in decreased absorption, decreased effect, increased effect (digitalis toxicity), or arrhythmias.

DRUG	INTERACTING DRUGS	POSSIBLE EFFECTS	NURSING IMPLICATIONS
digoxin, digitoxin	rifampin, barbiturates, phenytoin (digitoxin only), cholestyramine resin, antacids, kaolin-pectin, sulfasalazine	Decrease digoxin or digitoxin effect	• Monitor the patient for indications of effectiveness: decreased edema and jugular venous distention, weight loss, elimination of S_3 and basilar crackles (rales), increased urine output, improvement in oxygenation and pulse rate and rhythm, and increased well-being. • Increase the cardiac glycoside dosage, if prescribed.
	calcium preparations, quinidine, verapamil, anticholinergics, amiodarone, spironolactone, hydroxychloroquin	Cause digitalis toxicity	• Monitor the patient for signs and symptoms of digitalis toxicity: gastrointestinal, neurologic, and cardiac disturbances. • Monitor the patient's ECG for arrhythmias or atrioventricular block.
	amphotericin B, potassium-wasting diuretics, steroids, broad-spectrum penicillins	Cause hypokalemia, digitalis toxicity	• Monitor the patient for signs and symptoms of hypokalemia: drowsiness, hypoperistalsis, depression, paresthesia, muscle weakness, anorexia, depressed reflexes, orthostatic hypotension, and polyuria. • Monitor the patient's serum digoxin or digitoxin level. • Monitor the patient's serum potassium level and administer a potassium supplement as prescribed; encourage the ingestion of dietary potassium.
	beta-adrenergic blockers	Produce excessive bradycardia and arrhythmias	• Monitor the patient's pulse rate frequently. • Monitor the patient's ECG as indicated. • Have resuscitation equipment available.
	succinylcholine, thyroid preparations	Cause arrhythmias	• Monitor the patient's pulse rate frequently. • Monitor the patient's ECG as indicated.

the digoxin dosage usually is decreased by 50% when quinidine is added to the patient's regimen.

Verapamil inhibits electrical impulse conduction through the AV node, thereby enhancing the pharmacologic effect of the cardiac glycoside. However, studies of other calcium channel blockers (nifedipine, isradipine, and diltiazem) have found no consistent pharmacokinetic or clinically significant pharmacodynamic interaction with cardiac glycosides.

Because intestinal flora plays a role in cardiac glycoside metabolism, antibiotics that influence intestinal flora may affect serum digoxin concentrations. (For more information, see *Drug interactions: Cardiac glycosides.*)

ADVERSE DRUG REACTIONS

Because cardiac glycosides have a narrow therapeutic index, they may produce digitalis toxicity. To prevent digitalis toxicity, the dosage should be individualized based on the patient's serum digitalis concentration. The therapeutic serum concentration of digoxin typically ranges from 0.5 to 2 ng/ml; of digitoxin, from 14 to 26 ng/ml. However, patients vary greatly in their response to cardiac glycosides; one patient may exhibit toxicity when the serum concentration falls within the therapeutic range, whereas another may require serum concentrations above the therapeutic range to achieve the desired effect.

The following conditions may predispose a patient to digitalis toxicity: hypokalemia, hypomagnesemia, hypothyroidism, hypoxemia, advanced myocardial disease, active myocardial ischemia, and altered autonomic (increased

Signs and symptoms of digitalis toxicity

Digitalis toxicity affects several body systems, most commonly the gastrointestinal tract. The most common early symptoms are anorexia, nausea, vomiting, and diarrhea.

Gastrointestinal

- anorexia
- nausea
- vomiting
- diarrhea
- abdominal pain

Neurologic

- headache
- restlessness
- irritability
- depression
- personality change
- lassitude
- confusion
- disorientation
- insomnia
- psychosis
- seizures
- coma
- blurred vision or blue-yellow color blindness
- flickering lights
- white borders on dark objects
- colored dots

Cardiac

- atrial arrhythmias
- ventricular arrhythmias
- sinoatrial arrest or block
- accelerated junctional rhythms
- atrial tachycardia with atrioventricular (AV) block
- second-degree AV block (Wenckebach)
- third-degree AV block (complete)

vagal) tone. Elevated sympathetic tone and hyperthyroidism may cause resistance to the drug's effect.

The effects of digoxin and digitoxin toxicity are similar and are known as digitalis toxicity. The signs and symptoms of digitalis toxicity fall primarily into three categories: GI, neurologic, and cardiac. (For a list of the most common ones, see *Signs and symptoms of digitalis toxicity*.) The GI and neurologic symptoms may precede or follow the potentially life-threatening cardiac symptoms. The GI symptoms are nonspecific and may result from the central nervous system (CNS) action of cardiac glycosides rather than local irritation of the intestinal mucosa. The CNS effects of cardiac glycosides vary widely and may produce neurologic, psychiatric, or visual changes.

Digitalis toxicity also can cause arrhythmias. Changes in automaticity may lead to increased atrial or ventricular ectopy (premature contractions). Effects on the sinoatrial (SA) or AV node may result in tachycardia or bradycardia. For patients who receive cardiac glycosides for atrial fibrillation, toxicity may manifest itself as regularization of the rate. Three mechanisms may account for this regularization: complete AV block with an AV junctional or ventricular escape rhythm, ventricular tachycardia, or accelerated junctional rhythm.

The drug's half-life affects the duration of adverse reactions. Because digoxin has a shorter half-life, many physicians prefer using it over digitoxin.

Treatment of digitalis toxicity includes cardiac glycoside discontinuation, correction of predisposing factors, and symptomatic treatment. It also may include administration of digoxin-immune Fab (Digibind), which contains antigen-binding (Fab) fragments that reverse toxicity by binding with digitalis. (For details, see *Treatment of digitalis toxicity with digoxin-immune Fab*.)

Less common and less severe adverse reactions to cardiac glycosides include gynecomastia and hypersensitivity reactions, such as rash, fever, and eosinophilia.

NURSING PROCESS APPLICATION

The following information assists the nurse in caring for a patient who is receiving a cardiac glycoside.

Assessment

- Review the patient's history for a preexisting condition that contraindicates the use of a cardiac glycoside, such as ventricular fibrillation, digitalis toxicity, or known hypersensitivity to these drugs.
- Review the patient's history for a preexisting condition that requires cautious use of a cardiac glycoside, such as renal failure, severe pulmonary disease, hypoxia, acute myocardial infarction, severe heart failure, damaged myocardium, incomplete heart block, frequent ventricular premature contractions, or ventricular tachycardia.
- Assess the patient for adverse reactions to the prescribed cardiac glycoside. Be particularly alert for GI, neurologic, or cardiac signs of digitalis toxicity, such as anorexia, nausea, vomiting, headache, restlessness, personality change, atrial arrhythmias, ventricular arrhythmias, and accelerated junctional rhythms.
- Review the patient's medication history to identify the use of drugs that may interact with the prescribed cardiac glycoside, such as barbiturates, antacids, antineoplastics, potassium-wasting diuretics, or penicillins.
- Assess the effectiveness of the prescribed cardiac glycoside periodically.

• Evaluate the patient for fluid volume deficit if nausea, vomiting, anorexia, or diarrhea occur.

• Assess the patient for sensory-perceptual alterations if digitalis toxicity is suspected.

• Monitor the patient for decreased cardiac output if arrhythmias occur.

• Evaluate the patient's and family's knowledge about the prescribed cardiac glycoside.

Nursing diagnoses

The following examples represent appropriate nursing diagnoses for a patient receiving a cardiac glycoside.

• Potential for injury related to a preexisting condition that contraindicates the use of a cardiac glycoside

• Potential for injury related to a preexisting condition that requires cautious use of a cardiac glycoside

• Potential for injury related to adverse drug reactions

• Potential fluid volume deficit related to the adverse GI effects of a cardiac glycoside

• Sensory-perceptual alterations (visual) related to the adverse CNS effects of a cardiac glycoside

• Decreased cardiac output related to the adverse effects of a cardiac glycoside

• Knowledge deficit related to the prescribed cardiac glycoside

Planning and implementation

• Do not administer a cardiac glycoside to a patient with a condition that contraindicates its use.

• Administer a cardiac glycoside cautiously to a patient at risk because of a preexisting condition.

• Monitor the patient regularly for adverse drug reactions.

• *Assess the patient's baseline apical heart rate and rhythm before starting cardiac glycoside therapy; thereafter, take the apical rate before administering each dose. Assess the apical pulse because weak or irregular beats may not be palpable at the radial pulse. Withhold the drug and notify the physician if the pulse rate is below 60 beats/minute or the minimum specified by the physician.*

• Monitor for electrolyte imbalance and increased creatinine level to detect renal dysfunction, especially in a patient receiving digoxin. Monitor liver function studies to detect liver dysfunction in a patient receiving digitoxin.

• *Monitor the patient's serum digoxin or digitoxin levels as prescribed. To avoid a falsely elevated serum level, draw blood at least 8 hours after the last oral dose and preferably immediately before administering the daily maintenance dosage (about 24 hours after the last dose).*

• *Monitor serum digoxin levels carefully in neonates, infants, and patients with such conditions as renal dysfunction, pregnancy, hepatic failure, and preeclampsia because their blood may contain DLIS, which interferes with the levels.*

Treatment of digitalis toxicity with digoxin-immune Fab

The development of digoxin-immune Fab (Digibind) revolutionized the treatment of life-threatening digitalis toxicity. Before digoxin-immune Fab was available, management of digitalis toxicity consisted primarily of supportive treatment. Bradyarrhythmia and atrioventricular block were managed with temporary pacemakers; ventricular ectopy, with lidocaine (Xylocaine) or phenytoin (Dilantin). Charcoal was administered orally to enhance drug elimination, but was only marginally successful.

Digoxin-immune Fab is derived from digoxin antibodies in sheep. It distributes rapidly and binds with digoxin, making it inactive. Then the bound complex is excreted by the kidneys. (Excretion is delayed in a patient with renal insufficiency.) Digoxin-immune Fab reverses the inotropic and arrhythmogenic properties of digoxin as well as digitoxin.

Because of its extremely high cost, however, digoxin-immune Fab is reserved for patients with life-threatening complications of digitalis toxicity, such as ventricular tachycardia, ventricular fibrillation, progressive bradyarrhythmias, or paroxysmal atrial tachycardia that does not respond to other therapies. These complications typically result from ingestion of more than 10 mg of digoxin in an adult (4 mg in a child), which lead to digoxin concentrations of 10 ng/ml and cardiac arrest. Digoxin-immune Fab also may be used in a patient with digitalis toxicity and elevated serum potassium concentration, because the prognosis is poor otherwise.

Before digoxin-immune Fab treatment, a patient with a known allergy or previous exposure to digoxin-immune Fab or other sheep-derived preparations should undergo skin testing to check for a hypersensitivity reaction to the drug. The digoxin-immune Fab dosage should be based on the amount of digoxin in the patient's body, which can be estimated from the number of tablets consumed or the steady-state concentration of digoxin in the serum. During digoxin-immune Fab treatment, epinephrine should be available at the bedside in case the patient develops an anaphylactic reaction to this drug.

• Expect to adjust the loading dose as prescribed for a pediatric or geriatric patient or one with renal failure, heart failure, or hypoalbuminemia, because these conditions affect the volume of drug distribution.

• Expect to administer a reduced dosage as prescribed for a patient with renal dysfunction.

• Expect to administer a reduced dosage of digoxin capsules or elixir as prescribed because these drug forms have a higher bioavailability than tablets.

• *Do not administer digoxin I.M. because it causes severe pain at the injection site and increases serum CPK levels, which complicates interpretation of enzyme elevation.*

• Administer digoxin in two divided doses as prescribed for maintenance in a pediatric patient to avoid a high peak serum concentration.

• *Do not administer concurrently any drugs that reduce digoxin absorption, such as antacids, kaolin, or pectin.*

• *Do not administer digoxin with meals because this slows the absorption rate.*

• Do not administer digoxin with a high-bran snack because it may decrease the amount of drug absorbed.

• Expect to administer cardiac glycosides I.V. when speed is essential, as in treating pulmonary edema, or when oral administration is impossible, as with vomiting or coma. As prescribed, administer the drug slowly (over 5 minutes), taking care to avoid extravasation, which can cause irritation, necrosis, and sloughing.

• Observe the patient closely for changes in cardiac glycoside effect, such as increased shortness of breath, edema, or digitalis toxicity, when antibiotics are prescribed. These drugs can alter intestinal flora and may affect the serum digoxin concentration.

• Expect to decrease the digoxin dosage by 50% when quinidine is added to the patient's drug regimen because quinidine decreases digoxin's volume of distribution and elimination rate.

• *Monitor for signs and symptoms of digitalis toxicity, such as GI, neurologic, and cardiac dysfunction, even in a patient whose serum drug level falls within the therapeutic range. Be especially alert for these signs in a patient with hypokalemia, hypomagnesemia, hypothyroidism, hypoxemia, advanced myocardial disease, active myocardial ischemia, or altered autonomic tone; these conditions increase tissue sensitivity to digoxin or digitoxin.*

• *Withhold the cardiac glycoside, notify the physician, and obtain a serum drug level as prescribed if digitalis toxicity is suspected.*

• Assess for signs of improvement in the patient's condition. Effective congestive heart failure therapy should produce decreased edema and jugular vein distention, weight loss, elimination of S_3 and basilar crackles (rales), increased urine output, improved oxygenation, improved heart rate and rhythm, and an increased sense of well-being.

• Measure the patient's daily fluid intake and output. Monitor for signs of fluid retention, including decreased urine output, jugular vein distention, edema, and weight gain. Weigh the patient daily before breakfast. Remember that 1 liter of fluid weighs approximately 1 kg.

• Notify the physician if the patient's condition does not improve or if adverse reactions occur.

• Monitor for the following signs of dehydration if the patient develops nausea, vomiting, diarrhea, or anorexia from digitalis toxicity: concentrated urine that is decreased in amount, poor skin turgor, dry mucous membranes, and sudden weight loss.

• Prepare to begin I.V. therapy and electrolyte replacement if dehydration occurs.

• Notify the physician if the patient's hydration status changes.

• *Tell the patient to alert the nurse or physician if blurred vision or blue-yellow color blindness occurs. Sudden visual changes can signal digitalis toxicity.*

• Notify the physician at once if the patient reports visual changes. Withhold the prescribed cardiac glycoside and obtain a serum level, as prescribed.

• Take safety precautions if blurred vision occurs. For example, keep the bed in a low position and supervise patient ambulation.

• Monitor the patient's pulse rate and rhythm regularly to detect cardiovascular signs of digitalis toxicity.

• Notify the physician if arrhythmias occur during cardiac glycoside therapy. Withhold the prescribed cardiac glycoside and obtain a serum drug level, as ordered.

• Monitor the patient with arrhythmias closely for signs of decreased cardiac output, such as hypotension, tachycardia, shortness of breath, and pulmonary edema.

• *Prepare for emergency treatment as prescribed. Expect to administer an antiarrhythmic drug, such as phenytoin or lidocaine, to treat ventricular arrhythmias caused by a cardiac glycoside. Keep atropine readily available to treat decreased cardiac output caused by bradycardia or AV conduction arrhythmias. Prepare for cardioversion in a patient with atrial fibrillation or flutter and a rapid ventricular response that significantly decreases the cardiac output.*

Patient teaching

• Teach the patient and family the name, dose, frequency, action, and adverse effects of the prescribed cardiac glycoside.

• *Stress the importance of taking the drug exactly as prescribed, even when the patient feels well. Instruct the patient not to take an extra dose if one dose is missed, but to notify the physician.*

• *Demonstrate how to take a pulse. Advise the patient to report a pulse rate below 60, a change in pulse regularity, or signs and symptoms of digitalis toxicity.*

• Instruct the patient to recognize and report the following signs of congestive heart failure: persistent cough; shortness of breath; weight gain of 1 to 2 pounds (0.45 to 0.90 kg) in 1 day or 5 pounds (2.25 kg) in a week; swelling of ankles, legs, or hands; anorexia; nausea; and the sensation of abdominal fullness.

• Teach the patient who was treated for supraventricular arrhythmia to recognize and report signs of recurrence, such as a rapid heart rate (above 100 beats/minute), excessive fatigue, light-headedness, or chest pain.

• Encourage the patient to eat high-potassium foods (orange juice, bananas, spinach, cantaloupe, watermelon, dates, raisins, soybeans, apples, prunes, beans, potatoes, molasses, squash) unless the patient is taking a potassium-sparing diuretic, ACE inhibitor (such as captopril or enalapril), or a potassium supplement.

- *Instruct the patient to store the drug in a tightly covered, light-resistant container and to consult the physician before taking any other drugs, including over-the-counter ones.*
- Instruct the patient to consult with the pharmacist before each drug refill to ensure that the prescribed cardiac glycoside comes from the same manufacturer. Different formulations can display differences in bioavailability.
- Refer an elderly or debilitated patient without adequate home supervision to a home health agency to ensure safe administration of the prescribed cardiac glycoside. Take periodic pill counts to evaluate compliance and detect accidental overdose.
- Reassure the patient that the GI distress should subside and vision should return to normal when the drug is eliminated from the body.
- Advise the patient to call the physician to discuss concerns about cardiac glycoside therapy. Give the patient written instructions about the drug for home use.

Evaluation

The following examples represent appropriate evaluation statements for a patient receiving a cardiac glycoside.
- The patient has no conditions that contraindicate cardiac glycoside therapy.
- The patient exhibits no signs of complications in the preexisting condition linked to the prescribed cardiac glycoside.
- The patient experiences no adverse reactions to the prescribed cardiac glycoside.
- The patient maintains adequate hydration during cardiac glycoside therapy.
- The patient denies visual changes during cardiac glycoside therapy.
- The patient maintains normal cardiac output during cardiac glycoside therapy.
- The patient and family express an accurate understanding of the points taught about the prescribed cardiac glycoside.
- The patient correctly identifies signs and symptoms of digitalis toxicity and describes what to do if they occur.

BIPYRIDINES

The bipyridines are nonglycoside, noncatecholamine agents that are used to manage heart failure because of their positive inotropic effect. Currently, amrinone lactate is the only bipyridine available in the United States for treating heart failure.

PHARMACOKINETICS

Amrinone is administered I.V., distributed rapidly, and metabolized by the liver. It is excreted by the kidneys as amrinone (10% to 40%) and several other derivatives, including N-acetyl-amrinone and N-glycolyl-amrinone.

Amrinone is rapid acting, but has a short duration of action. After a single I.V. bolus dose of 0.5 to 1.5 mg/kg, cardiac output increases within 5 minutes. The peak effect occurs in about 10 minutes, decreasing by about half in 30 to 40 minutes. Residual effects continue for about 2 hours. Amrinone's half-life is 3.6 hours in stable patients and 6 hours in patients with congestive heart failure. The normal therapeutic plasma level of amrinone is approximately 0.5 to 7 mcg/ml.

PHARMACODYNAMICS

Amrinone improves cardiac output by increasing contractility and decreasing systemic vascular resistance (afterload) and venous return (preload). Although the mechanism of action has not been determined fully, amrinone probably increases intracellular cyclic adenosine monophosphate (cyclic AMP) levels, which facilitates calcium entry. It also relaxes the vascular smooth muscle. With increased cardiac output, renal blood flow improves and urine output increases. Amrinone's only effect on the conduction system is to facilitate AV nodal conduction.

PHARMACOTHERAPEUTICS

Amrinone is indicated for the short-term management of congestive heart failure in patients who have not responded adequately to treatment with digitalis preparations, diuretics, and vasodilators. The nurse should monitor the patient's hemodynamics closely.

amrinone lactate (Inocor). The only bipyridine clinically available, amrinone is administered I.V.
Usual adult dosage: 0.75 mg/kg I.V. over 2 to 3 minutes initially, followed by a maintenance dosage of 5 to 10 mcg/kg/minute by continuous I.V. infusion. An additional bolus of 0.75 mg/kg may be administered 30 minutes after therapy begins. The administration rate and duration of therapy depend on the patient's therapeutic responses and adverse reactions.

Drug interactions

Amrinone interacts negatively with disopyramide, causing hypotension. In a patient with atrial flutter or fibrillation with rapid ventricular response, concomitant therapy with amrinone and cardiac glycosides is recommended because amrinone may enhance AV conduction and increase the ventricular response rate.

ADVERSE DRUG REACTIONS

Adverse drug reactions are uncommon and usually occur only in patients receiving prolonged therapy. Amrinone can produce arrhythmias, thrombocytopenia, nausea, vomiting, abdominal pain, anorexia, fever, liver enzyme alterations, chest pain, and burning at the injection site. Mild increases in heart rate also may occur. These effects, however, occur in only a small percentage of patients. Excessive vasodilation may occur with amrinone therapy, producing hypotension, which requires a dosage reduction or discontinuation.

Patients on prolonged amrinone therapy have experienced hypersensitivity reactions to the drug. Signs and symptoms include pericarditis, pleuritis, and ascites.

NURSING PROCESS APPLICATION

The following information assists the nurse in caring for a patient who is receiving amrinone.

Assessment
• Review the patient's history for a preexisting condition that contraindicates the use of amrinone, such as known hypersensitivity to bipyridines or bisulfites or acute myocardial infarction.
• Review the patient's history for a preexisting condition that requires cautious use of amrinone, such as pregnancy or lactation.
• Assess the patient for adverse reactions to amrinone, such as arrhythmias, thrombocytopenia, nausea, vomiting, abdominal pain, anorexia, hypotension, or fever.
• Review the patient's medication history to identify the use of drugs that may interact with amrinone, such as disopyramide or cardiac glycosides.
• Assess the effectiveness of amrinone frequently.
• Evaluate the patient's and family's knowledge about amrinone.

Nursing diagnoses
The following examples represent appropriate nursing diagnoses for a patient receiving amrinone.
• Potential for injury related to a preexisting condition that contraindicates the use of amrinone
• Potential for injury related to a preexisting condition that requires cautious use of amrinone
• Potential for injury related to adverse drug reactions
• Knowledge deficit related to amrinone

Planning and implementation
• Do not administer amrinone to a patient with a condition that contraindicates its use.

• Administer amrinone cautiously to a patient at risk because of a preexisting condition.
• Monitor the patient regularly for adverse drug reactions.
• *Obtain baseline platelet counts and liver enzyme, electrolyte, blood urea nitrogen, and creatinine levels before starting amrinone therapy. Monitor these values throughout therapy.*
• Monitor the patient's heart rate and rhythm and blood pressure frequently to detect arrhythmias or hypotension. Also monitor the patient's ECG to detect arrhythmias. If the patient develops hypotension or arrhythmias, expect to decrease the amrinone dosage or discontinue the drug as prescribed.
• Take bleeding precautions for a patient with thrombocytopenia. This adverse reaction can be reversed by decreasing the amrinone dosage or discontinuing the drug as prescribed.
• *Measure blood pressure frequently to detect hypotension in a patient receiving amrinone and disopyramide concurrently.*
• *Dilute amrinone in normal saline solution before administration. Do not mix amrinone with dextrose because amrinone-dextrose solutions result in 11% to 13% activity loss after 24 hours. Use diluted solutions within 24 hours.*
• Administer I.V. infusions with an infusion pump. Amrinone produces burning but not tissue sloughing at the injection site; inject the drug using a central or peripheral line.
• Determine the effectiveness of amrinone therapy by monitoring the patient for increased blood pressure; decreased pulmonary venous congestion, pulmonary artery pressure, and pulmonary capillary wedge pressure; decreased systemic venous congestion and central venous pressure; increased urine output; decreased weight, peripheral edema, and dyspnea; and elimination of S_3 and basilar crackles.
• Notify the physician if the patient responds inadequately to amrinone or develops adverse drug reactions.

Patient teaching
• Teach the patient and family the name, dose, frequency, action, and adverse effects of amrinone.
• Instruct the patient to report any dyspnea, chest pain, palpitations, burning at injection site, nausea, vomiting, abdominal pain, or anorexia.

Evaluation
The following examples represent appropriate evaluation statements for a patient receiving amrinone.
• The patient has no conditions that contraindicate amrinone therapy.

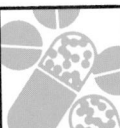

SELECTED MAJOR DRUGS

Cardiac glycoside agents and bipyridines

This table summarizes the major cardiac glycosides and bipyridines currently in clinical use.

DRUG	MAJOR INDICATIONS	USUAL ADULT DOSAGES	CONTRAINDICATIONS AND PRECAUTIONS
Cardiac glycosides			
digoxin	Congestive heart failure, supraventricular arrhythmias	Loading dose: 10 to 15 mcg/kg I.V. or P.O. Maintenance dosage: 0.125 to 0.5 mg daily I.V. or P.O.	• Know that digoxin is contraindicated in a patient with ventricular fibrillation, digitalis toxicity, or known hypersensitivity to digoxin. • Administer with extreme caution to a patient with idiopathic hypertrophic subaortic stenosis. • Administer with caution to a pregnant or lactating patient or one with renal failure, severe pulmonary disease, hypoxia, myxedema, acute myocardial infarction, severe heart failure, acute myocarditis, other myocardial damage, chronic constrictive pericarditis, incomplete heart block, increased carotid sinus sensitivity, frequent ventricular premature contractions, or ventricular tachycardia. Also administer cautiously to a hypertensive patient receiving the drug I.V. or one with atrial fibrillation or flutter and an anomalous conduction pathway disorder, such as Wolff-Parkinson-White syndrome.
digitoxin	Congestive heart failure, supraventricular arrhythmias	Loading dose for slow digitalization: 0.2 mg P.O. b.i.d. for 4 days Loading dose for rapid digitalization: 0.6 mg P.O. initially, followed by 0.4 mg and then 0.2 mg at 4- to 6-hour intervals Maintenance dosage: 0.05 to 0.3 mg P.O. daily	• Know that digitoxin is contraindicated in a patient with ventricular fibrillation, digitalis toxicity, or known hypersensitivity to digitoxin. • Administer with extreme caution to a patient with idiopathic hypertrophic subaortic stenosis. • Administer with caution to a pregnant or lactating patient or one with severe pulmonary disease, hypoxia, myxedema, acute myocardial infarction, severe heart failure, acute myocarditis, other myocardial damage, chronic constrictive pericarditis, incomplete heart block, increased carotid sinus sensitivity, frequent ventricular premature contractions, or ventricular tachycardia. Also administer cautiously to a hypertensive patient receiving the drug I.V. or one with atrial fibrillation or flutter and an anomalous conduction pathway disorder, such as Wolff-Parkinson-White syndrome.
Bipyridines			
amrinone	Congestive heart failure	Loading dose: 0.75 mg/kg I.V. over 2 to 3 minutes Maintenance dosage: 5 to 10 mcg/kg/minute by continuous I.V. infusion	• Know that amrinone is contraindicated in a patient with acute myocardial infarction or known hypersensitivity to bipyridines or bisulfites. • Administer with caution to a pregnant or lactating patient.

• The patient exhibits no signs of complications in the preexisting condition linked to amrinone.
• The patient displays no adverse reactions to amrinone.
• The patient and family express an accurate understanding of the points taught about amrinone.
• The patient agrees to report dyspnea, chest pain, and other symptoms to the nurse or physician.

CHAPTER SUMMARY

Chapter 29 discussed the cardiac glycosides and bipyridines used to increase cardiac output in congestive heart failure. Here are the highlights of the chapter.

• Cardiac glycosides are positive inotropic agents with electrophysiologic effects; these drugs (digoxin and digitoxin) are used to treat congestive heart failure and supraventricular arrhythmias. Cardiac glycosides are administered orally or I.V.

• Cardiac glycosides exert negative chronotropic and dromotropic effects.

• A small percentage of digoxin is metabolized; the remainder is excreted unchanged, primarily by the kidneys. Digitoxin is metabolized extensively by the liver and is eliminated by the kidneys.

• In a patient with acute myocardial infarction, cardiac glycosides are used with caution.

• Because cardiac glycosides have a narrow therapeutic range, their use may cause digitalis toxicity. Hypokalemia, hypoxemia, and other conditions may predispose a patient to digitalis toxicity.

• The signs and symptoms of digitalis toxicity fall primarily into three categories: GI, neurologic, and cardiac.

• When caring for a patient who receives cardiac glycosides, the nurse uses the nursing process. Care focuses on teaching the patient how to measure the pulse rate; recognize signs of digitalis toxicity, congestive heart failure, and hypokalemia; and identify high-potassium foods.

• Amrinone is the only FDA-approved bipyridine that is available clinically. It is administered I.V. for short-term treatment of congestive heart failure in patients who do not respond to digitalis compounds, diuretics, and vasodilators. It is contraindicated in a patient with acute myocardial infarction.

• Amrinone is metabolized by the liver and excreted by the kidneys.

• Adverse reactions to amrinone are uncommon and usually occur only in patients receiving prolonged therapy.

• For a patient receiving amrinone, nursing care emphasizes close monitoring of cardiovascular status, regular assessment for such adverse drug reactions as hypotension and arrhythmias, and evaluation of the drug's effectiveness in treating congestive heart failure.

STUDY QUESTIONS

See Appendix 1 for answers.

1. Miriam Drett, age 55, is admitted to the critical care unit with atrial fibrillation and rapid ventricular response. Her physician prescribes a digoxin loading dose of 0.5 mg I.V., followed by a daily maintenance dosage of 0.25 mg P.O. daily. The nurse could expect to adjust the digoxin dosage if Ms. Drett had which disorder?

(a) chronic obstructive pulmonary disease
(b) cerebrovascular accident
(c) hyperalbuminemia
(d) renal failure

2. The physician could have prescribed digitoxin for Ms. Drett. How does digitoxin differ from digoxin?
(a) Digitoxin is less lipid-soluble than digoxin.
(b) Digitoxin has a longer half-life than digoxin.
(c) Digitoxin is not as readily absorbed as digoxin.
(d) Digitoxin requires larger doses than digoxin.

3. Because the therapeutic range is relatively narrow for digoxin, the nurse must monitor Ms. Drett's digoxin level periodically. What is the therapeutic serum concentration of digoxin?
(a) 0.125 to 0.25 ng/ml
(b) 0.25 to 0.5 ng/ml
(c) 0.5 to 2.0 ng/ml
(d) 2.0 to 3.0 ng/ml

4. Why does Ms. Drett need to receive a loading dose of digoxin?
(a) A loading dose is required to treat ventricular fibrillation.
(b) A loading dose provides an immediate drug effect.
(c) A loading dose reduces the risk of digitalis toxicity.
(d) A loading dose minimizes the risk of arrhythmias.

5. During digoxin therapy, Ms. Drett displays signs of digitalis toxicity, such as nausea, confusion, and blurred vision. If she were to develop a life-threatening arrhythmia from digitalis toxicity, her physician probably would prescribe which drug?
(a) lidocaine
(b) bertyllium
(c) digoxin-immune Fab
(d) quinidine

6. Because Ms. Drett must take a maintenance dosage of digoxin at home, the nurse should teach her about which topic?
(a) pulse rate measurement
(b) blood pressure measurement
(c) use of potassium supplements
(d) dietary restrictions

7. Under which circumstances might the physician prescribe amrinone (Inocar) for Ms. Drett?
(a) if her condition stabilizes and she needs long-term maintenance
(b) if she can return only infrequently for follow-up visits
(c) if her serum potassium level decreases significantly
(d) if she does not respond adequately to digoxin therapy

SELECTED REFERENCES

AHFS drug information 90. (1990). Bethesda, MD: American Society of Hospital Pharmacists.

Carr, P. (1988). Cardiovascular drugs. *Home Health Care Nurse,* 6(5), 37-38.

Curran, C., and Mathewson, M. (1987). Use of cardiac glycosides in the critically ill. *Critical Care Nurse,* 7(6), 31-42.

Few, B. (1987). Digoxin immune Fab. *MCN,* 12(6), 431.

Friedman, P. (1988). Factors in individual sensitivity to cardiac glycosides and recognition of digitalis intoxication. *Primary Cardiology,* Special edition, (1), 13-17.

Gheorghiade, M., Rosman, H., Mahdyoon, H., and Goldstein, S. (1988). Incidence of digitalis intoxication. *Primary Cardiology,* Special edition, (1), 5-11.

Goodman and Gilman's the pharmacological basis of therapeutics (8th ed.; 1990). Elmsford, NY: Pergamon Press.

Hansten, P., and Horn, J. (1988). *Drug interactions: Clinical significance of drug-drug interactions* (6th ed.). Philadelphia: Lea & Febiger.

Hartshorn, E., and Hartshorn, J. (1988). Factors affecting digoxin action and kinetics. *Journal of Cardiovascular Nursing,* 2(4), 12-19.

Karboski, J., Godley, P., Frohna, P., Horton, M., and Reitmeyer, J. (1988). Marked digoxin-like immunoreactive factor interference with an enzyme immunoassay. *Drug Intelligence and Clinical Pharmacy,* 22(9), 703-705.

Kimmelstein, C., and Benotti, J. (1988). How effective is digitalis in the treatment of congestive heart failure? *American Heart Journal,* 116(4), 1063-1070.

Mercer, M. (1989). Myths and facts about cardiac drugs. *Nursing89,* 19(4), 31.

North American Nursing Diagnosis Association. (1990). *Taxonomy I - Revised, with official diagnostic categories.* St. Louis: NANDA.

Poole-Wilson, P. (1988) Digitalis: Dead or alive? *Cardiology,* 75(Suppl. 1), 103-109.

Rakel, R. (1989). *Conn's current therapy 1989.* Philadelphia: Saunders.

Rodin, S., and Johnson, B. (1988). Pharmacokinetic interactions with digoxin. *Clinical Pharmacokinetics,* 15(4), 227-244.

Salem, D., Berner, S., Eichorn, E., Sherman, L., Konstam, M. (1988). Digitalis therapy for congestive heart failure: Is the jury still out? *Pharmacotherapy,* 8(6), 319-323.

Smith, T. (1988). Digitalis: Mechanisms of action and clinical use. *New England Journal of Medicine,* 318(6), 358-365.

USPDI. (1991). *Drug information for the health care professional* (Vol. I, 11th ed.). Rockville, MD: United States Pharmacopeial Convention.

USPDI. (1991). *Advice for the patient* (Vol. II, 11th ed.). Rockville, MD: United States Pharmacopeial Convention.

ANTIARRHYTHMIC AGENTS

OBJECTIVES

After reading and studying this chapter, the student should be able to:

1. Explain the concepts of automaticity, excitability, contractility, and conductivity as they relate to myocardial pacemaker and muscle cells.

2. Differentiate between the action potential of a myocardial pacemaker cell and that of a myocardial muscle cell.

3. Describe the course of a normally conducted impulse from the sinus node to the ventricular myocardium.

4. Describe the mechanism of action for each class of antiarrhythmics.

5. Identify important pharmacokinetic differences among the agents in each class of antiarrhythmics.

6. Identify the clinical indications for treatment with each class of antiarrhythmics.

7. Identify adverse effects of the agents in each class of antiarrhythmics.

8. Describe how to apply the nursing process when caring for a patient receiving an antiarrhythmic agent.

INTRODUCTION

Antiarrhythmic drugs are used to treat abnormal electrical activity of the heart. The drugs discussed in this chapter limit cardiac electrical activity to normal conduction pathways and decrease abnormally fast heart rates. (For drugs used to increase abnormally slow heart rates, see Chapter 14, Cholinergic Blocking Agents, and Chapter 15, Adrenergic Agents; for a discussion of the negative chronotropic action of digitalis, see Chapter 29, Cardiac Glycoside Agents and Bipyridines.)

An overview of the normal electrophysiology and conduction system in the heart will help the nurse understand the action of antiarrhythmic drugs. Abnormalities of cardiac electrical activity can be diagnosed by electrocardiogram (ECG). (For more information about ECG patterns, see the Introduction to Unit Seven.)

Cardiac muscle, or myocardium, is made up of specialized cells. These cells have certain inherent characteristics that make them different from all other body cells. Myocardial cells exhibit *automaticity,* the ability to initiate or propagate an action potential (change in intracellular charge); *excitability,* the ability to respond to an electrical impulse; *conductivity,* the ability to transmit electrical impulses to the next cell; and *contractility,* the ability to shorten (contract) when stimulated.

Although all myocardial cells share the same characteristics, certain specialized cells generate electrical impulses. These pacemaker cells are located in the sinoatrial (SA) node, intranodal pathways, the atrioventricular (AV) node, the bundle of His, the right and left bundle branches, and the Purkinje fibers. Changes in ion concentrations within the cell initiate electrical stimulation that depolarizes and repolarizes the myocardial cell.

Myocardial contraction occurs when myocardial cells depolarize. Immediately before depolarization, the concentration of sodium ions (Na^+) outside the cell is greater than that inside it. The myocardial intracellular charge changes when Na^+ and calcium ions (Ca^{++}) flow into the cell, and potassium ions (K^+) flow out. This change is called the *action potential.*

The mechanism that initiates the stimulus for rapid change in cell membrane permeability remains unknown. Theories suggest that certain channels (fast and slow) allow Na^+ and Ca^{++} to enter the cell in large concentrations. When intracellular concentrations of Na^+ and Ca^{++} reach threshold levels, depolarization (contraction) occurs. Immediately after depolarization, Na^+ and Ca^{++} move slowly into the cell—the plateau phase. The concentration of K^+ remains unchanged. Repolarization occurs when K^+ flows out of the cell. The cell returns to its resting state through the action of an ion-transport system called the sodium-potassium pump.

Depolarization causes the myocardial cell to contract; repolarization causes relaxation. Because the specialized pacemaker cells have the most rapid automaticity or fastest discharge rate, electrical stimulation of the heart originates

Normal conduction and unidirectional block

The following illustrations show how normal conduction occurs and how it is affected by ischemia, as in a unidirectional block.

NORMAL CONDUCTION

Normal electrical impulse conduction flows through the left (L) and right (R) branches of the Purkinje fibers to the connecting branch (C). At the point where the impulses meet, the muscle contracts.

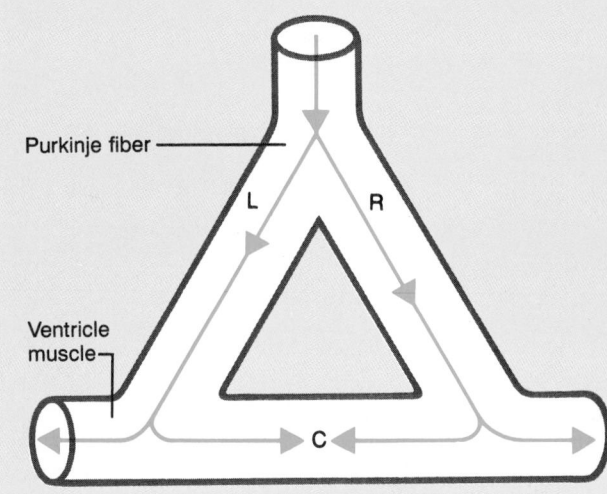

UNIDIRECTIONAL BLOCK

An ischemic area of conductive tissue blocks forward conduction. The impulse travels retrograde and reenters the fiber before the next normal beat.

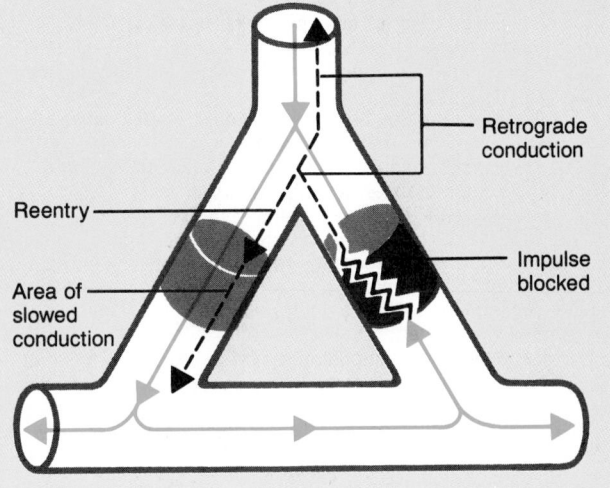

in the SA node. The impulses then spread throughout both atria and collect in the AV node, which delays the impulses slightly to allow the ventricles to fill with blood from the atria. From the AV node, the impulses travel along the bundle of His, both bundle branches, and upward through the Purkinje fibers to stimulate the ventricles to contract, ejecting blood into the pulmonary artery and aorta.

In the atria and the ventricles, pacemaker cells also conduct impulses to the other type of myocardial cells—muscle cells that relax and contract to move blood through the heart. When impulses activate the muscle cells, the cells contract in a synchronized manner, producing atrial and ventricular contractions. The ECG records atrial depolarization (contraction) as P waves, ventricular depolarization (contraction) as QRS complexes, and ventricular repolarization (relaxation) as T waves.

When stimulated, sympathetic fibers enhance excitability (bathmotropic effect), pacemaker firing rate (chronotropic effect), conduction speed (dromotropic effect), and contractility (inotropic effect). Parasympathetic stimulation depresses these effects.

Although the sympathetic and the parasympathetic branches of the autonomic nervous system stimulate myocardial cells, the SA node itself can generate an impulse. The SA node generates 60 to 100 impulses/minute, the

normal pulse rate. Other myocardial pacemaker cells exhibit automaticity at rates slower than 60 impulses/minute; myocardial muscle cells do not exhibit automaticity, unless they are damaged. Myocardial cell damage can cause abnormalities in the conduction of electrical impulses necessary for the heart to pump blood efficiently. In coronary artery disease, for example, blood flow to the myocardium is reduced. If it is reduced significantly, insufficient oxygen will be available for the cells to survive. An area of myocardium receiving less than an adequate oxygen supply is ischemic. When an area of myocardium dies, the result is an infarction.

Ischemic cells behave in at least two abnormal ways. First, they may have increased automaticity. For example, in the atria the SA node may fire at a rapid rate. This firing also may occur in several other cells in the atria (ectopic beats) until no effective or synchronized pattern exists. This chaotic electrical pattern, called *atrial fibrillation,* appears on the ECG as an irregular atrial pattern and loss of definitive P waves. In this state, the atrial muscle cells do not contract; they quiver. Although the AV node screens out some of these rapid impulses, many reach the ventricles, possibly causing the heart rate to exceed 200 beats/minute. At this rate, the ventricles do not fill sufficiently before contraction.

SELECTED NURSING DIAGNOSES

Antiarrhythmic agents

The following nursing diagnoses address representative problems and etiologies that a nurse may encounter when caring for a patient who is receiving an antiarrhythmic agent. Some of these nursing diagnoses contain generalized etiologies, which the nurse must individualize based on the patient's needs. (For some common nursing diagnoses and related interventions for each drug class, see the "Nursing Process Application" sections of this chapter.)

- Altered health maintenance related to amiodarone-induced thyroid dysfunction
- Altered health maintenance related to ineffectiveness of the prescribed antiarrhythmic agent
- Altered peripheral tissue perfusion related to the adverse cardiac effects of an antiarrhythmic agent
- Altered protection related to quinidine-induced cinchonism
- Altered protection related to the adverse hematologic effects of an antiarrhythmic agent
- Altered protection related to the risk of arrhythmias caused by the antiarrhythmic agent
- Altered sexuality patterns related to decreased libido caused by a class II antiarrhythmic agent
- Altered thought processes related to confusion caused by an antiarrhythmic agent
- Constipation related to the anticholinergic effects of an antiarrhythmic agent
- Decreased cardiac output related to moricizine-induced development of new arrhythmias or exacerbation of existing arrhythmias
- Diarrhea related to the adverse gastrointestinal effects of an antiarrhythmic agent
- Fatigue related to the adverse central nervous system (CNS) effects of an antiarrhythmic agent
- Fluid volume excess related to the adverse myocardial effects of the prescribed class IV antiarrhythmic
- Fluid volume excess related to antiarrhythmic-induced congestive heart failure

- Fluid volume excess related to fluid retention caused by the prescribed antiarrhythmic agent
- Hyperthermia related to fever caused by flecainide hypersensitivity
- Impaired gas exchange related to the adverse pulmonary effects of an antiarrhythmic agent
- Ineffective breathing pattern related to amiodarone-induced pulmonary toxicity
- Knowledge deficit related to the prescribed antiarrhythmic agent
- Noncompliance related to long-term use of an antiarrhythmic agent
- Pain related to headache caused by an antiarrhythmic agent
- Potential for injury related to a preexisting condition that contraindicates the use of an antiarrhythmic agent
- Potential for injury related to a preexisting condition that requires cautious use of an antiarrhythmic agent
- Potential for injury related to adverse drug reactions
- Potential for injury related to drug interactions
- Potential for trauma related to the adverse CNS effects of an antiarrhythmic agent
- Sensory-perceptual alterations (auditory, tactile, and visual) related to the adverse effects of the class IB antiarrhythmic agent
- Sensory-perceptual alterations (visual) related to corneal microdeposits caused by amiodarone
- Urinary retention related to the anticholinergic effects of an antiarrhythmic agent

Damaged myocardial cells in the ventricles can initiate a stimulus to contract on their own. Whether they contract singly or in pairs, they are referred to as *premature ventricular contractions.* More than four consecutive ventricular stimulated contractions is referred to as ventricular tachycardia. This conduction pattern indicates an irritable area (foci) in the ventricle that can progress to ventricular fibrillation, similar to atrial fibrillation.

Because no pulse or circulation is generated in ventricular fibrillation, the patient will die without treatment.

Ischemic pacemaker cells also can decrease conductivity greatly. For example, an ischemic cell in the Purkinje fibers may block normally conducted impulses. If this block is complete, the cell will not excite or conduct an impulse. If the block is incomplete, the cell will not excite an impulse from the normal pathway. The cell will excite from the opposite side and may conduct the impulse backward, resulting in an arrhythmia. These blocks are called *unidirectional.* Some antiarrhythmic agents can convert them to bidirectional blocks, preventing retrograde (backward) im-

pulse and ectopic beats, which originate in ischemic myocardial muscle cells. (For an illustration, see *Normal conduction and unidirectional block,* page 485.) Unidirectional block often sets up a circular impulse pattern, known as *reentry,* by which the impulse passes around the unidirectional block, travels back through the ischemic cell, and reenters the normal pathway.

Although ischemia is the most common cause of arrhythmias, other contributing factors occur singly or together with ischemia. These factors include congenital cardiac conditions, cardiac trauma or surgery, cardiomyopathy, electrolyte or acid-base imbalances, adverse drug reactions, emboli, invasive cardiac diagnostic procedures, cardiac valvular diseases, alcoholism, respiratory diseases, and viral infections. Thus, while an antiarrhythmic is used to treat an arrhythmia, the physician also attempts to correct the underlying condition, because doing so may eliminate the need for continued antiarrhythmic therapy.

Antiarrhythmics are categorized into four classes. Class I consists of four subgroups: class I contains moricizine;

class IA contains disopyramide phosphate; procainamide hydrochloride; and quinidine sulfate, gluconate, or polygalacturonate; class IB contains lidocaine hydrochloride, mexiletine hydrochloride, and tocainide hydrochloride; and class IC contains encainide, flecainide acetate, indecainide hydrochloride, and propafenone hydrochloride. Class II contains the beta-adrenergic blockers acebutolol hydrochloride, esmolol hydrochloride, and propranolol hydrochloride. Class III contains amiodarone hydrochloride and bretylium tosylate. Class IV contains the calcium channel blockers diltiazem hydrochloride and verapamil hydrochloride. The newest antiarrhythmic agent, adenosine, does not fall into any of these classes, but pharmacologically is most like the calcium channel blockers. The mechanisms of action of these drugs vary widely, but a few drugs exhibit properties common to more than one class.

The drugs discussed in this chapter are used to treat, suppress, or prevent three major mechanisms of arrhythmias: increased automaticity, decreased conduction, and reentry. Although mainly prescribed for adults, these drugs occasionally are prescribed for children.

For a summary of representative drugs, see *Selected major drugs: Antiarrhythmic agents,* pages 512 and 513. For a listing of applicable nursing diagnoses that the nurse may formulate when caring for a patient receiving these agents, see *Selected nursing diagnoses: Antiarrhythmic agents.*) For detailed information on applying the nursing process, see Chapter 6, The Nursing Process and Drug Therapy.

CLASS I ANTIARRHYTHMICS

Moricizine is a new class I antiarrhythmic agent with potent local anesthetic activity and myocardial membrane stabilizing effects.

PHARMACOKINETICS

After oral administration, approximately 38% of moricizine is absorbed and reaches a peak plasma concentration within 2 hours. Moricizine undergoes extensive metabolism with less than 1% of a dose excreted unchanged in the urine. The plasma half-life is about 3 hours. Plasma protein binding is about 95%.

PHARMACODYNAMICS

A class I antiarrhythmic with local anesthetic and myocardial membrane stabilizing effects, moricizine is thought to decrease the fast inward current in cardiac tissue caused by sodium ions. This depresses the depolarization rate and decreases the action potential duration and effective refractory period.

PHARMACOTHERAPEUTICS

Moricizine is the only class I antiarrhythmic agent currently in use. It is contraindicated in a lactating patient or one with second- or third-degree AV block, right bundle branch block associated with left hemiblock (unless a pacemaker is present), known hypersensitivity to the drug, or cardiogenic shock. It must be used with caution in a patient with severe hepatic or renal dysfunction, sick sinus syndrome, or congestive heart failure (CHF).

moricizine hydrochloride (Ethmozine). Moricizine is used to manage life-threatening ventricular arrhythmias, such as sustained ventricular tachycardia.
Usual adult dosage: 200 to 300 mg P.O. every 8 hours, individually titrated based on the patient's response and tolerance. The dosage may be adjusted in increments of 150 mg per day at 3-day intervals.

Drug interactions

Administration of cimetidine may increase the moricizine plasma level. Therefore, a patient receiving cimetidine should begin moricizine therapy at a low dosage. Propranolol administration may increase the PR interval on an ECG, but the clinical significance of this interaction is unknown. During clinical trials, patients receiving moricizine showed increased theophylline clearance with decreased half-life.

ADVERSE DRUG REACTIONS

The appearance of proarrhythmias (arrhythmia that occurs when another already is present) or exacerbation of existing arrhythmias is the most serious adverse reaction reported. Adverse reactions reported in more than 2% of patients in clinical trials include sustained ventricular tachycardia, hypesthesia, abdominal pain, dyspepsia, vomiting, sweating, cardiac chest pain, CHF, cardiac arrest, asthenia, nervousness, paresthesia, musculoskeletal pain, diarrhea, dry mouth, sleep disorders, and blurred vision. Those reported in more than 5% of patients include dizziness, nausea, headache, fatigue, palpitations, and dyspnea.

NURSING PROCESS APPLICATION

The following information assists the nurse in caring for a patient receiving the class I antiarrhythmic moricizine.

Assessment
• Review the patient's history for a preexisting condition that contraindicates the use of moricizine, such as second- or third-degree AV block, right bundle branch block associated with left hemiblock (unless a pacemaker is present), known hypersensitivity to the drug, cardiogenic shock, or lactation.
• Review the patient's history for a preexisting condition that requires cautious use of moricizine, such as severe hepatic or renal dysfunction, sick sinus syndrome, or CHF.
• Assess the patient for adverse reactions to moricizine, such as hypesthesia, gastrointestinal (GI) distress, cardiac dysfunction, or central nervous system (CNS) disturbances.
• Review the patient's medication history to identify the use of drugs that may interact with moricizine, such as cimetidine, propranolol, or theophylline.
• Assess the effectiveness of moricizine periodically.
• Assess the patient for arrhythmias frequently during moricizine therapy.
• Evaluate the patient's and family's knowledge about moricizine.

Nursing diagnoses
The following examples represent appropriate nursing diagnoses for a patient receiving moricizine.
• Potential for injury related to a preexisting condition that contraindicates the use of moricizine
• Potential for injury related to a preexisting condition that requires cautious use of moricizine
• Potential for injury related to adverse drug reactions
• Decreased cardiac output related to moricizine-induced development of new arrhythmias or exacerbation of existing arrhythmias
• Knowledge deficit related to moricizine

Planning and implementation
• Do not administer moricizine to a patient with a condition that contraindicates its use.
• Administer moricizine cautiously to a patient at risk because of a preexisting condition.
• Monitor the patient closely for adverse reactions during moricizine therapy.
• *Keep standard emergency equipment nearby when moricizine therapy begins because cardiac arrest can occur.*
• Monitor hydration if the patient develops nausea, vomiting, or diarrhea during moricizine therapy. Administer an antiemetic or antidiarrheal agent, as needed. Notify the physician if GI distress interferes with oral drug intake.

• *Monitor the patient for signs and symptoms of CHF, such as jugular vein distention, crackles (rales), sudden weight gain, and dyspnea. If the patient displays any of these signs or symptoms, notify the physician immediately and restrict the patient's sodium and fluid intake.*
• Take safety precautions if the patient develops dizziness or blurred vision. For example, keep the bed rails raised and supervise ambulation.
• Provide assistance if the patient develops fatigue or dyspnea.
• Monitor the patient for moricizine-induced headache or abdominal, chest, or musculoskeletal pain. Consult with the physician about appropriate pain management measures.
• Offer the patient ice chips or sugarless candy or gum if dry mouth occurs.
• Monitor the patient for CNS disturbances, such as hypesthesia, nervousness, paresthesia, or sleep disturbances. Protect the patient from injury if hypesthesia or paresthesia occurs. If the patient has insomnia, obtain a prescription for a sedative.
• Notify the physician if the patient experiences adverse drug reactions.
• *Monitor the patient's ECG for new arrhythmias or exacerbation of existing ones.*
• *Observe the patient with arrhythmias for signs of decreased cardiac output, such as weak pulse, hypotension, and dizziness.*
• Notify the physician if arrhythmias occur. Prepare to begin treatment immediately, as prescribed.

Patient teaching
• Teach the patient and family the name, dose, frequency, action, and adverse effects of moricizine.
• *Inform the patient that moricizine may cause headache or abdominal, cardiac chest, or musculoskeletal pain. Advise the patient to report such pain — especially cardiac chest pain — immediately because prompt treatment is necessary.*
• *Instruct the patient to report signs and symptoms of CHF, such as shortness of breath or sudden weight gain.*
• Encourage the patient to limit sodium and fluid intake during moricizine therapy.
• Advise the patient that blurred vision is drug-related and should subside when moricizine is discontinued.
• Instruct the patient to report any other adverse reactions.

Evaluation
The following examples represent appropriate evaluation statements for a patient receiving moricizine.
• The patient has no conditions that contraindicate moricizine therapy.
• The patient exhibits no signs of complications in the preexisitng condition linked to moricizine.

• The patient experiences no adverse reactions to moricizine.

• The patient maintains adequate cardiac output during moricizine therapy.

• The patient and family express an accurate understanding of the points taught about moricizine.

• The patient correctly identifies adverse reactions that must be reported to the physician during moricizine therapy.

CLASS IA ANTIARRHYTHMICS

Class IA antiarrhythmics include disopyramide phosphate, procainamide hydrochloride, and quinidine sulfate, gluconate, or polygalacturonate. Class IA antiarrhythmics are used to treat various atrial and ventricular arrhythmias. Commonly given orally, the class IA drugs are fairly safe; however, some GI and cardiovascular adverse reactions may result.

PHARMACOKINETICS

After oral administration, class IA drugs undergo fairly rapid absorption and metabolism. Because of this, researchers have developed sustained-release forms of these drugs to help maintain therapeutic levels. The nurse should monitor the patient's serum drug level closely during therapy with the class IA drugs.

Absorption, distribution, metabolism, excretion

When administered orally, quinidine is absorbed almost completely, and procainamide and disopyramide are about 90% absorbed from the GI tract. Food and extremes in gastric pH hasten or delay absorption; delay also occurs from use of sustained-release forms of these three drugs. Quinidine's absorption rate also depends on the salt with which it is combined: quinidine polygalacturonate and quinidine gluconate, although not sustained-release forms, are absorbed more slowly than quinidine sulfate.

Quinidine rarely is given intramuscularly (I.M.) or intravenously (I.V.). Procainamide, which is available in I.V. form, rarely is given I.M. Disopyramide is available only in oral form.

The three drugs are distributed through all body tissues except, in the case of quinidine, the brain. Disopyramide and quinidine also enter red blood cells. Plasma protein binding is 90% for quinidine, 20% for procainamide, and, depending on the concentration, 30% to 65% for disopyramide.

All class IA antiarrhythmics are metabolized in the liver. The metabolites of these drugs provide some antiarrhythmic activity—especially the procainamide metabolite N-acetylprocainamide (NAPA), which researchers are investigating as a separate antiarrhythmic. The amount of procainamide metabolized to NAPA varies depending on the patient's rate of acetylation (the metabolic process by which an acetyl group is introduced into a molecule of an organic compound).

All three drugs are excreted unchanged by the kidneys in the following amounts: 50% of disopyramide; 10% to 50% of quinidine, the percentage decreasing as urine pH increases; and 40% to 70% of procainamide, depending on the patient's rate of acetylation. The metabolites of each drug also are excreted in the urine. A small percentage of disopyramide is excreted in the feces.

Onset, peak, duration

Each class IA drug has an onset of action of 30 minutes to 3 hours after oral administration, depending in part on the dose given. Sustained-release forms may have a later onset. I.M. procainamide produces effects in 10 to 30 minutes, and the onset of I.V. procainamide is immediate. The immediate onset from the I.V. route makes it the practical choice in acute situations.

Disopyramide reaches a peak concentration level in 1 to 2 hours. Quinidine and oral procainamide capsules attain peak concentrations in 60 to 90 minutes. The sustained-release forms of these agents reach peak concentrations as follows: disopyramide in 5 hours, quinidine in 3 to 4 hours, and procainamide in 1½ to 2 hours. I.M. procainamide reaches peak concentrations in 15 to 60 minutes—one reason it is used infrequently.

The nurse must monitor the patient's serum concentration closely during therapy with a class IA drug to prevent toxicity. Normal therapeutic ranges are as follows: disopyramide, 2 to 6 mcg/ml; quinidine, 2 to 6 mcg/ml; and procainamide, 4 to 10 mcg/ml. NAPA levels resulting from procainamide metabolism usually range from 2 to 8 mcg/ml.

In healthy individuals, the half-life of disopyramide is from 5 to 12 hours; of quinidine, 6 to 8 hours; of procainamide, 3 hours; of NAPA, about 7 hours in a patient with normal renal function.

PHARMACODYNAMICS

Class IA antiarrhythmics exert their effects by altering the myocardial cell membrane and interfering with autonomic nervous system control of pacemaker cells. The drugs partially block the fast channel in the myocardial cell membrane, reducing the influx of Na^+. This reduction alters the action potential by depressing the depolarization rate, prolonging the plateau and repolarization and depressing

Action potentials of myocardial pacemaker and muscle cells

The intracellular charge of a myocardial cell is changed when Na$^+$ and Ca^{++} flow into the cell and K$^+$ flows out. This change in intracellular charge is referred to as *action potential*. Depolarization (contraction) occurs as the usual negative resting state of the cell changes to zero in the pacemaker cell or to slightly positive in the muscle cell. Repolarization (relaxation) occurs when the cell returns to its usual negative charge. This diagram shows the different action potentials of pacemaker and muscle cells. The pacemaker cell undergoes more gradual excitation, whereas the muscle cell has a steeper slope of depolarization and rapid excitation (phase 0). The pacemaker cell also does not have an early rapid repolarization (phase 1) or a plateau (phase 2) and exhibits final rapid repolarization (phase 3) and spontaneous depolarization at rest (phase 4).

Once a muscle cell has been depolarized, it is not susceptible to a second depolarization until a certain time period has elapsed. This time period is the effective refractory period (ERP), roughly equal to the action potential duration (APD).

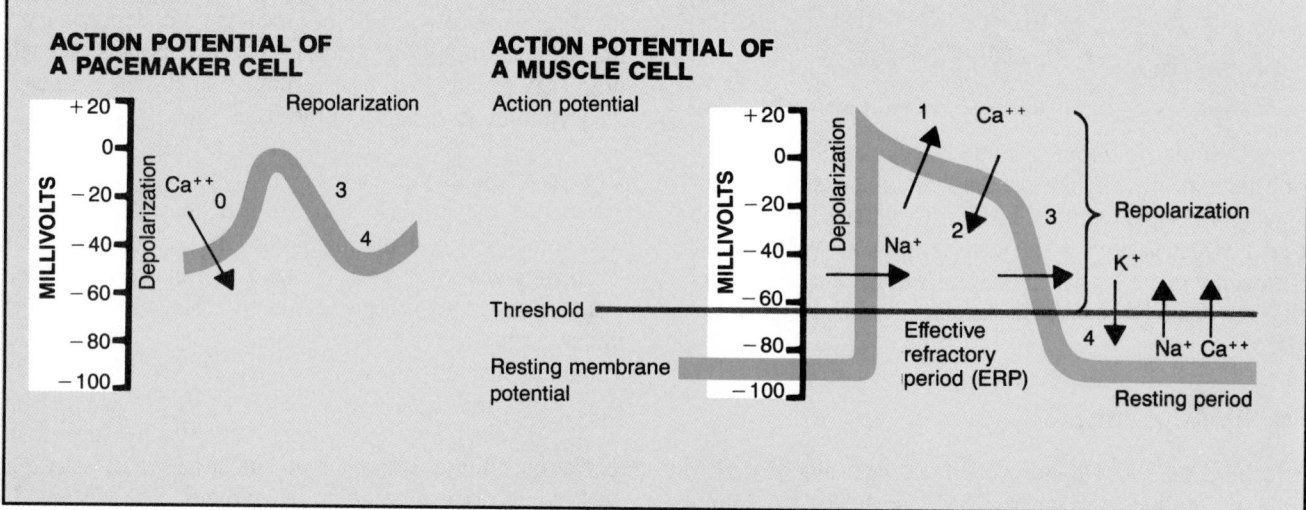

the slope of the resting period. These changes reduce the rate of automaticity in ectopic foci, increase the effective refractory period (ERP), and reduce the speed of conductivity. (For an illustration of these effects, see *Action potentials of myocardial pacemaker and muscle cells.*)

All three drugs also block parasympathetic nervous system discharges to the SA and AV nodes, thereby increasing the conduction rate of the AV node. This anticholinergic effect can produce dangerous increases in the ventricular heart rate if rapid atrial activity, as in atrial fibrillation, is present. In turn, the increased ventricular heart rate can offset the ability of the antiarrhythmics to convert atrial arrhythmias to a regular rhythm.

Disopyramide produces peripheral vasoconstriction, and procainamide and quinidine decrease peripheral vascular resistance (afterload). Disopyramide causes significant depression of myocardial contractility; procainamide and quinidine produce slight depression.

PHARMACOTHERAPEUTICS

Based on their differing therapeutic and adverse effects, class IA antiarrhythmics are prescribed to treat various atrial and ventricular arrhythmias. The drugs (especially quinidine) are synergistic with digoxin. Thus, because of decreased AV conduction time with digoxin, quinidine can be added to convert atrial fibrillation to regular rhythm.

disopyramide phosphate (Norpace, Norpace CR). Used to treat atrial and ventricular arrhythmias, disopyramide suppresses the frequency of ectopic ventricular beats as well as the frequency and duration of self-limiting bursts of ventricular tachycardia. Available only in oral form, disopyramide is not useful in acute situations, which require parenteral administration.

Usual adult dosage: for the immediate-release form, 100 to 200 mg P.O. every 6 hours; for the sustained-release form, 300 mg P.O. every 12 hours. In a patient with severe renal failure, the usual dosage is 100 mg given at intervals based on creatinine clearance: every 8 hours for a clearance of 30 to 40 ml/min, every 12 hours for a clearance of 15 to 30 ml/min, every 24 hours for a clearance of less than 15 ml/min.

Usual pediatric dosage: for infants under age 1, 10 to 30 mg/kg/day P.O. in equally divided doses every 6 hours; for children ages 1 to 4, 10 to 20 mg/kg in equally divided doses every 6 hours; for children ages 4 to 12, 10 to 15 mg/kg in equally divided doses every 6 hours; for children ages 12 to 18, 6 to 15 mg/kg in equally divided doses every 6 hours.

procainamide hydrochloride (Procan SR, Pronestyl). Used to prevent the recurrence of atrial fibrillation and other atrial arrhythmias, procainamide is only moderately effective in converting these arrhythmias to regular rhythm. Procainamide suppresses the frequency and duration of self-limiting bursts of atrial and ventricular tachycardia; it also suppresses ventricular ectopic beats. Parenteral procainamide is used to treat persistent ventricular tachycardia. Dosage is adjusted carefully to the patient's response.

Usual adult dosage: to convert atrial fibrillation, 1.25 grams P.O., if necessary 750 mg 1 hour later, then 500 mg to 1 gram every 2 hours until conversion or toxic signs appear; to prevent recurrence, 500 mg to 1 gram every 4 hours, or up to 1 gram of the sustained-release form every 6 hours; for ventricular ectopic beats, a 1-gram loading dose followed by 500 mg every 3 to 4 hours or 500 mg to 1 gram of sustained-release form every 6 hours; for frequent ventricular ectopic beats or ventricular tachycardia, 17 mg/kg of ideal body weight I.V. infused at a maximum rate of 50 mg/minute, followed by an infusion of 2.8 to 3 mg/kg of actual body weight per hour. A patient with moderate renal or cardiac failure requires a reduced infusion rate of 2 mg/kg/hour; with severe renal or cardiac failure, a loading dose of 12 mg/kg and an infusion rate of 1 mg/kg/hour; with renal failure or severe CHF, a reduced oral maintenance dosage. Dosage adjustments must be based on serum concentration.

Usual pediatric dosage: 50 mg/kg or 1.5 grams/m² P.O. daily divided into four to six doses, or 2 to 5 mg/kg (not to exceed 100 mg) I.V. over 5 minutes, every 15 minutes (not to exceed 30 mg/kg in 24 hours); or 3 to 6 mg/kg I.V. over 5 minutes followed by continuous infusion at 0.02 to 0.08 mg/kg/minute. Total dosage should not exceed 1 gram.

quinidine sulfate (CinQuin, Quinidex, Quinora), **quinidine gluconate** (Duraquin, Quinaglute), and **quinidine polygalacturonate** (Cardioquin). After converting atrial fibrillation to regular rhythm, quinidine prevents recurrence of the atrial fibrillation. It also suppresses atrial and ventricular ectopic beats as well as the frequency and duration of self-limiting bursts of atrial and ventricular tachycardia. Quinidine gluconate 267 mg or quinidine polygalacturonate 275 mg is equivalent to quinidine sulfate 200 mg.

Usual adult dosage: to convert atrial fibrillation, 300 to 400 mg P.O. of immediate-release quinidine sulfate every 6 hours, then 200 to 400 mg every 6 hours to maintain regular rhythm; to suppress atrial or ventricular ectopic beats, 200 to 300 mg quinidine sulfate P.O. every 6 to 8 hours or 300 to 600 mg of sustained-release quinidine sulfate every 8 to 12 hours; for maintenance of regular rhythm, 324 to 660 mg of sustained-release quinidine gluconate or 275 mg of quinidine polygalacturonate every 8

to 12 hours. A patient with congestive heart failure or cirrhosis may require a lower dosage.

Usual pediatric dosage: 30 mg/kg or 900 mg/m² P.O. daily, divided into five doses.

Drug interactions

Class IA antiarrhythmics may exhibit additive or antagonistic effects with other antiarrhythmics as well as with anticholinergic drugs. Quinidine used with oral anticoagulants can cause hypoprothrombinemia. Anticonvulsants may affect the metabolism of quinidine. Digoxin and alkalinizing agents also may interact with quinidine. (For more information, see *Drug interactions: Class IA antiarrhythmics.*)

ADVERSE DRUG REACTIONS

Adverse reactions to class IA antiarrhythmics include anticholinergic effects, GI changes, and reactions unique to quinidine's source, cinchona. Also, antiarrhythmic drugs themselves can produce arrhythmias.

The anticholinergic property of disopyramide commonly produces dry mouth, blurred vision, constipation, urinary hesitancy, and urine retention. The drug's negative inotropic effect combined with increased peripheral vasoconstriction sometimes results in CHF, hypotension, chest pain, edema, and dyspnea.

The class IA antiarrhythmics, especially quinidine, may produce diarrhea and other GI symptoms, such as cramping, nausea, vomiting, anorexia, and bitter taste.

Cinchonism, a reaction to the cinchona alkaloids, describes a set of quinidine-related reactions consisting of tinnitus, headache, vertigo, fever, light-headedness, and visual disturbances. Cinchonism may appear after the first dose or with quinidine toxicity. Quinidine syncope also may occur and probably is from transient ventricular tachycardia or ectopy.

Procainamide, especially the I.V. form, can produce hypotension. The drug's negative inotropic effect less commonly leads to CHF. Because I.V. quinidine may lead to severe hypotension and cardiovascular collapse, the drug rarely is administered by this route.

All class IA antiarrhythmics can *induce* arrhythmias, especially conduction delays that may compound existing heart blocks. Apparent conduction through the AV node may be increased, precipitating a dangerously high ventricular rate. As the ERP and the action potential duration (APD) increase, the ECG reflects a prolonged QT interval. This is a precursor to a special form of ventricular tachycardia known as Torsades de Pointes.

Up to 30% of patients using procainamide experience an adverse reaction that mimics systemic lupus erythematosus. Signs and symptoms include pain in small joints,

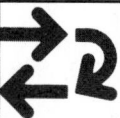

DRUG INTERACTIONS

Class IA antiarrhythmics

Class IA antiarrhythmics interact with several commonly administered drugs. The nurse must be aware of these interactions to implement appropriate assessment and intervention strategies.

DRUG	INTERACTING DRUGS	POSSIBLE EFFECTS	NURSING IMPLICATIONS
disopyramide	anticholinergic agents	Produce additive anticholinergic effects	• Observe the patient for adverse reactions, such as dry mouth, wheezing, urine retention, and orthostatic hypotension.
	verapamil	Causes myocardial depression	• Do not administer these drugs within 24 hours of each other. • Monitor for signs of congestive heart failure or decreased peripheral perfusion, if concurrent administration is necessary.
procainamide	cimetidine, amiodarone	Increase serum procainamide levels	• Monitor for therapeutic levels of procainamide. • Assess the patient for signs and symptoms of procainamide overdose, such as tachycardia, confusion, drowsiness, nausea, and vomiting.
quinidine	neuromuscular blockers	Increases skeletal muscle relaxation	• Observe the patient for hypoventilation when administering a class IA antiarrhythmic in the immediate postoperative period.
	oral anticoagulants	Produce hypoprothrombinemia	• Observe the patient for increased bruising, bleeding, or I.V. site oozing; monitor the patient's prothrombin time.
	digoxin	Increases serum digoxin level	• Monitor the patient's serum digoxin level; assess for signs of digitalis toxicity: anorexia, nausea, vomiting, headache, malaise, visual disturbances, or changes in pulse rate or regularity.
	urine-alkalinizing agents	Increase serum quinidine levels	• Assess the patient for signs of quinidine toxicity, such as arrhythmias, hypotension, and syncope.
	cimetidine, amiodarone	Increase serum quinidine levels	• Assess the patient for signs of quinidine toxicity, such as arrhythmias, hypotension, and syncope.
quinidine, disopyramide	rifampin, phenytoin, phenobarbital	Increase metabolism of quinidine and disopyramide	• Monitor the patient's pulse rate and ECG for signs of decreased therapeutic effect. • Monitor the patient's quinidine and disopyramide levels.

pleuritic pain, dyspnea, fever, headache, pericardial effusion, blood dyscrasias, and positive serum antinuclear antibody titers. This reaction, called *drug-induced systemic lupus,* is not dose-dependent and resolves when procainamide is discontinued. Rarely, quinidine also can cause lupus-like symptoms and hypersensitivity reactions manifested by fever, blood dyscrasias, skin eruptions, liver disorders, and anaphylaxis. All three of the class IA antiarrhythmics can precipitate CHF and can produce confusion in elderly patients.

NURSING PROCESS APPLICATION

The following information assists the nurse in caring for a patient who is receiving a class IA antiarrhythmic.

Assessment
• Review the patient's history for a preexisting condition that contraindicates the use of a class IA antiarrhythmic, such as digitalis intoxication with an AV conduction disorder or other severe intraventricular conduction defect, ectopic impulses and abnormal rhythms due to escape mechanisms, myasthenia gravis, or known hypersensitivity to these drugs.

• Review the patient's history for a preexisting condition that requires cautious use of a class IA antiarrhythmic, such as marginally compensated cardiovascular disease; renal, cardiac, or hepatic insufficiency; pregnancy; or lactation.

• Assess the patient for adverse reactions to the prescribed class IA antiarrhythmic, such as anticholinergic effects, GI disturbances, arrhythmias, severe hypotension, or cardiovascular collapse.

• Assess for signs of drug-induced systemic lupus, such as pain in small joints, pleuritic pain, dyspnea, fever, headache, blood dyscrasias, or pericardial effusion, during procainamide therapy.

• Assess for signs of cinchonism, such as tinnitus, headache, vertigo, fever, light-headedness, or visual disturbances, during quinidine therapy.

• Review the patient's medication history to identify the use of drugs that interact with the prescribed class IA antiarrhythmic, such as other antiarrhythmics, anticholinergic agents, oral anticoagulants, or alkalinizing agents.

• Assess the effectiveness of the prescribed class IA antiarrhythmic periodically.

• Evaluate the patient's and family's knowledge about the prescribed class IA antiarrhythmic.

Nursing diagnoses

The following examples represent appropriate nursing diagnoses for a patient receiving a class IA antiarrhythmic.

• Potential for injury related to a preexisting condition that contraindicates the use of a class IA antiarrhythmic

• Potential for injury related to a preexisting condition that requires cautious use of a class IA antiarrhythmic

• Potential for injury related to adverse drug reactions

• Knowledge deficit related to the prescribed class IA antiarrhythmic

Planning and implementation

• Do not administer a class IA antiarrhythmic to a patient with a condition that contraindicates its use.

• Administer a class IA antiarrhythmic cautiously to a patient at risk because of a preexisting condition.

• Monitor the patient frequently for adverse reactions.

• *Assess for early signs of congestive heart failure, such as hypotension, edema, and irregular heartbeat, by taking the patient's vital signs and auscultating breath sounds regularly, recording the patient's fluid intake and output, and weighing the patient daily.*

• *Monitor the patient's ECG for increased ventricular rate, a QT interval 50% greater than normal, and conduction disturbances.*

• Monitor electrolyte levels closely at the beginning of therapy and when administering diuretics with a class IA agent. Electrolyte abnormalities, especially hypokalemia, can predispose the patient to arrhythmias.

• *Monitor the patient's serum drug concentration closely to detect early toxicity. Notify the physician if the concentration falls outside of the therapeutic range.*

• Send a blood sample to the laboratory to determine the serum drug concentration as prescribed. Note on a laboratory slip the time when the last dose was given.

• Give around-the-clock doses (when appropriate and prescribed) rather than following a traditional t.i.d. or q.i.d. schedule to maintain therapeutic drug concentration.

• Take safety precautions if blurred vision or confusion occurs. For example, keep the bed in a low position and supervise ambulation.

• Offer small amounts of fluids and ice chips or hard candy to a patient with dry mouth.

• Encourage the patient to increase fluid and fiber intake, if permissible, to prevent or relieve constipation. Ask the physician to prescribe a laxative, if needed.

• Monitor the patient for urine retention.

• Monitor the patient's hydration status if nausea, vomiting, or anorexia occurs. Obtain a prescription for an antiemetic agent, if needed.

• *Observe for signs of drug-induced systemic lupus during procainamide therapy.*

• Monitor for signs of cinchonism during quinidine therapy.

• Administer a digoxin loading dose, if prescribed, before the first dose of the prescribed class IA antiarrhythmic for the patient starting treatment for atrial tachycardia or fibrillation.

• *Do not administer a class IA antiarrhythmic with food unless prescribed because food may affect absorption.*

• *Expect to adjust the disopyramide dosage for a patient with renal impairment; the quinidine dosage for a patient with congestive heart failure or liver dysfunction; and the procainamide dosage for a patient with renal or cardiac failure, as prescribed.*

• Monitor the patient's complete blood count, leukocyte count, and platelet count periodically during the first 3 months of procainamide therapy.

• Be aware that procainamide I.M. takes 15 to 60 minutes to reach peak concentration.

• *Expect to administer a reduced dosage of procainamide I.V. for a patient with renal or cardiac failure, as prescribed.*

• Administer procainamide I.V. by using an infusion pump and monitoring the patient's ECG and blood pressure frequently. When switching from the I.V. to the oral route, continue the infusion for 2 hours, or as prescribed, after the first oral dose.

• Notify the physician if adverse reactions occur.

Patient teaching

• Teach the patient and family the name, dose, action, frequency, and adverse effects of the prescribed class IA antiarrhythmic.

• *Instruct the female patient to notify the physician if she is pregnant or plans to become pregnant.*

• *Instruct the patient to obtain a daily weight at the same time of day in similar clothes to detect fluid retention. Advise the patient to notify the physician of sudden weight gain (2 pounds or more in one day), shortness of breath, or peripheral edema.*

• Stress the importance of having drug concentration tests and ECGs done regularly to detect abnormalities.

• Instruct the patient to take the prescribed class IA antiarrhythmic around the clock rather than just during the day to maintain therapeutic drug levels.

• *Advise the family that a class IA agent may cause confusion in an elderly patient. Instruct them to take safety measures, such as continual supervision, and to notify the physician if confusion occurs.*

• Teach the patient how to manage anticholinergic effects, such as dry mouth and constipation. Also advise the patient to report signs of urine retention, such as urinary frequency and a sensation of bladder fullness after voiding.

• Teach the patient to recognize and report to the physician the signs of drug-induced systemic lupus before taking the next dose of procainamide.

• Teach the patient to recognize signs of infection and bleeding, especially with procainanide therapy.

• Teach the patient to recognize and report to the physician signs of cinchonism before taking the next dose of quinidine.

• Instruct the patient not to take the class IA antiarrhythmic with food, unless otherwise directed.

• Advise the patient receiving sustained-release tablets or capsules that the wax matrix may be excreted intact in the stool. Provide reassurance that this is normal and that all of the drug has been extracted in the intestines.

• *Demonstrate how to take a pulse. Tell the patient to measure the pulse before taking the prescribed class IA antiarrhythmic. Advise the patient to notify the physician if the pulse is irregular or slow (below 60 beats/minute or the rate selected by the physician).*

• Instruct the patient to notify the physician if any other adverse reactions occur.

Evaluation

The following examples represent appropriate evaluation statements for a patient receiving a class IA antiarrhythmic.

• The patient has no conditions that contraindicate class IA antiarrhythmic therapy.

• The patient exhibits no signs of complications in the preexisting condition linked to the prescribed class IA antiarrhythmic.

• The patient has no adverse reactions to the prescribed class IA antiarrhythmic.

• The patient and family express an accurate understanding of the points taught about the prescribed class IA antiarrhythmic.

• The patient correctly demonstrates how to take a pulse and states when to take it.

CLASS IB ANTIARRHYTHMICS

Class IB antiarrhythmics include lidocaine hydrochloride, mexiletine hydrochloride, and tocainide hydrochloride. Lidocaine is one of the most widely used antiarrhythmics in acute care. Mexiletine and tocainide were developed recently. Although they have fewer clinical indications than class IA antiarrhythmics, the class IB antiarrhythmics, especially lidocaine, are more effective for treating acute ventricular arrhythmias and cause fewer adverse reactions. Phenytoin, which resembles the class IB antiarrhythmics, also may be used to treat arrhythmias. (For details, see *Phenytoin for digitalis toxicity.*)

PHARMACOKINETICS

The class IB antiarrhythmics exhibit considerable variation in their metabolism. These differences have important implications for their use.

Absorption, distribution, metabolism, excretion
All class IB antiarrhythmics are absorbed well from the GI tract after oral administration; however, lidocaine is not available in oral form because most of an absorbed dose undergoes first-pass metabolism in the liver. When given I.M., lidocaine is absorbed best from the deltoid muscle.

Lidocaine is distributed widely throughout the body, including the brain. Distribution data for mexiletine and tocainide are incomplete, but distribution of these drugs may resemble that of lidocaine. Class IB antiarrhythmics are bound to plasma proteins in the following amounts: lidocaine, 65%; mexiletine, 55%; and tocainide, 15%.

Lidocaine is metabolized by deethylation to various metabolites, some with mild antiarrhythmic properties. After minimal first-pass metabolism, mexiletine is methylated to several metabolites with minimal antiarrhythmic properties. Tocainide undergoes little first-pass metabolism; oxidative deamination converts tocainide into inactive metabolites.

Less than 10% of lidocaine, about 10% of mexiletine, and about 50% of tocainide are excreted unchanged in the urine. Metabolites of each drug also appear in the urine. Mexiletine also is secreted in breast milk.

Phenytoin for digitalis toxicity

Phenytoin sometimes is given intravenously to correct acute arrhythmias caused by digitalis toxicity. (For further details, see Chapter 29, Cardiac Glycoside Agents and Bipyridines.)

Phenytoin is distributed throughout the body and is 95% protein bound. The drug is metabolized in the liver by oxidation to an inactive metabolite, which then is excreted in the urine. Onset of action occurs within 5 minutes of I.V. administration. (Peak or therapeutic serum concentrations usually are not important when phenytoin is used to treat arrhythmias.) The duration of action is 4 to 6 hours, although the half-life of phenytoin usually is about 22 hours.

The mechanism of action of phenytoin in treating digitalis-induced arrhythmias resembles that of the class IB antiarrhythmics. The drug shortens the effective refractory period of the atrioventricular (AV) node and depresses the automaticity of ectopic myocardial cells. Phenytoin is used to shorten prolonged AV conduction time and to suppress premature ventricular beats.
Usual adult dosage: 100 mg I.V. push, repeated every 5 minutes until the arrhythmia disappears; if the total dosage reaches 1 gram without effect, another antiarrhythmic should be used.

Adverse reactions include pain at the infusion site, hypotension with cardiovascular collapse, a decreased level of consciousness, ventricular fibrillation, rash, and fever.

When administering phenytoin, the nurse should note the following considerations:
- Infuse the drug through a central line to avoid pain and phlebitis. If a peripheral site must be used, inject the drug into an I.V. line infusing normal saline solution.
- Do not dilute phenytoin; administer by I.V. push only at a rate of less than 50 mg/minute.
- Closely monitor the patient's heart rate and rhythm and blood pressure.
- Have emergency equipment or a code cart available.

Onset, peak, duration

Lidocaine exerts its antiarrhythmic effect in 1 to 2 minutes after I.V. bolus administration. Onset of action for mexiletine is 30 minutes to 2 hours; for tocainide, less than 30 minutes. Lidocaine reaches a peak concentration level 10 minutes after I.M. injection. After oral administration, peak concentration for mexiletine occurs in 2 to 3 hours; for tocainide, in 30 minutes to 2 hours.

Lidocaine provides antiarrhythmic effects for only 15 minutes after the I.V. infusion is stopped, although its half-life is 90 minutes. The durations of action for mexiletine and tocainide remain undetermined. The half-life of mexiletine is 10 to 12 hours; that of tocainide is 11 to 15 hours.

PHARMACODYNAMICS

Class IB antiarrhythmics are used only to treat ventricular arrhythmias. These drugs slightly depress depolarization in myocardial cells. Class IB antiarrhythmics are cell membrane stabilizers, but do not affect the automaticity of the SA node or conductivity through the AV node.

As their major action, class IB antiarrhythmics decrease the APD and to a lesser extent the ERP. The drugs especially affect the Purkinje fibers and myocardial cells in the ventricles. By shortening the ERP, class IB antiarrhythmics eliminate unidirectional block, which can trigger a reentry arrhythmia. The drugs also decrease ventricular ectopy by blocking the slow influx of sodium during plateau (phase 2) and by decreasing the slope of phase 4 depolarization. Class IB antiarrhythmics neither block nor mimic autonomic control of the heart.

PHARMACOTHERAPEUTICS

Class IB antiarrhythmics are used to treat ventricular ectopic beats, ventricular tachycardia, and ventricular fibrillation. Because class IB antiarrhythmics do not usually produce serious adverse reactions, they are the drugs of choice in acute care.

lidocaine hydrochloride (Xylocaine). Used to suppress frequent ventricular ectopic beats in acute ischemia, lidocaine also is used to treat ventricular arrhythmias related to digitalis toxicity and other acute conditions, to convert ventricular tachycardia in the absence of cardiovascular collapse, and to reduce the frequency and duration of abrupt, self-limiting ventricular tachycardia. The drug also is used to maintain sinus rhythm once ventricular fibrillation has been defibrillated electrically. Controversy exists over the use of lidocaine to prevent ventricular arrhythmias in patients with suspected myocardial infarction (MI). Usually given intravenously, lidocaine may be given intramuscularly, but the resultant striated muscle damage interferes with the measurement of cardiac enzymes during diagnosis of acute MI.
Usual adult dosage: an initial I.V. bolus of 50 to 100 mg, followed by a second bolus of 50 to 100 mg given 5 minutes after the first; then continuous I.V. infusion at 1 to 4 mg/minute. No more than 300 mg should be given per hour. Lidocaine can be given as a 300 mg dose I.M. and repeated in 60 to 90 minutes if necessary. If continuous administration is needed, I.V. infusion is the preferred route. In a patient with severe congestive heart failure or cardiogenic shock, the total bolus dosage should be reduced by half. In a patient with CHF or liver disease, the maintenance infusions should be reduced by a third to a half.
Usual pediatric dosage: 0.5 to 1 mg/kg I.V. bolus, which may be repeated but should not exceed 5 mg/kg; then a continuous infusion of 10 to 50 mcg/kg/minute.

mexiletine hydrochloride (Mexitil). Mexiletine is used to suppress frequent ventricular ectopy and to reduce the frequency and duration of abrupt self-limiting ventricular tachycardia.

Usual adult dosage: 200 to 300 mg P.O. every 8 hours; the daily dosage may be divided into two doses. Sometimes a loading dose of 400 mg P.O. is required to initiate therapy. A patient with severe liver disease may require a lower dosage and close monitoring. No data for pediatric dosages are available.

tocainide hydrochloride (Tonocard). Considered by some physicians to be the oral equivalent of lidocaine, tocainide is used to suppress frequent ventricular ectopy and to reduce the frequency and duration of abrupt self-limiting ventricular tachycardia. Tocainide sometimes is used when a patient is switched from I.V. lidocaine to an oral antiarrhythmic.

Usual adult dosage: 400 to 600 mg P.O. every 8 hours; the daily dosage may be divided into two doses. In a patient with severe renal or hepatic impairment, the dosage may be reduced; adequate response may occur with dosages of less than 1.2 grams daily. No data for pediatric dosages are available.

Drug interactions

Class IB antiarrhythmics may exhibit additive or antagonistic effects when administered with other antiarrhythmics, such as phenytoin, propranolol, procainamide, and quinidine. Lidocaine toxicity may result from concurrent administration of propranolol or cimetidine. Phenytoin may reduce mexiletine concentrations, requiring a dosage increase; rifampin may reduce mexiletine or tocainide concentrations, requiring a dosage increase to maintain a therapeutic effect.

ADVERSE DRUG REACTIONS

All class IB antiarrhythmics have a relatively high incidence of CNS disturbances, especially drowsiness, confusion, light-headedness, paresthesia, slurred speech, vision and hearing disturbances, tremor, seizures, and coma. Lowering the dose or stopping the drug reverses these reactions. Hypotension and bradycardia sometimes occur. Up to 40% of patients taking mexiletine or tocainide experience upper GI distress, which usually is relieved by taking the drug with food or antacids.

Tocainide can lead to two rare but serious reactions: blood dyscrasias and pulmonary fibrosis. These disappear when the drug is discontinued. Drug fever and hepatitis have occurred after tocainide therapy. Tocainide or mexiletine may produce allergic skin reactions. Generally, mexiletine is tolerated better than tocainide.

NURSING PROCESS APPLICATION

The following information assists the nurse in caring for a patient who is receiving a class IB antiarrhythmic.

Assessment
• Review the patient's history for a condition that contraindicates the use of a class IB antiarrhythmic, such as Stokes-Adams syndrome; Wolff-Parkinson-White syndrome; SA, AV, or intraventricular heart block in the absence of an artificial pacemaker; or known hypersensitivity to local amide-type anesthetics.
• Review the patient's history for a condition that requires cautious use of a class IB antiarrhythmic, such as hypovolemia, severe CHF, shock, or malignant hyperthermia.
• Assess the patient for adverse reactions to the prescribed class IB antiarrhythmic, such as CNS disturbances, hypotension, bradycardia, GI distress, blood dyscrasias, or pulmonary fibrosis.
• Review the patient's medication history to identify the use of drugs that may interact with the prescribed class IB antiarrhythmic, such as phenytoin, propranolol, procainamide, quinidine, or rifampin.
• Assess the effectiveness of the prescribed class IB antiarrhythmic periodically.
• Assess the patient for sensory-perceptual changes.
• Evaluate the patient's and family's knowledge about the prescribed class IB antiarrhythmic.

Nursing diagnoses
The following examples represent appropriate nursing diagnoses for a patient receiving a class IB antiarrhythmic.
• Potential for injury related to a preexisting condition that contraindicates the use of a class IB antiarrhythmic
• Potential for injury related to a preexisting condition that requires cautious use of a class IB antiarrhythmic
• Potential for injury related to adverse drug reactions
• Sensory-perceptual alterations (auditory, tactile, and visual) related to the adverse CNS effects of the class IB antiarrhythmic
• Knowledge deficit related to the prescribed class IB antiarrhythmic

Planning and implementation
• Do not administer a class IB antiarrhythmic to a patient with a condition that contraindicates its use.
• Administer a class IB antiarrhythmic cautiously to a patient at risk because of a preexisting condition.
• Monitor the patient closely for CNS disturbances and other adverse reactions.
• *Observe for signs of lidocaine toxicity, such as confusion and restlessness, when administering propranolol or cimetidine concurrently with the class IB agent.*

• Watch for signs of blood dyscrasias, such as changes in the patient's blood count, and signs of pulmonary fibrosis, such as respiratory changes, when administering tocainide. If these adverse reactions occur, expect to discontinue the drug.

• *Monitor the patient's serum potassium level because hypokalemia exacerbates arrhythmias.*

• *Take safety precautions if adverse CNS reactions occur. For example, keep the bed in a low position and supervise ambulation.*

• Administer lidocaine I.M. in the deltoid muscle to enhance absorption. Keep in mind, however, that I.M. administration of lidocaine interferes with cardiac enzyme measurements used to help diagnose an acute MI.

• Use the 100-mg prefilled syringe of lidocaine for an I.V. push bolus. Use the 1- or 2-gram prefilled syringe for mixing in 250 or 500 ml dextrose 5% in water.

• *Do not use lidocaine solutions containing epinephrine when lidocaine is prescribed to treat arrhythmias; such solutions are for local anesthesia only.*

• Administer continuous I.V. infusions using an infusion pump and monitor the patient's ECG constantly.

• *Expect to reduce the dosage of the class IB antiarrhythmic, as prescribed, in a patient with CHF, cardiogenic shock, liver disease, or severe renal or hepatic impairment.*

• Expect to adjust the dosage as prescribed in a patient receiving a drug that may interact with the class IB antiarrhythmic.

• Expect to switch the patient from I.V. lidocaine to tocainide, as prescribed, if an oral antiarrhythmic is needed.

• *Administer mexiletine or tocainide with food or antacids to reduce GI distress.*

• Notify the physician if adverse reactions occur.

• *Monitor the patient for sensory-perceptual alterations, such as vision or hearing disturbances or paresthesias.*

• Notify the physician if sensory-perceptual alterations occur. Reassure the patient that these alterations should disappear with dosage reduction or drug discontinuation.

Patient teaching

• Teach the patient and family the name, dose (if appropriate), frequency, action, and adverse effects of the prescribed class IB antiarrhythmic.

• Advise the patient not to perform activities that require alertness if adverse CNS reactions occur.

• *Instruct the family that the class IB antiarrhythmic may cause confusion.*

• *Teach the patient and family to recognize and report to the physician signs of toxicity, such as change in level of consciousness, seizures, or vision or hearing disturbances. Reassure them that these reactions will disappear with dosage reduction or drug discontinuation.*

• Instruct the patient to take mexiletine or tocainide with food or antacids.

• Instruct the patient to notify the physician if adverse reactions occur.

Evaluation

The following examples represent appropriate evaluation statements for a patient receiving a class IB antiarrhythmic.

• The patient has no conditions that contraindicate class IB antiarrhythmic therapy.

• The patient exhibits no signs of complications in the preexisting condition linked to the prescribed class IB antiarrhythmic.

• The patient demonstrates no adverse reactions to the prescribed class IB antiarrhythmic.

• The patient's sensory perception remains normal during therapy with the class IB antiarrhythmic.

• The patient and family express an accurate understanding of the points taught about the prescribed class IB antiarrhythmic.

• The patient correctly identifies signs of toxicity and describes what to do if they occur.

CLASS IC ANTIARRHYTHMICS

The Food and Drug Administration (FDA) has approved four class IC antiarrhythmics—encainide hydrochloride, flecainide acetate, indecainide hydrochloride, and propafenone hydrochloride—for use in treating certain types of severe, refractory ventricular arrhythmias. Encainide, flecainide, indecainide, and propafenone are local anesthetics that act to stabilize the cell membrane.

PHARMACOKINETICS

After oral administration, class IC antiarrhythmics are absorbed well, distributed in varying degrees, probably metabolized by the liver, and excreted primarily by the kidneys, except for propafenone, which is excreted primarily in the feces.

Absorption, distribution, metabolism, excretion

Flecainide, indecainide, and propafenone are absorbed rapidly and almost completely from the GI tract after oral administration. Absorption of encainide from the GI tract varies from 76% to 85%. However, its bioavailability is reduced to about 30% by extensive first-pass hepatic metabolism. First-pass metabolism also affects propafenone's bioavailability, which is dose-dependent and ranges from 5% to 40% for patients with normal hepatic function and up to 60% in those with severe liver disease.

Flecainide and indecainide are distributed widely, with about 50% bound to plasma protein. In contrast, encainide and propafenone display more limited distribution, but more extensive plasma protein binding.

Flecainide probably is metabolized in the liver, although the exact site has not been determined. It forms two major dealkylated metabolites, which exert only minor antiarrhythmic effects. The kidneys excrete about 30% of the unchanged drug and all of the metabolites; less than 5% of the drug is excreted in the feces.

The speed and degree of metabolism of encainide and propafenone is related to the patient's genetic ability to metabolize the drugs via oxidation. Encainide is demethylated rapidly in the liver to form at least two active metabolites, which are excreted in the urine. Propafenone is metabolized almost completely in the liver, producing at least 11 metabolites, two of which have electrophysiologic effects similar to the parent drug. Propafenone and its metabolites are excreted primarily in the feces.

Indecainide is metabolized partially, and about 80% of an oral dose is excreted in the urine.

Onset, peak, duration

Encainide begins to act in 1 to 2 hours when given orally. Data are incomplete, but its half-life is known to be 1 to 3 hours, and that of its metabolites, much longer. Its duration of action is 14 hours or longer.

Onset of action data are incomplete for flecainide, which reaches a peak concentration level in 30 minutes to 6 hours, with 2 to 3 hours the average. The therapeutic plasma level ranges from 0.2 to 1 mcg/ml. Its duration is undetermined, but its half-life ranges from 7 to 25 hours in healthy adults, with 13 to 16 hours as the average. The half-life may be increased in elderly patients or those with premature ventricular contraction or severe renal impairment.

Indecainide's peak concentration occurs about 4 hours after administration. Normally, its half-life varies from 6 to 12 hours; it is higher in patients with renal disease.

Propafenone reaches its peak concentration about 3.5 hours after oral administration in most patients. In patients who metabolize propafenone extensively, the half-life is 2 to 10 hours; in those who metabolize the drug poorly, the half-life ranges from 10 to 32 hours. Although the therapeutic concentration for propafenone is incompletely defined, it seems to range from 0.06 to 1.0 mcg/ml.

PHARMACODYNAMICS

Encainide, flecainide, and propafenone primarily block influx of sodium in the cell membrane fast channel during phase 0 of the action potential, thereby decreasing depolarization. Indecainide's mechanism of action is uncertain, but probably involves its ability to block the sodium current in Purkinje and myocardial cells.

Mechanism of action

At low dosages, encainide slows intracardiac conduction, but has relatively little effect on ERP or repolarization. It may increase APD slightly in atrial and ventricular muscle and decrease APD in Purkinje fibers. Its active metabolites also may decrease intracardiac conduction and may increase ERP to a greater extent than the parent drug. The effect on intracardiac conduction is reflected on the ECG by dose-related increases in PR, QRS, and to a lesser extent QT intervals. Encainide may depress normal SA and AV node function somewhat, especially in patients with preexisting sinus node dysfunction.

Encainide has little potential to increase endocardial pacing thresholds and may have a mild negative inotropic effect. In patients with compensated congestive heart failure, long-term encainide therapy usually does not affect ventricular function. However, long-term therapy occasionally causes or worsens congestive heart failure, although its myocardial depressant effect seems to be less than that of flecainide.

Flecainide produces a dose-related decrease in intracardiac conduction, minor effects on ERP, and little effect on repolarization and APD. Its effect on intra-atrial and AV conduction is less pronounced than its effect on intraventricular conduction. Although flecainide has little effect on normal SA and AV nodes or atrial cells, it depresses conduction and function in dysfunctional cells. Flecainide's effects on intracardiac conduction are reflected on ECGs by dose-related increases in PR, QRS, and to a lesser degree, QT intervals.

Flecainide also increases endocardial pacing thresholds and exerts some negative inotropic effect. It does not interfere with sympathetic or parasympathetic nervous system control of the heart.

As a class IC antiarrhythmic, indecainide may act by blocking the inward sodium current in Purkinje and myocardial cells.

Structurally similar to beta-adrenergic blocking agents, propafenone possesses a weak beta-adrenergic blocking activity. Like all type IC agents, propafenone prolongs intracardiac conduction, produces minor effects on refractoriness (inability of the heart to be restimulated), and has little effect on normal sinus node function. However, it may suppress function in a diseased sinus node. It also prolongs AV nodal functioning and ERP.

On ECG tracings, propafenone's conduction effects are reflected by prolonged PR and QRS intervals with little or no change in the QT interval.

Propafenone can alter pacing and sensing thresholds of artificial pacemakers. It also produces a mild, probably dose-related depression of ventricular function. Occasionally, propafenone has been reported to cause or worsen congestive heart failure, but as with encainide, its cardiac depressant effect seems to be less than that of flecainide.

PHARMACOTHERAPEUTICS

Like class IB antiarrhythmics, class IC drugs are used to treat life-threatening ventricular arrhythmias. Some arrhythmias respond better to class IC agents than to the class IB drugs. The class IC drugs also are being investigated for use in treating paroxysmal atrial fibrillation and supraventricular tachycardia.

encainide hydrochloride (Enkaid). This drug is indicated for treatment of documented life-threatening ventricular arrhythmias, such as ventricular tachycardia.
Usual adult dosage: initially, 25 mg P.O. every 8 hours, increasing to 35 mg, then to 50 mg, and finally to a maximum of 50 mg P.O. every 6 hours to control the arrhythmia. A 3- to 5-day interval between dosage increments is recommended. Patients with renal or hepatic impairment may require dosage adjustments.

flecainide acetate (Tambocor). Indications for this class IC antiarrhythmic are the same as for encainide.
Usual adult dosage: 100 to 200 mg P.O. every 12 hours; dividing the daily dosage into three doses given at 8-hour intervals sometimes is necessary. Patients with renal or hepatic impairment may require dosage adjustments.

indecainide hydrochloride (Decabid). Indecainide is used to manage life-threatening ventricular arrhythmias, such as sustained ventricular tachycardia.
Usual adult dosage: initially, 50 mg P.O. every 12 hours; increased as needed, based on patient response and tolerance, after at least 4 days to 75 mg P.O. every 12 hours, and then 4 days later to 100 mg P.O. every 12 hours. If higher dosages (up to 200 mg every 12 hours) are needed, the patient should be hospitalized during titration.

propafenone hydrochloride (Rythmol). This antiarrhythmic is used to manage life-threatening ventricular arrhythmias, such as sustained ventricular tachycardia.
Usual adult dosage: initially, 150 mg P.O. every 8 hours; increased as needed, based on patient response and tolerance, after at least 3 days to 225 mg P.O. every 8 hours, and then to 300 mg P.O. every 8 hours. The safety and efficacy of dosages above 900 mg/day have not been established.

Drug interactions

Class IC antiarrhythmics may exhibit additive effects with other antiarrhythmics. When used with digoxin, flecainide and propafenone can increase the serum digoxin concentration and predispose the patient to digitalis toxicity. When given with oral anticoagulants, propafenone can increase the patient's prothrombin time. (For more information, see *Drug interactions: Class IC antiarrhythmics,* page 500.)

ADVERSE DRUG REACTIONS

Class IC antiarrhythmics can produce serious adverse reactions, including proarrhythmias, which limit the use of these drugs.

All class IC agents cause adverse CNS reactions, which may include dizziness, headache, paresthesia, fatigue, and blurred vision. They also may produce adverse GI reactions, such as nausea and vomiting and constipation or diarrhea. A metallic or bitter taste may result from propafenone use and, to a lesser extent, from flecainide use. Indecainide may cause dyspepsia. The CNS and GI reactions may be dose-related in some patients and may abate with dosage reduction.

Adverse cardiovascular reactions to these agents include conduction abnormalities, exacerbation of CHF, arrhythmias, and hypotension. Paradoxically, class IC agents can aggravate existing arrhythmias. These proarrhythmic effects must not be misinterpreted as recurrence or spontaneous worsening of the original arrhythmia. Some data suggest these effects usually occur 1 to 4 weeks after starting therapy, but they may occur at any time during therapy.

Each class IC agent has some negative inotropic potential and can cause or worsen CHF. This effect is most pronounced with flecainide.

Because propafenone possesses beta-blocking properties, it may cause bronchospasm, although only a few cases have been reported. Rarely, flecainide, indecainide, and propafenone have been associated with hematologic disturbances. More commonly, flecainide causes fever, rash, and allergic reactions.

NURSING PROCESS APPLICATION

The following information assists the nurse in caring for a patient who is receiving a class IC antiarrhythmic.

Assessment
• Review the patient's history for a preexisting condition that contraindicates the use of a class IC antiarrhythmic, such as second- or third-degree AV block or right bundle branch block with a left hemiblock in the absense of a pacemaker, lactation, or known hypersensitivity to class IC antiarrhythmics.
• Review the patient's history for a preexisting condition that requires cautious use of a class IC antiarrhythmic, such as sick sinus syndrome; CHF; myocardial dysfunction; prolonged PR, QRS, or QT intervals; use of a permanent pacemaker or temporary pacing electrodes; or pregnancy.
• Assess the patient for adverse reactions to the prescribed class IC antiarrhythmic, such as CNS, cardiovascular, or GI disturbances.
• Review the patient's medication history to identify the use of drugs that may interact with the prescribed class IC

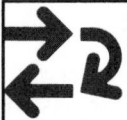

DRUG INTERACTIONS

Class IC antiarrhythmics

Class IC antiarrhythmics interact with several commonly administered drugs. To provide the best possible patient care, the nurse should be aware of these interactions and their implications.

DRUG	INTERACTING DRUGS	POSSIBLE EFFECTS	NURSING IMPLICATIONS
encainide	cimetidine	Decreases hepatic metabolism of encainide	• Assess the patient for signs of encainide toxicity, such as conduction disturbances, hypotension, and bradycardia.
	antiarrhythmics, beta-adrenergic blockers, verapamil, diltiazem	Cause additive effects on conduction system	• Monitor the patient for increased cardiac conduction effects.
flecainide, propafenone	digoxin	Increase serum digoxin concentration	• Monitor the patient's serum digoxin concentration. • Assess the patient for signs of digitalis toxicity, such as central nervous system, cardiovascular, and gastrointestinal disturbances.
flecainide	alkalinizing agents, cimetidine, propranolol	Increase serum flecainide concentration	• Assess the patient for signs of flecainide toxicity, such as conduction disturbances, hypotension, and bradycardia.
	disopyramide, verapamil, diltiazem, beta-adrenergic blockers	Cause additive negative inotropic effects	• Assess the patient for signs of congestive heart failure, such as shortness of breath and edema.
indecainide	other antiarrhythmic agents	Increase serum concentration and effects of indecainide	• Monitor the patient's cardiac status carefully.
propafenone	warfarin	Increases prothrombin time	• Observe the patient for increased bruising, bleeding, or I.V. site oozing. • Monitor the patient's prothrombin time.
	metoprolol, propranolol	Increases serum concentrations and effects of metoprolol and propranolol	• Observe the patient for signs of increased beta-blocking effect, such as hypotension, bradycardia, intensified atrioventricular block, congestive heart failure, or bronchoconstriction.
	quinidine	Inhibits propafenone metabolism	• Avoid concomitant administration.

antiarrhythmic, such as other antiarrhythmics, digoxin, or alkalinizing drugs.
• Assess the effectiveness of the prescribed class IC antiarrhythmic frequently.
• Assess the patient's fluid balance regularly during therapy with a class IC antiarrhythmic.
• Evaluate the patient's and family's knowledge about the prescribed class IC antiarrhythmic.

Nursing diagnoses
The following examples represent appropriate nursing diagnoses for a patient receiving a class IC antiarrhythmic.
• Potential for injury related to a preexisting condition that contraindicates the use of a class IC antiarrhythmic

• Potential for injury related to a preexisting condition that requires cautious use of a class IC antiarrhythmic
• Potential for injury related to adverse drug reactions
• Fluid volume excess related to antiarrhythmic-induced CHF
• Knowledge deficit related to the prescribed class IC antiarrhythmic agent

Planning and implementation
• Do not administer a class IC antiarrhythmic to a patient with a condition that contraindicates its use.
• Administer a class IC antiarrhythmic cautiously to a patient at risk because of a preexisting condition.

• *Monitor the patient closely for adverse reactions, especially CNS, cardiovascular, or GI disturbances. Reassure the patient that a dosage reduction may relieve adverse CNS reactions.*

• Monitor the ECG continuously for a critical care patient when beginning or adjusting antiarrhythmic therapy. Notify the physician if the original arrhythmia worsens, proarrhythmia occurs, or PR, QRS, or QT intervals become excessively prolonged because the drug's arrhythmogenic effects may be misinterpreted as recurrence or spontaneous worsening of the original arrhythmia.

• *Monitor the patient's vital signs regularly, particularly noting an irregular heartbeat or hypotension.*

• *Monitor for additive effects in a patient who receives another antiarrhythmic agent concurrently.*

• *Observe the patient receiving digoxin with flecainide or propafenone for signs of digitalis toxicity.* (For more information, see *Signs and symptoms of digitalis toxicity* in Chapter 29, Cardiac Glycoside Agents and Bipyridines.)

• Observe closely for increased bruising or spontaneous bleeding in a patient receiving propafenone and an oral anticoagulant if the patient's prothrombin time increases. Monitor the prothrombin time closely.

• Monitor the hydration status for a patient who develops nausea, vomiting, or diarrhea. Obtain a prescription for an antiemetic or antidiarrheal, if needed. If constipation occurs, encourage the patient to increase fluid and fiber intake (if permissible), and obtain a prescription for a laxative, if needed.

• Take safety measures if dizziness or blurred vision occurs. For example, keep the bed in a low position and supervise ambulation.

• Make dosage adjustments several days apart, as prescribed, when administering a class IC antiarrhythmic.

• *Expect to administer a lower dosage of encainide or flecainide, as prescribed, to a patient with renal or hepatic impairment.*

• Notify the physician if adverse reactions occur.

• *Monitor the patient closely for signs of CHF, such as increasing shortness of breath, crackles, jugular vein distention, and peripheral edema.*

• Record the patient's fluid intake and output to detect fluid retention.

• Limit the patient's fluid and salt intake to decrease fluid retention.

• Notify the physician if fluid retention occurs.

Patient teaching

• Teach the patient and family the name, dose, frequency, action, and adverse effects of the prescribed class IC antiarrhythmic.

• *Demonstrate how to take a pulse and tell the patient to do this before taking each dose of the prescribed class IC antiarrhythmic. Advise the patient to notify the physician if the pulse is irregular or lower than 60 beats/minute.*

• Stress the importance of taking the drug exactly as prescribed. Instruct the patient to notify the physician if a dose is inadvertently forgotten.

• *Teach the patient who must take digoxin concurrently with flecainide or propafenone to watch for and report signs of digitalis toxicity.*

• Instruct the patient taking propafenone and an oral anticoagulant to return regularly for prothrombin time testing to detect bleeding problems.

• Reassure the patient taking propafenone that adverse CNS reactions, such as altered taste, may disappear if the dosage is reduced.

• Instruct the patient to avoid activities that require mental alertness if dizziness, blurred vision, or other CNS reactions occur.

• Instruct the patient to notify the physician and obtain a prescription for an antiemetic or antidiarrheal if nausea, vomiting, or diarrhea occurs. Suggest ways to relieve or prevent constipation, if necessary.

• *Inform the patient that class IC antiarrhythmics can cause or worsen CHF. Review the signs and symptoms of this disorder and advise the patient to notify the physician if fluid retention occurs. Instruct the patient to limit fluid and salt intake to minimize fluid retention.*

• Instruct the patient to notify the physician if adverse reactions occur.

Evaluation

The following examples represent appropriate evaluation statements for a patient receiving a class IC antiarrhythmic.

• The patient has no conditions that contraindicate class IC antiarrhythmic therapy.

• The patient exhibits no signs of complications in the preexisting condition linked to the prescribed class IC antiarrhythmic.

• The patient demonstrates no adverse reactions to the prescribed class IC antiarrhythmic agent.

• The patient maintains a normal fluid balance.

• The patient and family express an accurate understanding of the points taught about the prescribed class IC antiarrhythmic.

• The patient correctly identifies signs and symptoms of CHF and describes how to prevent them.

CLASS II ANTIARRHYTHMICS

Class II antiarrhythmics are the beta-adrenergic blockers. Acebutolol, esmolol, and propranolol are FDA-approved antiarrhythmics. (For their antianginal effects, see Chapter 31, Antianginal Agents; for the overall effects of propranolol and acebutolol, Chapter 16, Adrenergic Blocking Agents; and for their antihypertensive effects, Chapter 32, Antihypertensive Agents.)

PHARMACOKINETICS

The pharmacokinetic properties of acebutolol, esmolol, and propranolol exhibit some similarities and some major differences.

Absorption, distribution, metabolism, excretion

Acebutolol and propranolol are absorbed almost entirely from the GI tract after oral administration. Although food may delay absorption slightly, it does not affect peak concentration levels significantly. Administered intravenously, esmolol is immediately available systemically.

Acebutolol, which has low lipid solubility, does not cross the blood-brain barrier. Distributed widely, propranolol has high lipid solubility and crosses readily. Esmolol is distributed rapidly and widely. Acebutolol is 26% protein bound in plasma; esmolol, about 55% protein bound; and propranolol, 90% protein bound.

Acebutolol and propranolol significantly bind to hepatic binding sites during first-pass metabolism. The major acebutolol metabolite of hepatic acetylation is very active. Propranolol is metabolized almost completely in the liver, and at least one metabolite is active. Esmolol is hydrolyzed rapidly by blood esterases. This occurs primarily in the cytosol of red blood cells (RBCs), and secondarily in highly perfused tissues that contain esterases.

About 35% of an acebutolol dose is excreted in the urine and 55% in the feces. Most of an esmolol dose is metabolized to an inactive metabolite, which is excreted in the urine. Only a small amount of unchanged drug is excreted in the urine (less than 2%) and possibly in the feces (less than 5%). Propranolol's metabolites are excreted in the urine.

Onset, peak, duration

After oral administration, the antiarrhythmic effects of acebutolol begin after 90 minutes; the onset of action of propranolol occurs in 30 minutes. Acebutolol reaches a peak concentration after 3 to 8 hours, whereas propranolol's peak concentration occurs in 60 to 90 minutes. After I.V. in-

fusion, esmolol has a rapid onset, usually less than 5 minutes. The drug achieves a steady-state blood concentration in 10 to 30 minutes, or if an I.V. loading dose is given, in about 5 minutes. Serum concentration assays have not been useful in monitoring the antiarrhythmic or toxic effects of acebutolol, esmolol, or propranolol.

With a long duration, acebutolol exerts some blocking capacity 24 to 30 hours after administration. Esmolol has a very short duration; its beta blockade reverses completely in 20 to 30 minutes. The duration of propranolol is 4 to 6 hours for tablets and up to 24 hours for long-acting capsules. The half-life of acebutolol is 3 to 4 hours; of esmolol, 5 to 23 minutes; of propranolol, 3.4 to 6 hours.

PHARMACODYNAMICS

Acebutolol, esmolol, and propranolol suppress arrhythmias by several different mechanisms of action. The drugs block receptor sites in the conduction system of the heart, thereby slowing SA node automaticity and the conductivity of the AV node and other cells. These effects probably convert unidirectional block to bidirectional block. The class II antiarrhythmics also exert a significant negative inotropic effect. By decreasing myocardial oxygen demand, this action also may decrease myocardial ischemia. As ischemia abates, myocardial cells lose their automaticity, and this effect suppresses atrial and ventricular ectopy.

PHARMACOTHERAPEUTICS

The class II drugs are not the drugs of choice to treat arrhythmias, in part because of their multiple effects and because of possible breakthrough ectopy. The use of these agents with other antiarrhythmics remains to be evaluated.

acebutolol hydrochloride (Sectral). In addition to its antihypertensive uses, acebutolol is used to suppress frequent ventricular ectopic beats.
Usual adult dosage: 200 to 600 mg P.O. every 12 hours.

esmolol hydrochloride (Brevibloc). This short-acting, beta$_1$-selective adrenergic blocker is used primarily to control the ventricular rate in patients with supraventricular tachycardia, atrial flutter, atrial fibrillation, paroxysmal supraventricular tachycardia, and supraventricular arrhythmias associated with Wolff-Parkinson-White syndrome. Because esmolol has a very short half-life and duration of action, it may be used to treat critically ill patients who require a beta-adrenergic blocker but cannot tolerate its prolonged adverse effects.
Usual adult dosage: initially, a loading dose of 500 mcg/kg/minute I.V. over 1 minute followed by a 4-minute maintenance infusion of 50 mcg/kg/minute. The heart rate and blood pressure must be monitored closely. The initial dose

may be repeated within 5 minutes if the rate has not slowed satisfactorily. The maintenance infusion is titrated up to 300 mcg/kg/minute at 50-mcg/kg/minute increments every 5 to 10 minutes until the desired response occurs.

propranolol hydrochloride (Inderal, Inderal LA). Possibly effective in various arrhythmias, including atrial and ventricular ectopy, propranolol also may be used to treat the sudden onset of self-limiting atrial or ventricular tachycardia. Propranolol is not used to terminate acute ventricular tachycardia. The drug is best used in patients with arrhythmias associated with excess catecholamines, ventricular or supraventricular tachyarrhythmias related to digitalis toxicity, or Wolff-Parkinson-White syndrome.
Usual adult dosage: for arrhythmias, 10 to 30 mg P.O. every 6 to 8 hours; for life-threatening arrhythmias, 0.5 to 3 mg I.V., followed by a second dose after 2 minutes, if needed, and additional I.V. doses at 4-hour intervals until oral therapy can begin. Because of insufficient data, propranolol is not recommended for use in pediatric patients.

Drug interactions
Class II antiarrhythmics interact with phenothiazines and antihypertensive drugs, which potentiate hypotension. Interactions with anticholinergics and cimetidine alter the effects of Class II antiarrhythmic drugs. (For details, see *Drug interactions: Class II antiarrhythmics,* page 504.)

ADVERSE DRUG REACTIONS

The most common adverse reactions to class II antiarrhythmics involve the cardiovascular system and usually occur when drugs are given initially. Because they inhibit sinus node stimulation, class II antiarrhythmics may produce bradycardia—a heart rate less than 60 beats/minute. Hypotension with peripheral vascular insufficiency also may occur, especially with esmolol. Syncope, angina, and shock may accompany these reactions. Occasionally, fluid retention and peripheral edema occur. Because class II antiarrhythmics reduce the force of myocardial contraction and increase preload, they may exacerbate or precipitate CHF. Arrhythmias, especially AV block, also may occur.

Adverse CNS reactions include dizziness, confusion, fatigue, lassitude, and decreased libido. Typical GI reactions, such as nausea, vomiting, mild diarrhea, or constipation, usually are transient.

Acebutolol and propranolol block bronchial beta receptors that otherwise dilate bronchioles; this action can lead to significant bronchoconstriction. Propranolol is more likely to cause this adverse reaction because it is a nonselective beta-adrenergic blocker. I.V. infusions of esmolol cause inflammation and induration at the injection site in about 80% of patients.

Other reactions to class II antiarrhythmics include rashes, blood dyscrasias, depression, and vivid dreams. These reactions, however, are rare.

NURSING PROCESS APPLICATION

The following information assists the nurse in caring for a patient who is receiving a class II antiarrhythmic.

Assessment
• Review the patient's history for a preexisting condition that contraindicates the use of a class II antiarrhythmic, such as cardiogenic shock, sinus bradycardia and greater than first-degree block, bronchial asthma, most types of congestive heart failure, or known hypersensitivity to class II antiarrhythmics.
• Review the patient's history for a preexisting condition that requires cautious use of a class II antiarrhythmic, such as a nonallergic bronchospastic disorder, diabetes mellitus, impaired hepatic or renal function, lactation, or pregnancy.
• Assess the patient for adverse reactions to the prescribed class II antiarrhythmic, such as cardiovascular dysfunction or bronchoconstriction.
• Review the patient's medication history to identify the use of drugs that may interact with the prescribed class II antiarrhythmic, such as phenothiazines, antihypertensive agents, anticholinergic agents, or cimetidine.
• Assess the effectiveness of the prescribed class II antiarrhythmic periodically.
• Assess the patient regularly for signs of fluid volume excess.
• Evaluate the patient's and family's knowledge about the prescribed class II antiarrhythmic.

Nursing diagnoses
The following examples represent appropriate nursing diagnoses for a patient receiving a class II antiarrhythmic.
• Potential for injury related to a preexisting condition that contraindicates the use of a class II antiarrhythmic
• Potential for injury related to a preexisting condition that requires cautious use of a class II antiarrhythmic
• Potential for injury related to adverse drug reactions
• Fluid volume excess related to fluid retention caused by the prescribed class II antiarrhythmic
• Knowledge deficit related to the prescribed class II antiarrhythmic

Planning and implementation
• Do not administer a class II antiarrhythmic to a patient with a condition that contraindicates its use.
• Administer a class II antiarrhythmic cautiously to a patient at risk because of a preexisting condition.
• *Monitor the patient closely for cardiovascular and other adverse reactions, especially when therapy first begins.*

DRUG INTERACTIONS
Class II antiarrhythmics

The interactions between class II antiarrhythmics and other drugs can be hazardous to the patient's well-being. The nurse must be aware of such interactions to provide quality patient care.

DRUG	INTERACTING DRUGS	POSSIBLE EFFECTS	NURSING IMPLICATIONS
acebutolol, esmolol, propranolol	phenothiazines	Increase hypotension	• Monitor the patient for dizziness and orthostatic hypotension.
	sympathomimetics (beta agonists)	Decrease effect of sympathomimetics	• Monitor the patient for decreased therapeutic effect.
	anticholinergics	Potentiate pressor effects, causing hypertension; reduce efficacy of the class II antiarrhythmics	• Monitor the patient's therapeutic response and heart rate and rhythm.
	antihypertensives	Increase hypotension	• Monitor the patient for dizziness and orthostatic hypotension.
	neuromuscular blockers	Enhance skeletal muscle relaxation	• Monitor the patient for hypoventilation when administering class II antiarrhythmics in the immediate postoperative period.
	verapamil	Increases cardiac depression	• Monitor the patient for decreased heart rate.
esmolol	digoxin	Increases serum digoxin concentration	• Monitor the patient's serum digoxin concentration. • Assess for signs of digitalis toxicity, such as cardiac, central nervous system, or gastrointestinal disturbances.
	morphine	Increases blood esmolol concentration	• Monitor the patient for esmolol toxicity, such as hypotension, bradycardia, and decreased level of consciousness.
propranolol	cimetidine	Decreases propranolol metabolism	• Observe the patient for adverse reactions even at a low dosage of propranolol.

• *Monitor the patient's ECG to detect arrhythmias, especially AV block and bradycardia.*
• Take the patient's vital signs, as prescribed. Particularly note decreased heart rate or blood pressure, especially during esmolol therapy.
• *Withhold the dose and notify the physician if the pulse is less than 60 beats/minute or the systolic blood pressure is less than 90 mm Hg.*
• *Auscultate the patient's breath sounds routinely to detect signs of bronchospasm, such as wheezing.*
• Take safety precautions if dizziness or confusion occurs. For example, keep the bed in a low position and supervise ambulation.
• Reassure the patient that decreased libido should return to normal when the drug is discontinued.
• Monitor hydration status if the patient develops adverse GI reactions, such as nausea, vomiting, or diarrhea. Request a prescription for an antiemetic or antidiarrheal agent, as

needed. If constipation occurs, obtain a prescription for a laxative. Reassure the patient that adverse GI reactions usually are transient.
• Observe the esmolol infusion site for signs of inflammation and induration.
• Use an infusion pump when administering esmolol to control dosage titration closely.
• *Inspect the esmolol solution carefully before administration. Discard the solution if it contains particles or is discolored.*
• Monitor the heart rate and blood pressure continuously during esmolol infusion.
• *Observe the patient receiving esmolol and digoxin concurrently for signs of digitalis toxicity.* (For a complete list, see *Signs and symptoms of digitalis toxicity* in Chapter 29, Cardiac Glycoside Agents and Bipyridines.)
• Monitor the patient for hypoventilation when administering a class II antiarrhythmic in the immediate postop-

erative period. Neuromuscular blockers used during surgery may interact with an antiarrhythmic agent.

• Notify the physician if adverse reactions occur.

• *Monitor the patient closely for signs of fluid retention, such as peripheral edema, crackles, weight gain, and shortness of breath.*

• Notify the physician if the patient displays signs of fluid retention.

Patient teaching

• Teach the patient and family the name, dose, frequency, action, and adverse effects of the prescribed class II antiarrhythmic.

• *Demonstrate how to take a pulse. Tell the patient to check the pulse before each dose of the prescribed antiarrhythmic. If the pulse is slow (below 60 beats/minute or the rate noted by the physician), advise the patient to withhold the dose and notify the physician.*

• Instruct the patient not to perform activities that require alertness if dizziness, fatigue, lassitude, or confusion occur.

• Reassure the patient that libido, which may decrease during drug therapy, should return to normal when the drug is discontinued.

• Instruct the patient to notify the physician if nausea, vomiting, diarrhea, or constipation occurs. A prescription for an antiemetic, antidiarrheal, or laxative agent may be needed.

• *Stress the importance of limiting fluid and salt intake to minimize fluid retention.*

• Advise the patient to notify the physician if adverse reactions occur.

Evaluation

The following examples represent appropriate evaluation statements for a patient receiving a class II antiarrhythmic agent.

• The patient has no conditions that contraindicate class II antiarrhythmic therapy.

• The patient exhibits no signs of complications in the preexisting condition linked to the prescribed class II antiarrhythmic.

• The patient experiences no adverse reactions to the prescribed class II antiarrhythmic.

• The patient maintains a normal fluid balance.

• The patient and family express an accurate understanding of the points taught about the prescribed class II antiarrhythmic.

• The patient describes appropriate dietary changes that should minimize fluid retention.

CLASS III ANTIARRHYTHMICS

The class III antiarrhythmics amiodarone and bretylium are used to treat ventricular arrhythmias. Both drugs significantly affect APD to produce their antiarrhythmic effect.

PHARMACOKINETICS

The two class III antiarrhythmics have quite different pharmacokinetic properties.

Absorption, distribution, metabolism, excretion

After oral administration, amiodarone is absorbed slowly at widely varying rates. The drug is distributed extensively and accumulates in many sites, especially in highly vascular organs and adipose tissue. It is 96% protein bound in plasma, mainly to albumin. Amiodarone probably is metabolized in the liver, and possibly in the intestinal lumen or GI mucosa, to at least one major metabolite with antiarrhythmic activity. The drug undergoes biliary excretion and is eliminated almost completely in feces.

Bretylium's erratic GI absorption mandates parenteral administration. Data about its distribution and protein binding are lacking. Bretylium is excreted unchanged by the kidneys over several days.

Onset, peak, duration

Amiodarone's onset of action may begin within 2 to 3 days in some patients, but usually does not occur for 1 to 3 weeks after therapy begins. After oral administration of amiodarone, the peak concentration level occurs within 3 to 7 hours. If a loading dose is not given, a steady-state concentration of amiodarone is not attained for at least 1 month and usually not for 5 months or longer. Although individuals show great variation between plasma amiodarone concentration and therapeutic effect, concentrations greater than 2.5 mcg/ml are linked to increased incidence of certain adverse reactions. Effects of amiodarone may persist for weeks or even months after discontinuation. Amiodarone has an initial half-life of 2.5 to 10 days and an average terminal half-life of 53 days.

In a patient with ventricular fibrillation, bretylium's onset begins within minutes of I.V. infusion. When the drug is given to suppress ventricular ectopy and ventricular tachycardia, however, onset takes 20 minutes to 6 hours. Peak plasma concentration of bretylium occurs immediately after I.V. infusion and within 1 hour of I.M. administration. The therapeutic serum level of bretylium is 0.5 to 1.5 mcg/

ml. The duration of action of bretylium is 6 to 24 hours; its half-life is 5 to 10 hours.

PHARMACODYNAMICS

Class III antiarrhythmics greatly prolong the APD and ERP of myocardial cells, thus decreasing the rate of automaticity of ventricular ectopic beats. The drugs may convert unidirectional block to bidirectional block, but they have little or no effect on depolarization. Amiodarone and bretylium inhibit sympathetic nervous system innervation of the heart; however, they increase circulating catecholamines. Both drugs produce some peripheral and coronary vasodilation.

Amiodarone may decrease intracardiac conduction, as shown by increased PR and QT intervals; the QRS interval may be unchanged or increased. Bretylium does not prolong these intervals. However, bretylium exerts a positive inotropic effect. The exact mechanism of action of class III antiarrhythmics that is most responsible for the antiarrhythmic effects remains uncertain.

PHARMACOTHERAPEUTICS

In part because of their adverse effects, class III antiarrhythmics are not the drugs of choice for antiarrhythmic therapy. The drugs produce synergistic effects when combined with any of several other antiarrhythmics.

amiodarone hydrochloride (Cordarone). Indicated for preventing life-threatening ventricular ectopy, amiodarone also is used to reduce the frequency and duration of persistent ventricular tachycardia unresponsive to other antiarrhythmics. Because large amounts of the drug are sequestered in various tissues, physicians usually order loading doses. Without the loading dose, steady-state plasma levels would take months to achieve. The dose must be titrated to the patient's requirements under close ECG monitoring.
Usual adult dosage: loading dose, 800 to 1,600 mg P.O. daily for 1 to 3 weeks or until a response occurs; reduced gradually to a maintenance dosage of 200 to 400 mg P.O. daily.

bretylium tosylate (Bretylol). Useful in preventing and treating ventricular fibrillation and ventricular tachycardia that are unresponsive to other treatment, bretylium is used only for short-term therapy in immediately life-threatening conditions.
Usual adult dosage: 5 mg/kg I.V. push over 1 minute, increased to 10 mg/kg I.V. push over 1 minute if necessary. Doses may be repeated every 1 to 2 hours, or a continuous I.V. infusion of 1 to 2 mg/minute can be used. Bretylium may be given 5 to 10 mg/kg I.M. and repeated every 1 to 2 hours.

Drug interactions

Significant interactions with other cardiovascular drugs, such as digoxin and antihypertensives, vary. Interactions are more serious with amiodarone than with short-term bretylium therapy. (For more information, see *Drug interactions: Class III antiarrhythmics.*)

ADVERSE DRUG REACTIONS

Adverse reactions to class III antiarrhythmics, especially amiodarone, vary widely and commonly lead to discontinuation of the drug.

Amiodarone may produce hypotension, nausea, and anorexia. It causes adverse CNS reactions in 20% to 40% of patients, including malaise, fatigue, tremor, involuntary movements, lack of coordination, abnormal gait, ataxia, dizziness, and paresthesia. Rarely, peripheral neuropathy and proximal myopathy occur.

Amiodarone causes several non-dose-related reactions. Pulmonary toxicity consisting of interstitial pneumonia and alveolitis occurs in 15% of patients and can be fatal; signs and symptoms include dyspnea, cough, and X-ray changes. Corneal microdeposits occur in almost all patients, but only 10% experience visual disturbances. The deposits disappear with dosage reduction or drug discontinuation. Skin photosensitivity occurs, sometimes producing a blue-gray discoloration of exposed skin. The metabolic effects of amiodarone can produce hypothyroidism or hyperthyroidism.

Like most antiarrhythmics, amiodarone and bretylium can aggravate arrhythmias, especially bradycardia, and increase ventricular ectopic beats.

Upon initial bretylium administration, orthostatic and supine hypotension commonly occur, producing dizziness. Nausea and vomiting commonly accompany rapid I.V. administration.

NURSING PROCESS APPLICATION

The following information assists the nurse in caring for a patient who is receiving a class III antiarrhythmic.

Assessment

• Review the patient's history for a preexisting condition that contraindicates the use of a class III antiarrhythmic, such as severe sinus node dysfunction, bradycardia-induced syncope (except in the presence of a pacemaker), or lactation.
• Review the patient's history for a preexisting condition that requires cautious use of a class III antiarrhythmic, such as pregnancy.
• Assess the patient for adverse reactions to the prescribed class III antiarrhythmic, such as cardiovascular, GI, CNS, or thyroid dysfunction.

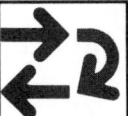

DRUG INTERACTIONS

Class III antiarrhythmics

The interactions between class III antiarrhythmics and other drugs may cause serious consequences for the patient. The nurse must be prepared to use appropriate assessment and intervention strategies in response to these interactions.

DRUG	INTERACTING DRUGS	POSSIBLE EFFECTS	NURSING IMPLICATIONS
bretylium, amiodarone	antihypertensives	Produce profound hypotension	• Monitor the patient for dizziness, orthostatic hypotension, and mental status changes.
amiodarone	warfarin	Increases hypoprothrombinemia	• Monitor the patient for increased bruising, bleeding, and I.V. site oozing; monitor prothrombin time.
	digoxin	Increases serum digoxin level	• Monitor the patient for signs of digitalis toxicity, such as anorexia, nausea, vomiting, diarrhea, visual disturbances, or arrhythmias.
	procainamide, quinidine, phenytoin	Increase serum antiarrhythmic concentration	• Monitor serum antiarrhythmic concentration; assess for increased antiarrhythmic effect.

• Review the patient's medication history to identify the use of drugs that may interact with the prescribed class III antiarrhythmic, such as an antihypertensive agent, warfarin, digoxin, procainide, quinidine, or phenytoin.
• Assess the effectiveness of the prescribed class III antiarrhythmic periodically.
• Monitor the patient's respiratory status during amiodarone therapy.
• Assess the patient for signs of thyroid dysfunction during amiodarone therapy.
• Evaluate the patient's and family's knowledge about the prescribed class III antiarrhythmic.

Nursing diagnoses
The following examples represent appropriate nursing diagnoses for a patient receiving a class III antiarrhythmic.
• Potential for injury related to a preexisting condition that contraindicates the use of a class III antiarrhythmic
• Potential for injury related to a preexisting condition that requires cautious use of a class III antiarrhythmic
• Potential for injury related to adverse drug reactions
• Ineffective breathing pattern related to amiodarone-induced pulmonary toxicity
• Altered health maintenance related to amiodarone-induced thyroid dysfunction
• Knowledge deficit related to the prescribed class III antiarrhythmic

Planning and implementation
• Do not administer a class III antiarrhythmic to a patient with a condition that contraindicates its use.

• Administer a class III antiarrhythmic cautiously to a patient at risk because of a preexisting condition.
• Monitor the patient closely for adverse reactions throughout antiarrhythmic therapy.
• *Monitor the patient's ECG. Be especially alert for bradycardia, increased ventricular ectopic beats, or, with amiodarone therapy, prolonged PR, QRS, and QT intervals.*
• *Take the patient's vital signs frequently, particularly noting a slow or irregular pulse or hypotension.*
• Observe the patient receiving a class III antiarrhythmic and another antiarrhythmic for additive effects.
• *Monitor the patient closely during concommitant therapy with a class III antiarrhythmic and another cardiovascular drug, such as digoxin or an antihypertensive agent.*
• Continue to monitor the patient for several months after amiodarone discontinuation; its effects may persist for weeks or months.
• Take safety precautions if dizziness, lack of coordination, abnormal gait, or ataxia occurs. For example, keep the bed in a low position and supervise ambulation.
• Monitor hydration if the patient develops nausea or vomiting. Obtain a prescription for an antiemetic, if needed.
• Titrate the amiodarone dosage as prescribed while monitoring the ECG closely.
• Notify the physician if adverse reactions occur.
• *Monitor the patient receiving amiodarone closely for signs of pulmonary toxicity, such as dyspnea, cough, and X-ray changes that show interstitial pneumonia or alveo-*

litis. If the patient displays these signs, notify the physician and expect to discontinue amiodarone.
• Place the patient with pulmonary toxicity in a position that enhances breathing.
• Prepare to treat pulmonary toxicity—for example, by administering oxygen and antibiotics.
• Assess the patient receiving amiodarone for signs of hypothyroidism, such as lethargy; weight gain; cool, dry skin; bradycardia; hypotension; and cold intolerance. Also check for signs of hyperthyroidism, such as nervousness, weight loss, warm and moist skin, tachycardia, and palpitations.
• Alert the physician if assessment findings suggest thyroid dysfunction.
• Prepare to treat thyroid dysfunction as prescribed.

Patient teaching

• Teach the patient and family the name, dose, frequency, action, and adverse effects of the prescribed class III antiarrhythmic.
• *Demonstrate how to take a pulse. Tell the patient to check the pulse before each dose of amiodarone and to notify the physician if the pulse falls below 60 beats/minute (or the rate set by the physician) or becomes irregular.*
• Instruct the patient receiving amiodarone to avoid activities that require alertness or coordination, if adverse CNS reactions occur.
• Advise the patient to consult with the physician about obtaining a prescription for an antiemetic if nausea or vomiting occurs.
• Inform the patient that the prescribed amiodarone dosage will be high for the first several weeks and then decreased gradually to a maintenance dosage.
• Instruct the patient taking amiodarone to notify the physician if signs of pulmonary toxicity occur, such as dyspnea or cough.
• Teach the patient to recognize and report to the physician any signs or symptoms of hypothyroidism or hyperthyroidism during amiodarone therapy.
• *Teach the patient taking amiodarone to use protective clothing and sunscreen products or to avoid sunlight to protect against photosensitivity.*
• Reassure the patient that corneal microdeposits produce visual disturbances in only 10% of all patients receiving amiodarone. However, tell the patient to notify the physician if visual changes occur.
• Advise the patient to notify the physician if any other adverse reactions occur during class III antiarrhythmic therapy.

Evaluation

The following examples represent appropriate evaluation statements for a patient receiving a class III antiarrhythmic.
• The patient has no conditions that contraindicate class III antiarrhythmic therapy.

• The patient exhibits no signs of complications in the preexisting condition linked to the prescribed class III antiarrhythmic.
• The patient experiences no adverse reactions to the prescribed class III antiarrhythmic.
• The patient maintains a normal respiratory rate and pattern during amiodarone therapy.
• The patient's thyroid function remains normal during amiodarone therapy.
• The patient and family express an accurate understanding of the points taughts about the prescribed class III antiarrhythmic.
• The patient correctly identifies signs and symptoms of thyroid dysfunctions and describes what to do if they occur.

CLASS IV ANTIARRHYTHMICS

Among the class IV antiarrhythmics, or calcium channel blockers, only verapamil is FDA-approved. Because diltiazem produces similar effects and is used to treat the same arrhythmias as verapamil, it also is included in this class, although FDA approval still is pending.

PHARMACOKINETICS

After oral administration, verapamil is about 90% absorbed, but its bioavailability is only 20% to 35% because of extensive first-pass metabolism. After oral or I.V. administration, the drug is 90% protein bound. It is metabolized rapidly and almost completely in the liver to numerous metabolites, including the only active one—norverapamil. Verapamil metabolites are excreted primarily in the urine and to a lesser extent in the feces.

After oral administration, diltiazem is about 80% absorbed. However, only 40% of the drug reaches the systemic circulation because of extensive first-pass metabolism. The drug is metabolized rapidly and almost completely to one active and numerous inactive metabolites. About 24% of the drug is excreted unchanged in urine; the remainder is eliminated as metabolites in urine and feces.

The antiarrhythmic effects of verapamil begin 3 to 5 minutes after I.V. administration and 30 minutes after oral administration. The peak concentration level occurs within 10 minutes after I.V. administration and within 1 to 2 hours after oral administration.

Diltiazem reaches its peak concentration 2 to 3 hours after administration of tablets; 6 to 11 hours after administration of extended-release capsules.

Verapamil's duration of action may be up to 6 hours but usually is less. Its half-life is 3 to 7 hours, but this may increase to 4.5 to 12 hours after long-term oral therapy, probably because of hepatic enzyme saturation. Diltiazem's half-life is 3.5 to 9 hours.

PHARMACODYNAMICS

Verapamil and diltiazem block the influx of calcium across the slow channels of myocardial electrical cells during the plateau (phase 2) and depolarization (phase 4) of the action potential. This blockade greatly increases the ERP of the AV node and slows the conduction rate between the atria and the ventricles. Although these agents rarely affect normal sinus node function, they may reduce the resting heart rate and produce sinus arrest or sinus block in patients with SA node disease.

PHARMACOTHERAPEUTICS

Verapamil and diltiazem are used to treat supraventricular arrhythmias with rapid ventricular response rates.

verapamil hydrochloride (Calan, Isoptin). I.V. verapamil is used to correct a rapid heart rate caused by reentry into the atria or the AV node. This rapid heart rate, called *paroxysmal supraventricular tachycardia (PSVT)*, has an abrupt onset and usually is self-limiting. Verapamil also is used when physical vagal stimulation is unsuccessful. The drug does not affect atrial ectopic beats. I.V. verapamil also decreases the ventricular response in patients with atrial flutter and atrial fibrillation by blocking AV conduction or converting the atrial rhythm—although the latter action is rare. Oral verapamil is used to prevent recurrent PSVT in adults.
Usual adult dosage: to correct PSVT, 5 to 10 mg I.V. push over 2 minutes (or over 3 minutes in elderly patients to minimize adverse reactions); followed by a second I.V. dose of 10 mg, 15 to 30 minutes after the initial dose if the patient tolerates but does not respond to it; to prevent recurrent PSVT, 240 to 480 mg P.O. daily in 3 or 4 divided doses; to control the ventricular response to chronic atrial fibrillation or flutter, 240 to 320 mg P.O. daily in 3 or 4 divided doses.
Usual pediatric dosage: in children under age 1, 0.75 to 2 mg I.V. push over 2 minutes; in children ages 1 and older, 2 to 5 mg I.V. bolus over 2 minutes.

diltiazem hydrochloride (Cardizem). This oral antiarrhythmic is used to prevent recurrent PSVT and to decrease the ventricular response in patients with chronic atrial fibrillation or flutter.
Usual adult dosage: 160 to 400 mg P.O. daily in 3 or 4 divided doses.

Drug interactions

Verapamil and diltiazem interact with other antiarrhythmics, producing additive effects. Interactions with antihypertensives potentiate hypotension and heart failure; with digoxin, an increased serum digoxin level and digitalis toxicity may result. Concomitant use of verapamil and other highly protein-bound drugs, such as hydantoins, salicylates, sulfonamides, and sulfonylureas, can cause adverse reactions associated with verapamil or the other drugs. Verapamil and diltiazem competitively inhibit liver enzyme metabolism of other drugs. Conversely, drugs that inhibit (cimetidine) or stimulate (rifampin) liver enzymes may interact with these agents. For example, concomitant use of cimetidine may decrease the antiarrhythmic's metabolism; rifampin may increase it.

ADVERSE DRUG REACTIONS

Verapamil and diltiazem may cause alterations in the cardiovascular system. These drugs sometimes causes hypotension, particularly orthostatic hypotension. Hypotension usually is associated with I.V. verapamil, especially with rapid I.V. bolus administration or administration to patients with rapid, narrow, complex arrhythmias, such as ventricular tachycardia. The class IV antiarrhythmics' effect on the SA and AV nodes causes arrhythmias, such as bradycardia, sinus block, and AV block. These drugs also depress myocardial contraction force, which may precipitate or exacerbate CHF.

Vasodilation produced by these agents occasionally causes dizziness, headache, flushing, weakness, and persistent peripheral edema. Other dose-related reactions include constipation and other GI disturbances, leg fatigue, and muscle cramps.

Hypersensitivity reactions include worsening of angina, skin eruptions, photosensitivity, pruritus, nasal congestion, and mood changes.

NURSING PROCESS APPLICATION

The following information assists the nurse in caring for a patient who is receiving a class IV antiarrhythmic.

Assessment
• Review the patient's history for a preexisting condition that contraindicates the use of a class IV antiarrhythmic, such as severe hypotension, cardiogenic shock, second- or third-degree AV block or sick sinus syndrome (except in the presence of an artificial pacemaker), severe congestive heart failure (unless the failure is from a supraventricular tachycardia that responds to verapamil), atrial flutter or fibrillation and accessory bypass tract (as in Wolff-Parkinson-White syndrome), or known hypersensitivity to class IV antiarrhythmics.

• Review the patient's history for a preexisting condition that requires cautious use of a class IV antiarrhythmic, such as pregnancy, lactation, or impaired hepatic or renal function.

• Assess the patient for adverse reactions to the prescribed class IV antiarrhythmic, such as cardiovascular or GI disturbances.

• Review the patient's medication history to identify the use of drugs that may interact with the prescribed class IV antiarrhythmic, such as other antiarrhythmics, antihypertensives, digoxin, hydantoins, or salicylates.

• Assess the effectiveness of the prescribed class IV antiarrhythmic regularly.

• Assess the patient closely for signs of fluid volume excess during class IV antiarrhythmic therapy.

• Evaluate the patient's and family's knowledge about the prescribed class IV antiarrhythmic.

Nursing diagnoses

The following examples represent appropriate nursing diagnoses for a patient receiving a class IV antiarrhythmic.

• Potential for injury related to a preexisting condition that contraindicates the use of a class IV antiarrhythmic

• Potential for injury related to a preexisting condition that requires cautious use of a class IV antiarrhythmic

• Potential for injury related to adverse drug reactions

• Fluid volume excess related to the adverse myocardial effects of the prescribed class IV antiarrhythmic

• Knowledge deficit related to the prescribed class IV antiarrhythmic

Planning and implementation

• Do not administer a class IV antiarrhythmic to a patient with a condition that contraindicates its use.

• Administer a class IV antiarrhythmic cautiously to a patient at risk because of a preexisting condition.

• *Monitor the patient closely for adverse cardiovascular and other reactions during antiarrhythmic therapy.*

• Be alert for interactions between verapamil and other highly protein-bound drugs, such as hydantoins, salicylates, sulfonamides, and sulfonylureas, during concomitant therapy.

• *Monitor the patient's vital signs frequently. Take a resting apical pulse in a patient with SA node disease because class IV antiarrhythmics can reduce the resting heart rate in such a patient.*

• *Monitor the ECG continuously while giving I.V. verapamil, being especially alert for SA or AV node effects, such as bradycardia, sinus block, and AV block.*

• *Be alert for hypotension or heart failure in a patient receiving a class IV antiarrhythmic and an antihypertensive agent; for digitalis toxicity in a patient receiving a class IV antiarrhythmic and digitalis.*

• *Have the patient sit up for a few minutes before standing to minimize the effects of orthostatic hypotension.*

• Take safety precautions if dizziness or weakness occurs. For example, place the bed in a low position and supervise ambulation.

• Obtain a prescription for an analgesic if the patient develops headache or muscle cramps.

• Increase the constipated patient's fluid and fiber intake; obtain a prescription for a laxative, as needed.

• Notify the physician if adverse reactions occur or if the class IV antiarrhythmic is ineffective.

• *Monitor the patient closely for signs of fluid retention, such as increasing shortness of breath, crackles, jugular vein distention, or persistent peripheral edema.*

• Limit the patient's salt and fluid intake to minimize fluid retention.

• Inform the physician immediately if the patient displays signs of fluid volume excess. Prepare to relieve fluid retention with the prescribed treatment, such as diuretic administration.

Patient teaching

• Teach the patient and family the name, dose, frequency, action, and adverse effects of the prescribed class IV antiarrhythmic.

• *Advise the patient to tell all personal physicians about class IV antiarrhythmic therapy to prevent drug interactions.*

• *Instruct the patient how to manage orthostatic hypotension.*

• Caution the patient to avoid activities that require alertness if dizziness or weakness occurs.

• Teach the patient how to manage constipation, headache, and muscle cramps.

• Teach the patient to minimize fluid retention by limiting fluid and salt intake and reporting signs of fluid retention, such as increasing shortness of breath or ankle swelling, to the physician.

• Instruct the patient to notify the physician of any adverse reactions.

Evaluation

The following examples represent appropriate evaluation statements for a patient receiving a class IV antiarrhythmic.

• The patient has no conditions that contraindicate class IV antiarrhythmic therapy.

• The patient exhibits no signs of complications in the preexisting condition linked to the prescribed class IV antiarrhythmic.

• The patient displays no adverse reactions to the prescribed class IV antiarrhythmic.

• The patient maintains a normal fluid balance during class IV antiarrhythmic therapy.

• The patient and family express an accurate understanding of the points taught about the prescribed class IV antiarrhythmic.

• The patient correctly identifies signs of fluid retention and describes how to minimize this problem.

OTHER ANTIARRHYTHMIC AGENTS

Adenosine is a new injectable antiarrhythmic agent indicated for acute treatment of PSVTs, including those associated with accessory bypass tracts, as in Wolff-Parkinson-White syndrome.

PHARMACOKINETICS

After I.V. administration, adenosine probably is distributed rapidly throughout the body, where it is removed from plasma by uptake into RBCs and vascular endothelial cells. Inside these cells, adenosine is metabolized rapidly to the inactive metabolite inosine, which is metabolized further to hypoxanthine and then to uric acid.

The half-life of adenosine is extremely short and may range from 0.6 to 10 seconds. An I.V. bolus of adenosine is removed completely from plasma in about 30 to 60 seconds.

Adenosine's onset of action is almost immediate. Most tachycardias terminate within 30 seconds after a dose, which may reflect adenosine's peak concentration level. The drug's duration of action is less than 2 minutes.

PHARMACODYNAMICS

Adenosine depresses SA node pacemaker activity and AV nodal conduction. It produces negative chronotropic (bradycardia) and negative dromotropic (AV block) effects on the heart. These actions make adenosine especially effective against reentry tachycardias that involve the AV node and more than 90% of PSVTs. Although I.V. infusion of adenosine also produces coronary and peripheral vasodilation, the bolus dosages used to treat arrhythmias appear to have little effect on systemic hemodynamics.

PHARMACOTHERAPEUTICS

Adenosine is available only as an I.V. preparation to treat arrhythmias.

adenosine. (Adenocard). Adenosine is indicated to convert PSVT (including that associated with accessory bypass tracts such as Wolff-Parkinson-White syndrome) to sinus rhythm.
Usual adult dosage: initially, 6 mg bolus given over 1 to 2 seconds directly into a vein or, if given through an I.V. line, as proximal as possible and followed by a rapid saline flush. If PSVT is not eliminated within 1 to 2 minutes after the first dose, give 12 mg as a rapid I.V. bolus. The 12-mg dose may be repeated a second time if required. Doses greater than 12 mg are not recommended.

Drug interactions
When adenosine is administered concurrently with carbamazepine, the additive cardiovascular effects may increase the degree of heart block. Dipyridamole potentiates the effects of adenosine; smaller doses of adenosine may be necessary. Methylxanthines, such as caffeine and theophylline, antagonize the effects of adenosine; larger doses of adenosine may be necessary.

ADVERSE DRUG REACTIONS

Adverse drug reactions reported during clinical trials in more than 5% of patients include facial flushing, shortness of breath, dyspnea, and chest pressure.

NURSING PROCESS APPLICATION

The following information assists the nurse in caring for a patient who is receiving adenosine.

Assessment
• Review the patient's history for a preexisting condition that contraindicates the use of adenosine, such as second- or third-degree AV block or sick sinus syndrome (except in the presence of an artificial pacemaker), atrial flutter, atrial fibrillation, ventricular tachycardia, or known hypersensitivity to adenosine.
• Review the patient's history for a preexisting condition that requires cautious use of adenosine, such as asthma or pregnancy.
• Assess the patient for adverse reactions to adenosine, such as facial flushing, shortness of breath, dyspnea, or chest pressure.
• Review the patient's medication history to identify the use of drugs that may interact with adenosine, such as carbamazepine, dipyridamole, or methylxanthines.
• Assess the effectiveness of adenosine regularly.

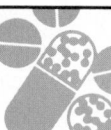

SELECTED MAJOR DRUGS

Antiarrhythmic agents

The following chart summarizes selected antiarrhythmic agents discussed in this chapter.

DRUG	MAJOR INDICATIONS	USUAL ADULT DOSAGES	CONTRAINDICATIONS AND PRECAUTIONS
Class IA			
quinidine	Conversion of atrial fibrillation to normal sinus rhythm Suppression of atrial or ventricular ectopic beats	300 to 400 mg quinidine sulfate P.O. every 6 hours, then 200 to 400 mg every 6 hours to maintain regular rhythm 200 to 300 mg quinidine sulfate P.O. every 6 to 8 hours	• Know that quinidine is contraindicated in a patient with digitalis intoxication with an atrioventricular (AV) conduction disorder or other severe intraventricular conduction defect, ectopic impulses and abnormal rhythms due to escape mechanisms, myasthenia gravis, or known hypersensitivity to quinidine. • Administer with extreme caution to a patient with incomplete AV block or digitalis intoxication in the absence of an AV conduction disorder or other severe intraventricular conduction defect. • Administer with caution to a pregnant or lactating patient or one with marginally compensated cardiovascular disease or renal, cardiac, or hepatic insufficiency.
Class IB			
lidocaine	Suppression of ventricular ectopic beats, conversion of ventricular tachycardia, prevention of ventricular arrhythmias	50 to 100 mg initial I.V. bolus, followed by a second bolus of 50 to 100 mg in 5 minutes, then continuous I.V. infusion at 1 to 4 mg/minute; or 300 mg I.M., repeated in 60 to 90 minutes, if needed	• Know that lidocaine is contraindicated in a patient with Stokes-Adams syndrome; Wolff-Parkinson-White syndrome; sinoatrial, AV, or intraventricular block in the absence of an artificial pacemaker; or known hypersensitivity to amide-type local anesthetics. • Administer with caution to a patient with hypovolemia, severe congestive heart failure, shock, or malignant hyperthermia.
Class IC			
flecainide	Prevention of sustained ventricular tachycardia	100 to 200 mg P.O. every 12 hours	• Know that flecainide is contraindicated in a lactating patient or one with second- or third-degree AV block or right bundle branch block when associated with a left hemiblock (unless a pacemaker is present), or known hypersensitivity to flecainide. • Administer with extreme caution to a patient with sick sinus syndrome. • Administer with caution to a pregnant patient or one with congestive heart failure; myocardial dysfunction; prolonged PR, QRS, or QT intervals; a permanent pacemaker; or temporary pacing electrodes.
Class II			
propranolol	Atrial or ventricular ectopy, sudden onset of self-limiting atrial or ventricular tachycardia	10 to 30 mg P.O. every 6 to 8 hours; 0.5 to 3 mg I.V. for life-threatening arrhythmias	• Know that propranolol is contraindicated in a patient with cardiogenic shock, sinus bradycardia and greater than first degree block, bronchial asthma, congestive heart failure unless the failure is secondary to a tachyarrhythmia treatable with propranolol, or known sensitivity to propranolol. • Administer with caution to a pregnant or lactating patient or one with a nonallergic bronchospastic disorder, diabetes mellitus, or impaired hepatic or renal function.

SELECTED MAJOR DRUGS

Antiarrhythmic agents (continued)

DRUG	MAJOR INDICATIONS	USUAL ADULT DOSAGES	CONTRAINDICATIONS AND PRECAUTIONS
Class III			
amiodarone	Ventricular tachycardia unresponsive to other antiarrhythmics	800 to 1,600 mg P.O. daily for 1 to 3 weeks as loading dose, reduced gradually to a maintenance dosage of 200 to 400 mg P.O. daily	• Know that amiodarone is contraindicated in a lactating patient or one with severe sinus node dysfunction; bradycardia-induced syncope (except in the presence of a pacemaker); or known hypersensitivity to amiodarone. • Administer with caution to a pregnant patient.
Class IV			
verapamil	Paroxysmal supraventricular tachycardia	5 to 10 mg I.V. push over 2 minutes, followed by a second dose of 10 mg I.V. push after 15 to 30 minutes if the patient tolerates but does not respond to the first dose	• Know that verapamil is contraindicated in a patient with severe hypotension or cardiogenic shock, second- or third-degree AV block or sick sinus syndrome (except in the presence of an artificial ventricular pacemaker), severe congestive heart failure (unless due to a supraventricular tachycardia that responds to verapamil therapy), atrial flutter or fibrillation and an accessory bypass tract (as in Wolff-Parkinson-White syndrome), or known hypersensitivity to verapamil.
	Ventricular rate control in atrial fibrillation or flutter	240 to 480 mg P.O. daily in three to four divided doses	• Administer with caution to a pregnant or lactating patient or one with impaired hepatic or renal function.

• Evaluate the patient's and family's knowledge about adenosine.

Nursing diagnoses

The following examples represent appropriate nursing diagnoses for a patient receiving adenosine.

• Potential for injury related to a preexisting condition that contraindicates the use of adenosine
• Potential for injury related to a preexisting condition that requires cautious use of adenosine
• Potential for injury related to adverse drug reactions
• Knowledge deficit related to adenosine

Planning and implementation

• Do not administer adenosine to a patient with a condition that contraindicates its use.
• Administer adenosine cautiously to a patient at risk because of a preexisting condition.
• Monitor the patient closely for adverse reactions during adenosine therapy.
• Administer adenosine as a rapid I.V. bolus only. If the drug must be given through an I.V. line, administer it as proximal as possible to the I.V. injection site and follow with a rapid saline flush.
• *Monitor the patient's respiratory rate and pattern continuously to detect changes during adenosine administration.*

• *Monitor the patient's ECG continuously during adenosine administration. Keep in mind that new rhythms may appear on the ECG during conversion to the normal sinus rhythm. These usually last for only a few seconds and do not require treatment. However, be prepared to treat heart block if it develops and persists. Be especially alert for heart block in a patient who also is receiving carbamazepine.*
• Expect to administer smaller doses of adenosine as prescribed if the patient also is receiving dipyridamole; higher doses as prescribed if the patient also is taking a methylxanthine.
• Inform the physician about the patient's cardiac status throughout adenosine therapy.

Patient teaching

• Teach the patient and family the name, dose, frequency, action, and adverse effects of adenosine.
• *Advise the patient to tell the nurse if shortness of breath, dyspnea, or chest pressure occurs.*

Evaluation

The following examples represent appropriate evaluation statements for a patient receiving adenosine.
• The patient has no conditions that contraindicate adenosine therapy.

• The patient exhibits no signs of complications in the preexisting condition linked to adenosine.

• The patient experiences no adverse reactions to adenosine.

• The patient and family express an accurate understanding of the points taught about adenosine.

• The patient correctly identifies symptoms, such as facial flushing, dyspnea, and chest pressure, that require immediate notification of the nurse.

CHAPTER SUMMARY

Chapter 30 discussed antiarrhythmic agents. These drugs are used to treat abnormal electrical activity in the heart by limiting cardiac electrical activity to normal conduction pathways and decreasing abnormally rapid heart rates. Here are the highlights of the chapter.

• Myocardial cells exhibit automaticity, excitability, contractility, and conductivity.

• Action potentials of myocardial muscle cells include rapid depolarization caused by rapid influx of Na^+ and Ca^{++} into the cell while potassium ions leave the cell. Cell depolarization causes the myocardial cell to contract. Repolarization occurs when potassium ions reenter the cell, causing the myocardial cell to relax.

• The normal conduction system of the heart consists of the SA node, atrial pathways, the AV node, the bundle of His, the right and left bundle branches, and the Purkinje fibers. Impulses travel along this system, leading to myocardial cell excitation and contraction.

• The four different classes of antiarrhythmics have widely varying mechanisms of action but also share some pharmacologic properties. They possess different pharmacokinetics and pharmacodynamics and are used to treat different arrhythmias. Class I antiarrhythmics are subdivided into four subclasses. Class I drugs include moricizine. Class IA agents include disopyramide phosphate; procainamide hydrochloride; and quinidine sulfate, gluconate, or polygalacturonate. Class IB includes lidocaine hydrochloride, mexiletine hydrochloride, and tocainide hydrochloride. Class IC includes encainide hydrochloride, flecainide acetate, indecainide hydrochloride, and propafenone hydrochloride. Class II contains the beta-adrenergic blockers acebutolol hydrochloride, esmolol hydrochloride, and propranolol hydrochloride. Class III includes amiodarone hydrochloride and bretylium tosylate. Class IV includes verapamil hydrochloride and diltiazem hydrochloride.

• Adenosine, the newest antiarrhythmic agent, does not fall into any of these classes, but pharmacologically resembles the calcium channel blockers verapamil and diltiazem.

• Administration of antiarrhythmics requires the nurse to monitor closely such data as heart rate and rhythm, blood pressure, plasma drug level (if appropriate), and interactions with other medications.

STUDY QUESTIONS

See Appendix 1 for answers.

1. Helen Jennings, age 70, is admitted to the critical care unit (CCU) with uncontrolled atrial fibrillation. Her physician prescribes the class IA antiarrhythmic quinidine as well as digoxin 0.125 mg P.O. Which of the following best describes quinidine's mechanism of action?
(a) It alters the myocardial cell membrane, interfering with control of pacemaker cells.
(b) It blocks beta-receptor sites in the conduction system of the heart.
(c) It prolongs the APD and ERP of myocardial cells.
(d) It acts as a calcium channel blocker.

2. During quinidine therapy, Ms. Jennings may experience cinchonism. What is cinchonism?
(a) quinidine-induced conversion of atrial fibrillation
(b) quinidine-related adverse reactions, such as tinnitus and visual disturbances
(c) quinidine-induced arrhythmia
(d) quinidine-induced asthma attack

3. While receiving quinidine and digoxin, Ms. Jennings develops an arrhythmia from digitalis toxicity. Which drug is likely to be prescribed to treat arrhythmias caused by digitalis toxicity?
(a) phenytoin
(b) lidocaine
(c) verapamil
(d) bretylium

4. Bob Johnson, age 51, is brought to the emergency department with ventricular tachycardia that progresses to ventricular fibrillation. After electrical defibrillation, the physician is most likely to prescribe which antiarrhythmic as part of the emergency treatment?
(a) propranolol
(b) acebutolol
(c) flecainide
(d) lidocaine

5. If Mr. Johnson does not respond to the antiarrhythmic and ventricular tachycardia persists, the physician is most likely to prescribe which drug?
(a) verapamil
(b) esmolol
(c) bretylium
(d) propranolol

6. Flecainide, a class IC antiarrhythmic, also may be used to treat ventricular tachycardia. What accounts for the limited use of class IC antiarrhythmic agents?
(a) They have a very short duration of action.
(b) They have a delayed onset of action.
(c) They can be administered I.V. only.
(d) They cause serious adverse reactions.

7. Ken Nobel, age 60, is admitted to the CCU with supraventricular tachycardia. His physician prescribes I.V. esmolol, a class II antiarrhythmic agent. What is the action of this drug?
(a) It blocks beta-adrenergic receptors.
(b) It blocks the calcium channel.
(c) It stabilizes the myocardial cell membrane.
(d) It acts as an anticholinergic agent.

8. To prevent the arrhythmia from recurring, Mr. Nobel's physician decides to change the antiarrhythmic agent to verapamil 240 mg P.O. daily. Which statement best describes the action of verapamil?
(a) It blocks sodium influx into myocardial cells.
(b) It blocks calcium influx into myocardial cells.
(c) It blocks potassium flow out of myocardial cells.
(d) It blocks beta-receptor sites on myocardial cells.

SELECTED REFERENCES

AHFS drug information 90. (1990). Bethesda, MD: American Society of Hospital Pharmacists.

Bachman, J., Bolton, E., and Cooke, D. (1989) The failing heart. *Patient Care,* 23(1), 132-144.

Belardinelli, L., Linden, J., and Berne, R. (1989). The cardiac effects of adenosine. *Progress in Cardiovascular Diseases,* 32(1), 73-97.

DiMarco, J. (1987). Adenosine and supraventricular tachycardia. In A. Pelleg, E. Michelson, and L. Dreifus (Eds.), *Cardiac electrophysiology and pharmacology of adenosine and ATP: Basic and clinical aspects* (pp. 271-282). New York: Liss.

Drug facts and comparisons. (1991). St. Louis: Facts and Comparisons Division.

Goodman and Gilman's the pharmacological basis of therapeutics (8th ed.; 1990). Elmsford, NY: Pergamon Press.

Hansten, P., and Horn, J. (1989). *Drug interactions* (6th ed.). Philadelphia: Lea & Febiger.

Marshall, J. (1988). Cardiopulmonary resuscitation: An update. *Current Reviews in Respiratory and Critical Care,* 10(13), 98-104.

Naccarelli, G., Rinkenberger, R., Dougherty, A., et al. (1988). Pharmacologic therapy of arrhythmias. *Hospital Practice,* 23(10), 183-195.

North American Nursing Diagnosis Association. (1990). *Taxonomy I-Revised, with official diagnostic categories.* St. Louis: NANDA.

Parker, R., McCollam, P., and Bauman, J. (1989). Propafenone: A novel type IC antiarrhythmic agent. *DICP The Annals of Pharmacotherapy,* 23(3), 196-202.

Rubin, J., and Bhandari, A. (1988). Premature ventricular complexes: How to avoid the risks and maximize the benefits of therapy. *Consultant,* 28(6), 35-39.

Sellers, T., Kirchhoffer, J., and Modesto, T. (1987). Adenosine: A clinical experience and comparison with verapamil for the termination of supraventricular tachycardias. In A. Pelleg, E. Michelson, and L. Dreifus (Eds.), *Cardiac electrophysiology and pharmacology of adenosine and ATD: Basic and clinical aspects* (pp. 283-299). New York: Liss.

Weiner, B. (1989). Second generation antidysrhythmic agents. *Critical Care Nursing Clinics of North America,* 1(2), 417-422.

ANTIANGINAL AGENTS

OBJECTIVES

After reading and studying this chapter, the student should be able to:

1. Discuss the physiology of myocardial ischemia, which results in angina.

2. Compare and contrast the three forms of angina.

3. Identify the mechanisms of action and clinical indications for the antianginal agents: nitrates, beta-adrenergic blockers, and calcium channel blockers.

4. Explain how routes of administration influence the onset of action and clinical uses of different nitrates.

5. List the most significant drug interactions and adverse reactions associated with various antianginal agents.

6. Describe how to apply the nursing process when caring for a patient who is receiving an antianginal agent.

INTRODUCTION

To pump effectively, the heart needs its own blood supply, which the coronary arteries provide. These arteries originate from the aorta at the ostia situated above the cusps of the aortic valve (the sinus of Valsalva). From there, the arteries branch out to cover and penetrate all parts of the cardiac muscle, or myocardium. After delivering oxygen and nutrients throughout the myocardium, the blood moves through large coronary veins and returns to the right atrium via the coronary sinus. The myocardium cannot extract oxygen from blood inside the chambers of the heart; instead, it depends on blood from the coronary arteries for its supply of oxygen and nutrients.

Even when the body is at rest, the percentage of oxygen extracted from coronary arterial blood by the myocardium is high, approximately 80%. During exercise or other exertion, the amount of blood flowing through the coronary arteries must increase significantly to meet the increased myocardial demand for oxygen. This additional oxygen is provided normally by an increase in aortic blood pressure and by local factors that dilate the coronary arteries during a process called *autoregulation.*

Exertion increases heart rate. At rest, the heart is in systole about one-third of the time and in diastole about two-thirds of the time. During diastole, the majority of blood flows through the coronary arteries. As heart rate increases, time in diastole shortens; thus, exertion increases oxygen demand while decreasing the time available for the coronary arteries to supply it. The coronary arteries help maintain the balance between oxygen supply and demand usually by dilating, allowing more blood to circulate to the myocardium.

Angina

In coronary artery disease, specifically atherosclerosis, the arteries may be unable to accommodate an increased blood flow such as that caused by exertion or may be unable to dilate. Atherosclerosis results from deposits of cholesterol, platelets, or other proteins and blood components in the interior, or lumen, of the artery, causing narrowing of the lumen.

When the myocardial oxygen demand exceeds the myocardial oxygen supply, areas become ischemic, causing chest pain. When the patient experiences symptoms from this myocardial ischemia, the condition is known as *angina* or *angina pectoris.* The patient may report a crushing sensation or a feeling of pressure behind the sternum, sometimes radiating into the neck, the jaw, and the shoulders and down the arms. Initially, symptoms may be mild: the patient may confuse the angina with indigestion, heartburn, chest muscle strain, or pain referred from other organs.

Angina's painful symptoms may result from decreased coronary artery blood flow, as from atherosclerosis or eating a heavy meal; decreased oxygen-carrying capacity of the blood, as from severe anemia; or increased myocardial work load, as from exertion.

Angina usually takes one of three main forms:

• Stable angina (also called predictable or chronic angina), in which pain occurs at a predictable level of physical or emotional stress, builds gradually, and reaches maximum intensity quickly.

How antianginal agents relieve angina

Angina occurs when the coronary arteries, the heart's primary source of oxygen, supply insufficient oxygen to the myocardium. This increases the heart's work load, increasing heart rate, preload, afterload, and force of myocardial contractility. The antianginal agents (nitrates, beta-adrenergic blockers, and calcium channel blockers) relieve angina by *decreasing* one or more of these four factors. Depending on the class of drug administered, myocardial oxygen demand may decrease or the myocardial blood supply may increase, or both. Also, nitrates and calcium channel blockers increase myocardial oxygen supply by producing coronary artery dilation. This diagram summarizes how antianginal agents affect the cardiovascular system.

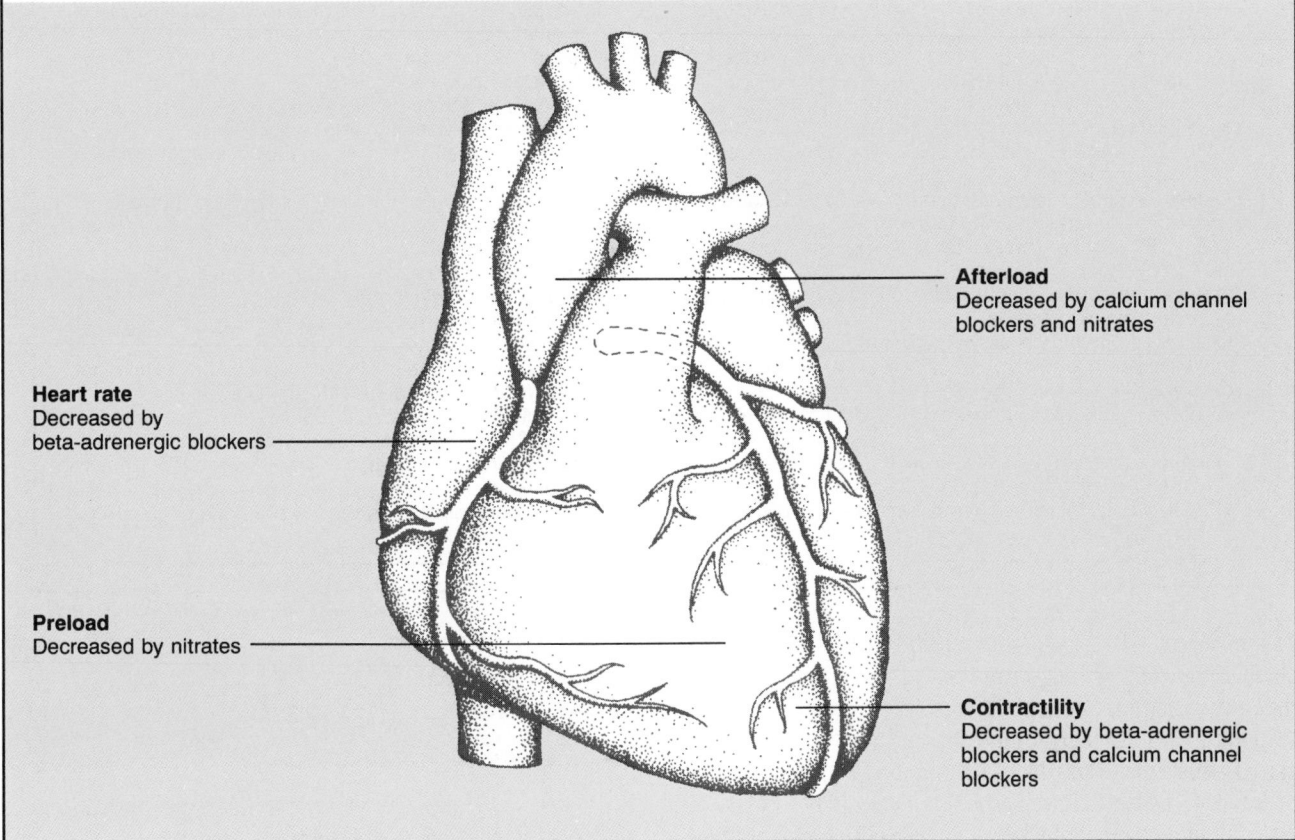

Afterload
Decreased by calcium channel blockers and nitrates

Heart rate
Decreased by beta-adrenergic blockers

Preload
Decreased by nitrates

Contractility
Decreased by beta-adrenergic blockers and calcium channel blockers

• Unstable angina (also called preinfarction or crescendo angina, acute coronary insufficiency, or impending myocardial infarction [MI]), in which pain takes an unpredictable course and is more severe than in stable angina.

• Prinzmetal's angina (also called variant angina), in which pain usually occurs while the patient is at rest and resembles that of unstable angina. Occasionally, a patient may have stable and Prinzmetal's angina.

Although angina's cardinal symptom is chest pain, the drugs used to treat angina are not analgesics. The antianginal agents discussed in this chapter are used to treat angina by reducing myocardial oxygen demand, by increasing myocardial oxygen supply, or by both mechanisms. (For a summary of how antianginal agents function, see *How antianginal agents relieve angina.*)

The antianginal agents are classified into the following groups: nitrates, including erythrityl tetranitrate, isosorbide dinitrate, nitroglycerin, and pentaerythritol tetranitrate; beta-adrenergic blockers, especially atenolol, nadolol, metoprolol tartrate, and propranolol hydrochloride; and calcium channel blockers, including diltiazem hydrochloride, nicardipine hydrochloride, nifedipine, and verapamil hydrochloride.

Combination antianginal therapy

Combination therapy with drugs from different classes of antianginal agents is indicated for symptoms that persist despite therapy with one or more drugs from a single class. Combining drugs from different classes provides antianginal effects from different mechanisms of action and reduces the risk of adverse reactions from high doses of any one drug.

Combination therapy also is used to control different types of angina occurring in one patient. For example, a

---

SELECTED NURSING DIAGNOSES

Antianginal agents

The following nursing diagnoses address representative problems and etiologies that a nurse may encounter when caring for a patient who is receiving an antianginal agent. Some of these nursing diagnoses contain generalized etiologies, which the nurse must individualize based on the patient's needs. (For some common nursing diagnoses and related interventions for each drug class, see the "Nursing Process Application" sections of this chapter.)

- Altered health maintenance related to ineffectiveness of the prescribed antianginal agent
- Altered nutrition: less than body requirements, related to the adverse GI effects of an antianginal agent
- Altered protection related to arrhythmias caused by an antianginal agent
- Altered protection related to blood dyscrasias caused by the beta-adrenergic blocking agent
- Altered sexuality patterns related to decreased libido caused by a beta-adrenergic blocker
- Altered thought processes related to alcohol intoxication caused by I.V. nitroglycerin
- Decreased cardiac output related to hypotension caused by an antianginal agent
- Decreased peripheral tissue perfusion related to peripheral vascular insufficiency caused by a beta-adrenergic blocker
- Diarrhea related to the adverse GI effects of an antianginal agent
- Fatigue related to the adverse central nervous system (CNS) effects of a beta-adrenergic blocker
- Fluid volume excess related to fluid retention caused by an antianginal agent

- Fluid volume excess related to the adverse cardiovascular effects of the beta-adrenergic blocker
- Impaired skin integrity related to skin eruptions caused by a calcium channel blocker
- Ineffective breathing pattern related to bronchoconstricting effects of the beta-adrenergic blocker
- Knowledge deficit related to the prescribed antianginal agent
- Noncompliance related to adverse reactions to the antianginal agent
- Pain related to nitrate-induced headache
- Pain related to the adverse CNS or muscular effects of the calcium channel blocker
- Potential for injury related to a preexisting condition that contraindicates the use of an antianginal agent
- Potential for injury related to a preexisting condition that requires cautious use of an antianginal agent
- Potential for injury related to adverse drug reactions
- Potential for injury related to drug interactions
- Potential for trauma related to the adverse CNS effects of the antianginal agent
- Sensory-perceptual alterations (visual) related to nitrate-induced blurred vision

---

patient might take a beta-adrenergic blocker or a calcium channel blocker for long-term control and supplement this therapy with rapid-acting nitrates for unusual exertional demands. Beta-adrenergic blockers prevent the reflex tachycardia sometimes reported with nitrates; nitrates, in turn, prevent the increased preload from beta-adrenergic blockers. Calcium channel blockers and beta-adrenergic blockers together more effectively treat Prinzmetal's angina that is unresponsive to beta-adrenergic blockers alone.

During combination therapy, the nurse should monitor the patient for adverse reactions, such as severe bradycardia, congestive heart failure, or excessive hypotension.

For a summary of representative drugs, see *Selected major drugs: Antianginal agents,* page 531. For a listing of applicable nursing diagnoses that the nurse may formulate when caring for a patient receiving these agents, see *Selected nursing diagnoses: Antianginal agents.* For detailed information on applying the nursing process, see Chapter 6, The Nursing Process and Drug Therapy.

NITRATES

Nitrates include erythrityl tetranitrate, isosorbide dinitrate, nitroglycerin, and pentaerythritol tetranitrate. Used for many years to relieve angina, these drugs are available in multiple forms with several routes of administration. Nitrates act primarily as vasodilators, working directly on vascular smooth muscle to reduce the degree of vasoconstriction. They act primarily on venous but also on arterial smooth muscle.

PHARMACOKINETICS

The many routes for administering nitrates account, in part, for the pharmacokinetic differences among these drugs.

Absorption, distribution, metabolism, excretion
Sublingual, buccal, and chewable tablets and lingual aerosols are absorbed almost completely through the richly vascularized oral mucosa. This vascularization enhances the direct absorption and transportation of nitrates through the internal jugular vein and superior vena cava into the

Pharmacokinetics of nitrates

The route of nitrate administration determines the extent of absorption and the rapidity of action, as shown below.

ROUTE OF ADMINISTRATION	EXTENT OF ABSORPTION	ONSET OF ACTION
Sublingual, buccal, or lingual	Almost 100% is absorbed through the richly vascularized oral mucous membranes.	1 to 3 minutes
Oral	50% to 60% is absorbed through the intestines.	20 to 60 minutes
Transdermal	Absorption rate varies among patients and types and sites of application.	30 to 60 minutes
I.V.	No absorption is necessary.	1 to 3 minutes

right atrium. In a patient whose mouth is dry, absorption may take longer, and some of the drug may return to the heart via the lymphatic circulation.

Nitrate capsules or tablets that are swallowed are absorbed through the gastric and intestinal mucosa. Orally administered nitrates are only about 50% to 60% absorbed.

Transdermal nitrates are absorbed slowly. The quantity of drug applied, the location and area of skin used for administration, and the amount of cutaneous circulation affect the percentage absorbed, which varies. Intravenous (I.V.) nitroglycerin, which does not require absorption, is delivered directly into the circulation.

Once in the body, nitrates are distributed widely, especially to the liver, heart, lungs, kidneys, spleen, and blood vessel walls. Nitroglycerin is approximately 60% bound to plasma proteins.

Nitrate metabolism occurs partly in the blood but mainly in the liver. The enzyme glutathione-organic nitrate reductase converts nitrates to metabolites that are much less active. This rapid conversion in the liver explains why higher doses are needed for oral nitrates, which undergo significant first-pass metabolism after absorption into the portal vein. Erythrityl tetranitrate is converted faster than nitroglycerin; isosorbide dinitrate and pentaerythritol tetranitrate are converted more slowly.

Metabolite excretion occurs via the kidneys.

Onset, peak, duration

Onset of the antianginal action of nitrates begins within 1 to 3 minutes of I.V., sublingual, buccal, or lingual administration. The onset of the nitrate forms that are swallowed occurs in 20 to 60 minutes. The onset of transdermal nitroglycerin occurs in 30 to 60 minutes. (For a summary of how the route of administration affects absorption and onset, see *Pharmacokinetics of nitrates*.)

Peak concentration levels of the nitrates occur almost simultaneously with their onset of action. Peak hemody-

namic effects of the transdermal and oral forms occur 1 to 2 hours after administration.

The rapidly acting nitrates absorbed in the mouth have the shortest duration of action: Sublingual nitroglycerin is 20 to 30 minutes; sublingual erythrityl tetranitrate and isosorbide dinitrate, up to 2 hours. Oral forms of the nitrates produce antianginal effects for up to 6 hours for erythrityl tetranitrate, isosorbide dinitrate, and nitroglycerin and for up to 5 hours for pentaerythritol tetranitrate. The half-life of isosorbide dinitrate is 45 minutes; however, the half-life of one of its active metabolites is 2 to 5 hours, prolonging its duration. The duration of sustained-release oral forms may persist for up to 12 hours.

For the various formulations of transdermal nitroglycerin, duration varies considerably. Nitroglycerin ointment exerts antianginal effects for 3 hours and hemodynamic effects for up to 6 hours. Longer-acting transdermal patches are replaced daily, although their actual duration may be somewhat less than 24 hours.

With a plasma half-life of only 1 to 4 minutes, I.V. nitroglycerin is active for only a short time after discontinuation of the infusion.

PHARMACODYNAMICS

Nitrates decrease preload and myocardial oxygen demand by dilating veins. They decrease afterload and also may increase myocardial oxygen supply by dilating arteries. In the coronary circulation, nitrates redistribute circulating blood flow, improving myocardial perfusion.

Mechanism of action

Nitrates act directly on vascular smooth muscle, producing relaxation and vessel dilation. These actions are independent of autonomic nervous system innervation of smooth muscle. Although veins have much less smooth muscle tissue than arteries have, nitrates dilate the veins considerably. Because the veins dilate, less blood is returned to the heart, decreasing the blood volume in the ventricles at the end of diastole, when the ventricles are full. (This blood volume in the ventricles and length of ventricular fibers at the end of diastole is called *preload.*) By decreasing preload, nitrates reduce ventricular size and wall tension, which reduces the myocardial demand for oxygen needed to pump blood out of the ventricles.

Nitrates also dilate arteries by direct action on arterial smooth muscle, independent of autonomic nervous system innervation. In the arterial system, most resistance to ejection of blood from the left ventricle occurs in the arterioles. The more the arterioles constrict, the more they resist left ventricular ejection. The amount of resistance is called *afterload.* Nitrates decrease afterload by dilating the arterioles, thereby decreasing the energy required for the heart to pump blood and reducing myocardial oxygen demand.

Besides decreasing myocardial oxygen demand, nitrates promote coronary artery autoregulation to improve blood flow to ischemic areas of the myocardium and to decrease blood flow to unaffected areas. This combined effect may explain their antianginal action. Dilation of coronary arteries by nitrates explains their effectiveness in relieving Prinzmetal's angina, which is caused by arterial spasm. Overall, their ability to decrease oxygen demand usually is more important than their ability to increase oxygen supply.

PHARMACOTHERAPEUTICS

Nitrates are indicated for immediate relief of angina, prevention of angina when an attack can be expected, and long-term prevention of chronic angina. These drugs are synergistic with certain beta-adrenergic blockers and with calcium channel blockers.

The rapidly absorbed nitrates, such as nitroglycerin, are the drugs of choice for relief of acute angina because of their rapid onset of action, ease of administration, and low cost. Daily application of the inconspicuous, long-acting nitroglycerin transdermal patch is convenient and effective for preventing chronic angina, especially for the patient who may have difficulty complying with a regimen requiring frequent doses. Oral nitrates have the advantage of seldom producing serious adverse reactions. I.V. nitroglycerin is most effective for relieving severe, acute angina because of its rapid onset of action and short half-life.

Most of the controversy about nitrates concerns the best route of administration and the drug tolerance that develops with prolonged, continuous use, rather than which nitrate to administer. Of the following nitrates, the efficacy of nitroglycerin is the best established.

erythrityl tetranitrate (Cardilate). Erythrityl tetranitrate is not used to relieve acute angina but to prevent expected and chronic angina attacks.
Usual adult dosage: for expected angina attacks, 10-mg chewable, sublingual, or buccal tablets; for long-term angina prevention, up to 100 mg/day in four or five doses.

isosorbide dinitrate (Isordil, Sorbitrate). Used to relieve acute angina and to prevent expected angina, isosorbide dinitrate is taken as sublingual, buccal, or chewable tablets or as sustained-release tablets or capsules.
Usual adult dosage: for acute angina or prevention of attacks, 2.5 to 10 mg sublingually or buccally or as a chewable tablet, repeated twice at 5- to 10-minute intervals if relief is not obtained. For angina prevention, the dosage may be repeated every 2 to 3 hours, but initial dosage of the chewable tablet should be no more than 5 mg. For long-term prevention, 10 to 20 mg P.O. t.i.d., or q.i.d., or 20 to 40 mg of sustained-release tablets or capsules every 6 to 12 hours, or 80 mg every 8 to 12 hours.

nitroglycerin (Nitro-Bid, Nitrostat). Used for relieving acute and persistent angina, nitroglycerin also is used for long-term angina prevention.
Usual adult dosage: for acute angina attacks, 0.15 to 0.6 mg sublingually, or 0.4 mg of a metered-dose aerosol spray onto or under the tongue, repeated up to three times at 5- to 10-minute intervals (this route also is used to prevent expected angina). For persistent angina, especially accompanying an acute MI, continuous I.V. infusion of 5 mcg/ minute, increased by 5 mcg every 3 to 5 minutes until pain is relieved. At higher doses, 10- to 20-mcg increases can be made at a time. Maximum dosage has not been established, and rates of up to 400 mcg/minute are used sometimes. For long-term prevention of angina, 1 to 3 mg of sustained-release tablets placed between the upper gum and lips t.i.d. or q.i.d.; 2.5 to 9 mg of sustained-release capsules or tablets P.O. b.i.d. to q.i.d. Long-term prevention also may be accomplished with nitroglycerin 2% ointment applied to the skin in ½" to 3" doses or unit-dose equivalents every 3 to 4 hours. Alternatively, sustained-release transdermal patches that release 2.5 to 15 mg over 24 hours are used daily.

pentaerythritol tetranitrate (Duotrate, Peritrate). Used only for long-term prevention of angina, pentaerythritol tetranitrate is taken orally.
Usual adult dosage: for long-term prevention of angina, 10 mg P.O. q.i.d. increased to 40 mg q.i.d., as needed; alternatively, sustained-release capsules or 30- to 80-mg tablets b.i.d.

Drug interactions

Severe hypotension can result when nitrates interact with alcohol. Delayed sublingual absorption across the oral membrane may occur when the patient's mouth is dry from using an anticholinergic agent.

ADVERSE DRUG REACTIONS

Most adverse reactions to nitrates are attributable to changes in the cardiovascular system. The reactions usually disappear when the dosage is reduced.

The decreased afterload produced by arteriolar dilation can cause hypotension that may be compounded by the reduced cardiac output after decreased preload. Hypotension is most noticeable when the patient assumes an upright position (orthostatic hypotension), because blood pressure is insufficient to perfuse the brain adequately. Besides a systolic blood pressure of less than 90 mm Hg, signs and symptoms of hypotension include syncope, dizziness, weakness, clammy skin, nausea, and vomiting. To compensate for the hypotension, the heart rate may increase to 150 or more beats/minute. However, this tachycardia may be counterproductive because the shortened diastolic time that results does not allow for adequate filling of the ventricles; therefore, cardiac output is reduced further.

Although rare, complete collapse of the cardiovascular system can occur even with normal doses. Signs of complete cardiovascular collapse include thready or absent peripheral pulses, loss of blood pressure, loss of consciousness, and urine and fecal incontinence.

Headache, the most common adverse reaction, probably is caused by blood vessel dilation in the meningeal layers between the brain and the skull. The pain may be severe and persistent but usually disappears after several days of nitrate administration. Headache may be relieved by acetaminophen. For patients receiving transdermal patch therapy, the application site does not affect the incidence of headache.

Transdermally applied nitrates occasionally cause local skin irritation. A generalized rash after any route of administration is uncommon. When such a rash occurs, it is most likely to result from pentaerythritol tetranitrate use. Many patients report a stinging sensation from the sublingual tablets, but the effect is not objectionable and even may indicate that the tablets are fresh. A few patients taking nitrates experience transient flushing of the face and neck.

Tolerance to nitrates may develop over time, especially with high-dose, long-term therapy. Patients appear to develop tolerance not just to specific nitrates but to the entire class. To minimize tolerance, nitrate therapy should be individualized, using the lowest effective dose and an intermittent dosage schedule. For example, a patient receiving transdermal nitroglycerin may need a 10- to 12-hour nitrate-free interval, which is accomplished by removing the trans-

dermal patch in the early evening and applying a new one the next morning. Another patient may need to omit the last daily dose of an oral, buccal, or topical preparation. Although such actions may minimize tolerance, they have some disadvantages. The minimum nitrate-free interval needed to maintain full nitrate effects is unknown, and symptoms may worsen in some patients at the end of the nitrate-free interval.

I.V. nitroglycerin can produce alcohol intoxication when large doses are administered for long periods. This reaction results from the alcohol used to preserve nitroglycerin in ampules or vials from which I.V. infusions are prepared. The most prominent alcohol intoxication signs are an additive hypotensive effect and depression of myocardial contractility.

Other reactions may include blurred vision, dry mouth, increased peripheral edema, and methemoglobinemia, which occurs with large, continuous doses of nitrates.

NURSING PROCESS APPLICATION

The following information assists the nurse in caring for a patient who is receiving a nitrate.

Assessment

• Review the patient's history for a preexisting condition that contraindicates the use of a nitrate, such as known hypersensitivity to nitrates or nitrites.
• Review the patient's history for a preexisting condition that requires cautious use of a nitrate, such as a depleted intravascular fluid volume, low systolic blood pressure, pregnancy, or lactation.
• Assess the patient for adverse reactions to the prescribed nitrate, such as hypotension, cardiovascular collapse, headache, alcohol intoxication, blurred vision, dry mouth, peripheral edema, or methemoglobinemia.
• Monitor the patient for decreased cardiac output if hypotension develops.
• Review the patient's medication history to identify the use of drugs that may interact with the prescribed nitrate, such as alcohol and anticholinergic agents.
• Assess the effectiveness of the prescribed nitrate regularly.
• Evaluate the patient's and family's knowledge about the prescribed nitrate.

Nursing diagnoses

The following examples represent appropriate nursing diagnoses for a patient receiving a nitrate.
• Potential for injury related to a preexisting condition that contraindicates the use of a nitrate
• Potential for injury related to a preexisting condition that requires cautious use of a nitrate
• Potential for injury related to adverse drug reactions
• Pain related to nitrate-induced headache

Applying nitroglycerin ointment

The supplies for administration are a tube of nitroglycerin ointment and a sheet of nitroglycerin measurement paper.

1. Identify the patient and explain the procedure and medication. Squeeze the prescribed amount of nitroglycerin ointment from the tube onto the special paper, allowing it to flow freely from the tube. The diameter of the ointment on the paper should approximate the diameter of the tube opening.

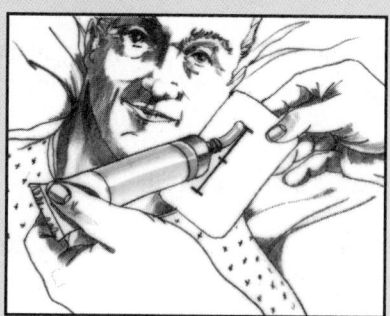

2. Place the paper on the skin medication-side-down against the skin. Spread the ointment evenly under the measurement paper. Do not rub the ointment into the skin.

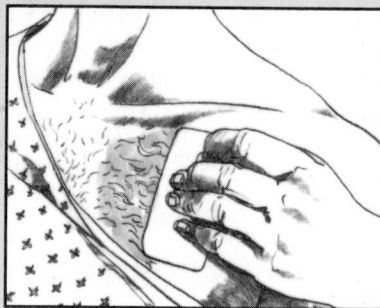

3. The chest, upper arm, and upper back are common administration sites. Other sites, such as the lower leg or abdomen, also are acceptable if cutaneous circulation is adequate. Administration sites should be rotated to decrease skin irritation. The sheet of plastic placed over the nitroglycerin ointment increases medication absorption.

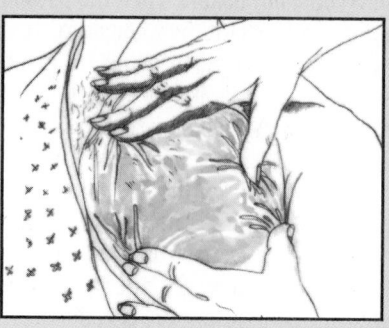

• Decreased cardiac output related to nitrate-induced hypotension
• Knowledge deficit related to the prescribed nitrate

Planning and implementation

• Do not administer a nitrate to a patient with a condition that contraindicates its use.
• Administer a nitrate cautiously to a patient at risk because of a preexisting condition.
• Monitor the patient frequently for cardiovascular and other adverse reactions during nitrate therapy.
• Do not administer erythrityl tetranitrate to relieve acute angina.
• Expect to repeat the isosorbide dinitrate dose twice at 5- to 10-minute intervals as prescribed if acute angina pain is not relieved, or to repeat the dose of sublingual or spray nitroglycerin up to three times.
• *Do not administer more than 5 mg of chewable isosorbide dinitrate as an initial dose.*
• Place nitroglycerin sustained-release tablets between the patient's upper gum and lips.
• *Administer the first nitrate dose by having the patient sit or lie down and taking the pulse and blood pressure before administration and again at the onset of action.*
• Apply a subsequent dose of nitroglycerin ointment by removing the ointment remaining from the preceding dose and selecting a new administration site to avoid skin irri-

tation. (For details, see *Applying nitroglycerin ointment.*) Remove a transdermal patch before electrical cardioversion.
• Prepare I.V. infusions of nitroglycerin cautiously. Mix the drug with dextrose 5% in water or normal saline solution in a glass bottle. Use administration tubing supplied by the manufacturer, if available, because nitroglycerin readily migrates into standard polyvinyl chloride tubing, greatly reducing the amount administered. (Some manufacturers add chemicals to the ampules to prevent such migration.)
• *Monitor the blood pressure and pulse every 5 to 15 minutes while titrating the dosage and every hour thereafter for a patient receiving I.V. nitroglycerin. Use an infusion pump and calculate the dose in mcg/minute in addition to ml/hour, using the manufacturer's tables.*
• Begin infusing I.V. nitroglycerin as prescribed at 5 mcg/minute and increase it by 5 mcg every 3 to 5 minutes until pain is relieved in a patient with persistent angina accompanied by acute MI. When higher doses are reached, 10- to 20-mcg increases can be made until pain is relieved.
• Monitor the patient closely for signs of alcohol intoxication, such as hypotension or depressed myocardial contractility, during high-dose, long-term, I.V. therapy with nitroglycerin.
• *Have the patient sit up for a few minutes before standing to minimize the effects of orthostatic hypotension.*

• Take safety measures if the patient develops blurred vision. For example, keep the bed in a low position and supervise ambulation.

• Notify the physician if adverse reactions occur or if the prescribed nitrate is ineffective.

• Monitor the patient for headache during nitrate therapy. Obtain a prescription for acetaminophen or another analgesic if the patient develops headache.

• Observe for signs of decreased cardiac output, such as hypotension, increased pulse rate, dizziness, and arrhythmias.

• *Take the patient's vital signs regularly and monitor closely for signs and symptoms of hypotension, such as a systolic blood pressure of less than 90 mm Hg, syncope, dizziness, weakness, clammy skin, nausea, vomiting, or tachycardia of 150 beats or more per minute.*

• Position the hypotensive patient to promote venous return, such as in a supine or legs-elevated position, and recheck the blood pressure. If hypotension persists, remove the nitrate ointment or slow the I.V. infusion rate, notify the physician, and continue to monitor the patient's heart rate and blood pressure every 5 to 15 minutes.

Patient teaching

• Teach the patient and family the name, dose, action, frequency, and adverse effects of the prescribed nitrate.

• *Instruct the patient to store sublingual nitroglycerin tablets in the original container away from heat, including body heat. Advise the patient to discard the cotton filler after opening the container, because cotton may absorb some of the drug. Also instruct the patient to replace the tablets with fresh ones every 3 months and to discard any unused tablets.*

• *Instruct the patient to go to the nearest emergency department (ED) if angina is not relieved by three tablets taken 5 minutes apart while resting. Explain that the pain may indicate an acute MI.*

• Inform the patient using an aerosol nitrate not to inhale the spray.

• Suggest that the patient use plastic wrap to cover the patch because nitroglycerin ointment may stain clothing.

• *Instruct the patient using long-acting patches to change them at the same time every day; for example, right after showering.*

• Encourage the patient to avoid drinking alcoholic beverages during nitrate therapy.

• *Instruct the patient to take nitrate tablets or capsules ½ hour before or 1 hour after meals, for better absorption.*

• Teach the patient with dry mouth to take a few sips of water before taking sublingual or buccal tablets because a dry mouth can inhibit absorption.

• *Instruct the patient not to stop taking nitrate medication without consulting the physician because vasospasm may follow abrupt discontinuation.*

• Instruct the patient to take a sublingual nitrate dose as prescribed a few minutes before engaging in activities known or expected to induce angina.

• Inform the patient that the stinging sensation from sublingual nitroglycerin tablets is normal and indicates drug freshness.

• Advise the patient with local skin irritation to apply transdermal nitrate patches in a different location until the irritation disappears.

• *Teach the patient to recognize and report signs and symptoms of hypotension. Also describe how to minimize the effects of orthostatic hypotension.*

• Instruct the patient to relieve nitrate-induced headache with a mild analgesic, such as acetaminophen, as prescribed.

• Reassure the patient that, although headache pain may be severe and persistent, it usually disappears after several days of nitrate administration.

• Advise the patient to notify the physician if adverse reactions occur or if the drug is ineffective.

Evaluation

The following examples represent appropriate evaluation statements for a patient receiving a nitrate.

• The patient has no conditions that contraindicate use nitrate therapy.

• The patient exhibits no complications in the preexisting condition linked to the prescribed nitrate.

• The patient experiences no adverse reactions to the prescribed nitrate.

• The patient denies having headaches.

• The patient maintains normal cardiac output during nitrate therapy.

• The patient and family express an accurate understanding of the points taught about the prescribed nitrate.

• The patient correctly identifies the signs and symptoms of hypotension and ways to minimize orthostatic hypotension.

BETA-ADRENERGIC BLOCKERS

Also called beta-adrenergic antagonists, beta-adrenergic blockers are used for long-term prevention of angina. Atenolol, metoprolol tartrate, nadolol, and propranolol hydrochloride are the antianginal agents approved by the Food and Drug Administration. (For more information on beta-adrenergic blockers, see Chapter 16, Adrenergic Blocking Agents.)

PHARMACOKINETICS

Only oral preparations of beta-adrenergic blockers are used to treat angina. These agents display varying pharmacokinetic properties.

Absorption, distribution, metabolism, excretion

Metoprolol and propranolol, having moderate to high lipid solubility, are absorbed almost entirely from the gastrointestinal (GI) tract. Because atenolol and nadolol have a low lipid solubility, less than 50% of a dose of either drug is absorbed.

These beta-adrenergic blockers are distributed widely, but only metoprolol and propranolol readily cross the blood-brain barrier and reach equilibrium rapidly in the central nervous system (CNS). The liver extracts and binds a large portion of metoprolol and propranolol doses. Each of the beta-adrenergic blockers is plasma protein bound as follows: propranolol, 90%; nadolol, 30%; atenolol, 16%; and metoprolol, 12%.

Propranolol is hydroxylated in the liver to form mildly active metabolites. Metoprolol also is hydroxylated but its metabolites are inactive. Atenolol and nadolol are unmetabolized.

Metabolites of metoprolol and propranolol are excreted in the urine. Unchanged, atenolol and nadolol are excreted in the urine and feces.

Onset, peak, duration

Because beta-adrenergic blockers are not used for relief of acute angina, their onset of action is difficult to measure. Metoprolol is present in the plasma within 10 minutes after oral administration. Propranolol usually appears in the plasma within 30 minutes; however, long-acting forms take longer. Corresponding data for atenolol and nadolol are unavailable.

The peak concentration level of metoprolol occurs within 90 minutes and is increased when the drug is taken with food. Peak concentration of propranolol occurs within 60 to 90 minutes for tablets and within 6 hours for long-acting capsules; if the drug is taken with food, peak concentration is delayed but not reduced. Nadolol and atenolol reach peak concentrations in 2 to 4 hours, regardless of food intake.

The duration of action of atenolol is about 24 hours and its half-life is 6 to 9 hours. The duration of nadolol also is about 24 hours and its half-life ranges from 10 to 24 hours. The duration of metoprolol is about 6 hours; its half-life varies from 3 to 7 hours. The duration of propranolol tablets is 4 to 6 hours; of the long-acting capsules, up to 24 hours. Propranolol's half-life ranges from 3 to 6 hours.

Serum levels are unreliable for monitoring the effectiveness or toxicity of beta-adrenergic blockers.

PHARMACODYNAMICS

Beta-adrenergic blockers decrease blood pressure through one or more mechanisms. (For more information, see Chapter 32, Antihypertensive Agents.) They also block beta-receptor sites in the myocardium and in the electrical conduction system of the heart. Subsequently, decreased heart rate and diminished force of myocardial contraction considerably reduce the oxygen requirements of the heart.

Beta-adrenergic blockers do not dilate veins. In fact, the heart rate becomes slower and weaker, allowing more blood to collect in the ventricles at the end of diastole. This process causes a slight increase in preload and myocardial oxygen demand. However, the combined actions of beta-adrenergic blockers decrease oxygen demand with little or no change in supply. The drugs also increase the patient's maximal exercise tolerance, because they prevent the angina that often accompanies exertion.

PHARMACOTHERAPEUTICS

Beta-adrenergic blockers are indicated for long-term prevention of angina, not for immediate relief of an angina attack or prevention of an imminent one. The drugs act synergistically with other antianginal agents. For example, because they decrease heart rate, the beta-adrenergic blockers are particularly useful for limiting the reflex tachycardia accompanying nitrate administration. However, because beta-adrenergic blockers also block peripheral vascular beta receptors and allow some unopposed alpha constriction, they are of limited use in treating Prinzmetal's angina.

atenolol (Tenormin). This drug is used for the long-term prevention of angina.
Usual adult dosage: 50 mg P.O. once daily; after 1 week, the dosage may be increased to 100 mg/day or even 200 mg/day in some patients.

metoprolol tartrate (Lopressor). Used for long-term prevention of angina, the effects of metoprolol vary considerably among patients.
Usual adult dosage: 50 to 100 mg P.O. b.i.d. or t.i.d.

nadolol (Corgard). This drug is used for long-term prevention of angina.
Usual adult dosage: 40 mg P.O. once daily as an initial dosage; if needed, the dosage is increased over several days up to 240 mg daily.

propranolol hydrochloride (Inderal, Inderal LA). Used for long-term prevention of angina, propranolol also is available in a long-acting form.
Usual adult dosage: 10 to 20 mg P.O. b.i.d. to q.i.d.; if needed, the dosage may be increased over several days up

to 320 mg divided into two to four doses; alternatively, 80 to 160 mg of the long-acting form is administered once daily.

Drug interactions

Beta-adrenergic blockers alter insulin and oral hypoglycemic agent requirements, and their effect of slowing the heart rate is additive when administered concurrently with digoxin. Increased hypotension may result from administering beta-adrenergic blockers with antiarrhythmics, antihypertensives, or phenothiazines. Aminophylline antagonizes beta-adrenergic blockers; cimetidine, flecainide, and propafenone inhibit the metabolism of some beta-adrenergic blockers. (For more information, see *Drug interactions: Beta-adrenergic blockers,* page 526.)

ADVERSE DRUG REACTIONS

The most common adverse reactions to beta-adrenergic blockers involve the cardiovascular system and occur when the drug is administered initially. Because they inhibit sinus node stimulation, beta-adrenergic blockers can cause bradycardia and hypotension with peripheral vascular insufficiency. Angina, syncope, or shock may accompany these reactions. Fluid retention and peripheral edema also may occur.

Because of decreased force of myocardial contractility and increased preload, congestive heart failure may be exacerbated or precipitated. Arrhythmias, especially atrioventricular (AV) block, also can occur.

Rapid discontinuation of a beta-adrenergic blocker may precipitate angina, hypertension, arrhythmias, or acute MI.

Adverse CNS reactions include dizziness, fatigue, lethargy, confusion or depression (especially in elderly patients), and decreased libido. They occur most commonly with propranolol therapy. GI reactions, such as nausea, vomiting, and diarrhea, usually are transient.

Significant bronchoconstriction can result from bronchial beta-receptor blockade, which otherwise dilates bronchioles. This adverse reaction is more likely to occur with nadolol and propranolol, which are nonselective beta-adrenergic blockers, but also can occur with high doses of atenolol and metoprolol.

Rashes, blood dyscrasias, depression, and vivid dreams occur rarely.

NURSING PROCESS APPLICATION

The following information assists the nurse in caring for a patient who is receiving a beta-adrenergic blocker.

Assessment

• Review the patient's history for a preexisting condition that contraindicates the use of a beta-adrenergic blocker, such as cardiogenic shock, sinus bradycardia and greater-than-first-degree heart block, bronchial asthma, known hypersensitivity to beta-adrenergic blockers, and congestive heart failure unless the failure is caused by a tachyarrhythmia treatable with propranolol.

• Review the patient's history for a preexisting condition that requires cautious use of a beta-adrenergic blocker, such as a nonallergic bronchospastic disorder, diabetes mellitus, impaired hepatic or renal function, pregnancy, or lactation.

• Assess the patient for adverse reactions to the prescribed beta-adrenergic blocker, such as bronchoconstriction or cardiovascular, CNS, or GI dysfunction.

• Review the patient's medication history to identify the use of drugs that may interact with the prescribed beta-adrenergic blocker, such as antacids, insulin, oral hypoglycemic agents, and anti-inflammatory agents.

• Assess the effectiveness of the prescribed beta-adrenergic blocker.

• Observe for signs of fluid volume excess, such as fluid retention, peripheral edema, jugular vein distention, or crackles.

• Assess the patient's breathing pattern for signs of bronchoconstriction.

• Evaluate the patient's and family's knowledge about the prescribed beta-adrenergic blocker.

Nursing diagnoses

The following examples represent appropriate nursing diagnoses for a patient receiving a beta-adrenergic blocker.

• Potential for injury related to a preexisting condition that contraindicates the use of a beta-adrenergic blocker

• Potential for injury related to a preexisting condition that requires cautious use of a beta-adrenergic blocker

• Potential for injury related to adverse drug reactions

• Fluid volume excess related to the adverse cardiovascular effects of the beta-adrenergic blocker

• Ineffective breathing pattern related to bronchoconstricting effects of the beta-adrenergic blocker

• Knowledge deficit related to the prescribed beta-adrenergic blocker

Planning and implementation

• Do not administer a beta-adrenergic blocker to a patient with a condition that contraindicates its use.

• Administer a beta-adrenergic blocker cautiously to a patient at risk because of a preexisting condition.

• Monitor the patient closely for adverse drug reactions, especially for cardiovascular dysfunction during initial administration.

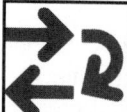

DRUG INTERACTIONS

Beta-adrenergic blockers

Drug interactions involving beta-adrenergic blockers primarily affect the cardiovascular and respiratory systems.

DRUG	INTERACTING DRUGS	POSSIBLE EFFECTS	NURSING IMPLICATIONS
atenolol, metopro-lol, nadolol, pro-pranolol	antacids	Delay absorption of drug from GI tract	• Administer several hours apart. • Monitor the patient for a decreased therapeutic effect.
	lidocaine	Increase plasma levels of li-docaine (potential toxicity); may cause additive cardiac depressant effects	• Monitor the patient for signs of lido-caine toxicity, such as confusion, rest-lessness, and tremors.
	insulin and oral hypoglycemic agents	May cause hypoglycemia or hyperglycemia; may mask tachycardia as a sign of hy-poglycemia (diaphoresis and agitation still present)	• Administer these drugs cautiously. • Monitor the patient's blood glucose levels frequently.
	anti-inflammatories (indo-methacin, salicylates)	Decrease hypotensive effects of beta-adrenergic blockers by inhibiting prostaglandin synthesis	• Monitor the patient for altered beta-adrenergic blocker effects.
	barbiturates	Stimulate metabolism of beta-adrenergic blockers that are metabolized extensively	• Monitor the patient for altered re-sponse to beta-adrenergic blockers that are metabolized by the liver (proprano-lol, metoprolol).
	cardiac glycosides	May cause additive bradycar-dia and depression of AV conduction	• Monitor the patient's blood pressure and heart rate frequently.
	calcium channel blockers	Increase pharmacologic and toxic effects of both agents	• Monitor the patient for adverse reac-tions.
	sympathomimetics (epineph-rine, dobutamine, dopamine, isoproterenol, terbutaline, me-taproterenol, albuterol, rito-drine)	May cause hypertension and reflex bradycardia from unop-posed alpha effects (vaso-constriction) and increased vagal tone	• Monitor the patient's blood pressure and heart rate frequently.
	cimetidine	Reduces metabolism of beta-adrenergic blockers; enhances ability of beta-adrenergic block-ers to reduce pulse rate	• Monitor the patient for altered re-sponse to beta-adrenergic blockers.
	rifampin	Inhibits therapeutic response to metoprolol and propranolol	• Monitor the patient for altered re-sponse to beta-adrenergic blockers.
	theophyllines	Impair bronchodilating effects of theophyllines by nonselec-tive beta-adrenergic blockers	• Monitor the patient's therapeutic re-sponse.
	clonidine	Enhances antihypertensive and bradycardic effects	• Monitor the patient's blood pressure closely.

• *Take the patient's vital signs regularly, particularly not-ing decreased blood pressure or heart rate or irregular rhythm.*
• *Withhold the dose and notify the physician if the pa-tient's apical pulse is less than 60 beats/minute or the systolic blood pressure is less than 90 mm Hg.*

• Monitor the patient closely for CNS reactions, such as dizziness, fatigue, lethargy, and decreased libido as well as depression and vivid dreams.
• Take safety precautions if the patient experiences dizzi-ness or lethargy. For example, keep the bed in a low position and supervise ambulation.

• Be alert for GI reactions, such as nausea, vomiting, and diarrhea. If these occur, monitor the patient's hydration and obtain a prescription for an antiemetic or antidiarrheal, if needed.

• Monitor the diabetic patient's blood glucose level regularly. Expect to adjust the insulin or oral hypoglycemic dose, as needed.

• *Do not administer metoprolol or propranolol with food because food delays their peak concentration.*

• *Do not administer a beta-adrenergic blocker to relieve an angina attack or prevent an imminent one.*

• Adjust the beta-adrenergic blocker dosage over several days, as prescribed, to prevent serious adverse reactions.

• Assess for signs of fluid volume excess, such as crackles, increasing dyspnea, elevated blood pressure, peripheral edema, and jugular vein distention.

• Notify the physician if fluid volume excess occurs; prepare to reduce fluid overload with such measures as diuretic administration.

• *Auscultate the lungs frequently and assess the ease of breathing to detect bronchoconstriction.*

• Notify the physician if bronchoconstriction occurs; prepare to administer bronchodilators and oxygen therapy.

Patient teaching

• Teach the patient and family the name, dose, frequency, action, and adverse effects of the prescribed beta-adrenergic blocker.

• *Instruct the patient taking metoprolol or propranolol to take the drug at the same time each day—but not with meals. Inform the patient taking atenolol or nadolol that the drug can be taken regardless of mealtimes.*

• *Instruct the patient not to discontinue a beta-adrenergic blocker abruptly. Such a drug should be tapered off over several days, as prescribed, to prevent angina, hypertension, arrhythmias, or acute MI.*

• Inform the patient that CNS effects may occur, especially during propranolol therapy. Advise the patient not to drive or operate heavy equipment if CNS effects occur.

• Reassure the patient that adverse GI effects usually are transient. If GI symptoms are severe or persistent, advise the patient to notify the physician who may prescribe an antiemetic or antidiarrheal agent.

• Teach the diabetic patient to test blood glucose regularly and to expect a change in the insulin or oral hypoglycemic dosage during beta-adrenergic blocker therapy.

• *Instruct the patient to notify the physician if adverse reactions occur, especially increasing dyspnea, wheezing, or peripheral edema.*

Evaluation

The following examples represent appropriate evaluation statements for a patient receiving a beta-adrenergic blocker.

• The patient has no conditions that contraindicate beta-adrenergic blocker therapy.

• The patient exhibits no signs of complications in the preexisting condition linked to the prescribed beta-adrenergic blocker.

• The patient displays no adverse reactions to the prescribed beta-adrenergic blocker.

• The patient maintains a normal fluid balance.

• The patient maintains a normal breathing pattern throughout beta-adrenergic blocker therapy.

• The patient and family express an accurate understanding of the points taught about the prescribed beta-adrenergic blocker.

• The patient schedules metoprolol administration at the appropriate time each day, avoiding mealtime administration.

CALCIUM CHANNEL BLOCKERS

A class of drugs consisting of diltiazem hydrochloride, nicardipine hydrochloride, nifedipine, and verapamil hydrochloride, calcium channel blockers produce antianginal effects by mechanisms different from those of the nitrates or the beta-adrenergic blockers. For this reason, these drugs often are used to prevent angina that is unresponsive to drugs in either of the other antianginal classes.

PHARMACOKINETICS

Although they produce similar effects, the various calcium channel blockers have very different chemical structures. These structural differences may explain the pharmacokinetic differences among these drugs.

Absorption, distribution, metabolism, excretion

When administered sublingually, nifedipine is absorbed quickly and almost completely. After oral administration, 80% of diltiazem, 90% of nifedipine and verapamil, and 100% of nicardipine is absorbed from the GI tract. Because of the first-pass effect, however, the bioavailability of these agents is much lower—only 20% for verapamil, 35% for nicardipine, 40% for diltiazem, and 65% to 70% for nifedipine. The calcium channel blockers are highly bound to plasma proteins in the following amounts: diltiazem, 80%; nifedipine, nicardipine, and verapamil, over 90%.

All calcium channel blockers are metabolized rapidly and almost completely in the liver. Some metabolites of diltiazem and verapamil are active, but those of nifedipine and nicardipine are inactive. The metabolites of all of these agents are excreted mostly in the urine and also in the feces. Only 2% to 4% of the drug is excreted unchanged in the urine.

Onset, peak, duration

The onset of action of oral diltiazem is 30 minutes; of nicardipine, 20 minutes; of nifedipine, 10 minutes; of verapamil, 30 to 60 minutes. The peak concentration level of oral diltiazem occurs within 2 to 3 hours; of nicardipine, in 0.5 to 2 hours; of nifedipine, within 30 minutes; and of verapamil, 30 to 60 minutes after an oral dose.

In the absence of significant hepatic disease, the half-lives of the calcium channel blockers are as follows: diltiazem, 3.5 to 6 hours; nicardipine and nifedipine, 2 to 4 hours; verapamil, 3 to 7 hours. The half-life of verapamil increases to 4.5 to 12 hours with long-term administration. Norverapamil, a metabolite of verapamil with less vasodilator properties, has a half-life of 8 to 12 hours.

PHARMACODYNAMICS

By blocking the flow of calcium ions into myocardial muscle cells and myocardial pacemaker cells, calcium channel blockers produce several effects in the heart. (For more information about these effects, see the section on calcium channel blockers in Chapter 30, Antiarrhythmic Agents.) Calcium channel blockers also act on vascular smooth muscle cells.

Mechanism of action

By preventing the influx of calcium ions into myocardial and vascular smooth muscle cells, calcium channel blockers inhibit the intracellular release of additional stores of calcium ions. These intracellular calcium ions otherwise would bind to the troponin-tropomyosin complex and allow actin and myosin to interact. The sliding of actin and myosin filaments past each other produces the contraction of a myocardial cell and ultimately of the whole ventricle. Thus, by inhibiting the release of intracellular calcium ions, calcium channel blockers decrease the force of myocardial contractility, thereby decreasing the oxygen demand.

Calcium channel blockers also prevent entry of calcium ions into arteriolar smooth muscle cells. This action decreases arteriolar constriction and so decreases systemic vascular resistance, or afterload. Decreasing afterload also decreases myocardial oxygen demand.

Myocardial oxygen demand also decreases when calcium channel blockers are used to slow the heart rate, regulated by the sinus node, and to decrease conduction velocity in the heart's conducting pathways, regulated by the AV node. This mechanism probably is significant only for patients with rapid heart rates.

Beside decreasing myocardial oxygen demand, calcium channel blockers increase the oxygen supply to the myocardium by dilating the coronary arteries. Because calcium channel blockers do not induce venous dilation appreciably, they have little effect on preload.

PHARMACOTHERAPEUTICS

Calcium channel blockers are indicated only for long-term prevention of angina. They are not used routinely to relieve acute attacks or to prevent expected ones. Calcium channel blockers are particularly effective in preventing Prinzmetal's angina, for which they are the drug of choice. Nicardipine and nifedipine produce the greatest arteriolar dilation, followed by verapamil and then diltiazem. Nifedipine also has little or no effect on the sinus and AV nodes. Calcium channel blockers do not promote bronchoconstriction and do not exacerbate peripheral vascular disease. They act synergistically with other antianginal agents.

diltiazem hydrochloride (Cardizem). This drug is used for long-term prevention of angina.
Usual adult dosage: initially, 30 mg P.O. before meals q.i.d.; if necessary, gradually increase to 60 mg q.i.d.; or 60 to 120 mg of sustained-release capsules P.O. b.i.d., adjusted up to 240 to 360 daily.

nicardipine hydrochoride (Cardene). This drug is used for long-term prophylaxis of chronic, stable angina.
Usual adult dosage: 20 mg P.O. t.i.d., increased every 3 days, if needed, to a maximum of 40 mg P.O. t.i.d.

nifedipine (Adalat, Procardia). This drug is used for long-term prevention of angina.
Usual adult dosage: 10 mg P.O. t.i.d., gradually increased up to 40 mg P.O. q.i.d., if needed; or 30 to 60 mg of sustained-release tablets P.O. once daily, increased up to a maximum of 120 mg P.O. daily in the morning.

verapamil hydrochloride (Calan, Isoptin). Verapamil is used for long-term prevention of angina.
Usual adult dosage: 240 to 480 mg P.O., divided into three or four doses daily; or 240 mg of sustained-release tablets P.O. daily in the morning, increased up to 240 mg P.O. b.i.d., as needed.

Drug interactions

Calcium channel blockers may interact with beta-adrenergic blockers, causing heart block or even congestive heart failure. They may increase digoxin serum concentrations, resulting in digitalis toxicity. These agents also can inhibit other drugs that are hepatically eliminated. Because all the calcium blockers are metabolized in the liver, they can interact with drugs that affect hepatic metabolism. Interaction with dietary calcium is possible; however this has not been established. (For more detailed information, see *Drug interactions: Calcium channel blockers,* page 530.)

ADVERSE DRUG REACTIONS

Undesirable alterations in the cardiovascular system are the most common and serious adverse reactions to calcium channel blockers. Because they decrease afterload and the force of ventricular contraction, calcium channel blockers sometimes predictably cause hypotension, including orthostatic hypotension. Arrhythmias, such as bradycardia, sinus block, and AV block, result from inhibition of the sinus and AV nodes, especially by diltiazem and verapamil. The depressant action on myocardial contractility may account for the onset or worsening of congestive heart failure.

Vasodilation can produce dizziness, headache, flushing, weakness, and persistent peripheral edema, especially with nicardipine and nifedipine. Other possible adverse reactions include GI disturbances, such as nausea, vomiting, and diarrhea, as well as muscle fatigue and cramps.

Other reactions to calcium channel blockers may include worsening of angina and skin eruptions, photosensitivity, pruritus, nasal congestion, and mood changes.

NURSING PROCESS APPLICATION

The following information assists the nurse in caring for a patient who is receiving a calcium channel blocker for angina.

Assessment
• Review the patient's history for a preexisting condition that contraindicates the use of a calcium channel blocker, such as known hypersensitivity to these drugs.
• Review the patient's history for a preexisting condition that requires cautious use of a calcium channel blocker, such as pregnancy.
• Assess the patient for adverse reactions to the prescribed calcium channel blocker, such as hypotension, arrhythmias, congestive heart failure, dizziness, headache, GI distress, or muscle cramps.
• Review the patient's medication history to identify the use of drugs that may interact with the calcium channel blocker, such as digoxin, beta-adrenergic blockers, and cimetidine.
• Assess the effectiveness of the prescribed calcium channel blocker regularly.
• Assess the patient regularly for headache or muscle cramps.
• Evaluate the patient's and family's knowledge about the prescribed calcium channel blocker.

Nursing diagnoses
The following examples represent appropriate nursing diagnoses for a patient receiving a calcium channel blocker.
• Potential for injury related to a preexisting condition that contraindicates the use of a calcium channel blocker
• Potential for injury related to a preexisting condition that requires cautious use of a calcium channel blocker
• Potential for injury related to adverse drug reactions
• Pain related to the adverse CNS or muscular effects of the prescribed calcium channel blocker
• Knowledge deficit related to the prescribed calcium channel blocker

Planning and implementation
• Do not administer a calcium channel blocker to a patient with a condition that contraindicates its use.
• Administer a calcium channel blocker cautiously to a patient at risk because of a preexisting condition.
• Monitor the patient frequently for adverse drug reactions, especially cardiovascular alterations.
• *Take the patient's vital signs regularly and monitor the electrocardiogram for arrhythmias, particularly when nicardipine or nifedipine are administered. Also monitor for fluid retention by auscultating the patient's lungs regularly and checking for persistent peripheral edema; for congestive heart failure, by noting jugular vein distention and increasing shortness of breath.*
• *Withhold the dose and notify the physician if the patient's heart rate is less than 60 beats/minute or if the systolic blood pressure is less than 90 mm Hg.*
• Expect to administer a calcium channel blocker as an antianginal agent when nitrates or beta-adrenergic blockers have been ineffective.
• *Do not administer a calcium channel blocker to relieve acute angina attacks or prevent an expected attack.*
• *Have the patient sit up for a few minutes before standing to minimize the effects of orthostatic hypotension.*
• Take safety precautions if dizziness occurs. For example, place the bed in the lowest position and supervise ambulation.
• Monitor hydration if the patient experiences GI distress, such as nausea, vomiting, or diarrhea. Ask the physician to prescribe an antiemetic or antidiarrheal agent, as needed.
• *Administer diltiazem before meals.*
• Administer the once-daily dosage of a sustained-release tablet in the morning.
• Notify the physician if adverse reactions occur.
• Monitor the patient for headaches or muscle cramps. Ask the physician to prescribe an analgesic, if needed.

Patient teaching
• Teach the patient and family the name, dose, frequency, action, and adverse effects of the prescribed calcium channel blocker.

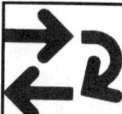

DRUG INTERACTIONS

Calcium channel blockers

Most drug interactions associated with calcium channel blockers result in adverse cardiovascular effects. The nurse must be aware of these interactions to monitor for these effects and to intervene appropriately.

DRUG	INTERACTING DRUGS	POSSIBLE EFFECTS	NURSING IMPLICATIONS
diltiazem, nicardipine, nifedipine, verapamil	cimetidine	Decreases hepatic clearance of the calcium channel blocker	• Monitor the patient for adverse reactions, which may occur more frequently. • Monitor the patient for orthostatic hypotension and for heart rate and rhythm changes.
	calcium salts, vitamin D	Reduce response to calcium channel blocker	• Do not administer concurrently; if necessary to do so, monitor the patient's therapeutic response and adjust the calcium channel blocker dosage, as prescribed.
diltiazem, verapamil	digoxin	Increase serum digoxin concentration	• Monitor the patient for bradycardia, nausea, and vomiting. • Monitor the patient's serum digoxin level.
verapamil	disopyramide phosphate, beta-adrenergic blockers	Cause myocardial depression	• Do not administer these drugs within 24 hours of each other; if concurrent administration is necessary, monitor the patient for signs of congestive heart failure or decreased peripheral perfusion.
	nondepolarizing blocking agents	Enhances muscle relaxant action	• Monitor the patient's respiratory function closely.
	carbamazepine	Enhances carbamazepine action	• Monitor the patient's carbamazepine levels.
diltiazem	cyclosporin	Enhances cyclosporin action	• Monitor the patient's renal function by recording the fluid intake and output and reviewing creatinine and blood urea nitrogen levels. • Monitor the patient's cyclosporin levels.

• Advise the female patient to tell the physician if she is pregnant or plans to become pregnant during calcium channel blocker therapy.

• Teach the patient to recognize and report to the physician the signs of fluid retention, such as peripheral edema or increasing shortness of breath.

• *Demonstrate how to take a pulse and tell the patient to do it before each dose of calcium channel blocker. Advise the patient to delay the dose and notify the physician if the pulse is less than 60 beats/minute.*

• *Emphasize that calcium channel blockers cannot relieve acute angina. If acute chest pain occurs, advise the patient to notify the physician immediately or go to the nearest ED.*

• Teach the patient how to manage orthostatic hypotension.

• Advise the patient not to perform activities that require alertness if dizziness occurs.

• Instruct the patient to notify the physician if nausea, vomiting, or diarrhea occur. If such GI problems occur, advise the patient to request an appropriate medication.

• *Instruct patient to take diltiazem before meals.*

• Instruct the patient to take a once-daily sustained-release tablet in the morning.

• Advise the patient with headaches or muscle cramps to take an analgesic, as prescribed.

• Instruct the patient to notify the physician if adverse reactions occur or if the drug is ineffective.

Evaluation

The following examples represent appropriate evaluation statements for a patient receiving a calcium channel blocker.

• The patient has no conditions that contraindicate calcium channel blocker therapy.

• The patient exhibits no signs of complications in the preexisting condition linked to the prescribed calcium channel blocker.

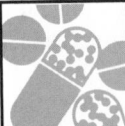

SELECTED MAJOR DRUGS

Antianginal agents

This chart summarizes the major antianginal agents currently in clinical use.

DRUG	MAJOR INDICATIONS	USUAL ADULT DOSAGES	CONTRAINDICATIONS AND PRECAUTIONS
Nitrate			
nitroglycerin	Relief of acute angina attack	0.15 to 0.6 mg sublingually repeated up to three times, or 5 mcg/min I.V., increased by 5 to 20 mcg every 3 to 5 minutes, up to a maximum of 400 mcg/minute, until pain is relieved	• Know that nitroglycerin is contraindicated in a patient with known hypersensitivity to it or other nitrates or nitrites. • Administer with caution to a pregnant or lactating patient or one with depleted intravascular fluid volume or low systolic blood pressure.
	Prevention of expected attack	0.15 to 0.6 mg sublingually repeated up to three times	
	Long-term prevention of angina	1 to 3 mg of a sustained-release tablet between the upper gum and lip t.i.d. or q.i.d., or a sustained-release transdermal patch that releases 2.5 to 15 mg over 24 hours	
Beta-adrenergic blocker			
propranolol	Long-term prevention of angina	10 to 20 mg P.O. b.i.d. to q.i.d., increased up to 320 mg in two to four divided doses, if needed; or 80 to 160 mg of the long-acting form P.O. daily	• Know that propranolol is contraindicated in a patient with cardiogenic shock, sinus bradycardia and greater-than-first-degree heart block, bronchial asthma, known hypersensitivity to propranolol, or congestive heart failure unless the failure is due to a tachyarrhythmia treatable with propranolol. • Administer with caution to a pregnant or lactating patient or one with a nonallergic bronchospastic disorder, diabetes mellitus, or impaired hepatic or renal function.
Calcium channel blocker			
nifedipine	Long-term prevention of angina, especially Prinzmetal's angina	10 mg P.O. t.i.d., gradually increased up to 40 mg P.O. q.i.d.; or 30 to 120 mg P.O. daily of the sustained-release form	• Know that nifedipine is contraindicated in a patient with known hypersensitivity to nifedipine. • Administer with caution to a pregnant patient.

• The patient experiences no adverse reactions to the prescribed calcium channel blocker.
• The patient reports no pain during calcium channel blocker therapy.
• The patient and family express an accurate understanding of the points taught about the prescribed calcium channel blocker.
• The patient correctly demonstrates how and when to take a pulse.

CHAPTER SUMMARY

Chapter 31 discussed nitrates, beta-adrenergic blockers, and calcium channel blockers as they are used to prevent or relieve angina. Here are the highlights of the chapter.
• The coronary arteries supply the heart with the blood it needs for nutrition and oxygen.

• Angina, a symptom of myocardial ischemia, may result from atherosclerosis, which causes narrowing of the coronary arteries. Sometimes coronary artery spasm (associated with Prinzmetal's angina) also contributes to angina.

• Antianginal agents prevent or relieve this ischemia by decreasing myocardial oxygen demand, increasing myocardial oxygen supply, or both.

• Factors affecting oxygen demand include heart rate, force of myocardial contractility, preload, and afterload.

• Nitrates are used for the immediate relief of angina, prevention of an expected angina attack, and long-term prevention of chronic angina.

• Nitrates dilate veins, thereby decreasing preload. To a lesser extent, nitrates also dilate arteries, thereby decreasing afterload. Although they may be administered by multiple routes, nitrates provide the fastest relief when given sublingually or buccally. Nitrates include erythrityl tetranitrate, isosorbide dinitrate, nitroglycerin, and pentaerythritol tetranitrate.

• Beta-adrenergic blockers, which include atenolol, metoprolol tartrate, nadolol, and propranolol hydrochloride, are used for long-term prevention of angina.

• Beta-adrenergic blockers depress myocardial contractility and heart rate, thereby decreasing myocardial oxygen demand. They also may cause hypotension.

• Calcium channel blockers include diltiazem hydrochloride, nicardipine hydrochloride, nifedipine, and verapamil hydrochloride. These drugs block the flow of calcium ions into the myocardial muscle cells and myocardial pacemaker cells, which decreases oxygen demand and contractility. They are especially useful in preventing Prinzmetal's angina. They may produce cardiovascular, GI, and other adverse reactions.

• Combination antianginal therapy often is the most effective means of relieving angina.

• When administering an antianginal agent, the nurse uses the nursing process to provide the best possible care, which includes prompt, skillful administration, close patient monitoring, and use of safety precautions.

STUDY QUESTIONS

See Appendix 1 for answers.

1. Phillip Connor, age 51, has just been admitted to the emergency department with chest pain, which developed an hour ago while he was working in the yard. The nurse administers nitroglycerin (Nitro-Bid) 0.4 mg sublingually stat, as prescribed. When should Mr. Connor expect to feel pain relief?
(a) 1 to 3 minutes
(b) 5 to 10 minutes
(c) 10 to 20 minutes
(d) 20 to 60 minutes

2. How does nitroglycerin exert its therapeutic effects?
(a) It decreases the heart rate, which reduces cardiac oxygen requirements.
(b) It diminishes the force of myocardial contractions, which reduces cardiac oxygen requirements.
(c) It acts directly on vascular smooth muscle, producing relaxation and vessel dilation.
(d) It prevents calcium influx into the smooth muscle cells to decrease arteriolar constriction.

3. The nurse assesses Mr. Connor frequently for adverse reactions to nitroglycerin. Which adverse reaction is most likely to occur?
(a) GI distress
(b) headache
(c) diarrhea
(d) dizziness

4. When Mr. Connor's condition improves, he is transferred to a medical-surgical unit. During his recovery, his physician prescribes nitroglycerin ointment and the beta-adrenergic blocker propranolol 10 mg P.O. t.i.d. Which beta-blocker effect counteracts an adverse reaction to nitroglycerin?
(a) decreased heart rate
(b) decreased preload
(c) increased heart contractility
(d) increased afterload

5. The nurse assesses Mr. Connor before administering each dose. Which findings should prompt the nurse to withhold propranolol and notify the physician?
(a) complaints of chest pain
(b) pulse greater than 60 beats/minute
(c) systolic blood pressure less than 70 mm Hg
(d) diastolic blood pressure more than 80 mm Hg

6. Before Mr. Connor's discharge, the physician replaces propranolol with diltiazem (Cardizem), 30 mg P.O. before meals q.i.d. How doess this calcium channel blocker affect the heart?
(a) It decreases preload.
(b) It increases heart rate.
(c) It increases afterload.
(d) It decreases contractility.

7. Calcium channel blockers are the drugs of choice for which type of angina?
(a) stable angina
(b) unstable angina
(c) preinfarction angina
(d) Prinzmetal's angina

8. When assessing Mr. Connor, the nurse is most likely to detect which adverse reaction to diltiazem?
(a) tachycardia
(b) congestive heart failure
(c) hypertension
(d) confusion

SELECTED REFERENCES

AHFS drug information 90. (1990). Bethesda, MD: American Society of Hospital Pharmacists.

Drug facts and comparisons. (1991). St. Louis: Facts and Comparisons Division, J.B. Lippincott.

Enger, E., and Schwertz, D. (1989). Mechanisms of myocardial ischemia. *Journal of Cardiovascular Nursing,* 3(4), 1-15.

Goodman and Gilman's the pharmacological basis of therapeutics (8th ed.; 1990). Elmsford, NY: Pergamon Press.

Hansten, P., and Horn, J. (1989). *Drug interactions.* (6th ed.). Philadelphia: Lea & Febiger.

Miller, C. (1988). Medications in angina. *Focus on Critical Care,* 15(4), 23-29.

North American Nursing Diagnosis Association. (1990). *Taxonomy I-Revised, with official diagnostic categories.* St. Louis: NANDA.

Parker, J. (1988). Pharmacologic treatment of angina: Nitrate tolerance. *Hospital Practice,* 23(11), 63-80.

Shapiro, W. (1989). Calcium channel blockers: Update on uses in ischemic heart disease. *Consultant,* 29(8), 132-136.

ANTIHYPERTENSIVE AGENTS

OBJECTIVES

After reading and studying this chapter, the student should be able to:
1. Describe the physiologic processes involved in homeostatic blood pressure regulation.
2. Differentiate between essential and secondary hypertension and describe the various types of hypertension.
3. Explain the use of antihypertensive agents in the stepped-care approach to antihypertensive therapy.
4. List at least three examples of sympatholytics, vasodilators, and angiotensin-converting enzyme (ACE) inhibitors.
5. Compare the mechanisms of action of drugs in the three classes of antihypertensive agents.
6. Identify the major adverse reactions that occur with each of the three major classes of antihypertensive agents.
7. Describe how to apply the nursing process when caring for a patient who is receiving an antihypertensive agent.

INTRODUCTION

Antihypertensive agents, which act to reduce blood pressure, are used to treat hypertension, a disorder characterized by elevation in systolic pressure, diastolic pressure, or both.

Affecting about 60 million Americans, hypertension is associated closely with certain risk factors, such as age-, gender-, and race-related factors, obesity, a positive family history, high sodium intake, excessive alcohol consumption, stress, diabetes mellitus, cigarette smoking, and hypercholesterolemia. For example, more men than women under age 50 develop hypertension, but men and women over age 50 have an approximately equal incidence. Hypertension also affects more blacks (27%) than whites (15%), with men and blacks developing cardiovascular complications more frequently than women and whites.

Early detection, effective treatment, and regular follow-up are critical in preventing the serious consequences of uncontrolled hypertension. Although hypertension produces few symptoms at first, the constant elevated pressure on the vessel walls can lead to cardiovascular complications that may affect the heart, eyes, kidneys, and central nervous system (CNS). Hemorrhagic and thrombotic stroke, ischemic heart disease including angina and myocardial infarction (MI), congestive heart failure (CHF), and chronic renal failure can result.

The American Heart Association (Haber, 1988) advocates the stepped-care approach to antihypertensive therapy. With this approach, the physician begins with nondrug treatments, if possible, as the first step in therapy, and then moves to step two if needed by adding the drug or combination of drugs least likely to produce adverse reactions. Subsequent steps involve adding to the initial drug (or drugs), or substituting another drug or drug combination, until the desired blood pressure or maximum effective dosage is reached, or intolerable adverse reactions are detected. (For more information, see *The stepped-care approach to antihypertensive therapy*.) In nonemergency circumstances, stepped-care therapy can reduce the blood pressure to an acceptable level in most patients within 6 months. If blood pressure remains controlled for at least 1 year in a patient who had mild hypertension, the antihypertensive drugs may be withdrawn.

Homeostatic blood pressure regulation

Several homeostatic mechanisms regulate blood pressure. Cardiac output (CO) primarily determines the systolic blood pressure; total peripheral resistance (TPR) chiefly determines the diastolic pressure (DP); and together, the cardiac output and total peripheral resistance determine the mean arterial pressure (MAP), which is expressed by the formula:

$$MAP = CO \times TPR$$

MAP also can be expressed in terms of pulse pressure, which is calculated by subtracting the diastolic from the systolic pressure. The following formula expresses this method of MAP determination:

$$MAP = DP + \tfrac{1}{3} (systolic - diastolic)$$

Short-term regulation of blood pressure involves the nervous and endocrine systems. A decrease in blood pres-

The stepped-care approach to antihypertensive therapy

In this approach, nondrug treatments are tried first if the diastolic blood pressure falls between 90 and 94 mm Hg. If the diastolic pressure exceeds 95 mm Hg or if nondrug treatments are ineffective, then a single, mild antihypertensive drug is prescribed, followed by an increased dosage of the same drug, if needed. Then the physician adds or substitutes one drug after another in gradually increasing dosages, as needed, until the patient achieves a predetermined blood pressure goal, experiences intolerable adverse reactions, or reaches the maximum dosage of each drug.

The patient on stepped-care therapy requires blood pressure monitoring. Depending on the results, the physician may adjust the patient's therapy, as appropriate, by stepping the regimen up or down. With some exceptions, therapy usually continues for life. After the patient has maintained good blood pressure control for more than 3 months, the physician will step the therapy down as long as this does not compromise control. If the patient is receiving a single drug and the diastolic pressure remains continuously below 80 mm Hg, the physician probably will stop the medication temporarily to see if the patient can maintain normal pressure.

STEP 1

Nondrug therapy should be tried first in a patient who has a diastolic pressure that falls between 90 and 94 mm Hg and is at low risk for developing cardiovascular disease. Nondrug therapies include sodium restriction, weight control, alcohol restriction, aerobic exercise, and control of other cardiovascular risk factors, such as smoking and fat consumption.

STEP 2

If the diastolic pressure remains above 90 mm Hg despite at least 6 months of vigorous nondrug treatments, the physician may elect to begin drug therapy. The Joint National Committee (1988) on Detection, Evaluation, and Treatment of High Blood Pressure recommends considering a thiazide diuretic, beta-adrenergic blocker, angiotensin-converting enzyme (ACE) inhibitor, or calcium channel blocker for initial therapy.

The physician probably will choose a diuretic or calcium channel blocker if the patient is over age 50, is black, or has peripheral vascular disease, asthma, or chronic pulmonary disease. Using the smallest effective diuretic dosage minimizes adverse reactions. If the patient is under age 50 or has ischemic heart disease, the physician may choose a beta blocker or ACE inhibitor. Beta blockers usually reduce blood pressure to the level achieved with diuretics.

If these drugs do not control the patient's blood pressure (or if adverse reactions limit the use of other drugs), the physician may consider three options for subsequent therapy: increase the dosage of the first drug if it is below recommended maximum; add a second drug from a different step-2 class; or discontinue the first drug and substitute a drug from a different step-2 class.

STEP 3

If the patient does not respond to diuretic therapy in step-2, the physician will add a low dosage of a sympatholytic (adrenergic-inhibitor) agent, such as a beta blocker. Similarly, if the patient began therapy with a beta blocker but did not respond, the physician will add a diuretic or substitute a diuretic for the beta blocker. If these measures do not control blood pressure, the physician may order a full dosage of the step-2 drug or may substitute another sympatholytic. Or, instead of increasing the step-2 drug dosage to the maximum, a direct vasodilator or calcium channel blocker may be added. Lower dosages of two drugs with different mechanisms of action may prove more effective than higher dosages of a single drug. This approach usually minimizes adverse reactions without significantly reducing effectiveness.

STEP 4

If a third drug is needed, a vasodilating agent may be added. Hydralazine and minoxidil are given most commonly, but a calcium channel blocker may be used instead. The drug chosen is administered with a sympatholytic agent (step 3) and a diuretic (step 2).

STEP 5

If the first four steps of therapy are ineffective and reasons other than drug failure have been ruled out, guanethidine may be added in increasing dosages, as needed, or substituted for one of the step-3 or step-4 drugs.

STEP 1	STEP 2	STEP 3	STEP 4	STEP 5
				Sympatholytics (guanethidine)
			Direct vasodilators	Direct vasodilators
		Sympatholytics	Sympatholytics	Sympatholytics
	Beta-adrenergic blockers	Beta-adrenergic blockers	Beta-adrenergic blockers	Beta-adrenergic blockers
	Diuretics	Diuretics	Diuretics	Diuretics
	ACE inhibitors	ACE inhibitors	ACE inhibitors	ACE inhibitors
	Calcium channel blockers	Calcium channel blockers	Calcium channel blockers	Calcium channel blockers
Sodium restriction	Sodium restriction	Sodium restriction	Sodium restriction	Sodium restriction
Weight control	Weight control	Weight control	Weight control	Weight control
Alcohol restriction	Alcohol restriction	Alcohol restriction	Alcohol restriction	Alcohol restriction
Aerobic exercise	Aerobic exercise	Aerobic exercise	Aerobic exercise	Aerobic exercise
Control of other cardiovascular risk factors	Control of other cardiovascular risk factors	Control of other cardiovascular risk factors	Control of other cardiovascular risk factors	Control of other cardiovascular risk factors

sure stimulates the sympathetic nervous system, promoting epinephrine and norepinephrine secretion. Epinephrine and norepinephrine increase the blood pressure by stimulating the beta$_1$ receptors in the heart to increase cardiac output. They also stimulate the alpha$_1$ receptors in the blood vessels, constricting and increasing their resistance to blood flow. Sympathetic nervous system stimulation also involves medullary vasomotor center control of blood pressure. With a decrease in blood volume, baroreceptors in the aorta and the carotid sinuses adjust the heart rate and blood vessel resistance, thus restoring normal blood pressure.

Hormonal regulation of blood pressure involves the renin-angiotensin-aldosterone system. When the blood pressure is decreased, the kidneys secrete renin, which acts on a plasma protein to produce angiotensin I. Then angiotensin I is converted to angiotensin II in the lungs by converting enzyme. Angiotensin II increases blood pressure by causing vasoconstriction, directly inhibiting the kidneys' excretion of salt and water (and thus increasing plasma volume) and stimulating the adrenal cortex to secrete aldosterone, a hormone that also acts on the kidneys to reduce salt and water excretion.

Types of hypertension

When homeostatic mechanisms fail to regulate blood pressure, essential (primary), or secondary hypertension may develop. In the early phases of essential hypertension, which affects about 95% of all hypertensive patients, CO may be normal or mildly elevated. But as hypertension progresses, peripheral resistance increases and CO decreases, possibly resulting in left ventricular hypertrophy and CHF.

Secondary hypertension affects about 5% of hypertensive patients and results from such underlying disorders as aortic regurgitation, renal stenosis, pheochromocytoma, and neurologic diseases. Treatment of the underlying disorder sometimes can cure secondary hypertension.

Either form of hypertension can occur to varying degrees. According to the World Health Organization's Expert Committee on Hypertension, hypertension is present when the systolic pressure is 160 mm Hg or higher and the diastolic pressure is 95 mm Hg or higher. The Report of the Joint National Committee (1988) on Detection, Evaluation, and Treatment of High Blood Pressure classifies hypertension based on an average of two or more readings on different patient visits.

Mild hypertension refers to a diastolic pressure between 90 and 104 mm Hg. Usually asymptomatic, the patient may not need medication if the diastolic pressure falls between 90 and 94 mm Hg, but will need to reduce risk factors, such as excessive sodium intake, excessive alcohol consumption, obesity, or smoking. However, if the diastolic blood pressure remains between 95 and 104 mm Hg, drug therapy may be initiated.

Moderate hypertension refers to a consistently elevated diastolic pressure, between 105 and 114 mm Hg. If it remains uncontrolled, this degree of hypertension will cause organ damage. Therefore, the patient probably will require therapy with an antihypertensive agent and a diuretic. Moderate hypertension may cause a few minor symptoms, including headache, dizziness, and epistaxis.

Severe hypertension refers to a diastolic pressure of 115 mm Hg or more. The patient typically is symptomatic and may experience damage to the heart, kidneys, and other organs as well as to the retinas. A patient with severe hypertension will require therapy with a potent antihypertensive agent and a diuretic.

Hypertensive crisis is a medical emergency manifested by a diastolic pressure above 140 mm Hg. Untreated, it is likely to result in severe tissue and organ damage—such as retinopathy, heart failure, renal failure, and encephalopathy. Hypertensive crisis requires aggressive parenteral treatment with a fast-acting vasodilator to reduce the diastolic pressure to 100 mm Hg or less.

Malignant hypertension also constitutes a medical emergency. It is characterized by a diastolic blood pressure greater than 140 mm Hg and papilledema. It also requires aggressive parenteral therapy with a potent, rapid-acting vasodilator.

Isolated systolic hypertension is characterized by a systolic blood pressure greater than 160 mm Hg and a diastolic pressure less than 90 mm Hg. Antihypertensive therapy to treat this condition is very individualized.

Assessment and treatment

While obtaining the patient's history, the nurse should identify all existing risk factors, such as high sodium intake, excessive alcohol consumption, stress, obesity, cigarette smoking, diabetes mellitus, hypercholesterolemia, or a family history of hypertension or early cardiac mortality. The nurse also should ask about previous antihypertensive therapy and symptoms of possible complications, such as chest pain, dyspnea, edema, or altered neurologic or renal function.

During the physical examination, the nurse should focus on the cardiovascular and target organ systems, monitoring the vital signs, examining the fundus of each eye, and assessing the heart, lungs, and neurologic system. Finally, the nurse should obtain baseline data from serum electrolyte determinations, renal function tests, electrocardiograms (ECGs), and chest X-rays.

After the diagnosis of hypertension has been confirmed, the nurse assists in implementing the prescribed nondrug or drug therapy.

Nondrug treatments—which should begin as soon as hypertension is diagnosed and continue throughout the course of antihypertensive treatment—include various lifestyle modifications. For example, through biofeedback, the

SELECTED NURSING DIAGNOSES

Antihypertensive agents

The following nursing diagnoses address representative problems and etiologies that a nurse may encounter when caring for a patient who is receiving an antihypertensive agent. Some of these nursing diagnoses contain generalized etiologies, which the nurse must individualize based on the patient's needs. (For some common nursing diagnoses and related interventions for each drug class, see the "Nursing Process Application" sections of this chapter.)

- Altered health maintenance related to ineffectiveness of the prescribed antihypertensive agent
- Altered nutrition: less than body requirements, related to the adverse GI effects of an antihypertensive agent
- Altered nutrition: more than body requirements, related to weight gain caused by a norepinephrine depletor
- Altered peripheral tissue perfusion related to exacerbation of peripheral vascular disease by an antihypertensive agent
- Altered protection related to masking of the early signs of hypoglycemia by a beta-adrenergic agent in a diabetic patient
- Altered protection related to the adverse hematologic effects of an antihypertensive agent
- Altered protection related to the increased risk of breast cancer associated with reserpine therapy
- Altered thought processes related to the adverse central nervous system (CNS) effects of an antihypertensive agent
- Altered urinary elimination related to guanadrel-induced nocturia
- Anxiety related to the adverse CNS effects of an antihypertensive agent
- Body image disturbance related to minoxidil-induced hypertrichosis
- Constipation related to the adverse GI effects of an antihypertensive agent
- Decreased cardiac output related to arrhythmias caused by an antihypertensive agent
- Diarrhea related to the adverse GI effects of an antihypertensive agent

- Fatigue related to the adverse CNS effects of a direct vasodilator
- Fluid volume excess related to antihypertensive-induced fluid retention
- Hyperthermia related to fever caused by an antihypertensive agent
- Ineffective breathing pattern related to the adverse respiratory effects of an antihypertensive agent
- Knowledge deficit related to the prescribed antihypertensive agent
- Noncompliance related to the adverse effects and duration of antihypertensive therapy
- Pain related to anginal attacks caused by an antihypertensive agent
- Pain related to vasodilator-induced headache, angina, or muscle cramps
- Potential for injury related to a preexisting condition that contraindicates the use of an antihypertensive agent
- Potential for injury related to a preexisting condition that requires cautious use of an antihypertensive agent
- Potential for injury related to adverse drug reactions
- Potential for injury related to drug interactions
- Potential for trauma related to the adverse CNS of the antihypertensive agent
- Sensory-perceptual alterations (tactile) related to paresthesia caused by an antihypertensive agent
- Sensory-perceptual alterations (visual) related to blurred vision caused by an antihypertensive agent
- Sexual dysfunction related to the adverse genitourinary effects of an antihypertensive agent
- Sleep pattern disturbance related to sleep alterations caused by an antihypertensive agent

patient can learn to relax to help control blood pressure. Regular aerobic exercise also can lower blood pressure and may help protect against coronary artery disease by elevating blood levels of high-density lipoproteins (HDLs), conjugated proteins that help protect the heart. Regular exercise also can help the patient maintain a normal weight or lose excess weight. Dietary modifications can help control hypertension in several ways. A well-balanced reducing diet can help an obese patient lose excess weight — a very significant risk factor. A low-sodium diet can help control fluid volume; a low-fat diet may help reduce cholesterol and the risk of coronary artery disease. The hypertensive patient should not smoke and should drink alcohol in moderation only.

Many patients require antihypertensive drug therapy. Antihypertensive agents do not cure hypertension; they only decrease the blood pressure. That is why some patients need long-term antihypertensive therapy.

Antihypertensive agents may be sympatholytics, vasodilators, ACE inhibitors, or thiazide diuretics. (For more information about the last drug category, see Chapter 33, Diuretic Agents.) Antihypertensive agents share the same therapeutic objective: to decrease the diastolic blood pressure below 90 mm Hg without producing undesirable adverse reactions.

For a summary of representative drugs, see *Selected major drugs: Antihypertensive agents,* pages 557 and 558. For a listing of applicable nursing diagnoses that the nurse may formulate when caring for a patient receiving these agents, see *Selected nursing diagnoses: Antihypertensive agents.* For detailed information on applying the nursing process, see Chapter 6, The Nursing Process and Drug Therapy.

SYMPATHOLYTIC AGENTS

The sympatholytics include various groups of drugs that reduce blood pressure by inhibiting or blocking motor and secretory action in the sympathetic nervous system. They are classified by their site or mechanism of action and include central-acting sympathetic nervous system inhibitors, ganglionic blocking agents, beta-adrenergic blocking agents, alpha-adrenergic blocking agents, mixed alpha- and beta-adrenergic blocking agents, and norepinephrine depletors.

Central-acting sympathetic nervous system inhibitors act in the CNS to reduce sympathetic activity and thus decrease arteriolar vasoconstriction. This group of sympatholytics includes clonidine hydrochloride, guanabenz acetate, guanfacine, and methyldopa.

Ganglionic blocking agents interfere with the transmission of sympathetic and parasympathetic nerve impulses through the ganglia, producing vasodilation and decreasing the blood pressure. Drugs in this group include mecamylamine hydrochloride and trimethaphan camsylate.

Beta-adrenergic blocking agents—acebutolol hydrochloride, atenolol, betaxolol hydrochloride, carteolol hydrochloride, metoprolol tartrate, nadolol, penbutolol sulfate, pindolol, propranolol hydrochloride, and timolol maleate—compete with epinephrine for beta-receptor sites, antagonizing the effect of epinephrine, a sympathetic neurotransmitter, and blocking sympathetic stimulation, resulting in decreased cardiac output.

Alpha-adrenergic blocking agents act on the sympathetic nervous system alpha receptors, preventing norepinephrine and epinephrine from occupying and activating them. With sympathetic stimulation blocked, vasodilation occurs. This class of drugs includes doxazosin mesylate, phentolamine, prazosin hydrochloride, and terazosin.

Labetalol is a mixed alpha- and beta-adrenergic blocking agent. This type of antihypertensive agent nonselectively blocks beta-adrenergic receptors and selectively blocks alpha$_1$ receptors.

Norepinephrine depletors interfere with the synthesis, storage, and release of norepinephrine from the nerve terminals. This interference leads to a loss of peripheral sympathetic tone, decreasing peripheral resistance and leading to a reduction in blood pressure. Norepinephrine depletors include guanadrel sulfate, guanethidine sulfate, and reserpine. (They sometimes are referred to as peripheral-acting sympatholytic agents.)

PHARMACOKINETICS

Most sympatholytics are absorbed well from the gastrointestinal (GI) tract, are distributed widely, metabolized in the liver, and excreted primarily in the urine. The pharmacokinetics of phentolamine are unknown.

Absorption

After oral administration, most central-acting nervous system inhibitors and the ganglionic blocking agents are absorbed well from the GI tract. However, absorption of the central-acting agent methyldopa is variable and incomplete. Because of this and the first-pass metabolism in the intestines and liver, its bioavailability averages about 25%. The ganglionic blocking agent trimethaphan must be administered I.V. because of erratic and incomplete absorption after oral administration. Although mecamylamine absorption is less erratic, the drug may decrease peristalsis, leading to delayed gastric emptying time and impaired absorption.

The beta-adrenergic blocking agents are absorbed well from the GI tract, except for atenolol and nadolol, which are absorbed rapidly but incompletely. The presence of food may increase propranolol and metoprolol bioavailability. Alpha-adrenergic blocking agents such as prazosin and doxazosin are absorbed well from the GI tract. Labetalol, the mixed alpha- and beta-adrenergic blocking agent, also is absorbed well and its bioavailability may be increased by ingestion of cimetidine or food or by chronic hepatic disease.

The absorption of norepinephrine depletors varies with each drug. Guanadrel is absorbed rapidly and almost completely; the absorption of guanethidine, however, usually is incomplete. Reserpine is absorbed slowly from the GI tract; its bioavailability is about 50%.

Distribution

The central-acting agents are distributed widely to body tissues. Clonidine and methyldopa are less than 20% bound to plasma proteins. Guanabenz, guanfacine, and methyldopa are distributed into the CNS, and clonidine passes into the cerebrospinal fluid and the CNS.

Ganglionic blocking agents also are distributed widely. Mecamylamine crosses the blood-brain barrier and reaches high concentrations in the liver, spleen, heart, and lungs. Because its ganglionic-blocking effects may decrease GI motility in the fetus, its use is contraindicated during pregnancy. It also may be secreted in breast milk.

All alpha- and beta-adrenergic blocking agents seem to achieve wide distribution. The beta-adrenergic blocking agents metoprolol and propranolol readily cross the blood-brain barrier and also appear in breast milk; propranolol is about 90% bound to plasma proteins. Protein binding is much lower with the other beta-adrenergic blocking agents:

11% to 25% with acebutolol, 16% with atenolol, about 50% with betaxolol, 23% to 30% with carteolol, 12% with metoprolol, 30% with nadolol, 80% to 98% with penbutolol, 40% to 60% with pindolol, and less than 10% with timolol. Protein binding for phetolamine is unknown. The alpha-adrenergic blocking agents doxazosin, prazosin, and terazosin also are highly protein bound. Labetalol, the mixed alpha- and beta-adrenergic blocking agent, has a 25% bioavailability after oral ingestion from first-pass effect, is distributed rapidly, and is about 50% protein bound. It crosses the placenta and is secreted in breast milk.

Norepinephrine depletors are distributed widely. Guanadrel is distributed widely and is about 20% protein bound. Guanethidine is distributed rapidly to storage sites in the liver, kidney, and lungs. Reserpine is distributed particularly well in adipose tissue, accounting for its long serum half-life in obese and elderly patients. It crosses the blood-brain barrier and the placenta and is secreted in breast milk.

Metabolism

As a rule, the central-acting, ganglionic-blocking, beta-adrenergic blocking, and mixed alpha- and beta-adrenergic blocking agents are metabolized extensively in the liver. However, some exceptions to this rule exist. For example, the ganglionic blocker trimethaphan is metabolized by pseudocholinesterase, and the metabolism of some beta-adrenergic blockers varies. Atenolol is not metabolized in the liver, for example, but about 95% of metoprolol is. Also, the liver's capacity to metabolize propranolol varies greatly from patient to patient.

Metabolism of prazosin occurs in the liver, primarily by demethylation and conjugation. Doxazosin also is metabolized extensively in the liver. Metabolism of the other alpha-adrenergic blocking agents, phentolamine and terazosin, is unknown.

The norepinephrine depletor guanadrel is 40% to 50% metabolized by the liver. Guanethidine's metabolism is variable with 25% to 60% excreted unchanged in the urine. Reserpine also undergoes metabolism in the liver.

Excretion

Most antihypertensive agents are excreted primarily in the urine. Among the central-acting agents, from 60% to 75% of clonidine and methyldopa is excreted this way, although methyldopa also is excreted in the feces and bile. Guanfacine is excreted 30% to 40% unchanged in the urine. The ganglionic blocker mecamylamine is excreted slowly by the kidneys as unchanged drug, and its rate of excretion increases in acidic urine and decreases in alkaline urine.

The amount of unchanged drug excreted varies among the beta-adrenergic blocking agents. For example, atenolol and nadolol appear to be excreted 100% unchanged; carteolol, 50% to 70% unchanged; pindolol, 40% unchanged;

and betaxolol, 15% unchanged. Only 6% to 10% of prazosin is excreted in the urine; the rest of this alpha-adrenergic blocking agent is excreted primarily in bile and the feces. (Its excretion may be decreased in a patient with CHF.) Doxazosin is excreted primarily in the feces. Terazosin is largely eliminated as metabolites, but some of it is excreted as unchanged drug in the urine (10%) and feces (20%). Labetalol metabolites are excreted in bile and urine.

About 85% of the norepinephrine depletor guanadrel is excreted primarily in the urine. Guanethidine's excretion occurs primarily in urine and feces. Reserpine also is excreted chiefly in the feces (60%) and in the urine.

Onset, peak, duration

The onset of action, peak concentration levels, and duration of action vary greatly among the sympatholytics. (For detailed information, see *Onset, peak, and duration of sympatholytic agents,* pages 540 and 541.)

PHARMACODYNAMICS

All sympatholytic agents inhibit stimulation of the sympathetic nervous system. They perform this function in different ways, but they all produce the same result: decreased blood pressure from peripheral vasodilation or decreased cardiac output.

Mechanism of action

Methyldopa, a central-acting agent structurally related to the catecholamines, acts as a false transmitter in the brain. Its central action involves its metabolism to the active compound alpha methylnorepinephrine. In the CNS, this compound stimulates the alpha-adrenergic receptors that inhibit sympathetic output. Output inhibition decreases vascular peripheral tone and arteriolar vasoconstriction. In this way, methyldopa lowers standing and supine blood pressures and reduces renal vascular resistance. Its action has little effect on cardiac output, however, and it produces less orthostatic hypotension than peripherally acting agents.

The other central-acting agents, clonidine, guanabenz, and guanfacine, reduce hypertension by activating alpha$_2$ receptors in the lower brain stem. This suppresses the outflow of sympathetic nervous activity from the brain. These drugs also may activate presynaptic (inhibitory) alpha$_2$ receptors in the peripheral nervous system. This stimulation decreases the sympathetic tone and resistance in the peripheral arterioles, lowering the standing and supine blood pressures and decreasing the heart rate and cardiac output. (Long-term guanabenz therapy, however, leaves the cardiac output unchanged). These drugs also produce peripheral vasodilation, and they produce less orthostatic hypotension than peripherally acting agents. They do not alter the glomerular filtration rate.

Onset, peak, and duration of sympatholytic agents

The pharmacokinetic properties of the major sympatholytic agents are summarized below.

DRUG	ROUTE	ONSET OF ACTION	PEAK CONCENTRATION	DURATION OF ACTION
Central-acting agents				
clonidine	P.O.	30 to 60 minutes	2 to 5 hours	Up to 8 hours (24 to 36 hours in some patients)
guanabenz	P.O.	1 hour	2 to 5 hours	10 to 12 hours
guanfacine	P.O.	1 to 2 hours	3 hours	15 to 20 hours
methyldopa	P.O. I.V.	3 to 6 hours Immediate	3 to 6 hours 4 to 6 hours	24 hours 10 to 16 hours
Ganglionic blocking agents				
mecamylamine	P.O.	30 minutes to 2 hours	3 to 5 hours	6 to 12 hours or more
trimethaphan	I.V. infusion	Immediate	Immediate	10 to 30 minutes after infusion stops
Beta-adrenergic blocking agents				
acebutolol	P.O.	60 to 90 minutes	2 to 2.5 hours	24 hours
atenolol	P.O.	1 hour	2 to 4 hours	24 hours
betaxolol	P.O.	1 hour	2 to 6 hours	24 hours
carteolol	P.O.	30 minutes	1 to 3 hours	48 hours
metoprolol	P.O.	10 minutes	90 minutes	12 to 18 hours
nadolol	P.O.	Unknown	2 to 4 hours	24 hours
penbutolol	P.O.	15 minutes	1 hour	24 hours
pindolol	P.O.	Rapid	1 to 2 hours	24 hours
propranolol	P.O.	30 minutes	60 to 90 minutes	8 to 12 hours
timolol	P.O.	30 minutes	1 to 2 hours	12 hours
Alpha-adrenergic blocking agents				
doxazosin	P.O.	1 to 2 hours	2 to 3 hours	Up to 36 hours
phentolamine	I.M.	Immediate	20 minutes	30 to 45 minutes
	I.V.	Immediate	2 minutes	15 to 30 minutes
prazosin	P.O.	1 to 2 hours	2 to 4 hours	6 to 24 hours
terazosin	P.O.	15 minutes	1 to 2 hours	18 hours

Onset, peak and duration of sympatholytic agents (continued)

DRUG	ROUTE	ONSET OF ACTION	PEAK CONCENTRATION	DURATION OF ACTION
Mixed alpha- and beta-adrenergic blocking agent				
labetalol	P.O.	20 minutes to 2 hours	1 to 4 hours	Dose-dependent: 8 to 12 hours (200 mg); 10 to 24 hours (300 mg)
	I.V. infusion or bolus	2 to 5 minutes	5 to 15 minutes	2 to 4 hours
Norepinephrine depletor				
guanadrel	P.O.	60 to 90 minutes	4 to 6 hours	4 to 14 hours
guanethidine	P.O.	Variable	6 to 8 hours	24 to 48 hours
reserpine	P.O.	Days	6 to 12 hours	6 to 24 hours

The ganglionic blocking agents mecamylamine and trimethaphan compete with acetylcholine to occupy cholinergic receptors on the autonomic ganglia. By thus interacting with the cholinergic receptors, these drugs interrupt transmission of parasympathic and sympathetic impulses. The resulting reduction in sympathetic tone and cardiac output increases vasodilation and lowers the blood pressure.

Beta-adrenergic blocking agents act by competing with epinephrine for beta-adrenergic receptor sites. By thus inhibiting or blocking sympathetic stimulation, they decrease heart rate and cardiac output and reduce the blood pressure. Carteolol, nadolol, penbutolol, pindolol, propranolol, and timolol are nonselective, blocking $beta_1$ (cardiac) and $beta_2$ (noncardiac) receptors. Acebutolol, atenolol, betaxolol, and metoprolol are selective, blocking primarily $beta_1$ receptors. By blocking the $beta_1$ receptors in the heart, these drugs decrease heart rate and myocardial contractility and ultimately lower cardiac output. Also, acebutolol, carteolol, penbutolol, and pindolol exhibit beta agonist (intrinsic sympathomimetic) activity in therapeutic dosages; they partially stimulate the receptor as they block it. This partial agonist activity causes a smaller reduction in cardiac output and resting heart rate than seen with drugs lacking agonist activity. Because renin release is mediated through $beta_1$ receptors in the kidney, beta blockers also decrease the effect of the renin-angiotensin-aldosterone system.

The alpha-adrenergic blocking agents doxazosin, prazosin, and terazosin selectively block $alpha_1$ receptors, interfering with sympathetic stimulation and directly relaxing arteriolar smooth muscle. This interference reduces peripheral vascular resistance and produces vasodilation without producing tachycardia or reducing cardiac output; maximum antihypertensive effects appear when the patient

is upright. Prazosin produces little or no increase in serum renin levels, cardiac output, renal blood flow, or glomerular filtration rate.

The nonselective alpha-adrenergic blocker phentolamine produces vasodilation in a slightly different way, by competitively blocking all alpha-adrenergic receptor sites and circulating epinephrine. This also increases gastric secretions, however, and may result in nausea, vomiting, and diarrhea. In addition, it produces reflex tachycardia as a result of direct cardiac stimulation and orthostatic hypotension from vasodilation.

Labetalol, the mixed alpha- and beta-adrenergic blocking agent, decreases total peripheral resistance, reduces plasma renin and aldosterone levels as well as renal vascular resistance, and may decrease cardiac output. Unlike nonselective alpha-adrenergic blockers, labetalol does not produce reflex tachycardia. In comparison with beta-adrenergic blocking agents, labetalol produces less bradycardia and reduction in blood flow as it decreases peripheral vascular resistance. It decreases standing blood pressure more than supine blood pressure. Besides its adrenergic activity, labetalol decreases plasma angiotensin II and aldosterone levels.

The norepinephrine depletors guanadrel, guanethidine, and reserpine exert antihypertensive effects by depleting the catecholamine stores in the sympathetic nerve endings and also may inhibit norepinephrine transport to storage sites. These actions reduce the sympathetic output, thus reducing vasomotor tone. The drugs also reduce total peripheral resistance, decrease cardiac output, and result in bradycardia; these effects contribute to blood pressure reduction.

Guanadrel exerts its strongest antihypertensive effects when the patient is standing. It does not decrease cardiac output or renal blood flow with long-term therapy, but it can decrease heart rate and may result in fluid retention.

Guanethidine selectively blocks the efferent peripheral sympathetic pathways, causing vasodilation with decreased peripheral resistance and leading to a prolonged decrease in the blood pressure. This drug reduces systolic blood pressure more than diastolic pressure and more effectively lowers standing blood pressure than supine blood pressure. Besides decreasing blood pressure, vasodilation may decrease renal, coronary, and cerebral blood flow as well as plasma renin activity.

PHARMACOTHERAPEUTICS

Sympatholytics typically are used to lower the blood pressure of patients with mild to severe essential hypertension. Using the stepped-care approach to antihypertensive therapy, the physician can change the type of drug used and alter the dosage to achieve effective therapeutic effects with the fewest adverse reactions.

clonidine hydrochloride (Catapres, Catapres-TTS). A central-acting nervous system inhibitor, clonidine is used as a step-3 drug to treat mild to moderate hypertension. It lowers the supine and standing blood pressures and usually is given with a diuretic or another antihypertensive agent to achieve the maximum blood pressure reduction. It is available as an oral preparation or transdermal patch system that delivers 0.1, 0.2, or 0.3 mg/day for seven days.
Usual adult dosage: initially, 0.1 mg P.O. b.i.d., increased by 0.1 to 0.2 mg/day every 2 to 4 days until the desired response is achieved; for maintenance, 0.1 to 0.2 mg b.i.d. to q.i.d. or up to a maximum of 2.4 mg/day. With a transdermal patch, the usual dosage is a 0.1 mg system, followed by another 0.1-mg or larger system if the blood pressure has not been reduced sufficiently after 1 or 2 weeks. Use of more than two 0.3-mg systems usually does not result in increased efficacy.

guanabenz acetate (Wytensin). A central-acting agent administered orally, guanabenz usually is considered a step-3 drug. Because it produces orthostatic hypotension in fewer than 1% of patients, guanabenz may be a useful substitute for guanethidine or adrenergic blocking agents when these drugs produce severe orthostatic hypotension.
Usual adult dosage: initially, 4 mg P.O. b.i.d., increased by 4 to 8 mg/day every 1 to 2 weeks as needed, up to a maximum of 32 mg b.i.d., although a dose this high rarely is needed.

guanfacine (Tenex). A central-acting agent, guanfacine also is considered a step-3 drug and is used to treat mild to moderate hypertension. It does not affect cardiac output but decreases total peripheral resistance. It usually is prescribed with a diuretic agent.
Usual adult dosage: 1 mg P.O. at bedtime may be increased to a maximum of 3 mg/day. Dosage adjustments may be required for renally impaired or elderly patients.

methyldopa (Aldomet). A central-acting agent, methyldopa usually is administered orally to control mild to moderate hypertension. It commonly is combined with a diuretic, because it can produce sodium and water retention. Usually used as a step-3 drug, methyldopa is useful for treating patients with impaired renal function. It may be administered I.V. to treat hypertensive crisis.
Usual adult dosage: initially, for mild to moderate hypertension, 250 mg P.O. b.i.d. or t.i.d., increased biweekly to a maintenance dosage of 500 mg to 2 grams/day in two to four divided doses or up to a maximum of 3 grams/day; for hypertensive crisis, 250 to 500 mg I.V. in 100 ml of dextrose 5% in water infused over 30 to 60 minutes, repeated every 6 hours if necessary.

mecamylamine hydrochloride (Inversine). A potent, long-acting ganglionic blocking agent, mecamylamine is used to treat moderate to severe hypertension. As an adjunct rather than a primary agent, it usually is used as a step-5 drug but can be substituted for one of the drugs used in steps 3 or 4. The required dosage varies widely according to patient factors, the time of day, and the season. Higher doses usually are required at night and in cold weather.
Usual adult dosage: initially, 2.5 mg P.O. b.i.d., increased by 2.5 mg every 2 or more days until the desired response is achieved. The average maintenance dosage is 25 mg/day given in three divided doses.

trimethaphan camsylate (Arfonad). A potent, short-acting ganglionic blocking agent, trimethaphan is administered I.V. to manage hypertensive crisis associated with pulmonary edema. Elderly patients may be unusually sensitive to its effects, necessitating dosage adjustments.
Usual adult dosage: 3 to 4 mg/minute I.V. of 500 mg diluted in 500 ml of dextrose 5% in water, adjusted according to the patient's response.

acebutolol hydrochloride (Sectral). A beta-adrenergic blocker, acebutalol is used as a step-2 or step-3 agent. It can be used alone or with other antihypertensive agents.
Usual adult dosage: 400 mg P.O. once daily or in two divided doses, increased gradually, as needed, to a maximum of 1,200 mg/day. Renal impairment requires the following dosage adjustment: with a creatinine clearance of 25 to 50 ml/minute, the daily dosage is reduced by 50%; with a clearance of less than 25 ml/minute, reduced by 75%.

atenolol (Tenormin). A selective beta-adrenergic blocking agent, atenolol produces maximum effects up to 3 days after the initial oral dose. It is used as a step-2 or a step-3 agent or sometimes with other drugs and should be given cautiously to a patient with chronic obstructive pulmonary disease (COPD), asthma, peripheral vascular disease (PVD), or diabetes.
Usual adult dosage: 50 to 100 mg P.O. once daily.

betaxolol hydrochloride (Kerlone). This beta-adrenergic blocking agent is used in step 2 or step 3 of hypertension treatment. It can be used alone or with other antihypertensive agents, particularly thiazide diuretics.
Usual adult dosage: 10 mg P.O. once daily, increased to 20 mg daily after 7 to 14 days if the desired response does not occur.

carteolol hydrochloride (Cartrol). A beta-adrenergic blocking agent, carteolol is indicated in step 2 or step 3 of hypertension therapy. This oral antihypertensive may be used alone or with other antihypertensive agents.
Usual adult dosage: 2.5 mg P.O. once daily, gradually increased to 10 mg daily, as needed. Renal impairment requires the following dosage adjustment: with a creatinine clearance of 20 to 60 ml/minute, the dosage interval is increased to 48 hours; with a clearance of less than 20 ml/minute, increased to 72 hours.

metoprolol tartrate (Lopressor). This cardioselective beta-adrenergic blocking agent may be used alone or with other antihypertensives as a step-2 or step-3 agent. It should be given cautiously to a patient with COPD or hepatic or renal disease.
Usual adult dosage: initially, 100 mg P.O. daily in single or divided doses, increased by 50 mg/day every week up to a maximum of 450 mg/day.

nadolol (Corgard). A beta-adrenergic blocking agent, nadolol is administered orally. Because of its long half-life, however, this step-2 agent may not reach therapeutic antihypertensive levels for up to 5 days after therapy begins.
Usual adult dosage: initially, 40 to 80 mg P.O. daily, increased by 40 to 80 mg every week, as needed and tolerated, up to a maximum of 320 mg/day. A patient with impaired renal function may require a lower dosage.

penbutolol sulfate (Levatol). A beta-adrenergic blocking agent, penbutolol is a step-2 or step-3 drug used to treat mild to moderate hypertension. Administered orally, it may be used alone or with other antihypertensive agents.
Usual adult dosage: initially 20 mg P.O. once daily.

pindolol (Visken). A beta-adrenergic blocking agent, pindolol is a step-2 or step-3 agent administered orally alone or with other antihypertensive agents.
Usual adult dosage: initially, 5 mg P.O. b.i.d., increased by 10 mg/day every 3 to 4 weeks up to a maximum dosage of 60 mg/day.

propranolol hydrochloride (Inderal, Inderal LA). A beta-adrenergic blocking agent, propranolol is used to treat mild to moderate hypertension. Administered orally, this step-2 or step-3 agent may be used alone, but it commonly is given with other antihypertensive agents, such as thiazide diuretics or vasodilators, to increase their efficacy and reduce their adverse effects.
Usual adult dosage: 40 mg P.O. b.i.d., or 80 mg of extended-release capsules once daily, increased gradually, as needed, up to a maximum of 640 mg/day.

timolol maleate (Blocadren). A beta-adrenergic blocking agent, timolol is a step-2 or step-3 drug used to treat mild to moderate hypertension. Administered orally, it may be used alone or with other antihypertensive agents.
Usual adult dosage: initially, 10 mg P.O. b.i.d., increased every week, as needed and tolerated, up to 30 mg b.i.d.; for maintenance, 20 to 40 mg/day.

phentolamine (Regitine). This alpha-adrenergic blocking agent is available as phentolamine hydrochloride and phentolamine mesylate and can be administered I.V. or I.M. It first was used to treat hypertension, but now is used to prevent or control hypertensive crisis associated with pheochromocytoma surgery and to aid in diagnosing pheochromocytoma.
Usual adult dosage: to diagnose pheochromocytoma, 5 mg I.V.; 1 to 2 hours before surgical removal of pheochromocytoma, 5 mg I.M. or I.V.; during surgery, 5 mg I.V.

doxazosin mesylate (Cardura). An alpha$_1$-receptor blocking agent, doxazosin resembles prazosin structurally and shares many of its pharmacologic effects. However, doxazosin's longer half-life (20 hours or more) permits once daily dosing. Doxazosin usually is considered a step-3 drug and can produce first-dose syncope.
Usual adult dosage: initially, 1 mg P.O. once daily, increased gradually based on patient tolerance and response, up to the maximum of 16 mg/day. Orthostatic hypotension increases substantially when the dosage exceeds 4 mg/day.

prazosin hydrochloride (Minipress). An alpha$_1$-adrenergic blocking agent, prazosin usually is considered a step-3 drug. Administered orally, it is most effective in reduced dosages given with a thiazide diuretic or a beta-adrenergic blocking agent. This drug may produce first-dose syncope.

Usual adult dosage: initially, 0.5 to 1 mg P.O. b.i.d to t.i.d., increased gradually to a maintenance dosage that meets the patient's requirements; for maintenance, 6 to 15 mg/day in divided doses when given alone or 1 to 2 mg P.O. t.i.d. when given with a diuretic or another antihypertensive agent. Dosages exceeding 20 mg/day usually do not produce increased effects, although a few patients may benefit from dosages up to 40 mg daily.

terazosin (Hytrin). An alpha₁-adrenergic blocking agent, terazosin is administered orally and indicated for treatment of patients with mild to moderate hypertension. This step-3 drug may be useful in a patient who cannot tolerate diuretics or beta-adrenergic blocking agents, but it is used more widely as an adjunct to these drugs.
Usual adult dosage: 1 to 20 mg P.O. daily in one or two doses, titrated according to the patient's response. Dosages that exceed 20 mg daily do not appear to lower the blood pressure further.

labetalol (Normodyne, Trandate). A mixed alpha- and beta-adrenergic blocking agent, labetalol is effective when used alone to treat mild to severe hypertension. It usually is administered orally as a step-3 antihypertensive agent, but also may be used as a step-2 drug. I.V. labetalol also is effective for treating hypertensive crisis. Labetalol is especially useful for treating hypertension in patients who are resistant to other forms of antihypertensive therapy and in those who have renal or cardiac diseases, COPD, or arterial insufficiency.
Usual adult dosage: for hypertension, 100 mg P.O. b.i.d., increased as needed up to 400 mg b.i.d.; for hypertensive crisis, 20 to 80 mg slow I.V. bolus every 10 minutes or 2 mg/minute by continuous I.V. infusion up to a maximum of 300 mg. By I.V. infusion, the effective dosage usually ranges from 50 to 200 mg.

guanadrel sulfate (Hylorel). A norepinephrine depletor, guanadrel is a step-3 drug administered orally to treat hypertension that has not responded sufficiently to thiazide diuretics alone.
Usual adult dosage: initially, 5 mg P.O. b.i.d., increased every week as needed to a maintenance dosage of 20 to 75 mg/day given in two to four divided doses.

guanethidine sulfate (Ismelin). A norepinephrine depletor administered orally, guanethidine can be used to treat moderate to severe hypertension but is not considered a primary agent. It usually is used as a step-5 drug along with another drug, but can be substituted for one of the drugs used in step 3 or step 4.
Usual adult dosage: initially, 10 to 12.5 mg P.O. once daily, increased by 10 to 12.5 mg every 5 to 7 days, as needed; for maintenance, 25 to 50 mg/day.

reserpine (Serpasil). A norepinephrine depletor, reserpine is used to treat mild to moderate hypertension. Not considered a primary agent in antihypertensive therapy, it often is combined with a diuretic or other antihypertensive agent as a step-3 drug. Its effects may not appear for up to several weeks.
Usual adult dosage: initially, 0.1 to 0.5 mg P.O. in a single daily dosage or in two divided doses; for maintenance, a maximum of 0.25 mg daily.

Drug interactions

Many different drugs can interact with sympatholytic agents, frequently producing blood pressure changes and other effects. (For detailed information, see *Drug interactions: Sympatholytic agents.*)

ADVERSE DRUG REACTIONS

Many sympatholytic agents cause adverse reactions in the CNS and the cardiovascular system. Additional reactions affecting other body systems vary with each drug.

Central-acting and ganglionic blocking agents typically produce CNS effects, such as sedation, drowsiness, and depression. Other common reactions include forgetfulness, inability to concentrate, and vivid dreams, that usually diminish after 2 to 3 weeks of therapy. Additional adverse reactions include sodium and water accumulation, edema, hepatic dysfunction, vertigo, paresthesias, weakness, fever, nasal congestion, and dry mouth. These drugs may decrease the libido and result in impotence, limiting their usefulness in men. They also may produce lactation in women and men.

Other adverse reactions vary according to the specific drug used. For example, clonidine is especially likely to cause dry mouth, because it decreases salivary flow. When the drug is discontinued, rebound hypertension to pretreatment levels may result.

Guanabenz may produce cardiovascular adverse reactions, such arrhythmias, chest pain, edema, and palpitations. Its other effects may include anxiety, ataxia, blurred vision, and nasal congestion. Like clonidine, guanabenz can produce rebound hypertension if it is discontinued suddenly. Because of its potential for producing serious adverse reactions, this drug requires cautious use in a patient with a recent MI or with cerebrovascular disease, severe coronary insufficiency, or hepatic or renal failure.

Shortness of breath, respiratory depression, and tachycardia can develop with mecamylamine therapy. The other ganglionic blocking agent, trimethaphan, can produce similar effects and may decrease serum potassium levels. Both of these agents should be used with extreme caution in a patient with prostatic hypertrophy, cardiovascular insufficiency, MI, fever or infection, hemorrhage, sodium depletion, glaucoma, or renal impairment. They also should be

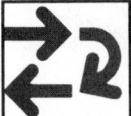

DRUG INTERACTIONS

Sympatholytic agents

The sympatholytic agents can interact with many drugs to produce blood pressure changes as well as other severe reactions.

DRUG	INTERACTING DRUGS	POSSIBLE EFFECTS	NURSING IMPLICATIONS
clonidine	tricyclic antidepressants	Increase blood pressure	• Avoid concomitant administration.
	beta-adrenergic blocking agents	Promote a paradoxical hypertensive response	• Monitor the patient's blood pressure frequently.
trimethaphan	nondepolarizing muscle relaxants, especially spinal anesthetics	Enhance hypotensive effects; cause prolonged apnea	• Monitor the patient's blood pressure frequently. • Avoid concomitant administration, if possible. • Monitor the patient's respiratory status.
labetalol	halothane anesthesia	Enhances the hypotensive effects of labetalol	• Monitor the patient's blood pressure frequently.
guanadrel	sympathomimetic agents	Inhibit antihypertensive effects of guanadrel	• Monitor the patient's blood pressure frequently.
guanethidine	sympathomimetic agents, phenothiazines, tricyclic antidepressants, amphetamines	Inhibit antihypertensive effects of guanethidine	• Avoid concomitant administration. • Monitor the patient's blood pressure frequently.
reserpine	levodopa	Depletes dopamine, inhibiting levodopa's effect	• Avoid giving reserpine to a patient receiving levodopa for Parkinson's disease.
acebutolol, atenolol, betaxolol, carteolol, metoprolol, nadolol, penbutolol, pindolol, propranolol, timolol	antacids	Delay absorption of drug from GI tract	• Administer several hours apart. • Monitor the patient for a decreased therapeutic effect.
	lidocaine	Increase plasma levels of lidocaine (potential toxicity); may cause additive cardiac depressant effects	• Monitor the patient for signs of lidocaine toxicity, such as confusion, restlessness, and tremors.
	insulin and oral hypoglycemic agents	May cause hypoglycemia or hyperglycemia; may mask tachycardia as a sign of hypoglycemia (diaphoresis and agitation still present)	• Administer these drugs cautiously. • Monitor the patient's blood glucose levels frequently.
	anti-inflammatories (indomethacin, salicylates)	Decrease hypotensive effects of beta-adrenergic blockers by inhibiting prostaglandin synthesis	• Monitor the patient for altered beta-adrenergic blocker effects.
	barbiturates, rifampin	Stimulate metabolism of beta-adrenergic blockers that are metabolized extensively	• Monitor the patient for altered response to beta-adrenergic blockers that are metabolized by the liver (propranolol, metoprolol).
	cardiac glycosides	May cause additive bradycardia and depression of AV conduction	• Monitor the patient's blood pressure and heart rate frequently.

(continued)

DRUG INTERACTIONS

Sympatholytic agents (continued)

DRUG	INTERACTING DRUGS	POSSIBLE EFFECTS	NURSING IMPLICATIONS
acebutolol, atenolol, betaxolol, carteolol, metoprolol, nadeolol, penbutolol, pindolol propranolol, timolol *(continued)*	calcium channel blockers	Increase pharmacologic and toxicologic effects of both agents	• Monitor the patient for adverse reactions.
	sympathomimetics (epinephrine, dobutamine, dopamine, isoproterenol, terbutaline, metaproterenol, albuterol, ritodrine)	May cause hypertension and reflex bradycardia from unopposed alpha effects (vasoconstriction) and increased vagal tone	• Monitor the patient's blood pressure and heart rate frequently.
	cimetidine	Reduces metabolism of beta-adrenergic blockers; enhances ability of beta-adrenergic blockers to reduce pulse rate	• Monitor the patient for altered response to beta-adrenergic blockers.
	theophyllines	Impair bronchodilating effects of theophyllines by nonselective beta-adrenergic blockers	• Monitor the patient's therapeutic response.
	clonidine	Attenuates or reverses antihypertensive effects and may produce a life-threatening increase in blood pressure	• Monitor the patient's blood pressure closely.

used cautiously in an elderly patient, who may be more sensitive to the antihypertensive effects. In addition, trimethaphan requires cautious use in a patient with Addison's disease, cerebrovascular insufficiency, diabetes mellitus, hepatic impairment, or respiratory insufficiency.

Because of their ability to penetrate the blood-brain barrier, beta-adrenergic blocking agents can produce the same CNS reactions as the central-acting and ganglionic blocking agents. (Atenolol, the least lipid-soluble beta-adrenergic blocking agent, appears to produce the fewest CNS effects.) Cardiovascular adverse reactions may include bradycardia, hypotension, congestive heart failure, and exacerbation of PVD. The beta-adrenergic blocking agents also may reduce HDL cholesterol levels and increase serum triglyceride, total cholesterol, low-density lipoprotein (LDL), and very-low-density lipoprotein (VLDL) levels.

Other adverse reactions to beta-adrenergic blocking agents include nausea, vomiting, diarrhea, nightmares, depression, insomnia, hallucinations, dry eyes, paresthesias, transient thrombocytopenia, agranulocytosis, sore throat, fever, and breathing difficulty. Because of these adverse reactions, beta-adrenergic blocking agents are contraindicated for a patient with asthma or emphysema and must be used with extreme caution in a patient with heart failure or hepatic or renal impairment.

In a patient with intermittent claudication or PVD, beta-adrenergic blocking agents may produce further symptoms of arterial insufficiency. In an insulin-dependent diabetic patient, beta-adrenergic blocking agents can mask the early warning signs of hypoglycemia, and rarely, produce hyperglycemia. They also may alter test results for alkaline phosphatase, blood urea nitrogen (BUN), LDL, serum creatinine, serum potassium, serum transaminase, serum triglycerides, serum uric acid, and serum glucose.

Alpha-adrenergic blocking agents tend to produce different adverse reactions than the beta-adrenergic blocking agents. For example, doxazosin and prazosin produce orthostatic hypotension more commonly than the beta-adrenergic blocking agents. They also produce first-dose syncope. Terazosin produces a few mild adverse reactions, including orthostatic hypotension and dizziness. It should be used cautiously in a patient with angina pectoris, because a decrease in blood pressure may precipitate an anginal attack. Phentolamine also can precipitate anginal attacks from rebound tachycardia and may produce hypotension as well as dizziness, weakness, flushing, palpitations, diarrhea, nausea, vomiting, and nasal congestion.

Adverse reactions to the mixed alpha- and beta-adrenergic blocking agent, labetalol, resemble those of the beta-adrenergic blocking agents. Other reactions may include scalp tingling, alopecia, orthostatic hypotension, intermittent claudication, bronchospasm, drug-induced systemic lupus erythematosus (SLE), eye irritation, myalgia, and rash. A patient with heart failure who is receiving a cardiac glycoside may be given labetalol with caution, but the drug is contraindicated in a patient with second- or third-degree heart block or cardiogenic shock.

Norepinephrine depletors produce a wide range of adverse reactions. The most clinically relevant adverse reaction to guanethidine and guanadrel is orthostatic hypotension, occurring primarily on awakening. Many patients also experience generalized weakness, especially early in therapy. A patient receiving guanadrel may faint upon exertion or standing and may develop nocturia and dyspnea, especially during the first 8 weeks of treatment. This drug is contraindicated for a patient with CHF and should be used cautiously in a patient with peptic ulcer disease.

Guanethidine can produce explosive diarrhea; failure to ejaculate; decreased myocardial contractility; fluid retention; increased BUN, aspartate aminotransferase (AST, formerly SGOT), and alanine aminotransferase (ALT, formerly SGPT) levels; and decreased prothrombin time and serum glucose and urine catecholamine levels. Because of the risk of these reactions, guanethidine is contraindicated in a patient with pheochromocytoma or CHF and must be used carefully in a patient with diarrhea, hepatic impairment, or bronchial asthma. (Catecholamine depletion can aggravate asthma.)

Common adverse reactions to reserpine include drowsiness, sleep alterations, weight gain, and nasal congestion. Increased GI motility, abdominal cramps, and diarrhea also may occur along with nightmares, depression, uterine contractions, and bronchoconstriction (in a patient with bronchitis). Reserpine also may increase the risk of breast cancer. When given to a lactating woman, it may result in increased respiratory secretions, nasal congestion, and cyanosis in the infant. Reserpine also may interfere with serum glucose and urine glucose test results, and may decrease urinary excretion of catecholamines, 17-hydroxycorticosteroid, 17-ketosteroid levels, and vanillylmandelic acid.

Despite these adverse reactions, reserpine remains useful because of its low cost. However, it is contraindicated in a patient with acute peptic ulcer disease or acute ulcerative colitis because it produces GI irritation. It must be given cautiously to a patient with renal or hepatic insufficiency, cardiac damage, or arrhythmias because it decreases peripheral vascular resistance and cardiac output.

Rare reactions to central-acting agents include anorexia, vomiting, parotid pain, and rash. Pruritus, abdominal discomfort, constipation, diarrhea, nausea, vomiting, and aches in the extremities also may occur. Guanabenz may result in headaches and sexual dysfunction. In rare instances, terazosin may produce diminished hearing, chest pain, insomnia, and GI distress. Reserpine may produce angina, bradycardia, blurred vision, impotence, and decreased libido.

NURSING PROCESS APPLICATION

The following information assists the nurse in caring for a patient who is receiving a sympatholytic agent.

Assessment

• Review the patient's history for a preexisting condition that contraindicates the use of a sympatholytic agent, such as asthma, sinus bradycardia, cardiogenic shock, greater-than-first-degree heart block, overt cardiac failure, or known hypersensitivity to these agents.

• Review the patient's history for a preexisting condition that requires cautious use of a sympatholytic agent, such as impaired hepatic function, pregnancy, or lactation.

• Assess the patient for adverse reactions to the prescribed sympatholytic agent, such as CNS or cardiovascular dysfunction.

• Review the patient's medication history to identify the use of drugs that may interact with the prescribed sympatholytic agent, such as tricyclic antidepressants, beta-adrenergic blockers, sympathomimetic agents, or levodopa.

• Assess the effectiveness of the sympatholytic agent regularly.

• Assess the patient's respiratory function regularly.

• Assess the patient periodically for fluid volume excess.

• Assess the patient for sexual dysfunction.

• Evaluate the patient's and family's knowledge about the prescribed sympatholytic agent.

Nursing diagnoses

The following examples represent appropriate nursing diagnoses for a patient receiving a sympatholytic agent.

• Potential for injury related to a preexisting condition that contraindicates the use of a sympatholytic agent

• Potential for injury related to a preexisting condition that requires cautious use of a sympatholytic agent

• Potential for injury related to adverse drug reactions

• Ineffective breathing pattern related to the adverse respiratory effects of a sympatholytic agent

• Fluid volume excess related to sympatholytic-induced fluid retention

• Sexual dysfunction related to the adverse genitourinary effects of a sympatholytic agent

• Knowledge deficit related to the prescribed sympatholytic agent

Planning and implementation

• Do not administer a sympatholytic agent to a patient with a condition that contraindicates its use.

• Administer a sympatholytic agent cautiously to a patient at risk because of a preexisting condition.

• Monitor the patient closely for adverse reactions throughout sympatholytic therapy.

• *Obtain baseline data before beginning sympatholytic therapy. Assess the patient's sitting, standing, and supine blood pressures and pulses. Monitor and record the patient's blood pressure and pulse when starting drug therapy, before administering each dose, and during peak concentration times.*

• Monitor the patient's vital signs, as instructed. For example, expect to monitor the patient's blood pressure and pulse every 15 to 30 minutes for at least the first 2 hours during initial administration of an alpha-adrenergic blocking agent.

• Monitor serum electrolyte levels, and correct any imbalances as prescribed before administering a norepinephrine-depletor.

• *Assess the patient's hepatic and renal function before beginning therapy with a beta-adrenergic blocker and at regular intervals. If the BUN or serum creatinine level is elevated, notify the physician.*

• *Observe the patient closely for syncope when administering the first dose of doxazosin, prazosin, or terazosin. To prevent severe first-dose orthostatic hypotension, have the patient lie down for at least 3 hours after taking it.*

• Take safety precautions if the patient develops CNS effects, such as sedation, vertigo, weakness, blurred vision, ataxia, or dizziness. For example, keep the bed in a low position and supervise ambulation.

• Relieve dry mouth by offering cool drinks, sugarless gum or hard candy, and frequent oral hygiene.

• Monitor hydration for a patient who experiences adverse GI reactions, such as nausea, vomiting, or diarrhea. Obtain a prescription for an antiemetic or antidiarrheal agent, if needed.

• Take bleeding precautions if the patient develops thrombocytopenia or an increased prothrombin time.

• *Monitor a diabetic patient's serum glucose level carefully, especially during beta-blocker or reserpine therapy.*

• Assist the patient with position changes and ambulation to prevent injury from orthostatic hypotension. Expect to substitute guanabenz for guanethidine or adrenergic blocking agents if these drugs produce severe orthostatic hypotension.

• Discontinue trimethaphan immediately and consult the physician if excessive hypotension occurs. Blood pressure usually is restored within 10 minutes.

• Monitor an elderly patient receiving a sympatholytic agent for signs of cerebral ischemia, such as syncope.

• Give labetalol, metoprolol, or propranolol between meals. If sedation occurs with a central-acting agent, give the drug in the evening. If the dosage is increased, start with an evening dose to minimize sedative effects.

• *Supervise a patient with a history of depression closely, because it may recur during antihypertensive therapy.*

• *Discontinue guanethidine for 72 hours before elective surgery, as prescribed, to prevent interaction with sympathomimetic agents that may be used during surgery.*

• Anticipate gradual discontinuation of a beta-adrenergic blocking agent over 3 to 14 days. During this time, the patient should avoid vigorous physical activity to prevent overtaxing the heart.

• Expect to decrease the guanfacine dosage for an elderly patient or one with renal impairment; the trimethaphan dosage for an elderly patient; and the atenolol, carteolol, or nadolol dosage for a patient with impaired renal function. Also expect to adjust the mecamylamine dosage according to various patient factors, time of day, and season.

• Administer I.V. trimethaphan as a secondary or piggyback solution in a primary I.V. line. Use an infusion pump or a microdrip regulator to allow precise adjustments to the flow rate. Do not mix trimethaphan with other medications. Monitor the patient closely during therapy to adjust the I.V. rate according to blood pressure response. Keep the patient supine during trimethaphan administration.

• *Do not discontinue clonidine or guanabenz abruptly to prevent rebound hypertension.*

• Interpret laboratory values with caution because sympatholytic agents affect many of them.

• Notify the physician if adverse reactions occur or if the drug is ineffective.

• *Monitor the patient closely for respiratory changes, especially noting respiratory depression (with ganglionic blocking agent therapy), breathing difficulty (with beta-adrenergic blocker therapy), bronchospasm (with mixed alpha- and beta-adrenergic blocker or norepinephrine depletor therapy) and bronchoconstriction (with norepinephrine depletor therapy in a patient with bronchitis).*

• Monitor the patient's respiratory rate and pattern before and after administration of each dose and auscultate breath sounds regularly. Particularly note wheezing, shortness of breath, or complaints of chest tightness or breathing difficulty.

• *Notify the physician if the patient's breathing pattern changes. Keep emergency respiratory equipment nearby, such as oxygen and bronchodilators. Help the patient into a position that promotes easier breathing.*

• *Monitor the patient regularly for signs of CHF, such as increasing dyspnea, crackles, jugular vein distention, fatigue, and pallor.*

• Monitor the patient's fluid intake and output to detect fluid retention. Keep in mind that a ganglionic blocker may cause oliguria with excessive hypotension.

• Limit the patient's salt intake. Restrict fluid consumption to less than 2 liters/day.

• Notify the physician if fluid retention occurs and expect to begin CHF treatment, such as diuretic administration and change in antihypertensive agents.

• Do not expect to see certain sympatholytic agents used in a young adult; central-acting and ganglionic blocking agents, guanethidine, and guanabenz can cause sexual dysfunction.

• Reassure the patient that sexual dysfunction is temporary and caused by drug therapy.

• Notify the physician if sexual dysfunction occurs and ask if the patient can be switched to a different agent.

Patient teaching
- Teach the patient and family the name, dose, frequency, action, and adverse effects of the prescribed sympatholytic agent.
- Review general instructions about use of the antihypertensive agent. (For a complete listing, see *Patient-teaching tips for antihypertensive agents.*)
- Inform the patient taking guanadrel of the possibility of fainting on exertion or standing and of developing nocturia and dyspnea, especially during the first 8 weeks of treatment.
- Inform the patient taking clonidine that vivid dreams may occur.
- Reassure the patient receiving a central-acting or ganglionic blocking agent that CNS effects usually diminish after 2 to 3 weeks of therapy.
- *Advise the patient taking methyldopa that the drug may darken the urine.*
- *Instruct the patient to take the first dose of doxazosin, prazosin, or terazosin at bedtime or to remain lying down for at least 3 hours after taking it to prevent severe first-dose orthostatic hypotension.*
- *Teach the patient on reserpine therapy to take the drug with food, milk, or 8 oz of water to minimize GI upset.*
- Instruct the patient and family about possible depression. Describe the early signs of depression, which may not occur for 6 months after therapy begins, and the risk of suicide if severe depression occurs.
- Instruct the patient to anticipate gradual discontinuation of the prescribed beta-adrenergic blocker and to avoid vigorous physical activity while the drug is being discontinued.
- Alert the patient on a sodium-restricted diet that noncompliance may result in fluid retention and edema.

Evaluation
The following examples represent appropriate evaluation statements for a patient receiving a sympatholytic agent.
- The patient has no conditions that contraindicate sympatholytic agent therapy.
- The patient exhibits no signs of complications in the preexisting condition linked to the prescribed sympatholytic agent.
- The patient experiences no adverse reactions to the prescribed sympatholytic agent.
- The patient maintains a normal breathing pattern.
- The patient maintains a normal fluid balance.
- The patient reports unchanged sexual function.
- The patient and family express an accurate understanding of the points taught about the prescribed sympatholytic agent.
- The patient correctly identifies techniques for minimizing the effects of orthostatic hypotension.

Patient-teaching tips for antihypertensive agents

The patient who will be taking an antihypertensive agent at home requires some general instructions. The nurse should provide these instructions orally and in writing so that the patient can take them home. The nurse also should provide more detailed information about the specific drug or drugs that the patient will be taking. Including the patient's family in the teaching sessions can help improve patient compliance.

After telling the patient the name, dosage, and schedule of the antihypertensive agent, the nurse should explain that its general action is to lower blood pressure. Then the nurse should provide the following instructions.
- Take the drug exactly as prescribed and do not stop taking it abruptly even if the patient feels well or has a normal blood pressure reading. Abrupt discontinuation may cause serious problems, such as severe hypertension, angina, or heart failure.
- Avoid delays in refilling prescriptions, and be prepared with enough medication for weekends and holidays. If a dose is missed accidentally, take it as soon as possible, but do not take a double dose or take the missed dose close to the time of the next scheduled dose.
- Avoid sudden changes in position to prevent dizziness, light-headedness, or fainting. If faintness occurs, lie down immediately.
- Avoid driving or operating potentially dangerous machinery until the drug's effects are known. (Some people become drowsy, light-headed, and dizzy.)
- Avoid physical exertion, especially in hot weather. It could cause dehydration and increase the risk of dizziness or fainting. Standing for a long time or taking a hot shower or bath can cause similar problems and should be avoided.
- Prevent complications and uncomfortable symptoms by avoiding excessive use of stimulants, such as coffee, tea, and other caffeinated beverages, and depressants, such as alcohol.
- Consult the physician before taking any over-the-counter medication, especially sympathomimetics and decongestants.
- Return for follow-up visits as directed.
- Store these drugs in tightly sealed containers away from light and moisture.
- Try to reduce the factors that tend to increase blood pressure, such as smoking, obesity, lack of exercise, stress, and excess salt intake. Overuse of salt also can cause excess fluid retention.

VASODILATING AGENTS

Two types of vasodilating agents exist: direct vasodilators and calcium channel blockers. Both types decrease systolic and diastolic blood pressure by relaxing arteriolar smooth muscle, leading to arteriolar dilation and decreasing peripheral resistance.

Direct vasodilators act on arteries, veins, or both. They include diazoxide, hydralazine hydrochloride, minoxidil, and sodium nitroprusside. Hydralazine and minoxidil usually are used to treat resistant or refractory hypertension as step-4 and step-5 agents, respectively. Diazoxide and nitroprusside are reserved for use in hypertensive crisis.

Calcium channel blockers produce arteriolar relaxation by preventing the entry of calcium into the cells, thus reducing the mechanical activity of vascular smooth muscle. They include diltiazem hydrochloride, nicardipine hydrochloride, nifedipine, and verapamil hydrochloride and may be used as step-2 and step-3 antihypertensive drugs.

PHARMACOKINETICS

Most of these drugs are absorbed rapidly and distributed well. They all are metabolized in the liver, and most are excreted by the kidneys.

Absorption, distribution, metabolism, excretion

I.V. diazoxide, which bypasses absorption, is 90% bound to plasma albumin, although the extent of binding is decreased in a patient with renal failure. It also crosses the placenta and is secreted in breast milk. The drug is metabolized in the liver to inactive metabolites and about one third of it is excreted unchanged by the kidneys.

After oral administration, hydralazine is absorbed readily from the GI tract, and administration with food can increase absorption. About 87% of a dose binds with plasma proteins. Hepatic metabolism occurs through acetylation, but the acetylation rate varies widely among individuals. Less than 15% of a hydralazine dose is excreted unchanged by the kidneys.

Minoxidil is absorbed rapidly and completely from the GI tract. It undergoes extensive metabolism in the liver to less active metabolites and is excreted by the kidneys.

After I.V. administration, nitroprusside is distributed rapidly. The ferrous ion in nitroprusside reacts with components of the vascular walls and red blood cells to form nitric oxide (the vasoactive component) and cyanide. The cyanide is metabolized in the liver to thiocyanate, which is excreted by the kidneys.

About 80% of a diltiazem dose is absorbed after oral administration. Extensive first-pass metabolism occurs with this drug, making it about 40% bioavailable. Diltiazem is 80% protein bound. Then it undergoes extensive metabolism to active metabolites and is excreted in the bile (65%) and the urine (35%). Only 2% to 4% of the unchanged drug appears in the urine.

Nicardipine is absorbed rapidly and almost completely after oral administration. However, first-pass metabolism reduces its bioavailability to about 35%. More than 95% of a nicardipine dose is bound to plasma proteins. The drug is metabolized extensively to inactive metabolites; less than

1% is excreted unchanged in the urine. The metabolites are excreted in urine and feces.

After oral administration, nifedipine is absorbed rapidly and completely. It undergoes first-pass metabolism to a free acid, reducing its bioavailability to 65% to 70%, and is then 90% protein bound. All metabolites are pharmacologically inactive and most are excreted in the urine; about 10% are excreted in the feces.

Verapamil is 90% absorbed from the GI tract after oral administration, but first-pass effect yields a bioavailability of only 20% to 35%. The drug is apprximately 90% protein bound. About 70% of the drug and its active metabolites are excreted in the urine, 16% in the feces.

Onset, peak, duration

Vasodilating agents vary widely in their pharmacokinetic processes. (For detailed information, see *Onset, peak, and duration of vasodilating agents.*)

PHARMACODYNAMICS

The direct vasodilators relax peripheral vascular smooth muscles, lowering blood pressure by increasing blood vessel caliber and reducing total peripheral resistance. Calcium channel blockers prevent calcium transport across the cell membrane, reducing the activity of the vascular smooth muscle, thus producing vasodilation and lowering the blood pressure.

Mechanism of action

A thiazide derivative, diazoxide directly affects the arteries, but its action remains unclear. Hydralazine dilates arterioles directly and promotes an increase in cardiac output and cerebral and renal blood flow. Minoxidil and diazoxide appear to alter cellular calcium metabolism and interfere with calcium movement. They do not decrease the glomerular filtration rate, but they seem to increase renin secretion. Nitroprusside rapidly forms nitric oxide, which directly relaxes arterial and venous smooth muscle.

Calcium channel blockers may act to relieve hypertension in several different ways. They all inhibit transport of calcium ions during cell membrane depolarization in cardiac and vascular smooth muscle. This inhibition reduces peripheral vascular resistance, decreasing the blood pressure. The same action dilates the coronary arteries, improving myocardial perfusion. Calcium channel blockers also may block norepinephrine-mediated vasoconstriction.

PHARMACOTHERAPEUTICS

Vasodilating agents usually are used as adjuncts in treating moderate to severe hypertension. They seldom are used as primary agents.

Onset, peak, and duration of vasodilating agents

The major pharmacokinetic properties of the direct vasodilators and the calcium channel blockers are summarized below.

DRUG	ROUTE	ONSET OF ACTION	PEAK CONCENTRATION	DURATION OF ACTION
Direct vasodilators				
diazoxide	I.V.	1 to 3 minutes	2 to 5 minutes	Usually 3 to 12 hours, but ranges from 1 to 72 hours
hydralazine	P.O.	20 to 30 minutes	2 hours	2 to 8 hours
	I.V.	5 to 20 minutes	10 to 80 minutes	2 to 6 hours
	I.M.	10 to 30 minutes	1 hour	2 to 6 hours
minoxidil	P.O.	30 minutes	2 to 8 hours	2 to 5 days
nitroprusside	I.V. infusion	Immediate	Immediate	1 to 10 minutes after infusion stops
Calcium channel blockers				
diltiazem	P.O.	30 to 60 minutes	2 to 3 hours	4 to 9 hours
nicardipine	P.O.	20 minutes	0.5 to 2 hours	8 hours
nifedipine	P.O.	20 minutes	30 minutes	6 to 8 hours
verapamil	P.O.	30 to 60 minutes	2 hours	6 to 8 hours

diazoxide (Hyperstat). This potent vasodilator is administered I.V., usually with a diuretic, to treat hypertensive crisis. It can decrease the blood pressure in 1 to 5 minutes. It also can be used to treat malignant hypertension. Its advantages include rapid action and a decreased tendency to produce sedation or extreme hypotension. It is contraindicated for use in a patient with MI, aortic aneurysm, or pulmonary edema because it increases the cardiac work load by reflex stimulation of the sympathetic nervous system.

Usual adult dosage: for hypertensive crisis and malignant hypertension, 1 to 3 mg/kg, up to a maximum of 150 mg I.V. bolus; may be repeated at 5- to 15-minute intervals until an adequate reduction in blood pressure is achieved and then repeated at 4- to 24-hour intervals to maintain the blood pressure reduction.

hydralazine hydrochloride (Apresoline). This direct vasodilator, which may be administered orally or parenterally, is used primarily as a step-4 drug and commonly is given with a thiazide diuretic or a beta-adrenergic blocking agent. It is indicated as an adjunct to treat malignant hypertension complicated by renal insufficiency or CHF. I.V. or I.M. hydralazine may be used to treat hypertensive crisis. Be-

cause it results in increased tachycardia and cardiac output, hydralazine should be used cautiously in an elderly patient or a patient with ischemic heart disease. In these individuals, the drug may produce anginal attacks, myocardial ischemia, cerebrovascular disease, or renal impairment.

Usual adult dosage: for moderate to severe hypertension, 40 mg P.O. daily for the first 2 to 4 days, increased to 100 mg/day for the rest of the week, then to 200 mg/day and up to a maximum of 300 mg/day, given in two to four doses; for hypertensive crisis, 10 to 40 mg I.V. or I.M., repeated as needed.

minoxidil (Loniten, Minodyl). A potent oral vasodilator, minoxidil is reserved for patients with target organ damage who have not responded to other drugs. This step-4 drug is most effective when use with a beta-adrenergic blocker to control tachycardia and a diuretic to counteract fluid retention. Topical minoxidil (Rogaine) is used to treat male pattern baldness. (For details about this use, see Chapter 73, Uncategorized and Other Agents.)

Usual adult dosage: 5 to 40 mg P.O. daily in one or two equal doses, increased up to a maximum of 100 mg/day.

sodium nitroprusside (Nipride). A potent I.V. vasodilator, nitroprusside is used in hypertensive crises for rapid reduction of blood pressure. It is preferred over diazoxide in patients with CHF because it does not produce water and sodium retention. Nitroprusside therapy requires continuous blood pressure monitoring by an arterial ine or, if an arterial line is not available, regular monitoring every 5 minutes.
Usual adult dosage: 0.5 to 10 mcg/kg/minute by I.V. infusion; average dosage is 3 mcg/kg/minute.

diltiazem hydrochloride (Cardizem SR). A calcium channel blocker, diltiazem may be administered orally as a step-2 or step-3 agent for controlling hypertension.
Usual adult dosage: 60 to 120 mg P.O. b.i.d. of sustained-release capsules, increased gradually as needed up to a maximum of 360 mg/day.

nicardipine hydrochloride (Cardene). The newest calcium channel blocker, nicardipine is used as part of step-2 or step-3 therapy for hypertension.
Usual adult dosage: 20 mg P.O. t.i.d., increased at 3-day intervals to a maximum of 40 mg P.O. t.i.d.

nifedipine (Procardia XL). As a part of step-2 or step-3 therapy, this calcium channel blocker may be given orally to treat hypertension. It also may be used to treat hypertensive crisis.
Usual adult dosage: 30 to 60 mg P.O. once daily of sustained-release tablets, increased to a maximum of 120 mg/day; for hypertensive crisis, 10 mg sublingually administered by placing the contents of a punctured capsule under the tongue or by having the patient bite and swallow the capsule.

verapamil hydrochloride (Calan, Calan SR, Isoptin, Isoptin SR, Verelan). An effective calcium channel blocker, verapamil may be administered orally as part of step-2 or step-3 therapy for hypertension.
Usual adult dosage: initially, 80 mg P.O. t.i.d., up to a maximum of 480 mg/day in divided doses; or 120 to 240 mg of sustained-release verapamil once daily, increased up to 240 mg b.i.d.

Drug interactions

Hydralazine and minoxidil produce additive effects when given with other antihypertensive drugs, such as methyldopa or reserpine. They also may produce additive effects when given with nitrates, such as isosorbide dinitrate or nitroglycerin. Few other drug interactions occur with the vasodilating agents. However, when given with digoxin, diltiazem and verapamil may promote digitalis toxicity; verapamil may produce a similar interaction with digitoxin. Diltiazem, nicardipine, and verapamil also may interact

with drugs that affect the hepatic microsomal system, altering the metabolism of either interacting drug. With concomitant administration, cimetidine may increase nicardipine plasma levels.

ADVERSE DRUG REACTIONS

Direct vasodilators commonly produce adverse reactions related to reflex activation of the sympathetic nervous system: palpitations, angina, tachycardia, increased myocardial work load, ECG changes, edema, breast tenderness, fatigue, headache, and rash. Severe pericardial effusions may develop. Alkaline phosphatase, BUN, and creatinine levels may increase. Unlike the other vasodilators, calcium channel blockers do not produce rebound tachycardia or significant edema. Other adverse reactions depend on the specific drug used.

Common adverse reactions to diazoxide include headache, anorexia, nausea, and diaphoresis. The following adverse reactions also may occur and usually require discontinuation of therapy: rash, drug fever, urticaria, polyneuritis, GI hemorrhage, anemia, and pancytopenia. Diazoxide also is especially likely to result in excessive hypotension and reflex sympathetic stimulation. It also may produce hyperglycemia in a diabetic patient. Because of these adverse reactions, the drug should be used cautiously in a patient with heart disease or renal failure.

Hydralazine commonly produces such adverse reactions as headache, diarrhea, constipation, dizziness or lightheadedness, orthostatic hypotension, facial flushing, shortness of breath, nasal congestion, urinary hesitancy, lacrimation, conjunctivitis, paresthesia, edema, tremor, and muscle cramps.

When hydralazine dosage exceeds 200 mg/day, the patient may develop drug-induced SLE. Initial symptoms of SLE include myalgias, arthralgias, and pleuritis. Later symptoms may include chest pain; generalized discomfort or weakness; blood dyscrasias (rare); joint pain; paresthesias, pain, or weakness in the hands or feet; skin rash or itching; sore throat; fever; swelling of the feet or lower legs; and lymphadenopathy.

Minoxidil commonly produces hypertrichosis (hair growth), especially on the face, arms, and back, 3 to 6 weeks after therapy begins. Minoxidil also is particularly likely to produce reflex tachycardia and fluid retention. Nitroprusside produces headache, dizziness, nausea, vomiting, and abdominal pain.

The most serious adverse reactions to diltiazem, hypotension and bradycardia, may be extensions of the drug's therapeutic effect. Other reactions may include flushing, palpitations, somnolence, tremor, insomnia, headache, edema, nausea, rash, and transient elevation of liver enzymes. Diltiazem is contraindicated in a patient with second- or third-degree heart block. It should be used cautiously in a patient with impaired renal or hepatic function.

When used in antihypertensive dosages, nicardipine commonly produces flushing, headache, and facial edema. Less common reactions include palpitations, dizziness, tachycardia, nausea, and somnolence. Allergic reactions are rare.

Nifedipine can produce the same reactions as diltiazem, along with peripheral edema and dizziness or light-headedness.

The most common adverse reaction to verapamil is constipation; other reactions include those listed for diltiazem along with atrioventricular heart block, peripheral edema, dizziness, light-headedness, and fatigue.

Hypersensitivity reactions (urticaria, rash, pruritus, fever, chills, arthralgia, eosinophilia, and rarely, obstructive jaundice and hepatitis) and blood dyscrasias (leukopenia, agranulocytosis, thrombocytopenia) also may occur with some of the antihypertensive vasodilators.

NURSING PROCESS APPLICATION

The following information assists the nurse in caring for a patient who is receiving a vasodilating agent.

Assessment
• Review the patient's history for a preexisting condition that contraindicates the use of a vasodilating agent, such as compensatory hypertension, MI, aortic aneurysm, pulmonary edema, or known hypersensitivity to these drugs.
• Review the patient's history for a preexisting condition that requires cautious use of a vasodilating agent, such as diabetes, impaired cerebral or cardiac circulation, or pregnancy.
• Assess the patient for adverse reactions to the prescribed vasodilating agent, such as palpitations, angina, tachycardia, ECG changes, GI distress, light-headedness, edema, breast tenderness, fatigue, headache, or rash.
• Review the patient's medication history to identify the use of drugs that may interact with the prescribed vasodilating agent, such as other antihypertensive agents, nitrates, and digoxin.
• Assess the effectiveness of the vasodilating agent periodically.
• Assess for fluid volume excess frequently during vasodilator therapy.
• Assess for pain regularly during vasodilator therapy.
• Evaluate the patient's and family's knowledge about the prescribed vasodilating agent.

Nursing diagnoses
The following examples represent appropriate nursing diagnoses for a patient receiving a vasodilating agent.
• Potential for injury related to a preexisting condition that contraindicates the use of a vasodilating agent
• Potential for injury related to a preexisting condition that requires cautious use of a vasodilating agent
• Potential for injury related to adverse drug reactions
• Fluid volume excess related to vasodilator-induced fluid retention
• Pain related to vasodilator-induced headache, angina, or muscle cramps
• Knowledge deficit related to the prescribed vasodilating agent

Planning and implementation
• Do not administer a vasodilating agent to a patient with a condition that contraindicates its use.
• Administer a vasodilating agent cautiously to a patient at risk because of a preexisting condition.
• Monitor the patient closely for adverse reactions throughout vasodilator therapy.
• *Monitor the patient's standing, sitting, and supine blood pressures, and assess the other vital signs during vasodilator therapy. Also monitor the blood pressure and pulse during peak concentration times.*
• Monitor the patient's blood pressure continuously during nitroprusside therapy by an arterial line or every 5 minutes if an arterial line is not available.
• Obtain baseline blood pressure and pulse rates before diazoxide administration. Then monitor the blood pressure and pulse rate at least every 15 minutes for 2 hours after the dose is given.
• Monitor the patient's blood pressure and pulse before administering hydralazine. During administration, monitor the blood pressure and pulse every 5 minutes for the first 30 minutes, then every 15 minutes for about 2 hours until the blood pressure stabilizes.
• *Monitor for signs of cerebral ischemia, such as sensory disturbances, anxiety, and slowed mental processes, as well as signs of impaired renal blood flow, such as decreased urine output. These signs are most likely to occur when vasodilator administration causes a rapid reduction in blood pressure. If any of these signs appear, help the patient into a supine position, elevate the patient's legs, and notify the physician immediately.*
• Monitor the patient's ECG for arrhythmias.
• Monitor the diabetic patient receiving diazoxide therapy for increases in serum glucose levels for up to 1 week after administration.
• Prevent orthostatic hypotension by keeping the patient in a supine position for 15 to 30 minutes after diazoxide or hydralazine administration.

• Observe for early signs of drug-induced SLE, such as myalgias, arthralgias, and pleuritis, when the hydralazine dosage exceeds 200 mg/day.

• Monitor hydration if the patient develops nausea, vomiting, diarrhea, or excessive diaphoresis. Obtain a prescription for an antiemetic or antidiarrheal agent as needed.

• Take safety precautions if dizziness or light-headedness occurs. For example, keep the bed in a low position and supervise ambulation.

• *Administer oral hydralazine with meals to promote absorption.*

• Administer diazoxide via a peripheral vein to prevent cardiac arrhythmias.

• Expect to discontinue diazoxide if the patient develops a rash, drug fever, urticaria, polyneuritis, GI hemorrhage, anemia, or pancytopenia.

• Watch for increases in alkaline phosphatase, BUN, and creatinine levels with direct vasodilator therapy and for transient elevation of liver enzymes with diltiazem therapy.

• Notify the physician if adverse reactions occur.

• *Monitor the patient closely for fluid volume excess. Weigh the patient daily and monitor fluid intake and output. Auscultate the patient's breath sounds regularly for crackles, and observe for jugular vein distention or peripheral edema.*

• Expect to administer a diuretic to counteract fluid retention, as prescribed.

• Notify the physician if the patient displays signs of fluid retention.

• Ask the patient to report headache, angina pain, or muscle cramps.

• Notify the physician if pain occurs and obtain a prescription for an appropriate agent, as needed.

Patient teaching

• Teach the patient and family the name, dose, frequency, action, and adverse effects of the prescribed vasodilating agent.

• Provide general information about vasodilator use. (For a complete listing, see *Patient-teaching tips for antihypertensive agents,* page 549.)

• *Advise a patient taking minoxidil that hypertrichosis is likely to occur 3 to 6 weeks after treatment begins. Reassure the patient that the extra hair growth should disappear 1 to 6 months after the drug is discontinued.*

• Advise the patient taking nifedipine to swallow the capsules whole.

• Instruct the patient to notify the physician if adverse reactions occur.

Evaluation

The following examples represent appropriate evaluation statements for a patient receiving a vasodilating agent.

• The patient has no conditions that contraindicate vasodilator therapy.

• The patient exhibits no signs of complications in the preexisting condition linked to the prescribed vasodilating agent.

• The patient experiences no adverse reactions to the prescribed vasodilating agent.

• The patient maintains normal fluid balance.

• The patient denies having pain.

• The patient and family express an accurate understanding of the points taught about the prescribed vasodilating agent.

• The patient correctly identifies adverse reactions that must be reported to the physician.

ANGIOTENSIN-CONVERTING ENZYME (ACE) INHIBITORS

Another class of antihypertensive agents, ACE inhibitors reduce blood pressure by interrupting the renin-angiotensin-aldosterone system. Three agents, captopril, enalapril, and lisinopril, block the conversion of angiotensin I to angiotensin II, a potent vasoconstrictor. A fourth agent, saralasin, competes with angiotensin II at tissue receptors, blocking its vascular, renal, adrenal, cardiac, and CNS effects.

Captopril, enalapril, or lisinopril may be used to treat hypertension in a patient who does not respond to the usual step-2 drugs. These agents are particularly useful in treating hypertension associated with high renin levels. The pharmacologic use of saralasin is limited almost exclusively to testing for angiotensin II-dependent hypertension associated with renal vascular disease. Because of its limited use, it is not included in the following discussion of ACE inhibitors.

PHARMACOKINETICS

Captopril, enalapril, and lisinopril are absorbed from the GI tract, distributed to most body tissues, metabolized somewhat in the liver, and excreted by the kidneys.

Absorption, distribution, metabolism, excretion

Captopril is absorbed well from the GI tract, although the presence of food reduces absorption. It is distributed to most body tissues but does not cross the blood-brain barrier. It is secreted in breast milk. About 25% to 30% of the circulating drug is bound to plasma protein. Captopril is metabolized in the liver and is excreted in the urine along with its metabolites. In a patient with normal renal function, more than 95% of an absorbed dose is excreted in the urine, 40% to 50% of it as unchanged drug.

After oral administration, about 60% of enalapril is absorbed. Because enalapril is a prodrug (precursor), it has little pharmacologic activity until hydrolyzed in the liver to enalaprilat. Distribution of enalapril and enalaprilat is not fully known. Enalaprilat is 50% to 60% protein bound in plasma. Enalapril crosses the blood-brain barrier poorly; enalaprilat does not cross it at all. About 60% of an absorbed dose of enalapril is metabolized to enalaprilat. It is excreted in urine and feces.

After oral administration, lisinopril is absorbed slowly and incompletely (only 25%). The drug undergoes little metabolism; 97% of the administered dose is excreted unchanged in the urine.

Onset, peak, duration

Captopril reaches a peak concentration level in 30 to 90 minutes and full therapeutic effectiveness in weeks. Its half-life probably is less than 2 hours, and its duration of action ranges from 6 to 12 hours.

Enalapril reaches peak concentration in 30 to 90 minutes after oral administration; enalaprilat in 3 to 4 hours. The drug produces initial antihypertensive effects in 1 hour and maximal effects in 4 to 8 hours. The estimated half-life of enalaprilat is 11 hours in healthy adults with normal renal function. Enalapril's duration is up to 24 hours.

Lisinopril begins to act in 1 hour and reaches peak concentration within 6 hours. Its half-life is 12 hours, and its duration is 24 hours.

PHARMACODYNAMICS

The ACE inhibitors act by interfering with the renin-angiotensin-aldosterone system. They do so by inhibiting the enzyme that converts angiotensin I to angiotensin II. This inhibition decreases aldosterone release by the adrenal cortex, preventing sodium and water retention. It also reduces peripheral arterial resistance without affecting the heart rate and cardiac output. The result, in a patient with hypertension, is a decreased blood pressure.

PHARMACOTHERAPEUTICS

ACE inhibitors are recommended for initial drug therapy of hypertension. They may be used alone or with another agent, such as a thiazide diuretic in mild to moderate hypertension.

captopril (Capoten). This agent is effective in treating hypertension associated with high or normal renin levels. It also is used to treat hypertension accompanied by low renin

levels, but requires adjunctive diuretic therapy. It is used as a step-2 drug in treating mild to moderate hypertension. *Usual adult dosage:* for hypertension, 12.5 to 25 mg P.O. t.i.d. initially, increased to 50 mg t.i.d. after 1 to 2 weeks up to a maximum of 450 mg/day.

enalapril maleate (Vasotec) or **enalaprilat** (Vasotec I.V.). A step-2 and step-3 drug, enalapril is administered orally to treat mild to moderate hypertension. If used with a diuretic, it may produce pronounced hypotension. The drug also is available for I.V. use in patients who cannot take it orally.
Usual adult dosage: initially, 5 mg P.O. once daily, increased to 10 to 40 mg/day, as needed, once a day or in divided doses; or 0.625 to 1.25 mg I.V. administered over 5 minutes every 6 hours. I.V. administration usually produces a response within 15 minutes and peak effects within 4 hours.

lisinopril (Prinivil, Zestril). This drug is used as a step-2 or step-3 agent in treating mild to moderate hypertension. A patient receiving a diuretic has an increased risk of hypotension after the initial dose of lisinopril.
Usual adult dosage: 10 mg P.O. once daily, increased to 20 to 40 mg/day as needed. A patient with renal impairment may require the following dosage reduction, which may be adjusted according to blood pressure response: with a creatinine clearance of 10 to 30 ml/minute, 5 mg daily; with a clearance of less than 10 ml/minute, 2.5 mg daily.

Drug interactions

All ACE inhibitors enhance the hypotensive effects of diuretics and other antihypertensives, such as beta-adrenergic blockers. They may be less effective when administered with nonsteroidal anti-inflammatory agents (NSAIDs).

ADVERSE DRUG REACTIONS

ACE inhibitors can produce a wide range of mild to severe adverse reactions. Severe adverse reactions, such as proteinuria, neutropenia, agranulocytosis, rash, and loss of taste (dysgensia), occur most commonly with captopril and may limit its use. Some of these reactions may be dose-related and may disappear during the first few weeks of therapy.

CNS reactions, which may be related to reduced blood pressure, can occur with all agents. These reactions may include headache, dizziness, fatigue, and syncope. GI reactions, such as abdominal pain, nausea, vomiting, and diarrhea, also can occur with the ACE inhibitors.

All ACE inhibitors may cause transient elevations of BUN and serum creatinine levels, especially in patients with hypertension caused by volume depletion, renal, or cardiovascular disease. Increases in serum potassium concentrations commonly occur, especially in patients with reduced renal function.

All ACE inhibitors can produce tickling in the throat and a dry, nonproductive, persistent cough. The cough, which occurs in about 15% of patients receiving ACE inhibitors, usually occurs in the first week of therapy and resolves when the drug is discontinued.

Angioedema may occur with all ACE inhibitors, producing flushing or pallor and swelling of the face, extremities, lips, tongue, glottis, or larynx. If angioedema affects the face, tongue, or glottis or causes laryngeal stridor, the nurse should discontinue the drug, notify the physician, and begin appropriate treatment, as prescribed.

NURSING PROCESS APPLICATION

The following information assists the nurse in caring for a patient who is receiving an ACE inhibitor.

Assessment
• Review the patient's history for a preexisting condition that contraindicates the use of an ACE inhibitor, such as known hypersensitivity to these agents.
• Review the patient's history for a preexisting condition that requires cautious use of an ACE inhibitor, such as impaired renal function, valvular stenosis, pregnancy, or lactation.
• Assess the patient for adverse reactions to the prescribed ACE inhibitor, such as CNS and GI disturbances.
• Review the patient's medication history to identify the use of drugs that may interact with the prescribed ACE inhibitor, such as diuretics, other antihypertensive agents, or NSAIDs.
• Assess the effectiveness of the ACE inhibitor periodically.
• Evaluate the patient's and family's knowledge about the prescribed ACE inhibitor.

Nursing diagnoses
The following examples represent appropriate nursing diagnoses for a patient receiving an ACE inhibitor.
• Potential for injury related to a preexisting condition that contraindicates the use of an ACE inhibitor
• Potential for injury related to a preexisting condition that requires cautious use of an ACE inhibitor
• Potential for injury related to adverse drug reactions
• Knowledge deficit related to the prescribed ACE inhibitor

Planning and implementation
• Do not administer an ACE inhibitor to a patient with a condition that contraindicates its use.
• Administer an ACE inhibitor cautiously to a patient at risk because of a preexisting condition.
• Monitor the patient closely for adverse reactions during treatment with an ACE inhibitor, especially captopril.

• *Obtain a baseline blood pressure and pulse rate before beginning ACE inhibitor therapy for later use in monitoring the patient.*
• Monitor supine and standing blood pressures during therapy to detect orthostatic hypotension.
• *Monitor the patient for hypotension when an ACE inhibitor is administered for the first time during concomitant diuretic therapy.*
• Document the patient's fluid intake and output and daily weight to assess renal function.
• Monitor the patient for proteinuria every 2 to 4 weeks for the first 3 months of therapy to detect decreased renal function.
• *Monitor the patient's liver function tests and serum BUN, creatinine, and potassium levels before treatment begins and monthly during the first 3 months of therapy.*
• Ask the patient taking an ACE inhibitor about taste impairment, because the patient may not associate it with drug therapy and so may not report it. If taste impairment occurs, monitor the patient's food intake to ensure adequate nutritional intake.
• Take safety precautions if dizziness or syncope occurs. For example, keep the bed in a low position and supervise ambulation.
• Request a prescription for a mild analgesic if the patient experiences headaches.
• Monitor hydration if the patient develops nausea, vomiting, or diarrhea. Obtain a prescription for an antiemetic or antidiarrheal agent as needed.
• *Observe for signs of angioedema, such as flushing or pallor and swelling of the face, extremities, lips, tongue, glottis, or larynx. If angioedema occurs, withhold the drug, notify the physician, and begin emergency treatment according to health care facility protocol.*
• Expect to decrease the dosage when administering an ACE inhibitor to a patient with renal impairment.
• *Administer captopril between meals for maximum effectiveness.*
• Evaluate ACE inhibitor effectiveness, especially when the patient also is receiving an NSAID, which can render these antihypertensives less effective.
• Notify the physician if adverse reactions occur.

Patient teaching
• Teach the patient and family the name, dose, frequency, action, and adverse effects of the prescribed ACE inhibitor.
• Provide general information about the use of ACE inhibitors. (For more information, see *Patient-teaching tips for antihypertensive agents,* page 549.)
• *Instruct the patient to notify the physician immediately if signs of angioedema occur.*
• *Advise the patient to take captopril on an empty stomach, preferably 1 hour before meals, for maximum effectiveness.*

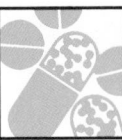

SELECTED MAJOR DRUGS

Antihypertensive agents

This chart summarizes the major antihypertensive drugs currently in clinical use.

DRUG	MAJOR INDICATIONS	USUAL ADULT DOSAGES	CONTRAINDICATIONS AND PRECAUTIONS
Sympatholytic agents			
Central-acting sympathetic nervous system inhibitors			
clonidine	Mild to moderate hypertension, as a step-3 drug	0.1 mg P.O. b.i.d. initially, increased by 0.1 or 0.2 mg/day every 2 to 4 days; maintenance dosage, 0.1 to 0.2 mg b.i.d. to q.i.d. up to a maximum of 2.4 mg/day	• Administer clonidine with caution to a pregnant or lactating patient or one with severe coronary insufficiency, recent myocardial infarction, cerebrovascular disease, or chronic renal failure.
methyldopa	Mild to moderate hypertension, as a step-3 drug	250 mg P.O. b.i.d. or t.i.d. initially, increased biweekly to a maintenance dosage of 500 mg to 2 grams/day in two to four divided doses or up to a maximum of 3 grams/day	• Know that methyldopa is contraindicated in a patient with active hepatic disease, a history of liver disorder associated with methyldopa use, or known hypersensitivity to the drug. • Administer with caution to a lactating patient or one with a history of liver disease or dysfunction.
	Hypertensive crisis	250 to 500 mg I.V. in 100 ml of dextrose 5% in water infused over 30 to 60 minutes, repeated every 6 hours, as needed	
Beta-adrenergic blockers			
metoprolol	Hypertension, alone or with other antihypertensives, as a step-2 or step-3 drug	100 mg P.O. daily in single or divided doses initially, increased by 50 mg/day every week up to a maximum of 450 mg/day	• Know that metoprolol is contraindicated in a patient with asthma, sinus bradycardia, greater-than-first-degree heart block, cardiogenic shock, or overt cardiac failure. • Administer with caution to a pregnant or lactating patient or one with hypertension or angina along with congestive heart failure controlled by digitalis or diuretics, bronchospastic diseases, diabetes mellitus, or impaired renal or hepatic function.
propranolol	Mild to moderate hypertension, alone or with other antihypertensives, as a step-2 or step-3 drug	40 mg P.O. b.i.d., or 80 mg P.O. daily of extended-release capsules, increased gradually to a maximum of 640 mg/day	• Know that propranolol is contraindicated in a patient with cardiogenic shock, sinus bradycardia and greater-than-first-degree heart block, bronchial asthma, congestive heart failure (CHF) unless the failure is due to a tachyarrhythmia that responds to propranolol, or known sensitivity to the drug. • Administer with caution to a pregnant or lactating patient or one with nonallergic bronchospasm disorder, diabetes mellitus, or impaired hepatic or renal function.
Alpha-adrenergic blockers			
prazosin	Hypertension, alone or with other antihypertensives, as a step-3 drug	0.5 to 1 mg b.i.d. to t.i.d. initially, increased gradually to a maintenance dosage of 6 to 15 mg/day when given alone or 1 to 2 mg P.O. t.i.d. when given with a diuretic or another antihypertensive agent	• Administer prazosin with caution to a pregnant or lactating patient.

(continued)

SELECTED MAJOR DRUGS

Antihypertensive agents (continued)

DRUG	MAJOR INDICATIONS	USUAL ADULT DOSAGES	CONTRAINDICATIONS AND PRECAUTIONS
Mixed alpha- and beta-adrenergic blockers			
labetalol	Mild to severe hypertension, alone or with other agents, as a step-2 or step-3 drug	100 mg P.O. b.i.d., increased as needed up to 400 mg b.i.d.	• Know that labetalol is contraindicated in a patient with bronchial asthma, overt cardiac failure, greater-than-first-degree heart block, cardiogenic shock, or severe bradycardia.
	Hypertensive crisis	20 to 80 mg slow I.V. bolus every 10 minutes or 2 mg/minute by continuous I.V. infusion up to a maximum of 300 mg	• Administer with caution to a pregnant or lactating patient or one with well-compensated heart failure, bronchospastic disease, pheochromocytoma, or impaired hepatic function.
Norepinephrine depletors			
guanethidine	Moderate to severe hypertension, as a step-5 drug	10 to 12.5 mg P.O. once daily initially, increased by 10 to 12.5 mg every 5 to 7 days, as needed, up to a maintenance dosage of 25 to 50 mg/day	• Know that guanethidine is contraindicated in a patient with known or suspected pheochromocytoma, CHF (not caused by hypertension), monoamine oxidase inhibitor therapy, or known hypersensitivity to the drug. • Administer with caution to a patient with bronchial asthma.
Vasodilating agents			
Direct vasodilators			
hydralazine	Moderate to severe hypertension	40 mg P.O. daily for the first 2 to 4 days, increased gradually to a maximum of 300 mg/day	• Know that hydralazine is contraindicated in a patient with mitral valve rheumatic heart disease or known hypersensitivity to the drug.
	Hypertensive crisis	10 to 40 mg I.V. or I.M., repeated as needed	• Administer with caution to a pregnant or lactating patient or one with renal or coronary insufficiency or a history of cerebrovascular accident.
Calcium channel blockers			
nifedipine	Hypertension, as a step-2 or step-3 drug	30 to 60 mg P.O. daily of sustained-release tablets, increased to a maximum of 120 mg/day	• Know that nifedipine is contraindicated in a patient with known hypersensitivity to the drug. • Administer with caution to a pregnant patient.
	Hypertensive crisis	10 mg sublingually, administered by placing the contents of a punctured capsule under the tongue or having the patient bite and swallow the capsule	
Angiotensin-converting enzyme (ACE) inhibitors			
captopril	Mild to moderate hypertension, alone or with a diuretic, as a step-2 drug	12.5 to 25 mg P.O. t.i.d. initially, increased to 50 mg P.O. t.i.d. after 1 to 2 weeks and up to a maximum of 450 mg/day	• Know that captopril is contraindicated in a patient with known hypersensitivity to the drug. • Administer with caution to a pregnant or lactating patient, one with impaired renal function or valvular stenosis, or one who is undergoing surgery or anesthesia.

• Reassure the patient that adverse reactions to captopril may disappear during the first few weeks of therapy.
• Instruct the patient to notify the physician if adverse reactions occur.

Evaluation

The following examples represent appropriate evaluation statements for a patient receiving an ACE inhibitor.
• The patient has no conditions that contraindicate ACE inhibitor therapy.
• The patient exhibits no signs of complications in the preexisting condition linked to the prescribed ACE inhibitor.
• The patient experiences no adverse reactions to the prescribed ACE inhibitor.
• The patient and family express an accurate understanding of the points taught about the prescribed ACE inhibitor.
• The patient correctly identifies signs of angioedema and describes what to do if they occur.

CHAPTER SUMMARY

Chapter 32 discussed sympatholytic agents, vasodilating agents, and ACE inhibitors as they are used to treat hypertension. Here are the highlights of the chapter.
• Hypertension is a common disease that may be controlled successfully with drug and nondrug therapy.
• Nondrug therapy should begin as soon as hypertension is diagnosed and should continue throughout the course of treatment. Nondrug interventions include sodium, alcohol, and saturated fat restriction; weight control; aerobic exercise; avoidance of smoking; and control of other cardiovascular risk factors.
• When necessary, drug treatment using the stepped-care approach is instituted to manage hypertension. This cumulative systematic approach to antihypertensive therapy begins with agents that are least likely to produce adverse reactions and adds to or substitutes for these agents, as needed, to achieve optimum blood pressure control.
• Many types of drugs can be used singly or in combination to treat hypertension, including sympatholytic agents, vasodilating agents, and ACE inhibitors.
• Sympatholytic agents reduce blood pressure by inhibiting or blocking motor and secretory action in the sympathetic nervous system. They are classified by their site or mechanism of action and include central-acting sympathetic nervous system inhibitors, ganglionic blocking agents, beta-adrenergic blocking agents, alpha-adrenergic blocking agents, mixed alpha- and beta-adrenergic blocking agents, and norepinephrine depletors.
• Two types of vasodilating agents exist: direct vasodilators and calcium channel blockers. Direct vasodilators act on arteries, veins, or both to reduce blood pressure. They include diazoxide, hydralazine, minoxidil, and nitroprusside. These drugs act by relaxing peripheral vascular smooth muscle, lowering blood pressure by increasing blood vessel caliber and reducing total peripheral resistance. Calcium channel blockers prevent calcium transport across the cell membrane, reducing the activity of the vascular smooth muscle, thus producing vasodilation and lowering the blood pressure. Calcium channel blockers include diltiazem, nicardipine, nifedipine, and verapamil.
• ACE inhibitors reduce blood pressure by interfering with the renin-angiotensin-aldosterone system. They inhibit the enzyme that converts angiotensin I to angiotensin II, a potent vasoconstrictor. ACE inhibitors also decrease aldosterone release, preventing sodium and water retention. They include captopril, enalapril, and lisinopril.
• When caring for a patient receiving an antihypertensive agent, the nurse should apply the nursing process. Nursing care typically includes regular blood pressure monitoring, fluid balance evaluation, and observation for CNS changes.

STUDY QUESTIONS

See Appendix 1 for answers.

1. Frank Ballard, age 40, recently has been diagnosed as having essential mild hypertension. Assessment findings include a blood pressure of 150/94 mm Hg, obesity, smoking of one pack of cigarettes per day, and a sedentary lifestyle. The physician prescribes step 1 of the stepped-care approach to antihypertensive therapy. What does step 1 include?
(a) weight control, sodium restriction, and aerobic exercise
(b) weight control, sodium restriction, and a diuretic
(c) weight control, aerobic exercise, and an ACE inhibitor
(d) weight control, sodium restriction, a diuretic, and a calcium channel blocker

2. After 6 months on step 1, Mr. Ballard returns for a follow-up visit. Because Mr. Ballard's blood pressure is 160/100 mm Hg, the physician prescribes the beta-adren-

ergic blocker propranolol 40 mg P.O. b.i.d. How does propranolol reduce blood pressure?
(a) It reduces sympathetic activity, thus decreasing arteriolar vasoconstriction.
(b) It interferes with transmission of sympathetic and parasympathetic nerve impulses, producing vasodilation.
(c) It competes with epinephrine for receptor sites, thereby blocking sympathetic stimulation.
(d) It alters the synthesis, storage, and release of norepinephrine, reducing peripheral vascular resistance.

3. Because Mr. Ballard also has type I diabetes, he takes 20 units of NPH insulin S.C. every morning. Why is propranolol used cautiously in an insulin-dependent diabetic patient?
(a) It may cause hyperglycemia.
(b) It may mask the signs of hypoglycemia.
(c) It may produce additive hypoglycemic effects.
(d) It may cause insulin tolerance.

4. Paul Robertson, age 70, is admitted to the critical care unit with severe hypertension. His blood pressure ranges from 170/110 to 180/140. The physician prescribes nitroprusside 0.5 mcg/kg/minute by I.V. infusion. How does nitroprusside reduce blood pressure?
(a) It directly relaxes arterial and venous smooth muscle.
(b) It inhibits calcium transport during depolarization.
(c) It depletes norepinephrine stores.
(d) It inhibits sympathetic activity.

5. When Mr. Robertson's blood pressure stabilizes, his medication is changed to the calcium channel blocker diltiazem 30 mg P.O. t.i.d. While Mr. Robertson is receiving diltiazem, the nurse should assess for which adverse reactions?
(a) hypotension and bradycardia
(b) hypertrichosis
(c) drug-induced SLE
(d) GI hemorrhage

6. Tom Perkins, age 34, has secondary hypertension caused by renal stenosis. Which antihypertensive agents are the treatment of choice for patients like Mr. Perkins, who have high renin levels?
(a) sympatholytic agents
(b) vasodilating agents
(c) ACE-inhibiting agents
(d) beta-blocking agents

7. For Mr. Perkins, the physician prescribes captopril 12.5 mg P.O. t.i.d. What other agent may be prescribed with captopril to increase the effectiveness of treatment?
(a) sympatholytic agent
(b) vasodilating agent
(c) calcium channel blocker
(d) thiazide diuretic

8. What should the nurse teach Mr. Perkins about captopril administration?
(a) Take the medication with meals.
(b) Take the medication at bedtime.
(c) Take the medication upon arising.
(d) Take the medication 1 hour before meals.

SELECTED REFERENCES

AHFS drug information 90. (1990). Bethesda, MD: American Society of Hospital Pharmacists.

Aspirin and antihypertensives. (1988). *Nurses Drug Alert,* 12(10), 75.

Beare, P. (1989). Calcium channel blockers: Nursing care for hypertension. *Critical Care Nurse,* 9(2), 37-42.

Buhler, R., and Kiowski, W. (1987). Age and antihypertensive response to calcium antagonists. *Journal of Hypertension,* 5(Suppl. 4), S111-S114.

Dix-Sheldon, D. (1989). Pharmacologic management of myocardial ischemia. *Journal of Cardiovascular Nursing,* 3(4), 17-30.

Freis, E. (1988). Age and antihypertensive drugs (hydrochlorothiazide, bendroflumethiazide, nadolol, and captopril). *American Journal of Cardiology,* 61(1), 117-121.

Gifford, R., Jr. (1989). Mild hypertension: Critical analysis of different therapeutic approaches. *Cleveland Clinic Journal of Medicine,* 56(4), 336-345.

Goodman and Gilman's the pharmacological basis of therapeutics (8th ed.; 1990). Elmsford, NY: Pergamon Press.

Gunnar, R., Mueller, H., Saksena, S., et al. (1988). Beta-blockers and nitrates in MI. *Patient Care,* 22(14), 88-97.

Haber, E. (ed.). (1988). *The proceedings of the seventh scientific meeting of the inter-American society. (Hypertension monographs: No. 4).* Dallas: American Heart Association, Inc.

Joint National Committee. (1988). Report on Detection, Evaluation, and Treatment of High Blood Pressure. *Archives of Internal Medicine,* 148(5), 1023-1038.

Just, P. (1989). The positive association of cough with ACE inhibitors. *Pharmacology,* 9(2), 82-87.

Kelleher, R. (1989). Cardiac drugs: New inotropes. *Critical Care Nursing Clinics of North America,* 1(2), 391-397.

MacMahon S., Cutler, J., and Stamler, J. (1989). Hypertensive drug treatment: Potential, expected, and observed effects on stroke and on coronary heart disease. *Hypertension,* 13(5), 145-150.

Moser, M. (1987). Diuretics in the management of hypertension. *Medical Clinics of North America,* 71(5), 935-946.

Moser, M. (1989). Lipid abnormalities and diuretics. *American Family Physician,* 40(4), 213-220.

Moser, M. (1989). Relative efficacy of, and some adverse reactions to, different antihypertensive regimens. *American Journal of Cardiology,* 63(4), 2B-7B.

Nicholson, J., Resnick, L., and Laragh, J. (1989). Hydrochlorothiazide is not additive to verapamil in treating essential hypertension. *Archives of Internal Medicine,* 149(1), 125-128.

North American Nursing Diagnosis Association. (1990). *Taxonomy I-Revised, with official diagnostic categories.* St. Louis: NANDA.

Packer, M., Lee, W., Medina, N., et al. (1987). Functional renal insufficiency during long-term therapy with captopril and enalapril in severe chronic heart failure. *Annals of Internal Medicine,* 106(3), 346-354.

Pollare, T., Lithell, H., and Berne, C. (1989). A comparison of the effects of hydrochlorothiazide and captopril on glucose and lipid metabolism in patients with hypertension. *New England Journal of Medicine,* 321(13), 868-873.

Prince, M., Stuart, C., Padia, M., et al. (1988). Metabolic effects of hydrochlorothiazide and enalapril during treatment of the hypertensive diabetic patient: Enalapril for hypertensive diabetics. *Archives of Internal Medicine,* 148(11), 2363-2368.

CHAPTER

33

DIURETIC AGENTS

OBJECTIVES

After reading and studying this chapter, the student should be able to:
1. Describe the absorption, distribution, metabolism, and excretion of thiazide and thiazide-like, loop, potassium-sparing, and osmotic diuretics.
2. Compare the mechanisms of action of the various types of diuretics.
3. Identify the major clinical indications for the various types of diuretics.
4. Describe the major drug interactions that can occur with the various types of diuretics.
5. Describe the fluid and electrolyte imbalances that commonly occur as a result of diuretic therapy.
6. Describe how to apply the nursing process when caring for a patient who is receiving a diuretic agent.

INTRODUCTION

Most diuretic agents promote renal excretion of water and electrolytes by increasing the glomerular filtration rate (GFR), decreasing sodium resorption, or increasing the rate of sodium excretion. Diuretics are used clinically to increase urine volume and the net excretion of solutes and water. These agents act at different sites within the nephrons (structural and functional units of the kidney) to produce diuresis. (For an illustration, see *Principal sites of diuretic action*.) The major diuretics discussed in this chapter are classified as thiazide and thiazide-like diuretics, loop, potassium-sparing, and osmotic diuretics. Other diuretics are discussed briefly, including the carbonic anhydrase inhibitors (which are used primarily to decrease intraocular pressure) and the mercurial diuretics.

For a summary of representative drugs, see *Selected major drugs: Diuretic agents,* pages 579 and 580. For a listing of applicable nursing diagnoses that the nurse may formulate when caring for a patient receiving these agents, see *Selected nursing diagnoses: Diuretic agents.* For detailed

Principal sites of diuretic action

Diuretics increase the urinary excretion of water and sodium, primarily by decreasing sodium chloride resorption in the renal tubules. Different diuretics act at different sites in the nephron, as illustrated below.

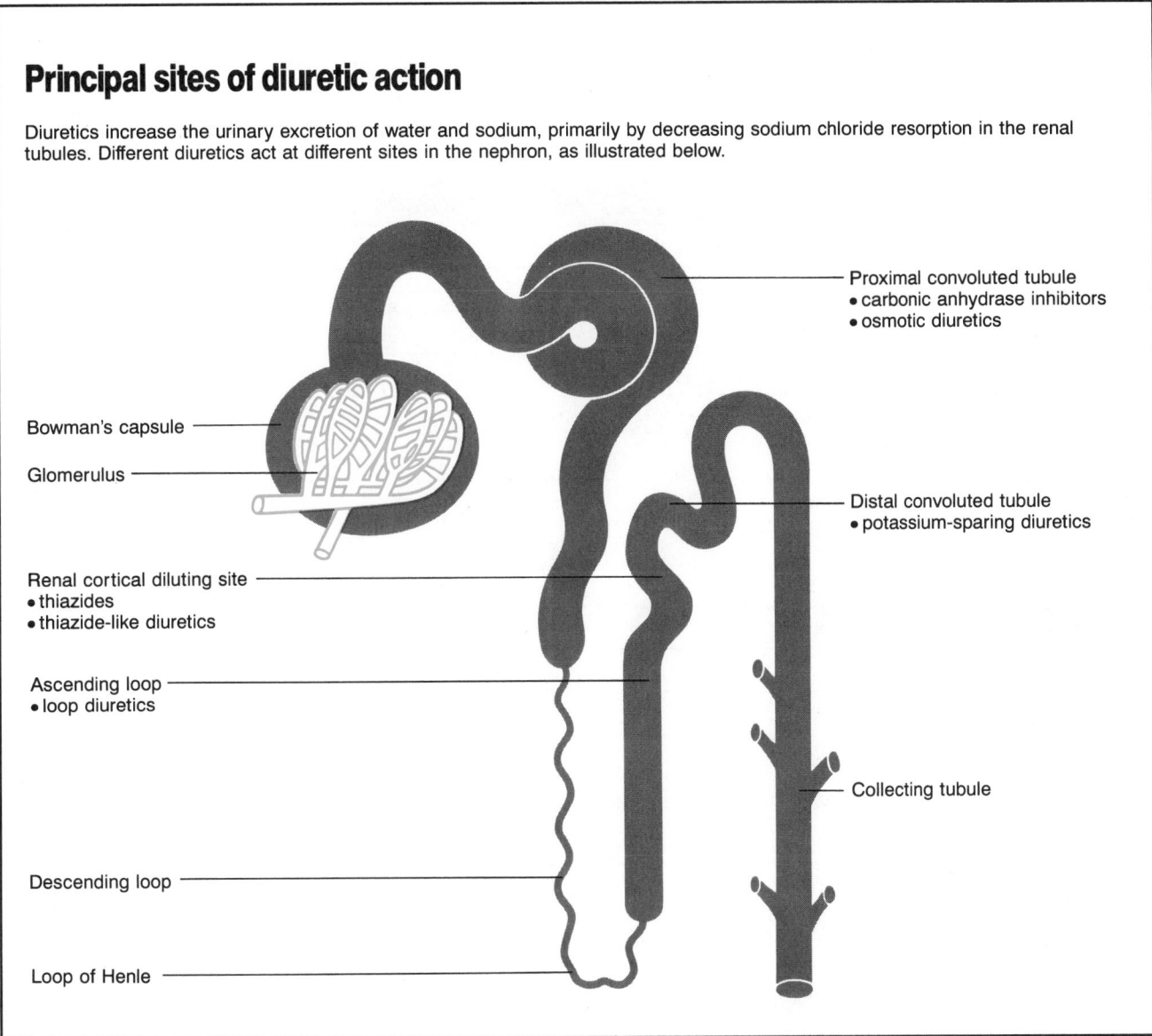

information on applying the nursing process, see Chapter 6, The Nursing Process and Drug Therapy.

THIAZIDE AND THIAZIDE-LIKE DIURETICS

Thiazide and thiazide-like diuretics are sulfonamide derivatives that inhibit sodium resorption, thereby increasing sodium and water excretion. These diuretics may induce a hypersensitivity reaction similar to sulfonamide's; they also increase the excretion of chloride, potassium, and bicar-

bonate ions, which can result in electrolyte imbalances, particularly hypokalemia. The thiazide diuretics include bendroflumethiazide, benzthiazide, chlorothiazide, hydrochlorothiazide, hydroflumethiazide, methyclothiazide, polythiazide, and trichlormethiazide. The thiazide-like diuretics include chlorthalidone, indapamide, metolazone, and quinethazone.

PHARMACOKINETICS

Thiazide diuretics are absorbed rapidly but incompletely after oral administration and are excreted in the urine. These drugs are particularly useful because of their rapid action.

Onset, peak, and duration of thiazide and thiazide-like diuretics

The onset of action, peak concentration levels, and duration of action of the thiazide and thiazide-like diuretics vary significantly. These differences will influence the nurse's plan of care for a specific patient.

DRUG	ONSET OF ACTION	PEAK CONCENTRATION	DURATION OF ACTION
Thiazide diuretics			
bendroflumethiazide	1 hour	4 hours	6 to 12 hours
benzthiazide	1 hour	4 to 6 hours	6 to 12 hours
chlorothiazide I.V.	15 minutes	30 minutes	2 hours
chlorothiazide P.O.	1 hour	4 hours	6 to 12 hours
hydrochlorothiazide	1 hour	4 to 6 hours	6 to 12 hours
hydroflumethiazide	1 hour	4 hours	6 to 12 hours
methyclothiazide	1 hour	6 hours	24 hours
polythiazide	1 hour	6 hours	24 to 48 hours
trichlormethiazide	1 hour	6 hours	24 hours
Thiazide-like diuretics			
chlorthalidone	2 hours	4 to 6 hours	24 to 72 hours
indapamide	1 hour	2 hours	8 to 12 hours
metolazone	1 hour	2 hours	12 to 24 hours
quinethazone	1 hour	6 hours	18 to 24 hours

Absorption, distribution, metabolism, excretion

Thiazide diuretics are absorbed rapidly but incompletely from the gastrointestinal (GI) tract after oral administration. Oral chlorothiazide is the most poorly absorbed (10% to 21%) thiazide diuretic. The protein binding of thiazide diuretics varies, ranging from 65% for hydrochlorothiazide to 95% for chlorothiazide. Thiazide diuretics cross the placenta and appear in breast milk. These agents differ in their degree of metabolism. Some agents, such as hydrochlorothiazide, are excreted basically unchanged in the urine; others, such as polythiazide and indapamide, are metabolized extensively.

The thiazides are eliminated rapidly by the kidneys because they are secreted actively by the proximal tubules. Minute quantities of these drugs usually appear in bile, but metolazone, which undergoes some enterohepatic metabolism, is present in higher quantities. Although 60% of indapamide is excreted in the urine as metabolites, 20% is excreted in the feces as metabolites and 5% in the urine as unchanged drug. Thiazide diuretic excretion is delayed in patients with congestive heart failure (CHF), impaired renal function, or any other disorder that reduces renal blood flow. (Thiazide diuretics are not effective in patients with renal impairment whose GFR is less than 20 ml/minute.)

Onset, peak, duration

Onset of action of the thiazide and thiazide-like diuretics usually occurs within 1 hour of oral administration. However, intravenous (I.V.) chlorothiazide will begin to act within 15 minutes of administration. Optimal antihypertensive effects of these agents, however, usually do not appear for 3 to 4 weeks after therapy begins—but they may appear within 3 or 4 days.

Peak concentration levels of thiazide and thiazide-like diuretics usually occur within 4 to 6 hours. I.V. chlorothiazide, indapamide, and metolazone are the exceptions: I.V. chlorothiazide reaches a peak concentration within 30 minutes; metolazone and indapamide, in 2 hours.

The duration of action of the thiazide and thiazide-like diuretics is 6 to 24 hours, depending on the drug excretion rate. I.V. chlorothiazide, polythiazide, and chlorthalidone are the exceptions. I.V. chlorothiazide has a duration of only 2 hours; polythiazide, of 24 to 48 hours; and chlorthalidone, of 24 to 72 hours. (For more details, see *Onset, peak, and duration of thiazide and thiazide-like diuretics.*)

PHARMACODYNAMICS

The thiazide and thiazide-like diuretics increase the excretion of sodium, chloride, and water by inhibiting sodium reabsorption. These drugs also increase the potassium ion excretion.

Mechanism of action

Thiazide and thiazide-like diuretics interfere with the transport of sodium ions across the renal tubular epithelium at the cortical-diluting, or distal, segments of the nephrons. Like the sulfonamides, thiazides create some minor carbonic anhydrase inhibition. These effects result in increased sodium, chloride, and water excretion with excretion of sodium and chloride in approximately equal amounts and concomitant excretion of magnesium, phosphate, bromide, and iodide. At the same time, the excretion of ammonium, urates, and calcium is decreased. Thiazide diuretics also may decrease the GFR.

Researchers currently believe that the action of the thiazide and thiazide-like diuretics is linked primarily to increased sodium excretion. Initially, these drugs decrease circulating blood volume, thus decreasing cardiac output. If the therapy is maintained, the cardiac output stabilizes, but extracellular fluid and plasma volume decrease.

PHARMACOTHERAPEUTICS

Thiazide and thiazide-like diuretics may be used alone or with other drugs; they are used primarily to treat hypertension and edema from mild or moderate CHF. Because these drugs decrease the urinary calcium level, they also are used alone or with other drugs to prevent the development and recurrence of calcium nephrolithiasis in hypercalciuric and normal calciuric patients.

Thiazides are used to treat the edema associated not only with CHF, but also with hepatic disease, renal disease, and corticosteroid and estrogen therapy. Although the thiazide and thiazide-like diuretics usually are not effective if the GFR is less than 20 ml/minute, one exception exists: metolazone, which remains effective even with a decreased GFR.

Thiazides may be used alone or with other drugs to treat hypertension. Although their antihypertensive effects may begin within 3 to 4 days after initiation of therapy, the drugs are most effective after 3 to 4 weeks of continued therapy. The thiazides commonly are used with other drugs for long-term control of hypertension.

In patients with diabetes insipidus, thiazides paradoxically decrease urine volume, possibly via sodium depletion and plasma volume reduction.

bendroflumethiazide (Naturetin). This thiazide diuretic is used to treat edema and hypertension.
Usual adult dosage: initially, 5 to 20 mg P.O. daily or in two divided doses; for maintenance, 2.5 to 5 mg P.O. daily.
Usual pediatric dosage: initially, 0.1 to 0.4 mg/kg/day in one or two doses; for maintenance, 0.05 to 0.1 mg/kg/day in one or two doses.

benzthiazide (Aquapres, Aquatag, Exna, Marazide, Proaqua, Urazide). This thiazide diuretic is used to treat edema and hypertension.
Usual adult dosage: for edema, 50 to 200 mg P.O. daily or in divided doses; for hypertension, 50 mg P.O. daily to b.i.d., depending on the patient's response.
Usual pediatric dosage: 1 to 4 mg/kg P.O. daily in three divided doses.

chlorothiazide (Diuril). A thiazide diuretic, chlorothiazide is used to treat edema and hypertension. It may be administered I.V. but not I.M. or S.C.
Usual adult dosage: for edema, 500 mg to 2 grams P.O. or I.V. daily or in two divided doses; for hypertension, 500 mg to 1 gram P.O. or I.V. daily or in divided doses.
Usual pediatric dosage: ages 6 months and over, 20 mg/kg P.O. or I.V. daily in divided doses; under age 6 months, up to 30 mg/kg P.O. or I.V. daily in divided doses.

hydrochlorothiazide (Esidrix, HydroDiuril, Oretic). This thiazide diuretic is used to treat edema and hypertension.
Usual adult dosage: for edema, 25 to 200 mg P.O. daily or intermittently; for hypertension, 25 to 100 mg P.O. daily or in divided doses; increased or decreased according to the patient's response.
Usual pediatric dosage: ages 6 months and over, 2.2 mg/kg P.O. daily divided in two doses; under age 6 months, 3.3 mg/kg P.O. daily divided in two doses.

hydroflumethiazide (Diucardin, Saluron). This thiazide diuretic is used to treat edema and hypertension.
Usual adult dosage: for edema, initially 25 to 100 mg P.O. daily in divided doses, then maintenance with 25 to 200 mg P.O. intermittently or on alternate days; for hypertension, 50 to 100 mg P.O. once or twice a day up to a maximum of 200 mg/day.
Usual pediatric dosage: 1 mg/kg P.O. daily.

methyclothiazide (Aquatensen, Enduron). This long-acting thiazide diuretic is used to treat edema and hypertension.
Usual adult dosage: 2.5 to 10 mg P.O. daily.

polythiazide (Renese). A long-acting thiazide diuretic, polythiazide is used to treat hypertension and edema from cardiac or renal failure.

Usual adult dosage: for hypertension, 2 to 4 mg P.O. daily; for edema, 1 to 4 mg P.O. daily.

trichlormethiazide (Metahydrin, Naqua). This long-acting thiazide diuretic is used to treat edema and hypertension. *Usual adult dosage:* for edema, 1 to 4 mg P.O. daily or in two divided doses; for hypertension, 2 to 4 mg P.O. daily.

chlorthalidone (Hygroton). This long-acting thiazide-like diuretic is used to treat edema and hypertension. *Usual adult dosage:* for edema, 50 to 100 mg P.O. daily or 100 mg on alternate days (up to 200 mg/day may be necessary for therapeutic effect); for hypertension, 25 to 50 mg P.O. daily, or 100 mg three times weekly or on alternate days (up to 200 mg/day may be necessary for therapeutic effect). *Usual pediatric dosage:* 2 mg/kg P.O. three times weekly.

indapamide (Lozol). This thiazide-like diuretic is used to treat edema and hypertension. *Usual adult dosage:* for edema or hypertension, 2.5 mg P.O. as a single daily dose, increased to 5 mg P.O. as a single daily dose, if needed.

metolazone (Diulo, Zaroxolyn). This thiazide-like diuretic is used to treat hypertension and the edema secondary to CHF, hepatic disease, or renal disease. It occasionally is used with other thiazides or furosemide. Unlike other thiazide and thiazide-like diuretics, metolazone is effective even when the patient's GFR is less than 20 ml/minute. *Usual adult dosage:* for edema from CHF, 5 to 10 mg P.O. daily; for edema from renal or hepatic disease, 5 to 20 mg P.O. daily; for hypertension, 2.5 to 5 mg P.O. daily; dosage may be increased or decreased to maintain the therapeutic effect.

quinethazone (Aquamox, Hydromox). This thiazide-like diuretic is used to treat edema. *Usual adult dosage:* 50 to 100 mg P.O. daily, as needed; dosage may be increased up to 200 mg/day.

Drug interactions
Drug interactions related to the thiazide and thiazide-like diuretics result in altered fluid volume, blood pressure, and serum electrolyte levels. (For more information, see *Drug interactions: Thiazide and thiazide-like diuretics.*)

ADVERSE DRUG REACTIONS

Numerous adverse reactions are associated with thiazide and thiazide-like diuretics. The most common are blood volume depletion, orthostatic hypotension, hyponatremia, and hypokalemia. Other dose-related adverse reactions include glucose intolerance, hypercalcemia, and hypophosphatemia, which may occur with prolonged therapy; hyperuricemia, especially in patients with a history of gout; and GI reactions, such as anorexia, nausea, and pancreatitis.

Hypersensitivity reactions may occur in the form of purpura, photosensitivity, rash, urticaria, necrotizing vasculitis, or blood abnormalities, which may include leukopenia, thrombocytopenia, aplastic anemia, or granulocytopenia.

NURSING PROCESS APPLICATION

The following information assists the nurse in caring for a patient who is receiving a thiazide or thiazide-like diuretic.

Assessment
• Review the patient's history for a preexisting condition that contraindicates the use of a thiazide or thiazide-like diuretic, such as anuria, lactation, or known hypersensitivity to these drugs.
• Review the patient's history for a preexisting condition that requires cautious use of a thiazide or thiazide-like diuretic, such as severe renal disease, impaired hepatic function, progressive liver disease, or pregnancy.
• Assess the patient for adverse reactions to the prescribed thiazide or thiazide-like diuretic, such as blood volume depletion, orthostatic hypotension, hypokalemia, or blood abnormalities.
• Review the patient's medication history to identify the use of drugs that may interact with the thiazide or thiazide-like diuretic, such as oral hypoglycemic agents, insulin, cardiac glycosides, or skeletal muscle relaxants.
• Assess the effectiveness of the thiazide or thiazide-like diuretic frequently.
• Assess the patient's urine elimination pattern throughout diuretic therapy.
• Assess the patient for signs and symptoms of dehydration, such as poor skin turgor and dry oral mucous membranes.
• Evaluate the patient's and family's knowledge about the prescribed thiazide or thiazide-like diuretic.

Nursing diagnoses
The following examples represent appropriate nursing diagnoses for a patient receiving a thiazide or thiazide-like diuretic
• Potential for injury related to a preexisting condition that contraindicates the use of a thiazide or thiazide-like diuretic
• Potential for injury related to a preexisting condition that requires cautious use of a thiazide or thiazide-like diuretic
• Potential for injury related to adverse drug reactions
• Altered urinary elimination related to the genitourinary effects of the prescribed thiazide or thiazide-like diuretic
• Potential fluid volume deficit related to use of a thiazide or thiazide-like diuretic

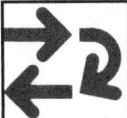 **DRUG INTERACTIONS**

Thiazide and thiazide-like diuretics

Drug interactions related to thiazide and thiazide-like diuretics may cause severe fluid and electrolyte imbalances and other potentially serious problems. The nurse needs to be aware of these interactions to plan appropriate nursing care.

DRUG	INTERACTING DRUGS	POSSIBLE EFFECTS	NURSING IMPLICATIONS
all thiazide and thiazide-like diuretics	oral hypoglycemic agents, insulin	May cause hyponatremia, thiazide resistance, hyperglycemia	• Monitor the patient's serum sodium and glucose levels. • Monitor the patient for signs and symptoms of hyponatremia, such as dizziness and weakness, and of hyperglycemia, such as polyuria, polydipsia, polyphagia, and weight loss.
	corticosteroids, ACTH	May cause hypokalemia	• Monitor the patient's serum potassium level. • Monitor the patient for the signs and symptoms of hypokalemia, such as weakness and flattened T wave on ECG.
	lithium carbonate	May cause lithium toxicity	• Monitor the patient for signs and symptoms of lithium toxicity, such as ataxia. • Monitor the patient's serum lithium level.
	skeletal muscle relaxants (tubocurarine, gallamine)	Increase responsiveness to the skeletal muscle relaxant	• Monitor the patient for the therapeutic effects of skeletal muscle relaxants. • Expect to adjust the muscle relaxant dosage.
	cardiac glycosides	May cause digitalis toxicity as a result of hypokalemia	• Monitor the patient for signs and symptoms of digitalis toxicity, such as GI, cardiovascular, or neurologic problems. • Monitor the patient's serum digitalis level. • Monitor the patient's serum electrolyte levels.
	probenecid	Decrease renal excretion of uric acid, which may precipitate or worsen gout	• Monitor the patient's fluid intake and output. • Monitor the patient's serum electrolyte levels.
	cholestyramine, colestipol	Decrease therapeutic effect of the diuretic	• Administer the thiazide or thiazide-like diuretic 2 hours before administering cholestyramine or colestipol. • Monitor the patient for the therapeutic effects of the diuretic.
	indomethacin, other non-steroidal anti-inflammatory drugs	Decrease antihypertensive effect	• Monitor the patient's vital signs, especially noting an increase in blood pressure. • Monitor the patient for the therapeutic effects of the diuretic.

• Knowledge deficit related to the prescribed thiazide or thiazide-like diuretic

Planning and implementation
• Do not administer a thiazide or thiazide-like diuretic to a patient with a condition that contraindicates its use.
• Administer a thiazide or thiazide-like diuretic cautiously to a patient at risk because of a preexisting condition.
• Monitor the patient frequently for adverse reactions to the prescribed thiazide or thiazide-like diuretic.
• Monitor the patient's serum electrolyte, creatinine, blood urea nitrogen (BUN), and glucose levels to detect imbalances.

• *Be especially alert for changes in the patient's serum potassium level, and observe for the signs and symptoms of hypokalemia, such as drowsiness, paresthesias, muscle cramps, and hyporeflexia.*
• *Administer potassium supplements as prescribed to maintain an acceptable serum potassium level.*
• Monitor the patient's pulse and serum digitalis level frequently during concomitant cardiac glycoside therapy to detect digitalis toxicity.
• Monitor the blood glucose level more frequently in a diabetic patient during long-term therapy with a thiazide or thiazide-like diuretic because these agents can cause glucose intolerance.

• *Weigh the patient daily under controlled conditions (at the same time each morning, after the patient voids, before the patient eats, with the patient wearing similar clothing at each weigh-in, and on the same scale).*

• Take the patient's vital signs and auscultate breath sounds frequently to assess the effectiveness of drug therapy.

• Do not administer chlorothiazide I.M. or S.C.

• Monitor the patient with a history of gout closely for hyperuricemia, which may be induced by a thiazide or thiazide-like agent.

• *Have the patient sit up for a few minutes before standing to minimize the effects of orthostatic hypotension.*

• Notify the physician if adverse reactions occur.

• Document the patient's fluid intake and output to detect alterations in urine elimination.

• Keep a urinal or bedpan within reach for a bedridden patient; ensure that the bathroom is easily accessible for an ambulatory patient.

• Expect a delay in urine elimination changes when administering a thiazide or thiazide-like agent to a patient with CHF, impaired renal function, or any other disorder that reduces renal blood flow.

• Expect to switch the patient to metolazone as prescribed if the GFR falls below 20 ml/minute.

• *Determine whether diuresis occurs at the appropriate time for the drug administered, based on its onset of action. If it does not, notify the physician because the drug may be ineffective.*

• *Administer the diuretic in the morning or early afternoon, if permissible, to prevent nocturia from upsetting the patient's normal sleep pattern.*

• Monitor the patient for signs of dehydration, such as poor skin turgor and dry oral mucous membranes.

• Monitor the patient's vital signs to detect evidence of hypovolemia, such as tachycardia, hypotension, and dyspnea. If such evidence appears, notify the physician.

• Monitor the patient's fluid intake and output. If extreme discrepancies occur, notify the physician and expect to decrease the diuretic dosage, as prescribed.

• Administer fluids, blood, blood products, or plasma expanders as prescribed to replace lost fluids and promote movement of extracellular fluid into the intravascular space.

Patient teaching

• Teach the patient and family the name, dose, frequency, action, and adverse effects of the prescribed thiazide or thiazide-like diuretic.

• Advise the female patient to tell the physician if she is pregnant or plans to become pregnant during diuretic therapy.

• Inform the patient that periodic blood tests must be performed to detect imbalances caused by diuretic therapy.

• *Teach the patient to recognize and report to the physician the signs of hypokalemia.*

• *Explain the importance of taking potassium supplements, if prescribed, and eating a potassium-rich diet. Give the patient a list of potassium-rich foods.* (For a list, see *Guide to potassium-rich foods.*)

• Teach the patient receiving concomitant cardiac glycoside therapy to identify the signs of digitalis toxicity, such as GI, cardiac, and neurologic disturbances.

• Instruct the diabetic patient receiving a thiazide or thiazide-like diuretic to monitor blood glucose levels closely. Advise this patient that diabetes treatment may require adjustment during diuretic therapy.

• *Instruct the patient to take the diuretic in the morning or early afternoon, if permissible, to avoid nocturia.*

• *Teach the patient to obtain a daily weight under the same conditions every time and to notify the physician of any sudden weight gain (greater than 2 pounds in 1 day), peripheral edema, or shortness of breath.*

• Instruct the patient how to minimize the effects of orthostatic hypotension.

• *Advise the patient to expect an increase in urinary frequency and amount voided.*

• Teach the patient to recognize and report to the physician the signs and symptoms of dehydration.

• Instruct the patient to notify the physician if adverse reactions occur or if concerns arise about the prescribed diuretic therapy.

Evaluation

The following examples represent appropriate evaluation statements for a patient receiving a thiazide or thiazide-like diuretic.

• The patient has no conditions that contraindicate the use of a thiazide or thiazide-like diuretic.

• The patient exhibits no signs of complications in the preexisting condition linked to the prescribed thiazide or thiazide-like diuretic.

• The patient displays no adverse reactions to the prescribed thiazide or thiazide-like diuretic.

• The patient urinates more frequently during thiazide or thiazide-like diuretic therapy.

• The patient displays no signs of dehydration during thiazide or thiazide-like diuretic therapy.

• The patient and family express an accurate understanding of the points taught about the prescribed thiazide or thiazide-like diuretic.

• The patient correctly identifies potassium-rich foods and plans to include them in the daily diet.

Guide to potassium-rich foods

The nurse should encourage the patient on diuretic therapy to eat potassium-rich foods. This chart can help provide information on foods the patient can include in the diet.

JUICES	mg per 8 fl. oz.
Tomato	533
Orange, fresh	496
Orange, reconstituted	474

VEGETABLES	mg per 100 grams
Potatoes	407
Lima beans	394
Carrots	341
Spinach	324
Radishes	322
Sweet potatoes	300
Brussels sprouts	295
Endive	294
Asparagus	238
Cabbage	233
Peppers	213

FRUITS	mg per 100 grams
Dates	648
Bananas	370
Raisins	355
Plums	299
Nectarines	294
Apricots	281
Prunes	262
Peaches	202
Oranges	200
Figs	152

FISH	mg per 100 grams
Sardines, canned	590
Halibut	525
Scallops	476
Salmon	421
Haddock	348
Flounder	342
Tuna	301
Perch	284
Bass	256
Oysters	203

MEATS	mg per 100 grams
Veal	500
Chicken	411
Turkey	411
Liver	380
Beef	370
Pork	326
Lamb	290

MISCELLANEOUS	mg per 100 grams
Milk, dry (nonfat solids)	1,745
Molasses (light)	917
Peanuts	674
Peanut butter	670
Gingersnaps	462
Graham crackers	384
Oatmeal cookies (with raisins)	370
Ice milk	195

LOOP DIURETICS

Loop, or high-ceiling, diuretics are highly potent agents. Very effective in treating edema, hypertension, and hypercalcemia, they also are valuable in treating patients who are resistant to less potent diuretics or who have decreased GFRs. Because of their potency, loop diuretics may produce profound diuresis, with water and electrolyte depletion. The loop diuretics include bumetanide, ethacrynate sodium, ethacrynic acid, and furosemide.

PHARMACOKINETICS

Loop diuretics usually are absorbed well and distributed rapidly. Extensively protein-bound, these agents undergo partial or complete metabolism in the liver except for fu-

rosemide, which is excreted primarily unchanged. Loop diuretics are excreted primarily by the kidneys.

Besides their greater potency, these diuretics have a more rapid onset of action and produce a much greater volume of diuresis than other types of diuretics.

Absorption, distribution, metabolism, excretion

Bumetanide is absorbed almost completely after oral or intramuscular (I.M.) administration. Also available for I.V. administration, it is more than 95% protein bound. Ethacrynate sodium and ethacrynic acid are absorbed rapidly from the GI tract after oral administration; available for I.V. administration as well, they also are about 95% protein bound. After oral administration, furosemide is 60% to 70% absorbed from the GI tract; taking the drug with food slows the absorption rate but has little effect on the total amount absorbed. Also available for I.V. administration, furosemide is over 95% protein bound.

Bumetanide is metabolized partially in the liver. About 80% of a dose is excreted in the urine, 50% as unchanged drug, and the remainder as conjugates and metabolites. About 15% is eliminated in the feces.

As ethacrynate sodium and ethacrynic acid accumulate in the liver, they are metabolized to active cysteine conjugate. About two-thirds of a dose is excreted in the urine, the remainder in the bile.

Furosemide is excreted primarily unchanged in the urine, accompanied by small amounts of a glucuronide. Amounts up to 30% may be excreted in the feces. Furosemide and bumetanide cross the placenta and appear in breast milk.

Onset, peak, duration

Bumetanide's onset of action occurs within 30 minutes after oral administration, within 40 minutes after I.M. administration, and within a few minutes after I.V. administration. The peak concentration level of bumetanide is reached within 1.5 to 2 hours after oral administration and within minutes after I.V. administration. The duration of action of bumetanide is from 3.5 to 4 hours, although it may increase to 6 hours with higher doses. Bumetanide's half-life is 1 to 1.5 hours.

Onset of ethacrynate sodium and ethacrynic acid occurs 30 minutes after oral administration and 5 minutes after I.V. administration. The duration is 6 to 8 hours after oral administration and 2 hours after I.V. administration. As with bumetanide, the duration of ethacrynate sodium and ethacrynic acid may increase with higher doses. The half-life of these drugs is 30 to 70 minutes.

Onset of furosemide occurs within 30 to 60 minutes after oral administration and 5 minutes after I.V. administration. Peak concentration occurs within 20 to 60 minutes; the drug's duration is about 2 hours after an I.V. dose and 6 hours after an oral dose. The half-life of furosemide usually is 30 to 60 minutes but may increase to 75 to 155 minutes in a patient with renal or hepatic insufficiency and to 20 hours in a patient with renal system dysfunction.

PHARMACODYNAMICS

The loop diuretics are the most potent diuretics available, producing the greatest volume of diuresis and having a high potential for causing severe adverse reactions. Producing maximal sodium excretion of 20% to 25% of the filtered load, loop diuretics inhibit sodium and chloride resorption in the renal tubules by direct action on the thick ascending limb of the loop of Henle. These drugs also may inhibit sodium, chloride, and water resorption in the proximal tubule while increasing the excretion of ammonium and titratable acids in the distal tubule. Increased potassium excretion from the distal tubule may result from the accelerated exchange with sodium ions caused by the increased sodium volume delivered to the distal tubule. Ethacrynate sodium and ethacrynic acid bind to sulfhydryl

groups in renal cellular protein. Bumetanide, the shorter-acting agent, is 40 times more potent than furosemide.

PHARMACOTHERAPEUTICS

Loop diuretics are used primarily to treat edema associated with CHF, hepatic or renal disease, or nephrotic syndrome. Loop diuretics also are used to treat mild hypertension, usually with a potassium-sparing diuretic or a potassium supplement to prevent hypokalemia. Bumetanide also has been used to treat edema related to menstruation and lymphedema. Ethacrynate sodium and ethacrynic acid also are used to treat cancer-related ascites, lymphedema, acute pulmonary edema, nephrogenic diabetes insipidus, and hypercalcemia. Furosemide also is used with mannitol to treat severe cerebral edema.

bumetanide (Bumex). Used to treat edema and hypertension, bumetanide may be substituted for furosemide in patients hypersensitive to that drug.
Usual adult dosage: 0.5 to 2 mg P.O. in a single daily dose or repeated at 4- to 5-hour intervals up to a total of 10 mg/day; maintenance dosages usually are given intermittently with 1- to 2-day rest periods; 0.5 to 1 mg I.M. or I.V., injected or infused slowly over 1 to 2 minutes; I.V. doses may be repeated every 2 to 3 hours up to a total of 10 mg/day.

ethacrynate sodium (Sodium Edecrin) and **ethacrynic acid** (Edecrin). These loop diuretics are used to treat acute pulmonary edema and other forms of edema.
Usual adult dosage: for acute pulmonary edema, 50 to 100 mg of ethacrynate sodium I.V., infused slowly over several minutes; for other forms of edema, 50 to 200 mg of ethacrynic acid P.O. once daily, after meals or on alternate days, or up to 200 mg b.i.d. if needed to obtain a therapeutic effect.
Usual pediatric dosage: for edema, initially, 25 mg of ethacrynic acid P.O. daily, gradually increased, if needed, in 25-mg increments until the therapeutic effect is obtained.

furosemide (Lasix). Used primarily to treat acute pulmonary edema and other forms of edema, furosemide also is used to treat hypertensive crisis, acute and chronic renal failure, hypertension, and hypercalcemia (because it promotes urinary calcium excretion). Furosemide can cause profound water and electrolyte depletion.
Usual adult dosage: for acute pulmonary edema, 40 mg I.V. injected slowly, then repeated every 2 hours as needed; for other forms of edema, 20 to 80 mg P.O. daily or b.i.d., up to 600 mg/day, or 20 to 40 mg I.M. or I.V. with repeated doses of 20 mg every 2 hours until the therapeutic effect is achieved; for hypertensive crisis and acute renal failure, 100 to 200 mg I.V. over 1 to 2 minutes; for chronic renal

failure, initially, 80 mg P.O. daily, increased up to 120 mg/day until the therapeutic effect is achieved; for hypertension, 20 to 80 mg P.O. daily.

Usual pediatric dosage: for edema, 2 mg/kg P.O. daily with an increase of 1 to 2 mg/kg in 6 to 8 hours if needed, up to 6 mg/kg/day; or 1 mg/kg I.V. or I.M., titrated as needed to a maximum of 6 mg/kg/day.

Drug interactions
Various drugs—including aminoglycosides, cardiac glycosides, oral hypoglycemics, and nonsteroidal anti-inflammatory drugs (NSAIDs)—interact with loop diuretics, causing altered renal function, fluid and electrolyte imbalances, and specific enhanced drug effects. (For details, see *Drug interactions: Loop diuretics,* page 572.)

ADVERSE DRUG REACTIONS

The adverse drug reactions to loop diuretics may be severe because of the potent effects of these drugs. The most severe reactions involve frequently occurring fluid and electrolyte imbalances.

Common adverse reactions to the loop diuretics include volume depletion (especially in elderly patients), orthostatic hypotension, hypokalemia, hypochloremia, hypochloremic alkalosis, asymptomatic hyperuricemia, hyponatremia, hypocalcemia, and hypomagnesemia. Transient deafness, abdominal discomfort or pain, diarrhea, impaired glucose tolerance, dermatitis, paresthesia, hepatic dysfunction, and thrombocytopenia also can occur. Furosemide toxicity may produce such adverse reactions as tinnitus, abdominal pain, sore throat, and fever.

Hypersensitivity reactions include purpura, photosensitivity, rash, pruritus, urticaria, necrotizing angiitis, exfoliative dermatitis, allergic interstitial nephritis, and erythema multiforme. Agranulocytosis also can occur.

NURSING PROCESS APPLICATION

The following information assists the nurse in caring for a patient who is receiving a loop diuretic.

Assessment
• Review the patient's history for a preexisting condition that contraindicates the use of a loop diuretic, such as anuria, hepatic coma, severe electrolyte depletion, or known hypersensitivity to loop diuretics.
• Review the patient's history for a preexisting condition that requires cautious use of a loop diuretic, such as pregnancy or severe renal disease.
• Assess the patient for adverse reactions to the prescribed loop diuretic, such as volume depletion, fluid and electrolyte imbalances, GI distress, or impaired glucose tolerance.

• Review the patient's medication history to identify the use of drugs that may interact with the loop diuretic, such as oral hypoglycemic agents, oral hypoglycemics, aminoglycosides, and NSAIDs.
• Assess the effectiveness of the loop diuretic periodically.
• Assess the patient's urine elimination pattern during loop diuretic therapy.
• Assess the patient frequently for signs and symptoms of dehydration, such as poor skin turgor and dry oral mucous membranes.
• Evaluate the patient's and family's knowledge about the prescribed loop diuretic.

Nursing diagnoses
The following examples represent appropriate nursing diagnoses for a patient receiving a loop diuretic.
• Potential for injury related to a preexisting condition that contraindicates the use of a loop diuretic
• Potential for injury related to a preexisting condition that requires cautious use of a loop diuretic
• Potential for injury related to adverse drug reactions
• Altered urinary elimination related to the genitourinary effects of a loop diuretic
• Potential fluid volume deficit related to use of a loop diuretic
• Knowledge deficit related to the prescribed loop diuretic

Planning and implementation
• Do not administer a loop diuretic to a patient with a condition that contraindicates its use.
• Administer a loop diuretic cautiously to a patient at risk because of a preexisting condition.
• Monitor the patient frequently for adverse reactions to the prescribed loop diuretic.
• Expect to switch to bumetanide as prescribed in a patient who experiences a hypersensitivity reaction to furosemide.
• Monitor the patient's serum electrolyte levels frequently.
• *Be especially alert for changes in the patient's serum potassium level and observe for signs and symptoms of hypokalemia, such as drowsiness, paresthesia, muscle cramps, and hyporeflexia.*
• *Administer potassium supplements as prescribed to maintain an acceptable serum potassium level.*
• Monitor the patient's pulse and serum digoxin or digitoxin level frequently during concomitant cardiac glycoside therapy to detect digitalis toxicity.
• *Weigh the patient daily under controlled conditions (at the same time in the morning, after the patient voids, before the patient eats, with the patient wearing similar clothing at each weigh-in, and on the same scale).*
• Take the patient's vital signs and auscultate breath sounds frequently to assess the effectiveness of loop diuretic therapy.

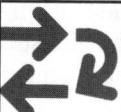

DRUG INTERACTIONS
Loop diuretics

Drug interactions with loop diuretics can alter renal function, cause fluid and electrolyte imbalances, and enhance certain effects of the drug.

DRUG	INTERACTING DRUGS	POSSIBLE EFFECTS	NURSING IMPLICATIONS
bumetanide, ethacrynate sodium, ethacrynic acid, furosemide	oral hypoglycemic agents	May cause hyperglycemia	• Monitor the patient's serum glucose level. • Monitor the patient for signs and symptoms of hyperglycemia, such as thirst and lethargy.
	aminoglycosides	May cause ototoxicity	• Exercise extreme caution when administering these drugs together. • Monitor the patient's auditory acuity.
	lithium carbonate	Decrease excretion, resulting in lithium toxicity	• Monitor the patient for signs and symptoms of lithium toxicity, such as ataxia. • Monitor the patient's serum lithium level.
	cisplatin	Causes additive ototoxicity	• Monitor the patient's auditory acuity.
	cardiac glycosides	Cause electrolyte disturbances that may predispose the patient to digitalis-induced arrhythmias	• Measure plasma levels of potassium and magnesium. • Monitor the patient's ECG and check the pulse rate and rhythm periodically.
	nonsteroidal anti-inflammatory agents	Inhibit antihypertensive and diuretic effects	• Monitor the patient's fluid intake and output, daily weight, and blood pressure.
furosemide	neuromuscular blocking agents	Enhances neuromuscular blockade	• Monitor for prolonged effects of the neuromuscular blocking agent. • Administer with caution to a patient with decreased renal function.
	phenytoin	Decreases furosemide absorption and effectiveness	• Monitor the patient's response to furosemide.

• Monitor uric acid levels for a patient with a history of gout to detect drug-induced hyperuricemia.

• *Have the patient sit up a few minutes before standing to minimize the effects of orthostatic hypotension.*

• Monitor a diabetic patient's blood glucose level carefully during loop diuretic therapy.

• Check the bumetanide dosage with extreme care; this drug is 40 times more potent than furosemide.

• Do not administer ethacrynate sodium or ethacrynic acid by I.M. or S.C. injection, to avoid tissue irritation.

• Administer I.M. furosemide using the Z-track method to minimize tissue irritation.

• *Administer an I.V. loop diuretic slowly over 1 to 2 minutes to prevent adverse reactions.*

• Store oral furosemide tablets and injectable furosemide in light-resistant containers to prevent discoloration.

• Refrigerate oral furosemide solutions to ensure stability. Do not use discolored (yellow) injectable furosemide solutions.

• Notify the physician if adverse reactions occur.

• Document the patient's fluid intake and output to detect alterations in urine elimination.

• Keep a urinal or bedpan within reach for a bedridden patient; ensure that the bathroom is easily accessible for an ambulatory patient.

• *Administer the loop diuretic in the morning or early afternoon, if permissible, to prevent nocturia from upsetting the patient's normal sleep pattern.*

• Monitor the patient for signs of dehydration, such as poor skin turgor and dry oral mucous membranes.

• Monitor the patient's vital signs to detect evidence of hypovolemia, such as tachycardia, hypotension, and dyspnea. If such evidence appears, notify the physician.

• Monitor the patient's fluid intake and output. If extreme discrepancies occur, notify the physician and expect to decrease the diuretic dosage, as prescribed.

• Administer fluids, blood, blood products, or plasma expanders as prescribed to replace lost fluids and facilitate movement of extracellular fluid into the intravascular space.

Patient teaching
• Teach the patient and family the name, dose, frequency, action, and adverse effects of the prescribed loop diuretic.
• Advise the female patient to tell the physician if she is pregnant or plans to become pregnant during loop diuretic therapy.
• Inform the patient that periodic blood tests must be performed to detect imbalances caused by loop diuretic therapy.
• *Teach the patient to recognize and report to the physician the signs of hypokalemia.*
• *Explain the importance of taking potassium supplements, if prescribed, and eating a potassium-rich diet. Give the patient a list of potassium-rich foods.* (For a list, see *Guide to potassium-rich foods,* page 569.)
• Teach the patient receiving concomitant cardiac glycoside therapy to identify the signs of digitalis toxicity, such as GI, cardiac, and neurologic disturbances.
• Instruct the diabetic patient receiving a loop diuretic to monitor the blood glucose level closely. Advise this patient that diabetes treatment may require adjustment during loop diuretic therapy.
• *Instruct the patient to take the diuretic in the morning or early afternoon, if permissible, to avoid nocturia.*
• *Teach the patient to obtain a daily weight under the same conditions every time and to notify the physician of any sudden weight gain (greater than 2 pounds in 1 day), peripheral edema, or shortness of breath.*
• Teach the patient how to minimize the effects of orthostatic hypotension.
• *Advise the patient to expect an increase in urinary frequency and amount voided.*
• Instruct the patient taking furosemide to report to the physician any signs of furosemide toxicity, such as tinnitus, abdominal pain, sore throat, and fever.
• Instruct the patient to store furosemide tablets in light-resistant containers to prevent discoloration.
• Instruct the patient to notify the physician if adverse reactions occur or if concerns arise about loop diuretic therapy.

Evaluation
The following examples represent appropriate evaluation statements for a patient receiving a loop diuretic.
• The patient has no conditions that contraindicate loop diuretic therapy.
• The patient exhibits no signs of complications in the preexisting condition linked to the prescribed loop diuretic.
• The patient experiences no adverse reactions to the prescribed loop diuretic.

• The patient urinates more frequently during loop diuretic therapy.
• The patient displays no signs of dehydration during loop diuretic therapy.
• The patient and family express an accurate understanding of the points taught about the prescribed loop diuretic.
• The patient correctly identifies signs of hypokalemia and describes what to do if they occur.

POTASSIUM-SPARING DIURETICS

Potassium-sparing diuretics have weaker diuretic and antihypertensive effects than other diuretics, but they have the advantage of conserving potassium. Therefore, they commonly are used with other antihypertensive agents. Whenever these diuretics are administered, however, the nurse must monitor the patient closely for hyperkalemia. The potassium-sparing diuretics include amiloride, spironolactone, and triamterene.

PHARMACOKINETICS

Potassium-sparing diuretics are administered orally and are absorbed in the GI tract. They are metabolized in the liver except for amiloride, which is not metabolized, and are excreted primarily in the urine and bile. These diuretics have a rapid onset of action, and their duration of action increases with multiple doses.

Absorption, distribution, metabolism, excretion
After oral administration, absorption of the potassium-sparing diuretics varies from more than 90% for spironolactone to 50% for triamterene and 20% for amiloride. Triamterene is absorbed erratically, depending on the dosage form, and has a variable bioavailability. The drugs are distributed widely in body fluids and tissues. Spironolactone is more than 90% bound to plasma proteins; triamterene is 60% protein bound, and amiloride is about 23% protein bound.

After extensive first-pass metabolism, spironolactone undergoes enterohepatic circulation. Triamterene also is metabolized extensively by the liver, but amiloride is not metabolized at all.

Spironolactone and triamterene are excreted as metabolites via the urine and feces, with very little of either drug being excreted unchanged. From 20% to 50% of amiloride is excreted unchanged in the urine, and 40% is excreted unchanged in the feces.

Onset, peak, duration

The onset of action for amiloride occurs in 2 hours; for spironolactone and triamterene, in 2 to 4 hours. Amiloride reaches a peak concentration level in 3 to 4 hours; spironolactone, in 1 to 2 hours; spironolactone metabolites, in 2 to 4 hours; and triamterene, in 2 to 4 hours. The duration of action of amiloride is 24 hours; of spironolactone, 48 to 72 hours; of triamterene, 12 to 16 hours. For all three drugs, duration may increase with multiple doses and prolonged therapy.

After a single oral dose in a healthy adult, spironolactone has an average half-life of 1.3 to 2 hours. The half-lives of its active metabolites canrenone and 7-thiomethyl spironolactone are 13 to 24 hours and 2.8 hours respectively. Amiloride's half-life is 6 to 9 hours; triamterene's, 100 to 150 minutes.

PHARMACODYNAMICS

The potassium-sparing diuretics act in the distal renal tubules. Water and sodium are excreted, and potassium is retained.

Mechanism of action

The direct action of the potassium-sparing diuretics on the distal renal tubules produces mild diuretic and antihypertensive effects that increase the urinary excretion of sodium, chloride, and calcium ions and reduce the excretion of potassium and hydrogen ions. These effects lead to increased serum potassium levels and urine pH. Amiloride and spironolactone do not depress the GFR, but triamterene does.

Amiloride and triamterene do not inhibit aldosterone or carbonic anhydrase, but spironolactone is an aldosterone antagonist. When hypovolemia, hyponatremia, hyperkalemia, or renin release leads to aldosterone secretion, metabolic alkalosis and potassium depletion may occur. Spironolactone counteracts these effects by competing with aldosterone for receptor sites and blocking the action of aldosterone on the distal tubules. As a result, sodium, chloride, and water are excreted and potassium is retained.

PHARMACOTHERAPEUTICS

Potassium-sparing diuretics commonly are used with other diuretics to potentiate their action or to counteract their potassium-wasting effects. Potassium-sparing diuretics are used primarily to treat edema (including refractory edema) and diuretic-induced hypokalemia in patients with CHF, cirrhosis, nephrotic syndrome, or hypertension. Spironolactone also is used to treat hyperaldosteronism and hirsutism, including hirsutism associated with polycystic ovary syndrome.

amiloride hydrochloride (Midamor). Amiloride usually is used with a thiazide or loop diuretic to treat hypertension or edema associated with CHF and to help restore normal serum potassium levels in patients with hypokalemia. Currently, researchers are investigating an amiloride aerosol to treat lung disease in cystic fibrosis.

Usual adult dosage: initially, 5 to 10 mg P.O. daily taken with food; increased up to 20 mg/day, if needed.

spironolactone (Aldactone). This diuretic is used to treat primary aldosteronism, essential hypertension, refractory edema, cirrhosis, nephrotic syndrome, and idiopathic edema. Spironolactone may be used with other drugs to potentiate their action or to decrease potassium loss. This drug also has been used investigationally to treat hirsutism in women with polycystic ovary syndrome or idiopathic hirsutism.

Usual adult dosage: for essential hypertension, initially, 50 to 100 mg P.O. daily; for edema, initially, 25 to 200 mg P.O. daily; the dosage may be given as a single dose or in two divided doses and may be adjusted up to 400 mg P.O. daily, according to the patient's response.

Usual pediatric dosage: for edema, initially, 3.3 mg/kg P.O. daily in divided doses.

triamterene (Dyrenium). This potassium-sparing diuretic usually is used with other diuretics to treat hypertension. Triamterene also is used to treat the edema associated with CHF, cirrhosis, and nephrotic syndrome as well as idiopathic edema, steroid-induced edema, and edema from hyperaldosteronism.

Usual adult dosage: initially, 100 mg P.O. b.i.d. after meals; the dosage may be adjusted for therapeutic effect but must not exceed 300 mg/day.

Usual pediatric dosage: initially, 4 mg/kg P.O. daily in two divided doses, increased to 6 mg/kg P.O. daily, if needed. The dosage should not exceed 30 mg/day.

Drug interactions

Few drug interactions are associated with the use of amiloride, spironolactone, and triamterene. Those that do occur are related to the potassium-sparing effects. (For details, see *Drug interactions: Potassium-sparing diuretics.*)

ADVERSE DRUG REACTIONS

Few adverse drug reactions occur with the potassium-sparing diuretics. However, their potassium-sparing effects can lead to hyperkalemia, especially if a potassium-sparing diuretic is given with a potassium supplement or a high-potassium diet.

Other dose-related reactions to potassium-sparing diuretics include megaloblastic anemia (especially with

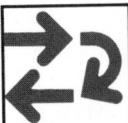

DRUG INTERACTIONS

Potassium-sparing diuretics

The drug interactions that occur with these diuretics may be related to their potassium-sparing effects. The nurse must observe patients receiving potassium-sparing diuretics for signs and symptoms of hyperkalemia.

DRUG	INTERACTING DRUGS	POSSIBLE EFFECTS	NURSING IMPLICATIONS
amiloride, spirono-lactone, triamterene	potassium supplements, other potassium-sparing diuretics, angiotensin-converting enzyme (ACE) inhibitors (captopril, enalapril, lisinopril)	May cause hyperkalemia	• Monitor the patient for signs and symptoms of hyperkalemia. Advise the patient not to use a potassium-based salt substitute.
spironolactone	cardiac glycosides	Decreases renal excretion of cardiac glycosides	• Monitor the patient for signs and symptoms of digitalis toxicity, such as nausea and yellow vision. • Monitor the patient's serum digoxin or digitoxin level.
	salicylates	Reduce clinical effects of spironolactone	• Monitor the patient's fluid intake and output and serum potassium level.

triamterene), dizziness, orthostatic hypotension, sore throat, dry mouth, nausea, and vomiting.

Amiloride may produce headache, nausea, vomiting, anorexia, diarrhea, muscle cramps, abdominal pain, constipation, impotence, and metabolic disturbances, including volume depletion, hyponatremia, a transient rise in the BUN level, and acidosis. Spironolactone may produce headache, abdominal cramps, diarrhea, gynecomastia in men, breast soreness and menstrual abnormalities in women, and rarely, agranulocytosis.

Hypersensitivity reactions to potassium-sparing diuretics include urticaria, pruritus, erythematous eruptions, rash, photosensitivity, and anaphylaxis.

NURSING PROCESS APPLICATION

The following information assists the nurse in caring for a patient who is receiving a potassium-sparing diuretic.

Assessment
• Review the patient's history for a preexisting condition that contraindicates the use of a potassium-sparing diuretic, such as anuria, hyperkalemia, impaired renal function, lactation, and known hypersensitivity to potassium-sparing diuretics.
• Review the patient's history for a preexisting condition that requires cautious use of a potassium-sparing diuretic, such as pregnancy or serious illness with increased risk of respiratory or metabolic acidosis.
• Assess the patient for adverse reactions to the prescribed potassium-sparing diuretic, such as hyperkalemia, mega-

loblastic anemia, dizziness, orthostatic hypotension, sore throat, dry mouth, and GI distress.
• Review the patient's medication history to identify the use of drugs that may interact with the potassium-sparing diuretic, such as potassium supplements, other potassium-sparing diuretics, angiotensin-converting enzyme (ACE) inhibitors, cardiac glycosides, or salicylates.
• Assess the effectiveness of the prescribed potassium-sparing diuretic periodically.
• Assess the patient's urine elimination pattern.
• Evaluate the patient's and family's knowledge about the prescribed potassium-sparing diuretic.

Nursing diagnoses
The following examples represent appropriate nursing diagnoses for a patient receiving a potassium-sparing diuretic.
• Potential for injury related to a preexisting condition that contraindicates the use of a potassium-sparing diuretic
• Potential for injury related to a preexisting condition that requires cautious use of a potassium-sparing diuretic
• Potential for injury related to adverse drug reactions
• Potential fluid volume deficit related to the adverse GI effects of the prescribed potassium-sparing diuretic
• Altered urinary elimination related to the genitourinary effects of the prescribed potassium-sparing diuretic
• Knowledge deficit related to the prescribed potassium-sparing diuretic

Planning and implementation

• Do not administer a potassium-sparing diuretic to a patient with a condition that contraindicates its use.

• Administer a potassium-sparing diuretic cautiously to a patient at risk because of a preexisting condition.

• Monitor the patient frequently for adverse reactions to the prescribed potassium-sparing diuretic.

• *Monitor the patient for signs and symptoms of hyperkalemia, such as confusion, hyperexcitability, muscle weakness, paresthesia, flaccid paralysis, arrhythmias, abdominal distention, diarrhea, and intestinal colic.*

• Monitor the patient's serum electrolyte levels for any imbalances.

• Monitor the patient's complete blood count for blood dyscrasias, such as megaloblastic anemia.

• *Weigh the patient daily under controlled conditions (at the same time each morning, after the patient voids, before the patient eats, with the patient wearing similar clothing at each weigh-in, and on the same scale).*

• Monitor the patient's vital signs and auscultate the lungs frequently to assess the effectiveness of the potassium-sparing diuretic.

• Monitor the patient's supine and standing blood pressures to assess for orthostatic hypotension.

• *Have the patient sit up for a few minutes before standing to minimize the effects of orthostatic hypotension.*

• Store spironolactone in a dark container away from light.

• Administer amiloride with food; give triamterene after meals.

• Notify the physician if adverse reactions occur.

• Observe the patient with nausea, vomiting, or diarrhea for signs of dehydration, such as dry mucous membranes, poor skin turgor, and decreased urine output.

• Give the patient sips of water or other fluids every hour to combat dehydration.

• Notify the physician if the patient experiences GI distress. Obtain a prescription for an antiemetic or antidiarrheal agent, if needed.

• Document the patient's fluid intake and output to detect alterations in urine elimination.

• Keep the urinal or bedpan within reach for a bedridden patient; ensure that the bathroom is easily accessible for an ambulatory patient.

• *Administer a potassium-sparing diuretic in the morning or early afternoon, if permissible, to avoid nocturia.*

Patient teaching

• Teach the patient and family the name, dose, frequency, action, and adverse effects of the prescribed potassium-sparing diuretic.

• Instruct the patient to expect an increase in urinary frequency and amount voided.

• Advise the female patient to tell the physician if she is pregnant or plans to become pregnant during potassium-sparing diuretic therapy.

• Inform the patient that periodic blood tests must be performed to detect imbalances caused by the potassium-sparing diuretic.

• *Teach the patient to recognize and report to the physician the signs of hyperkalemia.*

• *Advise the patient to avoid eating potassium-rich foods because these diuretics conserve potassium.*

• *Instruct the patient to take the potassium-sparing diuretic in the morning or early afternoon, if permissible, to avoid nocturia.*

• *Teach the patient to obtain a daily weight under the same conditions every time and to notify the physician of any sudden weight gain (greater than 2 pounds in 1 day), peripheral edema, or shortness of breath.*

• Teach the patient how to minimize the effects of orthostatic hypotension.

• Teach the patient how to manage minor adverse reactions, such as dry mouth (by chewing sugarless gum or sucking on sugarless hard candy) and constipation (by increasing fiber intake and exercise).

• Instruct the patient to ask the physician to recommend an analgesic if headaches occur.

• Inform the patient that amiloride-induced impotence may occur but should subside when the drug is discontinued.

• Instruct the patient to notify the physician if adverse reactions occur or if concerns arise about diuretic therapy.

Evaluation

The following examples represent appropriate evaluation statements for a patient receiving a potassium-sparing diuretic.

• The patient has no conditions that contraindicate the use of a potassium-sparing diuretic.

• The patient exhibits no signs of complications in the preexisting condition linked to the prescribed potassium-sparing diuretic.

• The patient experiences no adverse reactions to the prescribed potassium-sparing diuretic.

• The patient remains well-hydrated during diuretic therapy.

• The patient urinates more frequently during potassium-sparing diuretic therapy.

• The patient and family express an accurate understanding of the points taught about the prescribed potassium-sparing diuretic.

• The patient schedules follow-up visits for blood tests, as instructed.

OSMOTIC DIURETICS

Osmotic diuretics are low-molecular-weight substances that increase the osmolality of the plasma, glomerular filtrate, and tubular fluid by remaining in high concentrations in the renal tubules. This action decreases sodium, chloride, and water resorption, thereby increasing their excretion. (Potassium excretion is increased slightly.)

The osmotic diuretics are used primarily to prevent oliguria and acute renal failure but also to reduce increased intracranial and intraocular pressure and to treat certain forms of drug intoxication. Because they remain effective in patients with compromised renal circulation, mannitol and urea are the primary osmotic diuretics used clinically today.

PHARMACOKINETICS

After I.V. administration, mannitol and urea are distributed rapidly and are excreted primarily unchanged in the urine.

Absorption, distribution, metabolism, excretion

Mannitol and urea are distributed rapidly to the extracellular fluid after I.V. administration. Only 7% to 10% of a mannitol dose is metabolized. About 7% of a mannitol dose and 50% of a urea dose are resorbed by the renal tubules. They are filtered primarily by the glomeruli and excreted largely unchanged in the urine. In a patient with severe renal insufficiency, the excretion rate is reduced; the resulting retention of the osmotic diuretic increases extracellular tonicity, expanding the extracellular fluid and inducing hyponatremia.

Onset, peak, duration

When administered in the dosages used to decrease intraocular pressure, the onset of action of mannitol and urea occurs within 15 minutes. The peak concentration level for mannitol is reached in 30 minutes to 1 hour; of urea, in 1 to 2 hours. The duration of action of mannitol is 4 to 8 hours; of urea, 5 to 6 hours.

Diuresis occurs in 1 to 3 hours after mannitol administration and in 1 to 2 hours after urea administration. When administered in the dosages used to reduce intracranial pressure, the duration of mannitol is 3 to 8 hours; of urea, 3 to 10 hours. The half-life of mannitol is from 15 to 100 minutes; of urea, about 70 minutes.

PHARMACODYNAMICS

Osmotic diuretics act by increasing the osmolality of the plasma, glomerular filtrate, and tubular fluid. That decreases the resorption of fluid and electrolytes, increasing the excretion of water, chloride, and sodium and slightly increasing the excretion of potassium.

Osmotic diuretics are therapeutically effective because they are filtered freely at the glomeruli and are resorbed somewhat by the renal tubules, thus maintaining high concentration levels there. The drugs also are inert pharmacologically and resistant to extensive metabolism.

PHARMACOTHERAPEUTICS

Mannitol and urea primarily are used to reduce intracranial pressure and to prevent acute renal failure. They are effective even in a patient with compromised renal circulation.

mannitol (Osmitrol). Used primarily to prevent oliguria and acute renal failure, mannitol also is used to treat oliguria, increased intracranial pressure, increased intraocular pressure, and drug intoxication from secobarbital, imipramine, aspirin, or carbon tetrachloride. Mannitol also is used with sorbitol as a urogenital irrigation for patients experiencing a transurethral prostatic resection; this combination minimizes the hemolytic effects of water. (For additional information on the use of mannitol for increased intraocular pressure, see Chapter 71, Ophthalmic Agents.)
Usual adult dosage: for oliguria and prevention of acute renal failure, 50 to 100 grams I.V. of 5% to 25% solution; to reduce intracranial or intraocular pressure, 1.5 to 2 grams/kg I.V. of 15% to 20% solution infused over 30 to 60 minutes; for preoperative intraocular medication, give 1 to 1½ hours before surgery; for drug intoxication, maximum dosage of 200 grams I.V. of 5% to 10% solution over a 24-hour period; for urogenital irrigation with sorbitol, a test dose of 200 mg/kg I.V. infused over 3 to 5 minutes to elicit a urine flow of 30 to 50 ml/hour, may be repeated once.

urea (Aquacara, Carbamide, Ureaphil, Ureuert). Urea is used primarily to reduce increased intracranial and intraocular pressure and to prevent acute renal failure during prolonged surgery or trauma.
Usual adult dosage: 1 to 1.5 grams/kg I.V. of 30% solution, infused over 1½ to 2 hours, up to a maximum dosage of 120 grams/day.
Usual pediatric dosage: over age 2, 0.5 to 1.5 grams/kg I.V. of a 30% solution infused over 1½ to 2 hours; ages 2 and under, 0.1 to 0.5 gram/kg I.V. of a 30% solution infused over 1½ to 2 hours.

Drug interactions

No significant drug interactions occur with the use of mannitol or urea.

ADVERSE DRUG REACTIONS

Common adverse reactions to the osmotic diuretics include transient expansion of plasma volume during infusion, resulting in circulatory overload and tachycardia, electrolyte imbalances, volume depletion, cellular dehydration, headache, nausea, and vomiting. These drugs can produce local irritation at the infusion site if extravasation occurs and may lead to thrombophlebitis. Mannitol may cause rebound increased intracranial pressure 8 to 12 hours after diuresis and anginalike chest pain, blurred vision, rhinitis, thirst, and urine retention. Other adverse reactions to the osmotic diuretics include hypersensitivity reactions and thrombophlebitis.

NURSING PROCESS APPLICATION

The following information assists the nurse in caring for a patient who is receiving an osmotic diuretic.

Assessment
• Review the patient's history for a preexisting condition that contraindicates the use of an osmotic diuretic, such as anuria, severe pulmonary congestion, severe CHF, severe dehydration, or known hypersensitivity to osmotic diuretics.
• Review the patient's history for a preexisting condition that requires cautious use of an osmotic diuretic, such as pregnancy.
• Assess the patient for adverse reactions to the prescribed osmotic diuretic, such as circulatory overload, electrolyte imbalances, volume depletion, headache, nausea, or vomiting.
• Assess the effectiveness of the prescribed osmotic diuretic hourly.
• Evaluate the patient's and family's knowledge about the prescribed osmotic diuretic.

Nursing diagnoses
The following examples represent appropriate nursing diagnoses for a patient receiving an osmotic diuretic.
• Potential for injury related to a preexisting condition that contraindicates the use of an osmotic diuretic
• Potential for injury related to a preexisting condition that requires cautious use of an osmotic diuretic
• Potential for injury related to adverse drug reactions
• Knowledge deficit related to the prescribed osmotic diuretic

Planning and implementation
• Do not administer an osmotic diuretic to a patient with a condition that contraindicates its use.
• Administer an osmotic diuretic cautiously to a patient at risk because of a preexisting condition.
• Monitor the patient closely for adverse drug reactions.
• Monitor the patient for imbalances of serum electrolytes, particularly sodium, potassium, chloride, creatinine, and BUN.
• Measure the patient's vital signs hourly during osmotic diuretic therapy.
• *Document the patient's fluid intake and output hourly because therapy is based on the hourly urine flow rate.*
• *Monitor the patient for circulatory overload if the urine output is less than 30 to 50 ml/hour.*
• Observe the patient receiving mannitol for at least 12 hours after diuresis to detect rebound increased intracranial pressure.
• Administer mannitol 1 to 1½ hours before surgery when it is used as a preoperative medication.
• Expect to give a test dose of mannitol as prescribed to a patient undergoing a transurethral prostatic resection. Infuse mannitol with sorbitol over 3 to 5 minutes to elicit a urine flow of 30 to 50 ml/hour for urogenital irrigation.
• Observe I.V. administration sites for local irritation, extravasation, or signs of thrombophlebitis.
• *Redissolve parenteral mannitol, which crystallizes at low temperatures, by warming it in a hot-water bath and shaking the container vigorously. Then let the solution return to room temperature before administration. Do not administer crystallized medication.*
• Administer mannitol at the prescribed rate using an in-line I.V. filter.
• *Do not add blood products to I.V. lines used for mannitol administration because they are incompatible.*
• Store mannitol at 59° to 86° F (15° to 30° C) unless otherwise directed, and do not allow it to freeze.
• Promote mouth care and offer ice chips to relieve the patient's thirst.
• Notify the physician if adverse reactions occur.

Patient teaching
• Teach the patient and family the name, dose, frequency, action, and adverse effects of the prescribed osmotic diuretic.
• *Instruct the patient to notify the nurse if anginalike chest pain occurs during mannitol therapy.*
• Reassure the patient that blurred vision, rhinitis, and thirst should subside when mannitol is discontinued.
• Advise the patient that vital signs will be checked and the urinary catheter will be drained every hour to monitor the effectiveness of diuretic therapy.
• Explain the need for frequent blood tests to monitor for diuretic-induced electrolyte imbalances.

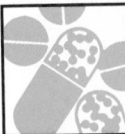

Diuretic agents

This chart summarizes the major diuretic agents currently in clinical use.

DRUG	MAJOR INDICATIONS	USUAL ADULT DOSAGES	CONTRAINDICATIONS AND PRECAUTIONS
Thiazide and thiazide-like diuretics			
benzthiazide	Edema Hypertension	50 to 200 mg P.O. daily or in divided doses 50 mg P.O. daily to b.i.d., depending on patient's response	• Know that benzthiazide is contraindicated in a patient with anuria or known hypersensitivity to this drug or other sulfonamide derivatives. • Administer with caution to a pregnant or lactating patient or one with severe renal disease, impaired hepatic function, or progressive liver disease.
chlorothiazide	Edema Hypertension	500 mg to 2 grams P.O. or I.V. daily or in two divided doses 500 mg to 1 gram P.O. or I.V. daily or in divided doses	• Know that chlorothiazide is contraindicated in a lactating patient or one with anuria or known hypersensitivity to this drug or other sulfonamide derivatives. • Administer with caution to a pregnant patient or one with severe renal disease, impaired hepatic function, or progressive liver disease.
hydrochlorothiazide	Edema Hypertension	25 to 200 mg P.O. daily or intermittently 25 to 100 mg P.O. daily or in divided doses	• Know that hydrochlorothiazide is contraindicated in a lactating patient or one with anuria or known hypersensitivity to this drug or other sulfonamide derivatives. • Administer with caution to a pregnant patient or one with severe renal disease, impaired hepatic function, or progressive liver disease.
metolazone	Edema from congestive heart failure (CHF) Edema from renal or hepatic disease Hypertension	5 to 10 mg P.O. daily 5 to 20 mg P.O. daily 2.5 to 5 mg P.O. daily	• Know that metolazone is contraindicated in a lactating patient or one with anuria, hepatic coma or pre-coma, or known hypersensitivity to this drug. • Administer with caution to a a pregnant patient or one with severely impaired renal function.
Loop diuretics			
bumetanide	Edema and hypertension	0.5 to 2 mg P.O. in a single daily dose or repeated at 4- to 5-hour intervals up to a total of 10 mg/day; maintenance dosages, usually given intermittently with 1- to 2-day rest periods, 0.5 to 1 mg I.M. or I.V. given over 1 to 2 minutes; I.V. doses may be repeated every 2 to 3 hours up to a total of 10 mg/day	• Know that bumetanide is contraindicated in a lactating patient or one with anuria, hepatic coma, severe electrolyte depletion, or known hypersensitivity to this drug. • Administer with caution to a pregnant patient or one with severe renal disease.
ethacrynate sodium, ethacrynic acid	Acute pulmonary edema Other forms of edema	50 to 100 mg of ethacrynate sodium I.V., infused slowly over several minutes 50 to 200 mg of ethacrynic acid P.O. once daily after meals or on alternate days; or up to 200 mg b.i.d. to obtain a therapeutic effect	• Know that ethacrynate sodium and ethacrynic acid are contraindicated in an infant, a lactating patient, or one with anuria or known hypersensitivity to these drugs. • Administer with caution to a pregnant patient, one with advanced cirrhosis of the liver, or one receiving potassium-depleting steroids. *(continued)*

SELECTED MAJOR DRUGS

Diuretic agents *(continued)*

DRUG	MAJOR INDICATIONS	USUAL ADULT DOSAGES	CONTRAINDICATIONS AND PRECAUTIONS
Loop diuretics *(continued)*			
furosemide	Acute pulmonary edema	40 mg I.V. injected slowly, then repeated every 2 hours as needed	• Know that furosemide is contraindicated in a patient with anuria or known hypersensitivity to this drug.
	Other forms of edema	20 to 80 mg P.O. daily or b.i.d., up to 600 mg/day, or 20 to 40 mg I.M. or I.V. with repeated doses of 20 mg every 2 hours until the therapeutic effect is reached	• Administer with caution to a pregnant or lactating patient.
	Hypertensive crisis and acute renal failure	100 to 200 mg I.V. over 1 to 2 minutes	
	Chronic renal failure	80 mg P.O. daily initially; increased up to 120 mg/day until the therapeutic effect is achieved	
	Hypertension	20 to 80 mg P.O. daily	
Potassium-sparing diuretics			
amiloride	Hypertension or edema associated with CHF	5 to 10 mg P.O. daily initially; increased up to 20 mg/day if needed	• Know that amiloride is contraindicated in a lactating patient or one with hyperkalemia, therapy with other drugs that prevent potassium excretion, potassium supplementation, impaired renal function, diabetes mellitus, or known hypersensitivity to amiloride. • Administer with caution to a pregnant patient or a severely ill patient who is prone to respiratory or metabolic acidosis.
spironolactone	Essential hypertension	50 to 100 mg P.O. daily in a single dose or two divided doses	• Know that spironolactone is contraindicated in a lactating patient or one with anuria, acute renal insufficiency, significantly impaired renal excretory function, hyperkalemia, therapy with other drugs that prevent potassium excretion, or known hypersensitivity to spironolactone. • Administer with caution to a pregnant patient.
	Edema	25 to 200 mg P.O. daily initially, in a single dose to two divided doses, with the total dosage adjusted according to the patient's response	
Osmotic diuretics			
mannitol	Oliguria or prevention of acute renal failure	50 to 100 grams I.V. of 5% to 25% solution	• Know that mannitol is contraindicated in a patient with severe pulmonary congestion, severe CHF, severe dehydration, metabolic edema associated with capillary fragility or membrane permeability, or known hypersensitivity to mannitol. It also is contraindicated in a patient with anuria caused by severe renal disease or impaired renal function who does not respond to a test dose of mannitol. • Administer with caution to a pregnant patient.
	Increased intracranial or intraocular pressure	1.5 to 2 grams/kg I.V. of 15% to 20% solution infused over 30 to 60 minutes; if preoperative medication, give 1 to 1½ hours before surgery	
	Drug intoxication from secobarbital, imipramine, aspirin, or carbon tetrachloride	Up to 200 grams I.V. of 5% to 10% solution over 24 hours	

• Encourage the patient and family to ask questions about the prescribed osmotic diuretic.

Evaluation

The following examples represent appropriate evaluation statements for a patient receiving an osmotic diuretic.

• The patient has no conditions that contraindicate osmotic diuretic therapy.

• The patient exhibits no signs of complications in the preexisting condition linked to the prescribed osmotic diuretic.

• The patient demonstrates no adverse reactions to the prescribed osmotic diuretic.

• The patient and family express an accurate understanding of the points taught about the prescribed osmotic diuretic.

• The patient agrees to notify the nurse if anginalike chest pain occurs.

OTHER DIURETICS

Carbonic anhydrase inhibitors and mercurial diuretics are other agents that may be used to induce diuresis.

Carbonic anhydrase inhibitors. These agents act as enzymatic blocking agents that reverse the hydration of carbon dioxide, producing a bicarbonate diuresis that promotes the excretion of sodium, potassium, and water. Sometimes given with miotics, carbonic anhydrase inhibitors (acetazolamide, dichlorphenamide, and methazolamide) primarily are used to decrease the formation of aqueous humor by the ciliary body and thereby to control the excessive intraocular pressure associated with glaucoma. (For more information, see Chapter 71, Ophthalmic Agents.) Carbonic anhydrase inhibitors also are used to treat edema related to cardiac disorders, periodic paralysis, and acute mountain sickness. They produce few significant drug interactions. Their major adverse reactions include fluid and electrolyte imbalances, especially potassium and bicarbonate depletion.

Mercurial diuretics. These drugs are fast-acting, effective diuretics that served as the major high-ceiling diuretics until the development of the less toxic, more effective loop diuretics in the 1960s. Because mercurial diuretics become inactive in an alkaline environment, acidifying agents often were used with them to enhance diuresis. After administration of a mercurial diuretic, sodium and chloride excretion and bicarbonate retention increase, leading to systemic alkalosis.

Mercurial diuretics no longer are used frequently because of their erratic oral absorption, which necessitates parenteral (usually I.M.) administration. As new diuretics have been introduced, they gradually have replaced the mercurial diuretics.

CHAPTER SUMMARY

Chapter 33 presented thiazide, thiazide-like, loop, potassium-sparing, osmotic, and other diuretic agents as they are used for therapeutic diuresis. Here are the chapter highlights.

• Thiazide and thiazide-like diuretics are sulfonamide derivatives that inhibit sodium resorption, thereby increasing the excretion of water, chloride, sodium, and potassium. They usually are used to treat hypertension and CHF-induced edema.

• Thiazides are ineffective if the patient's GFR is less than 20 ml/minute and therefore usually are ineffective in patients with renal insufficiency. Metolazone, the exception, is effective for patients with mild renal insufficiency.

• Loop diuretics, the most potent diuretics, are effective in treating edema, hypertension, and hypercalcemia and for patients who are resistant to less potent diuretics or who have decreased GFRs. They act directly on the thick ascending loop of Henle, inhibiting sodium and chloride resorption.

• Because of the powerful diuretic qualities associated with the loop diuretics, the risk of hypokalemia is great.

• Potassium-sparing diuretics are less potent than the other diuretics but have the advantage of conserving potassium. Potassium-sparing diuretics usually are used with other diuretic or antihypertensive agents.

• Because the patient may develop hyperkalemia during therapy with potassium-sparing diuretics, the nurse should monitor the patent's serum potassium level; the patient may need a low-potassium diet.

• The osmotic diuretics act by increasing the osmolality of the plasma, glomerular filtrate, and tubular fluid. That decreases the resorption of fluid and electrolytes, increasing the excretion of water, chloride, and sodium and slightly increasing the excretion of potassium. Osmotic diuretics are used to prevent acute renal failure and to reduce increased intracranial or intraocular pressure. Patients receiving osmotic diuretics should be monitored closely for signs of fluid and electrolyte imbalances.

• Other diuretics include carbonic anhydrase inhibitors and mercurial diuretics. Carbonic anhydrase inhibitors are used primarily to treat glaucoma. In most cases, mercurial diuretics have been replaced by newer, safer, more potent diuretics.

• For a patient receiving a diuretic agent, the nurse organizes care according to the nursing process. Care typically includes close monitoring of electrolyte levels, prevention of nocturia, and accurate assessment and documentation of fluid intake, output, and other signs of fluid balance.

STUDY QUESTIONS

See Appendix 1 for answers.

1. Rita Castillo, age 65, has a history of mild hypertension. Her physician prescribes the thiazide diuretic hydrochlorothiazide (HydroDiuril) 25 mg P.O. daily. How do thiazide and thiazide-like diuretics work?
(a) by inhibiting sodium resorption in the distal renal tubule
(b) by acting directly on the ascending limb of the loop of Henle
(c) by increasing the osmotic pressure in the glomerular filtrate
(d) by reversing the hydration of carbon dioxide, causing bicarbonate diuresis

2. After taking hydrochlorothiazide for a month, Ms. Castillo reports muscle cramps, weakness, and drowsiness. These symptoms may signal which adverse reaction?
(a) hyperuricemia
(b) hypophosphatemia
(c) hypokalemia
(d) hypernatremia

3. Alex Goettner, age 63, has been admitted to the hospital for treatment of acute renal failure. Which type of diuretic would be most effective in treating Mr. Goettner?
(a) potassium-sparing diuretic
(b) thiazide diuretic
(c) osmotic diuretic
(d) loop diuretic

4. Mr. Goettner's physician prescribes furosemide (Lasix) 100 mg I.V. over 2 minutes. Because Mr. Goettner also takes an oral hypoglycemic agent for diabetes, the nurse should assess for which potential drug interaction?
(a) hypoglycemia
(b) hyperglycemia
(c) hypersensitivity
(d) hyperosmolarity

5. Arnold Irving, age 55, has cirrhosis of the liver, ascites, and primary aldosteronism. After developing breathing difficulty, he is admitted to the hospital for a paracentesis. His physician prescribes spironolactone (Aldactone) 50 mg P.O. b.i.d. and furosemide (Lasix) 40 mg P.O. b.i.d. Why is spironolactone an ideal diuretic for Mr. Irving?
(a) It reduces potassium levels.
(b) It acts as an aldosterone antagonist.
(c) It is not metabolized in the liver.
(d) It is excreted in the bile.

6. While Mr. Irving is receiving spironolactone, the nurse should assess for which adverse reaction?
(a) hyperkalemia
(b) hypernatremia
(c) hyperglycemia
(d) hypercalcemia

7. Benjamin Horton, age 50, is rushed to the emergency department with head trauma from an automobile accident. To reduce Mr. Horton's intracranial pressure, the physician prescribes mannitol (Osmitrol) 1.5 grams/kg I.V. infused over 60 minutes. While preparing the mannitol, the nurse notices crystals in the solution. How should the nurse proceed?
(a) Warm and shake the bottle to dissolve the crystals.
(b) Administer the solution just as it is.
(c) Send the crystallized solution back to the pharmacy.
(d) Filter out the crystals before administration.

8. Shortly after receiving mannitol, Mr. Horton improves significantly. Twelve hours later, however, his neurologic status begins to deteriorate. What is the most likely cause for this change?
(a) cerebral dehydration
(b) epidural hematoma
(c) hyperosmolality
(d) rebound effect

SELECTED REFERENCES

AHFS drug information 90. (1990). Bethesda, MD: American Society of Hospital Pharmacists.

Culpepper, R. (1987). Which diuretic for which patient? *Patient Care,* 21(20), 103-112.

Drug facts and comparisons. (1991). St. Louis: Facts and Comparisons Division, J.B. Lippincott.

Goodman and Gilman's the pharmacological basis of therapeutics (8th ed.; 1990). Elmsford, NY: Pergamon Press.

Hansten, P., and Horn, J. (1989). *Drug interactions: Clinical significance of drug-drug interactions* (6th ed.). Philadelphia: Lea & Febiger.

Jacobson, J. (1987). Diuretics: Mechanisms of action and uses. *Hospital Practice, 22*(12), 129-149.

Knowles, M., et al. (1990). A pilot study of aerosolized amiloride for the treatment of lung disease in cystic fibrosis. *New England Journal of Medicine, 322*(17), 1189-1194.

North American Nursing Diagnosis Association. (1990). *Taxonomy I-Revised, with official diagnostic categories.* St. Louis: NANDA.

Todd, B. (1989). Diuretics' dangers. Geriatric Nursing, 10(4), 212-214.

ANTILIPEMIC AGENTS

OBJECTIVES

After reading and studying this chapter, the student should be able to:
1. Describe the blood lipid components and lipoproteins.
2. Identify the three major classes of antilipemic drugs and give an example of a drug found in each class.
3. Explain the mechanisms of action for each of the three major classes of antilipemic agents: bile-sequestering agents, fibric acid derivatives, and cholesterol synthesis inhibitors.
4. Describe how the bile-sequestering agents and fibric acid derivatives interact with other drugs.
5. Identify the major adverse reactions for each of the three major classes of antilipemic drugs.
6. Describe how niacin acts as an antilipemic agent, and identify its major adverse reactions.
7. Describe how to apply the nursing process when caring for a patient who is receiving an antilipemic agent.

INTRODUCTION

Antilipemic agents are used to lower abnormally high blood levels of lipids (fatty substances). In normal amounts, lipids help produce energy, maintain body temperature, and provide the chemical precursors of certain body constituents. In abnormally high amounts, lipids allow excess cholesterol to form and deposit in the blood vessels as atherosclerotic plaques. These plaques contribute to hypertension, slow the flow of oxygenated blood to the heart and other body organs, and increase the risk of coronary artery disease (CAD), which kills more than 500,000 people in the United States each year. The risk of CAD directly increases with the blood cholesterol level. (For more information, see *Cholesterol and coronary artery disease.*) Fortunately, reduced cholesterol levels also can reduce the risk of CAD.

Lipids are composed of several different chemicals: free fatty acids (FFAs), triglycerides (glycerol esters of FFAs), sterols (cholesterol and cholesterol esters), and phospholipids (phosphoric acid esters of lipid substances). Lipids

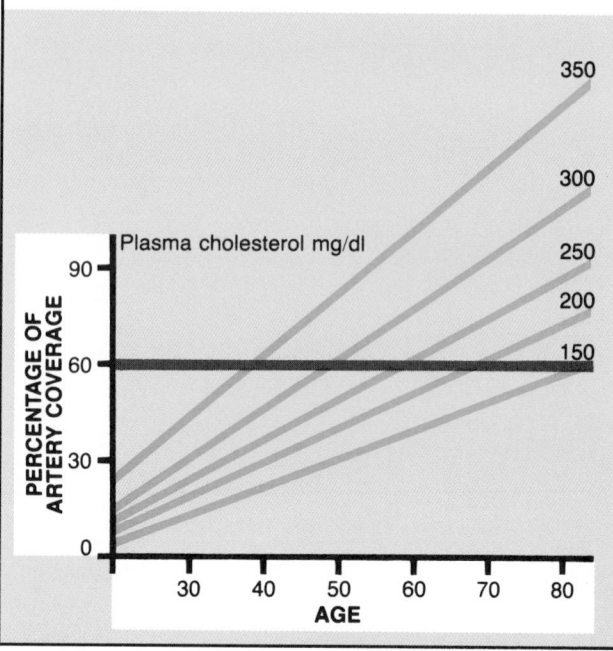

Cholesterol and coronary artery disease

When atherosclerotic plaque occludes 60% or more of the coronary arteries, the risk of coronary artery disease increases dramatically. The graph below shows how artery coverage with plaque increases with age and plasma cholesterol levels.

can be exogenous (derived from the diet) or endogenous (produced by the liver from the end products of lipid and carbohydrate breakdown, or catabolism). The body also produces endogenous lipids through anabolism, a constructive metabolic process that combines substances, such as cholesterol, with other substances.

Combinations of these lipids form various lipoproteins that transport lipids throughout the body: chylomicrons, chylomicron fragments, very-low-density lipoproteins

Lipoprotein synthesis and metabolism

Lipoprotein formation can be exogenous or endogenous. During exogenous formation, lipids enter the circulation from the intestine. During endogenous formation, lipids enter the circulation from the liver. The diagram below illustrates the other differences between exogenous and endogenous lipoprotein formation.

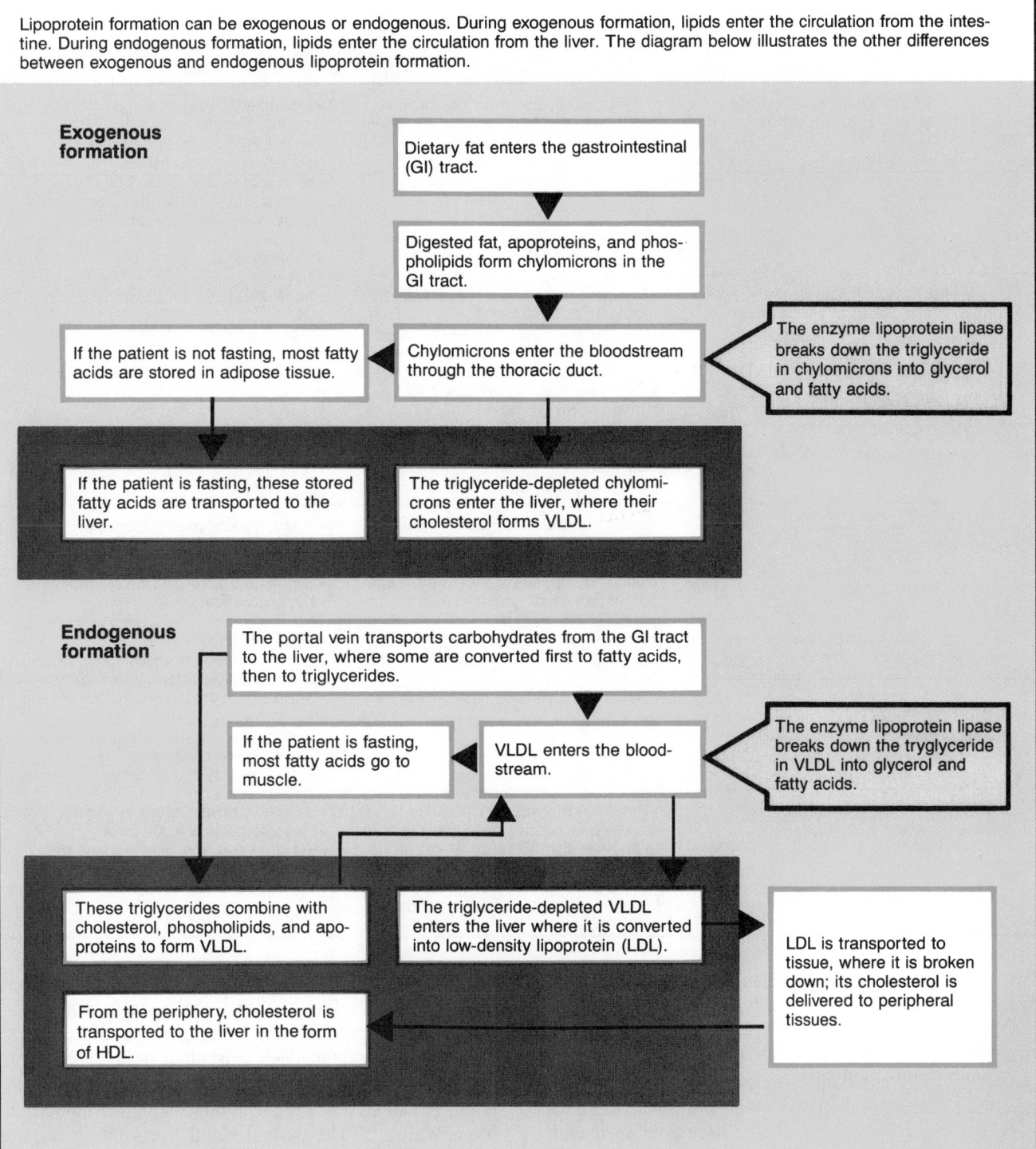

Exogenous formation

Dietary fat enters the gastrointestinal (GI) tract.

Digested fat, apoproteins, and phospholipids form chylomicrons in the GI tract.

If the patient is not fasting, most fatty acids are stored in adipose tissue.

Chylomicrons enter the bloodstream through the thoracic duct.

The enzyme lipoprotein lipase breaks down the triglyceride in chylomicrons into glycerol and fatty acids.

If the patient is fasting, these stored fatty acids are transported to the liver.

The triglyceride-depleted chylomicrons enter the liver, where their cholesterol forms VLDL.

Endogenous formation

The portal vein transports carbohydrates from the GI tract to the liver, where some are converted first to fatty acids, then to triglycerides.

If the patient is fasting, most fatty acids go to muscle.

VLDL enters the bloodstream.

The enzyme lipoprotein lipase breaks down the tryglyceride in VLDL into glycerol and fatty acids.

These triglycerides combine with cholesterol, phospholipids, and apoproteins to form VLDL.

The triglyceride-depleted VLDL enters the liver where it is converted into low-density lipoprotein (LDL).

LDL is transported to tissue, where it is broken down; its cholesterol is delivered to peripheral tissues.

From the periphery, cholesterol is transported to the liver in the form of HDL.

Types of hyperlipoproteinemia

The causes, incidence, and diagnostic findings vary with the type of hyperlipoproteinemia, as shown in the chart below.

TYPE	CAUSES AND INCIDENCE	DIAGNOSTIC FINDINGS
I (Frederickson's, exogenous hyperlipemia, idiopathic familial hyperlipoproteinemia)	• Deficient or abnormal lipoprotein lipase, resulting in decreased or absent postheparin lipolytic activity • Relatively rare	• Increased chylomicrons; decreased very-low-density lipoproteins (VLDLs), low-density lipoproteins (LDLs), high-density lipoproteins (HDLs) • High serum chylomicron and triglyceride levels; slightly elevated serum cholesterol level; lower serum lipoprotein lipase level • Leukocytosis
IIa (familial hyperbetalipoproteinemia, essential familial hypercholesterolemia)	• Deficient cell surface receptor that regulates LDL degradation and cholesterol synthesis, resulting in increased levels of plasma LDL over joints and pressure points • Onset between ages 10 and 30	• Increased plasma concentrations of LDL • Increased serum cholesterol and triglyceride levels • Amniocentesis shows increased LDL level
IIb (familial combined lipidemia)	• Severe forms are like type IIa; milder forms are associated with obesity or diabetes • Relatively common	• Elevated LDL and VLDL levels
III (familial broad beta disease, xanthoma tuberosum)	• Unknown underlying defect results in deficient conversion of triglyceride-rich VLDL to LDL • Uncommon; usually occurs after age 20 but can occur earlier in men	• Abnormal serum betalipoprotein level • Elevated cholesterol and triglyceride levels • Slightly elevated glucose tolerance • Hyperuricemia
IV (endogenous hypertriglyceridemia, hyperbetalipoproteinemia)	• Usually occurs secondary to obesity, alcoholism, diabetes, or emotional disorders • Relatively common, especially in middle-aged men	• Elevated VLDL level • Abnormal levels of triglycerides in plasma; variable increase in serum • Normal or slightly elevated serum cholesterol level • Mildly abnormal glucose tolerance • Positive family history • Early coronary artery disease
V (mixed hypertriglyceridemia, mixed hyperlipidemia)	• Defective triglyceride clearance causes pancreatitis; usually secondary to another disorder, such as obesity or nephrosis • Uncommon; onset usually occurs in late adolescence or early adulthood	• Increased chylomicrons in plasma • Elevated plasma VLDL level • Elevated serum cholesterol and triglyceride levels

(VLDLs), low-density lipoproteins (LDLs), intermediate-density lipoproteins (IDLs), and high-density lipoproteins (HDLs). HDLs, unlike other lipoproteins, may serve a protective role, clearing cholesterol from body tissues. Chylomicrons are minute lipid particles produced in the small intestine through emulsification with bile salts. Lipoproteins are larger lipid particles that have combined with proteins. (For more information, see *Lipoprotein synthesis and metabolism,* page 585.)

Excess of any type of lipid in the blood is known as hyperlipidemia. Hyperlipoproteinemia, an excess of lipoproteins in the blood, occurs in several forms. (For more information, see *Types of hyperlipoproteinemia.*) Hypercholesterolemia refers to excess cholesterol and its derivatives; hypertriglyceridemia refers to excess triglycerides. Any of these conditions may exist alone or in combination. Any can be familial (hereditary) and exist from early childhood, or can be nonfamilial, producing higher blood lipid levels with age. The normal blood levels for cholesterol and triglycerides vary for men and women of different ages, so the nurse must consider the patient's age and sex when interpreting blood lipid levels.

Drug therapy can reduce cholesterol and other lipid levels, but is not the first treatment of choice. Experts agree

SELECTED NURSING DIAGNOSES

Antilipemic agents

The following nursing diagnoses address representative problems and etiologies that a nurse may encounter when caring for a patient who is receiving an antilipemic agent. Some of these nursing diagnoses contain generalized etiologies, which the nurse must individualize based on the patient's needs. (For some common nursing diagnoses and related interventions for each drug class, see the "Nursing Process Application" sections of this chapter.)

- Altered cardiopulmonary tissue perfusion related to clofibrate-induced thromboembolic events
- Altered health maintenance related to ineffectiveness of the prescribed antilipemic agent
- Altered nutrition: less than body requirements, related to the adverse GI effects of an antilipemic agent
- Altered nutrition: more than body requirements, related to weight gain caused by the fibric acid derivative
- Altered peripheral tissue perfusion related to clofibrate-induced intermittent claudication
- Altered protection related to the adverse hematologic effects of the fibric acid derivative
- Altered protection related to the increased risk of malignant tumors caused by clofibrate therapy
- Body image disturbance related to alopecia, dry skin, brittle hair, and weight gain caused by the fibric acid derivative
- Constipation related to the adverse GI effects of the prescribed antilipemic agent
- Decreased cardiac output related to clofibrate-induced arrhythmias
- Diarrhea related to the adverse GI effects of an antilipemic agent

- Fatigue related to the adverse effects of the bile-sequestering agent
- Impaired physical mobility related to weakness caused by the bile-sequestering agent
- Impaired tissue integrity related to peptic ulceration caused by a bile-sequestering agent
- Knowledge deficit related to the prescribed antilipemic agent
- Noncompliance related to the adverse reactions to and duration of therapy with the antilipemic agent
- Pain related to biliary colic from drug-induced cholelithiasis
- Potential fluid volume deficit related to the adverse GI effects of an antilipemic agent
- Potential for injury related to a preexisting condition that contraindicates the use of an antilipemic agent
- Potential for injury related to a preexisting condition that requires cautious use of an antilipemic agent
- Potential for injury related to adverse drug reactions
- Potential for injury related to drug interactions
- Sensory-perceptual alterations (visual) related to lovastatin-induced lens opacities or blurred vision
- Sexual dysfunction related to the adverse genitourinary effects of the fibric acid derivative

that a patient should follow an initial regimen that combines proper diet, weight loss, appropriate antihypertensive therapy, and exercise. Then, if this regimen does not lower blood lipid levels sufficiently, therapy with antilipemic agents may begin.

The antilipemic agents discussed in this chapter include bile-sequestering agents (cholestyramine and colestipol hydrochloride), fibric acid derivatives (clofibrate and gemfibrozil), cholesterol synthesis inhibitors (lovastatin and probucol), and miscellaneous drugs, such as niacin.

For a summary of representative drugs, see *Selected major drugs: Antilipemic agents,* page 597. For a listing of applicable nursing diagnoses that the nurse may formulate when caring for a patient receiving these agents, see *Selected nursing diagnoses: Antilipemic agents.* For detailed information on applying the nursing process, see Chapter 6, The Nursing Process and Drug Therapy.

BILE-SEQUESTERING AGENTS

Cholestyramine and colestipol are large polymers (combinations of many small molecules) containing negative (anionic) groups. These bile-sequestering agents are anion-exchange resins, because they exchange their anionic groups for similar groups from other molecules that contain carboxylic acid and phenolic acid groups. This chemical activity allows the bile-sequestering agents to remove excess bile acids in the fat depots under the skin.

PHARMACOKINETICS

Because bile-sequestering agents have a high molecular weight, they are not absorbed from the gastrointestinal (GI) tract. Instead, they remain in the GI tract where they combine with bile acids for about 5 hours. Eventually, they are excreted in the feces.

PHARMACODYNAMICS

The bile-sequestering agents lower blood levels of LDL. As these agents form insoluble complexes with the bile acids in the GI tract, the bile acid levels in the gallbladder decrease. This triggers the liver to synthesize more bile acids from their precursor, cholesterol. As cholesterol leaves the bloodstream and other storage areas to replace the lost bile acids, blood cholesterol levels decrease. Because the small intestine needs bile acids to emulsify lipids and form chylomicrons, absorption of all lipids and lipid-soluble drugs decreases until the bile acids are replaced.

PHARMACOTHERAPEUTICS

Bile-sequestering agents are the drugs of choice for treating type IIa hyperlipoproteinemia (familial hypercholesterolemia) in patients who do not respond to dietary management. A patient whose blood cholesterol levels indicate a severe risk of CAD is most likely to require one of these agents to supplement the diet.

Cholestyramine does not appear to offer any advantages over colestipol in treating hypercholesterolemia. Although some reports show that it is more effective in heterozygotes (those who inherit the trait from one parent) than in homozygotes (those who inherit the trait from both parents), other reports show variable effects.

cholestyramine (Questran, Questran Light, Cholybar). Cholestyramine is used to treat type IIa hyperlipoproteinemia (hypercholesterolemia) when dietary changes fail to produce the desired response. Available as a powder or chewable flavored bar, each scoop, packet, or bar contains 4 grams of cholestyramine resin. The powder must be mixed with 120 to 180 ml of liquid, such as water, carbonated beverage, soup, cereal, or a pulpy fruit with a high moisture content, such as applesauce, pineapples, or peaches. It must not be taken in dry form because the patient may inhale the powder accidentally.
Usual adult dosage: 4 grams of resin P.O. one to six times daily mixed with liquid; or one chewable bar P.O. one to six times daily, followed by consumption of adequate fluids.

colestipol hydrochloride (Colestid). To treat hypercholesterolemia that is unresponsive to diet, granulated colestipol is available in 5-gram packets. However, it must not be taken in its dry form, because accidental inhalation or esophageal distress could result. Instead, colestipol should be dissolved in liquid, such as water, milk, fruit juice, or soup or a pulpy fruit with a high moisture content, such as applesauce, pineapples, or peaches. It also can be baked in cookies for the patient who finds other forms of administration unpalatable.

Usual adult dosage: 15 to 30 grams P.O. daily in two to four divided doses.

Drug interactions

Because bile-sequestering agents are anion-exchange resins, they may bind with acidic drugs in the GI tract, decreasing their absorption and effectiveness. (For information on drugs that commonly interact with these agents, see *Drug interactions: Bile-sequestering agents.*) Other acidic drugs that are likely to be affected include barbiturates, phenytoin, penicillins, cephalosporins, thyroid hormones, thyroid derivatives, chenodiol, digitoxin, and digoxin. Bile-sequestering agents also may reduce absorption of lipid-soluble vitamins, such as vitamins A, D, E, and K; poor absorption of vitamin K can affect prothrombin times significantly. Many other drugs that normally are absorbed from the GI tract — including tetracyclines — also may have decreased absorption and may need supplemental doses during therapy with bile-sequestering agents.

ADVERSE DRUG REACTIONS

Short-term adverse reactions to these drugs are relatively mild. More severe reactions can result from long-term use. Because of this, a patient receiving a bile-sequestering agent requires careful monitoring.

With long-term therapy, these drugs commonly produce GI reactions, which can be minimized by introducing and titrating them slowly to a maximum dosage. Patients who are over age 60 or who take more than 24 grams per day of cholestyramine are particularly likely to develop GI reactions. Constipation affects 1 patient in 10, but usually is not serious. Severe fecal impaction, however, may occur. In 1 patient in 30, GI adverse reactions may include abdominal pain, distention, flatulence, belching, nausea, vomiting, diarrhea, or hemorrhoid irritation. Peptic ulceration and bleeding, cholelithiasis, and cholecystitis are much less common, affecting only 1 patient in 100.

Miscellaneous reactions to bile-sequestering agents include headache, dizziness, anorexia, weakness, and fatigue.

NURSING PROCESS APPLICATION

The following information assists the nurse in caring for a patient who is receiving a bile-sequestering agent.

Assessment
• Review the patient's history for a preexisting condition that contraindicates the use of a bile-sequestering agent, such as complete biliary obstruction or known hypersensitivity to these agents.
• Review the patient's history for a preexisting condition that requires cautious use of a bile-sequestering agent, such as constipation, pregnancy, or lactation.

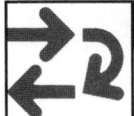

DRUG INTERACTIONS

Bile-sequestering agents

When given concomitantly, bile-sequestering agents will counteract the effects of acidic substances. But beta-adrenergic blocking agents will counteract the effects of the bile-sequestering agents, decreasing their effectiveness and increasing blood lipid levels.

DRUG	INTERACTING DRUGS	POSSIBLE EFFECTS	NURSING IMPLICATIONS
cholestyramine, colestipol	oral anticoagulants	Increase risk of clotting	• Administer an oral anticoagulant 1 hour before or 6 hours after administering a bile-sequestering agent. • Monitor the patient's prothrombin time carefully, and expect to increase the anticoagulant dosage, as needed. • Assess the patient for signs of thromboembolism (pain, swelling, or redness in the calf) or of pulmonary embolism (shortness of breath, chest pain, or anxiety).
	corticosteroids	Decrease effect of corticosteroids by decreasing absorption from the GI tract	• Administer a corticosteroid 1 hour before or 6 hours after administering a bile-sequestering agent. • Monitor the patient carefully for therapeutic effects of these drugs and expect to increase the corticosteroid dosage, as needed. • Assess the patient's weight and blood pressure regularly. • Monitor the patient's serum electrolyte levels.
	acetaminophen	Lessen pain relief by decreasing absorption from the GI tract	• Administer acetaminophen 1 hour before or 6 hours after administering a bile-sequestering agent. • Monitor the patient carefully for therapeutic effects of these drugs, and expect to increase the acetaminophen dosage, as needed.
	cardiac glycosides	Decrease effect of glycosides by decreasing absorption from the GI tract	• Administer cardiac glycosides 1 hour before or 6 hours after administering a bile-sequestering agent. • Monitor the patient's cardiac glycoside level carefully, and expect to increase the cardiac glycoside dosage, as needed. • Assess the patient for signs of congestive heart failure, such as tachycardia, peripheral edema, and hypotension.
	iron preparations	Reduce serum iron levels by decreasing absorption from the GI tract	• Administer an iron preparation 1 hour before or 6 hours after administering a bile-sequestering agent. • Monitor the patient's serum iron and hemoglobin levels, and expect to increase the iron dosage, as needed. • Inform the patient to expect that stools may become black.
	thiazide diuretics	Reduce diuretic effect by decreasing absorption from the GI tract	• Administer a thiazide diuretic 1 hour before or 6 hours after administering a bile-sequestering agent. • Monitor the patient carefully for therapeutic effects of these drugs, and expect to increase the thiazide diuretic dosage, as needed. • Assess the patient for peripheral edema. • Monitor the patient's serum electrolyte levels.

(continued)

DRUG INTERACTIONS

Bile-sequestering agents (continued)

DRUG	INTERACTING DRUGS	POSSIBLE EFFECTS	NURSING IMPLICATIONS
cholestyramine, colestipol (continued)	thyroid hormones	Reduce T_3 and T_4 levels by decreasing absorption of thyroid hormone from the GI tract	• Administer a thyroid hormone 1 hour before or 6 hours after administering a bile-sequestering agent. • Monitor the patient's T_3 and T_4 levels, and expect to increase thyroid hormone dosage, as needed.
	methotrexate	Decrease absorption of methotrexate from the GI tract	• Administer methotrexate 1 hour before or 6 hours after administering a bile-sequestering agent.

• Assess the patient for adverse reactions to the prescribed bile-sequestering agent, such as GI disturbances, headache, dizziness, weakness, and fatigue.
• Review the patient's medication history to identify the use of drugs that may interact with the prescribed bile-sequestering agent, such as oral anticoagulants, corticosteroids, acetaminophen, or cardiac glycosides.
• Assess the effectiveness of the bile-sequestering agent periodically.
• Assess the patient regularly for constipation.
• Determine the patient's compliance with the prescribed bile-sequestering agent regimen.
• Evaluate the patient's and family's knowledge about the prescribed bile-sequestering agent.

Nursing diagnoses
The following examples represent appropriate nursing diagnoses for a patient receiving a bile-sequestering agent.
• Potential for injury related to a preexisting condition that contraindicates the use of a bile-sequestering agent
• Potential for injury related to a preexisting condition that requires cautious use of a bile-sequestering agent
• Potential for injury related to adverse drug reactions
• Constipation related to the adverse GI effects of the prescribed bile-sequestering agent
• Noncompliance related to adverse reactions to and duration of therapy with a bile-sequestering agent
• Knowledge deficit related to the prescribed bile-sequestering agent

Planning and implementation
• Do not administer a bile-sequestering agent to a patient with a condition that contraindicates its use.
• Administer a bile-sequestering agent cautiously to a patient at risk because of a preexisting condition.
• *Obtain baseline blood cholesterol levels before therapy begins. Then monitor blood cholesterol levels every 3 to 6 months for a patient receiving long-term therapy.*

• Monitor the patient regularly for adverse drug reactions. Know that adverse reactions typically are mild with short-term therapy, more severe with long-term therapy, and more likely to occur in patients who are over age 60 or who take more than 24 grams per day of cholestyramine.
• *Introduce and titrate the bile-sequestering agent slowly as prescribed to minimize adverse GI reactions.*
• Take safety precautions if dizziness or weakness develops. For example, keep the bed in a low position and supervise ambulation.
• Mix the powder form with 120 to 180 ml of liquid, such as water, carbonated beverage, or soup, or a pulpy fruit with a high moisture content, such as applesauce. Never administer the dry powder because the patient may inhale it accidentally.
• Have the patient chew a cholestyramine bar and then drink at least 1 glass of water or other liquid.
• *Monitor prothrombin times regularly for a patient who also is receiving an oral anticoagulant.*
• Assess the patient receiving long-term bile-sequestering agent therapy for signs of vitamin A and D deficiencies, such as night blindness or rickets, and of vitamin K deficiency, such as tendency to bleed.
• *Administer drugs that bind with bile-sequestering agents 1 hour before or 6 hours after giving the agent.*
• Expect to increase the dosage, as prescribed, for drugs that normally are absorbed from the GI tract, such as tetracyclines, during therapy with a bile-sequestering agent.
• Observe the patient after withdrawing a bile-sequestering agent. Particularly note increased effects and possible overdose of acidic drugs that were given concurrently.
• Notify the physician of any adverse reactions.
• Monitor the patient's bowel habits throughout therapy to detect constipation.
• *Encourage the patient to drink 2 to 3 liters of fluid daily, (unless contraindicated) increase the dietary fiber intake, and get plenty of exercise to prevent constipation.*

• Notify the physician and request a prescription for a laxative if constipation develops.

• Stress the importance of adhering to the prescribed regimen. Be aware that drug noncompliance usually is higher in patients who receive long-term therapy or develop adverse reactions.

• Reassure the patient that adverse GI reactions should diminish as the GI tract adjusts to the increased bulk.

• Alert the physician if noncompliance occurs.

Patient teaching

• Teach the patient and family the name, dose, frequency, action, and adverse effects of the prescribed bile-sequestering agent.

• *Advise the patient to have blood cholesterol levels checked every 3 to 6 months to evaluate the effectiveness of therapy.*

• Advise the patient not to take the drug in its powder form. Demonstrate how to mix the agent in a suitable liquid, fruit, or other food.

• Instruct the patient to chew a cholestyramine bar thoroughly and then drink at least 1 glass of water or other liquid.

• Advise the patient not to drive or perform activities that require alertness if dizziness or weakness develops.

• Instruct the patient taking a drug that binds with the prescribed bile-sequestering agent to take it 1 hour before or 6 hours after taking the bile-sequestering agent.

• *Instruct the patient to inform all other physicians of the use of a bile-sequestering agent; the dosages of the other agents may need to be adjusted.*

• Teach the patient how to prevent constipation.

• Reassure the patient that adverse GI reactions usually diminish as therapy continues.

• Stress the importance of following the prescribed regimen for the bile-sequestering agent.

• Instruct the patient to notify the physician if adverse reactions occur or concerns arise about the bile-sequestering agent.

Evaluation

The following examples represent appropriate evaluation statements for a patient receiving a bile-sequestering agent.

• The patient has no conditions that contraindicate bile-sequestering agent therapy.

• The patient exhibits no signs of complications in the preexisting condition linked to the bile-sequestering agent.

• The patient experiences no adverse reactions to the prescribed bile-sequestering agent.

• The patient maintains normal bowel function.

• The patient complies with the bile-sequestering agent regimen.

• The patient and family express an accurate understanding of the points taught about the prescribed bile-sequestering agent.

• The patient schedules follow-up visits at appropriate intervals to have blood cholesterol levels checked.

FIBRIC ACID DERIVATIVES

Fibric acid, a branched-chain propionic acid with a phenyl group, is produced by several fungi. Derivatives of this acid are used to reduce high triglyceride levels and, to a lesser extent, high cholesterol levels. Currently, two fibric acid derivatives are available for clinical use: clofibrate and gemfibrozil.

PHARMACOKINETICS

Clofibrate and gemfibrozil are absorbed readily from the GI tract. After absorption, both drugs are 95% bound to plasma proteins. Then, clofibrate is hydrolyzed to free carboxylic acid derivative, the active ingredient. Gemfibrozil undergoes extensive metabolism in the liver, producing active and inactive metabolites. Both agents are excreted in the urine as unchanged drugs and as conjugates of glucuronic acid. A higher percentage of clofibrate is excreted as conjugate.

Onset, peak, duration

Both of these antilipemic agents begin to reduce VLDL levels in 2 to 5 days. Clofibrate's action peaks in 4 weeks, and its duration of action in unknown. Gemfibrozil's action peaks in 3 weeks and has a 3-week duration. Clofibrate's half-life is 12 to 35 hours; gemfibrozil's is 1.5 hours.

PHARMACODYNAMICS

Researchers have not established the exact mechanism of action for these drugs. They believe that the drugs may reduce cholesterol formation early in the biosynthetic process, mobilize cholesterol from the tissues, increase sterol excretion, decrease lipoprotein synthesis and secretion, and decrease triglyceride synthesis. The decreased triglyceride synthesis probably results from inhibition of lipolysis in adipose tissue.

Gemfibrozil produces two other effects. It increases HDL levels in the blood by increasing the synthesis of certain apoproteins (substances derived from proteins), and it increases the serum's capacity to dissolve additional cholesterol.

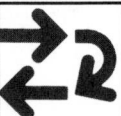

DRUG INTERACTIONS
Fibric acid derivatives

Drug interactions with fibric acid derivatives usually involve acidic drugs, such as oral anticoagulants and sulfonylureas.

DRUG	INTERACTING DRUGS	POSSIBLE EFFECTS	NURSING IMPLICATIONS
clofibrate, gemfibrozil	oral anticoagulants	Increase anticoagulant effect by displacing oral anticoagulants from binding sites in the serum albumin	• Monitor the patient's prothrombin time closely, and expect to adjust the anticoagulant dosage, as needed. • Assess the patient for signs of internal bleeding, such as hematuria and easy bruising. • Monitor the patient for signs of GI bleeding, such as hematemesis and melena.
	sulfonylureas	Increase hypoglycemic effect by displacing sulfonylurea from serum albumin sites, increasing insulin secretion, and competing for renal secretion	• Monitor the patient's blood glucose level and expect to adjust the sulfonylurea dosage, as needed.

PHARMACOTHERAPEUTICS

These drugs are used primarily to reduce triglyceride levels—especially very-low-density triglycerides—and secondarily to reduce blood cholesterol levels. Therefore, they should be used primarily in patients with types II, III, IV, and mild type V hyperlipoproteinemia. However, these agents should be used only in patients at severe risk for CAD who have not responded adequately to diet changes, who have premature CAD or a family member with the disease, who are hypercholesterolemic or have a family member with the disease, who have marked hypertriglyceridemia, or who smoke or exhibit other risk factors, such as hypertension or obesity. Fibric acid derivatives are most effective for patients with no previous history of CAD or angina.

In patients with types IIa, IIb, and IV hyperlipoproteinemia, niacin is used as adjunct therapy. Fibric acid derivatives are used with these patients when niacin does not produce an adequate response, is poorly tolerated, or is contraindicated. They also may be added to niacin and bile-sequestering agent therapy, if these two agents do not produce an adequate response.

clofibrate (Atromid-S). Available in 500-mg capsules, clofibrate is used primarily to treat type V hyperlipoproteinemia (mixed hyperlipidemia, mixed hypertriglyceridemia) and sometimes to treat types II and IV.
Usual adult dosage: 500 mg P.O. q.i.d.

gemfibrozil (Lopid). Available in 300-mg capsules, gemfibrozil is used to treat type III hyperlipoproteinemia as well as types II, IV, and V.

Usual adult dosage: 1,200 mg P.O. daily in two divided doses 30 minutes before the morning and evening meals. (Patient response can vary widely, so the actual dose may range from 900 to 1,500 mg/day.)

Drug interactions
Because clofibrate and gemfibrozil bind strongly with plasma proteins, they can displace anticoagulants in the plasma when given concurrently. This usually requires an anticoagulant dosage reduction and close monitoring of prothrombin times to prevent an anticoagulant overdose. Although no studies have shown that these antilipemic agents displace other acidic drugs, such as barbiturates, phenytoin, thyroid derivatives, and cardiac glycosides, the possibility of displacement exists when these drugs are administered concurrently. (For more information, see *Drug interactions: Fibric acid derivatives.*)

ADVERSE DRUG REACTIONS

The most common reactions to fibric acid derivatives are GI effects, which resemble those of the bile-sequestering agents.

Several studies show that clofibrate increases the incidence of cholelithiasis and the need for cholecystectomy. The drug is associated with benign and malignant liver tumors in rodents and malignant tumors in humans. Because of these potential reactions, clofibrate is not recommended for long-term use. This antilipemic can cause other adverse reactions, including pancreatitis, cardiac arrhythmias, intermittent claudication, thromboembolic events, and angina. It also may produce flulike symptoms and an increased creatinine phosphokinase (CPK) level.

Like clofibrate, gemfibrozil produces cholelithiasis. It does not seem to cause the other reactions related to clofibrate, but its use should be monitored closely because of the chemical similarities of the two agents.

Fibric acid derivatives may produce a wide range of hypersensitivity reactions. These may include skin rash, alopecia, urticaria, dry skin, brittle hair, hepatomegaly, impotence, decreased libido, leukopenia, weight gain, muscle pain, and abnormal liver function test results.

NURSING PROCESS APPLICATION

The following information assists the nurse in caring for a patient who is receiving a fibric acid derivative.

Assessment
• Review the patient's history for a preexisting condition that contraindicates the use of a fibric acid derivative, such as significant hepatic or renal dysfunction, primary biliary cirrhosis, lactation, or known hypersensitivity to fibric acid derivatives.
• Review the patient's history for a preexisting condition that requires cautious use of a fibric acid derivative, such as pregnancy or peptic ulcer.
• Assess the patient for adverse reactions to fibric acid derivatives, such as GI disturbances, cholelithiasis, arrhythmias, angina, leukopenia, or abnormal liver function tests.
• Assess the patient receiving clofibrate for warning signs of cancer: a change in bowel or bladder habits, a sore that does not heal, unusual bleeding or discharge, a thickening or lump, indigestion or difficulty swallowing, obvious change in a wart or mole, or a nagging cough or hoarseness.
• Review the patient's medication history to identify the use of drugs that may interact with the prescribed fibric acid derivative, such as an oral anticoagulant or sulfonylurea.
• Assess the effectiveness of the prescribed fibric acid derivative periodically.
• Assess the patient for biliary colic, which may cause the sudden onset of severe abdominal pain, increase in intensity, last for several hours, and be accompanied by nausea and vomiting.
• Assess the patient receiving clofibrate for signs of altered peripheral tissue perfusion, such as a color or temperature change, and signs of altered cardiopulmonary tissue perfusion, such as shortness of breath, chest pain, or anxiety.
• Evaluate the patient's and family's knowledge about the prescribed fibric acid derivative.

Nursing diagnoses
The following examples represent appropriate nursing diagnoses for a patient receiving a fibric acid derivative.
• Potential for injury related to a preexisting condition that contraindicates the use of a fibric acid derivative
• Potential for injury related to a preexisting condition that requires cautious use of a fibric acid derivative
• Potential for injury related to adverse drug reactions
• Pain related to biliary colic from drug-induced cholelithiasis
• Altered peripheral tissue perfusion related to clofibrate-induced intermittent claudication
• Altered cardiopulmonary tissue perfusion related to clofibrate-induced thromboembolic events
• Knowledge deficit related to the prescribed fibric acid derivative

Planning and implementation
• Do not administer a fibric acid derivative to a patient with a condition that contraindicates its use.
• Administering a fibric acid derivative cautiously to a patient at risk because of a preexisting condition.
• *Monitor liver function studies and white blood cell (WBC) count, as prescribed, to detect abnormalities.*
• *Monitor blood triglyceride and cholesterol levels, as prescribed, to assess the drug's effectiveness.*
• Interpret the CPK level carefully for a patient receiving clofibrate.
• Monitor the patient regularly for adverse reactions throughout the course of therapy. Particularly note warning signs of cancer and adverse GI effects.
• Monitor the electrocardiogram (ECG) and pulse for arrhythmias in a patient receiving clofibrate.
• Expect to reduce the anticoagulant dosage by as much as one half, as prescribed, and monitor the prothrombin time for a patient who must receive an anticoagulant and a fibric acid derivative.
• Take infection control precautions if leukopenia occurs. If leukopenia is severe, expect to place the patient in reverse isolation.
• Administer gemfibrozil in two divided doses daily 30 minutes before morning and evening meals as prescribed.
• Notify the physician if adverse reactions occur.
• *Monitor for biliary colic, which may be the first sign of cholelithiasis in a patient receiving a fibric acid derivative.*
• Notify the physician if biliary colic occurs and request an order for an analgesic.
• Expect to prepare the patient with biliary colic for diagnostic studies, such as ultrasonography and oral cholecystography, to diagnose cholelithiasis.
• *Monitor the patient regularly for signs of decreased peripheral tissue perfusion from intermittent claudication, such as color or temperature changes in leg or leg pain*

when walking, or from a peripheral thromboembolic event, such as leg pain, swelling, or redness.

• *Monitor the patient regularly for signs of decreased cardiopulmonary tissue perfusion from a pulmonary embolism, such as sudden onset of shortness of breath, chest pain, or anxiety.*

• Notify the physician immediately if decreased tissue perfusion is suspected.

• *Take emergency measures if pulmonary embolism occurs, such as raising the head of the bed, administering oxygen, and transferring the patient to the intensive care unit.*

• Notify the physician if deep vein thromboembolism is suspected, and keep the patient in bed until the physician performs an examination. Then maintain bed rest, if prescribed.

• Expect to administer heparin S.C. or I.V. and take bleeding precautions in a patient with thrombosis.

• Prepare the patient for diagnostic studies, as prescribed, such as a lung scan or pulmonary angiography to detect pulmonary emboli, or venography to confirm deep vein thrombosis.

• Expect to discontinue clofibrate if decreased tissue perfusion occurs.

Patient teaching

• Teach the patient and family the name, dose, frequency, action, and adverse effects of the prescribed fibric acid derivative.

• *Stress the importance of regular liver function studies and triglyceride and cholesterol level tests. Explain the purpose of these tests and tell the patient that they require a blood sample after fasting from midnight the previous night.*

• Teach the patient to recognize the warning signs of cancer and to report them or any other unusual symptoms to the physician.

• Reassure the patient that adverse GI reactions are the most common. Teach the patient how to manage GI disturbances. For example, urge the patient to increase the fluid and fiber intake and amount of exercise (unless contraindicated) to relieve constipation.

• *Instruct the patient who also takes an anticoagulant to notify the physician about fibric acid derivative therapy because the anticoagulant dosage may need to be reduced to prevent bleeding. Teach the patient to take bleeding precautions, such as avoiding cuts and bruises, using a soft toothbrush, and using an electric razor when shaving.*

• Instruct the patient with a decreased WBC count to prevent infection by avoiding crowds and people who are ill and by getting plenty of rest.

• Advise the patient receiving gemfibrozil to take it in two divided doses daily 30 minutes before morning and evening meals.

• Instruct the patient to notify the physician of biliary colic, which typically appears as abdominal pain or nausea and vomiting that subsides, with or without treatment, after several hours. Explain that diagnostic tests may be needed to check for cholelithiasis.

• *Instruct the patient to notify the physician if leg pain occurs when walking or if pain, swelling, or redness develops in either calf. Instruct the patient to go to the nearest emergency department if shortness of breath suddenly develops.*

• Tell the patient to notify the physician if any other adverse reactions occur.

Evaluation

The following examples represent appropriate evaluation statements for a patient receiving a fibric acid derivative.

• The patient has no conditions that contraindicate fibric acid derivative therapy.

• The patient exhibits no signs of complications in the preexisting condition linked to the prescribed fibric acid derivative.

• The patient develops no adverse reactions to the prescribed fibric acid derivative.

• The patient reports no pain.

• The patient maintains adequate peripheral and cardiopulmonary tissue perfusion throughout fibric acid derivative therapy.

• The patient and family express an accurate understanding of the points taught about the prescribed fibric acid derivative.

• The patient returns for regular liver function studies and triglyceride and cholestrol level tests, as scheduled.

CHOLESTEROL SYNTHESIS INHIBITORS

This section presents two other antilipemic agents: probucol and lovastatin. These drugs lower lipid levels by interfering with cholesterol synthesis.

PHARMACOKINETICS

Only 2% to 8% of probucol is absorbed from the GI tract. Absorption improves somewhat if probucol is given with food. This highly lipid-soluble drug is distributed mainly in fatty acid depots. Although its method of metabolism is unknown, probucol passes through the bile duct for elimination in the feces.

Probucol begins to produce effects 2 to 4 weeks after therapy begins. The effects peak in 20 to 50 days. When therapy ends, some probucol remains in the body for up to 6 months.

After oral administration, lovastatin is absorbed incompletely and undergoes extensive first-pass metabolism in the liver. Less than 5% of a single oral dose reaches the systemic circulation as active enzyme inhibitors. Food may increase the drug's systemic absorption. Distribution of lovastatin and its metabolites is not fully known. However, lovastatin and its major metabolite are more than 95% protein bound.

Lovastatin is metabolized extensively to four active metabolites, including mevinolinic acid, a 6-hydroxy metabolite, and 2 unidentified active metabolites. Lovastatin's half-life is unknown; the plasma half-life of mevinolinic acid ranges from 1.1 to 1.7 hours. Lovastatin and its metabolites are excreted in the urine and feces.

Little is known about lovastatin's onset of action, peak concentration level, and duration of action. Usually, lovastatin produces a therapeutic response within 2 weeks. Maximal changes in lipoprotein and cholesterol concentrations occur within 4 to 6 weeks.

PHARMACODYNAMICS

Although probucol's exact mechanism of action is unknown, researchers believe that it acts in one or more ways by inhibiting cholesterol transport from the intestine, inhibiting cholesterol synthesis, and increasing the secretion of cholesterol and bile acid. Probucol primarily reduces blood cholesterol levels, but it also lowers LDL levels.

Lovastatin and its metabolites inhibit hydroxymethylglutaryl-CoA (HMG-CoA) reductase. This reduces the conversion of HMG-CoA to mevalonic acid, a precursor of cholesterol, thus reducing cholesterol biosynthesis. The mechanisms by which lovastatin reduces LDL cholesterol are not understood fully. However, the drug may enhance the clearance of serum LDLs by liver receptors and may inhibit LDL production.

PHARMACOTHERAPEUTICS

The cholesterol synthesis inhibitors are used to treat various types of hyperlipoproteinemia.

probucol (Lorelco). Primarily used to treat type IIa hyperlipoproteinemia (hypercholesterolemia), this agent often is used to augment colestipol therapy when colestipol alone fails to reduce cholesterol levels.
Usual adult dosage: 500 mg P.O. b.i.d. with morning and evening meals.

lovastatin (Mevacor). Lovastatin is used with dietary therapy to decrease serum levels of total and LDL cholesterol in familial types IIa and IIb hyperlipoproteinemia, including hypercholesterolemia. This drug may be used with a bile-sequestering agent in a hypercholesterolemic patient who cannot tolerate or does not respond adequately to either drug separately.
Usual adult dosage: initially, 20 mg P.O. daily with the evening meal, or 40 mg P.O. daily for a patient with a serum cholesterol level greater than 300 mg/dl; increased, as needed, at intervals of 4 weeks or more up to a maximum of 80 mg P.O. daily until the desired effect is achieved. In a patient who falls below the desired target cholesterol range, the lovastatin dosage may be reduced.

Drug interactions

Unlike the bile-sequestering agents and fibric acid derivatives, the cholesterol synthesis inhibitors appear to interact with few other drugs. Probucol, however, can produce additive effects when given with clofibrate. This interaction markedly reduces the HDL level and prohibits the combined use of these agents. Probucol should not be used with drugs that prolong the QT interval, affect the atrial rate, or produce atrioventricular block because additive effects can occur. When lovastatin is administered with an immunosuppressant (especially cyclosporin), gemfibrozil, or niacin (in antilipemic dosages), the interaction may increase the risk of myopathy.

ADVERSE DRUG REACTIONS

In animals, probucol has affected cardiac nerve conduction. It also has prolonged the QT interval of the cardiac cycle. Because the drug is intended for long-term use, an ECG should be taken when treatment begins and after 6 months and 12 months of treatment to detect any cardiac effects. Additional adverse reactions to probucol, especially the GI effects, resemble those of the other antilipemic agents. Although the drug's teratogenic effects have not been established, women receiving probucol should avoid becoming pregnant for at least 6 months after treatment ends.

Lovastatin is well tolerated and has a low incidence of adverse reactions. The most common adverse reactions are GI disturbances (flatulence, abdominal pain or cramps, diarrhea or constipation, nausea, and dyspepsia) and headache. Increases in liver enzymes have been reported in 2% of patients receiving long-term lovastatin therapy. Additional adverse reactions include elevated an CPK level, myalgia, muscle cramps, myopathy, lens opacities, blurred vision, rash, or pruritus.

NURSING PROCESS APPLICATION

The following information assists the nurse in caring for a patient who is receiving a cholesterol synthesis inhibitor.

Assessment

• Review the patient's history for a preexisting condition that contraindicates the use of a cholesterol synthesis inhibitor, such as active liver disease, persistently elevated serum transaminase levels, pregnancy, lactation, or known hypersensitivity to these agents.

• Review the patient's history for a preexisting condition that requires cautious use of a cholesterol synthesis inhibitor, such as high alcohol consumption or a history of liver disease.

• Assess the patient for adverse reactions to the prescribed cholesterol synthesis inhibitor, such as cardiac nerve conduction dysfunction, diarrhea or other GI disturbances, myalgia, muscle cramps, myopathy, visual disturbances, rash, or pruritus.

• Review the patient's medication history to identify the use of drugs that may interact with the prescribed cholesterol synthesis inhibitor, such as clofibrate, immunosuppressants, or gemfibrozil.

• Assess the effectiveness of the cholesterol synthesis inhibitor.

• Assess the patient regularly for diarrhea during cholesterol synthesis inhibitor therapy.

• Evaluate the patient's and family's knowledge about the prescribed cholesterol synthesis inhibitor.

Nursing diagnoses

The following examples represent appropriate nursing diagnoses for a patient receiving a cholesterol synthesis inhibitor.

• Potential for injury related to a preexisting condition that contraindicates the use of a cholesterol synthesis inhibitor

• Potential for injury related to a preexisting condition that requires cautious use of a cholesterol synthesis inhibitor

• Potential for injury related to adverse drug reactions

• Diarrhea related to the adverse GI effects of the prescribed cholesterol synthesis inhibitor

• Knowledge deficit related to the prescribed cholesterol synthesis inhibitor

Planning and implementation

• Do not administer a cholesterol synthesis inhibitor to a patient with a condition that contraindicates its use.

• Administer a cholesterol synthesis inhibitor cautiously to a patient at risk because of a preexisting condition.

• *Do not administer probucol with clofibrate to prevent a significant decrease in the HDL level.*

• Monitor the patient for adverse drug reactions throughout antilipemic therapy.

• *Obtain an ECG when probucol treatment begins and after 6 months and 12 months of treatment, as prescribed, to detect any adverse cardiac effects, such as a prolonged QT interval.*

• *Obtain liver function tests before lovastatin therapy begins, every 4 to 6 weeks during the first 12 to 15 months of therapy, and periodically thereafter to detect liver function abnormalities.*

• *Monitor the patient's cholesterol level, as prescribed, to assess the drug's effectiveness.*

• Take safety precautions, such as assisting with ambulation, if blurred vision or lens opacities occur.

• Administer probucol with morning and evening meals and lovastatin with the evening meal to enhance absorption.

• Expect to reduce the lovastatin dosage as prescribed for a patient who falls below the desired target cholesterol range.

• Notify the physician if adverse reactions occur.

• Monitor the patient's bowel patterns to detect diarrhea.

• Notify the physician if diarrhea occurs and request a prescription for an antidiarrheal agent.

Patient teaching

• Teach the patient and family the name, dose, frequency, action, and adverse effects of the prescribed cholesterol synthesis inhibitor.

• *Inform the patient that an ECG must be obtained before and periodically during probucol therapy.*

• *Inform the patient who must take lovastatin that blood must be drawn for liver function studies before and periodically during lovastatin therapy.*

• *Inform the patient that the cholesterol level must be checked periodically to assess the drug's effectiveness.*

• Advise the patient to take probucol with morning and evening meals or lovastatin with evening meals to enhance absorption.

• Describe the adverse GI reactions to cholesterol synthesis inhibitors. Instruct the patient to notify the physician if these reactions become severe or persistent.

• Instruct the patient to notify the physician of any other adverse drug reactions.

• *Advise the female patient to avoid becoming pregnant for at least 6 months after discontinuation of probucol therapy.*

Evaluation

The following examples represent appropriate evaluation statements for a patient receiving a cholesterol synthesis inhibitor.

• The patient has no conditions that contraindicate cholesterol synthesis inhibitor therapy.

• The patient exhibits no signs of complications in the preexisting condition linked to the prescribed cholesterol synthesis inhibitor.

• The patient demonstrates no adverse reactions to the prescribed cholesterol synthesis inhibitor.

• The patient maintains normal bowel function.

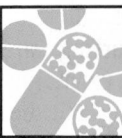

SELECTED MAJOR DRUGS

Antilipemic agents

This chart summarizes the major antilipemic agents currently in clinical use.

DRUG	MAJOR INDICATIONS	USUAL ADULT DOSAGES	CONTRADICTIONS AND PRECAUTIONS
Bile-sequestering agent			
cholestyramine	Type IIa hyperlipoproteine-mia (hypercholesterol-emia)	4 grams of resin P.O. one to six times daily mixed with 120 to 180 ml of fluid, soups, cereal, or pulpy fruits; or one chewable bar P.O. one to six times daily followed by consumption of adequate fluid	• Know that cholestyramine is contraindicated in a patient with complete biliary obstruction or known hypersensitivity to this drug. • Administer with caution to a pregnant or lactating patient or one with constipation.
Fibric acid derivative			
gemfibrozil	Type III hyperlipoproteine-mia; types II, IV, and V hyperlipoproteinemia	1,200 mg P.O. daily in two divided doses	• Know that clofibrate is contraindicated in a lactating patient or one with significant hepatic or renal dysfunction, primary biliary cirrhosis, or known hypersensitivity to this drug. • Administer with caution to a pregnant patient, one with peptic ulcer, or one receiving an anticoagulant.
Cholesterol synthesis inhibitor			
lovastatin	Primary type IIa and IIb hyperlipoproteinemia	20 to 80 mg P.O. daily	• Know that lovastatin is contraindicated in a pregnant or lactating patient or one with active liver disease, persistent transaminase elevations, or known hypersensitivity to this drug. • Administer with caution to a patient with high alcohol consumption or a history of liver disease.

• The patient and family express an accurate understanding of the points taught about the prescribed cholesterol synthesis inhibitor.
• The patient returns as scheduled for reassessment of the cholesterol level.

OTHER ANTILIPEMIC AGENTS

Several other drugs occasionally are used to treat hyperlipoproteinemia. However, they have not received approval from the Food and Drug Administration for this indication, so they rarely are used. These drugs include ethinyl estradiol, norethindrone acetate, nandrolone and other anabolic agents, and neomycin. (For information about these drugs, see Chapter 53, Androgenic and Anabolic Steroid Agents;

Chapter 54, Estrogens, Progestins, and Oral Contraceptive Agents; and Chapter 59, Antibacterial Agents.) Dextrothyroxine sodium, another antilipemic agent, has been approved to treat hypercholesterolemia. Its serious cardiovascular effects, however, limit its use to pediatric patients with no history of CAD. One additional agent, niacin, may be used to treat certain kinds of hyperlipoproteinemia.

niacin [nicotinic acid] (Nicolar, Nicobid). A vitamin, niacin decreases blood levels of LDL, VLDL, and phospholipids and increases the HDL level, especially in types II, III, IV, and V hyperlipoproteinemia. Its adverse reactions, however, limit its usefulness. After oral administration, it is absorbed readily and distributed throughout the body. In doses required to reduce cholesterol levels, it is excreted unchanged in the urine. Niacin's antilipemic effects normally begin in 7 to 14 days, peak in 6 to 8 weeks, and last 6 to 8 weeks after therapy ends. Although researchers have not discovered niacin's exact mechanism of action, they theorize that it inhibits the release of FFAs from lipid tissues.

Niacin commonly produces skin flushing that may be reduced if the drug is administered with antacids, aspirin, or food. It also may produce GI effects similar to those of the other antilipemic agents. The flushing and GI symptoms usually disappear in 2 to 6 weeks. This agent can cause other adverse reactions, including abnormal liver function test results, jaundice, abnormal prothrombin times, hypo-albuminemia, hyperglycemia, and hyperuricemia. For these reasons, it is contraindicated in a patient with arterial hemorrhage, severe hypotension, liver disease, or active peptic ulcer disease, and should be administered with caution to a patient with gallbladder disease, jaundice, diabetes, or gout. (For more information, see Chapter 45, Vitamin, Mineral, and Other Nutritional Agents.)

CHAPTER SUMMARY

Chapter 34 discussed the antilipemic agents. Here are the highlights of this chapter.
• Blood lipids consist of FFAs, triglycerides, sterols (cholesterol and cholesterol esters), and phospholipids.
• These blood lipids form various lipoproteins, including chylomicrons, chylomicron fragments, VLDLs, LDLs, IDLs, and HDLs.
• Hyperlipoproteinemia, or excess blood lipoproteins, is a major cause of CAD in the United States. Reduction of blood lipoprotein levels greatly reduces the risk of CAD.
• Antilipemic agents should be used only when other measures, such as proper diet, weight loss, appropriate anti-hypertensive therapy, and exercise, have failed to lower blood lipid levels sufficiently.
• The three major classes of antilipemic agents are bile-sequestering agents, fibric acid derivatives, and cholesterol synthesis inhibitors. The bile-sequestering agents include cholestyramine and colestipol. When given concomitantly, these agents counteract the effects of acidic substances, or are rendered less effective by beta-adrenergic blocking agents.
• The fibric acid derivatives include clofibrate and gemfibrozil. These agents commonly interact with acidic drugs, such as oral anticoagulants and sulfonylureas. Because clofibrate may produce cholelithiasis and some types of cancer, it is not indicated for long-term use.
• Cholesterol synthesis inhibitors include probucol and lovastatin. These agents produce few drug interactions. However, they have not been administered for long periods.
• Niacin also acts as an antilipemic agent. Its most common adverse reaction is flushing, but it can produce more severe adverse reactions that can limit its usefulness.

• When caring for a patient who is receiving an antilipemic agent, the nurse uses the nursing process. Nursing care includes regular monitoring of cholesterol levels, promoting compliance, and teaching the patient about drug and diet therapy.

STUDY QUESTIONS

See Appendix 1 for answers.

1. After a routine physical examination, blood tests reveal that Jim Blake, age 48, has hypercholesteremia. His plasma cholesterol level is 350 mg/dl. After 6 months of following a low-fat diet and exercise program, Mr. Blake's cholesterol level has not changed significantly. The physician prescribes the bile-sequestering agent cholestyramine (Questran) 9 grams P.O. q.i.d. What is the site of action for bile-sequestering agents?
(a) blood
(b) GI tract
(c) urinary tract
(d) liver

2. What should the nurse teach Mr. Blake about taking cholestyramine powder?
(a) Take the powder on an empty stomach.
(b) Swallow the powder dry for optimal effects.
(c) Mix the powder in a liquid or semi-liquid food.
(d) Take the powder on a full stomach.

3. Mr. Blake also takes a thiazide diuretic to treat hypertension. To minimize the interaction between the thiazide diuretic and cholestyramine, what should the nurse tell Mr. Blake to do?
(a) Discontinue the thiazide diuretic immediately.
(b) Take the thiazide diuretic 1 hour before or 6 hours after taking cholestyramine.
(c) Take the thiazide diuretic immediately before taking cholestyramine.
(d) Alternate administration of the thiazide diuretic with that of cholestyramine.

4. Karl Jones, age 40, has type IV hyperlipoproteinemia. After 6 months, a low-fat diet and 20-pound weight loss have not reduced his lipid levels. Which type of antilipemic agent is most effective in treating type IV hyperlipoproteinemia?
(a) bile-sequestering agent
(b) fibric acid derivative
(c) cholesterol synthesis inhibitor
(d) niacin derivative

5. For Mr. Jones, the physician prescribes clofibrate (Atromid-S) 500 mg P.O. q.i.d. Clofibrate administration would have to proceed with caution if Mr. Jones also were receiving which drug?
(a) penicillin
(b) thiazide diuretic
(c) alkalinizing agent
(d) oral anticoagulant

6. Gordon Kelly, age 30, has type II hyperlipoproteinemia. In addition to diet therapy, his physician prescribes the cholesterol synthesis inhibitor lovastatin 20 mg P.O. daily. How are cholesterol synthesis inhibitors different from other antilipemic agents?
(a) They produce more severe adverse reactions.
(b) They cause fewer significant drug interactions.
(c) Their GI absorption is higher.
(d) Their effectiveness is lower.

7. While Mr. Kelly is receiving lovastatin, what should the nurse expect to monitor periodically?
(a) liver function test results
(b) electrolyte levels
(c) results of GI ultrasonography
(d) thyroid hormone levels

8. Why is niacin used rarely as an antilipemic agent?
(a) Its therapeutic effects are minimal.
(d) It produces allergic reactions.
(c) It causes serious adverse reactions.
(d) It has a delayed onset of action.

SELECTED REFERENCES

AHFS drug information 90. (1990). Bethesda, MD: American Society of Hospital Pharmacists.

Drug facts and comparisons. (1991). St. Louis: Facts and Comparisons Division, J.B. Lippincott.

Goodman and Gilman's the pharmacological basis of therapeutics, (8th ed.; 1990). Elmsford, NY: Pergamon Press.

Guido, B., and Mocogni, F. (1989). Hypercholesterolemia as a cardiovascular risk factor: Nursing implications. *Critical Care Nursing Quarterly,* 12(2), 73-91.

Gwynne, J. (1988). Advances in lowering plasma cholesterol: Lipoprotein structure and metabolism. *Consultant,* 28(6), 6-14.

Hansten, P., and Horn, J. (1989). *Drug interactions: Clinical significance of drug-drug interactions* (6th ed.). Philadelphia: Lea & Febiger.

Lovastatin plus nicotinic acid: Possible interaction. (1989). *Nurses Drug Alert,* 13(1), 6-7.

Memmer, M. (1989). Hypercholesterolemia: Prevention and control. *Progress in Cardiovascular Nursing,* 4(2), 40-48.

North American Nursing Diagnosis Association. (1990). *Taxonomy I - Revised, with official diagnostic categories.* St. Louis: NANDA.

USPDI. (1991). *Drug information for the health care professional.* (Vol. I, 11th ed.). Rockville, MD: United States Pharmacopeial Convention.

DRUGS AFFECTING THE HEMATOLOGIC SYSTEM

Unit Eight covers drugs that affect red blood cell (RBC) formation, or erythropoiesis (hematinic agents), alter the coagulation properties of the blood (anticoagulant agents), and dissolve thrombi, or blood clots (thrombolytic agents) in acute situations. The unit introduction includes a brief overview of drugs used to control bleeding, whole blood, and blood derivatives.

ERYTHROPOIESIS

Blood is composed of plasma, which is the liquid component, and blood cells, which are formed elements including the RBCs, white blood cells (WBCs), and platelets. An RBC, or erythrocyte, transports oxygen to tissues. A WBC, or leukocyte, defends the body against invading organisms. Platelets aid in hemostasis, stopping bleeding.

Hematinic agents provide essential building blocks for RBC production (erythropoiesis) by increasing hemoglobin, the necessary element for oxygen transportation.

Normally, an RBC is small—about 7 microns in diameter. Shaped like a biconcave disk, the RBC has a large surface area relative to its volume. It can change shape as it moves through narrow blood vessels and can withstand the turbulence in small capillaries. RBCs are the most numerous of the formed elements of the blood. Normal RBC count is approximately 5,500,000 per cubic millimeter of blood.

RBCs carry oxygen to cells and exchange it for carbon dioxide. They carry most of these gases in combination with hemoglobin. Each RBC contains 200 to 300 million molecules of hemoglobin. One hemoglobin molecule contains four iron atoms, enabling the molecule to combine with four oxygen molecules and form oxyhemoglobin. The globin (protein) part of the hemoglobin molecule combines with carbon dioxide to form carbaminohemoglobin.

RBC maturation occurs in red bone marrow and involves nucleated cells called hemocytoblasts, or stem cells. The stem cells divide by mitosis and evolve through several stages to a mature erythrocyte. When an RBC leaves the bone marrow and enters the blood, it contains hemoglobin.

The life span of an RBC is 105 to 120 days, after which time the blood cell breaks down—usually in the capillaries and in the reticuloendothelial cells in the lining of the hepatic blood vessels. Phagocytes in the spleen and bone marrow envelop and destroy the fragments of the RBC, a process known as phagocytosis. During phagocytosis, iron is released from hemoglobin and a pigment called bilirubin is formed. The iron and bilirubin are transported to the liver, where the iron is stored and the bilirubin is excreted in bile. The bone marrow then reuses the stored iron to produce new RBCs. (For an illustration, see *Life cycle of a red blood cell*.) In healthy individuals, the number of

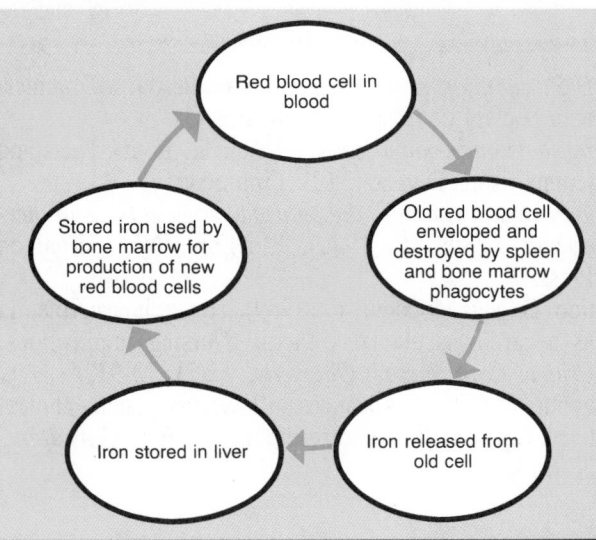

Life cycle of a red blood cell

Red blood cells are involved in a cyclic life of 105 to 120 days, which enables old cells to contribute to the formation of new cells.

Red blood cell in blood

Old red blood cell enveloped and destroyed by spleen and bone marrow phagocytes

Iron released from old cell

Iron stored in liver

Stored iron used by bone marrow for production of new red blood cells

Glossary

Activated partial thromboplastin time (APTT): screening test to evaluate the intrinsic coagulation pathway (except Factor VII and Factor XIII) and the common pathway and to monitor heparin therapy.

Anticoagulant: substance that suppresses, delays, or negates blood coagulation.

Antiplatelet: substance that interferes with activity of blood platelets.

Antithrombin III: alpha globulin that neutralizes the thrombin action and thus inhibits blood coagulation.

Coagulation: conversion of blood from a liquid, free-flowing state to a semisolid gel. Although coagulation, or clotting, can occur within an intact vessel, the process usually starts with tissue damage and exposure of the blood to air.

Embolus: clot or other plug (composed of fat, bone, or another substance foreign to blood) that is totally or partially dislodged from its site of origin and moved by blood flow to a more distant narrow site in the circulatory system, where it may obstruct flow.

Erythropoiesis: production of red blood cells (RBCs).

Erythropoietin: glycoprotein produced by the kidneys that stimulates RBC production.

Ferritin: one of the complexes in which iron is stored in the body.

Fibrin: insoluble protein formed from fibrinogen by thrombin action; fibrin is the major element of a blood clot.

Fibrin degradation products (FDPs): substances that result from plasmin action on fibrin; also called fibrin split products (FSPs).

Fibrinogen: high-molecular-weight plasma protein that is converted to fibrin through thrombin action; also called coagulation Factor I.

Fibrinolysis: breakdown of fibrin by the proteolytic enzyme, plasmin.

Hematinic: an agent capable of improving blood quality by increasing hemoglobin level and number of RBCs.

Hemoglobin: oxygen-carrying pigment of the RBCs.

Hemolytic anemia: disorder characterized by the premature destruction of RBCs. Anemia may be minimal if the bone marrow can increase RBC production.

Hemostasis: termination of bleeding by mechanical or chemical means or by the body's complex coagulation process, which consists of vasoconstriction, platelet aggregation, and thrombin and fibrin synthesis.

Hypercoagulability: state of abnormally increased coagulation.

Hypochromic anemia: disorder characterized by decreased hemoglobin in the RBCs.

Macrocytic anemia: disorder characterized by abnormally large, fragile RBCs, usually from vitamin B_{12} or folic acid deficiency.

Megaloblastic anemia: disorder characterized by immature, large, dysfunctional RBCs.

Microcytic anemia: disorder characterized by abnormally small, incompletely hemoglobinized RBCs in the bone marrow.

Normocytic anemia: disorder characterized by too few RBCs.

Partial thromboplastin time (PTT): screening test to evaluate the intrinsic coagulation pathway (except Factors VII and XIII) and the common pathway and to monitor heparin therapy; less sensitive than APTT.

Plasmin: highly specific proteolytic enzyme that dissolves fibrin clots.

Plasminogen: inactive precursor of plasmin.

Prothrombin: glycoprotein converted to thrombin by extrinsic thromboplastin during the second stage of blood coagulation; also called coagulation Factor II.

Prothrombin time (PT): screening test to evaluate the extrinsic coagulation and common pathways, and to monitor oral anticoagulant therapy.

Thrombin: enzyme derived from prothrombin that converts fibrinogen to fibrin.

Thrombin time: qualitative test to measure the functional fibrinogen level.

Thrombocytopenia: decrease in the number of platelets.

Thromboembolism: blood vessel obstruction by a thrombus dislodged from its site of origin.

Thrombolysis: breakdown of preformed thrombin by local plasmin action.

Thromboplastin: factor necessary for thrombin production.

Thrombosis: process of forming or developing a thrombus.

Thromboxane A_2: prostaglandin that increases the stickiness of platelets and fosters aggregation.

Thrombus: solid mass, clot, or plug formed in the circulatory system from the coagulation of blood constituents.

Tissue plasminogen activator (TPA): substance that converts inactive plasminogen to plasmin.

Tissue thromboplastin: lipoprotein peptidase released from injured tissues that stimulates coagulation; also called coagulation Factor III.

RBCs remains constant, with RBC production balancing destruction.

Erythropoiesis becomes more rapid when more RBCs are needed. For example, cell production increases when RBCs are lost in hemorrhage and when tissue hypoxia exists. Hemorrhage and hypoxia stimulate the kidneys to produce the hormone erythropoietin, which accelerates RBC production in the bone marrow.

The bone marrow requires adequate supplies of iron, vitamin B_{12}, amino acids, copper, and cobalt to produce erythrocytes.

Anemia represents a significant decrease in RBC or hemoglobin concentration in the circulating blood. Although many types of anemia exist, the two major types are microcytic anemia, from iron deficiency, and macrocytic anemia, from vitamin B_{12} or folic acid deficiency.

BLOOD COAGULATION

The pathways involved in blood coagulation include the intrinsic (intravascular) and the extrinsic (extravascular). The intrinsic pathway is activated by injury to the endothelial layer of the blood vessel, disrupting blood flow. The disrupted blood flow initiates a chain of events that forms a thrombus, or clot. Atherosclerotic plaque formation is a condition that activates this type of clotting.

The extrinsic pathway is activated by injury to tissues and vessels, such as surgical wounds or burns, releasing tissue thromboplastin into the circulation. The thromboplastin, a powerful procoagulant, stimulates a chain of events that forms a thrombus. (For details, see *Coagulation factors and pathways*.)

The body also produces blood clots to repair damage in blood vessel walls from normal wear and tear. Platelets adhere to the damaged vessel area and release adenosine diphosphate, which produces platelet stickiness that helps a clot form. Vasoconstriction in the damaged blood vessel reduces blood flow and produces blood stasis, allowing time for the clot to form.

The body maintains a delicate balance between clot formation (coagulation) and clot destruction (fibrinolysis). Coagulation is inhibited by (1) the liver and reticuloendothelial system, which remove clotting factors from the blood, (2) antithrombins, which neutralize thrombin, (3) adequate blood flow, which dilutes clotting factors, and (4) the fibrinolytic system, which interferes with the action of thrombin on fibrinogen.

Certain diseases are characterized by abnormal coagulation. Thrombus formation can occur in the venous system, causing venothrombosis (such as a pulmonary embolus), or in the arterial system, causing arterial thrombosis (such as a cerebrovascular thrombosis from a diseased mitral valve). Drugs that are used to treat or prevent thrombotic disorders are known as anticoagulant and antiplatelet drugs. They act by inhibiting formation of thrombin and of Factors II, VII, IX, and X (oral anticoagulants) and II, Xa, XIa, and XII (heparin) in the liver or by interfering with platelet aggregation.

FIBRINOLYSIS

Conditions such as blood stagnation or blood vessel damage trigger the coagulation mechanism and activate the fibrinolytic system. The fibrinolytic system restricts clot propagation in the general circulation, breaks down the thrombus (fibrinolysis), and removes the fibrin networks as the injured area heals.

When the fibrinolytic system is activated, tissue plasminogen activator (TPA) is released from stored areas in the endothelium. TPA is released during stress reactions, vigorous exercise, hypoglycemia, and anabolic steroid use.

TPA binds to fibrin and converts inactive circulating plasminogen to plasmin, the proteolytic enzyme that digests fibrin threads, fibrinogen, Factor V, Factor VIII, Factor XII, and prothrombin. The plasmin then can cause clot lysis.

Plasmin normally is inactivated in the circulation by alpha$_2$-antiplasmin, a physiologic inhibitor that prevents too much circulating plasmin, which can cause blood hypocoagulability. However, plasmin bound to fibrin is resistant to alpha$_2$-antiplasmin. Normally, fibrinolysis is restricted to a thrombus area, preventing generalized fibrinolysis and bleeding.

Fibrinolysis of a thrombus produces fibrin degradation products (FDPs). FDPs, which are not present normally in the bloodstream, interfere with platelet aggregation and produce an anticoagulant effect.

AGENTS TO CONTROL BLEEDING

Because bleeding is the major adverse effect of anticoagulant and thrombolytic agents, the nurse must be aware of the appropriate hemostatic agents. If bleeding results from a deficiency in the body's clotting factors, as in hemophilia, prescribed hemostatic agents, such as antihemophilic factor (Factor VIII) and Factor IX complex, would be administered. If the patient's bleeding is caused by fibrinolytic therapy, aminocaproic acid (Amicar) might be administered. Excessive bleeding from heparin or oral anticoagulant therapy is treated with protamine sulfate or vitamin K, respectively. Also, several agents can be applied locally to a wound or puncture site to control bleeding and capillary oozing. (For more information, see *Agents to control bleeding*, pages 604 and 605.)

BLOOD DERIVATIVES

Whole blood or one of its component fractions may be administered to replace blood volume lost in hemorrhage or to control bleeding. Some components of whole blood that can be separated are packed red cells, plasma, normal serum albumin, plasma protein fraction, and platelets. Using component transfusions provides therapy for specific deficiencies, expands the usefulness of a single blood donation, eases chronic shortages of blood supplies, and reduces the patient's risks of viral hepatitis and exposure to sensitizing agents and drugs.

Blood derivatives are used primarily to provide plasma expanders in patients with hypovolemic shock and other conditions. (For details, see *Whole blood and blood derivatives*, pages 606 and 607.)

(Text continues on page 608.)

Coagulation factors and pathways

Along with blood platelets, coagulation factors control clotting. In the intrinsic and extrinsic pathways, coagulation results from the activation of factors leading to thrombin inhibition that significantly affect coagulation.

Coagulation factors

The following chart lists the factors by number, name, and location.

FACTOR	SYNONYM	LOCATION
Factor I	Fibrinogen	Plasma
Factor II	Prothrombin	Plasma
Factor III	Tissue thromboplastin	Tissue cells
Factor IV	Calcium ion	Plasma
Factor V	Labile factor	Plasma
Factor VII	Stable factor	Plasma
Factor VIII	Antihemophilic globulin (AHG) or antihemophilic factor (AHF)	Plasma
Factor IX	Plasma thromboplastin component (PTC) or Christmas factor	Plasma
Factor X	Stuart-Prower factor	Plasma
Factor XI	Plasma thromboplastin antecedent (PTA)	Plasma
Factor XII	Hageman factor	Plasma
Factor XIII	Fibrin stabilizing factor	Plasma

Coagulation pathways

Various factors can affect coagulation via the intrinsic and extrinsic pathways. A naturally occurring protein, antithrombin III neutralizes thrombin. Heparin increases the thrombin-neutralizing action of antithrombin III, so its effect on coagulation is multiple. Oral anticoagulants diminish the action of vitamin K, which is responsible for the formation of Factors II, VII, IX, and X in the liver.

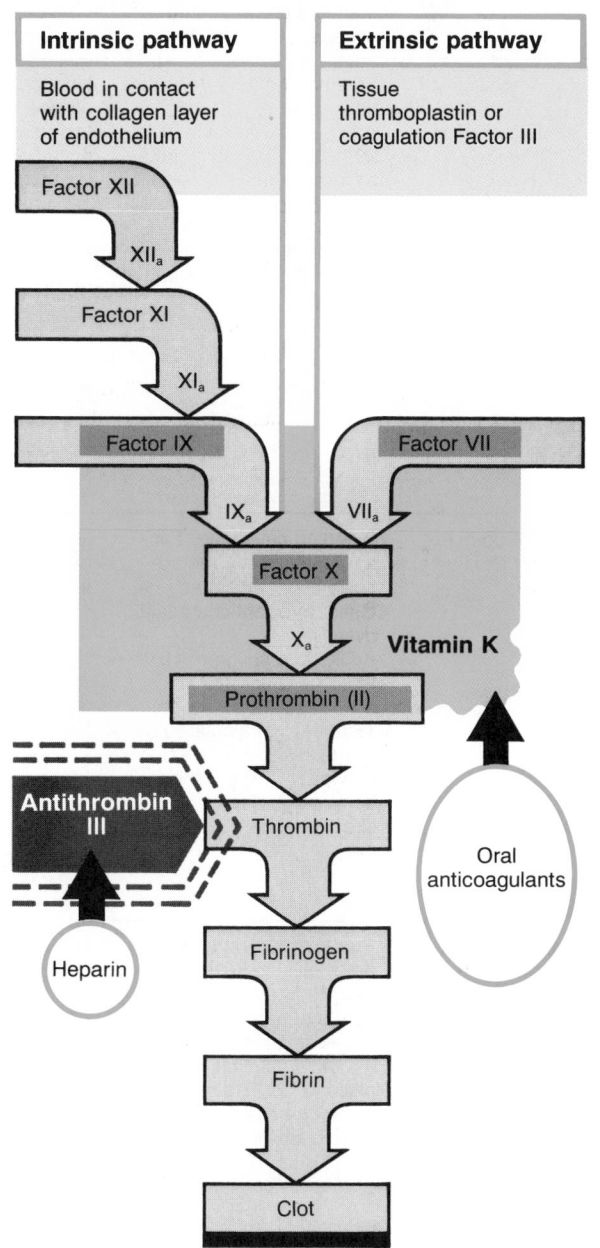

Agents to control bleeding

Bleeding is a major adverse reaction to anticoagulant therapy. When bleeding occurs, the nurse must be prepared to administer the prescribed controlling agents. Aminocaproic acid interacts with oral contraceptives. The other agents listed here have no significant interactions with other drugs.

DRUG	INDICATIONS AND USUAL DOSAGES	ADVERSE REACTIONS	NURSING IMPLICATIONS
aminocaproic acid (Amicar)	Excessive bleeding resulting from hyperfibrinolysis Adults: initially 5 grams P.O. or slow I.V. infusion followed by 1 to 1.25 grams/hour; maximum dosage, 30 grams/day	Generalized thrombosis, dizziness, malaise, headache, hypotension, bradycardia, arrhythmias, tinnitus, nasal stuffiness, nausea, cramps, diarrhea, skin rash	• Dilute with sterile water, normal saline, D_5W, or Ringer's solution. • Monitor coagulation study results. • Know that aminocaproic acid is contraindicated in conditions associated with active intravascular clotting.
antihemophilic factor (AHF, Factor VIII [Hemofilm, Koãte-HS, Koãte-HT, Monoclate])	Bleeding from Factor VIII deficiency Adults and children: 10 to 20 IU/kg I.V. push or infusion every 8 to 24 hours, calculated by this formula: AHF dosage = body weight (in kg) x desired Factor VIII (% of normal) x 0.5	Headache, paresthesias, altered consciousness, tachycardia, hypotension, disturbed vision, nausea, vomiting, erythema, urticaria, hypersensitivity	• Ensure that the patient's blood is typed and crossmatched as prescribed for possible transfusion. • Monitor the patient's vital signs frequently. If tachycardia develops, reduce the flow rate or stop administration, and notify the physician. • Monitor the patient for hypersensitivity reactions. • Use only a plastic syringe to administer I.V. Drug may interact with a glass syringe. • Monitor coagulation study results before and during therapy. • Refrigerate concentrate until use but not after reconstitution. Before reconstituting, bring concentrate and diluent bottles to room temperature. Use the reconstituted solution within 3 hours. • Do not mix with other I.V. solutions.
Factor IX complex (Konyne, Profilnine, Proplex)	Bleeding caused by Factor IX deficiency (hemophilia B or Christmas disease) or anticoagulant overdose Adults and children: 10 to 20 units/kg/day; for anticoagulant overdose, 15 units/kg, calculated by this formula: Factor IX dosage = 1 unit/kg x body weight (in kg) x desired increase (% of normal).	Headache, thromboembolic reactions, hypersensitivity	• Ensure that the patient's blood is typed and crossmatched as prescribed to treat possible hemorrhage. • Observe the patient for hypersensitivity reactions. • Monitor the patient's vital signs frequently. • Avoid rapid infusion, which may cause such adverse reactions as tingling sensations, fever, chills, or headache. • Slow the infusion and notify the physician if a hypersensitivity reaction occurs. • Reconstitute with 20 ml sterile water. Keep refrigerated until ready to use but warm to room temperature before reconstituting. Use within 3 hours of reconstituting. • Do not administer with other I.V. solutions.
absorbable gelatin sponge, film, or powder (Gelfoam)	Pressure ulcers: apply aseptically to wound. Adjunct to hemostasis in surgery: saturate with normal saline solution injection or thrombin solution, hold in place 10 to 15 seconds; when bleeding is controlled, leave in place	Localized infection, abscess formation	• Know that this agent is contraindicated in a patient with active infection. • Avoid overpacking. • Do not remove the sponge, film, or powder. It is systemically absorbed in 4 to 6 weeks.

Agents to control bleeding *(continued)*

DRUG	INDICATIONS AND USUAL DOSAGES	ADVERSE REACTIONS	NURSING IMPLICATIONS
microfibrillar collagen hemostat (Avitene)	Adjunct to hemostasis in surgery: apply drug directly to bleeding site for 1 to 5 minutes, gently remove excess, and reapply as needed	Hematoma, exacerbation of wound dehiscence, abscess formation, foreign body reaction, adhesion formation, enhanced infection in contaminated wounds, mediastinitis, hypersensitivity	• Know that this agent is contraindicated for closure of skin incisions. • Do not inject this drug. • Do not dilute; apply dry. • Handle with smooth, dry forceps and avoid contact with nonbleeding sites because the substance adheres to any wet surface. • Apply directly to bleeding site.
oxidized cellulose (Oxycel, Surgicel)	Adjunct for surgical hemostasis and control of external bleeding at tumor sites: apply using sterile technique, as needed	Headache after nasal packing or application to surface wounds, sneezing, epistaxis or burning, nasal membrane necrosis or septal perforation after packing for rhinologic procedures, encapsulation of fluid, foreign body reaction, burning or stinging, possible prolonged drainage in cholecystectomies	• Know that this agent is contraindicated in controlling hemorrhage from large arteries, in treating serious oozing surfaces, and in implantation for bone defects. • Apply loosely against the bleeding site. • Apply dry for best hemostatic effect. • Apply sparingly to area and remove excess. • Do not use as permanent packing because cyst formation may result.
anti-inhibitor coagulant complex (Autoplex T, Feiba VH immuno)	Bleeding or surgery in a patient with Factor VIII inhibitors 25 to 100 Factor VIII correctional units/kg I.V., repeated after 6 hours if the patient shows no improvement	Hypersensitivity reactions that range from a mild rash to anaphylaxis; headache; flushing; rapid pulse; disseminated intravascular coagulation (DIC) with dosages over 100 units/kg per single infusion or 200 units/kg per day	• Know that this agent is contraindicated in a patient with signs of fibrinolysis and in those with DIC or normal coagulation. • Assess fibrinogen levels before the infusion begins, and then monitor them periodically. • Administer the drug at the prescribed infusion rate, which may be as fast as 10 ml/minute. If headache, flushing, and rapid pulse occur, however, decrease the rate to 2 ml/min. • Keep epinephrine 1:1000 available to manage an acute hypersensitivity reaction.
tranexamic acid (Cyklokapron)	Reduction or prevention of hemorrhage in hemophilia patients; reduction of need for replacement therapy for tooth extraction 10 mg/kg I.V. immediately before tooth extraction or 25 mg/kg P.O. t.i.d. to q.i.d. for 1 day before tooth extraction; then 25 mg/kg P.O. t.i.d. to q.i.d. for 2 to 8 days afterwards	Nausea, vomiting, diarrhea, hypotension (with rapid I.V. injection), giddiness, retinal degeneration (with long-term use)	• Know that this agent is contraindicated in a patient with subarachnoid hemorrhage or defective color vision that prevents detection of toxicity. • Be aware that I.V. tranexamic acid is compatible with most I.V. solutions. • Do not mix with blood or penicillin.
topical thrombin (Thrombinar, Thrombostat)	Adjunct to hemostasis in surgery: apply dry powder or solution, as needed	Hypersensitivity reactions	• Know that this agent is contraindicated in a patient with an allergy to bovine products. • Do not inject this drug. • Prepare the solution with sterile distilled water or normal saline solution for irrigation. Solutions with a concentration of 100 units/ml commonly are used, but concentrations of 1,000 to 2,000 units/ml may be required to stop bleeding from liver or spleen lacerations.

Whole blood and blood derivatives

Because whole blood and blood derivatives frequently are used, the nurse should be aware of their indications, contraindications, and related information.

DESCRIPTION	INDICATIONS	CONTRAINDICATIONS	CROSSMATCHING
Whole blood			
Blood complete with all plasma and cell constituents	Inadequate blood volume in hemorrhaging, trauma, or burn patients	The patient does not need blood volume increase, and a specific component is available.	Necessary
Red blood cells (packed, frozen)			
Whole blood with 80% of plasma removed	Red blood cell (RBC) deficiency, inadequate oxygen-carrying capacity of blood, organ transplant, repeated febrile transfusion reactions (frozen RBCs)	The patient's anemia results from a deficiency of the hematopoietic nutrients; for example, iron, vitamin B_{12}, or folic acid.	Necessary
White blood cells (leukocyte concentrate)			
Whole blood with RBCs and 80% of plasma removed	Life-threatening granulocytopenia from intensive chemotherapy, especially infections that do not respond to antibiotics	The patient's health depends on the recovery of bone marrow function.	Must be ABO compatible
Plasma (fresh, fresh-frozen)			
Uncoagulated plasma separated from whole blood	Clotting factor deficiency, hypovolemia, or severe hepatic disease in a patient with limited synthesis of plasma coagulation factors; prevention of dilutional hypocoagulability	Blood coagulation can be corrected with available specific therapy; the patient needs albumin only.	Unnecessary
Platelets			
Platelet sediment from platelet-rich plasma, resuspended in 30 to 50 ml of plasma	Thrombocytopenia when bleeding is caused by decreased platelet production, increased platelet destruction, functionally abnormal platelets, or massive transfusions of stored blood (dilutional thrombocytopenia)	Bleeding is unrelated to decreased number or abnormal function of platelets; the patient experiences post-transfusion purpura or thrombotic thrombocytopenic purpura.	Unnecessary (donor plasma and recipient's RBCs should be ABO compatible)
Plasma protein fraction			
5% selected proteins solution, pooled plasma in buffered, stabilized saline diluent	Hypovolemic shock or hypoproteinemia. Shock in infants; dehydration or electrolyte deficiencies in children	The patient has severe anemia or heart failure, or has had cardiac bypass surgery.	Unnecessary
Normal serum albumin 5%, normal serum albumin 25%			
Heat-treated, aqueous, chemically processed fraction of pooled plasma	Shock; prevention of marked hemoconcentration; maintenance of electrolyte balance; hypoproteinemia; hyperbilirubinemia in infants	The patient has severe anemia or heart failure.	Unnecessary

SHELF LIFE	ADMINISTRATION TECHNIQUES	SPECIAL CONSIDERATIONS
21 days at 5° C (41° F)	Straight line set, Y-set, or microaggregate recipient set	• Whole blood seldom is transfused: components are extracted from it. • Plasma protein fraction or normal serum albumin usually is given as a volume expander until component needs are known.
For stored fresh-packed cells, 21 days; 24 hours after opening. For stored frozen cells, 3 years; 24 hours after thawing	Straight line set, Y-set, or microaggregate recipient set	• RBCs have the same oxygen-carrying capacity as whole blood without the volume overload hazards. Their use prevents the potassium and ammonia buildup that can occur in stored plasma. Frozen RBCs are expensive.
24 hours after collection at 5° C (41° F)	Straight line set with standard in-line filter Dosage: one unit daily until infection clears (usually within 5 days)	• Infusion induces fever and can cause mild hypertension, severe chills, disorientation, and hallucinations.
For fresh plasma, within 6 hours after collection. For fresh-frozen plasma, 12 months at −18° C (−0.4° F); 2 hours after thawing	Any straight line set; administer as rapidly as possible	• Normal saline solution is not needed for Y-set because the component contains no RBCs that otherwise would be damaged by nonisotonic solutions.
Up to 72 hours after whole blood collection	Syringe or component drip set only; administer as rapidly as possible (uninterrupted) Must use a nonwettable filter Dosage: 2 units/kg of body weight to raise platelet count, at least 50,000/mm³	• Platelets are usually given when the platelet count falls below 10,000/mm³. • Give antihistamines before transfusion if the patient has a history of adverse reactions. Slow administration may prevent overload. • Platelets are least hazardous when given fresh.
5 years if refrigerated; 3 years at room temperature	Any straight line set with the rate and volume based on the patient's condition and response	• Do not mix in same line with protein hydrolysates or alcohol solutions. • Plasma protein fraction frequently is used as a volume expander while crossmatching is done.
5 years at 2° C (35.6° F); 3 years at room temperature	Administration set provided with albumin Give undiluted, or diluted with normal saline solution or D₅W. Administer slowly (1 to 3 ml/minute) in hypoproteinemia to prevent rapid volume expansion; as rapidly as possible in shock.	• Albumin cannot transmit hepatitis because it is heat-treated at 60° C (140° F) for 10 hours. • It frequently is used as a volume expander while crossmatching is done.

OVERVIEW OF CHAPTERS

The chapters in Unit Eight discuss drugs that affect the hematologic system, including hematinic, anticoagulant, and thrombolytic agents.

Chapter 35
Hematinic Agents

Chapter 35 covers drugs that are used to improve blood quality (iron, vitamin B_{12}, and folic acid) and quantity (epoetin alfa). It emphasizes the clinical uses of hematinic agents in treating various anemias. It also highlights patient teaching and other aspects of nursing care for the patient receiving a hematinic agent.

Chapter 36
Anticoagulant Agents

This chapter discusses heparin, oral anticoagulants, and antiplatelet agents. It discusses clinical situations that reuire the use of anticoagulants and laboratory values that the nurse uses to monitor the various therapies. Chapter 36 stresses appropriate administration techniques and drug dosages for various clinical conditions. For each type of anticoagulant agent, it details the related nursing interventions.

Chapter 37
Thrombolytic Agents

Agents used to dissolve clots are the focus of Chapter 37. The chapter begins by discussing the clinical consequences of thromboembolic conditions for patients. Then it describes the thrombolytic agents, including alteplase, anistreplase, streptokinase, and urokinase, as well as the adverse effects of thrombolytic therapy. The chapter concludes with a discussion of associated nursing care, emphasizing appropriate laboratory values for monitoring the therapy and interventions for treating adverse reactions in the patient.

HEMATINIC AGENTS

OBJECTIVES

After reading and studying this chapter, the student should be able to:

1. Describe the function of iron, vitamin B_{12}, and folic acid in normal red blood cell (RBC) production.

2. Discuss the pharmacokinetics of iron, vitamin B_{12}, and folic acid preparations.

3. Explain the mechanisms of action for the major hematinic agents.

4. Discuss the use of iron to treat iron deficiency anemia and the use of vitamin B_{12} and folic acid to treat megaloblastic anemias.

5. Identify the major drug interactions and adverse reactions for iron, vitamin B_{12}, and folic acid.

6. Discuss the pharmacokinetics and therapeutic uses of epoetin alfa.

7. Describe how to apply the nursing process when caring for a patient who is receiving a hematinic agent.

INTRODUCTION

This chapter discusses the hematinic agents that are used to treat microcytic and macrocytic anemias: iron, vitamin B_{12} and folic acid. It also briefly describes the use of epoetin alfa to treat the normocytic anemia associated with chronic renal failure.

Microcytic hypochromic (iron-deficiency) anemia, characterized by small, incompletely hemoglobinized RBCs, results from inadequate dietary intake of iron or excessive blood loss, which may occur with slow, insidious gastrointestinal (GI) bleeding and heavy menstrual bleeding. Iron-deficiency anemia occurs worldwide and is a health problem, particularly for women. Treatment focuses on replacing depleted iron.

Macrocytic (megaloblastic) anemia, characterized by abnormally large RBCs, results from vitamin B_{12} or folic acid deficiency. Vitamin B_{12} and folic acid are essential elements for normal erythropoiesis (RBC production). Some

---

SELECTED NURSING DIAGNOSES

Hematinic agents

The following nursing diagnoses address representative problems and etiologies that a nurse may encounter when caring for a patient who is receiving a hematinic agent. Some of these nursing diagnoses contain generalized etiologies, which the nurse must individualize based on the patient's needs. (For some common nursing diagnoses and related interventions for each drug class, see the "Nursing Process Application" sections of this chapter.)

- Altered health maintenance related to ineffectiveness of the prescribed hematinic agent
- Altered nutrition: less than body requirements, related to the adverse gastrointestinal (GI) effects of a hematinic agent
- Altered peripheral tissue perfusion related to vitamin B_{12}-induced peripheral vascular thrombosis
- Constipation related to the adverse GI effects of iron
- Diarrhea related to the adverse GI effects of a hematinic agent
- Fluid volume excess related to vitamin B_{12}-induced pulmonary edema or congestive heart failure
- Impaired tissue integrity related to inflammation at the iron injection site
- Knowledge deficit related to the prescribed hematinic agent
- Noncompliance related to lifelong vitamin B_{12} therapy
- Pain related to discomfort from parenteral iron administration
- Potential altered body temperature related to febrile episodes caused by iron therapy
- Potential for injury related to a preexisting condition that contraindicates the use of a hematinic agent
- Potential for injury related to a preexisting condition that requires cautious use of a hematinic agent
- Potential for injury related to adverse drug reactions
- Potential for injury related to drug interactions
- Potential for poisoning related to accidental iron ingestion by a child
- Potential for trauma related to the adverse central nervous system effects of a hematinic agent
- Sensory-perceptual alterations (tactile) related to iron dextran-induced paresthesias

patients develop anemia from inadequate dietary intake or from insufficient GI tract absorption.

The symptoms of microcytic and macrocytic anemia include pallor, fatigue, rapid pulse, shortness of breath, irritability, and cardiac irregularities. Iron is used to treat iron-deficiency anemia; vitamin B_{12} or folic acid, or both, are used to treat macrocytic anemia.

An adequate, well-balanced diet usually provides sufficient amounts of these vitamins and minerals for normal RBC production. Meats, legumes, and green vegetables provide iron. Fish and meat supply vitamin B_{12}, and fresh green vegetables supply folic acid primarily as folate.

Characterized by a decrease in the number of RBCs, normocytic anemia results from erythropoietin deficiency. Normally, RBC production is stimulated by erythropoietin, a plasma protein that is converted into a hormone by the enzyme, renal erythropoietic factor. Chronic renal failure and other conditions that affect this enzyme's production or release can reduce erythopoietin levels, which leads to normocytic anemia. To treat this type of anemia, the RBC production stimulant epoetin alfa is used to increase the number of RBCs.

For a summary of representative drugs, see *Selected major drugs: Hematinic agents,* page 621. For a listing of applicable nursing diagnoses that the nurse may formulate when caring for a patient receiving these agents, see *Selected nursing diagnoses: Hematinic agents,* page 609. For detailed information on applying the nursing process, see Chapter 6, The Nursing Process and Drug Therapy.

IRON

Iron preparations are used to treat the most common form of anemia—iron-deficiency anemia—which results from inadequate iron ingestion, absorption, or utilization; increased iron requirement or excretion; or metabolic destruction of iron. Iron preparations discussed in this chapter include ferrous fumarate, ferrous gluconate, ferrous sulfate, and iron dextran.

PHARMACOKINETICS

An essential mineral, iron is a component of hemoglobin, myoglobin, and certain enzymes. Although 80% of the iron in the body is used for RBC production, iron also is important in muscle metabolism and in cognitive functions of children.

Absorption, distribution, metabolism, excretion

Iron is absorbed primarily from the duodenum and upper jejunum by an active transport mechanism that moves the iron into plasma as heme or into storage as ferritin. The amount of iron absorbed depends partially on the body stores of iron; when body stores are low or erythropoiesis is accelerated, iron absorption may increase by 20% to 30%. When total iron stores are large, only about 5% to 10% of iron is absorbed. The ferrous salt form is absorbed three times more readily than the ferric form. Ferrous fumarate, ferrous gluconate, and ferrous sulfate are absorbed almost equally although they contain different amounts of elemental iron. Enteric-coated preparations decrease iron absorption because the iron is released past the duodenum. Larger doses of iron will result in increased amounts being absorbed but by a reduced percentage. The lymphatic system absorbs the parenteral form of iron from intramuscular (I.M.) sites, which results in 60% absorption in 3 days and 90% absorption after 1 to 3 weeks.

Iron is transported by the blood and bound to transferrin, the plasma iron-transport protein. About 30% of the iron is stored primarily as hemosiderin or ferritin in the reticuloendothelial cells of the liver, spleen, and bone marrow. About two-thirds of the total body iron is contained in hemoglobin.

Iron is excreted in feces, sweat, urine, breast milk, and through intestinal cell sloughing. The daily loss amounts to 0.5 to 1 mg in a normal male and up to 2 mg in a menstruating female.

Onset, peak, duration

Within 3 days after the patient starts oral iron therapy, the reticulocyte count rises; after 1 week of therapy, the hemoglobin level and hematocrit increase. The peak concentration level occurs in about 4 weeks. When iron is given I.V. or I.M., the hemoglobin level rises approximately 1 gram/week, with the peak concentration occurring in 4 to 8 weeks.

PHARMACODYNAMICS

Iron is used by the body in erythropoiesis and is transported to intracellular sites by the protein transferrin.

Mechanism of action

Although iron serves as a component of myoglobin and various intracellular enzymes (such as cytochrome oxidase, peroxidase, and catalase), its most important role is in the normal production of hemoglobin. About 80% of iron in plasma goes to the erythroid marrow, where it is used for erythropoiesis. RBCs normally circulate for about 120 days; then they are catabolized by the reticuloendothelium. Part of the iron from the destroyed RBCs is bound to transferrin;

part is incorporated into ferritin stores in the reticuloendothelial cells.

Iron is absorbed as heme or inorganic iron from food in the intestine. After absorption, iron immediately combines with apotransferrin, a beta globulin, to form transferrin. Transferrin transports iron to all tissues, but especially to hepatic tissue. There it is stored as ferritin (a water-soluble complex) and hemosiderin (an insoluble complex). Transferrin also transports iron directly to the mitochondria of erythroblasts (immature RBCs) in the bone marrow, where it is used to synthesize hemoglobin.

PHARMACOTHERAPEUTICS

Iron therapy is used to prevent and treat iron-deficiency anemia. It also is used to prevent anemias in infants ages 6 months to 2 years—periods of rapid growth. Pregnant women may need iron therapy to replace the iron used by the developing fetus.

Iron-deficiency anemias can be treated successfully with oral drug therapy in most individuals. Hundreds of iron preparations are commercially available, ranging from simple water-soluble iron salts to sustained-release enteric-coated preparations to multivitamins with iron. These products vary in their iron content, absorption rate, adverse effects, and cost. Adults typically require 150 to 200 mg daily of elemental iron in three divided doses; children, 4 to 6 mg/kg in three divided doses. However, the dosage may vary depending on the iron salt prescribed.

Parenteral drug therapy is used for patients who cannot absorb oral preparations, are noncompliant with oral therapy, or have such bowel disorders as ulcerative colitis. The only currently available parenteral iron is iron dextran, which builds up iron stores more rapidly than oral preparations but does not correct anemia any faster.

The duration of iron therapy varies. The goal is to restore normal hemoglobin levels and replenish iron stores. The rate of hemoglobin repair is 0.2 grams/day per deciliter of whole blood, so the RBC mass usually is reconstituted in 1 to 2 months. The replenishment of iron stores may take several months. The individual with an inadequate diet may require continued low-dose therapy, whereas one with an adequate diet should not require further treatment when the hemoglobin is restored to normal. The average length of iron therapy for deficiency anemias is 6 months.

ferrous fumarate (Feostat, Fumerin). Ferrous fumarate contains 33% elemental iron and comes in tablets, sustained-release tablets, and suspension forms. It is used to prevent and treat iron-deficiency anemia.
Usual adult dosage: 100 to 400 mg P.O. daily to q.i.d.
Usual pediatric dosage: 3 to 6 mg/kg P.O. t.i.d.

ferrous gluconate (Fergon). Ferrous gluconate contains 11.6% elemental iron and comes in tablets, capsules, and elixir preparations. The indications for use are the same as for ferrous fumarate.
Usual adult dosage: 325 to 650 mg P.O. q.i.d.
Usual pediatric dosage: 100 to 300 mg (16 mg/kg) P.O. t.i.d. for a child age 2 or older

ferrous sulfate (Feosol, Fer-In-Sol, Fer-Iron). Ferrous sulfate contains 20% elemental iron (percentage of pure iron in the compound), or 65 mg of elemental iron per 325-mg tablet. The most widely used form of iron and the most economical, it is indicated to prevent and treat iron-deficiency anemia and is available in tablets, elixirs, capsules, and sustained-release preparations.
Usual adult dosage: 300 mg to 1.2 grams P.O. daily, depending on the severity of the anemia.
Usual pediatric dosage: 150 to 600 mg P.O. daily for a child who weighs 33 to 66 lb (15 to 30 kg); 5 mg/kg P.O. daily for a child who weighs less than 33 lb. A child over 66 lb can receive the adult dosage.

iron dextran (Imferon). One milliliter of iron dextran contains 50 mg of elemental iron. Iron dextran is used to treat iron-deficiency anemia in patients who cannot tolerate oral therapy, are noncompliant with oral therapy, or have a bowel disorder, such as ulcerative colitis.
Usual adult dosage: 0.5 ml I.M. or I.V. initially as a test dose, then 2 ml (100 mg) I.M. daily for a patient under 110 lb (50 kg) or 5 ml (250 mg) I.M. daily for a patient over 110 lb; or 2 ml I.V. daily at a rate of 1 ml/minute infused slowly. No single dose should exceed 100 mg I.V.
Usual pediatric dosage: 0.5 ml I.M. or I.V. initially as a test dose, then 0.5 ml (25 mg) for an infant under 11 lb (5 kg); or 1 ml (50 mg) for a child between 11 and 20 lb (5 and 9 kg). A child over 20 lb can receive the adult dosage.

Drug interactions

Few drugs interact with iron, but some antibiotics, antacids, and vitamin preparations, such as ascorbic acid, may alter the absorption rate of iron. Similarly, a few foods may interfere with iron absorption. (For details, see *Drug interactions: Iron,* page 612.)

ADVERSE DRUG REACTIONS

The major adverse reaction to iron therapy is gastric irritation. Accidental iron poisoning may be a danger when children have access to iron preparations, because iron tablets that are brightly colored and sugarcoated can be mistaken for candy. Parenteral iron dextran may elicit an acute hypersensitivity reaction that can be fatal.

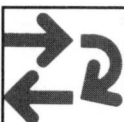

DRUG INTERACTIONS

Iron

A complete drug and food history must be obtained to maximize benefits of iron therapy and to decrease possible drug and food interactions.

DRUG	INTERACTING DRUGS AND FOODS	POSSIBLE EFFECTS	NURSING IMPLICATIONS
ferrous fumarate, ferrous gluconate, ferrous sulfate	tetracycline, oxytetracycline, methacyline, doxycycline	Decrease absorption of tetracycline and related drugs	• Instruct the patient to take these drugs at least 2 hours apart.
	antacids	Decrease the rate or extent of iron absorption by binding with it in the gastrointestinal tract	• Do not administer within 2 hours of each other. • Encourage the patient to use foods to buffer gastric effects, such as nausea.
	penicillamine	Decrease penicillamine absorption	• Instruct the patient not to take these drugs together.
	methyldopa	May reduce absorption and inhibit the antihypertensive effects of methyldopa	• Do not administer at the same time. • Expect to administer a different antihypertensive agent if blood pressure control is inadequate.
	vitamin E	Impairs the therapeutic response to iron therapy in children	• Monitor the patient's response to iron therapy. • Avoid concurrent use, if possible.
	cholestyramine, colestipol	Reduce serum iron levels	• Administer iron preparation 1 hour before or 6 hours after cholestyramine or colestipol. • Monitor the patient's serum iron and hemoglobin levels.
	coffee, tea	Inhibit iron absorption	• Teach the patient to avoid drinking coffee or tea for at least 1 hour after an iron dose.
	eggs, milk	Inhibit iron absorption	• Teach the patient not to use eggs or milk to buffer the gastric effects of iron therapy.

Because iron salts irritate the gastric mucosa, iron preparations often cause GI distress, such as anorexia, nausea, vomiting, constipation, and diarrhea. Iron preparations also darken the stool, and liquid preparations can stain the teeth.

Oral preparations that contain tartrazine yellow may produce allergic reactions, such as bronchospasm, especially in patients with aspirin hypersensitivity.

When iron dextran is given I.M., the patient may experience soreness, inflammation, and skin discoloration at the injection site. The Z-track administration technique can help prevent skin discoloration. Rapid I.V. administration may result in lymphadenopathy, local phlebitis at the infusion site, and peripheral vascular reddening (flushing).

Iron dextran injection also may cause acute hypersensitivity reactions, including anaphylaxis, dyspnea, urticaria and other rashes, pruritus, arthralgia and myalgia, febrile episodes, sweating, and allergic purpura. Therefore, a test dose of iron dextran should be administered before initiating therapy. Hypotension, seizures, arthritic reactivation, leu-

kocytosis, headache, backache, dizziness, malaise, transitory paresthesias, and shivering also have been reported.

NURSING PROCESS APPLICATION

The following information assists the nurse in caring for a patient who is receiving an iron preparation.

Assessment

• Review the patient's history for a preexisting condition that contraindicates the use of iron, such as primary hemochromatosis, infectious kidney disease during the acute phase, peptic ulcer, regional enteritis, ulcerative colitis, or known hypersensitivity to iron.

• Review the patient's history for a preexisting condition that requires cautious use of iron dextran, such as severely impaired liver function, significant allergies or asthma, pregnancy, or lactation.

• Assess the patient for adverse reactions to iron, such as GI distress, hypersensitivity reactions, hypotension, or seizures.

• Review the patient's medication history to identify the use of drugs that may interact with iron, such as certain antibiotics, antacids, methyldopa, vitamin E, cholestyramine, or colestipol.

• Obtain a dietary history to identify the use of foods that may interact with iron, such as coffee, tea, eggs, or milk.

• Assess the effectiveness of iron therapy regularly.

• Assess the patient for constipation regularly during iron therapy.

• Evaluate the patient's and family's knowledge about the prescribed iron preparation.

Nursing diagnoses

The following examples represent appropriate nursing diagnoses for a patient receiving an iron preparation.

• Potential for injury related to a preexisting condition that contraindicates the use of iron

• Potential for injury related to a preexisting condition that requires cautious use of iron dextran

• Potential for injury related to adverse drug reactions

• Constipation related to the adverse GI effects of iron

• Knowledge deficit related to the prescribed iron preparation

Planning and implementation

• Do not administer an iron preparation to a patient with a condition that contraindicates its use.

• Administer iron dextran cautiously to a patient at risk because of a preexisting condition.

• Monitor the patient closely for adverse reactions during iron therapy.

• Monitor hydration if the patient experiences GI distress. Obtain a prescription for an antiemetic or antidiarrheal agent, as needed.

• *Monitor the patient's blood pressure regularly to detect hypotension.*

• *Take seizure precautions, such as padding the bed rails. If the patient experiences seizures, notify the physician.*

• Expect to monitor the patient's serum iron levels and complete blood count with differential regularly to evaluate the drug's effectiveness. Increased iron and hemoglobin levels indicate effective therapy; decreased white blood cells indicate leukocytosis, an adverse reaction.

• Take infection control measures if leukocytosis occurs. For example, isolate the patient from people with infections.

• Obtain a prescription for an analgesic if the patient experiences headache or backache.

• *Take safety precautions if dizziness occurs. For example, keep the bed in a low position and supervise ambulation.*

• *Administer oral iron preparations between meals and at least 2 hours before or after giving an antacid.*

• Check the oral preparation's product listing for tartrazine yellow, which may produce bronchospasm and other allergic reactions, especially in patients with aspirin hypersensitivity.

• *Monitor the patient receiving iron dextran closely for an acute hypersensitivity reaction, such as anaphylaxis, dyspnea, urticaria and other rashes, pruritus, arthralgia and myalgia, febrile episodes, sweating, and allergic purpura. An acute reaction can be fatal. Keep standard emergency equipment nearby.*

• Give a test dose of iron dextran before beginning therapy, as instructed, to assess the patient's response. If no adverse reactions occur within 1 hour, give the total dosage.

• *Infuse iron dextran I.V. slowly at a rate of 1 ml/minute. More rapid infusion may cause phlebitis and peripheral vascular reddening (flushing) at the infusion site. Do not administer a single dose of more than 100 mg I.V.*

• Assess the patient for signs of hypersensitivity reactions during iron dextran I.V. infusion. Use only single-dose vials for I.V. therapy. Multidose vials contain the preservative phenol, which can cause serious adverse reactions.

• *Administer iron dextran I.M. by the Z-track technique to avoid leakage into subcutaneous tissue.*

• Notify the physician if adverse reactions occur.

• Encourage the patient to drink at least 2 liters of fluid daily (unless contraindicated), increase fiber intake, and exercise regularly to prevent constipation. If constipation occurs, obtain a prescription for a laxative.

Patient teaching

• Teach the patient and family the name, dose, frequency, action, and adverse effects of the prescribed iron preparation.

• Inform the patient of the daily iron requirement. (For more information, see *Daily iron requirements*.)

Daily iron requirements

Pregnant women have the highest daily iron requirements, necessitating plenty of iron-rich foods in their diet.

Children ages 6 months to 10 years	10 mg
Adolescents ages 11 to 18 • male • female	 12 mg 15 mg
Adult females • pregnant • nonpregnant	 30 mg 15 mg
Adult males	10 mg

Iron-rich foods

The nurse should teach the patient with iron-deficiency anemia that the following foods are high in iron.

- liver
- beef
- veal
- lamb
- pork
- turkey
- chicken
- oysters
- eggs
- peanut butter
- soybeans

- greens
- dried apricots
- peaches
- prunes
- figs
- dates
- raisins
- molasses
- dried navy and lima beans
- enriched breads and cereals

- Help the patient explore possible causes of anemia, such as inadequate diet or excessive menstrual bleeding, to prevent recurrence.
- Advise the patient to include iron-rich foods in the diet. (For more information, see *Iron-rich foods*.)
- *Teach the patient how to prevent accidental poisoning in small children.* (For information about this drug-related emergency, see *Accidental iron poisoning in children*.)
- Teach the patient to take liquid preparations with a straw to prevent tooth stains.
- Teach the patient to recognize the signs and symptoms of anemia, such as fatigue, weakness, shortness of breath, intermittent glossitis, and pallor.
- Inform the patient that the average duration of therapy for iron-deficiency anemia is 6 months.
- *Inform the patient that iron preparations normally darken the stool. However, the patient should notify the physician if bloody stool or abdominal cramping or pain occurs.*
- Reassure the patient with paresthesias that this adverse reaction is transitory.
- Inform the patient receiving I.M. iron dextran that soreness, inflammation, and skin discoloration may occur at the injection site.
- Instruct the patient to notify the physician if arthritic pain recurs.
- *Advise the patient not to perform activities that require alertness if dizziness or malaise develops.*
- Instruct the patient to take an oral iron preparation between meals.
- Instruct the patient to take an oral iron preparation 2 hours before or after taking an antacid, if prescribed.

- Teach the patient how to prevent or relieve constipation. For example, suggest that the patient increase fluid intake to 2 liters daily, increase fiber intake, and exercise regularly.
- *Stress the importance of returning for blood tests, as prescribed, to monitor the effectiveness of iron therapy and to detect leukocytosis. If leukocytosis occurs, teach the patient how to prevent infection.*
- Instruct the patient with headache or backache to take a mild analgesic, as prescribed.
- *Instruct the patient who develops seizures to withhold the next iron dose until the physician has been notified.*
- *Advise the patient to check with the physician or pharmacist before taking any new prescription or over-the-counter drugs.*
- *Instruct the patient to notify the physician if adverse reactions occur.*

Evaluation

The following examples represent appropriate evaluation statements for a patient receiving an iron preparation.
- The patient has no conditions that contraindicate iron therapy.
- The patient exhibits no complications in the preexisting condition linked to iron dextran use.
- The patient experiences no adverse reactions to the prescribed iron preparation.
- The patient's bowel function remains normal.
- The patient and family express an accurate understanding of the points taught about the prescribed iron preparation.
- The patient modifies the home environment to prevent accidental iron poisoning in children.

Accidental iron poisoning in children

Signs and symptoms of accidental iron poisoning include nausea, vomiting, and abdominal pain leading to shock. Shock is caused by gastrointestinal hemorrhage and high concentrations of unbound ionic iron in the plasma. Death may result from cardiovascular collapse in a few hours to 2 days. A child who survives the poisoning episode may have end-organ damage, including pyloric and antral stenosis, hepatic cirrhosis, and central nervous system damage.

Accidental iron poisoning is treated with vasopressor drugs, oxygen, and systemic alkalinizing agents. A specific antidote, deferoxamine, may be given if serum iron levels are greater than 300 mg/dl. Deferoxamine converts free and tissue-bound iron to a harmless chelate complex, which is excreted by the kidneys. It can be given via nasogastric tube or I.V. If the I.V. route is used, the infusion rate should not exceed 15 mg/kg of body weight per hour.

VITAMIN B$_{12}$

Megaloblastic anemias result from defective deoxyribonucleic acid (DNA) synthesis. Defective DNA synthesis usually results from a vitamin B$_{12}$ or folic acid deficiency. The anemia is caused by decreased RBC formation and the immaturity, fragility, and early destruction of these cells. As a result, the bone marrow contains large erythroid precursors with immature nuclei and mature hemoglobin-containing cytoplasm (megaloblasts). Large oval RBCs and neutrophils with six or more lobes appear in a peripheral blood smear. This section discusses the vitamin B$_{12}$ preparations cyanocobalamin and hydroxocobalamin.

PHARMACOKINETICS

Vitamin B$_{12}$ is available in oral and injectable forms. Its absorption depends on an intrinsic factor in the gastric mucosa, and most cases of vitamin B$_{12}$-deficiency megaloblastic anemia result from the patient's inability to absorb vitamin B$_{12}$. Therefore, the injectable form most commonly is used to treat this form of anemia.

Absorption, distribution, metabolism, excretion

Vitamin B$_{12}$ absorption depends on intrinsic factor, which is secreted by parietal cells in the body of the stomach. It binds with intrinsic factor, a glycoprotein, and is absorbed in the ileum. Vitamin B$_{12}$ is abundant in a diet of normal protein sources (for example, meat, seafood, milk, eggs, and liver). It even appears in a strict vegetarian diet, which usually includes legumes contaminated with bacteria that synthesize vitamin B$_{12}$, so most cases of this anemia result from malabsorption. The intrinsic factor is secreted by the same cells that secrete hydrochloric acid (HCl). Because parietal cells are stimulated to produce HCl and intrinsic factor by histamine, histamine analogues, and gastrin, an increase in stimulation by any of these will produce an increase in intrinsic factor. Maximal absorption of 1 mcg of vitamin B$_{12}$ requires 500 to 1,000 units of intrinsic factor.

When cyanocobalamin is injected I.M. or subcutaneously (S.C.), it is absorbed and binds to transcobalamin II for transport to the tissues. Vitamin B$_{12}$ is transported in the bloodstream to the liver, where 90% of the body's supply is stored. Although hydroxocobalamin is absorbed more slowly from the injection site, its uptake in the liver may be greater than that of cyanocobalamin. With either agent, the liver slowly releases vitamin B$_{12}$ as needed for cellular metabolic functions. It is excreted in breast milk during lactation. About 3 to 8 mcg of vitamin B$_{12}$ are secreted in bile each day and then reabsorbed in the ileum. Within 48 hours after injection of 100 to 1,000 mcg of vitamin B$_{12}$, 50% to 98% of the dose appears in urine. The major portion is excreted in the first 8 hours.

Onset, peak, duration

The onset of action is quite rapid; mature RBCs appear in a blood smear within 3 days. Patients usually feel better within 24 hours of therapy. The first objective change is the disappearance of the megaloblastic morphology of the bone marrow. The plasma iron concentration dramatically decreases, and the reticulocyte count increases on the second or third day and peaks 6 to 8 days later. By the tenth day, the platelet count is higher than normal, and the granulocyte count reverts to normal within 2 weeks. (For details, see *Effects of vitamin B$_{12}$ therapy on blood,* page 616.)

PHARMACODYNAMICS

The following are some of the known and speculated functions of vitamin B$_{12}$ in the body.

Mechanism of action

When vitamin B$_{12}$ is taken orally or by injection, it replaces vitamin B$_{12}$ that the body normally would absorb from the diet. This vitamin is essential for cell growth and replication and for the maintenance of normal myelin throughout the nervous system. When the vitamin B$_{12}$ supply is inadequate, folate becomes trapped as methyltetrahydrofolate and thus results in a functional deficiency of other intracellular forms of folic acid.

Vitamin B$_{12}$ also may be involved in lipid and carbohydrate metabolism. Impairment of this metabolism may interfere with synthesis of the lipid portion of the myelin sheath and contribute to the neurologic damage that occurs in patients with vitamin B$_{12}$ deficiency. Neurologic deficits also may result from the concurrent abnormality in folate metabolism.

PHARMACOTHERAPEUTICS

Two vitamin B$_{12}$ drugs, cyanocobalamin and hydroxocobalamin, are used to treat vitamin B$_{12}$-deficiency anemia. Vitamin B$_{12}$ usually is administered by the I.M. route, because vitamin B$_{12}$-deficiency anemia often is related to an inability to absorb dietary sources. A vitamin B$_{12}$ deficiency is diagnosed by determination of plasma concentrations of vitamin B$_{12}$ and gastric function tests. Measurement of gastric acidity can be an indirect measure of gastric function because the same cell secretes HCl and intrinsic factor. The Schilling test quantifies ileal absorption of vitamin B$_{12}$.

cyanocobalamin [vitamin B$_{12}$] (Betalin-12, Rubramin PC). Cyanacobalamin is indicated for vitamin B$_{12}$ deficiency caused by malabsorption syndrome, as seen in per-

Effects of vitamin B₁₂ therapy on blood

After administration, vitamin B₁₂ increases erythropoiesis almost immediately. It affects the hematocrit and reticulocyte count within days, as shown in the graphs below.

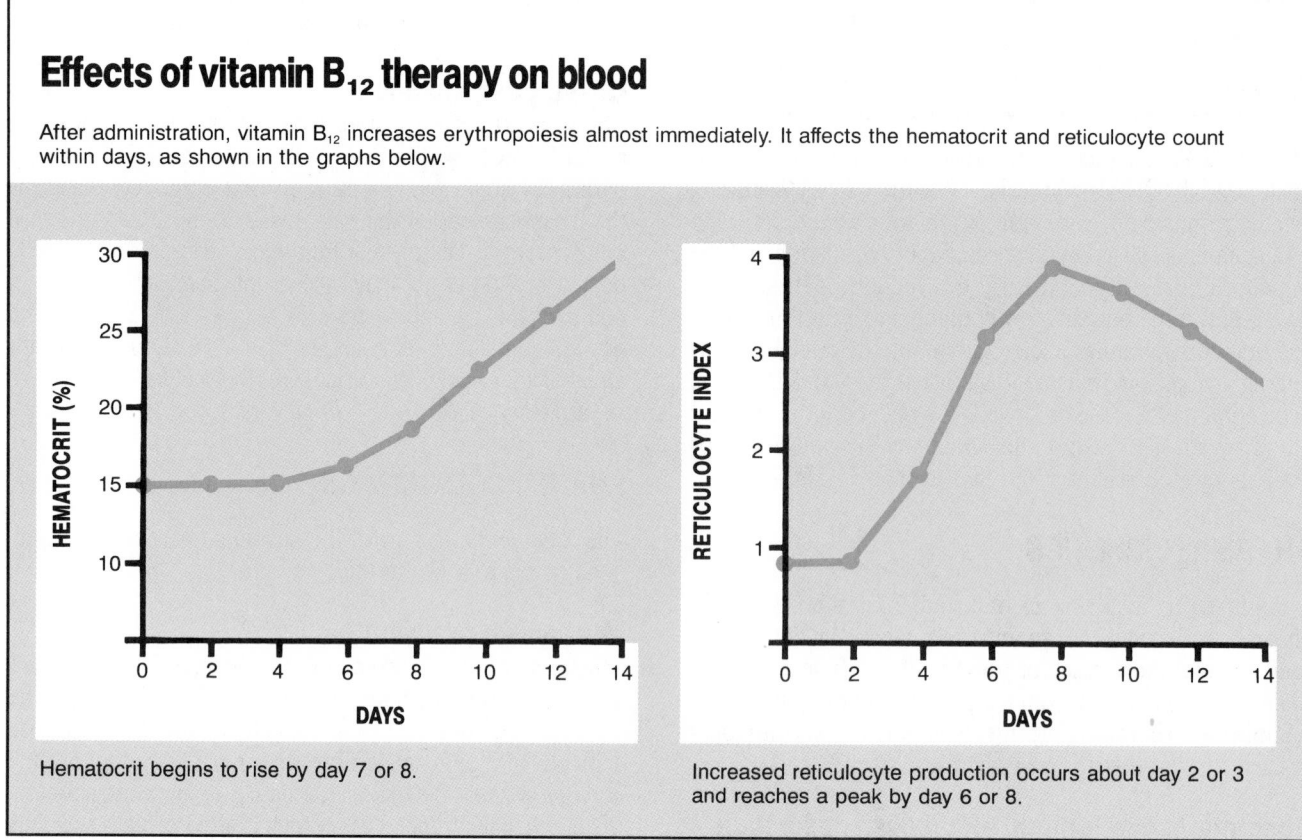

Hematocrit begins to rise by day 7 or 8.

Increased reticulocyte production occurs about day 2 or 3 and reaches a peak by day 6 or 8.

nicious anemia; GI pathology, dysfunction, or surgery; or inadequate dietary intake. Cyanacobalamin usually is given I.M. because in many cases the lack of intrinsic factor prevents absorption in the stomach. For patients with pernicious anemia, parenteral therapy is recommended and required for life.

Usual adult dosage: 100 to 1,000 mcg as a nutritional supplement, 15 mcg in an oral multivitamin preparation; 100 mcg I.M. or S.C. daily for 10 to 30 days or 100 mcg daily for 14 days followed by 100 mcg monthly. Considerably higher doses may be required for critically ill patients with neurologic or infectious diseases or hyperthyroidism.

hydroxocobalamin [vitamin B₁₂] (Alphamin, Alpha Redisol). Hydroxocobalamin is indicated for the same conditions as cyanocobalamin. Hydroxocobalamin is administered I.M. only. It is absorbed more slowly than cyanocobalamin and produces higher blood concentrations. It may be preferred for initial treatment of vitamin B₁₂ deficiency because it produces a more sustained increase in plasma vitamin B₁₂ concentrations. However, it offers no therapeutic advantage over cyanocobalamin when used for monthly maintenance.

Usual adult dosage: 30 mcg I.M. daily for 5 to 10 days followed by 100 to 200 mcg monthly.

Drug interactions

No significant drug interactions are associated with vitamin B₁₂.

ADVERSE DRUG REACTIONS

No dose-related adverse reactions occur with vitamin B₁₂ therapy. However, some uncommon reactions may occur when vitamin B₁₂ is administered parenterally. These include hypersensitivity reactions that could result in anaphylaxis and death, cardiovascular reactions (pulmonary edema, congestive heart failure, and peripheral vascular thrombosis), hematologic reactions (polycythemia vera), dermatologic reactions (itching, transient exanthema, and urticaria), and GI reactions (mild diarrhea). Severe, swift optic nerve atrophy has been reported in patients with hereditary optic nerve atrophy. Some patients report a feeling of swelling throughout the entire body.

NURSING PROCESS APPLICATION

The following information assists the nurse in caring for a patient who is receiving a vitamin B₁₂ preparation.

Assessment

• Review the patient's history for a preexisting condition that contraindicates the use of vitamin B$_{12}$, such as early Leber's disease or known hypersensitivity to the vitamin or cobalt.

• Assess the patient for adverse reactions to vitamin B$_{12}$, such as hypersensitivity, cardiovascular, hematologic, dermatologic, or GI reactions.

• Assess the effectiveness of vitamin B$_{12}$ regularly.

• Assess the patient's compliance with vitamin B$_{12}$ therapy periodically.

• Evaluate the patient's and family's knowledge about the prescribed vitamin B$_{12}$ preparation.

Nursing diagnoses

The following examples represent appropriate nursing diagnoses for a patient receiving a vitamin B$_{12}$ preparation.

• Potential for injury related to a preexisting condition that contraindicates the use of vitamin B$_{12}$

• Potential for injury related to adverse drug reactions

• Noncompliance related to lifelong vitamin B$_{12}$ therapy

• Knowledge deficit related to vitamin B$_{12}$

Planning and implementation

• Do not administer vitamin B$_{12}$ to a patient with a condition that contraindicates its use.

• Monitor the patient closely for adverse reactions.

• *Monitor appropriate laboratory tests, such as hematocrit and reticulocyte count, to determine effectiveness of therapy. Expect to see the hematocrit begin to rise by day 7 or 8 and the reticulocyte count begin to increase by day 2 or 3 and peak by day 6 or 8.*

• *Monitor blood folate levels for a patient who is receiving more than 10 mcg/day of vitamin B$_{12}$. In such a patient, the hematologic picture may seem normal but may mask a folate deficiency, which may be the true cause of megaloblastic anemia.*

• Monitor the patient's hematologic studies for signs of polycythemia vera, an adverse reaction to vitamin B$_{12}$.

• *Keep standard emergency equipment readily available because of the risk of anaphylaxis.*

• *Monitor the patient's vital signs and auscultate breath sounds regularly to detect signs and symptoms of pulmonary edema or congestive heart failure, such as shortness of breath, increased respiratory or heart rate, or crackles.*

• *Check the patient's extremities routinely for signs of decreased circulation, such as decreased or absent pulse or color and temperature or sensory changes. These signs may suggest peripheral vascular thrombosis.*

• Expect to administer the injectable form of vitamin B$_{12}$ as prescribed to a patient who cannot absorb vitamin B$_{12}$ orally.

• Expect to administer an intradermal test dose as prescribed to a patient with cobalt sensitivity who requires vitamin B$_{12}$.

• Expect to administer a higher dosage of cyanocobalamin as prescribed to a critically ill patient with a neurologic or infectious disease or hyperthyroidism.

• Store the parenteral form of the drug in a light-resistant container at room temperature.

• Encourage the patient to eat foods rich in vitamin B$_{12}$, such as meat, seafood, milk, eggs, and liver.

• Notify the physician if adverse reactions occur.

• Monitor the degree of compliance by reviewing the results of appropriate laboratory tests, especially for the patient who needs lifelong therapy.

• Stress the importance of monthly B$_{12}$ injections to the patient with pernicious anemia.

• *Stress the importance of treatment to the patient receiving long-term therapy with I.M. injections because neurologic damage can occur (degenerative spinal cord lesions, for example) as soon as 3 months after a vitamin B$_{12}$ deficiency develops.*

• Alert the physician if noncompliance occurs.

Patient teaching

• Teach the patient and family the name, dose, frequency, action, and adverse effects of the prescribed vitamin B$_{12}$ preparation.

• Explain that the patient should start to feel better 24 hours after therapy begins.

• *Inform the patient that initial parenteral therapy requires daily injections of cyanocobalamin for up to 30 days or of hydroxocobalamin for up to 10 days. Then monthly maintenance therapy is needed until the deficiency resolves or, in the case of pernicious anemia, for life.*

• Teach the patient and family how to administer the vitamin S.C. or I.M., as prescribed, if long-term vitamin B$_{12}$ therapy is necessary.

• Teach the patient how to store the parenteral drug properly.

• *Stress the importance of regular laboratory testing to monitor the effectiveness of therapy or to detect adverse hematologic reactions.*

• *Emphasize the importance of compliance with the drug regimen.*

• Teach the patient that a well-balanced diet can eliminate vitamin deficiencies.

• Instruct the patient to eat foods that are rich in vitamin B$_{12}$, such as meat, seafood, milk, eggs, liver, or legumes.

• Reassure the patient with exanthema that it is transitory.

• Reassure the patient with diarrhea that it usually remains mild. If it becomes troublesome, obtain a prescription for an antidiarrheal agent, as needed.

• Instruct the patient to notify the physician if adverse reactions occur.

Evaluation
The following examples represent appropriate evaluation statements for a patient receiving vitamin B_{12}.
• The patient has no conditions that contraindicate vitamin B_{12} therapy.
• The patient demonstrates no adverse reactions to the prescribed vitamin B_{12} preparation.
• The patient complies willingly with vitamin B_{12} therapy.
• The patient and family express an appropriate understanding of the points taught about the prescribed vitamin B_{12} preparation.
• The patient correctly demonstrates S.C. administration of vitamin B_{12}.

FOLIC ACID

The second cause of megaloblastic anemia is folic acid deficiency. Like vitamin B_{12}, folic acid, as folate, is available in sufficient quantities in the average diet. Fresh green vegetables, meat, and eggs are particularly rich in folates. Because most of the folate is absorbed in the proximal portion of the GI tract, folic acid deficiency may accompany pathology in the jejunum. Nontropical or tropical sprue, liver disease, or alcoholism also are common causes of folic acid deficiency and megaloblastic anemia.

PHARMACOKINETICS

Folate is required for nucleoprotein synthesis and the maintenance of normal erythropoiesis. Present in many foods, it must undergo hydrolysis, reduction, and methylation in the GI tract before it can be absorbed.

Absorption, distribution, metabolism, excretion
Folates present in food mostly take the form of reduced polyglutamates. Folate absorption requires transport and the action of an enzyme in the mucosal cell membranes. The mucosa of the duodenum and upper jejunum are rich in dihydrofolate reductase and can methylate most of the reduced folate.

Once absorbed, folate is transported rapidly to the tissues. It is distributed to all body tissues, but the largest amounts are found in the cerebrospinal fluid. Folate supplies are maintained from food and by the enterohepatic cycle. The liver actively reduces and methylates the folate components, which then are transported to bile for resorption by the gut and subsequently delivered to the tissues.

This pathway may provide as much as 200 mcg of folate daily for recirculation to the tissues.

Folates are excreted in urine and feces and secreted in breast milk.

Adults need 50 to 100 mcg of folic acid daily from food to balance the normal daily losses. However, because about 10 to 20 mg of folic acid are stored in the liver and other tissues, an unreplenished body supply could last for 3 to 6 months.

Onset, peak, duration
Within 48 hours after the patient starts folic acid therapy, megaloblastic erythropoiesis disappears, the plasma iron level falls, and erythropoiesis becomes more efficient. The reticulocyte count begins to rise by the second day and reaches a peak concentration level by the fifth or seventh day. The hematocrit begins to rise by the second week.

PHARMACODYNAMICS

Folic acid is an essential component for normal RBC production and growth. A deficiency results in megaloblastic anemia and low serum and RBC folic acid levels. Neurologic abnormalities do not result from folic acid deprivation but commonly accompany it in patients suffering from alcoholism or liver disease.

PHARMACOTHERAPEUTICS

Folic acid is used to treat folic acid deficiency. Parenteral folic acid seldom is required except to reverse the effect of antifolates during cancer chemotherapy or during a therapeutic trial to determine the hematopoietic response before oral therapy begins. Patients who are pregnant or undergoing treatment for liver disease, hemolytic anemia, alcoholism, skin disease, or renal failure will need prophylactic folic acid therapy.

folic acid [folate, vitamin B_9] (Folvite). Folic acid is used to treat megaloblastic anemia from folic acid deficiency as seen in sprue, nutritional anemias, pregnancy, alcoholism, and liver disease. Folic acid is available in many multivitamin and iron preparations in doses of 100 mcg to 1 mg. Folic acid dosages above 400 mcg require a prescription. *Usual adult dosage:* 100 to 400 mcg/day P.O.; 1 mg P.O. 1 to 3 times daily for severe malabsorption. Folic acid may be administered I.M., I.V., or S.C. if oral administration is not possible.

leucovorin calcium (Wellcovorin). Leucovorin calcium is given as an I.M. injection to prevent and treat the undesired hematopoietic effects of folic acid antagonists, such as methotrexate, used in cancer chemotherapy. Dosage varies with the chemotherapeutic agent being used. Leucovorin calcium also may be given P.O. or I.V. (For more information, see Chapter 67, Antimetabolite Agents.)

Drug interactions

Antifolates that inhibit dihydrofolate reductase include methotrexate (antimetabolite), antimalarial agents, triamterene (diuretic), pentamidine (antiprotozoal), and trimethoprim (urinary antimicrobial). These antifolates may cause a deficiency of active folate compounds, which can lead to megaloblastic anemia. Leucovorin calcium may be required to minimize interference.

In large doses, folic acid may increase seizure activity because it counteracts the effects of anticonvulsant agents, such as phenytoin, phenobarbital, and primidone. Such drugs as glutethimide, isoniazid, cycloserine, and oral contraceptives may interfere with folic acid absorption. Folic acid may interfere with the antimicrobial action of pyrimethamine.

ADVERSE DRUG REACTIONS

Allergic responses (erythema, rash, itching) have been reported after folic acid and leucovorin calcium administration.

NURSING PROCESS APPLICATION

The following information assists the nurse in caring for a patient who is receiving a folic acid preparation.

Assessment

• Review the patient's history for a preexisting condition that requires cautious use of folic acid, such as anemia when the cause has not been diagnosed yet.
• Assess the patient for adverse reactions to folic acid, such as erythema, rash, or itching.
• Review the patient's medication history to identify the use of drugs that may interact with the prescribed folic acid preparation, such as methotrexate, triamterine, trimethoprim, phenytoin, phenobarbital, or oral contraceptives.
• Assess the effectiveness of folic acid therapy periodically.
• Evaluate the patient's and family's knowledge about the prescribed folic acid preparation.

Nursing diagnoses

The following examples represent appropriate nursing diagnoses for a patient receiving a folic acid preparation.
• Potential for injury related to a preexisting condition that requires cautious use of a folic acid preparation
• Potential for injury related to adverse drug reactions
• Knowledge deficit related to the prescribed folic acid preparation

Planning and implementation

• *Administer folic acid cautiously to a patient at risk because of a preexisting condition.*
• Monitor the patient closely for adverse reactions during folic acid therapy.
• Expect to administer folic acid to a patient who is pregnant or undergoing treatment for liver disease, hemolytic anemia, alcoholism, skin disease, or renal failure. Expect to administer leucovorin calcium to a patient receiving an antifolate, such as methotrexate, antimalarial agents, triamterene, pentamidine, or trimethoprim, to prevent megaloblastic anemia.
• Monitor the effectiveness of folic acid therapy, particularly during the first 2 weeks. Check for a rise in the reticulocyte count that peaks by the fifth or seventh day and a rise in the hematocrit by the second week.
• *Take seizure precautions in a patient receiving large doses of folic acid during concomitant anticonvulsant therapy.*
• *Monitor closely for recurrence of megaloblastic anemia if the patient takes drugs that interfere with folic acid absorption, such as glutethimide, isoniazid, cycloserine, or an oral contraceptive.*
• Provide the patient with foods that are high in folate, such as fresh green vegetables, eggs, and meat.
• Notify the physician if adverse reactions occur or if folic acid effectiveness decreases.

Patient teaching

• Teach the patient and family the name, dose, action, frequency, and adverse effects of the prescribed folic acid preparation.
• Assess the patient's dietary habits. The diet of an elderly, alcoholic, or indigent patient may lack folate-rich foods.
• Teach the patient the dietary sources of folate. Instruct the patient not to overcook vegetables because this may destroy folic acid compounds.
• Teach the female patient about the increased need for folic acid during pregnancy.
• *Instruct the patient to inform all personal physicians about folic acid therapy to prevent drug interactions.*
• Advise the patient to notify the physician if adverse reactions occur or if signs of megaloblastic anemia recur.

Evaluation

The following examples represent appropriate evaluation statements for a patient receiving a folic acid preparation.
• The patient exhibits no signs of complications in the preexisting condition linked to the prescribed folic acid preparation.
• The patient displays no adverse reactions to the prescribed folic acid preparation.

• The patient and family express an accurate understanding of the points taught about the prescribed folic acid preparation.

• The patient correctly identifies folate-rich foods and describes how to prepare them.

OTHER HEMATINIC AGENTS

A new hematinic agent, epoetin alfa stimulates RBC production. It is used to treat patients with normocytic anemia caused by chronic renal failure (CRF).

PHARMACOKINETICS

After S.C. administration to patients with CRF, epoetin reaches the peak plasma level within 24 hours. It has a circulating half-life from 4 to 13 hours in patients with CRF. No difference in half-life is apparent in patients on dialysis and patients not on dialysis whose serum creatinine level is greater than 3. Small amounts of the drug have been recovered in plasma and urine after administration. The exact metabolic pathway has not been determined yet.

PHARMACODYNAMICS

Erythropoietin is an amino acid polypeptide that regulates RBC production in the bone marrow. Normally, erythropoietin is formed in the kidneys in response to hypoxia and anemia and stimulates erythropoiesis. Patients with CRF have decreased production of erythropoietin, resulting in chronic normocytic anemia.

PHARMACOTHERAPEUTICS

Like the other hematinic agents, epoetin alfa is used to replace a substance that is essential to the hematologic system.

epoetin alfa (Epogen). Epoetin is used to treat anemia associated with CRF. It elevates or maintains the RBC levels (as manifested by hematocrit or hemoglobin determinations) and decreases the need for transfusions. This drug is not intended for patients who require immediate correction of severe anemia. It is contraindicated in patients with uncontrolled hypertension or known hypersensitivity to mammalian cell-derived albumin or albumin-containing products. Epoetin alfa must be used with caution in pregnant or lactating patients and ones with porphyria.

Usual adult dosage: initially, 50 to 100 units/kg I.V. three times weekly in patients on dialysis (I.V. or S.C. for other patients); then reduced when the target range is reached or the hematocrit increases above 4 points in a 2-week period. The dosage should be increased if the hematocrit does not increase by 5 to 6 points after 8 weeks of therapy and remains below the target range of 30% to 33% of blood volume (maximum 36%). The maintenance dosage should be titrated based on the individual's response.

Drug interactions
No known drug interactions exist.

ADVERSE DRUG REACTIONS

Hypertension is the most common adverse reaction to epoetin alfa. It even may occur in previously hypotensive patients. Hypertension may result from increased hematocrit and blood viscosity, which increases peripheral vascular resistance.

Other adverse reactions reported in more than 5% of patients during clinical trials include headache, arthralgias, nausea, edema, fatigue, diarrhea, vomiting, chest pain, skin reactions at the administration site, asthenia, and dizziness. Other significant reactions during clinical trials include seizures (1.1%), cerebrovascular accident or transient ischemic attack (0.4%), and myocardial infarction (0.4%). Seizures are more likely to occur during the first 90 days of therapy, especially if the patient experiences a rapid rise in hematocrit.

NURSING PROCESS APPLICATION

The following information assists the nurse in caring for a patient who is receiving epoetin alfa.

Assessment
• Review the patient's history for a preexisting condition that contraindicates the use of epoetin alfa, such as uncontrolled hypertension or known hypersensitivity to mammalian cell-derived albumin or albumin-containing products.
• Review the patient's history for a preexisting condition that requires cautious use of epoetin alfa, such as porphyria, pregnancy, or lactation.
• Assess the patient for adverse reactions to epoetin alfa, such as hypertension, headache, GI distress, edema, dizziness, or seizures.
• Assess the effectiveness of epoetin alfa regularly.
• Evaluate the patient's and family's knowledge about epoetin alfa.

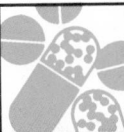

SELECTED MAJOR DRUGS

Hematinic agents

This chart summarizes drugs used to treat iron-deficiency anemia and megaloblastic anemia.

DRUGS	MAJOR INDICATIONS	USUAL ADULT DOSAGES	CONTRAINDICATIONS AND PRECAUTIONS
Iron preparations			
ferrous sulfate (20% elemental iron)	Prevention and treatment of iron-deficiency anemia	300 mg to 1.2 grams P.O. daily	• Know that ferrous sulfate is contraindicated in a patient with primary hemochromatosis, peptic ulcer, regional enteritis, ulcerative colitis, or known hypersensitivity to ferrous sulfate.
iron dextran	Treatment of iron-deficiency anemia in patients who cannot tolerate oral therapy	0.5 ml I.M. or I.V. initially as a test dose, then 2 ml I.M. daily for a patient under 110 lb (50 kg) or 5 ml I.M. daily for a patient over 110 lb; or 2 ml I.V. daily at a rate of 1 ml/minute infused slowly	• Know that iron dextran is contraindicated in a patient with any anemia other than iron-deficiency anemia, infectious kidney disease during the acute phase, or known hypersensitivity to iron dextran. • Administer with extreme caution to a paient with severely impaired liver function. • Administer with caution to a pregnant or lactating patient or one with significant allergies or asthma.
Vitamin B$_{12}$			
cyanocobalamin	Treatment of vitamin B$_{12}$-deficiency anemia caused by malabsorption syndrome, as seen in pernicious anemia; GI pathology, dysfunction, or surgery; or inadequate dietary intake	100 mcg I.M. or S.C. daily for 10 to 30 days, or 100 mcg daily for 14 days followed by 100 mcg monthly	• Know that cyanocobalamin is contraindicated in a patient with early Leber's disease or known hypersensitivity to vitamin B$_{12}$ or cobalt.
Folic acid			
folic acid	Treatment of megaloblastic anemia from folic acid deficiency	100 to 400 mcg P.O. daily; 1 mg P.O. 1 to 3 times daily for severe malabsorption	• Administer folic acid with extreme caution to a patient with anemia when the cause has not been diagnosed yet.

Nursing diagnoses

The following examples represent appropriate nursing diagnoses for a patient receiving epoetin alfa.

• Potential for injury related to a preexisting condition that contraindicates use of epoetin alfa

• Potential for injury related to a preexisting condition that requires cautious of epoetin alfa

• Potential for injury related to adverse drug reactions

• Knowledge deficit related to epoetin alfa

Planning and implementation

• Do not administer epoetin alfa to a patient with a condition that contraindicates its use.

• Administer epoetin alfa cautiously to a patient at risk because of a preexisting condition.

• Monitor the patient closely for adverse reactions during epoetic alfa therapy.

• Monitor the patient's blood pressure regularly to detect hypertension.

• *Take seizure precautions and monitor the patient's neurologic status closely because of the risk of seizures, especially during the first 90 days of therapy.*

• *Notify the physician if the patient experiences headache, arthralgias, or chest pain. Obtain a prescription for medication to relieve the discomfort. Expect to obtain an electrocardiogram immediately, as prescribed, if chest pain occurs.*

• Notify the physician if the patient develops nausea, vomiting, or diarrhea. Obtain a prescription for an antiemetic or antidiarrheal agent, as needed.

• *Take safety precautions if dizziness occurs. For example, keep the bed in a low position and supervise ambulation.*
• Evaluate the patient's hemoglobin level and hematocrit regularly as prescribed to monitor the effectiveness of epoetin alfa therapy.
• Expect to decrease the dosage as prescribed when the hematocrit reaches the target range or rises above 4 points in a 2-week period. Expect to increase the dosage as prescribed if the hematocrit does not increase by 5 to 6 points after 8 weeks of therapy and remains below the target range of 30% to 33% of blood volume (maximum 36%).
• Notify the physician if adverse reactions occur or if epoetin alfa therapy is ineffective.

Patient teaching
• Teach the patient and family the name, dose, action, frequency, and adverse effects of epoetin alfa.
• Inform the dialysis patient that the initial drug dosage will be given I.V. three times weekly; the nondialysis patient that it will be given I.V. or S.C. three times weekly. Then a maintenance dosage will be established.
• Stress the importance of having blood tests as prescribed to assess the effectiveness of epoetin alfa.
• *Inform the patient and family that seizures may occur, especially during the first 90 days of therapy.*
• *Caution the patient not to perform activities that require alertness if dizziness occurs.*
• Advise the patient to have the blood pressure checked regularly.
• *Instruct the patient to notify the physician immediately or go to the nearest emergency department if chest pain occurs.*
• Advise the patient to tell the physician if any other adverse reactions occur.

Evaluation
The following examples represent appropriate evaluation statements for a patient receiving epoetin alfa.
• The patient has no conditions that contraindicate epoetin alfa therapy.
• The patient exhibits no signs of complications in the preexisting condition linked to epoetin alfa.
• The patient experiences no adverse reactions to epoetin alfa.
• The patient and family express an accurate understanding of the points taught about epoetin alfa.
• The patient returns for regularly scheduled blood tests and blood pressure measurements.

CHAPTER SUMMARY

Chapter 35 primarily discussed two major types of anemias: microcytic hypochromic anemia, or iron-deficiency anemia, and macrocytic (megaloblastic) anemia caused by vitamin B_{12} or folic acid deficiencies. Both anemias generally can be prevented with adequate dietary intake and may result from conditions that produce inadequate absorption or use. The chapter also discussed epoetin alfa, an RBC production stimulant used to treat normocytic anemia associated with CRF. Here are the highlights of the chapter.
• Iron, vitamin B_{12}, and folic acid are all important for normal RBC production, and all three elements are present in a diet that includes meat and green leafy vegetables.
• Iron-deficiency anemia results from inadequate iron ingestion, absorption, or utilization; increased iron requirement or excretion; or metabolic destruction of iron.
• Iron-deficiency anemia is correctable with oral administration of an iron preparation, such as ferrous fumarate, ferrous gluconate, or ferrous sulfate. Therapy, which lasts about 6 months, restores normal hemoglobin levels and creates iron stores in the body.
• Parenteral iron therapy is indicated for a patient who cannot absorb oral preparations, is noncompliant with oral therapy, or has a bowel disorder, such as ulcerative colitis. The patient should receive a test dose of iron dextran before therapy begins to detect any adverse reactions.
• Malabsorption in the GI tract usually causes megaloblastic anemia. Proper absorption of vitamin B_{12} requires intrinsic factor, which is secreted by gastric cells.
• Patients who cannot absorb vitamin B_{12} from their diet will require monthly I.M. injections for life to ensure proper cellular metabolic functioning. Cyanocobalamin and hydroxocobalamin are used in vitamin B_{12} therapy.
• Folic acid deficiencies are seen most commonly in patients with liver disease, sprue, alcoholism, or malabsorption syndrome.
• Treating a folic acid deficiency with 1 mg of oral folic acid daily will reverse the anemia.
• Epoetin alfa, which has no known drug interactions, is used to treat anemia associated with CRF in patients who are undergoing dialysis and those who are not.
• When caring for a patient receiving a hematinic agent, the nurse uses the nursing process. Key aspects of nursing care include observing the patient closely for adverse reactions, minimizing such discomfort as iron-induced constipation, monitoring patient compliance during lifelong therapy, teaching the patient about hematinic drug administration, and reviewing nutritional principles to help prevent recurrence of anemia.

STUDY QUESTIONS

See Appendix 1 for answers.

1. Nina Lightner, age 20, is 16 weeks pregnant with her first child. When she comes to the clinic for her first prenatal visit, tests reveal that her hemoglobin is 10.5 grams/dl. The physician prescribes ferrous sulfate (Feosol) 300 mg P.O. t.i.d. When should the nurse expect to see an increase in Ms. Lightner's hemoglobin level?
(a) 3 days
(b) 1 week
(c) 4 weeks
(d) 8 weeks

2. If Ms. Lightner could not absorb oral iron, the physician probably would have prescribed iron dextran (Imferon) I.M. Why should the nurse use the Z-track technique when administering this drug?
(a) to prevent pain
(b) to prevent necrosis
(c) to prevent skin discoloration
(d) to prevent extravasation

3. At the next prenatal visit, Ms. Lightner reports having constipation. What should the nurse tell Ms. Lightner to relieve this common adverse reaction?
(a) Take the iron preparation with an antacid
(b) Discontinue the iron preparation.
(c) Take the iron preparation at bedtime.
(d) Increase her fluid and fiber intake.

4. James Hurley, age 35, has pernicious anemia. His physician prescribes I.M. cyanocobalamin. Why should Mr. Hurley receive cyanocobalamin by the I.M. route?
(a) Lack of intrinsic factor prevents absorption of oral cyanocobalamin.
(b) Oral cyanocobalamin is too irritating to the GI mucosa.
(c) Oral cyanocobalamin has an extremely slow onset of action.
(d) Absorption is too erratic when oral cyanocobalamin is administered.

5. When teaching Mr. Hurley about cyanocobalamin, the nurse stresses the importance of compliance with therapy. What may result if Mr. Hurley is noncompliant?
(a) severe fatigue
(b) hypotension
(c) hypokalemia
(d) neurologic damage

6. Bart Cramer, age 50, is an alcoholic who recently received a diagnosis of megaloblastic anemia caused by folic acid deficiency. His physician prescribes folic acid replacement therapy. What is the usual adult dosage?
(a) 50 to 100 mcg/day
(b) 100 to 400 mcg/day
(c) 1 to 3 mg/day
(d) 3 to 5 mg/day

7. Evelyn White, age 35, is receiving the chemotherapeutic agent methotrexate to treat breast cancer. Which drug probably will be ordered to inhibit this drug's antifolate effects?
(a) iron dextran
(b) leucovorin calcium
(c) vitamin B_{12}
(d) epoetin alfa

SELECTED REFERENCES

AHFS drug information 90. (1990). Bethesda, MD: American Society of Hospital Pharmacists.

Arthur, C., and Isbister, J. (1987). Iron deficiency: Misunderstood, misdiagnosed, and mistreated. *Drugs, 33*(2), 171-182.

Drug facts and comparisons. (1991). St. Louis: Facts and Comparisons Division, J.B. Lippincott.

Faulds, D., and Sorkin, E. (1989). Epoetin. *Drugs, 38*(6), 863-899.

Flaharty, K., Grimm, A., and Vlasses, P. (1989). Epoietin: Human recombinant therapy. *Clinical Pharmacy,* 8(11), 769-779.

Goodman and Gilman's the pharmacological basis of therapeutics (8th ed.; 1990). Elmsford, NY: Pergamon Press.

Hansten, P., and Horn, J. (1989). *Drug interactions: Clinical significance of drug-drug interactions* (6th ed.). Philadelphia: Lea & Febiger.

Harju, E. (1989). Clinical pharmacokinetics of iron preparations. *Clinical Pharmacokinetics,* 17(2), 69-89.

Iron, folic acid, and depletion of zinc: Prenatal supplements. (1987). *Nurses' Drug Alert,* 11(6), 45.

Iron supplements interact with methyldopa. (1988). *Nurses' Drug Alert,* 12(7), 51-52.

North American Nursing Diagnosis Association. (1990). *Taxonomy I - Revised, with official diagnostic categories.* St. Louis: NANDA.

Spurhill, W., and Wade, W. (1989). Anemias. In J. DiPiro and R. Talbert, et al. (Eds.), *Pharmacotherapy: A pathophysiologic approach.* New York: Elsevier.

CHAPTER

36

ANTICOAGULANT AGENTS

OBJECTIVES

After reading and studying this chapter, the student should be able to:
1. Describe how heparin, oral anticoagulants, and antiplatelet drugs produce their effects.
2. Discuss the indications for heparin, oral anticoagulants, and antiplatelet drugs.
3. Compare the drug interactions associated with heparin, oral anticoagulants, and antiplatelet drugs.
4. Describe how to monitor therapy with heparin, oral anticoagulants, and antiplatelet drugs.
5. Describe how the nurse should assess for bleeding complications in a patient receiving an anticoagulant agent.
6. Explain important points the nurse should include in patient teaching about anticoagulant therapy.
7. Describe how to apply the nursing process when caring for a patient who is receiving an anticoagulant agent.

INTRODUCTION

A delicate balance exists in the body between blood clotting and clot breakdown (lysis). Under normal physiologic conditions, little or no clotting occurs. However, certain diseases, such as thromboembolism, cause an abnormal tendency toward clotting. The resultant clots, or thrombi, may severely obstruct venous or arterial circulation. Anticoagulant drugs are prescribed to reduce clotting and thereby prevent further coagulation in high-risk patients. Three types of anticoagulants are discussed in this chapter: heparin, oral anticoagulants, and antiplatelet drugs.

Heparin, a naturally occurring substance, is administered parenterally to prevent a clot from enlarging during an acute thromboembolic event. The drug also is used to prevent thromboembolism in selected high-risk patients, such as those undergoing pelvic surgery. Heparin most frequently is used in inpatient settings but may be used in well-supervised home care settings.

The major oral anticoagulants are warfarin sodium and dicumarol. These drugs are used prophylactically in pa-

---

SELECTED NURSING DIAGNOSES

Anticoagulant agents

The following nursing diagnoses address representative problems and etiologies that a nurse may encounter when caring for a patient who is receiving an anticoagulant agent. Some of these nursing diagnoses contain generalized etiologies, which the nurse must individualize based on the patient's needs. (For some common nursing diagnoses and related interventions for each drug class, see the "Nursing Process Application" sections of this chapter.)

- Altered oral mucous membrane related to oral anticoagulant-induced mouth ulcers
- Altered protection related to the adverse hematologic effects of an anticoagulant agent
- Altered urinary elimination related to sulfinpyrazone-induced renal dysfunction
- Body image disturbance related to heparin-induced alopecia
- Constipation related to the adverse GI effects of aspirin used as an antiplatelet agent
- Diarrhea related to the adverse GI effects of an oral anticoagulant
- Impaired skin integrity related to skin necrosis caused by an oral anticoagulant
- Impaired tissue integrity related to aspirin-induced damage to the gastric mucosa
- Ineffective breathing pattern related to a hypersensitivity reaction to the antiplatelet agent
- Knowledge deficit related to the prescribed anticoagulant agent
- Noncompliance related to long-term use of an anticoagulant agent
- Pain related to aspirin-induced stomach pain
- Potential fluid volume deficit related to anticoagulant-induced bleeding
- Potential for injury related to a preexisting condition that contraindicates the use of an anticoagulant agent
- Potential for injury related to a preexisting condition that requires cautious use of an anticoagulant agent
- Potential for injury related to adverse drug reactions
- Potential for injury related to drug interactions
- Potential for trauma related to the adverse central nervous system effects of dipyridamole

tients at high risk for developing venous thromboembolism and are taken orally most commonly by outpatients requiring prolonged therapy.

Antiplatelet drugs currently used clinically include aspirin, dipyridamole, and sulfinpyrazone. (The uses of ticlopidine are under investigation). They may be used alone or with an oral anticoagulant to disrupt platelet aggregation, reducing arterial thromboembolism. The antiplatelet drugs currently are receiving extensive clinical trials to document their usefulness in preventing arterial clotting.

For a summary of representative drugs, see *Selected major drugs: Anticoagulant agents,* pages 639 and 640. For a listing of applicable nursing diagnoses that the nurse may formulate when caring for a patient receiving these agents, see *Selected nursing diagnoses: Anticoagulant agents*. For detailed information on applying the nursing process, see Chapter 6, The Nursing Process and Drug Therapy.

HEPARIN

Found naturally in body tissues, heparin also is prepared commercially from animal tissue for use in preventing clot formation and treating thromboembolism. Heparin impairs blood coagulation inside the body (in vivo) and outside it (in vitro) — such as in a test tube — but does not affect the synthesis of clotting factors. Thus, the drug cannot dissolve clots, an action performed by the body's own fibrinolytic system or hastened by thrombolytic agents, which are discussed in Chapter 37.

Heparin is prepared commercially from extractions of bovine lung and porcine intestinal mucosa; it also can be extracted from sheep and whales. Although all forms of heparins are biologically equivalent, porcine mucosal heparin produces a lower incidence of heparin-induced thrombocytopenia.

PHARMACOKINETICS

Heparin must be administered parenterally to achieve distribution to the intravascular compartments. It is metabolized in the liver, and its metabolites are excreted in the urine. Its onset of action and peak concentration level varies according to the route of administration. Although intravenous (I.V.) administration allows immediate distribution, the subcutaneous (S.C.) route is used in low doses to prevent thromboembolism in high-risk patients.

Absorption, distribution, metabolism, excretion

Because of its polarity and large molecular size, heparin is not absorbed well from the gastrointestinal (GI) tract, so it must be administered parenterally. The I.V. route is preferred for high-dose treatment of acute thrombotic episodes; the S.C. route, for low-dose prophylactic therapy. Distribution is immediate after I.V. administration, using I.V. bolus or continuous I.V. infusion, but it is much less predictable with an S.C. injection. The intramuscular (I.M.) route should be avoided because of the danger of local bleeding.

After I.V. administration, heparin is distributed to the intravascular compartments with little of the drug reaching the tissues. It then is taken up by the endothelium of the vascular and lymphatic system and by the cells of the reticuloendothelial system. After administration, heparin concentration levels in the epithelium can be 1,000 times greater than in the plasma, demonstrating a highly specific uptake by the endothelium. Heparin does not cross the placenta or pass into breast milk. The enzyme heparinase metabolizes heparin in the liver. Half-life, approximately 1 to 1.5 hours, is dose-related. The anticoagulant effect is measured by the activated partial thromboplastin time (APTT) test and the partial thromboplastin time (PTT) test.

Metabolites are excreted in the urine. (With a large dose, heparin itself appears in the urine.) Patients with hepatic or renal disease excrete heparin more slowly, prolonging its half-life and thus its anticoagulant effect. Patients with pulmonary embolism display rapid heparin excretion and may require increased doses.

Onset, peak, duration

With I.V. administration, heparin's onset of action is almost immediate, and the peak concentration level occurs within minutes. The patient's clotting time will return to normal within 2 to 6 hours after administration of a one-time I.V. bolus. With S.C. administration, onset is delayed for about 2 hours. The duration of action is extended with higher doses.

PHARMACODYNAMICS

Heparin interferes with clotting and reduces the triglyceride concentration level in the plasma. Heparin also has anticomplement properties and a slight antihistaminic effect.

Mechanism of action

Heparin indirectly inactivates thrombin by accelerating the interaction between thrombin and antithrombin III, a thrombin-inactivating glycoprotein found in the blood. Factors IXa, Xa, XIa, and XIIa are inactivated also. (For an illustration, see *Coagulation factors and pathways* in the introduction to this unit.) Low heparin doses increase the activity of antithrombin III against Factor Xa and thrombin and can inhibit the initiation of clotting. Much larger doses are necessary to inhibit fibrin formation once a clot has been formed. This relationship between dose and effect is the rationale for using low-dose heparin to prevent clotting. Whole blood clotting time, thrombin time, PTT, and APTT are prolonged during heparin therapy. However, these times may be prolonged only slightly with low or ultra-low prophylactic doses.

Heparin's effect on triglycerides and platelets may impede development of atherosclerotic plaques in blood vessels. For example, heparin has been shown to reduce triglyceride levels by releasing lipid-hydrolyzing enzymes from tissues into blood. These enzymes break down the triglycerides of chylomicrons and very-low-density lipoproteins bound to capillary endothelial cells. Extrahepatic tissues then metabolize the hydrolyzed fatty acids and partial glycerides.

By maintaining the electronegativity of the blood vessel surface, heparin also decreases platelet adhesiveness and release of platelet-derived growth factor. Heparin demonstrates many immune-mediating effects in laboratory experiments. It activates macrophages, increases the migration of B lymphocytes, and inhibits T and B lymphocytes. It also inhibits sensitivity reactions, such as anaphylaxis and antigen-antibody reactions.

PHARMACOTHERAPEUTICS

Heparin is prescribed to prevent and treat venous thromboembolisms, characterized by inappropriate or excessive intravascular activation of blood clotting. Venous thromboembolism results from venous stasis (slow blood flow). The clot consists of a fibrin network enmeshed with erythrocytes and platelets. It also has a long tail that can detach and travel to distant sites, such as the lungs, and cause pulmonary embolism. Immediate I.V. heparin administration is indicated for treating acute thromboembolism.

Heparin also is used whenever the patient's blood must circulate outside the body through a machine. Thus the patient undergoing open-heart surgery receives heparin so that the blood does not clot while the patient is on the cardiopulmonary bypass machine. Similarly, the patient undergoing hemodialysis receives heparin during each treatment.

Heparin may be used for a patient with disseminated intravascular coagulation (DIC) when massive clotting is the primary manifestation of the disorder. In this situation, the heparin halts further clotting, allowing the body to restore its clotting factors and prevent bleeding. Heparin also is used to treat arterial clotting and to prevent embolus formation in patients atrial fibrillation. (During atrial fibrillation, the inefficient and inadequate pumping of the atria may cause clots to form that can detach and travel to the lungs or brain.)

Heparin is used in orthopedic surgery, which in many cases activates the coagulation mechanisms excessively. A patient undergoing total hip or knee replacement may receive a postoperative heparin dosage of 15,000 to 20,000 units/day to prevent venous thromboembolism.

Heparin is the drug of choice to treat thromboembolism and to prevent clot formation in the venous system because of its immediate anticoagulant effect after I.V. administration. The nurse can monitor the anticoagulant effect by monitoring the patient's APTT and PTT. The APTT is more sensitive than the PTT and more common for monitoring heparin therapy and screening for clotting factor deficiencies in the intrinsic coagulation system. When the APTT is maintained at 1½ times the control, the risk of recurrent venous thromboembolism is about 3%. (For a summary of appropriate tests, see *Laboratory tests to monitor anticoagulant effects*.)

The effects of heparin can be reversed easily by administering protamine sulfate, which has a specific affinity for heparin and forms a stable nondissociable salt with it. (For more information on this drug, see *Protamine sulfate*, page 628.) Heparin produces relatively few adverse reactions when the APTT is maintained within the therapeutic range.

heparin sodium (Liquaemin). Used to treat thromboembolism, heparin also is used to prevent clot formation in the venous system. Low-dose S.C. heparin is used to prevent thromboembolism in high-risk patients, including patients immobilized on bed rest for long periods, those undergoing pelvic surgery, and those with a preoperative history of clot formation.
Usual adult dosage: to treat pulmonary embolism or thromboembolism, 5,000 to 10,000 units as a bolus, followed by continuous I.V. infusion of 1,000 to 2,000 units/hour. For intermittent I.V. treatment, 5,000 to 10,000 units every 6 hours; for S.C. administration to prevent thromboembolism in high-risk patients, 10,000 to 12,000 units every 8 hours, or 14,000 to 20,000 units every 12 hours. For low-dose S.C. therapy, 5,000 units 2 hours before surgery, then 5,000 units every 8 to 12 hours for 7 days or until the patient is fully ambulatory. Hip surgery patients may receive as much as 30,000 units/day to maintain the APTT at the upper end of the normal range.
Usual pediatric dosage: for continuous I.V. infusion, 50 units/kg I.V. bolus, followed by infusion of 100 units/kg over 4 hours; for intermittent I.V. treatment, 50 to 100 units/kg every 4 hours.

Drug interactions

Because heparin acts synergistically with all the oral anticoagulants, the risk of patient bleeding increases when both types of drugs are administered. The prothrombin time (PT), used to monitor the effects of oral anticoagu-

Laboratory tests to monitor anticoagulant effects

The following chart provides the laboratory tests and normal values for different types of anticoagulants. It also lists typical therapeutic ranges. The nurse should be aware, however, that each hospital determines its own therapeutic range to reflect its laboratory's specific reagents, instrumentation, and personnel.

DRUG CLASS	APPROPRIATE LABORATORY TEST	NORMAL VALUES	THERAPEUTIC RANGE DURING ANTICOAGULANT THERAPY
heparin	Activated partial thromboplastin time (APTT)	16 to 25 seconds	1½ to 2½ times control
	Partial thromboplastin time (PTT)	30 to 45 seconds	
oral anticoagulants (coumarin compounds)	Prothrombin time (PT)	12 seconds	PT ratio of 1.2 to 1.5; PT ranges from 14 to 18 seconds.*
antiplatelet drugs	Bleeding time test	3 to 10 minutes	Bleeding time may be 2 times control in 95% of patients. May increase more in children or in adults with bleeding disorders, such as hemophilia.

*Reduced ranges as recommended by The American College of Chest Physicians and the National Heart, Lung & Blood Institute, 1986, for selected conditions such as venous clots. May need to be in range of 1.5 to 1.8 for other conditions, such as mechanical heart valves or rheumatic mitral valve disease.

lants, may be prolonged if the patient also takes heparin. Similarly, the risk of bleeding increases when the patient takes an antiplatelet drug, such as aspirin or dipyridamole, while receiving heparin. Drugs that antagonize or inactivate heparin include antihistamines, digitalis, nicotine, phenothiazines, tetracycline hydrochloride, quinidine, neomycin sulfate, and I.V. penicillin. Some of these drugs are incompatible with highly acidic heparin and should not be mixed in the same solution. The nurse should check with the pharmacist for incompatibilities before mixing drugs with heparin. (For a summary, see *Drug interactions: Heparin,* page 629.)

ADVERSE DRUG REACTIONS

One advantage of heparin is that it produces relatively few adverse reactions, of which bleeding is the most common. Bleeding usually can be prevented if the patient's APTT is maintained within the therapeutic range (1½ to 2½ times the control). The drug may cause hypersensitivity reactions in some patients.

The potential for bleeding exists in all patients receiving high doses of heparin to treat thromboembolism. The nurse should monitor the patient's urine, stool, and emesis for blood and watch for bleeding from the gingiva or nose, at injection sites, and in subcutaneous tissue (hematoma).

Bleeding leads to more serious consequences if it occurs in the brain (subdural hematoma), at arterial puncture sites, or in or behind the peritoneum (intraperitoneal or retroperitoneal hemorrhage). The severity of this bleeding can be reduced by omitting or decreasing the heparin dose, and the risk of bleeding usually can be reduced by carefully maintaining the APTT at the prescribed level. The hemoglobin and hematocrit should be monitored regularly for indications of bleeding.

Heparin may depress the platelet count, resulting in thrombocytopenia, depending on the type of heparin used: bovine heparin may have a greater tendency than porcine heparin to produce thrombocytopenia. The nurse should monitor the patient's platelet count regularly during heparin therapy. If thrombocytopenia occurs, heparin should be discontinued as prescribed to return the platelet count to normal.

Because heparin is procured from animal sources, it can produce hypersensitivity reactions. Although such reactions are rare, heparin should be administered cautiously to a patient with a history of allergies. Administering a trial dose of 1,000 units can determine the patient's allergic potential. Hypersensitivity reactions can produce such signs and symptoms as chills, fever, urticaria, rash, and anaphylaxis, which are reversible upon discontinuation of treatment.

Alopecia may occur if therapy lasts for more than 6 months. Osteoporosis and spontaneous fractures may occur in patients who have been on long-term heparin therapy. (For the nursing implications associated with adverse reactions to this drug, see *Heparin: Summary of adverse reactions,* page 630.)

Protamine sulfate

Protamine sulfate is a strong base that neutralizes acidic heparin by binding with it to form a stable compound with no anticoagulant effect. However, protamine sulfate administered in the absence of heparin can produce an anticoagulant effect.

Protamine sulfate is available in a 1% solution or a 50-mg powder form. One milligram will neutralize approximately 100 units of heparin. The calculated dose should equal that required to neutralize half the previous heparin dose.

Administer protamine sulfate by I.V. only and slowly over 1 to 3 minutes (not more than 50 mg per single injection in a 10-minute period, unless additional monitoring of clotting times is performed). Rapid injection can cause such complications as dyspnea, flushing, bradycardia, and hypotension. Because protamines are proteins that occur in the sperm of salmon and some other fish, hypersensitivity reactions may occur in patients with allergies to fish.

NURSING PROCESS APPLICATION

The following information assists the nurse in caring for a patient who is receiving heparin.

Assessment

• Review the patient's history for a preexisting condition that contraindicates the use of heparin, such as severe thrombocytopenia, uncontrollable active bleeding state (unless caused by DIC), or known hypersensitivity to heparin.
• Review the patient's history for a preexisting condition that requires cautious use of heparin, such as pregnancy, a history of allergies, or a disease that increases the risk of hemorrhage.
• Assess the patient for adverse reactions to heparin, such as bleeding or hypersensitivity reactions.
• Review the patient's medication history to identify use of drugs that may interact with heparin, such as oral anticoagulants, antiplatelet agents, antihistamines, digitalis, tetracycline, or quinidine.
• Assess the effectiveness of heparin regularly.
• Assess for alopecia in a patient receiving long-term heparin therapy.
• Evaluate the patient's and family's knowledge about heparin.

Nursing diagnoses

The following examples represent appropriate nursing diagnoses for a patient receiving heparin.
• Potential for injury related to a preexisting condition that contraindicates the use of heparin
• Potential for injury related to a preexisting condition that requires cautious use of heparin
• Potential for injury related to adverse drug reactions

• Body image disturbance related to heparin-induced alopecia
• Knowledge deficit related to heparin

Planning and implementation

• Do not administer heparin to a patient with a condition that contraindicates its use.
• Administer heparin cautiously to a patient at risk because of a preexisting condition.
• *Monitor the patient closely for bleeding and other adverse reactions during heparin therapy.*
• Monitor the patient's APTT before each heparin dose during the early stages of intermittent therapy until the therapeutic level is reached. Then monitor the APTT every 12 hours for 3 days, or as prescribed.
• Monitor the patient's APTT every 4 hours during early stages of continuous I.V. therapy until the therapeutic range is achieved. Then monitor the APTT every 12 hours for 3 days, and daily thereafter or as prescribed. Notify the physician if the patient's APTT level exceeds the therapeutic range (1½ to 2½ times the control).
• Monitor the PTT and platelet count daily, as prescribed. Be aware that use of porcine mucosal heparin lowers the risk of heparin-induced thrombocytopenia.
• *Monitor the patient's vital signs, hemoglobin level, and hematocrit for indications of bleeding.*
• Use a flow chart to record the time and results of pertinent laboratory studies, such as PT, APTT, hemoglobin, and platelet count, and the administration time, dose, and injection site of heparin.
• *Assess the patient for early signs of bleeding, such as epistaxis, gingival bleeding, hematuria, hematemesis, or injection-site oozing, especially during high-dose heparin therapy.*
• *Assess wounds, drainage tubes, and I.V. sites frequently for signs of bleeding.*
• Observe for purpura, a sign of subcutaneous bleeding.
• *Check the patient's urine, stool, and emesis for occult blood.*
• *Notify the physician immediately if the patient develops neurologic dysfunction, a sign of intracranial bleeding. Expect to omit or decrease the heparin dose to reduce the severity of intracranial bleeding or bleeding at arterial puncture sites or in or behind the peritoneum.*
• *Take safety precautions for a patient with osteoporosis from long-term heparin therapy. For example, keep the bed in the lowest position, raise the bed rails, and assist with ambulation to prevent injury.*
• Expect to administer low-dose S.C. heparin to a patient at high risk for thromboembolism, such as one who is immobilized, must undergo pelvic surgery, or has a preoperative history of clot formation.
• Expect to increase the heparin dose for a patient with pulmonary embolism because of rapid heparin excretion.

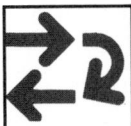

DRUG INTERACTIONS
Heparin

Many interactions involving heparin increase the risk of bleeding or clot formation.

DRUG	INTERACTING DRUGS	POSSIBLE EFFECTS	NURSING IMPLICATIONS
heparin	oral anticoagulants (warfarin, dicumarol)	Increase risk of bleeding	• Monitor the patient's activated partial thromboplastin time (APTT) regularly. • Assess the patient for signs of bleeding in gums, urine, I.V. and injection sites, nasogastric drainage, and wounds.
	antiplatelet agents (aspirin, dipyridamole)	Increase risk of bleeding	• Teach the patient about the dangers of taking aspirin-containing drugs during heparin therapy. • Assess the patient for signs of bleeding.
	digitalis, quinidine, tetracycline, neomycin, penicillin, phenothiazines, antihistamines	Inactivate heparin if mixed in same solution	• Do not add any of these drugs to heparin solutions. • Administer I.V. forms through separate or flushed I.V. lines.
	nicotine	May inactivate heparin	• Monitor APTT closely if the patient uses tobacco.
	nitroglycerin	Inhibits the effects of heparin	• Monitor APTT closely if nitroglycerin infusion is added to or deleted from the regimen.

• Administer heparin I.V. for high-dose treatment of acute thrombotic episodes or S.C. for low-dose prophylactic therapy, as prescribed.

• Administer S.C. heparin as prescribed into the anterior abdominal wall fold above the iliac crest and 2″ or more from the umbilicus to avoid risk of bleeding.

• Avoid aspirating and massaging after administering an S.C. injection of heparin to prevent risk of S.C. bleeding.

• *Do not administer heparin I.M., and avoid other I.M. injections, if possible.*

• Expect to administer a trial dose of 1,000 units of heparin to a patient with a history of allergies. During the trial, observe for signs of hypersensitivity, such as chills, fever, urticaria, rash, and anaphylaxis, which are reversible.

• Use an infusion pump for continuous I.V. infusion to ensure correct dosage, as prescribed.

• Check the drug label carefully before administering, because heparin is available in different strengths. Keep in mind that heparin is prescribed in units rather than in milligrams.

• Check with the pharmacist before mixing any other drug with a heparin infusion to prevent a drug interaction.

• Do not freeze or refrigerate heparin; it is stable at room temperature.

• Inspect all heparin vials for particulate matter or discoloration. If either is present, discard the vial.

• *Have the antidote protamine sulfate readily available in case of severe bleeding.*

• Notify the physician if adverse reactions occur.

• Determine how alopecia affects the body image of a patietn receiving prolonged heparin therapy.

• Support the patient's efforts to maintain a positive body image. For example, suggest wearing an attractive scarf, hat, or wig.

Patient teaching

• Teach the patient and family the name, dose (if administered at home), frequency, action, and adverse effects of heparin.

• Teach the patient and family about home care heparin therapy, if appropriate, including how to administer the drug properly and how to observe for signs of bleeding.

• Help the home care patient schedule necessary APTT tests. Keep in mind, however, that these tests may not be necessary if the APTT is maintained at the lower end of the therapeutic range (1½ times the control).

• Advise the patient that all normal activities of daily living may be performed if the platelet count is normal.

• Encourage the patient to use an electric razor and a soft toothbrush to avoid the risk of bleeding from cuts or irritated gums.

Heparin: Summary of adverse reactions

Heparin interferes with the normal human clotting cascade. Although this effect has therapeutic uses, it also has dangerous potential to cause bleeding.

ADVERSE REACTION	NURSING IMPLICATIONS
Bleeding	• Monitor the patient's activated partial thromboplastin time or partial thromboplastin time daily. • Assess the patient for bleeding. • Monitor the patient's platelet count daily.
Hypersensitivity reactions—rash, hives, chills, fever	• Question the patient about an allergy history. Document the patient's response. • Monitor the patient's response to a test dose of heparin before beginning therapy. • Assess the patient for signs of hypersensitivity during treatment.
Alopecia	• Explain to the patient that hair loss may occur with long-term therapy (more than 6 months), but that it is reversible. • Support the patient's efforts to maintain body image. For example, suggest wearing an attractive scarf, hat, or wig.
Osteoporosis, bone fractures	• Take safety precautions for elderly patients on long-term heparin therapy. For example, keep the bed in the lowest position, raise bed rails, and assist with ambulation.

• *Advise the patient to avoid all over-the-counter drugs, including aspirin preparations and antihistamines, unless the physician or pharmacist is consulted first.*
• Teach the hospitalized patient the signs and symptoms of bleeding and precautions to take after venipuncture.
• Reassure the patient with alopecia that it is reversible.
• Instruct the patient and family to notify the physician immediately if bleeding or other adverse reactions occur.

Evaluation
The following examples represent appropriate evaluation statements for a patient receiving heparin.
• The patient exhibits no signs of complications in the preexisting condition linked to heparin therapy.
• The patient has no condition that contraindicates heparin therapy.
• The patient develops no adverse reactions to heparin.
• The patient copes effectively with altered body image.

• The patient and family express an accurate understanding of the points taught about heparin.
• The patient schedules APTT tests as needed.

ORAL ANTICOAGULANTS

The coumarin compounds warfarin sodium and dicumarol are the oral anticoagulants widely used in the United States. These compounds inhibit liver synthesis of the vitamin K-dependent clotting factors prothrombin (Factor II) and Factors VII, IX, and X. The drugs are used to prevent recurrence of thromboembolism in patients requiring long-term management. They also are prescribed for patients at high risk for developing thromboembolism, such as a patient with prosthetic heart valves.

PHARMACOKINETICS

The oral anticoagulants produce their effect only in vivo, as opposed to heparin, which also produces in vitro. Therefore, they are referred to as *indirect anticoagulants.* Warfarin sodium is the major coumarin compound and the oral anticoagulant most commonly used in the United States.

Absorption, distribution, metabolism, excretion
Warfarin is absorbed rapidly and almost completely after oral administration; food decreases the absorption rate but not the total amount absorbed. Dicumarol is absorbed more slowly and erratically.

Warfarin and dicumarol usually are found in the plasma about 1 hour after administration. They are bound extensively to plasma albumin. Because warfarin is 99% bound to plasma protein, it does not diffuse into red blood cells, cerebrospinal fluid, or urine. Warfarin and dicumarol can cross the placenta and may cause fetal deformities and hemorrhagic diseases.

The oral anticoagulants are converted to inactivated metabolites in the liver (first-pass effect). These metabolites are secreted in bile, then into the duodenum, where they are reabsorbed partially before being excreted in urine. Unabsorbed dicumarol may be excreted unchanged in feces. Warfarin and dicumarol also are secreted into breast milk, so breast-feeding is not recommended, although it usually does not change the PT of infants.

Onset, peak, duration
Onset of action of the oral anticoagulants occurs within 24 to 72 hours. Their peak concentration levels are measured by the PT. The period of peak concentration for warfarin is ½ to 3 days; for dicumarol, 3 to 5 days.

Although the oral anticoagulants appear quickly in the plasma after administration, therapeutic anticoagulation does not occur until the blood has been depleted of clotting factors. Factor VII, with the shortest half-life, is the first clotting factor to be depleted. Significant depletion of Factor X and prothrombin (Factor II) may take 2 to 3 days. Thus, maximum anticoagulation and antithrombotic effects may not be achieved for 3 to 5 days after initiation of therapy.

The duration of action of warfarin is 2 to 5 days; of dicumarol, 2 to 10 days. The half-life of the oral anticoagulants varies from 0.5 to 2 days for warfarin and 1 to 2 days for dicumarol.

PHARMACODYNAMICS

The oral anticoagulants are vitamin K antagonists. Their administration results in production of biologically inactive precursor coagulation proteins.

Mechanism of action

The oral anticoagulants alter the synthesis of vitamin K-dependent clotting factors, including prothrombin and Factors VII, IX, and X. The alteration does not impede the synthesis of these factors (which remain immunologically detectable); instead, it makes them dysfunctional. The resulting therapeutic anticoagulant effect does not occur until the already circulating clotting factors are depleted; this takes from several hours for Factor VII to 2 to 3 days for prothrombin. Thus, optimal PT response is achieved in 1 to 4 days.

The anticoagulant effects of these agents are enhanced in patients with inadequate dietary intake of vitamin K or fat, and in patients with deficient vitamin K absorption. The anticoagulant effects are decreased in patients with increased intake of vitamin K. Patients with hepatic disease experience an increased anticoagulant effect because the disease causes impaired hepatic synthesis of clotting factors. Hypermetabolic states, such as fever and hyperthyroidism, also increase the response to oral anticoagulants; hypometabolic states reduce it.

Pregnancy appears to decrease response to the oral anticoagulants because of the increased activity of Factors VII, VIII, IX, and X. The oral anticoagulants can cross the placenta and seriously damage the fetus; thus heparin, which does not cross the placenta, is the anticoagulant of choice during pregnancy.

PHARMACOTHERAPEUTICS

Oral anticoagulants are prescribed to treat thromboembolism after initial treatment with heparin. Warfarin, however, may be started without heparin in outpatients at high risk for thromboembolism. The oral anticoagulants are the drugs of choice for the prophylactic therapy of deep vein thrombosis and for patients with prosthetic heart valves or diseased mitral valves. They sometimes are combined with an antiplatelet drug, such as dipyridamole, to decrease risk of arterial clotting.

The oral anticoagulants offer several advantages. They can be taken on an outpatient basis and monitored easily using the patient's PT. (For more information, see *Laboratory tests to monitor anticoagulant effects,* page 627.) Their major disadvantage is that they interact with numerous drugs, producing an increased risk of bleeding or clotting. Overall, the oral anticoagulants produce relatively few adverse reactions except for bleeding, which occurs in 20% to 30% of patients. Warfarin is the most commonly prescribed oral anticoagulant. The effects of the oral anticoagulants can be reversed with adequate doses of phytonadione (vitamin K_1).

dicumarol (Dicumarol Pulvules). Available for oral administration, dicumarol is difficult to use clinically because of slow and incomplete absorption. Dicumarol is used for the same clinical indications as warfarin.
Usual adult dosage: 200 to 300 mg P.O. the first day, then 25 to 200 mg/day, depending on PT results.

warfarin sodium (Coumadin). Warfarin sodium is the only oral anticoagulant that can be administered orally and by I.M. or I.V. injection; however, parenteral injection offers no clinical advantage, so warfarin usually is administered orally. It is used to treat thromboembolism after initial treatment with heparin. Long-term prophylactic warfarin therapy is used for patients with artificial heart valves and frequently is combined with such antiplatelet drugs as dipyridamole to prevent thromboembolism resulting from mitral stenosis and atrial fibrillation. It may be used after heparin therapy in patients with anterior or apical myocardial infarction (MI) accompanied by mural endocardial thrombosis.

Warfarin may be used instead of S.C. heparin to prevent venous thromboembolism in patients undergoing total hip and knee replacement surgery.
Usual adult dosage: for venous thrombosis, 10 mg P.O. daily for the first 2 to 3 days, adjusted to PT results, then a maintenance dosage of 2 to 10 mg P.O. daily. Patients with prosthetic heart valves, recurrent embolism, or rheumatic mitral valve disease may require higher PT ratios of 1.5 to 2.

Drug interactions

Many patients on oral anticoagulant therapy are treated with other drugs. The hazards of serious interactions between oral anticoagulants and other drugs are ever present, and many clinically significant interactions occur. The most commonly prescribed drugs that interact with the oral anticoagulants include barbiturates, salicylates, and phenylbutazone. Many foods, especially those high in vitamin K, also interact with the oral anticoagulants. However, only a diet containing high amounts of vitamin K is likely to cause problems.

The PT of a patient taking oral anticoagulants must be reevaluated whenever a drug is added to or deleted from the drug regimen. Reevaluating the PT helps monitor the many possible interactions involving drugs. The mechanisms underlying these interactions include inhibition of vitamin K production or absorption, displacement of the anticoagulant from its albumin-binding sites, inhibition or induction of enzymes responsible for metabolizing warfarin, and other mechanisms that are less well understood. (For more informaiton, see *Drug interactions: Oral anticoagulants*.)

ADVERSE DRUG REACTIONS

The use of oral anticoagulants may produce bleeding complications from inappropriate dosage adjustments (according to the PT), from drug interactions that increase the anticoagulant effect of the drugs, or from the patient's noncompliance. Elderly patients who respond more sensitively to oral anticoagulants are at increased risk for bleeding.

Other common causes of bleeding include peptic ulcers and occult GI tumors. Bleeding from these causes may be apparent only when the patient's urine, stool, or emesis is tested for occult blood. More obvious bleeding may appear as epistaxis, gingival bleeding, or ecchymoses.

Minor bleeding, the primary reaction to oral anticoagulant therapy, usually can be controlled by reducing the anticoagulant dosage. Severe bleeding may occur in the GI tract, urinary tract, or uterus. Ecchymoses and hematomas may form at arterial puncture sites (for example, after a blood gas sample is taken). Severe bleeding may occur as intraperitoneal hemorrhage from a ruptured corpus luteum, retroperitoneal hemorrhage, hemopericardium, intracranial hemorrhage, and adrenal hemorrhage.

Patients receiving oral anticoagulants must be assessed frequently for minor and major bleeding, and their PT responses must be monitored regularly. Bleeding can occur, however, even when the patient's PT falls within the therapeutic range.

Treating minor bleeding includes immediate discontinuation of the oral anticoagulant and, if necessary, administration of oral or parenteral vitamin K as prescribed. Several hours will elapse before vitamin K returns the PT time to normal. Severe bleeding requires vitamin K therapy and administration of plasma or fresh whole blood to replace the vitamin K-dependent clotting factors.

Vitamin K should be used cautiously to reverse anticoagulant therapy, because it can produce a rebound hypercoagulable state that is a threat to patients with artificial heart valves who are prone to clot formation. The patient with an artificial valve is best treated with fresh frozen plasma to provide clotting factors.

Red-orange urine, nausea, vomiting and diarrhea, abdominal cramping, priapism, mouth ulcers, and nephropathy rarely may occur. Other rare adverse reactions to the oral anticoagulants include alopecia, urticaria, dermatitis, skin necrosis, hepatitis, jaundice, fever, hypersensitivity reactions, agranulocytosis, leukopenia, and eosinophilia.

NURSING PROCESS APPLICATION

The following information assists the nurse in caring for a patient who is receiving an oral anticoagulant.

Assessment
• Review the patient's history for a preexisting condition that contraindicates the use of an oral anticoagulant, such as pregnancy; hemorrhagic tendencies; blood dyscrasias; recent central nervous system surgery; overt bleeding of the GI, genitourinary, or respiratory tract; or cerebrovascular hemorrhage.
• Review the patient's history for a preexisting condition that requires cautious use of an oral anticoagulant, such as lactation, moderate to severe hepatic or renal insufficiency, moderate to severe hypertension, polycythemia vera, or severe diabetes.
• Assess the patient for adverse reactions to the prescribed oral anticoagulant, such as obvious or occult bleeding.
• Review the patient's medication history to identify the use of drugs that may interact with the oral anticoagulant, such as barbiturates, salicylates, or phenylbutazone.
• Assess the effectiveness of the prescribed oral anticoagulant periodically.
• Determine the patient's compliance with long-term oral anticoagulant therapy by monitoring the PT value daily or as prescribed.
• Evaluate the patient's and family's knowledge about the prescribed oral anticoagulant.

Nursing diagnoses
The following examples represent appropriate nursing diagnoses for a patient receiving an oral anticoagulant.
• Potential for injury related to a preexisting condition that contraindicates the use of an oral anticoagulant
• Potential for injury related to a preexisting condition that requires cautious use of an oral anticoagulant
• Potential for injury related to adverse drug reactions
• Noncompliance related to long-term use of an oral anticoagulant
• Knowledge deficit related to the prescribed oral anticoagulant

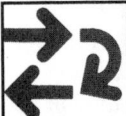

DRUG INTERACTIONS
Oral anticoagulants

This chart illustrates the wide range of potential interactions between oral anticoagulants and other drugs and between oral anticoagulants and food.

DRUG	INTERACTING DRUGS OR FOODS	POSSIBLE EFFECTS	NURSING IMPLICATIONS
warfarin, dicumarol	salicylates, phenylbutazone, sulfinpyrazone, indomethacin, clofibrate, anabolic and androgenic steroids, chloral hydrate, chloramphenicol, disulfiram, heparin, gemfibrozil, meclofenamate, mefenamic acid, metronidazole, miconazole, nalidixic acid, piroxicam, allopurinol, cimetidine, dextrothyroxine, erythromycin, glucagon, co-trimoxazole (sulfamethoxazole-trimethoprim), sulindac, thyroid hormones	Increase risk of bleeding	• Monitor the patient's prothrombin time (PT) frequently after any new drug is added to the drug regimen. • Assess the patient for signs of bleeding, such as epistaxis, bleeding gums, hematuria, or bruising. • Advise the patient to avoid using any over-the-counter product containing aspirin.
	barbiturates, glutethimide, ethchlorvynol, griseofulvin, carbamazepine, rifampin, vitamin K, cholestyramine, colestipol, aminoglutethimide, propylthiouracil, methimazole	Increase risk of clotting	• Assess the patient for signs of thromboembolism (increased pain, swelling, or redness in calf) or pulmonary embolism (increased shortness of breath, chest pain, or fever). • Monitor the patient's PT frequently after any of these drugs is administered.
	phenytoin	Increase risk of phenytoin toxicity; may increase or decrease anticoagulant effect	• Monitor the patient frequently for signs of phenytoin toxicity, such as nystagmus, ataxia, slurred speech, or confusion. • Assess the patient for signs of bleeding or thromboembolism.
	foods high in vitamin K (cabbage, cauliflower, broccoli, asparagus)	Increase clotting	• Obtain a dietary history from the patient to evaluate the amount of vitamin K-rich foods in the daily diet. • Caution the patient against sudden changes in ingestion of vitamin K-rich foods.
	alcohol	Increases risk of clotting with chronic abuse; increases risk of bleeding with acute intoxication	• Obtain a history from the patient and family about the extent of alcohol use. • Monitor the patient for bleeding. • Monitor the patient's PT frequently.

Planning and implementation

• Do not administer an oral anticoagulant to a patient with a condition that contraindicates its use.
• Administer an oral anticoagulant cautiously to a patient at risk because of a preexisting condition.
• *Monitor closely for bleeding and other adverse reactions throughout oral anticoagulant therapy, especially in an elderly patient.*
• Monitor PT responses daily for inpatients and every 1 to 4 weeks for outpatients; be aware that for venous throm-

boembolism, the therapeutic range established by the American College of Chest Physicians and the National Heart, Lung, and Blood Institute is a PT ratio of 1.2 to 1.5 times the control. Also be aware that bleeding can occur even when a patient's PT falls within the therapeutic range.
• Expect to see a higher PT ratio (1.5 to 2) in a patient with prosthetic heart valves, recurrent embolism, or rheumatic mitral valve disease.

- Reevaluate the patient's PT as prescribed whenever a drug is added to or deleted from the therapeutic regimen to detect drug interactions.
- Check and record the PT results before administering an oral anticoagulant dose. When the patient is changed from heparin to warfarin, expect heparin therapy to continue for several days until warfarin produces therapeutic effects.
- *Notify the physician immediately if the therapeutic range is exceeded, and withhold the next dose as prescribed.*
- *Monitor the patient for bleeding, such as epistaxis, gingival bleeding, or ecchymoses. Also test the patient's urine, stool, or emesis for occult bleeding, even when the PT is within the therapeutic range.*
- *Monitor the patient's vital signs frequently for any indications of severe internal bleeding. Use extra care in assessing elderly patients for signs of bleeding.*
- Treat minor bleeding by omitting one or more doses as instructed until the PT returns to the therapeutic range. If minor bleeding continues, administer vitamin K_1 (phytonadione) 1 to 10 mg P.O. as prescribed.
- *Administer 5 to 50 mg of vitamin K parenterally as prescribed if frank bleeding occurs. Small doses (1 to 15 mg) are recommended to prevent hypercoagulation.*
- *Administer 250 to 500 ml of fresh frozen plasma or give commercial Factor IX complex as prescribed if severe bleeding occurs. Be aware that plasma concentrates are associated with a high risk of hepatitis and are used cautiously when no alternative exists.*
- Monitor hydration if the patient experiences nausea, vomiting, or diarrhea. Obtain a prescription for an antiemetic or antidiarrheal agent, as needed.
- Support the patient's efforts to maintain a positive body image if alopecia occurs. For example, suggest wearing an attractive scarf, hat, or wig.
- Take infection control measures if the patient's white blood cell count decreases. For example, isolate the patient from people with infections.
- *Assess the patient regularly for signs of thrombophlebitis, such as the calf pain, tenderness, and redness.*
- *Notify the physician immediately if the patient displays any sign of pulmonary embolism, such as shortness of breath, chest pain, decreased oxygen in arterial blood gases, fever, or tachypnea.*
- Notify the physician if adverse reactions occur.
- Assess the patient's compliance with oral anticoagulant therapy regularly.
- Stress the importance of adhering to the prescribed oral anticoagulant regimen.
- Notify the physician if noncompliance occurs.

Patient teaching

- Teach the patient and family the name, dose, frequency, action, and adverse effects of the prescribed oral anticoagulant.

- Advise the patient to follow the written instructions for dosage; encourage the patient to keep a daily log to reinforce taking the correct dosage.
- *Instruct the patient receiving warfarin to take it in the evening and to have blood drawn for PT in the morning for accurate results. Teach the patient the importance of having blood drawn for PT (usually monthly after stabilization).*
- *Instruct the patient not to take any prescription or over-the-counter drug without first contacting the physician who ordered the anticoagulant therapy. Provide the patient and family members with written information about the interactions between oral anticoagulants and other drugs or food.*
- *Instruct the patient to avoid increased amounts of green leafy vegetables and all medications containing aspirin.*
- *Teach the patient the importance of reporting immediately to the physician any bruising or blood in the stool or urine.*
- Encourage the patient to wear a medical identification bracelet to alert medical personnel in case of trauma or sudden illness.
- Encourage the patient to avoid activities with high risk of physical injury.
- *Advise the female patient to inform the physician if she is pregnant or planning to become pregnant.*
- Reassure the patient with drug-induced alopecia that hair loss is reversible.
- Advise the patient to notify the physician if adverse reactions occur.

Evaluation

The following examples represent appropriate evaluation statements for a patient receiving an oral anticoagulant.
- The patient has no conditions that contraindicate oral anticoagulant therapy.
- The patient exhibits no signs of complications in the preexisting conditions linked to the prescribed oral anticoagulant.
- The patient experiences no adverse reactions to the prescribed oral anticoagulant.
- The patient demonstrates compliance with oral anticoagulant therapy, as prescribed.
- The patient and family express an accurate understanding of the points taught about the prescribed oral anticoagulant.
- The patient keeps a daily log of oral anticoagulant doses and times administered.

ANTIPLATELET DRUGS

The antiplatelet drugs have shown some potential for preventing arterial thromboembolism, particularly in patients at risk for MI and cerebrovascular accidents from arteriosclerosis. These drugs, with varying mechanisms of action, are currently the subject of many clinical research trials. The antiplatelet drugs include aspirin, dipyridamole, and sulfinpyrazone.

Dextrans, clofibrate, indomethacin, and other drugs show some antiplatelet activity. Dextrans are partially hydrolyzed polymers of glucose that usually are used as plasma expanders. Although they do not alter platelet aggregation in vitro, dextrans may alter bleeding time and fibrin polymerization, thus exerting antiplatelet action in vivo. Dextrans reduce platelet adhesiveness by coating platelets and the blood vessel endothelium. They also lower the level of circulating von Willebrand factor, increase the susceptibility of clots to fibrinolysis, and reduce erythrocyte aggregation, blood viscosity, and venous stasis. Dextrans also may dilute clotting factors through their oncotic effect.

Clofibrate, an antilipemic drug, may reduce platelet adhesiveness in vitro and increase abnormally short survival of platelets in some patients with coronary artery disease.

Indomethacin, an anti-inflammatory analgesic commonly used to treat rheumatoid arthritis, inhibits platelet aggregation but has a shorter duration of action than aspirin.

Other drugs that interfere with platelet function are tricyclic antidepressants, penicillin and related antibiotics, nitroprusside, chloroquine, and alcohol. However, these drugs are not used clinically as antiplatelet agents. Ticlopidine, available in Europe, is under investigation but is not available commercially in the United States.

The potential of antiplatelet drugs to prevent arterial thromboembolism is under study; they may interfere with platelet aggregation in atherosclerotic plaque development. When damage occurs to the endothelial lining of an artery, platelets adhere to the site of injury. Circulating platelets converge on the wound site, first touching and then adhering to the collagen fibers of the torn vessel lining (endothelium). This contact of platelets with collagen stimulates the platelets to secrete adenosine diphosphate (ADP), which causes them to break down and become adhesive, sticking together in clumps. Additional ADP activates greater numbers of platelets, which also collect at the site. This aggregation loosely plugs the wound to prevent further blood loss. Serotonin, also secreted by platelets, causes smooth muscle contraction, which facilitates vascular constriction and hemostasis. Thus, platelet adhesion rather than fibrin formation is the predominant hemostatic reaction.

PHARMACOKINETICS

The pharmacokinetic properties of aspirin, dipyridamole, and sulfinpyrazone vary, although all three are administered orally.

Absorption, distribution, metabolism, excretion

Aspirin is absorbed rapidly in the stomach and upper intestine (more slowly with enteric-coated preparations or food), then is distributed quickly into the bloodstream. After metabolism in the liver, aspirin is eliminated by the excretion of salicylic acid in the kidneys and by the oxidation and conjugation of metabolites.

Dipyridamole is absorbed from the GI tract; it is almost completely plasma protein bound (91% to 97%). The drug is distributed widely in body tissues and can cross the placenta in small amounts. Dipyridamole is metabolized in the liver and excreted in bile. This drug may undergo enterohepatic cycling before partial excretion in the feces. Small amounts may be excreted in the urine.

Sulfinpyrazone is absorbed well after oral administration and is 98% to 99% protein bound. After rapid but incomplete metabolism in the liver, yielding active and inactive metabolites, about 45% of the drug is excreted unchanged in the urine.

Onset, peak, duration

Aspirin's onset of action and peak concentration level as an antiplatelet drug still are being investigated. The duration of action of aspirin's platelet-inhibitor effect is the life span of the platelet, approximately 10 days. The half-life of low dosages of aspirin is about 3 hours.

The peak plasma concentration of dipyridamole occurs 2 to 2½ hours after oral administration. Sulfinpyrazone's onset, peak concentration, and duration as an antiplatelet drug still are being investigated. The drug may require several days of administration; some effects persist after withdrawal.

PHARMACODYNAMICS

The antiplatelet drugs interfere with platelet activity in different drug-specific and dose-related ways. The antithrombotic effects of these drugs have not been proven but have been suggested by tests of platelet function in patients receiving the drugs.

Mechanism of action

Low dosages of aspirin (325 mg per day) appear to inhibit clot formation by blocking prostaglandin synthetase action, which in turn prevents formation of the platelet-aggregating substance thromboxane A_2.

In vitro studies of dipyridamole have shown that this drug can inhibit platelet aggregation. However, in vivo studies have not shown the same effects.

Sulfinpyrazone appears to inhibit several platelet functions. At dosages of 400 to 800 mg/day, sulfinpyrazone lengthens platelet survival; dosages of more than 600 mg/day prolong the patency of arteriovenous shunts used for hemodialysis. A single dose produces rapid inhibition of platelet aggregation, suggesting that the drug directly affects circulating platelets.

PHARMACOTHERAPEUTICS

The antiplatelet drugs are under investigation today because evidence exists that platelet aggregation significantly promotes atherosclerotic plaque development. For example, at injured endothelial sites, platelet aggregation and subsequent fibrin formation can create arterial clots. Also, certain patient-related factors, such as a history of gout, diabetes, hypertension, hyperlipidemia, or cigarette smoking, may contribute to plaque development by promoting platelet aggregation.

The antiplatelet drugs, especially aspirin, act synergistically with heparin and the oral anticoagulants, thus increasing the risk of bleeding when these drugs are used together. Adverse reactions to some of these drugs may limit their usefulness in preventing arterial clotting.

The patient's bleeding time and platelet aggregation studies can measure the effectiveness of the antiplatelet ability of these agents. (For information on these two tests, see *Platelet activity tests*.)

aspirin. Although varying studies have evaluated aspirin dosages to prevent arterial clotting, no convincing evidence exists that one dosage is more effective than another. Although no dosages have been established, low dosages of aspirin have shown some effectiveness in preventing aortocoronary bypass shunt thrombosis. Aspirin also has shown some effectiveness in reducing clot formation in arteriovenous shunts in patients on hemodialysis and in patients with unstable angina. In some studies with male patients, aspirin has been effective in reducing the risk of recurring transient ischemic attacks. Aspirin also may be used to help prevent reinfarction and sudden death in men with acute MI and possibly to prevent postoperative venous thrombosis in patients who undergo elective hip and knee surgery.
Usual adult dosage: to prevent clot formation in arteriovenous shunts in hemodialysis patients, 160 mg P.O. daily; to prevent clot formation in patients with unstable angina, 325 mg P.O. daily; to help prevent reinfarction and sudden death in men with acute MI, 300 to 1,500 mg P.O. daily; for men with cerebral ischemic disease, 325 mg P.O. q.i.d. or 650 mg P.O. b.i.d.; to help prevent cerebral ischemic disease, 80 to 325 mg P.O. daily.

Platelet activity tests

Two of the platelet activity tests used to monitor antiplatelet therapy are bleeding time and platelet aggregation studies.

The *bleeding time* test measures the duration of bleeding after a standardized skin incision. Bleeding time depends on the elasticity of the blood vessel wall and on the number and functional capacity of platelets. Bleeding time may be measured by one of four methods: Duke, Ivy, template, or modified template. The template methods are used most commonly and are the most accurate.

After vascular injury, platelets gather at the injury site and clump together to form an aggregate—a plug—that helps maintain hemostasis and promote healing. The *platelet aggregation* test, an in vitro procedure, measures the rate at which the platelets in a sample of citrated platelet-rich plasma form a clump after the addition of an aggregating reagent (adenosine diphosphate, epinephrine, thrombin, collagen, or ristocetin). Because evenly suspended platelets aggregate and fall to the bottom of the tube, the greater the aggregation, the less turbid the sample. A spectrophotometer measures changes in turbidity and prints a graphic record of the results.

dipyridamole (Persantine). Used with warfarin, dipyridamole may help prevent thromboembolism in patients with prosthetic heart valves. Combined with aspirin, the drug may be effective in patients with cerebral ischemic attacks or who undergo coronary bypass graft surgery. Controversy concerning these combination therapies still exists, however. Some physicians advocate giving dipyridamole and aspirin 2 days preoperatively to decrease platelet adhesiveness at the site of aortosaphenous vein anastomosis. Physicians seem to agree that dipyridamole should be used with warfarin in patients with prosthetic heart valves who develop thromboembolic complications while receiving therapeutic warfarin dosages.
Usual adult dosage: for graft patency after coronary artery bypass surgery, 300 to 400 mg P.O. daily in divided doses (at this dosage, the drug may act as a vasodilator rather than as an antiplatelet agent); for patients with prosthetic heart valves who develop complications while receiving warfarin, 225 mg P.O. daily.

sulfinpyrazone (Anturane). This drug may be used to decrease platelet aggregation and increase platelet survival time in various cardiovascular disorders, including angina, MI, transient cerebral ischemic attacks, amaurosis fugax, peripheral arterial atherosclerosis, and deep vein and recurrent venous thrombosis. It also may be ordered for patients with arteriovenous dialysis shunts or prosthetic mitral valves.
Usual adult dosage: for prophylaxis in thromboembolic disorders, 600 to 800 mg P.O. daily. Dosages for other indications are highly individualized.

Drug interactions

Low dosages of aspirin prescribed for its antiplatelet activity should produce few adverse reactions. The risk of bleeding increases in patients receiving heparin and high dosages of aspirin because aspirin's effect on platelets increases bleeding time. Aspirin can antagonize the uricosuric effect of sulfinpyrazone. It also increases the risk of methotrexate or valproic acid toxicity.

The additive effect of dipyridamole with aspirin has been used to prevent thromboembolic disorders in patients with aortocoronary bypass grafts or prosthetic heart valves. When administered concurrently with many other drugs, sulfinpyrazone can cause some serious adverse reactions. (For some interactions and related nursing implications, see *Drug interactions: Antiplatelet drugs,* page 638.)

ADVERSE DRUG REACTIONS

In the dosage prescribed to prevent arterial clotting, aspirin most commonly produces GI signs and symptoms, such as stomach pain, heartburn, nausea, constipation, hematemesis, melena, and slight gastric blood loss. Rarely, it may cause significant GI bleeding or peptic ulcer disease.

Aspirin produces its principal adverse reaction by damaging the gastric mucosa. Because this damage requires acid in the stomach, it can be minimized by large dosages of antacids. The gastric damage also may be minimized by using enteric-coated tablets. Although aspirin usually is administered in fairly low dosages as an antiplatelet agent, repeated administration of large dosages of aspirin may cause salicylism, with symptoms including dizziness, tinnitus, difficulty hearing, nausea, vomiting, diarrhea, confusion, and lethargy. Aspirin overdose may result in respiratory alkalosis from hyperpnea, tachypnea, and metabolic acidosis.

Dipyridamole, usually well tolerated, produces minimal adverse reactions that may include headache, dizziness, nausea, flushing, weakness, syncope, and mild GI distress. These disappear when the drug is discontinued.

The major adverse reaction to sulfinpyrazone is epigastric discomfort, which may aggravate or reactivate peptic ulcer disease. Taking the drug with food, milk, or an antacid usually reduces this discomfort.

Hypersensitivity reactions to the antiplatelet drugs, particularly anaphylaxis, can occur; the most common is the induction of bronchospasm with asthmalike symptoms. Dipyridamole may cause a skin rash. Other reactions to sulfinpyrazone may include skin rash, blood dyscrasias (anemia, leukopenia, agranulocytosis, thrombocytopenia, or aplastic anemia), and bronchoconstriction. Some patients have experienced reversible renal dysfunction after sulfinpyrazone therapy.

NURSING PROCESS APPLICATION

The following information assists the nurse in caring for a patient who is receiving an antiplatelet agent.

Assessment

• Review the patient's history for a preexisting condition that contraindicates the use of an antiplatelet agent, such as known hypersensitivity to these drugs or a bleeding disorder.
• Review the patient's history for a preexisting condition that requires cautious use of antiplatelet agents, such as impaired renal function, hypoprothrombinemia, vitamin K deficiency, thrombocytopenia, or lactation.
• Assess the patient for adverse reactions to the antiplatelet agent, such as GI distress, salicylism, headache, dizziness, flushing, weakness, or syncope.
• Review the patient's medication history to identify the use of drugs that may interact with the antiplatelet agent, such as heparin, oral anticoagulants, other antiplatelet agents, methotrexate, or valproic acid.
• Assess the effectiveness of antiplatelet therapy regularly.
• Assess the patient's respiratory status frequently.
• Evaluate the patient's and family's knowledge about the prescribed antiplatelet agent.

Nursing diagnoses

The following examples represent appropriate nursing diagnoses for a patient receiving an antiplatelet agent.
• Potential for injury related to a preexisting condition that contraindicates the use of an antiplatelet agent
• Potential for injury related to a preexisting condition that requires cautious use of an antiplatelet agent
• Potential for injury related to adverse drug reactions
• Ineffective breathing pattern related to a hypersensitivity reaction to the antiplatelet agent
• Knowledge deficit related to the prescribed antiplatelet agent

Planning and implementation

• Do not administer an antiplatelet agent to a patient with a condition that contraindicates its use.
• Administer an antiplatelet agent cautiously to a patient at risk because of a preexisting condition.
• Monitor the patient closely for adverse reactions throughout antiplatelet therapy.
• *Monitor the patient for signs of GI distress, including stomach pain, heartburn, nausea, constipation, hematemesis, melena, and gastric blood loss (with aspirin); nausea (with dipyridamole); or epigastric distress (with sulfinpyrazone).*
• *Administer aspirin or sulfinpyrazone with milk, food, or an antacid because these drugs commonly produce GI*

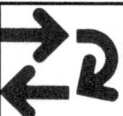

DRUG INTERACTIONS

Antiplatelet drugs

Antiplatelet drugs cause clinically significant interactions with any drugs that may cause bleeding. The chart below discusses some of the most clinically significant drugs.

DRUG	INTERACTING DRUGS	POSSIBLE EFFECTS	NURSING IMPLICATIONS
aspirin	heparin, oral anticoagulants	Increase risk of bleeding	• Monitor the patient's activated partial thromboplastin time, prothrombin time (PT), and bleeding times daily. Report any prolonged results to the physician. • Assess the patient for signs of minor or major bleeding.
	dipyridamole	Increases risk of bleeding	• Assess the patient's bleeding times closely if dipyridamole is added to or deleted from the drug regimen. • Assess the patient for signs of minor or major bleeding.
	sulfinpyrazone	Antagonizes uricosuric properties of sulfinpyrazone	• Assess the patient for increased signs and symptoms of gout, such as joint pain or swelling.
	methotrexate	Increases risk of methotrexate toxicity	• Do not administer aspirin to a patient receiving methotrexate.
	valproic acid	Increases risk of valproic acid toxicity	• Monitor valproic acid levels closely if aspirin is added to or deleted from the drug regimen. • Assess for signs of valproic acid toxicity, such as nausea, vomiting, sedation, or ataxia.
dipyridamole	aspirin	Increases risk of bleeding	• Assess the patient's bleeding time closely if aspirin is added to or deleted from the drug regimen. • Assess the patient for signs of minor or major bleeding.
sulfinpyrazone	aspirin	Antagonizes uricosuric properties of sulfinpyrazone	• Assess the patient for increased signs and symptoms of gout, such as joint pain or swelling.
	oral anticoagulants	Increase risk of bleeding	• Monitor the patient's PT closely if sulfinpyrazone is added to or deleted from the drug regimen. • Assess the patient for signs of minor or major bleeding.

distess. If distress persists during aspirin therapy, ask the physician to prescribe enteric-coated tablets.
• *Do not administer aspirin if it has a strong vinegarlike odor, which indicates drug deterioration. Give dipyridamole 1 hour before meals with 8 oz of water.*
• *Assess the patient for signs of minor bleeding, such as epistaxis, gingival bleeding, hematuria, hematemesis, or melena; and major bleeding, such as frank bleeding from the stomach or a wound, hematoma formation, hypotension, or tachycardia.* Bleeding is especially likely during concomitant therapy with heparin or an oral anticoagulant.

• Monitor the APTT, PTT, or PT as prescribed if the patient is receiving heparin or an oral anticoagulant.
• Expect to reduce the oral anticoagulant dosage as prescribed if aspirin is added to the patient's drug regimen.
• *Monitor for salicylism in a patient receiving high dosages of aspirin: dizziness, tinnitus, difficulty hearing, nausea, vomiting, diarrhea, confusion, and lethargy.*
• Consult the physician about a prescription for an analgesic if the patient receiving dipyridamole experiences a headache.

SELECTED MAJOR DRUGS

Anticoagulant agents

This chart summarizes the major anticoagulant agents currently in clinical use.

DRUG	MAJOR INDICATIONS	USUAL ADULT DOSAGES	CONTRAINDICATIONS AND PRECAUTIONS
Parenteral anticoagulant			
heparin	Pulmonary embolism or thromboembolism	5,000- to 10,000-unit bolus followed by a continuous I.V. infusion of 1,000 to 2,000 units/hour, or 5,000 to 10,000 units every 6 hours for intermittent I.V. therapy	• Know that heparin is contraindicated in a patient with known hypersensitivity to heparin, severe thrombocytopenia in whom suitable blood-coagulation tests cannot be performed at appropriate intervals, or uncontrollable active bleeding except when caused by disseminated intravascular coagulation. • Administer with extreme caution to a patient with a disease that carries a high-risk of hemorrhage, such as subacute bacterial endocarditis, severe hypertension, hemophilia, thrombocytopenia, some vascular purpuras, ulcerative lesions, or liver disease with impaired hemostasis. Administer with extreme caution to a patient undergoing a spinal tap procedure; spinal anesthesia; major surgery especially involving the brain, spinal cord, or eye; or continuous tube drainage of the stomach or small intestine. • Administer with caution to a pregnant patient or one with renal failure or allergies.
Oral anticoagulants			
warfarin	Venous thrombosis after initial treatment with heparin; prevention of deep vein thromboembolism in patients with artificial heart valves or diseased mitral valves	10 mg P.O. daily for 2 to 3 days, adjusted to prothrombin time (PT) results; maintenance dosage, 2 to 10 mg P.O. daily	• Know that warfarin is contraindicated in a patient with a condition in which the risk of hemorrhage might be greater than the drug's benefit, such as pregnancy; hemorrhagic tendency or blood dyscrasias; recent or contemplated central nervous system surgery or eye or traumatic surgery resulting in large open surfaces; bleeding tendency associated with active ulceration; overt bleeding of the GI, genitourinary, or respiratory tract; cerebrovascular hemorrhage; aneurysm; pericarditis; pericardial effusion; subacute bacterial endocarditis; threatened abortion; eclampsia or preeclampsia; inadequate laboratory facilities; senile dementia or cognitive impairment; alcoholism; psychosis; lack of patient cooperation; spinal puncture or other diagnostic or therapeutic procedures with potential for uncontrollable bleeding; major regional lumbar block anesthesia; or malignant hypertension. • Administer with caution to a lactating patient or one with a condition that increases the risk of hemorrhage or necrosis, such as moderate to severe hepatic or renal insufficiency; infectious disease; intestinal flora disturbance; trauma; large exposed raw surfaces from surgery; indwelling catheter use; moderate to severe hypertension; known or suspected hereditary, familial, or clinical deficiency of protein C; polycythemia vera; vasculitis; severe diabetes; or severe allergic or anaphylactic disorder. *(continued)*

SELECTED MAJOR DRUGS

Anticoagulant agents (continued)

DRUG	MAJOR INDICATIONS	USUAL ADULT DOSAGES	CONTRAINDICATIONS AND PRECAUTIONS
Oral anticoagulants (continued)			
dicumarol	Same indications as warfarin	200 to 300 mg P.O. the first day, then 25 to 200 mg/day, depending on PT results	• Know that dicumarol is contraindicated in a patient with the same conditions that contraindicate the use of warfarin. It also is contraindicated in a patient with open wounds, visceral carcinoma, vitamin K deficiency, or severe liver or kidney disease. • Administer with caution to a lactating or postpartal patient or one with a condition that increases the risk of hemorrhage or necrosis, such as mild to moderate hepatic or renal insufficiency; infectious disease; disturbance of intestinal flora; trauma; surgery resulting in large exposed raw surfaces; use of an indwelling catheter or drainage tube in any orifice; mild to moderate hypertension; known or suspected hereditary, familial, or clinical deficiency of protein C; polycythemia vera; vasculitis; severe diabetes; severe allergic or anaphylactic disorder; active tuberculosis; or history of ulcerative disease of the GI tract.
Antiplatelet agents			
aspirin	Prevention of clot formation in arteriovenous shunts in hemodialysis patients	160 mg P.O. daily	• Know that aspirin is contraindicated in a pregnant patient during the last trimester, a child or teenager with varicella or influenza (unless directed by a physician), or one with a bleeding disorder, known hypersensitivity to aspirin, or history of acute asthmatic attacks, urticaria, or rhinitis precipitated by aspirin. • Administer with caution to a lactating patient or one with impaired renal function or a history of GI lesions. • Administer with extreme caution to a patient with advanced chronic renal insufficiency, hypoprothrombinemia, vitamin K deficiency, thrombocytopenia, thrombotic thrombocytopenic purpura, severe hepatic impairment, or anticoagulant therapy. • Administer highly buffered aspirin preparations with extreme caution to a patient with congestive heart failure or any other condition in which high sodium intake is harmful.
	Prevention of clot formation in patients with unstable angina	325 mg P.O. daily	

• *Take safety precautions if dizziness, weakness, or syncope occurs. For example, keep the bed rails up, keep the bed in a low position, and supervise ambulation.*

• Monitor the patient's hematologic studies for blood dyscrasias during dipyridamole therapy.

• Monitor the patient's bleeding time and platelet aggregation studies to assess the effectiveness of antiplatelet therapy.

• Notify the physician if adverse reactions occur or if antiplatelet therapy is ineffective.

• *Observe for bronchospasm, asthmalike symptoms, or bronchoconstriction in a patient receiving aspirin or dipyridamole.*

• Auscultate the patient's breath sounds regularly, and assess for changes in the patient's respiratory rate or pattern.

• *Notify the physician immediately if breathing difficulty occurs; place the patient in a high Fowler's position to maximize breathing effectiveness.*

• *Prepare to administer oxygen and drugs, as prescribed, to relieve respiratory symptoms of a hypersensitivity reaction.*

Patient teaching

• Teach the patient and family the name, dose, action, frequency, and adverse effects of the prescribed antiplatelet agent.

• Instruct the patient taking aspirin or sulfinpyrazone to take it with milk, food, or an antacid and to report any severe gastric pain to the physician. Also tell the patient to take enteric-coated tablets, as prescribed.

• *Instruct the patient not to take aspirin if it has a strong vinegarlike odor, but to purchase a new container.*

• *Advise the patient to take dipyridamole 1 hour before meals with 8 oz of water.*

• Stress the importance of returning for laboratory tests, as instructed, to monitor the effectiveness of therapy or detect adverse reactions.

• *Teach the patient and family to recognize the signs of bleeding and report them to the physician.*

• *Instruct the patient taking aspirin to consult the physician before taking additional over-the-counter products that contain aspirin.*

• Teach the patient to avoid sports that pose a high risk of injury that could lead to bleeding.

• *Instruct the patient on high-dose aspirin therapy to recognize and report signs of salicylism.*

• Advise the patient not to perform activities that require alertness if dizziness, weakness, or syncope occurs.

• Instruct the patient to notify the physician immediately if adverse reactions occur.

Evaluation

The following examples represent appropriate evaluation statements for a patient receiving an antiplatelet agent.

• The patient has no conditions that contraindicate antiplatelet therapy.

• The patient exhibits no signs of complications in the preexisting condition linked to the prescribed antiplatelet agent.

• The patient experiences no adverse reactions to the prescribed antiplatelet agent.

• The patient maintains a normal breathing pattern throughout antiplatelet therapy.

• The patient and family express an accurate understanding of the points taught about the prescribed antiplatelet agent.

• The patient correctly identifies signs of bleeding and salicylism and describes what to do if they occur.

CHAPTER SUMMARY

Chapter 36 focused on heparin, the oral anticoagulants, and the investigational use of the antiplatelet drugs in anticoagulant therapy. Here are the chapter highlights.

• Heparin is the drug of choice to treat and prevent venous thromboembolism because of its immediate anticoagulant effect when administered I.V.

• Heparin arrests clot formation by accelerating the interaction between antithrombin III and thrombin. However, it does not dissolve existing clots.

• The anticoagulant effect of heparin is monitored best by the APTT or PTT, which should be maintained at 1½ to 2½ times the control.

• Low-dose S.C. heparin often is used to prevent thromboembolism in high-risk patients.

• Patients on high-dose continuous or intermittent heparin therapy need frequent nursing assessment for signs of minor and major bleeding. Those on home therapy need to have laboratory access for monitoring APTT or PTT values.

• Because heparin is synergistic with all oral anticoagulants, the risk of bleeding is increased in patients receiving both drugs.

• In patients with severe bleeding, protamine sulfate is used to neutralize heparin.

• The coumarin compounds, the most commonly used oral anticoagulants in the United States, are the drugs of choice for long-term management of patients with deep vein thrombosis and patients at high risk, such as those with prosthetic heart valves or diseased mitral valves. The oral anticoagulants alter liver synthesis of the vitamin K-dependent clotting factors—Factors II, VII, IX, and X.

• Oral anticoagulants are monitored by the patient's PT.

• The major adverse reactions to oral anticoagulants are bleeding complications. Treatment may include discontinuing the drug, reducing the dosage, or administering oral or parenteral vitamin K as prescribed.

• The nurse should teach patients receiving oral anticoagulants about drug interactions with other drugs and with food, ways to check for signs of bleeding, and the need for having blood drawn for PT results as prescribed.

• Researchers are studying antiplatelet drugs for prevention of arterial clotting, especially in patients with MI or cerebral ischemic disease. Aspirin currently is the most widely researched antiplatelet drug; dipyridamole and sulfinpyrazone also are under investigation.

• Although many drugs are known to alter platelet function, the clinical efficacy of these drugs in preventing arterial clotting remains the subject of intense clinical trials.

• Bleeding times and platelet aggregation studies are the best indicators of the effectiveness of antiplatelet therapy.

• When administering antiplatelet drugs, the nurse should monitor the patient regularly for GI signs and symptoms and hypersensitivity reactions.

STUDY QUESTIONS

See Appendix 1 for answers.

1. Lisa Bonner, age 47, is admitted to the medical-surgical unit for acute thrombophlebitis in her left calf. She has no previous history of thrombophlebitis. The physician orders heparin 5,000 units as an I.V. bolus, followed by continuous I.V. infusion of 1,000 units/hour. How does heparin exert its anticoagulant effect?
(a) by altering the synthesis of vitamin K-dependent clotting factors
(b) by lysing already formed thrombi, thus reestablishing circulation
(c) by accelerating the interaction between antithrombin III and thrombin
(d) by reducing platelet aggregation

2. To evaluate the anticoagulant effects of heparin on Ms. Bonner, the nurse should review the results of which laboratory test?
(a) bleeding time
(b) prothrombin time (PT)
(c) red blood cell (RBC) count
(d) activated partial thromboplastin time (APTT)

3. If Ms. Bonner started bleeding excessively during heparin therapy, which antidote is likely to be prescribed?
(a) vitamin K
(b) Factor VIII
(c) protamine sulfate
(d) sulfinpyrazone

4. While Ms. Bonner is receiving heparin, her physician prescribes the oral anticoagulant warfarin (Coumadin) 10 mg P.O. daily. Why is heparin administered concurrently with warfarin?
(a) Warfarin's therapeutic effects do not occur until clotting factors are depleted.
(b) Heparin activates warfarin.
(c) Warfarin and heparin have a synergistic effect.
(d) Heparin hastens the onset of action of warfarin.

5. How does warfarin produce its anticoagulant effects?
(a) It acts as a vitamin K antagonist.
(b) It prevents platelet aggregation.
(c) It promotes lysis of existing thrombi.
(d) It accelerates the thrombin-antithrombin III interaction.

6. While Ms. Bonner is receiving warfarin, the nurse should expect to monitor the results of which laboratory test to evaluate the drug's anticoagulant effects?
(a) bleeding time
(b) partial thrombin time (PTT)
(c) APTT
(d) PT

7. Because Ed Bernhardt, age 60, has arteriosclerosis and coronary artery disease, he is at risk for myocardial infarction (MI). To reduce Mr. Bernhardt's risk of MI, the physician prescribes aspirin 325 mg P.O. daily. How does aspirin prevent arterial thromboembolism?
(a) It prevents platelet aggregation.
(b) It dissolves atherosclerotic plaques.
(c) It causes clot lysis on atherosclerotic plaques.
(d) It prevents atherosclerotic plaque formation.

8. While Mr. Bernhardt is receiving low dosage aspirin therapy, the nurse should assess him for which common adverse reaction?
(a) fever
(b) GI distress
(c) skin rash
(d) dizziness

SELECTED REFERENCES

AHFS drug information 90. (1990). Bethesda, MD: American Society of Hospital Pharmacists.

Aledort, L. (1989). New approaches to management of bleeding disorders. *Hospital Practice,* 24(2), 207-221.

Drug facts and comparisons. (1990). St. Louis: Facts and Comparisons Division, J.B. Lippincott.

Goodman and Gilman's the pharmacological basis of therapeutics (8th ed.; 1990). Elmsford, NY: Pergamon Press.

Hematuria during anticoagulant therapy deserves workup. (1987). *Nurses Drug Alert,* 11(10), 77-78.

Hirsh, J., Poller, L., Deykin, D., et al. (1989). Optimal therapeutic range for oral anticoagulants. *Chest,* 95(Suppl. 2), 5s-11s.

North American Nursing Diagnosis Association. (1990). *Taxonomy I - Revised, with official diagnostic categories.* St. Louis: NANDA.

Wilson, J. (1988). Avoiding errors in intravenous heparin therapy. *AD Nurse,* 3(3), 31-32.

THROMBOLYTIC AGENTS

OBJECTIVES

After reading and studying this chapter, the student should be able to:
1. Discuss the pharmacokinetics of the thrombolytic agents.
2. Describe the mechanisms of action by which these drugs dissolve thrombi.
3. Identify the approved clinical indications for thrombolytic agents.
4. Explain why patients undergoing thrombolytic therapy are at increased risk for bleeding.
5. Identify the drug interactions that occur when thrombolytic agents are used with heparin, oral anticoagulants, or antiplatelet drugs.
6. Identify the adverse reactions to the thrombolytic agents.
7. Describe how to apply the nursing process when caring for a patient who is receiving a thrombolytic agent.

INTRODUCTION

Thromboembolic occlusion of an artery may result in the necrosis (death) of tissue distal to the obstruction, and the patient may lose the function of part or all of the affected organ. Although thrombi will disintegrate in 7 to 10 days by the action of the fibrinolytic system, tissue death can occur in hours.

If emboli that acutely occlude the major artery or vein are dissolved quickly, blood flow may be reestablished to distal tissues, and necrosis may be minimized or prevented. Thrombolytic therapy may be indicated for a coronary artery thrombus, pulmonary embolus, or deep vein thrombosis to dissolve the thrombus and reestablish circulation. Thrombolytic agents convert plasminogen to plasmin, allowing the hydrolysis (chemical alteration of a compound with water) of the fibrin that forms the clot.

Thrombolytic therapy still is somewhat controversial. In the last decade, researchers have conducted many clinical trials to determine the indications for therapy, the benefits and risks, and the appropriate route and dosage. In the trials, serious, unpredictable bleeding from the therapy has

SELECTED NURSING DIAGNOSES

Thrombolytic agents

The following nursing diagnoses address representative problems and etiologies that a nurse may encounter when caring for a patient who is receiving a thrombolytic agent. Some of these nursing diagnoses contain generalized etiologies, which the nurse must individualize based on the patient's needs. (For some common nursing diagnoses and related interventions for each drug class, see the "Nursing Process Application" section of this chapter.)

- Altered oral mucous membrane related to bleeding caused by the thrombolytic agent
- Altered protection related to bleeding caused by the thrombolytic agent
- Anxiety related to the risk of bleeding during thrombolytic agent therapy
- Decreased cardiac output related to arrhythmias from intracoronary administration of streptokinase
- Fluid volume excess related to anistreplase-induced lung edema
- Ineffective breathing pattern related to anistreplase-induced breathing difficulty
- Ineffective breathing pattern related to streptokinase-induced bronchospasm
- Knowledge deficit related to the prescribed thrombolytic agent
- Pain related to anistreplase-induced headache or chest pain
- Potential altered body temperature related to a febrile episode caused by the thrombolytic agent
- Potential fluid volume deficit related to blood loss caused by the thrombolytic agent
- Potential for injury related to a preexisting condition that contraindicates the use of a thrombolytic agent
- Potential for injury related to a preexisting condition that requires cautious use of a thrombolytic agent
- Potential for injury related to adverse drug reactions
- Potential for injury related to drug interactions
- Potential for trauma related to the adverse central nervous system effects of anistreplase
- Sensory-perceptual alterations (tactile) related to anistreplase-induced paresthesia

overwhelmed all other issues, and subsequent research is directed toward developing thrombolytic agents that are more selective in their actions.

For a summary of representative drugs, see *Selected major drugs: Thrombolytic agents,* page 648. For a listing of applicable nursing diagnoses that the nurse may formulate when caring for a patient receiving these agents, see *Selected nursing diagnoses: Thrombolytic agents,* page 643. For detailed information on applying the nursing process, see Chapter 6, The Nursing Process and Drug Therapy.

THROMBOLYTIC AGENTS

The major thrombolytic drugs discussed in this chapter include alteplase, anistreplase, streptokinase, and urokinase. Another thrombolytic agent, single-chain urokinase-type plasminogen activator (pro-urokinase), has shown promise in experimental trials but has not been approved yet for clinical use. This drug may act more specifically at the thrombus site, but via a different mechanism of action. Its pharmacokinetics, indications, and dosages remain to be determined.

PHARMACOKINETICS

The thrombolytic agents vary in their pharmacokinetic properties. Little is known about the pharmacokinetics of the newer thrombolytic agents, alteplase and anistreplase.

Absorption, distribution, metabolism, excretion
After intravenous (I.V.) or intracoronary administration, thrombolytic agents are distributed immediately throughout the circulation, quickly activating plasminogen. Alteplase is cleared rapidly from circulating plasma primarily by the liver. Little is known about the pharmacokinetics of anistreplase. Streptokinase is removed rapidly from the circulation by antibodies and the mononuclear phagocytic system (reticuloendothelial system). It does not appear to cross the placenta. Urokinase is metabolized rapidly by the liver, and small amounts are excreted in bile and urine. Research has not determined yet if it crosses the placenta.

Onset, peak, duration
The onset of action of the thrombolytic agents is almost immediate, with rapid plasminogen activation after I.V. or intracoronary administration.

The half-life of alteplase is unknown; of the activated fibrinolytic compound of anistreplase, 70 to 120 minutes. In clinical studies, streptokinase demonstrates a biphasic decline in plasma concentration, with an initial half-life of 18 minutes and a subsequent half-life of 83 minutes. The serum half-life of urokinase is 20 minutes.

After therapy is discontinued, the thrombolytic effects of all four agents disappear within a few hours, but the systemic effect on coagulation and the risk of bleeding may persist for 12 to 24 hours. The effect of these drugs on systemic coagulation is noted by decreased plasma levels of fibrinogen and plasminogen and increased levels of circulating fibrin degradation products (FDPs). (For a discussion of normal coagulation, see the introduction to this unit.) For 4 hours, thrombin time is decreased to less than twice the normal control value.

PHARMACODYNAMICS

The thrombolytic agents convert plasminogen to the enzyme plasmin, which lyses (dissolves) thrombi, fibrinogen, and other plasma proteins.

Mechanism of action
An active protease, alteplase produces limited conversion of plasminogen in the absence of fibrin. It binds to fibrin in a thrombus and converts the trapped plasminogen to plasmin. This initiates local fibrinolysis and limited systemic proteolysis. After alteplase administration, circulating fibrinogen decreases by 16% to 36%.

A derivative of a fibrinolytic enzyme, anistreplase is inactive in the presence of an anisoyl group. Immediately after administration, it is activated by deacylation of the anisoyl group. This results in plasmin production from plasminogen, which leads to thrombolysis.

Streptokinase indirectly activates plasminogen by forming an activator complex that later converts residual plasminogen into the proteolytic (protein-splitting) enzyme plasmin. Therapeutic dosages of streptokinase introduce a high level of activator into the bloodstream but relatively little plasmin. As the circulating activator diffuses into the thrombus, it activates adsorbed preplasmin II, which hydrolyzes fibrin. This action leads to endogenous lysis (dissolution). Plasmin generated in the circulation binds to antiplasmin and is released at the thrombus site, resulting in the external lysis of the clot.

During the first few hours of treatment, rapidly activated plasminogen can produce hyperplasminemia (excessive plasmin in the blood) and possible coagulation defects from increased hydrolysis and depleted fibrinogen and coagulation Factors V and VII. These changes, combined with fibrin dissolution, increase the risk of bleeding.

Streptokinase also decreases blood and plasma viscosity as well as the tendency for erythrocytes and platelets to aggregate. These actions increase blood flow and produce a perfusion of collateral blood vessels. Because streptokinase is highly antigenic, repeated administration produces antibodies that diminish the drug's effect and may promote allergic reactions.

Urokinase, an active protease, directly converts plasminogen to plasmin within and on the surface of thrombi and emboli. The plasmin breaks down fibrin, fibrinogen, and other procoagulant plasma proteins. Urokinase also produces an anticoagulant effect by dissolving fibrinogen and increasing the level of FDPs. With a greater affinity than streptokinase for fibrin-bound plasminogen, urokinase produces a milder systemic coagulation effect. Urokinase is nonantigenic and does not produce allergic reactions.

PHARMACOTHERAPEUTICS

The Food and Drug Administration (FDA) has approved the thrombolytic agents for treating certain thromboembolic disorders. These drugs also have been used to dissolve thrombi in arteriovenous cannulas to reestablish blood flow. The thrombolytic agents are the drugs of choice to break down newly formed thrombi. They seem most effective when administered immediately after thrombosis and up to 6 hours after the onset of symptoms. Alteplase and anistreplase also can be used to treat acute myocardial infarction (MI).

alteplase (Activase). Used to manage acute (MI), alteplase lyses thrombi obstructing coronary arteries, reduces infarct size, improves ventricular function after acute MI, and reduces the incidence of congestive heart failure and mortality associated with acute MI. Treatment should begin as soon as possible after the onset of acute MI symptoms.

Alteplase also is used to manage acute massive pulmonary embolism in adults. It lyses acute pulmonary emboli that obstruct blood flow to a lobe or multiple segments of the lungs, and pulmonary emboli accompanied by unstable hemodynamics, as in a patient who cannot maintain blood pressure without supportive measures.

Usual adult dosage: For acute MI, 60 mg I.V. in the first hour (of which 6 to 10 mg is given as a bolus), followed by 20 mg over the second hour and 20 mg over the third hour; for pulmonary embolus, 100 mg I.V. infused over 2 hours.

anistreplase (Eminase). This drug is used to manage acute MI, lyse thrombi obstructing coronary arteries, reduce infarct size, improve ventricular function after acute MI, and reduce mortality associated with acute MI.

Usual adult dosage: 30 units I.V. infused over 2 to 5 minutes.

streptokinase (Kabikinase, Streptase). The first thrombolytic agent introduced, streptokinase is used to treat deep vein thrombosis, pulmonary embolism, arterial thrombosis and embolism, and acute evolving transmural MI and to dissolve thrombi in arteriovenous cannulas. Patients who have had previous streptococcal infections will have antistreptokinase antibodies in their systems. To overcome these antibodies, a large loading dose may be administered or a different thrombolytic agent may be used if blood tests do not indicate lysis after 4 hours of therapy. A loading dose of 250,000 IU overcomes the antibody level in 90% to 95% of the patients and initiates fibrinolysis.

Usual adult dosage: for pulmonary embolus, the dosage is the same as for deep vein thrombosis, but the infusion continues for only 24 hours. For deep vein thrombosis and arterial thrombosis and emboli, an I.V. loading dose of 250,000 IU given over 30 minutes, followed by an I.V. infusion of 100,000 IU/hour for up to 72 hours, depending on clinical results. For arterial thrombosis and emboli, drug treatment may be used with surgery (arterial embolectomy). For arteriovenous cannula clearance, 100,000 to 250,000 IU by I.V. instilled slowly into occluded cannula. For acute evolving transmural MI, 1,500,000 IU by I.V. infusion over 60 minutes, or 140,000 IU by intracoronary infusion (20,000 IU by bolus followed by 2,000 IU/minute for 60 minutes).

urokinase (Abbokinase). Approved by the FDA for dissolving acute pulmonary emboli and coronary thromboses as well as for clearing clotted arteriovenous catheters, urokinase provides some advantages over streptokinase. Because it is nonantigenic, urokinase does not cause allergic reactions, and it has a greater affinity for fibrin-bound plasminogen than for plasma plasminogen — limiting its effect on systemic plasminogen. Despite these advantages, urokinase does not have greater clinical efficacy or cause less bleeding than streptokinase. Urokinase is much more expensive. It is indicated for patients who cannot tolerate streptokinase.

Usual adult dosage: for pulmonary embolism, 4,400 IU/kg/hour I.V. for 10 minutes as a loading dose, then 4,400 IU/kg/hour as a constant infusion over 12 to 24 hours. For coronary thrombosis, a bolus of 2,500 to 10,000 units of heparin I.V. followed with urokinase at 6,000 IU/minute for up to 2 hours via intracoronary catheter. For a clot in a central catheter or shunt, 5,000 IU/ml of I.V. fluid equal to the volume of the catheter is inserted and kept in the catheter for 5 to 60 minutes before being aspirated. If the clot cannot be dislodged, the procedure should be repeated in 5 minutes. If the catheter still is not clear after 30 minutes, it should be capped and the urokinase should remain in the catheter for up to 1 hour. Then clot aspiration should be tried again.

After the patient completes urokinase therapy, heparin and an oral anticoagulant should be infused to prevent rethrombosis. Before starting the heparin infusion, the nurse should expect to verify the patient's thrombin time, the best indicator of thrombolytic therapy. The thrombin time should be less than twice the normal control (usually about 4 hours after the cessation of urokinase).

Drug interactions

Thrombolytic agents interact with heparin, oral anticoagulants, antiplatelet drugs, and nonsteroidal anti-inflammatory drugs (NSAIDs), increasing the patient's risk of bleeding. Heparin and oral anticoagulants often are instituted after thrombolytic therapy, but not until the patient's thrombin time is less than twice the control. During concomitant therapy, the nurse must monitor the patient's thrombin time; assess for signs of bleeding, especially at puncture sites and invasive line insertion sites; and assess vital signs for indications of hemorrhage.

Aminocaproic acid (Amicar) inhibits streptokinase and can be used to reverse its fibrinolytic effects. (For more information, see *Aminocaproic acid [Amicar]*.)

ADVERSE DRUG REACTIONS

The major reactions associated with the thrombolytic agents are bleeding and allergic responses, especially with streptokinase and anistreplase. During and after treatment, the nurse must assess the patient closely for signs of bleeding,

which occur frequently with thrombolytic therapy. Thrombolytic agents dissolve fibrin deposits at all sites, not just at the arterial thrombus obstructing coronary or pulmonary circulation. Thus, bleeding can occur at a sutured wound or any puncture site, such as an arterial line or central line catheter site. Pressure dressings applied to the oozing areas usually will control bleeding so that the dosage does not have to be reduced.

Major bleeding may occur in some patients, resulting from a systemic bleeding disturbance. Hemorrhaging may occur intracranially, in the gastrointestinal (GI) or urinary tract, in the vagina, or retroperitoneally. The infusion of thrombolytic agents may be discontinued and blood replacement begun, as prescribed, in such instances.

Allergic reactions to streptokinase are common, because most patients possess circulating streptococcal antibodies. Anistreplase also has caused allergic reactions. Symptoms include urticaria, itching, flushing, nausea, headache, or musculoskeletal pain.

When administered by intracoronary catheter, streptokinase can produce hemorrhagic infarction at the site of myocardial necrosis as well as reperfusion arrhythmias. The reperfusion arrhythmias usually are premature ventricular contractions that require no treatment. Occasionally, more serious arrhythmias, such as complex or grouped premature ventricular contractions, ventricular tachycardia, and fibrillation occur and may require emergency antiarrhythmic therapy or defibrillation. Bradycardia after intracoronary thrombolytic therapy may warrant treatment with atropine or a pacemaker.

Some patients experience fever (an average of 1.5° F [0.8° C] increase) after therapy, particularly after receiving streptokinase or anistreplase. The cause of this response has not been established.

Anistreplase may cause conduction disorders and hypotension. Less common adverse reactions to anistreplase include chills, sweating, shock, cardiac rupture, chest pain, dyspnea, lung edema, emboli, purpura, nausea, vomiting, thrombocytopenia, elevated transaminase levels, arthralgia, headache, agitation, dizziness, vertigo, paresthesias, and tremor.

An anaphylactic response to streptokinase or anistreplase represents a serious, although rare, reaction. Symptoms range from minor breathing difficulties to bronchospasm, periorbital swelling, or angioneurotic edema.

NURSING PROCESS APPLICATION

The following information assists the nurse in caring for a patient who is receiving a thrombolytic agent.

Aminocaproic acid (Amicar)

Although its effectiveness is not well documented, aminocaproic acid is used as an antidote to streptokinase.

Action

- Inhibits plasminogen activator substances and, to a lesser degree, plasminic activity, thereby inhibiting thrombolysis

Administration and dosage

- Oral or I.V. loading dose of 5 grams followed by 1 gram/hour for the next 4 to 8 hours to a maximum of 30 grams in 24 hours
- For I.V. infusion, 4 to 5 grams diluted in 250 ml of diluent (normal saline solution, D_5W, or lactated Ringer's solution) for the first hour of treatment, followed by a continuous infusion of 1 gram/hour in 50 ml of diluent

Adverse reactions

- GI: nausea, cramps, diarrhea
- Cardiovascular: hypotension, especially if infused undiluted
- CNS: dizziness, tinnitus, headache, delirium, seizures
- Miscellaneous: conjunctival suffusion, nasal stuffiness, acute renal failure, thrombophlebitis, prolonged menstruation

Assessment

• Review the patient's history for a preexisting condition that contraindicates the use of a thrombolytic agent, such as active internal bleeding, cerebrovascular accident in the past 2 months, intracranial or intraspinal surgery, intracranial neoplasm, severe uncontrolled hypertension, or known hypersensitivity to thrombolytic agents.

• Review the patient's history for a preexisting condition that requires cautious use of a thrombolytic agent, such as major surgery in the past 10 days, organ biopsy, severe GI bleeding, recent trauma, hypertension, subacute bacterial endocarditis, hemostatic defects, or diabetic hemorrhagic retinopathy.

• Assess the patient for adverse reactions to the thrombolytic agent, such as bleeding and allergic reactions.

• Review the patient's medication history to identify the use of drugs that may interact with the prescribed thrombolytic agent, such as heparin, oral anticoagulants, antiplatelet drugs, or NSAIDs.

• Assess the effectiveness of the thrombolytic agent during administration and for several hours after.

• Evaluate the patient's and family's knowledge about the prescribed thrombolytic agent.

Nursing diagnoses

The following examples represent appropriate evaluation statements for a patient receiving a thrombolytic agent.

• Potential for injury related to a preexisting condition that contraindicates the use of a thrombolytic agent

• Potential for injury related to a preexisting condition that requires cautious use of a thrombolytic agent

• Potential for injury related to adverse drug reactions

• Knowledge deficit related to the prescribed thrombolytic agent

Planning and implementation

• Do not administer a thrombolytic agent to a patient with a condition that contraindicates its use.

• Administer a thrombolytic agent cautiously to a patient at risk because of a preexisting condition.

• *Monitor the patient closely for bleeding and other adverse reactions, especially during concomitant heparin therapy.*

• *Monitor the patient's coagulation studies during thrombolytic therapy. Coagulation studies are recommended before and 4 hours after systemic administration of a thrombolytic agent.* These studies should indicate lysis by demonstrating prolonged partial thromboplastin time (PTT), reduced fibrinogen levels, and the appearance of FDPs. If these effects do not occur, the patient probably is resistant to the drug, and fibrinolysis of the thrombus is not occurring. Prothrombin time, thrombin time, activated partial thromboplastin time, quantitative fibrinogen, euglobulin clot lysis, and plasminogen levels can be used. Each of these studies measures different factors and times along the coagulation cascade. The PTT measures how quickly a clot forms after thrombin is added to a patient's plasma sample. Thrombin converts fibrinogen to a fibrin clot, and the time that elapses until clot formation provides an estimation of plasma fibrinogen levels.

• *Monitor the patient closely for signs of bleeding during thrombolytic therapy, especially at puncture and wound sites.*

• *Monitor the patient's vital signs frequently to assess for signs of internal bleeding and to detect hypotension, significant pulse or respiratory changes, or fever.*

• *Treat severe bleeding complications by stopping the infusion and infusing fresh whole blood, packed red cells, or fresh frozen plasma, as prescribed. Prepare to administer aminocaproic acid, which may be prescribed as an antidote.*

• Continue to assess the patient for bleeding complications for 24 hours after thrombolytic therapy.

• *Assess the patient's chest pain if the intracoronary route is used; a decrease may signal myocardial reperfusion. Also evaluate the patient's electrocardiogram pattern, especially the ST segment and any ventricular arrhythmias or conduction disorders.*

• *Keep antiarrhythmic drugs, such as lidocaine, and a defibrillator easily accessible at all times.*

• Observe the patient for signs of microembolism, such as skin mottling, pallor, or cyanosis.

• Observe the patient for signs of an allergic reaction to streptokinase or anistreplase: nausea, pruritus, flushing, fever, musculoskeletal pain, dyspnea, bronchospasm, or angioneurotic edema.

• *Leave the femoral venous and arterial sheaths in place for 24 hours after intracoronary thrombolytic therapy. Immobilize the patient's entire leg for 24 hours to prevent bleeding. If bleeding occurs at the femoral insertion site, apply direct pressure with a pressure dressing or Amicar-soaked sponges. Monitor the patient's color, temperature, and femoral, popliteal, and dorsalis pedis pulses every 15 minutes for 1 hour, then every 30 minutes for 8 hours, and then once each shift.*

• Expect to administer a large loading dose of streptokinase as prescribed to a patient who has had a streptococcal infection.

• Expect to discontinue streptokinase therapy and use a different thrombolytic agent as prescribed if the thrombin time or other test does not indicate lysis after 4 hours of therapy.

• *Do not administer I.M. injections or insert new arterial lines during therapy or for 24 hours after therapy.*

• *Administer medications through existing I.V. sites, orally, or by nasogastric tube, as prescribed.*

• Administer acetaminophen rather than aspirin for a fever, as prescribed, to decrease the patient's risk of bleeding.

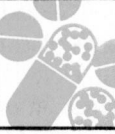

Thrombolytic agents

Thrombolytic agents are used to dissolve thrombi in deep vein thrombosis, pulmonary embolism, arterial thrombosis and emboli, and acute myocardial infarction (MI). They also are used to dissolve clots in arteriovenous catheters. This chart summarizes the major thrombolytic agents currently in clinical use.

DRUG	MAJOR INDICATIONS	USUAL ADULT DOSAGES	CONTRAINDICATIONS AND PRECAUTIONS
alteplase	Acute MI	60 mg I.V. in the first hour (of which 6 to 10 mg is given as a bolus), then 20 mg over the second hour, and 20 mg over the third hour	• Know that alteplase is contraindicated in a patient with active internal bleeding, history of cerebrovascular accident (CVA), intracranial or intraspinal surgery or trauma in the past 2 months, intracranial neoplasm, arteriovenous malformation, aneurysm, known bleeding diathesis, severe uncontrolled hypertension, or known hypersensitivity to alteplase.
	Pulmonary embolism	100 mg I.V. infused over 2 hours	• Administer with extreme caution to a pregnant patient, a patient over age 75, or one with major surgery in the past 10 days; cerebrovascular disease; gastrointestinal (GI) or genitourinary bleeding in the past 10 days; trauma, including trauma caused by cardiopulmonary resuscitation, in the past 10 days; hypertension (systolic blood pressure over 180 mm Hg or diastolic blood pressure over 110 mm Hg); high likelihood of left heart thrombus; subacute bacterial endocarditis; acute pericarditis; hemostatic defects, such as those caused by severe hepatic or renal disease; diabetic hemorrhagic retinopathy or other hemorrhagic ophthalmic condition; significant liver dysfunction; septic thrombophlebitis; occluded arteriovenous (AV) cannula at seriously infected site; concurrent administration of an oral anticoagulant; or any other condition in which bleeding constitutes a significant hazard or would be difficult to manage because of its location.
anistreplase	Acute MI	30 units I.V. over 2 to 5 minutes	• Know that anistreplase is contraindicated in a patient with any of the conditions that contraindicate the use of alteplase. • Administer with extreme caution to a patient with any of the conditions that require extremely cautious use of alteplase (except for significant liver dysfunction).
streptokinase	Deep vein thrombosis, arterial thrombosis and emboli	250,000 IU I.V. as a loading dose given over 30 minutes, then 100,000 IU/hour I.V. for up to 72 hours	• Know that streptokinase is contraindicated in a patient with active internal bleeding, CVA in the past 2 months, intracranial or intraspinal surgery, intracranial neoplasm, severe uncontrolled hypertension, or known hypersensitivity to streptokinase.
	Pulmonary embolus	250,000 IU I.V. as a loading dose given over 30 minutes, then 100,000 IU/hour I.V. for 24 hours	• Administer with extreme caution to a pregnant patient, a patient over age 75, or one with major surgery in the past 10 days; undergoing childbirth or organ biopsy; with previous puncture of noncompressible vessels, severe GI bleeding; recent trauma, including trauma caused by cardiopulmonary resuscitation; hypertension (systolic blood pressure over 180 mm Hg or diastolic blood pressure over 110 mm Hg); high likelihood of left heart thrombus, as in mitral stenosis with atrial fibrillation; subacute bacterial endocarditis; hemostatic defects, such as those caused by severe hepatic or renal disease; cerebrovascular disease; diabetic hemorrhagic retinopathy; septic thrombophlebitis; occluded AV cannula at seriously infected site; or any other condition in which bleeding constitutes a significant hazard or would be difficult to manage because of its location.
	Acute evolving transmural MI	1,500,000 IU by I.V. infusion over 60 minutes, or 140,000 IU by intracoronary infusion (20,000 IU by bolus followed by 2,000 IU/minute for 60 minutes)	
	Clot dissolution in arteriovenous cannula	100,000 to 250,000 IU instilled slowly into the occluded cannula	

• Monitor the patient's thrombin time after thrombolytic therapy is stopped; it should be less than twice the control before beginning heparin therapy.
• Notify the physician immediately if adverse reactions occur.

Patient teaching

• Teach the patient and family the name, dose, action, frequency, and adverse effects of the prescribed thrombolytic agent.
• Encourage the patient and family to ask questions about the drug regimen.
• *Instruct the patient to inform the nurse if adverse reactions occur or if initial symptoms, such as chest pain, improve or worsen.*

Evaluation

The following examples represent appropriate evaluation statements for a patient receiving a thrombolytic agent.
• The patient has no conditions that contraindicate thrombolytic agent therapy.
• The patient exhibits no signs of complications in the preexisting condition linked to the prescribed thrombolytic agent.
• The patient displays no adverse reactions to the prescribed thrombolytic agent.
• The patient and family express an accurate understanding of the points taught about the prescribed thrombolytic agent.
• The patient correctly identifies adverse reactions to thrombolytic therapy and agrees to notify the nurse if they occur.

CHAPTER SUMMARY

Chapter 37 presented the thrombolytic agents. These drugs activate and convert plasminogen to plasmin, which dissolves thrombi. The major disadvantage of the thrombolytic agents is lack of specificity; they activate not only the plasminogen bound to the fibrin clot but also plasma plasminogen, creating a generalized systemic thrombolytic state that increases the risk of bleeding at puncture and wound sites. Here are the chapter highlights.
• Thrombolytic agents currently approved for clinical use include alteplase, anistreplase, streptokinase, and urokinase. Another thrombolytic agent (single-chain urokinase-type plasminogen activator) has shown promise in experimental trials but has not been approved yet for clinical use.
• Thrombolytic agents are used to dissolve thrombi in deep vein thrombosis, pulmonary embolism, arterial thrombosis

and emboli, acute MI, and coronary thrombosis and to clear clotted arteriovenous cannulas. These drugs are infused parenterally into the general circulation or directly into the thrombosed blood vessel.
• Patients must be selected carefully for thrombolytic therapy, which should begin as soon as possible after thrombosis. Bleeding complications are reduced significantly if patients are free of blood dyscrasias, fresh surgical wounds, and intracranial and GI disorders.
• When administering the thrombolytics, the nurse must assess the patient carefully for signs of bleeding and allergic reactions. Such complications as arrhythmias and peripheral circulation disturbances after intracoronary reperfusion also must be assessed closely. The nurse must be prepared to intervene quickly in hemorrhagic or arrhythmic complications and should keep appropriate emergency drugs and equipment available.
• If bleeding occurs, the nurse may have to stop the thrombolytic infusion and administer fresh whole blood, packed red cells, or fresh frozen plasma, as prescribed.
• Aminocaproic acid (Amicar) may be used as an antidote, although this use is not well documented.

STUDY QUESTIONS

See Appendix 1 for answers.

1. On admission to the emergency department, Everett Carson, age 52, reports severe, crushing, substernal chest pain that has lasted for 1 hour. An electrocardiogram reveals an acute inferior wall myocardial infarction (MI). Because the pain persists after Mr. Carson receives oxygen, I.V. nitroglycerin, and I.V. morphine, his physician prescribes streptokinase 140,000 units by intracoronary infusion. Before administering this thrombolytic agent, the nurse obtains a thorough history. Which condition contraindicates the use of thrombolytic agents?
(a) acute pulmonary thromboembolism
(b) history of previous MI
(c) cerebrovascular accident in the past 2 months
(d) age 60 or older

2. Why is streptokinase ordered for Mr. Carson?
(a) to dissolve already formed clots
(b) to decrease platelet aggregation
(c) to prevent further thrombus formation
(d) to suppress vitamin K-dependent clotting factors

3. During streptokinase therapy, the nurse assesses Mr. Carson for bleeding. How do thrombolytic agents cause this common adverse reaction?
(a) They deplete coagulation factors.
(b) They cause a systemic thrombolytic state.
(c) They form thrombi, causing thrombocytopenia.
(d) They displace oral anticoagulants from protein-binding sites.

4. The nurse should assess Mr. Carson for which other adverse reaction to streptokinase?
(a) dizziness
(b) drowsiness
(c) cardiac rupture
(d) allergic reaction

5. If Mr. Carson begins to bleed severely, the physician probably will prescribe which drug?
(a) protamine sulfate
(b) aminocaproic acid
(c) Factor VIII
(d) vitamin K

6. The physician has prescribed morphine for Mr. Carson's chest pain. Which administration route should be avoided for 24 hours after thrombolytic therapy?
(a) I.V.
(b) oral
(c) I.M.
(d) rectal

7. If Mr. Carson displays a fever during streptokinase therapy, which drug is the physician most likely to prescribe?
(a) aspirin
(b) dipyridamole
(c) aminocaproic acid
(d) acetaminophen

SELECTED REFERENCES

Anistreplase for acute coronary thrombosis. (1990). *Medical Letter on Drugs and Therapeutics, 32*(812), 15-16.

Drug facts and comparisons. (1991). St. Louis: Facts and Comparisons Division, J.B. Lippincott.

Marder, V., and Sherry, S. (1988). Thrombolytic therapy: Current status. *New England Journal of Medicine, 318*(23), 1512-1520.

Marder, V., and Sherry, S. (1988). Thrombolytic therapy: Current status. *New England Journal of Medicine, 318*(24), 1585-1594.

North American Nursing Diagnosis Association. (1990). *Taxonomy I - Revised, with official diagnostic categories.* St. Louis: NANDA.

Rodriguez, S., and Reed R. (1987). Thrombolytic therapy for MI. *AJN, 87*(5), 631-640.

Rodvold, K., Quandt, C., and Friedenberg, W. (1989). Thromboembolic disorders. In J. DiPiro, R. Talbert, et al. (Eds.), *Pharmacotherapy: A pathophysiologic approach.* New York: Elsevier.

Verstraete, M. (1989). Use of thrombolytic drugs in noncoronary disorders. *Drugs, 38*(5), 801-821.

U N I T

▽
9

DRUGS TO IMPROVE RESPIRATORY FUNCTION

Unit Nine discusses pharmacologic agents used to improve respiratory function, including methylxanthines, expectorants, antitussives, mucolytics, and decongestants. These drugs are used to relieve constricted airways, mucosal edema, cough, abnormally viscid secretions, and nasal congestion. Other agents that improve respiratory function include cromolyn sodium, an agent that prevents acute asthmatic attacks, and pirbuterol, a new aerosolized bronchodilator. (For information about these drugs, see *Cromolyn sodium,* page 652, and *Pirbuterol acetate,* page 654.)

RESPIRATORY FUNCTION

The respiratory system extends from the nose to the pulmonary capillaries. It oxygenates tissue, removes carbon dioxide, regulates acid-base balance, and provides defense against infection.

Glossary

Antitussive: agent that suppresses or inhibits cough.

Bronchoconstriction: narrowing of the bronchi, resulting in increased airway resistance and decreased airflow in conducting airways.

Bronchodilatation: state of relaxed bronchiolar smooth muscle cells, resulting in a widened lumen of the bronchi and bronchioles.

Bronchodilator: substance that relaxes the bronchioles.

Bronchorrhea: excessive secretions from the bronchial mucous membrane.

Bronchospasm: paroxysmal bronchoconstriction from smooth muscle constriction.

Cilia: minute, vibrating, hairlike projections attached to the free surface of cells.

Coryza: profuse discharge from the nasal mucosa.

Cough (tussis): sudden noisy expulsion of air from the lungs.

Decongestant: agent that reduces swelling of mucous membranes and relieves congestion.

Expectorant: agent that promotes the expulsion of respiratory secretions.

Goblet cells: unicellular mucous glands found especially in respiratory and gastrointestinal epithelium.

Inspissated: thickened or dried out; used to describe mucus.

Methylxanthine: drug classification that includes caffeine and theophylline, whose actions include central nervous system stimulation, smooth muscle relaxation, vasodilation, diuresis, and cardiac stimulation.

Minute ventilation: amount of air breathed in during a 1-minute period; can be calculated by multiplying the exhaled tidal volume by the respiratory rate; also called total ventilation.

Mucin: mucopolysaccharide or glycoprotein that is the chief constituent of mucus.

Mucociliary clearance mechanism: defense mechanism of the respiratory tract, consisting of ciliated epithelial cells and mucus secretions that trap debris and bacteria and facilitate their removal; also called mucociliary escalator mechanism.

Mucokinesis: movement of mucus in the respiratory tract.

Mucokinetic agent: drug that facilitates mucokinesis.

Mucolytic: having the ability to break down the composition of mucus.

Mucus: coating of the mucous membranes containing glandular secretions, various inorganic salts, desquamated cells, and leukocytes.

Respiratory insufficiency: impaired ability to oxygenate and remove carbon dioxide from the blood.

Rhinitis: inflammation of the nasal mucosa.

Vasoconstrictor: agent that constricts or narrows the lumen of blood vessels.

Viscid: sticky.

Cromolyn sodium

Cromolyn sodium was synthesized to enhance the bronchodilator properties of the chromone drug khellin. Structural modification of khellin yielded cromolyn, which lacks bronchodilator activity but prevents allergic bronchospasm.

Cromolyn sodium prevents the release of histamine and slow-reacting substances of anaphylaxis by stabilizing the mast cell membrane, thereby preventing further cell degranulation. This reduces the stimulus for bronchospasm and bronchoconstriction.

Cromolyn sodium is used primarily as prophylactic treatment of bronchial asthma. It is not useful, however, in treating acute asthmatic attacks or status asthmaticus.

Cromolyn sodium usually is tolerated well by patients, even with prolonged continuous therapy. Adverse reactions are infrequent and minor. The most frequently seen adverse reactions are bronchospasm, sneezing, wheezing, cough, nasal congestion, and pharyngeal irritation. Dizziness, dysuria, joint swelling, joint pain, nausea, headache, and skin rash also may occur.

Cromolyn sodium is given by inhalation because it is absorbed poorly after oral administration. The drug is not metabolized and is excreted unchanged, 50% in urine and 50% in bile.

Two of the commonly used forms of cromolyn sodium include a metered-dose aerosol inhaler and a turbo inhaler. The aerosol delivers a small dose in a fine white mist. The turbo inhaler delivers a larger dose of dry white powder. Clinical trials have shown both delivery systems to be of equal efficacy. The aerosol requires the patient to synchronize breathing with dose delivery. The turbo inhaler is less likely to be confused with the bronchodilators that are available and used for acute asthmatic attacks. The two types of devices are illustrated below.

When administering cromolyn sodium for bronchial asthma, monitor the patient's respiratory patterns and the integrity of the patient's nasal and oral passages before and after therapy. Also inform the patient that throat irritation and cough may be decreased by gargling or drinking after each treatment.

Metered-dose aerosol inhaler

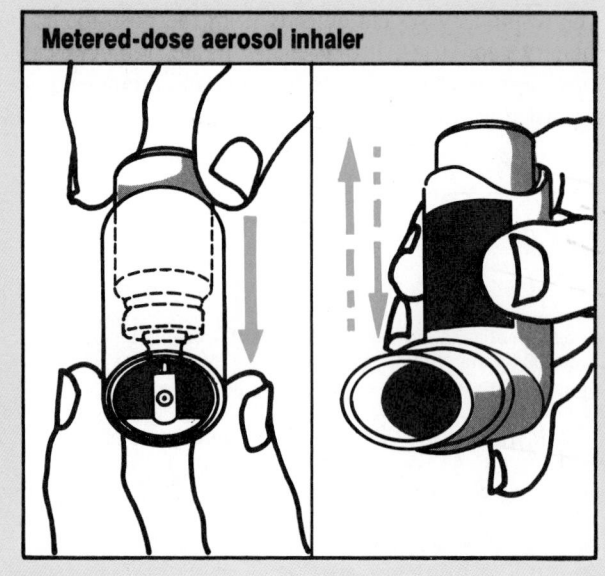

Turbo inhaler

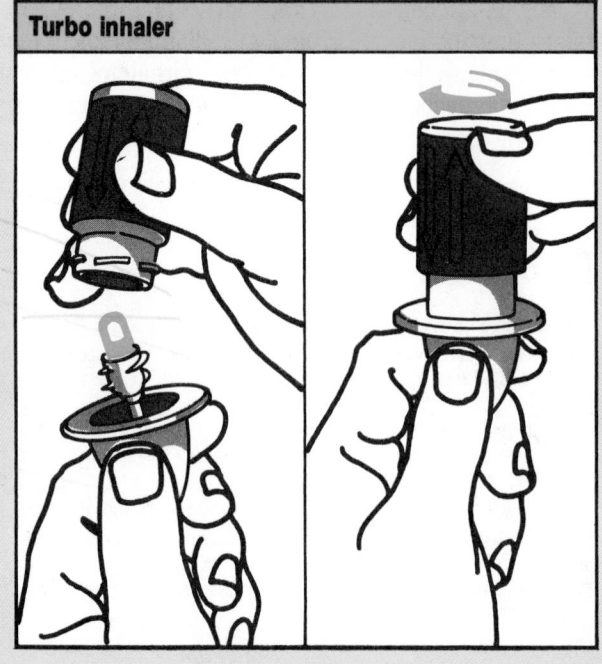

Oxygen-carbon dioxide exchange

Air flows into the lungs via the conducting airways (nose to bronchioles) and reaches the alveoli, where gas exchange occurs. Oxygen diffuses from the alveoli into the pulmonary capillaries, where most of the oxygen is bound to the hemoglobin in the red blood cells (RBCs). Only a small percentage is dissolved in the plasma. Then the RBCs are transported to all tissues, where oxygen is diffused from the blood into the cell to be used for cellular metabolism. Carbon dioxide, a by-product of cellular metabolism, is returned to the lungs to be eliminated. After diffusing from the blood into the alveoli, the carbon dioxide is exhaled from the lungs. (For an illustration of this process, see *Normal respiratory anatomy and physiology.*) Such conditions as mucosal edema, alveolar damage, bronchoconstriction, or a disrupted mucociliary clearance mechanism affect the integrity of the respiratory structures and can alter oxygen-carbon dioxide gas exchange.

Acid-base balance

The respiratory system is a major regulator of acid-base balance; the blood-buffer system and the kidneys are the other regulators. Normal arterial blood pH ranges from 7.35 to 7.45; blood pH can be lowered or raised by the

Normal respiratory anatomy and physiology

A knowledge of intrapulmonary blood circulation and gas exchange will help the nurse understand the actions of the drugs discussed in this unit. The respiratory system's major structures are illustrated below. The insert below right shows intrapulmonary blood circulation around the alveolus; the insert below left shows the partial pressures of the carbon dioxide and oxygen exchanged.

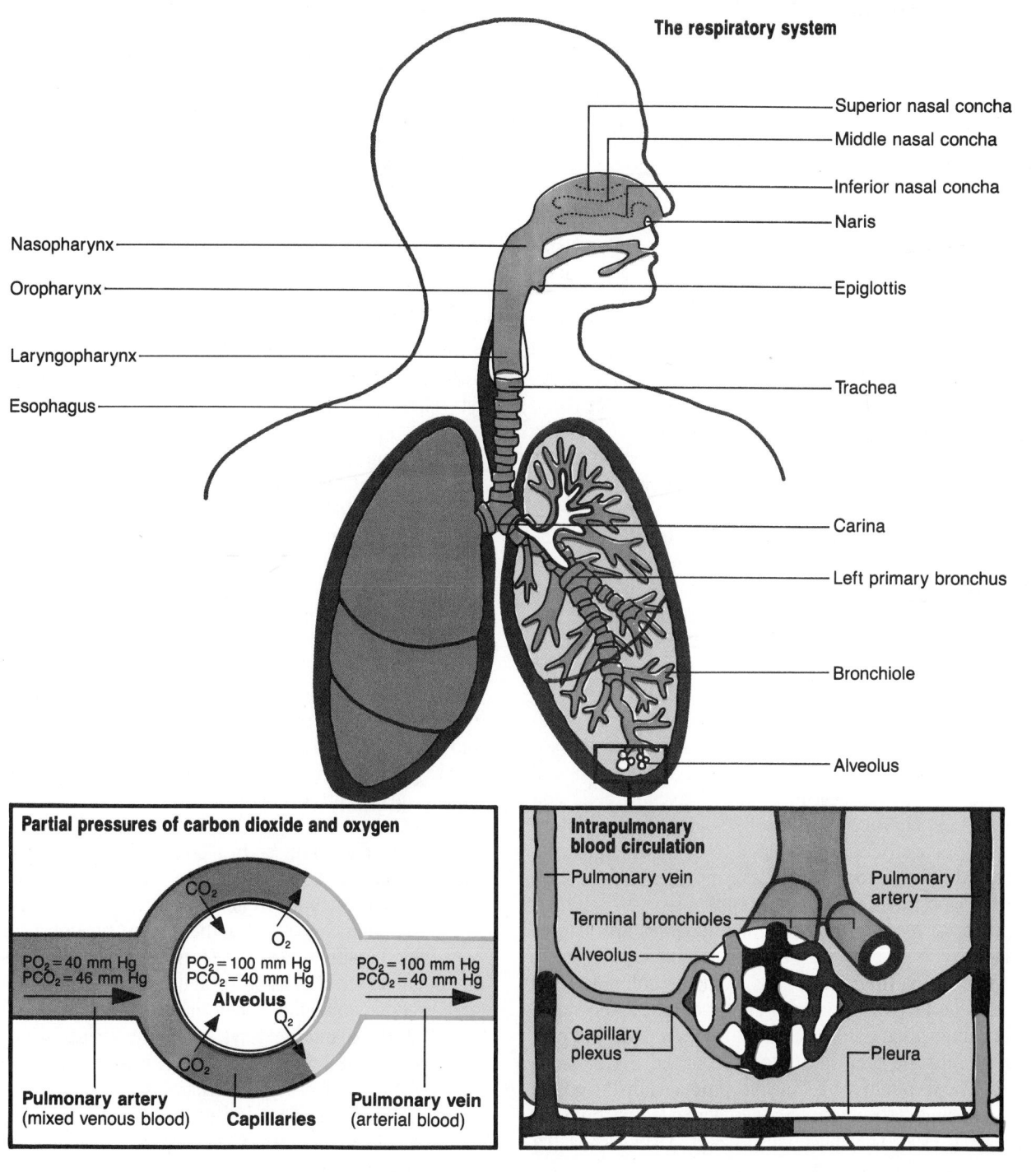

The respiratory system

- Superior nasal concha
- Middle nasal concha
- Inferior nasal concha
- Naris
- Epiglottis
- Trachea
- Carina
- Left primary bronchus
- Bronchiole
- Alveolus

Nasopharynx
Oropharynx
Laryngopharynx
Esophagus

Partial pressures of carbon dioxide and oxygen

CO_2
O_2
$PO_2 = 40$ mm Hg
$PCO_2 = 46$ mm Hg
$PO_2 = 100$ mm Hg
$PCO_2 = 40$ mm Hg
Alveolus
$PO_2 = 100$ mm Hg
$PCO_2 = 40$ mm Hg
O_2
CO_2

Pulmonary artery
(mixed venous blood)
Capillaries
Pulmonary vein
(arterial blood)

Intrapulmonary blood circulation
- Pulmonary vein
- Terminal bronchioles
- Alveolus
- Capillary plexus
- Pulmonary artery
- Pleura

Pirbuterol acetate

A new aerosolized bronchodilator, pirbuterol acetate (Maxair) acts as a beta$_2$-adrenergic receptor agonist. It is used to prevent and reverse bronchospasm in patients with reversible bronchospasm, including that caused by asthma. Pirbuterol may be used alone or with theophylline or steroid therapy.

For adults and children age 12 and older, the usual pirbuterol dosage is two inhalations (0.2 mg each), followed by one or two inhalations repeated every 4 to 6 hours. The patient may use a maximum of 12 inhalations daily. Adverse reactions to pirbuterol include nervousness, tremors, headache, palpitations, tachycardia, chest pain or tightness, nausea, diarrhea, and dry mouth.

retention or excretion of hydrogen ions and bicarbonate ions. Carbon dioxide and water combine in the presence of carbonic anhydrase (a catalyst) to form carbonic acid, as follows: $CO_2 + H_2O \rightleftharpoons H_2CO_3 \rightleftharpoons H + HCO_3$

This reaction, which is reversible, is affected by respiratory and renal function. In patients with compromised respiratory function, carbon dioxide retention increases hydrogen ion levels in the blood, thereby decreasing the blood pH; this state is known as respiratory acidosis. Similarly, carbon dioxide elimination by the respiratory system causes the blood to become more alkaline; this is known as respiratory alkalosis. The alterations in carbon dioxide levels are regulated by breathing frequency and the depth of the breaths, which is measured as minute ventilation. The respiratory system can restore normal arterial blood pH in minutes; however, dysfunction of the system can be the primary cause of an acid-base imbalance.

Defense mechanism

The nose filters, humidifies, and warms air during inhalation. It also traps particles in the mucosa to prevent their deposition lower in the respiratory tract. The mucosa and its secretions are influenced by the parasympathetic and sympathetic nervous systems. Sympathetic stimulation causes vasoconstriction of the nasal vascular structures and decreased mucus production. Parasympathetic stimulation has the opposite effect: It narrows the airway by vascular engorgement of mucosal tissues and increases mucus production.

Cilia are hairlike projections from the columnar epithelial cells that line the nasal and tracheal passageways. Ciliary undulations project respiratory secretions and particles toward the oropharynx to be coughed out or swallowed. The respiratory tract mucus, produced by the goblet cells, contains lysosomes and other elements that fight invading bacteria. The mucus also clears particles via the "mechanical" mucociliary escalator.

The cough is a protective mechanism that rapidly expels air and particles from the airways. The sneeze clears the nasal passageway. Should particles evade the mucociliary defense mechanism and reach the lower respiratory tract, alveolar macrophages can phagocytize and detoxify them.

OVERVIEW OF CHAPTERS

The chapters in Unit Nine present drugs that are used to improve respiratory function in disorders that range from emphysema and neonatal apnea to sinusitis and the common cold.

Chapter 38
Methylxanthine Agents

Chapter 38 explores the methylxanthine agents, including theophylline, its salts (aminophylline, oxtriphylline, and theophylline sodium glycinate), dyphylline, and caffeine. It describes their use in treating asthma, chronic bronchitis, emphysema, and neonatal apnea. It carefully details their dosages, which should be based on serum drug concentration, patient response, and the occurrence of adverse reactions. The chapter also compares the various methylxanthine preparations, routes, and uses. For example, the parenteral route is used to treat acute bronchoconstriction; the oral route, for long-term maintenance therapy. The chapter concludes with a discussion of nursing activities related to methylxanthine administration based on application of the nursing process.

Chapter 39
Expectorant, Antitussive, and Mucolytic Agents

This chapter begins by investigating expectorant agents, which purportedly facilitate removal of viscid mucus, although their efficacy is unknown. After explaining how expectorants may promote mucokinesis, the chapter explores the therapeutic uses of guaifenesin, the most widely used expectorant and an ingredient in many over-the-counter cough and cold preparations; the iodides, iodinated glycerol and potassium iodide; and terpin hydrate. It touches on combined expectorant and mucolytic therapy for patients with chronic respiratory diseases and associated mucus accumulation, such as bronchitis and emphysema. Then it focuses on nursing care for the patient receiving an expectorant, highlighting nursing process application and such nursing interventions as postural drainage, deep breathing, and effective coughing to help increase mucokinesis.

Next, the chapter features antitussive agents, which are used to suppress or inhibit coughing. It compares the pharmacokinetics and pharmacodynamics of the narcotic and nonnarcotic agents. Then it describes how these agents are used to help relieve an exhausting, dry, hacking cough, rather than a productive cough. It also details the drug interactions, adverse reactions, and nursing care related to antitussive administration.

Chapter 39 concludes with a discussion of acetylcysteine, the only mucolytic agent clinically available to treat patients with abnormally viscid, inspissated mucous secretions. The chapter describes acetylcysteine's use as a mucolytic and as a treatment for acetaminophen overdose. It also details application of the nursing process for a patient receiving this agent, highlighting patient teaching.

Chapter 40
Decongestant Agents

The focus of Chapter 40 is the sympathomimetic amines and local vasoconstrictors that are used to treat nasal congestion associated with colds or allergic rhinitis. The chapter discusses systemic and topical decongestants, which can be administered to improve nasal airway patency by shrinking the respiratory mucosa. It contrasts their duration of action, intensity of vasoconstriction, and potential for rebound congestion. For each type of decongestant, it also describes administration techniques, such as nasal drop instillation, and nursing process application related to decongestant therapy.

METHYLXANTHINE AGENTS

OBJECTIVES

After reading and studying this chapter, the student should be able to:

1. Identify the clinical indications for theophylline, its derivatives, and caffeine.

2. Describe the pharmacokinetic properties of the various methylxanthine agents, and explain their effects on drug administration.

3. Explain the actions of methylxanthine agents when they are used to treat asthma, chronic bronchitis, emphysema, and neonatal apnea.

4. Discuss the interactions associated with the methylxanthine agents and other drugs.

5. Describe the adverse reactions to methylxanthine therapy, including the signs and symptoms of methylxanthine toxicity.

6. Describe how to apply the nursing process when caring for a patient who is receiving a methylxanthine agent.

INTRODUCTION

The methylxanthine agents (also called xanthines) are used extensively to treat asthma, chronic bronchitis, emphysema, and neonatal apnea. Theophylline and its derivatives and caffeine are the agents used to treat these disorders. Theophylline also is used for its diuretic effect in treating congestive heart failure (CHF) and Cheyne-Stokes respiration; however, this chapter does not cover these uses. Chapter 38 focuses on the methylxanthine agents as they are used to treat respiratory diseases.

For a summary of representative drugs, see *Selected major drugs: Methylxanthine agents,* page 666. For a listing of applicable nursing diagnoses that the nurse may formulate when caring for a patient receiving these agents, see *Selected nursing diagnoses: Methylxanthine agents.* For detailed information on applying the nursing process, see Chapter 6, The Nursing Process and Drug Therapy.

SELECTED NURSING DIAGNOSES

Methylxanthine agents

The following nursing diagnoses address rpresentative problems and etiologies that a nurse may encounter when caring for a patient who is receiving a methylxanthine agent. Some of these nursing diagnoses contain generalized etiologies, which the nurse must individualize based on the patient's needs. (For some common nursing diagnoses and related interventions for each drug class, see the "Nursing Process Application" section of this chapter.)

- Altered cerebral tissue perfusion related to methylxanthine-induced hypotension
- Altered health maintenance related to ineffectiveness of the prescribed methylxanthine agent
- Altered protection related to methylxanthine-induced arrhythmias
- Anxiety related to the adverse central nervous system effects of the methylxanthine
- Altered renal tissue perfusion related to methylxanthine-induced hypotension
- Diarrhea related to the adverse GI effects of the methylxanthine agent
- Fluid volume deficit related to the adverse GI effects of the methylxanthine agent
- Knowledge deficit related to the prescribed methylxanthine agent
- Pain related to methylxanthine-induced headache
- Potential fluid volume deficit related to the adverse GI effects of the methylxanthine agent
- Potential for injury related to a preexisting condition that contraindicates the use of a methylxanthine agent
- Potential for injury related to a preexisting condition that requires cautious use of a methylxanthine agent
- Potential for injury related to adverse drug reactions
- Potential for injury related to drug interactions
- Potential for trauma related to seizures cause by a high serum concentration of the methylxanthine agent
- Sleep pattern disturbance related to methylxanthine-induced insomnia

THEOPHYLLINE, THEOPHYLLINE DERIVATIVES, AND CAFFEINE

The methylxanthine agents are used primarily to treat asthma, chronic bronchitis, emphysema, and neonatal apnea. The nurse should be aware, however, that some controversy exists regarding certain clinical uses for these agents, such as the use of beta$_2$-adrenergic agonists with theophyline to treat acute asthma. This chapter discusses the following methylxanthine agents: anhydrous theophylline, its salts (aminophylline, oxtriphylline, and theophylline sodium glycinate), dyphylline, and caffeine.

PHARMACOKINETICS

The methylxanthine agents vary pharmacokinetically according to the agent administered, its dosage form, and the administration route. The pharmacokinetic differences are particularly significant with the theophylline salts, developed to increase the solubility of theophylline, which is only slightly water-soluble. When administered orally or parenterally, the salts appear as theophylline in the blood. (For the amount of theophylline contained in each agent, see *Theophylline salts.*)

Dyphylline is freely water-soluble, and is not dissociated to theophylline in blood. Caffeine is more soluble than theophylline in water and lipids and, because caffeine is a weak base, its solubility can be increased in the presence of citric and benzoic acids.

Absorption

Theophylline's rate and extent of absorption depend on the dosage form administered. When theophylline is given as an oral solution, a rapid-release tablet, or a retention enema, it is absorbed rapidly and completely. However, rectal suppositories are absorbed erratically and are used less commonly. Absorption of some of the slow-release products (Theolair-SR and Theo-24) depends on gastric pH, which affects the dissolution rate and extent of absorption. Administering other slow-release products (Theo-Dur Sprinkle, Uniphyl) with meals can alter absorption significantly. Because of these factors, slow-release theophylline products should be administered with a small amount of food or when the patient's stomach is empty. Also, substituting one slow-release theophylline product for another is inadvisable, because their rate and extent of absorption may vary.

Dyphylline is absorbed incompletely after oral or I.M. administration and is about 75% bioavailable.

Theophylline salts

Theophylline is only slightly water-soluble. Its solubility can be increased by mixing it with other elements to form theophylline salts.

FORMULATION	THEOPHYLLINE CONTENT	EQUIVALENT DOSE FOR 100 MG THEOPHYLLINE
anhydrous theophylline (Slo-bid Gyrocaps, Theo-Dur, Theo-24)	100%	100 mg
aminophylline (Aminophyllin Injection, Somophyllin-DF Oral Liquid, Somophyllin Rectal Solution)	85%	118 mg
oxtriphylline (Brondecon, Choledyl)	64%	156 mg
theophylline sodium glycinate (Asbron G, Synophylate)	46%	217 mg

Caffeine is absorbed well after oral administration; however, rectal preparations may be absorbed slowly and erratically. Caffeine should not be given intramuscularly because of the irritating effect of the solution.

Distribution

The volume of distribution for theophylline ranges from 0.3 liter/kg to 0.7 liter/kg of body weight, averaging 0.5 liter/kg. These values remain relatively constant from infants to adults, even when other diseases are present. Theophylline is not distributed well into adipose tissue, so theophylline dosage should be based on the patient's ideal or actual body weight, whichever is less. Theophylline is approximately 60% protein bound in adults but only about 36% protein bound in the neonate. It readily crosses the placenta, producing similar serum concentrations in the mother and fetus. Theophylline also crosses into breast milk.

No information on dyphylline's distribution and protein-binding capacity is available.

Caffeine is distributed rapidly and widely. The volume of distribution is approximately 0.5 liter/kg in adults and 0.8 liter/kg in neonates. Less than 20% of a caffeine dose is protein bound in the plasma. Caffeine readily crosses the blood-brain barrier and the placenta, and small amounts appear in breast milk.

Metabolism and excretion

Theophylline is metabolized primarily in the liver. Because theophylline's metabolism rate varies greatly among patients, dosages need to be individualized and serum concentrations monitored. Liver disease, CHF, cor pulmonale, pulmonary edema, and prolonged high fever can decrease theophylline's metabolism and prolong half-life. Certain drugs also can increase or decrease theophylline's elimination. (For details, see *Drug interactions: Theophylline, theophylline derivatives, and caffeine,* page 663.) Also, smoking and high-protein diets increase the theophylline excretion rate, whereas high-carbohydrate diets decrease it. In children and adults, about 10% of a dose is excreted unchanged in the urine; in neonates and infants, as much as 50% of a dose may be excreted unchanged in the urine because the immature liver has limited metabolizing ability. The major metabolites also are excreted in the urine.

Dyphylline is not metabolized by the liver. Approximately 83% of a dose is excreted unchanged in the urine. Because dyphylline is not converted to theophylline, the nurse cannot use serum theophylline concentrations to monitor therapy. Dyphylline should not be used in neonates because information concerning such use is lacking.

Although caffeine can be a significant metabolite of theophylline in neonates, it is not a major metabolite in older infants or adults. Like theophylline, caffeine is metabolized extensively by the liver. In an adult, about 2% of a dose is excreted unchanged in the urine; in the neonate, however, about 85% of a dose is excreted this way.

Onset, peak, duration

Theophylline's onset and duration of action are related to the patient's serum theophylline concentration, which in turn depends on the drug's absorption and excretion rates. The excretion rate varies greatly from patient to patient. (For averages among different patient groups, see *Theophylline half-life.*) To treat respiratory disease, a serum concentration of 10 to 20 mcg/ml is considered therapeutic. To treat neonatal apnea, a serum concentration of 5 to 10 mcg/ml is required.

To achieve a therapeutic serum concentration of theophylline rapidly, a loading dose usually is administered as a rapid-release tablet or oral solutioin or an aminophylline I.V. injection. Using these preparations and administration routes produces theophylline's onset within 1 hour. Subsequently, a maintenance dose is started to keep theophylline's serum concentration within the therapeutic range. If no loading dose is administered, the maximum benefit from theophylline therapy occurs when the amount of drug excreted and the amount of drug absorbed is the same

---

Theophylline half-life

The half-life of theophylline can vary greatly from patient to patient. Therefore, serum theophylline concentrations should be monitored to provide useful clinical information for proper dosage and patient monitoring.

PATIENT POPULATION	AVERAGE HALF-LIFE*
Neonates	20 to 30 hours
Children ages 1 to 12	3 to 4 hours
Nonsmoking adults	7 to 8 hours
Nonsmoking elderly adults	9 to 10 hours
Smoking adults	4 to 5 hours

*In patients without diseases that can alter theophylline pharmacokinetics.

(steady state). For example, the average half-life of theophylline administered to a child age 2 is 4 hours. Steady state occurs after the patient has begun maintenance therapy and five half-lives have passed—that is, in 20 hours (5 × 4 hours) or approximately 1 day. After this point, serum concentrations are similar when drawn at the same time after each dose.

The nurse should monitor peak serum concentrations because they correlate with peak effectiveness and drug toxicity. (See "Adverse drug reactions" on page 664.) When an oral rapid-release tablet or solution is administered, peak concentrations are achieved about 1 to 2 hours after a dose. (For more information, see *Maintaining serum theophylline concentration levels.*) As theophylline concentrations decrease to below the therapeutic range, the drug effects also decrease. Duration of action is influenced by the half-life of the product used. In general, the half-life averages 3.5 hours for young children and 8 to 9 hours for adults.

Dyphylline's half-life is 2 to 2.5 hours. In anuric patients, the half-life may increase to 3 to 4 times the normal range. After oral or I.M. administration, peak serum concentrations occur in about 1 hour. Dyphylline's onset and duration remain unknown because therapeutic serum concentrations have not been determined.

Caffeine's onset usually occurs within 30 minutes after administration and peak concentrations within 1 to 2 hours. Caffeine's duration depends on the patient's serum concentration. In treating neonatal apnea, serum caffeine concentrations of 5 to 20 mcg/ml are considered therapeutic. Caffeine's half-life in neonates ranges from 31 to 144 hours, averaging more than 60 hours. The half-life decreases with age, averaging 3 to 6 hours in adults.

Maintaining serum theophylline concentration levels

This chart provides suggested theophylline dosage changes for maintaining a peak serum concentration when drawn with the patient at a steady-state level. To ensure the patient is at a steady-state level, theophylline doses should be administered at regular intervals, with no doses missed for 48 to 72 hours.

CONCENTRATION	SUGGESTED DOSAGE CHANGES
< 7.5 mcg/ml	Increase daily dosage by up to 25%; recheck serum concentrations during steady state before further dosage changes.
7.5 to 10 mcg/ml	Increase daily dosage by up to 25%; recheck serum concentrations within at least 6 months.
10 to 20 mcg/ml	No dosage change; if patient is on long-term oral treatment, recheck serum concentrations every 6 to 12 months or if adverse reactions to theophylline occur; if steady-state concentrations are in the upper therapeutic range, a 10% dosage decrease may be ordered if adverse reactions occur.
20 to 25 mcg/ml	Decrease the daily dosage by 10%, as ordered, even if no adverse reactions occur; recheck serum theophylline concentrations within at least 6 months.
25 to 30 mcg/ml	Omit the next dose and decrease daily dosage by 25%, as prescribed; recheck serum theophylline levels during steady state.
> 30 mcg/ml	Omit the next two doses and decrease the dosage by 50%, as prescribed; recheck serum theophylline concentrations during steady state.

Adapted with permission from Weinberger, M. (March 31, 1983). Slow-release theophylline rationale and basis for product selection. *New England Journal of Medicine,* 308(13), 760-764.

PHARMACODYNAMICS

The methylxanthine agents display similar pharmacologic activity but may differ in the intensity of their effects on the target organs.

Because most methylxanthine agents are powerful central nervous system (CNS) stimulants, they decrease drowsiness and fatigue and stimulate more rapid thinking. These agents also increase awareness of sensory stimuli and decrease reaction time. In the medulla, these agents stimulate the respiratory center; in the spinal cord, they increase reflex excitability. After CNS excitation by methylxanthine agents, the patient usually experiences a slight depression.

The methylxanthine agents also act on the cardiovascular system, directly stimulating the myocardium and increasing myocardial contractility. By directly relaxing vascular smooth muscle, these agents dilate coronary, pulmonary, and systemic blood vessels. They also strengthen skeletal muscle contractions and reduce muscle fatigability. Methylxanthine agents also cause diuresis, partly the result of improved cardiac function, from increased renal blood flow and glomerular filtration rate. These agents appear to have a direct action at the renal tubules, increasing sodium and chloride excretion.

Of all the methylxanthine agents, theophylline provides potent cardiac stimulation, smooth muscle relaxation, and diuresis. Caffeine provides the most potent CNS and skeletal muscle stimulation.

Methylxanthine agents stimulate gastric acid secretion; this may explain, in part, the adverse gastrointestinal (GI) reactions they can cause.

Mechanism of action

Although methylxanthine agents decrease nonspecific airway reactivity and, in the presence of bronchospasm, relax bronchial smooth muscle, their specific mechanism of action in reversible obstructive airway disease, such as asthma, is understood incompletely. Researchers believe that these agents inhibit the enzyme phosphodiesterase, causing decreased degradation of adenosine 3′,5′ monophosphate (cyclic AMP), an apparent bronchodilator. However, theophylline inhibits this enzyme at in vitro concentrations considerably higher than are considered clinically safe. Thus, this enzyme-inhibiting action does not account for the actions of these agents. A more likely explanation for the action of the methylxanthine agents is the inhibition of adenosine receptors. Other proposed mechanisms of action include the antagonism of prostaglandins as well as the intracellular translocation of ionized calcium, which causes myocardial stimulation and CNS excitation.

In nonreversible obstructive airway disease (chronic bronchitis, emphysema, and apnea), the methylxanthine agents appear to increase the central respiratory center's sensitivity to carbon dioxide and stimulate the respiratory drive. In chronic bronchitis and emphysema, these agents decrease diaphragmatic fatigue and improve cardiac ventricular function.

PHARMACOTHERAPEUTICS

Theophylline, its salts (aminophylline, oxtriphylline, and theophylline sodium glycinate), and dyphylline are indicated to treat asthma, chronic bronchitis, and emphysema. Caffeine is used primarily as a CNS stimulant and may be found in many over-the-counter preparations, prescription antihistamines, and barbiturates (to offset the sedative effects of these drugs), and with ergot alkaloids to produce cerebrovascular constriction in treating migraine headaches. Theophylline and caffeine also are used to treat neonatal apnea, although their use for this condition is unapproved by the Food and Drug Administration.

Theophylline acts as a bronchodilator, assists in ventricular emptying, decreases diaphragmatic fatigue, and increases mucociliary clearance. Theophylline relieves the bronchospasm associated with asthma better than dyphylline does. On a milligram-for-milligram basis, theophylline appears to have about 5 to 10 times the potency of dyphylline; however, it also causes more adverse reactions. Concomitant use of beta$_2$-adrenergic stimulants, such as albuterol, terbutaline, and metaproterenol, with theophylline or dyphylline produces additive bronchodilation in patients with chronic stable asthma but is controversial as therapy for patients with acute asthma. Beta$_2$-adrenergic stimulants relieve acute bronchospasm better than theophylline does. Combined use of these drugs to treat acute asthma is still common, although it does not appear to produce additive effects.

Treating chronic bronchitis and emphysema with theophylline or dyphylline also is controversial because bronchospasm is not a major component of these diseases: thus, the methylxanthine agents' activity is related to their effects on nonspecific airway reactivity, the diaphragm, ventricular function, and mucus clearance. To date, theophylline has produced subjective improvements—for example, the patient claims to feel less breathless—but researchers have not substantiated them objectively. Anticholinergic agents (atropine and ipratropium), beta$_2$-adrenergics, and theophylline are used to provide symptomatic relief for patients with chronic bronchitis and emphysema.

In patients with neonatal apnea (with or without bradycardia), theophylline and caffeine are equally effective. Theophylline is more readily available, but caffeine has a longer half-life, making a once-daily dosage possible. Caffeine also may have a wider therapeutic index.

anhydrous theophylline (Slo-bid Gyrocaps, Theo-24, Theo-Dur). Available in various oral formulations, anhydrous theophylline is used to treat asthma, chronic bronchitis, and emphysema. Therapy should be guided by monitoring serum theophylline concentrations, patient response, and the occurrence of adverse reactions.
Usual adult dosage: for asthma, chronic bronchitis, and emphysema, dosage varies and is calculated based on actual or ideal body weight, whichever is less. Usually the initial maximum dosage for adults is 13 mg/kg/day or a total of 800 mg/day, whichever is less. (For suggested amounts, see *Long-term oral theophylline dosages.*) For instituting oral therapy after administering I.V. aminophylline, the total

Long-term oral theophylline dosages

The theophylline dose is based on ideal body weight or actual body weight, whichever is less. (Actual weight up to 25% over ideal weight also is safe.) To determine the effects of a particular dosage on serum concentration, obtain peak concentration levels after no doses have been missed for 48 to 72 hours.

When changing dosages based on serum concentrations, divide the daily dose into an appropriate dosage interval for the product used. For patients age 1 or older, start at 16 mg/kg/day or a maximum of 400 mg/day, whichever is less. After 3 days with no adverse reactions, increase to 20 mg/kg/day for ages 1 to 9 and 16 mg/kg/day for ages 9 and older, but no more than 600 mg/day. The dosage should not exceed 800 mg/day without serum theophylline concentration monitoring. After an additional 3 days without adverse reactions, increase the dosage to the following:

AGE	DOSAGE
1 to 9 years	22 mg/kg/day
9 to 12 years	20 mg/kg/day
12 to 16 years	18 mg/kg/day
16 years and older	13 mg/kg/day

Adapted with permission from Weinberger, M. (March 31, 1983). Slow-release theophylline rationale and basis for product selection. *New England Journal of Medicine, 308*(13), 760-764.

daily dosage of oral theophylline should equal the aminophylline hourly infusion rate multiplied by 24 hours × 0.8 (aminophylline is 85% theophylline). When switching a patient from I.V. to oral therapy, the I.V. administration should be discontinued when the oral administration begins. (For suggested intervals for different preparations, see *Dosage intervals for theophylline.*)
Usual pediatric dosage: for neonatal apnea, the therapeutic serum concentration is 5 to 10 mcg/ml; loading dose, 5 mg/kg P.O. or I.V. (if I.V., administer over 20 to 30 minutes); maintenance dosage, 2 mg/kg every 12 hours; final dosage is determined by serum theophylline concentrations and patient response.

aminophylline (Aminophyllin, Somophyllin). Available in an oral solution, a rectal solution, an injectable solution, tablets, and suppositories, aminophylline is used to treat asthma, chronic bronchitis, and emphysema. Dosage should be based on the theophylline content of the preparation as well as the serum theophylline concentration, patient response, and occurrence of adverse reactions.
Usual adult dosage: a loading dose may be given first. If the patient has received no aminophylline or theophylline

Dosage intervals for theophylline

Each type of theophylline product has its own recommended dosage interval that should be maintained to ensure optimal efficacy. If the theophylline dosage for a 24-hour period is divided by the prescribed dosage interval, the dose can be determined.

DRUG	PATIENT POPULATION	
	Children and smoking adults	Nonsmoking adolescents and adults
Anhydrous theophylline		
Slow-release tablets		
Constant-T	q 8 hr	q 12 hr
LABID	q 8 hr	q 12 hr
Quibron-T/SR	q 8 hr	q 12 hr
*Respbid	q 8 hr	q 12 hr
Sustaire	q 12 hr	q 12 hr
Theo-Dur	q 12 hr	q 12 to 24 hr
*Theolair-SR	q 8 hr	q 12 hr
*Uniphyl	–	q 12 to 24 hr
Slow-release capsules		
Bronkodyl S-R	q 8 hr	q 12 hr
Elixophyllin SR	q 8 hr	q 12 hr
Slo-bid Gyrocaps	q 12 hr	q 12 hr
Slo-Phyllin Gyrocaps	q 8 hr	q 12 hr
Somophyllin-CRT	q 8 hr	q 12 hr
*Theo-24	–	q 12 to 24 hr
Theobid Duracaps	q 8 hr	q 12 hr
Theoclear L.A.	q 8 hr	q 12 hr
*Theo-Dur Sprinkle	q 12 hr	q 12 hr

DRUG	PATIENT POPULATION	
	Children and smoking adults	Nonsmoking adolescents and adults
Slow-release capsules (continued)		
Theophyl-SR	q 8 hr	q 12 hr
Theospan-SR	q 8 hr	q 12 hr
Theovent	q 8 hr	q 12 hr
Rapid-release oral liquids, tablets		
regardless of brand used	q 6 hr	q 6 to 8 hr
Aminophylline		
Rapid-release oral tablets, liquids, or rectal solutions		
regardless of brand used	q 6 hr	q 6 to 8 hr
Slow-release tablets		
Phyllocontin	q 8 hr	q 12 hr
Oxtriphylline		
Rapid-release tablet or liquids		
Choledyl	q 6 hr	q 6 to 8 hr
Slow-release tablets		
Choledyl SA	q 8 hr	q 12 hr
Theophylline sodium glycinate		
Rapid-release liquid		
Synophylate	q 6 hr	q 6 to 8 hr

*The rate and extent of absorption can be significantly affected when theophylline is given with food.

in the previous 24 hours, the loading dose is 5 to 6 mg/kg I.V. over 20 to 30 minutes to avoid cardiac toxicity. If the patient has received aminophylline or theophylline in the previous 24 hours, the serum theophylline concentration should be determined before giving any additional aminophylline. This serum concentration serves as the basis for calculating the loading dose. If the serum theophylline concentration cannot be determined quickly, some physicians elect to give half the normal loading dose, or 2.5 to 3 mg/kg. After the loading dose, a maintenance dosage of 0.4 to 0.7 mg/kg/hr is administered I.V. or the patient is switched to the oral dosage form.

Intravenous aminophylline should be given as a constant infusion via an infusion pump. If the patient has been on oral theophylline long-term in therapeutic dosages, the hourly infusion rate can be determined by dividing the daily dose by 24 hours. For example, a patient who has been receiving 600 mg/day of oral theophylline should be given an aminophylline infusion of 31 mg/hr (600 mg ÷ 24 hr = 25 mg/hr ÷ 0.8 = 31 mg/hr of aminophylline). For oral administration, calculate the daily maintenance dosage of oral theophylline and divide by 0.8. (For adult and pediatric dosage schedules, see *Long-term oral theophylline dosages,* page 660; *Dosage intervals for theophylline,* page 661; and *Guidelines for suggested theophylline dosage for infants.*) Some aminophylline products state the amount of theophylline in each dosage unit.

Rectal administration of theophylline may be accomplished using aminophylline rectal solutions; however, because of erratic and incomplete absorption, rectal suppositories are not recommended. Retention enemas have limited patient acceptability because of the retention volume required. Dosages and dosage intervals are the same as those for rapid-release oral theophylline products.

oxtriphylline (Brondecon, Choledyl). This agent is used to treat asthma, chronic bronchitis, emphysema, and similar chronic obstructive pulmonary diseases. To calculate the oxtriphylline dosage, divide the anhydrous theophylline dose by 0.64 because oxtriphylline is about 64% anhydrous theophylline. The specific dosage is based on the serum theophylline concentration, patient response, and occurrence of adverse reactions.
Usual adult dosage: 200 mg P.O. every 6 to 8 hours.
Usual pediatric dosage: for ages 2 to 12, 3.7 mg/kg P.O. every 6 hours. (For appropriate dosage intervals for the product used, see *Dosage intervals for theophylline,* page 661.)

theophylline sodium glycinate (Asbron G, Synophylate). This theophylline salt, containing approximately 46% the-ophylline, is used to treat asthma, chronic bronchitis, and emphysema.
Usual adult dosage: 330 to 600 mg P.O. every 6 to 8 hours.
Usual pediatric dosage: for ages 6 to 12, 220 to 330 mg P.O. every 6 to 8 hours; for ages 3 to 6, 110 to 165 mg P.O. every 6 to 8 hours; for ages 1 to 3, 55 to 110 mg P.O. every 6 to 8 hours.

dyphylline (Dylline, Lufyllin). Dyphylline is used to treat acute and chronic bronchial asthma and reversible bronchospasms associated with chronic bronchitis and emphysema.
Usual adult dosage: up to 15 mg/kg P.O. every 6 hours, or 250 to 500 mg I.M. up to a maximum of 15 mg/kg every 6 hours.
Usual pediatric dosage: 4.4 to 6.6 mg/kg/day in divided doses.

caffeine. Physicians usually prescribe caffeine as caffeine citrate, which contains a 50% caffeine base. This preparation must be compounded extemporaneously, because it is unavailable commercially. The I.V. caffeine and sodium benzoate solution available commercially should not be used in neonates, because the benzoate will displace bound bilirubin.
Usual pediatric dosage: in neonatal apnea, a loading dose of 10 mg/kg P.O. of caffeine base, followed by a maintenance dosage of 2.5 mg/kg/day P.O. of caffeine base started 24 hours after the loading dose.

Drug interactions

Some interactions that can occur between theophylline or its salts and food or other drugs can produce dangerously elevated or subtherapeutic drug levels and subsequent loss of effectiveness. (For a summary of interactions, see *Drug interactions: Theophylline, theophylline derivatives, and caffeine.*)

Smoking cigarettes or marijuana also increases theophylline elimination, thereby decreasing serum drug concentrations. Taking some theophylline products near mealtimes can decrease their rate and extent of absorption. As discussed previously, diet also can affect the rate of theophylline excretion from the body.

Probenecid inhibits renal excretion of dyphylline, increasing its half-life and prolonging its action. Drugs that alter theophylline's metabolism and excretion do not affect dyphylline; however, drugs that affect theophylline's excretion also may affect caffeine's excretion. Concomitant administration of adrenergic stimulants or consumption of caffeinated beverages may result in additive adverse reactions or signs and symptoms of methylxanthine toxicity.

Guidelines for suggested theophylline dosage for infants

Because the theophylline half-life is longer in infants compared with older children and adults, theophylline dosage must be conservative. Guidelines suggest theophylline be given 1 to 3 mg/kg every 6 to 12 hours as listed below.

INFANT (UP TO AGE 6 MONTHS)	MAINTENANCE DOSAGE
Preterm (younger than 40 weeks postconception)	1 mg/kg every 12 hours
Term (birth or 40 weeks postconception) Up to 4 weeks postnatal	1 to 2 mg/kg every 12 hours
Ages 4 to 8 weeks	1 to 2 mg/kg every 8 hours
Ages 8 weeks and older	1 to 3 mg/kg every 6 hours

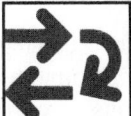

DRUG INTERACTIONS

Theophylline, theophylline derivatives, and caffeine

In many cases, interactions between theophylline and other drugs increase the risk of toxicity or subtherapeutic levels.

DRUG	INTERACTING DRUGS	POSSIBLE EFFECTS	NURSING IMPLICATIONS
anhydrous the-ophylline, amino-phylline, oxtriphyl-line, theophylline sodium glycinate	cimetidine	Increases the theophylline concentration level by inhibit-ing theophylline's rate of me-tabolism, resulting in a potentially toxic concentration	• Avoid concomitant cimetidine administration. If an H_2-antagonist is desired, ranitidine or famotidine can be used instead, because they do not alter theoph-ylline's metabolism significantly.
	erythromycin	Increases the theophylline concentration by altering theophylline's rate of metab-olism	• Decrease the theophylline dosage by 25%, as pre-scribed, if administered concomitantly, and monitor the patient for adverse reactions to theophylline.
	troleandomycin	Increases the theophylline concentration by altering the-ophylline's rate of metabolism	• Avoid concomitant administration with theophylline.
	allopurinol (high dose), disulfiram, thia-bendazole	Increase the theophylline concentration, probably by altering theophylline's rate of metabolism	• Observe the patient for signs and symptoms of theophylline toxicity, such as palpitations and rest-lessness.
	oral contraceptives	May increase the serum theophylline concentration, probably by inhibiting the cytochrome P-450 system	• Encourage the patient to use an alternative contra-ceptive method, if possible. • Monitor the theophylline concentration closely when adding or deleting oral contraceptives from the regimen.
	beta-adrenergic block-ing agents	Increase the theophylline con-centration by altering the drug's rate of metabolism, and antagonize theophylline bron-chodilating effect	• Avoid concomitant administration with theophylline. • Use a cardioselective agent, if a beta-adrenergic blocker is required.
	phenobarbital, phenyt-oin, rifampin, carba-mazepine	Decrease the serum theoph-ylline concentration probably by increasing theophylline's rate of metabolism	• Monitor the serum theophylline concentration and expect to adjust the theophylline dosage.
	halothane, enflurane, isoflurane, methoxyflu-rane	Increase the risk of cardiac toxicity	• Administer concomitantly with extreme caution.
	lithium	Increase lithium clearance	• Monitor the serum lithium concentration and ex-pect to adjust the lithium dosage.
	thyroid hormones, an-tithyroid agents	Increase or decrease the-ophylline metabolism	• Assess for signs and symptoms of theophylline toxicity or ineffectiveness. • Monitor the theophylline concentration closely if initiat-ing thyroid or antithyroid therapy. • Know that hyperthyroidism increases theophylline metabolism and hypothyroidism decreases theoph-ylline metabolism. Correction of either condition may affect the serum theophylline concentration in a pa-tient whose theophylline dosage previously had been stabilized.
	ciprofloxacin, norfloxa-cin	Increase the serum theophyl-line concentration by inhibiting theophylline's rate of metabo-lism, resulting in a potentially toxic concentration	• Administer concomitantly with caution. • Observe the patient for signs and symptoms of theophylline toxicity, such as palpitations and rest-lessness. • Monitor the serum theophylline concentration and expect to adjust the theophylline dosage.

ADVERSE DRUG REACTIONS

The adverse reactions to the methylxanthine agents can be transient or symptomatic of toxicity. These reactions commonly affect the central nervous, cardiac, and GI systems.

Administering methylxanthine agents, particularly theophylline, first may produce toxicity and other adverse reactions rather than therapeutic effects. These transient adverse reactions can occur (1) when a patient who has not taken the drug previously begins methylxanthine therapy; (2) when a patient who has taken the drug previously, but not recently, restarts the therapy; or (3) when the dosage is increased for a patient who already is taking the drug and is experiencing a change in health or altered dietary intake. These adverse reactions, which usually occur shortly after administration of the first dose, can affect the GI tract and CNS. GI tract irritation and increased gastric acid secretion may cause nausea, vomiting, abdominal cramping, epigastric pain, anorexia, or diarrhea. Adverse CNS reactions include headache, irritability, restlessness, anxiety, insomnia, and dizziness (rarely).

Methylxanthine agents also can produce adverse reactions when a dose results in a high serum concentration. (For theophylline and caffeine, this concentration usually is above 20 mcg/ml.) After administration of a rapid-release product, such adverse reactions can occur within 1 to 2 hours; after an I.V. loading dose, they can occur shortly after the infusion is completed, usually within 1 hour. With slow-release theophylline preparations, adverse reactions can occur 3 to 8 hours after administration. The adverse reactions that may occur include nausea, vomiting, diarrhea, and such CNS symptoms as irritability, insomnia, anxiety, headache, and seizures (with very high serum concentrations).

Although theophylline crosses into breast milk, its use (except for oxtriphylline) is not contraindicated in a lactating patient. The nurse, however, should be aware that the neonate may experience tachycardia or vomiting. Monitoring the neonate for these adverse reactions is important. Methylxanthine agents also can irritate the myocardium, producing such cardiovascular symptoms as tachycardia, palpitations, extrasystoles, or arrhythmias. Also, these drugs can cause peripheral vasodilation and hypotension.

Although hypersensitivity reactions to methylxanthine agents can occur, they are extremely rare and typically are associated with the base of the theophylline salt formulations. For example, the ethylenediamine component of aminophylline can produce a type of contact dermatitis. Some patients may not tolerate methylxanthine agents very well; usually less than 1% of children and 4% of adults receiving theophylline will develop these severe reactions. These hypersensitivity reactions can occur even with a dosage too low to achieve a therapeutic effect. Shortly after receiving the drug, the patient may display severe signs and symptoms of theophylline toxicity, which may include nausea, vomiting, diarrhea, headache, and occasionally anxiety and dizziness. This indicates intolerance.

NURSING PROCESS APPLICATION

The following information assists the nurse in caring for a patient who is receiving a methylxanthine agent.

Assessment
• Review the patient's history for a preexisting condition that contraindicates the use of a methylxanthine agent, such as known hypersensitivity to these agents.
• Review the patient's history for a preexisting condition that requires cautious use of a methylxanthine agent, such as severe cardiac disease, hypertension, acute myocardial injury, peptic ulcer disease, or pregnancy.
• Assess the patient for adverse reactions to the prescribed methylxanthine agent, such as CNS, cardiac, or GI dysfunction.
• Determine the patient's hydration status during methylxanthine therapy.
• Review the patient's medication history to identify the use of drugs that may interact with the prescribed methylxanthine agent, such as cimetidine, erythromycin, troleandomycin, oral contraceptives, or phenobarbital.
• Assess the effectiveness of the prescribed methylxanthine agent periodically.
• Assess the patient regularly for insomnia.
• Evaluate the patient's and family's knowledge about the prescribed methylxanthine agent.

Nursing diagnoses
The following examples represent appropriate nursing diagnoses for a patient receiving a methylxanthine agent.
• Potential for injury related to a preexisting condition that contraindicates the use of a methylxanthine agent
• Potential for injury related to a preexisting condition that requires cautious use of a methylxanthine agent
• Potential for injury related to adverse drug reactions
• Fluid volume deficit related to the adverse GI effects of the methylxanthine agent
• Potential for injury related to drug interactions
• Altered health maintenance related to ineffectiveness of the prescribed methylxanthine agent
• Sleep pattern disturbance related to methylxanthine-induced insomnia
• Knowledge deficit related to the prescribed methylxanthine agent

Planning and implementation

• Do not administer a methylxanthine agent to a patient with a condition that contraindicates its use.

• Administer a methylxanthine agent with caution to a patient at risk because of a preexisting condition.

• *Monitor the patient closely for adverse CNS, cardiac, or GI reactions during methylxanthine therapy, especially when the serum theophylline or caffeine concentration exceeds 20 mcg/ml, when therapy is initiated or restarted, or when the dosage is changed.*

• Withhold the drug and ask the physician about a dosage alteration, if adverse reactions occur.

• Monitor the patient's serum theophylline concentration when theophylline products are used or the serum caffeine concentration when caffeine products are used. When theophylline is administered to a neonate, monitor theophylline and caffeine serum concentrations because theophylline is metabolized to caffeine in the neonate.

• *Do not use the serum theophylline concentration to monitor dyphylline therapy because dyphylline is not metabolized to theophylline in vivo.*

• Use the peak serum concentration to monitor therapy with oral methylxanthine preparations. The peak concentration of rapid-release products occurs 1 to 2 hours after administration; of slow-release products, about 4 hours after administration. If no adverse reactions occur, measure the peak serum concentration when the steady-state level has been reached. Reaching the steady-state level requires that the patient receive the drug at regular intervals for 48 to 72 hours.

• *Consult the physician before repeating a dose of an oral methylxanthine preparation, if vomiting occurs shortly after administration. If the patient misses a dose, do not increase or double subsequent doses without first consulting the physician.*

• Obtain a prescription for an analgesic if the patient experiences a methylxanthine-induced headache.

• *Take seizure precautions if the serum theophylline or caffeine concentration becomes very high.*

• *Monitor the patient's blood pressure for hypotension and pulse for changes in the rate or pattern.*

• *Monitor the patient's electrocardiogram, as ordered, to detect arrhythmias.*

• Mix the loading dose for I.V. aminophylline in 5% dextrose or normal saline solution. Administer this dose over 20 to 30 minutes.

• Administer the I.V. maintenance dosage by constant infusion, using an infusion pump. Use a standard concentration, and do not vary the volume administered unless the patient is volume-restricted.

• *Change a patient from I.V. to oral theophylline or dyphylline by stopping the infusion when starting the oral drug as prescribed.*

• *Do not administer the I.V. caffeine and sodium benzoate solution to a neonate, because benzoate displaces bound bilirubin.*

• *Do not administer a rectal methylxanthine solution or suppository if rectal irritation or infection is present.*

• Encourage the patient receiving a theophylline enema or rectal solution to retain it as long as possible.

• Administer a methylxanthine oral preparation with a full glass of water and on an empty stomach or with only a small amount of food. Bead-filled capsules may be taken apart and their contents scattered on small amounts of soft food for administration to a patient who cannof swallow tablets. Slow-release products should not be chewed or crushed.

• *Administer a dyphylline injection by the I.M. route only.*

• Notify the physician if adverse reactions occur or if the methylxanthine agent is ineffective.

• Assess the patient with adverse GI reactions for signs of fluid volume deficit, such as poor skin turgor, dry mucous membranes, and increased urine concentration with decreased volume.

• Request a prescription for an antiemetic or antidiarrheal agent, as needed.

• Monitor the patient's serum drug concentration and observe for toxic drug interactions when theophylline is administered with such drugs as cimetidine or erythromycin.

• *Observe the patient for signs and symptoms of theophylline toxicity, such as palpitations and restlessness.*

• *Monitor the patient's serum theophylline or caffeine concentration, as instructed, to assess the effectiveness of therapy. For a patient with asthma, emphysema, or chronic bronchitis, the therapeutic serum theophylline concentration ranges from 10 to 20 mcg/ml; for neonatal apnea, from 5 to 10 mcg/ml. The therapeutic serum caffeine concentration ranges from 5 to 20 mcg/ml.*

• Encourage the patient with methylxanthine-induced insomnia to try relaxation techniques, such as taking a warm bath before bed, reading, or listening to soothing music.

• Notify the physician if insomnia persists and discuss measures that may relieve it, such as a dosage adjustment or change in administration time.

Patient teaching

• Teach the patient and family the name, dose, frequency, action, and adverse effects of the prescribed methylxanthine agent.

• *Stress the importance of returning for drug level testing, as prescribed, to detect toxicity or drug ineffectiveness (except with dyphylline therapy).*

• Advise the patient to withhold the drug and consult the physician if an adverse reaction occurs.

• *Instruct the patient to inform all personal physicians about methylxanthine therapy to prevent drug interactions.*

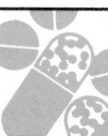

SELECTED MAJOR DRUGS

Methylxanthine agents

This chart summarizes the major methylxanthine agents currently in clinical use.

DRUG	MAJOR INDICATIONS	USUAL ADULT DOSAGES	CONTRAINDICATIONS AND PRECAUTIONS
anhydrous theophylline	Asthma, bronchitis, and emphysema. The rapid-release oral liquids are used to treat neonatal apnea.	The specific dosage is based on serum theophylline concentration, patient response, and occurrence of adverse reactions. The daily dosage is divided into 6- or 8-hour doses for rapid-release products and 8-, 12-, or 24-hour doses for slow-release products. Initial maximum dosage in adults is 13 mg/kg/day or a total of 800 mg/day, whichever is less.	• Know that theophylline is contraindicated in a patient with hypersensitivity to methylxanthine agents. • Administer with extreme caution to a patient with congestive heart failure. • Administer with caution to a neonate; an elderly, pregnant, or lactating patient; or one with severe cardiovascular disease, severe hypoxemia, hypertension, hyperthyroidism, acute myocardial injury, obstructive lung disease, or liver disease.
aminophylline	Asthma, chronic bronchitis, and emphysema	Adult dosage should be based on theophylline content. The specific dosage is based on serum theophylline concentration, patient response, and occurrence of adverse reactions. The daily dosage is divided into 6- or 8-hour doses for rapid-release products and 8- or 12-hour doses for slow-release products. After an I.V. loading dose of 5 to 6 mg/kg is given over 20 to 30 minutes, the patient may receive a maintenance dosage of 0.4 to 0.7 mg/kg/hr. Initial maximum dosage in adults is 13 mg/kg/day of theophylline or a total of 800 mg/day, whichever is less.	• Know that aminophylline is contraindicated in a patient with active peptic ulcer disease, known hypersensitivity to methylxanthine agents, or concurrent administration of other xanthine preparations. • Administer with caution to a neonate, a pregnant or lactating, an elderly (especially male) patient, or one with severe cardiac disease, hypertension, hyperthyroidism, acute myocardial injury, cor pulmonale, severe hypoxemia, hepatic impairment, alcoholism, history of peptic ulcer, or congestive heart failure.
oxtriphylline	Asthma, chronic bronchitis, emphysema, and similar chronic obstructive pulmonary diseases	200 mg P.O. every 6 to 8 hours. The daily dosage should be divided into 6- or 8-hour doses for rapid-release products and 8- or 12-hour doses for slow-release products. The specific dosage is based on serum theophylline concentration, patient response, and occurrence of adverse reactions. The initial maximum dosage in adults is 13 mg/kg/day of theophylline or a total of 800 mg/day, whichever is less.	• Know that oxtriphylline is contraindicated in a lactating patient or one with active peptic ulcer disease, a seizure disorder (unless the patient is receiving anticonvulsant medication), or known hypersensitivity to oxtriphylline's components. • Administer with caution to a pregnant patient or one with hypoxemia, hypertension, or a history of peptic ulcer.
dyphylline	Asthma, chronic bronchitis, and emphysema	Up to 15 mg/kg P.O. every 6 hours, or 250 to 500 mg I.M., up to a maximum of 15 mg/kg, every 6 hours	• Know that dyphylline is contraindicated in a patient with known hypersensitivity to dyphylline or related xanthine compounds. • Administer with caution to a pregnant or lactating patient or one with severe cardiac disease, hypertension, hyperthyroidism, acute myocardial injury, or peptic ulcer.

• *Teach the patient who misses a dose to consult the physician before increasing or doubling the next scheduled dose.*

• Instruct the patient to take a mild analgesic, as prescribed, for methylxanthine-induced headache.

• Advise the patient that aminophylline given I.M. produces severe pain at the injection site.

• *Instruct the patient to take an oral preparation with an 8-oz glass of water and preferably on an empty stomach. Advise the patient taking a slow-release product not to chew or crush it.*

• *Advise the patient to avoid using products that contain methylxanthine during methylxanthine therapy. The additional agents may not contribute to the therapy's effectiveness and may cause adverse reactions.*

Evaluation

The following examples represent appropriate evaluation statements for a patient receiving a methylxanthine agent.

• The patient has no conditions that contraindicate methylxanthine agent therapy.

• The patient exhibits no signs of complications in the preexisting condition linked to the prescribed methylxanthine agent.

• The patient experiences no adverse reactions to the prescribed methylxanthine agent.

• The patient remains well hydrated during methylxanthine therapy.

• The patient's regimen includes no drugs that interact with the methylxanthine agent.

• The patient's serum theophylline concentration remains within the therapeutic range.

• The patient's sleep pattern remains unchanged during methylxanthine therapy.

• The patient and family express an accurate understanding of the points taught about the prescribed methylxanthine agent.

• The patient schedules follow-up visits for serum drug testing.

CHAPTER SUMMARY

Chapter 38 covered the methylxanthine agents used clinically in the United States, including theophylline and its salts, dyphylline, and caffeine. Here are the highlights of the chapter.

• Theophylline, its salts, and dyphylline are prescribed to treat asthma, chronic bronchitis, and emphysema. Theophylline and caffeine are used to treat neonatal apnea.

• The therapeutic response of asthma patients to methylxanthine agents is bronchodilation. Theophylline and its salts are more potent bronchodilators than dyphylline. As a bronchodilator, theophylline assists in ventricular emptying, decreases diaphragmatic fatigue, and increases mucociliary clearance.

• Theophylline, administered as an oral solution, a rapid-release tablet, or a rectal solution, is absorbed rapidly and completely. Slow-release preparations are absorbed at varying rates and degrees. Dyphylline is absorbed incompletely. Caffeine is absorbed well after oral administration.

• Dosages of methylxanthine agents should be individualized based on serum drug concentration level, patient response, and occurrence of adverse reactions.

• Drug interactions involving methylxanthine agents can result in toxicity or reduced effectiveness.

• Adverse reactions to methylxanthine agents may affect the GI tract (nausea, vomiting, abdominal cramping, anorexia, and diarrhea), CNS (headache, anxiety, irritability, restlessness, dizziness, and, rarely, seizures), and cardiovascular system (arrhythmias, peripheral vasodilation, and hypotension).

• When caring for a patient receiving a methylxanthine agent, the nurse applies the nursing process and focuses on monitoring the patient closely for adverse reactions, administering the methylxanthine agent carefully, protecting the patient from injury, and teaching the patient and family about the prescribed agent.

STUDY QUESTIONS

See Appendix 1 for answers.

1. After determining that Alice Larkin, age 54, has emphysema, the physician prescribes anhydrous theophylline 200 mg P.O. every 8 hours. To arrive at this dosage, the physician had to consider which patient factor?
(a) blood count
(b) weight
(c) age
(d) sex

2. During theophylline therapy, the nurse monitors Ms. Larkin's serum theophylline concentration. When treating a respiratory disorder, what is the therapeutic theophylline concentration?
(a) 1 to 2 mcg/ml
(b) 2 to 5 mcg/ml
(c) 5 to 10 mcg/ml
(d) 10 to 20 mcg/ml

3. How does anhydrous theophylline correct a nonreversible obstructive airway disease, such as emphysema?
(a) It increases the central respiratory center's sensitivity to carbon dioxide and stimulates the patient's respiratory drive.
(b) It inhibits the enzyme phosphodiesterase, which decreases degradation of cyclic AMP, a bronchodilator.
(c) It stimulates adenosine receptors, causing bronchodilation.
(d) It alters diaphragmatic movement, increasing chest expansion and the lungs' capacity for gas exchange.

4. One month later, Ms. Larkin develops acute respiratory insufficiency. She is brought to the emergency department, where she receives I.V. anhydrous theophylline. After Ms. Larkin's condition stabilizes, the physician switches her to oral anhydrous theophylline. When should the nurse discontinue I.V. administration of this drug?
(a) when the oral administration begins
(b) 24 hours before oral therapy begins
(c) 24 hours after oral therapy begins
(d) after administering three oral doses

5. Ms. Larkin has smoked two packs of cigarettes a day for 30 years. How can cigarettes interact with anhydrous theophylline?
(a) They may decrease theophylline absorption.
(b) They may increase theophylline elimination.
(c) They may inhibit theophylline metabolism.
(d) They may produce additive effects.

6. Throughout Ms. Larkin's hospitalization, the nurse should monitor her closely for which adverse reactions to anhydrous theophylline?
(a) nausea, vomiting, and diarrhea
(b) congestive heart failure
(c) lethargy and drowsiness
(d) urine retention and proteinuria

SELECTED REFERENCES

AHFS drug information 90. (1990). Bethesda, MD: American Society of Hospital Pharmacists.

Anderson, M. (1989). The pharmacology of intervention for respiratory emergencies. *Emergency Care Quarterly,* 5(1), 23-36.

Bronchodilator aerosol deaths? (1987). *Nurses Drug Alert,* 11(11), 85.

Drug facts and comparisons. (1991). St. Louis: Facts and Comparisons Division, J.B. Lippincott.

Goodman and Gilman's the pharmacological basis of therapeutics (8th ed.; 1990). Elmsford, NY: Pergamon Press.

Hansten, P., and Horn, J. (1989) *Drug interactions* (6th ed.). Philadelphia: Lea & Febiger.

Janson-Bjerklie, S., and Shnell, S. (1988). Effect of peak flow information on patterns of self-care in adult asthma, *Heart & Lung,* 17(5), 543-549.

Krohmer, J. (1988). Asthma out of control. *Emergency Medicine,* 20(9), 96-105.

North American Nursing Diagnosis Association. (1990). *Taxonomy I—Revised, with official diagnostic categories.* St. Louis: NANDA.

Tinkelman, D. (1988). Theophylline: Use and misuse in pediatric asthma. *Hospital Practice,* 23(2), 179-184.

USPDI. (1991). *Drug information for the health care professional* (Vol. I, 11th ed.). Rockville, MD: United States Pharmacopeial Convention.

Weinberg, H. (1988). Long-term management of asthma. *Physician Assistant,* 12(6), 30-42.

EXPECTORANT, ANTITUSSIVE, AND MUCOLYTIC AGENTS

OBJECTIVES

After reading and studying this chapter, the student should be able to:

1. Describe the physiology of the cough mechanism.

2. Differentiate among the different actions of expectorants, antitussives, and mucolytics.

3. Describe the purported mechanisms of action for the expectorants, including the iodides and guaifenesin.

4. Identify the adverse reactions associated with the iodides.

5. Explain the difference between centrally acting and peripherally acting antitussives.

6. Identify the potential risks involved for the patient when using antitussives.

7. Explain why acetylcysteine is the only mucolytic used clinically in the United States.

8. Describe how to apply the nursing process when caring for a patient who is receiving an expectorant, antitussive, or mucolytic agent.

INTRODUCTION

Respiratory tract secretions, which originate from goblet cells and bronchial glands, combine to form mucus. Approximately 100 ml of mucus is produced daily; mucus is composed of water, lipids, glycoproteins, carbohydrates, and deoxyribonucleic acid. Mainly protective in nature, mucus acts as a barrier to prevent water loss from the epithelium. Mucus also plays an important role in the mucociliary clearance mechanism, protecting the epithelium from mechanical irritants, noxious agents, and microorganisms. (For an illustration of these defense mechanisms, see *Respiratory tract lining* in the introduction to this unit.) Inhaled particles are trapped in the mucus, and the debris is propelled to the oropharynx via the mucociliary clearance mechanism to be swallowed or expectorated.

The mucociliary clearance mechanism is compromised by inhibited ciliary function. Ciliary inhibition can result from chronic exposure to cigarette smoke or from a change in mucus viscosity or amount, which occurs in bronchitis and cystic fibrosis. Expectorants may assist clearance by increasing mucus output or altering mucus composition. Although the efficacy of expectorants is unsubstantiated, they are found in many over-the-counter (OTC) preparations and are advertised widely. The mucolytic acetylcysteine reduces the viscosity of tenacious secretions in the airway.

Like the mucociliary clearance mechanism, the cough facilitates removal of respiratory secretions. The cough is triggered by stimulating nerve receptors that are sensitive to chemicals and other irritants. These cough receptors are located throughout the respiratory tract as well as in the stomach, pleura, and diaphragm. Once the receptors are stimulated, the impulse travels through the afferent pathway, mainly via the vagus nerve, to the cough center in the medulla. Then the cough reflex is processed and coordinated in the brain stem.

The muscular contractions that constitute the cough are initiated via the efferent nervous pathways. The cough mechanism consists of three phases: inspiratory phase, compressive phase, and expiratory phase. After the deep inhalation of the inspiratory phase, the glottis closes and the expiratory muscles contract against the closed glottis. The compressive phase ends with the sudden opening of the glottis, producing a flow rate necessary for an effective cough by releasing the high intrathoracic pressure. The expiratory phase allows for the removal of debris from the respiratory tract.

Expiratory muscles contract even further during this phase, compressing the tracheobronchial tree. This compression contributes to an effective cough by decreasing the diameters of the airways, thus increasing the velocity and shearing forces of the gas in the airways. The cough

---

SELECTED NURSING DIAGNOSES

Expectorant, antitussive, and mucolytic agents

The following nursing diagnoses address representative problems and etiologies that a nurse may encounter when caring for a patient who is receiving an expectorant, antitussive, or mucolytic agent. Some of these nursing diagnoses contain generalized etiologies, which the nurse must individualize based on the patient's needs. (For some common nursing diagnoses and related interventions for each drug class, see the "Nursing Process Application" sections of this chapter.)

- Altered cerebral tissue perfusion related to hypotension caused by toxic dosages of a narcotic antitussive
- Altered health maintenance related to ineffectiveness of the prescribed expectorant, antitussive, or mucolytic agent
- Altered oral mucous membrane related to acetylcysteine-induced stomatitis
- Altered protection related to iodide-induced thyroid disorder
- Altered protection related to thrombocytopenic purpura caused by iodide hypersensitivity
- Altered renal tissue perfusion related to circulatory collapse caused by toxic dosages of a narcotic antitussive
- Altered role performance related to physical dependence on codeine
- Altered thought processes related to central nervous system (CNS) depression caused by extremely high dosages of dextromethorphan
- Constipation related to the adverse gastrointestinal (GI) effects of an expectorant or antitussive agent
- Diarrhea related to the adverse GI effects of guaifenesin
- Hyperthermia related to serum sickness caused by iodide hypersensitivity

- Impaired gas exchange related to the adverse respiratory effects of an antitussive or mucolytic agent
- Knowledge deficit related to the prescribed expectorant, antitussive, or mucolytic agent
- Pain related to guaifenesin-induced abdominal pain
- Potential fluid volume deficit related to the adverse GI effects of the expectorant, antitussive, or mucolytic agent
- Potential for injury related to a preexisting condition that contraindicates the use of an expectorant, antitussive, or mucolytic agent
- Potential for injury related to a preexisting condition that requires cautious use of an expectorant, antitussive, or mucolytic agent
- Potential for injury related to adverse drug reactions
- Potential for injury related to drug interactions
- Potential for suffocation related to laryngeal edema caused by iodide hypersensitivity
- Potential for trauma related to the adverse CNS effects of an expectorant or antitussive agent
- Potential impaired skin integrity related to benzonatate-induced skin eruptions
- Sensory-perceptual alterations (tactile) related to benzonatate-induced chilly sensations and numbness

---

serves as an important protective mechanism when the cilia prove ineffective against abnormal quantities or types of materials in the respiratory tract.

The numerous causes of the cough include congenital anomalies, infections, diseases such as cystic fibrosis, foreign body aspiration, reactive airway disease, irritants, and psychogenic reactions. A condition frequently associated with a transient cough is the common cold. Coughs can be productive or nonproductive of sputum. They also may be described as chronic, paroxysmal, or recurrent.

Although coughing is useful, protective, and beneficial, it can be irritating and exhausting and can interfere with an individual's activities of daily living. Coughing also can cause further complications. The intrathoracic pressures generated during the compressive phase can lead to rib fractures, ruptured rectus abdominis muscles, pneumothorax, bradycardia, or syncope.

Treatment of a cough depends on its cause. The cessation of smoking usually improves the cough associated with chronic bronchitis. Bronchodilators relieve the cough caused by reactive airway disease. If the cough disrupts an individual's sleep or activities of daily living, antitussives, which suppress the cough mechanism, may be an acceptable risk. Antitussives, however, are contraindicated in suppurative lung disease or a condition in which sputum is

increased, because they might promote atelectasis or pneumonia.

This chapter discusses the expectorant and mucolytic agents, which purport to enhance mucokinesis (mucus removal), and drugs that act to suppress coughing, the narcotic and nonnarcotic antitussives.

For a summary of representative drugs, see *Selected major drugs: Expectorant, antitussive, and mucolytic agents,* page 682. For a listing of applicable nursing diagnoses that the nurse may formulate when caring for a patient receiving these agents, see *Selected nursing diagnoses: Expectorant, antitussive, and mucolytic agents.* For detailed information on applying the nursing process, see Chapter 6, The Nursing Process and Drug Therapy.

EXPECTORANTS

Expectorants facilitate mucokinesis. Most drugs purported to remove mucus liquefy viscid secretions and thereby aid in mobilizing and evacuating secretions.

Providing adequate hydration of 2 or 3 liters of fluid per day also enhances mucokinesis. Overhydration, however, does not thin mucus and actually may impair its clearance. Deep-breathing exercises and frequent position changes also may help increase mucokinesis.

Some frequently used expectorants that are discussed in this chapter include guaifenesin, iodinated glycerol, potassium iodide, and terpin hydrate.

PHARMACOKINETICS

Because expectorants have not been researched thoroughly, data on peak concentration levels, duration of action, and half-life remain unavailable.

Absorption, distribution, metabolism, excretion

Guaifenesin, iodinated glycerol, potassium iodide, and terpin hydrate are absorbed via the gastrointestinal (GI) tract and distributed to the bronchial glands. The iodides also are distributed to the salivary, lacrimal, and thyroid glands, as well as across the placenta. Guaifenesin is metabolized by the liver. The metabolic fates of iodinated glycerol and terpin hydrate are unknown. Potassium iodide is not metabolized and is excreted basically unchanged. Excretion of expectorants is primarily renal, although the iodides also are excreted in breast milk.

Onset, peak, duration

The onset of action for expectorants is immediate to 30 minutes. Data remain unavailable on the peak concentrations, duration, and half-life of the expectorants.

PHARMACODYNAMICS

Expectorants are thought to increase mucus by acting on the bronchial glands or by reducing the adhesiveness and surface tension of the mucus. Expectorants also may provide a soothing demulcent effect on respiratory tract mucosa. The use of expectorants remains controversial because their efficacy has not been clearly established.

Mechanism of action

Guaifenesin supposedly increases mucus secretion by reducing mucus adhesiveness and surface tension. The increased flow of less viscid secretions promotes ciliary action, thus facilitating mucus removal.

The iodides, iodinated glycerol and potassium iodide, are thought to enter the bronchial glands of the tracheobronchial mucosa via the bloodstream and stimulate gland cells to secrete a watery mucus. The iodides also appear to stimulate ciliary activity and the salivary glands, causing rhinorrhea and salivation.

Terpin hydrate appears to act directly on lower respiratory secretory glands, stimulating them to increase fluid output.

PHARMACOTHERAPEUTICS

Expectorants are used for the symptomatic relief of cough from colds, as well as for minor bronchial irritations, bronchitis, influenza, sinusitis, bronchial asthma, emphysema, and other respiratory disorders. Guaifenesin, the most popular expectorant, is used to relieve a dry, hacking cough and is safe if taken as directed. It can be used alone or with antitussives, analgesics, or antihistamines. (For some commonly prescribed combination products containing guaifenesin, see *Combination products,* page 672.)

The iodides are prescribed less frequently because of the potential for toxic effects (especially on the thyroid gland) if they are taken in excessive amounts or used in prolonged therapy. Patients may tolerate iodinated glycerol better than the inorganic iodide because the iodine and glycerol are bound organically; as a result, no iodine is free to cause GI irritation.

Although potassium iodide may be used to liquefy tenacious mucus in conditions such as chronic bronchiectasis and bronchial asthma, it is used most frequently when preparing patients for thyroidectomy. When given preoperatively, potassium iodide reduces vascularity, firms glandular tissue, and shrinks cells in the thyroid gland; these effects facilitate thyroidectomy. (For more information, see Chapter 50, Thyroid and Antithyroid Agents.)

Iodinated glycerol and potassium iodide are contraindicated in patients with iodide sensitivity. Pregnant and lactating women should not receive iodides because abnormal thyroid function or goiter may occur in the fetus or neonate. The iodides also are contraindicated in patients with thyroid disease, tuberculosis, or acute bronchitis.

Patients with renal disease or hyperkalemia and patients taking potassium supplements should not take potassium iodide because increased serum potassium concentrations can cause cardiac arrhythmias and death.

Researchers have not clearly established the efficacy of terpin hydrate. Because of its high alcohol content, terpin hydrate is contraindicated in patients with peptic ulcer or severe diabetes mellitus. Also the high-alcohol elixir is contraindicated during pregnancy, because the alcohol can cross the placenta, causing congenital abnormalities in the fetus.

Many of the expectorants are found in OTC combination preparations. Therefore, the nurse must be aware of all the ingredients in combination cough and cold products and the usual dosage range for children. Pediatric dosages for these products vary, but the nurse usually can rely on the following general guidelines: children ages 6 to 12, give one-half the adult dosage; children ages 2 to 6, give

Combination products

Combination products contain varying amounts of different ingredients. The nurse must be aware of these ingredients to understand their potential effects on the therapeutic regimen. This chart is only a sampling. Other combinations, such as Benylin DM, combine antitussives and decongestants. The following chart lists readily available combination products that the nurse should know about.

DRUG	EXPECTORANT	ANTITUSSIVE	OTHER INGREDIENTS
Cheracol	guaifenesin, 20 mg/ml	codeine phosphate, 2 mg/ml	alcohol, 4.75%
Conar Expectorant Syrup	guaifenesin, 20 mg/ml	dextromethorphan hydrobromide, 3 mg/ml	phenylephrine hydrochloride, 2 mg/ml
Formula 44D	guaifenesin, 13 mg/ml	dextromethorphan hydrobromide, 2 mg/ml	pseudoephedrine hydrochloride, 4 mg/ml alcohol, 10%
Robitussin-DM	guaifenesin, 20 mg/ml	dextromethorphan hydrobromide, 3 mg/ml	alcohol, 1.4%
Vicks Children's Cough Syrup	guaifenesin, 10 mg/ml	dextromethorphan hydrobromide, 0.7 mg/ml	saccharin sucrose

one-fourth the adult dosage. No recommended dosage has been established for children under age 2. The nurse should check with the pharmacist or physician if the correct dose to give is not available in floor stock or the patient's medication drawer.

guaifenesin (Breonesin, Robitussin). Guaifenesin relieves the dry, hacking cough associated with the common cold as well as with other upper respiratory infections, such as bronchitis, laryngitis, pharyngitis, and influenza.
Usual adult dosage: 200 to 400 mg P.O. every 4 hours, not to exceed 2.4 grams/day.

iodinated glycerol (Organidin). This drug serves as adjunctive therapy in respiratory conditions, such as bronchial asthma, bronchitis, and emphysema. Iodinated glycerol is contraindicated in a pregnant or lactating patient or one with known hypersensitivity to iodides or a thyroid disease.
Usual adult dosage: 60 mg P.O. q.i.d.

potassium iodide (Pima, SSKI). Potassium iodide is used to liquefy tenacious mucus in such conditions as chronic bronchiectasis and bronchial asthma. It must not be used in a patient who is hypersensitive to the drug.
Usual adult dosage: for expectorant action, 300 to 650 mg P.O. t.i.d. to q.i.d. Potassium iodide also is available in saturated solution with 1 gram potassium iodide per milliliter. The solution dose is 0.3 to 0.6 ml, which must be measured with a calibrated dropper and then diluted in water, fruit juice, or milk.

terpin hydrate. This drug appears to increase mucus production. The increased mucus helps liquefy and reduce the viscosity of thick secretions. Terpin hydrate is contraindicated in a patient with known hypersensitivity to the drug or who uses disulfiram concomitantly.
Usual adult dosage: 5 to 10 ml P.O. t.i.d. or q.i.d. The elixir is not recommended for pediatric use because of its high alcohol content.

Drug interactions
Few interactions between drugs or between drugs and food occur with the expectorants. Guaifenesin administered with anticoagulants may increase the risk of bleeding. Iodinated glycerol and potassium iodide administered with lithium or the antithyroid drugs may potentiate hypothyroid and goitrogenic effects. Potassium iodide combined with potassium-sparing diuretics or potassium-containing drugs may increase the serum potassium level and lead to cardiac arrhythmias and cardiac arrest. Terpin hydrate should not be administered to patients taking disulfiram because they may experience an alcohol-disulfiram reaction.

ADVERSE DRUG REACTIONS

Adverse reactions to guaifenesin rarely or infrequently occur. However, the drug may produce vomiting if taken in doses larger than necessary for the expectorant action. Diarrhea, drowsiness, nausea, vomiting, and abdominal pain also may occur. Guaifenesin also may interfere with urinary 5-hydroxyindoleacetic acid (5-HIAA) and urinary vanillylmandelic acid (VMA) tests, resulting in falsely increased determinations.

Of the expectorants, the iodides produce the most potentially toxic adverse reactions. The prolonged use of large doses of iodides can cause thyroid gland hyperplasia, hypothyroidism, goiter, thyroid adenoma, or skin eruptions. It also may cause iodism, which is characterized by unpleasant brassy taste, burning in the mouth and throat, soreness of gums and teeth, increased salivation, coryza, sneezing, and eye irritation. Mild iodism can simulate a head cold. Gastric irritation commonly occurs; however, iodinated glycerol is less irritating to the GI tract than inorganic iodide. Patients with cystic fibrosis may experience an increased susceptibility to the goitrogenic effect of iodine, and adolescents with acne may find their condition aggravated. Potassium toxicity may occur in some patients taking potassium iodide.

Patients with iodide hypersensitivity may experience angioedema (submucosal swelling), laryngeal edema (swelling of the larynx), cutaneous and mucosal hemorrhage, and signs and symptoms of serum sickness, including fever, arthralgia (joint pain), lymph node enlargement, and eosinophilia (increase of eosinophils). Other manifestations attributed to iodide hypersensitivity include urticaria (pruritic skin eruptions), thrombocytopenic purpura (a bleeding disorder), and fatal periarteritis (an inflammatory condition of the arteries).

Terpin hydrate often causes drowsiness. It also may produce nausea and vomiting.

NURSING PROCESS APPLICATION

The following information assists the nurse in caring for a patient who is receiving an expectorant.

Assessment
• Review the patient's history for a preexisting condition that contraindicates the use of an expectorant, such as known hypersensitivity to the drug (guaifenesin, potassium iodide, or terpin hydrate); known hypersensitivity to iodides, pregnancy, lactation, or thyroid disease (iodinated glycerol); or concurrent use of disulfiram (terpin hydrate).
• Review the patient's history for a preexisting condition that requires cautious use of an expectorant, such as ineffective cough reflex, respiratory insufficiency, pregnancy, or lactation.
• Assess the patient for adverse reactions to the prescribed expectorant, such as GI distress, drowsiness, or thyroid dysfunction.
• Review the patient's medication history to identify the use of drugs that may interact with the prescribed expectorant, such as anticoagulants, lithium, antithyroid drugs, or potassium-sparing diuretics.

• Evaluate the patient's and family's knowledge about the prescribed expectorant.

Nursing diagnoses
The following examples represent appropriate nursing diagnoses for a patient receiving an expectorant.
• Potential for injury related to a preexisting condition that contraindicates the use of an expectorant
• Potential for injury related to a preexisting condition that requires cautious use of an expectorant
• Potential for injury related to adverse drug reactions
• Potential for injury related to drug interactions
• Knowledge deficit related to the prescribed expectorant

Planning and implementation
• Do not administer an expectorant to a patient with a condition that contraindicates its use.
• Administer an expectorant cautiously to a patient at risk because of a preexisting condition.
• Monitor the patient closely for adverse reactions during expectorant therapy.
• *Monitor the patient for dyspnea or ineffective cough.*
• *Keep suction equipment readily available during expectorant therapy.*
• *Monitor the patient on high-dose or long-term iodide expectorant therapy for signs of iodism, such as unpleasant brassy taste, burning in the mouth and throat, soreness of gums and teeth, increased salivation, coryza, sneezing, and eye irritation. Notify the physician if iodism occurs.*
• Monitor for hypothyroidism in a patient receiving an iodide expectorant.
• Administer guaifenesin in doses no higher than necessary to produce expectorant effects without causing vomiting.
• Monitor hydration if the patient develops nausea, vomiting, or diarrhea. Obtain a prescription for an antiemetic or antidiarrheal agent, as needed.
• *Take safety measures if drowsiness occurs. For example, place the bed in the low position, keep the bed rails up, and supervise ambulation.*
• *Monitor the patient closely for signs of iodide sensitivity, such as angioedema, laryngeal edema, cutaneous and mucosal hemorrhage, and serum sickness, during iodide expectorant therapy.*
• Interpret 5-HIAA and VMA tests cautiously in a patient receiving guaifenesin because this drug may cause falsely elevated determinations.
• *Increase the patient's fluid intake to 8 to 13 8-oz glasses (2 to 3 liters) per day (unless contraindicated) to help thin and mobilize respiratory secretions. To prevent fluid overload, document all fluid intake and ensure that it does not exceed 3 liters.*
• Mix potassium iodide solution with a glass of water, fruit juice, or other liquid. Administer the solution after meals or at bedtime with food to minimize GI distress.

• Dilute potassium iodide well and give the patient a glass drinking straw to help prevent tooth staining.
• *Discard any potassium iodide solution that has turned brown; such discoloration indicates decomposition.*
• Warm a crystallized potassium iodide solution and shake it gently before administration.
• Notify the physician if adverse reactions occur.
• *Observe for signs of bleeding in a patient receiving guaifenesin concomitantly with an anticoagulant.*
• Monitor closely for signs of hypothyroidism in a patient receiving an iodide expectorant during concomitant therapy with lithium or an antithyroid drug.
• *Monitor the patient's serum potassium level closely if potassium iodide is administered with a potassium-sparing diuretic or potassium-containing drug.*
• Notify the physician if the patient shows signs of drug interactions.

Patient teaching
• Teach the patient and family the name, dose, frequency, action, and adverse effects of the prescribed expectorant.
• Stress the importance of taking the drug exactly as prescribed.
• *Teach the patient receiving high-dose, long-term iodide expectorant therapy to recognize and report to the physician signs of iodism.*
• *Inform the patient taking terpin hydrate about the expectorant's high alcohol content.*
• *Advise family members purchasing an expectorant for a child to check with the pharmacist or physician if the pediatric dosage is unclear to them.*
• *Instruct the patient to avoid activities that require alertness if drowsiness occurs.*
• *Encourage the patient to increase fluid intake to 8 to 13 8-oz glasses (2 to 3 liters) per day.*
• Teach the patient to perform deep-breathing exercises and change positions frequently to help increase mucokinesis.
• Instruct the patient to mix potassium iodide solution with a glass of water, juice, or other liquid; use a glass drinking straw; and take the solution after meals or at bedtime with food.
• *Advise the patient to discard any potassium iodide solution that has turned brown.*
• Instruct the patient to warm and gently shake potassium iodide if crystallization occurs.
• Instruct the patient to notify the physician if adverse reactions occur or the expectorant is ineffective.

Evaluation
The following examples represent appropriate evaluation statements for a patient receiving an expectorant.
• The patient has no conditions that contraindicate expectorant therapy.

• The patient exhibits no signs of complications in the preexisting condition linked to the prescribed expectorant.
• The patient demonstrates no adverse reactions to the prescribed expectorant.
• The patient uses no drugs that interact with the prescribed expectorant.
• The patient and family express an accurate understanding of the points taught about the prescribed expectorant.
• The patient correctly describes how to measure, dilute, and self-administer potassium iodide solution.

ANTITUSSIVES

An antitussive is any agent that suppresses or inhibits coughing. Centrally acting antitussives suppress cough by depressing the cough center in the medulla. Narcotics are centrally acting antitussives that effectively suppress cough. Peripherally acting antitussives act on the cough receptors located throughout the airway. A number of peripherally acting antitussives, such as local anesthetics, bronchodilators, and mucokinetic drugs, can alleviate many types of cough. Home remedies, such as honey and whiskey, cough drops, and rock candy, also may relieve cough.

Because the cough acts as a protective mechanism by removing accumulated mucus and irritants, it should not be suppressed under normal circumstances. However, a persistent cough can begin to act as an irritant and can lead to a cough-irritant-cough cycle. Such a cycle can prove exhausting and can interrupt an individual's ability to sleep or talk.

The major antitussives include benzonatate, codeine, dextromethorphan hydrobromide, and hydrocodone bitartrate. Other drugs that provide antitussive activity include diphenhydramine hydrochloride and lidocaine hydrochloride.

PHARMACOKINETICS

The antitussives are absorbed well through the GI tract, metabolized in the liver, and excreted in the urine.

Absorption, distribution, metabolism, excretion
The narcotic antitussives codeine and hydrocodone bitartrate are absorbed via the GI tract, metabolized in the liver, and excreted in the urine. They are distributed across the placenta in pregnant women and are excreted in the breast milk of lactating women. No such data are available for benzonatate or dextromethorphan.

Onset, peak, duration

The onset of action for codeine occurs in 30 minutes. Codeine and hydrocodone bitartrate reach peak concentrations in about 1 hour. Duration of action varies: codeine lasts about 4 hours, and hydrocodone bitartrate lasts between 4 and 6 hours. Codeine has a half-life of 2.5 to 3 hours; hydrocodone bitartrate, of 4 hours.

Benzonatate and dextromethorphan provide an onset in about 15 to 30 minutes. The duration for benzonatate ranges from 3 to 8 hours; for conventional dosage forms of dextromethorphan, duration ranges from 3 to 6 hours.

PHARMACODYNAMICS

Benzonatate is a peripherally acting antitussive. Dextromethorphan is a methylated dextro isomer of levorphanol (an opiate analgesic) that acts centrally to suppress cough. Unlike codeine and hydrocodone bitartrate, dextromethorphan produces no analgesia, addiction, or central nervous system (CNS) depression.

Chemically classified as phenanthrenes, the narcotic antitussives codeine and hydrocodone bitartrate are opium alkaloids. These antitussives suppress the cough reflex by a direct effect on the cough center in the medulla. They also exert a drying effect on the respiratory tract mucosa, which increases the viscosity of bronchial secretions. Codeine and hydrocodone bitartrate produce sedative and constipating effects. (For more details about these drugs, see Chapter 22, Narcotic Agonist and Antagonist Agents.)

Mechanism of action

Benzonatate, the peripherally acting antitussive, acts by anesthetizing cough receptors of vagal afferent fibers throughout the bronchi, alveoli, and pleura. Codeine, dextromethorphan, and hydrocodone bitartrate suppress the cough reflex by directly affecting the sensitivity of the cough center in the medulla to incoming stimuli. (For an illustration, see *Location of action: Antitussives.*)

PHARMACOTHERAPEUTICS

The treatment of a cough should be directed at the cause. Treatment may include removing an irritant, such as cigarette smoke; administering antihistamines for postnasal drip; administering a bronchodilator to relieve bronchospasm; or administering an antitussive. Antitussives are used to treat a serious, nonproductive cough that interferes with a patient's ability to rest or carry out activities of daily living.

Benzonatate, a nonnarcotic antitussive, relieves cough associated with respiratory conditions such as pneumonia, bronchitis, and the common cold, as well as with chronic pulmonary diseases such as emphysema. At recommended dosages, benzonatate does not depress respiration. It also

Location of action: Antitussives

Codeine, hydrocodone bitartrate, and dextromethorphan act directly on the cough center in the medulla. The peripherally acting benzonatate acts on the bronchi, alveoli, and pleura.

can be used as adjunctive treatment during bronchial diagnostic tests, such as bronchoscopy, when the patient must avoid coughing during the procedure. Benzonatate does not pose the risk of addiction that codeine does.

The nonnarcotic antitussive dextromethorphan is the most widely used cough suppressant in the United States. Some data suggest that dextromethorphan may provide better antitussive activity than codeine. The popularity of dextromethorphan also may stem from the fact that the drug produces few adverse reactions and is nonaddictive.

The narcotic antitussives effectively suppress cough; however, they act centrally and can cause respiratory depression, which may be detrimental in patients with pulmonary disease. Narcotics also possess the potential for abuse; however, if the narcotic is used in antitussive dosages and for a short time, addiction liability is low. Potent narcotics are reserved for treating intractable cough, usually associated with lung cancer. Opiates taken with other CNS depressants can be fatal. (For a comparison of these drugs, see *Characteristics of antitussives,* page 676.)

Characteristics of antitussives

The following chart compares four antitussives. The nurse must know these comparisons to plan appropriate follow-up care for the patient.

DRUG	MECHANISM OF ACTION	EFFECTIVENESS	DEPENDENCE POTENTIAL	C.N.S. DEPRESSION
benzonatate	Peripherally acting	Equal to codeine	No	Sedation
codeine	Centrally acting	Less than morphine	Yes	Sedation
dextromethorphan	Centrally acting	Equal to codeine	No	Not at recommended dosage
hydrocodone bitartrate	Centrally acting	Greater than codeine	Yes	Sedation

benzonatate (Tessalon). This drug provides symptomatic relief of cough associated with respiratory conditions. Benzonatate can be administered before bronchial diagnostic tests to suppress cough during the procedure.
Usual adult dosage: 100 mg P.O. every 4 to 6 hours, not to exceed 600 mg/day.

codeine. A Schedule II drug, codeine is used to suppress the nonproductive cough that interferes with the patient's activities or leads to exhaustion.
Usual adult dosage: 10 to 20 mg P.O. every 4 to 6 hours, not to exceed 120 mg/day.

dextromethorphan hydrobromide (Robitussin-DM). This drug is used to treat nonproductive cough from minor throat and bronchial irritation.
Usual adult dosage: 10 to 20 mg P.O. every 4 hours, or 30 mg every 6 to 8 hours, not to exceed 120 mg/day. The long-acting preparation (60 mg) can be taken every 12 hours.

hydrocodone bitartrate (Hycodan). A Schedule II drug, hydrocodone bitartrate is used with other antitussives or expectorants to relieve nonproductive cough.
Usual adult dosage: 5 to 10 mg P.O. every 4 to 6 hours. Initiate therapy with a 5-mg dose.

Drug interactions
Benzonatate produces no significant drug interactions. Dextromethorphan may cause excitation and hyperpyrexia when taken with monoamine oxidase (MAO) inhibitors. The narcotic antitussives potentiate the depressant effects of MAO inhibitors, alcohol, and other CNS depressants. (For details, see *Drug interactions: Antitussives.*)

ADVERSE DRUG REACTIONS

Benzonatate can cause dizziness, sedation, headache, nasal congestion, burning eyes, nausea, GI upset, constipation, and skin rash. "Chilly" sensations, skin eruptions, pruritus, and numbness in the chest also have been reported.

Overdose of dextromethorphan can result in euphoria, hyperactivity, a sense of intoxication, nystagmus, staggering gait, lethargy, uncoordinated movements, stupor, and shallow breathing. CNS depression may occur with extremely high doses of dextromethorphan. At recommended doses, adverse reactions rarely occur. Patients most commonly complain of drowsiness and GI upset.

Toxic doses of the narcotic antitussives can produce miosis, bradycardia, tachycardia, hypotension, narcosis, seizures, circulatory collapse, and respiratory arrest.

Antitussive doses of codeine seldom cause respiratory depression. However, the patient may experience an impaired ability to perform activities that require alertness or coordination. Repeated doses of codeine increase the chance for nausea, vomiting, constipation, dizziness, sedation, palpitations, pruritus, excessive perspiration, and agitation. Long-term use of codeine may result in physical dependence.

Usual oral antitussive doses of hydrocodone bitartrate do not produce adverse reactions in most cases. However, ambulatory patients may experience dizziness, sedation, nausea, and vomiting more so than nonambulatory patients. Rash, pruritus, constipation, euphoria, and dysphoria also can occur with hydrocodone bitartrate use.

Hypersensitivity reactions to benzonatate, codeine, and dextromethorphan are rare; however, urticaria, pruritus, rash, and facial swelling can result from codeine use. Hypersensitivity reactions to hydrocodone bitartrate can occur.

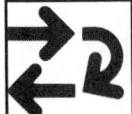

DRUG INTERACTIONS

Antitussives

Drug interactions involving centrally acting antitussives can be serious. The nurse must give special attention to patient teaching to prevent problems.

DRUG	INTERACTING DRUGS	POSSIBLE EFFECTS	NURSING IMPLICATIONS
codeine, hydroco-done bitartrate	monoamine oxidase (MAO) inhibitors (isocar-boxazid, phenelzine, tranylcypromine)	Cause excitation, hyper-tension or hypotension, coma	• Instruct the patient to avoid concomitant use of these drugs.
codeine	central nervous system (CNS) depressants (alco-hol, barbiturates, sedative-hypnotics, phenothiazines)	May increase CNS de-pressant effects (drowsi-ness, lethargy, stupor, respiratory depression, coma, death)	• Monitor the patient closely for CNS depres-sion. • Instruct the patient to avoid concomitant use of these drugs.
dextromethorphan	MAO inhibitors (isocarbox-azid, phenelzine, tranylcy-promine)	Cause excitation, hyperpy-rexia, hypotension, coma	• Instruct the patient to avoid concomitant use of these drugs.

NURSING PROCESS APPLICATION

The following information assists the nurse in caring for a patient who is receiving an antitussive.

Assessment
• Review the patient's history for a preexisting condition that contraindicates the use of an antitussive, such as known hypersensitivity to the drug, pregnancy, or lactation.
• Review the patient's history for a preexisting condition that requires cautious use of an antitussive, such as prostatic hypertrophy, debilitation, thoracotomy, laparotomy, or a history of drug or alcohol abuse.
• Assess the patient for adverse reactions to the prescribed antitussive, such as dizziness, sedation, nausea, vomiting, constipation, palpitations, pruritus, excessive perspiration, and agitation.
• Review the patient's medication history to identify the use of drugs that may interact with the antitussive, such as MAO inhibitors or CNS depressants.
• Assess the patient's bowel elimination pattern for constipation.
• Evaluate the patient's and family's knowledge about the prescribed antitussive.

Nursing diagnoses
The following examples represent appropriate nursing diagnoses for a patient receiving an antitussive.
• Potential for injury related to a preexisting condition that contraindicates the use of an antitussive
• Potential for injury related to a preexisting condition that requires cautious use of an antitussive

• Potential for injury related to adverse drug reactions
• Potential for injury related to drug interactions
• Constipation related to the adverse GI effects of the prescribed antitussive
• Knowledge deficit related to the prescribed antitussive

Planning and implementation
• Do not administer an antitussive to a patient with a condition that contraindicates its use. Also do not administer an antitussive to a patient with a productive cough or one who can benefit from coughing, such as a postoperative patient.
• Administer an antitussive cautiously to a patient at risk because of a preexisting condition.
• Monitor the patient closely for adverse reactions during antitussive therapy.
• *Monitor for signs of respiratory depression, such as decreased respiratory rate, depth of respiration, and level of consciousness, in a patient receiving codeine.*
• Monitor for hypersensitivity reactions in a patient taking codeine or hydrocodone bitartrate.
• Monitor hydration if the patient experiences nausea, vomiting, or excessive perspiration. Obtain a prescription for an antiemetic agent, as needed.
• *Take safety precautions if dizziness, sedation, or agitation occurs. For example, place the bed in the low position, keep the bed rails up, and supervise ambulation.*
• Request a prescription for an analgesic agent if the patient reports headache during benzonatate therapy.
• Question the patient who has taken codeine for a prolonged time about the need for this drug. Encourage patient

honesty because physical dependence can occur with prolonged use.

• *Monitor the patient closely for toxic effects of a narcotic antitussive (miosis, bradycardia, tachycardia, hypotension, narcosis, seizures, circulatory collapse, or respiratory arrest), dextromethorphan (euphoria, hyperactivity, a sense of intoxication, nystagmus, staggering gait, lethargy, uncoordinated movements, stupor, or shallow breathing) or benzonatate (dizziness, drowsiness, headache, nasal congestion, burning eyes, nausea, constipation, or skin rash).*

• Assess the effectiveness of the prescribed antitussive periodically.

• Notify the physician if adverse reactions occur or if the antitussive is ineffective.

• Avoid concomitant administration of the prescribed antitussive and MAO inhibitors.

• *Administer codeine with caution to a patient who also is receiving a CNS depressant; the combination can be fatal. Closely monitor the patient's level of consciousness to detect increased CNS depression.*

• Notify the physician if drug interactions occur.

• Monitor for constipation in a patient who takes an antitussive daily.

• Encourage the patient to drink 8 to 13 8-oz glasses (2 to 3 liters) of fluid daily, increase dietary fiber intake, and exercise regularly to prevent constipation.

• Obtain a prescription for a laxative if constipation occurs.

Patient teaching

• Teach the patient and family the name, dose, frequency, action, and adverse effects of the prescribed antitussive.

• Stress the importance of taking the antitussive exactly as prescribed. Tell the patient not to exceed the prescribed or recommended dosage to prevent toxicity.

• *Caution the patient not to perform activities that require alertness if sedation or dizziness occurs.*

• Instruct the patient to take a mild analgesic, as prescribed, if headache results from benzonatate use.

• *Inform the patient that prolonged use of codeine can cause physical dependency.*

• *Teach the patient to recognize the signs of toxicity and, if these signs appear, to withhold the drug and notify the physician.*

• *Instruct the patient to swallow benzonatate capsules whole; the patient should not chew these capsules because the release of benzonatate in the mouth can anesthetize the oral mucosa.*

• Instruct the patient to report persistent cough (lasting longer than 7 days) or a cough that changes from nonproductive to productive.

• *Advise the patient to keep the antitussive out of the reach of children.*

• *Warn the patient about the potentially fatal additive effects of CNS depressants, such as alcohol, when combined with an antitussive.*

• Teach the patient how to prevent constipation.

• Instruct the patient to notify the physician if adverse reactions occur or if the antitussive is ineffective.

Evaluation

The following examples represent appropriate evaluation statements for a patient receiving an antitussive.

• The patient has no conditions that contraindicate antitussive therapy.

• The patient exhibits no signs of complications in the preexisting condition linked to the prescribed antitussive.

• The patient experiences no adverse reactions to the prescribed antitussive.

• The patient uses no drugs that interact with the prescribed antitussive.

• The patient maintains a normal bowel elimination pattern during antitussive therapy.

• The patient and family express an accurate understanding of the points taught about the prescribed antitussive.

• The patient correctly lists the signs of toxicity and the actions to take if they appear.

OTHER ANTITUSSIVES

Diphenhydramine hydrochloride and lidocaine hydrochloride also provide antitussive effects. However, these drugs are used infrequently for this purpose.

diphenhydramine hydrochloride (Benadryl, Benylin). This drug is effective in suppressing cough. Although it is an antihistamine, diphenhydramine is thought to have a central and peripheral mechanism of action. Adverse reactions include the typical reactions to other antihistamines, including sedation and anticholinergic effects. (For a discussion of antihistamines, see Chapter 56, Antihistaminic Agents.) The nurse should administer diphenhydramine cautiously to a patient who takes sedatives or tranquilizers or ingests alcohol because of the additive CNS depressant effect.

lidocaine hydrochloride (Xylocaine). This drug is a local anesthetic that physicians can prescribe to suppress the cough reflex associated with tracheal intubation. Lidocaine also is administered topically for diagnostic procedures, such as bronchoscopy. (For further discussion, see Chapter 24, Local and Topical Anesthetic Agents.)

MUCOLYTICS

The epithelial tissues and bronchial glands of the respiratory tract continuously produce mucus, which the mucociliary clearance mechanism removes. If the mucus becomes excessive or so viscid that it interferes with the ciliary action, it can obstruct the airways. Mucolytics are drugs that purportedly alter mucus composition and thereby reduce its viscosity.

The two types of mucolytics include thiol compounds and proteolytic enzymes. Many thiol compounds have been studied for their mucolytic activity. Although some may provide mucolytic activity, most are toxic for use in vivo. Acetylcysteine is the only thiol compound used clinically in the United States to treat patients with abnormal, viscid, or inspissated (thick, hard) mucus. It also is used to treat acetaminophen overdose

Health care professionals rarely use the proteolytic enzymes because the expense and toxicity of these enzymes outweigh their minor therapeutic benefits. Proteolytic enzymes include deoxyribonuclease, trypsin, chymotrypsin, and leucine aminopeptidase.

PHARMACOKINETICS

Acetylcysteine is absorbed from the pulmonary epithelium and metabolized in the liver.

Absorption, distribution, metabolism, excretion

Acetylcysteine acts directly on the mucus. After the drug-mucus reaction, the remaining acetylcysteine is absorbed from the pulmonary epithelium and metabolized in the liver. Researchers do not know if acetylcysteine is excreted in the breast milk of lactating women; controlled studies of the use of acetylcysteine in pregnant women are unavailable.

Onset, peak, duration

The onset of action of acetylcysteine occurs 1 minute after inhalation and immediately after direct application or instillation. Maximal effect occurs in 5 to 10 minutes after inhalation. Additional data about peak concentration levels, duration of action, and half-life remain unavailable.

PHARMACODYNAMICS

Acetylcysteine decreases the viscosity of respiratory tract secretions by altering the molecular composition of mucus. Deoxyribonucleic acid and glycoproteins contribute to the mucus viscosity. The glycoprotein molecular complexes are bridged by disulfide bonds. When acetylcysteine splits these disulfide bonds, mucus viscosity decreases.

Mechanism of action

The mechanism of action of acetylcysteine depends on the sulfhydryl group in the drug. Drugs such as acetylcysteine that contain a free sulfhydryl group split the disulfide bridges between glycoprotein molecular complexes. The action alters the molecular composition of mucus and decreases mucus viscosity. (For an illustration, see *Action of acetylcysteine.*)

The mechanism of action when acetylcysteine is used for acetaminophen (acetylcysteine metabolite) overdose has not been determined fully. Evidence suggests that a sulfhydryl-containing compound inactivates the hepatotoxic metabolite.

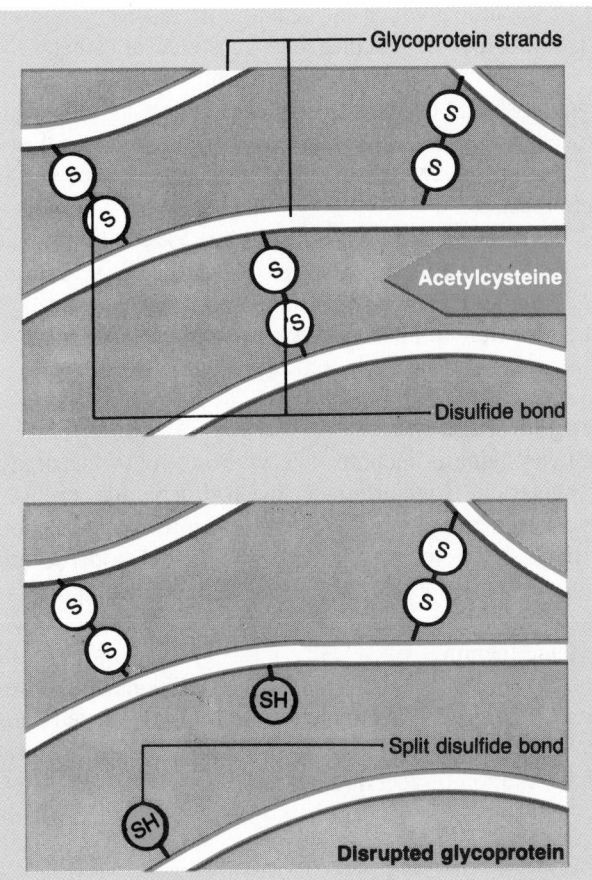

Action of acetylcysteine

Acetylcysteine's free sulfhydryl group splits the disulfide bridge between glycoprotein molecular complexes, disrupting the glycoprotein strands and changing mucus viscosity.

Glycoprotein strands

Acetylcysteine

Disulfide bond

Split disulfide bond

Disrupted glycoprotein

PHARMACOTHERAPEUTICS

Mucolytics are used as adjunctive therapy to treat patients with abnormal, viscid, or inspissated mucus secretions. Mucolytic therapy may benefit patients with bronchitis, emphysema, or pulmonary complications related to cystic fibrosis, as well as patients who develop atelectasis secondary to mucus obstruction, as may occur in pneumonia, bronchiectasis, or chronic bronchitis. Mucolytics also may be used to prepare patients for bronchograms and other bronchial studies. Acetylcysteine is the antidote for acetaminophen overdose; however, it does not provide full protection from hepatic damage caused by the overdose. This drug also is used for tracheostomy care.

acetylcysteine (Mucomyst). This agent reduces mucus viscosity. Acetylcysteine can be used for lung disorders in which mucus overproduction in the respiratory tract causes an accumulation of secretions. This accumulation may interfere with gas exchange and provide a medium for infection. Acetylcysteine usually is administered via a nebulizer.
Usual adult dosage: via nebulizer, 3 to 5 ml of a 20% solution, t.i.d. or q.i.d., or 6 to 10 ml of a 10% solution, t.i.d. or q.i.d.; for direct instillation, 1 to 2 ml of a 10% to 20% solution, which can be administered every hour via a tracheal tube or percutaneous transtracheal catheter.

For tracheostomy care, 1 to 2 ml of a 10% to 20% solution should be given every 1 to 4 hours; for diagnostic procedures, 1 to 2 ml of a 20% solution or 2 to 4 ml of a 10% solution—two to three doses should be given before the procedure.

To treat acetaminophen overdose, a 5% solution should be used, with a loading dose of 140 mg/kg P.O. followed by 70 mg/kg P.O. every 4 hours for 17 doses. If the patient vomits within an hour after receiving a dose of acetylcysteine, the dose should be repeated.

Drug interactions

Acetylcysteine is incompatible with the following drugs: amphotericin B, chlortetracycline hydrochloride, erythromycin lactobionate, oxytetracycline hydrochloride, ampicillin sodium, tetracycline hydrochloride, iodized oil, hydrogen peroxide, chymotrypsin, and trypsin. The nurse should not administer any of these drugs during acetylcysteine therapy.

Activated charcoal decreases acetylcysteine's effectiveness. Therefore, in acetaminophen overdose, activated charcoal should be removed by gastric lavage before the oral administration of acetylcysteine.

ADVERSE DRUG REACTIONS

Acetylcysteine provides a wide margin of safety; however, its "rotten egg" odor during administration may lead to nausea. With prolonged or persistent use, acetylcysteine may produce stomatitis, nausea, vomiting, drowsiness, and severe rhinorrhea.

Hypersensitivity rarely occurs; however, a rash can develop with prolonged or frequent exposure to acetylcysteine. Patients may have bronchorrhea, which may cause increased airway obstruction for those who cannot expectorate effectively. Bronchospasm can occur, particularly in asthmatic patients. The frequency of this adverse reaction increases with the 20% solution. Because bronchospasm can occur unpredictably, the nurse must monitor patients closely during inhalation therapy.

NURSING PROCESS APPLICATION

The following information assists the nursing in caring for a patient who is receiving acetylcysteine.

Assessment
• Review the patient's history for a preexisting condition that contraindicates the use of acetylcysteine, such as known hypersensitivity to the drug.
• Review the patient's history for a condition that requires cautious use of acetylcysteine, such as pregnancy, lactation, asthma, or advanced age or debilitation in a patient with severe respiratory insufficiency.
• Assess the patient for adverse reactions to acetylcysteine, such as stomatitis, nausea, vomiting, drowsiness, severe rhinorrhea, bronchospasm, or hypersensitivity reactions.
• Assess the effectiveness of acetylcysteine periodically.
• Review the patient's medication history to identify the use of drugs that may interact with acetylcysteine, such as amphotericin B, chlortetracycline, erythromycin, other antibiotics, or activated charcoal.
• Inspect the patient's oral cavity frequently for stomatitis.
• Evaluate the patient's and family's knowledge about acetylcysteine.

Nursing diagnoses
The following examples represent appropriate nursing diagnoses for a patient receiving acetylcysteine.
• Potential for injury related to a preexisting condition that contraindicates the use of acetylcysteine
• Potential for injury related to a preexisting condition that requires cautious use of acetylcysteine
• Potential for injury related to adverse drug reactions
• Potential for injury related to drug interactions
• Altered oral mucous membrane related to acetylcysteine-induced stomatitis
• Knowledge deficit related to acetylcysteine

Planning and implementation

• Do not administer acetylcysteine to a patient with a condition that contraindicates its use.

• Administer acetylcysteine cautiously to a patient at risk because of a preexisting condition.

• Monitor the patient closely for adverse reactions during acetylcysteine therapy.

• Prepare the patient for the drug's "rotten egg" smell, which may cause nausea.

• Monitor hydration if the patient develops stomatitis, nausea, or vomiting. Obtain a prescription for an antiemetic agent, as needed.

• *Take safety precautions if drowsiness occurs. For example, place the bed in the low position, keep the bed rails up, and supervise ambulation.*

• Inspect the patient's skin regularly for a rash during frequent or long-term acetylcysteine therapy.

• *Be prepared to administer a beta$_2$-adrenergic agonist by aerosol, as prescribed, if the patient experiences bronchospasm.*

• *Administer acetylcysteine via nebulizer. Because acetylcysteine reacts with iron, copper, and rubber, frequently monitor the patient's nebulizer equipment for reactive effects. The drug does not react with glass, plastic, aluminum, or stainless steel.*

• Use 10% and 20% acetylcysteine solutions undiluted, as prescribed. If further dilution is needed, use normal saline (0.9% sodium chloride) solution or sterile water for injection. During continuous nebulization with dry gas, when three-fourths of the initial volume has been nebulized, dilute the remaining solution with an equal volume of sterile water for injection.

• *Avoid contamination of the solution and refrigerate an opened vial; acetylcysteine does not contain an antimicrobial agent. Discard opened vials after 96 hours.*

• Administer discolored acetylcysteine, if needed. The drug may discolor to a light purple, which does not significantly affect the drug's mucolytic efficacy or safety.

• *Assess the patient's respiratory status before and after each administration, particularly noting any breathing difficulty, ineffective cough, or dyspnea. Follow acetylcysteine administration with chest physiotherapy and postural drainage if prescribed, and encourage coughing and deep breathing to facilitate removal of respiratory secretions. Suction the patient as needed.*

• Have the patient gargle after the respiratory treatments to relieve the unpleasant odor and dryness; wash the patient's face to eliminate stickiness caused by the drug.

• Clean the equipment after use because any drug residue may clog or corrode the equipment parts.

• Notify the physician if adverse reactions occur or if acetylcysteine is ineffective.

• Do not administer drugs that are incompatible with acetylcysteine.

• *Remove previously administered activated charcoal by gastric lavage before administering acetylcysteine to treat acetaminophen overdose as prescribed. If the patient vomits within 1 hour of acetylcysteine administration, repeat the dose.*

• Notify the physician if drug interactions occur.

• *Monitor the patient closely for signs of stomatitis, such as swollen, tender gums that bleed easily, papulovesicular ulcers in the mouth and throat, malaise, irritability, or fever.*

• Rinse the patient's mouth with warm, water mouth solutions if stomatitis occurs. Avoid antiseptic mouthwashes, which are irritating. Obtain a prescription for a topical anesthetic to relieve mouth ulcer pain. Change the patient's diet to a bland or liquid diet until symptoms subside.

• Notify the physician if stomatitis occurs; acetylcysteine therapy may need to be discontinued.

Patient teaching

• Teach the patient and family the name, dose, frequency, action, and adverse effects of acetylcysteine.

• *Advise the patient not to perform activities that require alertness if drowsiness occurs.*

• Show the patient how to use and maintain the nebulizer.

• *Teach the patient and family how to avoid contamination of the solution. Tell them that acetylcysteine may discolor to a light purple, but is still usable. Instruct the patient and family to refrigerate an opened vial and to discard it after 96 hours.*

• Stress the importance of gargling after treatment to relieve odor; also inform the patient about effective coughing before and after each treatment. Teach the patient and family to perform chest physiotherapy and postural drainage after acetylcysteine administration, if prescribed.

• Teach the patient to recognize signs of stomatitis and, if they occur, to manage symptoms appropriately.

• *Instruct the patient to seek medical help if the respiratory condition becomes progressively worse or if adverse reactions occur.*

Evaluation

The following examples represent appropriate evaluation statements for a patient receiving acetylcysteine.

• The patient has no conditions that contraindicate acetylcysteine therapy.

• The patient exhibits no signs of complications in the preexisting condition linked to acetylcysteine.

• The patient displays no adverse reactions to acetylcysteine.

• The patient uses no drugs that interact with acetylcysteine.

• The patient maintains normal integrity of the oral mucosa during acetylcysteine therapy.

• The patient and family express an accurate understanding of the points taught about acetylcysteine.

SELECTED MAJOR DRUGS

Expectorant, antitussive, and mucolytic agents

The following chart summarizes the major expectorant, antitussive, and mucolytic agents currently in clinical use.

DRUG	MAJOR INDICATIONS	USUAL ADULT DOSAGES	CONTRAINDICATIONS AND PRECAUTIONS
Expectorant			
guaifenesin	Cough associated with common cold and upper respiratory tract infection	200 to 400 mg every 4 hours, not to exceed 2.4 grams/day	• Know that guaifenesin is contraindicated in a patient with known hypersensitivity to the drug. • Administer with caution to a pregnant or lactating patient or one with an ineffective cough reflex or respiratory insufficiency.
Antitussives			
codeine	Nonproductive cough	10 to 20 mg every 4 to 6 hours, not to exceed 120 mg/day	• Know that codeine is contraindicated in a pregnant or lactating patient, one with a productive cough or known hypersensitivity to codeine, or one who can benefit from coughing, such as a postoperative patient. • Administer with caution to a debilitated patient, one who has undergone thoracotomy or laparotomy, or one with a history of drug or alcohol abuse.
dextromethorphan	Nonproductive cough	10 to 20 mg every 4 hours or 30 mg every 6 to 8 hours, not to exceed 120 mg/day; long-acting preparations, 60 mg every 12 hours	• Know that dextromethorphan is contraindicated in a patient with a productive cough or known hypersensitivity to the drug, one who is receiving an MAO inhibitor, or one who can benefit from coughing, such as a postoperative patient. • Administer with caution to a pregnant or lactating patient or one with prostatic hypertrophy.
Mucolytic			
acetylcysteine	Bronchopulmonary diseases (chronic bronchitis, emphysema, bronchiectasis, pneumonia, atelectasis, cystic fibrosis)	Nebulization: 3 to 5 ml (20% solution) t.i.d. or q.i.d., or 6 to 10 ml (10% solution) t.i.d. or q.i.d. Direct instillation: 1 to 2 ml of a 10% to 20% solution every hour	• Know that acetylcysteine is contraindicated in a patient with known hypersensitivity to this agent. • Administer with caution to an asthmatic, pregnant, or lactating patient or an elderly or debilitated patient with severe respiratory insufficiency.

• The patient demonstrates effective coughing, and the family demonstrates correct chest physiotherapy and postural drainage techniques.

CHAPTER SUMMARY

Chapter 39 focused on expectorants, antitussives, and mucolytics. It began with a discussion of mucus production in the respiratory tract, the mucociliary clearance mechanism, and cough. Here are the chapter highlights.

• Expectorants are administered to patients who experience difficulty expectorating sputum or who retain respiratory tract secretions. Although expectorants may enhance secretion clearance from the tracheobronchial tree, the efficacy of these agents has not been established.

• Guaifenesin, the most frequently used expectorant, is safe when given in recommended dosages. Many combination products that include expectorants are available over the counter. The iodides, iodinated glycerol and potassium iodide, are used less frequently because of their potential for toxicity.

• Narcotic and nonnarcotic antitussives are used to treat a nonproductive cough that is irritating and exhausting.

- The narcotic antitussives act centrally by depressing the cough center in the medulla.
- The most widely used antitussive in the United States, dextromethorphan also acts centrally and rarely causes adverse reactions. Benzonatate, a peripherally acting nonnarcotic antitussive, is as effective as codeine in suppressing the cough reflex and does not cause dependence.
- The antihistamine diphenhydramine has shown effective antitussive action. The local anesthetic lidocaine also is useful in suppressing cough associated with intubation procedures.
- If used in recommended dosages, antitussives are safe. However, the nurse must use caution when administering centrally acting antitussives with other CNS depressants. The nurse should monitor elderly and debilitated patients carefully.
- Antitussive agents should not be used in patients with a productive cough or in situations in which coughing is beneficial.
- Mucolytics reduce the mucus viscosity and elasticity. They are used to facilitate sputum expectoration and to unblock airways that are plugged with mucus.
- Acetylcysteine is the only thiol compound mucolytic clinically used in the United States.
- Aerosol administration of acetylcysteine can produce bronchospasm; prolonged or persistent use may produce stomatitis, nausea, vomiting, drowsiness, or severe rhinorrhea.
- Acetylcysteine is the antidote for acetaminophen overdose.
- When administering an expectorant, antitussive, or mucolytic agent, the nurse should apply the nursing process, providing care that includes monitoring for adverse drug reactions, screening for drug interactions, and using appropriate administration procedures.

STUDY QUESTIONS

See Appendix 1 for answers

1. Leonard Cantwell, age 53, seeks care for the fatigue, fever, and cough of influenza. His physician prescribes guaifenesin (Breonesin) 200 mg P.O. every 4 hours. What is the mechanism of action of this expectorant?
(a) cough reflex suppression
(b) production of mucostasis
(c) salivary gland stimulation
(d) promotion of mucus removal

2. The physician could have prescribed an iodide expectorant for Mr. Cantwell. What accounts for the limited use of iodide expectorants?
(a) potential for toxic effects
(b) limited efficacy as expectorants
(c) wide range of drug interactions
(d) potential for dependence

3. If Mr. Cantwell were receiving an iodide expectorant, the nurse would have to assess for functional changes in which organ?
(a) thymus
(b) kidneys
(c) lower intestine
(d) thyroid gland

4. Della Drake, age 38, has mycoplasmic pneumonia associated with a harsh, persistent, productive cough. Her physician prescribes hydrocodone bitartrate (Hycodan) 5 mg P.O. every 6 hours. For which type of cough are antitussives used?
(a) occasional cough
(b) nonproductive cough
(c) persistent cough that is exhausting
(d) productive cough

5. Hydrocodone bitartrate is a centrally acting antitussive. How do centrally acting and peripherally acting antitussives differ?
(a) Centrally acting antitussives are nonaddictive; peripherally acting antitussives are.
(b) Centrally acting antitussives depress the cough center in the medulla; peripherally acting antitussives do not.
(c) Centrally acting antitussives are less effective than peripherally acting antitussives.
(d) Centrally acting antitussives require larger doses than peripherally acting antitussives to achieve desired effects.

6. Michael Evans, age 21, has developed pulmonary complications of cystic fibrosis. His physician prescribes acetylcysteine (Mucomyst) 3 ml of a 20% solution t.i.d. via nebulizer. How does acetylcysteine improve respiratory status?
(a) It alters the molecular composition of mucus, which decreases its viscosity.
(b) It promotes ciliary activity, which increases secretion removal.
(c) It stimulates the cough reflex, which increases secretion expectoration.
(d) It dries up secretions, which improves respirations.

7. Before administering acetylcysteine, the nurse checks Mr. Evans's history for asthma. Why must acetylcysteine be used cautiously in an asthmatic patient?
(a) It acts as a respiratory depressant.
(b) It acts as a respiratory stimulant.
(c) It may produce bronchospasm.
(d) It inhibits the cough reflex.

8. Acetylcysteine also may be used to treat what other condition?
(a) acetaminophen overdose
(b) severe rhinorrhea
(c) hepatic tumor
(d) stomatitis

SELECTED REFERENCES

AHFS drug information 90. (1990). Bethesda, MD: American Society of Hospital Pharmacists.

Bardana, E., Braman, S., and Johnson, J. (1989). Chronic cough in a nonsmoker. *Patient Care,* 23(2), 42-56.

Brown, L. (1988). The effective cough. *Critical Care Nurse,* 8(2), 77-82.

Goodman and Gilman's the pharmacological basis of therapeutics (8th ed.; 1990). Elmsford, NY: Pergamon Press.

Hansten, P., and Horn, J. (1989). *Drug interactions* (6th ed.). Philadelphia: Lea & Febiger.

Kim, M., and Larson, J. (1987). Ineffective airway clearance and ineffective breathing patterns: Theoretical and research base for nursing diagnosis. *Nursing Clinics of North America,* 22(1), 125-134.

North American Nursing Diagnosis Association. (1990). *Taxonomy I-Revised, with official diagnostic categories.* St. Louis: NANDA.

USPDI. (1991). *Drug information for the health care professional* (Vol. I, 11th ed.). Rockville, MD: United States Pharmacopeial Convention.

DECONGESTANT AGENTS

OBJECTIVES

After reading and studying this chapter, the student should be able to:
1. Differentiate between the pharmacokinetic properties of the systemic and topical decongestants.
2. Explain the mechanism of action of systemic and topical decongestants in relieving upper respiratory tract signs and symptoms.
3. Compare the major drug interactions that can occur with systemic decongestants and topical decongestants.
4. Contrast the adverse drug reactions associated with systemic decongestants and topical decongestants.
5. Describe the physiologic mechanisms that produce rebound nasal congestion.
6. Describe how to apply the nursing process when caring for a patient who is receiving a decongestant agent.

INTRODUCTION

Decongestants provide their major benefit by helping to relieve upper respiratory tract signs and symptoms associated with the common cold. Reviewing the physiologic mechanisms by which these respiratory signs and symptoms develop will aid in understanding the use of the decongestants discussed in this chapter.

The respiratory system serves as one of the first lines of defense against microbial invasion of the body. Hairs located in the nasal turbinates filter out the largest invading particles. Smaller particles become trapped in the nasal mucus or mix with acidic nasal secretions. The cilia in the epithelium lining the nose move the trapped particles toward the pharynx, where they are swallowed or coughed to the exterior. Particles that manage to reach the lower respiratory tract become trapped in mucus secreted by the goblet cells and bronchial glands. Cilia in the lower respiratory passages then sweep the mucus up toward the phar-

ynx where it and the trapped particles are swallowed or expectorated. (For an illustration of these defense mechanisms, see *Respiratory tract lining* in the introduction to this unit.) Particles or microorganisms not removed in this manner are carried lower into the alveoli where macrophages ingest them.

Organisms entering the mouth come in contact with saliva, which acts as a cleanser of the oral cavity. Saliva contains IgA antibodies and, even more important, lysozyme, which breaks down the cell walls of bacteria. Swallowed saliva as well as swallowed mucus secretions from the respiratory passages force the trapped organism into contact with gastric acids, enzymes, and bile.

When invading organisms elude the respiratory and oropharyngeal barriers, infection results. As the infecting organism acts on invaded structures, cellular disruption and neutrophil migration occur. Histamine, released from circulating basophils, connective tissue, mast cells, and platelets, causes local vasodilation and increased permeability to protein. The neutrophils release active kallikrein, which passes through the permeable capillaries, splitting kininogen into kinins. Potent vasodilators, the kinins cause further vasodilation and permeability to protein. As these changes occur, fluid leaks from capillaries into the surrounding tissues, resulting in edema and swelling of the nasal passages. The use of decongestants relieves the swelling in clogged nasal passages associated with the common cold. Primarily synthetic versions of epinephrine, most decongestants are termed sympathomimetic in action and are used systemically or topically.

For a summary of representative drugs, see *Selected major drugs: Decongestant agents,* page 694. For a listing of applicable nursing diagnoses that the nurse may formulate when caring for a patient receiving these agents, see *Selected nursing diagnoses: Decongestant agents,* page 686. For detailed information on applying the nursing process, see Chapter 6, The Nursing Process and Drug Therapy.

SYSTEMIC DECONGESTANTS

As sympathomimetic amines, the systemic decongestants activate the sympathetic division of the autonomic nervous system. The three major systemic decongestants are ephedrine, phenylpropanolamine, and pseudoephedrine. These three drugs stimulate alpha receptors in vascular smooth muscle, thereby constricting arterioles of the nasal mucosa while reducing blood flow and edema. These actions open the nasal passages, increase airflow, and promote sinus drainage.

PHARMACOKINETICS

The systemic decongestants prove clinically effective when taken orally. They are distributed widely throughout the body and are excreted primarily unchanged in the urine.

Absorption, distribution, metabolism, excretion

The systemic decongestants discussed in this chapter are absorbed readily from the gastrointestinal (GI) tract after oral intake. The drugs are distributed widely throughout the body into various tissues and fluids, including the cerebrospinal fluid, placenta, and breast milk. Slowly and incompletely metabolized by the liver, the drugs are excreted largely unchanged in the urine within 24 hours after oral administration.

From 55% to 75% of ephedrine and pseudoephedrine and 80% to 90% of phenylpropanolamine is excreted unchanged. Acidic urine accelerates excretion of ephedrine and pseudoephedrine. Conversely, alkaline urine with a pH of about 8 decreases the excretion rate, increasing reabsorption in the renal tubules.

Onset, peak, duration

After oral administration of the systemic decongestants, the onset of nasal decongestion is 15 to 30 minutes, peaking within 60 to 90 minutes. The duration of action is 3 to 6 hours for tablets and syrups, and 8 to 12 hours for sustained-release capsules and tablets.

For ephedrine and pseudoephedrine, the half-life is 3 hours with a urine pH of 5, and about 6 hours with a pH of 6.3. Phenylpropanolamine has a half-life of 3 to 4 hours.

PHARMACODYNAMICS

The systemic decongestants are used for their vasoconstrictor effects in reducing nasal congestion associated with the common cold and other upper respiratory disorders. Drug effects result from direct or indirect action on target receptors.

Mechanism of action

Ephedrine, phenylpropanolamine, and pseudoephedrine act directly and indirectly. When taken orally, the drugs act directly on alpha-adrenergic receptors in the nasal mucosa and elsewhere, causing contraction of urinary and GI sphincters, mydriasis, and decreased pancreatic beta cell secretion. The major activity of these drugs, however, occurs indirectly and results in norepinephrine release from storage sites. The release of norepinephrine, a catecholamine, together with the direct action on receptors, produces vasoconstriction and nasal decongestion.

Additional effects of the drugs result primarily from stimulation of beta-adrenergic receptors. The effects of this indirect drug action include increased heart rate, force of myocardial contraction, and cardiac output, as well as relaxation of bronchial smooth muscle.

PHARMACOTHERAPEUTICS

Systemic decongestants are indicated for the symptomatic relief of swollen nasal membranes resulting from hay fever, allergic rhinitis, vasomotor rhinitis, acute coryza, sinusitis, and the common cold. Ephedrine, phenylpropanolamine, and pseudoephedrine are administered orally, frequently with other drugs, such as antihistamines, antimuscarinics, antipyretic-analgesics, caffeine, and antitussives.

The systemic decongestants offer the advantages of lengthy symptom relief and over-the-counter (OTC) availability. The major disadvantage is the systemic stimulation that occurs primarily as a result of alpha- and beta-receptor stimulation combined with norepinephrine release from the indirect action. The topical decongestants serve as alternatives to these systemic drugs. Although the topical drugs produce fewer systemic adverse effects, equally distressing effects do occur. (For details, see the "Adverse drug reactions" sections of this chapter.)

ephedrine sulfate. Ephedrine rarely is prescribed because of rebound hyperemia of the nasal mucosa, central nervous system (CNS) stimulation, transient hypertension, and palpitations associated with the drug's use. Effective orally, ephedrine is available in capsules and syrup.
Usual adult dosage: 25 to 50 mg P.O. every 3 to 4 hours.

phenylpropanolamine (Propagest, Rhindecon, Sucrets Cold Decongestant Formula). An extensively used oral nasal decongestant, phenylpropanolamine resembles ephedrine pharmacologically, but produces fewer adverse effects. The use of phenylpropanolamine can relieve nasal congestion associated with acute and chronic rhinitis, sinusitis, the common cold, hay fever, and other allergies. Available as a single-ingredient decongestant and in combination products, phenylpropanolamine is available OTC.
Usual adult dosage: 25 mg P.O. every 4 hours, or 75 mg P.O. of the sustained-release preparation every 12 hours. Dosage should not exceed 150 mg P.O. daily.

pseudoephedrine hydrochloride (Novafed, Sudafed), **pseudoephedrine sulfate** (Afrinol Repetabs). Similar to ephedrine in its uses and properties, pseudoephedrine is used more frequently because of the infrequent occurrence of CNS stimulation and hypertension associated with its use. Associated rebound congestion is minimal to absent. Available without a prescription, pseudoephedrine is used to treat nasal congestion and serous otitis media accompanied by eustachian tube congestion.
Usual adult dosage: 60 mg P.O. every 4 to 6 hours, or 120 mg P.O. of the sustained-release preparation every 12 hours.

Drug interactions

When given concurrently with other drugs, systemic decongestants may result in one of three different types of drug interactions. The first type of interaction may occur with the simultaneous administration of two or more drugs having opposing effects. Under these circumstances, the effects of one drug override the intended effects of the second.

A second type of interaction between drugs occurs when systemic decongestants are administered with other sympathomimetic amines. This interaction causes additive or cumulative drug effects, and potentiates the adverse effects of both drugs.

The third type of drug interaction occurs with concurrent administration of drugs that interfere with the excretion of sympathomimetic amines. Because the excretion of pseudoephedrine and ephedrine sulfate depends on urine acidity, the nurse needs to monitor drugs that alter urine pH. In the presence of alkaline urine, renal tubular reabsorption of these sympathomimetic amines increases. (For a detailed summary, see *Drug interactions: Systemic decongestants,* page 688.)

ADVERSE DRUG REACTIONS

The systemic decongestants produce primarily dose-related adverse reactions associated with norepinephrine action; however, not all of the reactions are dose-related. Other reactions associated with systemic decongestants include drug hypersensitivity and teratogenic effects.

The incidence and severity of adverse reactions depend on the patient's sensitivity to systemic decongestants. Patients who are hypersensitive to other sympathomimetic amines also may be hypersensitive to the systemic decongestants. The nurse should discourage the use of systemic decongestants by patients exhibiting this kind of drug sensitivity.

For nonsensitive patients, the incidence of adverse reactions is low. The most common adverse reactions result from CNS stimulation and include nervousness, restlessness, and insomnia. Nausea, palpitations, increased difficulty in urinating, and dose-related elevations in blood pressure occasionally occur.

Less dose-related reactions to systemic decongestants include first-time drug hypersensitivity reactions, teratogenic effects, and effects in breast-feeding infants. Other reactions include irregular heartbeat or tachycardia, feeling of tightness in the chest, hallucinations, seizures, headache, and greatly elevated blood pressure.

Because of the unpredictable and unknown effects of systemic decongestants on the fetus, a pregnant patient should avoid these drugs. Furthermore, these decongestants distribute to breast milk and result in high risk to the breast-feeding infant.

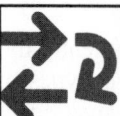

DRUG INTERACTIONS

Systemic decongestants

Systemic decongestants potentiate the effect of sympathetic nervous system stimulating drugs and interact with monoamine oxidase (MAO) inhibitors, releasing large amounts of stored norepinephrine.

DRUG	INTERACTING DRUGS	POSSIBLE EFFECTS	NURSING IMPLICATIONS
ephedrine, phenylpropanolamine, pseudoephedrine	other sympathomimetic amines, including epinephrine, norepinephrine, dopamine, dobutamine, isoproterenol, metaproterenol, terbutaline, phenylephrine, tyramine	Increase central nervous system stimulation	• Do not administer drugs concurrently because the interaction can be life-threatening.
	MAO inhibitors	May cause severe hypertension or hypertensive crisis	• Do not administer drugs concurrently because the interaction can be life-threatening.
pseudoephedrine	alkalinizing agents	Decrease urinary excretion of pseudoephedrine	• Monitor the patient for signs of increased pseudoephedrine effect, such as excessively dry nasal passages.

NURSING PROCESS APPLICATION

The following information assists the nurse in caring for a patient who is receiving a systemic decongestant.

Assessment
• Review the patient's history for a preexisting condition that contraindicates the use of a systemic decongestant, such as pregnancy, lactation, monoamine oxidase (MAO) inhibitor therapy, porphyria, severe coronary artery disease, cardiac arrhythmias, narrow-angle glaucoma, psychoneurosis, or known hypersensitivity to systemic decongestants.
• Assess the patient's history for a preexisting condition that requires cautious use of a systemic decongestant, such as advanced age, hypertension, hyperthyroidism, cardiovascular disease, or prostatic hypertrophy.
• Assess the patient for adverse reactions to the prescribed systemic decongestant, such as drug hypersensitivity, CNS stimulation, nausea, difficulty in urinating, hypertension, headache, or arrhythmias.
• Review the patient's medication history to identify the use of drugs that may interact with the prescribed systemic decongestant, such as other sympathomimetic amines, MAO inhibitors, hypoglycemic agents, or alkalinizing agents.
• Assess the patient regularly for signs of urine retention during systemic decongestant therapy.
• Evaluate the patient's and family's knowledge about the prescribed systemic decongestant.

Nursing diagnoses
The following examples represent appropriate nursing diagnoses for a patient receiving a systemic decongestant.
• Potential for injury related to a preexisting condition that contraindicates the use of a systemic decongestant
• Potential for injury related to a preexisting condition that requires cautious use of a systemic decongestant
• Potential for injury related to adverse drug reactions
• Potential for injury related to drug interactions
• Urine retention related to the adverse genitourinary effects of the systemic decongestant
• Knowledge deficit related to the prescribed systemic decongestant

Planning and implementation
• Do not administer a systemic decongestant to a patient with a condition that contraindicates its use.
• Administer a systemic decongestant cautiously to a patient at risk because of a preexisting condition.
• Monitor the patient closely for adverse reactions during systemic decongestant therapy.
• *Discourage the use of OTC systemic decongestants in a patient who is hypersensitive to other sympathomimetic amines. Such a patient also may be hypersensitive to systemic decongestants.*
• *Monitor the patient's blood pressure, pulse, and electrocardiogram (ECG), as instructed, particularly noting hypertension and an irregular heartbeat or tachycardia.*
• Reassure the patient who experiences nervousness, restlessness, insomnia, nausea, or palpitations that these dose-related adverse reactions should disappear when the drug is discontinued.

• *Take seizure precautions during systemic decongestant therapy.*

• Obtain a prescription for an analgesic if the patient develops a headache.

• *Take safety precautions and notify the physician if the patient experiences hallucinations. For example, place the bed in a low position, keep the bed rails up, and closely supervise the patient's activities.*

• Notify the physician if adverse reactions occur.

• *Do not administer other sympathomimetic amines concomitantly because increased CNS stimulation can occur.*

• *Notify the physician if the patient uses drugs that alter urine pH because alkaline urine increases renal tubular reabsorption of sympathomimetic amines.*

• Assess the effectiveness of the systemic decongestant periodically.

• *Encourage the patient to report difficulty urinating, which is especially common in patients with prostatic hypertrophy.*

• Palpate the bladder after the patient voids to detect urine retention.

• Notify the physician if the patient develops urine retention.

Patient teaching

• Teach the patient and family the name, dose, frequency, action, and adverse effects of the prescribed systemic decongestant.

• Teach how to use the systemic decongestant correctly. Instruct the patient to recognize and report any adverse reactions because a dosage change may be needed.

• Encourage avoidance of systemic decongestants if the patient is pregnant or lactating or has a condition that contraindicates their use. Such a patient should ask the physician to recommend an appropriate decongestant.

• *Inform the patient that the systemic decongestant may interfere with sleep, and suggest taking the drug a few hours before bedtime to minimize any insomnia. Also, remind the patient not to take more than the recommended amount and to consult with the physician before taking OTC products.*

• *Instruct the patient to use the drug in its complete form when taking sustained-release capsules or long-acting tablets. The patient should not break, cut, crush, or chew the capsule or tablet.*

Evaluation

The following examples represent appropriate evaluation statements for a patient receiving a systemic decongestant.

• The patient has no conditions that contraindicate systemic decongestant therapy.

• The patient exhibits no signs of complications in the preexisting condition linked to the prescribed systemic decongestant.

• The patient exhibits no adverse reactions to the prescribed systemic decongestant.

• The patient uses no drugs that interact with the prescribed systemic decongestant.

• The patient maintains a normal voiding pattern.

• The patient and family express an accurate understanding of the prescribed systemic decongestant.

• The patient correctly demonstrates how to use the prescribed systemic decongestant.

TOPICAL DECONGESTANTS

Selected sympathomimetic amine decongestants provide immediate relief from nasal congestion and swollen mucous membranes when applied directly to the nasal mucosa. Because these drugs, referred to as topical decongestants, are applied directly to the mucous membranes only and are not administered orally, they are discussed separately.

The mechanism of action of topical decongestants resembles that of the systemic decongestants; however, the topical decongestants display more receptor specificity and usually provide a faster onset of action, shorter duration, and fewer systemic effects. Topical decongestants include sympathomimetic amines (ephedrine, epinephrine, phenylephrine, and propylhexedrine) and imidazoline derivatives of sympathomimetic amines (naphazoline, oxymetazoline, tetrahydrozoline, xylometazoline).

PHARMACOKINETICS

Topical application of the sympathomimetic amines and imidazoline derivatives of the sympathomimetic amines provides immediate relief of nasal congestion and restricts drug absorption. The duration of symptom relief, however, usually is short.

Absorption, distribution, metabolism, excretion

Topical decongestants act directly on the alpha receptors of the nasal vascular smooth muscle, thereby constricting arterioles and reducing blood flow in the edematous membranes. As a result of this direct vasoconstriction, vascular absorption becomes negligible.

If topical decongestants are administered accidentally in greater than therapeutic dosage or are administered so that a large amount of the drug enters the nasopharynx and is swallowed, drug absorption will occur and systemic sympathetic stimulation will follow. When swallowed, epinephrine and phenylephrine are absorbed irregularly from the GI tract and metabolized in the liver by the enzymes catechol-O-methyltransferase (COMT) and MAO. By-products of metabolism are excreted in the urine. Furthermore, epinephrine is distributed to the placenta and breast milk. Information on the absorption, distribution, metabolism, and excretion of other topical decongestants is unavailable.

Onset, peak, duration
Onset of action rapidly follows the application of topical decongestants. Drug action then peaks quickly. Sympathomimetic agents provide symptomatic relief within seconds, peaking in 2 to 4 minutes with a 30-minute to 2-hour duration of action. Imidazoline derivatives of the sympathomimetic amines provide relief from nasal congestion within 5 to 10 minutes after application. Their effects last 3 to 10 hours, depending on the preparation.

PHARMACODYNAMICS

Topical decongestants act as local vasoconstrictors to provide rapid relief of nasal congestion.

Mechanism of action
The stimulation of alpha-adrenergic receptors in nasal vascular smooth muscle results in increased alpha-adrenergic activity and vasoconstriction. The subsequent reduction in nasal mucosal blood flow, together with decreased capillary permeability, decreases the edema associated with inflammation. The action of topical decongestants also helps drain sinuses, clear nasal passages, and open eustachian tubes, temporarily improving aeration.

PHARMACOTHERAPEUTICS

The fact that topical decongestants act directly on the alpha-adrenergic receptors in the nose helps explain their narrow scope of use, in contrast to the systemic decongestants, which act on alpha-adrenergic receptors throughout the body. The topical decongestants provide two major advantages: minimal adverse reactions and rapid relief of symptoms.

The rebound nasal congestion that occurs with frequent or long-term use of these drugs is their main disadvantage. This rebound congestion results from an alteration in the vasomotor stability of the nasal mucous membranes caused by repeated and prolonged sympathetic stimulation from the vasoconstrictors. Compensatory parasympathetic activation produces vasodilation and increased secretion. Temporary relief of rebound congestion occurs with even more frequent use of the drugs. When rebound congestion occurs, the patient should discontinue the drug treatment.

ephedrine (Efedron Nasal, Vatronol Nose Drops). This drug is used infrequently because of rebound hyperemia or congestion of the nasal mucosa and tachyphylaxis. Ephedrine is available in 0.5% to 0.6% drops and jelly.
Usual adult dosage: 2 to 3 drops or a small amount of jelly in each nostril every 4 hours, for no more than 4 days.

epinephrine 0.1% (Adrenalin). This endogenous catecholamine is available in drops or spray. Epinephrine drops usually are applied by physicians, who use the drug to control epistaxis or to control bleeding during nasal surgery. Because of the systemic sympathetic stimulating effects of epinephrine, use of the drug as a decongestant is limited.
Usual adult dosage: for decongestant effects, 1 to 2 drops every 4 to 6 hours; for control of epistaxis, not to exceed 1 ml over 15 minutes.

naphazoline (Privine). An imidazoline derivative sympathomimetic amine, naphazoline is applied topically to the nasal mucosa to relieve nasal congestion associated with the common cold, acute or chronic rhinitis, sinusitis, hay fever, and other allergies.
Usual adult dosage: 2 drops or sprays of 0.05% solution in each nostril, repeated every 3 to 6 hours. Duration of therapy should not exceed 5 days because longer use may cause rebound nasal congestion.

oxymetazoline (Afrin, Duration, Dristan Long Lasting). This drug is applied topically to the nasal mucosa to relieve nasal congestion associated with the common cold, acute or chronic rhinitis, sinusitis, hay fever, and other allergies. The duration of action for oxymetazoline, an imidazoline derivative sympathomimetic amine, is longer than that of the other imidazoline derivatives.
Usual adult dosage: 2 to 3 drops or 1 to 2 sprays of 0.05% solution in each nostril b.i.d., morning and evening. As with other topical decongestants, oxymetazoline should be used for short-term relief of symptoms because long-term use can lead to rebound congestion.

phenylephrine (Nōstril, Sinex, Neo-Synephrine). One of the most widely prescribed topical nasal decongestants, phenylephrine provides effects less potent than those of epinephrine but of longer duration. Phenylephrine is recommended for use in patients with otic inflammation or infection because application to the nasal mucosa may open obstructed eustachian tubes. Phenylephrine also helps shrink swollen nasal and pharyngeal membranes, thus increasing visualization of the membranes, which makes the drug useful before surgery. Available in 0.125% to 1% solution and in 0.5% jelly, phenylephrine is inhaled or applied to each nostril.
Usual adult dosage: 1 to 2 sprays or a small amount of jelly in each nostril every 4 hours. Because rebound congestion can occur, duration of therapy should not exceed 3 days.

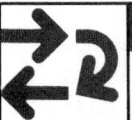

DRUG INTERACTIONS

Topical decongestants

Drug interactions associated with topical decongestants are few but can cause major problems for the patient.

DRUG	INTERACTING DRUGS	POSSIBLE EFFECTS	NURSING IMPLICATIONS
ephedrine, epinephrine, naphazoline, oxymetazoline, phenylephrine, propylhexedrine, tetrahydrozoline, xylometazoline	monoamine oxidase inhibitors	Increase central nervous system stimulation, increase hypertension, and may cause hypertensive crisis	• Do not administer drugs concurrently.
	beta-adrenergic blocking agents, methyldopa, reserpine, guanethidine	Decrease hypotensive drug action	• Do not administer drugs concurrently. • Monitor the patient for changes in blood pressure control.

propylhexedrine (Benzedrex Inhaler). Available in inhalers, propylhexedrine is used topically to relieve nasal congestion associated with the common cold, acute or chronic rhinitis, sinusitis, hay fever, and other allergies. Because propylhexedrine provides a wider margin of safety than ephedrine or epinephrine, it can be used when an increased pressor effect is undesirable. As with other topical decongestants, propylhexedrine should be used only for short-term relief of symptoms because prolonged use can cause rebound congestion.
Usual adult dosage: 2 inhalations in each nostril from the 250-mg inhaler.

tetrahydrozoline (Tyzine). An imidazoline derivative sympathomimetic amine, tetrahydrozoline is applied topically to the nasal mucosa to relieve nasal congestion associated with the common cold, acute or chronic rhinitis, sinusitis, hay fever, and other allergies.
Usual adult dosage: 2 to 4 drops or sprays of 0.1% solution in each nostril, repeated every 3 hours, if needed. Long-term use can cause rebound congestion.

xylometazoline (Otrivin). Another imidazoline derivative sympathomimetic amine, xylometazoline is applied topically to the nasal mucosa to relieve nasal congestion associated with the common cold, acute or chronic rhinitis, sinusitis, hay fever, and other allergies.
Usual adult dosage: 2 or 3 drops or sprays of 0.1% solution in each nostril every 8 to 10 hours, not to exceed three times in 24 hours. Long-term use can lead to rebound congestion.

Drug interactions
Because of the topical drug route and vasoconstrictor action, which decrease drug absorption, drug interactions involving topical decongestants seldom occur. Nonetheless,

if topical decongestants are swallowed, they can cause drug interactions.

One type of interaction may occur after the simultaneous administration of topical decongestants and other drugs having opposing effects. This interaction causes the effects of one drug to override the intended effects of the second.

A second type of interaction between drugs occurs when topical decongestants are administered with similarly acting drugs. This interaction causes additive or cumulative drug effects and may potentiate the adverse effects of both drugs. (For details, see *Drug interactions: Topical decongestants.*)

ADVERSE DRUG REACTIONS

The incidence and severity of adverse reactions depends primarily on the patient's sensitivity to topical decongestants and on the duration of action and frequency of drug use.

The most commonly reported adverse reaction associated with the use of topical decongestants is rebound nasal congestion. The disorder is characterized by hyperemia of the nasal mucosa, which appears red, boggy, and swollen. The rebound nasal congestion usually resolves spontaneously within a few days after discontinuation of the topical decongestant. Upon discontinuation of the drug, however, some patients may require supportive therapy using an oral decongestant and a normal saline spray.

The second most frequent adverse reaction is a transient burning and stinging of the nasal mucosa on application. Patients also report sneezing and mucosal dryness or ulceration.

Less common adverse reactions result from CNS stimulation and include nervousness, restlessness, and insomnia. Occasionally, nausea, palpitations, increased difficulty in urinating, and dose-related elevations in blood pressure occur. Similar to the systemic effects caused by an overdose of most adrenergic drugs, these effects more commonly are associated with administration of epinephrine, ephedrine, phenylephrine, and propylhexedrine. As a result, physicians carefully evaluate the use of topical vasoconstrictor decongestants for patients with cardiovascular disease, diabetes mellitus, increased intraocular pressure, hypertension, hyperthyroidism, or prostatic hypertrophy.

Less predictable adverse reactions may include first-time drug hypersensitivity reactions, teratogenic effects, and effects in breast-feeding infants. Patients who display hypersensitivity to sympathomimetic amines also may be sensitive to the topical decongestants; the nurse should discourage use of these drugs by these patients.

Other reactions are irregular heartbeat or tachycardia, feeling of tightness in the chest, hallucinations, seizures, headache, and greatly elevated blood pressure.

Safe use of topical decongestants during pregnancy and lactation has not been determined. Because of the unpredictable or unknown effect of decongestants on the fetus, pregnant patients should consider carefully the risk versus the benefit of these drugs. Lactating patients should use these decongestants cautiously because of the drugs' distribution in breast milk and the unknown risk to the infant.

NURSING PROCESS APPLICATION

The following information assists the nurse in caring for a patient who is receiving a topical decongestant.

Assessment
• Review the patient's history for a preexisting condition that contraindicates the use of a topical decongestant, such as narrow-angle glaucoma, pregnancy, or known hypersensitivity to topical decongestants.
• Review the patient's history for a preexisting condition that requires cautious use of a topical decongestant, such as hypertension, diabetes mellitus, cardiovascular disease, hyperthyroidism, prostatic hypertrophy, or lactation.
• Assess the patient for adverse reactions to the prescribed topical decongestant, such as rebound nasal congestion, mucosal discomfort or ulceration, CNS stimulation, arrhythmias, or nausea.
• Review the patient's medication history to identify the use of drugs that may interact with the prescribed topical decongestant, such as MAO inhibitors, beta-adrenergic blocking agents, methyldopa, reserpine, or guanethidine.
• Assess the patient's oral and nasal mucosa for signs of dryness or ulceration.
• Evaluate the patient's and family's knowledge about the prescribed topical decongestant.

Nursing diagnoses
The following examples represent appropriate nursing diagnoses for a patient receiving a topical decongestant.
• Potential for injury related to a preexisting condition that contraindicates the use of a topical decongestant
• Potential for injury related to a preexisting condition that requires cautious use of a topical decongestant
• Potential for injury related to adverse drug reactions
• Potential for injury related to drug interactions
• Impaired tissue integrity related to mucosal dryness and ulceration caused by a topical decongestant
• Knowledge deficit related to the prescribed topical decongestant

Planning and implementation
• Do not administer a topical decongestant to a patient with a condition that contraindicates its use.
• Administer a topical decongestant cautiously to a patient at risk because of a preexisting condition.
• Monitor the patient closely for adverse reactions during topical decongestant therapy.
• *Discourage topical decongestant use in a patient with known hypersensitivity to sympathomimetic amines because such a patient is likely to be sensitive to the topical decongestant also.*
• *Inspect the patient for signs of rebound nasal congestion, such as red, swollen, boggy nasal mucosa. If rebound nasal congestion occurs, withhold the drug and notify the physician. Obtain a prescription for normal saline nasal spray, if needed.*
• Warn the patient that transient burning and stinging of the nasal mucosa may occur during administration of the topical decongestant.
• *Monitor the patient's blood pressure, pulse, and ECG, as instructed, to detect hypertension and an irregular heart rate or tachycardia.*
• Reassure the patient who experiences nervousness, restlessness, insomnia, nausea, or palpitations that these dose-related adverse reactions should disappear when the drug is discontinued.
• *Take seizure precautions during topical decongestant therapy.*
• *Take safety precautions and notify the physician if the patient experiences hallucinations. For example, place the bed in the low position, keep the bed rails up, and closely supervise the patient's activities.*
• Encourage the patient to report difficulty urinating, which is especially common in patients with prostatic hypertrophy.
• Palpate the bladder after the patient voids to detect urine retention. If urine retention is present, notify the physician.
• *Administer topical decongestant drops correctly.* (For details, see *Patient positioning for instilling nasal and sinus drops.*)

Patient positioning for instilling nasal and sinus drops

Obtain a box of tissues and the ordered medication. After identifying the patient and explaining the procedure and medication, help the patient assume the appropriate position. The illustrations below show proper head positioning based on the area of congestion. For drops, place the patient in the head low or supine position with the head supported by a pillow. With incorrect patient positioning, the drops will run down the back of the throat and be ineffective. When instilling sprays, the patient should be upright. For drops, place the dropper ⅓ to ½ inch inside the nostril, being careful to avoid touching the dropper to the nostril. Squeeze the dropper bulb to deliver the prescribed number of drops. Instruct the patient to remain in this position for 5 minutes to prevent the medication from running out of the nostrils. Repeat on opposite side if necessary.

Eustachian tubes. Have the patient turn the head laterally to the affected side.

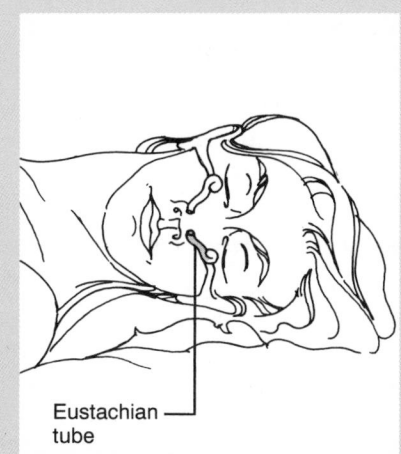

Eustachian tube

Sphenoid or ethmoid sinuses. Have the patient hyperextend the neck over a pillow.

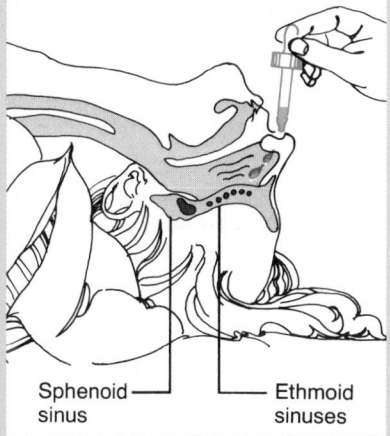

Sphenoid sinus — Ethmoid sinuses

Maxillary and frontal sinuses. Have the patient rotate the head laterally after hyperextension.

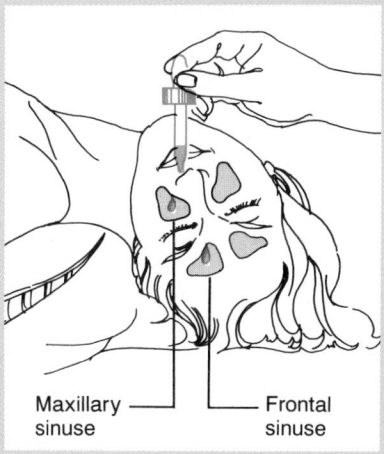

Maxillary sinuse — Frontal sinuse

• Notify the physician if adverse reactions occur.

• *Do not administer an MAO inhibitor, beta-adrenergic blocking agent, methyldopa, reserpine, or guanethidine concomitantly with a topical decongestant.*

• Assess the effectiveness of the topical decongestant periodically.

• *Inspect the patient's oral and nasal mucosa for ulceration regularly.*

• Encourage the patient to use a humidifier if nasal dryness occurs.

• Withhold the topical decongestant if the patient's tissue integrity becomes impaired and notify the physician.

Patient teaching

• Teach the patient and family the name, dose, frequency, action, and adverse effects of the prescribed topical decongestant.

• Teach the patient to recognize and report to the physician any adverse reactions because a dosage change may be needed.

• *Remind the patient not to exceed the recommended amount, frequency, and duration of use. Duration of therapy should not exceed 4 days. Caution the patient about*

taking other OTC products that may interact with the topical decongestant.

• Encourage avoidance of topical decongestants if the patient is pregnant or has narrow-angle glaucoma or hypersensitivity to sympathomimetic agents.

• *Teach the patient to minimize CNS-stimulating effects through proper administration: in the lateral head low position for drops, in the upright position for sprays. Instruct the patient who is using a decongestant to relieve blocked eustachian tubes to instill the drops by lying supine with the head turned 15 degrees toward the affected ear. Explain that the drops instilled in the affected nasal passage should be allowed to flow along the floor of the nose to the low point, where they will collect. The low point marks the entrance of the eustachian tube. Instruct the patient to remain in this position for 5 minutes. When both sides require treatment, advise the patient to repeat the procedure on the second side after the 5-minute wait.*

• Instruct the patient to use a humidifier if nasal dryness occurs, and to discontinue the drug if mucosal ulceration occurs.

• Advise the lactating patient to consult with her physician before taking a topical decongestant.

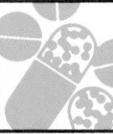

SELECTED MAJOR DRUGS

Decongestant agents

The drugs summarized in this chart are frequently used (and representative) decongestants.

DRUG	MAJOR INDICATIONS	USUAL ADULT DOSAGES	CONTRAINDICATIONS AND PRECAUTIONS
Systemic decongestants (sympathomimetic amines)			
phenylpropanol-amine	Nasal congestion associated with acute or chronic rhinitis, sinusitis, the common cold, hay fever, or other allergies	25 mg P.O. every 4 hours or 75 mg P.O. of the sustained-release preparation every 12 hours, not to exceed 150 mg P.O. daily	• Know that systemic decongestants are contraindicated in a pregnant or lactating patient, a patient receiving a monoamine oxidase inhibitor, or one with porphyria, severe coronary artery disease, cardiac arrhythmias, narrow-angle glaucoma, psychoneurosis, or known hypersensitivity to systemic decongestants.
pseudoephedrine		60 mg P.O. every 4 to 6 hours or 120 mg P.O. of the sustained-release preparation every 12 hours	• Administer with caution to an elderly patient or one with hypertension, hyperthyroidism, cardiovascular disease, or prostatic hypertrophy.
Topical decongestants (local vasoconstrictors)			
naphazoline	Nasal congestion associated with acute or chronic rhinitis, sinusitis, the common cold, hay fever, or other allergies	2 drops or sprays of 0.05% solution in each nostril, repeated every 3 to 6 hours	• Know that topical decongestants are contraindicated in a pregnant patient or one with narrow-angle glaucoma or known hypersensitivity to topical decongestants.
phenylephrine		1 to 2 sprays or small amount of jelly in each nostril, repeated every 4 hours	• Administer with caution to a lactating patient or one with hypertension, diabetes mellitus, cardiovascular disease, hyperthyroidism, or prostatic hypertrophy.
oxymetazoline		2 to 3 drops or 1 to 2 sprays of 0.05% solution in each nostril b.i.d.	
tetrahydrozoline		2 to 4 drops or sprays of 0.1% solution in each nostril, repeated every 3 hours, if needed	
xylometazoline		2 or 3 drops or sprays of 0.1% solution in each nostril every 8 to 10 hours, not to exceed three times in 24 hours	

Evaluation

The following examples represent appropriate evaluation statements for a patient receiving a topical decongestant.

• The patient has no conditions that contraindicate topical decongestant therapy.

• The patient exhibits no signs of complications in the preexisting condition linked to the prescribed topical decongestant.

• The patient displays no adverse reactions to the prescribed topical decongestant.

• The patient experiences no drug interactions during topical decongestant therapy.

• The patient's nasal mucosa remains intact.

• The patient and family express an accurate understanding of the points taught about the prescribed topical decongestant.

• The patient demonstrates the proper administration technique for the prescribed topical decongestant.

CHAPTER SUMMARY

Chapter 40 presented decongestants and their use in relieving nasal congestion, rhinitis, and eustachian tube occlusion associated with sinusitis, the common cold, hay fever, and other allergies. The chapter explained how the sympathomimetic action of decongestants, acting primarily on alpha-adrenergic receptors, promotes vasoconstriction of the nasal mucosa, thereby decreasing inflammation, congestion, and edema. Here are the highlights of the chapter.

• Decongestants are discussed according to their route of administration: systemic or topical. As sympathomimetic amines, systemic decongestants activate the sympathetic division of the autonomic nervous system. They are administered orally. Topical decongestants are powerful vasoconstrictors. They include sympathomimetic amines and imidazoline derivatives of sympathomimetic amines.

• Systemic decongestants promote nasal decongestion through stimulation of alpha-adrenergic receptors in the nasal mucosa (direct action) and stimulation of norepinephrine release (indirect action). Systemic decongestants include ephedrine, phenylpropanolamine, and pseudoephedrine. The mild adverse reactions that occur resemble those resulting from sympathetic nervous system stimulation. Systemic decongestants provide a longer duration of action than topical decongestants.

• Topical decongestants promote nasal decongestion through direct stimulation of the alpha-adrenergic receptors in the vascular smooth muscle of the nasal mucosa.

• Topical decongestants provide almost immediate relief of symptoms. Sympathetic nervous system stimulation rarely occurs when these agents are taken in the recommended doses and frequencies of administration. More prominent and bothersome is the frequent occurrence of rebound nasal congestion, which prompts drug dependence. Limiting drug use to 3 to 4 days helps prevent the rebound-dependence phenomenon.

• When caring for a patient receiving a decongestant, the nurse should apply the nursing process. Appropriate care includes observing the patient for adverse drug reactions and providing comprehensive information to the patient and family about the prescribed decongestant.

STUDY QUESTIONS

See Appendix 1 for answers.

1. Linda Osborne, age 35, has sinusitis. Her physician prescribes pseudoephedrine (Sudafed) 60 mg P.O. every 6 hours. How does this systemic decongestant work in treating sinusitis?
(a) It stimulates alpha-adrenergic receptors, resulting in vasoconstriction and nasal decongestion.
(b) It inhibits alpha-adrenergic receptors, resulting in vasoconstriction and nasal decongestion.
(c) It inhibits beta-adrenergic receptors, resulting in vasoconstriction and nasal decongestion.
(d) It stimulates beta$_1$-adrenergic receptors, resulting in vasoconstriction and nasal decongestion.

2. The physician could have prescribed ephedrine sulfate for Ms. Osborne. However, use of ephedrine increases the risk of which adverse reaction?
(a) addiction to decongestants
(b) blood pressure decrease
(c) CNS depression
(d) rebound hyperemia of nasal mucosa

3. Like ephedrine, phenylpropanolamine also is a systemic nasal decongestant. How does phenylpropanolamine differ from ephedrine?
(a) It has a more rapid onset of action.
(b) Its duration of action is longer.
(c) It produces fewer adverse reactions.
(d) It is less potent.

4. Carla Lane, age 57, has allergic rhinitis. Her history includes coronary artery disease and a myocardial infarction 2 years ago. For Ms. Lane, the physician prescribes a topical decongestant. Compared to systemic decongestants, topical decongestants offer which advantage?
(a) longer duration of action
(b) fewer adverse reactions
(c) easier administration
(d) less expensive

5. The nurse assesses Ms. Lane for adverse reactions to the topical decongestant. Which adverse reaction is the most common?
(a) rebound nasal congestion
(b) hypertension
(c) cardiac arrhythmias
(d) nausea

6. The physician recommends oxymetazoline for John LaGrange, age 44, to treat sphenoid sinus congestion. If Mr. LaGrange develops rebound nasal congestion, what action should the nurse suggest?
(a) Use the topical decongestant more frequently.
(b) Switch to another brand of decongestant.
(c) Use the decongestant less frequently and consult the physician.
(d) Discontinue the decongestant and consult the physician.

7. The nurse must teach Mr. LaGrange how to instill oxymetazoline nose drops. Which statement should be part of the teaching session?
(a) Sit upright and tilt the head forward immediately after instilling the drops.
(b) Lie supine with the head supported by a pillow during and for 5 minutes after instillation.
(c) Make sure the drops run down the back of the throat after instillation to ensure effectiveness.
(d) Hang the head over the edge of the bed and inhale deeply while instilling the drops.

SELECTED REFERENCES

AHFS drug information 90. (1990). Bethesda, MD: American Society of Hospital Pharmacists.

Drug facts and comparisons (1991). St. Louis: Facts and Comparisons Division, J.B. Lippincott.

Goodman and Gilman's the pharmacological basis of therapeutics (8th ed.; 1990). Elmsford, NY: Pergamon Press.

Hansten, P., and Horn, J. (1989). *Drug interactions* (6th ed.). Philadelphia: Lea & Febiger.

Jacobs, R., et al. (1989). Rhinitis: Not just hay fever. *Patient Care,* 23(6), 168-184.

Mazow, J. (1989). Allergic rhinitis: Formulating the best treatment plan. *Consultant,* 29(4), 143-155.

North American Nursing Diagnosis Association. (1990). *Taxomomy I-Revised, with official diagnostic categories.* St. Louis: NANDA.

USPDI. (1991). *Drug information for the health care professional* (Vol. I, 11th ed.). Rockville, MD: United States Pharmacopeial Convention.

10

DRUGS TO IMPROVE GASTROINTESTINAL FUNCTION

The gastrointestinal (GI) tract has three major functions: digestion of foods and fluids, absorption of foods and fluids, and excretion of metabolic waste. In the GI tract, various hormones and enzymes break down food into particles that are small enough to permeate cell membranes and be used for cellular energy. The GI tract itself helps prevent infection by maintaining mucous membrane integrity, secreting immunoglobulins, and destroying pathogens.

GI disorders frequently disrupt activities of daily living, interrupt work schedules, and lead to hospital admissions. Many are pathologic, such as benign or malignant tumors, peptic ulcer disease, gastroesophageal reflux, regional ileitis (Crohn's disease) and ulcerative colitis, malabsorption, intestinal obstruction, and diverticulosis. Others are psychophysiologic disorders. Whether the cause is pathologic or psychophysiologic, however, GI disorders usually produce similar signs and symptoms that typically are so vague and nonspecific that many patients delay seeking treatment.

SIGNS AND SYMPTOMS

Common signs and symptoms of GI tract disorders include anorexia, dysphagia, nausea, vomiting, dyspepsia, epigastric or abdominal pain, abdominal distention, flatulence, diarrhea, constipation, and rectal bleeding. These findings may suggest many possible causes. GI tract disorders may cause fluid and electrolyte imbalances with resultant cardiac arrhythmias and hypovolemia, extended areas of inflammation or infection, abscesses or fistulas, malnutrition, perforated structures with resultant peritonitis, and altered body image. Medical management of GI disorders usually is conservative, symptomatic, and supportive. Initial treatment usually consists of diet therapy, rest, and stress management. If these measures prove ineffective, drug therapy or surgery may be used.

OVERVIEW OF CHAPTERS

The chapters in Unit Ten discuss drugs that are used to manage GI tract disorders. They present the major drug categories, including adsorbents, antiflatulents, digestive agents, antidiarrheals, laxatives and cathartics, emetics, antiemetics, antacids, histamine$_2$-receptor antagonists, and other peptic ulcer agents. Because many of the drugs in these categories are available over the counter, self-medication is common.

This unit also presents two general categories of drug therapy: (1) treatment of specific diseases such as digestive enzyme deficiencies, portal-systemic encephalopathy, acute toxic poisoning, peptic ulcer disease, and esophageal reflux; and (2) control of symptoms of specific diseases such as nausea, vomiting, epigastric pain, dyspepsia, flatulence, diarrhea, and constipation.

Chapter 41
Adsorbent, Antiflatulent, and Digestive Agents
After reviewing normal GI tract function, Chapter 41 explores activated charcoal, an adsorbent agent used to treat acute poisoning. Then it discusses simethicone, an antiflatulent used to treat conditions that promote excess gas formation, and the digestive agents dilute hydrochloric acid, glutamic acid hydochloride, bile acids and bile salts, and the pancreatic enzymes pancreatin and pancrelipase. For each type of agent, it discusses appropriate nursing care through application of the nursing process.

Chapter 42
Antidiarrheal and Laxative Agents
Chapter 42 discusses diarrhea and constipation and presents the drugs used to treat them. It explores antidiarrheal agents, including opium tincture, paregoric, loperamide, difenoxin, diphenoxylate, and kaolin and pectin mixtures, as well as various laxatives, including hyperosmolar laxatives, dietary fiber and bulk-forming agents, emollient laxatives, stimulant laxatives, and lubricant laxatives. The chapter also

Glossary

Adsorbent: drug that inhibits the gastrointestinal (GI) absorption of various drugs, toxins, and chemicals by attracting and holding them to its surface.

Antacid: drug that neutralizes gastric acids.

Antidiarrheal: drug that decreases the frequency of defecation and water content of the stools.

Antiemetic: drug that relieves nausea and vomiting.

Antiflatulent: drug that decreases GI gas.

Cathartic: agent that promotes evacuation of the bowels.

Constipation: decreased movement of fecal matter through the large intestine.

Diarrhea: increased frequency or weight and liquidity of stools produced by the rapid movement of fecal matter through the large intestine.

Digestant: drug that enhances digestion in the GI tract.

Emetic: drug that induces vomiting.

Emollient: drug that softens the stool by increasing the water content of fecal material through a reduction in surface tension of bowel contents.

Gastrin: hormone secreted by the pyloric mucosa that increases the flow of gastric juices.

Histamine$_2$-receptor antagonist: drug that decreases gastric acid secretion by blocking gastric histamine (H_2) receptors.

Laxative: drug that stimulates defecation by forming bulk, stimulating peristalsis, or providing lubrication or chemical irritation.

Nausea: unpleasant epigastric or abdominal sensation that, in many cases, leads to vomiting.

Pepsin: proteolytic enzyme in gastric juice that acts as a catalyst in protein hydrolysis.

Ulcer: cutaneous or mucosal lesion caused by gradual erosion, disintegration, and necrosis of underlying tissue.

Vomiting: forcible expulsion of gastric contents through the mouth.

discusses nursing activities related to the administration of antidiarrheal and laxative agents.

Chapter 43
Emetic and Antiemetic Agents

Chapter 43 examines the physiology of nausea and vomiting and the conditions that stimulate them. Next, it explains the use of emetics, such as apomorphine and ipecac syrup, to induce vomiting after ingestion of toxic substances. Then it discusses the various antiemetic agents, including antihistamines, phenothiazines, benzquinamide, scopolamine, metoclopramide, diphenidol, and dronabinol. For each emetic and antiemetic drug class, the chapter discusses appropriate nursing care.

Chapter 44
Peptic Ulcer Agents

Chapter 44 presents the pathophysiology of peptic, duodenal, and gastric ulcers. Then it explores antacids, histamine$_2$-receptor antagonists, and other peptic ulcer agents used to treat ulcers, emphasizing their clinical use, safety, and effectiveness. The chapter also discusses general application of the nursing process for a patient receiving a peptic ulcer agent.

ADSORBENT, ANTIFLATULENT, AND DIGESTIVE AGENTS

OBJECTIVES

After reading and studying this chapter, the student should be able to:

1. Describe the physiology of digestion from the stomach to the large intestine, explaining how enzymes and hormones from the stomach, liver, pancreas, and duodenum aid digestion.

2. Explain how an adsorbent works to treat an acute poisoning.

3. Describe the mechanism of action by which antiflatulents work in the gastrointestinal (GI) tract.

4. Identify the purpose of each of the three major groups of digestive agents.

5. Discuss the pharmacokinetic properties of dilute hydrochloric acid, bile salts, and pancreatic enzymes.

6. Identify adverse reactions associated with digestive agents.

7. Describe how to apply the nursing process when caring for a patient who is receiving an adsorbent, antiflatulent, or digestive agent.

INTRODUCTION

The GI tract's primary function is to provide the human body with fluids and nutrients. Before the cells can use these fluids and nutrients, various absorptive, peristaltic, and digestive functions must occur.

The stomach mucosa consists of two sets of tubular glands: gastric glands and pyloric glands. The gastric glands secrete hydrochloric acid, pepsinogen, intrinsic factor, and mucus; the pyloric glands secrete mucus, pepsinogen, and the hormone gastrin. At a pH of approximately 0.8, hydrochloric acid is extremely acidic. When pepsinogen comes in contact with the hydrochloric acid, active pepsin, a proteolytic enzyme, is formed. Pepsin digests protein when the pH of the pepsin is less than 3.5.

As food enters the antrum of the stomach, the pyloric glands secrete gastrin, which aids digestion by stimulating (1) secretion of hydrochloric acid and pepsin, (2) secretion of intrinsic factor and pancreatic enzymes, (3) release of insulin and flow of hepatic bile, and (4) gastric and intestinal motility.

Hepatocytes (liver cells) continually produce bile, which ultimately is secreted into the common bile duct. From the common bile duct, bile is emptied directly into the duodenum or concentrated and stored in the gallbladder. Substances secreted in the bile include bile salts, bilirubin, cholesterol, lecithin, and electrolytes. As bile is concentrated in the gallbladder, the gallbladder mucosa reabsorbs large amounts of fluid and electrolytes. In the intestines, bile salts serve two major functions: they act as a detergent on fat particles, dispersing them into small globules (emulsification); and they help absorb cholesterol, fatty acids, monoglycerides, and other lipids from the intestinal tract. As fats are absorbed in the intestines, the fat-soluble vitamins A, D, E, and K also are absorbed.

The major functions of the pancreas include insulin production by the beta islet cells and production of pancreatic juice, which is released into the duodenum. Pancreatic juice includes specific enzymes that aid in the digestion of proteins, carbohydrates, and fats. The major proteolytic enzymes include trypsin (the most abundant), chymotrypsin, carboxypolypeptidase, ribonuclease, and deoxyribonuclease. Pancreatic amylase is the major digestive enzyme for carbohydrates; pancreatic lipase is the major digestive enzyme for fats. Secretin and cholecystokinin are hormones that increase pancreatic enzyme secretion. The acid content of the stomach releases secretin from the duodenum; food content stimulates the release of cholecystokinin.

Parasympathetic stimulation via the vagus nerve also increases enzyme release into the acinar cells of the pancreas. The combined result of these hormonal and neuronal

Major digestive substances and hormones

Digestive substances and hormones are essential for the body to use ingested foods. Each substance functions in a specific way on specific food components to produce usable nutrients. Each hormone stimulates or inhibits digestive functions that affect digestive substances.

DIGESTIVE SUBSTANCES

Substance	Source	Food component	Product
pepsin	Gastric glands	Proteins	Polypeptides, peptides, proteoses (partially digested proteins)
gastric acid	Gastric juice	Emulsified fats	Fatty acids, glycerol
bile	Liver (stored in and released from gallbladder)	Unemulsified fats	Emulsified fats
trypsin	Pancreatic juice	Proteins, polypeptides	Proteoses, peptides, amino acids
chymotrypsin	Pancreatic juice	Proteins, polypeptides	Polypeptides, amino acids
lipase	Pancreatic juice	Bile-emulsified fats	Fatty acids, glycerol
amylase	Pancreatic juice	Starch	Maltose, isomaltose
ribonuclease	Pancreatic juice	Nucleic acids	Nucleotides
deoxyribonuclease	Pancreatic juice	Nucleic acids	Nucleotides
carboxypolypeptidase	Pancreatic juice	Polypeptides	Smaller polypeptides

DIGESTIVE HORMONES

Hormone	Source	Activating substances	Action
gastrin	Gastric mucosa of the pylorus	Partially digested proteins in the pylorus	• Stimulates release of gastric juice rich in pepsinogen and hydrochloric acid
secretin	Duodenal mucosa	Partially digested proteins, fats, and acids in the duodenum	• Stimulates secretion of low-enzyme, high-bicarbonate pancreatic juice • Stimulates secretion of bile by liver • May enhance cholecystokinin activity in producing pancreatic enzymes; may inhibit gastric motility, acid secretion, and pyloric sphincter contraction
cholecystokinin	Duodenal mucosa	Partially digested proteins, fats, and acids in the duodenum	• Stimulates secretion of high-enzyme pancreatic juice • Inhibits gastric emptying and secretion and intestinal motility • Stimulates gallbladder contractions leading to bile release

actions is the increased secretion of pancreatic fluid, bicarbonate, and enzymes (trypsin, amylase, and lipase) into the small intestine to aid digestion. (For more information, see *Major digestive substances and hormones.*)

Adsorbent agents are used when toxins have been ingested. Toxins ingested through the GI tract that may cause poisoning or overdose include such drugs as amphetamines, aspirin, barbiturates, cocaine, morphine, opium, and tricyclic antidepressants. Ingested poisonous mushrooms also produce toxins.

Two major disturbances of digestion in the GI tract include gastric bloating with or without flatulence, and inadequate or incomplete digestion. Antiflatulents commonly are indicated for patients with functional gastric

SELECTED NURSING DIAGNOSES

Adsorbent, antiflatulent, and digestive agents

The following nursing diagnoses address representative problems and etiologies that a nurse may encounter when caring for a patient who is receiving an adsorbent, antiflatulent, or digestive agent. Some of these nursing diagnoses contain generalized etiologies, which the nurse must individualize based on the patient's needs. (For some common nursing diagnoses and related interventions for each drug class, see the "Nursing Process Application" sections of this chapter.)

- Altered health maintenance related to drug interactions with pancreatin or pancrelipase
- Altered health maintenance related to ineffectiveness of the prescribed digestive agent
- Constipation related to the adverse gastrointestinal (GI) effects of activated charcoal
- Diarrhea related to the adverse GI effects of a digestive agent
- Health-seeking behaviors related to GI discomfort caused by ineffectiveness of simethicone
- Knowledge deficit related to the prescribed adsorbent, antiflatulent, or digestive agent
- Noncompliance related to long-term use of a digestive agent
- Pain related to abdominal cramps or biliary colic caused by a bile salt or bile acid
- Potential for injury related to a preexisting condition that contraindicates the use of an adsorbent or digestive agent
- Potential for injury related to a preexisting condition that requires cautious use of a digestive agent
- Potential for injury related to adverse drug reactions
- Potential for poisoning related to ineffectiveness of activated charcoal
- Potential for poisoning related to massive overdose of hydrochloric acid
- Potential for trauma to tooth enamel related to hydrochloric acid administration

This chapter covers natural and synthetic adsorbents, antiflatulents, and digestants. For a summary of representative drugs, see *Selected major drugs: Adsorbent, antiflatulent, and digestive agents,* page 707. For a listing of applicable nursing diagnoses that the nurse may formulate when caring for a patient receiving these agents, see *Selected nursing diagnoses: Adsorbent, antiflatulent, and digestive agents.* For detailed information on applying the nursing process, see Chapter 6, The Nursing Process and Drug Therapy.

ADSORBENT AGENTS

An adsorbent is an agent that attracts molecules of a liquid, gas, or dissolved substance to its surface. The attracted molecules concentrate in a thin layer over the surface of the adsorbent. Adsorbents are prescribed in acute situations to prevent the absorption of drugs or toxins from the GI tract. The major adsorbent used clinically is activated charcoal, a black powder residue obtained from the distillation of various organic materials.

PHARMACOKINETICS

Adsorbent agents belong to the class of drugs known as protective agents of the GI mucosa, which are designed to prevent contact with possible irritants.

Absorption, distribution, metabolism, excretion
Activated charcoal is a chemically inert powder that attracts dissolved or suspended substances, such as gases, toxins, and bacteria, thereby preventing absorption of these substances in the GI tract. Activated charcoal, which is not absorbed nor metabolized by the body, is excreted unchanged in the feces.

Onset, peak, duration
Activated charcoal must be administered soon after poison ingestion because it only can bind drugs or toxins that have not been absorbed from the GI tract yet. Duration of action depends on the poison's transit time through the bowel and the resultant contact time for adsorption to occur. After initial absorption, some poisons move back into the bowel, where they are reabsorbed. Activated charcoal may be administered over time to break this cycle. The particle size of the charcoal also influences its duration. Activated charcoals composed of small particles prove the most effective because the small particles provide a larger total surface area for the toxin to adhere to.

bloating. Under normal physiologic conditions, gases collect in the GI tract from swallowed air, bacterial action, and gas diffusion from the blood into the lumen. Nitrogen and oxygen are the primary gases found in the stomach. Approximately 10 liters of gas enter or are formed daily in the large intestine. This GI gas may be absorbed or expelled through belching or flatus.

Digestive agents (digestants) are used in these clinical situations involving incomplete digestion: hydrochloric acid for hypochlorhydria and achlorhydria, bile salts as replacement therapy for conditions that cause bile salt deficiencies in the upper intestines, and pancreatic enzymes for conditions that decrease pancreatic juice production (pancreatitis or cystic fibrosis).

PHARMACODYNAMICS

Adsorbents attract and bind toxins in the intestinal lumen, thus inhibiting toxin absorption from the GI tract. This nonspecific GI binding delays or blocks further absorption of the poison, but does not alter systemic toxicity caused by earlier absorption of the toxin. Intended as an adjunct in poisoning management, adsorbents may be used in addition to dialysis, antidote administration, or gastric lavage.

PHARMACOTHERAPEUTICS

Activated charcoal is a general-purpose antidote used for acute episodes of oral poisoning. The adsorbent's effectiveness depends on its quick administration after toxin ingestion and its total surface area, which is determined by particle size.

Although activated charcoal is not effective for all toxins, it is indicated in many types of acute oral poisoning. (For a partial list, see *Common toxins treated by activated charcoal.*) However, activated charcoal is not indicated in acute poisoning from cyanide, ethanol, methanol, iron, sodium chloride alkalies, inorganic acids, or organic solvents.

activated charcoal (Charcocaps, Digestalin). Activated charcoal is an odorless, tasteless black powder obtained from the destructive distillation of several organic substances treated to increase their adsorptive power.
Usual adult dosage: 5 to 10 times the estimated weight of the drug or chemical ingested, or a minimum dose of 30 grams, mixed in 250 ml of water. For maximum effect, give activated charcoal P.O. within 30 minutes of the poisoning. The dose may be repeated every 2 hours when used for drugs that undergo enterohepatic recycling (such as phenobarbital) or for drugs that are resecreted into the stomach (such as tricyclic antidepressants).

Common toxins treated by activated charcoal

Activated charcoal is used to treat poisoning by numerous toxins. Knowing which toxins are susceptible to activated charcoal helps the nurse plan patient care and teaching.

- amphetamines
- antimony
- aspirin
- atropine
- barbiturates
- camphor
- carbon tetrachloride
- cardiotoxic glycosides
- cocaine
- phenothiazines
- potassium permanganate
- propoxyphene
- quinine
- sulfonamides
- tricyclic antidepressants

Drug interactions

Do not administer activated charcoal simultaneously with ipecac syrup; the activated charcoal will adsorb the ipecac, rendering it inactive. Give emetics, such as ipecac, and allow emesis to occur before administering activated charcoal because emesis enhances the effectiveness of the activated charcoal by decreasing the amount of toxin in the GI tract to be adsorbed. The result is more complete toxin removal.

ADVERSE DRUG REACTIONS

Adverse reactions to activated charcoal administration include black stools and constipation. A laxative such as sorbitol usually is given with activated charcoal to prevent constipation. No known hypersensitivity reactions exist. Furthermore, toxicity does not occur with activated charcoal, even at the maximum dose.

NURSING PROCESS APPLICATION

The following information assists the nurse in caring for a patient who is receiving activated charcoal.

Assessment
- Review the patient's history for a preexisting condition that contraindicates the use of activated charcoal, such as corrosive or petroleum distillate ingestion.
- Assess the effectiveness of activated charcoal.
- Assess the patient for adverse reactions to activated charcoal, such as constipation or black stools.
- Evaluate the patient's and family's knowledge about activated charcoal.

Nursing diagnoses
The following examples represent appropriate nursing diagnoses for a patient receiving activated charcoal.
- Potential for injury related to a preexisting condition that contraindicates the use of activated charcoal
- Potential for poisoning related to ineffectiveness of activated charcoal
- Constipation related to the adverse GI effects of activated charcoal
- Knowledge deficit related to activated charcoal

Planning and implementation
- Do not administer activated charcoal to a patient with a condition that contraindicates its use.
- *Do not administer activated charcoal to a patient who has ingested a poison for which activated charcoal is ineffective, such as cyanide, ethanol, methanol, iron, sodium chloride alkalies, inorganic acids, or organic solvents.*

• *Expect to administer large doses of activated charcoal to treat the poisoning if food is present in the patient's stomach.*
• Add fruit juice to the charcoal and water mixture to make it more palatable.
• *Administer activated charcoal within 30 minutes of the poisoning for maximum effect.*
• Prepare to administer activated charcoal every 2 hours to treat poisoning by drugs that undergo enterohepatic recycling or are resecreted into the stomach.
• *Do not administer activated charcoal simultaneously with ipecac syrup. Allow emesis to occur before administering activated charcoal because emesis enhances the effectiveness of the activated charcoal by decreasing the amount of toxin in the GI tract to be absorbed.*
• Expect to administer a laxative, such as sorbitol, to prevent adsorbent-induced constipation.

Patient teaching
• Teach the patient and family about the action, frequency of administration, and adverse effects of activated charcoal.
• Advise the patient to avoid eating ice cream after activated charcoal administration because ice cream decreases the drug's adsorbent capacity.
• Caution the patient to anticipate black stools from the activated charcoal.

Evaluation
The following examples represent appropriate evaluation statements for a patient receiving activated charcoal.
• The patient has no conditions that contraindicate the use of activated charcoal.
• The patient demonstrates no signs or symptoms of poisoning from the ingested drug or toxin after treatment with activated charcoal.
• The patient maintains normal bowel function after activated charcoal administration.
• The patient and family express an accurate understanding of the points taught about activated charcoal.
• The patient correctly describes the adverse GI reactions to activated charcoal.

ANTIFLATULENT AGENTS

Antiflatulents are mixtures of liquid dimethylpolysiloxanes and silica gel that possess antifoaming and water-repellent properties. Antiflatulents disperse gas pockets in the GI tract. They are available alone or in combination with antacids. This section discusses the major antiflatulent agent simethicone.

PHARMACOKINETICS

Antiflatulents are physiologically inactive and are not absorbed in the GI tract. Because antiflatulents are not absorbed, they do not interfere with gastric secretion or nutrient absorption. Antiflatulents are distributed only in the intestinal lumen and are eliminated intact in the feces. They provide an immediate onset of action, with a duration of approximately 3 hours.

PHARMACODYNAMICS

Antiflatulents are physiologically inactive substances that provide defoaming action in the GI tract. Simethicone, a pale gray transparent liquid, displays specific defoaming and water-repellent properties. By producing a film in the intestines that can collapse gas bubbles, simethicone disperses and helps prevent the formation of mucus-enclosed gas pockets.

PHARMACOTHERAPEUTICS

Antiflatulents are prescribed to treat conditions in which excess gas is a problem, such as functional gastric bloating, postoperative gaseous bloating, diverticulitis, spastic or irritable colon, air swallowing, and peptic ulcer. Although simethicone has been employed frequently to decrease gas shadows during bowel radiography and to improve visualization during gastroscopy, clinical research trials have not supported this use.

simethicone (Mylicon). Simethicone is available in drops, as an oral suspension (40 mg in 0.6 ml), in chewable tablets (40 to 125 mg), in tablets (50 to 95 mg), or in capsules (125 mg).
Usual adult dosage: 160 to 500 mg P.O. daily in divided doses, given after each meal and at bedtime.

Drug interactions
Simethicone does not produce any significant drug interactions.

ADVERSE DRUG REACTIONS

Simethicone does not cause any known adverse reactions.

NURSING PROCESS APPLICATION

The following information assists the nurse in caring for a patient who is receiving simethicone.

Assessment
• Assess the effectiveness of simethicone regularly.
• Evaluate the patient's and family's knowledge about simethicone.

Nursing diagnoses
The following examples represent appropriate nursing diagnoses for a patient receiving simethicone.
• Health-seeking behaviors related to GI discomfort caused by ineffectiveness of simethicone
• Knowledge deficit related to simethicone

Planning and implementation
• Ask the patient periodically about the degree of GI discomfort during simethicone therapy.
• Shake the antiflatulent suspension before administering the dose to ensure adequate mixing.
• Use a calibrated dropper to administer the medication in drops.
• *Administer simethicone after each meal and at bedtime for maximum effectiveness.*
• Notify the physician if simethicone is ineffective.

Patient teaching
• Teach the patient and family the name, dose, frequency, and action of simethicone.
• *Instruct the patient to take simethicone after meals and at bedtime.*
• Teach the patient to shake the simethicone suspension before preparing the dose.
• *Advise the patient that chewable tablets must be chewed thoroughly before swallowing.*
• Encourage a patient with functional gastric bloating to increase activity and exercise, if clinically advisable.
• Instruct the patient to notify the physician if simethicone is ineffective.

Evaluation
The following examples represent appropriate evaluation statements for a patient receiving simethicone.
• The patient reports relief of GI discomfort during simethicone therapy.
• The patient and family express an accurate understanding of the points taught about simethicone.
• The patient begins a moderate exercise program.

DIGESTIVE AGENTS

Digestive agents (digestants) aid digestion in patients who lack one or more of the specific substances that naturally digest food. This section discusses digestants that function in the GI tract, liver, and pancreas.

Bile salts (sodium salts of bile acids) and bile acids, such as dehydrocholic acid, are used to initiate bile flow from the liver. The precursor of bile salts is cholesterol, which is supplied in the diet or produced by the liver. Bile salts are converted to cholic acid and chenodeoxycholic acid. These acids conjugate with glycerine and taurine to form bile acids. Then the salts of the bile acids are secreted in the bile.

Glutamic acid hydrochloride and dilute hydrochloric acid replace natural gastric acids and are used to treat gastric hypochlorhydria (diminished hydrochloric acid in gastric juice), achlorhydria (absence of hydrochloric acid in gastric juice), and gastric achylia (absence of proteolytic enzymes and hydrochloric acid).

Pancreatin and pancrelipase are used to supplement or replace exocrine pancreatic secretions. These agents aid the digestion of proteins, carbohydrates, and fats. (For an illustration of the organs that contribute digestive secretions, see *Sites of enzyme and hormone formation.*)

PHARMACOKINETICS

The digestants are natural body substances. As such, they are absorbed, distributed, metabolized, and excreted as they would be if they were produced by the patient rather than taken therapeutically.

Absorption, distribution, metabolism, excretion
Approximately 80% of the bile salts are reabsorbed from the terminal ileum of the small intestine where they enter the enterohepatic circulation. Bile salts and bile acids eventually are excreted through the GI tract as bile end products in the feces.

Glutamic acid hydrochloride and hydrochloric acid are absorbed in the GI tract and distributed in the distal portion of the stomach. These digestants are excreted as a part of normal GI tract elimination.

Pancreatic enzymes are absorbed in the GI tract. They are distributed in the intestinal lumen and excreted as part of normal GI elimination.

Sites of enzyme and hormone formation

This anatomic illustration shows where various enzymes and hormones are produced in the gastrointestinal tract. Most digestive enzymes and hormones are formed at sites near their locus of physiologic action.

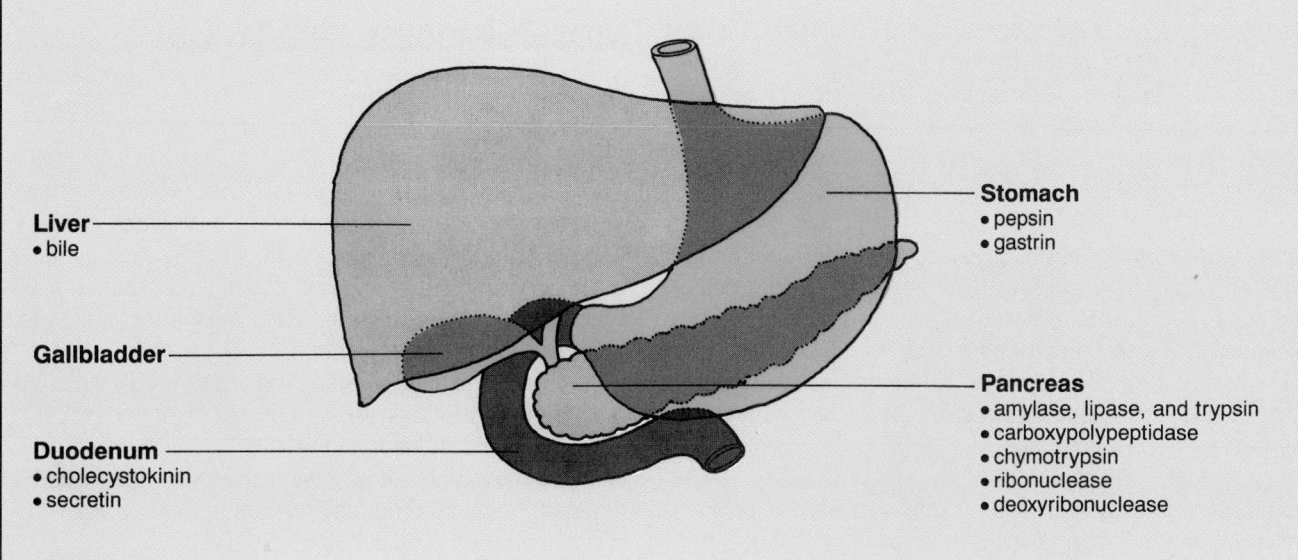

Liver
• bile

Gallbladder

Duodenum
• cholecystokinin
• secretin

Stomach
• pepsin
• gastrin

Pancreas
• amylase, lipase, and trypsin
• carboxypolypeptidase
• chymotrypsin
• ribonuclease
• deoxyribonuclease

Onset, peak, duration

The onset of action, peak concentration level, and duration of action of the digestants resemble those of the body substances they replace. Onset and duration depend on the type and amount of food ingested.

PHARMACODYNAMICS

The action of digestants resembles the action of the body substances they replace. Bile acids, referred to as choleretic drugs, stimulate bile production in the liver. Bile salts, however, provide little choleretic action. Bile salts emulsify fats, dispersing them into small globules. These salts also help in the absorption of fatty acids, fat-soluble vitamins, cholesterol, and other lipids from the intestinal tract, thereby promoting normal digestion. As a hydrocholeretic agent, dehydrocholic acid increases bile output without increasing the solids in it.

When administered, glutamic acid hydrochloride and hydrochloric acid convert pepsinogen in the stomach into pepsin. The hydrochloric acid and pepsin initiate the digestion of the stomach contents by beginning protein digestion in the lower third of the stomach.

The pancreatic enzymes pancreatin and precrelipase replace the normal exocrine pancreatic enzymes. These agents digest proteins via trypsin, carbohydrates via amylase, and fats via lipase.

PHARMACOTHERAPEUTICS

Bile acids and bile salts may be administered to (1) increase cholesterol solubility, thereby preventing accumulation of recurrent biliary calculi, (2) replace the natural substances in patients with conditions in which the bile component concentration in the small intestine is low, and (3) promote drainage of the common bile duct via a T-tube in post-cholecystectomy patients.

Clinical indications for the gastric digestants include conditions in which the patient produces none or insufficient amounts of the normally occurring gastric acids. For example, dilute hydrochloric acid is indicated for patients with hypochlorhydria or achlorhydria.

Pancreatic enzymes are used in clinical situations characterized by an insufficiency of pancreatic enzymes (specifically, pancreatitis and cystic fibrosis). Pancreatic enzymes also are used to treat steatorrhea, a disorder of fat metabolism.

bile salts (Bilron, Ox-Bile Extract Enseals). Once used to treat patients with biliary fistula and resection of the ileum, bile salts are used infrequently today.
Usual adult dosage: 1 to 2 enteric-coated tablets (324 mg each) P.O. t.i.d. after meals, or 150- to 600-mg capsules with or after meals.

dehydrocholic acid (Decholin, Cholan). This agent is given to stimulate bile flow from the liver. The hydrocholeretic activity of this bile acid also promotes T-tube drainage in postcholecystectomy patients.
Usual adult dosage: 244 to 500 mg P.O. t.i.d. after meals for 4 to 6 weeks.

glutamic acid hydrochloride (Acidulin). This agent is used to treat hypochlorhydria, achlorhydria, and gastric achylia.
Usual adult dosage: 1 to 3 capsules (340 mg to 1 gram) P.O. t.i.d. before meals. The capsule form of this digestant prevents damage to teeth, but glutamic acid hydrochloride is not as effective as dilute hydrochloric acid.

hydrochloric acid (dilute). In diluted form (10% solution), hydrochloric acid is used to treat hypochlorhydria, achlorhydria, and gastric achylia.
Usual adult dosage: 5 to 10 ml in 125 to 250 ml of water P.O. in several divided doses at 15-minute intervals. The patient must sip the solution through a glass straw to prevent damage to tooth enamel.

pancreatin (Dizymes). A natural substance obtained from fresh porcine or bovine pancreas, pancreatin is a combination of the enzymes amylase, trypsin, and lipase. Pancreatin replaces endogenous exocrine pancreatic enzymes and aids in digestion of carbohydrates, fats, and protein.
Usual adult dosage: 1 to 3 tablets P.O. after meals.

pancrelipase (Cotazym, Ilozyme, Pancrease, Viokase). Pancrelipase is derived from porcine pancreas. The lipase activity of pancrelipase is greater than that of pancreatin, making pancrelipase useful in treating steatorrhea and exocrine pancreatic secretion insufficiency associated with diseases such as cystic fibrosis.
Usual adult dosage: 1 to 3 capsules or tablets P.O. before or with meals, and 1 capsule or tablet P.O. with snacks, or 0.7 grams of powder P.O. before meals and snacks.

Drug interactions
No significant drug interactions occur with the administration of bile salts, the bile acid dehydrocholic acid, glutamic acid hydrochloride, or hydrochloric acid. However, antacids negate the effects of pancreatin and pancrelipase. Therefore, concomitant administration of these agents should be avoided.

ADVERSE DRUG REACTIONS

Bile salts and bile acids can produce abdominal cramping and diarrhea. Bile salts also may reduce the resistance of the mucosal barrier of the stomach and esophagus to acid. If a dislodged gallstone is obstructing a biliary duct, the choleretic bile acids can produce biliary colic.

Hydrochloric acid can damage tooth enamel. For this reason, it always should be administered through a glass straw. A massive overdose of hydrochloric acid can cause acid-base abnormalities (specifically, metabolic acidosis).

Administration of the pancreatic enzymes typically causes nausea and diarrhea.

NURSING PROCESS APPLICATION

The following information assists the nurse in caring for a patient who is receiving a digestant.

Assessment
• Review the patient's history for a preexisting condition that contraindicates the use of a digestant, such as peptic ulcer disease, gastric hyperacidity, marked hepatic dysfunction, biliary obstruction, nausea, vomiting, abdominal pain, or known hypersensitivity to hog protein.
• Review the patient's history for a preexisting condition that requires cautious use of pancreatin or pancrelipase, such as pregnancy or lactation.
• Assess the patient for adverse reactions to the prescribed digestant, such as abdominal cramping, nausea, diarrhea, biliary colic, or damaged tooth enamel.
• Review the patient's medication history to identify the use of drugs that may interact with pancreatin or pancrelipase, such as antacids.
• Evaluate the patient's and family's knowledge about the prescribed digestant.

Nursing diagnoses
The following examples represent appropriate nursing diagnoses for a patient receiving a digestant.
• Potential for injury related to a preexisting condition that contraindicates the use of a digestant
• Potential for injury related to a preexisting condition that requires cautious use of a digestant
• Potential for injury related to adverse drug reactions
• Altered health maintenance related to drug interactions with pancreatin or pancrelipase
• Knowledge deficit related to the prescribed digestant

Planning and implementation
• Do not administer a digestant to a patient with a condition that contraindicates its use.
• Administer pancreatin or pancrelipase cautiously to a patient at risk because of a preexisting condition.
• Monitor the patient frequently for adverse reactions during digestant therapy.
• *Monitor for abdominal pain in a patient receiving bile salts or bile acids. Also monitor for biliary colic in a patient receiving bile salts. Notify the physician if the patient experiences pain.*

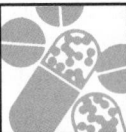

SELECTED MAJOR DRUGS

Adsorbent, antiflatulent, and digestive agents

The following chart summarizes selected adsorbents, antiflatulents, and digestive agents currently in clinical use.

DRUG	MAJOR INDICATIONS	USUAL ADULT DOSAGES	CONTRAINDICATIONS AND PRECAUTIONS
Adsorbent agents			
activated charcoal	Acute toxic poisoning	5 to 10 times the estimated weight of the drug or chemical ingested, or a minimum dose of 30 grams P.O. mixed in 250 ml of water	• Know that activated charcoal is contraindicated in a patient who has ingested a corrosive agent or petroleum distillate.
Antiflatulent agents			
simethicone	Excess GI tract gas	160 to 500 mg P.O. daily in divided doses, given after each meal and at bedtime	• Know that simethicone has no known contraindications or precautions.
Digestive agents			
bile salts	Insufficient bile production	1 to 2 enteric-coated tablets (324 mg each) P.O. t.i.d. after meals; or 150- to 600-mg capsules P.O. with or after meals	• Know that bile salts are contraindicated in a patient with marked hepatic dysfunction, biliary obstruction, nausea, vomiting, or abdominal pain.
dehydrocholic acid	Insufficient bile production	244 to 500 mg P.O. t.i.d. after meals for 4 to 6 weeks	• Know that dehydrocholic acid is contraindicated in a patient with biliary obstruction, nausea, vomiting, or abdominal pain.
glutamic acid hydrochloride	Hypochlorhydria and achlorhydria	1 to 3 capsules (340 mg to 1 gram) P.O. t.i.d. before meals	• Know that glutamic acid hydrochloride is contraindicated in a patient with gastric hyperacidity or peptic ulcers.
hydrochloric acid (dilute)	Hypochlorhydria and achlorhydria	5 to 10 ml in 125 to 250 ml of water P.O. in several divided doses at 15-minute intervals	• Know that hydrochloric acid is contraindicated in a patient with peptic ulcer disease.
pancreatin	Insufficient pancreatic enzymes	1 to 3 tablets P.O. after meals	• Know that pancreatin is contraindicated in a patient who is hypersensitive to hog protein. • Administer with caution to a pregnant or lactating patient.
pancrelipase	Insufficient pancreatic enzymes and steatorrhea	1 to 3 capsules or tablets P.O. before or with meals and 1 capsule or tablet P.O. with snacks; or 0.7 grams of powder P.O. before meals and snacks.	• Know that pancrelipase is contraindicated in a patient with known hypersensitivity to hog protein. • Administer with caution to a pregnant or lactating patient.

• Monitor hydration if the patient develops diarrhea. Obtain a prescription for an antidiarrheal agent, if needed.

• *Administer dilute hydrochloric acid through a glass straw to prevent damage to tooth enamel.*

• Administer the digestant before, with, or after meals, as prescribed.

• *Do not administer antacids with pancreatin or pancrelipase because antacids negate the effects of these agents.*

Patient teaching

• Teach the patient and family the name, dose, frequency, action, and adverse effects of the prescribed digestant.

• Inform the patient that hydrochloric acid tastes sour.

• *Instruct the patient to take dilute hydrochloric acid at 15-minute intervals in divided doses, as prescribed, and to use a glass straw.*

• *Instruct the patient taking a pancreatic enzyme to balance fat, protein, and carbohydrate intake to avoid indigestion.*

• Inform the patient that the number of bowel movements will decrease during digestant therapy and that the stool consistency will improve when replacement therapy reaches a therapeutic level. *Advise the patient, however, to report diarrhea to the physician.*

• Instruct the patient to store the digestant in a tight container at room temperature to prevent deterioration.

• *Advise the patient not to take a pancreatic enzyme with an antacid.*

• Stress the importance of taking the digestant before, with, or after meals, as prescribed, to enhance effectiveness.

Evaluation

The following examples represent appropriate evaluation statements for a patient receiving a digestant.

• The patient has no conditions that contraindicate digestant therapy.

• The patient exhibits no signs of complications in the preexisting condition linked to the prescribed digestant.

• The patient experiences no adverse reactions to the prescribed digestant.

• The patient discontinues use of antacids during digestant therapy.

• The patient and family express an accurate understanding of the points taught about the prescribed digestant.

• The patient makes appropriate food choices to balance fat, protein, and carbohydrate intake.

CHAPTER SUMMARY

Chapter 41 began with a discussion of the enzymes and hormones involved in digestion. The chapter then presented the pharmacokinetics, pharmacodynamics, pharmacotherapeutics, adverse drug reactions, and nursing process application related to adsorbents, antiflatulents, and digestants. Here are the chapter highlights.

• Enzymes and hormones secreted by the liver, pancreas, stomach, and duodenum work together to digest food in the body.

• Major disturbances of digestion in the GI tract include gastric bloating with or without flatulence, and inadequate or incomplete digestion.

• An adsorbent attracts molecules of a liquid, gas, or dissolved substance to its surface. Adsorbents are used to prevent drug or toxin absorption in the GI tract in acute poisonings.

• The adsorbent activated charcoal is a chemically inert powder that is not absorbed or metabolized by the body. It is excreted unchanged in the feces. Activated charcoal binds the toxin and thus inhibits its absorption.

• The nurse should keep in mind that an adsorbent is most effective when administered within 30 minutes of the poisoning.

• Antiflatulents are mixtures of liquid dimethylpolysiloxanes and silica gel that disperse and prevent the formation of mucus-enclosed gas pockets in the GI tract.

• The antiflatulent simethicone is a physiologically inactive substance that provides defoaming action in the GI tract. It is clinically safe when used to treat conditions in which excess gas is a problem.

• To promote the effectiveness of simethicone therapy, the nurse should teach the patient how to take the drug correctly and should assess the drug's effectiveness regularly.

• Specific digestants include bile salts, dehydrocholic acid, glutamic acid hydrochloride, hydrochloric acid (dilute), pancreatin, and pancrelipase.

• Digestants aid digestion in the patient who lacks one or more of the specific digestive substances produced by the body.

• When caring for a patient receiving a digestant, the nurse should provide specific instructions about the purpose of the drug and the precautions to take during administration.

STUDY QUESTIONS

See Appendix 1 for answers.

1. Carolyn Bevis, age 27, is admitted to the emergency department with a cocaine overdose. The physician orders immediate administration of activated charcoal. How does activated charcoal exert its therapeutic effect?
(a) by exerting an anabolic effect on toxins in the GI tract
(b) by enhancing the metabolism of toxins in the GI tract
(c) by absorbing the metabolic end products of toxins, thereby preventing their effects
(d) by attracting and binding with toxins, preventing their absorption in the GI tract

2. Which calculation is used to estimate the dose of activated charcoal?
(a) 5 to 10 times the patient's age
(b) 2 to 5 times the patient's weight
(c) 5 to 10 times the weight of the drug ingested
(d) 10 to 15 times the weight of the drug ingested

3. The nurse should expect which type of drug to be prescribed after activated charcoal is administered?
(a) an emetic
(b) an antacid
(c) an antiflatulent
(d) a laxative

4. Ken Carver, age 30, complains of abdominal fullness and bloating caused by an irritable colon. His physician prescibes simethicone (Mylicon) tablets 320 mg P.O. daily. How does simethicone relieve abdominal fullness?
(a) It disperses and prevents gas pocket formation.
(b) It facilitates expulsion of gas pockets.
(c) It neutralizes gastric contents, decreasing gas.
(d) It absorbs gas bubbles.

5. How should the nurse instruct Mr. Carver to take his medication?
(a) Take all the tablets at bedtime.
(b) Take each tablet on an empty stomach.
(c) Take one tablet after each meal and one at bedtime.
(d) Take half the tablets after breakfast and the other half at bedtime.

6. To help prevent gastric bloating, what else should the nurse teach Mr. Carver?
(a) Avoid concomitant use of antacids.
(b) Reduce activity to a minimum.
(c) Decrease fluid intake.
(d) Increase activity and exercise.

7. Diane Kellogg, age 40, had a cholecystectomy 3 days ago. Her physician prescribes dehydrocholic acid (Decholin) 244 mg P.O. t.i.d. to facilitate drainage of the common bile duct via the T-tube. How should the nurse administer this digestant?
(a) after meals
(b) with an antacid
(c) on an empty stomach
(d) with plenty of fluid

8. The nurse should monitor Ms. Kellogg for which adverse drug reaction?
(a) constipation
(b) diarrhea
(c) metabolic alkalosis
(d) flatulence

SELECTED REFERENCES

Activated charcoal alone for acute toxic ingestions. (1989). *Nurses Drug Alert,* 13(6), 48.

AHFS drug information 90. (1990). Bethesda, MD: American Society of Hospital Pharmacists.

Fardy, J., and Sullivan, S. (1988). Gastrointestinal gas. *Canadian Medical Association Journal,* 139(12), 1137-1142.

Hansten, P., and Horn, J. (1988). *Drug interactions: Clinical significance of drug-drug interactions* (6th ed.). Philadelphia: Lea & Febiger.

Krenzelok, E. (1987). Management of acute poisoning emergencies. *Emergency Medical Services,* 16(6), 26-33.

Levy, D. (1988). Activated charcoal update. *Emergency,* 20(6), 16-18.

North American Nursing Diagnosis Association. (1990). *Taxonomy I - Revised, with official categories.* St Louis: NANDA.

USPDI. (1991). *Drug information for the health care professional* (Vol. I, 11th ed.). Rockville, MD: United States Pharmacopeial Convention.

CHAPTER

42

ANTIDIARRHEAL AND LAXATIVE AGENTS

OBJECTIVES

After reading and studying this chapter, the student should be able to:

1. Identify the antidiarrheal agents indicated for acute, non-specific diarrhea and chronic diarrhea.

2. Explain the mechanism of action of opium tincture in alleviating diarrhea.

3. Discuss the potential adverse effects of opium tincture and paregoric.

4. Explain how loperamide, difenoxin, and diphenoxylate decrease gastrointestinal (GI) motility.

5. Describe the effectiveness of kaolin and pectin in treating different kinds of diarrhea.

6. Identify the contraindications and precautions the nurse should be aware of when administering antidiarrheals.

7. Describe the general mechanism of action of laxatives.

8. Compare the clinical indications for hyperosmolar, bulk-forming, emollient, stimulant, and lubricant laxatives.

9. Identify the fluid and electrolyte imbalances associated with hyperosmolar laxatives.

10. Describe how to apply the nursing process when caring for a patient who is receiving an antidiarrheal or laxative agent.

INTRODUCTION

Diarrhea and constipation represent the two major symptoms related to disturbances of the large intestine. Diarrhea refers to the increased frequency or weight and liquidity of stools produced by the rapid movement of fecal material through the large intestine. Constipation refers to the decreased movement of fecal matter through the large intestine.

Significant disorders involving diarrhea include ulcerative colitis, enteritis, and psychogenic diarrhea. Ulcerative colitis, a nonspecific inflammatory disease of the large intestine, is characterized by multiple ulcerations throughout the mucosal and submucosal linings of the intestine as well as repeated diarrheal stools. Although the cause of ulcerative colitis remains unclear, emotional factors as well as specific infectious bacteria may contribute to it. Enteritis is an infection of the large intestine caused by a virus or bacteria. Enteritis typically is an acute problem resulting in diarrhea, whereas ulcerative colitis usually is chronic, marked by acute exacerbations and remissions. Psychogenic diarrhea is characterized by excessive activation of the parasympathetic branch of the autonomic nervous system resulting in enhanced motility and secretion in the large intestine. This acute condition triggers a brief episode of self-limiting diarrhea.

Over time, the decreased peristaltic movements that characterize constipation may cause the production and accumulation of hard feces in the lower bowel, producing a decreased frequency, weight, and volume of stool passed. Most cases of constipation arise from poor bowel habits established in childhood and maintained through adulthood. This voluntary inhibition of normal defecation reflexes can weaken normal intestinal action. Long-term laxative abuse also impairs normal intestinal tone and peristaltic response, leading to an atonic bowel. Bowel retraining programs emphasize the gastrocolic and duodenocolic reflexes that are activated after a meal high in solid intake and fluids. Poor dietary habits also are a major cause of constipation, and constipation occasionally occurs from spasm of the sigmoid colon wall. The nurse may detect chronic constipation in patients who complain of repeated patterns of constipation and mucoid diarrhea. Constipation and diarrhea are common effects of many drugs.

Diarrhea and constipation involve debilitating physiologic sequelae that may interfere with an individual's ability to perform activities of daily living. Diarrhea may precipitate abdominal discomfort, malaise, and lethargy from dehydration. Constipation may be harmful in patients who

SELECTED NURSING DIAGNOSES

Antidiarrheal and laxative agents

The following nursing diagnoses address representative problems and etiologies that a nurse may encounter when caring for a patient who is receiving an antidiarrheal or laxative agent. Some of these nursing diagnoses contain generalized etiologies, which the nurse must individualize based on the patient's needs. (For some common nursing diagnoses and related interventions for each drug class, see the "Nursing Process Application" sections of this chapter.)

- Activity intolerance related to hyperosmolar laxative-induced weakness and lethargy
- Altered health maintenance related to ineffectiveness of the prescribed antidiarrheal or laxative agent
- Altered nutrition: less than body requirements, related to impaired absorption of nutrients and fat-soluble vitamins caused by long-term use of mineral oil or a stimulant laxative
- Altered protection related to electrolyte imbalance caused by a hyperosmolar or stimulant laxative
- Constipation related to the adverse gastrointestinal (GI) effects of an antidiarrheal or laxative agent
- Diarrhea related to the adverse GI effects of an antidiarrheal or laxative agent
- Fatigue related to the adverse effects of an antidiarrheal agent
- Hyperthermia related to the adverse central nervous system (CNS) effects of atropine
- Impaired skin integrity related to seepage of mineral oil after rectal administration
- Knowledge deficit related to the prescribed antidiarrheal or laxative agent
- Pain related to rectal administration of bisacodyl

- Potential fluid volume deficit related to decreased intake caused by the adverse GI effects of an antidiarrheal agent
- Potential fluid volume deficit related to hypovolemia caused by lactulose or a saline compound
- Potential for injury related to a preexisting condition that contraindicates the use of an antidiarrheal or laxative agent
- Potential for injury related to a preexisting condition that requires cautious use of an antidiarrheal or laxative agent
- Potential for injury related to adverse drug reactions
- Potential for injury related to drug interactions
- Potential for trauma related to cathartic colon caused by habitual use of a stimulant laxative
- Potential for trauma related to CNS depression caused by an antidiarrheal agent
- Potential for trauma related to hypoperistalsis or intestinal or esophageal obstruction caused by an antidiarrheal agent
- Sensory-perceptual alterations (visual) related to the adverse CNS effects of atropine
- Urinary retention related to the adverse genitourinary effects of atropine in difenoxin or diphenoxylate

should not strain, such as those with recent myocardial infarction. For patients with these problems, drugs designed to control diarrhea and constipation are invaluable.

Antidiarrheals reduce the fluidity of the stool and the frequency of defecation. They act systemically or locally. Opium tincture, paregoric, loperamide, difenoxin, and diphenoxylate are systemic agents. The combination of kaolin and pectin is a local agent.

Laxatives and cathartics include various drugs that stimulate defecation. Laxatives exert their effects by increasing the water content of the feces and increasing the movement of intestinal materials from the colon and rectum. The term *cathartic* implies a fluid evacuation in contrast to the term *laxative,* which implies the elimination of a soft, formed stool.

The major classes of laxatives include the hyperosmolar agents, dietary fiber and related bulk-forming substances, emollients, stimulants, and lubricants. The U.S. Food and Drug Administration Advisory Review Panel for Over-the-Counter Drugs has approved various laxative-cathartic agents as nonprescription drugs. Some patients abuse laxatives, which can cause physical dependence for maintenance of bowel pattern.

For a summary of representative drugs, see *Selected major drugs: Antidiarrheal and laxative agents,* pages 729 and 730. For a listing of applicable nursing diagnoses that the nurse may formulate when caring for a patient receiving these agents, see *Selected nursing diagnoses: Antidiarrheal and laxative agents.* For detailed information on applying the nursing process, see Chapter 6, The Nursing Process and Drug Therapy.

ANTIDIARRHEALS: OPIUM PREPARATIONS

Opium tincture and camphorated opium tincture (paregoric) are effective in treating acute, nonspecific diarrhea. However, these drugs should not be used for diarrhea caused by toxic chemicals or pathogens. These antidiarrheals, which are absorbed well, produce some of the systemic effects of morphine in high doses.

PHARMACOKINETICS

Opium tincture and paregoric have similar pharmacokinetic properties. Both are absorbed systemically, metabolized by the liver, and excreted by the kidneys. The onset of action occurs within 1 hour of administration.

Absorption, distribution, metabolism, excretion

When administered orally, opium tincture and paregoric are absorbed quickly from the GI tract. After absorption, the drugs are distributed to various parenchymatous tissues, specifically the kidneys, lungs, liver, and spleen. Metabolism and detoxification via conjugation with glucuronic acid occur in the liver. Approximately 90% of the opioid metabolites are excreted by the kidneys; the remainder is excreted as bile products in the feces.

Onset, peak, duration

When given orally, opium tincture and paregoric have an onset that occurs within the first hour and concentrations that peak within 2 to 3 hours. The duration of action is about 4 hours.

PHARMACODYNAMICS

The morphine in opium tincture and paregoric decreases GI motility and peristaltic movements.

Mechanism of action

The binding or receptor sites for opium tincture and paregoric are found in the nerve plexuses and exocrine glands of the stomach and large and small intestines. The morphine decreases hydrochloric acid secretion and stomach motility, and increases antral tone. It also decreases propulsive contractions in the small intestine.

Opium tincture and paregoric exert an antidiarrheal effect by (1) slowing the effects of the mesenteric plexus of the intestine, (2) inhibiting intestinal peristalsis by direct central action on the brain, (3) decreasing propulsive contractions, (4) enhancing anal sphincter tone, and (5) enhancing ileocecal valve tone.

PHARMACOTHERAPEUTICS

Opium tincture and paregoric are used to treat acute, nonspecific diarrhea. They commonly are used with kaolin, pectin, and bismuth salts because these three drugs offer adsorbent and protective effects. Also, opium tincture may be added to enteral feeding preparations to prevent the diarrhea that they typically cause. In large doses, opium tincture may affect the central nervous system (CNS).

opium tincture. A Schedule II drug, opium tincture is used to treat acute, nonspecific diarrhea.

Usual adult dosage: 0.6 ml (range 0.3 to 1 ml) P.O. q.i.d. The dosage should not exceed 6 ml daily.

paregoric or camphorated opium tincture. A Schedule III drug, paregoric is used to treat diarrhea. This drug is more dilute than opium tincture and is easier to measure.
Usual adult dosage: 5 to 10 ml P.O. daily to q.i.d., until acute diarrhea subsides.
Usual pediatric dosage: 0.25 to 0.5 ml/kg/day daily to q.i.d., until diarrhea subsides.

Drug interactions

Opium tincture and paregoric can enhance the depressant effects of alcohol, barbiturates, tranquilizers, and other CNS depressants. The drugs have an additive effect of constipation when used with anticholinergic drugs.

ADVERSE DRUG REACTIONS

Some adverse reactions to opium tincture and paregoric occur. However, reactions to usual doses typically are mild. Dose-related reactions to opium tincture and paregoric include nausea, vomiting, dizziness, dysphoria, constipation, and increased biliary tract pressure.

Hypersensitivity reactions include allergic reactions, such as urticaria and contact dermatitis. Anaphylactoid reactions are rare. Patients over age 60 experience more frequent allergic reactions and decreased sensitivity to pain.

NURSING PROCESS APPLICATION

The following information assists the nurse in caring for a patient who is receiving an antidiarrheal opium preparation.

Assessment

• Review the patient's history for a preexisting condition that contraindicates the use of an opium preparation, such as known hypersensitivity to the drug.
• Review the patient's history for a preexisting condition that requires cautious use of an opium preparation, such as asthma, severe prostatic hypertrophy, narcotic dependence, liver or kidney dysfunction, pregnancy, or lactation.
• Assess the patient for adverse reactions to the opium preparation, such as nausea, vomiting, dizziness, dysphoria, constipation, increased biliary tract pressure, or hypersensitivity reactions.
• Review the patient's medication history to identify the use of drugs that may interact with the opium preparation, such as CNS depressants and anticholinergic drugs.
• Assess the effectiveness of the opium preparation regularly.
• Assess the patient's bowel pattern regularly.
• Evaluate the patient's and family's knowledge about the prescribed opium preparation.

Nursing diagnoses

The following examples represent appropriate nursing diagnoses for a patient receiving an opium preparation.
• Potential for injury related to a preexisting condition that contraindicates the use of an opium preparation
• Potential for injury related to a preexisting condition that requires cautious use of an opium preparation
• Potential for injury related to adverse drug reactions
• Potential for injury related to drug interactions
• Altered health maintenance related to ineffectiveness of the opium preparation
• Constipation related to the adverse GI effects of the opium preparation
• Knowledge deficit related to the prescribed opium preparation

Planning and implementation

• Do not administer an opium preparation to a patient with a condition that contraindicates its use. Also do not administer an opium preparation to treat diarrhea caused by toxic chemicals or pathogens.
• Administer an opium preparation with caution to a patient at risk because of a preexisting condition.
• *Monitor the patient closely for adverse reactions during treatment with an opium preparation. Be especially alert for allergic reactions and decreased sensitivity to pain in a patient over age 60.*
• Monitor hydration if the patient experiences nausea and vomiting. Obtain a prescription for an antiemetic agent, as needed.
• *Take safety precautions if the patient experiences dizziness. For example, place the bed in a low position, keep the side rails up, and supervise ambulation.*
• *Do not interchange opium tincture with paregoric because the opium content of opium tincture is 25 times greater.*
• Expect a milky fluid to form when paregoric is added to water.
• Notify the physician if adverse reactions occur.
• *Monitor for enhanced CNS depression if the patient receives an opium preparation and another CNS depressant.*
• Monitor the patient's GI response to the drug. Record the frequency and amount of bowel movements per day, and replace fluid as needed.
• *Consult with the physician if the patient's diarrhea lasts longer than 48 hours or if fever and abdominal pain develop during opium preparation therapy. If the opium preparation is ineffective, the patient may require a change in the therapeutic regimen.*
• Monitor for constipation during treatment with an opium preparation, especially if the patient also is receiving an anticholinergic drug.
• Notify the physician if constipation occurs.

Patient teaching

• Teach the patient and family the name, dose, frequency, action, and adverse effects of the prescribed opium preparation.
• *Counsel the patient to take the drug as prescribed to avoid dependence.*
• *Instruct the patient to notify the physician if diarrhea lasts longer than 48 hours or if fever and abdominal pain develop during treatment with the opium preparation.*
• Instruct the patient to drink additional fluids to replace those lost through diarrhea.
• *Advise the patient to avoid activities that require mental alertness if dizziness occurs.*
• Inform the patient that paregoric normally appears milky when added to water.
• Instruct the patient to notify the physician if adverse reactions occur.

Evaluation

The following examples represent appropriate evaluation statements for a patient receiving an opium preparation.
• The patient has no conditions that contraindicate the use of an opium preparation.
• The patient exhibits no signs of complications in the preexisting condition linked to the prescribed opium preparation.
• The patient displays no signs of adverse reactions to the prescribed opium preparation.
• The patient uses no drugs that interact with the opium preparation.
• The patient demonstrates reduced diarrhea within 24 hours.
• The patient resumes a normal bowel pattern.
• The patient and family express an accurate understanding of the points taught about the prescribed opium preparation.
• The patient correctly describes conditions that require physician notification during treatment with an opium preparation.

ANTIDIARRHEALS: DIFENOXIN, DIPHENOXYLATE, AND LOPERAMIDE

Difenoxin, diphenoxylate, and loperamide are synthetic drugs related to meperidine. These drugs decrease peristalsis in the intestines. Loperamide produces less severe CNS effects than do difenoxin or diphenoxylate, which are combined with atropine to prevent abuse.

PHARMACOKINETICS

Difenoxin and diphenoxylate have better absorption, a faster onset of action, and a shorter duration of action than loperamide.

Absorption, distribution, metabolism, excretion

At the usual dosage, difenoxin and diphenoxylate are absorbed readily into the GI tract. When extremely high doses (40 to 60 mg) are administered inadvertently, these drugs penetrate well into the brain. Loperamide, which is not absorbed well after oral administration, does not penetrate well into the brain. After oral administration, these drugs enter the GI tract to bind with receptor sites in the mucosal layers of the large and small intestines. These medications are distributed in the serum. Metabolism occurs with the detoxification process in the liver. Diphenoxylate is metabolized to difenoxin, its biologically active, major metabolite. All three drugs are excreted primarily in the feces.

Onset, peak, duration

The peak concentration level of difenoxin probably occurs 40 to 60 minutes after administration; of diphenoxylate, 2 to 3 hours after administration. Diphenoxylate has a half-life of about 2.5 hours; its active metabolite difenoxin has a half-life of 3 to 12 hours. The duration of action of difenoxin and diphenoxylate is 3 to 4 hours.

The loperamide concentration peaks in 4 to 5 hours after oral administration. Loperamide has a longer duration and half-life than difenoxin and diphenoxylate. Loperamide's duration is 7 to 10 hours; its half-life, 7 to 14 hours.

PHARMACODYNAMICS

Difenoxin, diphenoxylate, and loperamide decrease peristalsis in the large and small intestine.

Mechanism of action

Difenoxin, diphenoxylate, and loperamide decrease GI motility by depressing the circular and longitudinal muscle action in the large and small intestines. These drugs also decrease propulsive contractions throughout the entire colon. Diphenoxylate may provide an antisecretory effect as well, but has little analgesic effect.

Difenoxin and diphenoxylate are combined with the anticholinergic agent atropine to discourage abuse of these agents. The addition of atropine is effective because the toxic effects of atropine occur before the narcotic effects of difenoxin or diphenoxylate. The symptoms of atropine toxicity (dry mouth, urine retention, tachycardia, and hyperthermia) tend to discourage abuse. Loperamide produces little CNS effect in usual dosages.

PHARMACOTHERAPEUTICS

Difenoxin, diphenoxylate, and loperamide are used to treat acute, nonspecific diarrhea. Loperamide also is used to treat chronic diarrhea. Large doses of difenoxin or diphenoxylate may affect the CNS, especially the brain; loperamide does not enter the CNS readily.

difenoxin hydrochloride (Motofen). A Schedule IV drug, difenoxin is given with atropine to adults for acute, nonspecific diarrhea. Little is known about the drug's safety and effectiveness in children.
Usual adult dosage: 2 mg P.O. initially, followed by 1 mg after every loose stool or 1 mg every 3 to 4 hours as needed up to a maximum of 8 mg daily. If no improvement occurs within 48 hours, the drug should be discontinued.

diphenoxylate hydrochloride (Lomotil). A Schedule V drug, diphenoxylate is given with atropine for acute, nonspecific diarrhea.
Usual adult dosage: for acute, nonspecific diarrhea, 5 mg P.O. q.i.d. initially; thereafter, the dosage is adjusted to the patient's response.
Usual pediatric dosage: 0.3 to 0.4 mg/kg daily, given in divided doses for children over age 2, in liquid form only; dosage may be reduced to as low as one-fourth the initial dose as soon as initial symptoms have been controlled.

loperamide (Imodium). This drug is used to treat acute, nonspecific diarrhea and chronic diarrhea.
Usual adult dosage: for acute, nonspecific diarrhea, 4 mg P.O. initially, then 2 mg after each unformed stool to a maximum dosage of 16 mg/day; for chronic diarrhea, 4 mg P.O. initially, then 2 mg after each unformed stool until diarrhea subsides. Then the dosage is adjusted to the patient's response.
Usual pediatric dosage: for acute diarrhea, initially 1 mg P.O. t.i.d. for children age 2 to 5, liquid form only; 2 mg P.O. b.i.d. for children age 6 to 8; 2 mg P.O. t.i.d. for children age 6 to 12 (over 30 kg); after the first day, 0.1 mg/kg is administered after a loose stool only.

Drug interactions

Difenoxin, diphenoxylate, and loperamide may enhance the depressant effects of barbiturates, alcohol, narcotics, tranquilizers, and sedatives.

ADVERSE DRUG REACTIONS

The adverse reactions to difenoxin, diphenoxylate, and loperamide include nausea, vomiting, abdominal discomfort or distention, drowsiness, fatigue, CNS depression, tachycardia, hypoperistalsis, and paralytic ileus. Allergic responses, such as rash and urticaria, may occur as hypersensitivity responses to difenoxin, diphenoxylate, and loperamide.

Adverse reactions to atropine include flushing, diminished secretions, hyperthermia, tachycardia, urine retention, miosis, nystagmus, and blurred vision.

NURSING PROCESS APPLICATION

The following information assists the nurse in caring for a patient who is receiving difenoxin, diphenoxylate, or loperamide.

Assessment
• Review the patient's history for a preexisting condition that contraindicates the use of difenoxin, diphenoxylate, or loperamide, such as known hypersensitivity to the drug or atropine sulfate, antibiotic-induced diarrhea or pseudomembranous colitis, diarrhea caused by infection with a certain organism (such as *Shigella, Salmonella,* or a particular strain of *Escherichia coli*), or a condition in which constipation must be avoided.
• Review the patient's history for a preexisting condition that requires cautious use of difenoxin, diphenoxylate, or loperamide, such as benign prostatic hypertrophy, narcotic dependence, liver dysfunction, pregnancy, lactation, or advanced hepatorenal disease.
• Assess the patient for adverse reactions to difenoxin, diphenoxylate, or loperamide, such as GI distress, CNS depression, or tachycardia. Also assess for signs of atropine toxicity, such as dry mouth, blurred vision, flushing, tachycardia, or urine retention.
• Review the patient's medication history to identify use of drugs that may interact with difenoxin, diphenoxylate, or loperamide, such as CNS depressants.
• Assess the effectiveness of difenoxin, diphenoxylate, or loperamide every 4 hours.

Signs of hypoperistalsis

The nurse should watch for the following signs and symptoms of hypoperistalsis during difenoxin, diphenoxylate, or loperamide therapy. If hypoperistalsis occurs, withhold the next dose of the drug and notify the physician.
• Anorexia and nausea in early stage
• Abdominal distention
• Auscultation of rushes or high-pitched sounds over the abdomen
• Eventually a "silent abdomen"—absent bowel sounds
• Possible percussion of air or fluid over abdomen
• Absence of flatus
• Absence of bowel movements
• Possible vomiting with resultant fluid and electrolyte imbalance

---

• Assess the patient receiving an antidiarrheal with atropine for signs of urine retention, such as urinary frequency or a sensation of fullness in the lower abdomen after voiding.
• Evaluate the patient's and family's knowledge about the prescribed antidiarrheal agent.

Nursing diagnoses
The following examples represent appropriate nursing diagnoses for a patient receiving difenoxin, diphenoxylate, or loperamide.
• Potential for injury related to a preexisting condition that contraindicates the use of difenoxin, diphenoxylate, or loperamide
• Potential for injury related to a preexisting condition that requires cautious use of difenoxin, diphenoxylate, or loperamide
• Potential for injury related to adverse drug reactions
• Urinary retention related to the adverse genitourinary effects of atropine in difenoxin or diphenoxylate
• Knowledge deficit related to the prescribed antidiarrheal agent

Planning and implementation
• Do not administer difenoxin, diphenoxylate, or loperamide to a patient with a condition that contraindicates its use.
• Administer difenoxin, diphenoxylate, or loperamide cautiously to a patient at risk because of a preexisting condition.
• Monitor the patient closely for adverse reactions to the prescribed antidiarrheal agent.
• *Observe for signs of atropine toxicity during difenoxin or diphenoxylate therapy, and reduce the dosage as prescribed.*
• Observe for signs of hypoperistalsis, and consult a physician if it occurs. (For details about this condition, see *Signs of hypoperistalsis.*)
• *Withhold the drug and consult the physician if the patient shows signs of abdominal distention, which may indicate toxic megacolon, especially in ulcerative colitis.*
• Monitor the patient's fluid and electrolyte status as well as the frequency and amount of bowel movements to ensure fluid and electrolyte balance.
• *Take safety precautions if drowsiness occurs. For example, place the bed in a low position, keep the side rails up, and supervise ambulation.*
• *Perform a neurologic check regularly to assess for CNS depression, especially during concomitant therapy with another CNS depressant.*
• Monitor the patient's heart rate regularly to detect tachycardia.
• *Withhold the drug and consult the physician if the patient with acute nonspecific diarrhea shows no improvement in 48 hours or if the patient with chronic diarrhea shows no improvement after 10 days.*

• Notify the physician if adverse reactions occur.
• *Monitor for urine retention regularly in a patient receiving difenoxin or diphenoxylate with atropine, especially if the patient has benign prostatic hypertrophy.*
• Ask the patient about urinary frequency and a sensation of fullness in the lower abdomen after voiding. If the patient reports these symptoms, palpate and percuss the bladder.
• Notify the physician if urine retention is suspected. Be prepared to catheterize the patient as prescribed. Expect to reduce the antidiarrheal dosage or administer a different antidiarrheal agent as prescribed.

Patient teaching

• Teach the patient and family the name, dose, frequency, action, and adverse effects of the prescribed antidiarrheal agent.
• *Advise the patient not to use alcohol or any other CNS depressant during difenoxin, diphenoxylate, or loperamide therapy.*
• *Teach the patient taking difenoxin or diphenoxylate with atropine to recognize and report the signs of atropine toxicity, which may require a dosage reduction.*
• *Instruct the patient to be alert for early warning signs of hypoperistalsis (nausea and anorexia) and toxic megacolon (abdominal distention). If these signs occur, tell the patient to notify the physician before taking the next dose of the prescribed antidiarrheal agent.*
• Encourage the patient to maintain a fluid intake of 8 to 13 8-oz glasses (2 to 3 liters) per day to replace the fluid lost through diarrhea.
• Caution the patient to avoid any activity that requires mental alertness if drowsiness occurs.
• *Teach the patient taking difenoxin or diphenoxylate with atropine to recognize and report signs or symptoms of urine retention.*
• Instruct the patient to consult the physician if acute nonspecific diarrhea does not improve in 48 hours, or if chronic diarrhea does not improve after 10 days.

Evaluation

The following examples represent appropriate evaluation statements for a patient receiving difenoxin, diphenoxylate, or loperamide.
• The patient has no conditions that contraindicate difenoxin, diphenoxylate, or loperamide therapy.
• The patient exhibits no signs of complications in the preexisting condition linked to the prescribed antidiarrheal agent.
• The patient experiences no adverse reactions to the prescribed antidiarrheal agent.
• The patient maintains a normal voiding pattern while receiving difenoxin or diphenoxylate with atropine.
• The patient and family express an accurate understanding of the points taught about the prescribed antidiarrheal agent.

• The patient correctly describes adverse reactions to the prescribed antidiarrheal agent and explains what to do if they occur.

ANTIDIARRHEALS: KAOLIN AND PECTIN

Kaolin and pectin, which are locally acting antidiarrheals, act as adsorbents. (For more information about adsorbents, see Chapter 41, Adsorbent, Antiflatulent, and Digestive Agents.) They are used to treat acute diarrhea from various causes. Although their effectiveness has not been established firmly through clinical studies, kaolin and pectin are sold over the counter and are used widely.

Kaolin is a hydrated aluminum silicate. Pectin is a purified carbohydrate product obtained from the acid extraction of citrus fruit rinds or from apple pomace.

PHARMACOKINETICS

Because kaolin and pectin are locally acting antidiarrheals, they are not absorbed and, therefore, not distributed throughout the body. Up to 90% of a dose is metabolized in the GI tract. The drugs and their metabolites are excreted in the feces.

The onset of action of kaolin and pectin occurs within 30 minutes after oral administration. Duration of action is 4 to 6 hours.

PHARMACODYNAMICS

Kaolin and pectin produce their antidiarrheal effects by acting as adsorbents and protectants on the intestinal mucosa.

Mechanism of action

Kaolin and pectin act as adsorbents, binding with bacteria, toxins, and other irritants on the intestinal mucosa. Pectin decreases the pH in the intestinal lumen and provides a soothing demulcent effect on the irritated mucosa. Both drugs protect the intestinal mucosa.

PHARMACOTHERAPEUTICS

Kaolin and pectin are used to relieve mild to moderate acute diarrhea. They also may be used to relieve chronic diarrhea temporarily until the cause has been determined and definitive treatment instituted. These agents are used safely to treat diarrhea of unknown cause, even if toxins or bacteria are suspected as the etiology. In the home, they commonly are used to treat simple gastroenteritis. Kaolin and pectin preparations are minimally effective for mild to moderate acute diarrhea, but are of little value in severe diarrhea. These drugs typically have a mild effect on the GI tract.

kaolin and pectin mixtures (Kaopectate, Pecto Kay). Available over the counter, kaolin and pectin mixtures are used to treat mild to moderate nonspecific diarrhea. Both drugs usually prove effective within 48 hours.
Usual adult dosage: for regular-strength suspension, 60 to 120 ml P.O.; for concentrated suspension, 45 to 90 ml P.O. Administer regular or concentrated suspension after each loose bowel movement, usually up to eight doses per day.
Usual pediatric dosage: for children age 3 to 5, 15 to 30 ml P.O. of regular suspension or 15 ml P.O. of concentrated suspension; for children age 6 to 11, 30 to 60 ml P.O. of regular suspension or 30 ml of concentrated suspension.

Drug interactions
Kaolin and pectin mixtures interfere with lincomycin absorption if administered within 2 hours before or 3 to 4 hours after lincomycin. These antidiarrheals also can interfere with absorption of digoxin or other drugs from the intestinal mucosa if administered concurrently.

ADVERSE DRUG REACTIONS

Kaolin and pectin mixtures cause few adverse reactions. Constipation may occur, especially in an elderly or debilitated patient, or with overdose and prolonged use, but the constipation usually is mild and transient. Rarely, fecal impaction occurs in infants and debilitated patients.

NURSING PROCESS APPLICATION

The following information assists the nurse in caring for a patient who is receiving a kaolin and pectin mixture.

Assessment
• Assess the patient for adverse reactions to kaolin and pectin, such as constipation or fecal impaction.
• Review the patient's medication history to identify the use of drugs that may interact with kaolin and pectin, such as lincomycin or digoxin.
• Assess the effectiveness of kaolin and pectin regularly.
• Evaluate the patient's and family's knowledge about kaolin and pectin.

Nursing diagnoses
The following examples represent appropriate nursing diagnoses for a patient receiving kaolin and pectin.
• Constipation related to the adverse GI effects of kaolin and pectin

• Knowledge deficit related to kaolin and pectin

Planning and implementation
• *Monitor the patient closely for constipation during kaolin and pectin therapy. Be aware that fecal impaction can result from severe constipation, especially in an infant or debilitated patient.*
• Withhold kaolin and pectin if the patient develops constipation, and notify the physician.

Patient teaching
• Teach the patient and family the name, dose, frequency, action, and adverse effects of kaolin and pectin.
• *Advise the patient to avoid self-medication for longer than 48 hours. Instruct the patient to consult a physician if diarrhea persists.*
• *Instruct the patient taking other medications to consult the physician because kaolin and pectin can interfere with the absorption of other drugs, making them ineffective.*
• Instruct the patient to drink at least 8 to 13 8-oz glasses (2 to 3 liters) of fluid daily to replace fluids lost through diarrhea.
• *Instruct the patient to take kaolin and pectin as prescribed; for example, a dose of kaolin and pectin after each loose bowel movement, but not more than eight doses per day. The patient who experiences more than eight bowel movements in one day should consult the physician.*

Evaluation
The following examples represent appropriate evaluation statements for a patient receiving kaolin and pectin.
• The patient resumes normal bowel patterns.
• The patient and family express an accurate understanding of the points taught about kaolin and pectin.
• The patient discusses other drug use with the physician.

HYPEROSMOLAR LAXATIVES

Hyperosmolar laxatives include glycerin, lactulose, and saline compounds (magnesium salts, sodium biphosphate, and sodium phosphate). These laxatives produce an osmotic effect in the intestinal lumen that causes fluid accumulation, intestinal distention, and eventual peristalsis. (For information about lactulose as an ammonia-detoxicating agent, see Chapter 48, Cation-Exchange Resin and Ammonia-Detoxicating Agents.)

PHARMACOKINETICS

These agents are absorbed poorly. They act within 30 minutes to 2 days.

Absorption, distribution, metabolism, excretion

Glycerin acts by osmotic fluid pressure shifts. Once inside the intestinal lumen, glycerin pulls water from the extraluminal spaces into the feces and stimulates reflex evacuation. Glycerin is introduced into the large intestine and is not absorbed systemically.

Lactulose enters the GI tract and is absorbed only to a minor degree; thus, the drug is distributed only in the intestine. Its site of action is the colon. Because lactulose is not hydrolyzed in the small intestine, it is not absorbed, and water and electrolytes are retained in the intestinal lumen because of the osmotic effect of the lactulose. In the distal ileum and colon, the unabsorbed lactulose is metabolized by the intestinal microflora into lactate and other organic acids, thereby significantly reducing the fecal pH. Blood ammonia concentrations are reduced 25% to 50% via the movement of the fluid and electrolytes into the intestinal lumen. This effect also is useful in treating systemic portal encephalopathy in patients with chronic liver disease. Lactulose is excreted in the feces.

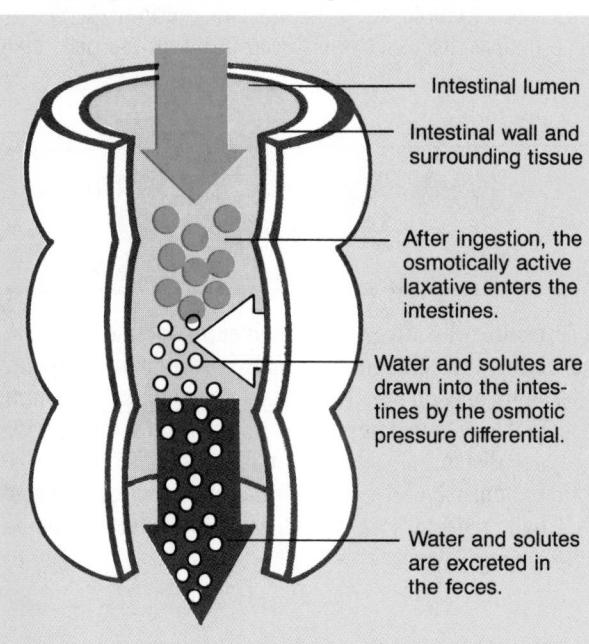

Effect of hyperosmolar laxatives on the intestine

Water and electrolytes increase the mass of the feces, distending the colon and causing bowel evacuation.

Intestinal lumen

Intestinal wall and surrounding tissue

After ingestion, the osmotically active laxative enters the intestines.

Water and solutes are drawn into the intestines by the osmotic pressure differential.

Water and solutes are excreted in the feces.

The saline compounds are natural substances used primarily for prompt bowel evacuation. Because saline compounds are hypernatremic solutions, they produce hypertonicity within the intestine. Once they are introduced into the GI tract, some absorption of the component ions occurs.

Approximately 20% of the magnesium in magnesium salts is absorbed systemically and excreted in the urine. The patient's renal function must be adequate or toxicity may occur.

Approximately 10% of the sodium in sodium phosphate and sodium biphosphate enemas may be absorbed and excreted in the urine.

Onset, peak, duration

Acting in the distal colon, glycerin usually causes bowel evacuation 15 to 30 minutes after administration. Bowel evacuation should occur 1 to 2 days after administration of lactulose. Saline cathartics produce a watery stool evacuation within 1 to 3 hours after administration.

PHARMACODYNAMICS

The hyperosmolar laxatives produce bowel evacuation by drawing water into the intestine. Distention of the bowel from fluid accumulation promotes peristalsis and bowel movement.

Mechanism of action

Like the other hyperosmolar laxatives, glycerin draws water into the intestinal lumen, producing bowel hypervolemia and a watery stool evacuation. (For a depiction of this mechanism of action, see *Effect of hyperosmolar laxatives on the intestine.*)

Lactulose usually produces a laxative effect by drawing water into the intestinal lumen. This drug promotes water and electrolyte retention in the intestine; unabsorbed, the drug is metabolized into lactate and other organic acids that decrease the fecal pH.

The laxative effect of saline cathartics, including magnesium salts and sodium phosphate, has two results: (1) hypertonicity within the lumen, which produces an osmotic effect; as a result, water rapidly enters the intestine, producing hypervolemia; and (2) stimulation of cholecystokinin secretion, which produces a spasm of Oddi's sphincter, the passage of bile into the duodenum, stimulation of intestinal motility, and inhibition of fluid and electrolyte absorption from the jejunum and ileum.

PHARMACOTHERAPEUTICS

Glycerin is helpful in bowel retraining. Lactulose is used to treat chronic constipation and reduce ammonia production and absorption from the intestines in liver disease.

Saline compounds are used when prompt and complete bowel evacuation is required.

glycerin. Suppositories are administered primarily to re-establish proper bowel patterns in laxative-dependent patients.
Usual adult dosage: 3 grams by suppository; 5 to 15 ml as an enema.

lactulose (Cephulac, Chronulac). Primarily used to reduce ammonia levels in liver dysfunction when the patient has systemic portal encephalopathy, lactulose also is used to manage chronic constipation.
Usual adult dosage: for constipation, 10 to 20 grams (15 to 30 ml) P.O. daily; for systemic portal encephalopathy, 20 to 30 grams (30 to 45 ml) P.O. t.i.d. or q.i.d., until two to three soft stools are produced daily, or 200 grams (300 ml) diluted in 700 ml of water or normal saline solution given via rectal balloon catheter and retained 30 to 60 minutes every 4 to 6 hours.

magnesium salts [magnesium citrate, magnesium hydroxide, magnesium sulfate] (Milk of Magnesia). Administered to relieve chronic constipation, magnesium salts also are used for complete bowel evacuation and as a general laxative.
Usual adult dosage: for chronic constipation and bowel evacuation, 10 to 15 grams of the sulfate salt P.O. in a glass of water, or 240 ml of the citrate salt P.O. h.s.; as a laxative, 15 to 40 ml of the hydroxide salt P.O. h.s.

sodium biphosphate or sodium phosphate (Fleet Enema, PhosphoSoda). These drugs are used as laxatives.
Usual adult dosage: oral solution, 20 to 30 ml mixed with a glass of water; enema, 120 ml (4 ounces).

Drug interactions
Hyperosmolar laxatives do not interact significantly with other drugs.

ADVERSE DRUG REACTIONS

The adverse reactions to hyperosmolar laxatives involve fluid and electrolyte imbalances. Glycerin administration, which is quite safe, produces relatively few adverse reactions. However, it may cause weakness and fatigue. Severe diarrhea and hypovolemia also may occur, but rarely.

Although lactulose administration has little risk of toxicity, predictable adverse reactions include abdominal distention, flatulence, and abdominal cramps in approximately 20% of patients taking full doses. Other adverse reactions include nausea, vomiting, diarrhea, hypokalemia, hypovolemia, increased blood glucose level in patients with impaired glucose tolerance, and increased systemic portal encephalopathy in patients with severe liver dysfunction.

Adverse effects of saline cathartics

The following electrolyte and fluid imbalances may occur with excessive use of saline cathartics. When caring for a patient receiving a saline cathartic, the nurse should monitor for the signs and symptoms of such imbalances.

Hypernatremia	• Tachycardia • Hypotension • Dry mucous membranes • Oliguria • Thirst • Dehydration • Coma
Hypermagnesemia	• Muscle weakness • Nausea • Vomiting • Diminished reflexes • Drowsiness • Tachycardia • Hypotension • Flaccid paralysis • Coma • Respiratory distress
Hypocalcemia	• Generalized neuromuscular irritability • Facial spasms • Grimace • Laryngospasm • Positive Chvostek's sign • Tetany • Seizures • Cardiac arrhythmias • Cardiac arrest
Hypovolemic shock	• Hypotension • Tachycardia • Oliguria • Decreased central venous pressure • Decreased cardiac output • Diminished vital organ perfusion

Adverse reactions to saline compounds include weakness, lethargy, dehydration from hypernatremia and resultant hypovolemia, hypermagnesemia, hyperphosphatemia, hypocalcemia, cardiac arrhythmias from electrolyte imbalance, and hypovolemic shock. (For the signs and symptoms of these imbalances, see *Adverse effects of saline cathartics.*)

NURSING PROCESS APPLICATION

The following information assists the nurse in caring for a patient who is receiving a hyperosmolar laxative.

Assessment

• Review the patient's history for a preexisting condition that contraindicates the use of a hyperosmolar laxative, such as congenital megacolon, imperforate anus, congestive heart failure, or any condition that requires a low-galactose diet.

• Review the patient's history for a preexisting condition that requires cautious use of a hyperosmolar laxative, such as diabetes mellitus, pregnancy, lactation, renal impairment, cardiac disease, colostomy, electrolyte imbalance, or a condition that predisposes the patient to electrolyte imbalance.

• Assess the patient for adverse reactions to the hyperosmolar laxative, such as fluid and electrolyte imbalances.

• Assess the effectiveness of the prescribed hyperosmolar laxative.

• Evaluate the patient's and family's knowledge about the prescribed hyperosmolar laxative.

Nursing diagnoses

The following examples represent appropriate nursing diagnoses for a patient receiving a hyperosmolar laxative.

• Potential for injury related to a preexisting condition that contraindicates the use of a hyperosmolar laxative

• Potential for injury related to a preexisting condition that requires cautious use of a hyperosmolar laxative

• Potential for injury related to adverse drug reactions

• Potential fluid volume deficit related to hypovolemia caused by lactulose or a saline compound

• Knowledge deficit related to the prescribed hyperosmolar laxative

Planning and implementation

• Do not administer a hyperosmolar laxative to a patient with a condition that contraindicates its use.

• Administer a hyperosmolar laxative cautiously to a patient at risk because of a preexisting condition.

• Monitor the patient for signs of adverse reactions to hyperosmolar laxative therapy.

• *Monitor the patient closely for fluid and electrolyte imbalances during hyperosmolar laxative therapy.* For example, assess the patient's vital signs regularly, being particularly alert for decreased blood pressure, tachycardia, irregular pulse, depressed respiratory rate, or a change in the respiratory pattern. Also monitor electrolyte levels as instructed to detect hypernatremia, hypermagnesemia, hypocalcemia, and other electrolyte imbalances.

• *Perform a neurologic assessment regularly to detect the CNS effects of an electrolyte imbalance.*

• *Take safety precautions if the patient develops weakness, drowsiness, or lethargy. For example, place the bed in a low position, keep the side rails up, and supervise ambulation.*

• *Monitor blood glucose levels once every shift or as prescribed for a patient with impaired glucose tolerance who is receiving lactulose. Also observe for signs of hyperglycemia, such as polyuria, polydipsia, polyphagia, and weakness.*

• Dilute lactulose with water or unsweetened juice before administration to reduce the sweetness and prevent nausea.

• Store lactulose below 86°F (30°C), but do not allow the drug to freeze.

• Encourage the patient to drink 8 to 13 8-oz glasses (2 to 3 liters) of fluid daily (unless contraindicated) during saline compound therapy.

• Monitor the patient's bowel patterns periodically throughout therapy to assess the drug's effectiveness or detect diarrhea.

• Notify the physician if adverse reactions occur or if the hyperosmolar laxative is ineffective.

• *Monitor hydration for the patient with nausea, vomiting, or diarrhea.* Obtain a prescription for an antiemetic agent as needed. Also expect to decrease the dosage or discontinue the hyperosmolar laxative as prescribed.

• Replace fluids as prescribed if diarrhea occurs.

• *Monitor the patient with a fluid volume deficit for signs of hypovolemic shock, such as hypotension, tachycardia, or oliguria. If these signs occur, notify the physician immediately.*

• *Be prepared to take supportive measures as needed. For example, place the patient in the Trendelenburg position and administer volume expanders as prescribed.*

Patient teaching

• Teach the patient and family the name, dose, frequency, action, and adverse effects of the prescribed hyperosmolar laxative.

• *Describe the proper use of laxatives and caution the patient about laxative dependence.*

• Discuss measures the patient can take to prevent constipation. (For details, see *Preventing constipation,* page 723.)

• Teach the patient with chronic constipation about bowel retraining, if prescribed. (For details, see *Bowel retraining program.*)

• *Stress the importance of taking the hyperosmolar laxative exactly as prescribed to help prevent fluid and electrolyte imbalances.*

• *Teach the patient to recognize the signs of fluid and electrolyte imbalances and, if they occur, to withhold the drug and notify the physician.*

• *Advise the patient to avoid activities that require mental alertness if weakness, drowsiness, or lethargy occurs.*

• *Instruct the patient with impaired glucose tolerance to be alert for signs of hyperglycemia and to monitor blood glucose levels regularly during lactulose therapy.*

• Teach the patient how to prepare and store lactulose properly.

Bowel retraining program

The nurse should follow these guidelines when instituting a bowel retraining program for a patient with chronic constipation.

See that the patient's meals are high in fluid content and adequate in solid bulk (especially breakfast).

⬇

Have the patient eat breakfast at approximately the same time each day.

⬇

Assist the patient to the toilet or onto the commode 15 to 30 minutes after the meal.

⬇

If reflex defecation does not occur, insert a lubricated glycerin suppository as prescribed.

⬇

If defecation does not follow suppository insertion, administer a Fleet enema as prescribed.

⬇

Eventually, the patient will defecate on a regular schedule on the basis of the meal plus the suppository.

⬇

The ultimate goal is reflex defecation based on the meal's content and the time of day, without the use of suppositories.

• Instruct the patient to drink adequate fluids during saline compound therapy.

• *Instruct the patient who experiences diarrhea to withhold the agent, notify the physician, and increase fluid intake (unless contraindicated).*

• Advise the patient to notify the physician if adverse reactions occur or if the prescribed hyperosmolar laxative is ineffective.

Evaluation

The following examples represent appropriate evaluation statements for a patient receiving a hyperosmolar laxative.

• The patient has no conditions that contraindicate hyperosmolar laxative therapy.

• The patient exhibits no signs of complications in the preexisting condition linked to the prescribed hyperosmolar laxative.

• The patient experiences no adverse reactions to the prescribed hyperosmolar laxative.

• The patient maintains adequate hydration throughout hyperosmolar laxative therapy.

• The patient and family express an accurate understanding of the points taught about the prescribed hyperosmolar laxative.

• The patient reports using various methods to prevent constipation, including a high-fiber diet and regular exercise.

DIETARY FIBER AND RELATED BULK-FORMING LAXATIVES

A high-fiber diet is the most natural way to prevent or treat constipation. Dietary fiber refers to the amount of plant food that is not digested in the small intestine. The bulk-forming laxatives, which resemble dietary fiber, contain natural and semisynthetic polysaccharides and cellulose. These laxatives include methylcellulose, polycarbophil, and psyllium hydrophilic mucilloid. Dietary fiber and bulk-forming laxatives increase fecal bulk and water content, thereby promoting peristalsis and elimination.

PHARMACOKINETICS

Dietary fiber and bulk-forming laxatives are not absorbed. The onset of action for both types of agents is slow.

Absorption, distribution, metabolism, excretion

Dietary fiber and related bulk-forming laxatives are ingested into the GI tract but are not absorbed systemically. Both act primarily in the small intestine and the colon. Polysaccharides in these agents are metabolized by intestinal bacterial flora into osmotically active metabolites. Dietary fiber and bulk-forming laxatives are excreted in the feces.

Onset, peak, duration

Fecal softening occurs 1 to 3 days after treatment begins. Continued administration of these agents results in a maximum effect in 3 to 4 days, and the duration of action depends on continued administration.

PHARMACODYNAMICS

Dietary fiber and bulk-forming laxatives increase stool mass, which in turn increases peristalsis.

Mechanism of action

The laxative effect of dietary fiber and bulk-forming laxatives depends on the hydrophilic bulk-forming properties of the polysaccharides in these agents. These bulk-forming properties increase the mass and water content of the stool, and form a viscous solution that promotes peristalsis and increases the elimination rate. The component polysaccharides are metabolized by the intestinal bacterial flora. Metabolism results in accumulation of osmotically active metabolites, which increase water and solute transport into the intestinal lumen.

PHARMACOTHERAPEUTICS

Bulk-forming laxatives are used to treat simple cases of constipation, especially for constipation from a low-fiber or low-fluid diet. These agents also are indicated for patients recovering from acute myocardial infarction or cerebral aneurysms who need to avoid Valsalva's maneuver and maintain soft feces. Bulk-forming laxatives also may be used to manage patients with irritable bowel syndrome and diverticulosis.

dietary fiber. To prevent constipation, adults should consume 6 to 10 grams of dietary fiber daily. Dietary fiber is a major component of bran, whole grain cereals, fresh fruits and vegetables, and legumes.

methylcellulose (Cologel, Citrucel, Maltsupex). This laxative is used to treat constipation in adults.
Usual adult dosage: 5 to 20 ml liquid P.O. t.i.d. with a full glass of water.

polycarbophil (Fibercon, Mitrolan). Adults use this laxative to treat constipation.
Usual adult dosage: 2 tablets P.O. up to q.i.d. with a full glass of liquid.

psyllium hydrophilic mucilloid (Metamucil, Syllact, Konsyl, Correctol). Adults use this laxative to treat constipation.
Usual adult dosage: 1 to 2 teaspoonfuls or 1 packet P.O. in a full glass of water b.i.d. or t.i.d. followed by a second glass of water.

Drug interactions

No significant drug interactions occur with the use of dietary fiber or bulk-forming laxatives.

ADVERSE DRUG REACTIONS

Use of dietary fiber or bulk-forming laxatives in the recommended amounts poses minimal risk of toxicity. Adverse reactions include flatulence, a sensation of abdominal fullness, intestinal obstruction, impaction, esophageal obstruction (if sufficient liquid has not been administered with the agent), and severe diarrhea. Allergic reactions rarely occur.

NURSING PROCESS APPLICATION

The following information assists the nurse in caring for a patient who is receiving dietary fiber or a bulk-forming laxative.

Assessment
• Review the patient's history for a preexisting condition that contraindicates the use of dietary fiber or a bulk-forming laxative, such as known hypersensitivity to the drug, intestinal obstruction, or fecal impaction.
• Assess the patient for adverse reactions to dietary fiber or the prescribed bulk-forming laxative, such as GI distress.
• Assess the effectiveness of dietary fiber or the prescribed bulk-forming laxative.
• Evaluate the patient's and family's knowledge about dietary fiber or the prescribed bulk-forming laxative.

Nursing diagnoses
The following examples represent appropriate nursing diagnoses for a patient receiving dietary fiber or a bulk-forming laxative.
• Potential for injury related to a preexisting condition that contraindicates the use of dietary fiber or a bulk-forming laxative
• Potential for injury related to adverse drug reactions
• Diarrhea related to the adverse GI effects of dietary fiber or the prescribed bulk-forming laxative

Preventing constipation

The nurse should review the following measures when teaching a patient how to avoid constipation and minimize laxative use.
• Maintain a regular diet with adequate amounts of dietary fiber and fluids.
• Maintain regularity of dietary consumption; consume meals at approximately the same time each day.
• Allow time each day to use the toilet; do not ignore the urge to defecate.
• Adhere to a regular daily exercise regimen.
• Avoid the habitual use of laxatives or cathartics.

• Knowledge deficit related to dietary fiber or the prescribed bulk-forming laxative

Planning and implementation
• Do not administer dietary fiber or a bulk-forming laxative to a patient with a condition that contraindicates its use.
• Monitor the patient closely for adverse GI effects during therapy.
• Evaluate the effects of dietary fiber intake or the bulk-forming laxative on the patient's bowel pattern. Notify the physician if these measures are ineffective.
• *Administer a bulk-forming laxative with an 8-oz glass of water to prevent esophageal obstruction. Ensure that the patient follows each dose of psyllium hydrophilic mucilloid with a second 8-oz glass of water.*
• *Notify the physician if assessment findings suggest a severe adverse reaction, such as intestinal obstruction, fecal impaction, or esophageal obstruction.*
• *Monitor the patient for diarrhea, which may become severe. Also monitor for laxative dependence.*
• *Monitor hydration if the patient develops diarrhea, and withhold dietary fiber or the bulk-forming laxative until the physician has been notified.*

Patient teaching
• Teach the patient and family the name, dose, frequency, action, and adverse effects of the prescribed bulk-forming laxative.
• Inform the patient and family about dietary sources of fiber, such as bran, whole grain cereals, fresh fruits and vegetables, and legumes. Tell the patient to consume 6 to 10 grams of dietary fiber daily to prevent constipation, but to increase consumption slowly to minimize GI upset.
• *Advise the patient with restricted sugar and salt intake against the frequent use of bulk-forming laxatives because most of these agents contain sugar and salt. Recommend sugar-free products to a diabetic patient.*
• *Teach the patient to take each dose of a bulk-forming laxative with an 8-oz glass of water and to increase fluid*

intake during the day to prevent impaction. Also tell the patient to follow each dose of psyllium hydrophilic mucilloid with a second 8-oz glass of water.
• Inform a patient with chronic constipation to use additional techniques to correct constipation. (For details, see *Preventing constipation.*)
• Explain that the patient may experience flatulence or a sensation of abdominal fullness when taking dietary fiber or a bulk-forming laxative.
• Instruct the patient to notify the physician if adverse reactions occur or if the dietary fiber or bulk-forming laxative is ineffective.

Evaluation
The following examples represent appropriate evaluation statements for a patient receiving dietary fiber or a bulk-forming laxative.
• The patient has no conditions that contraindicate the use of dietary fiber or a bulk-forming laxative.
• The patient experiences no adverse reactions to dietary fiber or the prescribed bulk-forming laxative.
• The patient's bowel pattern returns to normal.
• The patient and family express an accurate understanding of the points taught about dietary fiber or the prescribed bulk-forming laxative.
• The patient includes foods in the diet that provide 6 to 10 grams of fiber daily.

EMOLLIENT LAXATIVES

Emollients also are known as stool softeners. Usually safe, emollients are used to prevent constipation in patients who should avoid straining during defecation. They reduce the surface tension of interfacing liquid bowel contents, thereby promoting fluid accumulation in the bowel and softening the stool. Emollients include the calcium, potassium, and sodium salts of docusate and poloxamer 188.

PHARMACOKINETICS

Administered orally, emollients are absorbed and excreted through bile in the feces. Stool softening occurs within several days after administration.

Absorption, distribution, metabolism, excretion
Emollients usually are surface-acting agents. The degree of absorption remains unknown, but some absorption through the duodenum and jejunum occurs after oral administration. Emollients concentrate in the liver, and excretion occurs through bile in the feces.

Onset, peak, duration

After oral administration, the onset of action is within 12 to 72 hours for docusate salts and within 3 to 5 days for poloxamer 188.

PHARMACODYNAMICS

Emollients soften the stool and ease defecation by emulsifying the fat and water components of feces in the small and large intestines. This detergent action allows water and lipids to penetrate the fecal material, thereby producing net fluid accumulation. Emollients also stimulate electrolyte and fluid secretion from intestinal mucosal cells.

PHARMACOTHERAPEUTICS

Emollients are the drugs of choice for softening stool in patients who should avoid straining during defecation. Such patients include those who recently have had a myocardial infarction or surgery and those with a disease of the anus or rectum, increased intracranial pressure, or hernias. Children with hard, dry stools can receive emollients safely. Emollients also may be given before rectal cathartics to treat fecal impaction.

docusate calcium (Surfak). Docusate calcium is used to soften the stool of patients who should not strain during defecation.
Usual adult dosage: 240 mg P.O. daily until bowel movements are normal.

docusate potassium (Kasof, Dialose). This stool softener is used to treat occasional constipation. It is contraindicated in patients with renal dysfunction.
Usual adult dosage: 100 to 300 mg P.O. daily until bowel movements are normal.

docusate sodium (Colace, Doxinate, Regutol). A stool softener, docusate sodium frequently is prescribed for hospitalized and nonhospitalized patients.
Usual adult dosage: 50 to 500 mg P.O. daily until bowel movements are normal.
Usual pediatric dosage: 1.25 mg/kg P.O. up to q.i.d.

poloxamer 188 (Alaxin). Poloxamer 188 also is a stool softener.
Usual adult dosage: 240 mg P.O. daily to t.i.d. until bowel movements are normal.

Drug interactions

The nurse should not administer oral emollients with oral mineral oil because they enhance the systemic absorption of mineral oil and may result in tissue deposition. Because emollients may enhance the absorption of many oral drugs, the nurse should not administer them concurrently with oral drugs having low therapeutic indexes.

ADVERSE DRUG REACTIONS

Although adverse reactions to emollients rarely occur, they may include mild, transient abdominal cramping; a bitter taste; diarrhea; and throat irritation.

NURSING PROCESS APPLICATION

The following information assists the nurse in caring for a patient who is receiving an emollient laxative.

Assessment
• Review the patient's history for a preexisting condition that contraindicates the use of docusate potassium, such as renal dysfunction.
• Review the patient's history for conditions that require cautious use of an emollient laxative, such as pregnancy or lactation.
• Assess the patient for adverse reactions to the prescribed emollient laxative, such as mild, transient abdominal cramping; a bitter taste; diarrhea; or throat irritation.
• Review the patient's medication history to identify the use of drugs that may interact with the emollient laxative, such as oral mineral oil or oral drugs with a low therapeutic index.
• Assess the effectiveness of the prescribed emollient laxative regularly.
• Evaluate the patient's and family's knowledge about the prescribed emollient laxative.

Nursing diagnoses
The following examples represent appropriate nursing diagnoses for a patient receiving an emollient laxative.
• Potential for injury related to a preexisting condition that contraindicates the use of an emollient laxative
• Potential for injury related to a preexisting condition that requires cautious use of an emollient laxative
• Potential for injury related to adverse drug reactions
• Knowledge deficit related to the prescribed emollient laxative

Planning and implementation
• Do not administer an emollient laxative to a patient with a condition that contraindicates its use.
• Administer an emollient laxative cautiously to a patient at risk because of a preexisting condition.
• Monitor the patient closely for adverse reactions during emollient laxative therapy.
• Store the emollient laxative at 59° to 86° F (15° to 30° C). Protect liquid preparations from light.

• Give a liquid emollient in milk or fruit juice to mask the bitter taste.
• *Monitor hydration and notify the physician if the patient develops diarrhea. Replace fluid and electrolytes lost through diarrhea as prescribed.*
• *Avoid administering an emollient laxative with oral mineral oil because of enhanced absorption of mineral oil.*
• *Avoid administering an emollient laxative with an oral drug that has a low therapeutic index because the emollient may enhance its absorption.*

Patient teaching
• Teach the patient and family the name, dose, frequency, action, and adverse effects of the prescribed emollient laxative.
• Discuss measures the patient can take to prevent constipation. (For details, see *Preventing constipation,* page 723.)
• *Instruct the patient how to store and administer the emollient laxative. For example, caution the patient to swallow the emollient capsules and not to chew or open them.*
• Tell the patient to notify the physician if adverse reactions occur or if the prescribed emollient is ineffective.

Evaluation
The following examples represent appropriate evaluation statements for a patient receiving an emollient laxative.
• The patient has no conditions that contraindicate emollient laxative therapy.
• The patient exhibits no signs of complications in the preexisting condition linked to the prescribed emollient laxative.
• The patient displays no adverse reactions to the prescribed emollient laxative.
• The patient and family express an accurate understanding of the points taught about the prescribed emollient laxative.
• The patient correctly identifies adverse reactions to the prescribed emollient laxative.

STIMULANT LAXATIVES

Stimulant laxatives, also known as irritant cathartics, may irritate the intestinal mucosa directly or activate the intramural nerve plexus of the intestinal smooth muscle, thus increasing intestinal motility. Stimulant laxatives also alter electrolyte and fluid absorption, and some cause active ion secretion by intestinal mucosal cells, leading to net fluid accumulation in the intestines. The stimulant laxatives include bisacodyl, cascara sagrada, castor oil, phenolphthalein, and senna. These laxatives are used in constipation

produced by medications, by neurologic disorders, by irritable bowel syndrome, and by prolonged bed rest or hospitalization. They also are used to empty the bowel before surgery, radiologic procedures, and endoscopy.

PHARMACOKINETICS

Stimulant laxatives are absorbed slightly and metabolized in the liver. The metabolites are excreted in the urine or the feces.

Absorption, distribution, metabolism, excretion
Bisacodyl and phenolphthalein represent the diphenylmethane group of stimulant laxatives. Both are absorbed minimally, distributed to breast milk, metabolized by the liver, and excreted in the feces or urine.

Cascara sagrada and senna are of the anthraquinone group of stimulant laxatives. They are absorbed only slightly from the small intestine. Unabsorbed drug is hydrolyzed by colonic flora, thus becoming pharmacologically active. Cascara sagrada and senna are metabolized by the liver and distributed into some body tissues, including breast milk. They are excreted through bile in the feces and in the urine.

Researchers do not know whether castor oil is absorbed significantly from the small intestine. In the small intestine, castor oil is hydrolyzed to ricinoleic acid, its active ingredient.

Onset, peak, duration
Bisacodyl and phenolphthalein produce evacuation within 6 to 8 hours of oral administration and within 15 minutes to 1 hour after rectal administration. The duration of a single dose of phenolphthalein may be several days.

Cascara sagrada and senna produce an onset of action within 6 to 12 hours of oral administration and within ½ to 2 hours of rectal administration. Castor oil acts more quickly, with loose bowel movements occurring 2 to 3 hours after oral administration.

PHARMACODYNAMICS

Stimulant laxatives have several mechanisms of action to produce effective laxation.

Mechanism of action
Stimulant laxatives stimulate peristalsis and induce defecation by irritating the intestinal mucosa or stimulating nerve endings of the intestinal smooth muscle. These drugs also alter fluid and electrolyte absorption. Some stimulant laxatives produce active ion secretion by first inducing colonic mucosal cells to produce a net fluid accumulation in the bowel and laxation. All stimulant laxatives act on the

colon. Castor oil and phenolphthalein increase the peristaltic activity of the small intestine as well.

PHARMACOTHERAPEUTICS

Stimulant laxatives are the preferred drugs for emptying the bowel before general surgery, sigmoidoscopic or proctoscopic procedures, and radiologic procedures such as barium studies of the GI tract. Stimulant laxatives also are used to treat constipation caused by prolonged bed rest, neurologic dysfunction of the colon, and constipating drugs such as narcotics. These drugs may be used to treat constipation associated with pregnancy or delivery, but other, milder laxatives usually are prescribed because these agents may stimulate uterine contractions. Stimulant laxatives are never used in lactating women.

bisacodyl (Dulcolax). Administered for chronic constipation, bisacodyl also is used before delivery, surgery, or rectal or bowel examination.
Usual adult dosage: for constipation, 10 to 15 mg P.O. in the evening or before breakfast or 10 mg as a rectal suppository or 1.25-ounce (37.5 ml) enema; for complete bowel evacuation before special procedures, up to 30 mg P.O.
Usual pediatric dosage: 5 to 10 mg P.O. in the evening or before breakfast; 10 mg rectally as a suppository for children age 2 and over, 5 mg for those under age 2.

cascara sagrada (Cas-Evac). Administer cascara sagrada for acute constipation or before bowel or rectal examination.
Usual adult dosage: one 325-mg tablet P.O. h.s.; 1 ml fluid extract P.O. daily; 5 ml aromatic fluid extract P.O. daily.

castor oil (Neoloid). Administer castor oil before rectal or bowel examination or surgery, or for acute constipation.
Usual adult dosage: 15 to 60 ml of liquid P.O., on an empty stomach for best results.

phenolphthalein (Alophen, Ex-Lax). Administer phenolphthalein for acute constipation.
Usual adult dosage: 60 to 194 mg P.O. h.s.

senna (Senokot, X-Prep). Administer senna for acute constipation or before bowel or rectal examination.
Usual adult dosage: 2 to 4 tablets P.O.; ½ to 4 teaspoons of granules added to liquid; 1 to 3 teaspoonfuls syrup; 1 to 2 suppositories h.s.

Drug interactions
No significant drug interactions occur with the stimulant laxatives. However, because stimulant laxatives produce increased intestinal motility, they reduce the absorption of concomitantly administered oral drugs, especially sustained-release agents.

ADVERSE DRUG REACTIONS

Stimulant laxatives provide relatively safe treatment of short-term or acute constipation. Adverse reactions to these laxatives include weakness, nausea, abdominal cramps, and mild proctitis. Rectal administration of bisacodyl can produce a burning sensation. Phenolphthalein can cause a reddish discoloration in alkaline urine. Cascara sagrada and senna cause a reddish-pink or brown discoloration of urine. Castor oil may cause pelvic congestion in menstruating women.

With long-term use or overdose, stimulant laxatives may cause electrolyte imbalances, including hypokalemia, hypocalcemia, metabolic alkalosis, or acidosis. Malabsorption and weight loss also may occur. Habitual use may lead to cathartic colon with atony and dilation.

Stimulant laxatives can cause allergic reactions such as rash and pruritus. Phenolphthalein allergy may result in renal, cardiac, and respiratory dysfunction.

NURSING PROCESS APPLICATION

The following information assists the nurse in caring for a patient who is receiving a stimulant laxative.

Assessment
• Review the patient's history for a preexisting condition that contraindicates the use of a stimulant laxative, such as intestinal obstruction, lactation, or an acute abdominal condition that requires immediate surgery.
• Review the patient's history for a preexisting condition that requires cautious use of a stimulant laxative, such as pregnancy.
• Assess the patient for adverse reactions to the prescribed stimulant laxative, such as weakness, nausea, abdominal cramps, mild proctitis, electrolyte imbalances, malabsorption, or weight loss.
• Assess the effectiveness of the prescribed stimulant laxative regularly.
• Evaluate the patient's and family's knowledge about the prescribed stimulant laxative.

Nursing diagnoses
The following examples represent appropriate nursing diagnoses for a patient receiving a stimulant laxative.
• Potential for injury related to a preexisting condition that contraindicates the use of a stimulant laxative
• Potential for injury related to a preexisting condition that requires cautious use of a stimulant laxative
• Potential for injury related to adverse drug reactions
• Knowledge deficit related to the prescribed stimulant laxative

Planning and implementation

- Do not administer a stimulant laxative to a patient with a condition that contraindicates its use.
- Administer a stimulant laxative cautiously to a patient at risk because of a preexisting condition.
- Monitor the patient closely for adverse reactions during stimulant laxative therapy.
- *Monitor the patient's fluid and electrolyte levels and notify the physician if any imbalance occurs.*
- Monitor the patient's bowel evacuation pattern and notify the physician if the stimulant laxative is ineffective.
- *Discontinue the drug and notify the physician if the patient develops a rash or pruritus.*
- *Monitor for renal, cardiac, or respiratory dysfunction in a patient receiving phenolphthalein. This may indicate an allergic reaction.*
- Administer castor oil on an empty stomach for best results.
- Mix castor oil with juice or a carbonated beverage to mask the preparation's oily taste. Tell the patient to hold ice in the mouth before taking castor oil to help decrease the taste.
- Store castor oil below 40° C (104° F), but do not freeze; shake the emulsion well.

Patient teaching

- Teach the patient and family the name, dose, frequency, action, and adverse effects of the prescribed stimulant laxative.
- *Alert the patient that phenolphthalein may cause a reddish discoloration in alkaline urine and that cascara sagrada and senna may cause a reddish-pink or brown discoloration of urine.*
- *Instruct the patient to take the stimulant laxative exactly as prescribed to prevent dependence, chronic use, and cathartic colon with atony and dilation.*
- *Advise the patient to discontinue the laxative and notify the physician if a rash or pruritus occurs.*
- Teach the patient how to administer and store the prescribed stimulant laxative.
- *Instruct the patient not to chew bisacodyl tablets because they are enteric coated to prevent GI irritation. Also advise the patient not to take them with antacids.*
- Discuss measures the patient can take to prevent constipation. (For details, see *Preventing constipation,* page 723.)
- Advise the patient to notify the physician if adverse reactions occur or if the stimulant laxative is ineffective.

Evaluation

The following examples represent appropriate evaluation statements for a patient receiving a stimulant laxative.

- The patient has no conditions that contraindicate stimulant laxative therapy.
- The patient exhibits no signs of complications in the preexisting condition linked to the prescribed stimulant laxative.
- The patient experiences no adverse reactions to the prescribed stimulant laxative.
- The patient and family express an accurate understanding of the points taught about the prescribed stimulant laxative.
- The patient includes bulk in the daily diet and begins a moderate exercise program.

LUBRICANT LAXATIVE

Mineral oil, a lubricant laxative, increases water retention in the stool by creating a barrier between the colon wall and feces. This barrier prevents colonic reabsorption of fecal water. Mineral oil is used to treat constipation in patients who must avoid straining, including patients with recent myocardial infarction, increased intracranial pressure, or fecal impaction.

PHARMACOKINETICS

In its nonemulsified form, mineral oil is absorbed minimally; in the emulsified form, about half is absorbed. Defecation occurs 6 to 8 hours after oral administration and within 2 hours of rectal administration.

Absorption, distribution, metabolism, excretion

Nonemulsified mineral oil is absorbed minimally after oral and rectal administration and is excreted in the feces. After oral administration, 30% to 60% of emulsified mineral oil is absorbed. Absorbed mineral oil is distributed to the mesenteric lymph nodes, intestinal mucosa, liver, and spleen. Mineral oil is metabolized by the liver and excreted in the feces.

Onset, peak, duration

The onset of action occurs in 6 to 8 hours after oral administration of mineral oil and in ½ to 2 hours after rectal administration. The duration of action depends on continuing administration of the agent.

PHARMACODYNAMICS

Mineral oil acts as a lubricant in the colon to produce laxation.

Mechanism of action

Mineral oil lubricates the feces and the intestinal mucosa by preventing water reabsorption from the lumen of the bowel. The increased fluid content of the feces increases peristalsis. Emulsified mineral oil provides slightly more effective action than the nonemulsified form. Rectal administration via an enema also produces laxation by physical distention.

PHARMACOTHERAPEUTICS

Mineral oil is used to treat constipation and maintain soft stools when straining is contraindicated (after recent myocardial infarction to avoid Valsalva's maneuver, after eye surgery to prevent increased intraocular pressure, and after cerebral aneurysm repair to avoid increased intracranial pressure). Administered orally or by enema, this lubricant laxative also is used to treat patients with fecal impaction. Bulk-forming laxatives and emollients are considered to provide milder action than mineral oil.

mineral oil (Agoral Plain, Fleet Mineral Oil Enema). Used to treat constipation, mineral oil also is used to maintain soft stools when straining during defecation is contraindicated.
Usual adult dosage: 15 to 30 ml P.O., usually h.s.; or 4-ounce (120-ml) enema.

Drug interactions

Mineral oil may impair the absorption of many oral medications, including fat-soluble vitamins, oral contraceptives, and anticoagulants. Mineral oil also may interfere with the antibacterial activity of nonabsorbable sulfonamides.

ADVERSE DRUG REACTIONS

Mineral oil may produce nausea, vomiting, diarrhea, and abdominal cramping. Seepage from the rectum after rectal administration may result in anal irritation, pruritus ani, infection, and impaired healing of lesions in the area. Chronic oral use of nonemulsified mineral oil may impair absorption of fat-soluble vitamins (A, D, E, and K), causing vitamin deficiency. Lipid pneumonitis may result from the aspiration of oral mineral oil.

Systemic absorption of emulsified mineral oil can lead to granulomatous reactions in the mesenteric lymph nodes, liver, and spleen.

NURSING PROCESS APPLICATION

The following information assists the nurse in caring for a patient who is receiving mineral oil.

Assessment

• Review the patient's history for a preexisting condition that contraindicates the use of mineral oil, such as advanced age, debilitation, pregnancy, esophageal or gastric retention, dysphagia, or hiatal hernia.
• Assess the patient for adverse reactions to mineral oil, such as GI distress, fat-soluble vitamin deficiency, or rectal irritation or infection.
• Review the patient's medication history to identify the use of drugs that may interact with mineral oil, such as fat-soluble vitamins, oral contraceptives, anticoagulants, or nonabsorbable sulfonamides.
• Assess the effectiveness of mineral oil regularly.
• Evaluate the patient's and family's knowledge about mineral oil.

Nursing diagnoses

The following examples represent appropriate nursing diagnoses for a patient receiving mineral oil.
• Potential for injury related to a preexisting condition that contraindicates the use of mineral oil
• Potential for injury related to adverse reactions to mineral oil
• Altered nutrition: less than body requirements, related to impaired absorption of fat-soluble vitamins with long-term use of mineral oil
• Knowledge deficit related to mineral oil

Planning and implementation

• Do not administer mineral oil to a patient with a condition that contraindicates its use.
• Administer mineral oil cautiously to prevent aspiration.
• Monitor the patient closely for adverse reactions during mineral oil therapy.
• *Monitor hydration, withhold the next dose of mineral oil, and notify the physician if the patient develops nausea, vomiting, or diarrhea.*
• *Inspect the anal area regularly for irritation, pruritus ani, infection, or impaired lesion healing in a patient who receives mineral oil rectally.*
• *Avoid administering mineral oil with other oral medications because it impairs the absorption of many oral medications.*
• Monitor the patient for decreased effectiveness of fat-soluble vitamins, anticoagulants, and nonabsorbable sulfonamides during concomitant mineral oil therapy.
• Monitor the patient's fluid status and the effectiveness of the laxative.
• Mix mineral oil with fruit juice or a carbonated beverage to disguise its taste.
• Notify the physician if adverse reactions occur or if mineral oil is ineffective.
• *Monitor the patient on long-term mineral oil therapy for early signs of fat-soluble vitamin deficiency: night blind-*

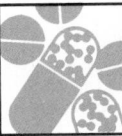

SELECTED MAJOR DRUGS

Antidiarrheal and laxative agents

The following chart summarizes the major antidiarrheals and laxatives currently in clinical use.

DRUG	MAJOR INDICATIONS	USUAL ADULT DOSAGES	CONTRAINDICATIONS AND PRECAUTIONS
Antidiarrheals			
opium tincture camphorated opium tincture (paregoric)	Acute, nonspecific diarrhea	0.6 ml (range 0.3 to 1 ml) P.O. q.i.d.; maximum dosage, 6 ml P.O. daily	• Know that opium tincture and paregoric are contraindicated in a patient with diarrhea caused by toxic chemicals or pathogens or known hypersensitivity to these drugs or atropine sulfate.
	Acute, nonspecific diarrhea	5 to 10 ml P.O. daily to q.i.d. until acute diarrhea subsides	• Administer with caution to a pregnant or lactating patient or one with asthma, severe prostatic hypertrophy, narcotic dependence, or liver or kidney dysfunction.
loperamide	Acute, nonspecific diarrhea; chronic diarrhea	4 mg P.O. initially, then 2 mg after each unformed stool; maximum dosage, 16 mg/day	• Know that loperamide is contraindicated in a patient with known hypersensitivity to the drug, antibiotic-induced pseudomembranous colitis or diarrhea, diarrhea caused by infection with certain organisms (such as *Shigella, Salmonella,* and some strains of *Escherichia coli),* or a condition in which constipation must be avoided. • Administer with caution to a pregnant or lactating patient or one with benign prostatic hypertrophy, liver dysfunction, or narcotic dependence.
diphenoxylate (with atropine) difenoxin (with atropine)	Acute, nonspecific diarrhea	5 mg P.O. q.i.d. initially; thereafter, the dosage is adjusted to individual response	• Know that difenoxin and diphenoxylate are contraindicated in a patient with known hypersensitivity to any of their components, jaundice, or antibiotic-induced diarrhea or pseudomembranous enterocolitis, or diarrhea caused by infection with certain organisms (such as *Shigella, Salmonella,* and some strains of *E. coli).*
	Acute, nonspecific diarrhea	2 mg P.O. initially, followed by 1 mg every 3 to 4 hours, as needed, up to a maximum of 8 mg P.O. daily	• Administer with extreme caution to a patient with advanced hepatorenal disease or abnormal liver function. • Administer with caution to a pregnant or lactating patient or one with narcotic dependence or benign prostatic hypertrophy.
kaolin and pectin mixtures	Mild to moderate nonspecific diarrhea	Regular-strength suspension: 60 to 120 ml P.O. after each loose bowel movement, usually up to eight doses per day Concentrated-strength suspension: 45 to 90 ml P.O. after each loose bowel movement, usually up to eight doses per day	• Be aware that no contraindications or precautions exist for kaolin and pectin.
Hyperosmolar laxatives			
glycerin	Reestablishment of proper bowel patterns in laxative-dependent adults	3 grams by suppository; 5 to 15 ml as an enema	• Be aware that no contraindications or precautions exist for glycerin used as a laxative.

(continued)

SELECTED MAJOR DRUGS

Antidiarrheal and laxative agents *(continued)*

DRUG	MAJOR INDICATIONS	USUAL ADULT DOSAGES	CONTRAINDICATIONS AND PRECAUTIONS
Hyperosmolar laxatives *(continued)*			
lactulose	Chronic constipation	10 to 20 grams (15 to 30 ml) P.O. daily	• Know that lactulose is contraindicated in a patient who requires a low-galactose diet. • Administer with caution to a pregnant or lactating patient or one with diabetes mellitus.
	Reduction of ammonia level in patients with systemic portal encephalopathy	20 to 30 grams (30 to 45 ml) P.O. t.i.d. or q.i.d. until two to three soft stools are produced daily, or 200 grams (300 ml) diluted in 700 ml of water or normal saline solution, given via rectal balloon catheter and retained 30 to 60 minutes every 4 to 6 hours	
saline compounds (magnesium salts, sodium phosphate, sodium biphosphate)	Prompt and complete bowel evacuation	10 to 15 grams of magnesium sulfate P.O. in a glass of water, 240 ml of magnesium citrate at bedtime, 20 to 30 ml of oral sodium phosphate or sodium biphosphate solution mixed with a glass of water, or 120 ml (4 oz) of sodium phosphate or sodium biphosphate enema	• Know that saline compounds are contraindicated in a patient with congenital megacolon, imperforate anus, or congestive heart failure. • Administer with caution to a patient with renal impairment, cardiac disease, colostomy, electrolyte disturbance, or a condition (such as dehydration or diuretic therapy) that predisposes to electrolyte disturbance.
Bulk-forming laxatives			
psyllium hydrophilic mucilloid	Treatment of constipation	1 to 2 teaspoonfuls or 1 packet P.O. dissolved in a glass of water b.i.d. or t.i.d. followed by a second glass of water	• Know that psyllium hydrophilic mucilloid and methylcellulose are contraindicated in a patient with known hypersensitivity to these drugs, intestinal obstruction, or fecal impaction.
methylcellulose	Treatment of constipation	5 to 20 ml liquid P.O. t.i.d. with a full glass of water	
Emollient laxative			
docusate sodium	Stool softening for patients who should not strain during defecation	50 to 500 mg P.O. daily until bowel movements are normal	• Administer docusate sodium with caution to a pregnant or lactating patient.
Stimulant laxative			
bisacodyl	Chronic constipation	10 to 15 mg P.O. in the evening or before breakfast, or 10 mg as a rectal suppository or 1.25 oz enema	• Know that bisacodyl is contraindicated in a lactating patient or one with intestinal obstruction or an acute abdominal condition that requires immediate surgery. • Administer with caution to a pregnant patient.
	Bowel evacuation before delivery, surgery, or rectal or bowel examination	Up to 30 mg P.O.	
Lubricant laxative			
mineral oil	Constipation or maintenance of soft stools when the patient should not strain during defecation	15 to 30 ml P.O., usually h.s., or 4-ounce enema	• Know that oral mineral oil is contraindicated in a geriatric, debilitated, or pregnant patient or one with esophageal or gastric retention, dysphagia, or hiatal hernia.

ness (vitamin A deficiency); profuse sweating, restlessness, and irritability (vitamin D deficiency); muscle weakness or intermittent claudication (vitamin E deficiency); or abnormal bleeding tendency (vitamin K deficiency).
• *Withhold mineral oil and notify the physician if fat-soluble vitamin deficiency is suspected.*
• *Do not administer mineral oil with or shortly after meals or with fat-soluble vitamins because it can interfere with vitamin absorption.*

Patient teaching

• Teach the patient and family the name, dose, frequency, action, and adverse effects of mineral oil.
• *Stress the importance of taking mineral oil exactly as prescribed because long-term use can cause fat-soluble vitamin deficiency.* Review the signs of the vitamin deficiencies with the patient as needed.
• *Advise the female patient taking an oral contraceptive that mineral oil can interefere with its absorption, reducing the contraceptive's effectiveness.*
• Teach the patient how to take mineral oil to disguise its taste.
• *Instruct the patient not to take mineral oil with or shortly after meals or medications.*
• Discuss measures the patient can take to prevent constipation. (For details, see *Preventing constipation,* page 723.)
• Advise the patient to notify the physician if adverse reactions occur or if mineral oil is ineffective.

Evaluation

The following examples represent appropriate evaluation statements for a patient receiving mineral oil.
• The patient has no conditions that contraindicate mineral oil therapy.
• The patient experiences no adverse reactions to mineral oil.
• The patient maintains adequate absorption of fat-soluble vitamins.
• The patient and family express an accurate understanding of the points taught about mineral oil.
• The patient correctly explains how and when to take mineral oil.

CHAPTER SUMMARY

Chapter 42 covered information about the antidiarrheal and laxative agents. Here are the highlights of the chapter.

• Diarrhea refers to the increased frequency or weight and liquidity of stools produced by the rapid movement of feces through the large intestine. Constipation refers to the decreased movement of fecal matter through the large intestine.
• Significant antidiarrheals include opium tincture, paregoric, difenoxin, diphenoxylate, loperamide, and kaolin and pectin mixtures. Antidiarrheals are used to treat acute, nonspecific diarrhea or chronic diarrhea.
• Opium tincture and paregoric (1) slow the effects of the mesenteric plexus of the intestine, (2) inhibit intestinal peristalsis by direct central action on the brain, (3) decrease propulsive contractions, (4) enhance anal sphincter tone, and (5) enhance the tone of the ileocecal valve.
• Difenoxin, diphenoxylate, and loperamide decrease GI motility by depressing the action of the circular and longitudinal muscles of the large and small intestine.
• Kaolin and pectin act as adsorbents, binding with irritants on the intestinal mucosa. These antidiarrheals are effective only for mild to moderate acute diarrhea.
• Antidiarrheals can cause nausea, vomiting, and constipation as well as other adverse reactions.
• When caring for a patient receiving an antidiarrheal, the nurse must monitor the patient's GI response to these drugs, documenting the frequency and consistency of bowel movements per day. Fluids and electrolytes should be replaced as needed.
• Laxatives exert their effect by increasing fecal water content and fecal movement from the colon and rectum.
• Hyperosmolar laxatives include glycerin, lactulose, and saline compounds. Glycerin is prescribed to reestablish proper bowel patterns. Lactulose is used to reduce ammonia levels in patients with liver dysfunction and to treat chronic constipation. Saline compounds are used for complete bowel evacuation and for chronic constipation.
• Adverse reactions to hyperosmolar laxatives include fluid and electrolyte imbalances.
• Dietary fiber intake is the most natural way to treat or prevent constipation. The bulk-forming laxatives (methylcellulose, polycarbophil, and psyllium hydrophilic mucilloid), which resemble dietary fiber, are used to treat constipation in patients who must avoid Valsalva's maneuver, who have irritable bowel syndrome or diverticulosis, or whose constipation is caused by a low-fiber or low-fluid diet.
• Administered orally, emollients are used to soften stools in patients who should avoid straining during defecation. These drugs are safe; however, they have a bitter taste.
• Stimulant laxatives are used for constipation produced by drugs, neurologic disorders, or prolonged bed rest. They also are used to empty the bowel before surgery.

• Mineral oil, a lubricant laxative, increases water retention in the stool by creating a barrier between the colon wall and feces.

• The excessive use of laxatives, especially in susceptible patients, may result in severe problems, such as habitual dependence, fluid and electrolyte imbalances, acid-base abnormalities, dehydration, and cardiac arrhythmias. For habitual users of laxatives, the nurse should institute bowel retraining and teach ways to prevent chronic constipation.

STUDY QUESTIONS

See Appendix 1 for answers.

1. John Conroy, age 42, is admitted to the emergency department with severe, uncontrollable diarrhea for the past 72 hours. He has a history of asthma and diabetes. Although opium tincture is an effective antidiarrheal, the physician decides not to prescribe it for Mr. Conroy. What is the most likely reason for the physician's decision?
(a) patient age
(b) history of asthma
(c) history of diabetes
(d) risk of addiction with short-term use

2. To control Mr. Conroy's diarrhea, the physician prescribes loperamide (Imodium) 4 mg P.O. initially. Where does loperamide exert its antidiarrheal action?
(a) the esophagus
(b) the stomach
(c) the intestines
(d) the CNS

3. For 24 hours, Rita Holmes, age 30, has had diarrhea caused by an intestinal virus. Her physician prescribes a kaolin and pectin mixture (Kaopectate) 60 ml after each loose bowel movement. What should the nurse tell Ms. Holmes about administration of this antidiarrheal agent?
(a) Take it on a full stomach.
(b) Take it on an empty stomach.
(c) Take it immediately before other drugs.
(d) Take it up to eight times a day, as needed.

4. Alan Bloom, age 59, is recovering from an acute myocardial infarction. To prevent Mr. Bloom from straining during defecation, the physician is most likely to prescribe which laxative?
(a) docusate sodium
(b) magnesium citrate
(c) lactulose
(d) diphenoxylate

5. The physician would not prescribe the saline cathartic sodium phosphate for Mr. Bloom because of the risk of which adverse reaction?
(a) CNS depression
(b) drug dependence
(c) anorexia and cachexia
(d) electrolyte imbalance

6. Before Mr. Bloom is discharged, the nurse teaches him how to prevent constipation. Which instruction should the nurse include in the teaching session?
(a) Limit exercise to twice per week.
(b) Take a mild laxative every day.
(c) Drink plenty of fluids every day.
(d) Eat a high-protein, low-fat diet.

7. Shirley Easton, age 50, is scheduled for a sigmoidoscopy. To prepare her for this test, which laxative is most likely to be prescribed?
(a) lactulose
(b) bisacodyl
(c) methylcellulose
(d) magnesium citrate

8. Edgar Smollet has just had eye surgery. To prevent Mr. Smollet from straining during defecation, the physician prescribes mineral oil 15 ml P.O. h.s. to maintain soft stools. When administering mineral oil to Mr. Smollet, the nurse should be alert for which adverse reaction?
(a) abdominal cramping
(b) leukocytosis
(c) rash or urticaria
(d) hypocalcemia

SELECTED REFERENCES

AHFS drug information 90. (1991). Bethesda, MD: American Society of Hospital Pharmacists.
Binder, H. (1988). Use of laxatives in clinical medicine. *Pharmacology,* 36(Suppl. 1), 226-229.

Bruckstein, A. (1988). Acute diarrhea. *American Family Physician,* 38(4), 217-228.

Goodman and Gilman's the pharmacological basis of therapeutics (8th ed.; 1990). Elmsford, NY: Pergamon Press.

Leung, A., and Robson, W. (1989). Acute diarrhea in children: What to do and what not to do. *Postgraduate Medicine,* 86(8), 161-174.

Ludan, A. (1988). Current management of acute diarrhoeas: Use and abuse of drug therapy. *Drugs,* 36(Suppl. 4), 18-25.

North American Nursing Diagnosis Association. (1990). *Taxonomy I - Revised, with official categories.* St. Louis: NANDA.

Sadler, C. (1988) The power of purgatives. *Community Outlook,* June 8, 11-12.

Tabibian, N. (1989). Diarrhea in critically ill patients. *American Family Physician,* 40(2), 135-140.

EMETIC AND ANTIEMETIC AGENTS

OBJECTIVES

After reading and studying this chapter, the student should be able to:
1. Explain the physiology of nausea and vomiting.
2. Describe the pharmacokinetic, pharmacodynamic, and pharmacotherapeutic properties of the emetic agents apomorphine hydrochloride and ipecac syrup.
3. Identify the drug interactions and adverse reactions associated with the emetic agents apomorphine and ipecac syrup.
4. List the components of patient teaching that should be included with the use of ipecac syrup in the home.
5. Compare the pharmacokinetic, pharmacodynamic, and pharmacotherapeutic properties of antihistamine, phenothiazine, and other antiemetics.
6. Identify the drug interactions and adverse reactions associated with antihistamine, phenothiazine, and other antiemetics.
7. Demonstrate the proper technique for administering transdermal scopolamine.
8. Describe how to apply the nursing process when caring for a patient who is receiving an emetic or antiemetic agent.

INTRODUCTION

The emetics and antiemetics represent two groups of drugs with opposing actions. The emetic drugs, which are derived from plants, produce vomiting upon administration. The antiemetic drugs decrease nausea and hence, the urge to vomit. For a summary of representative drugs, see *Selected major drugs: Emetic and antiemetic agents,* page 750. For a listing of applicable nursing diagnoses that the nurse may formulate when caring for a patient receiving these agents, see *Selected nursing diagnoses: Emetic and antiemetic agents.* For detailed information on applying the nursing process, see Chapter 6, The Nursing Process and Drug Therapy.

Emetics are prescribed primarily to induce vomiting in the emergency treatment of acute poisonings. The induced vomiting empties the stomach and prevents absorption of the ingested toxin. Generally, emetics should be administered immediately after a poisoning is discovered; however, they may prove effective even with delayed administration if the ingested toxin is one that empties slowly from the stomach.

Although usually safe, emetics should not be used indiscriminately. Vomiting should not be induced in poisoning by a caustic substance, such as lye, or petroleum distillate, such as gasoline, because the vomiting may cause further injury. Also, emetics should not be used by those with anorexia nervosa or bulimia.

The emergency use of emetics combined with other measures can be lifesaving in treating acute poisonings. The American Academy of Pediatrics recommends that parents of young children keep emetics on hand in case of accidental poisoning.

Antiemetics relieve nausea and vomiting from various causes. Although the physiology of vomiting is understood relatively well, the complex physiology of nausea is not. The vomiting, or emetic, center, located in the reticular formation of the medulla, integrates the nausea response and coordinates the resulting vomiting reflex. The nausea response can be initiated when the upper gastrointestinal (GI) tract sends nerve impulses to the vomiting center along the vagus and the sympathetic nerves. Several conditions stimulate these nerve impulses. Irritation of mucosal receptors in the GI tract may provide input to the vomiting center. The emetic ipecac, which directly irritates the gastric mucosa; radiation therapy injury to the GI mucosa; and malignant disease of the GI tract all may stimulate nausea and vomiting via the vomiting center pathway.

SELECTED NURSING DIAGNOSES

Emetic and antiemetic agents

The following nursing diagnoses address representative problems and etiologies that a nurse may encounter when caring for a patient who is receiving an emetic or antiemetic agent. Some of these nursing diagnoses contain generalized etiologies, which the nurse must individualize based on the patient's needs. (For some common nursing diagnoses and related interventions for each drug class, see the "Nursing Process Application" sections of this chapter.)

- Altered nutrition: less than body requirements, related to anorexia caused by long-term use of an antihistamine antiemetic
- Altered protection related to the adverse hematologic effects of an antiemetic agent
- Altered thought processes related to central nervous system (CNS) depression caused by an emetic or antiemetic agent
- Altered tissue perfusion (renal) related to apomorphine-induced circulatory depression
- Anxiety related to the adverse CNS effects of a phenothiazine antiemetic
- Constipation related to the anticholinergic effects of an antiemetic agent
- Diarrhea related to the adverse gastrointestinal (GI) effects of ipecac syrup
- Impaired physical mobility related to the extrapyramidal effects of trimethobenzamide or a phenothiazine antiemetic
- Ineffective breathing pattern related to apomorphine-induced respiratory depression
- Knowledge deficit related to the prescribed emetic or antiemetic agent
- Pain related to antiemetic-induced headache

- Potential fluid volume deficit related to ineffectiveness of an antiemetic agent
- Potential fluid volume deficit related to prolonged vomiting induced by an emetic agent
- Potential for injury related to a preexisting condition that contraindicates the use of an emetic or antiemetic agent
- Potential for injury related to a preexisting condition that requires cautious use of an emetic or antiemetic agent
- Potential for injury related to adverse drug reactions
- Potential for injury related to ipecac-induced generalized myopathy or cardiomyopathy
- Potential for trauma related to esophageal tears caused by ipecac syrup abuse
- Potential for trauma related to the adverse CNS effects of the antiemetic agent
- Sensory-perceptual alterations (visual or auditory) related to the anticholinergic effects of an antiemetic agent
- Sexual dysfunction related to impotence caused by an antihistamine antiemetic
- Sleep pattern disturbance related to insomnia caused by a phenothiazine antiemetic
- Urinary retention related to the anticholinergic effects of an antiemetic agent

---

Nausea and vomiting also may be induced via a second, more complex pathway. Another nucleus of cells, called the chemoreceptor trigger zone (CTZ), also is located in the medulla, close to the vomiting center. By itself, the CTZ cannot mediate the act of vomiting. However, activation of the CTZ can stimulate the vomiting center, which in turn initiates emesis. The CTZ contains dopamine receptors that can be activated by many stimuli, including narcotics, chemotherapeutic drugs, vestibular motion or inflammation, ketoacidosis, and uremia.

Nausea and vomiting are listed almost universally as adverse effects of many drugs. These symptoms also occur frequently after surgery from anesthetic and surgical manipulation.

Whether or not the nausea and vomiting originate inside or outside the GI tract, the underlying cause should be identified and treated directly. For example, parasitic intestinal disease, acute appendicitis, and migraine headache cause nausea. Each of these conditions can be identified and treated medically.

However, the underlying cause of nausea cannot always be treated, making symptomatic treatment necessary. For example, the nausea from a viral illness may require treatment for the duration of the disease.

Motion sickness results from stimulation of the vestibular apparatus of the ear. During motion sickness, stimulation of the CTZ activates the vomiting center. People who know that they may experience motion sickness under certain circumstances can use an antiemetic prophylactically to prevent nausea and vomiting.

Another cause of nausea that results from stimulation of the vestibular apparatus of the ear is labyrinthitis. With labyrinthitis, inflammation of the vestibular apparatus causes nausea, vomiting, dizziness, and hearing loss. Ménière's disease, which involves a dilation of the endolymphatic channels in the cochlea, also produces nausea as well as dizziness, tinnitus, and hearing loss. The symptoms of Ménière's disease may last from several days to months and may recur without warning. During exacerbations of the disease, an antiemetic drug is indicated.

Cancer chemotherapy can stimulate the vomiting center directly or indirectly (through the CTZ), causing severe nausea and vomiting. As with motion sickness, the administration of antiemetic drugs before the chemotherapy may prevent or decrease the severity of these symptoms.

Narcotics, such as morphine and meperidine, stimulate two pathways to produce nausea and vomiting. The drugs not only stimulate the CTZ directly, which in turn activates the vomiting center, but they also sensitize the vestibular apparatus of the ear. As a result, nausea occurs more frequently in ambulatory patients taking narcotics than among bedridden patients. Narcotic-induced nausea may be mild, occurring only with the first dose of the narcotic, or it may be more severe, resulting in vomiting that requires antiemetic medication. In anticipation that they will cause severe narcotic-induced nausea, some narcotics are premixed with an antiemetic. Mepergan, for example, is a combination of the narcotic meperidine and the antiemetic promethazine.

Many women experience nausea and vomiting during early pregnancy (morning sickness), a condition that poses treatment problems. The dilemma arises from the belief that any drug used during the first trimester of pregnancy may act teratogenically. Supportive measures usually are prescribed as the initial therapy. Drug use is reserved for the point at which the potential benefits of antiemetic therapy outweigh the risk to the mother and fetus. That point usually occurs when the nausea and vomiting so incapacitate the patient that a nutritional deficiency is possible.

Nausea and vomiting may lead to many other deleterious conditions. Vomiting, for example, may lead to esophageal injury or, postoperatively, to disrupted sutures. Prolonged vomiting may lead to dehydration and the loss of gastric secretions, which in turn causes electrolyte, acid-base, nutritional, and fluid abnormalities. While vomiting, a person also may aspirate gastric contents into the lungs, resulting in aspiration pneumonitis. Finally, nausea and vomiting can interrupt the absorption of some drugs, thus preventing the benefits of certain drug therapies.

EMETICS

Emetics are used to induce vomiting after the ingestion of toxic substances. Although many substances were used in the past to induce vomiting, only two drugs, apomorphine and ipecac syrup, now are available for use as emetics. Ipecac syrup is considered the emetic of choice to treat toxic ingestions because the drug is the most effective and is less likely to cause problems than other emetics or mechanical stimulation. Household emetics, such as sodium chloride (salt) solutions, can cause fatalities from electrolyte imbalances (hypernatremia). Researchers have not determined the safety and efficacy of soaps and detergents as emetics. Studies of mechanically stimulated vomiting, such as placing a finger or spoon in the throat to cause a gag reflex, have shown this method to be much less effective than the administration of ipecac syrup.

PHARMACOKINETICS

Very little information exists concerning the absorption, distribution, and excretion of ipecac syrup. Apomorphine, which is absorbed well from the injection site, provides a quicker onset of action than ipecac.

Absorption, distribution, metabolism, excretion
Researchers have noted some absorption of ipecac. In one study, the alkaloids of ipecac administered to patients were found later in the serum of those patients; however, the amount of the drug present in the serum varied considerably among patients.

Apomorphine administered by intramuscular (I.M.) or subcutaneous (S.C.) injection produces an emetic action that is more predictable than that produced by oral administration. The drug is absorbed well from the injection site and metabolized by the liver. Drug metabolites are excreted by the kidneys. Ipecac syrup and apomorphine distribute to breast milk.

Onset, peak, duration
After administration of ipecac syrup, a delay of approximately 10 minutes usually occurs before the onset of vomiting. About 50% of the patients receiving ipecac will begin vomiting in less than 20 minutes; about 90% will vomit within 30 minutes.

The onset of action of apomorphine is very fast. Most patients vomit within 5 minutes after S.C. administration; about 90% vomit within 15 minutes. The onset of apomorphine may occur more rapidly than that of ipecac syrup because apomorphine reaches its site of action more quickly. The narcotic sedative effect of apomorphine occurs within several minutes and lasts for about 2 hours after a dose.

PHARMACODYNAMICS

Ipecac syrup and apomorphine induce vomiting by stimulating the vomiting center located in the medulla of the brain.

Mechanism of action
Ipecac syrup induces vomiting by producing a local effect on the gastric mucosa and a central effect on the CTZ. After administration of ipecac syrup, the initial episode of vomiting probably is caused by the local effect of the ipecac on the stomach, although subsequent episodes of vomiting may result from CTZ stimulation. Ipecac produces regurgitation of the contents of the stomach and upper duodenum, but not of any contents further along the GI tract. Most patients vomit two or three times during the first hour after administration and can resume normal eating in several hours.

Apomorphine produces its emetic effect by directly stimulating the dopamine receptors located in the CTZ. Like ipecac, apomorphine induces regurgitation of the contents of the stomach and upper duodenum, but not of any contents in the lower GI tract. Excitation of vestibular centers also may be involved in producing apomorphine-induced vomiting, because movement intensifies the emetic effect of the drug.

Apomorphine produces some of the same pharmacologic effects as other narcotics. It may cause central nervous system (CNS) stimulation or depression. The drug also produces respiratory depression, hypotension, and sedation similar to those same effects produced by the other narcotics.

PHARMACOTHERAPEUTICS

Because most poisonings and overdoses involve toxin ingestion, the primary objective in treatment is to prevent the ingested substance from being absorbed into the body. To attain this goal, treatment involves one of three mechanisms: gastric emptying, binding of the substance in the stomach, and to a lesser extent, stimulating GI motility, which decreases the time the toxin travels through the GI tract. Gastric emptying involves physical removal of the toxic substance from the stomach, using an emetic or gastric lavage. Administered activated charcoal binds with the toxic substance and prevents its absorption. Cathartics stimulate GI motility and help the system quickly eliminate any unabsorbed poison in the feces.

Ipecac syrup is considered the therapy of choice for emptying the stomach because of its effectiveness and low incidence of adverse effects. It can be purchased without a prescription and can be stored in the home for emergencies.

Although the parenteral route of administration for apomorphine limits its use in the home, the drug is used occasionally in the emergency department. Apomorphine is as effective as ipecac syrup in removing toxic substances from the stomach, and has a slightly more rapid onset of action. However, the more rapid action may be outweighed by the longer time required for the patient to reach the emergency department to receive the drug.

ipecac syrup. This drug is available for use without a prescription in 1-ounce (30-ml) containers.
Usual adult dosage: 15 to 30 ml P.O. followed by 200 to 300 ml of water.
Usual pediatric dosage: for children age 1 and over, 15 ml P.O. followed by 200 ml of water or other clear liquid; for children under age 1, 5 to 10 ml P.O. followed by 100 ml of water or other clear liquid.

If vomiting does not occur within 30 minutes, repeat the initial dose. If the second dose does not produce emesis, initiate other measures, such as gastric lavage and activated charcoal, to minimize absorption and prevent toxicity from ipecac syrup and the poison.

apomorphine hydrochloride. A Schedule II drug, apomorphine is used to induce vomiting in poisoning. If emesis does not follow the initial dose of apomorphine, *do not* administer a subsequent dose because it is not likely to be any more effective.
Usual adult dosage: 5 to 6 mg S.C. or I.M. preceded by 200 to 300 ml of water.
Usual pediatric dosage: 0.07 to 0.1 mg/kg S.C. or I.M. preceded by 100 to 200 ml of water. The I.V. dose, which is used rarely, is 0.01 mg/kg for children and adults.

Drug interactions
Because ipecac syrup and apomorphine are used only in acute situations, drug interactions rarely occur. If poisoning is from ingestion of a phenothiazine, the phenothiazine's antiemetic effect on the CTZ may decrease the emetic effect of ipecac syrup or apomorphine. The administration of activated charcoal should be delayed until emesis has occurred because activated charcoal must remain in the GI tract to be effective. If activated charcoal and ipecac syrup are administered together, the activated charcoal may be vomited or become bound with the ipecac syrup, inactivating it.

ADVERSE DRUG REACTIONS

Like other narcotics, apomorphine directly affects the CNS. The drug may cause euphoria, restlessness, tachypnea, tremors, and profound CNS depression ranging from stupor to coma. Apomorphine also may produce acute circulatory depression, usually manifested by orthostatic hypotension, especially in elderly and debilitated patients. Respiratory depression occurs when large or repeated doses of apomorphine are administered. Administering the narcotic antagonist naloxone may relieve the CNS and respiratory depressant effects as well as the protracted emesis produced by apomorphine.

Ipecac syrup rarely produces adverse reactions when used in the recommended dosages. Almost all reports of problems from ipecac involved massive overdose, chronic use, a congenital abnormality, complications in elderly patients, or poisoning with phenothiazine ingestion. Adverse reactions may include prolonged vomiting for more than 1 hour or repeated vomiting involving more than six episodes in 1 hour, lethargy, and diarrhea. Ipecac contains a specific cardiotoxin that, in high doses, may cause cardiac arrhythmias or fatal myocarditis, especially in elderly patients. Heart failure usually is the cause of death after ipecac overdose.

Because the effects of ipecac syrup or apomorphine during pregnancy remain unknown, the drugs should be administered only when clearly indicated. Both drugs distribute to breast milk, so caution should be exercised when administering either drug to a lactating woman.

People with eating disorders (such as anorexia nervosa and bulimia) who abuse ipecac syrup can have serious, potentially fatal adverse reactions. These adverse reactions usually include generalized myopathy or cardiomyopathy. Other adverse reactions include fixed eruptions and toxic epidermal necrolysis as well as tears in the esophagus (Mallory-Weiss syndrome) from protracted, severe vomiting.

NURSING PROCESS APPLICATION

The following information assists the nurse in caring for a patient who is receiving an emetic agent.

Assessment
• Review the patient's history for a preexisting condition that contraindicates the use of an emetic, such as semicoma, unconsciousness, severe inebriation, seizures, shock, bulimia, anorexia nervosa, or absent gag reflex.
• Review the patient's history for a preexisting condition that requires cautious use of an emetic, such as impaired cardiac function, lactation, pregnancy, or sclerotic or other pathologic changes in blood vessels.
• Assess the patient for adverse reactions to the emetic, such as CNS stimulation or depression, respiratory depression, orthostatic hypotension, prolonged vomiting, lethargy, or diarrhea.
• Review the patient's medication history to identify the use of drugs that may interact with the emetic, such as phenothiazines or activated charcoal.
• Assess the effectiveness of the emetic shortly after administration.
• Evaluate the patient's and family's knowledge about the administered emetic.

Nursing diagnoses
The following examples represent appropriate nursing diagnoses for a patient receiving an emetic agent.
• Potential for injury related to a preexisting condition that contraindicates the use of an emetic
• Potential for injury related to a preexisting condition that requires cautious use of an emetic
• Potential for injury related to adverse drug reactions
• Potential fluid volume deficit related to prolonged vomiting caused by the administered emetic
• Knowledge deficit related to the administered emetic

Planning and implementation
• Do not administer an emetic to a patient with a condition that contraindicates its use.
• Administer an emetic cautiously to a patient at risk because of a preexisting condition.
• Monitor the patient closely for adverse reactions to the administered emetic.
• *Perform a neurologic assessment frequently after apomorphine administration to detect CNS stimulation or depression.*
• *Monitor the blood pressure and assess for signs of decreased tissue perfusion to detect acute circulatory depression in a patient receiving apomorphine, especially if the patient is elderly or debilitated.*
• *Assess the patient's respiratory rate and pattern, and auscultate breath sounds frequently to detect respiratory depression, which may occur with large or repeated doses of apomorphine.*
• *Keep the narcotic antagonist naloxone on hand to reverse respiratory or adverse CNS reactions or prolonged vomiting caused by apomorphine.*
• *Take safety precautions if sedation or lethargy occurs after emetic administration. For example, place the bed in a low position, keep the side rails up, and supervise ambulation.*
• *Monitor for cardiac arrhythmias in a patient receiving high doses of ipecac syrup, especially if the patient is elderly.*
• Precede apomorphine administration with 200 to 300 ml of water for an adult or 100 to 200 ml of water for a child.
• Be aware that the pharmacist prepares apomorphine for S.C. administration as follows: A 6-mg soluble tablet is dissolved in 1 to 2 ml of 0.9% saline solution or sterile water for injection. Then the solution is purified by passing it through a 0.22-micron filter before administration.
• Protect apomorphine tablets from air and light. *Do not use apomorphine solution if it turns green or brown.*
• Follow administration of ipecac syrup with the proper amount of water or other clear liquid based on the patient's age.
• Induce early emesis after drug administration by moving an adult or gently bouncing a child.
• *Do not administer a second dose of apomorphine if emesis does not occur after the initial dose. A repeat dose is not likely to be any more effective.*
• *Repeat the initial dose of ipecac syrup as prescribed, if vomiting does not occur within 30 minutes. If the second dose does not produce emesis, prepare to take other measures as prescribed, such as gastric lavage or activated charcoal administration.*
• Inform the physician frequently about the patient's condition. Notify the physician if adverse reactions occur.
• Monitor hydration if the patient experiences prolonged vomiting or diarrhea.

Home use of ipecac syrup

The nurse should include poison prevention counseling for family members as part of the 6-month or 1-year well-child examination for all children. Advise family members to purchase a 1-ounce (30-ml) bottle of ipecac syrup for poisoning emergencies, and teach them how to use the drug. Include the following points in the teaching:

• Keep ipecac syrup and all other medications out of the child's reach.
• Before using ipecac syrup to induce vomiting after poisoning, contact the physician, a poison control center, or emergency department. (Give the family the appropriate telephone numbers.)
• Do not give ipecac syrup to an unconscious or very drowsy child because vomited material may enter the lungs and cause pneumonia.
• Have the poisoned child drink a glass of water (approximately 6 to 8 ounces) immediately after taking ipecac syrup to help induce vomiting.
• Do not give the child milk unless otherwise instructed because milk will bind with the ipecac and prevent its vomiting effect.
• If the child does not vomit within 30 minutes, repeat the dose, and take the child to an emergency department. If the child does vomit, seek the physician's advice about follow-up medical care.

• Prepare to replace lost fluid and electrolytes as prescribed if a fluid volume deficit occurs. Continue to monitor the patient's hydration until vomiting or diarrhea ceases.

Patient teaching
• Teach the patient and family the name, dose, frequency, action, and adverse effects of the emetic to be administered.
• *Teach family members not to administer ipecac syrup to a child unless advised by a poison control center or other qualified health care personnel.* (For specific information to include in teaching, see *Home use of ipecac syrup.*)
• Explain that the patient may resume eating in several hours after ipecac administration.
• Encourage the patient and family to ask questions as concerns arise.

Evaluation
The following examples represent appropriate evaluation statements for a patient receiving an emetic agent.
• The patient has no conditions that contraindicate emetic administration.
• The patient exhibits no signs of complications in the preexisting condition linked to the administered emetic.
• The patient experiences no adverse reactions to the administered emetic.
• The patient maintains adequate hydration.
• The patient and family express an accurate understanding of the points taught about the prescribed emetic.

• The family members correctly describe how to administer ipecac syrup to their child.

ANTIHISTAMINE ANTIEMETICS

The antihistamine antiemetics consist of drugs that are related closely in chemical structure, all of which block the histamine (H_1) receptors and decrease nausea, vomiting, and vertigo. A number of antihistamine derivatives exist. However, those groups with the greatest antiemetic activity are the ethanolamine derivatives, including dimenhydrinate and diphenhydramine hydrochloride, and the piperazine derivatives, including buclizine hydrochloride, cyclizine hydrochloride, hydroxyzine hydrochloride, hydroxyzine pamoate, and meclizine hydrochloride. Trimethobenzamide is related structurally to the ethanolamine antihistamines.

PHARMACOKINETICS

Antihistamines are absorbed well from the GI tract and are metabolized primarily by the liver. Their inactive metabolites are excreted in the urine.

Absorption, distribution, metabolism, excretion
Most antihistamines are absorbed well from the GI tract. Little is known about the distribution, metabolism, and excretion of most antihistamines, but information about the few drugs studied may apply to all of the antihistamine antiemetics. Diphenhydramine, which has been studied widely, is distributed well to the CNS and throughout the body. Researchers believe that most antihistamine antiemetics also are distributed to breast milk. The antihistamine antiemetics are metabolized almost completely to inactive metabolites by the liver. The inactive metabolites are excreted by the kidneys within 24 hours.

Onset, peak, duration
The antihistamine antiemetics usually produce an onset of action 30 minutes after oral administration. The drug effects peak within 1 to 2 hours and last up to 6 hours. Some of the antihistamine antiemetics provide longer durations of action. For example, hydroxyzine and meclizine may provide a duration of up to 24 hours.

With trimethobenzamide, the onset of antiemetic action is 10 to 40 minutes, and drug action lasts up to 4 hours after oral administration. The onset and duration from rectal administration should be similar to that from oral administration. After I.M. injection of trimethobenzamide, the onset of antiemetic action is 15 to 35 minutes, and the duration is from 2 to 3 hours.

PHARMACODYNAMICS

The antihistamine antiemetics exert several biochemical and physiologic effects. All bind with the H_1 receptors to prevent histamine action during allergic reactions, and as antiemetics, these drugs penetrate the CNS, where they exert antiemetic and some adverse effects. Most of the antihistamine antiemetics also inhibit the response to acetylcholine at the muscarinic receptors and, therefore, produce anticholinergic effects, such as dry mouth, blurred vision, urine retention, and constipation.

Mechanism of action

The mechanism of action that produces the antiemetic effect of the antihistamines remains unclear. The drugs have been shown to inhibit vestibular stimulation of the ear, one of the primary causes of motion sickness. Also, the anticholinergic effects of antihistamines in the CNS may play an important role. Cholinergic stimulation in the vestibular and reticular systems may cause the nausea and vomiting of motion sickness. The antihistamines, through their anticholinergic action, block this stimulation and produce an antiemetic effect that helps treat motion sickness.

Finally, all antihistamine antiemetics produce generalized CNS depression, which probably accounts for some of their antiemetic effect.

Of the major antihistamine antiemetics, only trimethobenzamide can inhibit the emetic effects of apomorphine: that is, direct stimulation of the CTZ. Therefore, researchers believe that trimethobenzamide produces its antiemetic effect differently from the other antihistamines by inhibiting stimuli to the CTZ. Because of its direct inhibitory ability, trimethobenzamide produces a less specific antiemetic effect on the vestibular system of the ear. As a result, trimethobenzamide provides a general antiemetic effect regardless of the underlying cause. (For an illustration of the mechanisms of action of this drug group, see *Mechanism of action of antihistamine antiemetics.*)

PHARMACOTHERAPEUTICS

With the exception of trimethobenzamide, the antihistamines are fairly specific antiemetics for the nausea and vomiting caused by inner ear stimulation. As a consequence, these drugs prevent and treat motion sickness. They usually prove effective when given prophylactically before activities that produce motion sickness; the drugs are much less effective when nausea or vomiting has begun. If administered after nausea or vomiting has begun, they probably will not alleviate further episodes.

Although scopolamine, which is not an antihistamine antiemetic, may be the most effective drug for motion sickness, its use may be limited by its anticholinergic adverse effects. Therefore, many physicians prefer the antihistamine antiemetics to treat motion sickness. Furthermore, antihistamine antiemetics provide a longer duration of action than does oral (not transdermal) scopolamine. (For more information about scopolamine, see the section on "Other antiemetics" later in this chapter.)

The antihistamine antiemetics are used extensively to treat diseases that produce vertigo by affecting the vestibular system. Such diseases include labyrinthitis and Ménière's disease. Although studies have not proven conclusively that antihistamine antiemetics benefit patients with these diseases, they relieve some of the symptoms and therefore are useful for preventing or treating an acute attack.

Trimethobenzamide, used to control nausea and vomiting, is not as effective as the phenothiazine antiemetics but may be less toxic. This drug may be preferable to the phenothiazine antiemetics for long-term therapy because the risk of extrapyramidal reactions in the patient is lower.

buclizine hydrochloride (Bucladin-S Softab). This drug is supplied as a chewable tablet, which the patient can swallow whole, dissolve in the mouth and swallow, or chew before swallowing.
Usual adult dosage: for control of vertigo, 50 mg P.O. b.i.d.; for motion sickness, 50 mg P.O., repeated in 4 to 6 hours if necessary.

cyclizine hydrochloride (Marezine), **cyclizine lactate** (Marezine). Cyclizine hydrochloride is for oral use; cyclizine lactate is the form for I.M. injection.
Usual adult dosage: 50 mg P.O. or I.M. every 4 to 6 hours, if necessary, up to a maximum of 200 mg daily.
Usual pediatric dosage: for children age 6 to 12, 25 mg P.O. given 30 minutes before exposure to motion and repeated every 4 to 6 hours, if necessary, up to a maximum of 75 mg daily. Cyclizine is not recommended for children under age 6.

dimenhydrinate (Dramamine). Given orally, dimenhydrinate probably is the most commonly used drug for motion sickness because of its relatively low incidence of adverse effects.
Usual adult dosage: 50 to 100 mg P.O. every 4 to 6 hours up to a maximum of 400 mg daily.
Usual pediatric dosage: for children age 6 to 12, 25 to 50 mg P.O. every 6 to 8 hours, up to a maximum of 150 mg daily; for children age 2 to 5, 12.5 to 25 mg P.O. every 6 to 8 hours, up to a maximum of 75 mg daily.

Mechanism of action of antihistamine antiemetics

The antihistamine antiemetics prevent nausea and vomiting by inhibiting impulses from the inner ear to the vestibular nuclei as well as by inhibiting cholinergic stimulation of the chemoreceptor target zone (CTZ) and vomiting center from the vestibular nuclei. The vestibular pathway produces the nausea and vomiting of motion sickness and other labyrinth disorders. Trimethobenzamide directly inhibits dopaminergic stimulation of the CTZ, thus providing a general antiemetic effect.

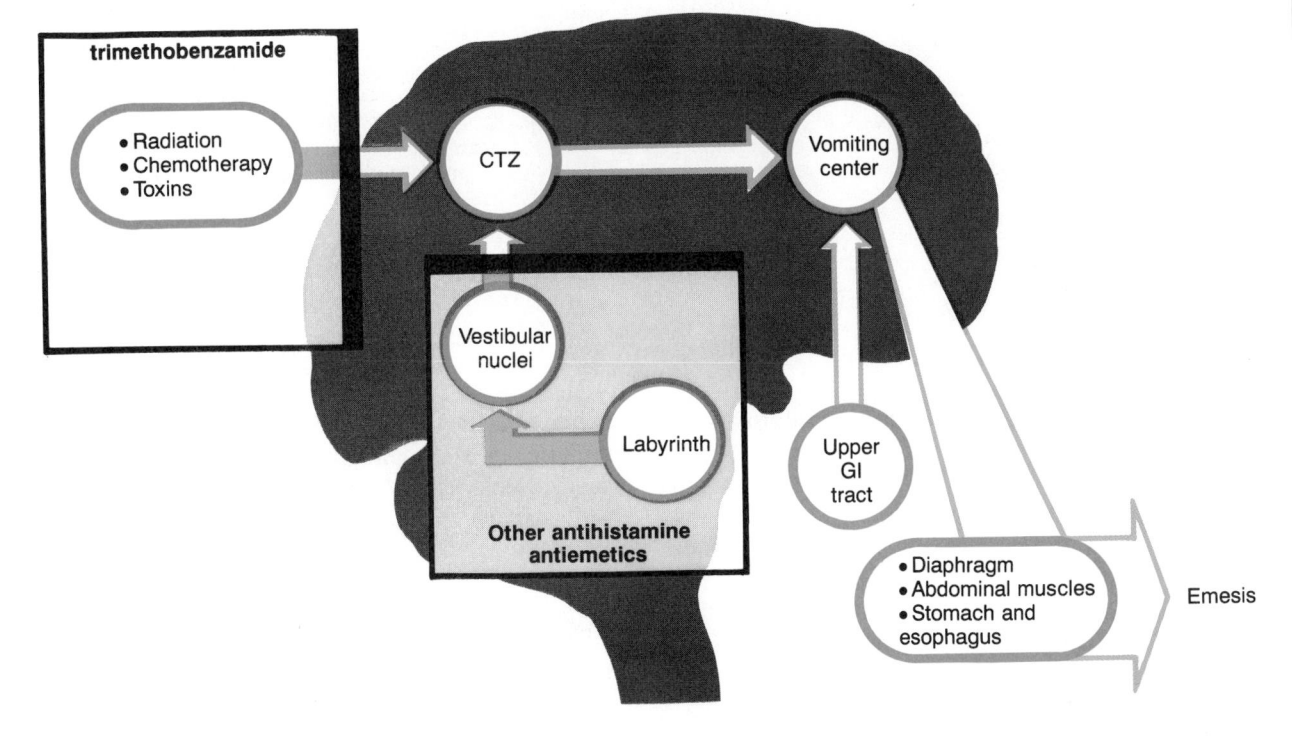

diphenhydramine hydrochloride (Benadryl). Although this drug produces an antiemetic effect, its use is limited by the sedation it usually produces.
Usual adult dosage: 25 to 50 mg P.O. or I.M. every 4 to 6 hours.
Usual pediatric dosage: for children who weigh more than 9 kg (20 lb), 12.5 to 25 mg P.O. t.i.d. or q.i.d.

hydroxyzine hydrochloride (Atarax), **hydroxyzine pamoate** (Vistaril). Also limited by its sedative effects, hydroxyzine produces a synergistic analgesic effect with narcotic analgesics and also decreases the nausea associated with narcotic administration.
Usual adult dosage: for antiemetic effects, 25 to 100 mg P.O. or I.M. t.i.d. or q.i.d.

meclizine hydrochloride (Antivert, Bonine). This drug provides a slower onset of action and longer duration of action than the other antihistamine antiemetics.

Usual adult dosage: for motion sickness, 25 to 50 mg P.O. daily at least 1 hour before travel; for vertigo, 25 to 100 mg P.O. daily in divided doses.

trimethobenzamide hydrochloride (Tigan). This drug is administered orally, rectally, or I.M. to treat nausea and vomiting. It is administered rectally or by I.M. injection to prevent postoperative nausea and vomiting.
Usual adult dosage: 250 mg P.O. t.i.d. or q.i.d, or 200 mg rectally or I.M. t.i.d. or q.i.d.
Usual pediatric dosage: for children who weigh 14 to 40 kg (31 to 88 lb), 100 to 200 mg P.O. or rectally t.i.d. or q.i.d.; for children who weigh less than 14 kg (31 lb), 100 mg rectally t.i.d. or q.i.d.

Drug interactions

Antihistamine antiemetics can produce an additive effect when they interact with other drugs that also produce an anticholinergic effect. The same is true for the sedative

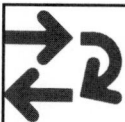

DRUG INTERACTIONS
Antihistamine antiemetics

The following chart presents the important drug interactions for the major antihistamine antiemetics discussed in this chapter.

DRUG	INTERACTING DRUGS	POSSIBLE EFFECTS	NURSING IMPLICATIONS
buclizine, cyclizine, dimenhydrinate, diphenhydramine, hydroxyzine, meclizine, trimethobenzamide	Central nervous system (CNS) depressants, including barbiturates, tranquilizers, alcohol, and opiates	Produce additive CNS depression	• Use caution when administering concurrently to avoid excessive CNS depression or sedation. • Inform ambulatory patients of the possible additive effect.
	anticholinergic drugs, including tricyclic antidepressants, phenothiazines, and antiparkinsonian drugs	Produce additive anticholinergic effects	• Assess for signs of increased anticholinergic activity, such as constipation, dry mouth, visual disturbances, and urine retention.
	ototoxic medications	Mask signs and symptoms of ototoxicity	• Monitor the patient for signs of hearing loss and conduct an audiometric test weekly or biweekly.

effect produced by antihistamines. (For more information, see *Drug interactions: Antihistamine antiemetics.*)

ADVERSE DRUG REACTIONS

Most adverse reactions to antihistamine antiemetics are predictable, mild, and usually easy to control. All antihistamine antiemetics produce some dose-related drowsiness. Reducing the dose may decrease the drowsiness without compromising the antiemetic effect. Paradoxical CNS stimulation has occurred, more often in children than adults. Symptoms of paradoxical CNS stimulation may range from restlessness, insomnia, and euphoria to tremors and even seizures. Other adverse CNS reactions include dizziness, headache, and lassitude.

The antihistamine antiemetics themselves may cause mild nausea or epigastric distress. Administering the drug with food or milk may decrease these symptoms. Anorexia also may occur and last for several weeks from long-term administration of an antihistamine antiemetic.

The anticholinergic effect of the antihistamines may cause constipation. Other anticholinergic effects include dry mouth and throat, dysuria, urine retention, and impotence. The anticholinergic action of antihistamines also may produce visual and auditory disturbances, such as blurred vision or tinnitus.

Besides the previously mentioned reactions, trimethobenzamide may produce extrapyramidal symptoms, such as acute dystonia and dyskinesis, that require discontinuation of the drug.

Hypersensitivity reactions, as manifested by rashes and photosensitivity, may occur. Blood dyscrasias have oc-

curred, but rarely. These include granulocytopenia, hemolytic anemia, leukopenia, thrombocytopenia, and pancytopenia. (For a list of reactions associated with the antihistamine antiemetics, see *Adverse reactions to antiemetics.*)

NURSING PROCESS APPLICATION

The following information assists the nurse in caring for a patient who is receiving an antihistamine antiemetic.

Assessment
• Review the patient's history for a preexisting condition that contraindicates the use of an antihistamine antiemetic, such as age (neonate), lactation, or known hypersensitivity to the drug.
• Review the patient's history for a preexisting condition that requires cautious use of an antihistamine antiemetic, such as a seizure disorder, narrow-angle glaucoma, prostatic hypertrophy, bronchial asthma, cardiac arrhythmias, or pregnancy.
• Assess the patient for adverse reactions to the prescribed antihistamine antiemetic, such as CNS stimulation or depression, GI distress, or anticholinergic effects.
• Review the patient's medication history to identify the use of drugs that may interact with the antihistamine antiemetic, such as CNS depressants, anticholinergic agents, or ototoxic medications.
• Assess the effectiveness of the prescribed antihistamine antiemetic regularly.
• Evaluate the patient's nutritional status regularly during long-term antihistamine antiemetic therapy.

Adverse reactions to antiemetics

The following table indicates the incidence of adverse drug reactions to the different kinds of antiemetics. The number and frequency of these reactions may vary according to the specific class of drug and may affect drug selection by the physician.

DRUG OR CLASS	NAUSEA AND VOMITING	ANTICHOLINERGIC REACTIONS	SEDATION	EXTRAPYRAMIDAL REACTIONS	DIZZINESS AND OTHER C.N.S. REACTIONS	DERMATOLOGIC REACTIONS
antihistamine antiemetics	+	+ +	+ + +	0	+ +	+
phenothiazine antiemetics	0	+ +	+ +	+ +	+	+ +
scopolamine	0	+ + +	+ + +	0	+ +	0

Key:
  0 = none
  + = low incidence
  + + = moderate incidence
  + + + = high incidence

• Assess for visual or auditory disturbances during antihistamine antiemetic therapy.

• Evaluate the patient's and family's knowledge about the prescribed antihistamine antiemetic.

Nursing diagnoses

The following examples represent appropriate nursing diagnoses for a patient receiving an antihistamine antiemetic.

• Potential for injury related to a preexisting condition that contraindicates the use of an antihistamine antiemetic

• Potential for injury related to a preexisting condition that requires cautious use of an antihistamine antiemetic

• Potential for injury related to adverse drug reactions

• Altered nutrition: less than body requirements, related to antiemetic-induced anorexia

• Sensory-perceptual alterations (visual and auditory) related to the anticholinergic effects of the prescribed antihistamine antiemetic

• Knowledge deficit related to the prescribed antihistamine antiemetic

Planning and implementation

• Do not administer an antihistamine antiemetic to a patient with a condition that contraindicates its use.

• Administer an antihistamine antiemetic cautiously to a patient at risk because of a preexisting condition.

• Monitor the patient closely for adverse reactions to the prescribed antihistamine antiemetic.

• *Take safety precautions if drowsiness or dizziness occurs. Expect to reduce the dosage as prescribed if the patient experiences drowsiness.*

• *Monitor a child for signs of paradoxical CNS stimulation, such as restlessness, insomnia, euphoria, tremors, or seizures, during antihistamine antiemetic therapy. Notify the physician if CNS stimulation occurs because the drug may need to be discontinued.*

• Obtain a prescription for a mild analgesic if the patient experiences a headache.

• Place the patient on a high-fiber diet and provide adequate fluids (unless contraindicated) to prevent constipation.

• Offer the patient hard sugarless candy or sips of water to relieve dry mouth.

• *Monitor closely for signs of urine retention,* such as urinary frequency and a sense of fullness in the lower abdomen after voiding, especially in a patient with prostatic hypertrophy. Palpate and percuss the bladder to assess for urine retention. If urine retention is present, notify the physician. Catheterize the patient and discontinue the antihistamine antiemetic, as prescribed.

• *Observe the patient for extrapyramidal symptoms,* such as acute dystonia and dyskinesia, during trimethobenzamide therapy. If these symptoms occur, expect to discontinue the drug.

• *Evaluate hematologic studies to detect signs of blood dyscrasias.* Alert the physician to any abnormalities.

• Administer an antihistamine antiemetic with food or milk to minimize nausea or epigastric distress.

• Consult the physician about giving a rectal suppository or I.M. injection if the patient vomits before drug administration.

• Expect a change in dosage or drug if one antihistamine antiemetic fails to produce the desired effects.

• Notify the physician if adverse reactions occur or if the prescribed antihistamine antiemetic is ineffective.

• *Monitor the patient for anorexia during and for several weeks after long-term antihistamine antiemetic therapy.*

• Weigh the patient regularly if anorexia occurs. Notify the physician if the patient loses more than 3 pounds (1.4 kg) in 1 week. Expect to administer a multivitamin supplement, as prescribed.

• Assess the patient regularly for visual disturbances, such as blurred vision, or auditory disturbances, such as tinnitus.

• *Take safety precautions if sensory or perceptual alterations occur. For example, place the bed in the low position, keep the side rails up, and supervise ambulation. Notify the physician if visual or auditory disturbances worsen or become troublesome.*

Patient teaching

• Teach the patient and family the name, dose, frequency, action, and adverse effects of the prescribed antihistamine antiemetic.

• Instruct the patient to take the prescribed drug with milk or food to minimize adverse GI reactions.

• *Advise the patient to ingest the drug 30 to 60 minutes before the activity that might produce motion sickness. Patients usually develop tolerance to motion sickness; therefore, only short-term therapy usually is needed.*

• *Alert the patient to the sedative effects, and advise the patient not to drive or participate in other activities that require mental alertness. Advise the patient not to drink alcohol or take other CNS depressants because doing so can result in the additive sedative effect of antihistamines.*

• *Advise family members that paradoxical CNS stimulation may occur in a child receiving an antihistamine antiemetic.*

• Teach the patient how to relieve the anticholinergic effects of these agents, such as constipation and dry mouth.

• *Advise the patient to notify the physician if urinary frequency and a sense of fullness in the lower abdomen occurs.*

• *Advise discontinuation of trimethobenzamide and physician notification if the patient develops extrapyramidal symptoms, such as slow, involuntary movements of large muscles in the limbs, trunk, and neck.*

• Instruct the patient to alert the physician if anorexia or a weight loss of more than 3 pounds in 1 week occurs during long-term antihistamine antiemetic therapy.

• Reassure the patient that visual and auditory disturbances are drug-related and should disappear when the drug is discontinued.

• Inform the male patient that impotence may occur with the antihistamine antiemetic.

• Instruct the patient to avoid prolonged exposure to sunlight or to wear protective clothing and a sunscreen because the antihistamine antiemetic may cause photosensitivity.

• Advise the patient to notify the physician if adverse reactions occur or if the drug is ineffective.

Evaluation

The following examples represent appropriate evaluation statements for a patient receiving an antihistamine antiemetic.

• The patient has no conditions that contraindicate antihistamine antiemetic therapy.

• The patient exhibits no signs of complications in the preexisting condition linked to the prescribed antihistamine antiemetic.

• The patient experiences no adverse reactions to the prescribed antihistamine antiemetic.

• The patient maintains adequate nutritional status.

• The patient develops no sensory or perceptual alterations.

• The patient and family express an accurate understanding of the points taught about the prescribed antihistamine antiemetic.

• The patient takes the prescribed antihistamine antiemetic with milk 60 minutes before traveling.

PHENOTHIAZINE ANTIEMETICS

The phenothiazines primarily are used to treat psychotic disorders. Yet, some of the phenothiazines are used to prevent and treat severe nausea and vomiting from various causes. Phenothiazine antiemetics are not as effective as the antihistamine antiemetics for nausea from motion sickness or vestibular dysfunction. The phenothiazines most commonly used for their antiemetic effect include chlorpromazine hydrochloride, perphenazine, prochlorperazine maleate, promethazine, and thiethylperazine.

PHARMACOKINETICS

The phenothiazine antiemetics are absorbed well, extensively metabolized by the liver, and excreted in the urine and feces.

Absorption, distribution, metabolism, excretion

Phenothiazines usually are absorbed well from the GI tract after oral and rectal administration. The drugs also are absorbed well after I.M. injection.

Phenothiazines are distributed to most body tissues and fluids, including breast milk. These drugs cross into the CNS with fairly high concentrations and become highly protein bound in the plasma.

Phenothiazines are metabolized by the liver to a number of metabolites, a few of which are pharmacologically active. After undergoing enterohepatic recirculation, these metabolites are excreted in the feces and urine.

Onset, peak, duration

The onset of action of chlorpromazine occurs shortly after oral, rectal, and parenteral administration. Concentration levels peak in about 1 to 2 hours, and duration of action is usually 4 to 5 hours. For other phenothiazines, onset and peak concentrations may not occur as quickly, although duration may be slightly longer.

PHARMACODYNAMICS

The biochemical and physiologic effects of the phenothiazines as antipsychotic drugs are well researched. Many of the effects of these drugs result from their antidopaminergic actions in the CNS. (For detailed information on the action of phenothiazines, see Chapter 28, Antipsychotic Agents.)

Mechanism of action

Phenothiazines produce their antiemetic effect by blocking the dopaminergic receptors in the CTZ. These drugs also may depress the vomiting center directly.

PHARMACOTHERAPEUTICS

Phenothiazine antiemetics control severe nausea and vomiting from various causes. When vomiting becomes severe and potentially hazardous, phenothiazines are the drugs of choice, providing effective treatment for postoperative nausea and vomiting and for the nausea and vomiting from viral illnesses. Phenothiazines are prescribed extensively to control the nausea and vomiting of cancer chemotherapy and radiotherapy. However, they are not as effective as the antihistamine antiemetics in controlling the nausea and vomiting from vertigo, motion sickness, or direct irritation of the stomach. Although not all the phenothiazines with antiemetic effects have been compared in controlled trials, those drugs that have been studied and compared displayed little difference in their antiemetic effects.

The phenothiazines are the most effective general antiemetics. However, their use is limited to short-term therapy because the potential for serious adverse reactions is higher with these drugs than with the antihistamine antiemetics. Although phenothiazine antiemetics are effective in treating morning sickness during pregnancy, their safety during pregnancy has not been established. As a result, phenothiazines should be used only when the potential benefits outweigh the potential risks.

The phenothiazines include several major drugs that share the same antiemetic use. The phenothiazine antiemetics are equally efficient in treating the nausea and vomiting from infection, uremia, cancer chemotherapy, radiotherapy, anesthesia, or drug toxicity. The choice of a phenothiazine antiemetic, therefore, depends on the drug's potential for adverse effects.

The parenteral route of administration for the phenothiazines is reserved for patients under direct observation. The rectal route is used more commonly in an outpatient setting, where parenteral administration proves less practical or when vomiting reduces the effectiveness of the oral preparations.

chlorpromazine hydrochloride (Thorazine). This drug is used to control nausea and vomiting.
Usual adult dosage: 10 to 25 mg P.O. or 25 mg I.M. every 4 to 6 hours; 100 mg rectally every 6 to 8 hours.
Usual pediatric dosage: 0.55 mg/kg P.O. every 4 to 6 hours; 1.1 mg/kg rectally every 6 to 8 hours; 0.55 mg/kg I.M. every 6 to 8 hours.

perphenazine (Trilafon). This antipsychotic agent also is used to treat severe nausea and vomiting.
Usual adult dosage: 8 to 16 mg P.O. daily in two to four divided doses; 5 mg I.M., repeated every 6 hours p.r.n.

prochlorperazine maleate (Compazine). This drug primarily is used to control nausea and vomiting. Although it is available as a sustained-release capsule, administered twice daily, sustained-release antiemetics offer no advantages and are more expensive than other forms.
Usual adult dosage: 5 to 10 mg P.O. or I.M. t.i.d. to q.i.d.; 25 mg rectally b.i.d.
Usual pediatric dosage: for a child who weighs 9 to 14 kg (20 to 31 lb), 2.5 mg P.O. or rectally once or twice a day; for a child who weighs 15 to 18 kg (33 to 40 lb), 2.5 mg b.i.d. or t.i.d.; 19 to 40 kg (42 to 88 lb), 2.5 mg P.O. or rectally t.i.d. or 5 mg b.i.d. The I.M. dosage is 0.132 mg/kg of body weight p.r.n.

promethazine (Phenergan). This drug often is used preoperatively and postoperatively or as an adjunct to narcotic analgesics for sedation and nausea control.
Usual adult dosage: 12.5 to 25 mg P.O., I.M., or rectally every 4 to 6 hours.
Usual pediatric dosage: 0.25 to 0.5 mg/kg rectally or 12.5 to 25 mg P.O. every 4 to 6 hours p.r.n.

thiethylperazine (Torecan). Thiethylperazine is another major phenothiazine used to relieve nausea and vomiting.
Usual adult dosage: 10 mg one to three times daily by oral, rectal, or I.M. administration.

Drug interactions

The drug interactions with the phenothiazine antiemetics resemble those of the antihistamine antiemetics. Phenothiazine antiemetics may produce an additive CNS depressant effect when given with other depressants, such as narcotics, sedatives, or alcohol. They also may have an additive anticholinergic effect when used with other drugs with anticholinergic action. (For details, see *Drug interactions: Phenothiazine antiemetics.*)

ADVERSE DRUG REACTIONS

Phenothiazines used in larger dosages as antipsychotics can produce numerous adverse reactions. When used as antiemetics, however, the drugs primarily produce sedation, hypotension, and extrapyramidal effects.

Adverse CNS reactions number among the major problems associated with phenothiazine antiemetics. Mild to moderate sedation occurs in 50% to 80% of the patients who receive these drugs, with chlorpromazine producing the greatest incidence. Tolerance to the sedative effect usually develops over several days of therapy. Confusion may occur, especially in elderly patients. Other adverse CNS reactions associated with phenothiazine antiemetics include anxiety, euphoria, agitation, depression, headache, insomnia, restlessness, and weakness. Because these drugs also can lower the threshold for seizures, they should be used with caution in patients who are predisposed to seizures.

Adverse anticholinergic reactions typically include dry mouth, blurred vision, constipation, and urine retention.

Hypotension and orthostatic hypotension with tachycardia, syncope, and dizziness frequently occur as adverse reactions to the phenothiazine antiemetics. Chlorpromazine produces the highest incidence of hypotensive effects; prochlorperazine and thiethylperazine, the lowest. Tolerance to the hypotensive effects usually develops.

Extrapyramidal reactions to phenothiazine antiemetics may occur. Such reactions usually are dose related and, therefore, relatively rare at antiemetic doses.

Hypersensitivity reactions can result when phenothiazines are used as antipsychotics, but rarely occur when the drugs are used as antiemetics. Granulocytopenia, although rare, is the most commonly reported adverse hematologic effect. The phenothiazines also produce many dermatologic effects, especially with long-term therapy. Hypersensitivity reactions manifested as cholestatic jaundice, blood dyscrasias, dermatologic reactions, and photosensitivity have occurred, usually within the first few months of phenothiazine therapy. (For the major adverse reactions to the phenothiazine antiemetics, see *Adverse reactions to antiemetics,* page 743.)

NURSING PROCESS APPLICATION

The following information assists the nurse in caring for a patient who is receiving a phenothiazine antiemetic.

Assessment

• Review the patient's history for a preexisting condition that contraindicates the use of a phenothiazine antiemetic, such as coma, CNS depression, bone marrow depression, brain damage, pediatric surgery, or known hypersensitivity to the drug.
• Review the patient's history for a preexisting condition that requires cautious use of a phenothiazine antiemetic, such as hepatic or cardiovascular disease, exposure to extreme heat or cold, a respiratory disorder, hypocalcemia, a seizure disorder, glaucoma, or prostatic hypertrophy.
• Assess the patient for adverse reactions to the prescribed azine antiemetic, such as CNS, cardiovascular, dermatologic, or hypersensitivity reactions.
• Review the patient's medication history to identify the use of drugs that may interact with the prescribed phenothiazine antiemetic, such as guanethidine, amphetamines, anticholinergics, or barbiturates.
• Assess the effectiveness of the prescribed phenothiazine antiemetic regularly.
• Evaluate the patient's and family's knowledge about the prescribed phenothiazine antiemetic.

Nursing diagnoses

The following examples represent appropriate nursing diagnoses for a patient receiving a phenothiazine antiemetic.
• Potential for injury related to a preexisting condition that contraindicates the use of a phenothiazine antiemetic
• Potential for injury related to a preexisting condition that requires cautious use of a phenothiazine antiemetic
• Potential for injury related to adverse drug reactions
• Knowledge deficit related to the prescribed phenothiazine antiemetic

Planning and implementation

• Do not administer a phenothiazine antiemetic to a patient with a condition that contraindicates its use.
• Administer a phenothiazine antiemetic cautiously to a patient at risk because of a preexisting condition.
• *Monitor the patient closely for adverse reactions to the phenothiazine antiemetic. Be aware that sedation, hypotension, and extrapyramidal effects are the most common reactions.*
• *Take safety precautions if sedation, dizziness, blurred vision, or confusion occurs. For example, place the bed in the low position, keep the side rails up, and supervise ambulation. Reassure the patient that tolerance to sedation usually develops over several days of therapy.*

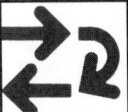

DRUG INTERACTIONS
Phenothiazine antiemetics

Drug interactions involving phenothiazines are relatively common and can be serious.

DRUG	INTERACTING DRUGS	POSSIBLE EFFECTS	NURSING IMPLICATIONS
chlorpromazine, perphenazine, prochlorperazine, promethazine, thiethylperazine	guanethidine	Inhibit uptake of guanethidine	• Monitor the patient's blood pressure frequently. • Expect to increase the guanethidine dosage, or replace guanethidine with another antihypertensive agent as prescribed.
	amphetamines, nonamphetamine anorexigenic agents	Inhibit effects of both drugs	• Do not administer these drugs concurrently.
	anticholinergics	Increase anticholinergic effects; decrease antiemetic effects	• Do not administer together routinely. If the drugs must be given concurrently, assess the patient for signs of reduced phenothiazine effects, such as continued vomiting. • Perform abdominal assessments to monitor the patient for diminished or absent bowel sounds, abdominal pain, constipation, and other abdominal problems.
	barbiturates	Increase CNS depressant effects; increase phenothiazine metabolism	• Observe the patient for erratic therapeutic effects, such as intermittent nausea and vomiting, and for increased depressant effects, such as stupor.
	levodopa	Reduce antiparkinsonian effects of levodopa when phenothiazines block dopamine receptors in the CNS	• Avoid concurrent administration, if possible. • Monitor the patient for an increase in Parkinson's symptoms.
	lithium	Increase chance of neurotoxicity, seizures, delirium, and encephalopathy in manic patients; can produce respiratory depression and hypotension	• Monitor the patient for reduced phenothiazine response and changes in neurologic status. • Monitor the patient's vital signs frequently.
	droperidol	Increases risk of extrapyramidal effects	• Monitor the patient for tremor.

• *Monitor the patient closely for other signs of adverse CNS reactions, such as anxiety, euphoria, agitation, depression, headache, insomnia, restlessness, or weakness.*
• *Take seizure precautions when administering a phenothiazide antiemetic to a patient who is predisposed to seizures because these drugs can lower the threshold for seizures.*
• Obtain a prescription for a mild analgesic if the patient experiences a headache.
• Place the patient on a high-fiber diet and provide adequate fluids to prevent constipation.
• Offer the patient hard sugarless candy or sips of water to relieve dry mouth.

• *Monitor closely for signs of urine retention, such as urinary frequency and a sense of fullness in the lower abdomen after voiding, especially in a patient with prostatic hypertrophy.* Palpate and percuss the bladder to assess for urine retention. If urine retention is present, notify the physician. Catheterize the patient and discontinue the phenothiazine antiemetic, if prescribed.
• *Monitor the patient's vital signs regularly to detect hypotension and tachycardia, especially in a patient receiving chlorpromazine.*
• *Evaluate hematologic studies for signs of blood dyscrasias. Alert the physician to any abnormalities.*

• *Avoid skin contact with oral solutions and injections when preparing or administering these drugs because they can cause dermatologic effects.*

• Notify the physician if adverse reactions occur or if the prescribed phenothiazine antiemetic is ineffective.

Patient teaching

• Teach the patient and family the name, dose, frequency, action, and adverse effects of the prescribed phenothiazine antiemetic.

• *Advise the patient that this drug is not effective for motion sickness.*

• *Alert the patient that the phenothiazine antiemetic may impair the ability to perform activities that require alertness or physical coordination, such as driving or operating machinery. Also inform the patient that alcohol or other sedatives will potentiate the sedative effect of the phenothiazine antiemetic.*

• *Inform the patient about the possibility of hypotension, and instruct the patient to remain recumbent for 30 to 60 minutes after receiving the drug.*

• Explain that the drug may make the patient's urine pink or red-brown but that this discoloration is harmless.

• Advise the patient to avoid prolonged exposure to sunlight or to wear protective clothing and sunscreen because the phenothiazine may produce photosensitivity.

• *Inform the seizure-prone patient that the phenothiazine antiemetic can lower the threshold for seizure. Instruct the patient to notify the physician if a seizure occurs because the drug may have to be discontinued.*

• Teach the patient how to relieve the anticholinergic effects of these agents, such as constipation and dry mouth.

• Advise the patient to notify the physician if urinary frequency and a sense of fullness in the lower abdomen after voiding occur. These may be symptoms of urine retention.

• Instruct the patient to notify the physician if other adverse reactions occur or if the prescribed agent is ineffective.

Evaluation

The following examples represent appropriate evaluation statements for a patient receiving a phenothiazine antiemetic.

• The patient has no conditions that contraindicate phenothiazine antiemetic therapy.

• The patient exhibits no signs of complications in the preexisting condition linked to the prescribed phenothiazine antiemetic.

• The patient develops no adverse reactions to the prescribed phenothiazine antiemetic.

• The patient and family express an accurate understanding of the points taught about the prescribed phenothiazine antiemetic.

• The patient takes appropriate measures to relieve dry mouth.

OTHER ANTIEMETICS

Other drugs, unrelated to the antihistamines or phenothiazines, also act effectively to prevent and treat nausea and vomiting.

benzquinamide hydrochloride (Emete-con). This drug is a benzquinoline derivative available as an antiemetic in parenteral form. Although unrelated chemically to the antihistamines and phenothiazines, benzquinamide does produce antiemetic, antihistamine, anticholinergic, vasopressor, and sedative effects. Benzquinamide probably produces its antiemetic effect by a direct depressant action on the CTZ.

Benzquinamide is used to prevent and treat nausea and vomiting associated with anesthesia and surgery. This drug may be preferred in some circumstances because it does not produce CNS or respiratory depression. Furthermore, benzquinamide does not produce the extrapyramidal effects or hypotension associated with the phenothiazines.

After I.M. injection, benzquinamide is absorbed rapidly. Its onset of action is within 15 minutes, and duration of action is from 3 to 4 hours. The drug is metabolized by the liver, and its metabolites are excreted in the urine and feces. Adverse reactions to benzquinamide usually involve the CNS, with drowsiness the most common. Anticholinergic adverse reactions commonly occur.

scopolamine (Triptone, Transderm-Scop). This drug has been used for years to prevent motion sickness. However, its use is limited because of its sedative and anticholinergic effects. One scopolamine transdermal preparation (Transderm-Scop) provides highly effective action without producing the drug's usual adverse effects. (For more information about transdermal scopolamine, see *Facts about scopolamine patches.*) Drowsiness and dry mouth from the anticholinergic action of scopolamine are the most common adverse reactions. Patients usually tolerate these reactions well because the reactions are not pronounced. (For more information, see *Adverse reactions to antiemetics,* page 743.) The nurse should observe the common anticholinergic precautions, such as administering scopolamine cautiously to a patient with glaucoma or GI or urinary tract obstruction.

metoclopramide hydrochloride (Reglan). This drug is used to manage GI motility disorders. Its effectiveness is attributed, in part, to its antagonistic effect on dopamine in the CNS. Apparently, metoclopramide also is antagonistic to dopamine in the CTZ, thereby suppressing the

Facts about scopolamine patches

Apply the transdermal scopolamine patch behind the ear. For optimal effect, apply the patch at least 4 hours before the need for its antiemetic action. Remove the patch after it no longer is needed or after 72 hours.

Why the transdermal route for motion sickness?
• The nerve fibers in the vestibular apparatus of the inner ear help people maintain balance. But for some, motion increases the activity of these fibers, causing dizziness, nausea, and vomiting. The transdermal scopolamine patch helps reduce the activity of these inner ear fibers.
• The patch releases minute amounts of scopolamine that permeate the intact skin at a programmed rate, minimizing adverse reactions. Scopolamine is absorbed directly into the bloodstream, quickly achieving and maintaining an optimal dose for up to 72 hours. That prevents the nausea and vomiting of motion sickness.
• The patch is a flexible, adhesive disk of four layers, as shown in the illustration.

• The priming dose of scopolamine rapidly achieves the required steady-state blood concentration. Over the 3-day lifetime of the patch, the drug is delivered at a nearly constant rate.
• The drug passes by diffusion through the membrane from the higher concentration inside the reservoir in the patch to the lower concentration outside the reservoir.
• The amount of drug delivered through diffusion is regulated by the membrane thickness, surface area and composition of the patch, and the drug concentration on each side of the membrane.

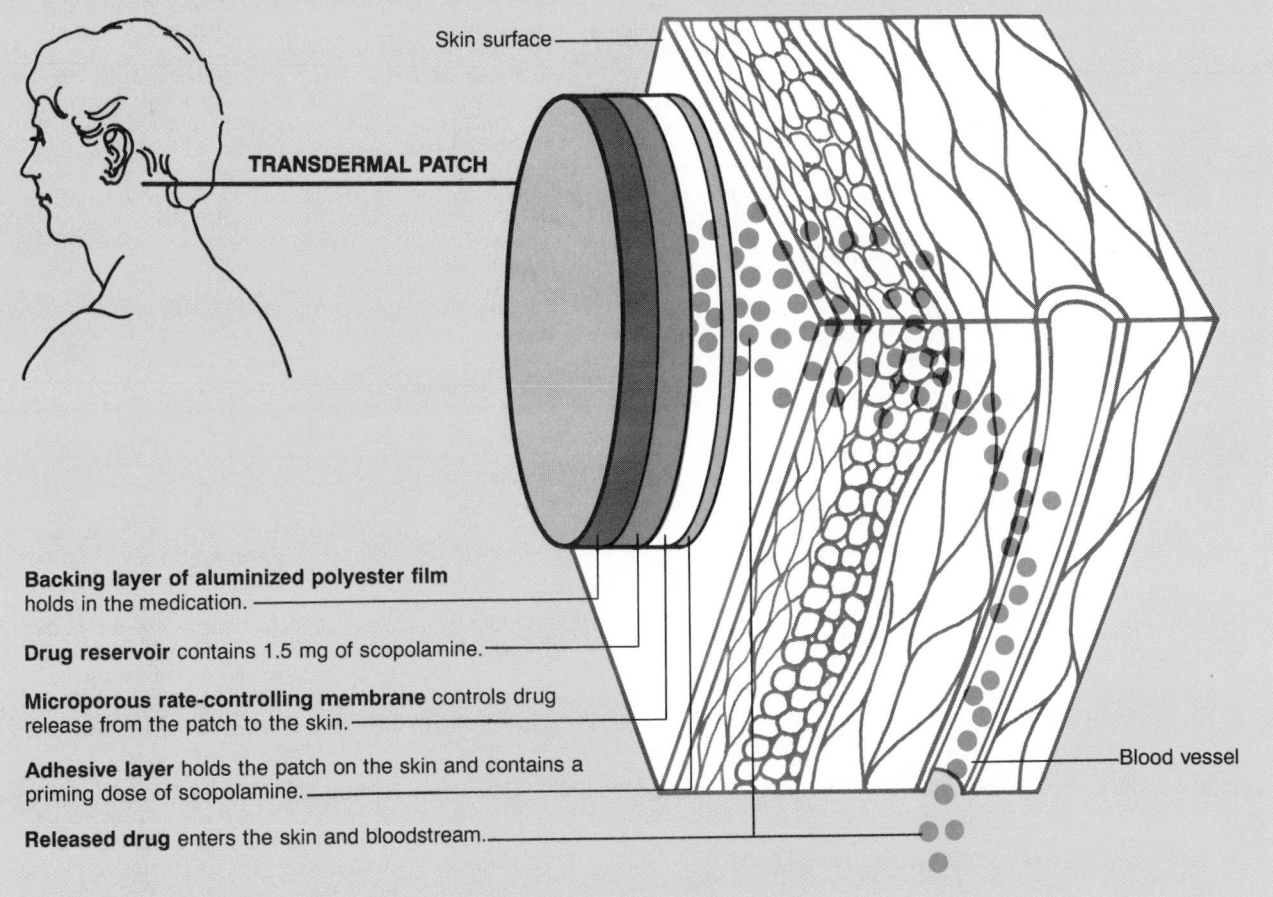

Skin surface

TRANSDERMAL PATCH

Backing layer of aluminized polyester film holds in the medication.

Drug reservoir contains 1.5 mg of scopolamine.

Microporous rate-controlling membrane controls drug release from the patch to the skin.

Adhesive layer holds the patch on the skin and contains a priming dose of scopolamine.

Released drug enters the skin and bloodstream.

Blood vessel

impulse to vomit. Metoclopramide also may decrease direct impulses from the GI tract to the vomiting center.

Used for many years in Europe to prevent motion sickness, metoclopramide currently is being used in the United States to prevent cancer chemotherapy-induced nausea and vomiting.

diphenidol (Vontrol). This drug appears to provide a dual effect, inhibiting impulse conduction from the vestibular area of the ear to the vomiting center and directly suppressing the CTZ. Thus, the drug not only effectively prevents vertigo, but also prevents and treats generalized nausea and vomiting. Diphenidol, which has a relatively

Emetic and antiemetic agents

The following chart summarizes the major emetic and antiemetic drugs currently in clinical use.

DRUG	MAJOR INDICATIONS	USUAL ADULT DOSAGES	CONTRAINDICATIONS AND PRECAUTIONS
Emetics			
ipecac syrup	Emesis of ingested poisons	15 to 30 ml P.O. followed by 200 to 300 ml of water; dose may be repeated in 30 minutes if vomiting is not induced	• Know that ipecac syrup is contraindicated in a semicomatose or unconscious patient or one with petroleum distillate or caustic substance poisoning, bulimia, anorexia nervosa, severe inebriation, seizures, shock, or absent gag reflex. • Administer with caution to a pregnant or lactating patient or one with impaired cardiac function or sclerotic or other pathologic changes in blood vessels.
Antihistamine antiemetics			
dimenhydrinate	Prevention of motion sickness	50 to 100 mg P.O. every 4 to 6 hours up to a maximum of 400 mg daily	• Know that dimenhydrinate is contraindicated in a neonate, a lactating patient, or one with known hypersensitivity to the drug. • Administer with caution to a pregnant patient or one with a seizure disorder, narrow-angle glaucoma, prostatic hypertrophy, bronchial asthma, or cardiac arrhythmias.
meclizine	Prevention of motion sickness	25 to 50 mg P.O. daily at least 1 hour before travel	• Know that meclizine is contraindicated in a patient with known hypersensitivity to the drug. • Administer with caution to a pregnant patient or one with asthma, glaucoma, or prostatic hypertrophy.
trimethobenzamide	Prevention and treatment of mild to moderate nausea and vomiting	250 mg P.O. t.i.d. or q.i.d. or 200 mg I.M. or rectally t.i.d. or q.i.d.	• Know that trimethobenzamide is contraindicated in a patient with known hypersensitivity to the drug. • Administer with caution in the treatment of vomiting in children.
Phenothiazine antiemetics			
prochlorperazine	Prevention and treatment of severe nausea and vomiting from various causes	5 to 10 mg P.O. or I.M. t.i.d. or q.i.d.; or 25 mg rectally b.i.d.	• Know that prochlorperazine is contraindicated in a patient undergoing pediatric surgery or any patient with known hypersensitivity to the drug, coma, central nervous system (CNS) depression, bone marrow depression, or brain damage. • Administer with caution to an elderly, debilitated, or pregnant patient or one with hepatic disease, cardiovascular disease, exposure to extreme heat or cold, a respiratory disorder, hypocalcemia, a seizure disorder, severe reaction to insulin or electroshock therapy, suspected brain tumor, intestinal obstruction, glaucoma, or prostatic hypertrophy.
promethazine	Prevention and treatment of severe nausea and vomiting from various causes	12.5 to 25 mg P.O., I.M., or rectally every 4 to 6 hours	• Know that promethazine is contraindicated in a patient undergoing pediatric surgery or any patient with known hypersensitivity to the drug, coma, CNS depression, bone marrow depression, or brain damage. • Administer with caution to an elderly, debilitated, or pregnant patient or one with hepatic disease, cardiovascular disease, exposure to extreme heat or cold, a respiratory disorder, hypocalcemia, a seizure disorder, severe reaction to insulin or electroshock therapy, suspected brain tumor, intestinal obstruction, glaucoma, or prostatic hypertrophy.

long half-life of 4 hours, is absorbed well from the GI tract and is metabolized by the liver. Its metabolites are excreted by the kidneys. The drug produces typical anticholinergic adverse reactions. Its use is limited because of the auditory and visual hallucinations, confusion, and disorientation that occur in 0.5% of patients. These adverse reactions occur within the first 3 days of therapy and usually disappear within 3 days after the therapy is discontinued.

dronabinol (Marinol). A Schedule II drug, dronabinol is the synthetic equivalent of the isomer of delta-9-tetrahydrocannabinol (THC), the principal psychoactive component in marijuana. Dronabinol is indicated for the nausea and vomiting from cancer chemotherapy in patients who do not respond adequately to conventional antiemetics. Although its use is controversial, dronabinol appears to be an effective antiemetic in cancer chemotherapy. After oral administration, dronabinol is metabolized extensively on its first pass through the liver. Some of the metabolites also are psychoactive. The serum concentration peaks within 3 hours after the oral dose, and excretion occurs primarily through the feces.

Dronabinol can accumulate in the body, and the patient can develop tolerance or physical and psychological dependence. The most prominent potential adverse reactions occur in the CNS and include mood changes (euphoria, panic, and paranoia), loss of memory, sleep disturbances, hallucinations, alterations of time perception, and poor impulse control. The nurse should advise the patient not to drive or participate in any activity requiring alertness. Furthermore, a responsible adult should monitor the patient taking the drug.

CHAPTER SUMMARY

Chapter 43 discussed the pharmacokinetics, pharmacodynamics, and pharmacotherapeutics of emetics and antiemetics, as well as the adverse reactions and nursing care associated with these drugs. Here are the highlights of the chapter.

• The emetics form the basis for the treatment of poisoning by ingestion. Drug-induced emesis removes the toxic substance from the stomach, thus preventing absorption.

• Ipecac syrup has become the emetic of choice because of its effectiveness in evacuating the stomach and relatively low incidence of adverse reactions. The American Academy of Pediatrics recommends that all families with small children keep ipecac syrup on hand for the emergency treatment of poisonings. When ipecac syrup is obtained, the nurse

should teach safe home use of the drug and instruct the family to contact the poison control center, physician, or other qualified health care professional before any use of the drug.

• The three basic groups of antiemetics include the antihistamines, the phenothiazines, and others, such as scopolamine. Some antiemetics control the nausea and vomiting from disturbances of the inner ear; others control generalized nausea and vomiting that arise from other causes.

• The antihistamine antiemetics and scopolamine commonly are used to prevent motion sickness. However, these drugs usually are not effective after the nausea has begun.

• Antihistamine antiemetics and scopolamine also are used to treat vertigo caused by disturbances of vestibular function. The symptomatic relief provided by these drugs for the vertigo of labyrinthitis or Ménière's disease varies among patients.

• The most pronounced adverse reactions to antihistamine antiemetics and scopolamine include drowsiness and anticholinergic effects.

• Generalized nausea and vomiting usually are treated with phenothiazine antiemetics. This nausea and vomiting, usually mediated through the CTZ of the medulla, may have various causes, including cancer chemotherapy and radiotherapy, infections, anesthesia and surgery, and drugs such as narcotics.

• The adverse reactions to phenothiazines resemble those of the antihistamines and include sedation and anticholinergic effects.

• Benzquinamide does not produce hypotensive effects, which sometimes makes its use preferable in postoperative conditions.

• Metoclopramide and dronabinal are used to prevent or treat cancer chemotherapy-induced nausea and vomiting.

• When caring for a patient receiving an emetic, the nurse should monitor the drug's effectiveness to prevent damage from the ingested toxin.

• For a patient receiving an antiemetic, the nurse should monitor the drug's effectiveness. The nurse also should monitor fluid and electrolyte levels to detect serious imbalances.

STUDY QUESTIONS

See Appendix 1 for answers.

1. Fred Barnes, age 42, is brought to the emergency department by a friend who tells the nurse that Mr. Barnes "took too many Valiums because he felt very depressed."

The physician orders an emetic for Mr. Barnes. When would an emetic agent be contraindicated?
(a) when the patient is a child
(b) when the patient is elderly
(c) when a caustic substance has been ingested
(d) when ingestion occurred more than 1 hour ago

2. To induce vomiting for Mr. Barnes, the physician is most likely to order which emetic agent?
(a) apomorphine
(b) ipecac syrup
(c) chlorpromazine hydrochloride
(d) activated charcoal

3. Mark Lewellan, age 35, is planning to go on an ocean cruise. Because Mr. Lewellan experiences motion sickness, he asks the physician to prescribe an antiemetic. Which antiemetic agent probably would be best for Mr. Lewellan?
(a) chlorpromazine hydrochloride
(b) dronabinol
(c) benzquinamide hydrochloride
(d) dimenhydrinate

4. When should Mr. Lewellan take the antiemetic agent?
(a) the day before leaving on his trip
(b) 30 to 60 minutes before traveling
(c) at the onset of motion sickness
(d) after vomiting occurs

5. The physician could have prescribed scopolamine for Mr. Lewellan. Which route of administration minimizes adverse reactions to scopolamine?
(a) I.M.
(b) oral
(c) rectal
(d) transdermal

6. Georgia DeWitt, age 40, is recovering from a cholecystectomy. To control postoperative nausea, her physician prescribes the phenothiazine agent promethazine (Phenergan) 12.5 mg P.O. every 6 hours. By which mechanism of action do phenothiazines prevent nausea and vomiting?
(a) CNS depression
(b) anticholinergic action
(c) inhibition of vestibular stimulation
(d) dopaminergic receptor blockade in the CTZ

7. Which adverse drug reaction occurs most commonly with phenothiazine administration?
(a) sedation
(b) hypertension
(c) pyramidal effects
(d) cardiac arrhythmias

8. Julia Brown, age 70, is receiving chemotherapy for ovarian cancer. To prevent the nausea and vomiting associated with cancer chemotherapy, her physician is most likely to prescribe which antiemetic agent?
(a) benzquinamide hydrochloride
(b) prochlorperazine maleate
(c) metoclopramide hydrochloride
(d) dronabinol

SELECTED REFERENCES

AHFS drug information 90. (1990). Bethesda, MD: American Society of Hospital Pharmacists.

Goodman and Gilman's the pharmacological basis of therapeutics (8th ed.; 1990). Elmsford, NY: Pergamon Press.

Eburn, E. (1989). Choosing the right antiemetic. *Nursing Times, 85*(24), 36-38.

Hansten, P., and Horn, J. (1988). *Drug interactions: Clinical significance of drug-drug interactions* (6th ed.). Philadelphia: Lea & Febiger.

Marin, J., Ibanez, M., and Arribas, S. (1990). Therapeutic management of nausea and vomiting. *General Pharmacology, 21*(1), 1-10.

Merrifield, K., and Chaffee, B. (1989). Recent advances in the management of nausea and vomiting caused by antineoplastic agents. *Clinical Pharmacology, 8*(3), 187-199.

North American Nursing Diagnosis Association. (1990). *Taxonomy I - Revised with official categories.* St. Louis: NANDA.

Nursing91 drug handbook. (1991). Springhouse, PA: Springhouse Corporation.

USPDI. (1991). *Drug information for the health care professional* (Vol. I, 11th ed.). Rockville, MD: United States Pharmacopeial Convention.

PEPTIC ULCER AGENTS

OBJECTIVES

After reading and studying this chapter, the student should be able to:

1. Explain peptic ulcer formation, concentrating on the role played by acetylcholine, prostaglandins, gastrin, and histamine.

2. Differentiate among the ways in which antacids, histamine$_2$ (H$_2$)-receptor antagonists, and other agents decrease peptic ulcer formation.

3. Describe the mechanism of action of antacids.

4. Explain why patients frequently are not compliant when taking antacids.

5. Describe the mechanism of action of H$_2$-receptor antagonists.

6. Discuss why H$_2$-receptor antagonists are the treatment of choice for duodenal and gastric ulcers.

7. Identify the major indications for oral and parenteral H$_2$-receptor antagonists.

8. Explain the mechanism of action of other agents, such as sucralfate, misoprostol, and omeprazole, in promoting peptic ulcer healing.

9. Describe how to apply the nursing process when caring for a patient who is receiving a peptic ulcer agent.

INTRODUCTION

A peptic ulcer is an open lesion of the epithelial, mucosal membranes of the lower esophagus, stomach, or duodenum. Between 5% and 10% of the U.S. population can expect to experience peptic ulcers; 3 to 4 million cases of active peptic ulcers occur each year. Several factors may contribute to the development of peptic ulcer disease, including smoking and the use of aspirin, nonsteroidal anti-inflammatory drugs (NSAIDs), or corticosteroids. Although stress and the consumption of coffee and alcohol are associated with peptic ulcer disease, health care professionals continue to debate the effect of these factors on peptic ulcer development.

Most experts believe that an imbalance between the damaging effects of acid and pepsin and the normal or decreased gastrointestinal (GI) tract defense mechanisms is the underlying cause of peptic ulcers. That imbalance damages the mucosal membranes and protective mechanisms. Some ulcers develop when increased acid secretions overcome the protective mechanisms of the GI tract; others develop from an impairment of those protective mechanisms. The combination of those two etiologies accounts for the development of peptic ulcers.

The rate of pepsin secretion usually is directly proportional to the rate of acid secretion, and many patients with duodenal ulcers display hypersecretion of acid and pepsin. Several factors contribute to hypersecretion of acid and pepsin. An increased cell mass of the parietal and chief cells, which are the secretory cells of the stomach, leads to higher-than-normal acid and pepsin output. Cholinergic stimulation via the vagus nerve and gastrin release in the postprandial state enhance gastric acid response. Gastrin, histamine, and acetylcholine stimulate acid secretion from the parietal cells and pepsin secretion from the chief cells. Furthermore, acid secretion from food stimulation increases, partially in response to an impaired feedback mechanism that permits gastrin release and partially in response to an increased sensitivity of the parietal cells to gastrin and possibly histamine.

The parietal cells of the stomach are the only cells that contain an acid pump, known as the proton pump. The proton pump relies on hydrogen/potassium adenosine triphosphatase (H$^+$/K$^+$ ATPase) to exchange hydrogen and potassium across the membrane to maintain gastric acidity. Blockage of this pump blocks acid secretion. This is therapeutic in peptic ulcer disease.

The timing of acid hypersecretion also is important in preventing peptic ulcer formation. Researchers have found nocturnal acid secretion to be higher in some individuals. Because nocturnal acid may be unopposed by food in the stomach, an ulcer can result. Nocturnal acid secretion also can inhibit ulcer therapy.

Mucosal defense mechanisms

Acetylcholine, gastrin, and histamine stimulate the release of hydrochloric acid from the parietal cells. Within the parietal cells, the proton pump maintains gastric acidity.

Acetylcholine is released after cholinergic stimulation from vagal fibers or from local neurons after distention of the stomach resulting from food ingestion. The released acetylcholine increases gastric acid directly by stimulating acid secretion and indirectly by sensitizing the parietal cells to the effects of gastrin and histamine and stimulating the release of gastrin. These effects can be decreased by blocking the cholinergic receptor with an anticholinergic such as atropine.

Gastrin is the most potent stimulant of gastric acid secretion. It is stored in the G cells, which are interspersed among the other epithelial cells of the stomach. Gastrin also stimulates pepsin secretion and gastrointestinal (GI) motility, promotes closure of the esophageal sphincter, and

stimulates hepatic bile flow and pancreatic secretions. Some researchers think that blocking the action of gastrin may serve as the goal for developing future antiulcer drugs.

Histamine in body tissues mediates many reactions, including allergic ones. Histamine is secreted by the gastric mucosa to stimulate the release of acid. However, the histamine receptors in the GI tract are not blocked by the typical antihistamine drugs. The GI tract receptors, the histamine$_2$ (H$_2$) receptors, are blocked only by H$_2$-receptor antagonists, drugs that represent a major advance in treating peptic ulcer disease.

Inside the parietal cells, the proton pump relies on hydrogen/potassium adenosine triphosphatase (H$^+$/K$^+$ ATPase) to maintain gastric acidity by exchanging hydrogen and potassium. Therefore, drugs that block the action of this pump can block acid secretion by the parietal cells.

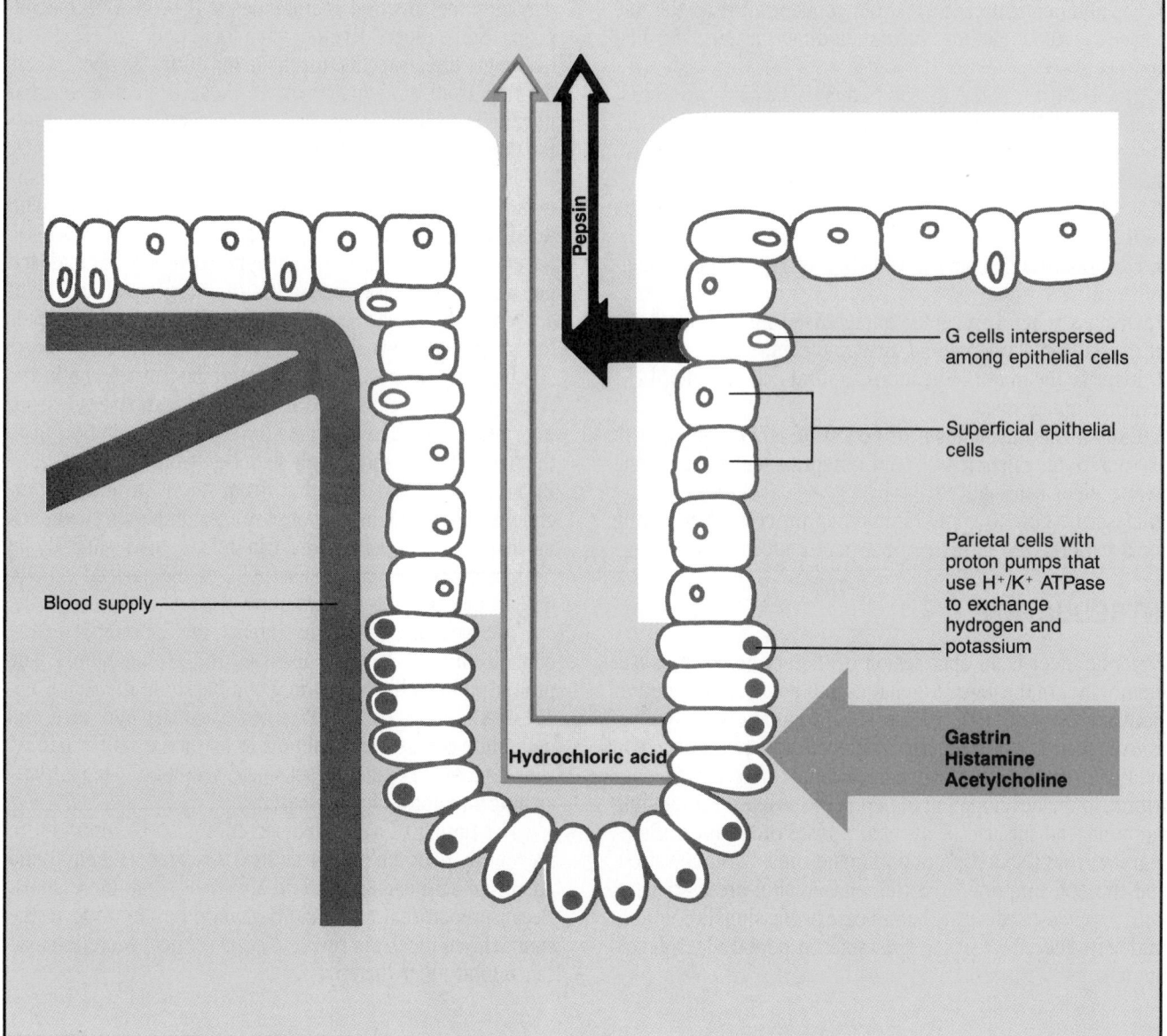

Pepsin

Hydrochloric acid

Blood supply

G cells interspersed among epithelial cells

Superficial epithelial cells

Parietal cells with proton pumps that use H$^+$/K$^+$ ATPase to exchange hydrogen and potassium

Gastrin
Histamine
Acetylcholine

SELECTED NURSING DIAGNOSES

Peptic ulcer agents

The following nursing diagnoses address representative problems and etiologies that a nurse may encounter when caring for a patient who is receiving a peptic ulcer agent. Some of these nursing diagnoses contain generalized etiologies, which the nurse must individualize based on the patient's needs. (For some common nursing diagnoses and related interventions for each drug class, see the "Nursing Process Application" sections of this chapter.)

- Altered protection related to omeprazole-induced gastric malignancy
- Altered protection related to the adverse hematologic effects of cimetidine
- Altered thought processes related to the adverse central nervous system effects of a histamine₂-receptor antagonist
- Altered tissue perfusion (cardiopulmonary) related to the cardiotoxic effects of a histamine₂-receptor antagonist
- Constipation related to the adverse gastrointestinal effects of a peptic ulcer agent
- Decreased cardiac output related to profound bradycardia caused by a histamine₂-receptor antagonist
- Diarrhea related to the laxative effects of a peptic ulcer agent
- Fluid volume excess related to sodium and fluid retention caused by a high-sodium antacid

- Knowledge deficit related to the prescribed peptic ulcer agent
- Noncompliance related to long-term antacid therapy
- Pain related to headache caused by a peptic ulcer agent
- Potential for injury related to a preexisting condition that contraindicates the use of a peptic ulcer agent
- Potential for injury related to a preexisting condition that requires cautious use of a peptic ulcer agent
- Potential for injury related to adverse drug reactions
- Potential for injury related to an electrolyte or mineral disturbance caused by an antacid
- Potential for trauma related to hemorrhoids, rectal fissures, or fecal impaction secondary to antacid-induced constipation
- Potential for trauma related to cimetidine-induced seizures
- Sexual dysfunction related to the adverse genitourinary effects of cimetidine or ranitidine

---

Not all patients with duodenal ulcers have hypersecretion of acid and pepsin. Some duodenal ulcers and most gastric ulcers are caused by a breakdown in the mucosal resistance to the effects of acid, pepsin, and other stomach contents. The gastric mucosal barrier is a complex defense system that allows hydrochloric acid to diffuse into the lumen of the stomach but prevents the return of such acid, thereby protecting the gastric mucosa from digesting itself. (For details about this protective system, see *Mucosal defense mechanisms.*) This protective response is referred to as cytoprotection. Cytoprotective drugs prevent mucosal damage and enhance the protective effect. Factors important to mucosal protection include mucus secretion, bicarbonate secretion, mucosal perfusion, and cellular repair.

In opposition to the parietal cells and chief cells, which secrete acid and pepsin, other epithelial cells in the stomach secrete mucus and bicarbonate. Brunner's glands and surface epithelial cells in the duodenum also secrete mucus and bicarbonate. The mucus secretion provides a protective layer along the walls of the stomach and duodenum. The bicarbonate secretion maintains the pH of the mucus layer at about 7, which protects the stomach from the acidic pH of 1 to 2 found in the gastric lumen. The mucus barrier also protects against pepsin and other injurious agents.

Endogenous prostaglandins also are important in maintaining normal mucosal defenses. Synthesized by the gastric mucosa, prostaglandins act to increase mucus and bicarbonate secretion, increase mucosal perfusion, and enhance cellular repair after injury. Therefore, prostaglandins are cytoprotective. The NSAIDs and aspirin may cause damage to the gastric mucosa because they inhibit prostaglandin synthesis.

If the mucosal defense system is impaired, peptic ulcer disease may occur. Pepsin, mechanical forces of the stomach, or other substances increasingly may damage the mucus layer. Hypersecretory states may thin and damage the mucus layer. Mucus or bicarbonate production may decline, thus thinning the mucus layer and presenting an inadequate buffer. The quality but not quantity of mucus may become abnormal, resulting in ulcers. Drugs that could correct these defects in the mucosal defense mechanisms would be important additions to peptic ulcer treatment.

Peptic ulcer therapy is directed at the imbalance between acid and pepsin secretion and the mucosal defense mechanisms. Peptic ulcer agents (1) neutralize acid in the GI tract, (2) reduce acid secretion, (3) bind to the ulcer, protecting it and neutralizing local acid, or (4) block the proton pump. Researchers currently are investigating new drugs that act by enhancing mucosal resistance to acid.

For a summary of representative drugs, see *Selected major drugs: Peptic ulcer agents,* page 767. For a listing of applicable nursing diagnoses that the nurse may formulate when caring for a patient receiving these agents, see *Selected nursing diagnoses: Peptic ulcer agents.* For detailed information on applying the nursing process, see Chapter 6, The Nursing Process and Drug Therapy.

756 UNIT TEN • DRUGS TO IMPROVE GASTROINTESTINAL FUNCTION

ANTACIDS

The antacids, which are over-the-counter medications, are used extensively alone and with other drugs to treat peptic ulcer disease. The subject of extensive advertising, antacids sometimes are used indiscriminately by the public for a wide variety of conditions.

Antacids are compounds that consist of a metallic cation (positively charged molecule) and a basic anion (negatively charged molecule). Commonly used cations are aluminum, magnesium, and calcium. The basic anion neutralizes acid, thereby producing the antacid's therapeutic effect. Hydroxide is the most commonly used anion; other anions include carbonate, bicarbonate, citrate, and trisilicate. Antacids discussed in this chapter include magnesium hydroxide and aluminum hydroxide with simethicone, magaldrate or aluminum-magnesium complex, and calcium carbonate.

PHARMACOKINETICS

Most modern antacids are formulated with aluminum, magnesium, and calcium cations. The effectiveness of antacids does not require their absorption.

Absorption, distribution, metabolism, excretion

The action of antacids takes place in the stomach. Absorption is neither necessary nor desired. Depending on the type of antacid and the patient's physical condition, problems may result if absorption takes place. For example, hypermagnesemia can occur if a patient with renal failure receives an antacid containing magnesium. Hypermagnesemia develops when the kidneys do not excrete the magnesium absorbed from the antacid. Acid-base abnormalities also may occur with antacid absorption. Antacids are distributed throughout the GI tract and are eliminated primarily in the feces.

Onset, peak, duration

Antacids usually provide a rapid to immediate onset of action. However, the speed at which antacids produce acid neutralization depends on their rate of solubility. Sodium bicarbonate is the most rapidly solubilized antacid, but is no longer recommended because of its high sodium content. Magnesium hydroxide is the second most rapidly solubilized antacid, followed by magnesium carbonate, calcium carbonate, and aluminum hydroxide. Because magnesium trisilicate is the least-soluble antacid, health care professionals question its usefulness.

The duration of action for antacids taken on an empty stomach is about 1 hour. Duration increases to 3 hours for antacids taken after a meal because food delays the gastric emptying time, which allows the antacid more time in the stomach to neutralize acid. Because of the short duration of action, frequent doses of antacids are needed.

PHARMACODYNAMICS

The acid-neutralizing action of antacids reduces the total acid load in the GI tract, which allows peptic ulcers to heal. Because pepsin acts more effectively in an acid medium, antacids also reduce its activity. Antacids do not coat the lining of peptic ulcers or the GI tract.

Mechanism of action

The anions of an antacid combine with the acidic hydrogen cations secreted by the stomach to form water, thereby increasing the pH of the stomach contents. Antacids do not neutralize all the stomach acid and usually do not increase the pH above 4.0 or 5.0. By increasing gastric pH from the normal 1.3 to 2.3, an antacid neutralizes about 90% of the gastric acid. By increasing the pH further to 3.3, the antacid neutralizes 99% of the gastric acid. This change in pH also affects the activity of pepsin. Pepsin activity is greatest at a pH of 1.5 to 2.5. By increasing the pH, the antacid decreases proteolytic activity, which becomes minimal at a pH above 4.0.

Increasing the pH and decreasing the pepsin activity provide symptomatic relief from peptic ulcer disease and, if adequately maintained, facilitate healing. Neither the amount nor the duration of neutralization for the optimal healing of peptic ulcer disease is known. However, most clinicians recommend that the pH be maintained at 3.0 to 3.5 throughout each 24-hour period. Therefore, regular, rather than p.r.n., doses of the antacid are needed to treat peptic ulcer disease.

PHARMACOTHERAPEUTICS

Antacids are used alone or combined with other drugs primarily to relieve pain and promote healing in peptic ulcer disease. Antacids also are used to relieve esophageal reflux, acid indigestion, heartburn, and dyspepsia. During times of severe physical stress in critically ill patients, antacids are used to prevent stress ulcers and GI bleeding. Aluminum hydroxide antacids are prescribed to control hyperphosphatemia in renal failure because the aluminum cation binds with phosphate in the GI tract, thus preventing phosphate absorption.

Antacids appear to treat gastric and duodenal ulcers effectively. When used alone in large doses over 4 weeks, they are as effective as any other therapy for peptic ulcer disease. They also may be used with histamine$_2$-receptor antagonists to help control or prevent pain.

Common over-the-counter antacids

The nurse administering antacids should be familiar with the ingredients of some commonly used over-the-counter antacids, their sodium content, and their acid-neutralizing effect.

TRADE NAME	INGREDIENTS	SODIUM CONTENT (mg/5 ml)	ACID NEUTRALIZING CAPACITY (mEq/5 ml)
ALternaGel	aluminum hydroxide	< 2.5	16
Gaviscon	magnesium carbonate, sodium alginate	13	3 to 4
Gelusil	magnesium and aluminum hydroxides, simethicone	0.7	12
Gelusil-II	magnesium and aluminum hydroxides, simethicone	1.3	24
Maalox	magnesium and aluminum hydroxides	1.4	13.3
Maalox TC	magnesium and aluminum hydroxides, simethicone	0.8	27.2
Mylanta	magnesium and aluminum hydroxides, simethicone	0.68	12.7
Mylanta-II	magnesium and aluminum hydroxides, simethicone	1.141	25.4
Riopan	magaldrate (aluminum-magnesium complex)	< 0.1	15
Riopan Plus	magaldrate (aluminum-magnesium complex)	< 0.3	30
Titralac Plus	calcium carbonate, simethicone	0.0005	11

Antacids commonly are combined with simethicone, a drug with antiflatulent properties. However, physicians usually do not use this combination to treat peptic ulcer disease unless concurrent symptoms require both effects. The combination of aluminum hydroxide and magnesium hydroxide often is used because one drug tends to offset the adverse effect of the other; that is, the aluminum hydroxide is constipating and the magnesium hydroxide has a laxative effect.

Antacids cause frequent and sometimes serious adverse effects. Patient acceptance and compliance may be lower than with other peptic ulcer medications because the patient must take the antacid frequently and use the liquid form. Palatability of the antacid also adversely affects compliance. For these reasons, antacids are no longer the first choice to treat peptic ulcer disease.

Not all antacids neutralize a given amount of gastric acid to the same extent. The known *in vivo* neutralizing capacity for each antacid must be considered when calculating the dosage of a specific antacid. Calcium carbonate antacids provide the most acid-neutralizing capacity, followed by those containing magnesium salts and aluminum salts.

In most cases, the adult dosage of an antacid should neutralize more than 1,000 mEq of acid daily. The large amount needed to accomplish this goal is administered in divided doses. A dose is given 1 hour after each meal, and again 3 hours after each meal, and at bedtime. The regimen requires seven doses. For example, using Mylanta-II, a dose of 30 ml would be given for each of these seven doses. The 30-ml dose is the usual dose for the concentrated forms of antacids, and a 60-ml dose is usual for the unconcentrated forms. The treatments continue from 4 to 6 weeks for duodenal ulcers and until healing is complete for gastric ulcers. (For information on other commonly used antacids, see *Common over-the-counter antacids.*)

calcium carbonate (Alka-Mints, Calcilac, Dicarbosil, Tums). This antacid is available as a suspension or chewable tablet.
Usual adult dosage: 1-gram tablet four to six times daily, chewed well and taken with water, or 1-gram suspension (5 ml of most products) 1 hour after meals and h.s.

magaldrate or aluminum-magnesium complex (Riopan, Riopan Plus). This antacid comes as a suspension, tablet, and chewable tablet.
Usual adult dosage: 540 to 1,080 mg (5 to 10 ml) of the suspension P.O. with water between meals and h.s., or 480 to 960 mg (1 to 2 tablets) P.O. with water between meals and h.s., or 480 to 960 mg (1 to 2 chewable tablets) chewed before swallowing between meals and h.s.

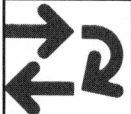

DRUG INTERACTIONS

Antacids

The nurse should be aware of the following drug interactions involving antacids, the possible effects of the interactions, and the nursing implications.

DRUG	INTERACTING DRUGS	POSSIBLE EFFECTS	NURSING IMPLICATIONS
antacids	digoxin, digitoxin, iron salts, isoniazid, quino-lones, tetracyclines	Decrease rate or extent of absorption of digoxin and other drugs by GI binding	• Do not administer the drugs within 2 hours of each other. • Monitor the patient for decreased therapeutic effects of the medication. • Monitor the patient's digoxin or digitoxin concentration level.
	amphetamines, quinidine	Increase urine pH; decrease excretion of weakly basic drugs, such as amphetamines and quinidine	• Do not administer the drugs within 1 hour of each other. • Monitor the patient for increased therapeutic effects of the medications. • Monitor the patient's quinidine concentration level.
	salicylates	Increase urine pH; increase excretion of weakly acidic drugs, such as salicylates	• Monitor the patient for decreased salicylate effects or decreased salicylate concentration level.
	methenamine compounds	Decrease activity of methenamine compounds	• Avoid concomitant use.

magnesium hydroxide and aluminum hydroxide with simethicone (Maalox TC, Mylanta-II, Gelusil-II). These drugs represent concentrated antacids.
Usual adult dosage: 10 to 30 ml P.O. 1 hour and 3 hours after each meal and h.s.

Drug interactions

All antacids can interfere with the absorption of concomitantly administered oral drugs by binding with them or changing the GI transit time. Some antacids also increase urine pH, which in turn increases the excretion of weakly acidic drugs and decreases the excretion of weakly basic drugs. However, aluminum and magnesium antacids do not affect urine pH. (For more information, see *Drug interactions: Antacids.*)

ADVERSE DRUG REACTIONS

The most common adverse reactions to antacids occur in the GI tract. Diarrhea and constipation commonly result from long-term antacid use. Aluminum hydroxide is particularly constipating. Constipation can be severe, and, if accompanied by dehydration or fluid restriction, may lead to intestinal obstruction. Hemorrhoids, rectal fissures, and fecal impaction may occur from hard stools. Conversely, magnesium-containing antacids produce a laxative effect and with frequent use can produce diarrhea and electrolyte

abnormalities. Aluminum hydroxide and magnesium-containing antacids usually are prescribed in combination, which usually produces a mild laxative effect.

Most antacid products have been reformulated to decrease their sodium content. Furthermore, all antacids that contain more than 0.2 mEq of sodium per dose must be labeled with the amount. Patients on a sodium-restricted diet because of hypertension, congestive heart failure, renal failure, or other conditions should pay particular attention to the sodium content of antacids. Some antacids also may possess a high potassium load, so patients on a potassium-restricted diet should note the product label.

When used in patients with renal failure, aluminum-containing antacids may produce a hyperaluminemia state, in which aluminum accumulates in bones, lungs, and nerve tissue. Osteomalacia and dementia may occur. Hypophosphatemia, with anorexia, malaise, and muscle weakness, also may occur from prolonged administration of aluminum-containing antacids.

Hypermagnesemia characterized by hypotension, nausea, vomiting, electrocardiogram changes, respiratory or mental depression, and coma has occurred in patients with renal failure taking magnesium-containing antacids.

Calcium-containing antacids usually are not recommended to treat peptic ulcer disease, but are recommended for short-term therapy for other GI conditions. When calcium carbonate is used, hypersecretion of gastric acid and acid rebound occur. Calcium carbonate also may cause the milk-alkali syndrome characterized by hypercalcemia, metabolic alkalosis, and renal impairment.

All adverse reactions to antacids are dose-related. No hypersensitivity reactions occur.

NURSING PROCESS APPLICATION

The following information assists the nurse in caring for a patient who is receiving an antacid.

Assessment
• Review the patient's history for a preexisting condition that contraindicates the use of a magnesium-containing antacid, such as renal failure.
• Review the patient's history for a preexisting condition that requires cautious use of an aluminum-containing antacid, such as renal failure.
• Assess the patient for adverse reactions to the antacid, such as diarrhea or constipation, hyperaluminemia, osteomalacia, dementia, hypophosphatemia, or hypermagnesemia.
• Review the patient's medication history to identify the use of drugs that may interact with the prescribed antacid, such as digoxin, amphetamines, or salicylates.
• Assess the effectiveness of the prescribed antacid regularly.
• Assess the patient's compliance with antacid therapy.
• Evaluate the patient's and family's knowledge about the prescribed antacid.

Nursing diagnoses
The following examples represent appropriate nursing diagnoses for a patient receiving an antacid.
• Potential for injury related to a preexisting condition that contraindicates the use of an antacid
• Potential for injury related to a preexisting condition that requires cautious use of an antacid
• Potential for injury related to adverse drug reactions
• Constipation related to the adverse GI effects of aluminum hydroxide
• Diarrhea related to the laxative effects of a magnesium-containing antacid
• Noncompliance related to long-term antacid therapy
• Knowledge deficit related to the prescribed antacid

Planning and implementation
• Do not administer an antacid to a patient with a condition that contraindicates its use.
• Administer an antacid cautiously to a patient at risk because of a preexisting condition.
• Monitor the patient closely for GI and other adverse reactions during antacid therapy.

• *Avoid administering calcium carbonate for long-term therapy of peptic ulcer disease because gastric hypersecretion and acid rebound may occur.*
• *Monitor for signs of hyperaluminemia, such as osteomalacia and dementia, in a patient with renal failure who is receiving an aluminum-containing antacid. For such a patient, take safety precautions to prevent fractures from osteomalacia or injury from dementia. For example, place the bed in the low position, keep the side rails up, and supervise ambulation.*
• *Monitor for signs of hypophosphatemia, such as anorexia, malaise, and muscle weakness, in a patient on long-term therapy with an aluminum-containing antacid. If hypophosphatemia is suspected, withhold the drug and notify the physician.*
• Shake the suspension well and give with a small amount of water.
• Have the patient thoroughly chew any chewable antacid tablets before swallowing and then drink 6 to 8 ounces of water. If a suspension or regular tablet is used, have the patient drink 6 to 8 ounces of water with it.
• *Do not give other oral medications within 1 to 2 hours of antacid administration because antacids impair the absorption of many other drugs.*
• *Separate the administration of antacids and enteric-coated drugs by 1 hour because antacids may cause premature release of enteric-coated drugs in the stomach.*
• Consider having the patient sample various antacids to determine individual taste preferences.
• Notify the physician if adverse reactions occur or if the antacid is ineffective.
• *Monitor the patient for constipation, which may become severe, especially with aluminum hydroxide use.*
• Place the patient on a high-fiber diet and encourage the patient to drink 8 to 13 8-oz glasses (2 to 3 liters) of fluid a day (if not contraindicated) to help prevent constipation.
• Request a prescription for a laxative if constipation occurs.
• *Expect to discontinue the antacid if constipation occurs in a dehydrated patient or one who must restrict fluids. Such a patient is at increased risk for intestinal obstruction.*
• Monitor for diarrhea in a patient who is receiving a magnesium-containing antacid because of the agent's laxative effect.
• Request a prescription for an antidiarrheal agent if the patient develops diarrhea. If diarrhea becomes severe, expect to discontinue the antacid as prescribed.
• Monitor for compliance with the prescribed antacid regimen. The need to take an unpalatable medication frequently may lower compliance.
• Notify the physician if noncompliance is suspected.

Patient teaching
• Teach the patient and family the name, dose, frequency, action, and adverse effects of the prescribed antacid.
• Reassure the patient that antacid therapy normally may make stools appear speckled or whitish.
• Teach the patient when and how to take the antacid for maximum effect.
• *Instruct the patient with renal failure not to take a magnesium-containing antacid to prevent hypermagnesemia.*
• *Advise the patient who must restrict sodium to avoid antacids with a high sodium content (greater than 0.2 mEq of sodium) because sodium and fluid retention may occur or increase.*
• *Instruct the patient who must restrict potassium to read antacid labels carefully because some antacids have a high potassium content.*
• Teach the patient how to prevent constipation during antacid therapy.
• Stress the importance of taking the antacid exactly as prescribed for maximum effectiveness.
• Instruct the patient to notify the physician if adverse reactions occur.

Evaluation
The following examples represent appropriate evaluation statements for a patient receiving an antacid.
• The patient has no conditions that contraindicate antacid therapy.
• The patient exhibits no signs of complications in the preexisting condition linked to the prescribed antacid.
• The patient experiences no adverse reactions to the prescribed antacid.
• The patient maintains normal bowel function during antacid therapy.
• The patient complies with the prescribed antacid regimen.
• The patient and family express an accurate understanding of the points taught about the prescribed antacid.
• The patient reports taking the antacid with water at the proper times.

HISTAMINE₂-RECEPTOR ANTAGONISTS

The histamine$_2$ (H$_2$)-receptor antagonists, used to treat duodenal and gastric ulcers, are the most commonly prescribed antiulcer drugs in the United States. The H$_2$-receptor antagonists act by blocking the histamine-receptor sites on the parietal cells of the stomach. These drugs inhibit not only histamine-stimulated acid secretion, but also basal-, postprandial-, and gastrin-stimulated acid secretion. The H$_2$-receptor antagonists available in the United States include cimetidine, famotidine, nizatidine, and ranitidine.

PHARMACOKINETICS

The H$_2$-receptor antagonists share a somewhat similar pharmacokinetic profile.

Absorption, distribution, metabolism, excretion
Cimetidine, nizatidine, and ranitidine are absorbed rapidly and completely from the GI tract; famotidine is absorbed incompletely. Food and antacids may impair the absorption of H$_2$-receptor antagonists. Three H$_2$-receptor antagonists undergo hepatic first-pass metabolism, with cimetidine displaying a bioavailability of 65% to 80%, famotidine 40%, and ranitidine 40% to 90%.

These drugs are distributed widely throughout the body, although ranitidine is distributed minimally into the central nervous system (CNS). The extent to which famotidine and nizatidine distribute into the CNS is unknown. All H$_2$-receptor antagonists are only mildly protein bound (approximately 20%).

Cimetidine and ranitidine are metabolized by the liver, but more than 50% of each drug is excreted unchanged in the urine. Famotidine and nizatidine also are metabolized by the liver, with over 70% and 65% of the dose, respectively, being excreted unchanged in the urine. Liver dysfunction increases the bioavailability and slightly prolongs the half-life of cimetidine and ranitidine. Liver dysfunction does not seem to affect nizatidine; its effects on famotidine's half-life are unknown. Nizatidine is metabolized only slightly and is more than 90% bioavailable. A decrease in renal function will prolong the half-lives of the H$_2$-receptor antagonists.

The H$_2$-receptor antagonists are excreted primarily in the urine.

Onset, peak, duration
Cimetidine, nizatidine, and ranitidine reach peak concentration levels in about 1 to 2 hours; famotidine, in 1 to 3.5 hours. The half-life of cimetidine is about 2 hours, of famotidine is 2.5 to 4 hours, of nizatidine is 1 to 2 hours, and of ranitidine is 2 to 3 hours.

PHARMACODYNAMICS

The H$_2$-receptor antagonists block the stimulant action of histamine on the acid-secreting parietal cells of the stomach.

Mechanism of action

Because the chemical structure of cimetidine resembles that of histamine, the drug readily binds with H$_2$ receptors on the parietal cells as well as with other histamine receptor sites throughout the body, including those located in androgen receptors, the hepatic oxidase system, and peripheral lymphocytes. The chemical structures of famotidine, nizatidine, and ranitidine differ from the structure of histamine, but they all bind competitively to the H$_2$ receptors. Unlike cimetidine, the other drugs in this class are specific and do not bind to other receptor sites. The specific binding may explain why the other H$_2$-receptor antagonists do not produce the same serious adverse effects that cimetidine does.

Acid secretion by the stomach depends on the binding of gastrin, acetylcholine, and histamine to their respective receptors on the parietal cells. If the binding of any one of these substances becomes blocked, acid secretion is reduced. Thus, by binding with H$_2$ receptors, the H$_2$-receptor antagonists reduce acid secretion. A cimetidine dose of 300 mg reduces basal acid output by 90% and reduces meal-stimulated acid secretion by 66%. The usual 150-mg dose of ranitidine twice daily reduces gastric acid by 70%. All H$_2$-receptor antagonists suppress nocturnal acid secretion by approximately 90% when given in appropriate dosages.

PHARMACOTHERAPEUTICS

As the drugs of choice to treat peptic ulcers, the H$_2$-receptor antagonists promote healing of duodenal and gastric ulcers. These drugs also are used for long-term treatment of pathologic GI hypersecretory conditions, such as Zollinger-Ellison syndrome or hyperhistaminemia. The H$_2$-receptor antagonists are prescribed to reduce gastric acid output and prevent stress ulcers in severely ill patients and in those with reflux esophagitis or upper GI bleeding. Although antacids may be used with the H$_2$-receptor antagonists to control pain, their addition does not appear to increase ulcer healing.

The final daily dose of the H$_2$-receptor antagonists should be given at bedtime. Although oral administration usually is as effective as parenteral administration, the parenteral route may be preferred for hospitalized patients with pathologic hypersecretory conditions, intractable ulcers, or an inability to take oral medication. To treat active gastric bleeding, an I.V. loading dose of the H$_2$-receptor antagonist followed by an I.V. infusion has been shown in experimental trials to be somewhat more effective than bolus injections.

cimetidine (Tagamet). This H$_2$-receptor antagonist is the least potent of the agents used to treat peptic ulcer disease.
Usual adult dosage: for active peptic ulcer disease, 800 mg P.O. daily h.s. (or 400 mg P.O. b.i.d. or 300 mg P.O. q.i.d.), or 300 mg I.V. every 6 to 8 hours up to a maximum of 2.4 grams in 24 hours; for maintenance after the ulcer has healed, 400 mg P.O. h.s.

famotidine (Pepcid). This drug is used primarily to treat peptic ulcer disease.
Usual adult dosage: for active peptic ulcer disease, 20 mg P.O. b.i.d. with the second dose h.s. (or 40 mg P.O. daily h.s.), or 20 mg I.V. every 12 hours; for maintenance after the ulcer has healed, 20 mg P.O. h.s.

nizatidine (Axid). Used to treat active peptic ulcer disease, this drug is the newest H$_2$-receptor antagonist on the market.
Usual adult dosage: for active peptic ulcer disease, 300 mg P.O. h.s. or 150 mg P.O. b.i.d.; for maintenance after the ulcer has healed, 150 mg P.O. h.s.

ranitidine (Zantac). Ranitidine is used primarily to treat peptic ulcer disease.
Usual adult dosage: for active peptic ulcer disease, 150 mg P.O. b.i.d., with the second dose h.s., or 300 mg P.O. daily h.s. increased to 400 mg in 24 hours, if needed; 50 mg I.V. or I.M. every 6 to 8 hours.

Drug interactions

The concomitant administration of antacids and H$_2$-receptor antagonists may decrease the absorption of the H$_2$-receptor antagonists. To prevent interactions, the nurse should not administer the drugs within 1 hour of each other. Cimetidine partially inhibits the hepatic cytochrome P450 enzyme system and consequently decreases the clearance or prolongs the half-lives of drugs that are metabolized by this system. Famotidine, nizatidine, and ranitidine do not produce this effect. (For details about these and other interactions, see *Drug Interactions: H$_2$-receptor antagonists,* page 762.)

ADVERSE DRUG REACTIONS

Cimetidine and ranitidine may produce headache, dizziness, malaise, myalgia, nausea, diarrhea or constipation, skin rashes, pruritus, loss of libido, and impotence. Cimetidine, however, is more likely to produce these adverse reactions. Cimetidine probably produces sexual dysfunction and gynecomastia through its binding to the androgen receptor. Substituting famotidine, nizatidine, or ranitidine decreases these adverse reactions. Famotidine and nizatidine produce very few adverse reactions, with headache being the most frequent (about 2% of patients), followed by constipation or diarrhea and skin rash.

Reversible confusion, agitation, depression, and hallucinations can result. However, these reactions occur much more commonly in patients receiving cimetidine, especially in severely ill or elderly patients. These reactions, which

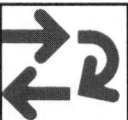

DRUG INTERACTIONS

H₂-receptor antagonists

The following chart contains information about drug interactions involving H₂-receptor antagonists, the possible effects from the interactions, and important nursing implications.

DRUG	INTERACTING DRUGS	POSSIBLE EFFECTS	NURSING IMPLICATIONS
cimetidine, famotidine, nizatidine, ranitidine	antacids	Inhibit H₂-receptor antagonist absorption	• Do not administer within 1 hour of one another. • Monitor the patient for decreased therapeutic effects.
cimetidine	oral anticoagulants, propranolol, possibly other beta blockers, benzodiazepines, tricyclic antidepressants, theophylline, procainamide, quinidine, lidocaine, phenytoin, calcium channel blockers, cyclosporine, carbamazepine, narcotic analgesics	Inhibits hepatic enzyme metabolism of these drugs, thereby increasing their levels and effects	• Avoid concurrent administration if possible. • Monitor the patient for increased sedation from the benzodiazepines. Oxazepam, lorazepam, and temazepam are eliminated differently and are not affected by cimetidine. • Monitor the patient for drug toxicity. • Monitor the patient's concentration levels of procainamide, phenytoin, quinidine, lidocaine, theophylline, and cyclosporine. • Monitor the patient's prothrombin time as prescribed when beginning or discontinuing cimetidine therapy during concomitant oral anticoagulant therapy.
	carmustine (BCNU)	Increases bone marrow toxicity	• Monitor the patient's blood cell counts carefully if concomitant use is necessary.
	ethyl alcohol	Increases alcohol absorption and decreases metabolism	• Caution the patient about the risk of increased alcohol effects.

usually are associated with decreased renal function, also may occur with overdose.

When given by rapid I.V. injection, H₂-receptor antagonists can produce profound bradycardia and other cardiotoxic effects. Pain at the injection site occasionally occurs.

The H₂-receptor antagonists rarely cause hypersensitivity reactions. Some patients develop increased hepatic enzyme levels, but this reaction also is rare. Cimetidine has been associated with adverse hematologic reactions, such as thrombocytopenia and granulocytopenia, and seizures if drug accumulation occurs. (For more information, see *Monitoring for adverse reactions to H₂-receptor antagonists.*)

NURSING PROCESS APPLICATION

The following information assists the nurse in caring for a patient who is receiving an H₂-receptor antagonist.

Assessment
• Review the patient's history for a preexisting condition that contraindicates the use of an H₂-receptor antagonist, such as lactation or known hypersensitivity to the drug.

• Review the patient's history for a preexisting condition that requires cautious use of an H₂-receptor antagonist, such as pregnancy or impaired renal or hepatic function.
• Assess the patient for adverse reactions to the prescribed H₂-receptor antagonist, such as headache, dizziness, malaise, myalgia, GI distress, skin rash, or pruritus.
• Review the patient's medication history to identify the use of drugs that may interact with the prescribed H₂-receptor antagonist, such as antacids, oral anticoagulants, carmustine, or ethyl alcohol.
• Assess the effectiveness of the prescribed H₂-receptor antagonist regularly.
• Assess for sexual dysfunction in a patient receiving cimetidine or ranitidine.
• Evaluate the patient's and family's knowledge about the prescribed H₂-receptor antagonist.

Nursing diagnoses
The following examples represent appropriate nursing diagnoses for a patient receiving an H₂-receptor antagonist.
• Potential for injury related to a preexisting condition that contraindicates the use of an H₂-receptor antagonist
• Potential for injury related to a preexisting condition that requires cautious use of an H₂-receptor antagonist

Monitoring for adverse reactions to H₂-receptor antagonists

The following should help the nurse assess and intervene while caring for a patient receiving an H₂-receptor antagonist.

ADVERSE REACTIONS	SIGNS AND SYMPTOMS	INTERVENTIONS
Headache	General headache, at times severe	Administer mild analgesics as prescribed.
Blood dyscrasias	Easy bruising, more frequent infections, granulocytopenia, leukopenia, or thrombocytopenia	Consult the physician to discontinue the drug.
Mental status changes	Confusion, agitation, depression, hallucinations, especially in severely ill or elderly patients or patients with renal failure	Consult the physician to substitute another H₂-receptor antagonist or to discontinue drug use for patients on cimetidine; discontinue drug use as prescribed for patients on famotidine, nizatidine, or ranitidine.
Anti-androgen effects	Gynecomastia, impotence	Consult the physician to discontinue the drug or alter the dosing schedule.
Changes in blood chemistry	Small increases in serum creatinine without increases in blood urea nitrogen	Continue to monitor the patient's renal function.
	Increases in hepatic enzymes	Monitor the patient for hepatotoxicity, especially in high-dose I.V. therapy.

• Potential for injury related to adverse drug reactions
• Sexual dysfunction related to the adverse genitourinary effects of cimetidine or ranitidine
• Knowledge deficit related to the prescribed H₂-receptor antagonist

Planning and implementation

• Do not administer an H₂-receptor antagonist to a patient with a condition that contraindicates its use.
• Administer an H₂-receptor antagonist cautiously to a patient at risk because of a preexisting condition.
• Monitor the patient closely for adverse reactions during H₂-receptor antagonist therapy.
• *Do not give an antacid within 1 hour of H₂-receptor antagonist administration because decreased absorption of the H₂-receptor antagonist may occur.*
• Obtain a prescription for a mild analgesic if the patient experiences a drug-induced headache.
• Take safety precautions if the patient develops dizziness, confusion, or other mental status changes. For example, place the bed in the low position, keep the side rails up, and supervise patient activity.
• Monitor hydration if the patient develops nausea or diarrhea. Obtain a prescription for an antiemetic or antidiarrheal agent as needed.
• Request a prescription for a laxative if the patient becomes constipated from H₂-receptor antagonist use.

• *Monitor the patient for profound bradycardia and other cardiotoxic effects when giving an H₂-receptor antagonist rapidly by I.V.*
• *Evaluate the results of hematologic studies for signs of abnormalities, such as thrombocytopenia and granulocytopenia, in a patient receiving cimetidine.*
• *Monitor blood chemistry results for changes in creatinine and hepatic enzymes, which may reflect changes in the patient's renal or hepatic function.*
• *Take seizure precautions if cimetidine accumulation occurs.*
• Expect to administer an I.V. H₂-receptor antagonist as prescribed to a critically ill patient to prevent GI bleeding.
• Administer an H₂-receptor antagonist as prescribed without regard to meals.
• *Dilute cimetidine, famotidine, and ranitidine before I.V. administration.* Dilute cimetidine in at least 50 ml, famotidine in at least 100 ml, and ranitidine in at least 20 ml of a compatible I.V. solution, such as 0.9% sodium chloride (normal saline), 5% or 10% dextrose (and combinations of these), lactated Ringer's, or 5% sodium bicarbonate. *Do not use sterile water for injection as a diluent.*
• Notify the physician if adverse reactions occur.
• Encourage the patient receiving cimetidine or ranitidine to express concerns about adverse genitourinary effects, such as loss of libido and impotence.

• Consult with the physician if the patient experiences sexual dysfunction. The patient may need to be changed to a different H$_2$-receptor antagonist.

Patient teaching

• Teach the patient and family the name, dose, frequency, action, and adverse effects of the prescribed H$_2$-receptor antagonist.
• *Instruct the patient not to take an antacid within 1 hour of taking the prescribed H$_2$-receptor antagonist.*
• *Advise the patient to avoid any activity that requires alertness if dizziness or mental changes occur.*
• Teach the patient how to prevent constipation.
• *Stress the importance of having laboratory studies done as instructed.*
• Instruct the patient to take the H$_2$-receptor antagonist as prescribed, without regard to meals.
• Inform the patient that sexual dysfunction may occur as an adverse reaction to cimetidine or ranitidine.
• Advise the patient to notify the physician if adverse reactions occur.

Evaluation

The following examples represent appropriate evaluation statements for a patient receiving an H$_2$-receptor antagonist.
• The patient has no conditions that contraindicate the use of an H$_2$-receptor antagonist.
• The patient exhibits no signs of complications in the preexisting condition linked to the prescribed H$_2$-receptor antagonist.
• The patient displays no adverse reactions to the prescribed H$_2$-receptor antagonist.
• The patient states that sexual activity remains unchanged.
• The patient and family express an accurate understanding of the points taught about the prescribed H$_2$-receptor antagonist.
• The patient returns for laboratory studies.

OTHER PEPTIC ULCER AGENTS

Besides antacids and H$_2$-receptor antagonists, misoprostol, omeprazole, and sucralfate may be used as peptic ulcer agents. Misoprostol is prescribed to prevent NSAID-induced gastric ulcers in patients at high risk for complications from gastric ulcers. Omeprazole has been approved to treat GI reflux disease and pathological hypersecretory conditions. Sucralfate is used for short-term treatment of duodenal ulcers.

Other agents currently are being investigated for their usefulness in treating peptic ulcer disease. For example, anticholinergic agents are being studied because they are known to reduce gastric acid secretion through parasympathetic blockade. Colloidal bismuth chelates with the base of the ulcer and protects it against the actions of acid, bile, and pepsin. This promotes the healing of duodenal and gastric ulcers. Two tricyclic antidepressants, doxepin hydrochloride and trimipramine maleate, are being tested for use in treating peptic ulcer disease. These agents produce an H$_2$-receptor antagonist effect and an anticholinergic effect that may be beneficial in ulcer treatment.

PHARMACOKINETICS

The pharmacokinetics of misoprostol, omeprazole, and sucralfate differ.

Absorption, distribution, metabolism, excretion

After oral administration, misoprostol is absorbed extensively and rapidly. It is metabolized by de-esterification to misoprostol acid, which is responsible for its clinical activity. Administration with food or antacids may decrease the plasma concentration and total bioavailability, but the decrease does not appear to be clinically significant. Misoprostol acid is 90% protein bound, has a half-life of 20 to 40 minutes, and does not accumulate with multiple doses. It is excreted primarily in the urine.

Omeprazole is absorbed rapidly after oral administration. Because omeprazole is affected by stomach acid, the capsules are formulated with delayed-release, enteric-coated granules so that drug absorption begins only after the granules leave the stomach. It undergoes some first-pass metabolism, which reduces the drug's bioavailability to 30% to 40%. About 95% of omeprazole is protein bound. The drug is metabolized almost completely, and most of its metabolites are excreted in urine.

The minimal absorption of sucralfate from the GI tract is appropriate because sucralfate exerts its effects locally, rapidly reacting with hydrochloric acid in the GI tract to form a highly condensed, viscous, adhesive, pastelike substance that adheres to the gastric mucosa and especially to ulcer sites. The drug is distributed minimally to other areas of the body and is excreted in the feces.

Onset, peak, duration

After oral administration, misoprostol reaches a peak plasma concentration level in approximately 12 minutes. The drug begins to inhibit gastric acid secretion about 30 minutes after administration. This action persists for at least 3 hours.

The plasma concentration of omeprazole peaks 0.5 to 3.5 hours after administration. The onset of action occurs within 1 hour; maximal effects occur within 2 hours. Gastric acid secretion is inhibited by about 50% at 24 hours and lasts for 72 hours. Omeprazole's half-life is short, only 0.5 to 1 hour. Secretion inhibition lasts far longer than would be expected for a drug with such a short half-life, apparently due to its prolonged binding to the H^+/K^+ ATPase. When omeprazole is discontinued, acid secretion returns to previous levels gradually over 3 to 5 days.

The onset of sucralfate is rapid once the drug reaches the GI tract. The duration of action for sucralfate depends on how long the drug remains in contact with its action site. The drug's viscosity, adhesiveness, and affinity for damaged mucosa prolong this contact. Usually, the duration is up to 6 hours after administration.

PHARMACODYNAMICS

Misoprostol's anti-ulcer activity may result from increased bicarbonate and mucus production in the GI tract or by inhibition of gastric acid secretion. Omeprazole is an acid pump inhibitor that blocks the action of H^+/K^+ ATPase in the parietal cells of the stomach. By binding to the ulcer site, sucralfate protects the ulcer from the damaging effects of acid and pepsin and permits healing.

Mechanism of action

Misoprostol is a synthetic prostaglandin E_1 analogue with antisecretory and mucosal protective properties. NSAIDs inhibit prostaglandin synthesis, which may diminish bicarbonate and mucus secretion and promote mucosal damage and ulcer formation in the GI tract. Misoprostol counteracts these effects by replacing the endogenous prostaglandins.

Omeprazole belongs to a unique class of antisecretory compounds known as the substituted benzimidazoles. It suppresses gastric acid formation by inhibiting H^+/K^+ ATPase enzyme in gastric parietal cells. This enzyme is part of the proton pump. Because omeprazole blocks this step in acid production, it is known as a proton pump inhibitor. The antisecretory effect is dose-related. Therapeutic doses almost totally block basal and stimulated gastric acid secretion.

In an acid environment, sucralfate becomes a pastelike material that is negatively charged, highly viscous, and adhesive. This material binds to the positively charged proteins, such as albumin, fibrinogen, damaged mucosal cells, and dead leukocytes, found at the base of an ulcer. By forming a barrier at the ulcer site, sucralfate protects the ulcer against the ulcerogenic effects of gastric acid, pepsin, and bile. Thus, the ulcer is allowed to heal. The action of sucralfate in actively inhibiting pepsin and in absorbing bile acids also may play a role in its mechanism of action.

PHARMACOTHERAPEUTICS

Misoprostol has been approved to prevent NSAID-induced gastric ulcers in patients at high risk for complications from gastric ulcer. It is under study for other uses, including the treatment and prevention of peptic ulcers.

Omeprazole is indicated for the short-term treatment of severe erosive esophagitis diagnosed by endoscopy or for short-term treatment of symptomatic esophagitis that responds poorly to usual treatments, such as use of an H_2-receptor antagonist. Omeprazole also is indicated for long-term treatment of pathologic hypersecretory conditions, such as Zollinger-Ellison syndrome, multiple endocrine adenomas, and systemic mastocytosis. In studies of peptic ulcer treatment, omeprazole has been shown to be at least as effective as the H_2-receptor antagonists.

Sucralfate is used for short-term treatment (up to 8 weeks) of duodenal ulcers. For this condition, sucralfate acts as effectively as H_2-receptor antagonists and antacids. Sucralfate also has been used successfully for the short-term treatment of gastric ulcers. The drug also may be prescribed to prevent recurrent ulcers, NSAID-induced ulcers, and stress ulcers.

Antacids may be used with sucralfate to relieve pain, but the antacids do not increase the ulcer healing. When combined with sucralfate, H_2-receptor antagonists increase the cost of therapy but do not offer any advantages. Therefore, the combination is not recommended.

Although sucralfate effectively treats ulcers, it is the least popular antiulcer agent. Compared to the H_2-receptor antagonists, sucralfate requires a cumbersome dosage schedule and produces a number of minor adverse reactions that lead to decreased patient compliance.

misoprostol (Cytotec). Misoprostol is used to prevent NSAID-induced gastric ulcers in patients at high risk for complications from gastric ulcer. Because the drug may induce miscarriage, a female patient should have a negative serum pregnancy test within 2 weeks before beginning misoprostol therapy.
Usual adult dosage: 200 mcg P.O. q.i.d. with food or, if the patient cannot tolerate this dosage, 100 mcg P.O. q.i.d.

omeprazole (Prilosec). Omeprazole is prescribed to treat GI reflux disease and pathological hypersecretory conditions.
Usual adult dosage: for severe erosive esophagitis or symptomatic esophagitis unresponsive to other treatments, 20 mg P.O. daily for 4 to 8 weeks; for pathological hypersecretory conditions, 60 mg P.O. daily initially and then individualized according to patient response up to a maximum of 120 mg P.O. t.i.d. Dosages in excess of 80 mg daily should be administered in divided doses.

sucralfate (Carafate). This agent is indicated for short-term treatment (up to 8 weeks) of duodenal ulcers. The timing of sucralfate administration is important because the drug is more active in the lower pH of an empty stomach than in the higher pH of a stomach buffered by food.
Usual adult dosage: 1 gram P.O. q.i.d. continued 4 to 8 weeks unless radiographic or endoscopic examination indicates healing.

Drug interactions

Concomitant antacid administration may bind with misoprostol or decrease its absorption, reducing the amount of misoprostol available for conversion to misoprostol acid. However, this effect does not appear to be clinically significant.

Omeprazole may interfere with the metabolism of diazepam, phenytoin, and warfarin, causing increased half-lives and elevated plasma concentrations of these agents. During concomitant administration of these drugs, the nurse should use caution and monitor the patient closely. Omeprazole may interfere with the absorption of drugs that depend on gastric pH for absorption, such as ketoconazole, ampicillin esters, and iron salts. Therefore, concomitant use should be avoided.

When given orally with sucralfate, some drugs bind with it in the GI tract, which decreases their absorption. Antacids, which increase the pH of the GI tract, display decreased activity when administered with sucralfate. Because sucralfate decreases the bioavailability of cimetidine, the nurse should give sucralfate 2 hours before or after the cimetidine dose.

ADVERSE DRUG REACTIONS

Misoprostol commonly causes adverse GI reactions. Diarrhea occurs in up to 40% of patients. It may be followed by abdominal pain, flatulence, dyspepsia, nausea, and vomiting. Because misoprostol is a prostaglandin, it also may affect the uterus, causing spotting, cramps, hypermenorrhea, and other menstrual disorders. In a pregnant patient, misoprostol therapy may induce miscarriage.

Omeprazole usually is tolerated well even in the higher dosages used to treat hypersecretory conditions. During clinical trials with omeprazole, the following dose-related adverse reactions were reported in more than 1% of patients: headache, diarrhea, abdominal pain, nausea, vomiting, upper respiratory tract infection, dizziness, rash, constipation, weakness, cough, and back pain. Omeprazole also has been linked to gastric malignancy when used in extremely high dosages in laboratory animals. Therefore, it is recommended only for short-term use.

Usually, sucralfate is well tolerated. Although typically minor, adverse reactions may become bothersome for the patient. Constipation is the most frequent dose-related adverse reaction, occurring in about 2% of all patients. Nausea and a metallic taste also may accompany the use of sucralfate. Less frequent reactions to this drug may include diarrhea, indigestion, dry mouth, back pain, dizziness, sleepiness, and vertigo. Sucralfate may produce a rash and pruritus, but these reactions are rare.

NURSING PROCESS APPLICATION

The following information assists the nurse in caring for a patient who is receiving misoprostol, omeprazole, or sucralfate.

Assessment
• Review the patient's history for a preexisting condition that contraindicates the use of misoprostol, omeprazole, or sucralfate, such as known hypersensitivity to the agent or its components.
• Review the patient's history for a preexisting condition that requires cautious use of sucralfate, such as chronic renal failure, pregnancy, or lactation.
• Assess the patient for adverse reactions to the peptic ulcer agent, such as GI distress, menstrual disorders, headache, dizziness, weakness, or rash.
• Review the patient's medication history to identify the use of drugs that may interact with the prescribed peptic ulcer agent, such as antacids, diazepam, warfarin, ketoconazole, or iron salts.
• Assess the effectiveness of the prescribed peptic ulcer agent periodically.
• Evaluate the patient's and family's knowledge about the prescribed peptic ulcer agent.

Nursing diagnoses
The following examples represent appropriate nursing diagnoses for a patient receiving misoprostol, omeprazole, or sucralfate.
• Potential for injury related to a preexisting condition that contraindicates the use of a peptic ulcer agent
• Potential for injury related to a preexisting condition that requires cautious use of a peptic ulcer agent
• Potential for injury related to adverse drug reactions
• Diarrhea related to the adverse GI effects of a peptic ulcer agent
• Knowledge deficit related to the prescribed peptic ulcer agent

Planning and implementation
• Do not administer a peptic ulcer agent to a patient with a condition that contraindicates its use.
• Administer a peptic ulcer agent cautiously to a patient at risk because of a preexisting condition.
• Monitor the patient closely for GI disturbances and other adverse reactions during peptic ulcer agent therapy.

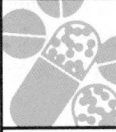

SELECTED MAJOR DRUGS

Peptic ulcer agents

The following chart summarizes the major peptic ulcer agents currently in clinical use.

DRUG	MAJOR INDICATIONS	USUAL ADULT DOSAGES	CONTRAINDICATIONS AND PRECAUTIONS
Antacids			
magaldrate or aluminum-magnesium complex	Symptomatic and therapeutic treatment of peptic ulcer disease	540 to 1,080 mg (5 to 10 ml) of suspension P.O. with water between meals and h.s., or 480 to 960 mg (1 to 2 tablets) P.O. with water between meals and h.s.	• Know that magnesium-containing antacids are contraindicated in a patient with renal failure. • Administer aluminum-containing antacids with caution to a patient with renal failure.
magnesium hydroxide and aluminum hydroxide with simethicone	Symptomatic and therapeutic treatment of peptic ulcer disease	10 to 30 ml P.O. 1 and 3 hours after each meal and h.s.	
Histamine$_2$-receptor antagonists			
cimetidine	Treatment and prevention of peptic ulcer disease	800 mg P.O. daily h.s.; 300 mg I.V. every 6 to 8 hours up to a maximum of 24 grams in 24 hours	• Know that cimetidine is contraindicated in a lactating patient or one with a known hypersensitivity to the drug. • Administer with caution to a pregnant patient or one with impaired renal or hepatic function.
famotidine	Treatment and prevention of peptic ulcer disease	20 mg P.O. b.i.d. with the second dose h.s., 40 mg P.O. h.s., or 20 mg I.V. every 12 hours	• Know that famotidine is contraindicated in a lactating patient or one with known hypersensitivity to the drug. • Administer with caution to a pregnant patient.
nizatidine	Treatment and prevention of peptic ulcer disease	300 mg P.O. h.s. or 150 mg P.O. b.i.d.	• Know that nizatidine is contraindicated in a lactating patient or one with known hypersensitivity to this drug or other H$_2$ receptor antagonists. • Administer with caution to a pregnant patient or one with impaired renal function.
ranitidine	Treatment and prevention of peptic ulcer disease	150 mg P.O. b.i.d. with the second dose h.s., 300 mg P.O. h.s., or 50 mg I.V. or I.M. every 6 to 8 hours	• Know that ranitidine is contraindicated in a patient with known hypersensitivity to the drug. • Administer with caution to a pregnant or lactating patient or one with hepatic dysfunction.
Other peptic ulcer agents			
misoprostol	Prevention of NSAID-induced gastric ulcers	200 mcg P.O. q.i.d. with food or, if the patient cannot tolerate this dosage, 100 mcg P.O. q.i.d.	• Know that misoprostol is contraindicated in a pregnant or lactating patient or one with a history of allergies to prostaglandins.
omeprazole	Treatment of severe erosive or symptomatic esophagitis Treatment of pathologic hypersecretory conditions	20 mg P.O. daily for 4 to 8 weeks 60 mg P.O. daily initially, then individualized based on the severity of the condition	• Know that omeprazole is contraindicated in a patient with known hypersensitivity to the drug or any of its components. • Administer with caution to a pregnant or lactating patient.
sucralfate	Short-term treatment of duodenal ulcers	1 gram P.O. q.i.d. for 4 to 8 weeks	• Administer sucralfate with caution to a pregnant or lactating patient or one with chronic renal failure.

• Increase the patient's fluid and fiber intake if constipation occurs. Request a prescription for a laxative if needed.

• *Take safety precautions if the patient develops dizziness, sleepiness, or vertigo. For example, keep the side rails up, place the bed in the low position, and supervise patient activity.*

• Request a prescription for a mild analgesic if the patient experiences headache during omeprazole therapy.

• *Do not administer an antacid at the same time as sucralfate or misoprostol; antacids decrease the activity of these peptic ulcer agents.*

• *Administer sucralfate 2 hours before or after cimetidine because sucralfate decreases the bioavailability of cimetidine.*

• *Administer omeprazole cautiously during concomitant therapy with diazepam, phenytoin, or warfarin. Omeprazole may interfere with the metabolism of these agents, causing elevated plasma concentrations.*

• *Monitor the effectiveness of ketoconazole, ampicillin esters, and iron salts during concomitant omeprazole therapy; omeprazole may interfere with their absorption.*

• Administer misoprostol with food.

• Administer sucralfate at least 1 hour before meals and at bedtime for best results.

• Notify the physician if adverse reactions occur.

• Monitor the patient's bowel function for diarrhea, especially during misoprostol therapy.

• Monitor hydration if the patient develops diarrhea. Obtain a prescription for an antidiarrheal agent.

• Consult the physician about discontinuing the peptic ulcer agent if diarrhea becomes severe.

Patient teaching

• Teach the patient the name, dose, frequency, action, and adverse effects of the prescribed peptic ulcer agent.

• Instruct the patient how to manage adverse reactions, such as constipation, diarrhea, and dry mouth.

• *Advise the patient not to perform activities that require alertness, if dizziness, sleepiness, or vertigo occurs.*

• *Instruct the patient not to take an antacid with sucralfate or misoprostol.*

• *Instruct the patient to take sucralfate 2 hours before or after cimetidine if both drugs are prescribed.*

• Teach the patient when and how to take the prescribed peptic ulcer agent.

• Alert the patient that nausea and a metallic taste may occur with sucralfate use.

• *Provide verbal and written warnings to a woman of childbearing age that misoprostol may induce miscarriage. To prevent miscarriage, advise such a patient to obtain a serum pregnancy test within 2 weeks before beginning therapy, to use an effective contraceptive method during therapy, and to notify her physician if she is preg-*

nant or plans to become pregnant. If pregnancy is suspected, misoprostol should be discontinued immediately.

• Instruct the patient to notify the physician if adverse reactions occur.

Evaluation

The following examples represent appropriate evaluation statements for a patient receiving misoprostol, omeprazole, or sucralfate.

• The patient has no conditions that contraindicate misoprostol, omeprazole, or sucralfate therapy.

• The patient exhibits no signs of complications in the preexisting condition linked to the prescribed peptic ulcer agent.

• The patient demonstrates no adverse reactions to the prescribed peptic ulcer agent.

• The patient maintains normal bowel function.

• The patient and family express an accurate understanding of the points taught about the prescribed peptic ulcer agent.

• The patient selects an appropriate form of contraception to use during misoprostol therapy.

CHAPTER SUMMARY

Chapter 44 discussed peptic ulcer drugs. Peptic ulcer therapy attempts to correct the unbalanced gastric acid and pepsin secretion and to repair inadequate mucosal defenses of the GI lining. Here are the highlights of the chapter.

• Peptic ulcer drugs (1) neutralize acid in the GI tract, (2) reduce acid secretion, (3) bind to the ulcer, protecting it and neutralizing local acid, or (4) block the proton pump.

• The antacids act in the stomach to neutralize acid, thereby reducing the acid load in the GI tract and permitting ulcers to heal.

• Antacids treat peptic ulcer disease safely and effectively. However, the unpleasant taste and the frequent doses required make their use as the first choice in treating peptic ulcer disease less attractive than the H$_2$-receptor antagonists.

• H$_2$-receptor antagonists used for 4 to 6 weeks with possible adjunctive antacid therapy for pain have become the treatment of choice for duodenal and gastric ulcers.

• H$_2$-receptor antagonists block histamine-receptor sites, thereby inhibiting histamine-stimulated acid secretion. The H$_2$-receptor antagonists include cimetidine, famotidine, nizatidine, and ranitidine. These drugs promote the healing of duodenal and gastric ulcers.

• The H$_2$-receptor antagonists (especially cimetidine) can produce headache, dizziness, malaise, nausea, diarrhea or constipation, skin rashes, loss of libido, and impotence.

• Misoprostol is a synthetic prostaglandin used to prevent NSAID-induced gastric ulcers in patients at high risk. It is contraindicated in pregnancy and in women of child-bearing age.

• Omeprazole is a proton pump inhibitor approved for short-term use in treating GI reflux disease and pathological hypersecretory conditions.

• Sucralfate binds to the ulcer site and produces a protective barrier. This agent is used for short-term treatment of duodenal and gastric ulcers.

• Researchers currently are investigating other peptic ulcer agents, including anticholinergic drugs, colloidal bismuth, and tricyclic antidepressants.

• When caring for a patient receiving a peptic ulcer agent, the nurse must monitor closely for adverse drug reactions and teach the patient about the prescribed agent.

STUDY QUESTIONS

See Appendix 1 for answers.

1. Roger Davis, age 47, seeks emergency medical care for severe upper abdominal pain and vomiting that has persisted for 2 days. According to his medical history, he has received intermittent treatment over the past 3 years for a duodenal ulcer. His usual treatment regimen consists of the antacid magaldrate (Riopan) and the H_2-receptor antagonist ranitidine (Zantac), taken during acute flare-ups. How do antacids treat peptic ulcer disease?
(a) They increase gastric pH and neutralize stomach contents.
(b) They form a protective coating over the ulcer.
(c) They inhibit the proton pump, decreasing acid secretion.
(d) They increase mucus and bicarbonate secretion.

2. What is the primary reason for administering an antacid to Mr. Davis?
(a) to relieve epigastric pain and discomfort
(b) to prevent the development of stress ulcers
(c) to alter the pH of the stomach and small intestine
(d) to coat the lining of the peptic ulcer

3. Mr. Davis also receives several other oral medications. Because he takes an antacid, how should the nurse administer these other medications?
(a) by an alternate route
(b) shortly before the antacid
(c) 30 minutes after the antacid
(d) 1 to 2 hours before or after the antacid

4. During acute flare-ups, Mr. Davis takes 150 mg of ranitidine P.O. b.i.d. How does this H_2-receptor antagonist exert its therapeutic effects?
(a) by increasing the absorption of stomach acid by the intestinal contents
(b) by decreasing the effectiveness of stomach alkalies in buffering acids
(c) by inhibiting the gastrocolic reflex, which is necessary for gastrin secretion
(d) by blocking the stimulant action of histamine on acid-secreting cells in the stomach

5. The nurse assesses Mr. Davis for adverse reactions to the prescribed peptic ulcer agent. Which H_2-receptor antagonist is *most* likely to cause adverse reactions, such as headache, diarrhea, and skin rash?
(a) cimetidine
(b) famotidine
(c) nizatidine
(d) ranitidine

6. Lucy Kenmore, age 35, takes large doses of an NSAID for rheumatoid arthritis. To prevent NSAID-induced ulcers, her physician prescribes sucralfate (Carafate) 1 gram P.O. q.i.d. How does sucralfate produce its therapeutic effects?
(a) It neutralizes the acid content of the stomach.
(b) It binds to the ulcer, forming a protective barrier.
(c) It decreases gastric acid secretion.
(d) It allows fluids to cleanse the ulcer site.

7. Ms. Kenmore's physician could have prescribed the synthetic prostaglandin misoprostol (Cytotec). How do synthetic prostaglandins prevent NSAID-induced ulcers?
(a) They stimulate mucus and bicarbonate secretion and suppress acid secretion.
(b) They neutralize the gastric content by increasing the pH.
(c) They provide a protective lining for the GI mucosa.
(d) They block histamine$_2$-receptor sites.

8. Which reason may explain why the physician did not prescribe misoprostol for Ms. Kenmore?
(a) It poses a high risk of adverse reactions.
(b) It has a cumbersome dosage schedule.
(c) It affects the uterus in childbearing women.
(d) It may produce severe allergic reactions.

SELECTED REFERENCES

AHFS drug information 90. (1990). Bethesda, MD: American Society of Hospital Pharmacists.

Dammann, H., Dreyer, M., Kangah, R., Muller, P., and Simon, B. (1988). Optimal reduction of gastric acid secretion in the treatment of peptic ulceration. *Drugs,* 35(suppl. 3), 106-113.

Goodman and Gilman's the pharmacological basis of therapeutics (8th ed.; 1990). Elmsford, NY: Pergamon Press.

Hansten, P., and Horn, J. (1988). *Drug interactions: Clinical significance of drug-drug interactions* (6th ed.). Philadelphia: Lea & Febiger.

North American Nursing Diagnosis Association. (1990). *Taxonomy I - Revised, with official categories.* St. Louis: NANDA.

Nostrant, T., and Barnett, J. (1989). Peptic ulcer disease: New developments. *Comprehensive Therapy,* 15(9), 45-51.

Ohning, G., and Soll, A. (1989). Medical treatment of peptic ulcer disease. *American Family Physician,* 39(4), 257-270.

USPDI. (1991). *Drug information for the health care professional* (Vol. I, 11th ed.). Rockville, MD: United States Pharmacopeial Convention.

DRUGS FOR FLUID, ELECTROLYTE, AND NUTRITIONAL BALANCE

Illness easily can disturb the homeostatic mechanisms that help maintain normal fluid, electrolyte, and nutritional balance. Such occurrences as loss of appetite, medication administration, vomiting, and diagnostic tests also can alter this delicate balance. Fortunately, numerous drugs can be used to correct fluid, electrolyte, acid-base, or nutritional imbalances. Unit Eleven provides a full range of information about these drugs.

FLUID AND ELECTROLYTE BALANCE

About 60% of an adult's body is made up of water: 60% of this body water is intracellular; 40% is extracellular. The ingestion of food and fluids and the metabolism of nutrients add water to the body—1,500 to 3,000 ml/day for an average adult. Ordinarily, the fluid intake equals the fluid output, but an illness can upset this delicate balance.

Intracellular and extracellular fluid compartments have specific chemical compositions of electrolytes. This unit addresses the major electrolytes: sodium, potassium, chloride, calcium, phosphorus, magnesium, and bicarbonate. (For detailed information, see *Normal electrolyte concentrations in intracellular and extracellular fluid.*)

Many disorders and diseases can alter electrolyte levels in the fluid compartments, profoundly affecting the body's water distribution, cell function, neuromuscular activity, and acid-base balance. When such imbalances occur, the agents discussed in this unit are used to reestablish homeostasis.

NUTRITIONAL BALANCE

Unit Eleven also includes agents used to maintain nutritional balance or to correct a nutritional imbalance. Maintaining nutrition is important because the body relies on exogenous sources of carbohydrate, fat, and protein to sustain life. Malnutrition must be corrected because it can decrease the ability of organ systems to function, complicating a patient's treatment.

Normal electrolyte concentrations in intracellular and extracellular fluid

Blood contains intracellular fluid (fluid in red blood cells) and extracellular fluid (plasma fluid). Because their cells allow different substances to permeate, intracellular and extracellular fluids contain different electrolyte concentration levels. For example, intracellular fluid contains about 30 times more potassium than extracellular fluid and extracellular fluid contains about 14 times more sodium than intracellular fluid.

Alterations in electrolyte balance will affect a patient's total physiologic functioning. Some drugs will alter that balance. Various electrolytes are prescribed to treat electrolyte imbalance.

In the clinical setting, the nurse will see values reflecting the components of extracellular fluid only.

Be aware that standards for these values vary among health care facilities.

ELECTROLYTE	INTRACELLULAR CONCENTRATION	EXTRACELLULAR CONCENTRATION
Sodium	10 mEq/liter	136 to 146 mEq/liter
Potassium	140 mEq/liter	3.5 to 5 mEq/liter
Calcium	10 mEq/liter	4.5 to 5.8 mEq/liter
Magnesium	40 mEq/liter	1.6 to 2.2 mEq/liter
Chloride	4 mEq/liter	96 to 106 mEq/liter
Bicarbonate	10 mEq/liter	24 to 28 mEq/liter
Phosphate	100 mEq/liter	1 to 1.5 mEq/liter

Glossary

Anion: negatively charged ion.

Beriberi: polyneuritis caused by a thiamine deficiency and characterized by spasmodic rigidity of the lower limbs, muscular atrophy, paralysis, anemia, and neuralgia.

Buffer: any substance in a solution that decreases the change in pH when an acid or base is added.

Carbonic anhydrase: enzyme that catalyzes the breakdown of carbonic acid to carbon dioxide and water, or the formation of carbon dioxide and water to carbonic acid.

Cation: positively charged ion.

Chelation: process of binding a metallic ion with an organic compound to form a compound that sequesters the metallic ion from other interactions.

Electrolyte: ion that can conduct electricity when dissolved in solution.

Extracellular fluid: fluid outside the cells that accounts for about 40% of total body water and includes functional plasma and interstitial fluid. Some of the components of extracellular fluid are protein, magnesium, potassium, chloride, calcium, and certain sulfates.

Hypercalcemia: excess calcium in the blood.

Hypercalciuria: excess calcium in the urine.

Hyperglycemia: excess glucose in the blood.

Hyperkalemia: excess potassium in the blood.

Hyperlipidemia: excess lipids in the blood.

Hypernatremia: excess sodium in the blood.

Hyperosmolality: excess solutes per unit of solvent.

Hyperphosphatemia: excess phosphate in the blood.

Hypervitaminosis: condition resulting from excessive intake of one or more vitamins.

Hypocalcemia: insufficient calcium in the blood.

Hypoglycemia: insufficient glucose in the blood.

Hypokalemia: insufficient potassium in the blood.

Hypomagnesemia: insufficient magnesium in the blood.

Hyponatremia: insufficient sodium in the blood.

Hypophosphatemia: insufficient phosphate in the blood.

Hypoprothrombinemia: insufficient prothrombin in the blood.

Hypovolemia: abnormally decreased volume of circulatory body fluid.

Intracellular fluid: fluid inside the cells that accounts for 60% of total body water, and includes intracellular and red blood cell fluid.

Lactic acidosis: decreased serum pH caused by the anaerobic metabolism of pyruvic acid to lactic acid.

Malabsorption: impaired absorption of nutrients.

Metabolic acidosis: decreased serum pH caused by an excess of hydrogen ions in the extracellular fluid.

Metabolic alkalosis: increased serum pH caused by excess bicarbonate in the extracellular fluid.

Mineral: naturally occurring inorganic substance with a distinctive chemical composition.

Nephrotoxic: poisonous or destructive to kidney cells.

Osmolality: solute concentration per unit of solvent.

Ossification: bone formation.

Osteodystrophy: defective bone formation.

pH: abbreviation for the relative hydrogen ion concentration (acidity or alkalinity) of a solution; a pH of 7 is neutral; below 7 is acid; above 7 is alkaline.

Systemic acidifier: agent that decreases serum pH level.

Systemic alkalinizer: agent that increases serum pH level.

Urinary acidifier: agent that decreases urine pH level.

Urinary alkalinizer: agent that increases urine pH level.

Vitamin: organic substance in food that is necessary for normal metabolism; classified as fat-soluble or water-soluble.

Nutritional assessment

Assessing the type and degree of malnutrition will help determine necessary nutritional support and the goals of therapy. To assess malnutrition, the nurse can use laboratory tests and daily clinical evaluations, including the patient's daily weight and other anthropometric measurements to help determine the status of protein and fat reserves. A triceps skinfold measurement estimates the body's fat reserve. Midarm muscle circumference indicates the protein deficit. The creatinine-height index helps evaluate muscle status. When assessing a patient, the nurse should compare the value of each measurement to the standard value to estimate the degree of depletion.

Certain laboratory tests can help assess visceral protein depletion. For example, a low serum albumin, serum transferrin, and total lymphocyte count may indicate this type of nutritional deficiency.

Nutritional supplements

A complete nutritional supplement will supply carbohydrates, proteins, lipids, electrolytes, vitamins, and trace elements. Patients need adequate nonprotein calories to allow optimal protein use, and carbohydrate calories should be given in amounts approximating the basal energy expenditure. Of the daily caloric requirements, 4% to 10% should include essential fatty acids. Daily protein requirements depend on the stress level because stress increases protein use. Maintenance therapy usually requires 0.5 to 1 gram of protein/kg/day; high-stress states or moderate protein repletion, 1.5 to 2 grams of protein/kg/day; extensive repletion, 2 to 4 grams of protein/kg/day. Two types of nutritional supplements may be prescribed: enteral agents, administered through the alimentary canal, and parenteral agents, administered through other routes.

Enteral nutrition

Many physicians prefer enteral nutrition to parenteral nutrition for patients with functional gastrointestinal tracts because it uses the normal metabolic pathways and processes. It allows the body to use nutrients more efficiently and tends to cause fewer metabolic problems. Enteral nutrition also is much less expensive, averaging approximately one-tenth the cost of parenteral nutrition.

The nurse can administer enteral nutrition by the bolus, gravity drip, or continuous drip method. The bolus method delivers 240 to 400 ml of feeding solution by gravity over several minutes and is repeated every 4 to 6 hours. Because most patients tolerate this method poorly, its use is limited. The gravity drip method infuses 240 to 400 ml of feeding solution over 30 to 60 minutes and is repeated every 4 to 6 hours. Patients usually tolerate this method better than the bolus method. The continuous drip method delivers the feeding solution continuously over 24 hours, usually at a rate of 50 to 125 ml/hour. Ideally, an infusion pump is used to control the infusion rate. Studies show that this method is the most reliable and best tolerated of the three enteral nutrition methods.

Parenteral nutrition

Patients who cannot tolerate oral feeding or enteral nutrition may need parenteral nutrition. Total parenteral nutrition (TPN) provides carbohydrates, proteins, lipids, electrolytes, vitamins, and trace elements intravenously. It supplies carbohydrate as a dextrose solution that provides 3.4 kcal/gram of dextrose. Concentrations of dextrose 5% to 10% may be given via a peripheral vein, but hypertonic solutions greater than 12.5% must be given via a central catheter. Parenteral nutrition supplies protein in amino acid solutions that provide 4 kcal/gram, and lipids in 10% or 20% fat emulsions that provide 1.1 kcal/ml or 2 kcal/ml, respectively.

The nurse typically initiates central TPN solutions slowly at about 40 to 50 ml/hour, increasing the rate over 24 to 48 hours to the maximum desired rate to avoid severe hyperglycemia. If a low dextrose concentration is used, the nurse may use a rate of 100 to 125 ml/hour. When discontinuing central TPN, the nurse must taper the rate gradually over 24 hours to avoid hypoglycemia.

Because some people are allergic to the egg protein in fat emulsions, therapy should begin with a test dose of 1 ml/minute for 30 minutes. If no adverse reactions occur, the rate may be advanced to the desired rate. The nurse may give fat emulsions through a central or peripheral catheter but should not use an in-line filter because the fat particles are too large to pass through the pores. (For a summary of these nutritional supplements, see *Comparing types of parenteral nutrition,* page 774.)

OVERVIEW OF CHAPTERS

Unit Eleven explores the drugs used to restore or maintain fluid, electrolyte, and nutritional balance. It presents vitamins, minerals, other nutritional agents, electrolyte replacement agents, alkalinizing and acidifying agents, a cation-exchange resin, and ammonia-detoxicating agents.

Chapter 45
Vitamin, Mineral, and Other Nutritional Agents

Chapter 45 focuses on vitamin, mineral, and other preparations used as nutritional supplements. It highlights the physiologic actions and clinical uses of fat-soluble vitamins, water-soluble vitamins, and minerals. It also discusses the new nutritional agent levocarnitine, which is used to treat carnitine deficiency. For each group of agents, the chapter presents related nursing care, including patient teaching.

Chapter 46
Electrolyte Replacement Agents

Chapter 46 discusses the primary intracellular fluid (ICF) electrolyte, potassium; a major extracellular fluid (ECF) electrolyte, calcium; and two other electrolytes essential for homeostasis: magnesium (in ICF) and sodium (in ECF). The chapter also demonstrates use of the nursing process related to electrolyte replacement therapy.

Chapter 47
Alkalinizing and Acidifying Agents

Chapter 47 explores the systemic and urinary alkalinizing and acidifying agents. It discusses the use of systemic agents, such as sodium bicarbonate and ammonium chloride, to treat metabolic acidosis and alkalosis. It also investigates the use of urinary alkalinizers, such as sodium bicarbonate and acetazolamide, to promote the excretion of certain weak acids and toxic drugs. It concludes with a discussion of ascorbic acid and ammonium chloride as urinary acidifiers. For each group of agents, the chapter delineates adverse reactions and related nursing care.

Chapter 48
Cation-Exchange Resin and Ammonia-Detoxicating Agents

Two types of agents are used to treat toxic imbalances: a cation-exchange resin and ammonia-detoxicating agents. Chapter 48 examines the cation-exchange resin, sodium polystyrene sulfonate, as a treatment for hyperkalemia. Then it investigates the use of lactulose and neomycin, two ammonia-detoxicating agents, to reduce the serum ammonia level in patients with hepatic encephalopathy. The chapter details the adverse and therapeutic effects of these agents and associated nursing responsibilities.

Comparing types of parenteral nutrition

This chart summarizes the uses and special considerations of the various forms of parenteral nutrition, which may be used for a patient who needs nutritional supplementation.

SOLUTION COMPONENTS PER LITER	USES	SPECIAL CONSIDERATIONS
Total parenteral nutrition (TPN) via central venous line		
• Dextrose 15% to 35% (1 liter dextrose 25% = 850 nonprotein calories) • Crystalline amino acids 2.5% to 5% • Electrolytes, vitamins, trace elements, insulin, and heparin as prescribed • Fat emulsion 10% to 20% (usually infused as a separate solution; can be given peripherally or centrally)	• 1 week or more (long term) • For patients with large caloric and nutrient needs • Provides needed calories, essential vitamins, electrolytes, minerals, and trace elements; restores nitrogen balance • Promotes tissue synthesis, wound healing, and normal metabolic function • Allows bowel rest and healing; reduces activity in the gallbladder, pancreas, and small intestine	**Basic solution** • Is nutritionally complete except for essential fatty acids • Requires minor surgical procedure for central line insertion • Delivers hypertonic solutions • May cause metabolic complications (glucose intolerance, electrolyte imbalances, essential fatty acid deficiency) **I.V. fat emulsion** • May not be used effectively in severely stressed patients (especially burn patients) • May interfere with immune mechanisms • Irritates peripheral vein in long-term use
Peripheral parenteral nutrition		
• Dextrose 5% to 10% • Crystalline amino acids 2.75% to 4.25% • Electrolytes, trace elements, and vitamins as prescribed • Fat emulsion 10% or 20% (1 liter dextrose 10% and amino acids 3.5% infused at same time with 1 liter 10% fat emulsion = 1,440 nonprotein calories: 340 from dextrose and 1,100 from fat emulsion) • Heparin as prescribed	• 1 week or less • Maintains nutritional state in patients who can tolerate relatively high fluid volume, those who usually resume bowel function and oral feedings in a few days, and those who are susceptible to catheter-related infections of central venous TPN	**Basic solution** • Short-term use only; cannot be used in nutritionally depleted patients • Cannot be used in volume-restricted patients because higher volumes of solution are needed than with central venous TPN • Avoids insertion and maintenance of central catheter, but patient must have good veins; I.V. site should be changed every 48 hours • Requires no surgery for peripheral line insertion • Delivers less hypertonic solutions than central venous TPN • May cause phlebitis **I.V. fat emulsion** • Is as effective as dextrose for caloric source • Irritates vein in long-term use • Diminishes phlebitis if infused at same time as basic nutrient solution
Protein-sparing therapy		
• Crystalline amino acids in same amounts as TPN • Electrolytes, vitamins, and minerals as prescribed	• 2 weeks or less • May preserve body protein in a stable patient • Augments oral or tube feedings	• Is nutritionally incomplete; may be initiated or stopped at any point in a patient's hospital stay • Allows administration of other I.V. fluids, some drugs, and blood by-products via same I.V. line • Is not as likely to cause phlebitis as peripheral parenteral nutrition
Standard I.V. therapy		
• Dextrose, water, electrolytes, and vitamins in varying amounts *Frequently used parenteral fluids include:* dextrose 5% = 170 calories/liter dextrose 10% = 340 calories/liter 0.9% NaCl (normal saline solution) = 0 calories	• Less than 1 week as nutrition source • Maintains hydration (main function) • Facilitates and maintains normal metabolic function	• Is nutritionally incomplete; does not provide sufficient calories to maintain adequate nutritional status

VITAMIN, MINERAL, AND OTHER NUTRITIONAL AGENTS

OBJECTIVES

After reading and studying this chapter, the student should be able to:

1. Explain the pharmacokinetics of the four fat-soluble vitamins (A, D, E, and K), including their routes of absorption, distribution, metabolism, and excretion.

2. Identify the signs of vitamin A and D toxicity.

3. Explain why vitamin K should not be administered undiluted by I.V. push.

4. Discuss the pharmacokinetics of the water-soluble vitamins (B and C), and explain why these preparations are less toxic than the fat-soluble vitamins.

5. Explain the rationale for water-soluble vitamin supplementation in a patient receiving dialysis for renal disease.

6. Identify the clinical uses of the other water-soluble vitamins.

7. Compare the pharmacokinetics, pharmacodynamics, and pharmacotherapeutics of the various minerals as well as their adverse effects.

8. Discuss the therapeutic uses of and the adverse reactions to the other nutritional agent levocarnitine.

9. Describe how to apply the nursing process when caring for a patient who is receiving a vitamin, mineral, or other nutritional agent.

INTRODUCTION

Since the early twentieth century, researchers have uncovered a wealth of information about the nutritional agents called vitamins and minerals. Evidence of the existence of vitamins and minerals was suggested by early research into the major nutritional-deficiency states, such as scurvy, night blindness, beriberi, and rickets. Despite years of study, however, experts possess incomplete knowledge about vitamins and minerals. Indeed, only recently have experts understood the roles of these chemicals in the maintenance of normal growth, development, and metabolic function. Knowledge of vitamins and minerals will grow as research related to these substances continues.

Vitamins are organic chemicals that do not fit into the categories of protein, fat, or carbohydrate. Although the human body requires only small amounts of these chemicals, they are essential for the normal operation of various metabolic functions. With two exceptions, the source of vitamins is from outside the body — from ingested foods or through an oral or parenteral supplement. The two exceptions are vitamin D, which can be formed within the body through the action of ultraviolet radiation in sunlight on 7-dehydrocholesterol in the skin, and one form of vitamin K, which is synthesized by bacteria in the gastrointestinal (GI) tract.

Vitamins and minerals are naturally occurring substances. However, many vitamins can be synthesized, and natural and synthetic forms are commercially available. Both forms function identically, and claims for the increased nutritional value of natural vitamins are unfounded.

Vitamins are divided into two categories based on their solubility: fat soluble and water soluble. Fat-soluble vitamins include A, D, E, and K. Water-soluble vitamins include B-complex vitamins and vitamin C.

Minerals are inorganic chemicals that are components of all living tissues. Like vitamins, they play a role in various metabolic functions. Because the body cannot manufacture minerals, they must be obtained from some exogenous source, usually food. This chapter discusses the trace minerals (or trace elements) chromium, copper, fluoride, iodine, manganese, molybdenum, selenium, and zinc.

Other minerals required by the body, such as calcium, sodium, and potassium, are discussed in Chapter 46, Electrolyte Replacement Agents. Iron is discussed in Chapter

---

SELECTED NURSING DIAGNOSES

Vitamin, mineral, and other nutritional agents

The following nursing diagnoses address representative problems and etiologies that a nurse may encounter when caring for a patient who is receiving a vitamin, mineral, or other nutritional agent. Some of these nursing diagnoses contain generalized etiologies, which the nurse must individualize based on the patient's needs. (For some common nursing diagnoses and related interventions for each drug class, see the "Nursing Process Application" sections of this chapter.)

- Altered growth and development related to skeletal changes caused by vitamin A or D toxicity
- Altered protection related to soft tissue calcification from high-dose vitamin D therapy
- Altered protection related to the adverse hematologic effects of a vitamin or mineral
- Altered protection related to the adverse thyroid effects caused by high concentrations of iodide
- Altered protection related to the vasodilating effects of nicotinic acid
- Altered peripheral tissue perfusion related to rapid parenteral administration of vitamin K
- Anxiety related to the adverse central nervous system effects of thiamine
- Body image disturbance related to hair loss or color change caused by vitamin E
- Body image disturbance related to levocarnitine-induced body odor
- Decreased cardiac output related to the adverse cardiovascular effects of parenteral vitamin K
- Diarrhea related to the adverse GI effects of a vitamin, mineral, or other nutritional agent
- Fatigue related to the adverse effects of vitamin A or E
- Fluid volume deficit related to the adverse GI effects of a vitamin, mineral, or other nutritional agent
- Hyperthermia related to iodide-induced fever
- Hypothermia related to the adverse effects of zinc
- Impaired gas exchange related to chromium-induced bronchospasm
- Impaired physical mobility related to Parkinson-like symptoms caused by manganese
- Impaired skin integrity related to sterile abscess formation caused by intramuscular injection of vitamin E

- Impaired tissue integrity related to the adverse integumentary effects of vitamin A
- Knowledge deficit related to the prescribed vitamin, mineral, or other nutritional agent
- Pain related to mouth, gum, and salivary gland tenderness caused by iodine therapy
- Personal identity disturbance related to copper-induced behavioral changes
- Potential for injury related to a preexisting condition that contraindicates the use of a vitamin, mineral, or other nutritional agent
- Potential for injury related to a preexisting condition that requires cautious use of a vitamin, mineral, or other nutritional agent
- Potential for injury related to adverse drug reactions
- Potential for injury related to drug interactions
- Potential for injury related to fluoride-induced hyperirritability or tetany
- Potential for injury related to increased intracranial pressure caused by vitamin A toxicity
- Potential for injury related to shock and cardiac or respiratory arrest caused by parenteral vitamin K therapy
- Potential for poisoning related to an overdose of the prescribed mineral
- Potential for trauma related to renal calculus formation or dental erosion caused by vitamin C therapy
- Sensory-perceptual alterations (gustatory) related to the metallic taste caused by iodine therapy
- Sensory-perceptual alterations (kinesthetic or tactile) related to the adverse effects of pyridoxine or fluoride
- Sensory-perceptual alterations (visual) related to the adverse effects of vitamin E or copper
- Sensory-perceptual alterations (visual) related to vitamin A toxicity

---

35, Hematinic Agents. Other minerals, especially the heavy metals lead, mercury, and arsenic, are nontherapeutic elements that are toxic even in trace amounts. A relatively new vitamin and mineral agent, levocarnitine, also is discussed. A naturally occurring substance composed of amino acids, levocarnitine is used to treat carnitine deficiency.

RECOMMENDED DAILY ALLOWANCE

In the United States, the Food and Nutrition Board of the National Academy of Sciences establishes recommended daily allowances (RDAs) for nutrients. These RDAs are updated periodically and serve as goals for good nutrition. Other countries have similar boards or committees that assess nutritional requirements.

RDAs are noted in the following discussion of each vitamin. The Food and Drug Administration requires that labels of all vitamin products indicate the amount of the vitamin and the proportion of the RDA each vitamin product provides.

For a summary of representative agents, see *Selected major drugs: Vitamin, mineral, and other nutritional agents*, pages 795 and 796. For a listing of applicable nursing diagnoses that the nurse may formulate when caring for a patient receiving these agents, see *Selected nursing diagnoses: Vitamin, mineral, and other nutritional agents*. For detailed information on applying the nursing process, see Chapter 6, The Nursing Process and Drug Therapy.

FAT-SOLUBLE VITAMINS

The fat-soluble vitamins A, D, E, and K require the presence of bile salts, pancreatic lipase, and dietary fat for absorption into the body. Although their mechanisms of absorption and storage potential in the body are similar, each performs different functions. Adequate amounts of vitamin A are necessary for vision in dim light, skin and mucous membrane development, normal growth, and reproduction. Vitamin D—actually two related substances, cholecalciferol (D_3) and ergocalciferol (D_2)—plays a role in regulating calcium and phosphorus balance. (For information about the vitamin D analogues calcifediol, calcitriol, and dihydrotachysterol as calcium regulators, see Chapter 51, Parathyroid Agents.) Vitamin E acts as an antioxidant and enzyme cofactor. Vitamin K stimulates the synthesis of clotting factors by the liver. (For a summary of the dietary sources and daily requirements of these vitamins, see *Fat-soluble vitamins: Food sources and RDAs.*)

PHARMACOKINETICS

Vitamin A exists as beta carotene, provitamin A, in plants and as the retinyl ester in animals. Both are converted to forms of retinol in the intestines, where they are absorbed. Vitamin D taken orally is absorbed readily from the GI tract in the presence of bile. Traveling in the blood bound to protein, vitamin D is stored mostly in fat and muscle, metabolized in the liver and kidneys, and excreted via bile in feces. A small amount is excreted in urine. Vitamin E exhibits poor absorption and wide distribution, is metabolized in the liver, and excreted via bile in feces. Vitamin K is absorbed from the GI tract and concentrates in the liver immediately after absorption. Metabolism occurs in the liver, and metabolites are excreted in bile and urine.

Absorption, distribution, metabolism, excretion

Physiologic doses of oral vitamin A preparations are absorbed readily and completely from the small intestine in the presence of bile salts, pancreatic lipase, protein, and dietary fat. Absorption is incomplete after the administration of large doses or in patients with fat malabsorption, low protein intake, intestinal infections, and hepatic or pancreatic disease. Absorption of vitamin A occurs via active transport and passive diffusion. Water-miscible preparations of vitamin A are absorbed more rapidly from the GI tract than oil solutions. Retinol is esterified in the intestines primarily to the retinyl palmitate form, which is carried by lymph to the liver and blood.

Vitamin A, existing as retinyl palmitate, retinol, and retinal, is distributed to and stored primarily in Kupffer's

Fat-soluble vitamins: Food sources and RDAs

To prevent chronic deficiencies, the nurse should teach the patient about dietary sources of and recommended daily allowances (RDAs) for vitamins A, D, E, and K. The chart below provides this information, with the RDAs grouped by age and condition.

VITAMIN	FOOD SOURCES	RDAs
vitamin A	Dairy products, liver, egg yolks, fish, and yellow or green fruits and vegetables	Infants to age 12 months: 375 mcg Children ages 1 to 10: 400 to 700 mcg Males ages 11 and older: 1,000 mcg Females ages 11 and older: 800 mcg Pregnant females: 1,300 mcg Lactating females: 1,200 to 1,300 mcg
vitamin D	Fortified milk and margarine	Infants to age 12 months: 7.5 to 10 mcg Children ages 1 to 10: 10 mcg Males ages 11 and older: 5 to 10 mcg Females ages 11 and older: 5 to 10 mcg Pregnant females: 10 mcg Lactating females: 10 mcg
vitamin E	Vegetable oils, margarine, milk, eggs, meats, green leafy vegetables, whole grains, and animal fats	Infants to age 12 months: 3 to 4 mg Children ages 1 to 10: 6 to 7 mg Males ages 11 and older: 10 mg Females ages 11 and older: 8 mg Pregnant females: 10 mg Lactating females: 11 to 12 mg
vitamin K	Liver, cheese, eggs, green leafy vegetables, tomatoes, meats, milk, and vegetable oils	Infants to age 12 months: 5 to 10 mcg Children ages 1 to 10: 15 to 30 mcg Males ages 11 and older: 45 to 80 mcg Females ages 11 and older: 45 to 65 mcg Pregnant females: 65 mcg Lactating females: 65 mcg

cells in the liver. Lesser amounts are stored in the kidneys, lungs, adrenal glands, retinas, and intraperitoneal fat. Beta-carotene is distributed widely in the body and is deposited in skin and body fat. Normal body stores of vitamin A are sufficient to supply body needs for up to 2 years. Vitamin A appears in breast milk, but it does not cross the placenta readily.

Retinal is released from the liver in response to physiologic needs and is transported in the blood bound to retinol-binding protein. Retinol is metabolized in the liver to a beta glucuronide, which undergoes enterohepatic circulation and oxidation to retinal and retinoic acid. Retinal, retinoic acid, and other water-soluble metabolites are excreted in the urine and in feces via bile.

Oral vitamin D is absorbed readily from the small intestine in the presence of bile. Vitamin D_3 may be absorbed more rapidly and completely than vitamin D_2. Gastrointestinal absorption is reduced in a patient with hepatic or biliary disease or a malabsorption syndrome.

Absorbed vitamin D circulates in the blood with vitamin D-binding protein. This protein is an alpha-globulin, specific for vitamin D. Vitamin D is stored primarily in fat and muscle. Although the plasma half-life is only 9 to 25 hours, vitamin D is stored in fat for prolonged periods of time.

Vitamin D is metabolized in the liver and kidneys. Ultraviolet light from the sun converts plant and animal steroidlike substances (sterols) to provitamin D. Vitamin D is converted into active metabolites in the liver and further metabolized in the kidneys to even more active metabolites.

Excretion of vitamin D occurs primarily in the feces via bile; a small amount is excreted in urine.

Absorption of vitamin E from the GI tract depends on the presence of bile. Only 20% to 60% of the vitamin obtained from dietary sources is absorbed. As the dosage of vitamin E increases, the fraction of vitamin E absorbed decreases. Water-miscible preparations are absorbed better than oil solutions.

After absorption, vitamin E is incorporated into lymphatic chylomicrons, which then are transported to the systemic circulation. Vitamin E circulates attached to beta-lipoproteins. It is distributed widely to all tissues and is stored in fat. Total body stores of vitamin E are estimated at 3 to 8 grams, which will meet the body's requirements for 4 years or more even if the diet is deficient in vitamin E. Placental transfer of vitamin E is incomplete, and neonates have low plasma tocopherol levels.

Vitamin E is metabolized in the liver. Excretion occurs via bile in feces, and small amounts of the metabolite are excreted in urine as glucuronides.

Phytonadione (vitamin K_1) and menaquinone (vitamin K_2) are absorbed from the GI tract only in the presence of bile. Absorption requires energy and occurs in the proximal

small intestine. Menadione (vitamin K_3), a synthetic product, is no longer commercially available. However, menadiol sodium diphosphate, a synthetic water-soluble derivative of menadione, is available. It is absorbed in the absence of bile, by diffusion in the distal portions of the small intestine and colon. After intramuscular (I.M.) injection, phytonadione is absorbed readily.

After absorption, phytonadione is concentrated in the liver, where it is metabolized to water-soluble metabolites. Only small amounts of phytonadione are stored in body tissues. Vitamin K crosses the placenta to a limited extent, but is secreted in breast milk.

Excretion of phytonadione occurs via bile and urine. A high fecal concentration level of vitamin K results from intestinal bacterial synthesis of the vitamin.

Onset, peak, duration

The onset of action of vitamin A depends on body requirements. In a patient with vitamin A deficiency, administration of vitamin A results in increased concentrations, first in the retinas, then in the liver. Retinal correction does not begin for 2 weeks to 2 months. Peak plasma concentration levels of retinol esters occur 4 to 5 hours after oral administration of retinol in oil solution; 3 to 4 hours after using water-miscible preparations.

After oral or I.M. administration of natural vitamin D, the onset is 10 to 24 hours. Peak concentration occurs about 4 weeks after daily administration of a fixed dosage, and the duration can be 2 months or longer.

Information on the onset, peak, and duration of vitamin E is unavailable.

Blood coagulation factors may increase in 6 to 12 hours after oral administration of phytonadione and in 1 to 2 hours after parenteral administration. Bleeding may be controlled in 3 to 8 hours, and a normal prothrombin time may be obtained 12 to 14 hours after parenteral administration. The onset of parenteral menadiol sodium diphosphate may require 8 to 24 hours.

PHARMACODYNAMICS

Vitamin A plays a role in preventing night blindness and is essential for growth and development of epithelial tissues, bone growth, human reproduction, and embryonic development. It also plays a role in many biochemical reactions, including steroid metabolism and cholesterol synthesis.

Active forms of vitamin D maintain calcium and phosphorus homeostasis in humans, primarily by facilitating their absorption, enhancing their mobilization from bone, and decreasing their renal excretion. (For actions of vitamin D in calcium regulation, see Chapter 51, Parathyroid Agents.)

Vitamin E may act as an antioxidant and help decrease platelet aggregation. It exists in foods, such as wheat germ oil, egg yolk, cereals, and beef liver, as alpha-, beta-, delta-, and gamma-tocopherols and tocotrienols. The most biologically active form is d-alpha-tocopherol.

After being produced by bacteria in the intestinal tract, vitamin K is used by the body to synthesize clotting factors and maintain hemostasis.

Mechanism of action

Vitamin A deficiency interferes with vision in dim light. This condition is known as night blindness, or nyctalopia. Adaptation to dark is a function of chemical reactions in the rods and cones of the retina. During the chemical reactions, photosensitive pigments in the retina initiate a receptor potential, allowing vision to occur. Primary adaptation occurs via the cones and takes place within several minutes. Secondary adaptation is a function of the rods and may take 30 minutes or longer.

A chemical reaction, the adaptation process results in formation of photosensitive pigments in the retina. The rod's photosensitive pigment, called rhodopsin, forms when the protein opsin combines with the vitamin A derivative 11-*cis*-retinal. The cone's photosensitive pigment forms when retinal combines with a protein similar to opsin. When these pigments are exposed to light, they undergo a chemical reaction that initiates a receptor potential in the retina, resulting in vision.

Vitamin A is essential for the growth and development of basal epithelial cells, which it stimulates to produce mucus-secreting or keratinizing tissues. Excessive retinol may inhibit keratinization by decreasing the number of mucus-producing goblet cells, leading to epithelial atrophy. The basal epithelial cells will continue to grow even without goblet cells, but the resulting keratinized epithelium is irritated and infected easily.

Vitamin D provides a different mechanism of action. Low serum calcium or phosphorus levels lead to the release of parathyroid hormone from the parathyroid gland. This hormone, as well as estrogen and prolactin, may increase the activity of enzymes in the kidneys that facilitate conversion of vitamin D to its active forms, 1,25-dihydroxy-ergocalciferol and calcitriol. Active vitamin D increases GI absorption of calcium and phosphorus from the jejunum and enhances the mobilization of calcium and phosphorus from bone. Active vitamin D also increases urinary retention of calcium and phosphorus by enhancing proximal tubular resorption of these substances. Thus, calcium and phosphorus are maintained at plasma concentrations necessary for normal neuromuscular activity, bone mineralization, and other calcium-dependent functions.

The exact biological function of vitamin E in humans is unknown. Vitamin E may act as an antioxidant, protecting fatty acids and other oxygen-sensitive substances, such as vitamin A and ascorbic acid, from oxidation. (The oxidation process uses oxygen to chemically alter a substance by freeing electrons, which results in energy production and an increased positive charge on the substance.) Vitamin E also may play a role in decreasing platelet aggregation.

Vitamin K_1, or phytonadione, is the only natural vitamin K available for therapeutic use. Vitamin K_2, or menaquinone, is the vitamin K produced by gram-positive bacteria in the intestines; menadiol sodium diphosphate is a synthetic form of vitamin K.

In normal individuals, phytonadione has no pharmacodynamic activity. In persons deficient in vitamin K, exogenous administration of phytonadione will promote the hepatic synthesis of vitamin K-dependent clotting factors. These include prothrombin (Factor II), proconvertin (Factor VII), plasma thromboplastin component (PTC, Christmas factor, or Factor IX), and the Stuart factor (Factor X).

Vitamin K-dependent clotting factors remain as inactive precursors in the liver in the absence of vitamin K or in the presence of coumarin-type anticoagulants. Vitamin K is an essential cofactor in activating these precursors. This is done by conversion of multiple peptide-bound residues of glutamic acid to gamma-carboxyglutamic acid in the completed precursor protein. Then this protein can bind calcium, a necessary event for clot formation.

PHARMACOTHERAPEUTICS

Vitamin A is used primarily to treat vitamin A deficiency, which rarely occurs in well-nourished individuals. Conditions that may lead to this deficiency include biliary tract or pancreatic disease, extreme dietary inadequacy, or malabsorption syndromes. The first step in treating vitamin A deficiency is correction of poor dietary habits. Because vitamin A deficiencies may be accompanied by other vitamin deficiencies, multivitamin preparations usually are administered. The use of water-miscible preparations of vitamin A may be beneficial in patients with GI disorders in which vitamin A absorption may be decreased.

Vitamin D is used most frequently as a dietary supplement. Nutritional rickets results from a lack of exposure to sunlight or a vitamin D-deficient diet. Because ergocalciferol is added to milk in the United States, rickets rarely occurs. Therefore, vitamin D is required as a supplement only in certain circumstances, as in persons with malabsorption syndrome, in breast-fed and premature infants, and in individuals receiving fewer than 10 mcg daily from food. Patients with vitamin D-dependent rickets usually respond best to calcitriol (one of the vitamin D analogues). Ergocalciferol and dihydrotachysterol have been used with oral calcium therapy to treat osteoporosis. However, further studies are needed to determine the efficacy of vitamin D therapy in osteoporosis.

Because vitamin E is abundant in normal diets, deficiency of this vitamin normally does not occur. Deficiencies may occur in persons with abetalipoproteinemia, abnormal fat absorption, or malabsorption syndromes. The only established use for vitamin E is for treating or preventing vitamin E deficiency.

Vitamin K deficiency can result from inadequate intake, lack of absorption or use of the vitamin by the body, or from the actions of a vitamin K antagonist, such as warfarin. The official RDAs have not been established.

Vitamin K is used to prevent and treat hypoprothrombinemia caused by vitamin K deficiency. Although vitamin K is the drug of choice for impending or actual hemorrhage, its long onset of action may necessitate the use of fresh frozen plasma or whole blood in an acute situation.

Vitamin K also is used to treat anticoagulant-induced hypoprothrombinemia. Phytonadione is the drug of choice for treating a moderate to severe hemorrhage caused by excessive dosages of coumarin anticoagulants. Menadiol sodium diphosphate is less effective in treating anticoagulant-induced hypoprothrombinemia. Vitamin K derivatives do not antagonize the effects of heparin. Excessive phytonadione dosages leading to normal prothrombin times may restore the condition that originally required administration of oral anticoagulant therapy. (For more details about anticoagulants, see Chapter 36, Anticoagulant Agents.)

Phytonadione is the drug of choice for treating and preventing hemorrhagic disease of the newborn. For several days after birth, neonates may be hypoprothrombinemic because of vitamin K deficiency. Menadiol sodium diphosphate can produce anemia, hyperbilirubinemia, kernicterus, and death in neonates and should not be used. Phytonadione also is effective in preventing neonatal hemorrhage resulting from anticonvulsants or anticoagulants used during pregnancy.

Other causes of hypoprothrombinemia, such as malabsorption syndromes and therapy with salicylates, sulfonamides, quinidine, coumarin anticoagulants, or broad-spectrum antibiotics, also are treated with phytonadione, which is more effective than synthetic vitamin K. Patients with hepatocellular damage may not be able to produce vitamin K-dependent clotting factors even with excessive vitamin K.

beta-carotene (Solatene). This preparation is used to reduce the severity of photosensitivity reactions in patients with erythropoietic protoporphyria, an inherited disorder characterized by production of large amounts of porphyrins (iron- or magnesium-free pyrrole derivatives) in the blood-forming tissue of the bone marrow. Dosage is adjusted according to the severity of symptoms and patient response.
Usual adult dosage: 30 to 300 mg P.O. daily, administered as a single dose or in divided doses, preferably with meals.
Usual pediatric dosage: 30 to 150 mg P.O. daily.

isotretinoin (Accutane). A retinoid preparation, isotretinoin is used to treat severe recalcitrant cystic acne by reducing sebum secretions. The dosage should be individualized according to clinical response, adverse reactions, and body weight.
Usual adult dosage: 0.5 to 2 mg/kg/day P.O. in two divided doses for 15 to 20 weeks.

vitamin A – as retinol, retinyl palmitate, or retinyl acetate (Aquasol A). These preparations are used to prevent and treat symptoms of vitamin A deficiency.
Usual adult dosage: for treatment of severe deficiency with corneal changes, 500,000 IU P.O. for 3 days, followed by 50,000 IU P.O. daily for 2 weeks and then a maintenance dosage of 10,000 to 20,000 IU P.O. daily for 2 months; for treatment of vitamin A deficiency without corneal changes, 10,000 to 25,000 IU P.O. daily for 1 to 2 weeks; for malabsorption syndromes, 10,000 to 50,000 IU P.O. daily.
Usual pediatric dosage: for children under age 1, 7,500 to 15,000 IU I.M. daily for 10 days; for children ages 1 to 8, 5,000 to 15,000 IU I.M. daily for 10 days or 5,000 IU/kg P.O. for 5 days or until recovery occurs; for children over age 8, use adult dosage.

cholecalciferol, or vitamin D₃. Available only in combination products, this vitamin is used for dietary supplementation and treatment or prevention of vitamin D deficiency.
Usual adult dosage: 400 to 1,000 IU P.O. daily or every other day. Dosage can be increased as needed every 4 weeks.

ergocalciferol, or vitamin D₂ (Calciferol). This vitamin is used to treat patients with familial hypophosphatemia (vitamin D-resistant rickets). Patients receiving long-term phenobarbital or phenytoin anticonvulsant therapy may develop low plasma concentrations of vitamin D and calcium. Rickets or osteomalacia rarely develop in these patients. If either occurs, treatment with ergocalciferol helps reverse the disorder. Ergocalciferol prophylaxis sometimes is used for patients on long-term anticonvulsant therapy.
Usual adult dosage: for familial hypophosphatemia, 0.25 to 1.5 mg P.O. daily; for hypoparathyroidism, 0.625 to 5 mg P.O. or I.M. daily; for renal osteodystrophy, 0.25 to 7.5 mg P.O. daily. Calcitriol and calcifediol (vitamin D analogues) also have been used because they function to a degree without being metabolized renally. If renal dysfunction becomes severe, dihydrotachysterol may be the drug of choice because it does not require renal conversion to the active form. For osteomalacia and rickets caused by dietary deficiency of vitamin D, 0.25 to 7.5 mg P.O. daily.

Usual pediatric dosage: for vitamin D deficiency, 0.25 to 0.625 mg P.O. daily; for hypoparathyroidism, 1.25 to 5 mg P.O. daily.

vitamin E (Aquasol E). Usually administered orally, the drug may be given I.M. when oral administration is not possible or malabsorption is suspected. Vitamin E should not be given I.V. Water-miscible oral vitamin E preparations are preferred for patients with malabsorption syndromes.

Because the potencies of the several forms of vitamin E vary, dosages are standardized into international units, based on activity. For example, 1 mg of *dl*-alpha-tocopheryl acetate equals 1 IU, whereas 1 mg of *d*-alpha-tocopherol is 1.49 IU.

Free tocopherols may be oxidized and destroyed when exposed to air and light. The ester and the acetate and succinate forms are stable in light and air.
Usual adult dosage: to treat vitamin E deficiency, 60 to 75 IU P.O. or I.M. daily; to prevent vitamin E deficiency, 30 IU P.O. daily with other vitamins.
Usual pediatric dosage: 5 IU P.O. daily to prevent vitamin E deficiency in premature, low-birth-weight neonates.

menadiol sodium diphosphate (Synkayvite). This drug is a synthetic, water-soluble form of vitamin K_3 that may be administered orally or by the S.C., I.M., or I.V. route. S.C. or I.M. administration may be contraindicated in a patient with hypoprothrombinemia because hemorrhage or hematoma may develop.
Usual adult dosage: for hypoprothrombinemia caused by obstructive jaundice and biliary fistulas, 5 mg P.O. daily; for bleeding caused by drug therapy, 5 to 10 mg P.O. daily. If the parenteral route is required, 5 to 15 mg may be given once or twice daily.

phytonadione (AquaMEPHYTON, Konakion, Mephyton). This drug is a derivative identical to the naturally occurring vitamin K_1. Although both forms may be given orally or I.M., only AquaMEPHYTON also may be given S.C. or I.V. In a patient with hypoprothrombinemia, I.M. or S.C. administration may be contraindicated because hemorrhage or hematoma may develop.

The rate of I.V. AquaMEPHYTON administration should not exceed 1 mg/minute, and slower rates may be safer. The drug always should be diluted in D_5W, normal saline solution, or dextrose 5% in normal saline solution. Never give AquaMEPHYTON undiluted by I.V. push. The I.V. route should be restricted for use with those patients for whom other routes are not feasible and the serious risk is justified.
Usual adult dosage: for anticoagulant-induced hypoprothrombinemia, 2.5 to 10 mg P.O., I.M., S.C., or slow I.V. Use the lowest dosage to minimize refractoriness to further anticoagulant treatment. If the initial response is not sat-

isfactory, the dose may be repeated in 12 to 48 hours after an oral dose or 6 to 8 hours after a parenteral dose. For hypoprothrombinemia resulting from other causes, 2 to 25 mg P.O., I.M., or S.C. Doses larger than 25 mg rarely are required, and 10 mg usually will suffice. To prevent hypoprothrombinemia associated with vitamin K deficiency in patients on prolonged total parenteral nutrition (TPN), 5 to 10 mg I.M. weekly.
Usual pediatric dosage: for hemorrhagic disease of the newborn, 0.5 to 1 mg I.M. or S.C. Higher dosages may be needed if the mother was taking an anticoagulant or anticonvulsant agent during pregnancy.

Drug interactions
Vitamin A interacts with mineral oil, resulting in decreased absorption of vitamin A. When Vitamin D is given concomitantly with cholestyramine, cholestipol hydrochloride, or mineral oil, the interaction may interfere with intestinal absorption of vitamin D. Large doses of vitamin E may increase the anticoagulant effects of warfarin by interfering with the synthesis of vitamin K-dependent clotting factors. Vitamin E also may impair the hematologic response to iron therapy in a patient with iron deficiency anemia. Vitamin K antagonizes the effect of coumarin anticoagulants by increasing the synthesis of vitamin K-dependent clotting factors.

ADVERSE DRUG REACTIONS

In most cases, the fat-soluble vitamins are relatively nontoxic when administered in the usual adult dosages. However, higher doses may cause various adverse reactions.

Because the primary functions of vitamin A relate to vision, development of epithelial tissues, and bone growth, adverse reactions to this drug tend to alter these functions. Changes in liver metabolism also are possible because the liver is the primary site of vitamin A storage.

Most adverse reactions to vitamin A appear to be dose-related. Toxicity, known as hypervitaminosis A, may be acute or chronic; signs of acute toxicity have occurred after administration of very large vitamin A doses over a short time or with a single dose. In adults, this results from doses in excess of 25,000 IU per kilogram.

In adults, chronic toxicity usually results from doses of 4,000 IU per kilogram for 6 to 15 months. Possible manifestations of toxicity include fatigue, malaise, lethargy, abdominal discomfort, anorexia, nausea, vomiting, and visual disturbances. Changes in epithelial tissues, including dry itchy skin, dry nose and mouth, inflammation of oral mucous membranes, or hair loss, may appear. Skeletal changes, including thickening of long bones, slowed growth, and migratory bone pain, also have been reported. Signs of increased intracranial pressure, such as headache and irritability, papilledema, and exophthalmos, may occur.

Other signs are hypoplastic anemia, a broad category of anemias characterized by a decrease in the number of red blood cells (RBCs), and leukopenia, an abnormal decrease in the number of white blood cells (WBCs). Also, because large amounts of vitamin A accumulate in the liver, an overdose may result in jaundice, hepatomegaly, and a rise in liver enzymes.

Adverse reactions to isotretinoin, a metabolite of vitamin A used to treat acne, are similar to those caused by other forms of the vitamin. Also, eye irritation, conjunctivitis, and cheilosis (scaly, cracked lips) tend to be prominent. Elevated serum triglyceride levels and photosensitivity also may result from use of isotretinoin. This drug also may cause fetal abnormalities and should not be used during pregnancy or in sexually active women of childbearing age.

Anaphylactic reactions and shock have occurred after I.V. administration of vitamin A. Parenteral vitamin A should be administered I.M. unless it is part of a multiple vitamin preparation used for total parenteral nutrition (TPN).

With vitamin D administration, the range between therapeutic and toxic levels is narrow. Maintenance of normal serum calcium and phosphorus levels, however, does not ensure the absence of adverse reactions.

High doses of vitamin D stimulate increased absorption of calcium and phosphorus from the GI tract and increase mobilization of calcium and phosphorus from bone. If serum levels of calcium and phosphorus rise to a particularly critical level, calcium phosphate precipitates and calcification of soft tissues results. The kidneys, heart, muscles, blood vessels, eyes, and lungs may be affected. This can result in renal insufficiency with polyuria, hypertension, arrhythmias, muscle pain, renal calculi, and conjunctivitis. Demineralization of bone can result in bone pain and osteoporosis in adults and growth retardation in children.

Other reactions associated with vitamin D toxicity include nausea, vomiting, anorexia, headache, weakness, and diarrhea or constipation. Elevations of aspartate aminotransferase (AST, formerly SGOT) and alanine aminotransferase (ALT, formerly SGPT) levels also may occur. Because some vitamin D preparations contain tartrazine, individuals susceptible to this chemical may develop an allergic response.

Vitamin E doses above 300 IU daily tend to result in such adverse GI reactions as nausea, vomiting, diarrhea, and abdominal cramping. Fatigue, weakness, headache, blurred vision, and rash also have been reported after vitamin E administration.

Vitamin E has been linked to increases in serum cholesterol and triglyceride levels and to decreases in serum thyroxine (T_4) and triiodothyronine (T_3) levels. Increases in urinary estrogen and androgen levels also have been noted.

At least two non-dose-related adverse reactions have been linked to vitamin E. Sterile abscesses have been documented after I.M. injection of vitamin E; for this reason, the oral route is preferred. White hair growth has been reported after oral administration of vitamin E for skin disorders accompanied by alopecia.

Adverse reactions to vitamin K primarily depend on the route of administration. Nausea, vomiting, and headache may occur with oral administration. Rapid parenteral administration may lead to transient flushing and, occasionally, dizziness, rapid and weak pulse, transient hypotension, dyspnea, cyanosis, or chest pain. Slow I.V. administration should help prevent these reactions. Infants may develop hyperbilirubinemia and jaundice with parenteral administration of phytonadione. This is particularly a problem in premature infants.

Allergic response may occur after vitamin K administration. Reactions can range from skin rashes and urticaria to severe and sometimes fatal anaphylactic reactions. Shock and cardiac or respiratory arrest have occurred with parenteral administration despite adequate dilution and slow administration.

NURSING PROCESS APPLICATION

The following information assists the nurse in caring for a patient who is receiving a fat-soluble vitamin.

Assessment
• Review the patient's history for a condition that contraindicates the use of a fat-soluble vitamin, such as hypersensitivity to the vitamin or its ingredients.
• Review the patient's history for a condition that requires cautious use of ergocalciferol, such as heart disease, renal calculus, arteriosclerosis, use of cardiac glycosides, or increased sensitivity to vitamin D analogues.
• Assess the patient for adverse reactions to the prescribed fat-soluble vitamin, such as toxicity, GI upset, headache, or skin rashes.
• Review the patient's medication history to identify the use of drugs that may interact with the fat-soluble vitamin, such as mineral oil or warfarin.
• Assess the effectiveness of the fat-soluble vitamin regularly.
• Assess the patient's skin integrity during vitamin A therapy.
• Assess the patient's serum calcium and phosphorus levels regularly during vitamin D therapy.
• Assess the patient for diarrhea during vitamin E therapy.
• Assess the patient for cardiovascular dysfunction during parenteral vitamin K therapy.
• Evaluate the patient's and family's knowledge about the prescribed fat-soluble vitamin.

Nursing diagnoses

The following examples represent appropriate nursing diagnoses for a patient receiving a fat-soluble vitamin.

• Potential for injury related to a preexisting condition that contraindicates the use of a fat-soluble vitamin
• Potential for injury related to a preexisting condition that requires cautious use of ergocalciferol
• Potential for injury related to adverse drug reactions
• Impaired tissue integrity related to the adverse integumentary effects of vitamin A
• Altered protection related to soft tissue calcification from high-dose vitamin D therapy
• Diarrhea related to the adverse GI effects of vitamin E
• Decreased cardiac output related to the adverse cardiovascular effects of parenteral vitamin K
• Knowledge deficit related to the prescribed fat-soluble vitamin

Planning and implementation

• Do not administer a fat-soluble vitamin to a patient with a condition that contraindicates its use.
• Administer ergocalciferol cautiously to a patient at risk because of a preexisting condition.
• Monitor the patient closely for adverse reactions, especially toxicity, because fat-soluble vitamins can accumulate in the body.
• *Monitor closely for hypersensitivity reactions during parenteral vitamin therapy. Keep emergency equipment nearby.*
• *Monitor the patient's fat-soluble vitamin intake from foods, dietary supplements, self-administered drugs, and prescription drugs to avoid possible toxicity.*
• Administer vitamin A with food to stimulate bile secretion, which aids absorption and decreases nausea.
• Avoid I.M. or S.C. administration of menadiol sodium diphosphate or phytonadione in a patient with hypoprothrombinemia because hemorrhage or hematoma may develop.
• *Do not administer vitamin E intravenously.*
• Inspect the patient's injection site for sterile abscess formation after administering vitamin E.
• *Monitor the patient for signs of continued bleeding, such as hematuria, oozing around I.V. catheters, petechiae, and bruising or bleeding from mucous membranes, during vitamin K therapy. Do so until prothrombin times return to normal. Apply pressure to control bleeding after I.M. administration.*
• Monitor bilirubin levels in a neonate receiving vitamin K.
• Take safety precautions if dizziness or lethargy occurs. For example, keep the bed in the low position and supervise patient activities.
• Store parenteral vitamin K in a light-resistant container.
• Notify the physician if adverse reactions occur.

• Monitor the patient receiving high-dose vitamin A therapy for changes in epithelial tissues, such as dry, itchy skin, dry nose and mouth, inflammation of oral mucous membranes, or hair loss.
• Apply a moisturizing cream to dry skin several times a day, if prescribed, to prevent skin breakdown.
• Offer the patient frequent sips of water to relieve dry mouth and apply petroleum jelly to dry lips and nostrils to prevent further drying.
• Consult the physician regarding discontinuation of vitamin A therapy if epithelial tissue changes become severe or persist.
• *Perform a baseline evaluation of the patient's usual patterns of diet and exposure to sunlight to avoid overadministration of vitamin D. Such foods as milk and cereals are fortified with vitamin D; sunlight also is an indirect source of vitamin D. Monitor the diet to ensure that the patient obtains sufficient amounts of calcium to enhance the effectiveness of vitamin D.*
• Monitor the patient's eating and bowel habits; dry mouth, nausea, vomiting, metallic taste, and diarrhea or constipation can be early indications of vitamin D toxicity.
• Monitor serum and urine calcium levels and serum levels of phosphorus, magnesium, blood urea nitrogen (BUN) and alkaline phosphatase for a patient receiving vitamin D therapy. The product of serum calcium and serum phosphorus levels (serum calcium level multiplied by serum phosphorus level) should remain below 70 to avoid calcification of soft tissue. A decrease in the serum level of alkaline phosphatase usually precedes hypercalcemia. Alert the physician if abnormalities occur.
• Monitor hydration if the patient develops diarrhea during vitamin E therapy. Obtain a prescription for an antidiarrheal agent, if needed.
• *Monitor the patient for severe adverse reactions to I.V. AquaMEPHYTON, particularly if it is given rapidly. This route is reserved for situations in which rapid correction of hypoprothrombinemia is necessary. If this drug must be given I.V., be sure to dilute it according to the manufacturer's guidelines and to administer it slowly: never faster than 1 mg/minute. Observe the patient closely for signs of allergic reactions, and notify the physician immediately if they appear. Be prepared to intervene if hypotension, bronchospasm, or cardiac or respiratory arrest occurs.*

Patient teaching

• Teach the patient and family the name, dose, frequency, action, and adverse effects of the prescribed fat-soluble vitamin.
• Inform the patient of the RDA and food sources for the prescribed fat-soluble vitamin.

• *Advise the patient that fat-soluble vitamins are potent drugs that can be toxic to anyone for whom they are not prescribed.*

• *Instruct the patient to take vitamin A with food to aid absorption and reduce nausea.*

• Instruct the patient to avoid using mineral oil during vitamin A therapy because it decreases absorption.

• *Teach the patient to identify and report the signs and symptoms of vitamin A toxicity.*

• Caution the patient receiving isotretinoin to avoid prolonged exposure to sunlight or to use a sunscreen to avoid photosensitivity reactions.

• *Inform the female patient that fetal abnormalities may occur if isotretinoin is taken during pregnancy. Advise her to use an effective contraceptive method and notify the physician if she becomes pregnant.*

• Instruct the patient to protect vitamin A preparations from light and heat to prevent deterioration.

• Teach proper storage procedures to avoid loss of vitamin A in food; 5% to 10% of vitamin A activity is lost when frozen foods are stored for 12 months at -23° C.

• *Instruct the patient to take vitamin D with food to prevent adverse GI reactions and promote absorption.*

• Teach the patient to identify and report the signs and symptoms of hypercalcemia.

• Caution the patient about the potential adverse effects of self-medication with high dosages of vitamin E.

• Instruct the patient to store vitamin E in a cool, dark place.

• *Caution the patient to take oral vitamin K with food to promote absorption and decrease nausea.*

• Instruct the patient receiving oral vitamin K for vitamin K deficiency to increase the dietary intake of vitamin K to decrease the risk of developing an ongoing deficiency.

• Instruct the patient to notify the physician if adverse reactions occur.

Evaluation

The following examples represent appropriate evaluation statements for a patient receiving a fat-soluble vitamin.

• The patient has no conditions that contraindicate fat-soluble vitamin therapy.

• The patient exhibits no complications in the preexisting condition linked to the prescribed fat-soluble vitamin.

• The patient exhibits no adverse reactions to the prescribed fat-soluble vitamin.

• The patient maintains normal tissue integrity during vitamin A therapy.

• The patient maintains normal calcium and phosphorus levels during vitamin D therapy.

• The patient maintains usual bowel patterns during vitamin E therapy.

• The patient remains free from cardiovascular problems during parenteral therapy with vitamin K.

• The patient and family express an accurate understanding of the points taught about the prescribed fat-soluble vitamin.

• The patient correctly identifies the signs and symptoms of vitamin toxicity.

WATER-SOLUBLE VITAMINS

Water-soluble vitamins include B-complex vitamins (thiamine, riboflavin, nicotinic acid, pyridoxine, para-aminobenzoic acid (PABA), pantothenic acid, biotin, choline, inositol, folic acid, and cyanocobalamin), and vitamin C (ascorbic acid). Although different in structure and function, the B-complex vitamins are grouped together because they originally were derived from all liver and yeast foods that contained antiberiberi properties. This section discusses thiamine (B_1), riboflavin (B_2), nicotinic acid or niacin (B_3), pyridoxine (B_6), and vitamin C in detail. (For information about folic acid and cyanocobalamin vitamin B_{12} and their roles in hematopoiesis, see Chapter 35, Hematinic Agents.) Although PABA is not considered a true vitamin, it is a precursor to folic acid. Therefore, it is discussed briefly in this section along with pantothenic acid, biotin, choline, and inositol.

The water-soluble vitamins are absorbed readily via the watery medium of the small intestine. They all function as coenzymes in various cellular enzymatic reactions, except vitamin C. Researchers believe that vitamin C participates in oxidation and reduction reactions used in cellular respiration. (For a summary of the dietary sources and daily requirements of these vitamins, see *Water-soluble vitamins: Food sources and RDAs.*)

PHARMACOKINETICS

Thiamine, riboflavin, nicotinic acid, pyridoxine, and vitamin C are absorbed well after administration and are distributed widely in the body, except for pyridoxine—which is stored primarily in the liver. Thiamine and nicotinic acid are metabolized in the liver; riboflavin and pyridoxine, in RBCs and the liver. Riboflavin also undergoes metabolism in GI mucosal cells. Vitamin C is oxidized reversibly to dehydroascorbic acid. All of these water-soluble vitamins are excreted in the urine, although some riboflavin also is excreted in the feces.

Absorption, distribution, metabolism, excretion

After administration of small oral doses, thiamine is absorbed readily. Absorption occurs through sodium-dependent active transport and usually is limited to 8 to 15 mg

Water-soluble vitamins: Food sources and RDAs

To prevent chronic deficiencies, the nurse should teach the patient about dietary sources of and recommended daily allowances (RDAs) for vitamins B and C. The chart below provides this information with the RDAs grouped by age and condition.

VITAMIN	FOOD SOURCES	RDAs
thiamine (B₁)	Yeast, whole grain and enriched cereals and breads, legumes, nuts, pork, and organ meats	Infants to age 12 months: 0.3 to 0.4 mg Children ages 1 to 10: 0.7 to 1.0 mg Males ages 11 and older: 1.2 to 1.5 mg Females ages 11 and older: 1.0 to 1.1 mg Pregnant females: 1.5 mg Lactating females: 1.6 mg
riboflavin (B₂)	Milk, cheese, organ meats, eggs, whole grain and enriched cereals and breads, and green leafy vegetables	Infants to age 12 months: 0.4 to 0.5 mg Children ages 1 to 10: 0.8 to 1.2 mg Males ages 11 and older: 1.4 to 1.8 mg Females ages 11 and older: 1.2 to 1.3 mg Pregnant females: 1.6 mg Lactating females: 1.7 to 1.8 mg
nicotinic acid (B₃)	Meats, liver, poultry, fish, eggs, yeast, whole grain and enriched cereals and breads, nuts, and legumes	Infants to age 12 months: 5 to 6 mg Children ages 1 to 10: 9 to 13 mg Males ages 11 and older: 15 to 20 mg Females ages 11 and older: 13 to 15 mg Pregnant females: 17 mg Lactating females: 20 mg
pyridoxine (B₆)	Meats, eggs, liver, whole grain cereals and breads, soybeans, and vegetables	Infants to age 12 months: 0.3 to 0.6 mg Children ages 1 to 10: 1.0 to 1.4 mg Males ages 11 and older: 1.7 to 2.0 mg Females ages 11 and older: 1.5 to 1.6 mg Pregnant females: 2.2 mg Lactating females: 2.1 mg
ascorbic acid (C)	Citrus fruits, tomatoes, strawberries, cabbage greens, and potatoes	Infants to age 12 months: 30 to 35 mg Children ages 1 to 10: 40 to 45 mg Males ages 11 and older: 50 to 60 mg Females ages 11 and older: 60 mg Pregnant females: 70 mg Lactating females: 90 to 95 mg

per day. At high concentrations, passive diffusion also occurs. Absorption may be improved by giving divided doses with food. Rapid and complete absorption occurs with I.M. administration.

Thiamine is distributed widely into body tissues. Body stores equal about 30 mg, and about 1 mg is lost each day from this supply. The body stores equal about 3 weeks' supply of the body's thiamine requirements.

Thiamine undergoes extensive metabolism in the liver. With physiologic doses, little or no thiamine is excreted unchanged in the urine. With large doses, unchanged thiamine and its metabolites are excreted in the urine after tissue stores are saturated.

GI absorption increases when riboflavin is taken with food and decreases in patients with hepatitis, cirrhosis, or biliary obstruction. Riboflavin, as flavin-adenine dinucleotide (FAD) and flavin mononucleotide (FMN), is distributed widely to body tissues. Limited amounts of the vitamin are stored in the liver, spleen, kidneys, and heart, mostly as FAD. Riboflavin crosses the placenta and appears in breast milk.

Riboflavin is metabolized to FMN in GI mucosal cells, RBCs, and the liver. FMN is metabolized to FAD in the liver. About 9% of a physiologic dose of riboflavin will appear in the urine. The fate of the remainder of the vitamin dose is unknown. Doses above the minimum requirement result in larger amounts excreted unchanged in the urine. Riboflavin also appears in the feces, probably as a result of synthesis by intestinal bacteria.

After oral administration, nicotinic acid and nicotinamide are absorbed readily from all portions of the GI tract. These drugs also are well absorbed from I.M. and S.C. injection sites. Nicotinic acid is distributed widely to all body tissues and is secreted in breast milk.

Nicotinic acid is converted to nicotinamide in the body, then metabolized in the liver. The metabolites of nicotinic acid are excreted in the urine. Normally, very little nicotinic acid is excreted unchanged, although greater amounts are excreted unchanged as the dose increases.

Pyridoxine is absorbed well from the GI tract after oral administration. Absorption may be decreased in patients with malabsorption syndromes or gastric resection. Pyridoxine is stored mainly in the liver, with smaller amounts in the muscle and brain. The physiologically active forms of vitamin B₆ are found in the blood as pyridoxal phosphate and pyridoxamine phosphate, which are highly protein-bound. Pyridoxine readily crosses the placenta and appears in breast milk.

Pyridoxine is converted to pyridoxal phosphate in RBCs and in the liver. Pyridoxamine phosphate is metabolized in the liver. Pyridoxine's metabolites are excreted in the urine.

Vitamin C is absorbed readily after oral administration. The absorption of dietary ascorbic acid is 80% to 90%

complete. Vitamin C is distributed widely into body tissues and is found in large concentrations in the liver, leukocytes, platelets, glandular tissues, and the lens of the eye. Ascorbic acid crosses the placenta and appears in breast milk.

Vitamin C is oxidized reversibly to dehydroascorbic acid and inactive compounds, which are eliminated in the urine as an oxalate. If high doses of ascorbic acid are administered, tissue stores become saturated and excess ascorbic acid is excreted unchanged in the urine.

Onset, peak, duration

For water-soluble vitamins, information about onset of action, peak concentration levels, and duration of action is incomplete. However, the following information is known.

The half-life of riboflavin is 66 to 84 minutes after oral or I.M. administration of a single dose. After oral administration, nicotinic acid-induced vasodilation may occur within 20 minutes and may persist for 20 to 60 minutes. Peak serum concentration occurs within 45 minutes, and the plasma half-life is 45 minutes. The half-life of pyridoxine is 15 to 20 days.

Vitamin C administration begins to reverse skeletal changes and hemorrhagic disorders in scurvy patients within 2 days to 3 weeks.

PHARMACODYNAMICS

Thiamine plays an important part in carbohydrate metabolism by acting as a coenzyme. However, it shows no pharmacodynamic activity when given in therapeutic doses to normal individuals. Riboflavin plays in important role in tissue respiration. Nicotinic acid is required for lipid metabolism, tissue respiration, and glycogenolysis (splitting of glycogen in the body, yielding glucose—the primary carbohydrate in the body). Pyridoxine is used in the metabolism of proteins, carbohydrates, and fats and acts as a coenzyme in many other metabolic reactions.

Vitamin C possesses few pharmacologic actions. However, it functions in many important biochemical reactions in the body.

Mechanism of action

Thiamine combines with adenosine triphosphate (ATP) to form thiamine pyrophosphate, the active form of vitamin B_1. Thiamine pyrophosphate acts as a coenzyme in carbohydrate metabolism. Related to metabolic rate, thiamine requirements increase as carbohydrate use increases. This may be important in patients maintained on TPN, who receive most of their calories as dextrose. Thiamine also may modulate neuromuscular transmission.

Humans require an exogenous source of riboflavin. Some riboflavin is produced by intestinal bacteria, but this is not absorbed systemically. FMN and FAD are the active forms of riboflavin. Functioning as coenzymes, they work

with respiratory flavoproteins, which are involved in the metabolism of organic substrates used in tissue respiration. Riboflavin also helps maintain RBC integrity.

The body converts nicotinic acid to nicotinamide. Nicotinamide subsequently is incorporated in nicotinamide-adenine dinucleotide (NAD) and nicotinamide-adenine dinucleotide phosphate (NADP). NAD and NADP function as coenzymes that carry hydrogen in tissue respiration, glycogenolysis, and lipid metabolism. Dosages of nicotinic acid greater than 1 gram per day decrease serum low-density lipoproteins (LDLs) and very-low-density lipoproteins (VLDLs).

All three forms of vitamin B_6 are converted to pyridoxal phosphate, the active form of vitamin B_6. Humans require exogenous pyridoxine for amino acid metabolism. Pyridoxine also is involved in carbohydrate and lipid metabolism. The active form of vitamin B_6 acts as a coenzyme in many metabolic reactions and serves as a cofactor in the production of several neurotransmitters and proteins.

Vitamin C functions in many oxidative biochemical reactions. It is involved in steroid synthesis, the conversion of folic acid to folinic acid, and microsomal drug metabolism. Vitamin C also plays a role in tyrosine metabolism and as an intracellular cement in the synthesis of many intracellular substances, such as collagen, tooth and bone matrix, and capillary endothelium.

PHARMACOTHERAPEUTICS

Thiamine is used primarily to prevent and treat thiamine deficiency syndromes, such as beriberi, Wernicke's encephalopathy, and peripheral neuritis associated with pellagra. Alcoholics deficient in thiamine may exhibit Wernicke's encephalopathy and Korsakoff's psychosis. Beriberi can lead to cardiac failure. Wernicke's encephalopathy and cardiac failure are medical emergencies. Thiamine malabsorption may occur in patients with alcoholism, cirrhosis, or GI disease, requiring supplementation. Increased thiamine requirements may be associated with pregnancy, increased physical activity, hyperthyroidism, infection, and hepatic disease. Because normal carbohydrate metabolism increases thiamine metabolism, glucose administration may precipitate symptoms of thiamine deficiency. However, because of increased intake of dietary thiamine or thiamine supplements, thiamine deficiency rarely is noted in these cases.

Riboflavin is used to prevent and treat riboflavin deficiency, which rarely is severe in humans but frequently is mild. Riboflavin deficiency seldom occurs alone. It usually is associated with deficiencies of the other B vitamins. It is characterized by digestive disturbances, burning sensations of the skin and eyes, inflammation and cracking at the corners of the mouth (cheilosis), inflammation of the tongue (glossitis), headache, scaly dermatitis around the nose, depression, and forgetfulness.

Nicotinic acid and nicotinamide are used to prevent and treat nicotinic acid deficiency and pellagra. Pellagra may result from dietary deficiency, isoniazid (INH) therapy, or certain neoplasms. Nicotamide is preferred by some users because it does not produce the vasodilating effects of nicotinic acid. Nicotinic acid also is used as an adjunct to dietary therapy in patients with hyperlipidemia.

Although vitamin B_6 exists as pyridoxine, pyridoxal, and pyridoxamine, the therapeutic preparation is called pyridoxine. Pyridoxine is used to prevent and treat vitamin B_6 deficiency. Deficiencies may occur in patients with uremia, alcoholism, cirrhosis, malabsorption syndromes, or therapy with INH, cycloserine, hydralazine, ethionamide, penicillamine, or an oral contraceptive. Clinical signs of deficiency are rare. Infants exposed to high amounts of pyridoxine in utero may become pyridoxine-dependent after birth. Pyridoxine is used to treat seizures unresponsive to standard therapy in these infants. It also is used as an adjunct to other measures in treating toxicity from INH, cycloserine, or hydralazine overdose. INH-induced seizures may be treated with pyridoxine and other anticonvulsants.

Vitamin C is used primarily as a dietary supplement to prevent or treat vitamin C deficiency. It also is used to treat scurvy, the result of severe vitamin C deficiency. Vitamin C also can be used as a urinary acidifier.

thiamine, or vitamin B₁ (Betalin S). This vitamin may be given P.O., I.M., or I.V.
Usual adult dosage: for dietary supplementation, 1 to 2 mg P.O. daily; for beriberi with cardiac failure (an emergency condition called wet beriberi), 30 mg I.V. t.i.d.; for beriberi alone, 10 to 20 mg I.M. t.i.d. for 2 weeks; for thiamine deficiency in patients who are not critically ill, 5 to 30 mg P.O. daily for 1 month; for Wernicke's encephalopathy, 100 mg I.V. daily.
Usual pediatric dosage: for dietary supplementation, 0.3 to 0.5 mg P.O. daily for infants, or 0.5 to 1 mg P.O. daily for older children.

riboflavin, or vitamin B₂. This drug is used to prevent or treat riboflavin deficiency.
Usual adult dosage: for dietary supplementation, 1 to 4 mg P.O. daily; for riboflavin deficiency, 5 to 30 mg P.O. daily in divided doses. Ocular and dermatologic manifestations may improve within several days.
Usual pediatric dosage: for riboflavin deficiency, 3 to 10 mg P.O. daily.

nicotinic acid, niacin, or vitamin B₃ (Nicobid, Nicolar). This drug may be given P.O., I.M., S.C., or I.V. For I.V. administration, the drug must be diluted to 10 mg/ml and infused slowly at a rate not to exceed 2 mg/minute. Oral administration should begin with small doses to avoid vasodilation reactions.
Usual adult dosage: for nicotinic acid deficiency, 10 to 20 mg P.O. daily; for pellagra, 300 to 500 mg P.O. daily in divided doses; for hyperlipidemia, 1.5 to 6 grams P.O. given in two to four divided doses.
Usual pediatric dosage: for pellagra, 100 to 300 mg P.O. daily, depending on the severity of the disease.

nicotinamide, or niacinamide. Used by the body as a source of nicotinic acid, nicotinamide does not possess the vasodilating or hypolipidemic effects of niacin. It is used to prevent and treat pellagra.
Usual adult dosage: for nicotinic acid deficiency, 10 to 20 mg P.O. daily; for pellagra, 300 to 500 mg P.O. daily in divided doses.

pyridoxine, or vitamin B₆ (Beesix, Hexa-Betalin). Requirements are higher in those receiving INH or an oral contraceptive. Pyridoxine may be given by the P.O., I.M., I.V., or S.C. route.
Usual adult dosage: to treat pyridoxine deficiency, 2.5 to 10 mg P.O. daily for 3 weeks, with recommended follow-up treatment with multivitamins containing 2 to 5 mg of pyridoxine; to prevent pyridoxine deficiency in patients receiving INH or penicillamine, 10 to 50 mg P.O. daily; to prevent seizures in patients receiving cycloserine, 100 to 300 mg P.O. daily in divided doses; to treat seizures induced by acute INH intoxication, 1 to 4 grams of pyridoxine I.V., followed by 1 gram I.M. every 30 minutes until the total dosage is given. The total pyridoxine dosage should approximate the amount of INH ingested and be used an an adjunct to other anticonvulsant therapy.
Usual pediatric dosage: for pyridoxine-dependent infants, 10 to 100 mg I.M. or I.V. for seizure activity. If the response to pyridoxine is positive, these infants may require 2 to 100 mg P.O. daily for life.

vitamin C, or ascorbic acid (Cecon, Cebid, Ce-Vi-Sol). This drug may be administered P.O., I.M., I.V., or S.C.
Usual adult dosage: to prevent scurvy, 75 to 150 mg P.O. daily; to treat scurvy, 100 mg to 500 mg P.O. daily in 1 or 2 divided doses for 2 to 3 weeks; to acidify the urine, 4 to 12 grams daily in divided doses.

Drug interactions

No clinically significant interactions occur with thiamine or riboflavin. Clonidine may block the flushing reaction associated with niacin. Combined therapy with niacin and lovastatin may cause rhabdomyolysis and myopathy. Pyridoxine accelerates the metabolism of levodopa, which decreases control of parkinsonian signs and symptoms.

Vitamin C may increase iron absorption and decrease warfarin effects. Concomitant administration of large doses of vitamin C may affect the excretion of acidic and basic drugs.

ADVERSE DRUG REACTIONS

In most cases, thiamine administration does not result in adverse reactions or toxicity; reactions that do occur seem to be non-dose-related. Because excess amounts are excreted in the urine, overdose cannot occur. Various nonspecific reactions that have been reported include nausea, anxiety, sweating, and sensations of warmth. Allergic reactions have occurred with parenteral administration, ranging from itching and urticaria to cardiovascular failure and death.

Riboflavin is considered nontoxic. Despite the administration of large quantities of the vitamin, no adverse reactions have been reported. This may be related to its short half-life in the body and the rapid excretion of excess amounts in the urine.

Although nicotinic acid and nicotinamide may be used interchangeably to correct niacin deficiency, nicotinamide produces fewer adverse reactions. The most common adverse reaction to nicotinic acid is vasodilation, which typically occurs with large doses. The cutaneous blood vessels of the face, neck, and chest are affected most. Tolerance to this effect may occur within 2 weeks. Sensations of flushing and warmth, itching, tingling, and hypotension have been reported with oral and parenteral administration. GI reactions also may occur, including nausea, vomiting, diarrhea, and abdominal pain. Hyperglycemia and hyperuricemia may occur with nicotinic acid therapy. Abnormalities of liver function tests, including increased serum bilirubin, have been documented. Nicotinic acid products that contain tartrazine may cause allergic-type responses in sensitive individuals.

In therapeutic doses, pyridoxine results in few if any adverse reactions. Very large doses, roughly 1,000 times the RDA, have resulted in nervous system damage. Patients have developed difficulty with balance and a sensory neuropathy after ingestion of 2 to 6 grams of pyridoxine. Other nervous system effects, such as drowsiness and paresthesia, have occurred with smaller doses of this vitamin.

Few adverse reactions are associated with ascorbic acid administration. However, because many people use large doses of vitamin C to treat such conditions as the common cold, the nurse should be aware of the adverse reactions. Dose-related reactions include diarrhea and the precipitation of oxalate or urate renal calculi. The development of renal calculi results from urine acidification. Dental erosion has occurred with the long-term use of chewable vitamin C. Patients may complain of tenderness at the injection site after I.M. administration. Rapid I.V. administration may cause brief dizziness. Ascorbic acid products that contain tartrazine may cause allergic responses in sensitive individuals.

NURSING PROCESS APPLICATION

The following information assists the nurse in caring for a patient who is receiving a water-soluble vitamin.

Assessment
• Review the patient's history for a preexisting condition that contraindicates the use of a water-soluble vitamin, such as known hypersensitivity to the agent or its ingredients, hepatic dysfunction, active peptic ulcer disease, severe hypotension, or arterial hemorrhage.
• Review the patient's history for a preexisting condition that requires cautious use of a water-soluble vitamin, such as gallbladder disease, diabetes mellitus, gout, coronary artery disease, or a history of renal calculi.
• Assess the patient for adverse reactions to the prescribed water-soluble vitamin, such as GI distress or allergic reactions.
• Review the patient's medication history to identify the use of drugs that may interact with the water-soluble vitamin, such as clonidine, lovastatin, levodopa, iron, or warfarin.
• Assess the effectiveness of the water-soluble vitamin periodically.
• Evaluate the patient's and family's knowledge about the prescribed water-soluble vitamin.

Nursing diagnoses
The following examples represent appropriate nursing diagnoses for a patient receiving a water-soluble vitamin.
• Potential for injury related to a preexisting condition that contraindicates the use of a water-soluble vitamin
• Potential for injury related to a preexisting condition that requires cautious use of a water-soluble vitamin
• Potential for injury related to adverse reactions to the prescribed water-soluble vitamin
• Knowledge deficit related to the prescribed water-soluble vitamin

Planning and implementation
• Do not administer a water-soluble vitamin to a patient with a condition that contraindicates its use.
• Administer a water-soluble vitamin cautiously to a patient at risk because of a preexisting condition.
• Monitor the patient closely for adverse reactions during therapy with a water-soluble vitamin.
• Inquire about tartrazine or aspirin hypersensitivity before administering nicotinic or ascorbic acid products with tartrazine. Patients who are aspirin-sensitive commonly are sensitive to tartrazine as well. The sensitive patient should

receive a test dose or another product. Monitor the patient closely for signs and symptoms of an allergic response.

• *Monitor the patient for allergic reactions to parenteral thiamine, which may range from itching and urticaria to cardiovascular failure and death. Keep emergency equipment nearby.*

• Check liver function tests, blood glucose levels, and serum uric acid levels frequently during nicotinic acid therapy to detect abnormalities.

• *Do not test a diabetic patient's urine for glucose with a cupric sulfate tablet (Clinitest) because a false-positive reaction can occur during therapy with nicotinic acid or large doses of vitamin C. Also, do not use glucose oxidase methods (Clinistix, Diastix, or Tes-Tape) for urine glucose testing during high-dose, vitamin C therapy because a false-negative result can occur.*

• Monitor hydration if the patient experiences nausea, vomiting, or diarrhea. Obtain a prescription for an antiemetic or antidiarrheal agent, as needed.

• Take safety precautions if the patient experiences balance problems or drowsiness during high-dose pyridoxine therapy. For example, keep the bed in the low position and supervise ambulation.

• *Administer thiamine in divided doses with food to improve absorption. Also administer riboflavin with food.*

• Expect to administer thiamine to a patient receiving TPN because thiamine requirements increase as carbohydrate use increases.

• Begin oral nicotinic acid therapy with small doses as prescribed to avoid vasodilation.

• Notify the physician if adverse reactions occur.

Patient teaching

• Teach the patient and family the name, dose, frequency, action, and adverse effects of the prescribed water-soluble vitamin.

• *Inform the patient of the RDA and food sources for the prescribed water-soluble vitamin.*

• Inform the patient that water-soluble vitamins are drugs, and stress the importance of adhering to the therapeutic regimen.

• Instruct the patient to store the water-soluble vitamin in a cool, dark place.

• *Teach the patient to check expiration dates and to avoid purchasing more than a 3-month supply because potency tends to diminish rapidly.*

• *Teach the patient to take thiamine or riboflavin with food.*

• Inform the patient that riboflavin colors the urine bright yellow. This may interfere with urinalysis based on spectrometry methods or color reactions.

• Teach the patient with diabetes mellitus or a history of renal calculi and who is receiving an oral anticoagulant to avoid large doses of ascorbic acid. Ascorbic acid can in-

terfere with urine testing for glucose or cause precipitation of renal calculi and may interfere with the action of warfarin.

• *Inform the patient that large doses of nicotinic acid can cause vasodilation of the face, neck, and chest. Reassure the patient that tolerance usually occurs within 2 weeks, returning the color in these areas to normal.*

• Inform the patient that dental erosion may occur with long-term use of chewable vitamin C.

• Advise the patient to avoid activities that require alertness if drowsiness or balance problems occur during pyridoxine therapy.

• Instruct the patient to notify the physician if adverse reactions occur.

Evaluation

The following examples represent appropriate evaluation statements for a patient receiving a water-soluble vitamin.

• The patient has no conditions that contraindicate therapy with a water-soluble vitamin.

• The patient exhibits no signs of complications in the preexisting condition linked to the use of the prescribed water-soluble vitamin.

• The patient experiences no adverse reactions to the prescribed water-soluble vitamin.

• The patient and family express an accurate understanding of the points taught about the prescribed water-soluble vitamin.

• The patient correctly identifies adverse reactions to the prescribed water-soluble vitamin.

OTHER WATER-SOLUBLE VITAMINS

Other water-soluble agents include the B-complex vitamins para-aminobenzoic acid, pantothenic acid, biotin, choline, and inositol.

Para-aminobenzoic acid (PABA) is not a true vitamin, but is part of the B-complex group because it is a precursor of folic acid. Present in small amounts in cereal, eggs, milk, and meats, PABA has no known nutrient value. However, it is used topically as a sunscreen agent.

Pantothenic acid is abundant in beef, egg yolks, and organ meats; therefore, deficiency in humans is rare. Although no clearly defined uses for this vitamin exist, it commonly is included in multivitamin preparations.

Biotin appears in yeast, grains, nuts, vegetables, fruits, organ meats, egg yolks, poultry, and seafood and is synthesized in the GI tract. It may play a role in fat and carbohydrate metabolism.

Choline, present in vegetable and animal fat and in egg yolks, is not considered an essential vitamin. It plays a role in fat metabolism and is a precursor of the neurotransmitter acetylcholine.

Inositol is present in plants, fruits, and whole-grain cereals and is synthesized in the GI tract. Inositol is not an essential vitamin. However, it plays some role in fat metabolism.

MINERALS (TRACE ELEMENTS)

This section discusses minerals that are used as nutritional supplements, including chromium, copper, fluoride, iodine, manganese, molybdenum, selenium, and zinc. (For a discussion of the mineral iron, see Chapter 35, Hematinic Agents.)

These minerals are inorganic chemicals found in all living tissues. Because most are required in very small quantities in the diet, they are known as *trace elements.* Usually, minerals are widely available in foods in the normal diet. (For more information, see *Food sources of trace minerals.*) Deficiencies are unusual unless some factor inhibits absorption or a patient requires long-term TPN and does not receive adequate supplementation. Research into the effects of trace mineral deficiencies has been difficult because of the small amounts of the minerals needed to maintain health and their widespread availability in the diet. For these reasons, RDAs for many minerals have not been established.

Minerals perform a wide variety of functions in the body. Many function as components of enzyme systems, regulating or enhancing enzyme reactions. Some act as building materials for cells, bones, and teeth. Others play a role in such essential body processes as nerve transmission, cellular respiration, glucose metabolism, or hormone functions. In some of these functions, the involved mineral is recognized as an essential component for normal functioning. For others, the evidence is not as clear. Additional research is needed to expand knowledge about these elements.

Food sources of trace minerals

To help prevent the development of nutritional deficiencies, the nurse should teach the patient about dietary sources of trace minerals. The nurse must remember, however, that the mineral content of foods depends on the mineral content of the soil, water, and grazing land.

VITAMIN	SOURCES
chromium	Yeast, cereal grains, meats
copper	Meats, seafood, legumes, whole grain cereals, liver
fluoride	Fluoridated water, seafood
iodine	Iodized salt, seafood
manganese	Green leafy vegetables, whole grains, legumes
molybdenum	Liver, milk, vegetables, legumes, cereal grains
selenium	Meats, seafood, dairy products, whole grains, vegetables
zinc	Whole grains, meats, dairy products, seafood

PHARMACOKINETICS

The pharmacokinetics of chromium, copper, fluoride, iodine, manganese, molybdenum, selenium, and zinc vary greatly.

Absorption, distribution, metabolism, excretion

Poorly absorbed after oral administration, chromium is distributed widely to many tissues. It is excreted in the urine.

After oral administration, copper is absorbed and is distributed mostly to the liver. It is excreted in the feces via bile.

Fluoride, as sodium fluoride, is absorbed completely from the GI tract after oral administration, but calcium fluoride and bone meal are absorbed slowly and variably. Fluoride is distributed mostly to bone and developing teeth. Fluoride is not metabolized and is excreted mainly in the urine.

Iodine is absorbed rapidly and completely from the GI tract as iodide. The highest concentration of iodine is in the thyroid gland. Iodine is not metabolized, but is incorporated into the tyrosine residues of thyroglobulin to produce thyroid hormones. When broken down, these hormones release iodine, which is reabsorbed by the thyroid. Unabsorbed iodine is 40% to 80% excreted in the urine.

Manganese is absorbed poorly from the GI tract. It is distributed widely to bone, the pituitary gland, liver, pineal gland, and lactating mammary glands. High concentrations are found in mitochondria and cell nuclei. Manganese is not metabolized and is excreted mainly in the feces via bile.

Molybdenum is absorbed well after oral administration and is distributed mostly to the liver, kidneys, spleen, lungs, brain, and muscle. Molybdenum is not known to undergo metabolism other than its incorporation into enzymes. It is excreted primarily in the urine, with small amounts lost in the feces via bile.

Selenium is absorbed well after oral administration and is distributed to the kidneys, liver, muscle, and skin. Selenium is incorporated into glutathione peroxidase but otherwise is not metabolized. It is excreted primarily in the urine, although significant losses occur in the feces.

Many factors influence zinc absorption. Amino acids and vitamin C increase zinc absorption; calcium and phosphate decrease it. High-fiber foods, such as bran, can interfere with zinc absorption. Zinc is distributed to bone and hepatic, pancreatic, retinal, and gonadal tissues. It is not metabolized and is excreted in urine, feces, and perspiration.

PHARMACODYNAMICS

The trace elements exhibit varying pharmacodynamic properties.

Mechanism of action

Chromium potentiates the action of insulin and is involved in the regulation of lipoprotein metabolism.

Copper functions as a component of enzymes involved in RBC formation, WBC formation, cellular energy production, elastin and collagen synthesis, and glucose and catecholamine metabolism.

Fluoride is incorporated into teeth and bone. Deposited in tooth enamel, it makes teeth resistant to acid dissolution and to formation of dental caries. Oral fluoride works best in developing teeth. After tooth calcification is complete, fluoride strengthens surface enamel. Fluoride also increases skeletal mass and density.

Iodine is essential in manufacturing thyroid hormones. By itself, it has no known metabolic function.

Manganese is involved in activating many metalloenzymes, such as pyruvate carboxylase and superoxide dismutase. Manganese and other metals activate enzymes involved in the metabolism of carbohydrates, proteins, and lipids.

Molybdenum functions as a component of xanthine oxidase, sulfite oxidase, and aldehyde oxidase, all enzymes integral to a number of metabolic reactions.

Selenium functions as an antioxidant. By incorporation into glutathione peroxidase, it helps protect cell membranes and structures from destruction by oxidation.

Zinc acts as a component of many zinc metalloenzymes and metalloproteins, such as alcohol dehydrogenase and carbonic anhydrase. It is involved in ribonucleic acid and protein metabolism, acts as a stabilizer of cell membranes, and interacts with insulin. Physiologic functions of zinc include cell growth and proliferation, sexual maturation and reproduction, taste, wound healing, and immune defenses.

PHARMACOTHERAPEUTICS

The trace elements chromium, copper, fluoride, iodine, manganese, molybdenum, selenium, and zinc may be used to treat specific nutritional deficiencies or to prevent deficiencies, such as in patients receiving TPN.

chromium (Chroma-Pak). This mineral is indicated primarily for patients receiving long-term TPN.
Usual adult dosage: 10 to 20 mcg I.V. daily or 50 to 200 mcg P.O. daily.

copper (Coppertrace). Used primarily as a supplement in TPN, copper also is used for patients on vegetarian diets and those with disease states that affect the absorption or excretion of copper, such as sprue, nephrosis, cancer, or burns. Copper deficiency also may result in patients receiving molybdenum. The daily dosage of copper varies with the patient's age and health.
Usual adult dosage: 0.5 to 1.5 mg I.V. daily or 2 to 3 mg P.O. daily.

fluoride (Luride, Pediaflor Drops). Used primarily to prevent dental caries and desensitize dentin, fluoride may be administered orally as sodium fluoride or topically onto teeth as stannous fluoride or sodium fluoride. Oral fluorides should be used by children if public water fluoride concentrations are 0.7 parts per million (ppm) or less. No guidelines for adult dosages exist. Topical fluorides, except those present in toothpaste or rinsing solutions, are applied by dental personnel only. Although sodium fluoride may be used to increase bone density and relieve bone pain in various metabolic and neoplastic bone diseases, it has not been approved for this use by the Food and Drug Administration.
Usual pediatric dosage: to prevent dental caries when the fluoride ion concentration in drinking water is less than 0.3 ppm, 0.25 mg P.O. daily for children under age 2, 0.5 mg P.O. daily for children ages 2 to 3, and 1 mg P.O. daily

for children ages 3 to 13; when the fluoride ion concentration ranges from 0.3 to 0.7 ppm, 0.25 mg P.O. daily for children ages 2 to 3 and 0.5 mg P.O. daily for children ages 3 to 13.

iodine (SSKI Solution). Used to treat goiter and hypothyroidism caused by iodine deficiency, iodine may suppress mild forms of hyperthyroidism and thyroid crisis. It is used to prepare hyperthyroid patients for thyroidectomy and may be used as an expectorant. The RDA for iodine is 150 mcg for adults, 175 mcg for pregnant females, and 200 mcg for lactating females.
Usual adult dosage: for patients on TPN, 1 to 2 mcg/kg/day; for thyroid crisis, 250 to 500 mg I.V. daily of sodium iodide or 50 to 250 mg P.O. t.i.d. of potassium iodide solution in water or juice; to prepare hyperthyroid patients for thyroidectomy, 3 to 5 drops of strong iodine solution t.i.d. for 10 days before surgery.

manganese (Manganese Gluconate). This mineral is used as a dietary supplement only. The need for manganese in human nutrition has been established; however, no RDA has been determined.
Usual adult dosage: as a dietary supplement, 5 to 50 mg P.O. daily. Those receiving TPN should receive 0.15 to 0.8 mg/day added to the solution.

molybdenum (Molypale, Molypen). This mineral is indicated primarily for patients receiving long-term TPN.
Usual adult dosage: 20 to 120 mcg I.V. daily. This may be increased to 163 mcg I.V. daily in deficiency states.

selenium (Selenitrace). Used primarily as a supplement in TPN, selenium also is used for patients with neoplasms.
Usual adult dosage: 40 to 100 mcg I.V. daily or 50 to 200 mcg P.O. daily.

zinc (Orazinc). This mineral is used to treat zinc deficiencies. The RDA is 15 mg for adults, 20 mg for pregnant females, and 25 mg for lactating females.
Usual adult dosage: for zinc deficiency, 200 to 220 mg P.O. t.i.d. (equal to 135 to 150 mg of elemental zinc daily, nine times the adult RDA). This amount may be increased for patients with diarrhea. Zinc may be added to solutions for patients receiving TPN, usually 2.5 to 6 mg I.V. daily.

Drug interactions
No significant drug interactions occur with minerals.

ADVERSE DRUG REACTIONS

With many minerals, the margin of safety between therapeutic and toxic levels is fairly narrow because of the body's limited ability to eliminate excess amounts. Most adverse reactions are related to administration of large dosages of minerals. Concentrated amounts of minerals also tend to irritate tissues they contact. GI symptoms may occur with oral administration. Phlebitis may develop if minerals are not diluted adequately before parenteral administration.

Overdose is the most common cause of adverse reactions to minerals. The patient should be monitored for toxicity any time a mineral is administered in amounts above the recommended dosage.

Chromium therapy may produce nausea, vomiting, gastric ulceration, rash, joint swelling, bronchospasm, convulsions, coma, or kidney and liver damage.

Copper therapy may produce diarrhea, lethargy, altered behavior, diminished reflexes, photophobia, or liver and kidney damage.

The patient on fluoride therapy may develop nausea, vomiting, diarrhea, abdominal pain, nervous system hyperirritability, tetany and paresthesia related to hypocalcemia, hypoglycemia, or cardiac and respiratory failure.

Iodine therapy may produce metallic taste, skin lesions, eyelid swelling, increased saliva production, iodide goiter (thyroid gland enlargement that results from ingestion of high concentrations of iodide), bloody diarrhea, fever, depression, or mouth, gum, and salivary gland tenderness.

Manganese therapy may cause anorexia, diarrhea, headache, or Parkinson-like symptoms, such as altered gait and speech impairment.

With molybdenum, goutlike symptoms can occur.

Adverse reactions to selenium therapy may include alopecia, skin lesions, GI irritation, depression, or garlic odor of breath and sweat. Acute poisoning has led to multiple organ failure and death.

Zinc therapy can result in stomach irritation, gastric ulceration, diarrhea, vomiting, elevated serum amylase levels, hypothermia, or hypotension accompanied by signs and symptoms of shock.

Hypersensitivity reactions have occurred after iodine administration. The use of stannous fluoride solutions has led to tooth discoloration. Allergy to fluoride has resulted in rash. Some products contain tartrazine, which may cause allergic-type reactions in sensitive individuals.

NURSING PROCESS APPLICATION

The following information assists the nurse in caring for a patient who is receiving a mineral.

Assessment
• Review the patient's history for a preexisting condition that contraindicates the use of a mineral, such as known hypersensitivity to the agent, acute bronchitis, tuberculosis, pregnancy, or lactation.

• Assess the patient for adverse reactions to the prescribed mineral, such as GI distress, skin lesions, CNS disturbances, or allergic reactions.

• Assess the effectiveness of the mineral periodically.

• Evaluate the patient's and family's knowledge about the prescribed mineral.

Nursing diagnoses

The following examples represent appropriate nursing diagnoses for a patient receiving a mineral.

• Potential for injury related to a preexisting condition that contraindicates the use of a mineral

• Potential for injury related to adverse reactions to the prescribed mineral

• Knowledge deficit related to the prescribed mineral

Planning and implementation

• Do not administer a mineral to a patient with a condition that contraindicates its use.

• Monitor the patient closely for adverse reactions, especially during high-dosage therapy.

• Monitor the patient for GI distress when administering an oral mineral preparation and for phlebitis when administering an I.V. preparation.

• *Dilute liquid preparations well before administration to improve the taste and decrease GI irritation.*

• Monitor hydration if the patient experiences nausea, vomiting, or diarrhea. Obtain a prescription for an antiemetic or antidiarrheal agent, as needed.

• *Dilute a parenteral mineral solution well and administer it via a central vein as prescribed to decrease vessel irritation. Discard a solution that contains minerals within 24 hours after mixing.*

• Consider the mineral content of the patient's diet in addition to the mineral supplements being taken to help prevent mineral toxicity. Watch for signs of toxicity, particularly if the patient has renal failure or hepatic disease. Monitor the patient for signs of adequate therapy so that the mineral dosage can be decreased or discontinued.

• *Document any patient history of allergy to iodine or shellfish before administering a preparation containing iodine. Be prepared to intervene if an allergic response occurs.*

• Take safety precautions if the patient displays CNS alterations, such as lethargy, hyperirritability, or altered gait.

• Obtain a prescription for an analgesic if the patient receiving manganese experiences a headache.

• Monitor the patient's vital signs regularly to detect a blood pressure decrease or a temperature increase or decrease.

• *Take seizure precautions for a patient receiving large dosages of chromium or fluoride.*

• Inspect for skin lesions in a patient receiving iodine or selenium.

• Provide a bland or pureed diet if the patient develops mouth or gum tenderness during iodine therapy.

• Monitor the patient's laboratory studies to detect decreased calcium or glucose levels, decreased amylase levels, or abnormal liver or renal function studies.

• Notify the physician if adverse reactions occur.

Patient teaching

• Teach the patient and family the name, dose, frequency, action, and adverse effects of the prescribed mineral.

• *Teach the patient that the best way to prevent mineral deficiencies is to eat a well-balanced diet of fresh foods, especially whole grain products, fruits, and vegetables. Deficiencies may develop if the patient usually eats large amounts of highly processed foods.*

• Teach the patient to preserve minerals by cooking foods in the smallest amount of water possible.

• *Teach the patient to avoid GI irritation by taking minerals with or immediately after meals, except for fluoride and zinc. These minerals should not be taken with dairy products, and zinc should not be taken with high-fiber foods, such as bran, which interfere with its absorption.*

• Teach the patient with small children to buy mineral preparations in containers with child-proof caps and to store them in a safe place, out of children's reach.

• Advise the patient to take the mineral only as prescribed to prevent toxicity.

• Teach the patient how to handle bothersome adverse reactions, such as mouth or gum tenderness.

• Caution the patient not to perform any activity that requires alertness if CNS alterations occur.

• Instruct the patient to notify the physician if adverse reactions occur.

Evaluation

The following examples represent appropriate evaluation statements for a patient receiving a mineral.

• The patient has no conditions that contraindicate mineral therapy.

• The patient experiences no adverse reactions to the prescribed mineral.

• The patient and family express an accurate understanding of the points taught about the prescribed mineral.

• The patient correctly describes how to manage adverse reactions.

OTHER NUTRITIONAL AGENTS

A relatively new nutritional agent, levocarnitine is used to treat deficiency of the amino acid carnitine.

PHARMACOKINETICS

The pharmacokinetics of levocarnitine have not been determined yet.

PHARMACODYNAMICS

A naturally occurring substance composed of amino acids that are required for mammalian energy metabolism, levocarnitine produces energy by facilitating long-chain fatty acid entry into cell mitochondria.

Primary systemic carnitine deficiency impairs fatty acid metabolism and leads to elevated triglyceride and fatty acid levels, decreased ketogenesis, and deposition of lipids in liver and muscle. Severe chronic deficiency can cause hypoglycemia, myasthenia, hypotonia, lethargy, hepatomegaly, encephalopathy, hepatic coma, cardiomegaly, congestive heart failure, cardiac arrest, neurologic disturbances, and impaired growth and development in infants.

PHARMACOTHERAPEUTICS

A new nutritional agent, levocarnitine is prescribed for patients with carnitine deficiency.

levocarnitine (Carnitor). Levocarnitine is used to treat primary systemic carnitine deficiency. It must be used with caution in a pregnant patient.
Usual adult dosage: 990 mg P.O. b.i.d. or t.i.d. as the 330-mg tablet, or 1 to 3 grams P.O. daily in evenly divided doses of the enteral liquid for a patient weighing 50 kg. For the enteral liquid form, dosage should begin with 1 gram daily and increase, as needed, to reflect patient tolerance and clinical response.
Usual pediatric dosage: 50 to 100 mg/kg/day P.O. in divided doses of the enteral liquid, with a maximum of 3 grams daily. Dosage should begin with 50 mg/kg/day and be titrated up according to tolerance and clinical response.

Drug interactions

No known interactions exist.

ADVERSE DRUG REACTIONS

The most common adverse reactions to levocarnitine include nausea, vomiting, abdominal cramps, diarrhea, and drug-related body odor. GI symptoms may be decreased by taking the drug slowly or by diluting the liquid form. Decreased dosage may diminish drug-related body odor as well as GI distress.

NURSING PROCESS APPLICATION

The following information assists the nurse in caring for a patient who is receiving levocarnitine.

Assessment
• Review the patient's history for a condition that requires cautious use of levocarnitine, such as pregnancy.
• Assess the patient for adverse reactions to levocarnitine, such as GI distress and drug-related body odor.
• Assess the effectiveness of levocarnitine periodically.
• Evaluate the patient's and family's knowledge about levocarnitine.

Nursing diagnoses
The following examples represent appropriate nursing diagnoses for a patient receiving levocarnitine.
• Potential for injury related to a preexisting condition that requires cautious use of levocarnitine
• Potential for injury related to adverse drug reactions
• Knowledge deficit related to levocarnitine

Planning and implementation
• Administer levocarnitine cautiously to a patient at risk because of a preexisting condition.
• Monitor the patient closely for adverse reactions during levocarnitine therapy.
• Monitor hydration if the patient experiences nausea, vomiting, or diarrhea. Obtain a prescription for an antiemetic or antidiarrheal agent, as needed.
• *Administer the drug slowly and dilute the liquid form or decrease the dosage as prescribed to minimize adverse reactions.*
• Monitor the patient's tolerance closely during the first week of administration and after any dosage increase.
• Monitor periodic blood chemistries, vital signs, and plasma carnitine concentrations as prescribed. Also monitor the patient's general clinical condition.
• *Use the entire or partial contents of each container immediately after opening. Discard unused contents of open containers.*
• *Do not administer levocarnitine parenterally.*
• Notify the physician if adverse reactions occur.

Patient teaching
• Teach the patient and family the name, dose, frequency, action, and adverse effects of levocarnitine.
• *Inform the patient that drug-related body odor may occur with levocarnitine use. If the odor becomes offensive, tell the patient to discuss dosage reduction with the physician.*
• Instruct the patient to take the drug slowly or dilute it to decrease GI distress.

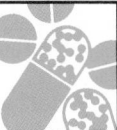

SELECTED MAJOR DRUGS

Vitamin, mineral, and other nutritional agents

The following chart summarizes the major vitamin, mineral, and other nutritional agents currently in clinical use.

DRUG	MAJOR INDICATIONS	USUAL ADULT DOSAGES	CONTRAINDICATIONS AND PRECAUTIONS
Fat-soluble vitamins			
vitamin A	Severe vitamin A deficiency with corneal changes	500,000 IU P.O. for 3 days, followed by 50,000 IU P.O. daily for 2 weeks, and then a maintenance dosage of 10,000 to 20,000 IU P.O. daily for 2 months	• Know that vitamin A is contraindicated in a patient with hypervitaminosis A or hypersensitivity to vitamin A or other ingredients in the commercial preparation.
ergocalciferol (vitamin D_2)	Familial hypophosphatemia	250 mcg to 1.5 mg P.O. daily	• Know that ergocalciferol is contraindicated in a patient with impaired renal function, hypercalcemia, or vitamin D toxicity. • Administer with extreme caution to a patient with heart disease, renal calculus, or arteriosclerosis. • Administer wtih caution to a patient receiving cardiac glycosides or one with increased sensitivity to vitamin D analogues.
menadiol sodium diphosphate (vitamin K)	Hypoprothrombinemia caused by obstructive jaundice or biliary fistulas	5 mg P.O. daily	• Know that menadiol sodium diphosphate is contraindicated in a neonate, any patient with known hypersensitivity to vitamin K, or in a pregnant patient to prevent physiologic hypoprothrombinemia or hemorrhagic disease of the newborn.
phytonadione (vitamin K)	Anticoagulant-induced hypoprothrombinemia	2.5 to 10 mg P.O., I.M., S.C., or slow I.V.	• Know that phytonadione is contraindicated in a patient with known hypersensitivity to this agent or other ingredients in the commercial preparation.
Water-soluble vitamins			
thiamine (vitamin B_1)	Thiamine deficiency	5 to 30 mg P.O. daily	• Know that thiamine is contraindicated in a patient with known hypersensitivity to thiamine or other ingredients in the commercial preparation.
riboflavin (vitamin B_2)	Riboflavin deficiency	5 to 30 mg P.O. daily	• Be aware that riboflavin has no known contraindications or precautions.
nicotinic acid (niacin, vitamin B_3)	Nicotinic acid deficiency Hyperlipidemia	10 to 20 mg P.O. daily 1 to 5 grams P.O. daily, given in two to four divided doses	• Know that nicotinic acid is contraindicated in a patient with hepatic dysfunction, active peptic ulcer disease, severe hypotension, arterial hemorrhage, or known hypersensitivity to the agent. • Administer with caution to a patient with gallbladder disease, diabetes mellitus, gout, or coronary artery disease.
pyridoxine (vitamin B_6)	Pyridoxine deficiency	2.5 to 10 mg P.O. daily for 3 weeks, followed by 2 to 5 mg P.O. daily	• Know that pyridoxine is contraindicated in a patient with known hypersensitivity to the agent and that the I.V. route is contraindicated in a patient with heart disease.
ascorbic acid (vitamin C)	Ascorbic acid deficiency Scurvy	70 to 150 mg P.O. daily 100 to 500 mg P.O. daily in divided doses for 2 to 3 weeks	• Administer long-term or high-dose ascorbic acid therapy with caution to a patient with a history of renal calculi.

(continued)

SELECTED MAJOR DRUGS

Vitamin, mineral and other nutritional agents *(continued)*

DRUG	MAJOR INDICATIONS	USUAL ADULT DOSAGES	CONTRAINDICATIONS AND PRECAUTIONS
Trace minerals			
iodine	Thyroid crisis	250 to 500 mg I.V. daily of sodium iodide or 50 to 250 mg P.O. t.i.d. of potassium iodide	• Know that iodine is contraindicated in a patient with known hypersensitivity to the agent, acute bronchitis, or tuberculosis.
	Additive to TPN solution	1 to 2 mcg/kg/day	
zinc	Zinc deficiency	200 to 220 mg P.O. t.i.d.	• Know that zinc is contraindicated in a pregnant or lactating patient.
	Additive to TPN solution	2.5 to 6 mg I.V. daily	

• *Advise the patient to use the contents of each container immediately after opening and discard unused contents of open containers.*
• Stress the importance of having periodic blood studies done to determine the drug's effectiveness.
• Instruct the patient to notify the physician if adverse reactions occur.

Evaluation

The following examples represent appropriate evaluation statements for a patient receiving levocarnitine.
• The patient exhibits no signs of complications in the preexisting condition linked to levocarnitine.
• The patient experiences no adverse reactions to levocarnitine.
• The patient and family express an accurate understanding of the points taught about levocarnitine.
• The patient schedules follow-up visits for blood studies.

CHAPTER SUMMARY

Chapter 45 presented the vitamins, minerals, and other agents that are used as nutritional supplements. The four categories of drugs highlighted are fat-soluble vitamins, water-soluble vitamins, minerals (trace elements), and other nutritional agents. Here are the highlights of the chapter.
• Fat-soluble vitamins, which are organic chemical substances required in the diet, include vitamins A, D, E, and K.
• Vitamin A is necessary for vision in dim light, healthy skin and mucous membranes, and normal growth and reproduction. Vitamin D plays a role in regulating calcium and phosphorus. Vitamin E acts as an antioxidant and en-

zyme cofactor. Vitamin K stimulates the synthesis of clotting factors by the liver.
• The fat-soluble vitamins are absorbed with dietary fats in the small intestine, so they require bile salts and pancreatic lipase for absorption.
• All fat-soluble vitamins are stored, but the amount stored varies with each vitamin.
• The primary clinical indication for fat-soluble vitamins is dietary supplementation to compensate for low levels of the vitamin, which may result from inadequate intake, decreased absorption, or increased excretion. Vitamin D also is used to treat calcium and phosphorus imbalances; vitamin K has been used to treat hypoprothrombinemia caused by vitamin K deficiency.
• Adverse reactions caused by fat-soluble vitamins vary; however, nausea and vomiting commonly occur with all of them. Vitamin A may produce changes in the skin and mucous membranes and congenital anomalies. Vitamin D may result in hypercalcemia. Vitamin E has been linked to increased serum cholesterol and triglyceride levels and decreased serum thyroxine and triiodothyronine levels. Severe hypersensitivity-like reactions and death have been noted after I.V. administration of vitamin K.
• Because fat-soluble vitamins can accumulate in the body, the nurse must monitor patients for signs of toxicity and teach them about the potential hazards.
• Water-soluble vitamins, which are organic chemical substances required in the diet, include B-complex vitamins and vitamin C.
• The water-soluble vitamins, except for vitamin C, all function as coenzymes in various metabolic functions. Vitamin C may function in many oxidative biochemical reactions in the body and is involved in the synthesis of intracellular substances.
• The water-soluble vitamins are absorbed readily from the small intestine.

• Because the water-soluble vitamins are not stored to a great extent, body supplies must be replenished frequently to avoid deficiency.

• Clinical indications for water-soluble vitamins include inadequate intake, impaired absorption, increased demand, or increased excretion.

• Although generally considered nontoxic, water-soluble vitamins can cause adverse reactions, including nausea, vomiting, diarrhea, flushing, rashes, and neuropathy.

• Water-soluble vitamins can be destroyed by heat and light and should be stored in a cool, dark place. Also, because they rapidly lose their potency, they should not be stored for long periods of time.

• Water-soluble vitamins should be taken with food to decrease adverse GI reactions and to improve absorption.

• Minerals are inorganic chemical substances that are components of all living tissues.

• Minerals cannot be manufactured by the body and therefore must be obtained from exogenous sources, usually food. Because all minerals are stored by the body, mineral levels may become toxic.

• Minerals function primarily as components of other substances, such as enzymes, hormones, bones, and teeth.

• The primary clinical indication for minerals is to treat deficiencies and as a nutritional supplement, particularly in patients receiving TPN.

• The most common adverse reaction to minerals is GI irritation, which usually can be prevented by administering them with food.

• Nurses should be aware of the symptoms of toxic levels of minerals. Toxicity usually can be prevented by limiting the patient's intake of minerals to those prescribed.

• When administering minerals parenterally, the nurse must ensure that they are diluted well and administered via a central vein to prevent phlebitis.

• A relatively new nutritional agent, levocarnitine, is used to treat carnitine deficiency. Its most common adverse reactions include nausea, vomiting, abdominal cramps, diarrhea, and drug-related body odor.

STUDY QUESTIONS

See Appendix 1 for answers.

1. Fran Loomis, age 81, lives alone and does all her own food shopping. Lately, she has been losing weight and states she has little appetite. Her physician, concerned with her nutritional status, prescribes various vitamin and mineral supplements. Why would the physician prescribe vitamin A for Ms. Loomis?
(a) to prevent glaucoma
(b) to prevent cataracts
(c) to correct color blindness
(d) to improve vision in dim light

2. If Ms. Loomis had a vitamin D deficiency, which function most likely would be affected?
(a) fat metabolism
(b) carbohydrate metabolism
(c) clotting factor synthesis
(d) calcium and phosphorus balance

3. After accidentally taking an overdose of warfarin, Ben Weaver, age 57, develops hypoprothrombinemia. Which vitamin agent is the drug of choice in treating anticoagulant-induced hypoprothrombinemia?
(a) phytonadione
(b) menaquinone
(c) calcitriol
(d) menadiol

4. Because Vera Peterson, age 65, has metastatic cancer, she is receiving TPN, which supplies most of her calories as dextrose. While Ms. Peterson is receiving TPN, she should receive which vitamin because it acts as a coenzyme in carbohydrate metabolism?
(a) thiamine
(b) riboflavin
(c) nicotinic acid
(d) pyridoxine

5. Jim Swift, age 40, has been taking large quantities of chewable vitamin C as a home remedy to treat a cold. What should the nurse teach Mr. Swift about chewable vitamin C?
(a) Vitamin C should be stored in a warm, well-ventilated place.
(b) Dietary sources of vitamin C include dairy products and green vegetables.
(c) Long-term use of chewable vitamin C may cause dental erosion.
(d) Vitamin C has a narrow margin of safety, so be alert for toxicity.

6. Ruth Hoover, age 61, has a poor nutritional status from chronic alcohol abuse. Because her diet lacks various minerals, the physician prescribes a multi-mineral supplement. Which of the following statements accurately characterizes mineral supplements?

(a) The risk of toxicity is low because the dosage is low.

(b) Toxicity may occur because minerals have a narrow margin of safety.

(c) Excesses of minerals are excreted readily from the body.

(d) Supplements rarely are needed because minerals are found in highly processed foods.

7. What instructions should the nurse give Ms. Hoover about mineral administration?

(a) Take the mineral preparation on an empty stomach to promote absorption.

(b) Take the mineral preparation with milk to minimize adverse CNS reactions.

(c) Take the mineral preparation with meals to minimize GI distress.

(d) Take the mineral preparation with high-fiber foods to enhance absorption.

8. Benny Slocum, age 3 months, has primary systemic carnitine deficiency. His physician prescribes levocarnitine 250 mg P.O. t.i.d. When caring for Benny, the nurse should be alert for which adverse reactions?

(a) vomiting and diarrhea

(b) restlessness and twitching

(c) peripheral edema and hypotension

(d) bronchospasm and shortness of breath

SELECTED REFERENCES

AHFS drug information 90. (1990). Bethesda, MD: American Society of Hospital Pharmacists.

Goodman and Gilman's the pharmacological basis of therapeutics (8th ed.; 1990). Elmsford, NY: Pergamon Press.

Hansten, P., and Horn, J. (1989). *Drug interactions: The clinical significance of drug-drug interactions* (6th ed.). Philadelphia: Lea & Febiger.

Margen, S., et al. (1989). Vitamin supplementation: Fact and fancy. *Hospital Medicine,* 25(4), 102-107.

North American Nursing Diagnosis Association. (1990). *Taxonomy-Revised, with official diagnostic categories.* St. Louis: NANDA.

Thomson, E., and Cordero, J. (1989). The new teratogens: Accutane and other vitamin-A analogs. *MCN,* 14(4), 244-248.

Trevelyan, J. (1988). A vital debate: Vitamins reclassified as medicines not food. *Nursing Times,* 84(47), 30-31.

Tsallas, G., Molgat, T., and Jeejeebhoy, K. (1988). Vitamins: Part 1. *Canadian Intravenous Nurses Association Journal,* 4(2), 4-19.

Vitamin D_3 and psoriasis. (1989). *Nurses Drug Alert,* 13(7), 55-56.

ELECTROLYTE REPLACEMENT AGENTS

OBJECTIVES

After reading and studying this chapter, the student should be able to:
1. Explain the physiology of fluid and electrolyte balance.
2. Identify the roles of the major electrolytes in maintaining homeostasis.
3. Describe the pharmacokinetics, pharmacodynamics, pharmacotherapeutics, and adverse effects of potassium.
4. Describe the pharmacokinetics, pharmacodynamics, pharmacotherapeutics, and adverse effects of calcium.
5. Explain the normal functions of magnesium and sodium, their causes of insufficiency, and replacement therapy.
6. Describe how to apply the nursing process when caring for a patient who is receiving an electrolyte replacement agent.

INTRODUCTION

Electrolyte replacement agents are mineral salts that increase depleted or deficient electrolyte levels, thus helping to maintain homeostasis, or stability in body fluid composition and volume. Chapter 46 discusses the primary intracellular fluid (ICF) electrolyte, potassium; a major extracellular fluid (ECF) electrolyte, calcium; and two other electrolytes essential for homeostasis: magnesium (in ICF) and sodium (in ECF).

Physiology of fluid and electrolyte balance

Homeostasis depends on a complex interrelationship among water, electrolyte, and acid-base metabolisms. Because they are related so closely, an alteration in any one of these factors can affect the others profoundly. (For a full discussion of acid-base balance, see Chapter 47, Alkalinizing and Acidifying Agents.)

Water makes up 45% to 75% of body weight. This water is present within the cells (ICF) or outside the cells (ECF). It must be present in sufficient volume for metabolic processes to take place.

ICF and ECF contain electrolytes, substances that separate into ions when in solution and conduct a weak electrical current—hence their name. For an environment conducive to proper cell functioning, fluid volume must be adequate, and ICF and ECF must be balanced electrically—that is, the number of negatively charged ions (anions) must equal the number of positively charged ions (cations). ICF and ECF differ in electrolyte composition: ICF primarily contains the cations potassium and magnesium and the anion phosphate. ECF primarily contains the cations sodium and calcium and the anions chloride and bicarbonate. Potassium is the main cation in ICF, whereas sodium is the main cation in ECF.

These electrolytes profoundly affect water distribution, osmolality, acid-base balance, and neuromuscular irritability. Normally, the body maintains fluid volume and electrolyte concentrations within narrow limits despite a varied diet and often-changing metabolic activity. When this balance is disturbed, it causes a profound change in cells' ability to function and in muscles' ability to respond to nerve transmission.

The four major electrolytes are potassium, sodium, calcium, and magnesium. Potassium is the electrolyte most often replaced, because it is not stored in the body, and the kidneys excrete almost all that is taken in daily. Replacement therapy for sodium depletion depends on the amount of water in the body. For example, in water intoxication, the amount of water taken in exceeds the amount excreted, thereby diluting the sodium in ECF. This can occur in patients with congestive heart failure or renal failure, or during intravenous (I.V.) fluid replacement. In these cases, the treatment is to restrict water intake rather than replace sodium. When sodium is lost through burns, diarrhea, vomiting, diuretics, salt-losing renal disorders, or adrenal insufficiency, its replacement is essential to electrolyte balance.

Calcium and magnesium are stored in bone and can be mobilized if needed. Even so, losses of these electrolytes can exceed the body's ability to mobilize them.

SELECTED NURSING DIAGNOSES

Electrolyte replacement agents

The following nursing diagnoses address representative problems and etiologies that a nurse may encounter when caring for a patient who is receiving an electrolyte replacement agent. Some of these nursing diagnoses contain generalized etiologies, which the nurse must individualize based on the patient's needs. (For some common nursing diagnoses and related interventions for each drug class, see the "Nursing Process Application" sections of this chapter.)

- Altered thought processes related to mental changes caused by potassium or calcium
- Constipation related to the adverse GI effects of calcium
- Decreased cardiac output related to calcium-induced cardiac arrhythmias
- Deceased cardiac output related to the adverse cardiovascular effects of potassium
- Decreased peripheral tissue perfusion related to potassium-induced peripheral vascular collapse
- Diarrhea related to the adverse GI effects of oral potassium
- Fluid volume deficit related to the adverse GI effects of the prescribed electrolyte
- Impaired physical mobility related to the adverse musculoskeletal effects of the prescribed electrolyte
- Impaired tissue integrity related to necrosis, tissue sloughing, or venous irritation from parenteral administration of calcium

- Impaired tissue integrity related to phlebitis caused by I.V. infusion of potassium
- Knowledge deficit related to the prescribed electrolyte
- Pain related to headache caused by hypercalcemia
- Potential for injury related to a preexisting condition that contraindicates the use of an electrolyte
- Potential for injury related to a preexisting condition that requires cautious use of an electrolyte
- Potential for injury related to adverse drug reactions
- Potential for injury related to drug interactions
- Potential for injury related to renal calculi caused by high calcium levels
- Sensory-perceptual alterations (tactile) related to potassium-induced paresthesia
- Sensory-perceptual alterations (gustatory) related to calcium-induced metallic taste

---

For a summary of representative drugs, see *Selected major drugs: Electrolyte replacement agents,* page 807. For a listing of applicable nursing diagnoses that the nurse may formulate when caring for a patient receiving one of these agents, see *Selected nursing diagnoses: Electrolyte replacement agents.* For detailed information on applying the nursing process, see Chapter 6, The Nursing Process and Drug Therapy.

POTASSIUM

Potassium is the major positively charged ion (cation) in ICF. It plays an important role in maintaining the electrical excitability of nerve and muscle cells, thus enhancing nerve impulse transmission and muscle contraction. Potassium also helps maintain acid-base balance, cellular function, and enzyme action necessary to change carbohydrates into energy and to reassemble amino acids into protein.

Because the body cannot store potassium, adequate amounts must be ingested daily. If this is not possible, potassium replacement can be accomplished orally or intravenously with potassium salts.

PHARMACOKINETICS

Oral potassium is absorbed readily from the gastrointestinal (GI) tract. Extended-release preparations embedded in a wax matrix are absorbed slowly as they move through the intestine, helping minimize small bowel ulcerations associated with potassium salts. I.V. potassium is effective immediately. After absorption into ECF, 98% of the potassium passes into ICF.

Normal serum levels of potassium are maintained by the kidneys, which excrete almost 90% of excessive potassium intake. The rest is excreted in feces (9%) and sweat (1%).

The onset of action of oral potassium (liquid or powder) usually is within 30 minutes. Extended-release forms have a slower onset, usually 1 to 2 hours.

PHARMACODYNAMICS

Potassium moves quickly into ICF to restore depleted potassium levels and reestablish homeostasis. Potassium is an essential element in determining cell membrane potentials and excitability. Therefore, it is necessary for proper functioning of all nerve and muscle cells and for nerve impulse transmission. Potassium also is essential for tissue growth and repair and maintenance of acid-base balance.

PHARMACOTHERAPEUTICS

Hypokalemia is a common occurrence in conditions that increase potassium excretion. These include malabsorption, excessive vomiting or diarrhea, polyuria, some kidney diseases, cystic fibrosis, burns, an excess of antidiuretic hormone (ADH), or therapy with a potassium-depleting diuretic. Other causes of potassium depletion include alkalosis, insufficient potassium intake from starvation, and administration of a glucocorticoid, I.V. amphotericin, or I.V. solutions that contain insufficient potassium.

Apart from its role in preventing or reversing hypokalemia, potassium also is used to decrease the toxic effects of digitalis. Because potassium inhibits the excitability of the heart, insufficient potassium enhances digitalis action, which may result in toxicity.

Potassium is available in several salts. These can be administered alone or with other potassium salts or electrolytes. (For information on commercially available combination products, see *Combination potassium replacement agents.*)

potassium bicarbonate (K-Lyte). Available as effervescent tablets for oral solution, potassium bicarbonate is used to treat symptomatic hypokalemia.

Combination potassium replacement agents

Several potassium salts are available as combination products to be given orally as electrolyte replenishers.

PRODUCT	DOSAGE	NURSING IMPLICATIONS
potassium bicarbonate and potassium chloride (Klorvess, K-Lyte/Cl)	20 mEq daily or b.i.d.	• Dissolve effervescent tablets or powder completely in 4 to 8 oz (120 to 240 ml) of cold water or juice.
potassium chloride, potassium bicarbonate, and potassium citrate (Kaochlor-Eff)	20 mEq daily to q.i.d.	• Dissolve effervescent tablets completely in 4 to 8 oz of cold water or juice.
potassium bicarbonate and potassium citrate (K-Lyte/CL 50)	50 mEq daily or b.i.d.	• Be careful not to confuse these double-strength tablets with regular-strength medications. • Dissolve effervescent tablets completely in 4 to 8 oz of cold water or juice.
potassium gluconate and potassium chloride (Kolyum)	20 mEq b.i.d. to q.i.d. (children, 20 to 40 mEq/m² or 2 to 3 mEq/kg/day in divided doses)	• Dissolve liquid or powder in 1 oz (30 ml) of cold water or juice.
potassium gluconate and potassium citrate (Bi-K, Twin-K)	20 mEq b.i.d. to q.i.d. (children, 20 to 40 mEq/m² or 2 to 3 mEq/kg/day in divided doses)	• Dilute in 4 oz of cold water or juice.
potassium gluconate, potassium citrate, and ammonium chloride (Twin-K-Cl)	15 mEq b.i.d. to q.i.d.	• Dilute in 4 to 8 oz of cold water or juice.
potassium acetate, potassium bicarbonate, and potassium citrate (Trikates, Tri-K)	15 mEq t.i.d. to q.i.d. (children, 15 to 30 mEq/m² or 2 to 3 mEq/kg/day in divided doses)	• Dilute in 4 oz of cold water or juice.
potassium and sodium phosphate tablets (Uro-KP-Neutral)	2 tablets q.i.d. in 8 oz of water	• Dissolve in 8 oz of water or juice. • Be aware that this agent is prescribed primarily to replace phosphorus.
potassium and sodium phosphate capsules for oral solution (Neutra-Phos)	1 to 8 capsules daily in divided doses	• Dissolve contents of capsule in 2½ oz (75 ml) of water or juice; patient must not swallow filled capsule. • Be aware that this agent is prescribed primarily to replace phosphorus.
potassium and sodium phosphate powder for oral solution (Neutra-Phos)	2½ to 20 oz (75 to 600 ml) of reconstituted solution daily in divided doses (children ages 4 and over, same as adult; under age 4, 2 oz [60 ml] q.i.d.)	• Do not dilute solution. • Be aware that this agent is prescribed primarily to replace phosphorus.

Usual adult dosage: 25 to 50 mEq P.O. dissolved in 4 to 8 oz of cold water once or twice daily.

potassium chloride (Kaochlor; Slow-K). Chloride depletion commonly occurs simultaneously with potassium depletion. Oral potassium chloride most commonly is used by patients taking potassium-depleting diuretics.
Usual adult dosage: to prevent hypokalemia, 20 to 60 mEq P.O. daily in one to three divided doses; to treat symptomatic hypokalemia, 40 to 96 mEq extended-release capsules P.O. daily in two to three divided doses, or 20 mEq P.O. diluted in 4 oz of cold water or juice once daily to q.i.d., or when oral replacement is not feasible or hypokalemia is life-threatening, 10 mEq I.V. hourly in concentration of 40 mEq/liter or less, to a maximum of 200 mEq daily based on the patient's serum potassium level.

potassium gluconate (Kaon). This potassium salt is used to replace and maintain potassium levels.
Usual adult dosage: to treat hypokalemia, 5 to 20 mEq P.O. b.i.d. to q.i.d. Further doses are based on serum potassium determinations.

potassium phosphate (Neutra-Phos-K). Recommended as an oral supplement for phosphorus deficiency, potassium phosphate also is used to treat hypokalemia.
Usual adult dosage: 1 capsule P.O. emptied and mixed into 75 ml of cold water q.i.d. (provides 14.25 mEq of potassium and phosphate and 250 mg of phosphorus) or when oral replacement is not feasible or hypokalemia is life-threatening, 3.3 ml/day of I.V. potassium phosphate preparation diluted in I.V. solution (supplies 14.5 mEq of potassium and 935 mg of phosphate).

Drug interactions
Potassium should be used cautiously in patients receiving potassium-sparing diuretics (such as amiloride, spironolactone, or triamterene) or angiotensin converting enzyme (ACE) inhibitors (such as captopril, endopril, or lisinopril) to avoid hyperkalemia.

ADVERSE DRUG REACTIONS

Administration of potassium preparations may produce hyperkalemia if the patient's serum potassium level is not monitored closely. Hyperkalemia causes listlessness, confusion, flaccid paralysis, and paresthesia, weakness, and limb heaviness. Cardiovascular signs may include electrocardiogram (ECG) changes (prolonged PR interval; wide QRS complex; depressed ST segment; and tall, tented T waves), peripheral vascular collapse with a fall in blood pressure, cardiac arrhythmias, heart block, and possible cardiac arrest.

Oral potassium sometimes causes nausea, vomiting, abdominal pain, and diarrhea. Enteric-coated tablets may cause small-bowel ulceration, stenosis, hemorrhage, and obstruction. Because wax-matrix tablets have largely replaced enteric-coated tablets, however, this adverse reaction no longer is common.

I.V. infusion of potassium preparations can cause pain at the site and phlebitis. Infusion of potassium in patients with decreased urine production increases the risk of hyperkalemia.

NURSING PROCESS APPLICATION

The following information assists the nurse in caring for a patient who is receiving potassium.

Assessment
• Review the patient's history for a preexisting condition that contraindicates the use of potassium, such as severe renal impairment, acute dehydration, hyperkalemia, metabolic acidosis, extensive tissue breakdown, or adrenal insufficiency.
• Review the patient's history for a preexisting condition that requires cautious use of potassium, such as pregnancy or lactation.
• Assess the patient for adverse reactions to potassium, such as hyperkalemia or GI distress.
• Review the patient's medication history to identify the use of drugs that may interact with potassium, such as potassium-sparing diuretics or ACE inhibitors.
• Assess the effectiveness of potassium replacement periodically.
• Evaluate the patient's and family's knowledge about the prescribed potassium preparation.

Nursing diagnoses
The following examples represent appropriate nursing diagnoses for a patient receiving potassium.
• Potential for injury related to a preexisting condition that contraindicates the use of potassium
• Potential for injury related to a preexisting condition that requires cautious use of potassium
• Potential for injury related to adverse reactions to potassium
• Potential fluid volume deficit related to the adverse GI effects of potassium
• Knowledge deficit related to the prescribed potassium preparation

Planning and implementation
• Do not administer a potassium preparation to a patient with a condition that contraindicates its use.
• Administer a potassium preparation cautiously to a patient at risk because of a preexisting condition.

• Monitor the patient closely for adverse reactions during potassium therapy.

• *Monitor serum potassium levels closely in a patient receiving potassium. Be particularly alert for hyperkalemia in a patient whose urine output decreases during potassium therapy.*

• Monitor the patient regularly for signs and symptoms of hyperkalemia, such as listlessness, confusion, flaccid paralysis, and paresthesia, weakness, and limb heaviness.

• *Monitor the patient's ECG for changes that suggest hyperkalemia, such as prolonged PR interval, wide QRS complex, depressed ST segment, and tall, tented T waves.*

• Monitor the patient's vital signs regularly. Particularly note any decrease in blood pressure or irregular heartbeat, which may suggest hyperkalemia.

• Review the patient's diet if hyperkalemia occurs. Evaluate the patient's intake of high-potassium foods.

• Use liquid potassium in a cardiac patient who has esophageal compression from an enlarged left atrium or one with esophageal stasis or obstruction. In such a patient, tablets in wax matrix sometimes lodge in the esophagus and cause ulceration.

• *Dilute an I.V. potassium preparation as prescribed before infusion; never give as a bolus or by intramuscular (I.M.) injection.*

• *Give diluted potassium slowly I.V.; potentially fatal hyperkalemia may result from too-rapid infusion.*

• Do not mix I.V. potassium phosphate in a solution that contains calcium or magnesium because precipitates will occur.

• *Inspect the patient's I.V. site regularly for signs of phlebitis, such as redness or swelling, and ask the patient about pain at the site. If phlebitis or pain occurs, change the I.V. site location.*

• Notify the physician if the patient shows signs of hyperkalemia.

• *Administer oral potassium with or after meals to minimize GI distress.*

• Perform an abdominal assessment if the patient reports GI distress. Particularly note decreased bowel sounds or other abnormalities that may reflect an obstruction. Notify the physician of any abnormalities.

• Monitor hydration if the patient experiences nausea, vomiting, or diarrhea. Obtain a prescription for an antiemetic or antidiarrheal agent, as needed.

Patient teaching

• Teach the patient and family the name, dose, frequency, action, and adverse effects of the prescribed potassium preparation.

• *Instruct the patient to take oral potassium with or after meals to minimize GI distress.*

• *Direct the patient to dissolve all powders and tablets in at least 4 oz of water or fruit juice, as directed, and to sip the solution slowly over 5 to 10 minutes.* Also advise the patient to take capsules or tablets with plenty of liquid.

• Remind the patient not to crush or chew extended-release tablets, which will defeat the purpose of the special coating.

• *Remind the patient that although remnants of the wax matrix may appear in feces, the drug will be absorbed.*

• Advise the patient that periodic blood tests will be needed to measure serum potassium levels.

• Teach the patient to recognize and report to the physician signs or symptoms of hyperkalemia or GI distress.

Evaluation

The following examples represent appropriate evaluation statements for a patient receiving potassium.

• The patient has no conditions that contraindicate potassium therapy.

• The patient exhibits no signs of complications in the preexisting condition linked to the prescribed potassium preparation.

• The patient demonstrates no adverse reactions to the prescribed potassium preparation.

• The patient maintains normal fluid balance throughout potassium therapy.

• The patient and family express an accurate understanding of the points taught about the prescribed potassium preparation.

• The patient correctly demonstrates dilution of the prescribed potassium preparation.

CALCIUM

Calcium is a major positively charged ion (cation) in ECF. Almost all the calcium in the body—99%—is stored in bone, where it can be mobilized if necessary. It is the small amount of extracellular ionized calcium that plays an essential role in normal nerve and muscle excitability. Calcium also is integral to normal functioning of the heart, kidneys, and lungs, and it affects the blood coagulation rate and cell membrane and capillary permeability. Calcium also is a factor in neurotransmitter and hormone activity, amino acid metabolism, vitamin B_{12} absorption, and gastrin secretion. It plays a major role in normal bone and tooth formation.

When dietary intake is insufficient to meet metabolic needs, calcium stores in bone are reduced. Chronic insufficient calcium intake can result in bone demineralization. Calcium is replaced orally or intravenously with calcium salts.

PHARMACOKINETICS

Oral calcium is absorbed readily from the duodenum and proximal jejunum. A pH of 5 to 7, parathyroid hormone, and vitamin D all aid calcium absorption. Absorption also depends on dietary factors, such as calcium binding to fiber, phytates, and oxalates and to fatty acids, with which calcium salts form insoluble soaps. Therefore, consumption of calcium with large amounts of spinach, rhubarb, bran, whole grain cereals and bread, and fresh fruits and vegetables will interfere with calcium absorption.

Calcium is distributed primarily in bone. About 80% of calcium salt is eliminated in feces; the rest is excreted in urine. Intravenous calcium infusion raises blood levels immediately; levels return to normal in 30 minutes to 2 hours.

PHARMACODYNAMICS

Calcium moves quickly into ECF to restore calcium levels and reestablish homeostasis. Its action is particularly crucial in the heart, nervous system, and bone.

PHARMACOTHERAPEUTICS

The major clinical indication for I.V. calcium is to treat acute hypocalcemia, in which a rapid increase in serum calcium levels is needed. Conditions that create this need are tetany, cardiac arrest, vitamin D deficiency, parathyroid surgery, and alkalosis. Intravenous calcium also is used to prevent a hypocalcemic reaction during exchange transfusions. Calcium is helpful in treating magnesium intoxication and in strengthening myocardial tissue after defibrillation or after a poor response to epinephrine.

Oral calcium commonly is used to supplement a calcium-deficient diet or to prevent osteoporosis. Pregnancy and lactation create a need for calcium replacement, as do periods of bone growth during childhood and adolescence. Chronic hypocalcemia from such conditions as chronic hypoparathyroidism, osteomalacia, rickets, and vitamin D deficiency also is treated with oral calcium.

Calcium is available in several salts, which can be administered alone or with other calcium salts.

calcium carbonate (Os-Cal 500). Available as regular and chewable tablets, calcium carbonate is the most efficient form of calcium. It contains 40% calcium by weight and also is used as an antacid and as a treatment for hyperphosphatemia.
Usual adult dosage: as a dietary supplement, 500 mg P.O. b.i.d. to q.i.d. 1 to 2 hours after meals.

calcium chloride. Available in injectable form, calcium chloride is used in acute situations that demand immediate increases in serum calcium levels. These include tetany and cardiac arrest.
Usual adult dosage: for hypocalcemia, 500 mg to 1 gram I.V. solution (1 gram equals 13.6 mEq of calcium) at a rate no faster than 1 ml/minute (repeated in 1 to 3 days as determined by serum calcium levels); for cardiac arrest, 500 mg to 1 gram I.V. or 200 to 400 mg injected directly into ventricle as a single dose.

calcium citrate (Citracal). Available in tablet form, calcium citrate is absorbed better from the GI tract than is calcium carbonate.
Usual adult dosage: as a dietary supplement, 950 mg to 1.9 grams P.O. t.i.d. or q.i.d. 1 to 2 hours after meals.

calcium glubionate (Neo-Calglucon Syrup). Calcium glubionate is used as a dietary supplement and as a replacement for calcium deficiency. In children, it is used as a dietary supplement during periods of bone growth.
Usual adult dosage: as a dietary supplement, 5.4 grams t.i.d. or q.i.d. before meals.
Usual pediatric dosage: as a dietary supplement in children up to age 1, 1.8 grams five times a day before meals; in children ages 1 to 4, 3.6 grams t.i.d. before meals; in children over age 4, same as adult dosage.

calcium gluconate (Kalcinate). Available in oral and I.V. forms, calcium gluconate has the same clinical indications as calcium glubionate and is used for magnesium toxicity as well.
Usual adult dosage: as a dietary supplement, 11 grams P.O. daily in divided doses after meals; for hypocalcemic tetany, 4.5 to 10 mEq I.V. at a rate not exceeding 5 ml/minute; for magnesium toxicity, 4.5 to 10 mEq I.V. at a rate no faster than 5 ml/minute.
Usual pediatric dosage: as a dietary supplement, 500 to 720 mg/kg of body weight P.O. daily in divided doses after meals.

calcium lactate. Calcium lactate is used primarily as a dietary supplement.
Usual adult dosage: 7.7 grams P.O. daily in divided doses after meals.
Usual pediatric dosage: 345 to 500 mg/kg of body weight P.O. daily in divided doses after meals.

Drug interactions

Calcium preparations interact with cardiac glycosides and calcium channel blockers. (For more information, see *Drug interactions: Calcium replacement agents.*)

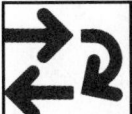

DRUG INTERACTIONS
Calcium replacement agents

Although the drug interactions involving calcium are few, they are potentially lethal and the nurse must be aware of them.

DRUG	INTERACTING DRUGS	POSSIBLE EFFECTS	NURSING IMPLICATIONS
calcium replacement agents	cardiac glycosides (digoxin, digitoxin)	Precipitate cardiac arrhythmias	• Administer calcium and cardiac glycosides simultaneously, if prescribed, by giving small amounts slowly.
	calcium channel blockers	Reduce response to calcium channel blockers	• Monitor the patient's therapeutic response to the calcium channel blocker, and expect to increase the calcium channel blocker dosage, as needed.

ADVERSE DRUG REACTIONS

Calcium preparations may produce hypercalcemia if the blood level is not monitored closely. Early signs of hypercalcemia include drowsiness, lethargy, muscle weakness, headache, constipation, and a metallic taste in the mouth. ECG changes include a shortened QT interval and heart block. Severe hypercalcemia can cause cardiac arrhythmias and arrest and, eventually, coma. Because calcium is excreted by the kidneys, high levels sometimes predispose patients to renal calculi.

Intravenous administration of calcium may cause venous irritation; I.M. injection may cause severe local reactions, such as burning, necrosis, and tissue sloughing.

NURSING PROCESS APPLICATION

The following information assists the nurse in caring for a patient who is receiving calcium.

Assessment
• Review the patient's history for a preexisting condition that contraindicates the use of calcium, such as hypercalcemia or ventricular fibrillation.
• Review the patient's history for a preexisting condition that requires cautious use of calcium, such as sarcoidosis, renal or cardiac disease, cor pulmonale, respiratory acidosis, or respiratory failure.
• Assess the patient for adverse reactions to calcium, such as hypercalcemia and tissue damage at injection sites.
• Review the patient's medication history to identify the use of drugs that may interact with calcium, such as cardiac glycosides and calcium channel blockers.
• Assess the effectiveness of calcium periodically.
• Evaluate the patient's and family's knowledge about the prescribed calcium preparation.

Nursing diagnoses
The following examples represent appropriate nursing diagnoses for a patient receiving calcium.
• Potential for injury related to a preexisting condition that contraindicates the use of calcium
• Potential for injury related to a preexisting condition that requires cautious use of calcium
• Potential for injury related to adverse drug reactions
• Knowledge deficit related to the prescribed calcium preparation

Planning and implementation
• Do not administer calcium to a patient with a condition that contraindicates its use.
• Administer calcium cautiously to a patient at risk because of a preexisting condition.
• Monitor the patient closely for adverse reactions to calcium therapy.
• Monitor the patient's serum calcium level.
• *Monitor the patient regularly for early signs of hypercalcemia, such as drowsiness, lethargy, muscle weakness, headache, constipation, and a metallic taste in the mouth.*
• *Monitor the patient's ECG for changes that suggest hypercalcemia, such as a shortened QT interval, heart block, or arrhythmias.*
• Administer I.V. calcium cautiously to prevent venous irritation. For example, warm the I.V. infusion to body temperature before administering it.
• *Administer an I.V. infusion slowly to prevent high concentrations from reaching the heart and causing cardiac arrhythmias and arrest.*
• Keep the patient recumbent for 15 minutes after injecting calcium.
• Discontinue the I.V. infusion if extravasation occurs. Also, infiltrate the area with 1% procaine and hyaluronidase to reduce vasospasm and dilute calcium, and apply warm, moist compresses to the area, as prescribed.

• Use the I.M. route in an emergency, only when the I.V. route is impossible to use. If the I.M. route is necessary, give the injection in the gluteal muscle in an adult or in the lateral thigh in an infant or small child.

• Administer an oral calcium supplement 1 to 2 hours after meals.

• *Notify the physician immediately if hypercalcemia occurs. Have emergency equipment nearby.*

• *Monitor the patient for signs of renal calculi, such as sudden flank pain and hematuria, which may occur when hypercalcemia is present.*

• Administer calcium and cardiac glycosides slowly and in small amounts to avoid precipitating arrhythmias during concomitant therapy.

• Monitor the patient's therapeutic response to the calcium channel blocker during concomitant therapy with calcium. If reduced response occurs, notify the physician and expect to increase the dosage of the calcium channel blocker as prescribed.

Patient teaching

• Teach the patient and family the name, dose, frequency, action, and adverse effects of the prescribed calcium preparation.

• *Advise the patient to avoid eating large amounts of spinach, rhubarb, bran, whole grain cereals and bread, and fresh fruits and vegetables when taking calcium because these foods interfere with calcium absorption. Or, unless instructed otherwise, the patient can take calcium tablets 1 to 2 hours after eating these foods.*

• *Suggest that the patient eat foods containing vitamin D, which enhances calcium absorption.*

• Stress the importance of having blood drawn to monitor calcium levels, as prescribed.

• Teach the patient to recognize and report the signs of hypercalcemia.

Evaluation

The following examples represent appropriate evaluation statements for a patient receiving calcium.

• The patient has no conditions that contraindicate calcium therapy.

• The patient exhibits no signs of complications in the preexisting condition linked to calcium therapy.

• The patient experiences no adverse reactions to the prescribed calcium preparation.

• The patient and family express an accurate understanding of the points taught about the prescribed calcium preparation.

• The patient correctly lists signs and symptoms of hypercalcemia.

OTHER ELECTROLYTES

Besides potassium and calcium, several other electrolytes are needed in proper amounts to maintain the body's acid-base balance and to ensure proper organ functioning. Magnesium and sodium are the most important of the other electrolytes.

Magnesium is the most common positively charged ion (cation) in ICF after potassium. It is essential in transmitting nerve impulses to muscle and in activating enzymes necessary for carbohydrate and protein metabolism. It also stimulates parathyroid hormone secretion, thus regulating ICF calcium levels, and aids in cell metabolism and in the movement of sodium and potassium across cell membranes.

Approximately 66% of the body's magnesium is stored in bone, 1% is in plasma and interstitial fluid, and the rest is in cells.

Magnesium stores may be depleted by malabsorption, chronic diarrhea, prolonged treatment with diuretics, nasogastric suctioning, prolonged therapy with parenteral fluids not containing magnesium, hyperaldosteronism, hypoparathyroidism, hyperparathyroidism, and excessive release of adrenocortical hormones.

Magnesium sulfate is the drug of choice for replacement therapy in magnesium deficiency. Severe cases can be treated using an I.V. infusion. The usual adult dosage is 5 grams in 1 liter of dextrose 5% in water (D_5W) or normal saline solution administered over 4 hours.

Intramuscular injection also may be used. For severe deficiency, the dosage is 250 mg/kg I.M. within 4 hours. For mild deficiency, the dosage is 1 gram as a 50% solution administered I.M. every 6 hours for a maximum of four doses per 24 hours.

Magnesium sulfate also is used to treat seizures, severe toxemia, and acute nephritis in children. (For more information on magnesium sulfate as an anticonvulsant, see Chapter 20, Anticonvulsant Agents.)

Sodium is the major positively charged ion (cation) in ECF. It maintains the osmotic pressure and concentration of ECF, acid-base balance, and water balance; contributes to nerve conduction and neuromuscular function; and plays a role in glandular secretion. Sodium is absorbed readily by the small intestine, and 90% of absorbed sodium can be found in ECF. It is excreted through the skin and by the kidneys.

Sodium replacement is necessary in conditions that rapidly deplete it, such as excessive loss of GI fluids or excessive perspiration. Diuretics and tap water enemas also can deplete sodium, particularly when fluids are replaced by plain water. Sodium can be lost in trauma or wound

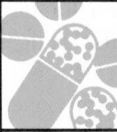

Electrolyte replacement agents

This chart summarizes the major electrolyte replacement agents currently in clinical use.

DRUG	MAJOR INDICATIONS	USUAL ADULT DOSAGES	CONTRAINDICATIONS AND PRECAUTIONS
potassium bicarbonate	Replacement electrolyte for symptomatic hypokalemia	25 to 50 mEq P.O. dissolved in 4 to 8 oz (120 to 240 ml) of cold water daily or b.i.d.	• Know that potassium bicarbonate is contraindicated in a lactating patient or one with severe renal impairment, acute dehydration, hyperkalemia, metabolic acidosis, extensive tissue breakdown, or adrenal insufficiency. • Administer with caution to a pregnant patient.
potassium chloride	Prevention of hypokalemia Replacement electrolyte for symptomatic hypokalemia	20 to 60 mEq P.O. daily in one to three divided doses 40 to 96 mEq extended-release capsules P.O. daily in two to three divided doses, or 20 mEq P.O. diluted in 4 oz of cold water or juice once daily to q.i.d., or 10 mEq I.V. hourly in concentration of 40 mEq/liter or less, to a maximum of 200 mEq daily based on patient's serum potassium level	• Know that potassium chloride is contraindicated in a patient with severe renal impairment, acute dehydration, hyperkalemia, systemic acidosis, extensive tissue breakdown, adrenal insufficiency, or therapy with a potassium-sparing diuretic. The solid form is contraindicated in a patient with a condition that can arrest or delay tablet passage through the gastrointestinal tract. • Administer with caution to a pregnant or lactating patient.
calcium carbonate	Dietary supplementation	500 mg P.O. b.i.d. to q.i.d. 1 to 2 hours after meals	• Know that calcium carbonate is contraindicated in a patient with hypercalcemia or ventricular fibrillation. • Administer with extreme caution to a patient with sarcoidosis or renal or cardiac disease.
calcium chloride	Replacement electrolyte for hypocalcemia Cardiac arrest	500 mg to 1 gram I.V. solution at a rate no faster than 1 ml/min 500 mg to 1 gram I.V. or 200 to 400 mg injected directly into ventricle as a single dose	• Know that calcium chloride is contraindicated in a patient with hypercalcemia or ventricular fibrillation. • Administer with extreme caution to a patient with sarcoidosis or renal or cardiac disease. • Administer with caution to a patient with cor pulmonale, renal disease, respiratory acidosis, or respiratory failure.
calcium glubionate	Dietary supplementation	5.4 grams t.i.d. or q.i.d. before meals	• Know that calcium glubionate is contraindicated in a patient with hypercalcemia or ventricular fibrillation. • Administer with extreme caution to a patient with sarcoidosis or renal or cardiac disease.
calcium gluconate	Dietary supplementation Replacement electrolyte for severe hypocalcemic tetany	11 grams P.O. daily in divided doses after meals 4.5 to 10 mEq I.V. at a rate no faster than 5 ml/min	• Know that calcium gluconate is contraindicated in a patient with hypercalcemia or ventricular fibrillation. • Administer calcium gluconate with extreme caution to a patient with sarcoidosis or renal or cardiac disease.

drainage, adrenal gland insufficiency, cirrhosis of the liver with ascites, inappropriate ADH secretion, and prolonged I.V. infusion of dextrose in water without other solutes.

Severe symptomatic sodium deficiency may be treated by I.V. infusion of 3% or 5% sodium chloride (NaCl) solution. Other I.V. solutions containing sodium chloride include D_5W and 0.9% NaCl; D_5W and 0.45% NaCl; dextrose 2.5% and 0.45% NaCl; and 0.9% NaCl. These solutions are used to prevent sodium depletion in those conditions that predispose the patient to sodium loss, such as severe vomiting, excessive perspiration, or fever.

Injectable sodium salts (sodium bicarbonate injection and sodium lactate injection) also are used to treat metabolic acidosis.

Intravenous solutions containing multiple electrolyte salts for treating dehydration with accompanying acidosis are available from various manufacturers.

CHAPTER SUMMARY

Chapter 46 presented the role of electrolyte replacement agents in maintaining homeostasis, or stability in body fluid composition and volume. Here are the chapter highlights.
• Fluid and electrolyte balance is essential for proper cell functioning. Water in ICF and ECF must be present in sufficient volume for metabolic processes to take place.
• Electrolytes are substances that separate into ions when in solution and conduct a weak electrical current. Those with a negative charge are anions; those with a positive charge are cations. To maintain homeostasis, the number of anions must equal the number of cations.
• Potassium, magnesium, and phosphate ions are found mainly in ICF; sodium, chloride, calcium, and bicarbonate are found mainly in ECF.
• Electrolytes profoundly affect water distribution, osmolality, acid-base balance, and neuromuscular irritability.
• Potassium is the main cation in ICF; sodium the main cation in ECF. Magnesium is the second most common cation in ICF; calcium is a major cation in ECF.
• Electrolytes are absorbed primarily through the GI tract and excreted by the kidneys. With the exception of calcium and magnesium, which are stored in bone, electrolytes are excreted by the kidneys within 24 hours. Any conditions that increase excretion or decrease absorption of electrolytes can lead to a deficiency state that disturbs homeostasis.
• Electrolytes can be replaced orally or parenterally. Calcium chloride can be injected directly into the ventricle in emergency situations.
• When administering a replacement electrolyte, the nurse must monitor for elevated blood levels of the electrolyte.

An excess of electrolytes can cause as serious an alteration in homeostasis as a deficit can. The nurse also should monitor the patient for adverse reactions to the electrolyte, attempt to determine the cause of the electrolyte deficiency (such as inadequate dietary intake), and teach the patient about the prescribed electrolyte replacement agent.

STUDY QUESTIONS

See Appendix 1 for answers.

1. Stewart Farmer, age 55, is admitted to the hospital with diabetic ketoacidosis (DKA). Laboratory tests reveal elevated blood glucose levels and seriously depressed serum potassium and bicarbonate levels. To correct Mr. Farmer's hypokalemia, the physician orders potassium chloride 40 mEq I.V. Why is hypokalemia a common occurrence in DKA and various other disorders?
(a) Large amounts of potassium are required to maintain normal ECF levels.
(b) Potassium is not readily available in food.
(c) The body cannot store potassium.
(d) Large amounts of potassium are required to maintain normal ICF levels.

2. How should the nurse administer the potassium chloride to Mr. Farmer?
(a) 20 mEq/hour by I.V. infusion
(b) 10 mEq/hour by I.V. infusion
(c) 40 mEq by I.V. bolus
(d) 20 mEq b.i.d by intermittent I.V. infusion

3. The nurse assesses Mr. Farmer for signs and symptoms of hyperkalemia, an adverse reaction to potassium. Which assessment findings suggest hyperkalemia?
(a) paresthesia, weakness, and confusion
(b) hyperexcitability, seizures, and confusion
(c) hallucinations, muscle rigidity, and clonic contractions
(d) numbness, muscle cramps, and nervousness

4. The nurse also monitors Mr. Farmer's ECG during potassium therapy. Which ECG changes suggest hyperkalemia?
(a) narrowed QRS complex and elevated ST segment
(b) elevated ST segments and tall, tented T waves
(c) widened QRS complex and elevated ST segments
(d) prolonged PR interval and tall, tented T waves

5. Michael Morgan, age 50, calls an ambulance because of severe chest pain. On the way to the emergency department (ED), he suffers cardiac arrest, and the paramedics begin cardiopulmonary resuscitation. On arrival to the ED, Mr. Morgan receives defibrillation for ventricular tachycardia. The physician administers sodium bicarbonate, epinephrine, and calcium chloride. Why is calcium chloride administered to Mr. Morgan?
(a) to enhance the effects of epinephrine
(b) to treat metabolic acidosis
(c) to strengthen myocardial tissue
(d) to prevent arrhythmias

6. Calcium chloride would have been used with caution if Mr. Morgan were receiving which drug?
(a) potassium chloride
(b) digitoxin
(c) norepinephrine
(d) magnesium sulfate

7. Cynthia Brown, age 30, is 9 months pregnant. She is admitted to the maternity unit with severe toxemia. Which of the following electrolytes is used to treat toxemia?
(a) sodium
(b) magnesium
(c) potassium
(d) calcium

SELECTED REFERENCES

AHFS drug information 90. (1990). Bethesda, MD: American Society of Hospital Pharmacists.

Farley, J. (1989). Myths and facts about electrolytes. *Nursing89, 19*(10), 80.

Goodman and Gilman's the pharmacological basis of therapeutics (8th ed.; 1990). Elmsford, NY: Pergamon Press.

Hansten, P., and Horn, J. (1989). *Drug interactions: Clinical significance of drug-drug interactions* (6th ed.). Philadelphia: Lea & Febiger.

Mathewson, M. (1989). Intravenous therapy. *Critical Care Nurse, 9*(2), 21-36.

Miller, J. (1989). Intravenous therapy in fluid and electrolyte imbalance. *Professional Nurse, 4*(5), 237-241.

North American Nursing Diagnosis Association. (1990). *Taxonomy-Revised, with official diagnostic categories.* St. Louis: NANDA.

Rutherford, C. (1989). Fluid and electrolyte therapy: Considerations for patient care. *Journal of Intravenous Nursing, 12*(3), 173-183.

ALKALINIZING AND ACIDIFYING AGENTS

OBJECTIVES

After reading and studying this chapter, the student should be able to:

1. Describe the homeostatic buffer systems and the compensatory mechanisms that maintain the acid-base balance in the blood.

2. Explain why sodium bicarbonate is used in cardiac arrest.

3. Explain how ammonium chloride, arginine chloride, and hydrochloric acid are used to treat metabolic alkalosis.

4. Explain the way acetazolamide acidifies the blood and alkalinizes the urine.

5. Discuss the action of urine-alkalinizing agents when they are used to treat drug overdose.

6. Explain why ascorbic acid is used to augment treatment of urinary tract infections.

7. Explain why the sodium content of certain alkalinizing agents must be monitored carefully in some patients.

8. Discuss the adverse reactions associated with each alkalinizing and acidifying agent.

9. Describe how to apply the nursing process when caring for a patient who is receiving an alkalinizing or acidifying agent.

INTRODUCTION

Alkalinizing and acidifying agents act to correct acid-base imbalances in the blood. They commonly are used to treat metabolic acidosis and alkalosis. An alkalinizing agent will increase the pH (hydrogen ion concentration) of the blood; an acidifying agent will decrease the pH. Some of these agents also alter urine pH, making them useful in treating some urinary tract infections and drug overdoses.

For a summary of representative drugs, see *Selected major drugs: Alkalinizing and acidifying agents,* page 819. For a listing of applicable nursing diagnoses that the nurse may formulate when caring for a patient receiving these agents, see *Selected nursing diagnoses: Alkalinizing and acidifying agents.* For detailed information on applying the

---

SELECTED NURSING DIAGNOSES

Alkalinizing and acidifying agents

The following nursing diagnoses address representative problems and etiologies that a nurse may encounter when caring for a patient receiving an alkalinizing or acidifying agent. Some of these nursing diagnoses contain generalized etiologies, which the nurse must individualize based on the patient's needs. (For some common nursing diagnoses and related interventions for each drug class, see the "Nursing Process Application" sections of this chapter.)

- Altered protection related to acid-base disturbances caused by administration of an alkalinizing or acidifying agent
- Altered protection related to bone marrow depression caused by acetazolamide
- Altered thought processes related to adverse effects of acetazolamide on the central nervous system
- Diarrhea related to adverse GI effects of acetazolamide or ascorbic acid
- Fluid volume deficit related to adverse GI effects of the prescribed alkalinizing or acidifying agent
- Fluid volume excess related to the high sodium content of sodium bicarbonate or sodium lactate
- Impaired tissue integrity related to tissue abnormalities from I.V. administration of an alkalinizing agent
- Ineffective breathing pattern related to tromethamine-induced respiratory depression
- Knowledge deficit related to the prescribed alkalinizing or acidifying agent
- Pain related to headache caused by an alkalinizing or acidifying agent
- Potential for injury related to a preexisting condition that contraindicates the use of an alkalinizing or acidifying agent
- Potential for injury related to a preexisting condition that requires cautious use of an alkalinizing or acidifying agent
- Potential for injury related to adverse drug reactions
- Potential for injury related to drug interactions
- Potential for injury related to tromethamine-induced hypoglycemia or hyperkalemia
- Sensory-perceptual alterations (tactile) related to acetazolamide-induced paresthesia
- Sleep pattern disturbance related to insomnia caused by high doses of ascorbic acid

Compensatory mechanisms

The lungs and kidneys work together closely to compensate for acid-base imbalances. When an imbalance is respiratory, the kidneys try to compensate by altering the formation or excretion of bicarbonate ions. When the imbalance is metabolic, the lungs try to compensate by altering the carbon dioxide concentration. The chart below shows the compensatory responses of these organ systems to the effects of various acid-base imbalances.

DISORDER AND CAUSE	EFFECTS	COMPENSATORY RESPONSE
Metabolic acidosis caused by diabetic ketoacidosis	Decreases HCO_3^- and blood pH	Lungs decrease P_{CO_2}.
Respiratory acidosis caused by chronic obstructive pulmonary disease	Increases P_{CO_2} and decreases blood pH	Kidneys increase HCO_3^-.
Metabolic alkalosis caused by excessive diuretic administration	Increases HCO_3^- and blood pH	Lungs increase P_{CO_2}.
Respiratory alkalosis caused by hyperventilation syndrome	Decreases P_{CO_2} and increases blood pH	Kidneys decrease HCO_3^-.

nursing process, see Chapter 6, The Nursing Process and Drug Therapy.

Acid-base balance and imbalance

The basis for all acid-base relationships is the pH. To maintain normal blood pH (between 7.35 and 7.45) and normal acid-base balance, the body constantly must engage in a delicate homeostatic process, balancing anions (negatively charged ions, such as bicarbonate [HCO_3^-]) with cations (positively charged ions, such as hydrogen [H^+]). The body of a person consuming the typical American diet produces 40 to 80 mEq of hydrogen ions every day from protein metabolism, and this excess easily is offset as part of the homeostatic process. However, disorders such as chronic obstructive pulmonary disease (COPD) and normal events such as exercise can disrupt this process, altering blood pH and causing an acid-base imbalance.

When an acid-base imbalance occurs, the body activates homeostatic buffer systems and compensatory mechanisms to counteract the problem. Blood buffer systems neutralize excess acids and alkalies by reducing high levels of hydrogen ions or by generating hydrogen ions when levels are too low. Blood buffer systems include the bicarbonate, phosphate, and sulfate systems; of these, perhaps the most important is the bicarbonate system. This system regulates shifting of bicarbonate and carbonic acid levels in the blood to offset shifts in the hydrogen ion concentration, or pH.

Besides the buffer systems, the respiratory and renal systems act as compensatory mechanisms to counteract acid-base imbalances. The lungs alter the carbon dioxide levels in the blood by increasing or decreasing the rate and depth of respirations, thus increasing or decreasing carbon dioxide elimination. The kidneys offset hydrogen ion levels by increasing or decreasing the resorption of bicarbonate ions. The two organ systems work together closely; if an acid-base imbalance occurs in one, the other will try to compensate for it. For example, if a disease such as COPD causes respiratory acidosis, the kidneys will try to compensate by retaining bicarbonate. (For more information, see *Compensatory mechanisms.*)

Despite the day-to-day reliability of the body's pH-regulating processes, which can function adequately even under the stress of a disorder such as COPD, alkalinizing or acidifying agents sometimes are needed to correct the acid-base disorders: respiratory or metabolic acidosis or alkalosis. They even may be given concomitantly to a severely ill patient who has a mixed acid-base disorder; for example, when a patient has respiratory acidosis from COPD complicated by metabolic alkalosis from excessive diuretic administration.

These agents also may be used to acidify or alkalinize the urine, which they do by affecting the buffer systems of the kidneys or hydrogen ion excretion.

This chapter covers the alkalinizing and acidifying agents as they are used to treat certain acid-base disorders.

ALKALINIZING AGENTS

Four alkalinizing agents are used to increase blood pH: sodium bicarbonate, sodium citrate, sodium lactate, and tromethamine. Sodium bicarbonate also is used to increase urine pH, as is the carbonic anhydrase inhibitor acetazolamide (which, paradoxically, lowers the blood pH).

PHARMACOKINETICS

All of the alkalinizing agents are absorbed well when given orally. Sodium citrate and sodium lactate are metabolized to the active ingredient, bicarbonate. Sodium bicarbonate is not metabolized. Tromethamine and acetazolamide undergo little or no metabolism and are excreted unchanged in the urine.

Absorption, distribution, metabolism, excretion

After oral administration, sodium bicarbonate is absorbed rapidly and completely. It is excreted as carbon dioxide from the lungs and as bicarbonate in the urine.

After oral administration of sodium citrate in Shohl's solution (a mixture of sodium citrate and citric acid) or in modified Shohl's solution (a mixture of sodium and potassium citrate with citric acid), the drug is metabolized by oxidation to form bicarbonate. Less than 5% of sodium citrate is excreted unchanged in the urine.

Sodium lactate is metabolized slowly in the liver to form bicarbonate (the alkalinizing metabolite) and glycogen. Conversion to bicarbonate usually occurs 1 to 2 hours after intravenous (I.V.) administration.

After I.V. administration, tromethamine combines with hydrogen ions and associated acid anions to form salts that are excreted by the kidneys.

When given orally, acetazolamide is absorbed well from the gastrointestinal (GI) tract, widely distributed in body tissues, and excreted unchanged by the kidneys.

Onset, peak, duration

Onset of action of the alkalinizing agents is rapid after oral administration and immediate after I.V. administration. The duration of action varies widely, however, depending on use and underlying disorders.

PHARMACODYNAMICS

Except for acetazolamide, all of the alkalinizing agents act by decreasing the hydrogen ion concentration and increasing the blood pH. Sodium bicarbonate and tromethamine do this directly; sodium lactate and citrate first must undergo conversion to bicarbonate. Acetazolamide decreases blood pH and increases urine pH.

Mechanism of action

Sodium bicarbonate dissociates in the blood to provide bicarbonate ions that are used in the bicarbonate blood buffer system to decrease the hydrogen ion concentration and raise the blood pH. As the bicarbonate ions are excreted in the urine, urine pH rises. Sodium citrate and lactate, after conversion to bicarbonate, alkalinize the blood and urine in the same way.

Tromethamine acts by combining with hydrogen ions to alkalinize the blood; the resulting tromethamine-hydrogen ion complex is excreted in the urine.

Acetazolamide promotes renal excretion of sodium, potassium, bicarbonate, and water. The bicarbonate ion excretion alkalinizes the urine and, by reducing blood bicarbonate levels, also acidifies the blood.

PHARMACOTHERAPEUTICS

Alkalinizing agents commonly are used to treat metabolic acidosis. Other uses include raising the urine pH to help remove certain substances, such as phenobarbital, after an overdose.

sodium bicarbonate. Administered I.V. or orally, this alkalinizing agent is used to treat metabolic acidosis related to cardiac arrest as well as metabolic acidosis from chronic renal failure and other disorders. The drug is used to alkalinize the urine and thus increase the excretion of weak acids, such as cystine or uric acid, that may accumulate as a result of gout or chemotherapy for soft-tissue cancer. Urine alkalinizing also is done to promote excretion of excess barbiturates, salicylates, and other toxic agents.

Sodium bicarbonate usually is not administered during cardiac arrest unless the patient's blood pH falls below 7.1 or the plasma bicarbonate level falls below 8 mEq/liter. When used to treat cardiac arrest, bicarbonate administration offsets the excess hydrogen ions (acidosis) generated by lactic acid produced during the arrest. It also helps prevent ventricular fibrillation, which tends to occur in patients with severe metabolic acidosis caused by cardiac arrest.

Mild metabolic acidosis may not require treatment, but oral or I.V. sodium bicarbonate can be used to treat severe acidosis. No matter which route is used, the dosage must be determined individually for each patient. The base-deficit formula provides the ideal method for dosage calculation. First, determine the patient's base deficit by subtracting the serum bicarbonate level from the desired one. Then use that figure in the following formula:

$$\text{sodium bicarbonate dosage (in mEq)} =$$
$$0.4 \times \text{body weight (kg)} \times \text{base deficit}$$

For example, if the patient's actual serum bicarbonate level is 8 mEq/liter and the desired level is 22 mEq/liter, the patient's base deficit is 14. If this patient weighs 70 kg, the calculation is:

$$\text{sodium bicarbonate dosage (in mEq)} = 0.4 \times 70 \times 14$$

Thus, the dosage would be 392 mEq of sodium bicarbonate.

Usual adult dosage: for severe metabolic acidosis in cardiac arrest, initially, half of the dosage calculated using the base-deficit formula, with subsequent dosages recalculated based on regularly monitored serum bicarbonate levels; or 1 mEq/kg I.V. initially, followed by 0.5 mEq/kg every 10 minutes; for less severe forms of metabolic acidosis, 2 to 5 mEq/kg I.V. infused over 4 to 8 hours; for acidosis related to chronic renal failure, 20 to 36 mEq P.O. daily in divided doses to achieve a serum bicarbonate level of 18 to 20 mEq/liter; for urine alkalinization, 48 mEq P.O. initially, followed by 12 to 24 mEq P.O. every 4 hours.

Usual pediatric dosage: for metabolic acidosis in cardiac arrest in a pediatric patient, 1 mEq/kg every 10 minutes; in a neonate, 1 mEq/kg by slow I.V. infusion of 1 part sodium bicarbonate and 1 part D_5W to avoid hypertonicity.

sodium citrate [Shohl's solution]. Usually administered orally as Shohl's solution for correction of metabolic acidosis, sodium citrate must be diluted with 60 to 90 ml of water. Refrigeration may help make the drug more palatable.

Usual adult dosage: for metabolic acidosis, 10 to 30 ml of Shohl's solution P.O. after meals and at bedtime.

Usual pediatric dosage: for metabolic acidosis, 5 to 15 ml of Shohl's solution P.O. after meals and at bedtime.

sodium lactate. This alkalinizing agent is administered I.V. to treat patients with moderate metabolic acidosis who cannot tolerate oral products. It cannot be used in a patient with an acute disorder or with hepatic impairment because the conversion of lactate to bicarbonate — its alkalinizing metabolite — occurs in the liver. The sodium lactate dosage should be determined using this formula:

$$\text{sodium lactate dosage (in ml of } \tfrac{1}{6} \text{ molar solution)} = 0.8 \times \text{body weight (lb)} \times (60 - \text{plasma } CO_2 \text{ value})$$

Usual adult dosage: for moderate metabolic acidosis, an individually calculated dosage based on the formula above I.V. as a $\frac{1}{6}$ molar solution at a rate no greater than 300 ml/hr; for alkalinizing the urine, 30 ml/kg of body weight of a $\frac{1}{6}$ molar solution, or P.O. in divided doses over 24 hours.

tromethamine (Tham). Tromethamine is administered I.V. to treat metabolic acidosis associated with cardiac bypass surgery, cardiac arrest, or cardiac disease. The drug is used to avoid the high sodium load that can occur with sodium bicarbonate, citrate, or lactate. (A high sodium load can cause water retention and expansion of the extracellular fluid compartment, worsening cardiac function in patients with these conditions.) This alkalinizing agent also may be used to treat metabolic acidosis in a patient with impaired ability to excrete sodium or carbon dioxide — for example, a patient with COPD.

Whether this drug is administered by slow I.V. infusion or with an infusion pump (during cardiac bypass surgery),

the dosage must be individualized. First, the patient's base deficit is determined by subtracting the serum bicarbonate level from the desired one. Then the base deficit is used in this formula:

$$\text{tromethamine dosage (in ml of 0.3 molar solution)} = \text{body weight (kg)} \times \text{base deficit (mEq/liter)}$$

Usual adult dosage: for metabolic acidosis associated with cardiac bypass surgery, cardiac arrest, or cardiac disease, an individually calculated dosage based on the base deficit and infused over 1 hour or more up to a maximum of 24 hours. The dosage may range from 3.5 to 6 ml/kg of the 0.3 molar solution in cardiac arrest. Additional therapy is based on serial determination of bicarbonate levels.

acetazolamide (Diamox). Acetazolamide may be used to alkalinize urine in treating phenobarbital or lithium overdose. Acetazolamide is not recommended to treat salicylate overdose, however, because both drugs can cause metabolic acidosis. (For information about other uses of acetazolamide, see Chapter 33, Diuretic Agents.)

Usual adult dosage: for urinary alkalinization in drug overdose, individualized oral or I.V. dosage based on the overdosed drug and pertinent laboratory results.

Drug interactions

Alkalinizing agents can interact with a wide range of drugs to increase or decrease their pharmacologic effects. (For details, see *Drug interactions: Alkalinizing agents,* page 814.)

ADVERSE DRUG REACTIONS

Alkalinizing agents may cause severe adverse reactions, which usually are related to overdose.

The most severe adverse reaction (causing hyperirritability, tetany, or both) is metabolic alkalosis related to sodium bicarbonate overdose. In a patient with diabetic ketoacidosis, rapid administration of sodium bicarbonate that corrects acidosis too quickly may cause cerebral dysfunction, tissue hypoxia, and lactic acidosis. The high sodium content (12 mEq or 276 mg/gram) in this drug may cause water retention and edema in some patients, especially those with renal disease, congestive heart failure (CHF), or other disorders that can cause fluid imbalance. Oral sodium bicarbonate may produce gastric distention and flatulence as it combines with hydrochloric acid in the stomach to release carbon dioxide. Shohl's solution, which produces less gastric upset than sodium bicarbonate, usually is preferred for this reason. Intravenous administration of sodium bicarbonate can cause extravasation that may result in tissue sloughing, ulceration, and necrosis.

Sodium citrate normally produces few adverse reactions, but an overdose may cause metabolic alkalosis or

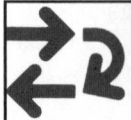

DRUG INTERACTIONS

Alkalinizing agents

Drug interactions involving alkalinizing agents may be severe and may increase or decrease the pharmacologic action of another drug.

DRUG	INTERACTING DRUGS	POSSIBLE EFFECTS	NURSING IMPLICATIONS
sodium bicarbonate, sodium citrate, sodium lactate	amphetamines	Decrease amphetamine excretion, resulting in increased stimulant effects	• Monitor the patient closely for signs of increased amphetamine effects, such as rapid heart rate, increased blood pressure, and restlessness.
	ketoconazole	Decrease ketoconazole absorption	• Avoid concomitant use with an oral alkalinizing agent.
	lithium	Increase lithium excretion	• Monitor the patient for signs of decreased lithium effectiveness, such as increased manic-depressive behavior. • Monitor the patient's lithium blood level regularly.
	methenamine	Decrease conversion of methenamine to formaldehyde, resulting in decreased antibacterial action	• Avoid concomitant use with an alkalinizing agent.
	quinidine	Decrease quinidine excretion, resulting in increased blood levels of quinidine	• Monitor the patient for signs of quinidine toxicity, such as tinnitus and a widened QT interval on ECG tracings.
	salicylates	Increase salicylate excretion if salicylate dosage exceeds 50 mg/kg/day	• Monitor the patient for signs of decreased salicylate effectiveness, such as increased pain and inflammation, at sites where relief had been obtained previously.
	pseudoephedrine	Decrease pseudoephedrine excretion	• Monitor the patient for adverse reactions to pseudoephedrine, such as increased heart rate and cardiac output.

tetany or may aggravate existing cardiac disease by decreasing serum calcium levels. Oral sodium citrate can have a laxative effect.

Sodium lactate also produces few adverse reactions except for metabolic alkalosis (from an overdose) and extravasation. Because the sodium content is high (8 to 9 mEq or 204 mg/gram), this agent may cause water retention and edema in a patient whose ability to excrete sodium is impaired, particularly by a renal disease or CHF.

Adverse reactions to tromethamine may be mild, such as phlebitis or irritation at the injection site, or severe, such as hypoglycemia, respiratory depression (especially in a patient who already has depressed respirations or is receiving drugs that depress respirations), extravasation, and hyperkalemia. In a patient with impaired renal function, this renally excreted drug may accumulate to toxic levels. In a severely ill neonate, hypertonic tromethamine given through the umbilical vein can cause hepatic necrosis. Be-

cause of these adverse reactions, tromethamine administration should not exceed 24 hours for most patients.

A wide range of adverse reactions can occur with acetazolamide. GI tract signs and symptoms include nausea, vomiting, diarrhea, anorexia, and weight loss. Central nervous system (CNS) reactions may include sedation, headache, confusion, and paresthesia. This drug also can elevate blood glucose levels in a diabetic patient; decrease uric acid excretion, leading to gout; cause metabolic acidosis; and precipitate hepatic coma in a patient with severe liver disease. Other adverse reactions to acetazolamide include hypersensitivity reactions, such as cholestatic jaundice, fever, rash, skin eruptions, and bone marrow depression (which may lead to aplastic anemia).

NURSING PROCESS APPLICATION

The following information assists the nurse in caring for a patient who is receiving an alkalinizing agent.

Assessment

- Review the patient's history for a preexisting condition that contraindicates the use of an alkalinizing agent, such as metabolic or respiratory alkalosis, excessive chloride loss, ingestion of a strong mineral acid, or severe renal impairment.
- Review the patient's history for a preexisting condition that requires cautious use of an alkalinizing agent, such as CHF, hypertension, renal dysfunction, peripheral or pulmonary edema, or toxemia of pregnancy.
- Assess the patient for adverse reactions to the alkalinizing agent, such as GI distress, metabolic alkalosis, tetany, extravasation, edema, hypoglycemia, or respiratory depression.
- Review the patient's medication history to identify the use of drugs that may interact with the alkalinizing agent, such as amphetamines, ketoconazole, lithium, methenamine, quinidine, salicylates, or pseudoephedrine.
- Assess the effectiveness of the alkalinizing agent regularly.
- Assess for fluid retention in a patient receiving sodium bicarbonate or sodium lactate.
- Evaluate the patient's and family's knowledge about the prescribed alkalinizing agent.

Nursing diagnoses

The following examples represent appropriate nursing diagnoses for a patient receiving an alkalinizing agent.
- Potential for injury related to a preexisting condition that contraindicates the use of an alkalinizing agent
- Potential for injury related to a preexisting condition that requires cautious use of an alkalinizing agent
- Potential for injury related to adverse drug reactions
- Fluid volume excess related to the high sodium content of sodium bicarbonate or sodium lactate
- Knowledge deficit related to the prescribed alkalinizing agent

Planning and implementation

- Do not administer an alkalinizing agent to a patient with a condition that contraindicates its use.
- Administer an alkalinizing agent cautiously to a patient at risk because of a preexisting condition.
- Monitor the patient closely throughout therapy for adverse reactions to the alkalinizing agent.
- Monitor the patient's serum pH and serum bicarbonate levels regularly to evaluate the effectiveness of therapy or detect problems.
- Monitor the patient's urine pH frequently when sodium bicarbonate or acetazolamide is used to alkalinize the urine.
- *Inspect the I.V. site regularly for extravasation in a patient receiving sodium bicarbonate, sodium lactate, or tromethamine. Observe for phlebitis or irritation in a patient receiving tromethamine.*

- Treat extravasation by elevating the affected limb, applying warm compresses, and administering lidocaine, hyaluronidase, or both, as prescribed.
- *Monitor the patient closely for signs and symptoms of alkalinizing agent overdose, such as hyperirritability and tetany (with sodium bicarbonate use) or metabolic alkalosis, tetany, or aggravation of existing cardiac disease (with sodium citrate use).*
- *Administer sodium bicarbonate slowly to a patient with diabetic ketoacidosis because cerebral dysfunction, tissue hypoxia, and lactic acidosis can occur.*
- Do not administer tromethamine for more than 24 hours to help prevent severe adverse reactions.
- Monitor hydration if the patient develops diarrhea, nausea, vomiting, or diarrhea. Obtain a prescription for an antiemetic or antidiarrheal agent, as needed.
- *Perform frequent respiratory assessment in a patient receiving tromethamine to detect respiratory depression.*
- Monitor glucose levels regularly in a patient receiving acetazolamide to detect hypoglycemia.
- Take safety precautions if the patient develops sedation or confusion during acetazolamide therapy. For example, keep the bed in a low position and supervise ambulation.
- Monitor for headaches in a patient receiving acetazolamide. Obtain a prescription for an analgesic if needed.
- Dilute Shohl's solution with 2 to 3 oz (60 to 90 ml) of water before administration, refrigerate it to improve the taste, and administer it after meals to prevent its laxative effects.
- Notify the physician if adverse reactions occur.
- *Monitor for signs of fluid retention, such as crackles, peripheral edema, and jugular vein distention in a patient receiving sodium bicarbonate or sodium lactate. The high sodium content of these drugs may cause fluid retention, especially in a patient with renal disease or CHF.*
- Notify the physician if fluid retention occurs.

Patient teaching

- Teach the patient and family the name, dose, frequency, action, and adverse effects of the prescribed alkalinizing agent.
- *Advise the patient receiving prolonged therapy with sodium bicarbonate tablets that GI distress and flatulence may occur and should be reported to the physician. Because GI distress can lead to noncompliance and subsequent acute acidosis, expect an alternate alkalinizing agent to be prescribed if the patient reports GI distress.*
- *Teach the patient to recognize the signs of fluid retention, such as ankle swelling and increasing tightness of rings. Emphasize the importance of reporting these signs immediately to the physician.*
- *Inform the diabetic patient that tromethamine can cause hypoglycemia or that acetazolamide can cause hypergly-*

cemia. Encourage the patient to monitor blood glucose levels closely.

• Advise the patient taking acetazolamide to avoid activities that require mental alertness if sedation or mental changes occur.

• Teach the patient how to prepare and administer Shohl's solution to improve its taste and prevent its laxative effects.

• Instruct the patient to notify the physician if adverse reactions occur.

Evaluation

The following examples represent appropriate evaluation statements for a patient receiving an alkalinizing agent.

• The patient has no conditions that contraindicate alkalinizing agent therapy.

• The patient exhibits no signs of complications in the preexisting condition linked to the prescribed alkalinizing agent.

• The patient experiences no adverse reactions to the prescribed alkalinizing agent.

• The patient maintains normal fluid balance during sodium bicarbonate or sodium lactate therapy.

• The patient and family express an accurate understanding of the points taught about the prescribed alkalinizing agent.

• The patient correctly identifies the signs of fluid retention and describes what to do if they occur.

ACIDIFYING AGENTS

Certain disorders cause alkalosis, or excess base in the blood. To correct this type of acid-base imbalance, the blood pH can be lowered by administering drugs that provide hydrogen ions or interfere with bicarbonate metabolism and decrease blood bicarbonate levels.

Three acidifying agents—ammonium chloride, arginine hydrochloride, and hydrochloric acid—are used to correct metabolic alkalosis. Ammonium chloride and ascorbic acid may serve as urine-acidifying agents. Because they acidify the urine, all these agents may be used to increase the effectiveness of certain urinary antibacterial agents and to enhance drug excretion in patients with overdoses of certain drugs.

PHARMACOKINETICS

Acidifying agents usually are administered I.V. (Ammonium chloride and ascorbic acid may be administered orally.) Ammonium chloride and arginine hydrochloride are metabolized and release hydrochloric acid, the acidifying agent.

Absorption, distribution, metabolism, excretion

When ammonium chloride is administered orally, it is absorbed completely in 3 to 6 hours. It is metabolized in the liver to form urea, which is excreted by the kidneys, and hydrochloric acid, the acidifying agent.

When used to treat metabolic alkalosis, arginine hydrochloride is administered I.V. The drug is metabolized in the liver to ornithine and urea, which are excreted by the kidneys, and to hydrochloric acid.

After I.V. administration, hydrochloric acid is broken down into hydrogen and chloride ions. The hydrogen ions are used as the acidifying agent.

After oral administration, ascorbic acid usually is absorbed well. However, absorption of a large dose may be limited because the body's stores fill and level off at the renal threshold and the excess is excreted. When this occurs, no additional ascorbic acid will be absorbed, even if more is administered. Ascorbic acid is distributed widely in body tissues and metabolized in the liver. Metabolites are excreted in the urine along with excess ascorbic acid, which is excreted unchanged.

PHARMACODYNAMICS

When alkalosis occurs, therapy must increase the hydrogen ion concentration to correct the acid-base imbalance. Acidifying agents can increase the concentration directly—by providing hydrogen ions from metabolic release of hydrochloric acid—or indirectly—by interfering with bicarbonate metabolism.

Mechanism of action

Ammonium chloride lowers the blood pH after being metabolized to urea and to hydrochloric acid, which provides hydrogen ions to acidify the blood or urine. Arginine hydrochloride also provides hydrogen ions via metabolism to hydrochloric acid. Hydrochloric acid lowers blood pH directly by acidifying the blood with hydrogen ions.

Ascorbic acid directly acidifies the urine, providing hydrogen ions and lowering the urine pH.

PHARMACOTHERAPEUTICS

A patient with metabolic alkalosis requires therapy with an acidifying agent that provides hydrogen ions; such a patient may need chloride ion therapy as well. Although the patient can receive both in a hydrochloric acid infusion, this infusion is difficult to prepare, and an overdose can produce severe adverse reactions. That is why most patients receive both types of ions in oral or parenteral doses of ammonium chloride—a safer drug that is easy to prepare.

A patient with a urinary tract infection or a drug overdose may benefit from receiving a urine-acidifying agent.

ammonium chloride. This acidifying agent is used to treat metabolic alkalosis related to chloride loss, which may result from vomiting, gastric suctioning, fistula drainage, pyloric stenosis, or the use of a chloride-wasting diuretic, such as hydrochlorothiazide or furosemide. It is effective for 3 to 4 days, until the compensatory responses of the kidneys take effect and they begin to excrete the same amount of acid as the patient receives.

This agent also may be used to acidify the urine of a patient with a urinary tract infection. This use is discouraged, however, because it can produce metabolic acidosis.

Ammonium chloride may be administered by the oral or I.V. route. The dosage should be calculated by using this formula:

$$\text{mEq of chloride (as ammonium chloride)} =$$
$$\text{chloride deficit in mEq/liter} \times (0.2 \times \text{body weight in kg})$$

For I.V. use, the 26.75% concentrate must be diluted in 0.9% sodium chloride (NaCl) before administration. A dilute solution may be prepared by adding 100 mEq of ammonium chloride (20 ml of the 26.75% injection) to 500 ml of 0.9% NaCl injection, or by adding 200 mEq of ammonium chloride (40 ml of the 26.75% injection) to 1,000 ml of 0.9% NaCl injection.
Usual adult dosage: for metabolic alkalosis, an individualized dosage based on the patient's chloride deficit and administered in a dilute solution I.V. at a rate not exceeding 5 ml/min; as a urine acidifying agent, 4 to 12 grams P.O. daily in divided doses every 4 to 6 hours.
Usual pediatric dosage: as an acidifying agent, 75 mg/kg/day in four divided doses.

arginine hydrochloride. Like ammonium chloride, arginine hydrochloride is used to treat metabolic alkalosis related to chloride loss. (For information about other uses of arginine, see Chapter 52, Pituitary Agents.) It is available as a 100 mg/ml I.V. solution. The correct dosage can be determined by using this formula:

$$\text{arginine dosage (in grams)} = \frac{\text{base deficit} \times \text{body weight (kg)}}{9.6}$$

Usual adult dosage: for metabolic alkalosis, dosage calculated using the patient's base deficit.

hydrochloric acid. In a dilute solution, hydrochloric acid can be used to treat metabolic alkalosis, but it must be given I.V. after preparation in the pharmacy under carefully controlled aseptic conditions. (For information about other uses of hydrochloric acid, see Chapter 41, Adsorbent, Antiflatulent, and Digestive Agents.)
Usual adult dosage: for metabolic alkalosis, 0.1 or 0.2 molar solution administered I.V. at a rate of 0.2 mEq/kg/hour or less through a central venous line. Subsequent doses must be based on arterial blood gas measurements taken every 4 hours during the infusion.

ascorbic acid [vitamin C] (Ascorbicap, Cebid). Administered orally, this drug is used to maintain the urine acidity needed for effective action of urinary antibacterial agents, such as methenamine mandelate (Mandelamine), which can only be converted to its active ingredient in an acidic environment. In addition, the acidic environment itself helps decrease bacterial growth in the urine. Some clinicians, however, question the effectiveness of ascorbic acid. (For information about the other uses of ascorbic acid, see Chapter 45, Vitamin, Mineral, and Other Nutritional Agents.)
Usual adult dosage: as a urine acidifier, 4 to 12 grams daily P.O. in divided doses.

Drug interactions

Acidifying agents do not cause any clinically significant drug interactions.

ADVERSE DRUG REACTIONS

Adverse reactions to acidifying agents usually are mild, such as GI distress. However, overdose can occur, especially with parenteral administration, and may lead to acidosis.

Oral administration of ammonium chloride may cause nausea, vomiting, anorexia, and thirst. Large doses may cause metabolic acidosis and loss of electrolytes, especially potassium. Rapid I.V. administration may cause pain and irritation at the infusion site. Ammonium toxicity also may occur, producing twitching and hyperreflexia.

Adverse reactions to arginine hydrochloride typically result from too-rapid I.V. administration and include flushing, nausea, vomiting, headache, numbness, and irritation at the infusion site. In some patients, arginine hydrochloride causes a hypersensitivity reaction consisting of a macular rash with redness and edema of the hands and face; these disappear when the drug is discontinued. This agent also may cause other hypersensitivity reactions, such as nasal obstruction and discharge, sweating, and increased pulse rate.

With hydrochloric acid administration, metabolic acidosis may occur with an overdose.

In high doses, ascorbic acid can produce GI distress, such as nausea, vomiting, diarrhea, and abdominal cramps, and flushing, headache, and insomnia. In a patient with glucose-6-phosphate dehydrogenase (G6PD) deficiency, hemolytic anemia may develop after administration of a high dose of ascorbic acid.

NURSING PROCESS APPLICATION

The following information assists the nurse in caring for a patient who is receiving an acidifying agent.

Assessment

• Review the patient's history for a preexisting condition that contraindicates the use of an acidifying agent, such as severe hepatic or renal dysfunction, primary respiratory acidosis, or high total carbon dioxide and buffer base.

• Review the patient's history for a preexisting condition that requires cautious use of an acidifying agent, such as pulmonary insufficiency, cardiac edema, or renal calculi.

• Assess the patient for adverse reactions to the acidifying agent, such as GI distress, metabolic acidosis, local reactions at the I.V. site, ammonium toxicity, flushing, headache, or insomnia.

• Assess the effectiveness of the acidifying agent periodically.

• Evaluate the patient's and family's knowledge about the prescribed acidifying agent.

Nursing diagnoses

The following examples represent appropriate nursing diagnoses for a patient receiving an acidifying agent.

• Potential for injury related to a preexisting condition that contraindicates the use of an acidifying agent

• Potential for injury related to a preexisting condition that requires cautious use of an acidifying agent

• Potential for injury related to adverse drug reactions

• Knowledge deficit related to the prescribed acidifying agent

Planning and implementation

• Do not administer an acidifying agent to a patient with a condition that contraindicates its use.

• Administer an acidifying agent cautiously to a patient at risk because of a preexisting condition.

• Monitor the patient closely for adverse reactions during acidifying agent therapy.

• *Monitor the patient for signs of metabolic acidosis, such as CNS depression, abnormal respirations, and abnormal laboratory values of arterial blood pH, serum bicarbonate, serum chloride, or serum potassium.*

• Monitor fluid balance if the patient experiences nausea, vomiting, anorexia, or thirst during acidifying agent therapy. Obtain a prescription for an antiemetic, as needed.

• *Observe for signs of ammonium toxicity, such as twitching and hyperreflexia, in a patient receiving ammonium chloride. If these signs appear, withhold the agent, notify the physician immediately, and switch the patient to a different acidifying agent if prescribed.*

• *Monitor the patient receiving large doses of ammonium chloride for signs of hypokalemia, such as anorexia, vomiting, drowsiness, muscle weakness or cramps, and orthostatic hypotension. Also monitor for other electrolyte imbalances. If an electrolyte imbalance is suspected, notify the physician. Expect to draw blood to determine*

electrolyte levels and to start therapy to correct the imbalance, as prescribed.

• Monitor the patient for headaches and insomnia during ascorbic acid therapy. Obtain a prescription for an analgesic or hypnotic agent, as needed.

• Monitor the complete blood count, as instructed, in a patient with G6PD who is receiving high doses of ascorbic acid. Particularly note changes that suggest hemolytic anemia.

• Expect an acidifying agent to be prepared for I.V. administration under aseptic conditions, preferably in a laminar airflow hood. Expect the pharmacy to prepare a hydrochloric acid infusion, because the acid is extremely caustic.

• *Administer an I.V. acidifying agent slowly to prevent pain or irritation at the infusion site as well as other adverse reactions.*

• Notify the physician if adverse reactions occur.

Patient teaching

• Teach the patient and family the name, dose, frequency, action, and adverse effects of the prescribed acidifying agent.

• *Inform the patient receiving ascorbic acid or oral ammonium chloride to take the agent exactly as prescribed, to report severe adverse GI reactions, and to monitor the urine pH regularly.*

• *Instruct the patient to withhold the next ammonium chloride dose and notify the physician if twitching occurs because twitching may indicate ammonium toxicity.*

• Advise the patient to take a mild analgesic for headache as prescribed when receiving high-dose ascorbic acid therapy. If the patient experiences insomnia, suggest relaxation techniques, such as a warm bath or reading before bedtime. If these techniques are ineffective, advise the patient to take a hypnotic agent, as prescribed.

• Advise the patient to notify the physician if adverse drug reactions occur.

Evaluation

The following examples represent appropriate evaluation statements for a patient receiving an acidifying agent.

• The patient has no conditions that contraindicate acidifying agent therapy.

• The patient exhibits no signs of complications in the preexisting condition linked to the prescribed acidifying agent.

• The patient experiences no adverse reactions to the prescribed acidifying agent.

• The patient and family express an accurate understanding of the points taught about the prescribed acidifying agent.

• The patient correctly describes conditions that must be reported to the physician during acidifying agent therapy.

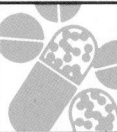

SELECTED MAJOR DRUGS

Alkalinizing and acidifying agents

This chart summarizes the major alkalinizing and acidifying agents currently in clinical use.

DRUG	MAJOR INDICATIONS	USUAL ADULT DOSAGES	CONTRAINDICATIONS AND PRECAUTIONS
Alkalinizing agents			
sodium bicarbonate	Severe metabolic acidosis in cardiac arrest	1 mEq/kg I.V. initially, followed by 0.5 mEq/kg every 10 minutes; or an individualized dosage	• Know that sodium bicarbonate is contraindicated in a patient with metabolic or respiratory alkalosis, hypocalcemia when alkalosis may induce tetany, excessive chloride loss, or predisposition to development of diuretic-induced hypochloremic alkalosis. Also know that oral sodium bicarbonate is contraindicated in a patient who has ingested a strong mineral acid.
	Less severe metabolic acidosis	2 to 5 mEq/kg I.V. infused over 4 to 8 hours	
	Urine alkalinization	48 mEq P.O. initially, followed by 12 to 24 mEq P.O. every 4 hours	• Administer sodium bicarbonate with extreme caution to a patient with congestive heart failure or other edematous or sodium-retaining condition, renal insufficiency, or who is undergoing corticosteroid or corticotropin therapy.
sodium citrate	Metabolic acidosis	10 to 30 ml of Shohl's solution P.O. after meals and at bedtime	• Know that sodium citrate is contraindicated in a patient with severe renal impairment or one who must follow a sodium-restricted diet. • Administer sodium citrate with extreme caution in a patient with congestive heart failure, hypertension, renal dysfunction, peripheral or pulmonary edema, or toxemia of pregnancy. • Administer sodium citrate with caution to a patient with low urine output.
Acidifying agents			
ammonium chloride	Metabolic alkalosis related to chloride loss	Up to 5 ml/minute I.V. of dilute solution based on the patient's chloride deficit	• Know that ammonium chloride is contraindicated in a patient with severe hepatic dysfunction, severe renal dysfunction when metabolic alkalosis is caused by vomiting and is accompanied by substantial sodium loss, primary respiratory acidosis, or high total carbon dioxide and buffer base.
	Urine acidification	4 to 12 grams P.O. daily in divided doses every 4 to 6 hours	• Administer ammonium chloride with caution to a patient with pulmonary insufficiency or cardiac edema.
ascorbic acid	Urine acidification	4 to 12 grams daily P.O. in divided doses	• Administer ascorbic acid with caution to a pregnant patient. Administer high doses with caution to a neonate or a patient with a history of gouty arthritis, deep vein thrombosis, or renal calculi.

CHAPTER SUMMARY

Chapter 47 covered alkalinizing and acidifying agents as they are used to treat certain acid-base disorders and to regulate blood and urine pH. Here are the highlights of the chapter.
• Homeostatic buffer systems and compensatory mechanisms help keep blood pH within a narrow normal range—between 7.35 and 7.45. Certain disorders can upset this delicate acid-base balance, which may be corrected by administering an alkalinizing or acidifying agent.
• Alkalinizing agents, such as tromethamine and sodium bicarbonate, citrate, and lactate, are used to treat metabolic acidosis by alkalinizing the blood. They do this by decreasing the hydrogen ion concentration.
• Some alkalinizing agents, such as sodium bicarbonate and acetazolamide, also can alkalinize the urine. They are useful for promoting the excretion of certain weak acids, such as uric acid, or toxic drugs, such as phenobarbital.

• Alkalinizing agents can interact with a wide variety of drugs, increasing or decreasing their pharmacologic action.

• Alkalinizing agents may cause severe adverse reactions, which usually are related to overdose. Sodium bicarbonate and lactate may cause water retention and edema in patients with impaired ability to excrete sodium from such disorders as CHF or renal dysfunction.

• Acidifying agents, such as ammonium chloride, arginine hydrochloride, and hydrochloric acid, are used to correct metabolic alkalosis by acidifying the blood. They do this by increasing the hydrogen ion concentration.

• Ammonium chloride and large doses of ascorbic acid may be used to acidify the urine in patients with urinary tract infections.

• Acidifying agents cause no clinically significant drug interactions. However, they may produce adverse reactions that range from mild, such as GI distress, to severe, such as acidosis.

• When administering an alkalinizing or acidifying agent, the nurse must monitor the patient's blood pH closely because overdose can occur when the pH falls outside of the narrow normal range of 7.35 to 7.45.

STUDY QUESTIONS

See Appendix 1 for answers.

1. Dorothy Blauvelt, age 60, is brought to the emergency department (ED) in cardiac arrest. On the way to the ED, the rescue squad began cardiopulmonary resuscitation, inserted a central venous line, and administered sodium bicarbonate to treat metabolic acidosis. How does sodium bicarbonate correct metabolic acidosis?
(a) by decreasing the hydrogen ion concentration
(b) by increasing the hydrogen ion concentration
(c) by decreasing uric acid excretion in urine
(d) by increasing uric acid excretion in urine

2. When monitoring Ms. Blauvelt during sodium bicarbonate administration, the nurse is likely to detect which severe adverse reaction?
(a) hepatic necrosis
(b) metabolic alkalosis
(c) respiratory depression
(d) hypersensitivity reaction

3. Alan Kominsky, age 50, has severe coronary artery disease and is scheduled for coronary bypass surgery. During bypass surgery, the physician prescribes tromethamine to treat metabolic acidosis. Why is tromethamine the preferred drug to treat Mr. Kominsky's metabolic acidosis?
(a) It has a faster onset of action than other alkalinizing agents.
(b) It avoids the high sodium load that can occur with other alkalinizing agents.
(c) It produces fewer adverse reactions than other alkalinizing agents.
(d) It is metabolized and excreted more readily than other alkalinizing agents.

4. Like most patients, Mr. Kominsky will receive tromethamine for only 24 hours. Why?
(a) Its effectiveness decreases with longer use.
(b) It produces rebound metabolic acidosis after 1 day.
(c) Severe adverse reactions occur with longer use.
(d) Larger doses are needed to achieve therapeutic effects after 1 day.

5. Martin Elfant, age 25, is brought to the ED after taking a phenobarbital overdose. The physician prescribes the alkalinizing agent acetazolamide (Diamox). For Mr. Elfant, what is the purpose of administering acetazolamide?
(a) to treat metabolic acidosis
(b) to neutralize phenobarbital in the vascular system
(c) to increase urinary output, preventing renal damage
(d) to alkalinize urine, promoting phenobarbital excretion

6. Gloria Benton, age 64, is admitted to the hospital for treatment of metabolic alkalosis caused by the chloride-wasting diuretic furosemide. The physician prescribes ammonium chloride, 1 ml/min. I.V. of a 2.14% solution. Why is ammonium chloride selected over hydrochloric acid to treat Mrs. Hahn's metabolic alkalosis?
(a) It is safer and easier to prepare.
(b) It provides hydrogen and chloride ions.
(c) It has a more rapid onset of action.
(d) It bypasses hepatic metabolism.

7. While administering ammonium chloride to Ms. Benton, the nurse should assess her carefully for signs of metabolic acidosis and what other common electrolyte imbalance?
(a) hyponatremia
(b) hypocalcemia
(c) hypokalemia
(d) hypomagnesia

SELECTED REFERENCES

Adinaro, D. (1987). Liver failure and pancreatitis: Fluid and electrolyte concerns. *Nursing Clinics of North America,* 22(4), 827-836.

AHFS drug information 90. (1990). Bethesda, MD: American Society of Hospital Pharmacists.

Butts, D. (1987). Fluid and electrolyte disorders associated with diabetic ketoacidosis and hyperglycemic hyperosmolar nonketotic coma. *Nursing Clinics of North America,* 22(4), 827-836.

Hansten, P., and Horn, J. (1989). *Drug interactions: The clinical significance of drug-drug interactions* (6th ed.). Philadelphia: Lea & Febiger.

Mathewson, M., and Mathewson, R. (1987). Establishing acid-base balance. *Critical Care Nurse,* 7(5), 77-85.

North American Nursing Diagnosis Association. (1990). *Taxonomy-Revised, with official diagnostic categories.* St. Louis: NANDA.

Stowe, K. (1988). Acid-base imbalances in the surgical patient. *Point of View,* 25(1), 8-10.

York, K. (1987). The lung and fluid-electrolyte and acid-base imbalances. *Nursing Clinics of North America,* 22(4), 805-814.

CHAPTER
48

CATION-EXCHANGE RESIN
AND AMMONIA-DETOXICATING AGENTS

OBJECTIVES

After reading and studying this chapter, the student should be able to:
1. Describe how the cation-exchange resin sodium polystyrene sulfonate acts to remove endogenous substances from the body.
2. Discuss the pharmacokinetics of sodium polystyrene sulfonate.
3. Describe how the acidification of the colon contents after lactulose therapy reduces ammonia absorption.
4. Discuss the pharmacokinetics of the ammonia-detoxicating agents.
5. Describe the adverse effects of the cation-exchange resin and ammonia-detoxicating agents.
6. Describe how to apply the nursing process when caring for a patient receiving a cation-exchange resin or ammonia-detoxicating agent.

INTRODUCTION

Chapter 48 describes drugs that decrease toxic levels of endogenous substances via the gastrointestinal (GI) tract. The body naturally contains potassium and ammonia. When the serum concentration levels of these substances are within the normal range, potassium and ammonia participate in the normal metabolic function of the internal environment. When the serum concentration levels increase, both of these substances can lead to harmful and potentially fatal reactions.

A cation-exchange resin, also called a potassium-removing resin, is an insoluble compound of high molecular weight, capable of exchanging sodium ions for potassium ions in surrounding solution. Sodium polystyrene sulfonate is a synthetic cation-exchange resin used to remove potassium from the body of a patient with hyperkalemia. Sodium polystyrene sulfonate may be used alone, if the potassium

concentration is elevated only slightly, or with other drugs to treat higher serum potassium concentrations.

Ammonia is formed in the body in several ways: (1) by the liver during deamination of amino acids; (2) by epithelial cells of the proximal and distal tubules and collecting duct of the nephron, as part of regulation of hydrogen ion; and (3) by bacteria in the GI tract acting on urea or dietary protein. A normally functioning liver then converts the absorbed ammonia to urea, a less toxic substance. Urea is excreted by the kidneys in the urine.

Liver damage or the shunting of blood flow around the liver can inhibit the conversion of ammonia to urea. The resulting elevated blood ammonia concentration can lead to a disorder known as hepatic encephalopathy, which may cause a decreased level of consciousness, an altered mental state, impaired neuromuscular functioning, or death.

Neomycin and lactulose help reduce the blood ammonia concentration. The antibiotic neomycin is formed naturally by a particular bacterial strain. When administered orally, neomycin also will eliminate the normal bacterial flora of the GI tract and may lead to superinfection. (For more information about the antimicrobial uses of neomycin, see Chapter 59, Antibacterial Agents.) Lactulose is a synthetic derivative of lactose. Lactulose also is used to treat constipation. (For more information about the use of lactulose as a laxative, see Chapter 42, Antidiarrheal and Laxative Agents.)

For a summary of representative drugs, see *Selected major drugs: Cation-exchange resin and ammonia-detoxicating agents,* page 830. For a listing of applicable nursing diagnoses that the nurse may formulate when caring for a patient receiving these agents, see *Selected nursing diagnoses: Cation-exchange resin and ammonia-detoxicating agents.* For detailed information on applying the nursing process, see Chapter 6, The Nursing Process and Drug Therapy.

SELECTED NURSING DIAGNOSES

Cation-exchange resin and ammonia-detoxicating agents

The following nursing diagnoses address representative problems and etiologies that a nurse may encounter when caring for a patient who is receiving a cation-exchange resin or ammonia-detoxicating agent. Some of these nursing diagnoses contain generalized etiologies, which the nurse must individualize based on the patient's needs. (For some common nursing diagnoses and related interventions for each drug class, see the "Nursing Process Application" sections of this chapter.)

- Altered nutrition: less than body requirements, related to nausea, vomiting, or anorexia caused by sodium polystyrene sulfonate
- Altered protection related to hypokalemia caused by sodium polystyrene sulfonate
- Altered protection related to lactulose-induced hyperglycemia in a patient with impaired glucose intolerance
- Altered protection related to superinfection caused by neomycin-induced destruction of normal bowel flora
- Constipation related to the adverse GI effects of sodium polystyrene sulfonate
- Diarrhea related to the adverse GI effects of the ammonia-detoxicating agent
- Fluid volume disturbance related to the adverse GI effects of the cation-exchange resin or ammonia-detoxicating agent
- Hyperthermia related to fever caused by the ammonia-detoxicating agent
- Impaired physical mobility related to muscle dysfunction caused by the cation-exchange resin or ammonia-detoxicating agent

- Ineffective breathing pattern related to neomycin-induced neuromuscular blockade
- Knowledge deficit related to the prescribed cation-exchange resin or ammonia-detoxicating agent
- Pain related to lactulose-induced gas formation in the GI tract
- Potential for injury related to a preexisting condition that contraindicates the use of a cation-exchange resin or ammonia-detoxicating agent
- Potential for injury related to a preexisting condition that requires cautious use of a cation-exchange resin or ammonia-detoxicating agent
- Potential for injury related to adverse drug reactions
- Potential for injury related to calcium or magnesium deficiency caused by sodium polystyrene sulfonate
- Potential for trauma related to neomycin-induced nephrotoxicity
- Sensory-perceptual alterations (auditory) related to neomycin-induced ototoxicity

---

CATION-EXCHANGE RESIN

Sodium polystyrene sulfonate is the only commercially available drug that is effective as a cation-exchange resin. The drug exchanges sodium ions for potassium ions in the GI tract. This action of sodium polystyrene sulfonate makes the resin useful for treating hyperkalemia.

PHARMACOKINETICS

Because sodium polystyrene sulfonate is insoluble, the resin remains available for binding potassium, which exists in high concentration in the large intestine.

Absorption, distribution, metabolism, excretion

Sodium polystyrene sulfonate is not absorbed from the GI tract. Theoretically, each gram of the resin may bind up to 3.1 mEq of potassium. However, because other cations, such as calcium and magnesium, also bind to sodium polystyrene sulfonate, an actual exchange capacity greater than 1 mEq of potassium per gram of resin is unlikely.

Each gram of sodium polystyrene sulfonate powder contains about 4.1 mEq of sodium. Although only 33% of the

resin's sodium content is distributed systemically, daily administration of 15 to 60 grams of the drug also may result in administration of 30 to 80 mEq of sodium.

Resin distribution is limited to the GI tract. Sodium polystyrene sulfonate is not metabolized to any extent, and nearly 100% of a dose is excreted from the intestinal tract in the feces, primarily as potassium polystyrene sulfonate.

Onset, peak, duration

The potassium-lowering effects of sodium polystyrene sulfonate are slow and unpredictable. Onset of action may not occur for 2 to 24 hours after oral administration. The onset after rectal administration is somewhat shorter. The duration of action for sodium polystyrene sulfonate is about 4 to 6 hours.

PHARMACODYNAMICS

Sodium polystyrene sulfonate is a cation-exchange resin used to reduce elevated potassium levels.

Mechanism of action

After oral administration of sodium polystyrene sulfonate, sodium ions are exchanged with hydrogen ions found in the stomach's acidic environment. As the resin passes through the GI tract, hydrogen ions are released in exchange for other cations present in higher concentrations. Because of the high concentration of potassium in the large intestine, potassium readily exchanges with hydrogen ions. Then the modified resin, which includes small amounts of other cations besides potassium, is eliminated in the feces. After rectal administration of sodium polystyrene sulfonate, sodium ions are released directly in exchange for potassium ions.

PHARMACOTHERAPEUTICS

Oral or rectal sodium polystyrene sulfonate is used to lower serum potassium concentrations in treating hyperkalemia when urgent reduction of potassium is not necessary. Because effective lowering of the serum potassium concentration with sodium polystyrene sulfonate may take hours to days, life-threatening hyperkalemia first is treated with prompt-acting, shorter-duration measures to reduce the serum potassium concentration. Therapies that rapidly lower the serum potassium concentration include I.V. sodium bicarbonate or glucose and insulin. These therapies produce a transient intracellular shift of potassium, thus lowering the plasma concentration. Intravenous calcium decreases myocardial irritability caused by hyperkalemia, but does not correct hyperkalemia. Hemodialysis also rapidly and effectively reduces the serum potassium concentration.

sodium polystyrene sulfonate (Kayexalate, SPS). During treatment, the dosage and duration of sodium polystyrene sulfonate therapy must be individualized and depends on the daily assessment of total body potassium.
Usual adult dosage: 15 grams P.O. one to four times daily, with each dose given as a suspension in 20 to 100 ml of water or syrup. Using 70% sorbitol as a vehicle for administering this agent may prevent constipation because of sorbitol's laxative effect. As a retention enema, 30 to 50 grams rectally every 1 to 2 hours initially, then every 6 hours, or as needed. The agent should be retained at least 20 to 30 minutes to be effective.
Usual pediatric dosage: 1 gram for each mEq of potassium to be removed.

Drug interactions

Antacids that contain certain cations (such as calcium or magnesium) tend to interfere with the effectiveness of sodium polystyrene sulfonate by competing for binding sites. Combined use also may result in systemic alkalosis. Foods or liquids that contain potassium also may reduce the effectiveness of sodium polystyrene sulfonate.

Some patients receiving sodium polystyrene sulfonate and aluminum hydroxide gel antacids concurrently have experienced intestinal obstruction when these drugs combine to form a hard mass in the intestinal tract. Correcting the problem may require surgical intervention.

ADVERSE DRUG REACTIONS

Sodium polystyrene sulfonate can cause numerous adverse reactions, requiring close patient monitoring. The most serious adverse reactions are electrolyte imbalances; the most common ones involve GI disturbances.

Because sodium polystyrene sulfonate works by exchanging sodium ions for potassium ions, this drug will alter levels of these electrolytes. The patient will retain sodium ions and lose potassium ions. Serious hypokalemia may develop from sodium polystyrene sulfonate therapy. Hypokalemia may cause disturbances of muscle function, cardiac rhythm, acid-base balance, and deep tendon reflexes, as well as potential digitalis toxicity. Sodium polystyrene sulfonate administration usually is discontinued when the serum potassium concentration begins to approach the normal range.

Although sodium polystyrene sulfonate primarily affects sodium and potassium balance, it also may affect other electrolytes. Calcium and magnesium deficiencies have been noted during therapy with the cation-exchange resin.

Patients may complain of GI tract disturbances, such as nausea, vomiting, or anorexia, during sodium polystyrene sulfonate therapy. These reactions may stem from the drug's taste, the patient's feelings of fullness, or slowing of GI motility. Constipation is a serious problem because it may cause fecal impaction. To help the patient avoid constipation, the nurse can mix the sodium polystyrene sulfonate with 70% sorbitol, which draws water into the GI tract, thereby helping to keep stools soft and promoting elimination. However, patients may develop diarrhea from taking the sorbitol.

NURSING PROCESS APPLICATION

The following information assists the nurse in caring for a patient who is receiving sodium polystyrene sulfonate.

Assessment
• Review the patient's history for a preexisting condition that contraindicates the use of sodium polystyrene sulfonate, such as hypokalemia or known hypersensitivity to the drug.
• Review the patient's history for a preexisting condition that requires cautious use of sodium polystyrene sulfonate, such as pregnancy, lactation, or sodium load intolerance (as in congestive heart failure [CHF]).
• Assess the patient for adverse reactions to sodium polystyrene sulfonate, such as GI distress and electrolyte imbalances.
• Review the patient's medication history to identify the use of drugs that may interact with sodium polystyrene sulfonate, such as calcium or magnesium antacids.

• Assess the effectiveness of sodium polystyrene sulfonate regularly.

• Assess the patient's elimination pattern daily throughout sodium polystyrene sulfonate therapy.

• Evaluate the patient's and family's knowledge about sodium polystyrene sulfonate.

Nursing diagnoses

The following examples represent appropriate nursing diagnoses for a patient receiving sodium polystyrene sulfonate.

• Potential for injury related to a preexisting condition that contraindicates the use of sodium polystyrene sulfonate

• Potential for injury related to a preexisting condition that requires cautious use of sodium polystyrene sulfonate

• Potential for injury related to adverse drug reactions

• Constipation related to the adverse GI effects of sodium polystyrene sulfonate

• Knowledge deficit related to sodium polystyrene sulfonate

Planning and implementation

• Do not administer sodium polystyrene sulfonate to a patient with a condition that contraindicates its use.

• Administer sodium polystyrene sulfonate cautiously to a patient at risk because of a preexisting condition.

• Monitor the patient for adverse reactions—especially GI distress and electrolyte imbalances—frequently during sodium polystyrene sulfonate therapy.

• *Monitor the patient's serum potassium level at least once daily, and observe for signs of hypokalemia, including irritability, confusion, cardiac arrhythmias, and muscle weakness.*

• Monitor electrocardiograms and the patient's clinical condition closely. Serum potassium levels may not reflect intracellular potassium deficiency.

• Identify and eliminate, if possible, any exogenous sources of potassium the patient may be receiving (in diet, medications, and blood products).

• *Monitor the patient with hypertension, CHF, or edema for signs of sodium and fluid overload. Also monitor the serum sodium level regularly.*

• Monitor hydration if the patient experiences nausea, vomiting, or anorexia. Obtain a prescription for an antiemetic, as needed.

• Avoid concurrent administration of a calcium or magnesium antacid. Such an antacid can decrease sodium polystyrene sulfonate effectiveness.

• *Monitor for signs of digitalis toxicity, such as GI, cardiac, or central nervous system disturbances, in a patient receiving a cardiac glycoside during therapy with sodium polystyrene sulfonate.*

• Administer a sodium polystyrene sulfonate enema by placing it at least 8″ (20 cm) into the colon. The patient should retain the enema for 20 to 30 minutes or as prescribed. If the patient has difficulty retaining the enema, elevate the patient's hips on pillows, have the patient assume a knee-chest position, or instill the enema through a catheter held in place with an inflatable balloon.

• Mix sodium polystyrene sulfonate with 20 to 100 ml of fruit juice, water, syrup, or a soft drink to increase its palatability for oral administration. However, avoid fluids with high potassium content, including citrus juices, prune juice, milk, and apricot nectar. Sodium polystyrene sulfonate should be given in suspension. Do not administer the drug as a paste because it is much less effective in that form.

• Notify the physician if adverse reactions occur or if the drug is ineffective.

• *Monitor bowel function frequently to ensure that the patient is eliminating the resin. For constipation, mix sodium polystyrene sulfonate in 70% sorbitol solution (rather than juice or other liquid) as prescribed to produce one or two soft stools daily.*

• *Consult the physician about withholding any prescribed aluminum hydroxide gel antacid until the sodium polystyrene sulfonate therapy has ended. Concurrent use can cause intestinal obstruction.*

• Notify the physician if constipation occurs or persists.

Patient teaching

• Teach the patient and family the name, dose, frequency, action, and adverse effects of sodium polystyrene sulfonate.

• Show the patient or a family member how to prepare and administer sodium polystyrene sulfonate correctly.

• *Teach the patient to recognize and report the signs and symptoms of sodium and potassium imbalances.*

• *Advise the patient to avoid high-sodium foods, such as processed foods and lunch meats, and high-potassium foods, such as orange juice and bananas.* (For more information, see *Guide to potassium-rich foods* in Chapter 33, Diuretic Agents.)

• *Instruct the patient to avoid calcium or magnesium antacids while taking sodium polystyrene sulfonate.*

• *Teach the patient to recognize the signs and symptoms of digitalis toxicity during concurrent therapy with a cardiac glycoside and sodium polystyrene sulfonate.*

• *Inform the patient of the constipating effects of sodium polystyrene sulfonate. Discuss ways to prevent or reduce constipation, such as eating a high-fiber diet and drinking 8 to 12 glasses (2 to 3 liters) of fluids per day.*

• Instruct the patient to take sodium polystyrene sulfonate mixed with sorbitol early in the day. Taking the drug early should prevent problems with diarrhea at night.

• Tell the patient to notify the physician if adverse reactions occur.

Evaluation

The following examples represent appropriate evaluation statements for a patient receiving sodium polystyrene sulfonate.

• The patient has no conditions that contraindicate sodium polystyrene sulfonate therapy.

• The patient exhibits no signs of complications in the preexisting condition linked to sodium polystyrene sulfonate.

• The patient displays no signs of adverse reactions to sodium polystyrene sulfonate.

• The patient maintains normal bowel function during sodium polystyrene sulfonate therapy.

• The patient and family express an accurate understanding of the points taught about sodium polystyrene sulfonate.

• The patient correctly demonstrates how to prepare and administer sodium polystyrene sulfonate.

AMMONIA-DETOXICATING AGENTS

The ammonia-detoxicating drugs lactulose and neomycin commonly are used to lower blood ammonia concentration levels in patients with hepatic encephalopathy. However, they lower these concentrations by different mechanisms. Lactulose acidifies the colon contents, thereby trapping ammonia in the GI tract. Neomycin, an aminoglycoside, eliminates colonic bacteria that form ammonia.

PHARMACOKINETICS

Lactulose remains in the GI tract, where it is absorbed and distributed. Neomycin also remains in the GI tract, where it undergoes GI distribution only.

Absorption, distribution, metabolism, excretion

After oral administration, lactulose is absorbed from the GI tract, but only to a minor degree. Distribution of lactulose then occurs throughout the GI tract.

The unabsorbed lactulose is metabolized by colonic bacteria to lactic, acetic, and formic acids. The small quantity of lactulose absorbed is not metabolized and is excreted unchanged in the urine, bile, and feces. Excretion of lactulose is complete within 24 hours.

About 1% to 3% of a neomycin dose is absorbed from the GI tract after oral or rectal administration. However, more may be absorbed in certain circumstances, such as impaired GI motility.

Because most of an oral or rectal dose of neomycin remains in the GI tract, drug distribution is limited to this area. The small amount of neomycin that is absorbed systemically is distributed mostly into the extracellular fluid. Neomycin is not metabolized, and 97% to 99% of a dose remains unchanged in the GI tract. This unabsorbed neomycin is excreted in the feces. The small percentage of absorbed neomycin is eliminated in the urine.

Onset, peak, duration

The onset of action for lactulose varies with the route of administration and the patient's condition. With rectal administration, lactulose may produce beneficial effects in 2 to 12 hours. Orally administered lactulose may not produce beneficial effects for 24 to 48 hours. The duration of action for a single dose may range from 6 to 8 hours.

The onset for neomycin to reduce the blood ammonia concentration also varies. Theoretically, neomycin should begin to decrease the number of ammonia-producing bacteria when the drug reaches the large intestine. Reaching this destination, however, may take up to several hours, depending on the activity in the patient's GI tract.

The peak plasma concentration from the absorbed portion of neomycin may occur 1 to 4 hours after oral or rectal administration.

The duration for neomycin to treat hepatic encephalopathy is about 4 to 6 hours. Administering the neomycin dose every 6 hours should maintain an adequate drug level in the bowel.

PHARMACODYNAMICS

Lactulose is a disaccharide sugar. When metabolized, the drug acts to decrease blood ammonia levels, thereby reducing the degree of hepatic encephalopathy. Neomycin is an aminoglycoside antibiotic used to sterilize the bowel.

Mechanism of action

The disaccharide sugar lactulose consists of galactose and fructose. The metabolism of lactulose by colonic bacteria produces lactic, acetic, and formic acids. These organic acids acidify the colon from its normal pH of 7 to a pH of 5. Acidification of the colon contents converts nonionized ammonia to ionized ammonia, preventing its absorption.

Nonionized ammonia can diffuse from the blood into the colon. In the colon, the nonionized ammonia is converted to relatively nonabsorbable ammonium ions. These ammonium ions remain trapped in the GI tract. The following represents the progress from nonionized ammonia to the nonabsorbable ammonium ion:

$$\text{Blood} \qquad \text{Intestine}$$
$$NH_3 \rightarrow NH_3 + H^+ \rightarrow NH_4^+$$

Colon acidification maintains the ammonium ion in its ionized state. The charged ions cannot be absorbed readily through the lipid layer of the intestine. Furthermore, colon acidification encourages the growth of weak ammonia-producing bacteria, such as *Lactobacillus acidophilus,* over such ammonia producers as *Escherichia coli.* Lactulose also may produce osmotic diarrhea, which decreases the intestinal transit time available for ammonia production and absorption.

Neomycin lowers the blood ammonia level by decreasing the number of such ammonia-producing bacteria as *E. coli* in the GI tract. As with other aminoglycosides, neomycin exerts its antibacterial activity directly on the ribosomes of susceptible organisms, among them *E. coli,* by inhibiting protein synthesis via direct action on ribosomal subunits. When these bacteria are present, they convert urea to ammonia. Neomycin is bactericidal in high concentrations and bacteriostatic in low concentrations.

PHARMACOTHERAPEUTICS

Lactulose serves as an adjunct to protein restriction and supportive therapy to prevent or treat hepatic encephalopathy. Lactulose also can be used to prevent or treat hepatic encephalopathy from surgical portocaval shunts and chronic hepatic diseases, such as cirrhosis. The drug may reduce ammonia levels by 25% to 50%, usually accompanied by improved mental status. Clinical responses occur in 75% to 85% of the patients undergoing lactulose therapy. Patients unresponsive to neomycin and protein restriction therapy also may respond to lactulose; however, studies have shown that lactulose and neomycin are about equally effective.

Because neomycin destroys bacteria and lactulose requires bacterial metabolism, some researchers theorize that concomitant use of these drugs may be counterproductive. In practice, however, lactulose seems to remain active even in the presence of neomycin. In fact, some evidence suggests that concomitant use of lactulose and neomycin may be more beneficial than using either drug alone.

Neomycin serves as an adjunct to protein restriction and lactulose therapy in treating hepatic encephalopathy. It also is used as a preoperative intestinal antiseptic and as a treatment for diarrhea caused by enteropathogenic *E. coli.*

Although clinical trials have shown neomycin to be as effective as lactulose in reducing elevated blood ammonia levels, toxicity from systemic absorption of neomycin may be significant, especially with prolonged therapy. Therefore, lactulose may be more suitable for patients who need more than 2 to 3 days of therapy or for those with compromised renal function. Lactulose also is used to treat constipation because it produces osmotic diarrhea.

lactulose (Cephulac, Chronulac). Lactulose can be given orally or rectally.
Usual adult dosage: 20 to 30 grams (30 to 45 ml) P.O. t.i.d. or q.i.d., adjusted every 1 to 2 days, as needed, to produce two to three soft stools daily. The dosage also may

be adjusted by measuring the stool pH (acidity of the colon contents), until the pH approximates 5. For most patients, typical dosages range from 60 to 100 grams (90 to 150 ml) daily. Hourly doses of 30 to 45 ml may induce rapid defecation in acute situations.

For rectal administration, dilute 200 grams (300 ml) in 700 ml of tap water or 0.9% sodium chloride solution. Repeat every 4 to 6 hours. If the patient does not retain the enema for 30 minutes, repeat immediately.

neomycin (Mycifradin Sulfate, Neobiotic). Neomycin therapy usually accompanies other methods of reducing blood ammonia levels. These methods include a low-protein diet and cleansing the GI tract of blood from GI bleeding.
Usual adult dosage: as adjunctive treatment of hepatic encephalopathy, 4 to 12 grams/day P.O. in four divided doses. Therapy should continue for 5 to 6 days. Chronic hepatic insufficiency may require 4 grams/day for an indefinite time.

Rectally, administer a 1% solution as a retention enema for 20 to 60 minutes q.i.d.

Drug interactions

Ammonia-detoxicating agents produce no clinically significant interactions with other drugs. However, a cleansing enema containing soapsuds or an alkaline agent may interact with rectally administered lactulose or neomycin, interfering with their effectiveness.

ADVERSE DRUG REACTIONS

Lactulose is administered via the GI tract, and little of the drug is absorbed systemically. Therefore, GI symptoms represent the most frequent adverse reactions to lactulose. As intestinal bacteria metabolize lactulose to lactic, acetic, and formic acid, hydrogen gas is released. As a result, patients may experience gaseous abdominal distention, abdominal pain, belching, or flatulence. Some patients have reported nausea and vomiting after lactulose ingestion,which may represent a reaction to the extremely sweet taste of the drug.

Diarrhea, sometimes accompanied by abdominal cramping, may result from too much lactulose because some metabolites of lactulose produce a laxative action. Lactulose also exerts an osmotic effect, drawing water into the large intestine. This effect, increased with large doses, may produce frequent, loose stools. If the patient exhibits severe hepatic encephalopathy with a high blood ammonia level, diarrhea may be considered an acceptable adverse reaction.

Because lactulose is a disaccharide, small amounts of the oral drug are converted to galactose and fructose, which may be absorbed from the small intestine. After large doses of lactulose, these sugars may be absorbed in amounts sufficient to produce hyperglycemia in patients with diabetes mellitus.

Like other aminoglycoside antibiotics, neomycin may produce nephrotoxicity and ototoxicity. Despite the limited absorption of oral neomycin, long-term therapy with high doses of the drug administered concurrently with other aminoglycoside antibiotics can lead to these serious adverse reactions.

Several factors may increase the risk of toxicity and other adverse reactions to neomycin. Patients with decreased GI motility or mucosal ulceration tend to absorb larger amounts of neomycin, thereby increasing their serum cocentrations of the drug. Most of the toxic effects relate directly to the concentration and duration of action of high blood concentrations of neomycin. Serum concentrations of neomycin also are likely to be higher in patients who are elderly, dehydrated, experiencing renal failure, or taking potent diuretic drugs.

Because nephrotoxicity can result from neomycin, the nurse should monitor the patient closely for signs of impaired renal function. Furthermore, the signs of nephrotoxicity may not appear until after neomycin therapy has been discontinued. The nephrotoxic changes from neomycin usually are reversible over time.

Ototoxicity from damage to the vestibular and auditory branches of the eighth cranial nerve also may result from neomycin therapy. Auditory changes are more common than vestibular changes, but vestibular effects tend to be more reversible. (For preventive measures for nephrotoxicity and ototoxicity, see *Identifying and preventing neomycin toxicity.*)

Nausea, vomiting, and diarrhea probably represent the most frequent adverse reactions to neomycin. Diarrhea may result from malabsorption of fat, xylose, glucose, or other substances. It also may stem from superinfection with bacteria after normal bowel flora destruction by neomycin. *Clostridium difficile* infection leading to pseudomembranous colitis can be a particularly devastating result.

The potential for neuromuscular blockade also exists after neomycin administration. This reaction occurs less commonly with oral administration, but the nurse never should discount the problem. Neuromuscular blockade probably results when the release of acetylcholine at the nerve synapse becomes inhibited. Most cases of neuromuscular blockade have occurred when high doses of neomycin were administered concurrently with neuromuscular blocking drugs (such as tubocurarine and succinylcholine) or with general anesthesia. Hypocalcemia or myasthenia gravis also seems to increase the risk of neuromuscular blockade. The effects of neuromuscular blockade usually include a decreased rate and depth of respiration and acute muscle paralysis. The administration of calcium gluconate and perhaps neostigmine usually reverses these effects.

Identifying and preventing neomycin toxicity

Because neomycin therapy produces nephrotoxicity and ototoxicity, the nurse must know the signs and symptoms of these adverse reactions and how to prevent them.

SIGNS AND SYMPTOMS	PREVENTION
Nephrotoxicity	
• Decreased specific gravity and osmolality of urine, indicating impaired urine concentrating ability • Protein or granular or hyaline casts in the urine • Increasing serum creatinine level	• Do not administer neomycin to a patient with decreased gastric motility or GI ulceration because these conditions cause increased neomycin absorption. Do not administer to a patient with dehydration or renal failure, or in combination with a potent diuretic. • Avoid concurrent use with other drugs that can produce nephrotoxicity. • Monitor the serum neomycin concentration level. • Monitor urine specific gravity, urinalysis, and serum creatinine level before, during, and after neomycin therapy. • Monitor intake, output, and body weight daily, remembering that renal failure from neomycin commonly is nonoliguric.
Ototoxicity	
• Onset of a high-pitched tinnitus, which may be initial symptom • Loss of high-frequency sounds • Hearing loss later in therapy • Headache followed by dizziness, nausea, vomiting, and difficulty with coordination, caused by vestibular damage	• Do not administer neomycin to a patient with decreased gastric motility or GI ulceration because these conditions lead to increased neomycin absorption. Do not administer to a patient with preexisting hearing loss. • Avoid concurrent administration of other drugs that might cause ototoxicity. • Instruct the patient to report ringing in the ears or headache. • Consider audiometric evaluation before, during, and after neomycin therapy.

Although hypersensitivity reactions to ammonia-detoxicating agents are uncommon, some reactions have resulted from neomycin. These include skin rashes, fever, angioedema, stomatitis, and anaphylactic shock.

NURSING PROCESS APPLICATION

The following information assists the nurse in caring for a patient who is receiving an ammonia-detoxicating agent.

Assessment

• Review the patient's history for a preexisting condition that contraindicates the use of an ammonia-detoxicating agent, such as a condition that requires a low-galactose diet, known hypersensitivity to the drug, GI ulceration, or intestinal obstruction.
• Review the patient's history for a preexisting condition that requires cautious use of an ammonia-detoxicating agent, such as diabetes mellitus, pregnancy, lactation, myasthenia gravis, renal failure, advanced age, dehydration, hearing impairment, or use of a neuromuscular blocking agent, general anesthetic, or nephrotoxic or ototoxic drug.
• Assess the patient for adverse reactions to the prescribed ammonia-detoxicating agent, such as GI distress, nephrotoxicity, or ototoxicity.
• Assess the effectiveness of the ammonia-detoxicating agent periodically.
• Assess the patient's bowel function regularly during ammonia-detoxicating agent therapy.
• Evaluate the patient's and family's knowledge about the prescribed ammonia-detoxicating agent.

Nursing diagnoses

The following examples represent appropriate nursing diagnoses for a patient receiving an ammonia-detoxicating agent.
• Potential for injury related to a preexisting condition that contraindicates the use of an ammonia-detoxicating agent
• Potential for injury related to a preexisting condition that requires cautious use of an ammonia-detoxicating agent
• Potential for injury related to adverse drug reactions
• Diarrhea related to the adverse GI effects of the ammonia-detoxicating agent
• Knowledge deficit related to the prescribed ammonia-detoxicating agent

Planning and implementation

• Do not administer an ammonia-detoxicating agent to a patient with a condition that contraindicates its use.
• Administer an ammonia-detoxicating agent cautiously to a patient at risk because of a preexisting condition.
• *Monitor the patient for adverse reactions frequently throughout therapy. Be especially alert for adverse reactions to neomycin in a patient who is elderly or dehydrated; has renal failure, decreased GI motility, or mucosal ulcerations; or takes a potent diuretic.*
• *Monitor the patient for signs of effectiveness of the ammonia-detoxicating agent by assessing the patient's level of consciousness, asterixis, muscle coordination, and blood*

ammonia level. All of these factors should improve as the blood ammonia level decreases.
• Test for muscle coordination by having the patient provide a signature or draw a five-pointed star each day. As hepatic encephalopathy improves, muscle coordination should improve, making the patient's signature and drawings clearer.
• Check the stool pH periodically. A pH of 5 or less indicates that the colon contents are acidic enough to trap ammonia ions, thereby reducing ammonia absorption.
• *Monitor the blood glucose level regularly in a diabetic patient receiving lactulose.*
• *Evaluate the patient's renal function before, during, and after neomycin therapy. Also, document information about the patient's auditory and vestibular function before neomycin therapy begins.*
• *Monitor the respiratory rate and depth and motor function in a patient at risk for neuromuscular blockade. Have calcium gluconate and neostigmine readily available if such a patient must receive neomycin.*
• Note that lactulose may be mixed in a beverage such as juice, a soft drink, milk, or water to improve its palatability and decrease nausea and vomiting.
• Administer rectal neomycin or lactulose via a catheter held in place with a large balloon for inflation. Administer the drug deep into the rectum, at least 8″ (20 cm). After administration, the patient should retain the drug for 30 to 60 minutes. Inflating the rectal catheter balloon improves retention. Do not use cleansing enemas containing soapsuds or alkaline agents with rectally administered lactulose or neomycin because the soapsuds and alkalines interfere with the drug's effectiveness.
• Monitor the number and consistency of the patient's stools during lactulose therapy. Normally, consider the dosage to be adequate if the patient has two to three soft stools per day.
• Notify the physician if adverse reactions occur or if the ammonia-detoxicating agent is ineffective.
• *Monitor the patient daily for diarrhea. In acute situations, the large amounts of prescribed lactulose may cause diarrhea. If diarrhea occurs, monitor the patient for fluid, electrolyte, and acid-base disturbances, particularly dehydration, hypokalemia, and acidosis. Take measures to protect the patient's perianal skin from the irritation caused by frequent defecation.*

Patient teaching

• Teach the patient and family the name, dose, frequency, action, and adverse effects of the prescribed ammonia-detoxicating agent.
• *Instruct the diabetic patient receiving lactulose to monitor blood glucose levels regularly and be alert for hyperglycemia.*
• *Advise the patient receiving neomycin to report hearing or equilibrium changes to the physician.*

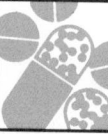

Cation-exchange resin and ammonia-detoxicating agents

The following chart summarizes the major cation-exchange resin and ammonia-detoxicating agents currently in clinical use.

DRUG	MAJOR INDICATIONS	USUAL ADULT DOSAGES	CONTRAINDICATIONS AND PRECAUTIONS
Cation-exchange resin			
sodium polystyrene sulfonate	Hyperkalemia	15 grams P.O. one to four times daily or 30 to 50 grams every 1 to 6 hours rectally	• Know that sodium polystyrene sulfonate is contraindicated in a patient with hypokalemia or known hypersensitivity to this agent. • Administer with caution to a pregnant or lactating patient or one who cannot tolerate sodium loads, such as one with congestive heart failure.
Ammonia-detoxicating agents			
lactulose	Hepatic encephalopathy	Initial dose of 20 to 30 grams (30 to 45 ml) P.O. t.i.d. to q.i.d.; for rectal administration, 200 grams (300 ml) in 700 ml water or 0.9% sodium chloride solution; for acute toxicity in hapatic encephalopathy, 30 to 45 ml every hour	• Know that lactulose is contraindicated in a patient who requires a low-galactose diet. • Administer with caution to a pregnant or lactating patient or one with diabetes mellitus.
neomycin	Hepatic encephalopathy	4 to 12 grams P.O. in four divided doses for 5 to 6 days; or rectal administration of a 1% solution retained for 20 to 60 minutes, q.i.d.	• Know that neomycin is contraindicated in a pregnant patient or one with known hypersensitivity to the agent, intestinal obstruction, or GI ulceration. • Administer with caution to a patient with myasthenia gravis, renal failure, advanced age, dehydration, hearing impairment, or hypocalcemia or to one who is receiving a neuromuscular blocking agent, general anesthesia, or a nephrotoxic or ototoxic drug.

• Teach the patient or a family member how to prepare and administer the prescribed ammonia-detoxicating agent.
• Instruct the patient to notify the physician if adverse reactions occur.

Evaluation
The following examples represent appropriate evaluation statements for a patient receiving an ammonia-detoxicating agent.
• The patient has no conditions that contraindicate ammonia-detoxicating agent therapy.
• The patient has no conditions that require cautious use of an ammonia-detoxicating agent.
• The patient demonstrates no adverse reactions to the prescribed ammonia-detoxicating agent.
• The patient does not experience severe diarrhea during ammonia-detoxicating agent therapy.
• The patient and family express an accurate understanding of the points taught about the prescribed ammonia-detoxicating agent.

• The patient correctly demonstrates how to prepare and administer the prescribed ammonia-detoxicating agent.

CHAPTER SUMMARY

Chapter 48 covered the cation-exchange resin and ammonia-detoxicating agents. Both kinds of drugs decrease toxic levels of endogenous substances by increasing their elimination via the GI tract or decreasing their production. Here are the highlights of the chapter.
• Sodium polystyrene sulfonate is a nonabsorbable resin that releases sodium and absorbs potassium in the GI tract. The drug is used to treat hyperkalemia.
• The onset of action of sodium polystyrene sulfonate is slow, and changes in the serum potassium level may not occur for 2 to 24 hours. This cation-exchange resin should

not be used alone in a patient with a life-threatening serum potassium level because it may not remove the excess potassium quickly enough.

• Sodium polystyrene sulfonate may be administered orally or rectally via retention enema.

• Sodium polystyrene sulfonate may absorb calcium, magnesium, and other electrolytes, causing imbalances. It also may release sufficient sodium to cause problems for a patient who cannot tolerate a sodium load. When caring for a patient receiving sodium polystyrene sulfonate, the nurse should monitor closely for signs and symptoms of fluid and electrolyte imbalance and should evaluate serum electrolyte levels regularly.

• Sodium polystyrene sulfonate tends to solidify in the GI tract, which can lead to fecal impaction. To prevent impaction, the nurse can administer the drug with 70% sorbitol, which forms softer stools and helps excrete the resin.

• Lactulose and neomycin reduce the blood ammonia level in patients with hepatic encephalopathy. Lactulose is a disaccharide sugar composed of galactose and fructose. Neomycin is an aminoglycoside antibiotic that is absorbed minimally from the GI tract.

• Lactulose is metabolized by colonic bacteria to lactic, acetic, and formic acid, thereby acidifying the colon contents. As the colon contents become more acidic, ammonia found within the bowel and diffused from the serum is trapped in the stool and excreted from the body.

• Effective lactulose therapy generally results in two to three soft stools per day. Diarrhea may result if large dosages are used to treat acute toxicity.

• Neomycin lowers the blood ammonia concentration by acting in the GI tract to eliminate bacteria that form ammonia from urea.

• As with all aminoglycoside antibiotics, neomycin can produce serious toxicity. Nephrotoxicity, ototoxicity, and neuromuscular blockade may result from prolonged use of neomycin.

• Before administering an ammonia-detoxicating agent, the nurse should assess the patient for preexisting conditions that increase the risk of adverse reactions, especially to neomycin. During therapy, the nurse should monitor the patient closely for adverse drug reactions.

STUDY QUESTIONS

See Appendix 1 for answers.

1. Mel Baker, age 65, was admitted to the hospital with acute renal failure. During Mr. Baker's admission assessment, the nurse noted skin pallor, irregular pulse, edema, weight gain, and decreased urine output. Laboratory tests revealed elevated potassium, blood urea nitrogen, and creatinine levels. To lower Mr. Baker's potassium, the physician prescribed sodium polystyrene sulfonate (Kayexalate). Where does this drug exert its primary action?
(a) serum
(b) kidneys
(c) liver
(d) GI tract

2. For administration of sodium polystyrene sulfonate, which administration route provides the fastest onset of action?
(a) oral
(b) rectal
(c) intravenous
(d) intramuscular

3. How does sodium polystyrene sulfonate reduce serum potassium levels?
(a) It exchanges sodium for hydrogen, which is exchanged for potassium.
(b) It produces a transient intracellular shift of potassium.
(c) It prevents the release of intracellular potassium.
(d) It prevents further absorption of potassium from the GI tract.

4. Sodium polystyrene sulfonate can cause constipation. To prevent this adverse reaction, the nurse combines which agent with with sodium polystyrene sulfonate for Mr. Baker?
(a) sorbitol
(b) neomycin
(c) calcium carbonate
(d) aluminum hydroxide

5. Will Davis, age 50, is admitted to the hospital with hepatic encephalopathy caused by cirrhosis of the liver. His serum ammonia level is 100 mcg/dl. Mr. Davis's physician prescribes lactulose (Cephulac) 30 grams P.O. q.i.d. How does lactulose reduce the serum ammonia level?
(a) It decreases the number of ammonia-producing bacteria in the bowel.
(b) It acidifies the colon, which prevents ammonia absorption.
(c) It increases the colon pH to neutralize the ammonia there.
(d) It creates a barrier in the GI tract that prevents ammonia absorption.

6. The physician could have selected neomycin instead of lactulose as an ammonia-detoxicating agent. Why is lactulose preferred over neomycin for prolonged therapy?
(a) Neomycin may cause toxicity when absorbed systemically.
(b) Neomycin is more expensive than lactulose.
(c) Neomycin is not as effective at lowering the ammonia level.
(d) Neomycin loses its effectiveness with prolonged use.

7. The nurse reviews Mr. Davis's history carefully before administering lactulose. Which condition would warrant cautious administration of lactulose?
(a) renal insufficiency
(b) congestive heart failure
(c) diabetes mellitus
(d) diabetes insipidus

8. After administering lactulose, the nurse assesses Mr. Davis for signs of the drug's effectiveness. Which assessment finding suggests a decreased blood ammonia level?
(a) increased level of consciousness
(b) increased asterixis
(c) decreased muscle strength
(d) hyperreflexia

SELECTED REFERENCES

AHFS drug information 90. (1990). Bethesda, MD: American Society of Hospital Pharmacists.

Goodman and Gilman's the pharmacological basis of therapeutics (8th ed.; 1990). Elmsford, NY: Pergamon Press.

Hagerty, J. (1989). The aminoglycosides. *Focus on Critical Care,* 16(2), 104-108.

Hansten, P., and Horn, J. (1989). *Drug interactions: Clinical significance of drug-drug interactions* (6th ed.). Philadelphia: Lea & Febiger.

Hepatic failure due to nicotinic acid. (1989). *Nurses Drug Alert,* 13(10), 80.

Johnson, C. (1988). Hearing loss following the application of topical neomycin. *Journal of Burn Care Rehabilitation,* 9(2), 162-164.

North American Nursing Diagnosis Association. (1990). *Taxonomy—Revised, with official diagnostic categories.* St. Louis: NANDA

DRUGS TO TREAT ENDOCRINE SYSTEM DISORDERS

Endocrine pharmacology encompasses a wide range of agents, including natural hormones and their synthetic analogues, hormonelike substances, and drugs that stimulate or suppress hormone secretion. To understand endocrine pharmacology, the nurse needs to know about the endocrine system and its hormones. (For an illustration of endocrine glands and the substances they secrete, see *Endocrine hormones,* page 835.)

PANCREATIC HORMONES

The pancreas secretes two hormones, insulin and glucagon, from special cells in the islets of Langerhans. The beta cells produce insulin; the alpha cells secrete glucagon.

Insulin promotes glucose uptake, storage, and use; glucagon increases glycogenolysis and gluconeogenesis. Insulin also inhibits lipolysis and promotes cellular uptake of amino acids and protein synthesis. The blood glucose level primarily controls insulin and glucagon secretion. At a normal fasting blood glucose level, (70 to 110 mg/dl), little insulin is secreted. When the blood glucose level rises above 110 mg/dl, insulin secretion rapidly increases. When it falls below 70 mg/dl, glucagon secretion increases, rapidly increasing hepatic glucose production. Thus, glucagon prevents hypoglycemia and insulin prevents hyperglycemia.

THYROID HORMONES

The thyroid gland secretes triiodothyronine (T_3) and thyroxine (T_4), which influence the body's metabolic rate, and calcitonin, which helps regulate calcium metabolism. Secretion of these thyroid hormones is controlled primarily by thyroid-stimulating hormone (TSH), which is secreted by the anterior pituitary gland.

The thyroid gland secretes more T_4 than T_3. Although the hormones function the same physiologically, they differ in onset and intensity of action. T_3 is about four times as potent as T_4 and produces effects much more rapidly. Yet both hormones increase protein synthesis, stimulate cellular enzyme activity, promote growth, and enhance carbohydrate and fat metabolism. They also increase cardiac output and heart rate, respiratory rate and depth, and gastrointestinal (GI) motility.

Calcitonin is secreted primarily by the thyroid gland. When the serum calcium level is high, calcitonin secretion increases. Calcitonin reduces the serum calcium level by inhibiting bone resorption, reducing osteoclast activity (bone absorption and removal), and increasing renal excretion of calcium.

PARATHYROID HORMONE

Secretion of parathyroid hormone by the parathyroid glands is regulated primarily by the plasma calcium concentration. Any physiologic or pathologic alteration that increases the serum calcium level will suppress parathyroid gland secretion. Any decrease in serum calcium level will increase parathyroid gland secretion.

Parathyroid hormone stimulates the resorption of calcium and phosphate from bone. It also increases GI absorption and decreases renal excretion of calcium.

ANTERIOR PITUITARY HORMONES

The anterior pituitary gland secretes six hormones that help control metabolic processes throughout the body: growth hormone (GH), adrenocorticotropic hormone (ACTH), TSH, prolactin, follicle-stimulating hormone (FSH), and luteinizing hormone (LH).

Also called somatotropic hormone or somatotropin, GH promotes growth by increasing protein synthesis, decreasing carbohydrate use, and increasing fat mobilization and use for energy.

ACTH, also called adrenocorticotropin or corticotropin, controls cortisol secretion and enhances androgen production by the adrenal gland. It also influences aldosterone secretion.

Glossary

Abortifacient: agent used to induce fetal expulsion.

Adrenocorticotropin: anterior pituitary hormone that stimulates the adrenal cortex.

Anabolic: promoting general body growth.

Androgenic: producing masculine characteristics.

Calcitonin: thyroid hormone that decreases the serum calcium level.

Chvostek's sign: facial muscle spasm elicited by tapping the muscles or facial nerve in a hypocalcemic patient.

Diabetes insipidus: metabolic disorder characterized by extreme polyuria and polydipsia from deficient secretion of antidiuretic hormone (ADH) or the inability of kidney tubules to respond to ADH.

Diabetes mellitus: metabolic disorder in which the ability to metabolize carbohydrates is lost because of decreased insulin secretion; characterized by hyperglycemia, glycosuria, polyuria, polydipsia, polyphagia, emaciation, and weakness.

Eclampsia: severe complication of pregnancy characterized by seizures, coma, hypertension, edema, and proteinuria.

Euthyroid: with a normal thyroid gland.

Gluconeogenesis: carbohydrate formation from protein molecules.

Glycogenolysis: breakdown of the polysaccharide glycogen in body tissues.

Gonadotropin: hormonal substance that stimulates the ovaries or testes.

Gynecomastia: excessive development of male mammary glands.

Hyperglycemia: abnormally high blood glucose level.

Hypoglycemia: abnormally low blood glucose level.

Hypogonadism: condition resulting from abnormally decreased functioning of the ovaries or testes, characterized by retarded growth and sexual development.

Hyposthenuria: excretion of urine with a low specific gravity.

Iodism: toxicity from excessive ingestion of iodine, characterized by glandular atrophy, coryza, frontal headache, emaciation, weakness, and skin eruptions.

Lipoatrophy: wasting of the body's fatty tissues.

Lipodystrophy: disturbance of fat metabolism involving regional loss of subcutaneous fat.

Lipohypertrophy: excessive enlargement of fatty tissues.

Lipolysis: fat breakdown.

Myxedema: condition resulting from hypothyroidism and characterized by dry, waxy, nonpitting edema; abnormal mucin deposits in the skin; swollen lips; and a thickened nose.

Paget's disease: progressive metabolic bone disease characterized by enlargement, bowing, destruction, or deformity of the bones; tenderness; and dull, aching pain.

Panhypopituitarism: pituitary insufficiency.

Preeclampsia: complication of late pregnancy characterized by hypertension, proteinuria, and edema.

Tetany: manifestation of abnormal calcium metabolism by sharp flexion of the wrist and ankle joints (carpopedal spasms), muscle twitching, muscle cramps, seizures, and stridor.

Thyroglobulin: iodine-containing protein in the colloid of thyroid gland follicles, which stores thyroid hormones.

Thyroiditis: thyroid gland inflammation.

Thyrotoxicosis: disorder caused by thyroid gland overactivity; hyperthyroidism.

Thyrotropin: anterior pituitary hormone that stimulates the thyroid gland.

Tocolytic agent: drug that inhibits uterine contractions, labor, or childbirth.

Trousseau's sign: carpopedal spasm elicited by putting pressure on large nerves in a hypocalcemic patient.

TSH, or thyrotropin, stimulates the thyroid gland to increase T_3 and T_4 production and secretion. Normally, the thyroid hormone level remains fairly constant because of an effective feedback mechanism. Increased levels of thyroid hormone inhibit TSH secretion from the pituitary gland; decreased levels stimulate TSH secretion. A hypothalamic hormone, thyrotropin-releasing hormone, regulates the increase in TSH secretion.

Prolactin promotes mammary gland development and milk production. Prolactin secretion predominantly is under the negative control of the hypothalamus, which synthesizes a hormone that suppresses its secretion from the pituitary gland. During lactation, however, formation of this prolactin inhibitory hormone is suppressed, and sucking or breast manipulation stimulates prolactin secretion.

FSH and LH are gonadotropic hormones secreted in response to a hypothalamic releasing hormone and regulated by plasma estrogen and progesterone levels. During each female reproductive cycle, FSH and LH plasma levels increase and decrease. During the first phase of the cycle, increased hormone secretion stimulates new follicle growth in the ovaries. Eventually, one follicle becomes more highly developed than the others and begins to secrete large amounts of estrogen, which triggers a feedback mechanism that inhibits FSH secretion by the anterior pituitary. This makes the other follicles stop growing and involute. The one large follicle continues to grow through the self-stimulating effect of the secreted estrogen. Shortly before ovulation, LH and FSH secretion by the anterior pituitary increases markedly, producing rapid swelling of the follicle that culminates in ovulation.

POSTERIOR PITUITARY HORMONES

The posterior pituitary gland secretes antidiuretic hormone (ADH) and oxytocin. Nerve impulses originating in the hypothalamus regulate the secretion of these hormones.

Endocrine hormones

In the endocrine system, various glands secrete different endocrine hormones, as shown below. These hormones stimulate or inhibit the activity of target glands or cells to maintain homeostasis.

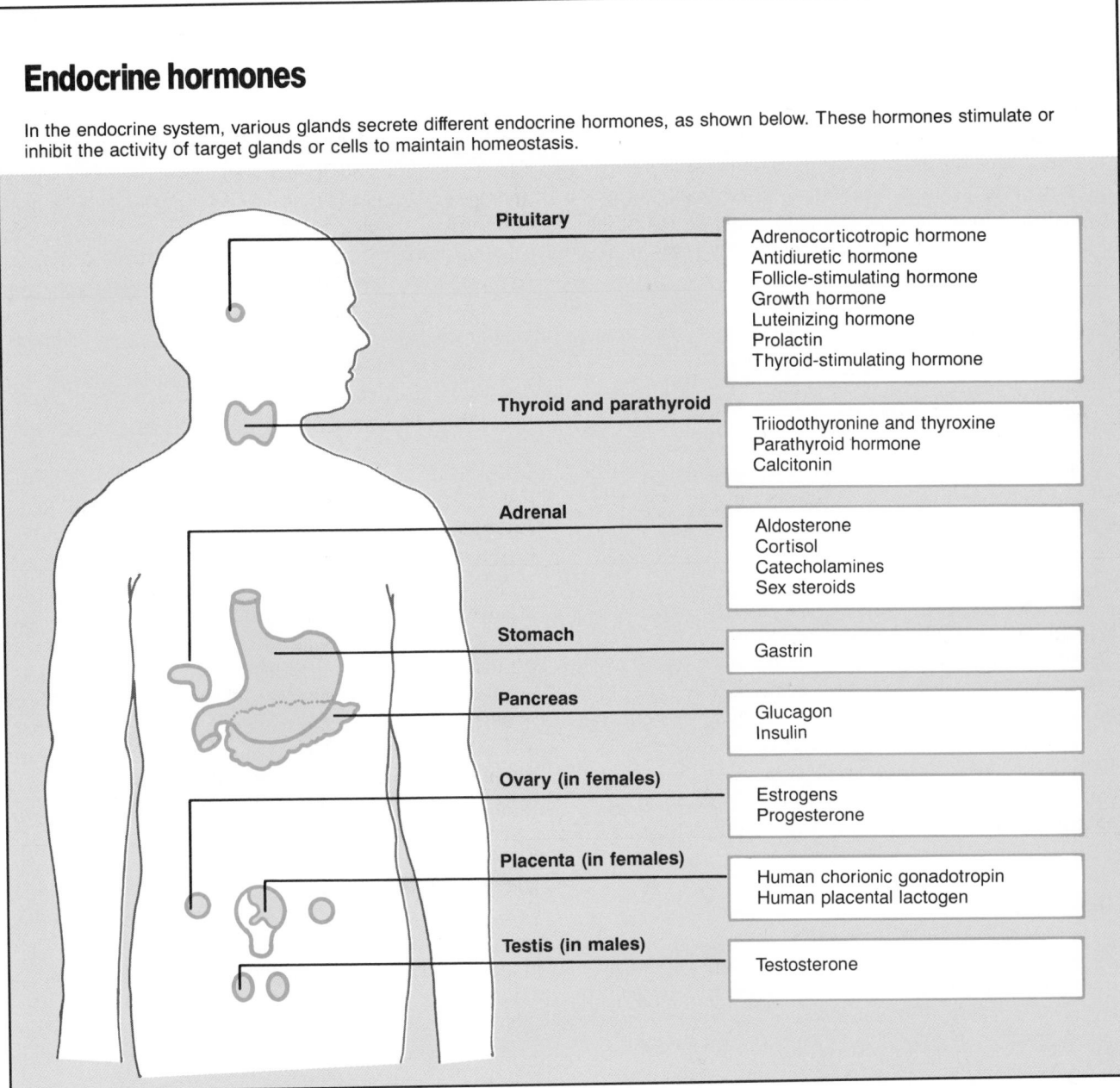

Pituitary

Adrenocorticotropic hormone
Antidiuretic hormone
Follicle-stimulating hormone
Growth hormone
Luteinizing hormone
Prolactin
Thyroid-stimulating hormone

Thyroid and parathyroid

Triiodothyronine and thyroxine
Parathyroid hormone
Calcitonin

Adrenal

Aldosterone
Cortisol
Catecholamines
Sex steroids

Stomach

Gastrin

Pancreas

Glucagon
Insulin

Ovary (in females)

Estrogens
Progesterone

Placenta (in females)

Human chorionic gonadotropin
Human placental lactogen

Testis (in males)

Testosterone

ADH, or vasopressin, increases water resorption in the collecting ducts of the nephrons. Its production is regulated by osmotic receptors and volume receptors. Concentration of body fluids stimulates the osmotic receptors in the hypothalamus, increasing the impulses transmitted to the posterior pituitary to stimulate ADH secretion, which increases the water permeability of the collecting ducts.

Blood loss stimulates the volume receptors (atrial stretch receptors and baroreceptors in the carotid, aortic, and pulmonary arteries). This precipitates a marked increase in ADH secretion. ADH also exerts a potent pressor effect to maintain arterial blood pressure.

Oxytocin produces uterine contractions and milk release from the breast alveoli into the milk ducts. At the end of pregnancy, stretching or irritation of the cervix transmits a neurogenic reflex to the posterior pituitary, which stimulates increased oxytocin secretion and, subsequently, uterine contraction.

GONADAL HORMONES

The testes secrete testosterone, the major male gonadal hormone, and other male sex hormones, or androgens. These hormones produce androgenic (masculinizing) effects but also exert some anabolic effects. The adrenal gland also secretes androgens, but they are much less potent and do not produce significant androgenic effects.

The ovaries secrete estrogens and progesterone in response to FSH and LH. Estrogens stimulate the cellular proliferation and growth of sex organs and related reproductive tissues. They also affect skeletal growth, fat deposition, skin vascularity, and various intracellular functions. Progesterone promotes secretory changes in the endometrium to prepare the uterus for implantation of the fertilized ovum. It also evokes secretory changes in the fallopian tubes and breasts.

Estrogen or progesterone can inhibit ovulation by a negative feedback effect on the hypothalamus and subsequent suppression of FSH and LH release.

OVERVIEW OF CHAPTERS

Unit Twelve presents agents that are used to treat endocrine system disorders. Many of these agents are used to replace missing hormones or to stimulate or suppress hormone secretion.

Chapter 49
Hypoglycemic Agents and Glucagon

Chapter 49 begins by differentiating between Type I and Type II diabetes mellitus. Then it presents the role of insulin and the oral hypoglycemic agents or sulfonylureas in treating hyperglycemic states. It concludes with a discussion of glucagon, a hyperglycemic agent used to treat hypoglycemic states. For each drug class, the chapter demonstrates application of the nursing process when administering these agents.

Chapter 50
Thyroid and Antithyroid Agents

Chapter 50 discusses the normal anatomy and physiology of the thyroid gland and the biosynthesis and physiologic effects of T_3 and T_4. Then it investigates the pharmacotherapeutic uses of thyroid and antithyroid agents. It also highlights nursing process activities related to administration of these agents.

Chapter 51
Parathyroid Agents

Chapter 51 presents the agents that regulate serum calcium levels: calcitonin, etidronate disodium, and the vitamin D analogues. It compares their actions and adverse effects, and highlights nursing process activities.

Chapter 52
Pituitary Agents

Chapter 52 first explores the normal functions of anterior and posterior pituitary hormones. Then it details the pharmacology of corticotropin, cosyntropin, somatrem, vaso-

pressin, and oxytocin. The chapter also discusses application of the nursing process when caring for a patient receiving an anterior or posterior pituitary agent.

Chapter 53
Androgenic and Anabolic Steroid Agents

Chapter 53 differentiates between agents used primarily as androgenic agents and those used mainly as anabolic ones. It discusses the pharmacologic properties of the predominantly androgenic agents, including, danazol, fluoxymesterone, methyltestosterone, and the testosterones; the predominantly anabolic agents, including oxandrolone, oxymetholone, and testolactone; and related agents. Throughout, the chapter emphasizes their pharmacotherapeutic uses, adverse effects, and appropriate nursing care using the nursing process.

Chapter 54
Estrogens, Progestins, and Oral Contraceptive Agents

Chapter 54 presents agents that mimic the physiologic effects of female gonadal hormones. After reviewing the physiology of the female reproductive cycle, it discusses estrogen and progestin agents. Then it explores specific administration procedures, including their therapeutic rationales, and details patient teaching information as well as other aspects of nursing care. The chapter also discusses oral contraceptives, which usually are estrogen-progestin combinations, delineating their other therapeutic uses, adverse effects, and nursing care through the nursing process.

Chapter 55
Uterine Motility Agents

Chapter 55 addresses the uterine-stimulating agents (the prostaglandins and ergot alkaloids) and the uterine-inhibiting, or tocolytic agents (magnesium sulfate, ritodrine, and terbutaline). It examines their actions, therapeutic uses, and adverse effects. The chapter also discusses nursing process activities related to administration of these agents.

HYPOGLYCEMIC AGENTS AND GLUCAGON

OBJECTIVES

After reading and studying this chapter, the student should be able to:

1. Differentiate between Type I and Type II diabetes mellitus and describe the patient's needs in each.

2. Identify the different sources of insulins and describe how they are classified.

3. Describe the mechanism of action by which insulin decreases the blood glucose level.

4. Explain the important points the nurse should teach a diabetic patient about taking insulin.

5. Explain why different insulin regimens exist.

6. Discuss the pharmacokinetics of oral hypoglycemic agents.

7. Describe the clinical uses of oral hypoglycemic agents.

8. Explain how glucagon increases the blood glucose level.

9. Describe how to apply the nursing process when caring for a patient who is receiving a hypoglycemic agent or glucagon.

INTRODUCTION

Scattered throughout the pancreas are cell clusters known as the islets of Langerhans. Beta cells in the islets of Langerhans produce insulin; alpha cells in the islets of Langerhans produce glucagon. Insulin decreases the blood glucose level, whereas glucagon increases it.

During normal carbohydrate metabolism, insulin facilitates cellular uptake of glucose as well as its storage (in the form of glycogen and fat) and metabolism. Insulin also plays an important role in the metabolism of protein and fat. During protein metabolism, insulin increases protein synthesis and inhibits protein breakdown. In fat metabolism, insulin stimulates triglyceride synthesis and inhibits fat breakdown. Without insulin, the body cannot metabolize glucose and must break down protein and fat for fuel.

Glucagon opposes the actions of insulin. It stimulates glycogenolysis (conversion of glycogen to glucose). It also stimulates gluconeogenesis (glucose production from plasma amino acids resulting from protein breakdown). Furthermore, glucagon increases lipolysis (fat breakdown) and inhibits triglyceride storage.

An absolute or relative insulin deficiency causes diabetes mellitus. This disorder is characterized by hyperglycemia. Diabetes mellitus is categorized into the following types:

• *Type I diabetes mellitus.* The etiology of Type I diabetes mellitus, also called insulin-dependent diabetes mellitus or IDDM, remains unknown. However, genetic factors, viral infections, and an autoimmune disease may play a role. In the initial stages of Type I diabetes mellitus, the pancreas cannot produce sufficient insulin. As the disease rapidly progresses, an absolute insulin deficiency occurs. A patient with this disorder depends on exogenous insulin for survival. Diet and exercise are other essential components of therapy for patients with Type I diabetes mellitus.

• *Type II diabetes mellitus.* Also called noninsulin-dependent diabetes mellitus or NIDDM, Type II diabetes mellitus is characterized by a relative deficiency of insulin and insulin resistance. With relative deficiency, the patient cannot produce sufficient insulin to meet the body's needs. With insulin resistance, the patient cannot maintain an adequate blood glucose level—despite normal or excessive insulin production—because of aberrant glucose metabolism. Relative insulin deficiency and insulin resistance cause an inability to maintain a normal blood glucose level. Patients with Type II diabetes mellitus need not depend on exogenous insulin for survival although they may at times require it to maintain a blood glucose level within acceptable limits.

Diet and exercise are essential for achieving blood glucose control in Type II diabetes mellitus. Therapy also may include oral hypoglycemic agents, insulin, or both if diet alone cannot the maintain the blood glucose level within

---

SELECTED NURSING DIAGNOSES

Hypoglycemic agents and glucagon

The following nursing diagnoses address representative problems and etiologies that a nurse may encounter when caring for a patient who is receiving a hypoglycemic agent or glucagon. Some of these nursing diagnoses contain generalized etiologies, which the nurse must individualize based on the patient's needs. (For some common nursing diagnoses and related interventions for each drug class, see the "Nursing Process Application" sections of this chapter.)

- Altered health maintenance related to ineffectiveness of the prescribed hypoglycemic agent
- Altered health maintenance related to the development of insulin resistance
- Altered protection related to hypoglycemia caused by a hypoglycemic agent
- Altered protection related to insulin-induced Somogyi or dawn phenomenon
- Altered protection related to the adverse hematologic or hepatic effects of an oral hypoglycemic agent
- Altered urinary elimination related to the adverse renal effects of an oral hypoglycemic agent
- Impaired tissue integrity related to a local reaction to insulin
- Knowledge deficit related to the prescribed hypoglycemic agent or glucagon
- Noncompliance related to long-term use of a hypoglycemic agent
- Potential fluid volume deficit related to the adverse gastrointestinal effects of an oral hypoglycemic agent
- Potential for injury related to a preexisting condition that contraindicates the use of a hypoglycemic agent or glucagon
- Potential for injury related to a preexisting condition that requires cautious use of a hypoglycemic agent or glucagon
- Potential for injury related to adverse drug reactions
- Potential for injury related to a systemic hypersensitivity reaction to insulin

---

acceptable limits. The etiology of Type II diabetes mellitus is unknown, although obesity seems to play a role in genetically predisposed persons. (For a comparison of characteristics, see *Type I and Type II diabetes mellitus.*)

• *Other types of diabetes mellitus.* Other types of diabetes mellitus may occur secondary to drug therapy or to another disease or condition. Such cases of diabetes may be temporary.

• *Gestational diabetes mellitus.* This type of diabetes occurs only during pregnancy and results from the stress of pregnancy, which increases insulin demands. It requires diet, exercise, and possibly insulin for blood glucose control. After the woman gives birth, gestational diabetes usually resolves. However, it may recur with other pregnancies and may lead to diabetes mellitus.

Patients with blood glucose levels that are above normal but not diagnostic for diabetes mellitus are considered to have impaired glucose tolerance.

Insulin and oral hypoglycemic preparations are classified as antidiabetic or hypoglycemic agents. Glucagon is classified as a hyperglycemic agent.

For a summary of representative drugs, see *Selected major drugs: Hypoglycemic agents and glucagon,* page 853. For a listing of applicable nursing diagnoses that the nurse may formulate when caring for a patient receiving one of these agents, see *Selected nursing diagnoses: Hypoglycemic agents and glucagon.* For detailed information on applying the nursing process, see Chapter 6, The Nursing Process and Drug Therapy.

INSULIN

Patients with Type I diabetes mellitus require exogenous insulin to control the blood glucose level. Insulin also may be given to patients with Type II and other types of diabetes mellitus. Insulin decreases the blood glucose level by facilitating glucose cellular uptake and metabolism during normal carbohydrate metabolism.

Four sources of insulin are available:
- beef insulin, from the bovine pancreas
- pork insulin, from the porcine pancreas
- "human" insulin, from a recombinant DNA process in which the insulin is synthesized in *Escherichia coli* bacteria that have been altered genetically by adding a human gene
- "human" insulin, from an enzymatic conversion of pork insulin through which the pork insulin molecule becomes identical to that produced by the human pancreas.

Three concentrations of insulin are available: U-40, or 40 units of insulin per milliliter; U-100, or 100 units of insulin per milliliter; and U-500, or 500 units of insulin per milliliter.

PHARMACOKINETICS

The absorption, distribution, metabolism, and excretion of different insulins are similar. However, their onset, peak, and duration of action vary considerably.

Absorption, distribution, metabolism, excretion

Insulin is *not* effective when taken orally because the gastrointestinal (GI) tract breaks down the protein molecule before it reaches the bloodstream. All insulins, however, may be given by subcutaneous (S.C.) injection. Absorption

Type I and Type II diabetes mellitus

The information in this table is for comparative purposes only. All patients do not fit the age and weight patterns.

PATIENT CHARACTERISTIC	TYPE I DIABETES MELLITUS	TYPE II DIABETES MELLITUS
Age	Usually diagnosed before age 20	Usually diagnosed after age 40
Weight	Usually underweight or thin	Usually overweight or obese
Endogenous insulin production	Decreased or absent	Slightly decreased, normal, or increased
Exogenous insulin requirement	Required for all Type I diabetics	May be required for 20% to 30% of Type II diabetics
Ketoacidosis	Probable	Unlikely, except during infection or stress
Genetic susceptibility	Related to human leukocyte antigen (HLA-DR3, -DR4, and others)	Related to family history, but unrelated to HLA
Symptoms	Sudden onset of acute polydipsia, polyuria, polyphagia, and weight loss accompanied by fatigue	Gradual onset of mild polydipsia, polyuria, polyphagia, and weight loss. Other signs and symptoms may include visual disturbances, skin abnormalities, and infections, especially vaginal infections. Symptoms may be so gradual and mild that the patient may not recognize them or may attribute them to aging.

of S.C. insulin varies according to the injection site and the vascular supply and degree of tissue hypertrophy at the injection site. (For details, see *Subcutaneous insulin injection,* page 840.)

Also, regular (unmodified) insulin may be given intravenously (I.V.) or intramuscularly (I.M.) as well as in dialysate fluid infused into the peritoneal cavity for patients on peritoneal dialysis therapy.

After absorption into the bloodstream, insulin is distributed throughout the body. Insulin-responsive tissues are located in the liver, adipose tissue, and muscle.

Insulin is metabolized primarily in the liver, to a lesser extent in the kidneys, and in the muscle tissue. Enzymes degrade the insulin protein into two amino acid chains, with a resulting loss of activity. Insulin is excreted in the feces and urine.

Onset, peak, duration

Insulins are categorized as rapid-acting, intermediate-acting, and long-acting. In general, after S.C. administration, rapid-acting insulins act in ½ to 1 hour, reach peak concentration levels in 2 to 10 hours, and have a duration of action of 5 to 16 hours. Intermediate-acting insulins act in 1 to 2 hours and reach peak concentrations in 4 to 15 hours. Duration of intermediate-acting insulins is from 22 to 28 hours. Long-acting insulins act in 4 to 8 hours, and reach peak concentrations in 10 to 30 hours. Their duration can be 36 or more hours. Without insulin-binding antibodies,

insulin circulating in the bloodstream has a half-life of 5 to 10 minutes.

The exact times for onset, peak, and duration, however, are not absolute. They vary not only from patient to patient, but also from injection to injection in the same patient. If insulin absorption is altered, insulin onset, peak, and duration also are altered. If insulin absorption occurs more rapidly, the onset and peak concentration times occur more rapidly. Conversely, if insulin absorption is prolonged, insulin onset and peak concentration are delayed and duration is prolonged.

PHARMACODYNAMICS

Insulin is an anabolic, or building, hormone. It promotes the storage of glucose as glycogen, increases protein and fat synthesis, and inhibits the breakdown of glycogen, protein, and fat. Although it has no antidiuretic effect, insulin can correct the polyuria and polydipsia associated with the osmotic diuresis of hyperglycemia by decreasing the blood glucose level. Insulin also facilitates the movement of potassium from the extracellular fluid into the cell.

Mechanism of action

Insulin decreases blood glucose by facilitating the uptake and metabolism of glucose by insulin-dependent cells. Insulin also inhibits hepatic glucose production and the breakdown of glycogen, protein, and fat while it promotes the

Subcutaneous insulin injection

Subcutaneous insulin is absorbed most rapidly at abdominal injection sites, more slowly at sites on the arms, and slowest at sites on the anterior thigh. Absorption of insulin into the subscapular areas and the upper-outer quadrant of the buttocks is less predictable.

The greater the degree of tissue hypertrophy at the injection site, the greater the time required for the tissue to absorb the insulin.

If the vascular supply to the injection site increases, the time required for the tissue to absorb the insulin decreases. The vascular supply can be altered by temperature, massage, and exercise. Insulin injection deeper into the tissue also increases the absorption rate.

storage of energy in the form of glycogen, protein, and triglycerides. When insulin and glucose levels are sufficient in the postprandial period, the body will use glucose for fuel rather than break down protein and fat. In a fasting state, however, fats are the primary energy source for the body. In muscle, insulin increases the active transport of amino acids, thereby increasing protein synthesis. In adipose tissue, insulin facilitates the uptake of glucose and its transformation to fat.

PHARMACOTHERAPEUTICS

Insulin is indicated for Type I diabetes mellitus. It also is administered to patients with gestational, Type II, and other types of diabetes mellitus when other methods of maintaining a normal blood glucose level are ineffective or contraindicated. Patients with Type II diabetes mellitus may find the usual methods of maintaining a normal blood glucose level ineffective during periods of emotional or physical stress (infection, surgery) or contraindicated because of pregnancy or hypersensitivity. These patients may need insulin to control blood glucose more stringently. Insulin also is indicated for two of the comas that are complications of diabetes: diabetic ketoacidosis (DKA), more common with Type I diabetes mellitus, and hyperosmolar nonketotic syndrome (HNKS), more common with Type II.

Sometimes, insulin is prescribed for patients who do not have diabetes mellitus. Because insulin stimulates cellular uptake of potassium, it may be administered with hypertonic glucose to patients with severe hyperkalemia. This insulin and glucose mixture produces a shift of serum potassium into cells and lowers the serum potassium level.

All insulins have the same effect in the body. The advantages or disadvantages of a particular kind of insulin reflect the differences in onset of action, peak concentration, and duration of action, as well as in concentration, source, and purity. Thirty-two different insulin preparations are available on the U.S. market. Several of these are available in more than one concentration. (For the manufacturer and species of the various preparations, see *Available insulins.*)

In most cases, an insulin is selected that will provide a normal or near-normal blood glucose level throughout the day with minimal risk and disruption to the patient's life. To achieve this goal, a particular insulin category (rapid-, intermediate-, or long-acting) or a combination of categories is chosen. For example, a patient with fairly predictable episodes of hyperglycemia might be put on a regimen involving multiple injections of rapid-acting insulin throughout the day and night. The patient, however, may prefer a different regimen that causes less disruption in lifestyle. For such a patient, an intermediate- or long-acting insulin or a combination of rapid-, intermediate-, and long-acting insulins may be recommended. (For some common regimens, see *Selected insulin regimens,* page 842.)

Insulin concentration is measured in units of insulin per milliliter (ml). Insulin is available as U-40 (40 units/ml), U-100 (100 units/ml), and U-500 (500 units/ml). Although U-100 is by far the most commonly used, U-40 and U-500 may be used for patients who take very small or very large amounts of insulin in one injection. For example, a patient might need 4 units of insulin for an injection. This amount would require 0.04 ml of U-100 or 0.10 ml of U-40. Because 0.04 ml could be difficult for the patient to withdraw accurately from the insulin vial, U-40, with its 0.10-ml dose, would be the preferable insulin. Another patient who needs 250 units of insulin for injection would require 2.5 ml of U-100 or 0.5 ml of U-500. Because a 2.5-ml dose is too large for one S.C. injection, the patient would use U-500.

Some insulins are made from a single animal species; others from a combination. Mixtures of beef and pork insulins may have slight batch-to-batch variations of beef and pork percentages. A small percentage of individuals may develop an allergy to animal insulins, with beef insulin considered more antigenic than pork insulin. Human insulin is the least antigenic. Beef insulin differs from human insulin by three amino acids. Pork insulin differs from human insulin by one amino acid.

Animal insulins are obtained by cleaving the insulin protein from a larger polypeptide called proinsulin. Standard insulins contain no more than 25 parts per million (ppm) of proinsulin and related contaminants that result from an incomplete conversion of proinsulin. Purified insulins contain less than 10 ppm of proinsulin and related contaminants. These contaminants may cause adverse reactions, including hypersensitivity reactions, antibody formation, and lipodystrophy. Such reactions, however, occur in only a few patients. Purified insulins, which cost more than standard forms, are indicated for patients with insulin allergy, severe insulin resistance from insulin antibodies, lipoatrophy, onset of diabetes during pregnancy, or an acute

Available insulins

The insulins currently available are divided into rapid-acting, intermediate-acting, and long-acting categories, with an additional division for standard and purified preparations.

Standard			Purified		
TRADE NAME	**MANUFACTURER**	**SPECIES**	**TRADE NAME**	**MANUFACTURER**	**SPECIES**
Rapid-Acting					
Regular Iletin I	Lilly	beef and pork	Regular Iletin II	Lilly	pork
Regular	Squibb-Novo	pork	Regular Purified Pork Insulin Injection (formerly Actrapid)	Squibb-Novo	pork
Semilente Iletin I	Lilly	beef and pork	Velosulin R	Nordisk	pork
Semilente Insulin	Squibb-Novo	beef	Semilente Purified Pork Prompt Insulin Zinc Suspension (formerly Semitard)	Squibb-Novo	pork
			Humulin R	Lilly	human*
			Novolin R (formerly Actrapid Human)	Squibb-Novo	human†
Intermediate-Acting					
NPH Iletin I	Lilly	beef and pork	NPH Iletin II	Lilly	beef
Lente Iletin I	Lilly	beef and pork	NPH Iletin II	Lilly	pork
NPH Isophane	Squibb-Novo	beef	Lente Iletin II	Lilly	beef
Lente	Squibb-Novo	beef	Lente Iletin II	Lilly	pork
			NPH Purified (formerly Protaphane)	Squibb-Novo	pork
			Lente Purified (formerly Monotard)	Squibb-Novo	pork
			Insulatard NPH	Nordisk	pork
			Mixtard‡	Nordisk	pork
			Humulin L	Lilly	human*
			Humulin N	Lilly	human*
			Novolin L	Squibb-Novo	human†
			Novolin N	Squibb-Novo	human†
Long-Acting					
Ultralente Iletin I	Lilly	beef and pork	Protamine Zinc & Iletin II	Lilly	beef
Protamine Zinc & Iletin I	Lilly	beef and pork	Protamine Zinc & Iletin II	Lilly	pork
Ultralente	Squibb-Novo	beef	Ultralente Purified	Squibb-Novo	beef

*Recombinant DNA alteration of *Escherichia coli*
†Enzymatic conversion of porcine insulin
‡30% Velosulin R, 70% Insulatard NPH

Selected insulin regimens

A patient receiving insulin may be placed on one of many regimens. The four most frequently encountered ones are detailed here.

REGIMEN	TYPES OF INSULIN	ADMINISTRATION TIMES
Single-dose	Intermediate-acting	30 minutes before breakfast.
Mixed-dose	Rapid-acting and intermediate-acting	30 minutes before breakfast.
	Rapid-acting, intermediate-acting, and long-acting	30 minutes before breakfast.
Split-mixed dose	Rapid-acting and intermediate-acting	In two injections: 30 minutes before breakfast and 30 minutes before dinner.
Multiple dose	Rapid-acting and intermediate-acting	In four injections: rapid-acting taken 30 minutes before each meal; intermediate-acting taken at bedtime.
	Rapid-acting and long-acting	In three injections: long-acting and rapid-acting taken 30 minutes before breakfast; rapid-acting taken 30 minutes before lunch and dinner.
	Rapid-acting	In multiple injections, usually before each meal and at bedtime, perhaps via an insulin pump.

problem that requires short-term or intermittent insulin therapy.

Adult dosages of insulin, which vary widely, represent the amount needed to keep the blood glucose at a normal or near-normal level. The dose varies from person to person as well as at different times for the same person. Insulin requirements are increased by growth, pregnancy, increased food intake, stress, surgery, infection, illness, increased insulin antibodies, and some medications. Insulin requirements are decreased by hypothyroidism, decreased food intake, exercise, and some medications.

The diagnosis of Type I or Type II diabetes mellitus gives no clue to dosage requirements. Although the individual with Type II diabetes mellitus does not depend on exogenous insulin for survival, that patient may receive a dosage exceeding 200 units/day if insulin resistance is present.

Insulin usually is administered by the S.C. route. However, it may be given via the I.V. route in certain situations or the I.M. route in an emergency.

Drug interactions
Some drugs interact with insulin to alter its ability to decrease the blood glucose level; other drugs directly alter the patient's blood glucose level. If a medication that produces hypoglycemia is added to the patient's drug regimen, the insulin dosage may need to be decreased. If a medication that produces hyperglycemia is added, the insulin dosage may need to be increased.

Because alcohol consumption is particularly risky for individuals with diabetes mellitus, they should not drink. Alcohol can contribute to hypoglycemia; its adverse effects may mask the symptoms of hypoglycemia. Moreover, patients who drink alcohol may be tempted not to eat to limit caloric intake, but this further increases the chance of hypoglycemia. If patients with diabetes mellitus do drink alcoholic beverages, they should eat adequately and include these beverages in their dietary exchanges. (For a list of drugs that lead to hypoglycemia and hyperglycemia, see *Drug interactions: Insulin.*)

ADVERSE DRUG REACTIONS

The patient may experience dose-related reactions or idiosyncratic reactions to contaminants in the insulin.

Hypoglycemia (below-normal blood glucose levels) is a relatively frequent adverse reaction to insulin. It usually results from too much insulin, too little food, too much exercise, or some combination of these. Although no absolute correlation exists between hypoglycemic symptoms and blood glucose levels, symptoms typically appear when the blood glucose level falls below 50 mg/dl.

Specific symptoms may vary and include nervousness or shakiness, diaphoresis, weakness, light-headedness, confusion, paresthesia, irritability, headache, hunger, tachycardia, and changes in speech, hearing, or vision. If untreated, symptoms may progress to unconsciousness, seizures, coma, and death. Symptoms of hypoglycemia result

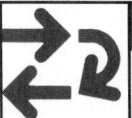

DRUG INTERACTIONS

Insulin

Insulin interactions with other drugs can increase or decrease its effect, resulting in an inappropriately altered blood glucose level for the patient. The nurse must be aware of these interactions.

DRUG	INTERACTING DRUGS	POSSIBLE EFFECTS	NURSING IMPLICATIONS
insulin	alcohol	Causes hypoglycemia	• Discourage the patient's consumption of alcohol. • Monitor the patient for signs and symptoms of hypoglycemia, such as hunger, diaphoresis, weakness, tremor, dizziness, and tachycardia. • Decrease the insulin dose as prescribed.
	anabolic steroids, salicylates, MAO inhibitors	Cause hypoglycemia	• Monitor the patient for signs and symptoms of hypoglycemia, such as hunger, diaphoresis, weakness, tremor, dizziness, and tachycardia. • Decrease the insulin dose as prescribed.
	corticosteroids, sympathomimetic agents, thiazide diuretics, dextrothyroxine	Cause hyperglycemia	• Monitor the patient for signs and symptoms of hyperglycemia, such as thirst, polyuria, rapid weak pulse, and stupor. • Increase the insulin dose as prescribed.
	beta blockers	Modify symptoms of hypoglycemia; delay recovery from hypoglycemia	• Teach the patient that concomitant use of these drugs may mask the signs and symptoms of hypoglycemia, except for diaphoresis which may be more profuse. • Monitor the patient for prolonged hypoglycemia.

from an adrenergic reaction as well as from cellular malnutrition, primarily at the neurologic level.

The Somogyi phenomenon occurs when hypoglycemia is followed by a compensatory period of rebound hyperglycemia as the body increases glucose production to correct the problem. The Somogyi phenomenon typically occurs during the late night or early morning when the patient is asleep. During this time, insulin continues to be absorbed from the S.C. injection site, although insufficient glucose may be present for it to act on. As a result, the blood glucose level drops rapidly. In response, the body secretes glucagon, norepinephrine, and corticosteroids to correct the hypoglycemia. An overshot phenomenon occurs, resulting in hyperglycemia. Although the patient awakens with symptoms of hyperglycemia, hypoglycemia is the condition that must be corrected.

The dawn phenomenon (an early morning rise in blood glucose) may result from uneven therapy. Unlike the Somogyi phenomenon, the dawn phenomenon is not preceded by hypoglycemia. It may result from nocturnal secretion of growth hormone, which causes insulin resistance. The dawn phenomenon must be differentiated from the Somogyi phenomenon because different adjustments in the insulin regimen are required for the two.

A patient can develop local or systemic hypersensitivity reactions to any type of insulin, but such reactions to pur-

ified and human insulin are unlikely. Local reactions are characterized by redness, itching, or burning at the injection site. Local hypersensitivity usually disappears after 1 or 2 months of continued insulin use. A patient who currently is using a standard insulin can be switched to a purified insulin. If the patient is uncomfortable, an antihistamine may be prescribed.

A systemic hypersensitivity reaction to insulin is characterized by generalized urticaria (hives), angioedema (swelling of submucosa), dyspnea, tachycardia, and possibly anaphylactic shock. Systemic hypersensitivity reactions rarely occur. Treatment involves discontinuing the offending insulin and introducing insulin from another source. Desensitization therapy also may be required.

Two kinds of lipodystrophy (disturbance in fat metabolism) can occur with insulin injections. Lipoatrophy (loss of fat tissue at the injection site) can be improved when purified insulins are injected into the area. Lipohypertrophy (thickening of subcutaneous fat tissue) is not influenced by the purity of the insulin. Rotation of insulin injection sites is essential to prevent lipoatrophy and lipohypertrophy.

Patients can develop a resistance to insulin. Although anti-insulin antibodies may play a role, insulin resistance usually results from a decreased number of insulin receptors, a postreceptor defect in insulin action, or an excess of hormones antagonistic to insulin. A characteristic of

Type II diabetes mellitus, insulin resistance also can occur in poorly controlled Type I diabetes mellitus, but improves with insulin therapy. Insulin resistance associated with Type II diabetes mellitus may be reversed at least partially with such treatments as a weight-reduction diet or the addition of exogenous insulin therapy. Insulin antibodies seem more likely to develop during episodic insulin therapy with Type II diabetes mellitus. Therefore, human insulin is preferred for episodic insulin therapy because it is the least antigenic.

NURSING PROCESS APPLICATION

The following information assists the nurse in caring for a patient receiving insulin.

Assessment
• Review the patient's history for a preexisting condition that contraindicates the use of insulin, such as hypoglycemia or known hypersensitivity to the particular insulin.
• Review the patient's history for a preexisting condition that requires cautious use of insulin, such as impaired renal or hepatic function.
• Assess the patient for adverse reactions to insulin, such as hypoglycemia, hypersensitivity reactions, lipodystrophy, or insulin resistance.
• Review the patient's medication history to identify the use of drugs that may interact with insulin, such as alcohol, anabolic steroids, salicylates, corticosteroids, or beta blockers.
• Assess the effectiveness of the prescribed insulin regularly.
• Assess the patient's compliance with the insulin regimen regularly.
• Evaluate the patient's and family's knowledge about the prescribed insulin.

Nursing diagnoses
The following examples represent appropriate nursing diagnoses for a patient receiving insulin.
• Potential for injury related to a preexisting condition that contraindicates the use of insulin
• Potential for injury related to a preexisting condition that requires cautious use of insulin
• Potential for injury related to adverse drug reactions
• Altered protection related to the development of insulin resistance
• Noncompliance related to long-term use of insulin
• Knowledge deficit related to the prescribed insulin therapy

Planning and implementation
• Do not administer insulin to a patient with a condition that contraindicates its use.

• Administer insulin cautiously to a patient at risk because of a preexisting condition.
• Monitor the patient for adverse reactions frequently during insulin therapy. *Be alert for signs and symptoms of hypoglycemia, such as nervousness or shakiness, diaphoresis, weakness, light-headedness, confusion, or irritability, especially when the insulin reaches its peak action.*
• *Monitor the patient's blood glucose level regularly and more frequently after the insulin dosage is increased. Expect to check the blood glucose level during the night and early morning if the Somogyi or dawn phenomenon is suspected.*
• *Avoid delays in the patient's mealtimes to prevent hypoglycemia.*
• Monitor the patient's intake to ensure that daily caloric requirements are met. Be sure to count the calories in I.V. solutions in the patient's daily caloric intake.
• *Keep a source of glucose or glucagon readily available to treat a hypoglycemic reaction. After such a reaction, provide a complex carbohydrate snack.*
• Notify the physician if the patient experiences hypoglycemia frequently and expect a dosage adjustment or dietary increase in calories.
• *Avoid dosage errors by measuring U-100 insulin in U-100 insulin syringes and U-40 insulin in U-40 insulin syringes.*
• *Prepare a U-500 dose with extreme caution. A small, inadvertent overdose of U-500 insulin could cause death.*
• *Do not shake insulin because the resulting froth prevents withdrawal of an accurate dose and may damage protein molecules.*
• *Mix insulins in the same order every time.*
• *Administer mixed insulins within 5 minutes after mixing.*
• *Do not administer regular insulin that appears cloudy or any insulin solution that contains particles.*
• Expect to administer insulin S.C. If prescribed, however, administer regular insulin I.V. or I.M., or mix it with dialysate and infuse it into the peritoneal cavity during peritoneal dialysis.
• Administer a once-daily a.m. dosage of insulin 30 minutes before breakfast or a split a.m. and p.m. dosage 30 minutes before breakfast and 30 minutes before dinner, unless otherwise prescribed.
• Rotate and document insulin injection sites.
• *Observe the S.C. or I.M. injection site for signs and symptoms of a local hypersensitivity reaction, such as redness, itching, or burning at the site.* If the reaction persists for more than 2 months or becomes worse in a patient who is taking a standard insulin, expect to switch the patient to a human or purified insulin.

• *Observe the patient closely during initial or episodic insulin therapy, particularly noting systemic hypersensitivity reactions, such as generalized urticaria, angioedema, dyspnea, tachycardia, and possibly anaphylactic shock. Have standard emergency equipment readily available. If such a reaction occurs, expect to switch the patient to an insulin from another source. If prescribed, begin desensitization therapy.*

• Inspect the injection sites regularly for lipoatrophy or lipohypertrophy. If lipoatrophy occurs, expect to inject purified insulins into the area to correct the problem. To prevent lipodystrophy, ensure that injection sites are rotated.

• *Observe the patient for signs and symptoms of hyperglycemia, such as polyuria, polydipsia, polyphagia, weight loss, and fatigue. These suggest a need to change the insulin regimen.*

• *Monitor the diabetic patient with hyperglycemia for signs of DKA or HNKS, such as Kussmaul's respirations or electrolyte imbalances, and test the patient's urine for ketones.* DKA or HNKS may cause dehydration and an intracellular potassium deficit, although the serum potassium level may be normal or high. Ketosis is present with DKA and absent or nearly absent with HNKS; dehydration usually is more severe with HNKS. Therefore, be prepared to administer I.V. fluids, insulin, and potassium as prescribed.

• Notify the physician if hyperglycemia or adverse reactions occur.

• *Monitor patient for signs of insulin resistance, such as hyperglycemia that persists despite adherence to the diabetic regimen, and a progressive increase in the amount of insulin needed to achieve blood glucose control.*

• *Administer only human insulin as prescribed for episodic insulin therapy.*

• Expect the obese patient with suspected insulin resistance to be placed on a weight-reduction diet. If weight reduction decreases the blood glucose level, insulin resistance probably is present.

• Adjust the insulin dosage as prescribed for the patient with suspected insulin resistance.

• Question the patient with uncontrolled diabetes mellitus about compliance with the prescribed insulin regimen.

• Notify the physician if the patient is noncompliant and try to determine the patient's reasons for noncompliance.

Patient teaching

• Teach the patient and family about the name, dose, frequency, action, and adverse effects of the prescribed insulin.

• Teach the patient and family how to draw up and administer the prescribed insulin.

• Instruct the patient to rotate vials of intermediate- and long-acting insulin gently before withdrawing the dose. This ensures proper dispersion of the suspension.

• *Advise the patient to use a U-40 insulin syringe with U-40 insulin and a U-100 syringe with U-100 insulin.*

• Inform the patient with impaired vision of the numerous aids available to help withdraw the correct amount of insulin into a syringe.

• *Instruct the patient who must mix insulins always to follow the same order when drawing the insulins into the syringe. Typically the rapid-acting insulin is drawn first.* (For the sequence for withdrawing two insulins into one syringe, see *Mixing insulins,* page 846.)

• *Instruct the patient using mixtures to withdraw and administer the mixture within 5 minutes or to store the mixture in the refrigerator and administer after the binding period (15 minutes for regular insulin with NPH insulin; 24 hours for regular insulin with lente insulin).*

• Teach the patient that proper rotation of S.C. injection sites helps prevent lipodystrophy.

• Instruct the patient to let insulin reach room temperature before injection to minimize pain on administration.

• *Instruct the patient to store insulin at a temperature less than 80° F (27° C) and greater than 36° F (2° C).* Unopened vials can be stored in the refrigerator, but insulin should never be frozen or left in direct sunlight.

• Instruct the patient using an insulin pump how to care for the device.

• *Instruct the patient not to change the manufacturer, type, purity, species, or dosage of insulin unless instructed to do so by the physician.*

• *Teach the patient the signs and symptoms of hypoglycemia and hyperglycemia and what to do if they occur.*

• *Teach the patient how to monitor the blood glucose level.* Monitoring blood glucose is especially important for a patient who needs rigid control of the blood glucose level or requires sliding-scale insulin coverage (dose varies according to the body's need). *Also instruct the patient to monitor the blood glucose level during times of stress or infection because the insulin requirement may increase.* Some patients may monitor the urine glucose level rather than the blood glucose level, although this indirect method for estimating the blood glucose level typically provides less accurate and less reliable information.

• *Teach the patient how to monitor urine acetone levels to detect ketosis, especially during illness or stress.*

• Review all aspects of diabetic care that may affect insulin therapy and predispose the patient to hypoglycemia or hyperglycemia, such as diet, exercise, and stress.

• Review sick day rules to follow during insulin therapy. For example, instruct the patient to contact the physician for insulin dosage adjustments and to test blood glucose more frequently when illness occurs.

Mixing insulins

The patient may withdraw two different types of insulin into the same syringe. In this series of diagrams, a rapid-acting insulin (R vial) is combined with an intermediate-acting insulin (I vial).

1 After cleaning the rubber stopper on both vials with an alcohol wipe, inject the amount of air equal to the dose of the intermediate-acting insulin into the I vial.

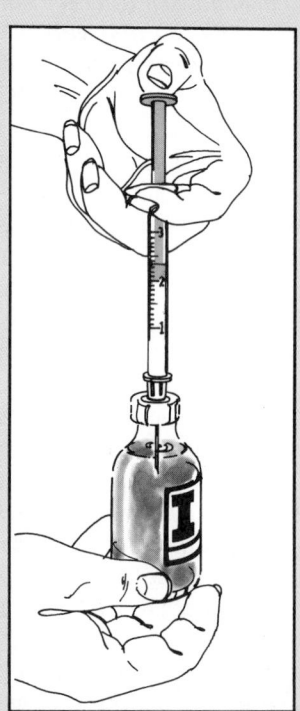

2 Inject the amount of air equal to the dose of the rapid-acting insulin into the R vial.

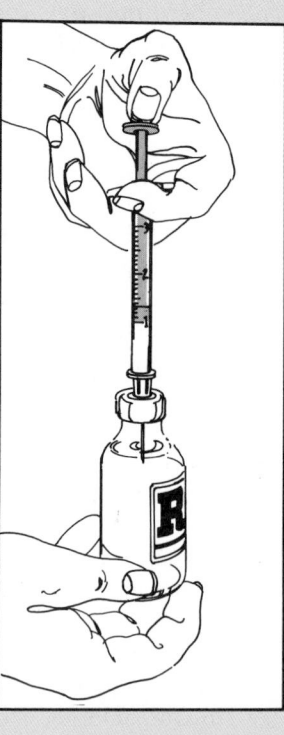

3 Withdraw the correct amount of rapid-acting insulin.

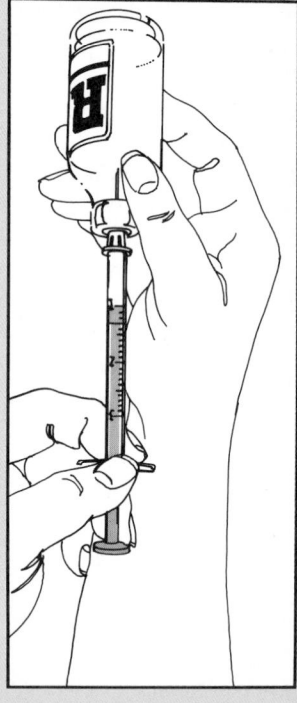

4 Withdraw the correct amount of intermediate-acting insulin. (Note: Pull the plunger down to the unit mark that equals the dose of rapid-acting insulin *plus* the dose of intermediate-acting insulin. The insulins will mix immediately in the syringe. If too large an amount of intermediate-acting insulin is withdrawn, the entire contents of the syringe must be discarded.)

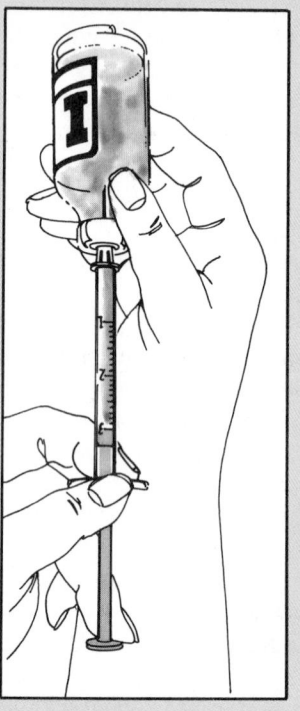

● *Advise the patient to obtain alcohol-use guidelines from the physician.*

● Stress the importance of adhering to the prescribed insulin regimen.

● *Instruct the patient receiving insulin to wear medical identification and to have ready access to a source of glucose, such as hard candy.*

● Advise the patient to notify the physician if hyperglycemia or adverse reactions occur.

Evaluation

The following examples represent appropriate evaluation statements for a patient receiving insulin.

● The patient has no conditions that contraindicate insulin therapy.

● The patient exhibits no signs of complications in the preexisting condition linked to the prescribed insulin.

● The patient experiences no adverse reactions to the prescribed insulin.

● The patient shows no signs of insulin resistance.

• The patient's blood glucose and glycosylated hemoglobin levels fall within the normal range.
• The patient and family express an accurate understanding of the points taught about the prescribed insulin.
• The patient and family correctly demonstrate how to draw up and administer insulin.

ORAL HYPOGLYCEMIC AGENTS

Oral hypoglycemic agents are given to patients with Type II diabetes mellitus when those patients cannot maintain normal or near-normal blood glucose levels with exercise and a controlled diet. All oral hypoglycemic agents approved for use in the United States are sulfonylureas. These drugs act to stimulate pancreatic beta-cell production of insulin and increase tissue sensitivity to insulin.

The initially developed drugs, known as first-generation sulfonylureas, include acetohexamide, chlorpropamide, tolazamide, and tolbutamide. Developed more recently, the second-generation sulfonylureas include glipizide and glyburide.

PHARMACOKINETICS

The absorption and distribution of oral hypoglycemic agents are similar. These drugs, however, vary in metabolism, excretion, onset of action, peak concentration levels, and duration of action as well as in the hypoglycemic activity of their metabolites.

Absorption, distribution, metabolism, excretion

Available only in oral forms, sulfonylureas are absorbed well after administration. Absorption varies, depending on whether the patient takes the drug while fasting or with food. Absorption occurs more rapidly when the patient is fasting.

Sulfonylureas are absorbed from the GI tract and distributed via the bloodstream throughout the body. First- and second-generation sulfonylureas rapidly bind to plasma proteins. Only a small portion of a sulfonylurea dose is left free to produce an effect.

The oral hypoglycemic agents are metabolized primarily in the liver, and the activity of their metabolites varies significantly. Of the first-generation sulfonylureas, only tolbutamide metabolites are inactive; tolazamide and chlorpropamide metabolites are weak, but the metabolites of acetohexamide are quite active. The acetohexamide metabolites provide a hypoglycemic effect 2½ times as potent

as acetohexamide itself. Metabolites of the second-generation agents are inactive.

The sulfonylureas are excreted primarily in the urine, with some biliary excretion. Glyburide is excreted equally in the urine and feces. Patients with renal dysfunction taking these drugs require careful monitoring for signs of hypoglycemia and metabolite accumulation.

Onset, peak, duration

The onset of action varies for the oral hypoglycemic agents. Acetohexamide and chlorpropamide begin to act in 1 hour; tolbutamide in ½ to 1 hour; glipizide in 1 to 1½ hours; glyburide in 2 hours; and tolazamide in 4 to 6 hours.

Oral hypoglycemic agents reach peak concentration levels within 2 to 6 hours of administration. The half-life and duration of action of these drugs vary considerably. (For specific peak, half-life, and duration times, see *Pharmacokinetics of sulfonylureas,* page 848.)

PHARMACODYNAMICS

First- and second-generation sulfonylureas stimulate insulin release and appear to work by the same mechanism of action, which is understood incompletely.

Mechanism of action

Generally accepted theory suggests that oral hypoglycemic agents provide pancreatic and extrapancreatic actions to regulate blood glucose. These drugs probably stimulate pancreatic beta cells to release insulin. Although the mechanism of stimulation remains unknown, the pancreas already must be functioning at a minimal level. Within a few weeks to a few months of the initial response to the sulfonylureas, pancreatic insulin secretion drops to pretreatment levels. However, blood glucose levels remain normal or near-normal. Extrapancreatic actions of oral hypoglycemic agents probably maintain this continued control of blood glucose.

The oral hypoglycemic agents may provide several extrapancreatic actions to decrease and control blood glucose. The drugs probably decrease glucose production by the liver. They also may increase the number of cellular insulin receptors. With more available receptors, the cells can bind insulin sufficiently to initiate the process of glucose metabolism. Oral hypoglycemic agents also may partially reverse the postreceptor deficit in insulin action, enabling the completion of intracellular glucose metabolism. The ability to restore tissue sensitivity to insulin at the receptor and postreceptor level is not restricted to sulfonylureas; weight reduction and exercise probably provide similar effects.

Pharmacokinetics of sulfonylureas

The following chart summarizes the peak serum concentration level, half-life, and duration of action of the first-generation and second-generation sulfonylureas.

	PEAK SERUM CONCENTRATION (HOURS)	HALF-LIFE (HOURS)	DURATION (HOURS)
First-generation sulfonylureas			
acetohexamide	2	5 to 8	10 to 24
chlorpropamide	4	32 to 40	36 to 72
tolazamide	6	6 to 8	12 to 24
tolbutamide	2	4 to 6	6 to 12
Second-generation sulfonylureas			
glipizide	2	2 to 4	18 to 24
glyburide	4	10	24

PHARMACOTHERAPEUTICS

Oral hypoglycemic agents are indicated for patients with Type II diabetes mellitus if diet and exercise do not maintain blood glucose at normal or near-normal levels. These agents are not indicated for patients with Type I diabetes mellitus because pancreatic beta cells are not functioning at a sufficient level. They are contraindicated in patients who are allergic to sulfonylureas.

Combining oral hypoglycemic agents and insulin may be indicated for some patients who do not respond to either therapy alone.

Compared to insulin, the oral hypoglycemic agents provide one major advantage — oral administration — and several disadvantages:
• The patient must have endogenous insulin; the beta cells must be functioning.
• Oral hypoglycemic agents cannot be used if the patient has been instructed not to take anything by mouth.
• Oral hypoglycemic agents may not control blood glucose sufficiently during periods of acute injury, stress, or infection.
• Oral hypoglycemic agents are contraindicated during pregnancy and lactation because their effects on the fetus and breast-feeding infant remain unknown.

acetohexamide (Dymelor). A first-generation sulfonylurea, acetohexamide is used to manage mild to moderately severe, stable Type II diabetes mellitus.

Usual adult dosage: 250 to 1,500 mg P.O. daily or divided into two doses during the day.

chlorpropamide (Diabinese, Glucamide). A first-generation sulfonylurea, chlorpropamide is used to manage mild to moderately severe stable Type II diabetes mellitus. Because chlorpropamide potentiates the action of antidiuretic hormone, it may be used to treat mild diabetes insipidus.
Usual adult dosage: 100 to 750 mg P.O. daily.

tolazamide (Tolinase). A first-generation sulfonylurea, tolazamide is used to manage mild to moderately severe, stable Type II diabetes mellitus.
Usual adult dosage: 100 to 1,000 mg P.O. daily or divided into two doses during the day.

tolbutamide (Orinase). Tolbutamide is a first-generation sulfonylurea used to manage mild to moderately severe, stable Type II diabetes mellitus.
Usual adult dosage: 250 to 3,000 mg P.O. divided into two or three doses during the day.

glipizide (Glucotrol). A second-generation sulfonylurea, glipizide is used as an adjunct to diet in managing Type II diabetes mellitus when hyperglycemia cannot be controlled by diet alone.
Usual adult dosage: 2.5 to 40 mg P.O. daily or divided into two doses during the day.

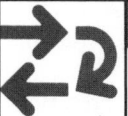

DRUG INTERACTIONS
Oral hypoglycemic agents

Numerous drugs can interact with the sulfonylureas to produce hypoglycemia or hyperglycemia.

DRUG	INTERACTING DRUGS	POSSIBLE EFFECTS	NURSING IMPLICATIONS
acetohexamide, chlorpropamide, tolazamide, tolbutamide, glipizide, glyburide	alcohol	Causes hypoglycemia or hyperglycemia	• Monitor the patient for signs and symptoms of hyperglycemia (thirst, polyuria, rapid weak pulse, and stupor) and hypoglycemia (hunger, diaphoresis, weakness, tremor, dizziness, and tachycardia). • Discourage alcohol consumption. • Teach the patient about the possibility of a disulfiram-like reaction with chlorpropamide.
	dicumarol	Causes hypoglycemia; increase anticoagulant effect	• Monitor the patient for signs and symptoms of hypoglycemia. • Monitor the patient for increased anticoagulant effect, such as epistaxis, bruises, and hematuria. • Change the patient to another medication for anticoagulant therapy, if prescribed.
	anabolic steroids, chloramphenical, clofibrate, gemfibrozil, monoamine oxidase inhibitors, phenylbutazone, salicylates, sulfonamides	Cause hypoglycemia	• Monitor the patient for signs and symptoms of hypoglycemia.
	corticosteroids, dextrothyroxine, rifampin, sympathomimetic agents, thiazide diuretics	Cause hyperglycemia	• Monitor the patient for signs and symptoms of hyperglycemia. • Increase the oral hypoglycemic agent as prescribed.
	beta blockers, clonidine	Produce modified signs of hypoglycemia	• Be aware that beta blockers will block the epinephrine-induced symptoms of hypoglycemia but not alter the hypoglycemia itself. • Monitor the patient for hypoglycemia by testing the blood glucose level. • Teach the patient that most typical signs and symptoms of hypoglycemia, such as tachycardia and tremor, may be masked, but that diaphoresis will be detectable and may be more profuse.

glyburide (DiaBeta, Micronase). A second-generation sulfonylurea, glyburide is used as an adjunct to diet in managing Type II diabetes mellitus.
Usual adult dosage: 1.25 to 20 mg P.O. daily or divided into two doses during the day.

Drug interactions
Some drugs interact with the oral hypoglycemic agents and alter their ability to decrease the blood glucose level, but other drugs directly alter the patient's blood glucose level. If a drug that produces hypoglycemia is added to the patient's medication regimen, the sulfonylurea dosage may need to be decreased. If a drug that produces hyperglycemia is added to the patient's medication regimen, the sulfonyl-

urea dosage may need to be increased. Although not all drug interactions involving oral hypoglycemic agents are serious, the nurse should use caution when giving a sulfonylurea with any interacting drug. (For details, see *Drug interactions: Oral hypoglycemic agents.*)

Alcohol consumption proves particularly risky for the patient receiving an oral hypoglycemic agent. Alcohol produces a hypoglycemic effect, but some alcoholic beverages may increase the blood glucose level because of their carbohydrate content. Alcohol and chlorpropamide can interact to cause a disulfiram (Antabuse)-like reaction. During such a reaction, the patient may experience such symptoms as flushing, nausea, vomiting, headache, syncope, dyspnea, and tachycardia.

ADVERSE DRUG REACTIONS

Patients may develop adverse reactions to sulfonylureas, but other than hypoglycemia and drug failure, these are uncommon

Hypoglycemia, the major adverse reaction to oral hypoglycemic agents, typically results from too little food or too much medication. Some patients, especially elderly ones, may decide to skip a meal because they are not hungry. Hypoglycemia also can occur after an incorrect dose or, more likely, from drug or metabolite accumulation in the body. Patients with decreased liver or kidney function and those taking chlorpropamide must be especially careful to note signs of hypoglycemia.

Other relatively uncommon reactions to oral hypoglycemic agents include GI effects (nausea, vomiting, cholestasis), skin reactions (rash, pruritus, photosensitivity), a diffuse pulmonary reaction, hematologic reactions (leukopenia, thrombocytopenia, hemolytic anemia), hepatic effects (abnormal liver function tests), and renal effects (severe diuretic or antidiuretic effect).

In 1970, the University Group Diabetes Project reported an increase in the incidence of cardiovascular mortality among patients using oral hypoglycemic agents. Since then, the finding has been disputed widely. Today, health care professionals generally consider the cardiovascular mortality reported by the Diabetes Project to have been caused by other individual risk factors related to cardiovascular disease.

Oral hypoglycemic agents may cause an allergic reaction.

When a patient does not respond initially to sulfonylurea therapy, the patient is said to exhibit primary failure. Primary failure occurs in about 20% of the patients on oral hypoglycemic agents; the mechanism of drug failure is unknown. In secondary failure, the sulfonylurea maintains a normal or near-normal blood glucose level for a time, but then, for unknown reasons, no longer can do so. Each year, secondary failure occurs in 5% to 10% of the patients taking oral hypoglycemic agents. However, 25% to 60% of patients with secondary failure to one oral hypoglycemic agent will respond to another agent. Therefore, trial with a different agent may be warranted.

NURSING PROCESS APPLICATION

The following information assists the nurse in caring for a patient who is receiving an oral hypoglycemic agent.

Assessment
• Review the patient's history for a preexisting condition that contraindicates the use of an oral hypoglycemic agent, such as pregnancy, lactation, diabetic ketoacidosis, or known hypersensitivity to the drug.

• Review the patient's history for a condition that requires cautious use of an oral hypoglycemic agent, such as impaired renal or hepatic function.
• Assess the patient for adverse reactions to the prescribed oral hypoglycemic agent, such as hypoglycemia, drug failure, GI distress, abnormal laboratory values, or diuretic or antidiuretic effects.
• Review the patient's medication history to identify the use of drugs that may interact with the oral hypoglycemic agent, such as alcohol, dicumarol, chloramphenical, corticosteroids, or beta blockers.
• Assess the effectiveness of the oral hypoglycemic agent regularly.
• Assess the patient's compliance with the prescribed oral hypoglycemic regimen.
• Evaluate the patient's and family's knowledge about the prescribed oral hypoglycemic agent.

Nursing diagnoses
The following examples represent appropriate nursing diagnoses for a patient receiving an oral hypoglycemic agent.
• Potential for injury related to a preexisting condition that contraindicates the use of an oral hypoglycemic agent
• Potential for injury related to a preexisting condition that requires cautious use of an oral hypoglycemic agent
• Potential for injury related to adverse drug reactions
• Noncompliance related to long-term use of the oral hypoglycemic agent
• Knowledge deficit related to the prescribed oral hypoglycemic agent

Planning and implementation
• Do not administer an oral hypoglycemic agent to a patient with a condition that contraindicates its use.
• Administer an oral hypoglycemic agent cautiously to a patient at risk because of a preexisting condition.
• Monitor the patient for adverse reactions frequently. *Be particularly alert for signs of hypoglycemia (nervousness, diaphoresis, weakness, confusion, irritability) and of drug failure (polyuria, polyphagia, polydipsia, weight loss, and fatigue).*
• Monitor the patient's blood glucose level regularly and more frequently after dosage is increased.
• *Avoid delays in the patient's mealtimes to prevent glucose alterations.*
• Monitor the patient's intake to ensure that daily caloric requirements are met. Be sure to include the calories in I.V. solutions in the patient's daily calorie count.
• *Keep a source of glucose or glucagon readily available to treat a hypoglycemic reaction. After such a reaction, provide a complex carbohydrate snack.*
• Notify the physician if the patient experiences hypoglycemia frequently and expect a dosage adjustment.

• Monitor hydration and the blood glucose level if the patient experiences nausea and vomiting. Obtain a prescription for an antiemetic, if needed. Expect to change the patient to a different oral hypoglycemic agent or to begin insulin therapy as prescribed.

• Monitor the patient's laboratory tests for results that indicate leukopenia, thrombocytopenia, hemolytic anemia, or liver dysfunction. Notify the physician of any abnormal test results.

• Record the patient's fluid intake and output. *Also observe the patient for severe diuretic effects (massive diuresis, dehydration, decreased blood pressure, electrolyte imbalance) or antidiuretic effects (fluid retention).* Alert the physician if fluid imbalance occurs.

• Give an oral hypoglycemic agent 30 minutes before breakfast; if the drug dose is divided, give the second dose 30 minutes before dinner. The patient taking tolbutamide three times a day should take a dose before each meal. Oral hypoglycemic agents should be taken on a regular schedule to minimize wide fluctuations in the blood glucose level.

• Notify the physician if adverse reactions occur.

• Question the patient about compliance with the prescribed drug regimen. If the patient is noncompliant, attempt to determine why.

• Notify the physician if noncompliance occurs or is suspected.

Patient teaching

• Teach the patient and family the name, dose, frequency, action, and adverse effects of the prescribed oral hypoglycemic agent.

• *Teach the patient the signs and symptoms of hypoglycemia and hyperglycemia and what to do if they occur.*

• Instruct the patient to eat meals on a regular schedule; skipping a meal increases the risk of hypoglycemia.

• *Advise the patient to adjust the sulfonylurea dosage* **only under medical supervision.** A change in body weight, diet, or amount of exercise may require a change in the drug dosage. Severe stress also may require a dosage change or the addition of insulin to the regimen.

• Teach the patient how to monitor the blood glucose level. Blood glucose determination better indicates diabetic management than urine glucose measurement because of individual variations in the renal threshold for glucose.

• *Instruct the patient to carry or wear medical identification and to have ready access to a source of glucose, such as hard candy.*

• *Advise the patient to notify the physician if increased diuresis or signs of fluid retention (ankle swelling, weight gain unrelated to caloric intake) occur.*

• *Inform the patient that the oral hypoglycemic agent may cause photosensitivity and to avoid exposure to the sun.* When this is not possible, the patient should use protective measures, such as sunglasses, sunscreen lotion, and a hat.

• *Advise the patient to obtain alcohol-use guidelines from the physician.*

• Advise the patient to notify the physician if adverse reactions occur.

Evaluation

The following examples represent appropriate evaluation statements for a patient receiving an oral hypoglycemic agent.

• The patient has no conditions that contraindicate oral hypoglycemic agent therapy.

• The patient exhibits no signs of complications in the preexisting condition linked to the prescribed oral hypoglycemic agent.

• The patient displays no signs of adverse reactions to the prescribed oral hypoglycemic agent.

• The patient's blood glucose level falls within or near the normal range, demonstrating compliance with the prescribed oral hypoglycemic regimen.

• The patient and family express an accurate understanding of the points taught about the prescribed oral hypoglycemic agent.

• The patient obtains a medical identification card and carries it at all times.

GLUCAGON

Unlike insulin and oral hypoglycemic agents, which decrease the blood glucose level, glucagon increases it. This hyperglycemic agent is a hormone normally produced by the alpha cells of the islets of Langerhans in the pancreas.

PHARMACOKINETICS

Glucagon increases blood glucose through glycogenolysis and gluconeogenesis. When the body is in a resting or near-resting state, the liver must replace about 10 grams of glucose each hour. The brain requires approximately 6 of these 10 grams of glucose per hour. Other tissues consume the remaining 4 grams. Hepatic glucose production must equal the glucose demands of the brain and other tissues. Except during meals and extended fasting, glucagon is responsible for hepatic glucose production. Glucagon also increases the breakdown of protein and fat, which provides additional fuel for cellular metabolism.

Absorption, distribution, metabolism, excretion

After S.C., I.M., or I.V. injection, glucagon is absorbed rapidly. It cannot be taken orally because it is a protein, and it would be destroyed in the GI tract. Glucagon is distributed throughout the body, although its effect occurs primarily in the liver, where it increases glycogenolysis and gluconeogenesis. The exact metabolic fate of glucagon is unknown, although it is degraded extensively in the liver. Glucagon is removed from the body by the liver and kidneys.

Onset, peak, duration
The blood glucose level begins to increase within 5 to 20 minutes of glucagon administration. The half-life of glucagon in plasma is about 3 to 6 minutes. The ability of glucagon to increase hepatic glucose production begins to decline after 1 to 2 hours, and glucose production returns to the original level. This decrease in hepatic glucose production results, in part, from the inhibitory effect of the hyperglycemia produced by the glucagon.

PHARMACODYNAMICS

Glucagon regulates the rate of glucose production through glycogenolysis, gluconeogenesis, and lipolysis. A glucagon deficiency results in hypoglycemia. Although glucagon stimulates insulin secretion, insulin antagonizes glucagon's actions through a negative feedback system.

PHARMACOTHERAPEUTICS

Glucagon is used for emergency treatment of severe hypoglycemia. It also is used during radiologic examination of the GI tract to produce a hypokinetic state.

glucagon. Used for emergency treatment of severe hypoglycemia, glucagon also serves as a diagnostic aid. *Usual adult dosage:* for hypoglycemia, 0.5 to 1 mg S.C., I.M. or I.V. If the patient does not awaken from the hypoglycemic coma within 5 to 20 minutes of the first injection, the dose should be repeated once or twice. As a diagnostic aid, the dose ranges from 0.25 to 2 mg I.M. or I.V.

Drug interactions
As a normal body protein, glucagon only interacts adversely with oral anticoagulants, increasing the anticoagulant effects.

Although glucagon does not interact adversely with any food, it is ineffective in poorly nourished or starving patients. If the patient has no glycogen stored in the liver, glycogenolysis cannot occur even with glucagon.

ADVERSE DRUG REACTIONS

Adverse reactions to glucagon are rare. Nausea and vomiting may occur occasionally. They may result from glucagon's inhibitory effect on GI motility or from hypoglycemia. Because of the short half-life of glucagon, overdose is unlikely. Also, no evidence of glucagon toxicity exists. With large doses or prolonged treatment with glucagon, hypokalemia can result.

Because glucagon is a protein, a patient can develop an allergy to it, but this reaction is rare. A patient also can develop antibodies to glucagon, although the effect of such antibodies remains unknown.

NURSING PROCESS APPLICATION

The following information assists the nurse in caring for a patient who is receiving glucagon.

Assessment
• Review the patient's history for a preexisting condition that contraindicates the use of glucagon, such as pheochromocytoma or known hypersensitivity to the drug.
• Review the patient's history for a preexisting condition that requires cautious use of glucagon, such as pregnancy, lactation, or a history that suggests insulinoma or pheochromocytoma.
• Assess the patient for adverse reactions to glucagon, such as nausea, vomiting, or an allergic reaction.
• Review the patient's medication history to identify the use of drugs that may interact with glucagon, such as an oral anticoagulant.
• Assess the effectiveness of glucagon after administration.
• Evaluate the patient's and family's knowledge about glucagon.

Nursing diagnoses
The following examples represent appropriate nursing diagnoses for a patient receiving glucagon.
• Potential for injury related to a preexisting condition that contraindicates the use of glucagon
• Potential for injury related to a preexisting condition that requires cautious use of glucagon
• Potential for injury related to adverse drug reactions
• Knowledge deficit related to glucagon

Planning and implementation
• Do not administer glucagon to a patient with a condition that contraindicates its use.
• Administer glucagon cautiously to a patient at risk because of a preexisting condition.
• Monitor the patient closely for adverse reactions to glucagon.
• Monitor hydration if the patient experiences nausea or vomiting after glucagon administration. Obtain a prescription for an antiemetic, if needed.
• *Observe the patient receiving high-dose or long-term glucagon therapy for signs of hypokalemia, such as de-*

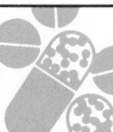

SELECTED MAJOR DRUGS

Hypoglycemic agents and glucagon

This chart summarizes the major hypoglycemic agents and glucagon currently in clinical use.

DRUG	MAJOR INDICATIONS	USUAL ADULT DOSAGES	CONTRAINDICATIONS AND PRECAUTIONS
Insulin			
insulin	Hyperglycemia	Individualized according to the patient's blood glucose level	• Know that insulin is contraindicated in a patient with hypoglycemia or known hypersensitivity to the drug. • Administer with caution to a patient with impaired renal or hepatic function.
Oral hypoglycemic agents			
chlorpropamide	Hyperglycemia	100 to 750 mg P.O. daily	• Know that chlorpropamide is contraindicated in a pregnant or lactating patient or one with diabetic ketoacidosis or known hypersensitivity to the drug. • Administer with caution to a patient with impaired renal or hepatic function.
glipizide	Hyperglycemia	2.5 to 40 mg P.O. daily	• Know that glipizide is contraindicated in a pregnant or lactating patient or one with diabetic ketoacidosis or known hypersensitivity to the drug. • Administer with caution to a patient with impaired renal or hepatic function.
glyburide	Hyperglycemia	1.25 to 20 mg P.O. daily	• Know that glyburide is contraindicated in a pregnant or lactating patient or one with diabetic ketoacidosis or known hypersensitivity to the drug. • Administer with caution to a patient with impaired renal or hepatic function.
tolbutamide	Hyperglycemia	250 to 3,000 mg P.O. daily	• Know that tolbutamide is contraindicated as sole treatment of Type I diabetes, in a pregnant or lactating patient, or in one with diabetic ketoacidosis or known hypersensitivity to the drug. • Administer with caution to a patient with impaired renal or hepatic function.
Glucagon			
glucagon	Emergency treatment of severe hypoglycemia	0.5 to 1 mg S.C., I.M., or I.V., repeated once or twice if patient does not awaken after the first injection	• Know that glucagon is contraindicated in a patient with pheochromocytoma or known hypersensitivity to the drug. • Administer with caution to a pregnant or lactating patient or one with a history that suggests insulinoma or pheochromocytoma.

creased potassium levels, arrhythmias, mental status changes, or irritability.
• *Monitor the patient for signs of bleeding, such as epistaxis, bleeding gums, hematuria, or bruising, during concomitant therapy with glucagon and an oral anticoagulant.* Notify the physician if bleeding occurs and expect to decrease the oral anticoagulant dosage, as prescribed.

• *Give the patient with Type I diabetes mellitus who requires glucagon a complex carbohydrate snack as soon as possible to restore the liver glycogen and prevent secondary hypoglycemia.* A patient with Type I diabetes mellitus typically has a limited amount of glycogen stored in the liver, and glycogen must be available before glucagon can act effectively.

• *Contact the physician immediately to obtain a prescription for I.V. glucose if the patient does not respond to glucagon because of the potential harmful effects of cerebral hypoglycemia.*

• *Administer I.V. glucose with glucagon as prescribed if the patient is in a deep coma or does not awaken from the coma after glucagon administration.*

• *Mix glucagon powder only with the diluent provided.*

• *Do not administer I.V. glucagon in a solution that contains calcium, potassium, or sodium chloride because precipitation can occur.*

• Notify the physician if adverse reactions occur.

Patient teaching

• Teach the patient and family the name, dose, conditions that require administration, action, and adverse effects of glucagon.

• *Teach the family to recognize the signs and symptoms of hypoglycemia. Also show them how to prepare and administer glucagon in an emergency.* Glucagon is supplied premixed or as a white powder with a vial of solution. Instruct the family to use only the diluent provided for glucagon preparation.

• *Instruct the family to provide a complex carbohydrate snack after the patient awakens from the coma.* Also advise them to notify the physician because the patient's medication regimen may need to be changed.

• *Advise the family to seek emergency help immediately if the patient does not respond to glucagon therapy.*

Evaluation

The following examples represent appropriate evaluation statements for a patient receiving glucagon.

• The patient has no conditions that contraindicate glucagon therapy.

• The patient exhibits no signs of complications in the preesixting condition linked to glucagon.

• The patient experiences no adverse reactions to glucagon.

• The patient and family express an accurate understanding of the points taught about glucagon.

• The family members correctly demonstrate how to prepare and administer glucagon to the patient.

CHAPTER SUMMARY

Chapter 49 examined insulin, oral hypoglycemic agents, and glucagon. Because these drugs are used to treat diabetes mellitus, the chapter also discussed this disease briefly. Here are the chapter highlights.

• The patient with Type I diabetes mellitus displays an absolute insulin deficiency and cannot maintain a normal blood glucose level. This patient depends on exogenous insulin for survival. The patient with Type II diabetes mellitus displays a relative insulin deficiency and insulin resistance. This patient does not require exogenous insulin, although the patient may need it during times of stress.

• Insulin is a normal body protein produced by the pancreas. With variations in manufacturer, source, purity, and concentration, 32 insulins are sold in the United States.

• Insulins may vary in onset, peak, and duration, but are similar in absorption, distribution, metabolism, and excretion. All insulins treat hyperglycemia by facilitating glucose uptake and metabolism.

• Hypoglycemia is the most common adverse reaction to insulin therapy.

• When caring for a patient receiving insulin, the nurse should help the patient balance diet, exercise, and insulin requirements and prevent complications of therapy.

• All oral hypoglycemic agents currently on the market in the United States are sulfonylureas. The sulfonylureas vary in pharmacokinetics and hypoglycemic activity.

• Sulfonylureas are used to treat hyperglycemia in the patient with Type II diabetes. Hypoglycemia and drug failure are the most common adverse reactions.

• For a patient receiving an oral hypoglycemic agent, the nurse should teach about diet, exercise and prevention of adverse reactions to the prescribed agent.

• Glucagon is a protein made by the pancreas and used in the emergency treatment of severe hypoglycemia.

• Glucagon regulates the rate of glucose production through glycogenolysis, gluconeogenesis, and lipolysis. It produces few adverse reactions.

• Nursing care for a diabetic patient should include teaching the patient and the patient's family how and when to administer glucagon.

STUDY QUESTIONS

See Appendix 1 for answers.

1. Katie Reibel, age 8, has Type I diabetes. She is admitted to the hospital for diabetes regulation with insulin. How does insulin lower the blood glucose level?
(a) It prevents glucose absorption from the GI tract.
(b) It increases glucose excretion from the GI tract.
(c) It promotes glucose storage as glycogen and inhibits glycogen breakdown.
(d) It promotes gluconeogenesis.

2. For Katie, the physician prescribes a combination of regular and NPH Iletin II insulin. What is the difference between regular and NPH insulin?
(a) Regular insulin is rapid-acting; NPH insulin is inter-mediate-acting.
(b) Regular insulin is purer than NPH insulin.
(c) Regular insulin is more concentrated than NPH insulin.
(d) Regular insulin is derived from beef; NPH insulin comes from pork.

3. The nurse assesses Katie carefully after insulin administration because insulin can cause an allergic reaction. Which type of insulin is the least antigenic?
(a) beef insulin
(b) beef and pork insulin
(c) pork insulin
(d) human insulin

4. The nurse teaches Katie and her parents to recognize signs of diabetic complications, especially hyperglycemia and hypoglycemia. Which of the following are signs and symptoms of hypoglycemia?
(a) polyuria, fatigue, and headache
(b) nervousness, diaphoresis, and confusion
(c) polydypsia, pallor, and irritability
(d) polyphagia and flushed, dry skin

5. Joe Tanner, age 50, has Type II diabetes. His physician prescribes glyburide (DiaBeta), a second-generation sulfonylurea. How does glyburide control diabetes?
(a) It mimics the action of insulin.
(b) It stimulates pancreatic beta-cell production of insulin.
(c) It promotes glycogen storage and inhibits glycogen breakdown.
(d) It stimulates gluconeogenesis.

6. When should the nurse instruct Mr. Tanner to take his oral hypoglycemic agent?
(a) with meals
(b) after meals
(c) 30 minutes before bedtime
(d) 30 minutes before breakfast

7. Ted Brown, a 56-year-old diabetic, has used insulin for 20 years. He is brought to the emergency department semiconscious, with diaphoresis and a blood glucose level of 40. The physician prescribes 0.5 mg of glucagon I.V. How does glucagon produce its therapeutic effects?
(a) It promotes glycogenolysis and gluconeogenesis.
(b) It acts as a competitive inhibitor at insulin receptor sites.
(c) It facilitates insulin metabolism.
(d) It blocks insulin production by the beta cells.

8. Mr. Brown receives glucagon by I.V. injection. Why isn't this drug administered by the oral route?
(a) It would irritate the GI tract too much.
(b) It would have a delayed onset of action.
(c) It would be destroyed by the GI tract.
(d) It would be absorbed unpredictably.

SELECTED REFERENCES

AHFS drug information 90. (1990). Bethesda, MD: American Society of Hospital Pharmacists.

American Diabetes Association. (1988) *Physician's guide to type I diabetes diagnosis and treatment* (2nd ed.). Alexandria, VA: American Diabetes Association.

American Diabetes Association. (1988). *Physician's guide to type II diabetes diagnosis and treatment* (2nd ed.). Alexandria, VA: American Diabetes Association.

Drug facts and comparisons. (1991). St. Louis: Facts and Comparisons Division, J.B. Lippincott.

Ferner, R. (1988). Oral hypoglycemic agents. *Medical Clinics of North America.* 72(6), 1323-1335.

Gerich, J. (1989). Oral hypoglycemic agents. *New England Journal of Medicine,* 321(18), 1231-1245.

Goodman and Gilman's the pharmacological basis of therapeutics (8th ed., 1990). Elmsford, NY: Pergamon Press.

Guthrie, D. (1988). What's wrong with this patient? *Nursing 88,* 19(4), 84-88.

Hansten, P., and Horn, J. (1989). *Drug interactions* (6th ed.). Philadelphia: Lea & Febiger.

Lumley, W. (1988). Controlling Hypoglycemia and Hyperglycemia. *Nursing88,* 18(10), 34-42.

North American Nursing Diagnosis Association. (1990). *Taxonomy I - Revised, with official diagnostic categories.* St. Louis: NANDA.

Wensing, G. (1989). Glipizide: An oral hypoglycemic drug. *American Journal of the Medical Sciences,* 298(1), 69-71.

THYROID AND ANTITHYROID AGENTS

OBJECTIVES

After reading and studying this chapter, the student should be able to:

1. Describe the normal anatomy and physiology of the thyroid gland, and explain how thyroid hormones function.

2. Describe how synthetic thyroid agents act as hormones.

3. Recognize the physiologic effects of insufficient hormone levels, and identify pharmacologic interventions.

4. Describe the pharmacokinetics, pharmacodynamics, and pharmacotherapeutics of thyroid USP (dessicated), levothyroxine sodium, liothyronine sodium, liotrix, and thyroglobulin.

5. Recognize the physiologic effects of excess hormone levels, and identify pharmacologic interventions.

6. Explain how antithyroid agents interfere with hormone secretion.

7. Describe the pharmacokinetics, pharmacodynamics, and pharmacotherapeutics of methimazole, propylthiouracil, iodine, and radioactive iodine.

8. Identify the major drug interactions and adverse reactions for the major classes of thyroid and antithyroid agents.

9. Describe how to apply the nursing process when caring for a patient who is receiving a thyroid or antithyroid agent.

INTRODUCTION

Thyroid and antithyroid agents are drugs that function to correct the thyroid hormone imbalances hypothyroidism and hyperthyroidism. This chapter discusses the use of thyroid agents as replacement therapy in patients with hypothyroidism (thyroid hormone deficiency). It also describes antithyroid agents and their ability to interfere with thyroid hormone synthesis in patients with hyperthyroidism (thyroid hormone excess).

Anatomy of the thyroid

The thyroid gland secretes two significant hormones, triiodothyronine (T_3) and thyroxine (T_4). Located just below the larynx and anterior to the trachea, the thyroid gland has two lateral lobes, one on each side of the trachea, that give it a butterfly shape. A narrow band of tissue, called the isthmus, connects the lobes. The parathyroid glands usually are located on the posterior surface of the lobes. Recurrent laryngeal nerves run medial to the lobes in the cleft between the trachea and the esophagus. Four major arteries supply blood to the thyroid gland, making it highly vascular.

On a cellular level, the gland is composed of many nodules, actually groups of closed follicles. Epithelial cells line the follicles and secrete a substance called colloid into them. Colloid contains a large glycoprotein, thyroglobulin, which contains thyroid hormones in its molecule. The release of colloid initiates thyroid hormone secretion.

Thyroid hormone production and function

Thyroid hormone secretion is controlled primarily by thyrotropin, the thyroid-stimulating hormone (TSH) secreted by the anterior pituitary gland. TSH is in turn stimulated by thyrotropin-releasing hormone (TRH) from the hypothalamus. Iodine and circulating thyroid levels are key factors in the storage and secretion of thyroid hormones. Iodine is essential for thyroid hormone formation, and circulating levels of thyroid hormone act as a feedback mechanism, telling the body to increase or decrease the hormone secretion rate.

Besides the two major thyroid hormones, the thyroid also secretes calcitonin to help regulate calcium. The thyroid's follicles include the parafollicular, or C, cells, which secrete calcitonin (thyrocalcitonin). Calcitonin and parathyroid hormone produce opposite effects on the blood calcium level. Calcitonin rapidly decreases the blood calcium level, but its effects last only a few days at most.

Thyroid hormone storage and release

Thyroid cells store a hormone precursor, colloidal iodinated thyroglobulin, which contains iodine and thyroglobulin. When stimulated by thyroid-stimulating hormone (TSH), a follicular cell takes up some of the stored thyroglobulin. The cell membrane extends fingerlike projections into the colloid, then pulls portions of it back into the cell. Lysosomes in the cell fuse with the colloid, which then is degraded by proteolysis into T_3 and T_4, which are released into the circulation and the lymphatic system by exocytosis.

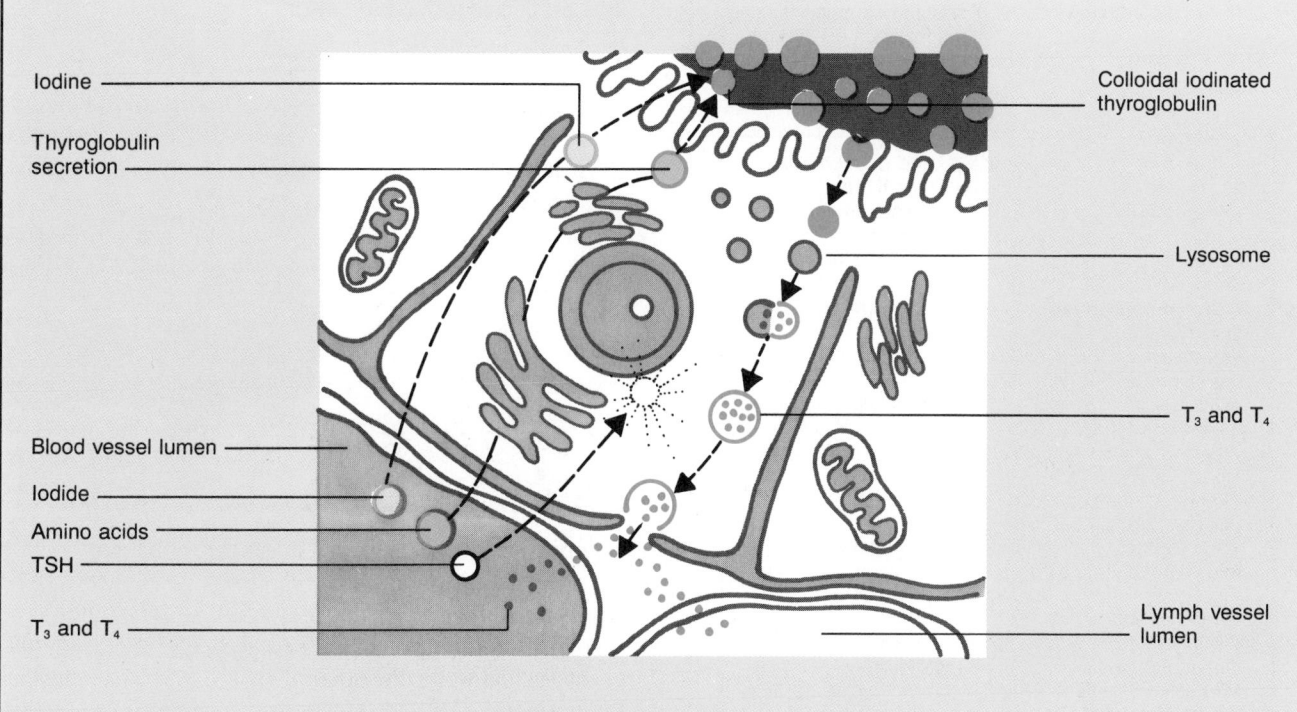

Parathyroid hormone, however, increases the blood calcium level for a long time.

Calcitonin's primary target site is bone. But T_3 and T_4 have as their primary target site almost all body tissue. Their primary function is to increase the metabolic processes throughout the body.

Iodine, a major component of T_3 and T_4, must be present in the body for thyroid hormone synthesis to occur. The optimum daily iodine requirement for adults is 150 to 300 mcg. In the United States, the average intake is 200 to 500 mcg daily from water, food, and medicine. Iodized table salt, iodine-rich foods such as shellfish, and foods such as milk that use iodophors (sterilizing agents with iodine) add iodine to the diet. After ingestion, iodine is broken down into iodide.

The process of thyroid hormone synthesis and release involves six steps: (1) entrapment of iodide, (2) oxidation of iodide, (3) combination of iodide with tyrosine to form monoiodotyrosine (MIT) and diiodotyrosine (DIT), (4) coupling of MIT and DIT to form T_3 and T_4, (5) storage of T_3 and T_4, and (6) hormone release.

After the synthesis process is complete, the thyroid hormone can be stored or released. (For more information, see *Thyroid hormone storage and release.*) Thyroglobulin molecules can store T_3 and T_4 for up to several months. This long-term storage explains why the effects of hormone deficiency may not appear for several months, even when hormone synthesis has ceased.

When the body needs thyroid hormones, TSH stimulates the release of T_3 and T_4. They diffuse through the base of the thyroid cell into the blood of the surrounding capillaries. The thyroid cell also releases MIT and DIT, which are deiodinated (iodine is cleaved from them by deiodinase enzyme) so that the iodine can be reused.

In the blood, most of the hormones combine with plasma proteins, mainly thyroxine-binding globulin (TBG), thyroxine-binding prealbumin (TBPA), and thyroxine-binding albumin (TBA). Very little of the hormone circulates freely in the blood. A bound hormone has a long half-life in circulation because it is protected from metabolism and excretion.

TBG, which is synthesized by the liver, transports about 75% of the T_3 and T_4 in the serum. T_4 is deiodinated in

---

the liver and kidneys to produce about 80% of the T_3, which is 3 to 4 times more potent than T_4. Breakdown of T_4 also produces metabolically inert reverse T_3 (rT_3). In the liver, T_3 and T_4 are conjugated (joined) with acids and excreted by the biliary tract. Then they are hydrolyzed in the intestines, and most of them reenter the blood by the hepatic portal vessel. About 20% of these thyroid hormones

is excreted unchanged in the feces. T_4 has a half-life of 6 to 7 days. T_3 has a half-life of 2 days or less because of its lower affinity for protein binding.

Thyroid hormones affect the body in various ways. For example, they regulate growth and development through their influence on the central nervous system and somatotropin (growth hormone); produce heat by increasing the metabolic rate of body tissues; stimulate the cardiovascular system; and increase protein, lipid, and carbohydrate metabolism.

For a summary of representative drugs, see *Selected major drugs: Thyroid and antithyroid agents,* page 869. For a listing of applicable nursing diagnoses that the nurse may formulate when caring for a patient receiving these agents, see *Selected nursing diagnoses: Thyroid and antithyroid agents.* For detailed information on applying the nursing process, see Chapter 6, The Nursing Process and Drug Therapy.

THYROID AGENTS

Thyroid agents can be natural or synthetic and may contain T_3, T_4, or both. Natural thyroid agents, which are derived from animal thyroid, include thyroid USP (dessicated) and thyroglobulin. Both contain T_3 and T_4. Synthetic thyroid agents actually are the sodium salts of the L-isomers of the hormones. These synthetic hormones include levothyroxine sodium, which contains T_4, liothyronine sodium, which contains T_3, and liotrix, which contains T_3 and T_4. All of these agents are used for exogenous replacement of thyroid hormone.

PHARMACOKINETICS

Thyroid hormones are absorbed variably from the gastrointestinal (GI) tract and distributed in plasma bound to serum proteins. They are metabolized through deiodination, primarily in the liver, and excreted unchanged in the feces.

Absorption, distribution, metabolism, excretion
The body absorbs natural and synthetic thyroid hormones in a similar way. About 50% to 80% of orally administered levothyroxine is absorbed from the GI tract, primarily in the ileum and colon. Absorption increases with fasting and decreases with malabsorption states. Two other factors may influence the absorption of different brands of levothyroxine sodium tablets: particle size and solubility. About 95% of orally administered liothyronine is absorbed from the GI tract. Thyroid USP displays variable absorption.

Therapeutic effectiveness of thyroid agents

In hypothyroidism, drug therapy includes triiodothyronine (T_3), thyroxine (T_4), or combinations of these hormones. Although most T_4 is converted to T_3, the prolonged action and long half-life of T_4 make it the treatment of choice. T_3, a short-acting drug, and combinations of T_3 and T_4 have varying durations of action, depending on their relative concentrations.

DRUG	EQUIVALENT DOSE	CONTENTS	RELATIVE DURATION
levothyroxine	100 mcg	T_4	Long (Effects occur in 1 to 3 weeks.)
liothyronine	25 mcg	T_3	Short (Effects occur in 24 to 72 hours.)
liotrix	62.5 to 75 mcg	T_4 and T_3 in 4:1 ratio	Intermediate*
thyroglobulin	65 mg	T_4 and T_3 in 2.5:1 ratio	Intermediate*
thyroid USP	65 mg	T_4 and T_3 in variable ratios	Intermediate*

*Those with higher T_4 concentrations are longer acting; those with lower T_4 concentrations are shorter acting.

After intramuscular (I.M.) administration, levothyroxine and liothyronine may demonstrate variable, even poor, absorption. Therefore, this route of administration is not recommended. When synthetic hormones must be given parenterally, intravenous (I.V.) administration is recommended and levothyroxine is preferred over liothyronine.

All thyroid agents are distributed in the plasma. They are bound reversibly to protein, mainly TBG.

The primary method of metabolism of the T_4 in these drugs is deiodination, which produces T_3 and physiologically inactive rT_3. Then T_3 and rT_3 are deiodinated to form an inactive metabolite in plasma. The thyroid gland uses the liberated iodine for hormone synthesis, or the body excretes the liberated iodine in feces, bile, or urine.

After conjugation in the liver, T_4 is distributed by the biliary system to the intestines. Although some of the T_4 is hydrolyzed and reabsorbed, 20% to 40% of it is excreted unchanged in the feces.

Onset, peak, duration
The fastest-acting thyroid agent is liothyronine. Maximum effects occur 24 to 72 hours after oral therapy is begun. The drug continues to work for up to 72 hours after discontinuation. Its half-life is short — 1 to 2 days.

Levothyroxine and thyroglobulin have a much slower onset of action and longer duration of action. Their full effects occur 1 to 3 weeks after therapy has begun. However, an initial I.V. dose of levothyroxine administered to a patient in hypothyroid coma will demonstrate effectiveness in 6 to 8 hours and will reach a peak concentration within 24 hours.

Levothyroxine, which has a great affinity for protein binding, is eliminated much more slowly from the body than liothyronine. Levothyroxine's half-life is 6 to 7 days, although the plasma half-life of any thyroid agent is de-

creased in patients with hyperthyroidism and increased in patients with hypothyroidism.

Liotrix is an intermediate-acting agent. (For a comparison of the effects of these agents, see *Therapeutic effectiveness of thyroid agents*.)

PHARMACODYNAMICS

Natural and synthetic thyroid agents act as essential hormones, affecting many physiologic processes.

Mechanism of action
Research continues to determine how thyroid agents work in the body. Some researchers believe that the mechanism of action is related to nucleoproteins that have an extremely high affinity for thyroid hormones.

In the adult, thyroid hormones act on tissues through various mechanisms, including intracellular transport of amino acids and electrolytes, synthesis of specific intracellular enzymes, and enhancement of intracellular processes that lead to changes in cell size and number.

The principal pharmacologic effect of exogenous thyroid hormones is an increased metabolic rate in body tissues. These hormones affect protein and carbohydrate metabolism and stimulate protein synthesis. They promote gluconeogenesis (carbohydrate formation from noncarbohydrate molecules) and increase the use of glycogen stores. By decreasing hepatic and serum cholesterol concentrations, thyroid hormones affect lipid metabolism. They stimulate the heart and increase cardiac output. They even may increase the heart's sensitivity to catecholamines and increase the number of myocardial beta-adrenergic receptors. Thyroid hormones may increase renal blood flow and the glomerular filtration rate in hypothyroid patients, producing diuresis within 24 hours after administration.

PHARMACOTHERAPEUTICS

Thyroid agents act as replacement or substitute hormones when the body's hormone level cannot meet its needs. Therefore, they are used to treat the many forms of hypothyroidism.

Primary hypothyroidism results from thyroid gland malfunction, which can be related to reduced functional thyroid tissue mass or to impaired synthesis or release of hormones. This malfunction can be congenital, as in cretinism, or acquired. The congenital malfunction may result from the absence or underdevelopment of the thyroid gland, resulting in cretinism if left untreated. Treatment with thyroid hormone replacement has the best results when begun in patients under age 3 months. Children metabolize thyroid hormone more quickly than adults, so pediatric dosages usually are higher. The acquired malfunction may result from neoplasms, thyroidectomy, radiation therapy, iodine deficiency, or excess consumption of antithyroid agents.

Secondary hypothyroidism results from pituitary dysfunctions, such as neoplasms, postpartal pituitary necrosis, or pituitary insufficiency that results in insufficient TSH secretion.

Tertiary hypothyroidism results from hypothalamic dysfunction. Myxedema is a severe form of hypothyroidism.

Thyroid agents also may be used with antithyroid agents to prevent goitrogenesis (goiter formation) and hypothyroidism. In diagnostic tests, these agents help differentiate between primary and secondary hypothyroidism. Treating papillary or follicular thyroid carcinoma also may require their use.

Although thyroid USP (dessicated) is the oldest thyroid agent, it presents the problem of variable absorption. Its potency also may vary from batch to batch. Levothyroxine is the drug of choice for thyroid hormone replacement and TSH suppression therapy. It is available in I.V. form and has a relatively long half-life, so that administration once a day is acceptable. Liothyronine has a faster onset of action. However, it has a short half-life and causes problems with laboratory monitoring. Therefore, it is recommended for short-term TSH suppression. The combination drug liotrix is expensive and may result in excess serum concentrations of T_3.

thyroid USP (dessicated) (S-P-T, Thyrar, Thyro-Teric). Used for thyroid hormone replacement in hypothyroidism, thyroid USP (dessicated) is cleaned, dried, and powdered thyroid gland obtained from domesticated animals, such as pigs, sheep, and cattle. It also is used to suppress thyrotropin secretion in patients with simple goiter or chronic lym-phocytic thyroiditis, to reduce goiter size, and to treat cretinism.

Usual adult dosage: for mild hypothyroidism, initially 60 mg P.O. daily, increased in 60-mg increments at 30-day intervals until the desired response is achieved; for severe hypothyroidism, initially 15 mg P.O. daily, increased to 30 mg/day after 2 weeks and to 60 mg/day after 4 weeks, then if laboratory results do not improve, increased to 120 mg/day, and finally to 180 mg/day; for maintenance, 60 to 180 mg P.O. daily; for adult myxedema, 16 mg P.O. daily, may be doubled every 2 weeks to a maximum of 120 mg daily.

Usual pediatric dosage: for cretinism and juvenile hypothyroidism, children ages 1 and older may approach adult dosage (60 to 180 mg P.O. daily), depending on response; children ages 4 to 12 months, 30 to 60 mg P.O. daily; children ages 1 to 4 months, initially, 15 to 30 mg P.O. daily, increased at 2-week intervals; for maintenance, 30 to 45 mg P.O. daily.

levothyroxine sodium [T₄ or L-thyroxine sodium] (Levothroid, Noroxine, Synthroid). Levothyroxine is the preferred agent for thyroid hormone replacement in primary hypothyroidism and cretinism. It also is used in secondary hypothyroidism. Its standard hormone content makes its effects predictable. Although usually administered orally, it can be given I.M. or I.V.

Usual adult dosage: for mild hypothyroidism, initially 50 mcg P.O. daily, increased every 2 to 4 weeks by 25 to 50 mcg until the desired effect is achieved; for an otherwise healthy adult with recent onset of hypothyroidism, initially 100 to 200 mcg P.O. daily; for severe hypothyroidism, initially 12.5 to 25 mcg P.O. daily, increased every 2 to 4 weeks by 25 to 50 mcg; for maintenance, 100 to 200 mcg P.O. daily; for an elderly hypothyroid patient, initially 12.5 to 50 mcg daily, increased every 3 to 8 weeks until the desired effect is achieved; for maintenance for an elderly patient, about 25% less than that for a younger adult; for parenteral administration, about half of the oral adult dose; for myxedema coma, initially 400 mcg I.V. in a concentration of 100 mcg/ml, increased by 100 to 300 mcg or more on the second day if improvement has not occurred; for parenteral maintenance, 50 to 200 mcg I.V. daily until the patient is stabilized and can take oral medication.

liothyronine sodium [T₃] (Cytomel). Because liothyronine has a rapid onset and short duration of action, it usually is preferred for a rapid effect. Used primarily in the T_3 suppression test, liothyronine can differentiate hyperthyroidism from euthyroidism in patients with borderline to high values on the ^{131}I thyroid uptake test. It usually is administered orally, but researchers are investigating a parenteral preparation.

Usual adult dosage: for mild hypothyroidism, initially 25 mcg P.O. daily, increased by 12.5 to 25 mcg every 1 to 2 weeks; for maintenance, 25 to 75 mcg P.O. daily; for severe hypothyroidism, initially 5 mcg P.O. daily, increased every 1 to 2 weeks by 5 to 10 mcg; for maintenance, 50 to 100 mcg daily; for an elderly patient, initially 5 mcg P.O. daily, increased every 1 to 2 weeks by 5 mcg; for myxedema coma, 200 mcg I.V. initially, followed by 10 to 25 mcg I.V. every 8 to 12 hours until the patient stabilizes; for use in the T_3 suppression test, 75 to 100 mcg P.O. daily for 7 days. (A ^{131}I uptake test is performed at the beginning and end of this medication regimen.)

liotrix (Euthroid, Thyrolar). Liotrix is a synthetic combination of T_4 and T_3 in a 4:1 ratio by weight and a 1:1 ratio in terms of physiologic activity. However, the total amount of hormone varies between drugs from different manufacturers. For example, Euthroid-1 contains 60 mcg of T_4 and 15 mcg of T_3; Thyrolar-1 contains 50 mcg of T_4 and 12.5 mcg of T_3. Liotrix may be used as a replacement agent in hypothyroidism, but its use remains controversial because it may result in excessive T_3 concentrations with normal T_4 concentrations.
Usual adult dosage: for hypothyroidism, Euthroid-½ (30 mcg T_4 and 7.5 mcg T_3) or Thyrolar-¼ (12.5 mcg T_4 and 3.1 mcg T_3) or Thyrolar-½ (25 mcg T_4 and 6.25 mcg T_3) P.O. daily initially, before breakfast, increased every 1 to 2 weeks, as needed. Dosages are individualized to approximate the deficit in the patient's thyroid secretion.

thyroglobulin (Proloid). Obtained from hog thyroid glands, the T_4 and T_3 content of this agent is standardized. Each 65 mg of thyroglobulin equals about 60 to 65 mg of thyroid USP, 100 mcg of levothyroxine, or 25 mcg of liothyronine. Although thyroglobulin is used as a replacement agent in hypothyroidism, it has no clinical advantage over thyroid USP.
Usual adult dosage: for hypothyroidism, initially 32 mg P.O. daily, increased gradually by 32 mg every 1 to 2 weeks; for maintenance, 65 to 200 mg P.O. daily.

Drug interactions

Thyroid agents interact with several common medications. For instance, they may increase the effect of anticoagulants. (For more information, see *Drug interactions: Thyroid agents,* page 862.)

ADVERSE DRUG REACTIONS

Most adverse reactions to thyroid agents result from toxicity. Discontinuation of the drugs will reverse the signs and symptoms.

Common GI signs and symptoms of thyroid toxicity include diarrhea, abdominal cramps, weight loss, and increased appetite. Cardiovascular signs and symptoms also may occur, including palpitations, diaphoresis, tachycardia, increased blood pressure, angina pectoris, and arrhythmias. Other manifestations of toxicity may include headache, tremor, insomnia, nervousness, fever, heat intolerance, and menstrual irregularities. These effects usually subside when the drug is discontinued temporarily. Thyroid USP, thyroglobulin, and levothyroxine should be discontinued for 2 to 7 days; liothyronine, for 2 to 3 days. When the patient starts to take the medication again, the dosage must be decreased.

Elderly patients beginning thyroid therapy require close monitoring because the cardiostimulatory effect of the thyroid agent may produce angina pectoris or a myocardial infarction (MI) if coronary artery disease is present.

A patient with adrenal insufficiency should receive corticosteroids to correct the insufficiency before thyroid therapy begins. Because thyroid agents increase tissue demand for adrenal hormones, thyroid therapy could precipitate an acute adrenal crisis in a patient with adrenal insufficiency.

Euthroid and Synthroid tablets contain tartrazine yellow dye, which may produce bronchial asthma and other hypersensitivity reactions in a susceptible individual. Although rare, these reactions are more likely to occur in an aspirin-sensitive patient. A lactose-sensitive patient may need to avoid levothyroxine because it contains lactose. A patient who is sensitive to pork may experience GI distress when taking thyroid USP or thyroglobulin.

NURSING PROCESS APPLICATION

The following information assists the nurse in caring for a patient who is receiving a thyroid agent.

Assessment
• Review the patient's history for a preexisting condition that contraindicates the use of a thyroid agent, such as thyrotoxicosis, acute MI uncomplicated by hypothyroidism, uncorrected adrenal insufficiency, or known hypersensitivity to the drug.
• Review the patient's history for a preexisting condition that requires cautious use of a thyroid agent, such as angina pectoris, hypertension, other cardiovascular disease, advanced age, or lactation.
• Assess the patient for adverse reactions to the prescribed thyroid agent, such as signs and symptoms of toxicity or hypersensitivity reactions.
• Review the patient's medication history to identify the use of drugs that may interact with the thyroid agent, such as oral anticoagulants, phenytoin, or digitalis.
• Assess the effectiveness of the thyroid agent regularly.
• Assess the elderly patient regularly for the sudden onset of chest pain.
• Evaluate the patient's and family's knowledge about the prescribed thyroid agent.

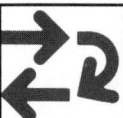

DRUG INTERACTIONS
Thyroid agents

Thyroid agents interact with several common drugs, including oral anticoagulants, cholestyramine, and phenytoin. The nurse should monitor for the effects of drug interactions in any patient who is receiving these drugs and taking thyroid agents.

DRUG	INTERACTING DRUGS	POSSIBLE EFFECTS	NURSING IMPLICATIONS
levothyroxine, liothyronine, liotrix, thyroglobulin, thyroid USP	oral anticoagulants	Increase risk of bleeding	• Monitor the patient for signs of bleeding, such as epistaxis, bleeding gums, hematuria, or easy bruising. • Monitor the patient's prothrombin time (PT) closely when thyroid therapy begins. • Reduce the anticoagulant dosage, as prescribed, when thyroid therapy begins. Readjust it as prescribed, according to the PT results.
	cholestyramine, colestipol	Bind T_3 and T_4 in the GI tract, preventing absorption and recirculation of hormones	• Administer these medications at least 4 hours apart. • Monitor the results of the patient's thyroid function tests.
	phenytoin	Increases metabolism of thyroid hormones; increases T_4 levels by displacing T_4 from plasma protein binding sites	• Monitor the results of the patient's thyroid function tests. • Adjust the thyroid dosage, as prescribed.
	cardiac glycosides	Decrease serum digitoxin or digoxin levels; increase risk of arrhythmias	• Monitor the patient's serum digitoxin or digoxin level. • Monitor the pulse and ECG as prescribed.
	carbamapazine	Increases metabolism of thyroid hormones	• Assess the patient for signs of ineffectiveness of thyroid therapy. • Monitor the results of the patient's thyroid function tests when beginning or ending carbamazepine therapy.
	theophylline	Decrease serum level of theophylline	• Monitor the patient's theophylline level closely when starting thyroid agent therapy. • Monitor the patient's respiratory status during concomitant therapy.

Nursing diagnoses
The following examples represent appropriate nursing diagnoses for a patient receiving a thyroid agent.
• Potential for injury related to a preexisting condition that contraindicates the use of a thyroid agent
• Potential for injury related to a preexisting condition that requires cautious use of a thyroid agent
• Potential for injury related to adverse drug reactions
• Pain related to angina pectoris or acute MI induced by the thyroid agent
• Knowledge deficit related to the prescribed thyroid agent

Planning and implementation
• Do not administer a thyroid agent to a patient with a condition that contraindicates its use.
• Administer a thyroid agent cautiously to a patient at risk because of a preexisting condition.

• *Monitor the patient frequently for toxicity and other adverse reactions during thyroid agent therapy.* If toxicity occurs, notify the physician. Also, expect to discontinue the drug temporarily and to decrease the dosage as prescribed when therapy begins again.
• Assess for any history of pork sensitivity before administering thyroid USP or thyroglobulin, lactose sensitivity before administering levothyroxine, and aspirin sensitivity before administering Euthroid or Synthroid. If the patient has a history of hypersensitivity to a thyroid agent, consult the physician about using a different thyroid preparation.
• Evaluate the patient's response to therapy regularly. Appropriate treatment should restore normal serum levels of T_3 and T_4. With thyroid USP or levothyroxine, expect to see a change in the patient's physical appearance and well-being in 1 to 3 weeks. With liothyronine, expect a change in 1 to 3 days.

Myxedema coma

Chronic untreated hypothyroidism or abrupt withdrawal of thyroid medication may lead to myxedema coma. Because its mortality is 50% to 80%, myxedema coma is a medical emergency. The following information presents the causes, signs and symptoms, treatment, and nursing implications of myxedema coma.

Causes

In a patient with a thyroid disorder, other causes of myxedema coma may include thyroidectomy, infection, decreased pituitary stimulation of the thyroid, sedatives, narcotics, anesthesia, hypothermia, stress, respiratory acidosis and carbon dioxide narcosis from hypoventilation, or hypoglycemia.

Signs and symptoms

- Lethargy, stupor, or a decreased level of consciousness
- Dry skin and hair
- Delayed deep-tendon reflexes
- Progressive respiratory center depression
- Decreased cardiac output, bradycardia, and hypotension
- Weight gain
- Progressive cerebral hypoxia
- Decreased serum levels of free T_4, dilutional hyponatremia (low sodium levels caused by excessive water in the bloodstream), serum hypoosmolality, and highly concentrated urine
- Hypothermia
- Hypoglycemia

Treatment

- Establish and maintain a patent airway.
- Assist with ventilation if respiratory failure occurs.
- Establish an I.V. line to administer fluids and medications and to maintain fluid volume as prescribed.
- Establish a normal thyroid hormone level by administering T_3 or T_4 I.V. or through a nasogastric tube as prescribed. (The usual dosage of liothyronine sodium is 200 mcg I.V. initially, and 10 to 25 mcg I.V. every 8 to 12 hours until the patient is stable. The usual dosage of levothyroxine sodium is 400 mcg I.V. initially, 100 to 300 mcg I.V. on the second day, and thereafter 50 to 200 mcg I.V. daily until the patient can take oral medication.)
- Administer glucocorticoids, if prescribed, after adrenal function laboratory work is complete.

Nursing implications

- Be aware that hypothermia can be present without shivering. Also know that the use of a hypothermia blanket is not recommended because active warming may cause peripheral vasoconstriction and shock in a patient with intense peripheral vasoconstriction.
- Be aware that aggressive replacement of thyroid hormones may cause serious cardiac arrhythmias and precipitate myocardial infarction.
- Be aware that dosage adjustment is necessary when administering narcotics or sedatives to the severely hypothyroid patient to avoid further compromise of the patient's respiratory status.

- Evaluate thyroid function test results carefully because thyroid agents can alter results.
- *Monitor the patient's prothrombin time and partial thromboplastin time, and adjust anticoagulant dosages, as prescribed. Instruct the patient to report any unusual bleeding or bruising.*
- *Reconstitute levothyroxine for injection immediately before administration. Do not add it to other I.V. fluids. Discard any unused portions.*
- *Ensure that a patient with adrenal insufficiency receives corticosteroid therapy as prescribed before beginning thyroid therapy.*
- Notify the physician if adverse reactions occur.
- *Monitor for cardiac problems if the patient is elderly or has a history of cardiac disease because T_4 may aggravate angina pectoris and lead to MI. Particularly note any chest pain.*
- *Do not withdraw a thyroid agent abruptly in a patient with myxedema because it may precipitate myxedema coma.* (For a summary of the causes and treatments of this disorder, see *Myxedema coma.*)
- *Notify the physician immediately if the patient experiences chest pain during thyroid agent therapy. Obtain a prescription for a drug to relieve pain, such as nitroglycerin. Also obtain an electrocardiogram, if prescribed.*

Patient teaching
- Teach the patient the name, dose, frequency, action, and adverse effects of the prescribed thyroid agent.
- *Teach the patient to recognize and report the signs and symptoms of hyperthyroidism, such as fatigue, breathlessness, and heat intolerance. Also instruct the patient to report any headaches, palpitations, or nervousness — symptoms of thyroid hormone overdose.*
- Discuss the prescribed medication regimen with the patient. A prescription for T_3 may require the patient to take it two to three times per day because of its rapid plasma half-life. A T_4 prescription usually specifies that it be taken once a day. Remind the patient to take levothyroxine on an empty stomach to promote regular absorption and to take it in the morning to help prevent insomnia and to mimic normal hormone release.
- Remind the patient to store the thyroid agent in a tightly capped, light-resistant container at 59° to 86° F (15° to 30° C) to prevent deterioration.
- *Teach the patient that different brands of thyroid agents may vary slightly in concentration.* Instruct the patient to check that the physician orders the drug by brand name and that the pharmacist does not substitute a different brand.

• *Stress the importance of returning for routine thyroid studies, as prescribed, to assess the drug's effectiveness and detect toxicity.*
• Instruct the patient to notify the physician if adverse reactions occur.

Evaluation

The following examples represent appropriate evaluation statements for a patient receiving a thyroid agent.
• The patient has no conditions that contraindicate thyroid agent therapy.
• The patient exhibits no complications in the preexisting condition linked to the prescribed thyroid agent.
• The patient demonstrates no adverse reactions to the prescribed thyroid agent.
• The patient does not experience chest pain during thyroid agent therapy.
• The patient and family express an accurate understanding of the points taught about the prescribed thyroid agent.
• The patient returns for follow-up thyroid studies as instructed.

OTHER THYROID AGENTS

Several thyroid agents are used in diagnostic tests. The most common ones — thyrotropin and protirelin — help differentiate between the various forms of hypothyroidism.

thyrotropin [thyroid-stimulating hormone or TSH] (Thytropar). Made from bovine pituitary glands, thyrotropin aids in the differential diagnosis of primary and secondary hypothyroidism. Parenteral administration of 10 IU of thyrotropin for 1 to 3 days precedes serum T_3 and T_4 measurements.

protirelin [thyrotropin-releasing hormone or TRH] (Relefact-TRH, Thypinone). A synthetic version of the natural hypothalamic tripeptide hormone, protirelin assists in the differential diagnosis of secondary and tertiary hypothyroidism. After blood is drawn to obtain a baseline TSH level, the patient receives 400 to 500 mcg of protirelin I.V. A second blood sample is drawn for a TSH level 30 minutes after administration and a third is drawn 30 minutes later. The patient requires careful monitoring for 1 hour after injection because complications can occur, including transient hypotension or hypertension.

ANTITHYROID AGENTS

A number of agents act as antithyroid agents, or thyroid antagonists. These agents function by interfering with hormone synthesis, modifying tissue response to hormones, or destroying the thyroid gland. Used for patients with hyperthyroidism (thyrotoxicosis), these agents include the thionamides (propylthiouracil and methimazole) and the iodides (stable iodine and radioactive iodine).

PHARMACOKINETICS

The thionamides and the iodides are absorbed through the GI tract, concentrated in the thyroid, metabolized by conjugation, and excreted in the urine.

Absorption, distribution, metabolism, excretion

Propylthiouracil is absorbed rapidly, but its bioavailability ranges from 50% to 80%. In contrast, methimazole is absorbed at variable rates, but its bioavailability approaches 100%. Both are distributed by the blood, concentrated in the thyroid, metabolized in the liver, and excreted by the kidneys. The kidneys excrete most of a propylthiouracil dose in 24 hours and 60% to 75% of a methimazole dose in 48 hours.

Stable iodine is reduced to iodide in the GI tract, absorbed in the small intestine, concentrated in the thyroid and epithelial cells, and excreted by the kidneys. Radioactive iodine is absorbed rapidly after oral administration, concentrated by the thyroid, and incorporated into storage follicles in the thyroid gland. It is excreted in the urine.

Onset, peak, duration

The thionamides inhibit the synthesis, rather than the release, of hormones. Therefore, their onset of action may take 3 to 4 weeks. A patient whose thyroid gland contains a relatively high concentration of iodine (from ingestion or from administration during a radiologic diagnostic test) may respond slowly to an antithyroid agent. The thionamides reach peak plasma concentration levels about 1 hour after administration. The plasma half-life of propylthiouracil is 1.5 to 2 hours; that of methimazole is 6 to 13 hours. Because the follicular cells of the thyroid accumulate these agents, their effective half-life is much longer than the serum half-life. Their duration of action varies; for example, 100 mg of propylthiouracil can inhibit hormone synthesis for 7 hours, and 10 mg of methimazole can inhibit most of it for 8 hours.

Because iodides inhibit hormone release, their onset is faster than that of the thionamides. A decrease in symptoms can occur with the iodides in 2 to 7 days; peak concentrations occur in 10 to 15 days. The serum half-life of plasma iodide is about 8 hours.

PHARMACODYNAMICS

The thionamides prevent thyroid hormone synthesis by blocking the combination of iodide and tyrosine. Stable iodine inhibits hormone synthesis through the Wolff-Chaikoff effect, in which above-critical concentrations of intracellular iodide seem to deter hormone synthesis. Radioactive iodine limits hormone secretion by destroying thyroid tissue.

Mechanism of action

The thionamides have distinct mechanisms of action in treating Graves' disease and other forms of hyperthyroidism. They inhibit hormone production by reducing the combination of iodide and tyrosine and the coupling of MIT and DIT. One thionamide, propylthiouracil, inhibits the peripheral conversion of T_4 to T_3. All thionamides act as immunosuppressants, which may help decrease the concentrations of thyroid-stimulating antibody (TSAb) acting on thyroid cells.

Pharmacologic doses of stable iodine rapidly produce a critical level of iodide in the thyroid. This results in the Wolff-Chaikoff effect, significantly decreasing the rate of thyroid hormone synthesis. However, this effect is temporary. In a few days, the thyroid begins to synthesize hormones again in spite of the high iodine intake. This phenomenon occurs because the body adapts to the high iodine levels by decreasing iodide transport and lowering the intracellular iodide concentration level. Iodine also can limit thyroid hormone release by inhibiting thyroglobulin endocytosis, which results in colloid accumulation in the follicles.

Radioactive iodine works in two ways: by inducing acute radiation thyroiditis and chronic gradual thyroid atrophy. These mechanisms destroy thyroid tissue. Acute radiation thyroiditis usually occurs 3 to 10 days after administering radioactive iodine. Chronic thyroid atrophy may take several years to appear.

PHARMACOTHERAPEUTICS

Antithyroid agents commonly are used to treat hyperthyroidism, especially in the form of Graves' disease, which accounts for 85% of all hyperthyroidism. (Other causes of hyperthyroidism that require therapy include toxic multinodular goiter, thyroiditis, excessive intake of thyroid hormones, and neoplasms.) Graves' disease is an autoimmune disorder that affects only the thyroid gland and may be caused by an inherited defect in the manufacture of TSAb. The goal of treatment is to produce a temporary euthyroid state that will allow the autoimmune response to recede

spontaneously or from the medication's immunosuppressive properties. Propylthiouracil, which lowers serum T_3 levels faster than methimazole, usually is used for rapid improvement of severe hyperthyroidism. It also is the thionamide of choice in pregnancy because its rapid action lessens placental transfer and because it does not cause aplasia cutis (a severe dermatologic disorder) in the fetus. Because methimazole blocks thyroid hormone formation for a longer time, it is better suited for administration once a day to patients with mild to moderate hyperthyroidism. Therapy may continue for 12 to 24 months before remission.

To help treat hyperthyroidism, the thyroid gland may be removed by surgery or destroyed by radiation. Preoperatively, stable iodine is used to prepare the gland for surgical removal by firming it and decreasing its vascularity. Stable iodine also is used after radioactive iodine therapy to control symptoms of hyperthyroidism while the radiation takes effect.

methimazole [thiamazole] (Tapazole). Used to treat hyperthyroidism, methimazole also can serve as an adjunct before thyroid surgery and with radioactive iodine therapy. It is about 10 times as potent as propylthiouracil.
Usual adult dosage: initially, for hyperthyroidism, 5 to 20 mg P.O. t.i.d.; for maintenance, 5 to 20 mg/day. Dosages for preoperative preparation are the same.

propylthiouracil [PTU] (Propyl-Thyracil). Because propylthiouracil takes effect faster than methimazole, it is used to treat severe hyperthyroidism. It also is used to treat thyroid crisis (thyroid or thyrotoxic storm) because it inhibits the conversion of T_4 to T_3. It also can be used to prepare the thyroid gland before surgery or radioactive iodine therapy. It is the agent of choice in pregnancy because it is safer for the fetus.
Usual adult dosage: 100 to 200 mg P.O. t.i.d.; for thyroid crisis, dosage may be increased up to 1,200 mg/day; for maintenance, 50 to 200 mg/day.

iodine (Potassium Iodide Solution, USP; Sodium Iodide, USP; Strong Iodine Solution, USP). Used for the rapid treatment of hyperthyroidism, iodine produces visible effects in 3 days. More commonly, it is used to prepare the thyroid gland for surgery because it firms the gland and reduces its vascularity. Iodine usually is administered orally as strong iodine solution or Lugol's solution (5 grams iodine and 10 grams potassium iodide per 100 ml of solution, yielding 6 mg iodine per drop) or as saturated solution of potassium iodide, or SSKI (100 grams potassium iodide per 100 ml of solution, yielding 50 mg iodide per drop).
Usual adult dosage: for hyperthyroidism, 3 to 5 drops of Lugol's solution t.i.d. or 1 drop of SSKI t.i.d.; as a preoperative agent, 3 to 5 drops of Lugol's solution t.i.d. or 1 to 5 drops of SSKI t.i.d. for 10 to 14 days before surgery;

for thyroid crisis, 1 gram I.V. of sodium iodide or 10 drops of SSKI every 8 hours or 30 drops of Lugol's solution P.O. or by nasogastric tube daily.

radioactive iodine [¹³¹I, sodium iodine-131]. Administering radioactive iodine often is the preferred treatment for hyperthyroidism. It exposes only the thyroid tissue to altering radiation, eliminates the problems of surgery, and allows the patient to be treated as an outpatient. However, the use of radioactive iodine can create problems for young adults because it may cause neoplastic changes in the gland later in life, may induce delayed hypothyroidism, and may require months to take effect. Therefore, it usually is used with older patients and those with cardiac disease rather than surgery. It is the treatment of choice when hyperthyroidism persists after a thyroidectomy or when drug therapy has not produced remission. Administered orally, it can be given as a capsule or dissolved in 4 oz of water. After a tracer dose is administered, the patient's optimal dosage can be calculated based on the iodine accumulated by the gland, the rate of iodine loss, and the estimated weight of the gland.

Usual adult dosage: for hyperthyroidism, 4 to 10 mCi P.O.; for thyroid cancer, 50 to 150 mCi P.O. Radioactive iodine is contraindicated in pregnant women because of the potential adverse effects on the fetus. It also is contraindicated in lactating women because it is secreted in breast milk and can affect the infant. Its use in children still is under investigation.

Drug interactions
Iodide preparations may react synergistically with lithium, causing hypothyroidism. Other interactions have not proven clinically significant.

ADVERSE DRUG REACTIONS

The most serious adverse reaction to thionamide therapy is potentially fatal granulocytopenia. It typically appears after 4 to 8 weeks of treatment and usually produces a precipitous drop in white blood cell count. The patient may develop a sore throat or fever, which should be reported immediately to the physician so that a roat culture and blood count with differential can be done. If the laboratory results reveal fewer than 1,500 granulocytes/mm³, the drug will be discontinued and the patient will begin taking antibiotics.

Hypersensitivity reactions to the thionamides commonly produce pruritus, rash, or fever in the first 3 weeks of treatment.

The iodides can cause iodism (chronic toxicity related to iodine therapy) which is dose-dependent. Iodism can produce an unpleasant brassy taste and burning sensation in the mouth and increased salivation and swelling of the parotid and submaxillary glands. Other signs and symptoms may include headache, rhinitis, conjunctivitis, gastric irritation, bloody diarrhea, anorexia, and depression. These reactions should disappear a few days after iodine therapy is discontinued.

Potassium iodide can cause tooth discoloration. Radioactive iodine can produce a feeling of fullness in the neck and a metallic taste and can increase the risk of birth defects and leukemia.

Rarely, I.V. iodine administration can cause an acute hypersensitivity reaction with angioedema, hemorrhagic skin lesions, and serum sickness. Radioactive iodine also can cause a rare — but acute — reaction 3 to 14 days after administration. During this time, thyroglobulin pours out of damaged follicles and can lead to acute exacerbation of hyperthyroidism and thyroid crisis. (For more information, see *Thyroid crisis.*) Thyroid crisis also may occur after propylthiouracil withdrawal or after administering iodine or iodinated contrast dye.

NURSING PROCESS APPLICATION

The following information assists the nurse in caring for a patient who is receiving an antithyroid agent.

Assessment
• Review the patient's history for a preexisting condition that contraindicates the use of an antithyroid agent, such as lactation or known hypersensitivity to the drug.
• Review the patient's history for a preexisting condition that requires cautious use of an antithyroid agent, such as tuberculosis or concurrent therapy with another drug known to cause granulocytopenia.
• Assess the patient for adverse reactions to the prescribed antithyroid agent, such as granulocytopenia, iodism, or hypersensitivity reactions.
• Review the patient's medication history to identify the use of drugs that may interact with the antithyroid agent, such as lithium.
• Assess the effectiveness of the antithyroid agent regularly.
• Assess the patient's compliance with the antithyroid regimen.
• Evaluate the patient's and family's knowledge about the prescribed antithyroid agent.

Nursing diagnoses
The following examples represent appropriate nursing diagnoses for a patient receiving an antithyroid agent.
• Potential for injury related to a preexisting condition that contraindicates the use of an antithyroid agent
• Potential for injury related to a preexisting condition that requires cautious use of an antithyroid agent
• Potential for injury related to adverse drug reactions

Thyroid crisis

A medical emergency, thyroid crisis occurs when a hyperthyroid patient becomes critically thyrotoxic. Its mortality ranges from 20% to 40%. Sometimes called thyroid storm, thyroid crisis has a rapid onset and may be triggered by excess intake of thyroid hormones, abrupt withdrawal of antithyroid agents, radioactive iodine therapy, infection, trauma, severe stress, and thyroidectomy, if antithyroid agents were not given preoperatively. Listed below are the signs and symptoms, treatment, and nursing implications of thyroid crisis.

Signs and symptoms
- fever
- hot, flushed skin
- tachycardia and tachyarrhythmia
- agitation and restlessness
- confusion and psychosis
- GI disturbances, such as diarrhea and abdominal pain
- apathy, severe myopathy, congestive heart failure, profound weight loss, and atrial fibrillation in elderly patients
- elevated serum levels of free T_4
- elevated T_3 levels
- elevated serum levels of total and free calcium
- abnormal results on liver function tests, especially in elderly patients
- a progression from stupor to coma, hypotension, and vascular collapse

Treatment
- Begin treatment quickly, or the patient could die within 48 hours.
- Initiate I.V. fluid replacement as prescribed.

- Block thyroid hormone release with sodium iodide as prescribed. (The usual dosage is initially 1 to 2 grams I.V. repeated every 12 to 24 hours, or 1 gram every 8 hours by continuous infusion.)
- Block thyroid hormone synthesis with propylthiouracil as prescribed. (The usual dosage is initially 600 to 1,000 mg P.O., then 300 mg P.O. every 6 hours.)
- Block the peripheral effects of thyroid hormones with propranolol as prescribed.
- Replace glucocorticoids with hydrocortisone as prescribed.
- Treat fever with a hypothermia blanket and nonsalicylate antipyretics as prescribed.

Nursing implications
- Be aware that aspirin may interfere with the binding of T_3 and T_4 to circulating protein.
- Be aware that excess thyroid hormones may increase glycogenolysis (carbohydrate breakdown), causing hyperglycemia.
- Be aware that excess thyroid hormones increase the metabolic rate.

- Noncompliance related to long-term use of the antithyroid agent
- Knowledge deficit related to the prescribed antithyroid agent

Planning and implementation
- Do not administer an antithyroid agent to a patient with a condition that contraindicates its use.
- Administer an antithyroid agent cautiously to a patient at risk because of a preexisting condition.
- Monitor the patient frequently for adverse reactions during antithyroid therapy.
- *Monitor the patient's complete blood count periodically to detect impending granulocytopenia, leukopenia, and thrombocytopenia.* Notify the physician if any of these conditions exist. Thionamide agents commonly cause these effects 4 to 8 weeks after therapy begins. If laboratory results reveal fewer than 1,500 granulocytes/mm³, expect to discontinue the drug and administer antibiotics as prescribed.
- *Monitor the patient receiving an iodide for signs and symptoms of iodism, such as increased salivation and swelling of the parotid and submaxillary glands, rhinitis, GI distress, and depression.* Expect to discontinue iodide therapy if iodism occurs.
- Observe the patient for hypersensitivity reactions to the antithyroid agent.

- *Monitor the patient for signs and symptoms of thyroid crisis after administering iodine, iodinated contrast dye, or radioactive iodine or after discontinuing propylthiouracil. Be prepared to begin emergency treatment if needed.*
- Evaluate the patient's response to treatment. With propylthiouracil, expect the serum T_4 level to return to normal 14 to 60 days after therapy begins. The average time to reach a euthyroid state is 42 to 49 days, but this can vary with drug dosage. Signs and symptoms of increased sympathetic activity, such as tachycardia, palpitations, and tremor, usually reverse rapidly. Signs and symptoms of increased catabolic activity, such as weight loss and myopathy, will take longer to improve.
- *Monitor the patient for signs of toxicity, such as thyroid gland enlargement. Also monitor for signs and symptoms of hypothyroidism, such as depression, cold intolerance, and nonpitting edema.*
- *Take full radiation precautions for 24 hours after a patient receives a dose of radioactive iodine for hyperthyroidism.* The patient will have slightly radioactive urine and saliva for 24 hours, and highly radioactive vomitus for 6 to 8 hours.
- *Isolate a patient who receives a dose of radioactive iodine for thyroid cancer because the patient will have radioactive urine, saliva, and perspiration for 3 days.* Observe the following precautions: Ensure that pregnant personnel do

not take care of the patient, use disposable eating utensils and linens, and have the patient save all urine in a lead container for 24 to 48 hours so that the laboratory can measure the amount of radioactive material excreted. Have the patient drink as much fluid as possible for 48 hours after drug administration to facilitate excretion. Limit contact with the patient to 30 minutes per person per shift on the first day and 1 hour on the second day.
• Question the patient about compliance with the prescribed antithyroid regimen. Notify the physician if noncompliance occurs.

Patient teaching

• Teach the patient and family the name, dose, frequency, action, and adverse effects of the prescribed antithyroid agent.
• *Instruct the patient receiving a thionamide agent to call the physician immediately if a sore throat and fever develop.* Explain that the patient may need blood tests and a throat culture if these symptoms appear. Inform the patient that these symptoms are most likely to occur 4 to 8 weeks after drug therapy begins.
• Teach the patient to recognize and report the signs and symptoms of iodism during iodide therapy.
• *Advise the patient who is discharged in fewer than 7 days after receiving radioactive iodine for thyroid cancer to avoid close prolonged contact with small children. Also instruct the patient not to sleep in the same room with anyone else for 7 days after treatment because of the risk of thyroid cancer to people exposed to radioactive iodine. Inform the patient that using the same bathroom as the rest of the family is safe.*
• Review radiation precautions with the patient receiving radioactive iodine for hyperthyroidism.
• Teach the patient to recognize the signs and symptoms of a hypersensitivity reaction, such as pruritus and a rash. Explain that these symptoms may occur during the first 3 weeks of therapy, and if they do, the physician may prescribe a different medication or treat the reaction with an antihistamine.
• Teach the patient to recognize the signs and symptoms of hypothyroidism, which may occur after radioactive iodine therapy.
• *Advise a pregnant patient that she should not receive radiation therapy. Also recommend that she wait several months after therapy before becoming pregnant. Advise a male patient not to father a child for several months after therapy.*
• Teach the patient to keep the antithyroid agent in a light-resistant container.
• Advise the patient to take the antithyroid agent with meals to prevent adverse GI reactions. Radioactive iodine, however, requires overnight fasting before administration. Instruct the patient to dilute potassium iodide with water, milk, or fruit juice to mask the salty taste, and to drink it through a straw to avoid tooth discoloration.
• Advise the patient to consult the physician before eating iodized salt and iodine-rich foods such as shellfish during treatment with an antithyroid agent. The patient also should consult the physician before using any over-the-counter cough medicines because they may contain iodine.
• Instruct the patient to notify the physician if adverse reactions occur.

Evaluation

The following examples represent appropriate evaluation statements for a patient receiving an antithyroid agent.
• The patient has no conditions that contraindicate antithyroid therapy.
• The patient exhibits no complications in the preexisting condition linked to the prescribed antithyroid agent.
• The patient experiences no adverse reactions to the prescribed antithyroid agent.
• The patient maintains full compliance with the antithyroid regimen.
• The patient and family express an accurate understanding of the points taught about the prescribed antithyroid agent.
• The patient correctly identifies the signs and symptoms of adverse reactions to the prescribed antithyroid agent.

OTHER ANTITHYROID AGENTS

Other agents may be used as thyroid antagonists, although they currently are not used as first-line drug therapy for hyperthyroidism. These agents include ionic inhibitors, primarily perchlorate; adrenergic blocking agents, primarily propranolol; and ipodate, a cholecystographic agent used experimentally to decrease serum T_3 levels.

Ionic inhibitors interfere with the ability of the thyroid gland to concentrate iodide ions. One of the ionic inhibitors, perchlorate, is concentrated in the thyroid gland and excreted unchanged by the kidneys. However, the occasional incidence of granulocytopenia has limited its use.

Researchers recently have recognized lithium as a cation-exchange agent that induces hypothyroidism. But they have not established indications yet for lithium therapy in hyperthyroidism.

Adrenergic blocking agents deplete catecholamines or prevent their release. These agents, which include propranolol, guanethidine, and reserpine, have been used to reduce the signs and symptoms of hyperthyroidism, such as nervousness, tremor, palpitations, tachycardia, and diaphoresis. Currently, propranolol is used as a short-term

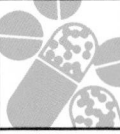

SELECTED MAJOR DRUGS

Thyroid and antithyroid agents

This chart summarizes the drugs most commonly used in treating hypothyroidism and hyperthyroidism.

DRUG	MAJOR INDICATIONS	USUAL ADULT DOSAGES	CONTRAINDICATIONS AND PRECAUTIONS
Thyroid agents			
thyroid USP	Mild hypothyroidism	60 mg P.O. daily initially, increased until desired response is achieved	• Know that thyroid USP is contraindicated in a patient with thyrotoxicosis, acute myocardial infarction (MI) uncomplicated by hypothyroidism, uncorrected adrenal insufficiency, or known hypersensitivity to the drug.
	Adult myxedema	16 mg P.O. daily; may double dosage every 2 weeks to a maximum of 120 mg daily	• Administer with extreme caution to a patient with angina pectoris, hypertension, or other cardiovascular disease. • Administer with caution to a geriatric or lactating patient.
levothyroxine	Mild hypothyroidism	50 mcg P.O. daily initially, increased by 25 to 50 mcg every 2 to 4 weeks; 100 to 400 mcg P.O. daily for maintenance	• Know that levothyroxine is contraindicated in a patient with thyrotoxicosis, acute MI uncomplicated by hypothyroidism, uncorrected adrenal insufficiency, or known hypersensitivity to the drug.
	Myxedema coma	400 mcg I.V. initially in a concentration of 100 mcg/ml, increased by 100 to 300 mcg or more, if needed	• Administer with extreme caution to a patient with angina pectoris, hypertension, or other cardiovascular disease. • Administer with caution to a geriatric or lactating patient or any patient with a history of lactose intolerance.
Antithyroid agents			
propylthiouracil	Hyperthyroidism, adjunct preparation before thyroid surgery or radioactive iodine therapy, thyroid crisis	100 to 200 mg P.O. t.i.d., increased up to 1,200 mg/day for thyroid crisis if needed; 50 to 200 mg P.O. daily for maintenance	• Know that propylthiouracil is contraindicated in a lactating patient or one with known hypersensitivity to the drug. • Administer with extreme caution to a pregnant patient or one who is receiving another drug known to cause granulocytopenia. • Administer with caution to a patient over age 40 because of the risk of heart disease.
iodine	Adjunct preparation before thyroid surgery	3 to 5 drops of Lugol's solution t.i.d. or 1 to 5 drops of SSKI t.i.d. for 10 to 14 days before surgery	• Know that iodine is contraindicated in a pregnant patient or one with acute bronchitis or known hypersensitivity to the drug. • Administer with extreme caution to a patient with tuberculosis.
	Thyroid crisis	1 gram I.V. of sodium iodide or 10 drops of SSKI every 8 hours, or 30 drops of Lugol's solution P.O. or by nasogastric tube daily	
	Hyperthyroidism	3 to 5 drops of Lugol's solution t.i.d. or 1 drop of SSKI t.i.d.	

adjunct treatment in hyperthyroidism when tachycardia is a problem. Although propranolol reduces conversion of T_4 to T_3, it is not effective when used alone. Also, because it tends to weaken myocardial contractions, propranolol is contraindicated in patients with low-output heart failure.

(It is not contraindicated in patients with right-sided heart failure or high-output failure caused by thyrotoxicosis.

Ipodate (Oragraffin) is an oral cholecystographic agent that has decreased serum T_3 levels in experiments. When given to a hyperthyroid patient, it can reduce serum T_3 levels by almost 70% in 48 hours. Researchers have discovered no toxic effects in the experimental group receiving ipodate therapy. Ipodate shows promise for use in the short-term management of hyperthyroidism, as an adjunct therapy after radioactive iodine administration, for more rapid control of hyperthyroidism when given with thionamides, and in preparation for thyroid surgery.

CHAPTER SUMMARY

Chapter 50 presented the normal anatomy of the thyroid gland as well as the physiology of the thyroid hormones. Then it discussed the thyroid agents used to treat hypothyroidism and antithyroid agents used to treat hyperthyroidism. Here are the chapter highlights.
• The body synthesizes thyroid hormones after ingestion of iodine, which is a natural part of the diet. The thyroid gland can store hormones for several months.
• The two major thyroid hormones are triiodothyronine (T_3) and thyroxine (T_4).
• Thyroid-stimulating hormone (TSH), or thyrotropin, primarily controls the release of thyroid hormones. TSH is secreted by the anterior pituitary gland, which is stimulated by thyrotropin-releasing hormone (TRH) from the hypothalamus.
• Thyroid agents are natural or synthetic preparations that contain T_3, T_4, or both. Although the onset of action varies widely among thyroid agents, their principal pharmacologic effect is the same: an increase in the metabolic rate of body tissues.
• Thyroid agents are used as replacements when the body's thyroid hormone level cannot meet its needs. These agents include thyroid USP, levothyroxine, liothyronine, liotrix, and thyroglobulin.
• Levothyroxine sodium usually is the drug of choice for thyroid hormone replacement and TSH suppression therapy.
• Liothyronine is used when rapid action is needed. It also is used in diagnostic tests to differentiate among primary, secondary, and tertiary hypothyroidism.
• Antithyroid agents are used to treat hyperthyroidism. Major drugs in this class include the thionamides (propylthiouracil and methimazole) and the iodides (stable iodine and radioactive iodine).
• Antithyroid agents function by interfering with hormone synthesis, modifying the tissue response to hormones, or destroying the thyroid gland.
• When caring for a patient receiving a thyroid or antithyroid agent, the nurse should teach the patient about the signs and symptoms of hypothyroidism and hyperthyroidism, the importance of compliance with the regimen, the

need for follow-up care, and the signs and symptoms of adverse drug reactions.

STUDY QUESTIONS

See Appendix 1 for answers.

1. Upon admission to the hospital, Ron Mooney, age 48, is overweight and lethargic and speaks in a slow monotone. After determining that Mr. Mooney has hypothyroidism, the physician prescribes levothyroxine 100 mcg daily. Which administration route ensures optimal absorption of this drug?
(a) oral
(b) rectal
(c) subcutaneous
(d) intramuscular

2. Levothyroxine has a relatively slow onset of action. Which thyroid agent has the fastest onset of action?
(a) liotrix
(b) liothyronine
(c) thyroglobulin
(d) thyroid USP

3. By which mechanism of action do thyroid agents correct hypothyroidism?
(a) by directly stimulating thyroid hormone secretion
(b) by stimulating the anterior pituitary to secrete TSH
(c) by stimulating the hypothalamus to secrete TRH
(d) by acting as the essential hormones that are lacking

4. The nurse instructs Mr. Mooney to take levothyroxine exactly as prescribed. What may occur if the drug is discontinued abruptly?
(a) myxedema coma
(b) hyperthyroidism
(c) myocardial infarction
(d) renal insufficiency

5. Annette Plummer, age 26, has Graves' disease, the most common form of hyperthyroidism. Her physician prescribes methimazole (Tapazole) 5 mg P.O. t.i.d. How does methimazole correct hyperthyroidism?
(a) It inhibits thyroid hormone synthesis.
(b) It inhibits thyroid hormone release.
(c) It destroys excess thyroid tissue.
(d) It inactivates thyroid hormones.

6. If Ms. Plummer develops a sore throat and fever during methimazole therapy, what should the nurse advise her to do?
(a) Take aspirin and see if her condition improves.
(b) Notify the physician immediately.
(c) Discontinue the medication immediately.
(d) Wait for this minor reaction to subside in a few days.

7. Luis Ramirez, age 70, continues to experience hyperthyroidism after a thyroidectomy. His physician prescribes treatment with radioactive iodine 4 mCi P.O. Which nursing intervention is appropriate after the initial dose of radioactive iodine?
(a) Restrict the patient's fluid intake.
(b) Provide complete oral care for the patient.
(c) Take full radiation precautions for 24 hours.
(d) Stay with the patient for 2 hours to detect adverse reactions.

8. Twelve days after radioactive iodine administration, Mr. Ramirez develops fever, flushed skin, tachycardia, and restlessness. What is the most likely cause of these signs and symptoms?
(a) iodine hypersensitivity
(b) thyroid crisis
(c) radiation sickness
(d) granulocytopenia

SELECTED REFERENCES

AHFS drug information 90. (1990). Bethesda, MD: American Society of Hospital Pharmacists.

Goodman and Gilman's the pharmacological basis of therapeutics (8th ed.; 1990). Elmsford, NY: Pergamon Press.

Katzung, B. (Ed.). (1987). *Basic and clinical pharmacology* (3rd ed.). Los Altos, CA: Lange Medical Publications.

Kreisberg, R., Rose, L., and Russo, G. (1989). Skin signs in endocrine disease. *Patient Care,* 23(6), 73-82.

Ladenson, P., and Ragland, G. (1988). Endocrine emergencies. *Patient Care,* 22(10), 36-48.

North American Nursing Diagnosis Association. (1990). *Taxonomy I-Revised, with official diagnostic categories.* St. Louis: NANDA.

Schneeberg, N. (1989). "Incurable" hyperthyroidism? *Consultant,* 29(4), 89-90.

Thyroxine overtreatment and bone loss. (1990). *Nurses Drug Alert,* 14(10), 75.

PARATHYROID AGENTS

OBJECTIVES

After reading and studying this chapter, the student should be able to:

1. Describe how parathyroid hormone functions physiologically to increase the serum calcium concentration.

2. Describe the absorption, distribution, metabolism, and excretion of calcitonin, etidronate disodium, and vitamin D analogues.

3. Describe the mechanism of action of calcitonin, etidronate disodium, and vitamin D analogues.

4. Identify the diagnostic and therapeutic uses of the calcium-regulating drugs.

5. Identify interactions among the calcium regulators, foods, and other drugs.

6. Explain why calcium-regulating drugs can cause hypercalcemia or hypocalcemia.

7. Identify adverse reactions associated with the calcium-regulating drugs.

8. Describe the procedures for checking Chvostek's and Trousseau's signs to help assess for hypocalcemia.

9. Describe how to apply the nursing process when caring for a patient who is receiving a parathyroid agent.

INTRODUCTION

Normally, the endocrine system maintains calcium homeostasis through the action of parathyroid hormone (PTH) and calcitriol, the active metabolite of vitamin D.

PTH and calcitriol formation

The serum concentration of ionized calcium serves as feedback to the parathyroid glands to release or retain PTH. When the serum calcium concentration is decreased, the parathyroid glands respond by secreting PTH. When the serum calcium concentration is elevated, the parathyroid glands reduce the rate of PTH secretion.

The body obtains inactive forms of vitamin D from vitamin synthesis in the epidermal layer of the skin and from ingestion of vitamin D-rich foods or supplements.

After these inactive forms of vitamin D enter the circulation, they are transported to the liver where they are metabolized to 25-hydroxy vitamin D. Then they are transported to the kidneys where they undergo further metabolism to 1,25-dihydroxy vitamin D (calcitriol, the active form of vitamin D). Calcitriol production is regulated by calcium, phosphorus, PTH, and calcitriol itself.

Calcium homeostasis

To maintain calcium homeostasis, PTH and calcitriol exert their effects on the intestines, kidneys, and bones. In these target tissues, PTH and calcitriol increase intestinal absorption of calcium, decrease renal clearance of calcium, and mobilize calcium from bone.

The action of PTH involves activation of adenylate cyclase, a membrane-bound enzyme that increases production of cyclic adenosine $3',5'$ monophosphate (cyclic AMP). (For more information, see *Cyclic AMP mechanism of action of parathyroid hormone.*) Most calcitriol-mediated actions result from the binding of calcitriol to intracellular receptors.

Understanding the importance of calcium metabolism requires knowing the vital role that calcium plays in the body's physiologic processes. Calcium, an important constituent of biological membranes, affects the permeability and electrical properties of those membranes. For example, calcium ions are instrumental in regulating heart rhythm. Calcium also acts to stabilize neuromuscular activity. An increase or decrease in the serum calcium concentration alters neuron permeability and nerve tissue excitability, resulting in altered muscle function. Calcium also is involved in the release of preformed hormones (hormones that are stored in glands in active form and do not require metabolism or cleavage to exert their effects) by endocrine cells and in the secretion of transmitter substances at synaptic junctions. Finally, calcium serves as an important component in the adhesive that binds cells, in enzyme activity, and in blood coagulation.

Under normal circumstances, the body obtains sufficient calcium to sustain these physiologic processes. When

Cyclic AMP mechanism of action of parathyroid hormone

Parathyroid hormone (PTH) uses the cyclic adenosine 3′5′ monophosphate (cyclic AMP) mechanism to stimulate target tissues. PTH binds with receptors on the cell membrane of target cells in the intestines, kidneys, and bone. The binding of PTH and the receptor activates the protein enzyme adenylate cyclase, which enters the cytoplasm and facilitates the conversion of adenosine triphosphate (ATP) to cyclic AMP. Cyclic AMP activates a cascade of enzymes and stimulates protein phosphorylation, thereby regulating calcium.

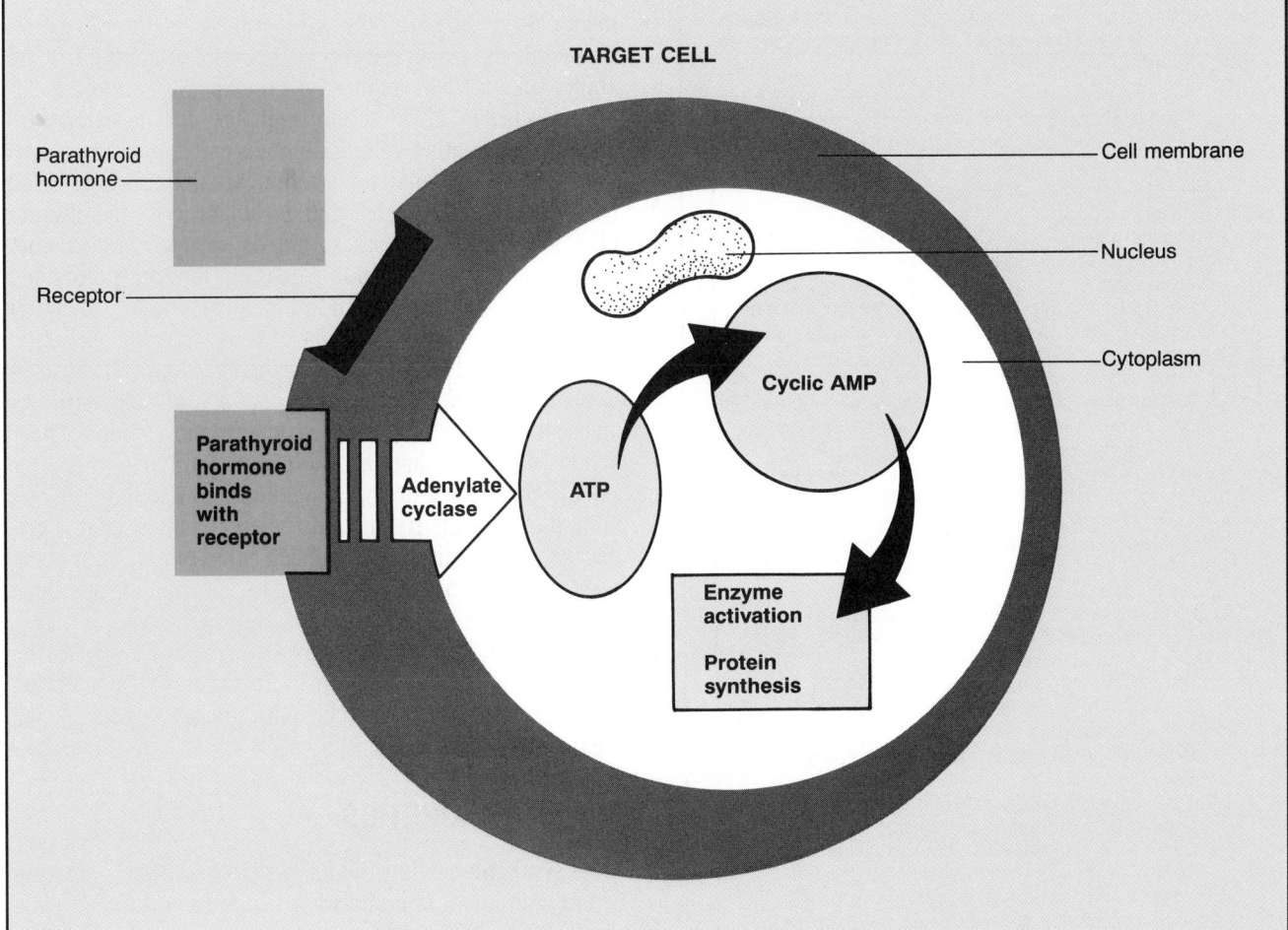

a calcium imbalance occurs, however, calcium regulators may be necessary. For example, calcium imbalance may result from hypoparathyroidism. This disorder, which may be caused by injury, disease, or surgical removal of the parathyroid glands, may decrease or halt PTH secretion. When this occurs, a calcium regulator is needed to maintain a normal calcium level.

This chapter discusses the following calcium-regulating drugs: PTH, calcitonin, etidronate disodium, and the vitamin D analogues calcifediol, calcitriol, and dihydrotachysterol. (For a discussion of vitamin D [cholecalciferol, vitamin D₂; and ergocalciferol, vitamin D₃], see Chapter 45, Vitamin, Mineral, and Other Nutritional Agents.)

Although no therapeutic use of exogenous PTH currently exists, the drug formerly was used to increase serum calcium concentrations. Today, PTH is available for diagnostic and research purposes only. The effects of vitamin D analogues on serum calcium concentrations resemble the effect of endogenous and exogenous PTH; however, other drugs discussed in this chapter—calcitonin and etidronate disodium—produce effects opposite to those of PTH.

For a summary of representative drugs, see *Selected major drugs: Parathyroid agents,* page 880. For a listing of applicable nursing diagnoses that the nurse may formulate when caring for a patient receiving a parathyroid agent, see *Selected nursing diagnoses: Parathyroid agents.* For detailed information on applying the nursing process, see Chapter 6, The Nursing Process and Drug Therapy.

CALCIUM REGULATORS

The calcium regulators include calcitonin, etidronate disodium, and vitamin D analogues, such as calcifediol, calcitrol, and dihydrotachysterol.

Calcitonin, a polypeptide hormone, is produced in mammals by the parafollicular C cells of the thyroid gland. Calcitonin is a single-chain polypeptide composed of 32 amino acids. When required for therapeutic purposes, calcitonin is isolated from salmon and pigs (porcine calcitonin) or prepared synthetically as human calcitonin. In salmon and other submammalian vertebrates, calcitonin is secreted from the ultimobrachial glands adjacent to the thyroid glands. (In mammals, these glands are incorporated into the thyroid gland.) Salmon calcitonin is more potent and lasts longer than porcine and human calcitonin. Calcitonin acts to inhibit bone resorption, increase the renal excretion of calcium, and decrease the gastrointestinal (GI) absorption of calcium. The regulating actions of calcitonin decrease the extracellular serum calcium concentration. These actions usually antagonize the actions of PTH.

Etidronate disodium, a synthetic compound, inhibits bone metabolism. It functions as a calcium regulator primarily by preventing PTH-induced bone resorption, slowing bone metabolism, and decreasing bone formation and bone turnover.

Along with PTH, vitamin D analogues regulate the serum calcium concentration by increasing GI absorption of calcium, mobilizing calcium from bone, and decreasing renal calcium clearance.

PHARMACOKINETICS

Most synthetic calcium regulators provide the advantages of oral administration and longer duration of action. As a result, the synthetic calcium regulators provide better long-term therapeutic effects than PTH, which no longer is used therapeutically.

Absorption, distribution, metabolism, excretion

After parenteral administration, calcitonin is absorbed directly into the circulation. It is metabolized rapidly by conversion to smaller inactive fragments, primarily in the kidneys, but also in the blood and peripheral tissues. A small amount of unchanged hormone and its inactive metabolites are excreted in the urine. Calcitonin does not cross the placental barrier, and its passage to cerebrospinal fluid and breast milk is uncertain. Salmon calcitonin is considerably more potent than the porcine or human variety; it also is cleared more slowly from the system.

Etidronate disodium absorption is dose-dependent and progressive. For example, on the average, about 1% of an oral dose of 5 mg/kg of body weight daily is absorbed. However, as the amount increases, so does the percent absorbed. At 20 mg/kg daily, approximately 6% is absorbed. Food in the GI tract reduces absorption. Etidronate disodium is distributed mainly into bone and is not metabolized. Unabsorbed drug is eliminated slowly in the feces. Within 24 hours, half of the absorbed drug is excreted unchanged in urine. Etidronate disodium does not cross the placental barrier. Its distribution into breast milk is uncertain.

Administered orally, the vitamin D analogues (calcifediol, calcitriol, and dihydrotachysterol) are absorbed well from the small intestine, although bile is essential for adequate intestinal absorption. The drugs are distributed throughout the body and are stored in fat deposits for long periods. Calcifediol is converted in the kidneys to calcitriol, the active form of vitamin D. Dihydrotachysterol is activated in the liver to 25-hydroxydihydrotachysterol and requires no further activation in the kidneys. Metabolism occurs in the liver. Excretion is primarily through bile in feces, with a small percentage of the drugs appearing in urine.

Onset, peak, duration

After intramuscular (I.M.) or subcutaneous (S.C.) administration, calcitonin produces an onset of action within 15 minutes, reaches a peak concentration level in 4 hours, and has a duration of action from 8 to 24 hours. The half-life of calcitonin is about 10 minutes.

The onset of etidronate disodium is slow, with therapeutic effects occurring as long as 1 to 3 months after initiation of therapy. Remissions (decreased bone pain and other symptoms) may last for 3 to 12 months after the drug is discontinued.

The vitamin D analogues calcifediol and calcitriol produce an onset in about 2 hours. The hypercalcemic effect of these drugs peaks in 10 hours. Duration is about 3 to 5 days. Dihydrotachysterol begins to act several hours after administration. The drug's hypercalcemic effect peaks within 1 to 2 weeks. With the discontinuation of therapy, the serum calcium concentration of dihydrotachysterol drops markedly within 4 to 5 days, and the drug's effect disappears after 2 weeks.

PHARMACODYNAMICS

A potent hypocalcemic agent, calcitonin reduces bone resorption and increases renal calcium clearance. Etidronate disodium decreases serum calcium primarily by reducing bone resorption. The vitamin D analogues produce their effects by promoting bone resorption, increasing GI absorption of calcium, and decreasing renal calcium clear-

---

Serum calcium regulation by parathyroid hormone

Homeostatic serum calcium concentration levels are maintained by an elaborate feedback system that begins with the stimulation or inhibition of parathyroid hormone (PTH) secretion. The increase or decrease of the PTH level elicits concurrent responses in the renal, gastrointestinal (GI), and skeletal systems. These responses return the serum calcium concentration to a normal level.

• Increase in serum calcium concentration level	• Decrease in serum calcium concentration level
• Decreased PTH secretion	• Increased PTH secretion
• Increase in kidney calcium excretion • Decrease in GI calcium absorption • Decrease in bone calcium resorption	• Decrease in kidney calcium excretion • Increase in GI calcium absorption • Increase in bone calcium resorption

• Concentration of serum calcium returns to normal (Normal = 4.5 to 5.8 mEq/liter or 8.5 to 10.5 mg/dl)

---

ance. (For a diagram, see *Serum calcium regulation by parathyroid hormone.*)

Mechanism of action

A rise in the blood calcium concentration stimulates secretion of naturally occurring calcitonin, which is thought to increase cyclic AMP in bone cells not activated by PTH. Calcitonin decreases osteoclastic activity as well as the rate at which mesenchymal stem cells convert to osteoclasts. By binding to specific receptor sites on the osteoclast cell membrane and decreasing the transmission of calcium and phosphorus, calcitonin acts antagonistically to PTH and its action. Initially, the use of exogenous calcitonin enhances the activity of the osteoblasts, but this effect decreases with prolonged use. Calcitonin increases renal excretion of calcium, phosphorus, sodium, and water. It also may inhibit intestinal absorption of calcium. The hypocalcemic effect of calcitonin is rapid but transitory. However, its effects on bone metabolism are more long-term.

Effects of parathyroid hormone on target tissues

Excessive secretion of endogenous parathyroid hormone (PTH) acts on bone, the kidneys, and the intestines to increase the calcium concentration in the extracellular fluid.

Bone

- Adenylate cyclase converts ATP to cyclic AMP.
- Osteoclastic activity increases calcium release.

Kidney

- Adenylate cyclase converts ATP to cyclic AMP.
- Tubular calcium reabsorption increases.

Intestines

- Calcium absorption increases when vitamin D is present.

Etidronate disodium decreases the number of osteoclasts, inhibits bone resorption and regeneration, and appears to reduce the rate of bone turnover. Therefore, it is used to treat Paget's disease (osteitis deformans), a disorder characterized by increased skeletal remodeling (increased bone resorption and bone formation), bone pain and deformity, neurologic disorders, and elevated cardiac output. Etidronate disodium lowers serum alkaline phosphatase and urinary hydroxyproline levels and reduces increased cardiac output by decreasing the bone vascularity. The drug also enhances hyperphosphatemia, which is reversible upon discontinuation of therapy.

Vitamin D analogues stimulate calcium absorption from the GI tract and promote calcium secretion from bone to blood, thereby raising the serum calcium concentration. (For an illustration of how increased naturally occurring parathyroid hormone secretion increases the serum calcium concentration, see *Effects of parathyroid hormone on target tissues*.)

PHARMACOTHERAPEUTICS

Calcitonin and etidronate disodium decrease serum alkaline phosphatase concentrations, urinary hydroxyproline levels, and blood flow in the bone. The action of calcitonin and etidronate disodium reduces the rate of bone turnover and restores normal bone structure. These effects make calcitonin and etidronate disodium the drugs of choice in the treatment of Paget's disease. One major disadvantage of calcitonin is that patients commonly develop resistance to the hormone. Safe use of calcitonin for children has not been established. Vitamin D analogues are the drugs of choice for increasing the serum calcium concentration.

calcitonin-salmon (Calcimar) and **calcitonin-human** (Cibacalcin). Calcitonin-salmon is used to treat hypercalcemia of infancy, vitamin D intoxication, postmenopausal osteoporosis, osteolytic bone metastases, and occasionally hyperphosphatemia. Calcitonin-salmon and calcitonin-human also are important therapeutic agents in relieving the bone pain and neurologic and biochemical complications that may accompany Paget's disease. They may be used with plicamycin to control Paget's disease. Calcitonin-salmon also may be prescribed to treat the severe hypercalcemia associated with cancer. Calcitonin-salmon is measured in international units (IU); calcitonin-human is measured in mg.

Usual adult dosage: for hypercalcemia, 4 IU/kg S.C. or I.M. every 12 hours, increased to 8 IU/kg every 12 hours if no response; for postmenopausal osteoporosis, 100 IU S.C. or I.M. daily; for Paget's disease, 100 IU S.C. or I.M. daily for the first few months, followed by 50 to 100 IU daily or every other day, or 0.5 mg S.C. daily followed by a maintenance dosage of 0.5 mg S.C. b.i.d to 0.5 mg two or three times weekly based on the patient's clinical and radiologic response and changes in biochemical parameters.

etidronate disodium (Didronel). A drug of choice for Paget's disease, etidronate disodium slows the accelerated bone turnover of the disease. Reduced bone pain usually accompanies the reduced bone turnover. Etidronate disodium also is used to prevent and treat heterotopic ossification (nonmalignant overgrowth of bone), which may occur for unknown reasons or may follow total hip replacement or spinal cord injury.

Usual adult dosage: for Paget's disease, 5 to 10 mg/kg P.O. daily for no more than 6 months, or 11 to 20 mg/kg P.O. daily for no more than 3 months. Dosages above 10 mg/kg P.O. daily for no more than 3 months are reserved for the prompt reduction of increased cardiac output or bone turnover suppression. (Treatment may be reinstituted after a drug-free interval of 3 months). In the treatment of heterotopic ossification with total hip replacement, the usual dosage is 20 mg/kg P.O. daily for 1 month preoperatively, then 20 mg/kg P.O. daily for 3 months postoperatively. In heterotopic ossification with spinal cord injury, the initial dosage is 20 mg/kg P.O. daily for 2 weeks, followed by 10 mg/kg P.O. daily for 10 weeks.

calcifediol (Calderol). This vitamin D analogue is used primarily to manage metabolic bone disease associated with renal failure.

Usual adult dosage: 50 to 100 mcg P.O. daily.

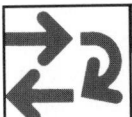

DRUG INTERACTIONS

Calcium regulators

Drug interactions involving calcium regulators can increase or decrease bone resorption, kidney resorption, and intestinal absorption of calcium. These interactions can produce hypercalcemia or hypocalcemia.

DRUG	INTERACTING DRUGS	POSSIBLE EFFECTS	NURSING IMPLICATIONS
calcitonin	theophylline, isoproterenol	Increase bone resorption, intestinal absorption, and kidney resorption of calcium	• Monitor the patient's calcium and phosphate levels. • Observe for signs and symptoms of calcium imbalance.
etidronate disodium	foods and drugs that contain calcium, iron, magnesium, or aluminum	Decrease absorption of etidronate disodium	• Administer the drug between meals. • Instruct the patient not to ingest interacting substances within 2 hours after administration of this drug. • Monitor for signs and symptoms of calcium imbalance.
vitamin D analogue (calcifediol)	cholestyramine, colestipol	Decrease calcifediol absorption	• Observe the patient closely for desired therapeutic effect of calcifediol if given with cholestyramine or colestipol.
	thiazide diuretics	Cause hypercalcemia in patients with hypoparathyroidism	• Observe for signs and symptoms of calcium imbalance. • Discontinue the vitamin D analogue, as instructed.

calcitriol [1,25-dihydroxycholecalciferol] (Rocaltrol). A vitamin D analogue, calcitriol is used primarily to treat hypocalcemia in patients undergoing long-term dialysis and in patients with hypoparathyroidism and pseudohypoparathyroidism.
Usual adult dosage: to treat hypocalcemia in patients undergoing long-term dialysis, 0.25 mcg P.O. daily, possibly increased by 0.25 mcg P.O. daily at 2- to 4-week intervals, with maintenance dosages of 0.25 mcg P.O. every other day, up to 0.5 to 1.25 mcg P.O. daily. For hypoparathyroidism or pseudohypoparathyroidism in adults and children ages 1 and older, 0.25 mcg P.O. daily, with dosages possibly increased at 2- to 4-week intervals. Maintenance dosages are 0.25 to 2 mcg P.O. daily for adults and children ages 6 and older, and 0.25 to 0.75 mcg P.O. daily for children ages 1 to 5.

dihydrotachysterol (DHT Intensol, DHT Oral Solution, Hytakerol). Major uses of this vitamin D analogue include treatment of hypocalcemia associated with hypoparathyroidism and pseudohypoparathyroidism and treatment of renal osteodystrophy in chronic uremia.
Usual adult dosage: for hypocalcemia caused by hypoparathyroidism or pseudohypoparathyroidism, 0.8 to 2.4 mg P.O. daily for several days, with maintenance dosages of 0.2 to 1 mg P.O. daily as required to maintain a normal serum calcium concentration. For renal osteodystrophy in chronic uremia, 0.1 to 0.6 mg P.O. daily.

Usual pediatric dosage: for hypocalcemia caused by hypoparathyroidism or pseudohypoparathyroidism, 1 to 5 mg P.O. for several days; for maintenance in children ages 6 and older, 0.5 mg to 2 mg; for maintenance in children ages 1 to 5, 0.25 to 0.75 mg daily as required to maintain a normal serum calcium concentration.

Drug interactions
Several types of drugs and some foods can interact with the calcium regulators to alter their therapeutic effects. (For details, see *Drug interactions: Calcium regulators.*)

ADVERSE DRUG REACTIONS

The use of these agents to regulate calcium and bone metabolism may produce hypercalcemia. However, because some of these drugs work in opposition to each other, hypocalcemia also may result. With the use of vitamin D analogues, vitamin D intoxication associated with hypercalcemia may occur.

Clinical use of calcitonin can cause flushing, nausea, vomiting, and urticaria. Because calcitonin also is a protein, a severe systemic reaction may occur. Long-term calcitonin therapy often produces swelling and tenderness of the hands. Diarrhea and neurologic symptoms, such as headache, also may occur. Calcitonin antibody formation may result from the activation of the body's antigen-antibody complex. A local inflammatory reaction at the injection site has been

Calcium regulators: Summary of adverse reactions

The primary adverse reactions to parathyroid hormone agents (calcium regulators) include hypersensitivity, hypercalcemia, and hypocalcemia, any of which can produce serious consequences. The nurse must observe for the early signs and symptoms of such reactions.

DRUG	REACTION
calcitonin	Hypersensitivity reaction, hypocalcemic tetany, facial flushing and urticaria, local inflammation at injection site, nausea
etidronate disodium	Increased bone pain, nausea, diarrhea
vitamin D analogues	Vitamin D intoxication associated with hypercalcemia (weakness, fatigue, lassitude, headache, nausea, vomiting, and diarrhea), altered renal function from hypercalcemia (possible polyuria, polydipsia, nocturia, hyposthenuria (excretion of urine with a low specific gravity), and proteinuria)

documented after long-term use. Rarely, hypocalcemic tetany has been observed.

Adverse reactions to etidronate disodium are dose-related and infrequent. Most commonly affecting the GI tract, adverse reactions include nausea, vomiting, abdominal cramps, and diarrhea. Also, an increased serum phosphate concentration may occur. Etidronate disodium may cause hypocalcemic crisis in which the threshold potential of the neuron is lowered, enabling the neurons to fire more easily. This enhanced motor nerve activity is accompanied by sensory symptoms, including numbness, tingling, muscle twitches, and cramps. Finally, suppressed bone mineralization in the uninvolved skeleton increases the risk of bone fractures in patients with Paget's disease. These patients also experience increased bone pain at the pagetic sites as well as at previously uninvolved sites.

Normal dosages of vitamin D analogues produce no significant dose-related adverse reactions. Adverse reactions associated with excessive amounts of vitamin D analogues and an increased responsiveness to normal amounts of vitamin D represent a clinical syndrome that probably results from deranged calcium metabolism. The syndrome involves vitamin D intoxication associated with hypercalcemia. Initial signs and symptoms include weakness, fatigue, lassitude, headache, nausea, vomiting, and diarrhea. Signs and symptoms caused by impaired renal function from

hypercalcemia include polyuria, polydipsia, nocturia, hyposthenuria (excretion of urine with a low specific gravity) and proteinuria. During chronic hypercalcemia, calcium deposits occur in soft tissue, especially the kidneys, which can lead to nephrolithiasis (kidney stones) and nephrocalcinosis (calcium deposits in the kidneys leading to infection, hematuria, renal colic, and decreased renal function). Osteoporosis may occur during vitamin D intoxication from the mobilization of calcium from bone. Some infants may exhibit hyperactivity even when small amounts of vitamin D are administered. (For a brief summary, see *Calcium regulators: Summary of adverse reactions.*)

NURSING PROCESS APPLICATION

The following information assists the nurse in caring for a patient who is receiving a calcium regulator.

Assessment
• Review the patient's history for a preexisting condition that contraindicates the use of a calcium regulator, such as lactation, hypercalcemia, vitamin D toxicity, or known hypersensitivity to fish or the gelatin in calcitonin-salmon diluent.
• Review the patient's history for a preexisting condition that requires cautious use of a calcium regulator, such as pregnancy, renal dysfunction, or digitalis use.
• Assess the patient for adverse reactions to the prescribed calcium regulator, such as calcium imbalances, vitamin D toxicity, or hypersensitivity reactions.
• Review the patient's medication history to identify the use of drugs that may interact with the prescribed calcium regulator, such as theophylline, cholestyramine, colestipol, thiazide diuretics, or drugs the contain calcium, iron, magnesium, or aluminum.
• Assess the effectiveness of the calcium regulator regularly.
• Assess for signs of dehydration, such as decreased urine output, dry mucous membranes, and poor skin turgor, in a patient with GI distress.
• Evaluate the patient's and family's knowledge about the prescribed calcium regulator.

Nursing diagnoses
The following examples represent appropriate nursing diagnoses for a patient receiving a calcium regulator.
• Potential for injury related to a preexisting condition that contraindicates the use of a calcium regulator
• Potential for injury related to a preexisting condition that requires cautious use of a calcium regulator
• Potential for injury related to adverse drug reactions
• Potential fluid volume deficit related to the adverse GI effects of the prescribed calcium regulator
• Knowledge deficit related to the prescribed calcium regulator

Assessing hypocalcemic tetany

Severe hypocalcemia may cause tetany and spasms of the skeletal muscles. The effects of severe hypocalcemia ultimately can progress to cardiac arrest. Chvostek's sign and Trousseau's sign are two methods of assessing hypocalcemic tetany.

Elicit Chvostek's sign by tapping or stroking the area over the facial nerve in front of the ear. Then observe the lips and cheek for twitching, a positive sign.

Evoke Trousseau's sign by applying a blood pressure cuff to the arm, inflating the cuff between diastolic and systolic blood pressure levels, and maintaining the inflation for 3 minutes. Then observe for carpal spasm as evidenced by palmar flexion, a positive sign.

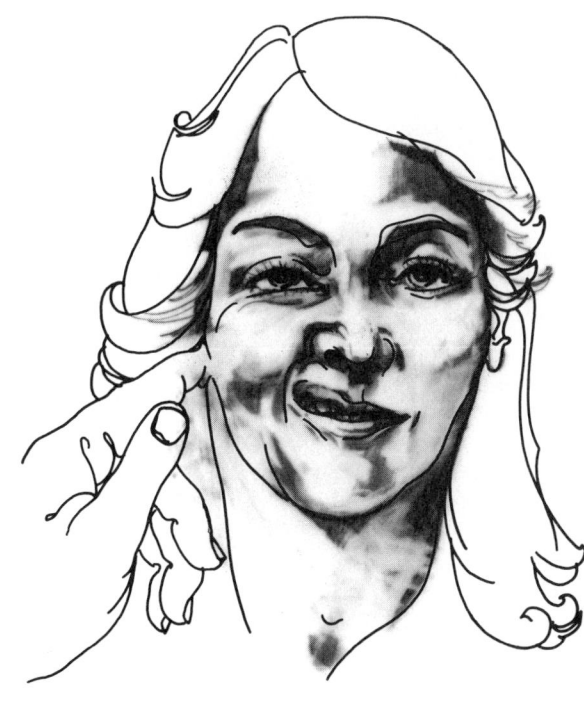
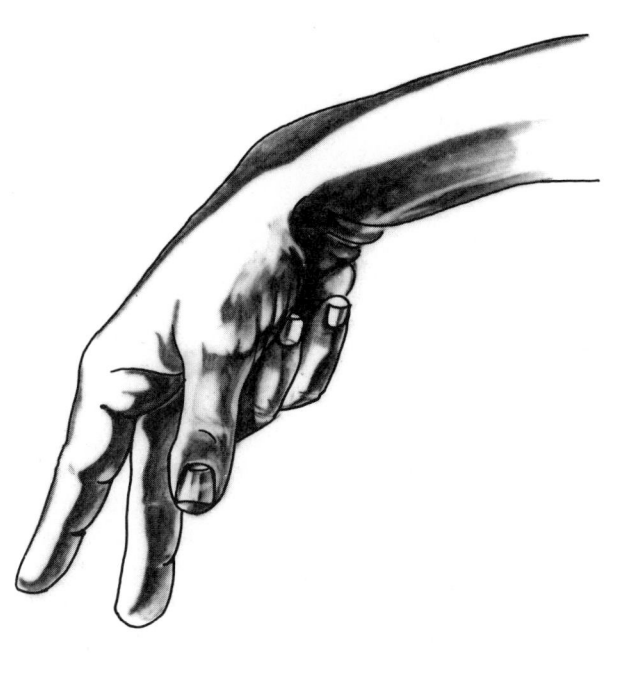

Planning and implementation

• Do not administer a calcium regulator to a patient with a condition that contraindicates its use.

• Administer a calcium regulator cautiously to a patient at risk because of a preexisting condition.

• Monitor the patient frequently for adverse reactions during calcium regulator therapy.

• *Monitor the serum calcium level closely, assess for signs of hypocalcemic tetany, report the earliest signs of tetany, and ascertain drug compliance if a relapse occurs.*

• *Monitor for signs of hypocalcemic tetany, such as a positive Chvostek's or Trousseau's sign and a serum calcium concentration of 7 to 8 mg/dl (latent tetany) or less than 7 mg/dl (manifest tetany).* (For more information, see *Assessing hypocalcemic tetany.*) Chvostek's and Trousseau's signs sometimes can be elicited in a patient with a normal calcium concentration. However, the strength of the muscle contraction will be much less severe in such a patient than in a hypocalcemic patient. Of the two tests, Trousseau's sign is more reliable.

• *Take seizure precautions until the calcium level is restored in a hypocalcemic patient.* For example, pad the bed rails, keep the bed in a low position, and have a suction setup nearby. Also, reduce sound and light stimuli by placing the hypocalcemic patient in a quiet room with dim lights.

• *Prevent vitamin D intoxication by administering the drug exactly as prescribed and by monitoring the serum calcium level.* (Serum calcium level multiplied by serum phosphate level should not exceed 70.) Ensure that the patient's daily calcium intake is adequate.

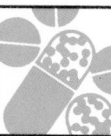

Parathyroid agents

This chart summarizes representative parathyroid agents (calcium regulators) currently in clinical use.

DRUG	MAJOR INDICATIONS	USUAL ADULT DOSAGES	CONTRAINDICATIONS AND PRECAUTIONS
calcitonin-salmon	Paget's disease	100 IU S.C. or I.M. daily for first few months, followed by 50 to 100 IU daily or every other day	• Know that calcitonin-salmon is contraindicated in a child, a pregnant or lactating patient, or one with hypersensitivity to fish or to the gelatin in the diluent. • Be aware that calcitonin-salmon has no known precautions.
etidronate disodium	Paget's disease	5 to 10 mg/kg P.O. daily for no more than 6 months, or 11 to 20 mg/kg P.O. daily for no more than 3 months	• Know that etidronate disodium has no known contraindications. • Administer with caution to a pregnant or lactating patient or one with renal dysfunction.
calcitriol	Hypoparathyroidism and pseudohypoparathyroidism	0.25 mcg P.O. daily, with dosages possibly increased at 2- to 4-week intervals	• Know that calcitriol is contraindicated in a lactating patient or one with hypercalcemia or vitamin D toxicity. • Administer with caution to a pregnant patient or one receiving digitalis.

• *Expect to perform or assist with a skin test before administering calcitonin because this drug can cause a systemic allergic reaction.* The appearance of more than mild erythema 15 minutes after injection constitutes a positive test, indicating that the drug should not be administered.

• *Keep emergency equipment and medications, such as oxygen, epinephrine, and steroids, readily available during calcitonin treatment to manage systemic allergic reaction. Also have calcium readily available for the emergency treatment of hypocalcemic tetany, which also may result from calcitonin use.*

• Be aware that calcitonin is commercially prepared in 200 MRC units per ml, packaged in gelatin. Refrigerate the reconstituted drug to maintain its potency.

• Administer etidronate disodium (oral tablet form) with 8 oz of water or juice to reduce GI distress. To enhance etidronate disodium absorption, administer the drug 2 hours before or after the patient consumes food, especially milk, or an antacid high in metals (calcium, iron, magnesium, or aluminum).

• Protect calcitriol and dihydrotachysterol from heat and light to prevent loss of potency. Do not refrigerate dihydrotachysterol.

• Notify the physician if adverse drug reactions occur.

• Monitor for signs and symptoms of dehydration in a patient with nausea, vomiting, or diarrhea caused by calcitonin or etidronate sodium. If the patient is dehydrated, notify the physician and obtain a prescription for an antiemetic or antidiarrheal agent, as needed.

Patient teaching

• Teach the patient and family the name, dose, frequency, action, and adverse effects of the prescribed calcium regulator.

• Teach the patient to self-administer calcitonin via the preferred S.C. route. If the calcitonin dose exceeds 2 ml, instruct the patient to use the I.M. route and to rotate the injection sites.

• Teach the patient how to use aseptic technique when reconstituting calcitonin and when administering the injection. Teach the patient to recognize and seek advice about local inflammation at injection sites.

• *Teach the patient receiving calcitonin to recognize the signs and symptoms of hypocalcemia.* Explain to the patient that the initial nausea and vomiting tend to disappear with continued therapy. Inform the patient that facial flushing and warmth occur in some patients within minutes of a calcitonin injection, and assure the patient that these effects usually last no longer than 1 hour. Stress the importance of having periodic laboratory tests to assess renal function.

• *Advise the patient taking calcitonin to consult the physician before using over-the-counter (OTC) preparations during treatment because some combination vitamins, hematinics, and antacids contain calcium.* The patient using calcitonin may have to reduce dietary calcium intake. High-calcium foods include green, leafy vegetables and milk and other dairy products.

• Teach the patient receiving etidronate disodium to maintain a well-balanced diet with an adequate intake of calcium and vitamin D. Advise the patient to include milk and other dairy products as well as green, leafy vegetables in the diet. However, advise the patient not to eat such foods within 2 hours of taking the drug.

• *Instruct the patient to report promptly the sudden onset of unexplained bone pain. Urge the patient to keep follow-up appointments for periodic testing.*

• *Advise the patient receiving a vitamin D analogue to maintain the prescribed diet and calcium supplementation and avoid OTC drugs. Teach the patient to report signs and symptoms of hypercalcemia and to store the drugs properly. Also, explain that although these drugs are vitamins, they are potent and must not be taken by anyone for whom they were not prescribed because serious toxicity may result.*

• Instruct the patient to contact the physician if adverse reactions occur.

Evaluation

The following examples represent appropriate evaluation statements for a patient receiving a calcium regulator.

• The patient has no conditions that contraindicate calcium regulator therapy.

• The patient exhibits no signs of complications in the preexisting condition linked to the prescribed calcium regulator.

• The patient experiences no adverse reactions to the prescribed calcium regulator.

• The patient maintains adequate hydration during calcium regulator therapy.

• The patient and family express an accurate understanding of the points taught about the prescribed calcium regulator.

• The patient correctly demonstrates self-administration of S.C. calcitonin.

• The major calcium regulators include calcitonin, etidronate disodium, and the vitamin D analogues. Vitamin D analogues increase the serum calcium concentration; calcitonin and etidronate disodium decrease the concentration.

• Most synthetic analogues provide more effective therapeutic results than PTH because the body metabolizes them more slowly and they provide a longer duration of action. Calcitonin is metabolized by the kidneys and is excreted in the urine. Etidronate disodium is excreted as unchanged drug, primarily in the urine. Vitamin D analogues are metabolized in the liver and eliminated through the bile in feces.

• Calcitonin is used to treat hypercalcemia, vitamin D intoxication, postmenopausal osteoporosis, osteolytic bone metastases, hyperphosphatemia, and Paget's disease. A drug of choice for Paget's disease, etidronate disodium also is used to treat heterotopic ossification after hip replacement or spinal cord injury. Uses of the vitamin D analogues vary with the specific agent and include metabolic bone disease, hypocalcemia, hypoparathyroidism, pseudohypoparathyroidism, and renal osteodystrophy.

• Most adverse reactions to calcium regulators are dose-dependent. Because some calcium regulators increase the serum calcium concentration while others decrease it, toxicity can result in hypercalcemia or hypocalcemia. A systemic allergic reaction may occur with calcitonin administration.

• When caring for a patient receiving a calcium regulator, the nurse should monitor the patient for allergic reactions, signs and symptoms of hypercalcemia or hypocalcemia, and kidney dysfunction. The nurse also should teach the patient about administering the specific drug, following a prescribed diet, and avoiding OTC products, especially those containing calcium.

CHAPTER SUMMARY

Chapter 51 discussed the major parathyroid agents (calcium regulators): calcitonin, etidronate disodium, and the vitamin D analogues. Here are the highlights of the chapter.

• The parathyroid glands secrete PTH into the blood. PTH acts as a calcium regulator, responding to the serum calcium concentration. Any decrease in the concentration stimulates the release of PTH to increase the circulating calcium. This hormonal action depends on the activation of cyclic AMP.

• Endogenous PTH regulates serum calcium by acting on the bone, kidneys, and GI system. The role of PTH in calcium regulation is vital to the body because calcium ions play an important part in cardiac and neuromuscular functioning, in cell binding, in enzyme activity, and in blood coagulation.

STUDY QUESTIONS

See Appendix 1 for answers.

1. Ellen Griffin, age 52, receives calcitonin (Calcimar) 100 IU S.C. daily for Paget's disease. What is the mechanism of action of calcitonin?

(a) It reduces bone resorption and increases renal calcium clearance.

(b) It increases bone resorption and decreases renal calcium clearance.

(c) It increases GI absorption of calcium.

(d) It increases osteoclastic activity.

2. Calcitonin increases the renal excretion of water and several electrolytes. Which electrolyte is likely to be affected by calcitonin?
(a) potassium
(b) chloride
(c) magnesium
(d) sodium

3. Although calcitonin commonly is used to treat Paget's disease, it poses which major disadvantage?
(a) development of hypercalcemia
(b) increased bone pain when therapy begins
(c) development of resistance to calcitonin
(d) high incidence of toxicity

4. Jennifer Pinsky, age 28, seeks care because she is experiencing neuromuscular irritability. Her laboratory tests show decreased serum and urine calcium concentrations and an increased phosphorous concentration. Suspecting hypoparathyroidism, her physician prescribes the vitamin D analogue calcitriol 0.25 mcg P.O. daily. How does calcitriol increase the calcium concentration?
(a) It reduces bone resorption.
(b) It increases GI absorption and bone resorption of calcium.
(c) It stimulates the parathyroid gland to secrete PTH.
(d) It decreases osteoclastic activity.

5. When caring for Ms. Pinsky, the nurse should be alert for which early signs and symptoms of vitamin D intoxication?
(a) numbness and tingling of the hands
(b) weakness, fatigue, nausea, and vomiting
(c) increased central nervous system activity, including seizures
(d) flushing, urticaria, and angioedema

6. Until Ms. Pinsky's calcium concentration returns to normal, which nursing intervention is appropriate?
(a) Take seizure precautions.
(b) Provide environmental stimuli.
(c) Assist with range-of-motion exercises.
(d) Monitor the fluid intake and output.

7. To monitor for vitamin D intoxication, the nurse assesses Ms. Pinsky's serum electrolyte concentrations. To be therapeutic, the serum calcium level multiplied by the serum phosphorous level should not exceed which number?
(a) 60
(b) 70
(c) 80
(d) 90

SELECTED REFERENCES

AHFS drug information 90. (1990). Bethesda, MD: American Society of Hospital Pharmacists.

Drug facts and comparisons. (1991). St. Louis: Facts and Comparisons Division, Lippincott.

Goodman and Gilman's the pharmacological basis of therapeutics (8th ed.; 1990). Elmsford, NY: Pergamon Press.

Hansten, P., and Horn, J. (1989). *Drug interactions: Clinical significance of drug-drug interactions* (6th ed.). Philadelphia: Lea & Febiger.

North American Nursing Diagnosis Association. (1990). *Taxonomy I - Revised, with official diagnostic categories.* St. Louis: NANDA.

Walpert, N. (1990). An orderly look at calcium metabolism disorders. *Nursing 90, 20*(7), 60-64.

Walworth, J. (1990). Parathyroidectomy: Maintaining calcium homeostasis. *Today's OR Nurse, 12*(4), 20-35.

Vitamin D in older women. (1990). *Nurses Drug Alert, 14*(2), 14.

CHAPTER

52

PITUITARY AGENTS

OBJECTIVES

After reading and studying this chapter, the student should be able to:
1. Identify the hormones secreted by the pituitary gland.
2. Compare the pharmacokinetic properties of the anterior pituitary hormones.
3. Describe several diagnostic and therapeutic uses of the anterior pituitary hormone drugs corticotropin, cosyntropin, and somatrem.
4. Explain why the patient must be monitored carefully for adverse reactions during adrenocorticotropic hormone therapy.
5. Identify the uses of the posterior pituitary hormone drugs.
6. Describe the interactions between posterior pituitary hormone drugs and other agents.
7. Discuss common adverse reactions to posterior pituitary hormones.
8. Describe how to apply the nursing process when caring for a patient who is receiving a pituitary agent.

INTRODUCTION

The pituitary gland, approximately ½ inch (1.25 cm) in diameter, lies buried in the sella turcica, a pouchlike sac at the base of the brain. The gland consists of an anterior lobe (adenohypophysis) and a posterior lobe (neurohypophysis). Between these two lobes is a small avascular area called the pars intermedia. The pars intermedia, almost absent in humans, remains functional in lower animals.

Also called the master gland, the anterior lobe of the pituitary secretes six major hormones, four of which regulate the functions of other endocrine glands. The major hormones include growth hormone (GH), adrenocorticotropic hormone (ACTH), thyroid-stimulating hormone (TSH), follicle-stimulating hormone (FSH), luteinizing

hormone (LH), and prolactin. The secretion of anterior lobe hormones is controlled by neurohormonal-stimulating and neurohormonal-inhibiting release factors secreted from the hypothalamus into the pituitary portal system.

Anterior pituitary hormones are secreted in minuscule amounts but produce important effects on the function and structure of the human body. These hormones also regulate the synthesis and secretion of other hormones in target organs and tissues.

The posterior pituitary gland secretes two hormones: antidiuretic hormone (ADH, vasopressin) and oxytocin. The secretion of ADH regulates fluid balance in the body and occurs in response to hypovolemia and increased serum osmolality. An increased secretion of oxytocin (in response to estrogen levels and nipple stimulation) stimulates smooth muscle contraction of the pregnant uterus and milk ejection during lactation.

Pituitary hormones are mammalian metabolites produced by the endocrine glands. When released into the bloodstream, these hormones elicit a biological effect on specific organs and tissues. The pituitary hormones are derived from amino acid chains, the building blocks of protein. Because the natural pituitary hormones extracted from animals contain proteins that can precipitate hypersensitivity reactions, synthetically prepared pituitary substances are preferable. In some instances, however, the natural hormones provide therapeutic effects superior to those of the synthetic analogues. That is particularly true for a synthetic extract that does not mirror exactly the natural hormone it is replacing.

For a summary of representative drugs, see *Selected major drugs: Pituitary agents,* page 894. For a listing of applicable nursing diagnoses that the nurse may formulate when caring for a patient receiving these agents, see *Selected nursing diagnoses: Pituitary agents,* page 884. For detailed information on applying the nursing process, see Chapter 6, The Nursing Process and Drug Therapy.

SELECTED NURSING DIAGNOSES

Pituitary agents

The following nursing diagnoses address representative problems and etiologies that a nurse may encounter when caring for a patient who is receiving a pituitary agent. Some of these nursing diagnoses contain generalized etiologies, which the nurse must individualize based on the patient's needs. (For some common nursing diagnoses and related interventions for each drug class, see the "Nursing Process Application" sections of this chapter.)

- Altered health maintenance related to iatrogenic Cushing's syndrome caused by long-term use of corticotropin
- Altered health maintenance related to ineffectiveness of the prescribed pituitary agent
- Altered health maintenance related to oxytocin-induced uterine problems and hypertensive disorders
- Altered health maintenance related to somatrem-induced endocrine imbalances
- Altered protection related to the adverse effects of corticotropin on wound healing
- Anxiety related to the adverse central nervous system effects of a natural antidiuretic hormone
- Body image disturbance related to corticotropin-induced hyperpigmentation
- Decreased cardiac output related to oxytocin-induced arrhythmias
- Diarrhea related to increased gastrointestinal (GI) motility caused by a natural antidiuretic hormone
- Fluid volume excess related to sodium and water retention caused by a pituitary agent
- Fluid volume excess related to water intoxication caused by a posterior pituitary agent
- Impaired tissue integrity related to nasal passage ulcerations caused by nasal administration of a posterior pituitary hormone
- Knowledge deficit related to the prescribed pituitary agent
- Pain related to abdominal and uterine cramps caused by a posterior pituitary agent
- Potential fluid volume deficit related to the adverse GI effects of the posterior pituitary agent
- Potential for infection related to corticotropin-induced immunosuppression
- Potential for injury related to a preexisting condition that contraindicates the use of a pituitary agent
- Potential for injury related to a preexisting condition that requires cautious use of a pituitary agent
- Potential for injury related to adverse drug reactions
- Potential for injury related to a hypersensitivity reaction to the pituitary agent
- Potential for injury related to drug interactions with the prescribed pituitary agent
- Potential for trauma related to oxytocin-induced uterine rupture

ANTERIOR PITUITARY HORMONES

The protein hormones produced in the anterior pituitary regulate growth, development, and sexual characteristics by stimulating the actions of other endocrine glands. The anterior pituitary hormone drugs may be used diagnostically or therapeutically. Anterior pituitary hormone drugs include the adrenocorticotropics (corticotropin, cosyntropin), growth hormone (somatrem), the gonadotropics (chorionic gonadotropin, menotropins), and the thyrotropics (TSH, or thyrotropin, and protirelin). (For a detailed discussion of the gonadotropics, see Chapter 73, Uncategorized and Other Agents. For a discussion of the thyrotropics, see Chapter 50, Thyroid and Antithyroid Agents.)

PHARMACOKINETICS

The anterior pituitary hormones have peptide links, which enable peptidases in the gastrointestinal (GI) tract to destroy the hormones. Therefore, oral administration proves ineffective. Some of these hormones can be administered topically, but most require injection. Although the precise pharmacokinetic fate of some anterior pituitary hormones remains unknown, these drugs produce rapid therapeutic results. Usually, natural hormones are absorbed, distributed, and metabolized rapidly. Some analogues, however, are absorbed and metabolized more slowly, providing a prolonged duration of action. Anterior pituitary hormones are metabolized at the receptor site and also by the liver and kidneys. The hormones are excreted primarily in urine.

Absorption, distribution, metabolism, excretion

Corticotropin (ACTH) is absorbed rapidly when administered parenterally. The drug usually is administered by intramuscular (I.M.) injection, but also is given intravenously (I.V.) or subcutaneously (S.C.) Repository corticotropin contains ACTH in gelatin, designed to delay absorption and extend the period of therapeutic effectiveness. Repository corticotropin usually is given I.M. or S.C. Corticotropin zinc hydroxide, a combination of ACTH and zinc, also is absorbed slowly. This drug, like repository corticotropin, provides extended effectiveness; it is administered I.M. The distribution information regarding these three drugs is imprecise, but all three are metabolized at the receptor site and by the liver and kidneys, and all are excreted in the urine.

After I.M. administration, cosyntropin is absorbed rapidly. The specific rate of cosyntropin metabolism remains

Control and effects of the anterior and posterior pituitary hormones

The hypothalamus (by the hypothalamic neurohormonal releasing factors) and stress stimulate the anterior pituitary to secrete hormones that act on various target organs in the endocrine system. The hypothalamus (by direct hypothalamic neurocontrol) stimulates the posterior pituitary to secrete hormones that act on specific target organs. This chart summarizes the specific action of each hormone and the target organs involved.

STIMULUS	HORMONE	TARGET ORGAN	ACTION
Anterior pituitary			
Hypothalamic neurohormonal releasing factors and stress	TSH	• Thyroid gland	• Synthesis and secretion of thyroid hormone • Metabolic rate control
	GH	• Body muscles • Adipose tissue	• Growth stimulation • Protein synthesis increase
	prolactin	• Mammary glands	• Lactation
	ACTH	• Adrenal cortex	• Growth stimulation • Cortisol (hydrocortisone) secretion • Increased protein, fat, and carbohydrate metabolism
	FSH	• Ovaries	• Ovulation • Testosterone and progesterone production
	LH	• Testes	• Spermatogenesis and estrogen production
Posterior pituitary			
Hypothalamic neurocontrol (direct)	oxytocin ADH oxytocin	• Mammary glands • Kidneys • Uterus	• Lactation • Water reabsorption • Uterine contractions

unknown. However, the drug is removed rapidly from the plasma by the tissues and is excreted in the urine.

Clinical tests have shown somatrem to be the pharmacokinetic equivalent of the natural pituitary growth hormone. When administered parenterally, somatrem is absorbed well, distributed, metabolized in the liver, and excreted in the urine.

Onset, peak, duration

When administered parenterally, corticotropin acts within 5 minutes and has a duration of action of 2 to 4 hours. The plasma level half-life is less than 20 minutes. For repository and zinc hydroxide preparations, onset of action is 6 hours, with a duration of 18 to 72 hours.

Cosyntropin acts in 5 minutes and peaks in 1 hour after I.V. administration. The duration is 2 to 4 hours. The action of cosyntropin can be monitored by plasma cortisol levels.

The effects of somatrem begin immediately and last several days. The plasma level half-life is 15 to 50 minutes.

PHARMACODYNAMICS

The anterior pituitary hormones exert a profound effect on the body's growth and development. Under the control of neurohormonal-stimulating and neurohormonal-inhibiting release factors from the hypothalamus, these hormones alter the functions of their target tissues. The concentration of hormones in the circulating blood helps determine hormone production rate. Increased hormone levels inhibit hormone production; decreased levels raise production and secretion. The relationship between hormone concentration and hormone production critically affects the regulation of hormone levels. (For a summary of the target organs and actions of these hormones, see *Control and effects of the anterior and posterior pituitary hormones.*)

Mechanism of action

Anterior pituitary hormones interact with specific plasma membrane receptors to produce enzymatic actions. The hormone-receptor interaction induces direct changes in membrane permeability or stimulates cyclic adenosine 3',5'-monophosphate (cyclic AMP) production, which transmits the hormone signal within the cell. Both effects of the hormone-receptor interaction affect the metabolic rate of target organs.

PHARMACOTHERAPEUTICS

The clinical indications for anterior pituitary hormone drugs are diagnostic and therapeutic. Because of their protein structure, pituitary tropic drugs (drugs that act on one of the target organs) prove ineffective when administered orally. As a result, they are not used routinely for hormone replacement in deficiency states. Instead, oral preparations of hormones normally produced by the target glands (corticosteroids and thyrotropic and gonadotropic hormones) are prescribed to maintain normal body function. Somatrem is an exception and is used to treat pituitary dwarfism. Corticotropin and cosyntropin are used diagnostically to differentiate between primary and secondary failure of the adrenal cortex. Finally, corticotropin is used to treat certain progressive diseases.

corticotropin [ACTH] (Acthar), **corticotropin repository** (ACTH Gel, Cortigel, Cortrophin Gel, H.P. Acthar Gel), **and corticotropin zinc hydroxide** (Cortrophin-Zinc). Used for the diagnostic testing of adrenocortical function, these drugs also are used to treat adrenal insufficiency from long-term use of corticosteroids. The drugs also are used like glucocorticoids, as anti-inflammatory and immunosuppressant agents, as well as for their effect on the hematopoietic and lymphatic systems. These characteristics make the corticotropins useful for treating dermatologic, allergic, ophthalmic, respiratory, edematous, hematologic, and GI diseases. Commonly referred to as ACTH, corticotropin also is used to treat the symptoms of acute episodes of multiple sclerosis and to increase muscle strength in patients with myasthenia gravis. It also may be used in treating collagen diseases, rheumatoid arthritis, and acute rheumatic fever. Miscellaneous uses include treating tubercular meningitis with subarachnoid block and hypercalcemia associated with cancer.

Usual adult dosage: for adrenal function tests, up to 80 units in a single injection or an I.V. infusion of 10 to 25 units (aqueous form) in 500 ml D_5W administered over 8 hours. Deficiency states require an I.M. or S.C. injection of 20 units q.i.d.; repository preparations, 40 to 80 units I.M. or S.C. every 24 to 72 hours; or zinc hydroxide preparations, 40 units I.M. every 12 to 24 hours. Multiple sclerosis episodes respond to 80 to 120 units I.M. per day for 2 to 3 weeks.

cosyntropin (Cortrosyn, Synacthen Depot). Cosyntropin is used strictly as a diagnostic drug to differentiate primary (adrenal) from secondary (pituitary) adrenal insufficiency. *Usual adult dosage:* for the rapid screening test, 0.25 to 0.75 mg I.M., or 0.25 mg in dextrose or sodium chloride solution I.V. over 4 to 8 hours at a rate of 40 mcg/hour over 6 hours.

somatrem (Protropin). Used in children to treat linear growth failure from hormonal deficiency, the drug also may be used as replacement therapy before epiphyseal closure in pediatric patients with GH deficiency. Somatrem produces an increase in the size and number of muscle cells, thereby affecting organ growth, as well as protein, carbohydrate, lipid, mineral, and connective tissue metabolism.

Usual pediatric dosage: up to 0.1 mg (0.2 IU) per kg of body weight I.M. three times weekly. To avoid adverse effects, do not exceed this dosage.

Drug interactions

When administered with aspirin, corticotropin decreases the blood level of the salicylate. Because of the hyperglycemic activity of corticotropin, diabetic patients may need increased insulin or oral antidiabetic agents. Corticotropin administered with a diuretic may cause increased electrolyte losses.

Amphetamines, estrogens, and lithium alter the cortisol level and, when taken with cosyntropin, may alter diagnostic test results. Radioactive scans should not be scheduled within 1 week of a cosyntropin test because cosyntropin may alter the results of the scan.

Concomitant glucocorticoid therapy may diminish the growth-stimulating potential of somatrem and act synergistically with it to increase the blood glucose level by producing insulin resistance. Thyroid hormone and androgens given simultaneously may precipitate epiphyseal closure, reducing the effectiveness of somatrem. (For a summary, see *Drug interactions: Anterior pituitary agents.*)

ADVERSE DRUG REACTIONS

Because of the polypeptide nature of all pituitary hormones, the major adverse drug reactions are hypersensitivity reactions. Short-term, intensive hormone therapy with animal preparations increases the possibility of a hypersensitivity reaction. However, these reactions occur less commonly when the therapy involves synthetic hormones. For example, hypersensitivity reactions to cosyntropin rarely occur, probably because it is produced synthetically and used only diagnostically. The incidence of hypersensitivity reactions has decreased because of advancements in bioassay, immunoassay, and radioimmunoassay techniques, which

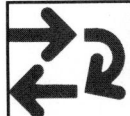

DRUG INTERACTIONS

Anterior pituitary agents

Drug interactions with anterior pituitary agents may reduce the effectiveness of therapy or create additional abnormalities.

DRUG	INTERACTING DRUGS	POSSIBLE EFFECTS	NURSING IMPLICATIONS
corticotropin	immunosuppressants	Cause neurologic complications	• Assess the patient's neurologic status.
	aspirin	Decreases salicylate levels	• Assess for decreased therapeutic effects of aspirin.
	diuretics	Cause electrolyte losses	• Monitor electrolyte levels, particularly potassium.
	barbiturates, phenytoin, rifampin	Decrease corticotropin effect	• Expect to increase the corticotropin dosage, as prescribed.
	estrogens	Potentiate the effects of corticotropin	• Adjust the corticotropin dosage as prescribed if estrogens are added or withdrawn from the patient's drug regimen.
cosyntropin	amphetamines, estrogens, lithium	Produce altered test results	• Obtain a complete and current drug history. • Consult with the physician to reschedule the test.
somatrem	thyroid hormone and androgens (concurrently)	Precipitate epiphyseal closure	• Assess the patient annually for bone age.
	corticosteroids	Cause diminished growth response; decreased hyperglycemia and sensitivity to insulin	• Document the patient's growth rate carefully for 6 to 12 months before treatment begins. • Instruct a family member to record the child's height accurately at regular intervals. • Monitor the patient continually for glycosuria or an increased blood glucose level.

have improved the quality, quantity, and refinement of natural protein hormones and synthetic analogue extracts.

Because the physiologic need for hormones fluctuates greatly with the patient's age, state of health, stress level, and other variables, dosages must vary. Continual assessment of the patient's response to therapy helps determine the hormone drug regimen. Because the dosage must vary, the number and types of adverse reactions vary also.

The most common dose-related reactions from corticotropin include sodium and water retention, impaired wound healing, dizziness, seizures, and euphoria. Less common dose-related reactions include hypokalemia, hypertension, ketosis, immunosuppression, skin hyperpigmentation, and mood elevation. Long-term use of corticotropin can cause iatrogenic Cushing's syndrome indistinguishable from the naturally occurring condition.

Cosyntropin administration can cause pruritus and flushing.

Somatrem may cause glucose intolerance and hypothyroidism. A large percentage of patients treated with somatrem develop antibodies to the hormone. However, the antibodies usually do not interfere with the effectiveness

of the therapy. (For a list of possible reactions, see *Anterior pituitary agents: Summary of adverse reactions,* page 888.)

NURSING PROCESS APPLICATION

The following information assists the nurse in caring for a patient who is receiving an anterior pituitary hormone.

Assessment
• Review the patient's history for a preexisting condition that contraindicates the use of an anterior pituitary hormone, such as adrenocortical hyperfunction, primary adrenal insufficiency, or known hypersensitivity to the drug.
• Review the patient's history for a preexisting condition that requires cautious use of corticotropin, such as latent tuberculosis, diabetes mellitus, or renal insufficiency.
• Assess the patient for adverse reactions to the prescribed anterior pituitary hormone, such as hypersensitivity reactions and electrolyte imbalances.
• Review the patient's medication history to identify the use of drugs that may interact with the prescribed anterior

Anterior pituitary agents: Summary of adverse reactions

Dose-related adverse reactions from anterior pituitary hormones vary greatly. Many of the reactions have long-term physiologic ramifications for the patient.

DRUG	REACTION
corticotropin	Hypersensitivity, iatrogenic Cushing's syndrome (with long-term therapy), electrolyte imbalances, hyperpigmentation, immunosuppression, impaired wound healing, mood elevation, hypertension
cosyntropin	Hypersensitivity, pruritus, facial flushing
somatrem	Pain at injection site, glucose intolerance, transient hypothyroidism during treatment, development of antibodies that may interfere with treatment (rare)

pituitary hormone, such as aspirin, insulin, amphetamines, or thyroid hormone.
• Assess the effectiveness of the anterior pituitary hormone regularly.
• Assess the patient for impaired wound healing, if applicable.
• Assess the patient for signs and symptoms of fluid retention.
• Evaluate the patient's and family's knowledge about the prescribed anterior pituitary hormone.

Nursing diagnoses
The following examples represent appropriate nursing diagnoses for a patient receiving an anterior pituitary hormone.
• Potential for injury related to a preexisting condition that contraindicates the use of an anterior pituitary hormone
• Potential for injury related to a preexisting condition that requires cautious use of corticotropin
• Potential for injury related to adverse drug reactions
• Altered protection related to the adverse effects of corticotropin on wound healing
• Fluid volume excess related to corticotropin-induced sodium and water retention
• Knowledge deficit related to the prescribed anterior pituitary hormone

Planning and implementation
• Do not administer an anterior pituitary hormone to a patient with a condition that contraindicates its use.

• Administer corticotropin cautiously to a patient at risk because of a preexisting condition.
• Monitor the patient frequently for hypersensitivity reactions, electrolyte imbalances, and other adverse reactions during therapy with the anterior pituitary hormone.
• *Perform a hypersensitivity skin test before administering any anterior pituitary hormone.* After the test, document the result. If it is negative, therapy can begin as prescribed. If it is positive, notify the physician.
• *Keep epinephrine 1:1,000 readily available for emergency treatment of an allergic reaction.*
• *Observe the patient closely for hypersensitivity reactions during the first 15 minutes of I.V. administration or immediately after I.M. or S.C. injection.*
• *Observe the patient for signs of hypersensitivity, such as urticaria, tachycardia, and pruritus, after the cosyntropin test (rapid ACTH test).*
• Monitor the patient's thyroid function and blood glucose, blood urea nitrogen, and electrolyte levels during somatrem administration.
• *Check the urinary and plasma corticosteroid values as instructed to measure the adrenal response before and after administering corticotropin to test adrenocortical function.*
• Place the patient on a high-potassium diet as prescribed to offset corticotropin-induced loss of potassium.
• *Take safety precautions if the patient experiences dizziness during corticotropin therapy. For example, place the bed in the lowest position, keep the bed rails raised, and supervise ambulation.*
• *Take seizure precautions, such as padding the bed rails, during corticotropin therapy.*
• *Use caution when matching the type of preparation to the administration method. I.V. infusions of corticotropin require aqueous solutions; I.M. and S.C. injections require suspension and gelatin solutions.*
• Be aware that corticotropin repository is viscid at room temperature. Corticotropin zinc and corticotropin repository are not suitable for I.V. use and should be shaken before injecting into the gluteal muscle.
• *Taper off high dosage levels of corticotropin as prescribed rather than suddenly withdrawing the drug because withdrawal usually causes 2 to 5 days of hypofunction.*
• Protect corticotropin solutions from heat, temperatures below freezing, and agitation to avoid denaturing the protein molecules in the drug.
• Reconstitute cosyntropin (a synthetic peptide powder) by adding 1 ml of normal saline solution to a 0.25-mg vial to provide 0.25 mg/ml. Reconstituted solutions have a pH of 5.5 to 7.5 and remain stable for 12 hours at room temperature or 21 days if refrigerated.

• Reconstitute each 5-mg vial of somatrem with 1 to 5 ml of bacteriostatic water for injection. Use only bacteriostatic water preserved with benzyl alcohol. To prepare the solution, inject the bacteriostatic water into the 5-mg vial, aiming the stream against the glass wall. Then rotate the vial gently without shaking it. The contents of the vial should be clear after reconstitution. Discard any drug that appears cloudy or contains particulate material. Use small syringes to validate the accuracy of the dose and a needle of adequate length (1 inch [2.5 cm] or greater) to ensure muscle insertion.

• Refrigerate the anterior pituitary agent for storage but avoid freezing. Use the contents of reconstituted vials within 1 week.

• Notify the physician if adverse reactions occur.

• Provide a high-protein diet as prescribed for a patient receiving corticotropin.

• *Monitor for poor wound healing in a patient receiving corticotropin.*

• Notify the physician if wound healing is delayed.

• *Monitor the patient for signs of fluid retention (such as ankle swelling, jugular vein distention, and crackles in the lungs on auscultation) during corticotropin therapy.*

• Provide a low-sodium diet and restrict fluids throughout corticotropin therapy, if appropriate.

• Weigh the patient daily, particularly noting any sudden increase of 2 pounds of more.

• Monitor the patient's blood pressure regularly to detect any increase. Also monitor the patient's fluid intake and output to identify any imbalance.

• Notify the physician if fluid retention occurs.

Patient teaching

• Teach the patient and family the name, dose, frequency, action, and adverse effects of the prescribed anterior pituitary hormone.

• *Inform the patient that a skin test must be performed before drug administration to assess for hypersensitivity reactions.*

• *Instruct the patient to report promptly any signs of hypersensitivity, such as hives or pruritus, during use of an anterior pituitary hormone.*

• Review the signs and symptoms of infection, peptic ulcer disease, Cushing's syndrome, hypothyroidism, hyperglycemia, and electrolyte imbalances with the patient, and discuss what to do if they occur. Stress the importance of returning for regular laboratory tests to detect these abnormalities.

• Encourage the patient to consume a low-sodium, high-protein, high-potassium diet during the therapy.

• *Warn the patient that corticotropin injections are painful.*

• *Caution the patient to avoid activities that require mental alertness if dizziness occurs.*

• *Inform the patient with a wound that healing may by delayed during corticotropin therapy.*

• Instruct the patient to record body weight daily and report a sudden weight gain of 2 pounds or more. Also teach the patient to recognize and report other signs of fluid retention. If appropriate, advise the patient not to drink more than eight 8-oz glasses (2 liters) of fluid daily.

• Explain the purpose of the cosyntropin test (rapid ACTH test) before administering it. *Advise the patient to fast for 12 hours, rest for 30 minutes before the test, and take no ACTH or steroids before the test.*

• Advise the patient to notify the physician as soon as an adverse reaction is noted.

Evaluation

The following examples represent appropriate evaluation statements for a patient receiving an anterior pituitary hormone.

• The patient has no conditions that contraindicate the use of an anterior pituitary hormone.

• The patient exhibits no signs of complications in the preexisting condition linked to corticotropin.

• The patient experiences no adverse reactions to the prescribed anterior pituitary hormone.

• The patient's wound continues to heal during anterior pituitary hormone therapy.

• The patient maintains normal fluid balance.

• The patient and family express an accurate understanding of the points taught about the prescribed anterior pituitary hormone.

• The patient correctly identifies signs of fluid retention and describes what to do if they occur.

POSTERIOR PITUITARY HORMONES

Protein hormones synthesized by the nerve bodies of the hypothalamus and stored in the posterior pituitary have a pressor effect from arteriole and capillary vasoconstriction, an antidiuretic action from increased resorption of water in the renal tubular and collecting duct, and a stimulation effect on smooth muscles in the body. These hormones are secreted into the blood by the pituitary gland. Posterior pituitary hormone drugs include all forms of ADH, such as desmopressin, lypressin, and vasopressin; and the oxytocic agents oxytocin and oxytocin citrate.

PHARMACOKINETICS

Because enzymes in the GI tract can destroy all protein hormones, oral administration of the hormones proves ineffective. Preparations of posterior pituitary hormones may be given by injection or topical intranasal spray. Blood peptidases destroy some of the administered hormone; some binds to receptors on the myometrium. Yet one-third to one-half of any given dose reaches the receptors of the renal tubules, where it stimulates water resorption. Target tissues degrade much of the hormone; less than 20% is excreted unchanged in the urine.

Absorption, distribution, metabolism, excretion

Desmopressin and lypressin are absorbed effectively after intranasal administration. Although quantitative absorption data for lypressin currently are unavailable, 10% to 20% of the desmopressin dose is absorbed via this route. Desmopressin and lypressin are distributed throughout the extracellular fluid, metabolized by the liver and kidneys, and excreted in the urine.

After absorption, vasopressin is distributed throughout the extracellular fluid, metabolized in the liver and kidneys, and excreted in the urine. After an S.C. dose of vasopressin, 5% is excreted unchanged in the urine after approximately 4 hours; after I.V. administration, 5% to 15% of the dose appears in the urine.

The precise pharmacokinetics of the oxytocic drugs remains unclear. Like other natural hormones, however, oxytocic drugs usually are absorbed, distributed, and metabolized rapidly. Parenterally administered oxytocin is absorbed rapidly, but when it is administered intranasally, absorption is erratic. Oxytocin is distributed throughout the extracellular fluid, rapidly metabolized by the liver and kidneys, and excreted in the urine. Oxytocinase, an enzyme produced in the placenta, helps to degrade oxytocin, thereby controlling the oxytocin concentration in the uterus.

Onset, peak, duration

Desmopressin and lypressin act within 1 hour. The desmopressin concentration level peaks in 1 to 4 hours and lasts 8 to 20 hours; lypressin concentration peaks in ½ to 2 hours and lasts 3 to 8 hours.

After S.C. administration, the onset of action of vasopressin is within 1 hour; the duration of action is 2 to 8 hours. With I.M. injection, the onset varies, and duration is 6 to 12 hours. After I.V. administration, vasopressin has an onset of 1 minute and a half-life of 1 to 20 minutes.

Uterine response to oxytocin occurs 3 to 7 minutes after I.M. administration and lasts 2 to 3 hours. After I.V. administration, the onset of oxytocin is 1 minute, with a shorter duration. Response occurs in 5 to 10 minutes after nasal spray administration. The plasma half-life of oxytocin is 3 to 5 minutes.

PHARMACODYNAMICS

The posterior pituitary hormones, under neural control, affect smooth muscle contraction in the uterus, bladder, and GI tract; fluid balance via renal reabsorption of water; and blood pressure via stimulation of the arterial wall muscles.

Mechanism of action

As with other protein hormones, an increase in cyclic AMP in the target cells mediates the effects of ADH. In the kidneys, ADH is bound by receptors on the surfaces of collecting duct cells, thereby regulating the threshold for water reabsorption by the distal tubules, collecting tubules, and collecting ducts. High dosages of ADH stimulate vessel contraction, producing pressor effects and increasing blood pressure. Desmopressin, which has an antidiuretic action, also increases the plasma level of Factor VIII (Anti-hemophilic Factor). Oxytocin may stimulate uterine contractions by increasing the permeability of uterine cell membranes to sodium ions.

PHARMACOTHERAPEUTICS

ADH is prescribed for hormone replacement therapy in patients affected by neurogenic diabetes insipidus. However, it does not treat nephrogenic diabetes insipidus effectively. ADH treatment is short-term for patients with transient diabetes insipidus after head injury or surgery, but may be lifelong for patients with idiopathic hormone deficiencies. The drugs of choice for chronic deficiency, the synthetic extracts desmopressin and lypressin are administered intranasally two to four times a day based on the degree of polyuria. These drugs prove particularly useful for patients allergic or refractory to vasopressin of animal origin. When given in large dosages by I.V., desmopressin is used to increase Factor VIII in patients with mild to moderate hemophilia A or B or Type I von Willebrand's disease. Used for short-term therapy, vasopressin elevates the blood pressure in patients with hypotension caused by lack of vascular tone. It also relieves postoperative gaseous distention.

The oxytocics are used to induce labor and complete incomplete abortions. The short biological half-lives of oxytocin and vasopressin can offer advantages or disadvantages, depending on the therapeutic objectives.

desmopressin acetate (DDAVP). This synthetic ADH is used to treat diabetes insipidus, hemophilia A or B, von Willebrand's disease, and temporary polyuria and polydipsia associated with pituitary trauma or surgery.
Usual adult dosage: for diabetes insipidus and polyuria with pituitary trauma, 0.1 to 0.4 ml daily intranasally, in single or divided doses (most patients require 0.2 ml daily in two

doses adjusted according to the patient's response); for hemophilia A or B or von Willebrand's disease, 0.3 mcg/kg of body weight diluted in 50 ml of normal saline solution, infused slowly by I.V. over 15 to 30 minutes.

lypressin (Diapid Nasal Spray). A synthetic ADH analogue that produces minimal vasopressor or oxytocic effect, lypressin is used primarily to treat neurogenic diabetes insipidus and is useful in patients allergic or refractory to vasopressin of animal origin.
Usual adult dosage: 1 or 2 sprays into each nostril q.i.d. Based on urine output and thirst, the dosage may range from 1 to 10 sprays into each nostril every 3 to 4 hours. However, 4 sprays in each nostril is the maximum that can be absorbed at any one time. One spray provides 2 posterior pituitary (pressor) units.

posterior pituitary intranasal (Posterior Pituitary). A natural hormone with antidiuretic properties, posterior pituitary intranasal can control the polyuria, polydipsia, and dehydration associated with diabetes insipidus from an ADH deficiency.
Usual adult dosage: individualized dosage t.i.d. to q.i.d., based on the patient's degree of polyuria, polydipsia, or dehydration.

vasopressin (Pitressin) A natural ADH, vasopressin is used to treat diabetes insipidus, to relieve postoperative intestinal gaseous distention, to dispel gas shadows appearing before abdominal X-rays, and to treat transient polyuria from an ADH deficiency following trauma.
Usual adult dosage: for abdominal distention, 5 units of vasopressin I.M. initially, followed by 10 units every 3 to 4 hours; for diabetes insipidus, 5 to 10 units S.C. or I.M., b.i.d. to t.i.d.; for abdominal X-rays, two injections of 10 units each, the first administered 2 hours and the second ½ hour before the films are exposed; for polyuria caused by ADH deficiency, 5 to 10 units intranasally, S.C., or I.M., every 8 to 12 hours.

oxytocin (Pitocin, Syntocinon) **and oxytocin citrate** (Pitocin Citrate). Synthetic compounds identical to the natural hormone, oxytocin and oxytocin citrate treat uterine inertia and induce labor in patients with erythroblastosis fetalis. These drugs also are used to treat preeclampsia, eclampsia, and premature rupture of membranes. Oxytocin also is prescribed to control postpartal hemorrhage and uterine atony, hasten uterine involution, and complete inevitable abortions after week 20 of pregnancy.
Usual adult dosage: for inducing labor or treating preeclampsia, eclampsia, or premature rupture of membranes, 1 to 2 mU/minute (0.001 to 0.002 units/minute) by I.V. drip infusion (drip), gradually increased by 1 to 2 mU/minute at 15- to 30-minute intervals until a normal con-

traction pattern is established or the maximum dosage (20 mU/minute) is reached. For reducing postpartal bleeding, 10 to 40 units added to 1,000 ml of physiologic electrolyte solution and infused at a rate necessary to control uterine atony. Also, 10 units may be administered I.M. after the delivery of the placenta. For treating incomplete abortion, 10 units in 500 ml of solution by I.V. infusion at a rate of 10 to 20 mU/ml/minute. For stimulating lactation, one nasal spray (40 units/ml) into one or both nostrils 2 to 3 minutes before breast-feeding.

Drug interactions
Drug interactions with posterior pituitary hormones include decreased antidiuretic properties when combined with alcohol, demeclocycline, and lithium; and increased antidiuretic activity when combined with cyclophosphamide, chlorpropamide, clofibrate, and carbamazepine. Also, barbiturate sedation or cyclopropane anesthesia may produce synergistic and additive effects. The resulting potentiation of the antidiuretic effect may lead to coronary insufficiency and cardiac arrhythmias.

When given with oxytocin, cyclophosphamide can increase the oxytocic effects. Ephedrine, methoxamine, and other vasopressors can potentiate the effects of oxytocin, possibly resulting in severe hypertension and postpartal rupture of cerebral blood vessels. (For more information, see *Drug interactions: Posterior pituitary agents,* page 892.)

ADVERSE DRUG REACTIONS

Hypersensitivity reactions are the most common adverse reactions to ADH drugs and oxytocics. These reactions occur more commonly with natural hormone extracts than with synthetic drug preparations. Large dosages of ADHs can cause GI distress and cardiovascular problems.

Common dose-related reactions to natural ADHs include circumoral and facial pallor, increased GI motility, and abdominal and uterine cramps. Other adverse reactions can include tinnitus, anxiety, hyponatremia, albuminuria, eclamptic attacks, mydriasis, and transient edema. Nasal preparations can cause irritation, rhinorrhea, and nasal passage ulceration. Accidental deep inhalation of the powder preparation into the bronchial passages may cause substernal tightness, coughing, and transient dyspnea. Large dosages may increase blood pressure. Anaphylaxis has occurred after injection.

Adverse reactions to synthetic drugs are rare, although high dosages can cause transient headaches, nausea, nasal congestion, rhinitis, flushing, mild abdominal cramps, and vulvar pain. Decreasing the dosage usually reduces such reactions.

Synthetic extracts have replaced natural oxytocics. Synthetic oxytocin, however, can cause adverse reactions for the pregnant patient, such as postpartal hemorrhage, GI

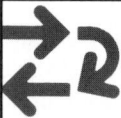

DRUG INTERACTIONS
Posterior pituitary agents

Drug interactions with posterior pituitary hormone can be antagonistic, synergistic, or potentiating. Patients receiving hormone therapy must be monitored continually for drug interactions that can alter the desired therapeutic effect.

DRUG	INTERACTING DRUGS	POSSIBLE EFFECTS	NURSING IMPLICATIONS
desmopressin, lypressin, posterior pituitary intranasal, vasopressin	alcohol, demeclocycline, lithium	Decrease antidiuretic hormone (ADH) activity	• Monitor for signs of dehydration, such as acute weight loss, increased pulse rate, dry skin and mucous membranes, decreased postural systolic blood pressure, decreased skin turgor, thirst, and fatigue. • Monitor urine output and specific gravity and serum osmolality. • Monitor vital signs and weight. • Monitor laboratory values for hematocrit, hemoglobin, red blood cell (RBC) count, and blood urea nitrogen.
	chlorpropamide, clofibrate, carbamazepine, cyclophosphamide	Increase ADH activity	• Monitor for signs and symptoms of water intoxication, such as drowsiness, increased blood pressure, dyspnea, headache, confusion, and weight gain. • Monitor urine output and specific gravity and serum osmolality. • Monitor vital signs and weight. • Monitor laboratory values for hematocrit, hemoglobin, and RBC counts.
	barbiturate or cyclopropane anesthetics	Produce synergistic effects leading to coronary insufficiencies or cardiac arrhythmias	• Monitor vital signs.
oxytocin	cyclophosphamide	Increases oxytocic effects	• Monitor uterine contractions. • Monitor for signs and symptoms of water intoxication.
	vasopressors (anesthetics, ephedrine, methoxamine)	Increase possibility of hypertensive crisis and postpartal rupture of cerebral blood vessels	• Monitor vital signs. • Monitor the patient for neurologic changes, such as decreased level of consciousness.

disturbances, diaphoresis, headache, dizziness, and tinnitus. Severe water intoxication has been associated with slow oxytocin infusion over 24 hours. Excessive dosages as well as hypersensitivity to the drug may result in uterine hypertonicity, tetany, or uterine rupture. Uterine hypertonicity can produce fetal asphyxia, which may lead to fetal bradycardia, neonatal jaundice, cardiac arrhythmias, or death. (For a summary, see *Posterior pituitary agents: Summary of adverse reactions.*)

NURSING PROCESS APPLICATION

The following information assists the nurse in caring for a patient who is receiving a posterior pituitary hormone.

Assessment

• Review the patient's history for a preexisting condition that contraindicates the use of a posterior pituitary hormone, such as known hypersensitivity to the drug, epilepsy, chronic nephritis with nitrogen retention, umbilical cord prolapse, placenta previa, or invasive cervical carcinoma.
• Review the patient's history for a preexisting condition that requires cautious use of vasopressin, such as epilepsy, migraine headaches, asthma, cardiovascular disease, or fluid overload.
• Assess the patient for adverse reactions to the prescribed posterior pituitary hormones, such as hypersensitivity reactions, GI distress, or cardiovascular dysfunction.
• Review the patient's medication history to identify the use of drugs that may interact with the prescribed posterior pituitary hormone, such as alcohol, lithium, cyclophosphamide, clofibrate, barbiturates, or methoxamine.

Posterior pituitary agents: Summary of adverse reactions

The major adverse reactions to posterior pituitary hormones include hypersensitivity, gastrointestinal (GI) disorders, and cardiovascular dysfunctions. Other significant adverse reactions can occur.

DRUG	REACTION
desmopressin acetate	Transient headaches, nausea, nasal congestion, rhinitis, flushing, abdominal cramps (rare and dose-dependent)
lypressin	Facial pallor, GI disturbances, water intoxication, hyponatremia, hypertension, hypersensitivity (high dosages), nasal congestion, pruritus, rhinorrhea, heartburn
vasopressin	Facial pallor, GI disturbances, water intoxication, hyponatremia, hypertension, hypersensitivity (high dosages)
oxytocin	Uterine contractions and ruptured uterus, cardiac arrhythmias, neurologic disorders, water intoxication, hyponatremia, GI disturbances, anaphylactic reactions, postpartal hemorrhage, fetal bradycardia, neonatal jaundice

• Assess the effectiveness of the prescribed posterior pituitary hormone regularly.

• Assess the patient regularly for signs of fluid overload, such as crackles in the lungs, ankle edema, and jugular vein distention.

• Evaluate the patient's and family's knowledge about the prescribed posterior pituitary hormone.

Nursing diagnoses

The following examples represent appropriate nursing diagnoses for a patient receiving a posterior pituitary hormone.

• Potential for injury related to a preexisting condition that contraindicates the use of a posterior pituitary hormone

• Potential for injury related to a preexisting condition that requires cautious use of vasopressin

• Potential for injury related to adverse drug reactions

• Fluid volume excess related to water intoxication caused by a posterior pituitary hormone

• Knowledge deficit related to the prescribed posterior pituitary hormone

Planning and implementation

• Do not administer a posterior pituitary hormone to a patient with a condition that contraindicates its use.

• Administer vasopressin cautiously to a patient at risk because of a preexisting condition.

• Monitor the patient frequently for hypersensitivity reactions, GI distress, cardiovascular dysfunction, and other adverse reactions during therapy.

• *Monitor the patient for hypersensitivity reactions to the posterior pituitary agent, and be prepared to deliver emergency treatment, as prescribed.*

• Monitor hydration if the patient experiences GI distress. Obtain a prescription for an antiemetic or antidiarrheal agent as needed.

• *Assess the patient's cardiovascular function frequently. Particularly note vital sign abnormalities, such as irregular heartbeat or increased blood pressure, as well as symptoms such as chest discomfort, shortness of breath, or skin color changes. Notify the physician if abnormalities occur.*

• Monitor the patient's urine output to assess the effectiveness of antidiuretic therapy used to treat diabetes insipidus.

• Inspect the nasal passages frequently when natural ADH is given nasally. Be alert for nasal irritation, ulcerations, or rhinorrhea.

• Monitor the patient for nausea, nasal congestion, headaches, rhinitis, flushing, mild abdominal cramps, and vulvar pain during high-dose therapy with a synthetic antidiuretic. If these adverse reactions become severe, decrease the dosage, as prescribed, to reduce the reactions.

• Assess the patient for bowel sounds, flatus passage, and resumption of bowel movements during ADH therapy used to improve peristalsis in the GI tract.

• *Check the expiration date on the desmopressin label before administering the drug. Nasal solutions expire 1 year after the date of manufacture.*

• Store parenteral and nasal desmopressin in a refrigerator at 39° F (4° C). Discard any cloudy or discolored solution.

• *Ensure that a physician is present during administration of oxytocin I.V. or I.M.*

• *Keep magnesium sulfate available during I.M. administration of oxytocin to produce endometrial relaxation, if needed.*

• Rotate the oxytocin solution container gently to distribute the drug throughout the solution during I.V. administration. Use a Y connection to the infusion tubing; this provides an alternate route for another solution and ensures patency of the vein if the oxytocin must be discontinued. *Always control oxytocin administration with an infusion pump and never administer it by more than one route at a time.*

• Administer oxytocin with an infusion of dextrose 5% with Ringer's, dextrose 5% with lactated Ringer's, D_5W, or D_5W with normal saline solution as prescribed.

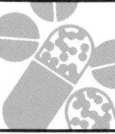

SELECTED MAJOR DRUGS

Pituitary agents

The following chart summarizes representative pituitary agents currently in clinical use.

DRUG	MAJOR INDICATIONS	USUAL ADULT DOSAGES	CONTRAINDICATIONS AND PRECAUTIONS
Anterior pituitary hormones			
corticotropin	Diagnostic testing of adrenal function	Up to 80 units in a single injection; 10 to 25 units in 500 ml D₅W over 8 hr I.V. Repository: 40 to 80 units I.M. or S.C. q 24 to 72 hr Zinc hydroxide preparation: 40 units I.M. q 12 to 24 hr	• Know that corticotropin is contraindicated in a patient with adrenocortical hyperfunction, primary adrenal insufficiency, systemic fungal infection, peptic ulcer disease, ocular herpes simplex, recent surgery, congestive heart failure, scleroderma, osteoporosis, uncontrolled hypertension, or known hypersensitivity to the drug or to porcine proteins. • Administer with extreme caution to a patient with myasthenia gravis. • Administer with caution to a woman of childbearing age, a pregnant or lactating patient, a patient being immunized, or one with latent tuberculosis, hypothyroidism, impaired hepatic function, diabetes mellitus, psychoses, diverticulitis, abscess or other pyogenic infection, thromboembolic disorder, seizures, or renal insufficiency.
cosyntropin	Diagnostic testing of adrenal function	0.25 to 0.75 mg I.M. or 0.25 mg I.V. over 4 to 8 hr	• Know that cosyntropin is contraindicated in a patient with known hypersensitivity to the drug or to corticotropin. • Be aware that cosyntropin has no known precautions.
Posterior pituitary hormones			
vasopressin	Diabetes insipidus	5 to 10 units S.C. or I.M., b.i.d. to t.i.d.	• Know that vasopressin is contraindicated in a patient with anaphylaxis, known hypersensitivity to the drug, or chronic nephritis with nitrogen retention. • Administer with caution to a pediatric, geriatric, pregnant, or lactating patient or one with epilepsy, migraine headaches, asthma, cardiovascular disease, or fluid overload.
oxytocin	Labor induction	1 to 2 mU/min I.V. initially, increased gradually to a maximum of 20 mU/min, if needed	• Know that oxytocin is contraindicated in a patient with significant cephalopelvic disproportion, unfavorable fetal position, fetal distress when delivery is not imminent, cord prolapse, placenta previa, fetal prematurity, uterine overdistention, grand multiparity, traumatic delivery, invasive cervical carcinoma, known hypersensitivity to the drug, or a history of cesarean delivery or uterine sepsis. • Be aware that oxytocin has no known precautions.

• Reconstitute oxytocin by adding 1 ml (10 units) to 1,000 ml of normal saline or other I.V. fluid to provide a solution containing 10 mU/ml (0.01 units/ml).

• *Assess the fetal heart rate and uterine contractions during oxytocin administration. Discontinue the I.V. infusion immediately, administer oxygen, and notify the physician if contractions become more frequent than every 2 minutes and last longer than 60 seconds without uterine relaxation; if contractions become excessively strong or exceed 50 mm Hg as measured on a monitor; or if the fetal heart rate indicates bradycardia, tachycardia, or irregular rhythm as measured on a monitor.*

• Assess the intrapartal patient's fundus and the postpartal patient's lochia frequently during oxytocin therapy.

• *Monitor the patient closely for signs and symptoms of a hypertensive crisis, such as a sudden severe increase in blood pressure above 200/120 mmHg, severe headache, visual disturbances, and epistaxis, if local or regional anesthesia is administered during oxytocin therapy.*

• Keep the plastic nasal tube for oxytocin administration clean and dry. Measure the nasal oxytocin dosage exactly because the drug is potent.

• Notify the physician if adverse reactions occur or if the drug is ineffective.

• *Monitor the patient closely for early signs of water intoxication, such as decreased level of consciousness, reduced orientation, headache, and vomiting, when administering a posterior pituitary hormone. Document the patient's fluid intake and output.*

• Notify the physician if the patient displays signs of water intoxication.

• *Be aware that no known specific antidote exists for water intoxication caused by ADH. However, use of a loop diuretic such as furosemide can induce diuresis.*

Patient teaching

• Teach the patient and family the name, dose, frequency, action, and adverse effects of the prescribed posterior pituitary hormone.

• Teach the patient how to administer the agent if needed.

• Instruct the patient to clear the nasal passages before administering a nasal preparation, to hold the squeeze bottle upright, and to spray into the nostril while sitting with the head vertical. *A nasal preparation must not be administered with the patient lying down or the head tilted back.*

• Teach the patient how to measure fluid intake and output and how to interpret 24-hour fluid measurements during ADH therapy.

• *Instruct the patient never to increase the number of intranasal vasopressin sprays without checking with the physician.*

• Explain the purpose of I.V. oxytocin administration to the patient and describe the expected outcome. Advise the patient that I.V. oxytocin always is administered under a physician's supervision.

• Instruct the patient to notify the physician if adverse reactions occur or if the drug is ineffective.

Evaluation

The following examples represent appropriate evaluation statements for a patient receiving a posterior pituitary hormone.

• The patient has no conditions that contraindicate posterior pituitary hormone therapy.

• The patient exhibits no signs of complications in the preexisting condition linked to vasopressin.

• The patient displays no adverse reactions to the prescribed posterior pituitary hormone.

• The patient maintains adequate fluid balance.

• The patient and family express an accurate understanding of the points taughts about the prescribed posterior pituitary hormone.

• The patient correctly demonstrates self-administration of desmopressin nasal spray.

CHAPTER SUMMARY

Chapter 52 discussed the pituitary gland and its hormones. It also presented the anterior and posterior pituitary hormones. Here are the chapter highlights.

• The pituitary gland is divided into the anterior lobe and the posterior lobe. Each lobe secretes different hormones that produce widespread physiologic effects on body structure and function. Hypothalamic release factors stimulate or inhibit secretion of pituitary hormones as needed.

• Anterior pituitary hormones act on other endocrine glands, such as the thyroid, adrenals, and gonads, to control their structure and function. These hormones also directly affect sexual maturity, reproduction, and linear growth. The three major anterior pituitary hormone drugs are corticotropin, cosyntropin, and somatrem.

• Posterior pituitary hormones regulate fluid volume, stimulate smooth muscle contraction, and affect blood pressure by stimulating the arterial wall muscles. These hormones include ADH and oxytocin. Posterior pituitary hormone drugs include posterior pituitary intranasal, vasopressin, desmopressin acetate, lypressin, oxytocin, and oxytocin citrate.

• Pituitary hormones are administered parenterally or, for some drugs, intranasally. Natural pituitary hormone drugs are absorbed rapidly, metabolized by the kidneys and liver, and excreted in the urine. They have a short duration of action. Synthetic analogues are metabolized more slowly, providing a longer therapeutic duration.

• Interactions between anterior pituitary hormones and other drugs can produce a wide variety of reactions. Interactions between posterior pituitary hormones and other drugs can alter ADH activity and can produce cardiovascular dysfunction and water intoxication.

• The most significant adverse reaction to these agents is hypersensitivity to the natural hormones. Administering synthetic ones decreases the risk of hypersensitivity.

• Nursing care for a patient receiving a pituitary hormone typically includes assessing for hypersensitivity reactions and providing emergency treatment and monitoring for signs and symptoms of other adverse reactions. It also includes patient teaching that explains hormone therapy, stresses accurate dosages, demonstrates correct administration, and emphasizes compliance with the prescribed drug regimen.

STUDY QUESTIONS

See Appendix 1 for answers.

1. Audrey McCallum, age 38, is admitted to the hospital with an acute episode of multiple sclerosis. Her physician prescribes corticotropin (Acthar) 80 units daily. Which administration route would render corticotropin ineffective?
(a) intravenous route
(b) intramuscular route
(c) subcutaneous route
(d) oral route

2. For Ms. McCallum, what is the onset of action of corticotropin?
(a) 5 minutes
(b) 15 minutes
(c) 30 minutes
(d) 60 minutes

3. Ms. McCallum must receive long-term corticotropin therapy. When teaching her about corticotropin, the nurse should discuss which potential adverse reaction?
(a) glucose intolerance
(b) orthostatic hypotension
(c) transient hypothyroidism
(d) iatrogenic Cushing's syndrome

4. Joyce Dugan, age 16, has just received a diagnosis of neurogenic diabetes insipidus. Which pituitary hormone is Joyce lacking?
(a) GH
(b) ADH
(c) TSH
(d) ACTH

5. For Ms. Dugan, the physician prescribes vasopressin 5 units S.C. b.i.d. During vasopressin therapy, Ms. Dugan is likely to develop which adverse reaction?
(a) dehydration
(b) hypokalemia
(c) hypernatremia
(d) water intoxication

6. Lois Chan, age 25, is admitted to the maternity unit with premature rupture of membranes. Her physician decides to induce labor. Which agent is most likely to be prescribed for labor induction?
(a) oxytocin
(b) lypressin
(c) vasopressin
(d) desmopressin

7. During labor induction, the nurse determines that Ms. Chan's contractions occur every 90 seconds and last 70 seconds. How should the nurse intervene?
(a) Continue the medication and notify the physician.
(b) Decrease the dosage and continue to monitor the patient.
(c) Stop the medication immediately and notify the physician.
(d) Increase the dosage until the cervix is dilated fully.

SELECTED REFERENCES

AHFS drug information 90. (1990). Bethesda, MD: American Society of Hospital Pharmacists.

Behi, R. (1989). Treatment and care of thyroid problems. *Nursing,* 3(41), 4-6.

Billups, N., and Billups, S. (1989). *American drug index 1989* (33rd ed.). Philadelphia: Lippincott.

Boylan, P., and MacDonald, D. (1988). Oxytocin: The need to distinguish between induction and augmentation and between multiparas and primiparas. *Birth,* 15(4), 203-204.

Curtis, P., and Safransky, N. (1988). Rethinking oxytocin protocols in the augmentation of labor. *Birth,* 15(4), 199-202.

Goodman and Gilman's the pharmacological basis of therapeutics (8th ed.; 1990). Elmsford, NY: Pergamon Press.

Hansten, P., and Horn, J. (1988). *Drug interactions: Clinical significance of drug-drug interactions* (6th ed.). Philadelphia: Lea & Febiger.

Jacoby, A., and Wiegman, M. (1990). Cardiovascular complications of intravenous vasopressin therapy. *Focus on Critical Care,* 17(1), 63-66.

Littlefield, L. (1988). Interactions of drugs and antidiuretic hormone. *Journal of Pediatric Health Care,* 2(6), 325-327.

North American Nursing Diagnosis Association. (1990). *Taxonomy I - Revised, with official diagnostic categories.* St. Louis: NANDA.

CHAPTER

53

ANDROGENIC AND ANABOLIC STEROID AGENTS

OBJECTIVES

After reading and studying this chapter, the student should be able to:

1. Differentiate between the effects of the androgenic and anabolic steroid agents.

2. Identify the androgenic and anabolic steroid agents that are associated with hepatic disorders.

3. Explain why these agents are used to treat hypogonadism and related disorders; breast engorgement, breast cancer, and related disorders; and osteoporosis, anemias, and tissue-development problems.

4. Describe the mechanisms of action of these agents.

5. Describe the major drug interactions that occur with androgenic and anabolic steroid agents.

6. Describe the common adverse reactions to these agents and explain how to manage them.

7. Describe how to apply the nursing process when caring for a patient receiving an androgenic or anabolic steroid agent.

INTRODUCTION

Androgenic steroids stimulate the growth of male accessory sex organs and produce masculinizing effects, such as facial hair growth and voice deepening. Anabolic steroids promote a positive nitrogen balance in the body, which stimulates tissue building and reverses tissue depletion.

In reality, these sharp distinctions are blurred. No purely androgenic or anabolic steroids exist. All androgenic steroids provide some anabolic effects, and all anabolic steroids provide some androgenic effects. Yet the distinctions remain useful because one effect always predominates. Predominantly androgenic steroid agents include danazol, fluoxymesterone, methyltestosterone, and all forms of testosterone. Predominantly anabolic steroid agents include ethylestrenol, nandrolone decanoate and phenpropionate, oxandrolone, oxymetholone, stanozolol, and testolactone.

Researchers derived many of the androgenic and anabolic steroid agents from testosterone, the male hormone secreted by the testes and, in smaller amounts, by the ovaries and adrenal cortex. They modified the base molecule of testosterone to try to minimize the androgenic effects and maximize the anabolic effects. Today, the search continues for an anabolic agent that can promote tissue building without producing masculinizing effects.

For a summary of representative drugs, see *Selected major drugs: Androgenic and anabolic steroid agents,* page 902. For a listing of applicable nursing diagnoses that the nurse may formulate when caring for a patient receiving these agents, see *Selected nursing diagnoses: Androgenic and anabolic steroid agents,* page 897. For detailed information on applying the nursing process, see Chapter 6, The Nursing Process and Drug Therapy.

ANDROGENIC AND ANABOLIC STEROIDS

These steroid agents have many clinical uses. In androgen-deficient males, predominantly androgenic agents can correct hypogonadism and related disorders. In females, they can prevent postpartal breast engorgement and may be used to treat certain types of breast cancer and related disorders. Predominantly anabolic agents can promote weight gain in underweight patients affected by a catabolic disorder or drug. They also may be used to treat certain types of osteoporosis and anemias.

PHARMACOKINETICS

Anabolic and androgenic steroids are absorbed rapidly and highly bound to plasma proteins. These lipid-soluble agents are distributed widely throughout the body, metabolized in the liver, and excreted mainly by the kidneys.

Absorption, distribution, metabolism, excretion

Although oral and parenteral forms of testosterone are absorbed readily, they undergo such rapid hepatic metabolism that they produce little response. To overcome this problem, researchers modified the testosterone molecule or placed it in a special vehicle. Today, alkylated steroids allow rapid absorption but retard hepatic metabolism, making oral administration possible. Testosterone cypionate and enanthate use an oil base to prolong absorption and allow effective parenteral administration. After absorption, all androgenic and anabolic steroids are distributed widely throughout the body and highly bound to plasma proteins.

Testosterone and all other androgenic and anabolic steroid agents are excreted in the urine or feces as metabolites or unchanged drug.

Onset, peak, duration

The onset of action, peak concentration level, and duration of action vary with the testosterone molecule modification. After oral administration, for example, the 17-alpha-alkylated steroids (oxymetholone, oxandrolone, ethylestrenol, and stanozolol) provide a short duration. After parenteral administration, the 17-beta esters (nandrolone decanoate and phenpropionate) offer a longer duration. Parenteral administration of testosterone cypionate and enanthate also provides an extended duration.

PHARMACODYNAMICS

Steroids produce predominantly androgenic or anabolic effects, depending on the agent used. A predominantly androgenic agent acts as an exogenous replacement, stimulating normal development in an androgen-deficient male. A predominantly anabolic agent stimulates cellular protein synthesis, promoting a positive nitrogen balance and tissue development.

Mechanism of action

Agents such as testosterone produce androgenic and anabolic effects by binding to androgen receptors in target organs, such as skeletal muscle, the prostate gland, and bone marrow. Receptor binding not only stimulates development in these organs, but also increases protein synthesis. These actions produce dramatic effects in androgen-deficient patients, such as castrated men, men with pituitary hormone deficiencies, and normal women.

Steroid agents may promote anabolic effects by blocking cortisol uptake in muscle and liver cells. Secreted by the adrenal gland, cortisol normally acts as a catabolic agent, increasing muscle breakdown and body stress mechanisms. By blocking cortisol uptake in muscle cells, steroid agents reduce muscle breakdown and increase muscle mass. By blocking cortisol uptake in liver cells, they maximize its effect on body stress reactions. Steroids also decrease plasma protein synthesis in the liver, which enhances their effects by increasing the amount of free, or unbound, drug in the plasma.

The anabolic steroid agents reduce urinary excretion of nitrogen and electrolytes, causing water retention and weight gain.

PHARMACOTHERAPEUTICS

Although each agent produces androgenic and anabolic effects, one effect always predominates and helps determine the agent's clinical indications.

Androgenic agents, such as testosterone cypionate and enanthate, best serve as androgen replacements for castrated and hypogonadal males. They produce pronounced effects in prepubertal males. Some predominantly anabolic agents, such as oxymetholone, can stimulate erythropoiesis (red blood cell production) in the bone marrow, which makes them effective against aplastic and other anemias in 25% of patients. Danazol and other agents can be used to treat hereditary angioedema (an immune disorder that causes transient attacks of subcutaneous, submucosal, or visceral edema) because they can stabilize the immune defect by increasing or restoring components in the complement system. Testosterone propionate and related agents can provide palliative treatment for some hormone-sensitive breast cancers. (For more information on androgens used to treat breast cancer, see Chapter 69, Hormonal Antineoplastic Agents.) Predominantly anabolic steroids, such as oxandrolone, sometimes are used to treat malnourished patients. For some, they can promote a positive nitrogen balance, enhance the appetite, and increase the sense of well-being.

Recently, healthy people have taken predominantly anabolic steroids to increase their muscle mass and enhance their athletic performance. However, medical studies have not provided evidence that these agents can enhance athletic performance, so these dubious claims of enhancement should be weighed against the adverse effects of these agents. (For more information, see the appendix on Substance Abuse.)

danazol (Danocrine). Administered primarily for its androgenic effects, danazol may be used to treat endometriosis and fibrocystic breast disease in women. It also can be used to prevent hereditary angioedema.
Usual adult dosage: for endometriosis, 100 to 200 mg P.O. b.i.d. for mild cases, or 400 mg P.O. b.i.d. for moderate to severe cases, uninterrupted for 3 to 6 months (may continue for 9 months); for fibrocystic breast disease, 100 to 400 mg P.O. daily in two divided doses for 2 to 6 months; for hereditary angioedema, 200 mg P.O. b.i.d. or t.i.d. until the desired response is achieved, then decreased by half every 1 to 3 months to determine lowest effective dosage.

fluoxymesterone (Halotestin). Because of its predominantly androgenic activity, fluoxymesterone is used to treat hypogonadism and impotence caused by a testicular deficiency. It also can reduce postpartal breast engorgement and act as a palliative treatment for breast cancer in women.
Usual adult dosage: for hypogonadism and impotence, 5 to 20 mg P.O. daily; for postpartal breast engorgement, 2.5 mg P.O. when active labor begins, followed by 5 to 10 mg daily for 5 days; for breast cancer, 10 to 40 mg P.O. daily in divided doses, adjusted to the individual's needs and reduced to a minimum when desired effects are noted.

methyltestosterone (Metandren). A predominantly androgenic agent, methyltestosterone can be used to treat eunuchoidism (deficient testicular secretion), eunuchism (underdeveloped sex organs), male climacteric symptoms (reduced sexual activity), and postpubertal cryptorchidism (failure of one or both testes to descend normally). In women, it is used to treat breast cancer 1 to 5 years after menopause and postpartal breast engorgement.
Usual adult dosage: for eunuchoidism, eunuchism, and male climacteric symptoms, 10 to 50 mg P.O. daily or 5 to 20 mg buccally daily; for postpubertal cryptorchidism, 30 mg P.O. daily or 15 mg buccally daily; for breast cancer, 50 to 200 mg P.O. daily or 25 to 100 mg buccally daily; for postpartal breast engorgement, 80 mg P.O. daily or 40 mg buccally daily.

testosterone (Histerone, Testoject). Used primarily for its androgenic effects, testosterone is indicated for eunuchoidism, eunuchism, and male climacteric symptoms. It also can be used to treat breast cancer in postmenopausal women and postpartal breast engorgement.
Usual adult dosage: for eunuchoidism and related disorders, 10 to 25 mg I.M. two or three times weekly; for breast cancer, 100 mg I.M. three times weekly as long as improvement is maintained; for postpartal breast engorgement, 25 to 50 mg I.M. daily for 3 to 4 days starting at delivery.

testosterone cypionate (Andro-Cyp, Depo-Testosterone). Also used primarily as an androgen, this form of testosterone can help treat eunuchism, male hormone deficiency after castration, and male climacteric symptoms. It also may be used to treat metastatic breast cancer in women.
Usual adult dosage: for eunuchism and related disorders, 50 to 400 mg I.M. every 2 to 4 weeks; for breast cancer, 200 to 400 mg I.M. every 2 to 4 weeks.

testosterone enanthate (Android-TLA, Andryl). Another agent used chiefly for its androgenic effects, this form of testosterone is indicated for eunuchism, eunuchoidism, male hormone deficiency after castration, and male climacteric symptoms. It also may be used to treat metastatic breast cancer in women and oligospermia (insufficient sperm in the semen).
Usual adult dosage: for eunuchism and related disorders, 50 to 400 mg I.M. every 4 weeks; for breast cancer, 200 to 400 mg I.M. every 2 to 4 weeks; for oligospermia, 100 to 200 mg I.M. every 4 to 6 weeks.

testosterone propionate (Androlan, Testex). This form of testosterone is used chiefly for its androgenic effects in treating eunuchism, eunuchoidism, male climacteric symptoms, and impotence. It also may be used to treat metastatic breast cancer in women.

Usual adult dosage: for eunuchism and related disorders, 10 to 25 mg I.M. two to four times weekly; for breast cancer, 50 to 100 mg I.M. three times weekly.

ethylestrenol (Maxibolin). Used primarily for its anabolic effects, ethylestrenol can promote weight gain and combat tissue depletion from refractory anemias, corticosteroid therapy, osteoporosis, prolonged immobilization, and various debilitated states. For an adult or child, therapy should not exceed 6 weeks. However, after a 4-week interval, treatment may be repeated.

Usual adult dosage: for weight gain, tissue depletion, and debilitation, 4 to 8 mg P.O. daily, decreased to the lowest effective maintenance dosage as soon as the desired response is achieved.

Usual pediatric dosage: for weight gain, tissue depletion, and debilitation, 1 to 3 mg P.O. daily, individualized to the patient's needs.

nandrolone decanoate (Deca-Durabolin). Predominantly used as an anabolic agent, nandrolone decanoate is indicated to treat refractory anemia and to build tissue.

Usual adult dosage: for refractory anemia, 50 to 200 mg deep I.M. weekly, preferably in the gluteal muscle; for tissue building, 50 to 100 mg deep I.M. every 3 to 4 weeks.

nandrolone phenpropionate (Durabolin). Also used primarily as an anabolic agent, nandrolone phenpropionate is indicated for control of metastatic breast cancer.

Usual adult dosage: 50 to 100 mg deep I.M. weekly, preferably in the gluteal muscle.

oxandrolone (Anavar). Used primarily for its anabolic effects, oxandrolone is indicated as an adjunct treatment to promote weight gain after extensive surgery, chronic infection, trauma, or other medically related weight loss. It also may be used to relieve bone pain in osteoporosis or to offset catabolism from long-term corticosteroid use.

Usual adult dosage: for weight gain, osteoporosis, or catabolism, 5 to 10 mg P.O. daily, increased to 20 mg daily for 2 to 4 weeks, if needed.

Usual pediatric dosage: for weight gain, osteoporosis, or catabolism, 0.1 to 0.25 mg/kg P.O. daily for 2 to 4 weeks. Continuous therapy should not exceed 3 months.

oxymetholone (Anadrol-50). A predominantly anabolic agent, oxymetholone is used to treat anemias caused by deficient red blood cell production, myelofibrosis, and myelotoxic drugs as well as acquired and congenital aplastic anemias.

Usual adult dosage: 1 to 5 mg/kg P.O. daily.

stanozolol (Winstrol). Primarily used for its anabolic activity, stanozolol can be used to treat hereditary angioedema.

Usual adult dosage: for hereditary angioedema, 2 mg P.O. t.i.d. initially, followed by a maintenance dosage of 2 mg P.O. daily.

testolactone (Teslac). This predominantly anabolic agent is indicated as an adjunct in treating advanced or disseminated postmenopausal breast cancer.

Usual adult dosage: 250 mg P.O. q.i.d.

Drug interactions

Although testosterone and its salts produce no significant drug interactions, other androgenic and anabolic steroid agents can cause a few. The oral anabolic agents methyltestosterone and oxymetholone may increase the effects of oral anticoagulants. Androgenic and anabolic steroid agents also may interact with high-sodium foods, causing sodium and fluid retention.

ADVERSE DRUG REACTIONS

Androgenic and anabolic steroid agents can cause many adverse reactions, ranging from changes in sexual characteristics to life-threatening liver failure.

In women, long-term or high-dosage use may cause masculinizing reactions, including hoarseness or voice deepening, male-pattern hair distribution, menstrual irregularities, acne, increased libido, and clitoral enlargement. Drug discontinuation may reverse many of these reactions.

In men, adverse reactions result from the conversion of steroids to female sex hormone metabolites in the body. This commonly causes gynecomastia — especially in adolescent males — and also may produce testicular atrophy, decreased levels of pituitary reproductive hormones, and prostatic hypertrophy. Other adverse reactions may include priapism (persistent erection), increased libido, and oligospermia.

In children, androgenic and anabolic steroid agents may cause premature epiphyseal closure (closure of the growth plate in the long bones), thus retarding growth. Prepubertal boys may develop secondary sex characteristics prematurely.

These agents can produce serious toxic effects. In many patients, they elevate liver enzyme levels, resulting in jaundice. In some patients, peliosis hepatis (blood-filled liver cysts) may occur, leading to liver failure. In others, long-term oral steroid use may cause liver cancer.

Androgenic and anabolic steroids can affect metabolism in several ways. They commonly increase the serum cholesterol level and decrease the high-density lipoprotein level, predisposing the patient to atherosclerotic heart disease. These agents may increase serum calcium to a dangerous level in a patient with metastatic bone disease or parathyroid hormone oversecretion. They also may cause sodium and water retention, leading to edema.

Androgenic and anabolic steroid agents do not appear to precipitate allergic or other hypersensitivity reactions.

NURSING PROCESS APPLICATION

The following information assists the nurse in caring for a patient who is receiving an androgenic or anabolic steroid.

Assessment
• Review the patient's history for a preexisting condition that contraindicates the use of an androgenic or anabolic steroid, such as pregnancy, lactation, known hypersensitivity to the drug, breast or prostate cancer in a male patient, or a serious cardiac, hepatic, or renal disease.
• Review the patient's history for a preexisting condition that requires cautious use of an androgenic or anabolic steroid, such as delayed puberty in a male patient.
• Assess the patient for adverse reactions to the prescribed androgenic or anabolic steroid, such as changes in sexual characteristics; increased liver enzyme, serum cholesterol, or serum calcium levels; decreased high-density lipoprotein level; or edema.
• Review the patient's medication history to identify the use of drugs that may interact with the androgenic or anabolic steroid, such as oral anticoagulants.
• Assess the effectiveness of the androgenic or anabolic steroid periodically.
• Assess the patient for changes in sexuality patterns.
• Assess the patient for fluid retention.
• Evaluate the patient's and family's knowledge about the prescribed androgenic or anabolic steroid.

Nursing diagnoses
The following examples represent appropriate nursing diagnoses for a patient receiving an androgenic or anabolic steroid.
• Potential for injury related to a preexisting condition that contraindicates the use of an androgenic or anabolic steroid
• Potential for injury related to a preexisting condition that requires cautious use of an androgenic or anabolic steroid
• Potential for injury related to adverse drug reactions
• Altered sexuality patterns related to the adverse genitourinary effects of the androgenic or anabolic steroid
• Fluid volume excess related to sodium and water retention caused by the androgenic or anabolic steroid
• Knowledge deficit related to the prescribed androgenic or anabolic steroid

Planning and implementation
• Do not administer an androgenic or anabolic steroid to a patient with a condition that contraindicates its use.
• Administer an androgenic or anabolic steroid cautiously to a patient at risk because of a preexisting condition.
• *Monitor the patient regularly for adverse reactions that can range from changes in sexual characteristics to life-threatening liver failure.*
• *Perform a complete physical and nutritional assessment before therapy begins to develop a baseline against which the drug's effects can be measured.* Include the patient's blood pressure, pulse rate, and respirations in the physical assessment. Monitor serum protein determinations, which indicate nitrogen and protein balance, as part of the nutritional assessment. Also monitor baseline values for the patient's complete blood count, serum cholesterol and serum calcium levels, and hepatic and cardiac function.
• *Inspect the patient's sclera and skin for jaundice in natural – not fluorescent or incandescent – light.* If jaundice exists, notify the physician.
• *Monitor the patient for and report other signs and symptoms of hepatotoxicity, such as nausea, vomiting, an increased prothrombin time, and increased bilirubin, aspartate aminotransferase (formerly SGOT), and alkaline phosphatase levels.*
• *Monitor for signs and symptoms of hypercalcemia, such as muscle weakness, arrhythmias, and bone pain, in a patient with metastatic bone cancer or parathyroid hormone oversecretion.* Monitor the patient's serum calcium level and administer fluids to decrease the risk of renal calculi, which may develop with hypercalcemia and cause flank pain, fever, and hematuria.
• Help the patient cope with body changes by providing emotional support and a positive attitude. Encourage the patient's family and friends to do the same.
• Ask the patient about changes in sexual activity during therapy with an androgenic or anabolic steroid. If altered sexuality patterns trouble the patient, notify the physician and provide a referral to an appropriate counselor or support group.
• *Monitor the patient's fluid intake and output and weigh the patient regularly during dosage determination.* Report to the physician any weight gain of more than 2 lb/week or any signs of edema, such as swelling in the feet or ankles. Expect to administer a diuretic and a low-sodium diet, as prescribed, to relieve water retention.

Patient teaching
• Teach the patient and family the name, dose, frequency, action, and adverse effects of the prescribed androgenic or anabolic steroid.
• *Teach the patient to take the drug exactly as prescribed for the specified duration. Advise the patient not to elim-*

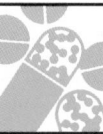

Androgenic and anabolic steroid agents

The following chart summarizes some of the major androgenic and anabolic steroids currently in clinical use.

DRUG	MAJOR INDICATIONS	USUAL ADULT DOSAGES	CONTRAINDICATIONS AND PRECAUTIONS
fluoxymesterone	Hypogonadism and impotence caused by testicular deficiency	5 to 20 mg P.O. daily	• Know that fluoxymesterone is contraindicated in a pregnant, suspected pregnant, or lactating patient; a male patient with breast or prostate cancer; or any patient with serious cardiac, hepatic, or renal disease or known hypersensitivity to the drug. • Administer with caution to a male patient with delayed puberty.
	Breast cancer in women	10 to 40 mg P.O. daily in divided doses, adjusted to individual's needs and reduced to minimum when effects are noted	
	Postpartal breast engorgement	2.5 mg P.O. when active labor begins, followed by 5 to 10 mg P.O. daily for 5 days	
testosterone cypionate	Eunuchism, male hormone deficiency after castration, and male climacteric symptoms	50 to 400 mg I.M. every 2 to 4 weeks	• Know that testosterone cypionate is contraindicated in a pregnant or lactating patient, a male patient with breast or prostate cancer, or any patient who is easily sexually stimulated or has serious cardiac, hepatic, or renal disease, hypercalcemia, or known hypersensitivity to the drug. • Administer with caution to a male patient with delayed puberty.
	Metastatic breast cancer in women	200 to 400 mg I.M. every 2 to 4 weeks	
testolactone	Adjunct in treating advanced or disseminated postmenopausal breast cancer	250 mg P.O. q.i.d.	• Know that testolactone is contraindicated in a male patient with breast cancer or any patient with known hypersensitivity to the drug.

inate any doses or discontinue the drug without consulting the physician.

• Advise the patient receiving a parenteral steroid to report irritation at the injection site.

• Teach the patient to store an oral steroid in a dry, light-resistant, tightly closed container.

• *Instruct the patient to carry a Medic Alert card or other drug information source.*

• Advise the patient to return as directed for follow-up laboratory tests and physician consultations.

• Help the patient maximize tissue building by establishing a diet that includes calcium, protein, vitamins, adequate calories, and ample fluids.

• *Warn the patient not to take an androgenic or anabolic steroid for bodybuilding or aphrodisiac effects. The risks outweigh the benefits.*

• Prepare the patient for changes in appearance, and encourage expression of concerns or fears about these changes.

• Advise the female patient to report to the physician any masculinizing effects, such as hoarseness or voice changes, facial hair growth, clitoral enlargement, acne, libido increase, and menstrual irregularities. Tell her to be alert particularly for a libido increase, which may be an early indication of toxicity.

• Reassure the female patient that such effects as facial hair growth and acne should disappear with drug discontinuation. Other effects, such as voice changes caused by structural alterations in the larynx, may be irreversible.

• Advise the male patient to report to the physician any libido increase, priapism, or urinary hesitancy. These reactions may require a dosage reduction or drug discontinuation.

• Advise the prepubertal boy and his family that steroid therapy may cause premature development of secondary sex characteristics, such as facial hair and phallic enlargement. The patient or family should report any of these changes to the physician.

• Instruct the patient to notify the physician if any adverse reactions or other concerns arise.

Evaluation

The following examples represent appropriate evaluation statements for a patient receiving an androgenic or anabolic steroid.

• The patient has no conditions that contraindicate androgenic or anabolic steroid therapy.

• The patient exhibits no signs of complications in the preexisting condition linked to the prescribed androgenic or anabolic steroid.

• The patient experiences no adverse reactions to the prescribed androgenic or anabolic steroid.

• The patient reports continued sexual satisfaction during androgenic or anabolic steroid therapy.

• The patient maintains normal fluid balance.

• The patient and family express an accurate understanding of the points taught about the prescribed androgenic or anabolic steroid.

• The patient correctly identifies adverse drug reactions and describes what to do if they occur.

CHAPTER SUMMARY

Chapter 53 investigated steroid agents, which produce a predominantly androgenic, or masculinizing, effect or a predominantly anabolic, or protein-sparing, effect. Here are the chapter highlights.

• Androgenic and anabolic steroid agents include testosterone—a hormone produced in the testes, ovaries, and adrenal glands—and its chemical derivatives. Predominantly androgenic steroids include danazol, fluoxymesterone, methyltestosterone, and all forms of testosterone. Predominantly anabolic steroids include ethylestrenol, nandrolone decanoate and phenpropionate, oxandrolone, oxymetholone, stanozolol, and testolactone.

• Oral and parenteral steroids are absorbed well and distributed throughout the body.

• The duration of action of an androgenic or anabolic steroid depends on its chemical structure.

• Androgenic and anabolic steroids are used in males to treat hypogonadism and related disorders, in females to treat breast cancer and related disorders, and in both sexes to stimulate weight gain and tissue and bone development.

• Testosterone and its salts produce no significant drug interactions, but oral anabolic agents may interact with oral anticoagulants.

• Androgenic and anabolic steroids can cause many adverse reactions, ranging from changes in sexual characteristics to life-threatening liver failure.

• When caring for a patient receiving an androgenic or anabolic steroid, the nurse should obtain baseline data, monitor closely for adverse reactions, teach the patient how to store and use the prescribed agent, and help the patient cope with drug-induced changes in the body or in sexuality patterns.

STUDY QUESTIONS

See Appendix 1 for answers.

1. Dolores Garner, age 57, has had a bilateral mastectomy to treat postmenopausal metastatic breast cancer. Her physician considers prescribing an androgenic steroid. Although androgenic and anabolic steroids produce similar effects, generally how do they differ?
(a) Androgenic steroids produce masculinizing effects; anabolic steroids stimulate tissue building.
(b) Androgenic steroids promote development of female sex characteristics; anabolic steroids suppress their development.
(c) Androgenic steroids promote a positive nitrogen balance; anabolic steroids stimulate cellular protein synthesis.
(d) Androgenic steroids promote tissue development; anabolic steroids stimulate growth in male accessory sex organs.

2. The physician is most likely to prescribe which agent for Ms. Garner?
(a) danazol
(b) stanozolol
(c) testosterone
(d) ethylestrenol

3. While Ms. Garner receives the androgenic steroid, the nurse should assess her for which adverse reaction?
(a) decreased libido
(b) voice deepening
(c) gynecomastia
(d) growth retardation

4. During androgenic steroid therapy, the nurse should assess Ms. Garner for which serious toxic effect?
(a) anaphylaxis
(b) liver failure
(c) blood dyscrasias
(d) cardiac arrhythmias

5. How may the androgenic steroid affect Ms. Garner's fat metabolism?
(a) It may increase serum cholesterol and decrease high-density lipoprotein (HDL) levels.
(b) It may decrease serum cholesterol and increase low-density lipoprotein (LDL) levels.
(c) It may decrease serum cholesterol and LDL levels.
(d) It may increase serum cholesterol and HDL levels.

6. The nurse teaches Ms. Garner to be alert for androgenic and anabolic effects. Which anabolic effect should Ms. Garner report to her physician?

(a) hirsutism

(b) gynecomastia

(c) urinary hesitancy

(d) weight gain and edema

7. Ron Barnes, age 18, is on the track team at school. He asks his physician about using anabolic steroids to improve his athletic performance. Which statement accurately characterizes this use of anabolic steroids?

(a) Anabolic steroids are prescribed widely to increase muscle mass and enhance athletic performance.

(b) Anabolic steroids have no effect on athletic performance.

(c) Anabolic steroids are safe when used in small amounts to improve athletic performance.

(d) Anabolic steroids should not be used to enhance performance because the risks outweigh the benefits.

SELECTED REFERENCES

Adjuvant therapy for breast cancer. (1990). *Emergency Medicine,* 22(2), 45-46.

AHFS drug information 90. (1990). Bethesda, MD: American Society of Hospital Pharmacists.

Danazol intracranial hypertension. (1987). *Nurses Drug Alert,* 11(9), 72.

Goodman and Gilman's the pharmacological basis of therapeutics (8th ed.; 1990). Elmsford, NY: Pergamon Press.

Goodman, M. (1988). Concepts of hormonal manipulation in the treatment of cancer. *Oncology Nursing Forum,* 15(5), 639-647.

Hansten, P., and Horn, J. (1988). *Drug interactions: Clinical significance of drug-drug interactions* (6th ed.). Philadelphia: Lea & Febiger.

Miller, R. (1988). Athletes and steroids: Playing a deadly game. *FDA Consumer,* 21(9), 16-21.

Nelson, M. (1989). Androgenic-anabolic steroid use in adolescents. *Journal of Pediatric Health Care,* 3(4), 175-180.

North American Nursing Diagnosis Association. (1990). *Taxonomy I-Revised, with official diagnostic categories.* St. Louis: NANDA.

Testosterone treatment for delayed growth. (1989). *Nurses Drug Alert,* 13(3), 23-24.

White, G., Richardson, G., and Grosshans, O., et al. (1987). Preventing steroid abuse in youth: The health educator's role. *Health Educator,* 18(4), 32-35.

Yelverton, G. (1989). Anabolic steroids. *Pediatric Nursing,* 15(1), 63.

ESTROGENS, PROGESTINS, AND ORAL CONTRACEPTIVE AGENTS

OBJECTIVES

After reading and studying this chapter, the student should be able to:
1. Describe the major physiologic actions of estrogen and progesterone.
2. Explain the relationship of first-pass metabolism to estrogen and progestin dosages.
3. Describe the therapeutic uses of estrogens, progestins, and oral contraceptives.
4. Identify the major adverse reactions to estrogens, progestins, and oral contraceptives.
5. Describe how oral contraceptives prevent pregnancy.
6. Compare the monophasic, biphasic, and triphasic oral contraceptives.
7. Describe how to apply the nursing process when caring for a patient who is receiving an estrogen, progestin, or oral contraceptive agent.

INTRODUCTION

Estrogens, progestins, and oral contraceptives mimic the physiologic effects of the naturally occurring female sex hormones, the estrogens and progesterone. The naturally occurring estrogens and progesterone serve a vital function in the development of the female reproductive tract and secondary sex characteristics. Also, estrogens and progesterone are responsible for the maturation of the ovum and its development after fertilization. Therapy with estrogens and progestins includes their use as contraceptives and as replacement therapy after menopause.

Hormonal control of the menstrual cycle

A woman's reproductive years are characterized by monthly rhythmic changes in estrogen and progesterone secretion. The hypothalamus and pituitary gland control the changing concentrations of these hormones. The gonadotropic hor-

mones—follicle-stimulating hormone (FSH) and luteinizing hormone (LH)—secreted by the anterior pituitary gland stimulate the ovaries to secrete estrogen and progesterone. Elevated estrogen and progesterone concentrations produce negative feedback to the hypothalamus and pituitary gland. This leads to reduced FSH and LH concentrations, ultimately reducing ovarian secretion of estrogens and progesterone. (For an illustration of how the various hormones interrelate, see *Female reproductive cycle,* page 906.)

Physiology of the menstrual cycle

Menstrual bleeding is caused by desquamation of the endometrium. The first day of menstrual bleeding represents the beginning of the female reproductive cycle. During the next few days, the FSH and LH concentrations rise, stimulating the growth of 6 to 12 follicles in the ovaries. One follicle becomes predominant and begins to secrete large amounts of estrogen, which reduces FSH and LH concentrations via a negative feedback mechanism. The diminished FSH and LH levels result in degeneration of the remaining follicles and stimulation of growth of a new endometrial lining. This process, known as the *proliferation phase,* occurs during the 2 weeks after menstruation.

After the proliferation phase and about 2 weeks after onset of menstruation, LH secretion rises sharply, signaling that ovulation is about to occur. At this time, the endometrial glands secrete a thin, stringy mucus, deposited mainly near the cervix, that helps channel sperm into the uterus.

After ovulation has occurred, the remaining cells of the estrogen-secreting follicle become the corpus luteum, which produces large quantities of estrogen, progesterone, and inhibin in the days after ovulation. Under the influence of these hormones, the endometrium undergoes a second developmental process. This is known as the *secretory phase,* when progesterone causes swelling and accumulation of secretory substances in the endometrial lining. These

Female reproductive cycle

The following information illustrates the interrelationships among hormones involved in the female reproductive cycle. The first panel shows the changes in follicle-stimulating hormone (FSH) and luteinizing hormone (LH) concentrations. The second panel displays the cyclic nature of estrogen and progesterone concentrations. The third panel illustrates the changes in the ovaries and endometrial tissue produced by FSH, LH, estrogens, and progesterone.

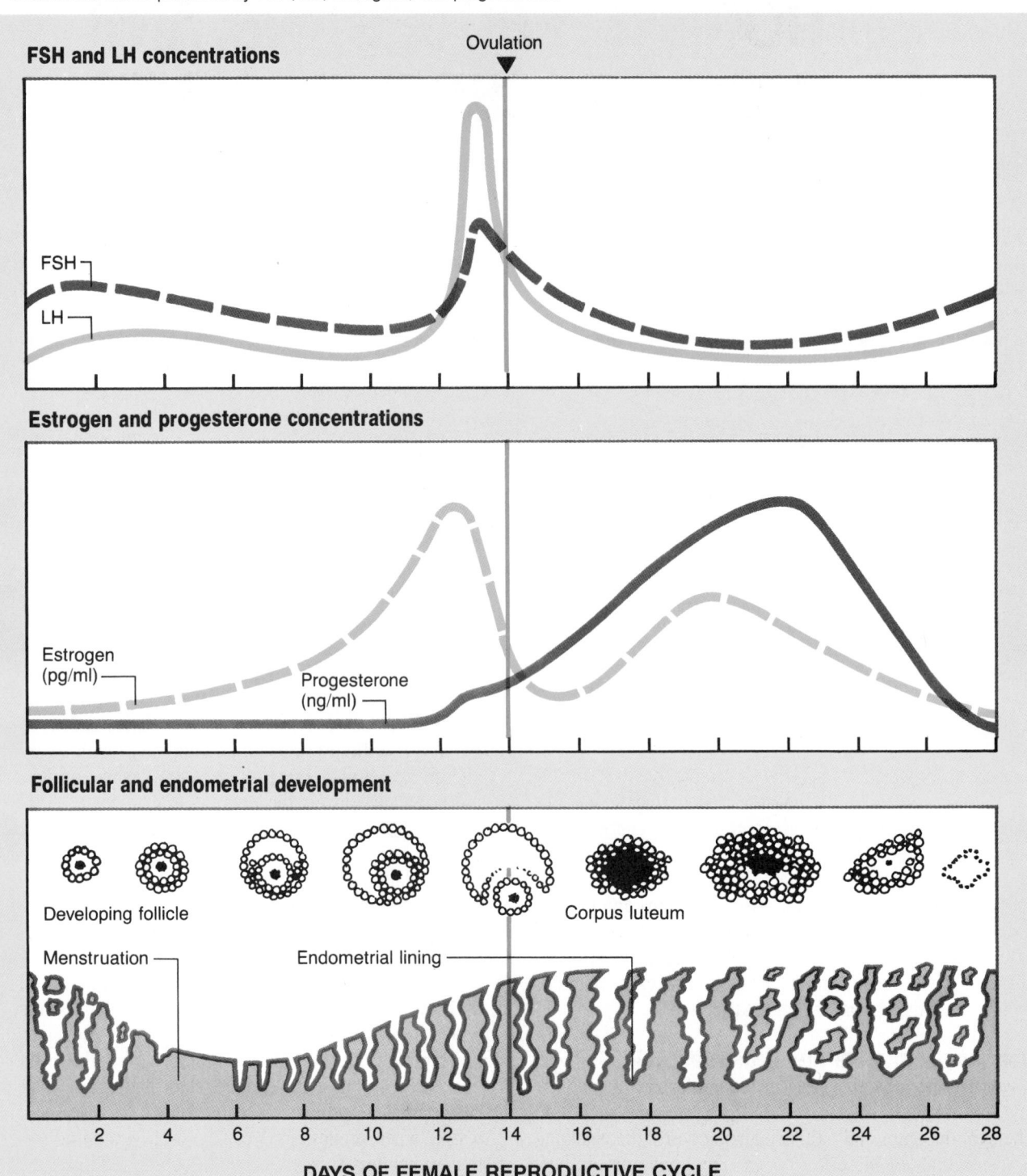

SELECTED NURSING DIAGNOSES

Estrogens, progestins, and oral contraceptive agents

The following nursing diagnoses address representative problems and etiologies that a nurse may encounter when caring for a patient who is receiving an estrogen, progestin, or oral contraceptive agent. Some of these nursing diagnoses contain generalized etiologies, which the nurse must individualize based on the patient's needs. (For some common nursing diagnoses and related interventions for each drug class, see the "Nursing Process Application" sections of this chapter.)

- Altered nutrition: less than body requirements, related to decreased folic acid absorption caused by an estrogen or oral contraceptive agent
- Altered nutrition: less than body requirements, related to progestin-induced weight loss
- Altered nutrition: more than body requirements, related to progestin-induced weight gain
- Altered protection related to the increased risk of cancer associated with estrogen or oral contraceptive use
- Altered protection related to metabolic abnormalities caused by an estrogen or oral contraceptive agent
- Altered cardiopulmonary tissue perfusion related to thromboembolism caused by an estrogen or progestin agent
- Altered sexuality patterns related to altered libido caused by an estrogen or oral contraceptive agent
- Altered thought processes related to depression caused by an estrogen or oral contraceptive agent
- Body image disturbance related to the adverse dermatologic effects of an estrogen, progestin, or oral contraceptive agent
- Constipation related to the adverse gastrointestinal (GI) effects of an oral contraceptive
- Diarrhea related to the adverse GI effects of an oral contraceptive
- Fatigue related to the adverse effects of a progestin
- Fluid volume excess related to fluid retention caused by an estrogen, progestin, or oral contraceptive agent
- Impaired tissue integrity related to progestin-induced cervical erosion

- Knowledge deficit related to the prescribed estrogen, progestin, or oral contraceptive agent
- Noncompliance related to adverse reactions to the prescribed estrogen, progestin, or oral contraceptive agent
- Pain related to breast tenderness caused by an estrogen, progestin, or oral contraceptive agent
- Pain related to migraine headache caused by an estrogen or oral contraceptive agent
- Potential fluid volume deficit related to the adverse GI effects of an oral contraceptive
- Potential for infection related to the increased risk of vaginal candidiasis associated with estrogen or progestin use
- Potential for injury related to a preexisting condition that contraindicates the use of an estrogen, progestin, or oral contraceptive agent
- Potential for injury related to a preexisting condition that requires cautious use of an estrogen, progestin, or oral contraceptive agent
- Potential for injury related to adverse drug reactions
- Potential for injury related to the adverse cardiovascular effects of an oral contraceptive agent
- Potential for trauma related to the adverse central nervous system effects of an estrogen or progestin agent
- Sensory-perceptual alterations (visual) related to vision disturbances caused by an estrogen or oral contraceptive agent
- Sleep pattern disturbance related to progestin-induced insomnia

changes allow accumulation of large stores of nutrients and provide appropriate conditions for the implantation of a fertilized ovum.

The postovulation surge in estrogen and progesterone production causes FSH and LH concentrations to decline sharply because of the negative feedback effect. The corpus luteum no longer can survive unless implantation of the fertilized ovum occurs. Degeneration of the corpus luteum results in sharply decreased estrogen and progesterone concentrations, causing desquamation of the superficial layers of the endometrium and menstrual bleeding. These hormonal decreases also cause cessation of the negative feedback effect on the pituitary, thereby allowing FSH and LH levels to increase and initiate a new cycle of follicular and endometrial growth.

If implantation occurs, the fertilized ovum secretes human chorionic gonadotropin, which prevents degeneration of the corpus luteum and thus promotes the continued secretion of estrogens and progesterone. The corpus luteum

continues its secretory action until about the twelfth week of pregnancy. At that point, the placenta secretes sufficient estrogens and progesterone to sustain the pregnancy on its own.

During pregnancy, elevated concentrations of estrogens and progesterone suppress LH and FSH secretion, thereby preventing ovulation and the development of follicles throughout the pregnancy.

This chapter details the natural and synthetic estrogens, used to correct estrogen-deficient states and to prevent pregnancy; the natural and synthetic progestins, used to restore or regulate the menstrual cycle and to treat premenstrual syndrome (PMS); and the oral contraceptives, used to prevent pregnancy.

For a summary of representative drugs, see *Selected major drugs: Estrogens, progestins, and oral contraceptive agents,* page 923. For a listing of applicable nursing diagnoses that the nurse may formulate when caring for a patient receiving these agents, see *Selected nursing diagnoses: Es-*

trogens, progestins, and oral contraceptive agents, page 907. For detailed information on applying the nursing process, see Chapter 6, The Nursing Process and Drug Therapy.

ESTROGENS

Estrogens are used to replace natural estrogen in estrogen-deficient states, to provide contraception, and to treat certain cancers, such as breast or prostate cancer.

The estrogens discussed in this section include the natural products (conjugated estrogenic substances, estradiol, and estrone) as well as the synthetic estrogens (chlorotrianisene, dienestrol, diethylstilbestrol, diethylstilbestrol diphosphate, esterified estrogens, estradiol cypionate and valerate, ethinyl estradiol, and quinestrol).

PHARMACOKINETICS

Estrogens are absorbed well and distributed throughout the body. Metabolism occurs in the liver, and the metabolites are excreted primarily by the kidneys.

Absorption, distribution, metabolism, excretion
After oral administration, natural estrogens and their derivatives are absorbed rapidly and well, but first-pass metabolism limits their potency by shortening their duration of action.

After absorption from the gastrointestinal (GI) tract, natural estrogens travel via the portal vein to the liver, where large amounts are metabolized rapidly to inactive compounds before entering the general circulation. Synthetic estrogens also are absorbed rapidly after oral administration, but they undergo less first-pass metabolism. As a result, they provide greater oral potency than the natural estrogens do. Estrogens also are absorbed rapidly and well after administration via the skin (transdermally) or mucous membranes. Because they do not undergo first-pass metabolism, estrogens administered by these routes reach higher levels in the body than orally administered preparations do.

Estrogens are distributed throughout most body tissues, but the highest concentrations are found in fat deposits. Estrogens are 50% to 80% bound to plasma proteins, primarily albumin. Natural estrogens are metabolized primarily in the liver. Most of an oral dose is inactivated via first-pass metabolism. The remaining unchanged drug and the metabolites are converted further in the liver to more water-soluble compounds.

The metabolic fate of synthetic estrogens has not been determined fully, but it appears to resemble that of the natural estrogens.

Estrogens and their metabolites are excreted primarily in urine, with small amounts excreted in feces.

Onset, peak, duration
Estrogens exert their pharmacologic effects via protein synthesis at the cellular level. The time required for this process varies greatly among the preparations.

Although estrogens reach peak plasma concentration levels within hours of administration, their onset of action may not occur for days, weeks, or even months after therapy begins. Their duration of action also is unrelated to their plasma concentration. Their plasma half-life is much shorter than their biological half-life.

PHARMACODYNAMICS

The estrogens primarily promote the growth and development of the female reproductive system. At puberty, estrogen secretion by the ovaries increases about twenty-fold, precipitating several major physiologic events — the female sex organs increase in size and become functional, the endometrium undergoes proliferation and becomes glandular in nature, and the vaginal epithelium becomes secretory. Furthermore, estrogen-induced metabolic changes result in the development of secondary female sex characteristics and cause increased fat deposition in the subcutaneous tissues. Estrogen also increases skeletal osteoblastic activity, causing a growth spurt as the woman reaches her reproductive years. After a few years, however, estrogen-stimulated fusion of the epiphysis and the shafts of the long bones halts further growth, which is why women usually do not reach the height of men.

Estrogen is responsible for the reepithelialization and proliferation of the endometrium before the ovulation phase of each reproductive cycle. The highly secretory endometrium contains large amounts of nutrients to support growth of a fertilized ovum. At the end of the reproductive cycle, estrogen and progesterone secretion declines, resulting in the abrupt breakdown of endometrial tissue and menstrual bleeding.

Mechanism of action
The exact mechanism of action of estrogen is not understood well but is believed to involve cytoplasmic receptor proteins found in estrogen-responsive tissues in the female breast and genitourinary tract. After estrogen binds to these cytoplasmic receptors, the resulting estrogen-receptor complex is transported into the nucleus. This action stimulates the synthesis of messenger ribonucleic acid (mRNA) and deoxyribonucleic acid (DNA), which in turn promotes the synthesis of specific proteins responsible for the actions of

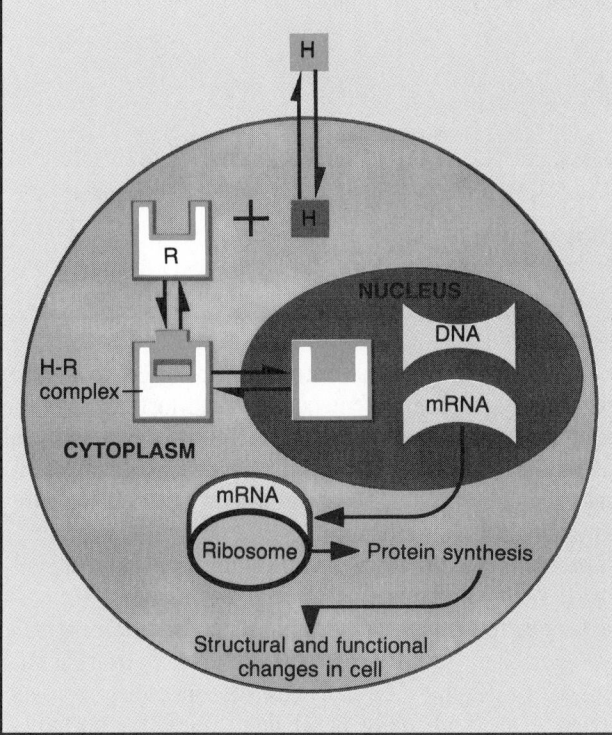

Mechanism of action of estrogens and progestins

This figure illustrates how estrogens and progestins exert their pharmacologic effects. The hormone (H) passes through the cell membrane into the cell cytoplasm, where it binds with a cytoplasmic receptor (R). The resulting hormone-receptor (H-R) complex is transported through the cytoplasm and into the cell nucleus, where it stimulates deoxyribonucleic acid (DNA) to produce messenger ribonucleic acid (mRNA). The mRNA contains the genetic coding for the production of specific proteins responsible for structural and functional changes in the cell. These changes produce the physiologic effects of the hormone.

the estrogens. (For a schematic representation, see *Mechanism of action of estrogens and progestins.*)

PHARMACOTHERAPEUTICS

Estrogens are prescribed primarily for hormonal replacement therapy in postmenopausal women to relieve symptoms caused by loss of ovarian function. Specific postmenopausal indications include the relief of vasomotor symptoms (hot flashes) and urogenital atrophy as well as the prevention of osteoporosis. Less commonly, estrogens are used for hormonal replacement therapy in patients with primary ovarian failure or female hypogonadism and in patients who have undergone surgical castration. Estrogens also are used to prevent postpartal breast engorgement in women who are not breast-feeding and palliatively to treat advanced, inoperable breast cancer in postmenopausal women and prostate cancer in men. (For more information about estrogen use in cancer patients, see Chapter 69, Hormonal Antineoplastic Agents.)

Estrogen therapy has been linked with increased risk of endometrial cancer, thromboembolism, hypertension, and other less serious adverse reactions. Adding progestin to estrogen therapy may reduce the risk of some of these reactions, particularly endometrial cancer. Because some data suggest an association between estrogen therapy and breast cancer, estrogenic agents are not recommended for women at high risk for breast cancer.

Estrogens are administered most commonly in a cyclic manner during 3 out of 4 weeks of a calendar month. However, this method can cause confusion because therapy may start or end on a different day each month. As an alternative, the patient may take the drug for the first 25 days of the month, not take the drug for the remaining 5 to 6 days, then resume the therapy. This regimen may prove easier to follow because it starts on the first day of the calendar month and always ends on day 25. If a progestin is added, it is administered during the last 10 days of each 25-day cycle. (For illustrations, see *Estrogen regimens*, page 910.)

Because orally administered estrogens undergo first-pass metabolism, they more commonly are associated with adverse reactions involving the liver, such as alterations in hepatic lipid metabolism thought to be responsible for thromboembolic diseases. To avoid first-pass metabolism, a transdermal delivery system for estradiol (Estraderm) has been developed.

chlorotrianisene (TACE). A synthetic estrogen, chlorotrianisene is administered P.O. or I.M. to relieve vasomotor symptoms of menopause and to treat atrophic vaginitis, female hypogonadism, and postpartal breast engorgement. *Usual adult dosage:* for menopausal symptoms, 12 to 25 mg P.O. daily in 21-day cycles; for atrophic vaginitis, 12 to 25 mg P.O. daily for 30 to 60 days; for female hypogonadism, 12 to 25 mg P.O. for 21 days, followed by one dose of 100 mg I.M. progesterone or 5 to 10 mg daily of medroxyprogesterone during the last 5 days of therapy; for postpartal breast engorgement, 72 mg P.O. b.i.d. for 2 days, 50 mg every 6 hours for six doses, or 12 mg q.i.d. for 7 days, starting within 8 hours after delivery.

conjugated estrogenic substances (Estrocon, Premarin). Administered P.O., I.M., I.V. or vaginally, these natural estrogenic substances are used to relieve vasomotor symptoms of menopause and to treat atrophic vaginitis, kraurosis vulvae, female hypogonadism, surgical castration, primary ovarian failure, postpartal breast engorge-

Estrogen regimens

In the traditional estrogen regimen, the patient receives 3 weeks of therapy followed by 1 drug-free week. In the example below, the second cycle starts on the 29th day and ends on the 18th day of the next month. In the alternative 25-day regimen, therapy starts on the first day and ends on the 25th day of each month, making it easier for the patient to follow month by month. In either regimen, progestin can be co-administered during the last 10 days of the cycle as a precaution against endometrial cancer.

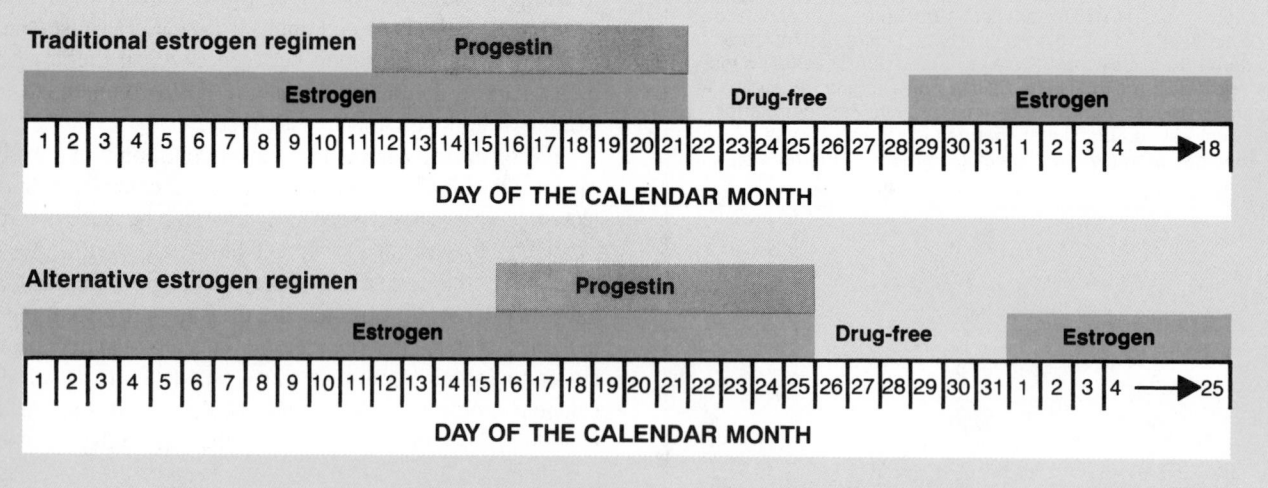

ment, osteoporosis, and abnormal uterine bleeding from hormonal imbalance.

Usual adult dosage: for atrophic vaginitis or kraurosis vulvae, 0.3 to 1.25 mg P.O. daily or 2 to 4 grams cream administered vaginally daily in 21-day cycles; for female hypogonadism, 2.5 mg P.O. b.i.d. or t.i.d. for 20 consecutive days each month; for surgical castration or primary ovarian failure, 1.25 mg P.O. daily in 21-day cycles; for menopausal symptoms, 0.3 to 1.25 mg P.O. daily in 21-day cycles; for postpartal breast engorgement, 3.75 mg P.O. every 4 hours for five doses or 1.25 mg P.O. every 4 hours for 5 days; for osteoporosis, 0.625 mg P.O. daily in 21-day cycles; for abnormal uterine bleeding caused by hormonal imbalance, 25 mg I.V. or I.M., repeated in 6 to 12 hours, as prescribed.

dienestrol (DV Cream, Ortho Dienestrol). A synthetic estrogen cream, dienestrol is administered vaginally to treat atrophic vaginitis and kraurosis vulvae (atrophy of the female external genitalia).

Usual adult dosage: for atrophic vaginitis or kraurosis vulvae, one to two applicatorsful of cream daily for 2 weeks, then half-doses for 2 weeks.

diethylstilbestrol [DES] and **diethylstilbestrol diphosphate** (Stilphostrol). Administered orally or by vaginal sup-

pository, these synthetic estrogens are used to relieve vasomotor symptoms of menopause and to treat atrophic vaginitis, kraurosis vulvae, female hypogonadism, surgical castration, primary ovarian failure, and postpartal breast engorgement. They also are used as a postcoital contraceptive ("morning-after" pill).

Usual adult dosage: for atrophic vaginitis or kraurosis vulvae, 0.1 to 1 mg by vaginal suppository daily for 10 to 14 days, or up to 5 mg/week by vaginal suppository; for female hypogonadism, surgical castration, or primary ovarian failure, 0.2 to 0.5 mg P.O. daily; for menopausal symptoms, 0.1 to 2 mg P.O. daily in 21-day cycles; for postcoital contraception, 25 mg P.O. b.i.d. for 5 days, starting within 72 hours after coitus; for postpartal breast engorgement, 5 mg P.O. daily or t.i.d., up to 30 mg.

esterified estrogens (Estratab, Estratest, Menest). These natural estrogen esters are administered orally to relieve postmenopausal symptoms and to treat female hypogonadism, surgical castration, and primary ovarian failure.

Usual adult dosage: for female hypogonadism, surgical castration, or primary ovarian failure, 2.5 mg P.O. daily to t.i.d. in 21-day cycles; for postmenopausal symptoms, 0.3 to 1.25 mg P.O. in 21-day cycles.

estradiol (Estrace, Estrace Vaginal Cream), **estradiol transdermal system** (Estraderm), **estradiol cypionate** (Depo-Estradiol Cypionate, Dura-Estrin, Estroject-LA), and **estradiol valerate** (Delestrogen, Duragen, Estradiol L.A., Valergen). Administered P.O., I.M., vaginally, or transdermally, these natural (estradiol) and synthetic estrogens are used to relieve vasomotor symptoms of menopause and to treat atrophic vaginitis, kraurosis vulvae, female hypogonadism, surgical castration, primary ovarian failure, and postpartal breast engorgement.

Usual adult dosage: for atrophic vaginitis or kraurosis vulvae, 2 to 4 grams estradiol cream administered vaginally daily for 1 to 2 weeks with a maintenance dosage of 1 gram one to three times weekly, or 1 to 2 mg estradiol P.O. daily in 21-day cycles; for female hypogonadism, surgical castration, primary ovarian failure, or menopausal symptoms, 1 to 2 mg estradiol P.O. daily in 21-day cycles, 1 to 5 mg estradiol cypionate I.M. monthly, 5 to 20 mg estradiol valerate I.M. every 4 weeks, or 0.05 to 0.1 mg daily estradiol transdermal patch twice weekly in 21-day cycles; for postpartal breast engorgement, 10 to 25 mg estradiol valerate I.M. at the end of the first stage of labor.

estrone (Bestrone, Kestrone-5, Theelin). A natural estrogen, estrone is administered I.M. to relieve menopausal symptoms and to treat atrophic vaginitis, kraurosis vulvae, female hypogonadism, and primary ovarian failure.

Usual adult dosage: for menopausal symptoms, atrophic vaginitis, and kraurosis vulvae, 0.1 to 0.5 mg I.M. two or three times weekly; for female hypogonadism and primary ovarian failure, 0.1 to 2 mg I.M. weekly.

ethinyl estradiol (Estinyl, Feminone). A synthetic estrogen administered orally, ethinyl estradiol is used to relieve menopausal symptoms and to treat female hypogonadism.

Usual adult dosage: for menopausal symptoms, 0.02 to 0.05 mg P.O. daily in 21-day cycles; for female hypogonadism, 0.05 mg P.O. daily to t.i.d. for 2 weeks per month, followed by 2 weeks of progesterone therapy, continued for 3 to 6 monthly cycles, followed by 2 months off therapy.

quinestrol (Estrovis). A long-acting synthetic estrogen, quinestrol is used to relieve menopausal symptoms and to treat female hypogonadism, primary ovarian failure, atrophic vaginitis, and kraurosis vulvae.

Usual adult dosage: for all indications, 100 mcg daily for 7 days, then no drug for 7 days, after which a maintenance dosage of 100 mcg weekly is begun; the dosage may be increased to 200 mcg weekly.

Drug interactions

Relatively few drugs interact with estrogens. Those that do, such as rifampin, barbiturates, carbamazepine, phenytoin, and primidone, typically result in decreased estrogenic activity, which may not be significant. Estrogens interfere with the absorption of dietary folic acid, which may result in a folic acid deficiency.

ADVERSE DRUG REACTIONS

Most adverse reactions to estrogens are mild and do not have serious or long-term consequences. However, endometrial and breast cancer may be more likely to occur in women taking estrogens. Most of the risk appears to be dose-related—higher dosages over longer periods increase the risk.

The risk of endometrial cancer increases fourfold to eightfold in women taking estrogens. However, mortality in this group does not seem to increase, probably because of the closer monitoring of patients on estrogen therapy and the less aggressive nature of these estrogen-induced cancers. An increased risk of breast cancer associated with low-dose estrogen replacement therapy has not been determined definitely. Evidence exists that progestin therapy (medroxyprogesterone 5 to 10 mg daily) added to the last 5 to 10 days of an estrogen therapy cycle may reduce the risk of endometrial and breast cancer.

Thromboembolic disorders have not been linked clearly to estrogen replacement therapy in postmenopausal women. However, the nurse should monitor such patients closely for thromboembolic disorders because they may occur.

The incidence of gallbladder disease increases with estrogen use. Increased blood pressure also may occur. Although such increases usually are minor and reversible, some women may develop hypertension.

Metabolic adverse reactions may include decreased glucose tolerance, altered thyroid and liver function test results, increased serum lipoprotein levels, fluid retention, decreased absorption of dietary folic acid, and cholestatic jaundice.

Adverse genitourinary reactions may include breakthrough bleeding, spotting, altered menstrual flow, dysmenorrhea, amenorrhea, and increased risk of vaginal candidiasis. Breast tenderness, enlargement, and secretions also can occur. Adverse central nervous system (CNS) reactions may include depression, migraine headaches, dizziness, and altered libido. Changed corneal curvature may cause vision disturbances or intolerance to hard or rigid gas-permeable contact lenses. Adverse reactions involving the skin include melasma and acne. Urticaria, skin rash, and very rare hypersensitivity reactions may occur.

NURSING PROCESS APPLICATION

The following information assists the nurse in caring for a patient who is receiving an estrogen.

Assessment

• Review the patient's history for a preexisting condition that contraindicates the use of an estrogen, such as known or suspected pregnancy, thrombophlebitis, a thromboembolic disorder, estrogen-dependent cancer of the breast or reproductive organs (except when used as palliative therapy for inoperable cancer in a postmenopausal woman), or undiagnosed abnormal uterine bleeding.

• Review the patient's history for a preexisting condition that requires cautious use of an estrogen, such as depression, a metabolic bone disease, blood dyscrasia, gallbladder disease, a seizure disorder, diabetes mellitus, amenorrhea, a family history of breast or genital cancer, or a condition aggravated by fluid retention.

• Assess the patient for adverse reactions to the prescribed estrogen, such as a thromboembolic disorder, gallbladder disease, metabolic changes, or genitourinary or CNS dysfunction.

• Assess the effectiveness of the prescribed estrogen periodically.

• Assess the patient for signs of fluid retention, such as jugular vein distention and swelling of the ankles, hands, and face.

• Evaluate the patient's and family's knowledge about the prescribed estrogen.

Nursing diagnoses

The following examples represent appropriate nursing diagnoses for a patient receiving an estrogen.

• Potential for injury related to a preexisting condition that contraindicates the use of an estrogen

• Potential for injury related to a preexisting condition that requires cautious use of an estrogen

• Potential for injury related to adverse drug reactions

• Fluid volume excess related to estrogen-induced fluid retention

• Knowledge deficit related to the prescribed estrogen

Planning and implementation

• Do not administer an estrogen to a patient with a condition that contraindicates its use.

• Administer an estrogen cautiously to a patient at risk because of a preexisting condition.

• Monitor the patient frequently for adverse reactions during estrogen therapy.

• Obtain a complete health history and perform a physical examination before estrogen therapy begins and every 6 to 12 months thereafter. During physical examinations, pay special attention to assessments of the patient's blood pressure, breasts, abdomen, pelvic organs, and hepatic function as well as to Papanicolaou (Pap) test results.

• *Determine if the patient is hypersensitive to natural oils (sesame, peanut, or castor oil) before estrogen adminis-*

tration because some I.M. products are dispersed in such oils.

• *Observe the patient closely for signs of a thromboembolic disorder, such as deep vein thrombosis (calf tenderness, redness, and warmth) or pulmonary embolism (sudden onset of shortness of breath, chest pain, and anxiety). Notify the physician immediately if they occur. Be prepared to administer treatment as prescribed.*

• *Monitor the patient's blood pressure frequently to detect estrogen-induced hypertension.*

• *Monitor the patient's blood glucose level regularly. For a diabetic patient, adjust the insulin or oral hypoglycemic agent dosage as prescribed.*

• Observe the patient for signs of folic acid deficiency, such as progressive fatigue, shortness of breath, weakness, irritability, or pallor.

• *Take safety measures if the patient experiences dizziness during estrogen therapy. For example, place the bed in the lowest position, keep the bed rails raised, and supervise ambulation.*

• Obtain a prescription for an analgesic if the patient develops headaches during estrogen therapy.

• Monitor the results of the following tests to detect estrogen-induced abnormalities: metyrapone test, platelet count, thyroid and liver function tests, prothrombin time (PT), and serum folate, serum triglyceride, and phospholipid level determinations. When any relevant specimen is submitted, inform the laboratory that the patient is receiving estrogen. Notify the physician of any abnormal test results.

• Roll the vial for I.M. administration between the palms to mix the contents completely.

• Administer an I.M. injection deeply into a large muscle.

• Notify the physician if adverse reactions occur.

• Monitor the patient for signs of fluid retention.

• Place the patient on a low-sodium diet and restrict fluid intake to no more than 2 liters a day, as prescribed, if fluid retention occurs.

• Notify the physician if fluid retention worsens.

Patient teaching

• Teach the patient and family the name, dose, frequency, action, and adverse effects of the prescribed estrogen.

• Advise the patient to read the estrogen package insert. Explain and reinforce this information, as needed. (For more information, see *Estrogen patient-teaching tips.*)

• *Instruct the patient to report signs and symptoms of disorders associated with estrogen use, such as abdominal pain or mass, severe headache, slurred speech, vomiting, dizziness, faintness, weakness, numbness, heaviness in the chest, shortness of breath, blurred vision, blind spots, breast lumps, yellow skin or sclera, dark urine, or light-colored stools.*

• *Counsel a sexually active woman of childbearing age to use an effective contraceptive method because estrogens*

Estrogen patient-teaching tips

The nurse should advise the patient to read the patient package insert before starting estrogen therapy. This insert provides information about the adverse reactions to estrogens and explains what precautions the patient should take during estrogen therapy. The patient should know the drug name, dosage, and schedule. The following material will help answer the patient's questions.

Why is this estrogen being prescribed?
• Estrogens are hormones produced by the body. When these natural hormones are deficient, synthetic estrogens are used in women to relieve unpleasant menopausal symptoms and medical problems (hot flashes, sweating, and brittle bones). Estrogens also are prescribed to treat some forms of cancer, including breast cancer and, in men, prostate cancer.

How should the estrogen be used?
• Estrogens are available in tablets, which should be swallowed whole.
• Estrogens also are available as vaginal creams or as suppositories to be inserted into the vagina. The physician, nurse, or pharmacist should explain to the patient exactly how to insert these products. The patient may want to use a sanitary napkin to avoid soiling clothing.
• Estrogens also are available as patches to be stuck on the skin like adhesive tape.
• Some estrogens are injected into muscle.

Which special instructions should the patient receive about using an estrogen?
• The patient should report known or suspected pregnancy to the physician immediately.

• The patient should keep all appointments for checkups so that the physician can check for any problems that may occur during estrogen therapy.
• The patient should inform the physician of the estrogen therapy before any type of laboratory test is performed.

How should estrogen be stored?
• The drug should be stored in its original container.
• The patient should keep this and all other medications out of the reach of children.

What should the patient do if she forgets to take a dose?
• The patient should take the dose as soon as she discovers the oversight but should not take two doses at the same time to make up for a missed dose.

What can the patient do about adverse reactions?
• The patient can eat a light snack to help relieve nausea, which should disappear after the estrogen has been taken for a while. However, the patient should inform her physician if nausea continues.
• The patient should not worry about breast tenderness or fullness, which is harmless.
• The patient should inform the physician about ankle swelling and weight gain, leg cramps, vaginal bleeding or discharge, or pain or tenderness in the groin or calf.

(especially diethylstilbestrol) can cause congenital fetal defects.
• Inform the patient that corneal curvature may change, causing vision disturbances or intolerance to hard or rigid gas-permeable contact lenses.
• Explain to the patient on cyclic therapy for postmenopausal symptoms that withdrawal bleeding may occur but does not indicate fertility restoration.
• *Instruct the diabetic patient to monitor the blood glucose level regularly and adjust the insulin or oral hyperglycemic agent dosage as prescribed if estrogen causes hyperglycemia.*
• Instruct the patient to avoid activities that require mental alertness if dizziness occurs.
• *Stress the importance of returning for follow-up examinations and laboratory tests as prescribed to detect adverse reactions, such as cancer.*
• *Teach the female patient how to perform breast self-examination.*
• Instruct the patient to notify the physician if any adverse reactions occur.

Evaluation

The following examples represent appropriate evaluation statements for a patient receiving an estrogen.
• The patient has no conditions that contraindicate estrogen therapy.
• The patient exhibits no signs of complications in the preexisting condition linked to the prescribed estrogen.
• The patient displays no signs of adverse reactions to the prescribed estrogen.
• The patient maintains normal fluid balance.
• The patient and family express an accurate understanding of the points taught about the prescribed estrogen.
• The patient correctly identifies adverse drug reactions that must be reported to the physician.

PROGESTINS

Progestins have pharmacologic properties similar to those of the natural female sex hormone progesterone, which acts primarily to prepare the endometrium for pregnancy and the breasts for lactation. Progestins are used to regulate or restore the menstrual cycle and to treat endometrial or renal cancer, endometriosis, and PMS. With estrogens, progestins also are used as oral contraceptives.

Progesterone is the major natural hormone in this drug class, but it has limited potency (a short duration of action) when administered orally because it undergoes rapid and extensive first-pass metabolism in the liver. To overcome this disadvantage, researchers have developed several synthetic progestins that remain active when administered orally. Of these, medroxyprogesterone acetate, norethindrone, and norethindrone acetate are used most commonly. Hydroxyprogesterone caproate is a synthetic agent that is administered I.M.

PHARMACOKINETICS

Progestins are absorbed well and distributed throughout the body. Metabolism occurs in the liver, and the metabolites are excreted primarily by the kidneys.

Absorption, distribution, metabolism, excretion

Natural and synthetic progestins are absorbed rapidly and well when administered orally. However, they have limited potency because first-pass metabolism shortens their duration of action. The natural progestin, progesterone, is most active when administered parenterally. Like natural progesterone, orally administered synthetic progestins also undergo first-pass metabolism but not as extensively as the natural agent does. Progestins are absorbed rapidly and well through the skin and mucous membranes.

Progestins are 80% to 95% bound to the plasma proteins albumin and sex hormone-binding globulin; small amounts are stored in body fat.

Progestins are metabolized primarily in the liver. Most of an oral dose is inactivated via first-pass metabolism. The remaining unchanged drug and the metabolites are converted further in the liver to more water-soluble compounds.

Progestins and their metabolites are excreted primarily in urine, with small amounts excreted in feces.

Onset, peak, duration

Like estrogens, progestins exert their pharmacologic effects via protein synthesis at the cellular level. Although these drugs reach peak plasma concentration levels within hours of administration, their onset of action may not occur for days or weeks after initiation of therapy. Their duration of action also is unrelated to their plasma concentrations. Hydroxyprogesterone has a long duration (7 to 14 days). Their plasma half-life is much shorter than their biological half-life.

PHARMACODYNAMICS

Progesterone commonly is called the "pregnancy hormone" because it functions primarily to prepare the uterus to receive and nourish the fertilized ovum. Under the influence of progesterone, the endometrium swells and becomes highly secretory. Progesterone also decreases the frequency of uterine muscle contractions, thereby preventing expulsion of the implanted ovum, and stimulates the secretory cells of the breast (the alveoli). Finally, the cyclic withdrawal of progesterone toward the end of the menstrual cycle leads to breakdown of the endometrium, beginning menstruation.

Mechanism of action

At the cellular level, progestins act on receptor proteins in cellular cytoplasm. The resulting progesterone-receptor complex is transported into the cell nucleus, where the synthesis of mRNA is stimulated. Under the direction of mRNA, the cell produces various proteins that are responsible for the pharmacologic effects of the progestins.

PHARMACOTHERAPEUTICS

Natural progesterone and its synthetic derivatives are used to treat ovarian disorders. The primary clinical indications for progestin therapy are amenorrhea and abnormal uterine bleeding caused by hormonal imbalance. These conditions are characterized by an absent or abnormal menstrual flow, so the goal of therapy is to restore a regular menstrual cycle. This goal is accomplished by administering estrogens and progestins in a cyclic pattern that resembles the natural secretion pattern of estrogen and progesterone.

Continuous progestin therapy is used to treat endometriosis by preventing menstruation for several months, thereby relieving the symptoms and promoting the regression of the ectopic endometrial growths.

Singly and in combination with estrogens, progestins also are used commonly as oral contraceptives. (For a complete discussion of this use, see the Oral Contraceptives section later in this chapter.) They are used less commonly to treat PMS and to provide palliative therapy for advanced metastatic endometrial and renal cancer. (For information about the use of progestins in cancer patients, see Chapter 69, Hormonal Antineoplastic Agents.)

Despite their therapeutic value, progestins have some disadvantages. For example, when they are used for prolonged periods, such as for endometriosis, ovulation may not resume for several months after discontinuation of therapy. Also, progestin use should be avoided during pregnancy because the drug can lead to congenital fetal defects.

hydroxyprogesterone caproate (Delalutin, Duralutin). A synthetic progestin administered I.M., hydroxyprogesterone is used to treat amenorrhea and abnormal uterine bleeding caused by hormonal imbalance.
Usual adult dosage: for amenorrhea or abnormal uterine bleeding, 375 mg I.M. every 4 weeks if needed, not to extend beyond four cycles.

medroxyprogesterone acetate (Amen, Curretab, Depo-Provera, Provera). A synthetic preparation, medroxyprogesterone is used to treat amenorrhea and abnormal uterine bleeding caused by hormonal imbalance.
Usual adult dosage: for amenorrhea or abnormal uterine bleeding, 5 to 10 mg P.O. daily for 5 to 10 days beginning on day 16 of the menstrual cycle; if the patient has received estrogen previously, 10 mg P.O. daily for 10 days beginning on day 16 of the menstrual cycle.

norethindrone (Norlutin). An orally active synthetic agent, norethindrone is used to treat amenorrhea, abnormal uterine bleeding caused by hormonal imbalance, and endometriosis. However, the drug must be used cautiously in a patient with cardiac or renal impairment because it causes fluid retention.
Usual adult dosage: for amenorrhea or abnormal uterine bleeding, 5 to 20 mg P.O. daily from day 5 through day 25 of the menstrual cycle; for endometriosis, 10 mg P.O. daily for 14 days, then increased by 5 mg daily at 14-day intervals up to a total of 30 mg daily.

norethindrone acetate (Aygestin, Norlutate). Twice as potent as norethindrone, this oral synthetic agent is used to treat amenorrhea, abnormal uterine bleeding caused by hormonal imbalance, and endometriosis.
Usual adult dosage: for amenorrhea or abnormal uterine bleeding, 2.5 to 10 mg P.O. daily from day 5 through day 25 of the menstrual cycle; for endometriosis, 5 mg P.O. daily for 14 days, then increased by 2.5 mg daily at 14-day intervals up to a total of 15 mg daily.

progesterone (Femotrone, Profac-O, Progelan, Progest-50, Progestaject-50). This natural progestin preparation is administered I.M. or by vaginal or rectal suppository to treat amenorrhea, abnormal uterine bleeding from hormonal imbalance, and PMS.
Usual adult dosage: for amenorrhea, 5 to 10 mg I.M. daily for 6 to 8 days starting 8 to 10 days before the anticipated start of menstruation; for abnormal uterine bleeding, 5 to 10 mg I.M. daily for 6 days, or as a single 50- to 100-mg I.M. dose; for PMS, 200- to 400-mg suppository once or twice a day, administered vaginally or rectally.

Drug interactions

Rifampin may increase the excretion rate of progestins.

ADVERSE DRUG REACTIONS

The progestins produce several minor adverse reactions, such as altered vaginal bleeding, breast tenderness, and edema. They rarely produce hypersensitivity reactions.

Breakthrough bleeding, spotting, changes in menstrual flow, and amenorrhea are the most common adverse reactions to the progestins. Cervical erosions or abnormal secretions, uterine fibromas, vaginal candidiasis, edema, weight gain or loss, depression, cholestatic jaundice, and melasma also may occur. Occasional adverse CNS reactions include migraine headaches, dizziness, nervousness, insomnia, and fatigue. Rare reactions include breast tenderness and galactorrhea.

Progestins and estrogens used in combination as oral contraceptives have been associated with an increased risk of thrombophlebitis, pulmonary embolism, and cerebral embolism. Because these disorders also may occur in patients receiving progestins alone, the nurse should monitor all patients receiving these agents for signs and symptoms of these disorders.

Hypersensitivity reactions, including urticaria, pruritus, angioedema, and generalized skin rash (with or without pruritus) have occurred. Anaphylaxis is rare.

NURSING PROCESS APPLICATION

The following information assists the nurse in caring for a patient who is receiving a progestin.

Assessment
• Review the patient's history for a preexisting condition that contraindicates the use of a progestin, such as known or suspected pregnancy, thrombophlebitis, a thromboembolic disorder, cancer of the breast or reproductive organs (except for palliative therapy for inoperable cancer in a postmenopausal woman), hepatic disease or dysfunction, undiagnosed abnormal uterine bleeding, or missed abortion.
• Review the patient's history for a preexisting condition that requires cautious use of a progestin, such as cardiac or renal impairment.
• Assess the patient for adverse reactions to the prescribed progestin, such as changes in vaginal bleeding patterns, breast tenderness, CNS reactions, thrombophlebitis, or pulmonary embolism.
• Review the patient's medication history to identify the use of drugs that may interact with the progestin, such as rifampin.
• Assess the effectiveness of the progestin periodically.
• Assess the patient's sleep pattern to detect insomnia.
• Assess the patient for signs of fluid retention, such as jugular vein distention and edema of the ankles, hands, or face.

• Evaluate the patient's and family's knowledge about the prescribed progestin.

Nursing diagnoses

The following examples represent appropriate nursing diagnoses for a patient receiving a progestin.
• Potential for injury related to a preexisting condition that contraindicates the use of a progestin
• Potential for injury related to a preexisting condition that requires cautious use of a progestin
• Potential for injury related to adverse drug reactions
• Sleep pattern disturbance related to progestin-induced insomnia
• Fluid volume excess related to progestin-induced fluid retention
• Knowledge deficit related to the prescribed progestin

Planning and implementation

• Do not administer a progestin to a patient with a condition that contraindicates its use.
• Administer a progestin cautiously to a patient at risk because of a preexisting condition.
• Monitor the patient frequently for adverse reactions during progestin therapy. Particularly note changes in vaginal bleeding patterns, such as breakthrough bleeding, spotting, changes in menstrual flow, or amenorrhea. Notify the physician if these changes persist or worsen.
• Obtain a prescription for an analgesic if the patient experiences a migraine headache.
• *Take safety precautions if the patient experiences dizziness. For example, place the bed in the lowest position, keep the bed rails raised, and supervise ambulation.*
• *Observe the patient for signs of thromboembolic disorders, such as thrombophlebitis (calf tenderness, redness, and warmth), pulmonary embolism (sudden onset of shortness of breath, chest pain, and anxiety), or cerebral embolism (abrupt change in consciousness). Notify the physician immediately if any of these signs or symptoms occur and prepare to administer treatment as prescribed.*
• *Determine if the patient is hypersensitive to natural oils (sesame, castor, or peanut oil) before progestin administration because I.M. solutions are dispersed in such oils.*
• *Keep standard emergency equipment nearby because anaphylaxis can occur. Observe the patient closely for signs of hypersensitivity reactions, such as urticaria, pruritus, angioedema, or generalized skin rash when beginning progestin therapy. If these signs occur, consult with the physician about discontinuing therapy.*
• Monitor the results of the following tests to detect progestin-induced abnormalities: urine pregnanediol determination and serum alkaline phosphatase, plasma amino acid, and urinary nitrogen levels. When any specimen is submitted for testing, inform the laboratory that the patient is receiving progestin.

• Roll the vial for I.M. administration between the palms to mix the contents completely.
• Administer an I.M. injection deeply into a large muscle.
• Notify the physician if adverse reactions occur.
• Obtain a prescription for a hypnotic agent if the patient experiences insomnia during progestin therapy.
• Monitor the patient for signs of fluid retention.
• Place the patient on a low-sodium diet and restrict fluid intake to no more than 2 liters a day, as prescribed, if fluid retention occurs.
• Notify the physician if fluid retention increases.

Patient teaching

• Teach the patient and family the name, dose, frequency, action, and adverse effects of the prescribed progestin.
• Advise the patient to read the progestin package insert. Explain and reinforce this information, as needed. (For more information, see *Progestin patient-teaching tips.*)
• Explain to the patient that routine follow-up examinations should be performed every 6 to 12 months, with special attention given to the breasts and pelvic organs, the Pap test, and liver function tests.
• *Teach the female patient how to perform breast self-examination.*
• Advise the patient to avoid activities that require mental alertness if dizziness occurs.
• *Teach the patient to report any signs of thromboembolic disorders, including pain in the chest, groin, or calf; headache or changes in vision; shortness of breath; or slurred speech.*
• *Counsel a sexually active woman of childbearing age to use an effective contraceptive method because progestins may cause congenital fetal defects.*
• Teach the patient with insomnia to use relaxation techniques, such as reading or taking a warm bath before bedtime, to promote sleep. If insomnia persists, advise the patient to consult the physician for a hypnotic agent.
• Instruct the patient to notify the physician if any adverse reactions occur or if concerns arise regarding progestin therapy.

Evaluation

The following examples represent appropriate evaluation statements for a patient receiving a progestin.
• The patient has no conditions that contraindicate progestin therapy.
• The patient exhibits no signs of complications in the preexisting condition linked to the prescribed progestin.
• The patient demonstrates no adverse reactions to the prescribed progestin.
• The patient reports undisturbed sleep patterns during progestin therapy.
• The patient maintains normal fluid balance.

Progestin patient-teaching tips

The nurse should see that the patient receives and reads the patient package insert, which provides information about adverse reactions to progestins and explains which precautions to take during progestin therapy. The patient should know the drug name, dosage, and schedule. The following material will help answer the patient's questions.

Why is this progestin being prescribed?
• Progestins are hormones produced by the body. They are used to regulate the menstrual cycle and to treat endometriosis and some cases of breast and kidney cancer.

How should the progestin be used?
• Some progestins are taken in tablet form; others are injected into the muscle.

Which special instructions should the patient receive while using a progestin?
• The patient should stop taking the drug and inform the physician immediately of known or suspected pregnancy.
• The patient should keep all appointments for checkups so that the physician can detect any problems that may occur during progestin therapy.
• The patient should inform the physician of the progestin therapy before any laboratory test is performed.

How should progestin be stored?
• The drug should be stored in its original container.
• The patient should keep this and all other medications out of the reach of children.

What should the patient do if she forgets to take a dose?
• The patient should take the dose as soon as she discovers the oversight but should not take two doses at the same time to make up for a missed dose.

What can the patient do about adverse reactions?
• The patient can eat a light snack to help relieve nausea.
• The patient should expect breast tenderness or fullness, which is harmless.
• The patient should inform the physician about any ankle swelling, weight gain, leg cramps, vaginal bleeding or discharge, or pain or tenderness in the groin or calf.

• The patient and family express an accurate understanding of the points taught about the prescribed progestin.
• The patient schedules routine follow-up examinations and tests, as recommended.

ORAL CONTRACEPTIVES

The oral contraceptives were the first drugs developed for use in healthy individuals. They are used not to cure disease, but to prevent a condition that arises from normal physiologic events. Currently available contraceptive agents are combination products containing 50 mcg or less of estrogen and 1 mg or less of progestin. The few progestin-only preparations are known as minipills.

This section discusses the following oral contraceptives: ethinyl estradiol-ethynodiol diacetate, ethinyl estradiol-levonorgestrel, ethinyl estradiol-norethindrone, ethinyl estradiol-norethindrone acetate, ethinyl estradiol-norgestrel, mestranol-norethindrone, mestranol-norethynodrel, norethindrone, and norgestrel.

PHARMACOKINETICS

The pharmacokinetic profiles of the oral contraceptives are the same as those of the estrogens and progestins described earlier in this chapter.

Absorption, distribution, metabolism, excretion

Oral contraceptives are absorbed well and are distributed throughout the body. Metabolism occurs in the liver, and the metabolites are excreted primarily by the kidneys.

Only two estrogens, ethinyl estradiol and mestranol, are used currently in oral contraceptives. Ethinyl estradiol, the more potent of the two agents, is used in nearly all low-dose preparations. Mestranol, found primarily in the high-dose products, is metabolized to ethinyl estradiol in the liver. Among the progestins used in the various oral contraceptives, norethynodrel, ethynodiol diacetate, and norethindrone acetate are metabolized to norethindrone by the liver.

Onset, peak, duration

The onset of action of the oral contraceptives is delayed somewhat because of their mechanisms of action. Full contraceptive benefits are not experienced until the contraceptive agents have been taken for at least 10 days. As a result, a woman starting contraceptive therapy should use a back-up contraceptive method, such as condoms, a diaphragm, or spermicidal foam, during the first month.

Oral contraceptives remain effective throughout the 21-day cycle. When the woman has taken all of the tablets properly, the contraceptive efficacy extends through the 7-day contraceptive-free period each month. If doses are missed immediately before or after the contraceptive-free period, however, the likelihood of breakthrough ovulation and contraceptive failure is great. This is especially true for low-dose products containing estrogen and progestin.

Ovulation usually resumes within three to six menstrual cycles after discontinuation of oral contraceptives. Women are advised to wait to become pregnant until three menstrual cycles have passed after discontinuation of oral contraceptives, because the endometrium may require up to 3 months to regain its normal physiology.

PHARMACODYNAMICS

Estrogens and progesterone are endogenous substances that are responsible for ovulation and the nurturing of the fertilized ovum after implantation. Exogenous estrogens and progestins can promote changes in the female reproductive organs that help prevent fertilization and implantation even if ovulation occurs.

Mechanism of action

Estrogens act as contraceptives by suppressing ovulation and inhibiting implantation of the fertilized ovum. Oral contraceptives create negative feedback to the hypothalamus and pituitary gland, reducing FSH and LH concentrations. The diminished FSH concentration prevents follicle development, and the absence of the midcycle surge of LH prevents ovulation. Although estrogens are 95% to 98% effective in inhibiting ovulation, the chance of ovulation increases when doses are missed and when low doses of estrogen are used.

Estrogens can interfere with implantation of the fertilized ovum by altering ovum transport and by inhibiting the normal secretory development of the endometrium. Alteration of ovum transport can cause the fertilized ovum to be delivered to the uterus at a time improper for implantation. Inhibited secretory development of the endometrium can result in unfavorable conditions for implantation. Interference with ovum implantation is the main mechanism of action of the estrogen-only postcoital contraceptives.

Progestins also inhibit ovulation via the negative feedback mechanism, making combinations of estrogen and progestin nearly 100% effective. However, noncompliance and low doses of progestin reduce the efficacy of these products.

Besides inhibiting ovulation, pharmacologically increased concentrations of progestin occurring during the first half of the female reproductive cycle promote changes in the endometrium that make it unsuitable for ovum implantation. Progestins also thicken cervical mucus, blocking sperm migration toward the ovum. Finally, progestins can slow ovum transport through the fallopian tubes. This may be why women taking the minipill have a higher incidence of tubal and ectopic pregnancies.

PHARMACOTHERAPEUTICS

Oral contraceptives are used primarily to prevent pregnancy and are the most effective form of reversible contraception available. With proper administration, the theoretical failure rate is less than one pregnancy per 100 women per year. Higher failure rates occur with irregular use, missed doses, and estrogen doses less than 20 mcg.

Oral contraceptives containing high doses of estrogen and progestin may be used to treat hypermenorrhea and endometriosis and to promote cyclic withdrawal bleeding. Progestin-dominant oral contraceptives (those providing mainly progestin effects) sometimes are used to treat dysmenorrhea. Because most of the severe adverse reactions to oral contraceptives are dose-related, the trend is toward use of lower-dose contraceptives.

Several types of combination oral contraceptives are available. Most are monophasic, providing fixed doses of estrogen and progestin throughout the 21-day cycle. One biphasic product delivers a constant amount of estrogen throughout the 21-day cycle but an increased amount of progestin for the last 11 days. The newest oral contraceptives are triphasic formulations. Two of these provide fixed doses of estrogen throughout the 21-day cycle, with progestin doses varying every 7 days. The others are tablets that vary the estrogen and progestin doses every 7 days throughout the 21-day cycle.

ethinyl estradiol-ethynodiol diacetate (Demulen 1/35-21, Demulen 1/50-21, Demulen 1/50-28). This monophasic oral contraceptive provides relatively well-balanced estrogen and progestin effects.
Usual adult dosage: for contraception with the 21-day products, one tablet P.O. daily, followed by 7 days without a dose before beginning the next cycle of tablets; for contraception with the 28-day product, one tablet P.O. daily.

ethinyl estradiol-levonorgestrel (Levlen, Nordette, Tri-Levlen, Triphasil). Levlen and Nordette are monophasic oral contraceptives with slightly progestin-dominant formulations. Tri-Levlen and Triphasil are triphasic products that provide relatively well-balanced estrogen and progestin activity throughout the 21-day cycle.
Usual adult dosage: for contraception with the 21-day products, one tablet P.O. daily, followed by 7 days without a dose before beginning the next cycle of tablets; for contraception with the 28-day products, one tablet P.O. daily.

ethinyl estradiol-norethindrone (Brevicon, Genora 1/35, ModiCon, N.E.E. 1/35, Nelova 1/35E, Norcept-E 1/35, Norethin 1/35E, Norinyl 1+35, Ortho-Novum 1/35, Ortho-Novum 7/7/7, Ortho-Novum 10/11, Ovcon-35, Ovcon-50, Tri-Norinyl). Ovcon, Brevicon, and ModiCon are slightly estrogen-dominant monophasic oral contraceptives. Genora, N.E.E. 1/35, Nelova 1/35E, Norcept-E 1/35, Norethin 1/35E, Norinyl, and Ortho-Novum 1/35 also are monophasic preparations, but they provide relatively well-balanced estrogen and progestin effects. A biphasic formulation, Ortho-Novum 10/11, provides estrogen-dominant effects during days 1 to 10, then relatively well-balanced estrogen and progestin effects during days 11 to 21 of the 21-day cycle. Ortho-Novum 7/7/7 and Tri-Norinyl are triphasic oral contraceptives that provide relatively well-balanced estrogen and progestin effects during the 21-day cycle. Both products are slightly estrogen-dominant during days 1 to 7 and slightly progestin-dominant during days 15 to 21.

Usual adult dosage: for contraception with the 21-day products, one tablet P.O. daily, followed by 7 days without a dose before beginning the next cycle of tablets; for contraception with the 28-day products, one tablet P.O. daily.

ethinyl estradiol-norethindrone acetate (Loestrin 1/20, Loestrin 1.5/30, Loestrin Fe 1/20, Loestrin Fe 21 1.5/30, Norlestrin 1/50, Norlestrin 2.5/50, Norlestrin Fe 1/50, Norlestrin Fe 2.5/50). These oral contraceptives are monophasic formulations. Loestrin products are progestin-dominant. Norlestrin products provide relatively well-balanced estrogen and progestin effects.

Usual adult dosage: for contraception with the 21-day products, one tablet P.O. daily, followed by 7 days without a dose before beginning the next cycle of tablets; for contraception with the 28-day products, 1 tablet P.O. daily.

ethinyl estradiol-norgestrel (Lo/Ovral, Ovral). These monophasic oral contraceptives include Ovral, a progestin-dominant formulation, which also is used for postcoital contraception. Lo/Ovral provides relatively well-balanced estrogen and progestin effects.

Usual adult dosage: for contraception with the 21-day products, one tablet P.O. daily, followed by 7 days without a dose before beginning the next cycle of tablets; for contraception with the 28-day products, one tablet P.O. daily; for postcoital contraception, two tablets P.O. within 24 to 72 hours of unprotected intercourse and two more tablets 12 hours later.

mestranol-norethindrone (Genora 1/50, Nelova 1/50M, Norinyl 1 + 50, Norinyl 1 + 80, Norinyl 2 mg, Ortho-Novum 1/50, Ortho-Novum 1/80, Ortho-Novum 2 mg). Norinyl 2 mg and Ortho-Novum 2 mg are monophasic progestin-dominant oral contraceptives also used to treat hypermenorrhea. Genora 1/50, Nelova 1/50M, Norinyl 1 + 50, and Ortho-Novum 1/50 provide relatively well-balanced estrogen and progestin effects. Norinyl 1 + 80 and Ortho-Novum 1/80 are estrogen-dominant products.

Usual adult dosage: for contraception with the 21-day products, one tablet P.O. daily, followed by 7 days without a dose before beginning the next cycle of tablets; for contraception with the 28-day products, 1 tablet P.O. daily; for hypermenorrhea, a 3-month course of therapy with Norinyl 2 mg, one tablet P.O. daily for 20 days, followed by 8 days without a dose before beginning the next cycle of tablets; or a 3-month course of therapy with Ortho-Novum 2 mg, one tablet P.O. daily for 21 days, followed by 7 days without a dose before beginning the next cycle of tablets.

mestranol-norethynodrel (Enovid, Enovid-E). These products are estrogen-dominant monophasic formulations. Enovid-E is used as a contraceptive; Enovid is used to treat endometriosis and hypermenorrhea.

Usual adult dosage: for contraception with Enovid-E, one tablet P.O. daily, followed by 7 days without a dose before beginning the next cycle of tablets; for severe hypermenorrhea, 20 to 30 mg of Enovid P.O. daily until bleeding is controlled, then 10 mg P.O. daily through day 24 of the cycle; for endometriosis, 5 or 10 mg of Enovid P.O. daily for 14 days, increased by 5 or 10 mg every 14 days until a daily dose of 20 mg is achieved, then 20 mg/day continuously for 6 to 9 months.

norethindrone (Micronor, Nor-Q.D.). This is a noncyclic, progestin-only oral contraceptive.

Usual adult dosage: one tablet P.O. daily on a continual basis.

norgestrel (Ovrette). This is a noncyclic, progestin-only oral contraceptive.

Usual adult dosage: one tablet P.O. daily on a continual basis.

Drug interactions
Relatively few interactions occur between oral contraceptives and other drugs. However, those few interactions are clinically significant. (For more information, see *Drug interactions: Oral contraceptives,* page 920.)

ADVERSE DRUG REACTIONS

The oral contraceptives can produce adverse reactions that range from severe to merely annoying. Many common adverse reactions are related to the estrogen content of oral contraceptives. The reactions tend to be most pronounced during the first cycle of oral contraceptive therapy and usually abate after three or four cycles.

The most common adverse reaction is nausea. Other GI reactions can include vomiting, abdominal cramping, diarrhea, and constipation.

Melasma is the most common dermatologic adverse reaction. Facial hyperpigmentation may develop 1 month to 2 years after the initiation of oral contraceptive therapy, fades very slowly, and may be permanent. Paradoxically, acne may improve or develop. Estrogen-dominant products tend to improve it; progestin-dominant products tend to cause or worsen it.

Serious cardiovascular reactions can result from oral contraceptive use. The incidence of hypertension in women using oral contraceptives is about two to three times that of nonusers. Researchers have not determined whether estrogen or progestin is primarily responsible. Women taking oral contraceptives also are at greater risk for developing

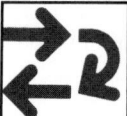

DRUG INTERACTIONS

Oral contraceptives

This chart summarizes the major interactions that can occur between the oral contraceptives and other drugs.

DRUG	INTERACTING DRUGS	POSSIBLE EFFECTS	NURSING IMPLICATIONS
all combination oral contraceptives, especially the low-dose monophasic and the biphasic and triphasic products	barbiturates, carbamazepine, phenylbutazone, phenytoin, primidone, rifampin	May cause rapid metabolism of oral contraceptives, leading to breakthrough bleeding and decreased contraceptive efficacy	• Advise the patient to use an alternative contraceptive method if therapy with known enzyme-inducers is necessary.
	ampicillin, penicillin V, tetracycline	May alter GI bacterial flora, leading to decreased contraceptive efficacy and breakthrough bleeding	• Advise the patient to use an alternative contraceptive method during anti-infective therapy and for 1 week after its discontinuation.
	benzodiazepines	Decrease metabolism of oxidatively metabolized benzodiazepines and increase elimination of benzodiazepines that undergo glucuronide conjugation	• Monitor the patient for enhanced therapeutic effects of oxidatively metabolized benzodiazepines (alprazolam, chlordiazepoxide, clorazepate, diazepam, flurazepam, halazepam, and prazepam). • Administer a higher dosage of a benzodiazepine eliminated via glucuronide conjugation (lorazepam, oxazepam, and temazepam), if prescribed.
	corticosteroids	Enhance anti-inflammatory actions of corticosteroids	• Observe the patient for signs of excessive corticosteroid effects. • Alter the corticosteroid dosage, if prescribed, when an oral contraceptive is started or discontinued.
	cyclosporine	Increase plasma concentration of cyclosporine	• Monitor the patient's plasma cyclosporine concentration. • Reduce the cyclosporine dosage, if prescribed.

myocardial infarction. This risk increases with age, duration of oral contraceptive use, and especially cigarette smoking.

Oral contraceptives also are associated with an increased risk of thromboembolic disorders because of their estrogen and progestin content. (The current lower-dose formulations, however, are less likely to cause thromboembolic disorders than the original formulations.) The risk of developing cerebrovascular accidents and subarachnoid hemorrhage, also increased in patients taking oral contraceptives, is increased further if the patient smokes or has hypertension.

Endocrine and metabolic adverse reactions can occur. Decreased glucose tolerance appears to be related primarily to estrogen, but progestin also may be involved. Estrogens can increase the concentration of high-density lipoprotein; progestins can decrease it. Thus, the overall effect of an oral contraceptive on cholesterol level depends on whether it is estrogen- or progestin-dominant. Oral contraceptive use also may lead to folate deficiency.

Oral contraceptives can affect several serum proteins produced by the liver, elevate the thyroxine-binding globulin concentration, and alter albumin and immunoglobulin concentrations. Oral contraceptive users also have an increased incidence of liver tumors, primarily benign hepatic adenomas, and gallbladder disease.

Recent epidemiologic studies indicate that oral contraceptives may not be as carcinogenic as was believed. For example, none of the currently available oral contraceptives increases the risk of endometrial cancer. However, they may increase the risk of cervical cancer. Recent studies have found no association between oral contraceptive use and breast cancer.

Adverse genitourinary reactions may occur, depending on the estrogen or progestin dominance of the oral contraceptive. Dizziness, headache, depression, lethargy, decreased libido, fluid retention, and edema also are associated

Oral contraceptives: Summary of adverse reactions

This table summarizes the adverse reactions to an excess or deficiency of estrogen or progestin, which may result from aging or oral contraceptive use.

Estrogen excess

General effects
- Nausea and vomiting
- Dizziness
- Cyclic headaches
- Irritability
- Edema and fluid retention
- Cyclic weight gain and bloating
- Altered fit of rigid contact lenses
- Hypertension
- Thromboembolic disorder

Reproductive effects
- Breast tenderness and cystic changes
- Uterine enlargement
- Leukorrhea
- Hypermenorrhea
- Suppressed lactation

Estrogen deficiency

General effects
- Spotting and breakthrough bleeding on days 1 through 7
- Amenorrhea or decreased menstrual flow

Menopause-like effects
- Irritability
- Nervousness
- Depression
- Decreased libido
- Hot flashes and other vasomotor symptoms
- Atrophic vaginitis
- Dyspareunia

Progestin excess

General effects
- Noncyclic weight gain and increased appetite
- Fatigue and weakness
- Decreased menstrual flow
- Monilial vaginitis

Androgenic effects
- Oily skin and scalp
- Acne
- Hirsutism
- Depression

Pill-free day effects
- Nausea and vomiting
- Dizziness
- Cyclic headaches
- Edema and bloating
- Cyclic weight gain
- Breast tenderness

Progestin deficiency

General effects
- Breakthrough bleeding on days 8 through 21
- Heavy menstrual flow and clotting
- Delayed withdrawal bleeding
- Weight loss

---

with oral contraceptive use. Oral contraceptives also may worsen myopia and astigmatism and may alter the fit of rigid contact lenses.

Some oral contraceptive users have experienced hypersensitivity reactions, such as skin rashes, urticaria, and pruritus. (For a summary of hormone-related effects, see *Oral contraceptives: Summary of adverse reactions.*)

NURSING PROCESS APPLICATION

The following information assists the nurse in caring for a patient who is receiving an oral contraceptive.

Assessment

- Review the patient's history for a preexisting condition that contraindicates the use of an oral contraceptive, such as known or suspected pregnancy, thrombophlebitis, a thromboembolic disorder, estrogen-dependent cancer of the breast or reproductive organs (except when used as palliative therapy for inoperable cancer in a postmenopausal woman), or undiagnosed abnormal uterine bleeding.
- Review the patient's history for a preexisting condition that requires cautious use of an oral contraceptive, such as depression, metabolic bone disease, gallbladder disease, a blood dyscrasia, a seizure disorder, diabetes mellitus, amenorrhea, any condition that may be aggravated by fluid retention, or a family history of breast cancer.
- Assess the patient for adverse reactions to the prescribed oral contraceptive, such as GI, dermatologic, cardiovascular, endocrine, metabolic, or genitourinary dysfunction.
- Review the patient's medication history to identify the use of drugs that may interact with the oral contraceptive, such as barbiturates, ampicillin, benzodiazepines, corticosteroids, or cyclosporine.
- Assess the effectiveness of the oral contraceptive periodically.

Oral contraceptive patient-teaching tips

The nurse should see that the patient receives and reads the patient package insert before taking an oral contraceptive. This insert provides information about adverse reactions to oral contraceptives and explains which precautions to take while using them. The patient should know the drug name, dosage, and schedule. The following information will help answer the patient's questions.

Why is this oral contraceptive being prescribed?
• Oral contraceptives (birth control pills) contain two female sex hormones that prevent the release of an egg from the ovaries each month, thus preventing pregnancy. Oral contraceptives, the most effective birth control method, can prevent unplanned pregnancy almost completely if taken correctly.

How should the oral contraceptive be used?
• Oral contraceptives are pills that should be swallowed whole.
• The patient should use an alternative contraceptive method (condoms, spermicides, or diaphragm) for the first cycle (3 weeks) to ensure full protection.
• Oral contraceptives come in packs that contain 21 or 28 pills. In the 28-pill pack, the last seven pills are colored differently and are inactive. The patient should expect her period to begin while taking these last seven pills. If the patient is using the 21-pill pack, her period should begin a few days after taking the last pill in the pack.
• The physician will tell the patient how to start the first cycle. One way is to start taking the pills on the day 5 of menstrual bleeding. The other way is to take the first pill on the first Sunday after the patient's period begins. If her period begins on Sunday, she should take the first pill on that day.
• The pills must be taken exactly on schedule to ensure effectiveness. The patient should take the pill at the same time each day—for example, at bedtime or with breakfast.

Which special instructions should the patient follow when using an oral contraceptive?
• The patient should stop taking the pills and contact the physician if pregnancy is suspected or confirmed.
• The patient should keep all appointments for checkups so that the physician can detect any problems that may occur.

What can the patient do about adverse reactions?
• Although spotting or bleeding may occur during the first two cycles of birth control pills, the patient should report to the physician any spotting or bleeding that persists after the second cycle. Mild reactions, including nausea, weight gain, breast tenderness, and skin blotching, are not unusual. They should not cause alarm.
• If headache or nausea occurs, the patient may take the pill at bedtime to reduce the severity of these reactions.
• Severe adverse reactions, such as blood clots, rarely occur. However, blood clots can produce pain in the chest, arms, or legs; numbness; dizziness; headaches; or vision changes. If any of these symptoms appear, the patient should contact the physician immediately.

How should oral contraceptives be stored?
• The oral contraceptives should be stored in their original container.
• The patient should keep this and all other medications out of the reach of children.

What should the patient do if she forgets to take a dose?
• If the patient misses one pill, she should take it as soon as she remembers. (If she does not remember it until the next day, she should take two pills—the one she forgot and the one scheduled for that day.)
• If the patient misses two pills in a row, she should take two pills daily for the next 2 days and use an alternative contraceptive method during the rest of the cycle.
• If the patient misses three or more pills in a row, she should not take any more pills from that cycle and should discard the pack. She should use an alternative contraceptive method until her period begins, then start a new pack on the regular schedule.

• Evaluate the patient's knowledge about the prescribed oral contraceptive.

Nursing diagnoses
The following examples represent appropriate nursing diagnoses for a patient receiving an oral contraceptive.
• Potential for injury related to a preexisting condition that contraindicates the use of an oral contraceptive
• Potential for injury related to a preexisting condition that requires cautious use of an oral contraceptive
• Potential for injury related to adverse drug reactions
• Knowledge deficit related to the prescribed oral contraceptive

Planning and implementation
• Do not administer an oral contraceptive to a patient with a condition that contraindicates its use.

• Administer an oral contraceptive cautiously to a patient at risk because of a preexisting condition.
• Monitor the patient frequently for adverse reactions during oral contraceptive use.
• Notify the physician if the patient reports or exhibits adverse reactions. Be prepared to implement treatment, as prescribed.

Patient teaching
• Teach the patient the name, dose, frequency, action, and adverse effects of the prescribed oral contraceptive.
• Advise the patient to read the oral contraceptive package insert. Explain and reinforce this information, as needed. (For more information, see *Oral contraceptive patient-teaching tips.*)

SELECTED MAJOR DRUGS

Estrogens, progestins, and oral contraceptive agents

This chart summarizes the major estrogens, progestins, and oral contraceptives currently in clinical use.

DRUG	MAJOR INDICATIONS	USUAL ADULT DOSAGES	CONTRAINDICATIONS AND PRECAUTIONS
Estrogens			
conjugated estrogenic substances	Atrophic vaginitis or kraurosis vulvae	0.3 to 1.25 mg P.O. daily or 2 to 4 grams cream administered vaginally daily in 21-day cycles	• Know that conjugated estrogenic substances are contraindicated in a patient with known or suspected pregnancy, thrombophlebitis or a thromboembolic disorder, estrogen-dependent cancer of the breast or reproductive organs (except when used as palliative therapy for inoperable cancer in a postmenopausal woman), or undiagnosed abnormal uterine bleeding.
	Female hypogonadism	2.5 mg P.O. b.i.d. or t.i.d. for 20 consecutive days each month	
	Surgical castration or primary ovarian failure	1.25 mg P.O. daily in 21-day cycles	
	Menopausal symptoms	0.3 to 1.25 mg P.O. daily in 21-day cycles	• Administer with caution to a patient with a condition that may be aggravated by fluid retention or one with depression, metabolic bone disease, a blood dyscrasia, gallbladder disease, a seizure disorder, diabetes mellitus, amenorrhea, or a family history of breast or genital cancer.
	Postpartal breast engorgement	3.75 mg P.O. every 4 hours for five doses or 1.25 mg P.O. every 4 hours for 5 days	
	Osteoporosis	0.625 mg P.O. daily in 21-day cycles	
	Abnormal uterine bleeding caused by hormonal imbalance	25 mg I.V. or I.M., repeated in 6 to 12 hours as prescribed	
Progestins			
medroxyprogesterone acetate	Amenorrhea or abnormal uterine bleeding caused by hormonal imbalance	5 to 10 mg P.O. daily for 5 to 10 days beginning on day 16 of the menstrual cycle; if the patient has received estrogen previously, 10 mg P.O. daily for 10 days beginning on day 16 of the menstrual cycle	• Know that medroxyprogesterone acetate is contraindicated in a patient with thrombophlebitis or a thromboembolic disorder, known or suspected pregnancy, cancer of the breast or reproductive organs (except for palliative therapy for inoperable cancer in a postmenopausal woman), hepatic disease or dysfunction, undiagnosed abnormal uterine bleeding, or missed abortion. The drug also is contraindicated as a test for pregnancy.
Oral contraceptives			
estrogen-progestin combination products	Contraception	*21-tablet therapy:* one tablet P.O. at the same time each day for 21 days beginning on day 5 of the menstrual cycle	• Know that estrogen-progestin combination products are contraindicated in a patient with known or suspected pregnancy, thrombophlebitis or a thromboembolic disorder, estrogen-dependent cancer of the breast or reproductive organs (except when used as palliative therapy for inoperable cancer in a postmenopausal woman), or undiagnosed abnormal uterine bleeding.
		28-tablet therapy: one active tablet P.O. at the same time each day for 21 days beginning on day 5 of the menstrual cycle, then one inactive tablet P.O. daily for 7 days; when all 28 tablets have been taken, the patient should start a new pill pack	• Administer with caution to a patient with a condition that may be aggravated by fluid retention or one with depression, a metabolic bone disease, a blood dyscrasia, gallbladder disease, a seizure disorder, diabetes mellitus, amenorrhea, or a family history of breast or genital cancer.
		Alternate 28-tablet therapy: one active or inactive tablet P.O. daily based on manufacturer's instructions	

• *Stress the importance of a semiannual Pap test and blood pressure check and an annual gynecologic examination.*
• *Teach the patient how to perform breast self-examination.*
• *Advise the patient who smokes to stop. Explain the increased risks of cardiovascular dysfunction and thromboembolic events associated with smoking while using an oral contraceptive.*
• Instruct the patient to weigh herself at least twice a week and to report any sudden weight gain or swelling to her physician.
• *Counsel the patient to use an alternate contraceptive method before surgery to decrease the risk of thromboembolism.*
• Ensure that the patient understands the sequence to follow in taking the pills.
• *Explain to the patient that if she misses one menstrual period after having taken all the pills on time, she should start her next cycle of pills at the regularly scheduled time. However, if she misses one menstrual period and has not taken all the pills on time, or if she misses two consecutive menstrual periods even though she has taken all the pills on time, she should stop taking the pills and have a pregnancy test. Explain to the patient that progestins and estrogens can cause birth defects if taken early in pregnancy.*
• *Explain to the patient that achieving pregnancy may be difficult for a short time after the oral contraceptive is discontinued.* Advise her to wait 3 months before trying to become pregnant, using an alternative contraceptive method in the interim, because the endometrium may take up to 3 months to return to normal.
• Advise the patient that oral contraceptive use may alter the fit of rigid contact lenses.
• Instruct the patient to notify the physician if adverse reactions occur or if other concerns arise.

Evaluation
The following examples represent appropriate evaluation statements for a patient receiving an oral contraceptive.
• The patient has no conditions that contraindicate oral contraceptive use.
• The patient exhibits no signs of complications in the preexisting condition linked to the prescribed oral contraceptive.
• The patient experiences adverse reactions to the prescribed oral contraceptive.
• The patient expresses an accurate understanding of the points taught about the prescribed oral contraceptive.
• The patient correctly demonstrates breast self-examination.

CHAPTER SUMMARY

Chapter 54 presented the estrogens, progestins, and oral contraceptives, which are used to regulate the function of the female reproductive tract, relieve menopausal and postmenopausal symptoms, treat diseases of the female reproductive organs, and prevent pregnancy. Here are the chapter highlights.
• Estrogens and progesterone are hormones that play a vital role in the development of the female reproductive tract and secondary sex characteristics. These hormones also are responsible for maturation of the ovum and its development after fertilization. Estrogen and progesterone are necessary for development of the endometrial lining during the female reproductive cycle and for the maintenance of pregnancy.
• Many oral estrogens and progestins undergo first-pass metabolism. After absorption from the GI tract, these agents are transported via the portal vein to the liver, where large amounts of both agents are metabolized rapidly to inactive compounds before entering the general circulation. To achieve therapeutic effects, oral dosages of estrogens and progestins must be much higher than parenteral dosages, which do not undergo first-pass metabolism.
• Estrogens are prescribed primarily for hormonal replacement therapy in postmenopausal women. They also are used as contraceptives, either alone or with progestins.
• Progestins are used to treat ovarian disorders, such as abnormal menstrual flow, endometriosis, PMS, and advanced metastatic endometrial or renal cancer. They also are used as contraceptives, either alone or with estrogens.
• Oral contraceptives are used to prevent pregnancy and to treat hypermenorrhea, endometriosis, and dysmenorrhea and to promote cyclic withdrawal bleeding.
• Oral contraceptives act primarily by inhibiting ovulation. Large dosages of estrogenic oral contraceptives (the so-called morning-after pills) interfere with implantation of the fertilized ovum. Progestins act by preventing sperm migration toward the ovum and creating a hostile environment in the uterus that is unsuitable for ovum implantation even if fertilization occurs.
• Most oral contraceptives contain estrogen and progestin. The monophasic preparations provide fixed doses of both hormones throughout the 21-day cycle. The biphasic preparations deliver a constant amount of estrogen throughout the 21-day cycle but an increased amount of progestin

during the last 11 days. The progestin dose in triphasic preparations varies every 7 days; the estrogen dose may remain fixed throughout the 21-day cycle or may vary every 7 days.

• Use of estrogens, progestins, and oral contraceptives is associated with various adverse reactions. The most severe involve the cardiovascular system and include hypertension, cerebrovascular accident, thromboembolism, and MI. Women who smoke while taking an oral contraceptive have a greatly increased risk of developing adverse cardiovascular reactions. Research has shown that the risk of cervical cancer also may increase with oral contraceptive use.

• The nurse should monitor the patient closely for adverse drug reactions and teach the patient how to take the drug safely and effectively.

STUDY QUESTIONS

See Appendix 1 for answers.

1. During menopause, Virginia May, age 45, experiences vasomotor symptoms. To relieve these symptoms, her physician prescribes conjugated estrogenic substances (Premarin) 0.3 mg P.O. daily. Before therapy begins, the nurse obtains a thorough medical history. Which condition would contraindicate estrogen therapy for Ms. May?
(a) hepatic dysfunction
(b) thromboembolic disorder
(c) diabetes insipidus
(d) gallbladder disease

2. During estrogen therapy, Ms. May is at greatest risk for developing which type of cancer?
(a) endometrial
(b) ovarian
(c) liver
(d) cervical

3. The nurse teaches Ms. May how to recognize and manage adverse reactions to estrogen. Which of the following reactions warrants physician notification?
(a) breast tenderness
(b) transient nausea
(c) leg cramps
(d) acne

4. Francine Fedder, age 25, receives progestin, as prescribed, for abnormal uterine bleeding from endometriosis. By which mechanism does progestin correct endometriosis?
(a) It regulates the menstrual cycle, preventing further ectopic endometrial growth.
(b) It prevents excessive bleeding from ectopic endometrial growths.
(c) It prevents menstruation for several months, allowing ectopic endometrial growths to regress.
(d) It promotes dissolution and excretion of ectopic endometrial growths.

5. The nurse should give Ms. Fedder which information about conception during progestin therapy?
(a) Conception should be avoided because progestin may cause congenital defects.
(b) Conception is safe during progestin therapy because progestin is a natural hormone.
(c) Conception is unlikely because progestin acts as a safe and effective contraceptive.
(d) Conception is common during therapy with progestin, the "pregnancy hormone."

6. Marianne Banyon, age 30, comes to the clinic for information about birth control methods. After Ms. Banyon considers her options, the physician prescribes the triphasic oral contraceptive Ortho-Novum 7/7/7. The nurse teaches Ms. Banyon about the oral contraceptive. Which problem may require immediate discontinuation of the oral contraceptive?
(a) nausea and constipation
(b) breast tenderness and fullness
(c) altered fit of rigid contact lenses
(d) two consecutive missed menstrual cycles

7. The nurse also teaches Ms. Banyon how to take the oral contraceptive. If Ms. Banyon misses a dose, what should she do?
(a) Abstain from sexual intercourse and call her physician immediately.
(b) Wait until the next scheduled dose and use an additional contraceptive method until then.
(c) Take the missed dose as soon as she remembers or take two pills the next day.
(d) Double the prescribed dosage for the next 7 days.

8. Two years later, Ms. Banyon decides to have another child. After discontinuing the oral contraceptive, when can she safely begin attempting to conceive?
(a) when she feels ready
(b) after at least 1 week
(c) after one normal menstrual cycle
(d) after at least three menstrual cycles

SELECTED REFERENCES

AHFS drug information 90. (1990). Bethesda, MD: American Society of Hospital Pharmacists.

Drug facts and comparisons. (1991). St. Louis: Facts and Comparisons Division, Lippincott.

Engel, N. (1989). Update on cancer risk and oral contraceptives. *MCN, 15*(1), 37.

Estrogen replacement and breast cancer. (1989). *Harvard Medical School Health Letter, 14*(12), 1-3.

Goodman and Gilman's the pharmacological basis of therapeutics (8th ed.; 1990). Elmsford, NY: Pergamon Press.

Hansten, P., and Horn, J. (1988). *Drug interactions: Clinical significance of drug-drug interactions* (6th ed.). Philadelphia: Lea & Febiger.

North American Nursing Diagnosis Association. (1990). *Taxonomy I - Revised, with official diagnostic categories.* St. Louis: NANDA.

Nursing91 Drug Handbook. (1991). Springhouse, PA: Springhouse Corporation.

USPDI. (1991). *Drug information for the health care professional* (Vol. I, 11th ed.). Rockville, MD: United States Pharmacopeial Convention.

UTERINE MOTILITY AGENTS

OBJECTIVES

After reading and studying this chapter, the student should be able to:

1. Distinguish between uterine-stimulating agents and uterine-inhibiting (tocolytic) agents.

2. Discuss the pharmacokinetics of each drug class that affects uterine motility.

3. Compare the mechanisms of action of the uterine-stimulating agents to those of the uterine-inhibiting agents.

4. Identify the major drug interactions and adverse reactions associated with the three classes of uterine motility agents.

5. Describe how to apply the nursing process when caring for a patient who is receiving a uterine motility agent.

INTRODUCTION

Uterine motility agents are drugs that stimulate or inhibit uterine contractions. Those that stimulate contractions are used primarily to induce or augment labor, to abort pregnancy, or to control postpartal hemorrhage. Those that inhibit contractions are used to prevent or stop preterm labor. Chapter 55 discusses the two classes of uterine-stimulating agents—the prostaglandins and the ergot alkaloids—and the single class of uterine-inhibiting agents, also known as tocolytic agents. A third class of uterine-stimulating agents, oxytocic agents, is discussed in Chapter 52, Pituitary Agents.

Physiology of labor and delivery

Although hormonal and mechanical factors produce uterine contractions during labor, the ratio of estrogen to progesterone appears to be crucial. Estrogen stimulates uterine contractions, and progesterone inhibits them. Until the seventh month of pregnancy, both hormones are secreted in progressively greater quantities. From that point on, however, estrogen secretion continues to increase, whereas progesterone secretion decreases slightly. This increasing estrogen-progesterone ratio promotes the onset of uterine contractions.

Oxytocin and the prostaglandins are other hormones that stimulate uterine contractions. Produced by the hypothalamus and stored in the pituitary gland, oxytocin is secreted in increasing amounts by the mother and fetus in late pregnancy. The fetal membranes release high concentrations of prostaglandins during labor.

The mechanical factors that stimulate uterine contractions include muscle stretch and cervical irritation. The uterine smooth muscles are stretched continuously as the fetus grows and intermittently as it moves. Apparently this stretching helps stimulate uterine contraction when labor begins.

How cervical irritation stimulates uterine contractions is unknown. One theory suggests that irritation of neuronal cells in the cervix sets up reflex contractions in the uterus.

Uterine motility agents are used to prevent or treat problems that occur during labor and delivery. Uterine-stimulating agents are used to induce labor when early vaginal delivery is desired, such as when the mother has Rh incompatibility, diabetes mellitus, preeclampsia near or at term, or premature rupture of the membranes. These agents also stimulate or reinforce contractions and help control severe bleeding in the third stage of labor and postpartal hemorrhage.

Uterine-inhibiting (tocolytic) agents are used to prevent or treat preterm labor.

For a summary of representative drugs, see *Selected major drugs: Uterine motility agents,* page 935. For a listing of applicable nursing diagnoses that the nurse may formulate when caring for a patient receiving these agents, see *Selected nursing diagnoses: Uterine motility agents,* page 928. For detailed information on applying the nursing process, see Chapter 6, The Nursing Process and Drug Therapy

SELECTED NURSING DIAGNOSES

Uterine motility agents

The following nursing diagnoses address representative problems and etiologies that a nurse may encounter when caring for a patient who is receiving a uterine motility agent. Some of these nursing diagnoses contain generalized etiologies, which the nurse must individualize based on the patient's needs. (For some common nursing diagnoses and related interventions for each drug class, see the "Nursing Process Application" sections of this chapter.)

- Altered peripheral tissue perfusion related to ergot poisoning
- Altered protection related to metabolic abnormalities caused by ritodrine or terbutaline
- Altered thought processes related to ergot poisoning
- Anxiety related to the adverse central nervous system effects of ritodrine or terbutaline
- Decreased cardiac output related to the adverse cardiovascular effects of a uterine motility agent
- Diarrhea related to the adverse gastrointestinal (GI) effects of a uterine motility agent
- Hyperthermia related to prostaglandin-induced fever
- Impaired gas exchange related to prostaglandin-induced bronchospasm
- Ineffective breathing pattern related to magnesium toxicity
- Ineffective breathing pattern related to the adverse bronchial effects of a prostaglandin
- Knowledge deficit related to the prescribed uterine motility agent
- Pain related to the adverse effects of a prostaglandin
- Potential fluid volume deficit related to the adverse GI effects of a uterine motility agent
- Potential for injury related to a preexisting condition that contraindicates the use of a uterine motility agent
- Potential for injury related to a preexisting condition that requires cautious use of a uterine motility agent
- Potential for injury related to adverse drug reactions
- Potential for trauma related to prostaglandin-induced seizures
- Potential for trauma to the neonate related to tocolytic agent use in the mother

PROSTAGLANDINS

Prostaglandins are derivatives of fatty acids (lipid acids) found in virtually every tissue and fluid in the body. As uterine-stimulating agents, clinically they are used mainly to abort pregnancy.

The endogenous prostaglandins available for use as abortifacients (agents that induce expulsion of the fetus) are carboprost tromethamine and dinoprostone.

PHARMACOKINETICS

The pharmacokinetics of the prostaglandins are not fully understood, even though they have been used clinically for about 20 years.

Absorption, distribution, metabolism, excretion
Carboprost is absorbed slowly after I.M. administration. After vaginal insertion of a dinoprostone suppository, the drug slowly diffuses across the vaginal wall into the maternal blood and is distributed widely.

Little is known about the metabolism and excretion of these agents, but dinoprostone appears to be metabolized rapidly to inactive metabolites in the maternal lungs and liver. After metabolism, the parent compound and metabolites are excreted primarily in the urine and small amounts in the feces.

Onset, peak, duration
With carboprost, the onset of action occurs about 16 hours after I.M. injection, but is shorter with increased gravidity (number of pregnancies) or parity (number of live births) and longer with increased gestational age. Onset with dinoprostone suppositories usually occurs within 10 minutes of administration. The half-life of dinoprostone usually ranges from less than 1 minute to 10 minutes.

PHARMACODYNAMICS

Although their mechanism of action has not been established completely, the abortifacient prostaglandins appear to act directly on the myometrium of the uterus. They stimulate uterine contractions similar to those that occur during labor, inducing fetal expulsion. They also facilitate cervical dilation and softening.

PHARMACOTHERAPEUTICS

The prostaglandins carboprost and dinoprostone are used primarily to terminate pregnancy.

carboprost tromethamine (Prostin/15M). The primary clinical indication for this drug is termination of pregnancy between weeks 13 and 20 of gestation. I.M. administration makes it the drug of choice for patients with profuse vaginal bleeding or ruptured placental membranes. It also is used to treat postpartal hemorrhage from uterine atony. Carboprost is available in 1-ml ampules containing 250 mcg/ml.

Usual adult dosage: for abortion, 250 mcg deep I.M., followed by 250 to 500 mcg I.M. every 1½ to 3½ hours if necessary, up to a maximum total dosage of 12 mg and for no more than 48 hours; for postpartal hemorrhage, 250 mcg deep I.M., repeated every 15 to 90 minutes, if necessary, up to a maximum total dosage of 2 mg.

dinoprostone (Prostin E$_2$). The primary indication for dinoprostone is termination of pregnancy from week 12 to 20 of gestation. Available as 20-mg intravaginal suppositories, dinoprostone stimulates uterine contractions similar to those of labor. It also is used to soften the cervix before labor induction. Continuous I.V. infusion of dilute oxytocin may be administered with dinoprostone to hasten the onset of uterine contractions, thus shortening the time required for uterine evacuation.

Usual adult dosage: one 20-mg suppository inserted high into the vagina; after insertion, the patient should remain supine for at least 10 minutes to allow adequate absorption; additional suppositories may be administered every 3 to 5 hours as necessary until abortion occurs or symptoms of intolerance develop.

Drug interactions

The major interactions between prostaglandins and other drugs involve alcohol and oxytocin. Alcohol antagonizes the action of dinoprostone. Oxytocin enhances the effect of carboprost and dinoprostone. Therefore, concomitant administration of these drugs requires extreme caution and frequent monitoring of uterine contractions and cervical dilation.

ADVERSE DRUG REACTIONS

Adverse reactions to exogenous prostaglandins are diverse, mimicking the effects that occur with natural prostaglandins.

Prostaglandins cause gastrointestinal (GI), vascular, bronchial, and uterine adverse reactions. GI stimulation causes the most common adverse reactions. Nausea and vomiting occur in 60%, and diarrhea in 20%, of patients receiving prostaglandins. Other adverse reactions include coughing, pain, and fever, which occur in more than half of all patients receiving the drugs.

Hypersensitivity reactions to prostaglandins are potentially life-threatening and include bronchospasm, seizures, hypotension, and cardiac arrest. The most severe reactions usually occur in patients with underlying cardiovascular disease, asthma, or seizure disorders.

NURSING PROCESS APPLICATION

The following information assists the nurse in caring for a patient who is receiving a prostaglandin.

Assessment

• Review the patient's history for a preexisting condition that contraindicates the use of a prostaglandin, such as known hypersensitivity to the drug or a history of pelvic inflammatory disease.
• Review the patient's history for a preexisting condition that requires cautious use of a prostaglandin, such as cervical lacerations or uterine rupture.
• Assess the patient for adverse reactions to the prescribed prostaglandin, such as GI, vascular, bronchial, or uterine dysfunction.
• Review the patient's medication history to identify the use of drugs that may interact with the prostaglandin, such as alcohol and oxytocin.
• Assess the effectiveness of the prostaglandin throughout administration.
• Assess the patient's respiratory status during prostaglandin therapy.
• Evaluate the patient's knowledge about the prescribed prostaglandin as well as the family's knowledge, if appropriate.

Nursing diagnoses

The following examples represent appropriate nursing diagnoses for a patient receiving a prostaglandin.
• Potential for injury related to a preexisting condition that contraindicates the use of a prostaglandin
• Potential for injury related to a preexisting condition that requires cautious use of a prostaglandin
• Potential for injury related to adverse drug reactions
• Ineffective breathing pattern related to the adverse bronchial effects of the prostaglandin
• Knowledge deficit related to the prescribed prostaglandin

Planning and implementation

• Do not administer a prostaglandin to a patient with a condition that contraindicates its use.
• Administer a prostaglandin cautiously to a patient at risk because of a preexisting condition.
• Monitor the patient frequently for adverse reactions during prostaglandin therapy.
• Monitor the patient for nausea, vomiting, or diarrhea during prostaglandin therapy. Premedicate the patient as prescribed with an antiemetic, such as prochlorperazine, and an antidiarrheal agent, such as a diphenoxylate, to decrease the risk of adverse GI reactions. Notify the physician if nausea, vomiting, or diarrhea persists.
• *Monitor the patient's vital signs regularly, particularly noting hypotension or fever.* Temperature increases occur in more than half of all patients taking prostaglandins; this drug fever may be misinterpreted for infection or may mask concomitant infection. It does not respond to antipyretics such as aspirin, but sponge baths with water or alcohol may be effective.

• Monitor the degree of discomfort caused by the uterine contractions. Consult the physician about prescribing an analgesic, as needed.

• *Observe the patient closely for hypersensitivity reactions, such as bronchospasm, seizures, hypotension, or cardiac arrest, after prostaglandin administration.* These reactions are more likely to occur in a patient with cardiovascular disease, asthma, or a seizure disorder.

• *Closely monitor a patient with a history of seizures. Take seizure precautions throughout drug use. For example, pad the patient's bed rails.*

• *Administer carboprost tromethamine deep I.M.*

• *Do not administer carboprost tromethamine repeatedly for more than 48 hours.*

• *Insert dinoprostone high into the vagina. After insertion, instruct the patient to remain supine for at least 10 minutes to allow adequate absorption.*

• Store carboprost in a refrigerator at 35.6° to 39.2° F (2° to 4° C). Store dinoprostone suppositories in a freezer at temperatures below −4° F (20° C), but bring them to room temperature before use.

• *Monitor the patient after pregnancy termination for signs of postabortion hemorrhage, such as decreased blood pressure, increased pulse and respiratory rate, and profuse, bloody vaginal discharge.*

• Inform the physician of the patient's progress during prostaglandin therapy and report any adverse reactions.

• Monitor the patient's breathing pattern frequently and auscultate lung fields regularly to detect prostaglandin-induced bronchospasm. Alert the physician if bronchospasm develops or if the patient complains of chest tightness or shortness of breath.

Patient teaching

• Teach the patient and family (if appropriate) the name, dose, frequency, action, and adverse effects of the prescribed prostaglandin agent.

• *Instruct the patient to notify the nurse immediately if she experiences GI distress, breathing difficulty, or chest discomfort.*

• Inform the patient that her vital signs will be monitored frequently during prostaglandin therapy to detect changes.

• Reassure the patient that pain from uterine contractions is normal and that an analgesic may be prescribed.

• Provide emotional support to the patient and refer her to a counselor or support group, if needed.

• Encourage the patient to express any concerns or ask questions about the prescribed prostaglandin.

Evaluation

The following examples represent evaluation statements for a patient receiving a prostaglandin.

• The patient has no conditions that contraindicate prostaglandin therapy.

• The patient exhibits no signs of complications in the preexisting condition linked to the prescribed prostaglandin.

• The patient experiences no adverse reactions to the prescribed prostaglandin.

• The patient maintains adequate respiratory function during prostaglandin therapy.

• The patient and family express an accurate understanding of the points taught about the prescribed prostaglandin.

• The patient asks appropriate questions about prostaglandin therapy.

ERGOT ALKALOIDS

Ergot alkaloids are naturally occurring substances that markedly increase the motor activity of uterine smooth muscle. They are used clinically to control postpartal or postabortion hemorrhage from uterine atony or subinvolution. Ergonovine maleate and its semisynthetic derivative, methylergonovine maleate, are the ergot alkaloids used as uterine motility agents.

PHARMACOKINETICS

Ergot alkaloids are absorbed and distributed rapidly and appear to be metabolized in the liver and excreted in feces.

Absorption, distribution, metabolism, excretion

Ergonovine and methylergonovine are absorbed rapidly after oral and I.M. administration. Bioavailability of oral methylergonovine is about 60%. Although their distribution is not understood fully, both ergot alkaloids are distributed rapidly to plasma and extracellular fluid. Methylergonovine has been detected in breast milk. However, concentrations are too low to affect a breast-feeding infant. The ergot alkaloids are thought to be metabolized in the liver and excreted in the feces.

Onset, peak, duration

After oral administration, the onset of action for both drugs usually occurs within 5 to 15 minutes. The peak concentration time varies from 30 minutes to 3 hours, and the duration of action lasts 3 hours or longer. With I.M. administration, the onset occurs in 2 to 5 minutes, and duration is at least 3 hours. I.V. administration causes immediate uterine contractions that last for 45 minutes.

PHARMACODYNAMICS

Ergonovine and methylergonovine are pharmacologically similar, directly stimulating uterine and vascular smooth muscle contractions. Both drugs increase the amplitude and frequency of uterine contractions, thus impeding uterine blood flow by vasoconstriction. Cervical smooth muscle contractions also are increased by both agents.

PHARMACOTHERAPEUTICS

The ergot alkaloids are used to prevent and treat postpartal and postabortion hemorrhage from uterine atony or sub-involution. They should *not* be used to induce or augment labor. Ergonovine also has been used to diagnose coronary artery spasm in patients with variant (Prinzmetal's) angina.

ergonovine maleate (Ergotrate Maleate). To treat post-partal and postabortion hemorrhage, ergonovine is available in oral and parenteral forms.
Usual adult dosage: for postpartal and postabortion hemorrhage, 0.2 mg I.M. every 2 to 4 hours, to a maximum of five doses; for severe vaginal bleeding, 0.2 mg I.V. over 1 minute while blood pressure and uterine contractions are monitored, diluting the I.V. dose to a volume of 5 ml with normal saline solution; after initial I.M. or I.V. dose, 0.2 to 0.4 mg P.O. every 6 to 12 hours for 2 to 7 days, decreasing the dosage if severe uterine cramping occurs.

methylergonovine maleate (Methergine). To treat post-partal and postabortion hemorrhage, methylergonovine is available in oral and parenteral forms.
Usual adult dosage: for postpartal and postabortion hemorrhage, 0.2 mg I.M. every 2 to 4 hours to a maximum of five doses; for severe vaginal bleeding, 0.2 mg I.V. over 1 minute while blood pressure and uterine contractions are monitored, diluting the I.V. dose to a volume of 5 ml with normal saline solution; after initial I.M. or I.V. dose, 0.2 to 0.4 mg P.O. every 6 to 12 hours for 2 to 7 days, decreasing the dosage if severe uterine cramping occurs.

Drug interactions

Few—but potentially harmful—drug interactions occur with the ergot alkaloids. The combined use of dopamine or other vasoconstrictors with ergot alkaloids may cause increased peripheral vasoconstriction, resulting in cyanosis and tissue necrosis. Hypertension may occur if an ergot alkaloid is administered concomitantly with a vasoconstrictor or a regional anesthetic.

ADVERSE DRUG REACTIONS

Most adverse reactions to the ergot alkaloids occur when the drugs are administered incorrectly—either in undiluted form or too rapidly.

The most common adverse reactions are nausea and vomiting. These may be minimized by administering pro-chlorperazine or another phenothiazine antiemetic before administering the ergot alkaloid, as prescribed.

Other adverse reactions include dizziness, headache, tinnitus, diaphoresis, palpitations, transient chest pain, and dyspnea. Hypertension also may occur, most commonly with ergonovine; its incidence increases if the ergot alkaloid is administered undiluted or too rapidly. Patients with a history of eclampsia or hypertension are at greater risk. With severe overdosage, ergot poisoning, characterized by seizures and gangrene, may occur. Other manifestations include numbness and coldness of the extremities, hyper-coagulability, and confusion. Hypersensitivity reactions, including shock, also have been reported.

NURSING PROCESS APPLICATION

The following information assists the nurse in caring for a patient who is receiving an ergot alkaloid.

Assessment

• Review the patient's history for a preexisting condition that contraindicates the use of an ergot alkaloid, such as known hypersensitivity or idiosyncratic reaction to the drug, threatened spontaneous abortion, hypertension, heart disease, venoatrial shunt, mitral valve stenosis, or obliterative vascular disease.
• Review the patient's history for a preexisting condition that requires cautious use of an ergot alkaloid, such as sepsis or hepatic or renal impairment.
• Assess the patient for adverse reactions to the prescribed ergot alkaloid, such as nausea, vomiting, hypertension, or ergot poisoning.
• Review the patient's medication history to identify the use of drugs that may interact with the ergot alkaloid, such as dopamine or other vasoconstrictors.
• Assess the effectiveness of the ergot alkaloid regularly.
• Evaluate the patient's and family's knowledge about the prescribed ergot alkaloid.

Nursing diagnoses

The following examples represent appropriate nursing diagnoses for a patient receiving an ergot alkaloid.
• Potential for injury related to a preexisting condition that contraindicates the use of an ergot alkaloid
• Potential for injury related to a preexisting condition that requires cautious use of an ergot alkaloid
• Potential for injury related to adverse drug reactions

• Knowledge deficit related to the prescribed ergot alkaloid

Planning and implementation
• Do not administer an ergot alkaloid to a patient with a condition that contraindicates its use. *Also do not administer an ergot alkaloid to induce or augment labor.*
• Administer an ergot alkaloid cautiously to a patient at risk because of a preexisting condition.
• *Monitor the patient frequently for nausea, vomiting, hypertension, ergot poisoning, and other adverse reactions during ergot alkaloid therapy.*
• Expect to administer prochlorperazine or another phenothiazine antiemetic, as prescribed, before administering the ergot alkaloid to minimize nausea and vomiting.
• *Monitor the patient's blood pressure, pulse, uterine contractions, and vaginal bleeding. Report sudden vital sign changes, frequent periods of uterine relaxation, and any change in the character or amount of vaginal bleeding.*
• *Observe the patient closely for signs of ergot poisoning, such as seizures, gangrene, numbness and coldness of extremities, or confusion.* If these signs appear, notify the physician immediately and expect to discontinue the ergot alkaloid.
• *Avoid concomitant administration of a vasoconstrictor, vasopressor, or regional anesthetic.*
• Dilute an I.V. preparation to a volume of 5 ml with normal saline solution, and administer over at least 1 minute.
• Store the ergot alkaloid in a tightly closed, light-resistant container. Discard any discolored solution.
• Notify the physician if other adverse reactions occur or if the ergot alkaloid is ineffective.

Patient teaching
• Teach the patient and family the name, dose, frequency, action, and adverse effects of the prescribed ergot alkaloid.
• *Instruct the patient to notify the nurse if she experiences nausea, vomiting, dizziness, headache, tinnitus, diaphoresis, palpitations, chest pain, dyspnea, or numbness or coldness of the extremities.*
• Encourage the patient to express concerns and ask questions about the prescribed ergot alkaloid.

Evaluation
The following examples represent appropriate evaluation statements for a patient receiving an ergot alkaloid.
• The patient has no conditions that contraindicate ergot alkaloid therapy.
• The patient exhibits no signs of complications in the preexisting condition linked to the prescribed ergot alkaloid.
• The patient develops no adverse reactions to the prescribed ergot alkaloid.
• The patient and family express an accurate understanding of the points taught about the prescribed ergot alkaloid.

• The patient correctly identifies reactions that require immediate notification of the nurse.

TOCOLYTIC AGENTS

Uterine-inhibiting (tocolytic) agents, most commonly magnesium sulfate and the beta-receptor agonists ritodrine hydrochloride and terbutaline sulfate, are used to inhibit uterine contractions in preterm labor. Ethyl alcohol also relaxes uterine smooth muscle, but it rarely is used in clinical practice.

PHARMACOKINETICS

The tocolytic agents readily cross the placenta and appear in breast milk. When administered I.V., they have a rapid onset of action.

Absorption, distribution, metabolism, excretion
After oral administration, terbutaline and ritodrine are absorbed from the GI tract, with a bioavailability of 30% to 50%, and 30%, respectively. Both agents cross the placenta and appear in breast milk. Magnesium sulfate is administered I.V. and distributed widely. The beta-receptor agonists are metabolized in the liver. All tocolytic agents and their metabolites are excreted in urine; 90% to 98% of a magnesium sulfate dose is excreted in urine and the remainder in feces.

Onset, peak, duration
After I.V. administration, tocolytic agents have a rapid onset of action. Ritodrine reaches a peak concentration level after 50 minutes; terbutaline, in 30 to 60 minutes. Terbutaline has a duration of action of 1.5 to 4 hours; magnesium sulfate, 30 minutes. The therapeutic blood level for magnesium sulfate is 6 mEq/liter. When this level falls, uterine contractions may recur.

After oral administration, ritodrine has an onset of 30 to 60 minutes and reaches peak concentration in 30 to 60 minutes. Oral terbutaline has an onset of 30 minutes and reaches peak concentration in 2 hours. Ritodrine's half-life is 15 to 17 hours after I.V. administration and 12 to 20 hours after oral administration.

PHARMACODYNAMICS

The mechanisms of action for the tocolytic agents vary. However, all three agents directly affect uterine muscle.

Mechanism of action

The beta-receptor agonists ritodrine and terbutaline interact with beta receptors in the uterus. This interaction stimulates release of adenylate cyclase, increasing the production of 3′,5′ cyclic adenosine monophosphate (AMP). The increased production of cyclic AMP causes an increased uptake and sequestration of intracellular calcium. The final result is inhibition of uterine smooth muscle contractions with decreased intensity and frequency of contractions.

Magnesium sulfate's mechanism of action as a tocolytic agent is unknown. The present theory is that magnesium sulfate competes with calcium in uterine smooth muscle, preventing calcium from triggering uterine contractions.

PHARMACOTHERAPEUTICS

The tocolytic agents initially are administered I.V. for rapid inhibition of uterine contractions. After contractions are under control, oral beta-receptor agonists are used to maintain the initial effect.

magnesium sulfate. Administered I.V., magnesium sulfate is used to prevent or control seizures in preeclampsia or eclampsia, to control preterm labor, and to treat hypomagnesemia. It must be administered with caution to a patient with renal impairment.
Usual adult dosage: for preventing or controlling seizures in preeclampsia or eclampsia, initially, 4 grams I.V. in 250 ml D₅W (not to exceed 3 ml per minute) and 4 grams deep I.M. into each buttock, then 4 grams deep I.M. into alternate buttock every 4 hours as needed or, alternatively, 4 grams I.V. as a loading dose followed by 1 to 2 grams hourly as an I.V. infusion; for controlling preterm labor, initially, 6 grams I.V. of a 10% solution as a loading dose, given slowly at a rate of 150 mg/minute until contractions stop or adverse reactions occur; maintenance dosage, 2 grams/hour I.V. infusion, keeping magnesium levels between 4 and 6 mEq/liter; for treating hypomagnesemia, 1 gram I.M. every 6 hours for four doses.

ritodrine hydrochloride (Yutopar). This is the beta-receptor agonist approved by the Food and Drug Administration for inhibition of preterm uterine contractions.
Usual adult dosage: initially, 50 to 100 mcg/minute I.V., increasing every 10 minutes by 50 mcg/minute to a maximum of 350 mcg/minute until contractions stop or adverse reactions occur; maintenance dosage, 10 mg P.O. 30 minutes before stopping the I.V. infusion, repeated every 2 hours for the first 24 hours, then 10 to 20 mg P.O. every 4 to 6 hours, not to exceed 120 mg/day.

terbutaline sulfate (Brethine, Bricanyl). Although it is not approved or labeled for use as a tocolytic agent, terbutaline commonly is used to treat preterm labor.
Usual adult dosage: initially, 2.5 mcg/minute I.V., increasing every 20 minutes by 2.5 mcg/minute to a maximum of 17.5 mcg/minute until contractions stop or adverse reactions occur; once contractions cease, continue I.V. infusion for 60 minutes to determine the lowest effective dosage; continue lowest effective dosage for at least 12 hours, then begin 15 mg P.O./day maintenance therapy.

Drug interactions

Tocolytic agents may interact with corticosteroids and beta-adrenergic blocking and neuromuscular blocking agents. (For details, see *Drug interactions: Tocolytic agents.*)

ADVERSE DRUG REACTIONS

Tocolytic agents cause many minor adverse reactions and several that can be severe, including cardiovascular reactions, electrolyte imbalances, and seizures.

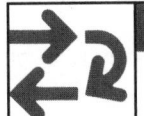

DRUG INTERACTIONS

Tocolytic agents

The chart below summarizes drug interactions involving the tocolytic agents.

DRUG	INTERACTING DRUGS	POSSIBLE EFFECTS	NURSING IMPLICATIONS
ritodrine, terbutaline	corticosteroids	Cause pulmonary edema	• Monitor the patient's respiratory status, if concomitant administration is unavoidable.
	beta-adrenergic blocking agents	Antagonize uterine-inhibiting action	• Avoid concomitant administration. • Monitor the patient's uterine contractions frequently.
magnesium sulfate	neuromuscular blocking agents	Enhances neuromuscular blockade	• Avoid concomitant administration. • Monitor the patient's vital signs frequently.

Most adverse reactions to the beta-receptor agonists ritodrine and terbutaline are extensions of their actions. Common maternal adverse reactions to these agents include an increase in heart rate by 20 to 40 beats/minute, increased cardiac output, hypotension, hyperglycemia, increased insulin secretion, increased free fatty acid release, hypokalemia, anxiety, headache, nausea, vomiting, nervousness, and tremor. They also can cause hypersensitivity reactions, such as pulmonary edema, chest tightness or pain, arrhythmias, palpitations, acute congestive heart failure, and hypertensive crisis.

Because these agents cross the placenta, the neonate also may experience adverse reactions, including increased heart rate, hypotension, and hypocalcemia as well as hypersensitivity reactions, including respiratory depression, paralytic ileus, and pulmonary edema (rare).

Adverse reactions to magnesium sulfate typically depend on the drug dosage, the rapidity of administration, and the serum magnesium level. (For a correlation between the magnesium blood level and the associated adverse reactions, see *Physiologic effects of magnesium levels*.) A mother who receives magnesium sulfate may give birth to a neonate with hypermagnesemia, hypotonia, or central nervous system (CNS) or respiratory depression.

Physiologic effects of magnesium levels

Maternal reactions to magnesium sulfate administration depend on the serum magnesium level. The list below indicates serum magnesium levels and their corresponding physiologic effects.

MAGNESIUM LEVEL (mEq/liter)	PHYSIOLOGIC EFFECTS
1.5 to 3	Normal serum level; no adverse physiologic effects
4 to 6	Therapeutic level for preventing or controlling seizures associated with preeclampsia or eclampsia and for controlling preterm labor contractions
7 to 10	Loss of deep tendon reflexes, hypotension, central nervous system depression (early signs of magnesium toxicity)
11 to 15	Respiratory paralysis
>15	Cardiac conduction arrhythmias
>25	Cardiac arrest

NURSING PROCESS APPLICATION

The following information assists the nurse in caring for a patient who is receiving a tocolytic agent.

Assessment
• Review the patient's history for a preexisting condition that contraindicates the use of a tocolytic agent, such as known hypersensitivity to the drug or any maternal or fetal condition in which pregnancy continuation is hazardous.
• Review the patient's history for a preexisting condition that requires cautious use of a tocolytic agent, such as renal impairment.
• Assess the patient for adverse reactions to the prescribed tocolytic agent, such as increased heart rate and cardiac output, hypotension, hyperglycemia, hypokalemia, or CNS, GI, respiratory, or cardiac dysfunction.
• Review the patient's medication history to identify the use of drugs that may interact with the tocolytic agent, such as corticosteroids, beta-adrenergic blocking agents, or neuromuscular blocking agents.
• Assess the effectiveness of the tocolytic agent throughout administration.
• Assess the neonate for adverse reactions, such as increased heart rate, hypotension, or hypocalcemia, if the mother received a tocolytic agent.
• Evaluate the patient's and family's knowledge about the prescribed tocolytic agent.

Nursing diagnoses
The following examples represent appropriate nursing diagnoses for a patient receiving a tocolytic agent.
• Potential for injury related to a preexisting condition that contraindicates the use of a tocolytic agent
• Potential for injury related to a preexisting condition that requires cautious use of a tocolytic agent
• Potential for injury related to adverse drug reactions
• Potential for trauma to the neonate related to tocolytic agent use in the mother
• Knowledge deficit related to the prescribed tocolytic agent

Planning and implementation
• Do not administer a tocolytic agent to a patient with a condition that contraindicates its use.
• Administer a tocolytic agent cautiously to a patient at risk because of a preexisting condition.
• Monitor the patient frequently for adverse reactions during tocolytic agent therapy.
• *Monitor maternal vital signs and a 20- to 30-minute fetal monitor strip before initiating beta-receptor agonist therapy. Also assess the maternal heart rate and blood pressure before increasing the infusion rate.*
• *Monitor uterine activity and fetal heart rate continuously during beta-receptor agonist therapy.*

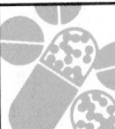

SELECTED MAJOR DRUGS

Uterine motility agents

This chart summarizes the major uterine motility agents currently in clinical use.

DRUG	MAJOR INDICATIONS	USUAL ADULT DOSAGES	CONTRAINDICATIONS AND PRECAUTIONS
Prostaglandins			
carboprost	Termination of pregnancy between weeks 13 and 20 of gestation	250 mcg deep I.M.; repeated doses of 250 to 500 mcg I.M. every 1½ to 3½ hours, if needed, up to a total dosage of 12 mg	• Know that carboprost is contraindicated in a patient with known hypersensitivity to the drug or a history of pelvic inflammatory disease. • Administer with caution to a patient with cervical lacerations or uterine rupture.
Ergot alkaloids			
ergonovine	Postpartal and postabortion hemorrhage from uterine atony or subinvolution	0.2 mg I.M. every 2 to 4 hours to a maximum of five doses followed by 0.2 to 0.4 mg P.O. every 6 to 12 hours for 2 to 7 days	• Know that ergonovine is contraindicated in a patient with threatened spontaneous abortion, hypertension, heart disease, venoatrial shunts, mitral valve stenosis, obliterative vascular disease, or known hypersensitivity or iodiosyncratic reaction to the drug. • Administer with caution to a patient with sepsis or hepatic or renal impairment.
	Severe vaginal bleeding	0.2 mg I.V. diluted in normal saline solution and administered over 1 minute followed by 0.2 to 0.4 mg P.O. every 6 to 12 hours for 2 to 7 days	
Tocolytic agents			
ritodrine	Inhibition of preterm uterine contractions	50 to 100 mcg/minute I.V. initially, increased every 10 minutes by 50 mcg/minute to a maximum of 350 mcg/minute until contractions stop or adverse reactions occur; maintenance dosage, 10 mg P.O. 30 minutes before stopping the infusion, followed by 10 mg every 2 hours for 24 hours, then 10 to 20 mg P.O. every 4 to 6 hours not to exceed 120 mg/day	• Know that ritodrine is contraindicated before week 20 of pregnancy, in a patient with known hypersensitivity to the drug, or in one with a condition that makes pregnancy continuation hazardous, such as antepartal hemorrhage that demands immediate delivery, eclampsia, severe preeclampsia, intrauterine fetal death, chorioamnionitis, maternal cardiac disease, pulmonary hypertension, maternal hyperthyroidism, or uncontrolled maternal diabetes mellitus. • Be aware the ritodrine has no known precautions.

• Monitor hydration carefully in a patient receiving a beta-receptor agonist to ensure that she is not hypovolemic or hypervolemic. *To prevent hypervolemia, ensure that the I.V. infusion rate does not exceed 150 ml/hour.*

• Administer an antiemetic agent, if prescribed, to a patient who experiences nausea or vomiting.

• *Be prepared to administer repeated I.V. doses of the beta-receptor agonist because standard dosages do not induce therapeutic effects in all cases and uterine contractions may recur.*

• Monitor potassium and blood and urine glucose levels for a patient before and regularly during therapy with a beta-receptor agonist.

• *Monitor the patient receiving a beta-receptor agonist for chest tightness and pain, palpitations, and dyspnea. Notify the physician immediately if these symptoms occur.*

• Monitor the patient's vital signs, knee jerk reflex, and fluid intake and output during magnesium sulfate therapy.

• Monitor the patient's magnesium level every 4 to 6 hours until it stabilizes.

• *Administer a bolus dose of magnesium sulfate slowly, at a rate of 150 mg/minute, to prevent nausea, vomiting, headache, palpitations, and flushing.*

• Notify the physician if adverse reactions occur or if the tocolytic agent is ineffective.

• *Monitor the neonate of a patient who received a beta-receptor agonist for increased heart rate, hypotension, and hypocalcemia.*

• *Monitor the neonate of a patient who received magnesium sulfate for hypermagnesemia, hypotonia, CNS depression, and respiratory depression.*

• Notify the physician if the neonate displays adverse reactions to the tocolytic agent and prepare to provide supportive treatment, as needed.

Patient teaching

• Teach the patient and family the name, dose, frequency, action, and adverse effects of the prescribed tocolytic agent.

• Advise the patient that laboratory studies, vital sign measurements, and fetal monitoring will be performed throughout tocolytic therapy to detect adverse reactions.

• Inform the patient receiving magnesium sulfate that blood will be drawn regularly to determine the effectiveness of the drug.

• *Instruct the patient to inform the nurse immediately if she experiences chest pain, palpitations, or dyspnea.*

• *Advise the patient receiving a beta-receptor agonist that drug-induced nervousness, tremor, or anxiety may occur.*

• Encourage the patient to express concerns and ask questions about tocolytic therapy.

Evaluation

The following examples represent appropriate evaluation statements for a patient receiving a tocolytic agent.

• The patient has no conditions that contraindicate tocolytic agent therapy.

• The patient exhibits no signs of complications in the preexisting condition linked to the prescribed tocolytic agent.

• The patient experiences no adverse reactions to the prescribed tocolytic agent.

• The neonate displays no adverse reactions to maternal tocolytic therapy.

• The patient and family express an accurate understanding of the points taught about the prescribed tocolytic agent.

• The patient expresses concern for the safety of her neonate and asks appropriate questions about tocolytic agent therapy.

CHAPTER SUMMARY

Chapter 55 discussed uterine motility agents as they are used to induce or augment labor, to terminate pregnancy, to control postpartal hemorrhage, and to stop preterm labor. Here are the chapter highlights.

• Uterine motility agents include uterine-stimulating agents and uterine-inhibiting (tocolytic) agents.

• Uterine-stimulating agents include prostaglandins and ergot alkaloids as well as oxytocin, which is discussed in Chapter 52, Pituitary Agents.

• Uterine-inhibiting agents include magnesium sulfate and the beta-receptor agonists ritodrine and terbutaline.

• The two endogenous prostaglandins used as abortifacients (agents that induce fetal expulsion) are carboprost and dinoprostone.

• Two ergot alkaloids are commercially available: ergonovine and its semisynthetic derivative, methylergonovine. Both are used to prevent and treat postpartal hemorrhage.

• The beta-receptor agonists ritodrine and terbutaline are considered the drugs of choice to stop uterine contractions in preterm labor, although the use of magnesium sulfate is increasing. Used correctly, these agents are safe and cause few major adverse reactions.

• When caring for a patient receiving a uterine motility agent, the nurse should monitor the patient closely for adverse reactions. During tocolytic agent therapy, the nurse also should monitor the fetus and neonate because of potential adverse reactions.

STUDY QUESTIONS

See Appendix 1 for answers.

1. At 14 weeks' gestation, Lisa Keller, age 20, experiences placental membrane rupture. To terminate the pregnancy, the physician is most likely to prescribe which drug?
(a) ritodrine
(b) ergonovine
(c) carboprost
(d) terbutaline

2. After administering the prescribed drug, the nurse should assess Ms. Keller for which adverse reaction?
(a) fever
(b) tinnitus
(c) tachycardia
(d) hypertension

3. Ms. Keller develops postabortion hemorrhage. Which drug might the physician prescribe to control the bleeding?
(a) carboprost
(b) ritodrine
(c) magnesium sulfate
(d) methylergonovine

4. Seven months pregnant, Hollie Brown, age 29, develops preterm labor. After she is admitted to the hospital, the physician prescribes terbutaline (Brethine) 2.5 mcg/minute I.V. How does this tocolytic agent inhibit uterine contractions?
(a) It acts as a beta-receptor agonist.
(b) It acts as a beta-receptor antagonist.
(c) It acts as an alpha-receptor agonist.
(d) It acts as an alpha-receptor antagonist.

5. Myrna Pappas, age 30, is admitted to the hospital with preterm labor. To control labor, the physician prescribes magnesium sulfate. This tocolytic agent may be used for which other indication?
(a) seizures in preeclampsia or eclampsia
(b) epileptic seizures
(c) status epilepticus during pregnancy
(d) atypical or absence seizures

6. The magnesium sulfate dosage for Ms. Pappas depends on her serum magnesium level. Which serum magnesium level is considered therapeutic?
(a) 1.5 to 3 mEq/liter
(b) 4 to 6 mEq/liter
(c) 8 to 10 mEq/liter
(d) 12 to 15 mEq/liter

7. During magnesium sulfate therapy, the nurse monitors Ms. Pappas closely. Which signs and symptoms should alert the nurse to magnesium toxicity?
(a) hyperreflexia and shortness of breath
(b) confusion and tachycardia
(c) absent deep tendon reflexes and hypotension
(d) hypertension and a positive Babinski sign

SELECTED REFERENCES

AHFS drug information 90. (1990). Bethesda, MD: American Society of Hospital Pharmacists.

Drug facts and comparisons. (1991). St. Louis: Facts and Comparisons Division, J.B. Lippincott.

Dudley, D., Gagnon, D., and Varner, M (1989). Long-term tocolysis with intravenous magnesium sulfate. *Obstetrics and Gynecology,* 73(3), 373-378.

Gupta, R., Foster, S., Romano, P., et al. (1989). Acute pulmonary edema associated with the use of oral ritodrine for premature labor. *Chest,* 95(2), 479-481.

Moncada, S., Flower, R., and Vane, J. (1990). Prostaglandins, prostacyclin, thromboxane A_2, and leukotrienes. In *Goodman and Gilman's the pharmacological basis of therapeutics* (9th ed.). (pp. 660-673). New York: Macmillan.

North American Nursing Diagnosis Association. (1990). *Taxonomy I-Revised, with official diagnostic categories.* St. Louis: NANDA.

Physicians' desk reference 1990. (44th ed.). (1990). Oradell, NJ: Medical Economics Co.

Roberts, J., Jenning, B., Franklin, K., et al. (1989). Use of prostaglandins in nurse-midwifery practice. *Journal of nurse midwifery,* 34(3), 137-143.

Severe hypermagnesemia due to dosing errors. (1989). *Nurses Drug Alert,* 13(4), 25-26.

USPDI. (1991). *Drug information for the health care professional* (Vol. I, 11th ed.). Rockville, MD: United States Pharmcopeial Convention.

DRUGS TO CONTROL INFLAMMATION, ALLERGY, AND ORGAN REJECTION

Some agents used to control inflammation, allergy, and organ rejection are used for more than one purpose. The glucocorticoids, for example, exert anti-inflammatory and immunosuppressant effects, and the antiallergy drugs block inflammation caused by antigen-antibody reactions. Immunosuppressant drugs, however, are used specifically to prevent organ rejection. To understand the mechanisms of action of these drugs, the nurse needs an overview of the immune and inflammatory responses.

IMMUNE AND INFLAMMATORY RESPONSES

Immune and inflammatory responses protect the body from foreign substances and insults. These responses usually help maintain homeostasis, but sometimes are inappropriate, as in a patient undergoing organ transplantation or experiencing autoimmune disease. In such instances, drugs are used to suppress these responses.

The immune system's complex network of specialized cells degrades and removes damaged or dead cells and prevents the growth and development of abnormal cells. The immune system generates two types of response: cell-mediated and humoral.

Cell-mediated response depends on the T lymphocyte (T cell) system. Stem cells in the bone marrow give rise to T cell precursors, which later are released from the thymus as mature T cells. (They are called T cells because they come from the thymus.) T cells may be helper or suppressor cells. Helper T cells enhance the body's immune response; suppressor T cells inhibit it. Helper T cells usually outnumber suppressor T cells by two to one. In a disease such as acquired immunodeficiency syndrome (AIDS), however, the number of helper T cells drops to almost zero.

In an autoimmune disease, such as systemic lupus erythematosus or rheumatoid arthritis, the cell-mediated response is activated by the individual's cells, which the immune system treats as foreign substances.

The humoral response depends on B lymphocyte (B cell) activity. B cells (lymphocytes that originate as stem cell precursors in the bone marrow) respond to an antigen by differentiating into plasma cells that secrete antigen-specific antibodies. This antigen-antibody reaction activates the complement system, which causes lysis of antigenic cells. (For a summary of cell-mediated and humoral responses, see *Immune responses.*)

Immune responses commonly result in inflammation, the local reaction of vascularized tissue to injury. When injury occurs, chemical reactions involving bradykinin, prostaglandins, and histamines ensue. These reactions cause vasodilation at the injury site, which increases blood flow, redness, and warmth. Capillary permeability also increases, causing edema (swelling). Pain results from the edema and the effects of histamine and bradykinin on nerve endings. Leukocyte migration to the area to remove cellular debris contributes to the edema and pain.

An exaggerated immune response, or hypersensitivity reaction, can occur in a sensitized individual. Reexposure to an allergen can cause such symptoms as rhinitis, wheezing, and red, tearing eyes.

OVERVIEW OF CHAPTERS

Unit Thirteen presents drugs that modify abnormal immune or inflammatory responses. These drugs are used in such diverse disorders as allergic rhinitis, gout, and kidney transplant rejection.

Chapter 56
Antihistaminic Agents

Chapter 56 investigates the antihistaminic agents: the ethanolamines, ethylenediamines, alkylamines, phenothiazines, piperidines, and miscellaneous agents. First, it describes the events that occur in a Type I hypersensitivity reaction and discusses the histamine (H_1)-receptor antagonists. For each class of antihistaminic agent, it explores the related mechanisms of action and clinical uses. It concludes with a discussion of nursing process application, which features patient teaching.

Immune responses

When an antigen stimulates the bone marrow stem cells, the immune system produces a cell-mediated or humoral response, as shown below.

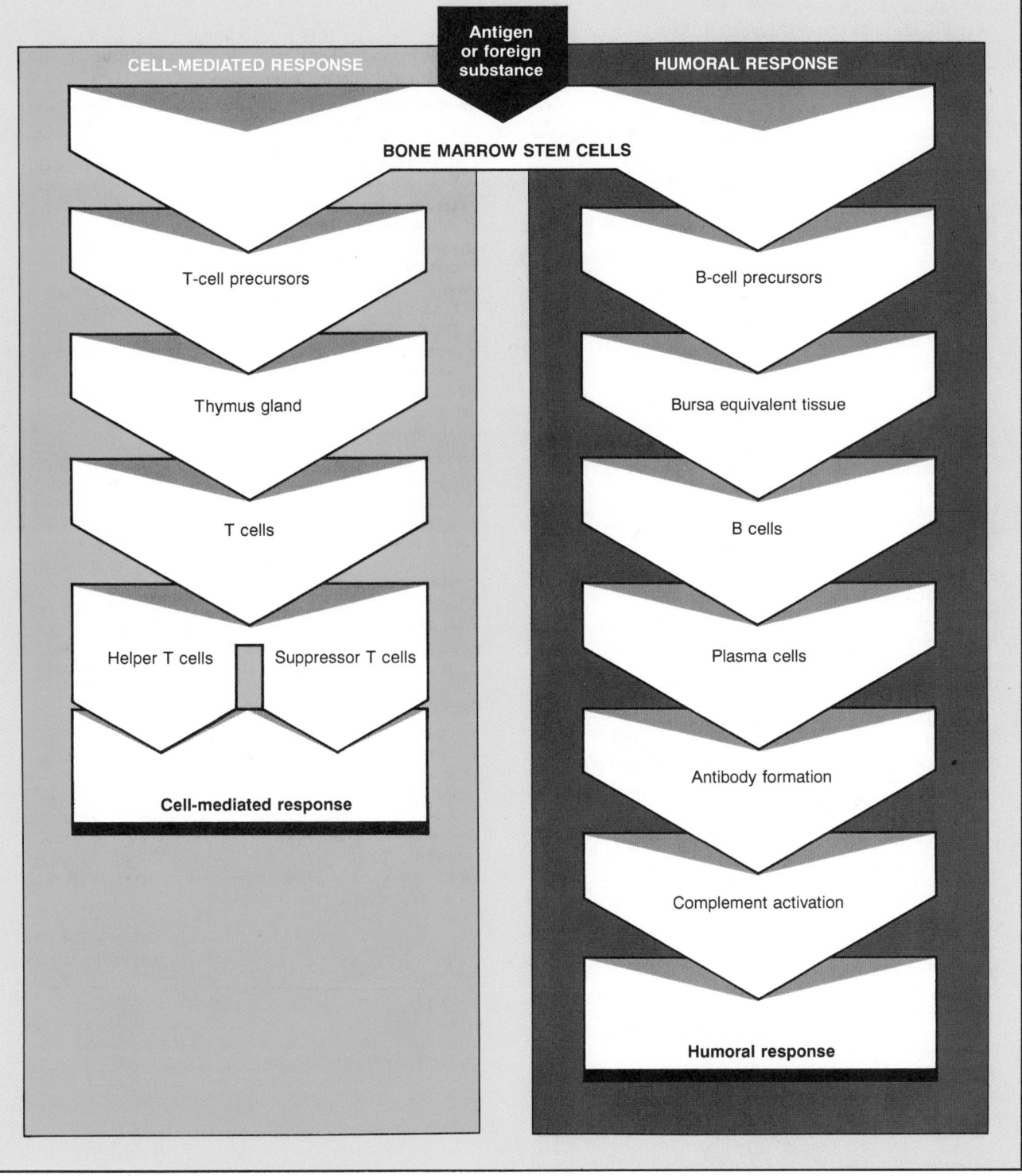

Glossary

Allergen: substance capable of producing a hypersensitivity reaction.

Allergy: hypersensitivity reaction acquired through exposure to an allergen that results in an increased reaction upon reexposure.

Allograft, allogenic graft, or **homograft:** tissue transplanted between genetically different individuals of the same species.

Antibody: immunoglobulin synthesized by lymphoid tissue in response to an antigenic stimulus.

Antigen: high-molecular-weight foreign protein or protein-polysaccharide complex that can stimulate the synthesis of a specific antibody.

Autoimmunity: abnormal reactivity of the body to its own tissue.

Basophil: granulocytic leukocyte characterized by a lobulated nucleus and coarse, large, round, irregular bluish cytoplasmic granules. In an allergic reaction, basophils release histamine, bradykinin, heparin, and serotonin.

B cell: bursal lymphocyte responsible for humoral immunity.

Chemotaxis: movement of an organism in response to a chemical stimulus.

Complement: serum substance that combines with an antibody-antigen complex, producing antigen lysis.

Conjunctivitis: inflammation of the mucous membrane lining the eyelids and covering the exposed surface of the eyeball.

Creatinine clearance: volume of plasma cleared of creatinine per unit of time; the total average value is 120 ml/minute.

Dyskinesia: impaired ability to execute voluntary movements.

Ecchymosis: skin discoloration caused by extravasation of blood into subcutaneous tissue; bruise.

Exocrine gland: gland that secretes externally through a duct to the skin.

Fibroblast: connective tissue cell.

Globulin: class of proteins characterized by solubility in saline solutions but not in water.

Glucocorticoid: adrenocortical hormone that increases gluconeogenesis, raising the concentration of liver glycogen and blood glucose, and inhibits the inflammatory response.

Gout: condition caused by abnormal purine metabolism, characterized by an increased serum uric acid level, acute arthritic episodes, and formation of chalky urate deposits in the joints.

Histamine: powerful tissue substance released during an allergic reaction that dilates capillaries, contracts most smooth muscles, increases heart rate, and stimulates gastric secretions.

Hypercalcemia: excess calcium in the blood.

Hyperglycemia: excess glucose in the blood.

Hypernatremia: excess sodium in the blood.

Hypersensitivity: exaggerated immune system reaction, with characteristic symptoms, to contact with certain substances (allergens) that are innocuous to nonsensitized individuals.

Hyperuricemia: excess uric acid in the blood.

Hypocalcemia: calcium deficiency in the blood.

Hypokalemia: potassium deficiency in the blood.

Immunology: study of the immune system and its reactions to antigens.

Immunosuppression: inhibition of the body's immune response to foreign substances.

Inflammation: tissue response to injury characterized by pain, heat, redness, edema, and sometimes loss of function.

Labyrinthitis: inner ear inflammation.

Lymphocyte: white blood cell with a single nucleus and nongranular protoplasm that arises from the reticular tissue of the lymph gland.

Lymphokine: soluble substance released by a lymphocyte when stimulated by an antigen.

Lysosome: minute cellular body containing hydrolytic enzymes that are released upon injury to the cell.

Macrophage: large mononuclear cell that ingests microorganisms, other cells, or foreign particles.

Mast cell: large connective tissue cell that secretes heparin, histamine, bradykinin, and serotonin in response to an allergic or inflammatory stimulus.

Mineralocorticoid: adrenocortical hormone that increases sodium retention and potassium excretion.

Myelosuppression: inhibition of blood cell production by the bone marrow.

Myopathy: skeletal muscle disorder.

Paresthesia: abnormal burning, prickling, or tingling sensation.

Phagocytosis: engulfment of microorganisms, cells, or foreign particles by reticuloendothelial cells, polymorphonuclear leukocytes, monocytes, or macrophages.

Polymorphonuclear leukocyte: white blood cell with a lobed nucleus that responds to allergic and inflammatory stimuli.

Proteolysis: enzymatic hydrolysis of proteins into proteose, peptone, and other by-products.

Rheumatoid arthritis: autoimmune disease characterized by connective tissue inflammation, especially in the muscles and joints.

Rhinitis: inflammation of nasal mucous membranes

Rhinorrhea: discharge of thin nasal mucus.

Seborrhea: sebaceous gland dysfunction characterized by excessive secretion of sebum that forms white or yellowish greasy scales or cheesy plugs.

T helper cell: cell released by T lymphocytes in response to an antigen that activates other T cells, B cells, and macrophages.

Tophi: chalky urate deposits in the tissue around joints that typically occur in individuals with gout.

T suppressor cell: cell released by T lymphocytes in response to an antigen that prevents other T cells from producing an excessive immune response that might damage the body severely.

Uricosuric: agent that promotes uric acid excretion.

Urticaria: skin reaction characterized by transient wheals that are paler or redder than the surrounding skin and commonly are accompanied by severe itching; also called hives.

Chapter 57
Corticosteroids and Other Immunosuppressant Agents

Chapter 57 focuses on anti-inflammatory and immunosuppressant agents, including the systemic and topical glucocorticoids, mineralocorticoids, and immunosuppressants (azathioprine, cyclosporine, lymphocyte immune globulin, antithymocyte globulin, and muromonab-CD3). It introduces adrenal anatomy and physiology and presents the pharmacologic properties of the drug classes, emphasizing the clinical uses of the agents and their long-term adverse effects. The chapter also demonstrates application of the nursing process related to these agents, highlighting ways to help a patient prevent secondary infection and recognize and cope with adverse reactions.

Chapter 58
Uricosurics, Other Antigout Agents, and Gold Salts

Chapter 58 presents the uricosurics (probenecid and sulfinpyrazone), other antigout agents (allopurinol and colchicine), and gold salts (auranofin, aurothioglucose, and gold sodium thiomalate). After discussing the causes and signs and symptoms of gout and rheumatoid arthritis, the chapter details the pharmacologic properties of the agents used to treat these disorders. It details related care through the nursing process, including patient teaching about detection, prevention, and response to adverse reactions.

ANTIHISTAMINIC AGENTS

OBJECTIVES

After reading and studying this chapter, the student should be able to:

1. Describe the sequence of physiologic events in a type I hypersensitivity reaction.

2. Explain the mechanism of action of H_1-receptor antagonists and explain how they relieve allergy symptoms.

3. Identify drugs in the six major antihistamine drug classes.

4. Describe the interactions between H_1-receptor antagonists and other drugs.

5. Discuss the major adverse reactions to the H_1-receptor antagonists.

6. Describe how to apply the nursing process when caring for a patient who is receiving an antihistaminic agent.

INTRODUCTION

Antihistamines primarily act to block histamine effects that occur in an immediate (type I) hypersensitivity reaction, commonly called an allergic reaction. A review of the immunologic sequence and the antigen-antibody reaction will aid in understanding the mechanism of action of the antihistamines.

The human immune system reacts to agents that it recognizes as foreign to the host. These foreign substances, or antigens, stimulate the production of antibodies that help defend the body against bacterial, viral, or other invasion. An allergy occurs when an individual has an antigen response to an ordinary substance in the environment. Most people with allergies have inherited an immune system deficiency that makes them more vulnerable than others to foreign substances.

Type I hypersensitivity develops after the first exposure to a protein or other substance that the host recognizes as foreign. This antigen, or allergen, stimulates production of unusual amounts of immunoglobulin E (IgE) antibodies,

SELECTED NURSING DIAGNOSES

Antihistaminic agents

The following nursing diagnoses address representative problems and etiologies that a nurse may encounter when caring for a patient who is receiving an antihistaminic agent. Some of these nursing diagnoses contain generalized etiologies, which the nurse must individualize based on the patient's needs. (For some common nursing diagnoses and related interventions for each drug class, see the "Nursing Process Application" section of this chapter.)

- Altered health maintenance related to ineffectiveness of the prescribed antihistaminic agent
- Constipation related to the adverse gastrointestinal (GI) effects of the antihistaminic agent
- Diarrhea related to the adverse GI effects of the antihistaminic agent
- Hyperthermia related to antihistamine-induced drug fever
- Ineffective airway clearance related to thick, tenacious bronchial secretions caused by the antihistaminic agent
- Knowledge deficit related to the prescribed antihistaminic agent
- Noncompliance related to long-term use of the antihistaminic agent
- Potential for injury related to a preexisting condition that contraindicates the use of an antihistaminic agent
- Potential for injury related to a preexisting condition that requires cautious use of an antihistaminic agent
- Potential for injury related to adverse drug reactions
- Potential for injury related to drug interactions
- Potential for poisoning related to use of an antihistaminic agent
- Potential for trauma related to the sedative effects of an antihistaminic agent
- Sensory-perceptual alterations (auditory or visual) related to the adverse sensory effects of an antihistaminic agent
- Sleep pattern disturbance related to antihistamine-induced insomnia or sedation
- Urinary retention related to the anticholinergic effects of the antihistaminic agent

Allergic response

This illustration traces the cellular and systemic events that occur in an allergic response, or type I hypersensitivity reaction.

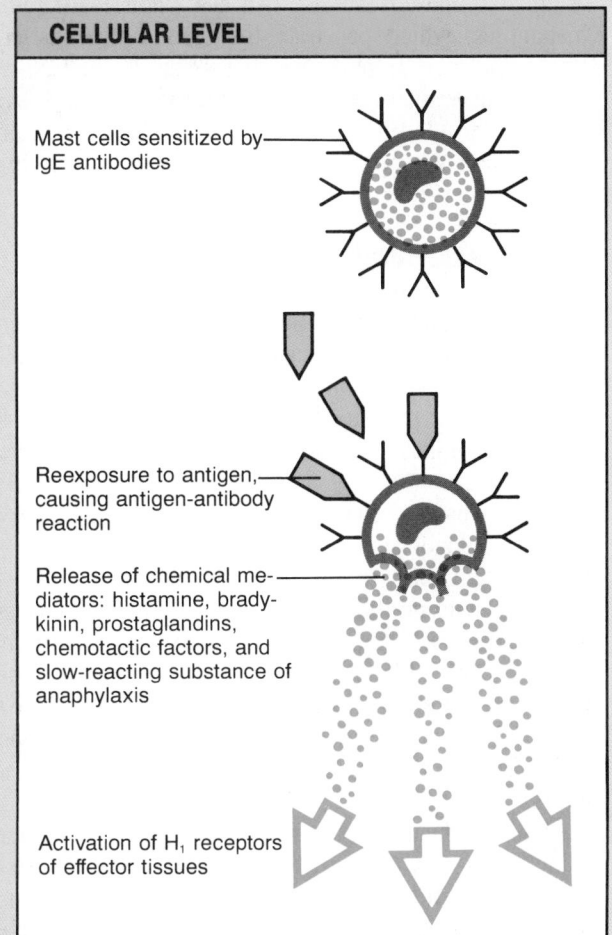

CELLULAR LEVEL

Mast cells sensitized by IgE antibodies

Reexposure to antigen, causing antigen-antibody reaction

Release of chemical mediators: histamine, bradykinin, prostaglandins, chemotactic factors, and slow-reacting substance of anaphylaxis

Activation of H_1 receptors of effector tissues

SYSTEMIC LEVEL

Oronasopharyngeal
- Rhinorrhea
- Sneezing
- Itching in the nose and throat

Skin
- Itching
- Angioedema
- Flushing
- Flares
- Wheals

Respiratory
- Contraction of bronchial smooth muscle
- Bronchial constriction with bronchospasm
- Increased mucus production
- Decreased vital capacity

Cardiovascular
- Increased heart rate
- Increased vasodilation
- Increased capillary permeability
- Decreased blood pressure

Gastrointestinal
- Increased smooth muscle contraction
- Increased parietal cell secretion

Endocrine
- Increased release of epinephrine and norepinephrine

which normally are present in very small quantities. These antibodies sensitize mast cells (connective tissue cells that contain histamine) and basophils (specialized leukocytes) by attaching to their surfaces. Later, when the sensitized cells are reexposed to the antigen, a reaction occurs between the antigen and the IgE antibodies. This antigen-antibody reaction stimulates the sensitized cells to release chemical mediators, including histamine, bradykinin, prostaglandins, chemotactic factors (substances that produce cell movement), and slow-reacting substance of anaphylaxis. The body responds to these mediators by dilating the veins and arteries, increasing capillary permeability, constricting smooth muscles (except arterioles), and increasing the secretions of exocrine glands, such as parietal cells and lacrimal glands.

Histamine, the major chemical mediator in this reaction, is responsible for producing most allergy symptoms. When histamine binds to H_1 receptors on effector tissues (tissues that contract or secrete in response to nerve impulses), it produces profound peripheral vasodilation and capillary permeability. This in turn leads to edema and constriction of bronchial smooth muscles. (For a summary of this process, see *Allergic response.*)

Antihistamine therapy works to block the binding of histamine to H_1 receptors. By doing this, antihistamines diminish most histamine effects and relieve the symptoms of a type I hypersensitivity reaction. They are available alone or in combination products, by prescription or over the counter (OTC).

For a summary of representative drugs, see *Selected major drugs: Antihistaminic agents,* pages 952 and 953. For a listing of applicable nursing diagnoses that the nurse may formulate when caring for a patient receiving these agents, see *Selected nursing diagnoses: Antihistaminic agents,* page 942. For detailed information on applying the nursing process, see Chapter 6, The Nursing Process and Drug Therapy.

H₁-RECEPTOR ANTAGONISTS

The term antihistamine refers to drugs that act as H₁-receptor antagonists. Drugs that antagonize H₂ receptors are not considered antihistamines and are discussed separately. (For a discussion of these drugs, see Chapter 44, Peptic Ulcer Agents.) Based on chemical structure, antihistamines are categorized into six major classes: ethanolamines, ethylenediamines, alkylamines, phenothiazines, piperidines, and miscellaneous agents.

The ethanolamines include clemastine fumarate, dimenhydrinate, diphenhydramine hydrochloride, and phenyltoloxamine citrate. The ethylenediamines are pyrilamine maleate and tripelennamine. The alkylamines include brompheniramine, chlorpheniramine maleate, dexchlorpheniramine maleate, and triprolidine hydrochloride. The phenothiazines include methdilazine hydrochloride, promethazine hydrochloride, and trimeprazine tartrate. The piperidine class consists of azatadine maleate, cyclizine lactate, cyproheptadine hydrochloride, hydroxyzine hydrochloride, hydroxyzine pamoate, meclizine hydrochloride, and phenindamine tartrate. Astemizole and terfenadine are miscellaneous antihistamines, which are longer-acting and produce fewer central nervous system (CNS) effects than the other antihistamines.

All classes of antihistamines competitively block the binding of histamine to H₁-receptor sites on effector tissues. This blocking action can halt the progression of a type I hypersensitivity reaction but cannot reverse effects that already are present. Certain H₁-receptor antagonists also can counteract motion sickness, vertigo, nausea, and vomiting.

PHARMACOKINETICS

Studies of three compounds—brompheniramine, chlorpheniramine, and diphenhydramine—have provided most of the information about the fate of antihistamines in the body. These studies show that antihistamines are metabolized by the liver and that most metabolites are excreted in the urine in 24 hours.

Absorption, distribution, metabolism, excretion

H₁-receptor antagonists are absorbed well after oral or parenteral administration. They are distributed widely throughout the body and CNS, with the highest concentration in the lungs and lower concentrations in the kidneys, brain, spleen, muscles, and skin. The only exceptions are astemizole and terfenadine, two new "nonsedating" antihistamines, which penetrate the blood-brain barrier so poorly that very little drug is distributed in the CNS.

Antihistamines are metabolized by hepatic enzymes and excreted in the urine, almost entirely as degradation products of metabolism. Small amounts are excreted in breast milk.

Onset, peak, duration

Onset of action, peak concentration level, and duration of action vary among the antihistamines. After oral administration of an H₁-receptor antagonist, symptom relief begins in about 30 minutes. Onset ranges from 15 to 60 minutes. After parenteral administration, onset occurs in 20 to 30 minutes. Effects of rectal suppositories develop 30 to 40 minutes after administration. Terfenadine and astemizole have a delayed onset compared to the other H₁-receptor antagonists. Terfenadine begins to act in 1 to 2 hours; astemizole in more than 4 hours.

Peak concentration usually occurs 1 to 2 hours after administration. Studies indicate that diphenhydramine reaches a peak blood concentration after about 2 hours, remaining there for another 2 hours before the level begins to fall. Terfenadine also achieves a peak concentration in about 2 hours but does not reach peak effects for 3 to 4 hours.

Usually, the duration varies from 4 to 8 hours, although some drugs have a longer duration. For instance, the antihistaminic effects of terfenadine and azatadine last 12 hours. The plasma half-life for most antihistamines is about 4 hours, but longer-acting drugs have longer half-lives. For example, the half-life of terfenadine is 20 hours; of astemizole, about 7 days.

PHARMACODYNAMICS

Most H₁-receptor antagonists are used to block the effects of histamine in allergic reactions. Their histamine-blocking action also makes them useful in treating other disorders.

Mechanism of action

H₁-receptor antagonists competitively antagonize histamine at H₁-receptor sites on effector cells in the small blood vessels, smooth muscles, peripheral nerves, adrenal medulla, exocrine glands, and brain. Through this antagonism, histamine binding on these target tissues is blocked, but the overall release of histamine continues. This action prevents further responses to histamine but does not reverse the present effects of histamine. That means that continued exposure to the allergen will cause continued histamine release. If the amount of histamine increases rapidly, antihistamines may not be able to block the numerous histamine molecules from the receptors. When that happens, epinephrine or another physiologic histamine antagonist must be administered to produce the opposite effects of histamine: constricting small blood vessels and relaxing bronchial smooth muscles.

H₁-receptor antagonists effectively block the action of histamine on the small blood vessels. They can decrease small arteriole dilation and engorgement of related tissues. They significantly reduce capillary permeability, decreasing interstitial leakage of plasma proteins and fluids and lessening edema.

H₁-receptor antagonists inhibit most smooth muscle responses to histamine. In particular, they block the constriction of bronchial, gastrointestinal (GI), and vascular smooth muscle. They are less effective on histamine-induced vasodilation. However, administration of an H₂-receptor antagonist may correct this problem.

H₁-receptor antagonists also relieve symptoms by acting on the terminal nerve endings in the skin. Nerve endings stimulated by histamine produce a flare (redness around an urticarial lesion) and itching. H₁-receptor antagonists suppress both symptoms, possibly by blocking histamine receptors that occupy nerve endings.

The drugs also selectively suppress adrenal medulla stimulation, autonomic ganglia stimulation, and exocrine gland secretion, such as lacrimal and salivary secretion. Although these anticholinergic properties may contribute to the adverse effects of the drug, they allow them to be used as antimuscarinics, which inhibit responses to acetylcholine. The drugs, however, do not affect parietal cell secretion, which is suppressed more effectively by H₂-receptor antagonists.

Several antihistaminic agents have a high affinity for H₁ receptors in the brain and are used for their CNS effects. The CNS effects of diphenhydramine make it useful as a sedative or hypnotic agent. Dimenhydrinate, diphenhydramine, promethazine, and various piperidine derivatives serve as effective antiemetic and antivertigo agents, although their exact mechanisms of action are unknown. Diphenhydramine can act as an antidyskinetic (a drug that corrects impaired involuntary movements) because of its ability to inhibit the responses to acetylcholine. Diphenhydramine also suppresses the cough center in the medulla, making it an effective antitussive agent. (For a summary of the effects of each class of antihistamine, see *Antihistamine effects*.)

PHARMACOTHERAPEUTICS

The ability of these drugs to block H₁ receptors throughout the body helps to explain their broad spectrum of activity and multiple indications for use. Antihistaminic agents are used to treat the symptoms of type I hypersensitivity reactions, such as allergic rhinitis, vasomotor rhinitis, allergic conjunctivitis, urticaria (hives), and angioedema (submucosal swelling in the hands, face, and feet). They also are used as adjunctive therapy to treat anaphylactic reactions after acute manifestations are controlled. Additional clinical indications include nausea, vomiting, motion sickness, vertigo, and preoperative sedation. In fact, some of these drugs are used primarily as antiemetics. (For more information on this use, see Chapter 43, Emetic and Antiemetic Agents.) Diphenhydramine can help treat Parkinson's disease (parkinsonism) and drug-induced extrapyramidal re-

Antihistamine effects

The effects of antihistamines vary among the classes of drugs and among the specific drugs in each class. The following chart summarizes the general effects for each pharmacologic class.

ANTIHISTAMINE CLASS	SEDATIVE EFFECTS	ANTICHOLINERGIC EFFECTS	ANTIEMETIC EFFECTS
ethanolamines	Moderate to high	High	Moderate to high
ethylenediamines	Low to moderate	None to low	Low
alkylamines	Low	Moderate	Low
phenothiazines	Low to high	High	Very high
piperidines	Low to moderate	Moderate	Low
Miscellaneous antihistamines (astemizole and terfenadine)	None to low	None to low	None

actions. Because of its antiserotonin qualities, cyproheptadine may be used to treat Cushing's disease, serotonin-associated diarrhea, vascular cluster headaches, and anorexia nervosa.

Most antihistamines lack specificity for selective H_1 receptors. Although nonspecificity promotes multiple use, it causes a major disadvantage: sedation. Most antihistamines readily cross the blood-brain barrier and bind to H_1 receptors in the brain. That leads to CNS depression, which can be an undesired effect, depending on the treatment goal. Ethanolamines, in particular, can produce extreme CNS depression and sedation.

clemastine fumarate (Tavist). An ethanolamine derivative, clemastine is used to relieve the symptoms of histamine-induced allergic reactions. Its most common adverse reaction is drowsiness.
Usual adult dosage: 1.34 mg P.O. b.i.d. or 2.68 mg P.O. one to three times a day, depending on the patient's age and condition. The lower dosage usually is indicated for an elderly patient or a patient with rhinitis and other allergy symptoms; the higher dosage, for a younger patient or one with a dermatologic condition. Dosage should not exceed 8.04 mg/day.

dimenhydrinate (Dimetabs, Dramamine, Dymenate, Marmine). An ethanolamine derivative, dimenhydrinate also is an anticholinergic that acts principally through CNS depression. Through its depressant action on hyperstimulated labyrinthine function, it can prevent and treat the nausea, vomiting, and vertigo associated with motion sickness. It also can relieve the symptoms of labyrinthitis, Ménière's disease, and other diseases affecting the vestibular system. Most oral forms of the drug are available over the counter, but parenteral forms require a prescription.
Usual adult dosage: 50 to 100 mg P.O. every 4 to 6 hours p.r.n., not to exceed 400 mg/day; 50 to 100 mg I.M. every 4 hours p.r.n.; 50 mg I.V. in 10 ml of normal saline solution injected over at least 2 minutes, every 4 hours p.r.n.

diphenhydramine hydrochloride (Benadryl, Benylin, Caladryl, Compoz, Genahist, Nordryl, Nytol, Sominex Formula 2). An ethanolamine derivative, diphenhydramine probably is the broadest-spectrum antihistamine. It has strong central and peripheral actions. Its central action makes it useful for preventing or treating motion sickness and nausea and vomiting associated with amphotericin administration and cancer chemotherapy. It is effective as a preoperative sedative and as a nighttime sleep aid, appearing in many OTC products, such as Nytol and Sominex. In syrup form, it is used to treat coughs related to colds or allergy. The central action of this drug may inhibit the action of acetylcholine mediated by muscarinic receptors. As a result, it is useful as an antidyskinetic and antimus-

carinic, especially in some elderly patients with Parkinson's disease or drug-induced dyskinesias who should not take stronger drugs.

Because of diphenhydramine's peripheral action, it can be used to relieve allergy symptoms and prevent transfusion reactions in sensitized patients who are receiving platelet transfusions.

Although oral administration is preferred, the drug may be given by deep I.M. or I.V. injection. The parenteral form is available in 10 and 50 mg per ml. Diphenhydramine also is available in topical 1% and 2% creams and lotions (Caladryl). In these forms, it temporarily relieves itching associated with skin conditions.
Usual adult dosage: for allergy symptoms or motion sickness, 25 to 50 mg P.O. t.i.d. or q.i.d., or 10 to 50 mg deep I.M. or I.V. For prophylaxis before transfusions, cancer chemotherapy, or amphotericin administration, 50 mg P.O. or I.V. For dyskinesias, 50 mg P.O. one to three times a day or 25 to 50 mg deep I.M. or I.V. For hypnotic effects, 25 to 50 mg P.O. at bedtime. For coughs, 12.5 to 25 mg of syrup P.O. every 4 hours. For itching, topical application t.i.d. or q.i.d.

phenyltoloxamine citrate (Naldecon). An ethanolamine derivative, phenyltoloxamine citrate works with chlorpheniramine maleate and two sympathomimetic amines, phenylpropanolamine hydrochloride and phenylephrine hydrochloride, to relieve congestion and the symptoms of hay fever and other allergies.
Usual adult dosage: to relieve allergy symptoms, 5 ml of syrup P.O. every 3 to 4 hours, not to exceed four doses in 24 hours; or one sustained-release tablet P.O. every 8 hours p.r.n. Tablets must be swallowed whole to be effective.

pyrilamine maleate (Dormarex, Quiet World). An ethylenediamine derivative, pyrilamine is available alone or in combination products and provides symptomatic relief for allergic reactions. In combination products, this drug also acts as a nighttime sleep aid.
Usual adult dosage: for allergies, 25 to 50 mg P.O. t.i.d. or q.i.d.; as a sleep aid, 50 mg P.O. at bedtime.

tripelennamine (PBZ, PBZ-SR, Pyribenzamine, Ro-Hist). An ethylenediamine, this drug comes in two forms: tripelennamine citrate and tripelennamine hydrochloride. Both forms can be given orally, but the hydrochloride salt also can be administered topically as a cream. Tripelennamine relieves allergy symptoms.
Usual adult dosage: 37.5 to 75 mg of tripelennamine citrate P.O. every 4 to 6 hours, not to exceed 900 mg/day; 25 to 50 mg of tripelennamine hydrochloride P.O. every 4 to 6 hours, not to exceed 600 mg/day; or 100 mg of sustained-release tripelennamine hydrochloride P.O. b.i.d. or t.i.d.

brompheniramine (Bromphen, Dimetane, Dimetane Extentabs, Veltane). An alkylamine, brompheniramine is available in an elixir, regular and sustained-release tablets, and injectable form to treat allergy symptoms. In combination with other drugs, it is used to treat seasonal and perennial allergic rhinitis and upper respiratory symptoms in the common cold.

Usual adult dosage: 4 mg P.O. every 4 to 6 hours, not to exceed 24 mg/day; 8 to 12 mg of sustained-release tablets P.O. every 8 to 12 hours; or 10 mg I.V., I.M., or S.C. every 6 to12 hours p.r.n., not to exceed 40 mg/day.

chlorpheniramine maleate and **dexchlorpheniramine maleate** (Chlor-Trimeton, Chlor-Trimeton Repetabs, Dexchlor, Polaramine, Teldrin). An alkylamine used to treat rhinitis and allergy symptoms, chlorpheniramine maleate is available in various forms: capsules; solutions; regular, chewable, and sustained-release tablets; parenteral injections; and in combination products. The parenteral form also is used to relieve symptoms of anaphylaxis and allergic reactions to blood or plasma. Dexchlorpheniramine is available in tablets, repeat-action tablets, and syrups.

Usual adult dosage: for rhinitis and allergy symptoms, 4 mg P.O. of chlorpheniramine maleate every 4 to 6 hours, not to exceed 24 mg/day; 2 mg of dexchlorpheniramine maleate P.O. every 4 to 6 hours, not to exceed 12 mg/day; 8 to 12 mg of sustained-release chlorpheniramine tablets P.O. b.i.d., not to exceed 24 mg/day; or 4 to 6 mg of sustained-release dexchlorpheniramine maleate tablets P.O. at bedtime or every 8 to 10 hours when awake. For anaphylaxis or severe allergic reactions, 10 to 20 mg of chlorpheniramine maleate I.V. or I.M.For uncomplicated allergic reactions or when oral administration is contraindicated, 5 to 20 mg of chlorpheniramine maleate I.V. or I.M. The maximum parenteral dosage is 40 mg/day.

triprolidine hydrochloride (Actidil). An alkylamine derivative, triprolidine is used to relieve symptoms of colds and allergies. It is available in solutions, tablets, and with pseudoephedrine hydrochloride in combination products, such as Actifed.

Usual adult dosage: 2.5 mg P.O. every 4 to 6 hours, not to exceed 10 mg/day.

methdilazine hydrochloride (Tacaryl). A phenothiazine derivative, this drug comes in tablets, chewable tablets, and solutions. It is used primarily to relieve symptoms of pruritus associated with urticaria.

Usual adult dosage: 8 mg P.O. b.i.d. to q.i.d.

promethazine hydrochloride (Pentazine, Phenergan). A phenothiazine derivative, promethazine commonly produces sedation, which limits its usefulness in allergy relief for an ambulatory patient. This action, however, makes promethazine useful as a preoperative and postoperative sedative, an adjunct to analgesics for controlling postoperative pain, an antianxiety agent, and a hypnotic. Although not understood fully, its actions on the CNS also make this drug useful in treating nausea, vomiting, and motion sickness. Dosage forms include tablets, syrups, rectal suppositories, and I.V. and I.M. injections. The preferred route of administration is oral.

Usual adult dosage: for motion sickness, initially, 25 mg P.O. 30 to 60 minutes before traveling; then 8 to 12 hours later p.r.n., and b.i.d. thereafter, taken upon arising and before the evening meal. For nausea and vomiting, initially, 25 mg P.O., I.M., or rectally, followed by 12.5 to 25 mg every 4 to 6 hours p.r.n. For preoperative and postoperative prevention of nausea and vomiting, initially, 25 mg P.O. or I.M., followed by 25 mg every 4 to 6 hours. For sedation or for postoperative sedation with analgesics, 25 to 50 mg P.O. For preoperative sedation, 50 mg P.O. the night before surgery.

trimeprazine tartrate (Temaril). A phenothiazine derivative, trimeprazine is a stronger histamine antagonist than promethazine but produces fewer anticholinergic and CNS depressant effects. It can alleviate histamine-induced urticaria and pruritus and is available in tablets, sustained-release capsules, and syrups.

Usual adult dosage: 2.5 mg P.O. q.i.d. p.r.n. for tablets or syrups; 5 mg P.O. every 12 hours p.r.n. for sustained-release capsules.

azatadine maleate (Optimine). A piperidine, azatadine relieves the symptoms of allergic rhinitis and chronic urticaria. In a fixed combination product with pseudoephedrine hydrochloride, azatadine can treat the symptoms of upper respiratory tract congestion associated with allergic rhinitis.

Usual adult dosage: 1 to 2 mg P.O. b.i.d.

cyclizine lactate (Marezine). A piperidine, cyclizine is used as an antiemetic to prevent or treat motion sickness. The drug probably acts indirectly on the medullary chemoreceptor trigger zone, diminishes vestibular stimulation, and depresses labyrinthine function. It is available in tablet and injection form.

Usual adult dosage: 50 mg P.O. or I.M. 30 minutes before traveling, repeated every 4 to 6 hours p.r.n.

cyproheptadine hydrochloride (Periactin). This piperidine is used primarily to relieve pruritus and cold urticaria (edema and wheals caused by exposure to cold). Research on its antiserotonin properties has promoted its unlabelled use in managing the symptoms of anorexia nervosa, carcinoid syndrome, vascular cluster headaches, galactorrhea-

amenorrhea syndrome, and other antiserotonin-responsive disorders.
Usual adult dosage: for allergy symptoms, 4 mg P.O. t.i.d. or q.i.d., not to exceed 0.5 mg/kg/day.

hydroxyzine hydrochloride (Atarax) and **hydroxyzine pamoate** (Vistaril). A piperidine, hydroxyzine acts on the subcortical areas of the CNS to produce sedation and relieve anxiety. The sedative effects may explain how it helps manage histamine-induced pruritus.
Usual adult dosage: for pruritus, 25 to 100 mg P.O. t.i.d. or q.i.d.; for preoperative and postoperative sedation, 25 to 100 mg I.M.

meclizine hydrochloride (Antivert, Bonine). A piperidine, meclizine is used to prevent and treat motion sickness and relieve vertigo associated with vestibular disturbances, such as Ménière's disease.
Usual adult dosage: for motion sickness, 25 to 50 mg P.O. 1 hour before traveling, repeated every 24 hours p.r.n.; for vertigo, 25 to 100 mg P.O. daily in divided doses.

phenindamine tartrate (Nolahist). The piperidine phenindamine is used to treat allergic reactions. It is available in tablet form over the counter.
Usual adult dosage: 25 mg P.O. every 4 to 6 hours, not to exceed 150 mg/day.

astemizole (Hismanal). A miscellaneous antihistaminic agent, astemizole is a new, "nonsedating" antihistamine. It is used to relieve symptoms associated with seasonal allergic rhinitis and chronic idiopathic urticaria.
Usual adult dosage: 10 mg P.O. once daily. With a single-dose regimen, astemizole plasma concentrations are dose-proportional. Administering a single dose of 30 mg P.O. on day 1, then 20 mg P.O. on day 2, followed by the 10-mg P.O. recommended daily maintenance dosage starting on day 3 can reduce the time required to reach steady-state plasma concentrations.

terfenadine (Seldane). This miscellaneous antihistaminic agent also is "nonsedating." Available in tablets, terfenadine effectively relieves rhinorrhea, sneezing, oronasopharyngeal irritation or itching, lacrimation, and red, irritated, or itching eyes associated with seasonal allergic rhinitis. It is less effective in relieving nasal congestion.
Usual adult dosage: 60 mg P.O. b.i.d.

Drug interactions

When given with other drugs, antihistamines may cause three types of interactions. The first type may occur when a patient simultaneously receives two or more drugs that have similar effects. The patient will display additive or cumulative drug effects characteristic of drug overdose.

Drugs that are likely to cause this interaction with antihistamines include CNS depressants, antimuscarinics, tricyclic antidepressants, and monoamine oxidase (MAO) inhibitors.

The second type of interaction may occur when an antihistamine blocks or reverses the effects of another drug. For instance, if epinephrine is administered to a patient receiving one of the phenothiazines, the antihistamine may block—or reverse—the intended vasopressor effect. If a vasopressor is required for a patient receiving phenothiazines, norepinephrine or phenylephrine should be used. Similarly, antihistamines may block H_1 receptors in the skin, suppressing the flare reaction to antigen skin testing. Therefore, antihistamines should be discontinued for 4 days before skin testing, whenever possible.

The third type of interaction occurs when antihistamine use masks the toxic signs and symptoms of another drug. For example, an antihistamine used to depress vestibular stimulation and labyrinthine function in motion sickness and vertigo can mask the signs of ototoxicity associated with aminoglycosides or large dosages of salicylates. If antihistamines must be given with aminoglycosides, the patient must be monitored closely for signs of ototoxicity. (For further details, see *Drug interactions: Antihistaminic agents.*)

ADVERSE DRUG REACTIONS

Used as antiallergy agents, antihistamines produce many adverse reactions, especially CNS depression. However, this adverse reaction and others have been exploited widely and now provide the pharmacologic basis for many other antihistamine uses. Because an adverse reaction may be a desired therapeutic response or a dose-related drug reaction, the goal of antihistaminic treatment should be considered before determining that an adverse reaction is undesirable. Not all adverse reactions are dose-related, however; sensitivity reactions to antihistamines include hematologic and hypersensitivity reactions.

The incidence and severity of adverse reactions vary among the antihistamines, but severe toxicity rarely occurs, and a dosage reduction or use of a different antihistamine usually will relieve a mild reaction. Susceptibility to adverse reactions varies among patients. For instance, an elderly patient is more likely than a younger adult to develop dizziness, sedation, and hypotension.

The most common adverse reaction is CNS depression, which can produce sedation and other symptoms. Occurring with usual dosages, sedation can range from mild drowsiness to deep sleep. Other CNS reactions may include dizziness, lassitude, disturbed coordination, and muscle weakness. After 2 to 3 days of antihistamine therapy, these adverse reactions may disappear spontaneously. Less com-

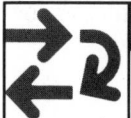

DRUG INTERACTIONS

Antihistaminic agents

Antihistamines can increase the anticholinergic effects of anticholinergic drugs and the sedative effects of CNS depressants, such as tricyclic antidepressants, tranquilizers, barbiturates, and alcohol. The combination of these drugs with antihistamines can cause life-threatening consequences.

DRUG	INTERACTING DRUGS	POSSIBLE EFFECTS	NURSING IMPLICATIONS
clemastine, dimenhydrinate, diphenhydramine, phenyltoloxamine, pyrilamine, tripelennamine, brompheniramine, chlorpheniramine, dexchlorpheniramine, triprolidine, methdilazine, promethazine, trimeprazine, cyclizine, hydroxyzine, meclizine, azatadine, cyproheptadine, phenindamine, astemizole	CNS depressants, including barbiturates, tranquilizers, alcohol, and opiates	Produce additive CNS depression	• Use caution when administering these drugs concurrently to avoid excessive CNS depression or sedation. • Inform an ambulatory patient of the possible additive effect.
	anticholinergic drugs, including tricyclic antidepressants, phenothiazines, and anti-parkinsonian drugs	Produce additive anticholinergic effects	• Assess for signs of increased anticholinergic activity, such as constipation, dry mouth, visual disturbances, and urine retention. • Notify the physician if anticholinergic effects occur.
	ototoxic drugs, including aminoglycosides and salicylates	Mask signs and symptoms of ototoxicity	• Monitor the patient for signs of hearing loss and conduct an audiometric test weekly or biweekly. • Notify the physician of changes in the patient's hearing.
	epinephrine	Reverse the vasopressor effect of epinephrine, causing vasodilation, increased heart rate, and decreased blood pressure	• Monitor the patient's heart rate and blood pressure. • Notify the physician if the patient displays abnormal vital signs.

mon reactions include CNS excitation, restlessness, insomnia, palpitations, and seizures.

The next most common adverse reactions are GI symptoms, including epigastric distress, loss of appetite, nausea, vomiting, constipation, and diarrhea. Taking the drug with meals or with milk may reduce these symptoms.

The third most common reactions are anticholinergic ones, which occur especially with the ethanolamines. Dryness of the mouth, nose, and throat and thickening of bronchial secretions commonly occur and may be desired. But in a patient with asthma or chronic obstructive pulmonary disease, they may lead to airway obstruction. Such a patient should use antihistamines with caution and only under a physician's direction. Other anticholinergic effects include urine retention and dysuria; vertigo, tinnitus, and labyrinthitis; vision disturbances, such as diplopia and blurred-vision; and cardiovascular effects, such as hypotension, hypertension, tachycardia, and extrasystoles. The anticholinergic effects of antihistamines can exacerbate some underlying conditions. Therefore, antihistamines—especially the ethanolamines—should be administered with extreme caution to a patient with narrow-angle glaucoma, peptic ulcer disease, pyloroduodenal obstruction, symptomatic prostatic hypertrophy, or bladder neck obstruction. They also should be used cautiously by a patient with cardio-

vascular disease, hypertension, bronchial asthma, or increased intraoccular pressure.

Sensitivity reactions to antihistamines occur much less commonly but may include hypersensitivity, drug fever, hematologic complications, and teratogenic effects (effects that interfere with fetal development). Hypersensitivity manifested by urticaria, drug rash, and photosensitivity may occur with oral drug administration, but usually results from topical application. Once local hypersensitivity has occurred, topical or systemic reuse of the drug or any drug in the same chemical class will produce a similar reaction.

Although rare, hematologic complications include leukopenia, granulocytopenia, hemolytic anemia, thrombocytopenia, and pancytopenia.

Antihistamines have been used extensively to control nausea and vomiting during pregnancy. However, evidence regarding their teratogenic effects is limited. Meclizine and dimenhydrinate offer the lowest risk of teratogenicity. The teratogenic effects of the other antihistamines are not known fully. Therefore, a pregnant patient should take antihistamines only under the direction of her physician. Because some antihistamines appear in breast milk, a breast-feeding patient should avoid using them.

Drug fever is a sign of a toxic reaction or overdose. Because of the wide use and ready availability of OTC antihistamines, acute poisoning commonly occurs, especially in children. The CNS effects of the drugs pose the greatest threat and account for most of the signs and symptoms of poisoning: hallucinations, excitement, ataxia, athetosis, involuntary movements, and seizures. Fever is more common in children than in adults. Fixed, dilated pupils accompany other anticholinergic effects and may be followed by coma and death. Because no specific therapy exists for H_1-receptor antagonist poisoning, the patient must receive symptom relief and supportive treatment.

NURSING PROCESS APPLICATION

The following information assists the nurse in caring for a patient receiving an antihistaminic agent.

Assessment
• Review the patient's history for a preexisting condition that contraindicates the use of an antihistaminic agent, such as lactation or known hypersensitivity to the drug.
• Review the patient's history for a preexisting condition that requires cautious use of an antihistaminic agent, such as narrow-angle glaucoma, stenosing peptic ulcer, pyloroduodenal obstruction, symptomatic prostatic hypertrophy, or bladder neck obstruction.
• Assess the patient for adverse reactions to the prescribed antihistaminic agent, such as CNS depression or excitement, GI dysfunction, anticholinergic effects, or hypersensitivity reactions.
• Review the patient's medication history to identify the use of drugs that may interact with the antihistaminic agent, such as CNS depressants, anticholinergic agents, ototoxic drugs, or epinephrine.
• Assess the effectiveness of the prescribed antihistaminic agent periodically.
• Assess the patient for sedative effects regularly.
• Assess the patient for visual or auditory disturbances throughout antihistaminic agent therapy.
• Evaluate the patient's and family's knowledge about the prescribed antihistaminic agent.

Nursing diagnoses
The following examples represent appropriate diagnoses for a patient receiving an antihistaminic agent.
• Potential for injury related to a preexisting condition that contraindicates the use of an antihistaminic agent
• Potential for injury related to a preexisting condition that requires cautious use of an antihistaminic agent
• Potential for injury related to adverse drug reactions
• Potential for trauma related to the sedative effects of an antihistaminic agent
• Sensory-perceptual alterations (auditory or visual) related to the adverse sensory effects of an antihistaminic agent

• Knowledge deficit related to the prescribed antihistaminic agent

Planning and implementation
• Do not administer an antihistaminic agent to a patient with a condition that contraindicates its use.
• Administer an antihistaminic agent cautiously to a patient at risk because of a preexisting condition.
• Monitor the patient frequently for adverse reactions during antihistamine therapy.
• Expect to decrease the dosage or use a different antihistaminic agent, as prescribed, if a mild adverse reaction occurs.
• *Monitor the patient — especially a pediatric patient — for signs of acute poisoning, such as hallucinations, excitement, ataxia, athetosis, involuntary movements, seizures, fever, and fixed, dilated pupils. Keep standard emergency equipment nearby. If acute poisoning occurs, discontinue the antihistamine and prepare for symptomatic and supportive treatment, such as mechanical ventilation. If acute poisoning is not recognized early, coma and death may occur.*
• Observe the patient for signs of a hypersensitivity reaction, such as urticaria, drug rash, and photosensitivity, especially when administering a topical antihistamine.
• *Take safety precautions if the patient develops dizziness, vertigo, lassitude, disturbed coordination, or muscle weakness. For example, keep the bed rails up and supervise ambulation. Keep in mind that these effects may disappear spontaneously after 2 or 3 days of antihistamine therapy.*
• Monitor the patient's vital signs regularly for signs of anticholinergic effects, such as changes in blood pressure, heart rate or rhythm, or respiratory rate or rhythm, or for signs of a toxic reaction or overdose, such as fever. Notify the physician of any vital sign changes.
• *Take seizure precautions as needed, especially in a patient with a history of seizures.*
• Monitor hydration if the patient experiences anorexia, nausea, vomiting, constipation, or diarrhea. Obtain a prescription for an antiemetic, antidiarrheal, or laxative agent, as needed. Also administer the prescribed antihistamine with meals or milk to decrease adverse GI reactions.
• Observe the patient for anticholinergic effects, such as dryness of the mouth, nose, and throat, and thickening of bronchial secretions. Ask the patient about signs of urine retention, such as bladder fullness after voiding, frequent voiding of small amounts, or dysuria. If urine retention occurs, prepare to catheterize the patient, as instructed.
• Monitor the patient's complete blood count for adverse hematologic reactions to the prescribed antihistaminic agent, such as leukopenia, granulocytopenia, hemolytic anemia, thrombocytopenia, or pancytopenia.

• Consult the physician about discontinuing the antihistamine for 4 days before the patient receives an allergy skin test to avoid masking positive results.

• Administer a parenteral antihistamine deep I.M., using the Z-track method to prevent subcutaneous irritation.

• Notify the physician if adverse reactions occur or if the prescribed antihistamine is ineffective.

• Monitor the patient for sedation, the most common adverse reaction to antihistamines, especially during concomitant administration of other CNS depressants.

• *Take safety precautions if sedation occurs.*

• Notify the physician if sedation is pronounced or does not disappear after 2 or 3 days of antihistamine therapy.

• Monitor the patient for hearing loss, tinnitus, or visual changes, such as diplopia and blurred vision.

• Conduct an audiometric test weekly or biweekly, as instructed, to unmask signs of ototoxicity if the patient is receiving an ototoxic drug during antihistamine therapy.

• *Take safety precautions if visual disturbances occur.*

• Notify the physician if auditory or visual disturbances occur.

Patient teaching

• Teach the patient and family the name, dose, frequency, action, and adverse effects of the prescribed antihistaminic agent.

• Review all contraindications with the patient to help prevent misuse of an OTC antihistaminic agent. Advise against using an antihistamine during pregnancy, while breast-feeding, or if the patient has a history of asthma, enlarged prostate, cardiovascular disease, hypertension, intestinal blockage, kidney disease, overactive thyroid, stomach ulcer, or urinary tract blockage. Caution the patient against taking an antihistamine concurrently with an antimuscarinic (muscle relaxant and antispasmodic), MAO inhibitor, or drug that can produce tinnitus or balance problems, such as aspirin, other salicylates, or aminoglycosides.

• *Advise a patient with a severe allergy to carry identification or wear an identification band that lists the type of allergy, the usual treatment, and the physician's name.*

• Review adverse CNS, anticholinergic, and GI reactions with the patient.

• Explain that the antihistamine can produce drowsiness and reduce alertness. Taking the drug at bedtime can minimize these symptoms but may cause continued drowsiness in the morning. These effects may lessen after 2 to 3 days of use. Advise the patient not to drive or engage in activities that require mental alertness until the reaction to the drug is known.

• Inform the patient that combining an antihistamine with alcohol or another CNS depressant adds to the sedative effects of these drugs. Advise the patient taking an antihistamine to consult the physician before taking any CNS depressants, such as narcotics, sedatives, barbiturates, OTC sleep aids, tranquilizers, tricyclic antidepressants, muscle relaxants, anesthetics, and alcohol.

• *Remind the patient to keep this and other drugs out of the reach of children. Instruct the patient to be alert for signs of an overdose, such as clumsiness, unsteadiness, seizures, severe drowsiness, and hallucinations. Advise the patient to get help immediately if an overdose is suspected.*

• Instruct the patient to drink fluids, chew sugarless gum, or suck on sugarless candy if the antihistamine produces mouth dryness.

• Advise the patient to avoid exposure to the sun or to wear sunscreen, sunglasses, and a hat when in the sun.

• Suggest that the patient take an oral antihistamine with food or milk to avoid adverse GI reactions.

• Instruct the patient to take an antihistamine prescribed for motion sickness at least 30 minutes — but preferably 1 to 2 hours — before traveling.

• Advise the patient to take a sustained-release capsule or long-acting tablet in whole form. Remind the patient not to break, cut, crush, or chew the medication.

• Instruct the patient to report adverse reactions to the physician because a change in dosage may be indicated.

Evaluation

The following examples represent appropriate evaluation statements for a patient receiving an antihistaminic agent.

• The patient has no conditions that contraindicate antihistamine therapy.

• The patient exhibits no signs of complications in the preexisting condition linked to the prescribed antihistaminic agent.

• The patient experiences no adverse reactions to the prescribed antihistaminic agent.

• The patient remains mentally alert during antihistamine therapy.

• The patient exhibits no changes in hearing or vision during antihistamine therapy.

• The patient and family express an accurate understanding of the points taught about the prescribed antihistaminic agent.

• The patient obtains and wears an identification band that lists the type of allergy, the usual treatment, and the physician's name.

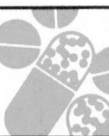

Antihistaminic agents

This chart summarizes the major antihistamines currently in clinical use.

DRUG	MAJOR INDICATIONS	USUAL ADULT DOSAGES	CONTRAINDICATIONS AND PRECAUTIONS
Ethanolamines			
dimenhydrinate	Nausea, vomiting, and vertigo associated with motion sickness; vestibular system diseases	50 to 100 mg P.O. every 4 to 6 hours, p.r.n., not to exceed 400 mg/day; 50 to 100 mg I.M. every 4 hours p.r.n.; or 50 mg I.V. in 10 ml of normal saline solution injected over 2 minutes every 4 hours, p.r.n.	• Know that dimenhydrinate is contraindicated in a lactating patient or one with known hypersensitivity to the drug. • Administer with extreme caution to a patient with narrow-angle glaucoma, stenosing peptic ulcer, pyloroduodenal obstruction, symptomatic prostatic hypertrophy, or bladder neck obstruction. • Administer with caution to a patient with bronchial asthma, increased intraocular pressure, hyperthyroidism, cardiovascular disease, or hypertension.
diphenhydramine	Motion sickness; rhinitis and other allergy symptoms Dyskinesias and Parkinson's disease Hypnotic effects	25 to 50 mg P.O. t.i.d. or q.i.d., or 10 to 50 mg deep I.M. or I.V. 50 mg P.O. one to three times a day or 25 to 50 mg deep I.M. or I.V. 25 to 50 mg P.O. at bedtime	• Know that diphenhydramine is contraindicated in a neonate or premature neonate, a lactating patient, or one with known hypersensitivity to this drug or any other antihistamine with a similar chemical structure. • Administer with extreme caution to a patient with narrow-angle glaucoma, stenosing peptic ulcer, pyloroduodenal obstruction, symptomatic prostatic hypertrophy, or bladder neck obstruction. • Administer with caution to a patient with bronchial asthma, increased intraocular pressure, hyperthyroidism, cardiovascular disease, or hypertension.
Ethylenediamines			
tripelennamine	Allergy symptoms	37.5 to 75 mg of tripelennamine citrate P.O. every 4 to 6 hours, not to exceed 900 mg/day; 25 to 50 mg of tripelennamine hydrochloride P.O. every 4 to 6 hours, not to exceed 600 mg/day; or 100 mg of sustained-release tripelennamine hydrochloride P.O. b.i.d. or t.i.d.	• Know that tripelennamine is contraindicated in a neonate or premature neonate, a pregnant or lactating patient, a patient who is undergoing MAO inhibitor therapy, or one with prostatic hypertrophy, bladder neck obstruction, narrow-angle glaucoma, bronchial asthma, stenosing peptic ulcer, pyloroduodenal obstruction, or known hypersensitivity to this drug or related compounds. • Administer with caution to a patient with increased intraocular pressure, hyperthyroidism, cardiovascular disease, hypertension, or a history of bronchial asthma.
Alkylamines			
brompheniramine	Allergy symptoms; seasonal and perennial allergic rhinitis	4 mg P.O. every 4 to 6 hours, not to exceed 24 mg/day; 8 to 12 mg of sustained-release tablets P.O. every 8 to 12 hours; 10 mg I.V., I.M., or S.C. every 6 to 12 hours, p.r.n., not to exceed 40 mg/day	• Know that brompheniramine is contraindicated in a pregnant or lactating patient or one with prostatic hypertrophy, bladder neck obstruction, narrow-angle glaucoma, or bronchial asthma.

SELECTED MAJOR DRUGS

Antihistaminic agents (continued)

DRUG	MAJOR INDICATIONS	USUAL ADULT DOSAGES	CONTRAINDICATIONS AND PRECAUTIONS
Alkylamines *(continued)*			
chlorpheniramine	Allergy symptoms	4 mg P.O. every 4 to 6 hours, not to exceed 24 mg/day; 8 to 12 mg of sustained-release tablets P.O. b.i.d.	• Know that chlorpheniramine is contraindicated in a patient with bronchial asthma, narrow-angle glaucoma, or prostatic hypertrophy.
	Uncomplicated allergic reactions	5 to 20 mg I.V. or I.M.	
	Anaphylactic reactions	10 to 20 mg I.V. or I.M.	
Miscellaneous antihistaminic agents			
astemizole	Allergic rhinitis	10 mg P.O. daily	• Know that astemizole is contraindicated in a patient with known hypersensitivity to the drug or any of its inactive ingredients. • Administer with caution to a pregnant or lactating patient or one with asthma or other lower airway disease, cirrhosis or other liver disease, or renal impairment.
terfenadine	Allergic rhinitis	60 mg P.O. b.i.d.	• Know that terfenadine is contraindicated in a lactating patient or one with known hypersensitivity to the drug or any of its ingredients. • Administer with caution to a pregnant patient or one with prostatic hypertrophy, bladder neck obstruction, narrow-angle glaucoma, or bronchial asthma.

CHAPTER SUMMARY

Chapter 56 discussed the antihistaminic agents, specifically H_1-receptor antagonists. Here are the highlights of the chapter.
• Antihistamines antagonize H_1 receptors, blocking the effects of histamine on target tissues. Most useful in exudative allergies, such as seasonal rhinitis and conjunctivitis, the drugs diminish most histamine effects and relieve symptoms of type I hypersensitivity reactions. Additional uses exploit the sedative, antiemetic, and antimuscarinic effects of these drugs.
• The classes of antihistamines include ethanolamines, ethylenediamines, alkylamines, phenothiazines, piperidines, and miscellaneous agents.
• Ethanolamines are potent and effective H_1-receptor antagonists that can produce extreme CNS depression and sedation. This class includes clemastine, dimenhydrinate, diphenhydramine, and phenyltoloxamine citrate.

• Ethylenediamines include pyrilamine and tripelennamine. In most cases, these drugs produce low to moderate sedative effects and low anticholinergic and antiemetic effects.
• Because alkylamines produce few CNS effects, they are more suitable for daytime use. Alkylamines include brompheniramine, chlorpheniramine, dexchlorpheniramine maleate, and triprolidine.
• Phenothiazines are used primarily for their antiemetic effects. The phenothiazines are methdilazine, promethazine, and trimeprazine.
• The piperidines are used to manage allergic pruritus and to prevent and treat motion sickness. This class consists of azatadine, cyclizine, cyproheptadine, hydroxyzine, meclizine, and phenindamine.
• The miscellaneous antihistaminic agents astemizole and terfenadine offer the benefits of a longer duration of action and significantly less sedation.
• In descending order of frequency, common adverse reactions to antihistamines include CNS depression, GI dysfunction, anticholinergic effects, and hypersensitivity reactions.
• When caring for a patient who is taking an antihistamine, the nurse should monitor closely for signs of acute poi-

soning—especially in a pediatric patient—because coma and death can result. No specific therapy exists for H_1-receptor antagonist poisoning. Therefore, the nurse should relieve symptoms and provide supportive treatment as prescribed for a patient with acute antihistamine poisoning.

STUDY QUESTIONS

See Appendix 1 for answers.

1. Edward Kemp, age 47, is admitted to the emergency department because he has been stung by a bee. His history reveals that a previous sting caused skin flushing, hives, and itching. Because the same symptoms have begun to appear, the physician holds Mr. Kemp for observation and prescribes diphenhydramine (Benadryl) 50 mg P.O. Mr. Kemp is exhibiting a type I hypersensitivity reaction. Which statement best describes what happens during a such a reaction?
(a) The body produces too few IgE antibodies.
(b) IgE antibodies release chemical mediators.
(c) IgE antibodies sensitize mast cells and basophils.
(d) The immune system fails to recognize a substance as foreign.

2. For Mr. Kemp, how does diphenhydramine exert its therapeutic effects?
(a) It acts as a competitive H_1-receptor antagonist to reverse histamine effects.
(b) It acts as a competitive H_1-receptor antagonist to prevent further response to histamine.
(c) It acts as a competitive H_2-receptor antagonist to reverse histamine effects.
(d) It acts as a competitive H_2-receptor antagonist to prevent further response to histamine.

3. Antihistamines most commonly produce which adverse reaction?
(a) drug fever
(b) GI distress
(c) CNS depression
(d) urine retention

4. Sandra Grant, age 50, is receiving platelet transfusions to correct thrombocytopenia caused by cancer chemotherapy. To prevent a transfusion reaction, the physician is most likely to prescribe which antihistamine?
(a) pyrilamine maleate
(b) triprolidine hydrochloride
(c) diphenhydramine hydrochloride
(d) methdilazine hydrochloride

5. Ms. Grant also receives meperidine every 4 hours, p.r.n. for pain. Which drug interaction is this CNS depressant likely to cause when given with an antihistamine?
(a) additive anticholinergic effects
(b) profound CNS depression
(c) extreme hyperexcitability
(d) paradoxical allergic response

6. While Ms. Grant is receiving an antihistamine, the nurse should assess her for adverse reactions. Which of the following may indicate a toxic reaction or overdose?
(a) polycythemia
(b) photosensitivity
(c) arrhythmias
(d) drug fever

SELECTED REFERENCES

AHFS drug information 90. (1990). Bethesda, MD: American Society of Hospital Pharmacists.

Drug facts and comparisons. (1991). St. Louis: Facts and Comparisons Division, J.B. Lippincott.

Fusaro, R. and Kingsley, D. (1986). Topical glucocorticoids: How they are used and misused. *Postgraduate Medicine,* 79(1), 283-291.

Goodman and Gilman's the pharmacological basis of therapeutics (8th ed., 1990.). Elmsford, NY: Pergamon Press.

Hansten, P., and Horn, J. (1989). *Drug interactions: Clinical significance of drug-drug interactions.* (6th ed.). Philadelphia: Lea & Febiger.

North American Nursing Diagnosis Association. (1990). *Taxonomy I - Revised, with official categories.* St. Louis: NANDA.

USPDI. (1991). *Drug information for the health care professional* (Vol. I, 11th ed.). Rockville, MD: United States Pharmacopeial Convention.

USPDI. (1991). *Advice for the patient* (Vol. II, 11th ed.). Rockville, MD: United States Pharmacopeial Convention.

CORTICOSTEROID AND OTHER IMMUNOSUPPRESSANT AGENTS

OBJECTIVES

After reading and studying this chapter, the student should be able to:

1. Discuss the mechanisms of action of the systemic and topical corticosteroids (glucocorticoids and mineralocorticoids).

2. Identify the common clinical uses of the systemic and topical corticosteroids.

3. Describe the most common adverse reactions to the systemic and topical corticosteroids.

4. Describe how to apply the nursing process when caring for a patient who is receiving a systemic or topical corticosteroid.

5. Discuss the mechanisms of action of the immunosuppressants.

6. Identify the common clinical uses of the immunosuppressants.

7. Describe the most common adverse reactions to the immunosuppressants.

8. Describe how to apply the nursing process when caring for a patient who is receiving an immunosuppressant.

INTRODUCTION

Corticosteroid drugs, which are available as natural or synthetic steroids, are used to suppress immune responses and to reduce inflammation. Natural corticosteroids are hormones produced by the adrenal cortex; most corticosteroid drugs are synthetic forms of these hormones. Natural and synthetic corticosteroids are classified according to their biological activities. The glucocorticoids, such as cortisone and dexamethasone, affect carbohydrate and protein metabolism; the mineralocorticoids, such as aldosterone and desoxycorticosterone acetate, regulate electrolyte and water balance.

Besides their primary uses as anti-inflammatory and immunosuppressant agents, glucocorticoids and mineralocorticoids are used for replacement therapy in patients with adrenocortical insufficiency (decreased secretion of endogenous corticosteroids) and for suppression of adrenocortical hyperfunction in patients with adrenogenital syndrome.

The noncorticosteroid immunosuppressant agents include antithymocyte globulin (ATG), azathioprine, cyclophosphamide, cyclosporine, and muromonab-CD3. Except for cyclophosphamide, they are used to prevent rejection of transplanted organs and experimentally to treat various autoimmune disorders. Cyclophosphamide is used primarily to treat cancer. (For information about this drug, see Chapter 66, Alkylating Agents.)

Physiology of the adrenal glands

The adrenal glands, which lie at the superior poles of the kidneys, consist of an inner medulla and an outer cortex. (For information about their composition and function, see *Anatomy of the adrenal glands,* page 956.) The medulla secretes the hormones epinephrine and norepinephrine. The three layers of the cortex secrete three classes of adrenocortical hormones: glucocorticoids, mineralocorticoids, and androgens.

The glucocorticoids, of which the most prominent is hydrocortisone (cortisol), are synthesized in the zona fasciculata, the middle layer of the adrenal cortex. (Their synthesis is controlled by another hormone, adrenocorticotropic hormone [ACTH], secreted by the pituitary gland.) Normally, the adrenal cortex produces about 30 mg of glucocorticoids a day. Acute stress, such as from infection, trauma, or surgery, may increase glucocorticoid production tenfold. This increase occurs because stress stimulates secretion of the hormone corticotropin-releasing factor by the hypothalamus, which in turn activates pituitary secretion of ACTH, thereby increasing glucocorticoid secretion.

Anatomy of the adrenal glands

The adrenal glands are paired structures located retroperitoneally, one atop each kidney. Each gland consists of an external layer, the capsule; a cortex, composed of three layers; and a medulla, as shown in the cross section on the right. The outer layer of the cortex, the zona glomerulosa, produces mineralocorticoids; the middle layer, the zona fasciculata, produces glucocorticoids; and the innermost layer, the zona reticularis, produces androgens. The medulla stores catecholamines (epinephrine and norepinephrine).

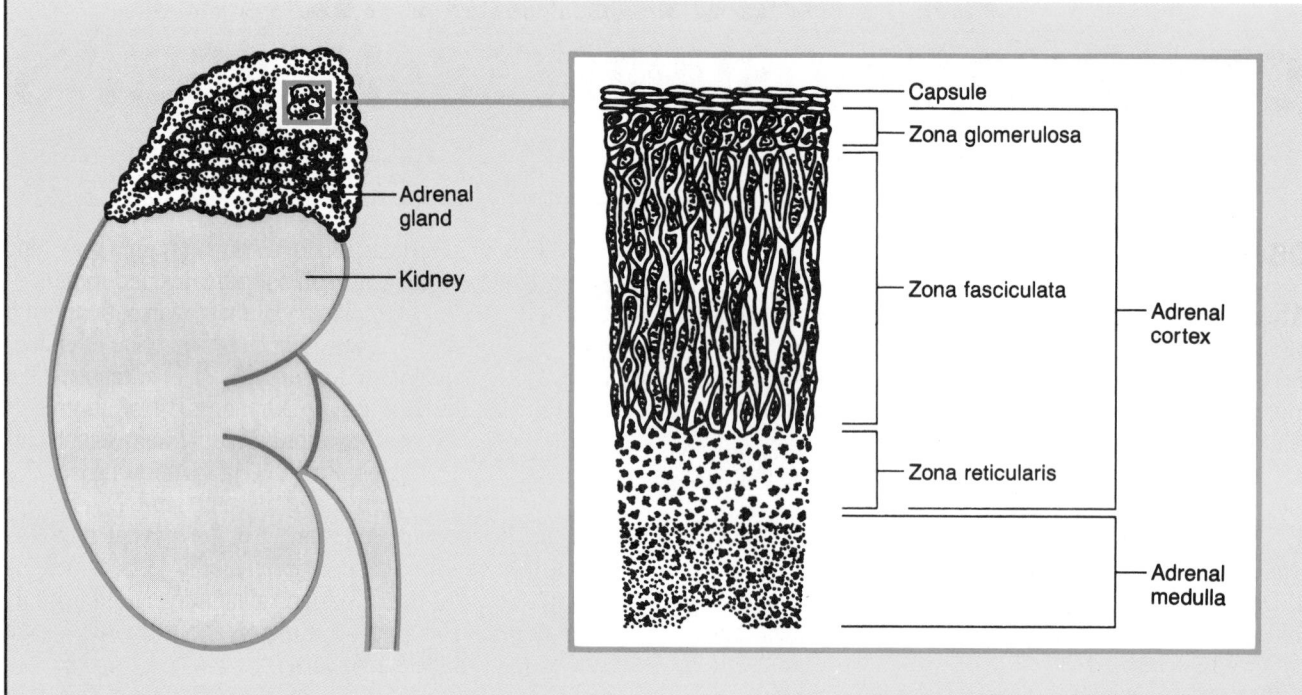

Acute stress also causes a sharp rise in levels of mineralocorticoids, which are synthesized in the zona glomerulosa—the outermost layer of the adrenal cortex. Production of these hormones is controlled by the potassium level in the blood and by the renin-angiotensin system. Aldosterone, the major mineralocorticoid, is secreted in response to sodium depletion rather than to ACTH secretion. Aldosterone increases sodium retention at the distal convoluted tubule of the kidney, thus maintaining extracellular fluid volume and adequate circulation. The mineralocorticoids and the glucocorticoids share many functions in maintaining the cardiovascular tone essential for homeostasis.

The amount of androgens synthesized in the zona reticularis, the innermost layer of the adrenal cortex, is far less than the amount secreted by the gonads. Although androgens are secreted by the adrenal gland, they are not considered corticosteroids. Androgens are used to treat endocrine system disorders. (For information about these agents, see Chapter 53, Androgenic and Anabolic Steroid Agents.)

For a summary of representative drugs, see *Selected major drugs: Corticosteroid and other immunosuppressant agents,* pages 976 to 978. For a listing of applicable nursing diagnoses that the nurse may formulate when caring for a patient receiving these agents, see *Selected nursing diagnoses: Corticosteroid and other immunosuppressant agents.* For detailed information on applying the nursing process, see Chapter 6, The Nursing Process and Drug Therapy.

SYSTEMIC GLUCOCORTICOIDS

Most glucocorticoids are synthetic analogues of hormones secreted by the zona fasciculata of the adrenal cortex. They exert anti-inflammatory, metabolic, and immunosuppressant effects. Drugs in this class include beclomethasone dipropionate, betamethasone, cortisone acetate, dexamethasone, hydrocortisone, methylprednisolone, parametha-

---

SELECTED NURSING DIAGNOSES

Corticosteroid and other immunosuppressant agents

The following nursing diagnoses address representative problems and etiologies that a nurse may encounter when caring for a patient who is receiving a corticosteroid or other immunosuppressant agent. Some of these nursing diagnoses contain generalized etiologies, which the nurse must individualize based on the patient's needs. (For some common nursing diagnoses and related interventions for each drug class, see the "Nursing Process Application" sections of this chapter.)

- Altered nutrition: more than body requirements, related to increased appetite caused by corticosteroid therapy
- Altered oral mucous membrane related to immunosuppressant-induced mouth ulcerations, gingival hyperplasia, or stomatitis
- Altered protection related to adrenocorticoid insufficiency caused by long-term corticosteroid therapy
- Altered protection related to immunosuppression caused by long-term corticosteroid or other immunosuppressant therapy
- Anxiety related to the adverse central nervous system effects of the corticosteroid or other immunosuppressant
- Body image disturbance related to abnormal fat distribution, exophthalmos, or adverse dermatologic effects caused by long-term corticosteroid therapy
- Diarrhea related to the adverse gastrointestinal effects of an immunosuppressant
- Fluid volume excess related to sodium and water retention caused by a corticosteroid or other immunosuppressant
- Hyperthermia related to immunosuppressant-induced fever
- Impaired skin integrity related to atrophic dermal and epidermal changes caused by a topical glucocorticoid
- Knowledge deficit related to the prescribed corticosteroid or other immunosuppressant
- Noncompliance related to long-term therapy with a corticosteroid or other immunosuppressant

- Pain related to corticosteroid-induced headache
- Potential activity intolerance related to proximal muscle weakness in the extremities, shoulders, and pelvic muscles caused by large doses of a corticosteroid
- Potential for injury related to a preexisting condition that contraindicates the use of a corticosteroid or other immunosuppressant
- Potential for injury related to a preexisting condition that requires cautious use of a corticosteroid or other immunosuppressant
- Potential for injury related to adverse drug reactions
- Potential for injury related to an electrolyte imbalance or hematologic disorder caused by a corticosteroid or other immunosuppressant
- Potential for injury related to altered metabolism caused by prolonged corticosteroid therapy
- Potential for injury related to drug interactions
- Potential for trauma related to corticosteroid-induced vertigo or seizures
- Potential for trauma related to the adverse dermatologic effects of the corticosteroid
- Sensory-perceptual alterations (auditory or tactile) related to cyclosporine-induced tinnitus, hearing loss, or paresthesia
- Sensory-perceptual alterations (visual) related to indiscriminate use of a topical glucocorticoid in or around the eye
- Sleep pattern disturbance related to corticosteroid-induced insomnia

---

sone, prednisolone, prednisone, and triamcinolone and their salts. The main active ingredient in all of these drugs is prednisone.

PHARMACOKINETICS

The glucocorticoids are absorbed well when administered orally or topically. After intramuscular (I.M.) administration, they are absorbed completely, but their onset and duration of action may vary. Glucocorticoids are bound to plasma proteins and distributed via the blood. They are metabolized in the liver and excreted by the kidneys.

Absorption, distribution, metabolism, excretion

After oral administration, most systemic glucocorticoids are absorbed well and quickly from the gastrointestinal (GI) tract. After parenteral administration (except intravenous [I.V.]), absorption varies. Glucocorticoids combined with freely soluble salts, such as sodium phosphate and sodium succinate, are absorbed rapidly; those com-

bined with poorly soluble esters, such as acetate and acetonide, are absorbed slowly but completely. The glucocorticoids are absorbed equally well from the mucous membranes and the skin when applied topically. Rectal absorption is less than 20% but can be increased to 50% if tissues are inflamed or damaged.

All glucocorticoids are distributed to the tissues by the blood bound to corticosteroid-binding globulin and corticosteroid-binding albumin. They cross the placenta and are distributed into breast milk. Metabolism of prednisone to the active drug prednisolone occurs in the liver; the kidneys excrete the inactive metabolites.

Onset, peak, duration

The systemic glucocorticoids have a rapid onset of action and reach peak concentration within 1 hour of oral administration. The onset for parenteral and topical forms varies with the drug and the administration route. The peak concentration for forms combined with sodium phosphate or sodium succinate are attained in 1 hour when given I.M.

For forms combined with acetate, the peak concentration is attained in 24 to 48 hours when given I.M. or intra-articularly. The duration of action of the glucocorticoids depends on the dosage form, administration route, and individual patient factors.

No positive correlation exists between the half-lives of these drugs and their biological effects. Glucocorticoid preparations may be short-acting (half-life of 8 to 12 hours), intermediate-acting (half-life of 18 to 36 hours), or long-acting (half-life of 36 to 54 hours), but their pharmacologic effects can last days, weeks, or longer. In fact, after prolonged therapy with high doses of these drugs, adrenal suppression of the ACTH response may persist for up to 12 months.

PHARMACODYNAMICS

Because the systemic glucocorticoids are distributed throughout the body, they enter all tissues and compartments, including the cerebrospinal fluid. They influence lipid, protein, and carbohydrate metabolism; suppress hypersensitivity and immune responses; and enhance sodium retention.

Mechanism of action

Glucocorticoids suppress hypersensitivity and immune responses through a process not entirely understood. Researchers believe that the glucocorticoids inhibit these responses by suppressing or preventing cell-mediated immune reactions; reducing the concentration of thymus-dependent leukocytes, monocytes, and eosinophils; decreasing the binding of immunoglobulins to cell surface receptors; and inhibiting interleukin synthesis. Unfortunately, this clinically useful process also may mask the signs and symptoms of serious concomitant infections.

Glucocorticoids suppress the redness, edema, heat, and tenderness associated with the inflammatory response. On the cellular level, the glucocorticoids stabilize the lysosomal membranes so that they do not release their store of hydrolytic enzymes into the cells. The drugs also prevent plasma exudation, suppress the migration of polymorphonuclear leukocytes, inhibit phagocytosis, decrease antibody formation in injured or infected tissues, and disrupt histamine synthesis, fibroblast development, collagen deposition, microvasculature dilation, and capillary permeability.

PHARMACOTHERAPEUTICS

Besides their use as replacement therapy for patients with adrenocortical insufficiency, the glucocorticoids are prescribed for their anti-inflammatory and immunosuppressant properties and their effects on the blood and lymphatic systems. Specific indications include suppression of adre-

nocortical hyperfunction in patients with adrenogenital syndrome and treatment of hypercalcemia in patients with cancer with bone metastases, such as breast cancer (glucocorticoids increase calcium excretion); multiple myeloma; and vitamin D intoxication. In patients with rheumatoid arthritis, osteoarthritis, rheumatic fever, nephrotic syndrome, inflammatory bowel disease, or collagen diseases, glucocorticoids are used for their anti-inflammatory effects. They may cause a rapid and marked reduction in symptoms but do not affect disease progression. The glucocorticoids also are used to relieve hypersensitivity reactions by suppressing the inflammatory response in patients with asthma, food and drug hypersensitivities, bee stings, hay fever, contact or exfoliative dermatitis, ulcerative colitis, or vasculitis. These drugs also contribute antilymphocytic effects in treating leukemias, lymphomas, and myelomas; reduce or prevent the cerebral edema associated with neoplasms, neurosurgery, and trauma; are used in chronic obstructive pulmonary disease; and are combined with other immunosuppressants to prevent or treat transplant rejection. Finally, glucocorticoids commonly are used to decrease ocular inflammatory processes.

Patient factors, such as response to therapy and occurrence and types of adverse reactions, must be taken into account in selecting glucocorticoids and dosages for individual patients.

beclomethasone dipropionate (Beclovent, Vanceril). A synthetic drug, beclomethasone is used primarily as an inhalant to treat bronchial asthma that has not responded to conventional therapy or as an alternative to oral systemic corticosteroids for patients who need reduced dosages to decrease the risk or severity of adverse reactions. It is a potent anti-inflammatory agent and is contraindicated in acute asthmatic episodes.
Usual adult dosage: 2 to 4 inhalations of 42 mcg each, t.i.d. or q.i.d., up to 20 sprays daily.

betamethasone (Celestone). A synthetic drug, betamethasone has potent anti-inflammatory and immunosuppressant properties. Because of its minimal mineralocorticoid effects, it cannot be used alone to manage adrenocortical insufficiency. It is used for its anti-inflammatory properties in local injections into affected joints. The administration route and the dosage depend on the patient's disorder and response.
Usual adult dosage: as an anti-inflammatory, initially, 0.6 to 7.2 mg P.O. daily or 0.5 to 9 mg I.M. daily, followed by individualized dosages for further therapy; for joint inflammation, 0.25 to 2 ml injected into the affected joint or bursa.

cortisone acetate (Cortone). Cortisone is usually the drug of choice for replacement therapy in patients with adrenocortical insufficiency. It has glucocorticoid and mineralocorticoid properties. Dosage varies greatly, depending on the nature and severity of the disease. The drug is not given I.V.

Usual adult dosage: initially, 25 to 300 mg P.O. or 20 to 300 mg I.M. daily; lower dosages may be used in patients with less severe forms of the disease.

dexamethasone (Decadron, Hexadrol). A potent anti-inflammatory agent, dexamethasone is used to treat acute self-limiting allergic disorders or exacerbation of chronic allergies. It also is used as a diagnostic aid to test for Cushing's syndrome and depression.

Usual adult dosage: 0.75 to 9 mg P.O. daily, usually in two to four divided doses.

dexamethasone acetate (Decadron-LA). A delayed-onset, long-acting salt of dexamethasone, dexamethasone acetate is not given when an immediate, short-term effect is needed. It is used to treat inflammatory conditions.

Usual adult dosage: for inflammatory conditions, 8 to 16 mg I.M. or 4 to 16 mg injected into the joint or soft tissue every 1 to 3 weeks.

dexamethasone sodium phosphate (Decadron Phosphate, Hexadrol Phosphate). Another salt of dexamethasone, dexamethasone sodium phosphate is used in emergencies, such as cerebral edema or unresponsive shock, or when oral therapy is not possible. It is available in oral, inhalant, and parenteral forms.

Usual adult dosage: for bronchospasm or asthma, initially 0.5 to 9 mg I.M. or I.V. daily, or three inhalations (300 mcg) b.i.d. to q.i.d., up to 1,200 mcg daily; for inflammatory conditions, 2 to 4 mg into large joints, 0.8 to 1 mg into small joints; for cerebral edema, initially 10 mg I.V., then 4 to 6 mg I.M. every 6 hours for 2 to 4 days, then tapered off.

hydrocortisone (Cortef, Hydrocortone). The prototype systemic glucocorticoid, hydrocortisone is used to treat adrenocortical insufficiency and severe inflammation. Dosage varies greatly depending on the nature and severity of the disease.

Usual adult dosage: 10 to 320 mg P.O. daily in three or four divided doses.

hydrocortisone acetate (Hydrocortone Acetate). A salt of hydrocortisone, hydrocortisone acetate is used to treat adrenocortical insufficiency and severe inflammation. The dosage depends on where the drug is administered: into soft-tissue lesions, bursae, joints, or ganglia. The drug is not given I.V.

Usual adult dosage: 25 to 75 mg into soft tissue; 5 to 12.5 mg into tendon sheath; 25 to 50 mg into bursae and large joints; 10 to 25 mg into ganglia and small joints. Injections may be repeated.

hydrocortisone sodium phosphate (Hydrocortone Phosphate). A salt of hydrocortisone, hydrocortisone sodium phosphate is a parenteral drug used to treat adrenocortical insufficiency and severe inflammation. Dosage varies greatly, depending on the nature and severity of the disease.

Usual adult dosage: initially, 15 to 240 mg I.M., I.V., or S.C. daily; further therapy must be individualized for each patient.

hydrocortisone sodium succinate (A-HydroCort, Solu-Cortef). A salt of hydrocortisone, hydrocortisone sodium succinate is a parenteral drug used to treat adrenocortical insufficiency and severe inflammation. Dosage varies greatly depending on the nature and severity of the disease.

Usual adult dosage: initially, 100 to 500 mg I.M. or I.V., then every 2 to 10 hours as needed; further therapy must be individualized for each patient.

methylprednisolone (Medrol). Methylprednisolone is used primarily as an anti-inflammatory or immunosuppressant agent. Because it produces minimal mineralocorticoid effects, it cannot be used alone to manage adrenocortical insufficiency.

Usual adult dosage: initially, 2 to 60 mg P.O. daily; further therapy must be individualized for each patient.

methylprednisolone acetate (Depo-Medrol, Medrol Acetate). The acetate salt of methylprednisolone is used for its anti-inflammatory properties. It is not given I.V.

Usual adult dosage: 10 to 80 mg I.M. or 4 to 80 mg injected into joints or soft-tissue lesions.

methylprednisolone sodium succinate (Solu-Medrol). Used with prednisone and prednisolone, this drug has been used in pulse therapy (intermittent high-dose therapy) for patients with severe lupus nephritis or incapacitating rheumatoid arthritis. Successful pulse therapy induces a temporary remission.

Usual adult dosage: 10 to 250 mg I.M. or I.V. every 4 to 6 hours.

paramethasone acetate (Haldrone). Paramethasone is used primarily as an anti-inflammatory or immunosuppressant agent; because it has minimal mineralocorticoid effects, it cannot be used alone to manage adrenocortical insufficiency.

Usual adult dosage: initially, 2 to 24 mg P.O. daily in three or four divided doses; further therapy must be individualized for each patient.

prednisolone (Delta-Cortef). Prednisolone is used primarily as an anti-inflammatory or immunosuppressant agent.

Usual adult dosage: initially, 5 to 60 mg P.O. daily in two to four divided doses; further therapy must be individualized for each patient.

prednisolone acetate (Key-Pred 25, Predcor-25). The acetate salt of prednisolone is used primarily as an anti-inflammatory or immunosuppressant agent. It is not given I.V.

Usual adult dosage: initially, 4 to 60 mg I.M. daily; further therapy must be individualized for each patient.

prednisolone sodium phosphate (Hydeltrasol). This drug is used primarily as an anti-inflammatory or immunosuppressant agent.

Usual adult dosage: 2 to 30 mg injected into joints, repeated every 3 days to 3 weeks, or 4 to 60 mg I.M. or I.V. daily initially; maintenance dosage, 10 to 400 mg I.M. or I.V. daily.

prednisolone tebutate (Hydeltra-TBA). Used for its anti-inflammatory effects, prednisolone tebutate is injected into joints, soft tissue, or lesions. It is not given I.V.

Usual adult dosage: 4 to 40 mg injected into joints, soft tissue, or lesions every 2 to 3 weeks.

prednisone (Deltasone, Orasone). Prednisone is the oral glucocorticoid of choice for anti-inflammatory or immunosuppressant effects.

Usual adult dosage: initially, 5 to 60 mg P.O. daily; further therapy must be individualized for each patient.

triamcinolone (Aristocort, Kenacort). Triamcinolone is used primarily as an anti-inflammatory or immunosuppressant agent. Because it has minimal mineralocorticoid effects, it cannot be used alone to manage adrenocortical insufficiency.

Usual adult dosage: 4 to 48 mg P.O. daily in one to four divided doses.

triamcinolone acetonide (Azmacort, Kenalog). A slowly absorbed derivative of triamcinolone, triamcinolone acetonide is available as an inhalant for long-term therapy for bronchial asthma. It also is used I.M. for its anti-inflammatory and immunosuppressant properties.

Usual adult dosage: for bronchial asthma, 600 to 800 mcg (100 mcg/spray) by oral inhalation daily divided into three or four doses, or 4 to 48 mg P.O. daily divided into two to four doses; for anti-inflammatory or immunosuppressant effects, 60 mg I.M. or 2.5 to 40 mg injected into the affected joint, bursa, or tendon sheath.

triamcinolone diacetate (Amcort, Aristocort Forte Parenteral). Triamcinolone diacetate is used for its anti-inflammatory and immunosuppressant properties.

Usual adult dosage: 40 mg I.M. weekly, or 2 to 40 mg injected into the joint, soft tissue, or lesion.

Drug interactions

Many drugs interact with the systemic glucocorticoids. (For more information, see *Drug interactions: Systemic glucocorticoids and mineralocorticoids.*)

ADVERSE DRUG REACTIONS

Because systemic glucocorticoids affect nearly every body system, they can cause widespread adverse reactions. Such reactions are unlikely to occur with short-term administration, even at high dosages. However, when glucocorticoids are given for more than a brief period, devastating reactions can occur. If long-term therapy with these drugs is necessary, alternate-day therapy may decrease the severity of adverse reactions.

Long-term therapy may cause some degree of adrenocortical insufficiency, depending on the dosage frequency and especially on the duration of therapy. For example, rapid withdrawal of glucocorticoids after long-term therapy will cause acute adrenocortical insufficiency. The withdrawal syndrome is characterized by arthralgia, myalgia, anorexia, lethargy, weakness, depression, hypotension, and hypoglycemia. To prevent this syndrome, the drug must be withdrawn gradually. Although the adrenal glands almost always return to normal after a period of glucocorticoid-induced adrenocortical insufficiency, the patient may need replacement therapy during stressful situations—such as surgery, severe infection, or trauma—for up to a year. (For a summary, see *Adverse reactions to systemic corticosteroids,* page 963.)

Weakness of the proximal muscles of the extremities, shoulders, and pelvis occurs occasionally in patients receiving large doses of glucocorticoids; this severe complication may force cessation of therapy. Even then, recovery typically is slow and incomplete.

Prolonged therapy with systemic glucocorticoids causes abnormal fat distribution, depleting it in the extremities and increasing its deposition in the face and abdomen and between the shoulder blades. (For more information, see *Cushingoid signs and symptoms,* page 964.) Glucocorticoids also can lead to catabolism (protein destruction) and inhibited protein synthesis, which results in muscle wasting, weakness, osteoporosis, poor wound healing, and immunosuppression.

These drugs alter carbohydrate metabolism by promoting glyconeogenesis and glycogenolysis and by antagonizing the action of insulin. This can result in diabetes mellitus in susceptible people. It also may cause hypergly-

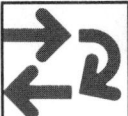

DRUG INTERACTIONS

Systemic glucocorticoids and mineralocorticoids

Corticosteroids interact with many other drugs. The nurse must be aware that these interactions affect electrolytes as well as medication dosages.

DRUG	INTERACTING DRUGS	POSSIBLE EFFECTS	NURSING IMPLICATIONS
systemic glucocorticoids, mineralocorticoids	barbiturates, phenytoin, rifampin	Decrease corticosteroid effect by speeding hepatic metabolism	• Increase the corticosteroid dosage, if prescribed.
	amphotericin B, chlorthalidone, ethacrynic acid, furosemide, thiazide diuretics	Increase the incidence or severity of hypokalemia	• Monitor the patient's serum potassium level, and observe for signs and symptoms of hypokalemia. • Administer potassium supplements, if prescribed. • Recommend high-potassium foods, such as bananas and grapes.
	erythromycin, troleandomycin	Decrease corticosteroid metabolism	• Observe for signs and symptoms of increased corticosteroid effects. • Decrease the corticosteroid dosage, if prescribed.
	salicylates	Increase the risk of GI ulceration; decrease plasma concentration and effects of salicylates	• Watch for signs and symptoms of GI irritation (heartburn) and ulceration (melena). • Increase the salicylate dosage, if prescribed, when administered concomitantly with a corticosteroid. • Observe the patient for signs and symptoms of salicylate intoxication, such as tinnitus or hyperventilation, when the corticosteroid dosage is decreased.
	nonsteroidal anti-inflammatory agents	Increase the risk of peptic ulcer	• Watch for signs and symptoms of GI irritation. • Administer these drugs at least 2 hours apart.
	vaccines, toxoids	Decrease the patient's response to vaccines and toxoids; may increase replication of attenuated viruses	• Administer with extreme caution and only as prescribed. • Observe for signs and symptoms of specific viral infection after vaccine or toxoid administration.
	estrogen, oral contraceptives that contain estrogen	Enhance corticosteroid effect	• Observe for signs and symptoms of increased corticosteroid effects. • Decrease the corticosteroid dosage, if prescribed.
	aminoglutethimide	May decrease corticosteroid effect by increasing metabolism	• Increase the corticosteroid dosage, if prescribed.
	hypoglycemic agents	May increase blood glucose level in patients with diabetes mellitus	• Monitor the patient's blood glucose level. • Monitor the patient for signs and symptoms of hyperglycemia, such as polyuria, polydipsia, polyphagia, and weight loss.
	cholestyramine	May decrease corticosteroid absorption	• Observe the patient for signs of reduced response to corticosteroid therapy. • Administer cholestyramine at least 2 hours before or after the corticosteroid.

(continued)

DRUG INTERACTIONS

Systemic glucocorticoids and mineralocorticoids (continued)

DRUG	INTERACTING DRUGS	POSSIBLE EFFECTS	NURSING IMPLICATIONS
Systemic glucocorticoids minealocorticoids (continued)	isoniazid	Reduce effect of isoniazid; reduces metabolism and increases effect of corticosteroid	• Monitor the patient for signs and symptoms of reduced response to isoniazid, such as exacerbation of tuberculosis, or enhanced corticosteroid effect. • Expect to increase the isoniazid dosage, if prescribed.
	antihypertensive agents	May antagonize the antihypertensive effect by increasing sodium retention	• Monitor the patient for increased blood pressure and edema. • Restrict the patient's sodium and fluid intake. • Increase the antihypertensive dosage, if prescribed.

cemia, glycosuria, and an increase in the severity of existing diabetes mellitus.

The immunosuppressant and anti-inflammatory effects of the glucocorticoids commonly delay detection of major infections and profoundly compromise patient resistance. The most common adverse reaction to oral inhalation therapy, for example, is fungal (Candida albicans) infection of the mouth and pharynx. Although usually of little clinical significance, such infections require antifungal therapy.

Adverse GI reactions to glucocorticoids include abdominal distention, pancreatitis, ulcerative esophagitis, gastric irritation, and weight gain caused by increased appetite. Occasionally, these drugs play a role in peptic ulcer formation, reactivation, perforation, hemorrhage, or delayed healing.

With prolonged glucocorticoid use, posterior subcapsular cataracts may occur, particularly in children. So may exophthalmos or increased intraocular pressure, occasionally causing glaucoma and damaging the optic nerve. Glucocorticoids also may induce secondary fungal or viral eye infections.

Various dermatologic effects are associated with glucocorticoid therapy. These include skin atrophy and thinning, acne, striae formation, excessive diaphoresis, hirsutism, facial erythema, petechiae, ecchymoses, and easy bruising. Parenteral therapy sometimes results in scarring, induration, and sterile abscesses.

Glucocorticoids may cause adverse neurologic reactions as well, including insomnia, vertigo, headache, increased motor activity, restlessness, and seizures. Alterations in behavior can range from mood swings, anxiety, depression, and euphoria to frank psychoses.

Fluid and electrolyte disturbances, such as sodium retention, may result in edema, weight gain, hypertension, and potassium loss, leading to hypokalemic alkalosis. Glu-

cocorticoids also promote calcium excretion, which may cause hypocalcemia.

Because glucocorticoids inhibit ACTH secretion by the pituitary gland, the adrenal glands are not stimulated and eventually may atrophy. The resulting decrease in adrenal function means the patient must receive increased amounts of glucocorticoids (and mineralocorticoids) during periods of stress, such as surgery.

Glucocorticoids also can increase red blood cell and hemoglobulin concentrations, leading to polycythemia; enhance coagulability, resulting in increased incidence of emboli and thrombi; and retard normal growth in children by its effect on the epiphyseal cartilage.

In children, even small doses of glucocorticoids can inhibit or even arrest growth by interfering with deoxyribonucleic acid (DNA) synthesis and cell division.

Reported anaphylactic reactions in patients receiving parenteral glucocorticoids may be from hypersensitivity to the preservative used in some parenteral formulations.

NURSING PROCESS APPLICATION

The following information assists the nurse in caring for a patient who is receiving a systemic glucocorticoid.

Assessment

• Review the patient's history for a preexisting condition that contraindicates the use of a systemic glucocorticoid, such as a systemic fungal infection or hypersensitivity to any component of the drug.
• Review the patient's history for a preexisting condition that requires cautious use of a systemic glucocorticoid, such as GI ulceration, renal disease, hypertension, osteoporosis, varicella, vaccinia, exanthema, diabetes mellitus, hypothyroidism, thromboembolic disorder, seizures, myasthenia gravis, congestive heart failure (CHF), tuberculosis,

Adverse reactions to systemic corticosteroids

Systemic corticosteroids—the systemic glucocorticoids and mineralocorticoids—affect almost all body systems, so they can cause widespread adverse reactions. The list below presents the most common of these reactions by body system.

Central nervous system

- Behavioral changes ranging from mood alterations to psychosis and suicidal behavior
- Insomnia
- Increased intracranial pressure
- Seizures
- Cerebral edema
- Blunted sensorium

Endocrine system (and metabolic functions)

- Diabetes mellitus
- Hyperlipidemia
- Adrenal atrophy
- Hypothalamic-pituitary axis suppression
- Dysmenorrhea
- Altered protein, fat, and carbohydrate metabolism and protein catabolism
- Cushingoid symptoms
- Increased serum cholesterol levels
- Inhibited protein synthesis

Urinary system

- Increased sodium and water retention
- Increased potassium excretion

Immune system

- Suppressed immune response
- Suppressed inflammation
- Increased susceptibility to infection
- Suppressed signs and symptoms of infection

Musculoskeletal system

- Osteoporosis
- Aseptic necrosis of bone
- Increased susceptibility to fractures
- Muscle wasting
- Myopathy
- Arthralgia

Gastrointestinal system

- Intestinal perforation
- Peptic ulcer
- Pancreatitis

Cardiovascular system

- Hypertension
- Edema
- Hypercoagulability
- Thrombophlebitis
- Embolism
- Atherosclerosis
- Polycythemia

Integumentary system

- Impaired wound healing
- Hirsutism
- Ecchymoses
- Acne
- Striae
- Thin, fragile skin

Ophthalmic system

- Glaucoma
- Posterior subcapsular cataracts

---

ocular herpes simplex, hypoalbuminemia, emotional instability, or psychosis.

- Assess the patient for adverse reactions to the prescribed systemic glucocorticoid, such as adrenocortical insufficiency, myopathy, cushingoid symptoms, altered carbohydrate metabolism, a fluid or electrolyte imbalance, or a hypersensitivity reaction to the drug.
- Review the patient's medication history to identify the use of drugs that may interact with the prescribed systemic glucocorticoid, such as barbiturates, salicylates, oral contraceptives, cholestyramine, or antihypertensive agents.
- Assess the effectiveness of the prescribed systemic glucocorticoid periodically.
- Assess the patient regularly for signs of infection, such as delayed wound healing and a decreased white blood cell

(WBC) count, because glucocorticoid use can mask other common signs of infection, such as fever and redness.

- Assess the patient's body image during long-term systemic glucocorticoid therapy.
- Evaluate the patient's and family's knowledge about the prescribed systemic glucocorticoid.

Nursing diagnoses

The following examples represent appropriate nursing diagnoses for a patient receiving a systemic glucocorticoid.

- Potential for injury related to a preexisting condition that contraindicates the use of a systemic glucocorticoid
- Potential for injury related to a preexisting condition that requires cautious use of a systemic glucocorticoid
- Potential for injury related to adverse drug reactions

• Altered protection related to immunosuppression caused by long-term systemic glucocorticoid therapy
• Body image disturbance related to abnormal fat distribution, exophthalmos, or adverse dermatologic effects caused by long-term systemic glucocorticoid therapy
• Knowledge deficit related to the prescribed systemic glucocorticoid

Planning and implementation

• Do not administer a systemic glucocorticoid to a patient with a condition that contraindicates its use.
• Administer a systemic glucocorticoid cautiously to a patient at risk because of a preexisting condition.
• Monitor the patient frequently for adverse reactions during systemic glucocorticoid therapy.
• *Observe the patient closely for an anaphylactic reaction after drug administration. Such a reaction may result from hypersensitivity to the preservative used in the systemic glucocorticoid. Keep standard emergency equipment nearby.*
• Obtain baseline data as instructed before a patient begins long-term glucocorticoid therapy. Such data may include an electrocardiogram (ECG), chest and spinal X-rays, a glucose tolerance test, a Mantoux test for tuberculosis, and measurements of blood pressure, body weight, and hypothalamic-pituitary-adrenal axis function.
• Monitor the following during systemic glucocorticoid therapy: the patient's serum glucose level, body weight, blood pressure, complete blood count (CBC), blood chemistries (particularly electrolytes), and ocular pressure. Also obtain chest and spinal X-rays regularly, as prescribed.
• Monitor the patient for signs of adrenocortical insufficiency, such as hypotension, dehydration, fatigue, hyponatremia, diarrhea, and anorexia, during and after glucocorticoid therapy.
• Monitor the patient for potential stressors, such as surgery, trauma, and infections, and adjust the dosage accordingly, as prescribed.
• Monitor the patient for signs of Cushing's syndrome. (For details, see *Cushingoid signs and symptoms.*)
• Monitor the patient's fluid and electrolyte balance and observe for signs and symptoms of hypernatremia, hypokalemia, and hypocalcemia.
• Prevent severe GI complications by assessing the patient for epigastric pain 1 to 3 hours after meals and for nausea, vomiting, bloody stools, hematemesis, "coffee-ground" vomitus, decreased hemoglobin level and hematocrit, and a positive guaiac stool test.
• *Observe for and report any emotional changes. Suicide precautions may be needed for severely depressed patients.*
• Monitor the patient for myopathy by assessing muscle strength and reported weakness.
• Measure the blood glucose level to detect alterations for a patient with diabetes mellitus. Assess all patients for signs

---

Cushingoid signs and symptoms

Prolonged corticosteroid therapy may result in the signs and symptoms associated with Cushing's syndrome—a condition marked by widespread abnormalities, including obvious fat deposits in the face, between the shoulders, and around the waist.
  During corticosteroid therapy, the nurse should assess the patient for the following cushingoid signs and symptoms:

• Acne
• Moon face
• Hirsutism and masculinization
• Cervicodorsal fat (buffalo hump)
• Protruding abdomen
• Girdle obesity
• Amenorrhea
• Purplish abdominal striae
• Edema
• Thinning and atrophy of extremities
• Muscle weakness or atrophy
• Hypertension
• Hyperglycemia
• Glycosuria
• Renal disorder
• Mental changes, ranging from euphoria to depression
• Lowered resistance to infection

---

and symptoms of hyperglycemia, such as polyuria, polydipsia, polyphagia, and decreased or blurred vision.
• Administer the daily dosage in four equally divided doses or in one single dose in the early morning for a patient who needs short-term oral therapy. Keep in mind that early-morning administration simulates the natural circadian rhythm of corticosteroid secretion—higher in the morning, lower in the evening.
• Expect to administer alternate-day therapy (a single dose administered every other morning) for a patient who needs long-term therapy (longer than a month). This minimizes the risk or severity of adverse reactions.
• Inject an I.M. glucocorticoid preparation deeply into gluteal muscle, and avoid using the same site for repeated injections to help prevent atrophy at injection sites. Know that S.C. injection usually is contraindicated.
• *Do not administer beclomethasone via oral inhalation to a patient with an acute asthmatic attack because the drug cannot stop bronchospasm.*
• Notify the physician if adverse reactions occur.
• *Monitor the patient closely for signs of infection, such as delayed wound healing and a decreased WBC count, because systemic glucocorticoids increase susceptibility to infection.*
• *Handle or dress all wounds, sites, tubes, and catheters with meticulous care to help prevent contamination and reduce the risk of infection.*
• Notify the physician if an infection is suspected.

• Observe the patient for changes in appearance that may affect body image.

• Encourage the patient to express feelings about changes in appearance.

• Reassure the patient that physical changes usually are not permanent.

• Help the patient find ways to enhance personal appearance.

Patient teaching

• Teach the patient and family the name, dose, frequency, action, and adverse effects of the prescribed systemic glucocorticoid.

• Ensure that the patient and family clearly understand why the systemic glucocorticoid has been prescribed and know the risks associated with it. *Advise the patient who is taking the drug for more than 1 week not to stop taking it abruptly. Explain that the dosage must be decreased gradually before the drug can be discontinued.*

• Instruct the patient about storage requirements.

• *Emphasize the importance of taking the drug exactly as prescribed.* (For more information, see *Answers to patients' questions about prednisone therapy.*)

• *Review guidelines for missed doses with the patient.* In general, a missed daily dose should be taken as soon as the patient remembers it (but not the next day — doses should never be doubled). The patient who misses one portion of a divided daily dose should take the next dose on schedule. A patient on alternate-day therapy should not take a missed dose, even if it is remembered that same morning. Instead, the patient should take the missed dose the next morning, skip a day, then resume alternate-day therapy on the following day.

• Review the signs and symptoms of adrenocorticoid insufficiency with the patient. Instruct the patient to notify the physician if they occur.

• Advise the patient to avoid the use of alcohol, cigarettes, caffeine, aspirin, or aspirin-containing compounds without consulting the physician.

• Teach the patient to recognize the signs and symptoms of GI disorders and to notify the physician immediately if they appear.

• Inform the patient that the glucocorticoid may cause emotional changes that should be reported to the physician.

• Instruct the patient about therapy-related dietary precautions, including adequate intake of proteins, vitamins, and calcium. Foods high in potassium and low in sodium also may be prescribed. Have the patient keep a weekly weight record and report any gain over 5 lb.

• Explain the need for the patient to keep active to prevent osteoporosis. (Periodic X-rays also may be required to monitor bone status.)

• Instruct the patient to take an oral glucocorticoid with food or milk to decrease the risk of gastric irritation.

• Teach the patient the correct way to use the beclomethasone oral inhaler: shake the inhaler well immediately before use; invert the inhaler; exhale completely; place the mouthpiece of the inhaler in the mouth and close the lips around it; while pressing the metal canister down with a finger, inhale slowly and deeply through the mouth; after

---

Answers to patients' questions about prednisone therapy

When teaching the patient about prednisone therapy, the nurse should explain why the medication is necessary, why it should be taken exactly as prescribed, and which adverse reactions it may cause. The following information can help the nurse answer questions that may arise during the teaching session.

Q. **My doctor has prescribed prednisone. Why?**

A. Prednisone is similar to a substance called cortisone that is made by your body. The drug helps decrease the pain, heat, or swelling that accompanies arthritis, so-called allergic reactions, and other inflammatory conditions.

Q. **How should I take prednisone?**

A. Your doctor will instruct you on how to take the medication. Follow the directions on the prescription's label. If you do not understand the directions, be sure to ask the pharmacist or your doctor to clarify them. Take the drug regularly with food or milk, as prescribed.

Q. **Is there anything special I need to know about taking prednisone?**

A. Yes. Follow these guidelines:
• Weigh yourself daily. Report any unusual weight gain to your doctor.
• Report to your doctor any sore throat, cold, or infection that lasts an unusually long time.
• Report to your doctor any changes in your appearance, moods, behavior, or (if female) menstrual periods.
• Report any muscle weakness, frequent heartburn, or black, tarry stools.
• Tell your dentist or any other doctor you consult that you are taking prednisone.
• Limit your salt intake and intake of sodium from other products, such as diet soda.
• Do not take aspirin or over-the-counter products that contain aspirin.
• Wear or carry medical alert identification that states you are taking prednisone.

Q. **Is it okay to stop taking the drug when I feel better?**

A. No. Do not stop taking your prednisone. When you no longer need the medication, your doctor will taper off your dosage gradually before discontinuing it completely.

holding the breath as long as possible, remove the mouthpiece and exhale as slowly as possible. Wait 1 minute (breathing normally) before inhaling again.

• Advise the patient to take extra medication along when traveling in case the trip lasts longer than expected. Also advise the patient not to pack the medication in a suitcase, but to carry it at all times.

• *Instruct the patient to wear a medical identification tag or to carry an identification card at all times. The patient also should notify any health care professional (dentists or oral surgeons, for example) about the glucocorticoid therapy before undergoing any other kind of treatment.*

• Help the patient reduce the risk of infection by teaching self-care practices to prevent skin injury and proper care of minor injuries.

• Instruct the patient to call the physician if signs or symptoms of infection, such as fever, develop.

• *Advise the patient to avoid people with infections, especially respiratory infections.*

• Stress the importance of scrupulous oral hygiene during oral inhalation therapy, especially immediately after treatment.

• Inform the patient receiving long-term glucocorticoid therapy about the possibility of changes in appearance, such as fat deposits in the face, acne, hirsutism, and truncal obesity. Reassure the patient that these changes are therapy-related.

• Instruct the patient to notify the physician if adverse reactions occur.

Evaluation

The following examples represent appropriate evaluation statements for a patient receiving a systemic glucocorticoid.

• The patient has no conditions that contraindicate systemic glucocorticoid therapy.

• The patient exhibits no signs of complications in the preexisting condition linked to the prescribed systemic glucocorticoid.

• The patient experiences no adverse reactions to the prescribed systemic glucocorticoid.

• The patient remains free from infection during systemic glucocorticoid therapy.

• The patient copes positively with body image changes during systemic glucocorticoid therapy.

• The patient and family express an accurate understanding of the points taught about the prescribed systemic glucocorticoid.

• The patient demonstrates proper use of an oral inhaler for beclomethasone therapy.

TOPICAL GLUCOCORTICOIDS

Topical glucocorticoids — available as creams, ointments, gels, aerosols, lotions, solutions, and drug-impregnated tape — are used to treat various skin diseases, principally for their anti-inflammatory and antiproliferative effects. The numerous preparations available have similar uses and actions and can cause similar adverse reactions.

PHARMACOKINETICS

The topical glucocorticoids are absorbed through the skin in varying degrees and enter the circulation. Then they are metabolized in the liver and excreted by the kidneys.

Absorption, distribution, metabolism, excretion

Topical glucocorticoids are applied for their local effects on the epidermis or dermis. The skin usually is an effective barrier against percutaneous absorption; however, some absorption does occur. The most important factors determining the amount of percutaneous absorption are the vehicle used in the formulation and the degree of skin moisture. For example, occlusive dressings that prevent air circulation keep the skin moist and promote drug penetration. Other factors affecting absorption include drug concentration (the mechanism for absorption is passive diffusion), breaks in the skin, the length of time the drug stays on the skin, the amount of drug applied, and the site of application (the face has the thinnest layer of skin, and the soles and palms have the thickest). Once the topical glucocorticoid enters the circulation, most of it is metabolized in the liver and excreted by the kidneys.

PHARMACODYNAMICS

The major actions of the topical glucocorticoids are anti-inflammatory and antiproliferative.

Mechanism of action

The anti-inflammatory effects of the topical glucocorticoids result partly from vasoconstriction, but the exact sequence of events is unknown. The vasoconstriction may be a direct or indirect effect exerted by the reduction of catecholamine, prostaglandin, or histamine levels at target cell sites. The anti-inflammatory effects of these drugs also may result from interference with the migration of polymorphonuclear leukocytes through the capillary walls and from decreased adherence of WBCs to the capillary endothelium.

The glucocorticoids also exert anti-inflammatory effects by interfering with the function of lymphocytes and macrophages and by decreasing the action of lymphokines. (Lymphokines are released in the presence of an antigen and play a role in macrophage activation, lymphocyte transformation, and cell-mediated immunity.) The glucocorticoids also decrease cell membrane permeability, impair the release of toxins or lysosomal enzymes, and inhibit the release or action of other chemical mediators during the inflammatory process.

Topical glucocorticoids that are more potent than hydrocortisone produce an antiproliferative effect on epidermal cells and dermal fibroblasts. In the epidermis, the drugs reduce ribonucleic acid (RNA) transcription, which decreases DNA synthesis. When used to treat psoriasis, the topical glucocorticoids may interfere with reformation of the granular layer.

PHARMACOTHERAPEUTICS

All topical glucocorticoids are used to treat acute and chronic inflammatory dermatoses, psoriasis, atopic eczema, pruritus ani, neurodermatitis, contact dermatitis, seborrheic dermatitis, and exfoliative dermatitis. Because glucocorticoid creams evaporate, they are used on acute, wet lesions. Because glucocorticoid ointments moisturize, they are used on chronic, dry, scaly lesions. Any specific indications are noted below.

amcinonide (Cyclocort).
Usual adult dosage: 0.1% cream or ointment applied b.i.d. or t.i.d.

betamethasone dipropionate (Diprosone, Diprolene).
Usual adult dosage: 0.05% cream, ointment, or lotion applied daily to q.i.d.; or one 3-second spray of 0.1% aerosol t.i.d. or q.i.d.

betamethasone valerate (Betatrex, Valisone).
Usual adult dosage: 0.1% cream, ointment, or lotion or 0.01% reduced-strength cream, applied b.i.d. or t.i.d.

clobetasol propionate (Temovate). To avoid percutaneous absorption, clobetasol should not be covered with an occlusive dressing.
Usual adult dosage: 0.05% cream or ointment applied b.i.d. to a maximum of 50 grams/week and a total treatment time of 14 days.

clocortolone pivalate (Cloderm). Besides the usual indications, clocortolone is used to treat corticosteroid-responsive dermatoses.
Usual adult dosage: 0.1% cream applied daily to q.i.d.

desonide (DesOwen, Tridesilon). Desonide is indicated for acne rosacea as well as seborrheic dermatitis.
Usual adult dosage: 0.05% cream or ointment applied b.i.d. to q.i.d.

desoximetasone (Topicort).
Usual adult dosage: 0.05% or 0.25% cream applied b.i.d., 0.05% gel applied b.i.d., or 0.25% ointment applied b.i.d.

dexamethasone (Aeroseb-Dex, Decaderm, Decaspray).
Usual adult dosage: 0.1% gel applied t.i.d. or q.i.d., or 0.01% or 0.04% aerosol b.i.d. to q.i.d. sprayed from 6 inches above the surface for 1 to 2 seconds.

diflorasone diacetate (Florone, Maxiflor).
Usual adult dosage: 0.05% cream or ointment applied b.i.d. to q.i.d.

fluocinolone acetonide (Fluonid, Synalar, Synemol).
Usual adult dosage: 0.01% to 0.2% cream, 0.025% ointment, or 0.01% solution applied b.i.d. to q.i.d.

fluocinonide (Lidex).
Usual adult dosage: 0.05% cream, ointment, solution, or gel applied t.i.d. or q.i.d.

flurandrenolide (Cordran).
Usual adult dosage: 0.05% or 0.025% cream or ointment applied b.i.d. or t.i.d., 0.05% lotion applied b.i.d. or t.i.d., or 4 mcg/cm^2 drug-impregnated tape applied daily or b.i.d.

halcinonide (Halog).
Usual adult dosage: 0.1% or 0.025% cream applied b.i.d. to t.i.d., or 0.1% ointment or solution applied b.i.d. or t.i.d.

hydrocortisone (Aeroseb-HC, Cort-Dome, Dermacort).
Usual adult dosage: 0.25% or 2.5% cream or lotion, 0.5% to 2.5% ointment, 1% gel, or 0.5% aerosol spray applied daily to q.i.d.

methylprednisolone acetate (Medrol Acetate).
Usual adult dosage: 0.25% or 1% ointment applied daily to q.i.d.

triamcinolone acetonide (Aristocort, Kenalog).
Usual adult dosage: 0.025% to 0.5% cream, ointment, or lotion applied b.i.d. to q.i.d.

Drug interactions

No significant interactions occur between other drugs and the topical glucocorticoids themselves. However, chemicals used in formulating the preparations may interact with certain drugs. Ethylenediamine, a stabilizer in certain preparations, interacts with systemic aminophylline, antazoline, antazoline hydrochloride ophthalmic solution, and edetate disodium, a preservative common in ophthalmic solutions. The interaction may cause allergic contact dermatitis, urticaria, and systemic eczematous contact-type dermatitis.

ADVERSE DRUG REACTIONS

Many adverse reactions can occur with use of topical glucocorticoids. These effects are more pronounced when fluorinated preparations (fluocinolone acetonide, fluocinonide, or flurandrenolide) are used or when glucocorticoids are used with occlusive dressings.

Long-term use of the more potent topical glucocorticoids can cause atrophic changes in the epidermis and dermis, including striae, telangiectasia, subcutaneous fat wasting or muscle wasting, ecchymoses, and increased skin fragility. These changes may result from decreased synthesis of fibrous tissue by fibroblasts and increased collagen breakdown. Facial skin eruptions usually result from improper use of fluorinated topical glucocorticoids. Steroid rosacea eruptions range from skin reddening to papulopustular lesions. Perioral dermatitis appears as a reddened papular eruption.

The anti-inflammatory action of topical glucocorticoids can mask the characteristic signs of certain conditions, such as tinea and scabies. Inappropriate use of these preparations may lead to superinfections. Indiscriminate use of topical glucocorticoids in or around the eye may result in periorbital swelling, glaucoma, or cataracts.

Percutaneous absorption of the topical glucocorticoids can cause the same adverse reactions as those occurring with systemic glucocorticoids. Allergic contact dermatitis usually is caused by chemicals added to the preparations.

NURSING PROCESS APPLICATION

The following information assists the nurse in caring for a patient receiving a topical glucocorticoid.

Assessment

• Review the patient's history for a preexisting condition that contraindicates the use of a topical glucocorticoid, such as known hypersensitivity to any component of the drug.
• Assess the patient for adverse reactions to the prescribed topical glucocorticoid, such as dermatologic changes, superinfection, allergic contact dermatitis, or eye disorder.
• Review the patient's medication history to identify the use of drugs that may interact with the prescribed topical glucocorticoid, such as systemic aminophylline, antazoline, antazoline hydrochloride ophthalmic solution, or edetate disodium.

• Assess the effectiveness of the prescribed topical glucocorticoid periodically.
• Assess the patient's skin for atrophic changes.
• Assess the patient's vision regularly.
• Evaluate the patient's and family's knowledge about the prescribed topical glucocorticoid.

Nursing diagnoses

The following examples represent appropriate nursing diagnoses for a patient receiving a topical glucocorticoid.
• Potential for injury related to a preexisting condition that contraindicates the use of a topical glucocorticoid
• Potential for injury related to adverse drug reactions
• Impaired skin integrity related to atrophic dermal and epidermal changes caused by a topical glucocorticoid
• Sensory-perceptual alterations (visual) related to indiscriminate use of a topical glucocorticoid in or around the eye
• Knowledge deficit related to the prescribed topical glucocorticoid

Planning and implementation

• Do not administer a topical glucocorticoid to a patient with a condition that contraindicates its use.
• Monitor the patient closely for adverse reactions during topical glucocorticoid therapy, especially when using a fluorinated preparation or an occlusive dressing.
• Wash the patient's skin before applying the medication.
• *Do not use a fluorinated glucocorticoid on the patient's face, except as prescribed.*
• *Do not apply a high-potency glucocorticoid to the patient's face, axilla, or groin, except as prescribed.*
• *Do not use a solution on dry lesions, except as prescribed, because it will cause further drying and itching.* Solutions also are contraindicated for use in the perineal area, where they can cause burning.
• Use a gel or lotion for glucocorticoid application to the scalp or other hairy areas, as prescribed.
• Apply a topical glucocorticoid in the smallest amount and the lowest concentration possible.
• Prevent skin damage by applying a cream, lotion, ointment, solution, or gel gently, leaving a thin coat. To apply medication to the scalp or other hairy areas, part the patient's hair and apply the medication directly to the lesion.
• Administer an aerosol preparation by spraying at least 6 inches above the site for 1 to 2 seconds. Also, prevent inhalation by protecting the patient's nose and mouth as well as those of others in the immediate area.
• Apply an occlusive dressing, when needed. To do this, first apply medication as indicated; cover the area with a light gauze dressing followed by a layer of impermeable plastic (such as plastic wrap); seal the edges with hypoallergenic or paper tape; secure the dressing with a stockinette or an elastic bandage; and leave it in place for as

long as prescribed. This technique usually is not used if infection is present or if the lesion is wet or exudative.
• *Remove the dressing and notify the physician if the patient's body temperature rises after an occlusive dressing is used.*
• *Do not cover clobetasol with an occlusive dressing.*
• *Report any infection, rash, pruritus, atrophic change, or purpura to the physician.*
• *Watch for and report signs of precutaneous absorption of the topical glucocorticoid, which can cause the same adverse reactions as a systemic glucocorticoid.* (For more information, see "Adverse drug reactions" in the section on systemic glucocorticoids earlier in this chapter.)
• Notify the physician if any adverse reactions occur.
• Monitor the patient's skin before each application for atrophic dermal and epidermal changes, such as striae, telangiectasia, subcutaneous fat wasting or muscle wasting, ecchymoses, or increased skin fragility.
• Handle the patient's skin gently to prevent trauma.
• Notify the physician if atrophic changes occur.
• *Use caution when applying a topical glucocorticoid in areas of thin or broken skin around the patient's eyes.*
• Report any vision changes or unusual appearance of the patient's eyes.

Patient teaching
• Teach the patient and family the name, dose, frequency, action, and adverse effects of the prescribed topical glucocorticoid.
• *Inform the patient that the topical glucocorticoid is for external use only and that overuse may cause adverse reactions.*
• Teach the patient the proper technique for applying the prescribed topical glucocorticoid and any dressing needed.
• *Emphasize that topical glucocorticoids should not be used for purposes other than those prescribed, nor should they be shared with other family members.*
• Caution the patient to handle the skin gently and to avoid vigorous rubbing of the application site when drying it after bathing.
• Provide additional information, as needed. (For more information, see "Nursing process application" in the section on systemic glucocorticoids earlier in this chapter.)
• Instruct the patient to notify the physician if adverse reactions occur.

Evaluation
The following examples represent appropriate evaluation statements for a patient receiving a topical glucocorticoid.
• The patient has no conditions that contraindicate topical glucocorticoid therapy.
• The patient experiences no adverse reactions to the prescribed topical glucocorticoid.
• The patient's skin remains intact at the application site.

• The patient reports no visual changes when the topical glucocorticoid is used around the eyes.
• The patient and family express an accurate understanding of the points taught about the prescribed topical glucocorticoid.
• The patient demonstrates correct application of the prescribed topical glucocorticoid.

MINERALOCORTICOIDS

The mineralocorticoid drugs—administered orally, I.M., or as implanted pellets—are synthetic analogues of hormones secreted by the zona glomerulosa layer of the adrenal cortex. These drugs affect electrolyte and water balance and typically are used for replacement therapy in patients with adrenocortical insufficiency. Drugs in this class include desoxycorticosterone acetate, desoxycorticosterone pivalate, and fludrocortisone acetate. Aldosterone, a natural mineralocorticoid, is the prototype drug in this class, but its use has been limited by its high cost, limited availability, and requirement of parenteral administration.

PHARMACOKINETICS

The mineralocorticoids are absorbed well and distributed to all parts of the body. These drugs are metabolized to inactive forms, in part, by the body tissues, but the liver is the major metabolic site. The mineralocorticoids are excreted by the kidneys, primarily as inactive metabolites.

Onset, peak, duration
The onset of action, peak concentration level, and duration of action of the mineralocorticoids vary widely—from minutes to months—depending on the preparation used, the dosage, and the administration route. The plasma half-life of desoxycorticosterone acetate injection is 70 minutes. The duration for the pellet form of this drug is 8 to 12 months; for the I.M. form, 1 to 2 days. The desoxycorticosterone pivalate repository injection has a duration of 4 weeks. After oral administration, fludrocortisone has an onset of 30 minutes and a duration of 1 to 2 days.

PHARMACODYNAMICS

The mineralocorticoids affect fluid and electrolyte balance by acting on the distal renal tubule to enhance sodium resorption and potassium and hydrogen secretion. The glomerular filtration rate is increased, favoring sodium excretion. However, the net effect of the mineralocorticoids usually is sodium retention.

PHARMACOTHERAPEUTICS

The mineralocorticoids are used as part of replacement therapy for patients with adrenocortical insufficiency. They also are used to treat salt-losing congenital adrenogenital syndrome after the patient's electrolyte balance has been restored.

desoxycorticosterone acetate (Doca Acetate, Percorten Acetate). The most potent mineralocorticoid, desoxycorticosterone acetate is used to treat salt-losing adrenogenital syndrome and, with glucocorticoids, adrenocortical insufficiency.
Usual adult dosage: 1 to 5 mg I.M. daily, may range up to 10 mg. Once a maintenance dosage has been established and administered for 2 to 3 months, one pellet (125 mg) may be implanted S.C. for each 0.5 mg of the daily maintenance dosage. Pellet implantation is repeated every 8 to 12 months.

desoxycorticosterone pivalate (Percorten Pivalate). This mineralocorticoid is used only for maintenance therapy in patients with salt-losing adrenogenital syndrome. With glucocorticoids, it also is used to treat adrenocortical insufficiency.
Usual adult dosage: 25 to 100 mg I.M. every 4 weeks.

fludrocortisone acetate (Florinef Acetate). Almost always given with cortisone or hydrocortisone, fludrocortisone is used to treat salt-losing adrenogenital syndrome and adrenocortical insufficiency.
Usual adult dosage: 0.1 to 0.2 mg P.O. daily, usually with 10 to 37.5 mg of cortisone P.O. daily or with 10 to 30 mg of hydrocortisone P.O. daily in three or four divided doses.

Drug interactions

The drug interactions associated with the mineralocorticoids are similar to those associated with the systemic glucocorticoids. (For detailed information, see *Drug interactions: Systemic glucocorticoids and mineralocorticoids,* pages 961 and 962.)

ADVERSE DRUG REACTIONS

Desoxycorticosterone has virtually no glucocorticoid effects. Therefore, its adverse effects are limited to fluid and electrolyte imbalances and their effects, such as edema, hypertension, congestive heart failure (CHF), hypernatremia, hypokalemia, and hypocalcemia.

Although it is a potent mineralocorticoid, fludrocortisone causes adverse reactions associated with glucocorticoids and mineralocorticoids. (For more information, see *Adverse reactions to systemic corticosteroids,* page 963.) The mineralocorticoids themselves do not cause hypersensitivity reactions, but chemicals used in their preparation may do so.

NURSING PROCESS APPLICATION

The following information assists the nurse in caring for a patient receiving a mineralocorticoid.

Assessment

• Review the patient's history for a preexisting condition that contraindicates the use of a mineralocorticoid, such as cardiac disease or known hypersensitivity to any component of the drug.
• Review the patient's history for a preexisting condition that requires cautious use of a mineralocorticoid, such as Addison's disease, GI ulceration, renal disease, osteoporosis, or diabetes mellitus.
• Assess the patient for adverse reactions to the prescribed mineralocorticoid, such as fluid and electrolyte imbalances and their effects.
• Review the patient's medication history to identify the use of drugs that may interact with the mineralocorticoid, such as barbiturates, salicylates, oral contraceptives, cholestyramine, or antihypertensive agents.
• Assess the effectiveness of the prescribed mineralocorticoid periodically.
• Assess the patient regularly for signs of fluid retention, such as increased blood pressure, sudden increase in body weight (greater than 2 lb in 24 hours) ankle edema, or crackles in the lung fields.
• Evaluate the patient's and family's knowledge about the prescribed mineralocorticoid.

Nursing diagnoses

The following examples represent appropriate nursing diagnoses for a patient receiving a mineralocorticoid.
• Potential for injury related to a preexisting condition that contraindicates the use of a mineralocorticoid
• Potential for injury related to a preexisting condition that requires cautious use of a mineralocorticoid
• Potential for injury related to adverse drug reactions
• Fluid volume excess related to sodium and water retention caused by a mineralocorticoid
• Knowledge deficit related to the prescribed mineralocorticoid

Planning and implementation

• Do not administer a mineralocorticoid to a patient with a condition that contraindicates its use.
• Administer a mineralocorticoid cautiously to a patient at risk because of a preexisting condition.
• *Monitor the patient regularly for fluid and electrolyte imbalances and other adverse reactions during mineralocorticoid therapy.*

• *Observe the patient closely for signs and symptoms of hypernatremia (such as fluid retention, irritability, confusion, and other mental changes) and hypocalcemia and hypokalemia (such as arrhythmias and muscle weakness) during mineralocorticoid therapy.*

• Monitor plasma sodium, potassium, and calcium levels periodically.

• *Inject I.M. desoxycorticosterone acetate only in the upper outer quadrant of the buttock. Rotate injection sites, but never use the patient's arms to administer the drug because of the increased risk of subcutaneous atrophy.*

• *Inject desoxycorticosterone pivalate in the upper outer quadrant of the buttock with a 20-gauge needle.*

• Monitor the patient for additional adverse reactions, which usually are associated with systemic glucocorticoids. (For more information, see "Adverse drug reactions" and "Nursing process application" in the section on systemic glucocorticoids earlier in this chapter.)

• Notify the physician if the patient develops adverse reactions.

• Monitor the patient closely for signs of fluid retention by daily measurements of blood pressure and body weight, inspection for edema, and auscultation of lung fields.

• Do not allow the patient to consume more than eight 8-oz glasses (2 liters) of fluid daily, unless prescribed.

• Provide a low-sodium, high-potassium diet for the patient, as prescribed.

• Notify the physician if fluid retention occurs.

Patient teaching

• Teach the patient and family the name, dose, frequency, action, and adverse effects of the prescribed mineralocorticoid.

• *Inform the patient of the importance of periodic evaluations of serum electrolyte levels and blood pressure.*

• *Advise the patient to control salt intake and to monitor daily weight. Teach the patient to recognize and report signs of edema, such as swollen ankles and feet.*

• Instruct the patient to consume high-potassium foods and to avoid high-sodium foods.

• Teach the patient to note and report adverse reactions typically associated with systemic glucocorticoids.

• Instruct the patient to notify the physician if adverse reactions occur.

Evaluation

The following examples represent appropriate evaluation statements for a patient receiving a mineralocorticoid.

• The patient has no conditions that contraindicate mineralocorticoid therapy.

• The patient exhibits no signs of complications in the preexisting condition linked to the prescribed mineralocorticoid.

• The patient experiences no adverse reactions to the prescribed mineralocorticoid.

• The patient maintains normal fluid and electrolyte balance.

• The patient and family express an accurate understanding of the points taught about the prescribed mineralocorticoid.

• The patient plans a diet that minimizes fluid retention by restricting sodium intake.

IMMUNOSUPPRESSANTS

Several drugs used for their immunosuppressant effects in patients undergoing allograft transplantation (for example, patients receiving kidney, bone marrow, heart, or skin allografts) also are used experimentally to treat autoimmune diseases. Drugs in this immunosuppressant class include azathioprine, cyclosporine, lymphocyte immune globulin, antithymocyte globulin (equine) (ATG), and muromonab-CD3. Cyclophosphamide, classified as an alkylating agent, also is used as an immunosuppressant, but it is used primarily to treat cancer. (For information about this agent, see Chapter 66, Alkylating Agents.)

PHARMACOKINETICS

Because the drugs in this category vary greatly in structure, their pharmacokinetics also vary widely.

Absorption, distribution, metabolism, excretion

Azathioprine and cyclosporine usually are administered orally, but may be administered I.V. Azathioprine is absorbed readily from the GI tract, whereas absorption of cyclosporine is varied and incomplete. ATG and muromonab-CD3 are administered I.V.

The distribution of azathioprine is not understood fully, but it is bound partially to serum protein; the unbound drug rapidly clears from the blood. Cyclosporine and muromonab-CD3 are distributed widely throughout the body, and about 90% of cyclosporine is protein bound mainly to lipoproteins. Azathioprine and cyclosporine cross the placenta. The distribution of ATG is not defined clearly, but it may be distributed in breast milk.

Azathioprine is metabolized in the liver, primarily to mercaptopurine. The metabolic pathway is unknown. Cyclosporine is metabolized in the liver. Muromonab-CD3 is consumed by T cells circulating in the blood; it does not react with other cells or tissues in the body. The metabolism of ATG is unknown.

Azathioprine and ATG are excreted in the urine; cyclosporine is excreted principally in the bile. The excretion of muromonab-CD3 is unknown.

Onset, peak, duration

After oral administration, azathioprine reaches a peak concentration level in 2 hours, cyclosporine in 3½ hours. The peak concentration of ATG depends on the patient's ability to catabolize foreign immunoglobulin G (IgG).

For muromonab-CD3, onset of action begins within minutes of I.V. administration. During treatment with 5 mg/day for 14 days, the patient's concentration of muromonab-CD3 rises over the first 3 days and levels off to 0.9 mcg/ml on days 3 through 14.

The estimated half-life of azathioprine is 5 hours, with 50% excreted in the urine within 24 hours. The immunosuppressant effects, however, may persist for long periods after the drug is eliminated. The half-life of cyclosporine ranges from 10 to 27 hours. The plasma half-life of ATG is about 6 days but may range from 1.5 to 12 days.

PHARMACODYNAMICS

Because of the varied structure of these drugs, they have a wide range of action.

Mechanism of action

The action of azathioprine has not been determined precisely. It antagonizes metabolism of the amino acid purine and therefore may inhibit RNA and DNA synthesis. The drug also may alter RNA and DNA in some way, resulting in chromosome breaks, malfunctioning of the nucleic acids, or manufacture of fraudulent proteins. It also may inhibit coenzyme formation and function, thus interfering with cellular metabolism, and may act to prevent mitosis. In patients receiving kidney allografts, the drug suppresses cell-mediated hypersensitivities and produces various alterations in antibody production.

The precise mechanism of action of cyclosporine also is unknown, but experimental data suggest that the drug inhibits the helper T cells and the suppressor T cells. Its effectiveness in suppressing B cells is controversial. Cyclosporine does not affect the nonspecific immune system (macrophages), nor does it cause significant leukopenia and lymphopenia. Unlike azathioprine, cyclosporine lacks myelosuppressive action.

Muromonab-CD3 is a monoclonal antibody that preferentially reacts with the T_3 complex and thus blocks the function of T cells. ATG has an unknown mechanism of action, but it may eliminate antigen-reactive T cells in peripheral blood, alter T-cell function, or both.

PHARMACOTHERAPEUTICS

The immunosuppressant drugs are used mainly to prevent rejection in patients who undergo organ transplantation.

azathioprine (Imuran). Used with corticosteroids, local radiation, and other cytotoxic agents, azathioprine helps prevent rejection of kidney allografts. It also is used to treat severe rheumatoid arthritis unresponsive to conventional therapies.

Usual adult dosage: for prevention of kidney allograft rejection, 3 to 5 mg/kg P.O. daily starting on the day of transplantation or 1 to 3 days before; after transplantation, the same dosage I.V. until the patient can tolerate oral dosing (usually in 1 to 4 days); for rheumatoid arthritis, 1 mg/kg P.O. daily, increased by 0.5 mg/kg/day P.O., if necessary after 6 to 8 weeks of therapy, up to a maximum of 2.5 mg/kg/day. If the patient exhibits no therapeutic response in 12 weeks, therapy should be discontinued.

cyclosporine (Sandimmune). Used to prevent organ allograft rejection, cyclosporine always is given with corticosteroids. The drug also is used to treat chronic rejection in patients previously treated with other immunosuppressant agents to prolong graft survival of allogenic transplants and prophylactically to ameliorate or prevent graft-versus-host disease after bone marrow transplantation.

Usual adult dosage: 15 mg/kg P.O. 4 to 12 hours before transplantation, followed by 15 mg/kg P.O. daily for 1 to 2 weeks postoperatively, and then by dosages decreased 5% per week to a maintenance level of 5 to 10 mg/kg/day. When cyclosporine cannot be administered orally, it may be given I.V. at one-third the oral dosage (5 mg/kg I.V. daily), but the patient should be switched to oral administration as soon as possible.

lymphocyte immune globulin, antithymocyte globulin (equine) (Atgam). ATG is used as adjunctive therapy to prevent and treat rejection of kidney allografts. However, controlled studies have shown that it effectively treats acute rejections as well. ATG also has been used to treat aplastic anemia, with good results. It has been used with some success to treat acute graft-versus-host disease in patients with bone marrow allografts, but corticosteroids are still the drugs of choice. Finally, ATG has been effective in preventing rejection of skin allografts and has had some success as part of immunosuppressive protocols for the prevention and treatment of heart allograft rejection.

Usual adult dosage: for prevention of kidney allograft rejection, 15 mg/kg I.V. daily for 14 days, starting within 24 hours before or after surgery, followed by alternate-day therapy with the same dosage for an additional 14 days; for management of acute rejection, 10 to 15 mg/kg I.V. daily for 14 days, followed by alternate-day therapy with the same dosage for up to another 14 days if necessary; for aplastic anemia, 10 to 15 mg/kg I.V. daily for 10 to 14 days, followed by alternate-day therapy with the same dosage for 14 additional days; for prevention of graft-versus-host disease in patients with bone marrow allografts, 7 to 10 mg/kg I.V. every other day for a total of six doses; for management of acute graft-versus-host disease, 7 mg/kg I.V. every other day for a total of six doses; for prevention of skin allograft rejection, 10 mg/kg I.V. 24 hours before the first allograft, followed by a maintenance dosage of 10 to 15 mg/kg every other day.

muromonab-CD3 (Orthoclone OKT3). Muromonab-CD3 is used as first-line therapy or to "rescue" allograft rejection that has not responded to other therapies. It also is effective in preventing allograft rejection.
Usual adult dosage: 5 mg I.V. daily for 10 to 14 days.

Drug interactions

Most drug interactions with this class of drugs involve other immunosuppressant and anti-inflammatory agents and various antibiotic and antimicrobial drugs. (For more information, see *Drug interactions: Immunosuppressants,* page 974.)

ADVERSE DRUG REACTIONS

The immunosuppressant drugs can produce multisystemic toxic reactions and should be administered only under close medical supervision.

The primary adverse reaction to azathioprine is bone marrow depression, evidenced by leukopenia, macrocytic anemia, pancytopenia, and thrombocytopenia. This may alter clotting mechanisms and cause hemorrhaging. Nausea, vomiting, anorexia, and diarrhea can occur with high dosages; mouth ulcerations, esophagitis, and steatorrhea are other adverse reactions. In a small number of patients, hepatic dysfunction has been reported. Other adverse reactions to azathioprine include alopecia, arthralgia, retinopathy, Raynaud's disease, and pulmonary edema.

The most severe adverse reaction to cyclosporine is nephrotoxicity, usually characterized by increased blood urea nitrogen (BUN) and serum creatinine levels. Thus, differentiating between allograft rejection and an adverse reaction to cyclosporine can be difficult. More common adverse reactions include hyperkalemia, hyperuricemia, decreased serum bicarbonate level, hypertension, tremor, gingival hyperplasia, hirsutism, diarrhea, nausea, vomiting, generalized abdominal discomfort, and infection. Less common reactions are gastritis, hiccups, and peptic ulcer. Occasional complaints include central nervous system effects (flushing, paresthesia, headache) and hepatotoxicity (usually occurring during the first month of therapy and with high dosages). Leukopenia, thrombocytopenia, and anemia are uncommon, and hematuria and psychiatric disorders are rare. In 3% of patients undergoing cyclosporine therapy, sinusitis and gynecomastia have been reported; conjunctivitis, hearing loss, tinnitus, hyperglycemia, edema, fever, and muscle pain have been reported in 2% or fewer.

With ATG therapy, the most common adverse reaction is fever accompanied by chills. Up to 20% of patients receiving kidney allografts experience leukopenia, thrombocytopenia, or both while receiving this drug. Early myelosuppression also may occur and force discontinuation of ATG. The immunosuppressant effects of ATG may lead to local and systemic infections. Nausea, vomiting, diarrhea, stomatitis, hiccups, epigastric pain, and abdominal distention also may occur. Rash, pruritus, urticaria, and erythema have been reported in 10% to 15% of patients. Adverse cardiovascular reactions to ATG, such as hypotension, hypertension, tachycardia, edema, pulmonary edema, iliac vein obstruction, and renal artery stenosis, are uncommon.

Most adverse reactions to muromonab-CD3 occur during the first 2 days of therapy. The most common reactions are fever and chills. Others include dyspnea, chest pain, vomiting, wheezing, nausea, diarrhea, and tremor. Severe — potentially fatal — pulmonary edema is reported in 2% or fewer of patients receiving this drug. The incidence of infection associated with muromonab-CD3 therapy is comparable to that associated with high dosages of corticosteroids. The most common infections, which involve cytomegalovirus and herpes simplex, occur during the first 45 days of therapy.

All drugs in this class can cause hypersensitivity reactions, which range from rash and serum sickness to anaphylaxis. Azathioprine may cause hypersensitivity pancreatitis.

NURSING PROCESS APPLICATION

The following information assists the nurse in caring for a patient receiving an immunosuppressant agent.

Assessment

● Review the patient's history for a preexisting condition that contraindicates the use of an immunosuppressant agent, such as fluid overload or known hypersensitivity to the drug.
● Review the patient's history for a preexisting condition that requires cautious use of an immunosuppressant agent, such as a systemic reaction to an ATG skin test or previous exposure to muromonab-CD3.
● Assess the patient for adverse reactions to the prescribed immunosuppressant, such as bone marrow depression, fluid and electrolyte imbalance, hypersensitivity, or GI dysfunction.

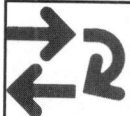

DRUG INTERACTIONS

Immunosuppressants

Interactions involving the immunosuppressants and other drugs can increase the patient's risk of infection greatly. The nurse should assess the patient carefully and continually for fever, malaise, and other signs and symptoms of infection.

DRUG	INTERACTING DRUGS	POSSIBLE EFFECTS	NURSING IMPLICATIONS
azathioprine	allopurinol	Increases the blood level of azathioprine by slowing its metabolism	• Decrease the azathioprine dosage, if prescribed, during concomitant administration of these drugs.
cyclosporine	acyclovir, aminoglycosides, amphotericin B	Increase potential for nephrotoxicity	• Monitor the patient's blood urea nitrogen (BUN) and serum creatinine levels. • Monitor the patient's fluid intake and output. • Decrease the dosage of both nephrotoxic drugs, if prescribed.
	other immunosuppressant agents (except corticosteroids)	Increase risk of infection and lymphoma	• Monitor the patient for signs and symptoms of infection.
	ketoconazole	Increases the serum cyclosporine concentration	• Monitor the patient for excessive cyclosporine effect (neurotoxicity). • Monitor the patient's BUN and serum creatinine levels. • Monitor the patient's fluid intake and output. • Decrease the cyclosporine dosage, if prescribed.
	barbiturates, rifampin, phenytoin, sulfonamides, trimethoprim	Decrease the plasma cyclosporine concentration	• Increase the cyclosporine dosage, if prescribed.
	calcium channel blockers, cimetidine	Increase the plasma cyclosporine concentration	• Decrease the cyclosporine dosage, if prescribed.
	anabolic steroids, oral contraceptives	Increase the serum cyclosporine concentration	• Monitor the patient's serum cyclosporine concentration. • Decrease the cyclosporine dosage, if prescribed. • Monitor the patient's BUN and serum creatinine levels. • Advise the patient to avoid concomitant use of oral contraceptives or anabolic steroids.
	cardiac glycosides	Increases the serum digoxin concentration	• Monitor for signs and symptoms of digitalis toxicity, such as cardiac, gastrointestinal, and neurologic dysfunction. • Monitor the patient's serum digoxin concentration. • Decrease the cardiac glycoside dosage, if prescribed.
	erythromycin, metoclopramide	Increase the serum cyclosporine concentration	• Monitor the patient's BUN and serum creatinine levels. • Monitor the serum cyclosporine concentration.
lymphocyte immune globulin, antithymocyte globulin (ATG)	other immunosuppressant agents	Increase risk of infection and lymphoma	• Monitor the patient's white blood cell count for leukocytosis.
muromonab-CD3	other immunosuppressant agents	Increase immunosuppressant effectiveness	• Monitor the patient for signs and symptoms of infection.

• Review the patient's medication history to identify the use of drugs that may interact with the prescribed immunosuppressant, such as other immunosuppressant agents, allopurinol, barbiturates, or cardiac glycosides.

• Assess the effectiveness of the prescribed immunosuppressant periodically.

• Assess the patient regularly for signs of infection, such as fever, chills, elevated WBC, and purulent drainage.

• Evaluate the patient's and family's knowledge about the prescribed immunosuppressant.

Nursing diagnoses

The following examples represent appropriate nursing diagnoses for a patient receiving an immunosuppressant.

• Potential for injury related to a preexisting condition that contraindicates the use of an immunosuppressant

• Potential for injury related to a preexisting condition that requires cautious use of an immunosuppressant

• Potential for injury related to adverse drug reactions

• Altered protection related to immunosuppression caused by long-term immunosuppressant therapy

• Knowledge deficit related to the prescribed immunosuppressant

Planning and implementation

• Do not administer an immunosuppressant to a patient with a condition that contraindicates its use.

• Administer an immunosuppressant cautiously to a patient at risk because of a preexisting condition.

• Monitor the patient frequently for adverse reactions during immunosuppressant therapy.

• *Monitor the patient closely for hypersensitivity reactions, which can range from a rash and serum sickness to anaphylaxis. Keep standard emergency equipment nearby.*

• Give the patient 1 mg/kg of methylprednisolone sodium succinate I.V., as prescribed, before administering muromonab-CD3 I.V. to reduce the risk of a first-dose reaction.

• Administer 100 mg of hydrocortisone sodium succinate I.V., as prescribed, 30 minutes after muromonab-CD3 I.V. administration to reduce the risk of a first-dose reaction.

• *Perform an intradermal skin test as prescribed before administering the first dose of ATG to assess the patient's risk for severe systemic adverse reactions.*

• Monitor the patient's CBC (including platelets) and liver function tests frequently during azathioprine therapy.

• Evaluate the patient's liver enzymes and BUN, serum creatinine, and bilirubin levels frequently during cyclosporine therapy.

• Monitor the cyclosporine blood concentration periodically for a patient receiving oral cyclosporine.

• *Document that the patient starting muromonab-CD3 therapy has had a chest X-ray 24 hours before receiving the first dose; the chest must be clear of fluid.*

• Monitor the patient's T-cell assays regularly as prescribed during muromonab-CD3 therapy.

• Monitor hydration if the patient develops anorexia, nausea, vomiting, or diarrhea during immunosuppressant therapy. Obtain a prescription for an antiemetic or antidiarrheal agent as needed.

• *Inspect the patient's oral cavity daily for signs of mouth ulceration, gingival hyperplasia, and stomatitis. If changes occur, notify the physician to discuss appropriate treatment.*

• *Monitor the patient's vital signs frequently.* ATG may cause fever and changes in the blood pressure or heart rate; muromonab-CD3 may cause fever and changes in the respiratory rate or pattern.

• *Take bleeding precautions if the patient's platelet level falls below normal.* For example, have the patient use an electric razor for shaving and avoid activities that can cause cuts and bruises.

• Monitor the patient for signs of fluid retention, such as increased blood pressure and body weight, ankle swelling, jugular vein distention, and crackles.

• Monitor the patient for paresthesia, tinnitus, and hearing loss during cyclosporine therapy. Notify the physician if these adverse reactions occur.

• Administer azathioprine in divided doses after meals, as prescribed, to reduce the risk or severity of adverse GI reactions.

• Administer azathioprine I.V., as prescribed, if the patient cannot tolerate the oral drug, but resume oral therapy as soon as possible.

• Give I.V. azathioprine as a bolus or diluted in normal saline (0.9% sodium chloride) solution or dextrose 5% in water (D_5W) and infuse over 30 to 60 minutes.

• Mix oral cyclosporine in a glass container with milk or orange juice at room temperature to increase its palatability. Stir it well with a metal spoon and administer the drink immediately. Then put a little more milk or orange juice in the container and have the patient drink it to receive the entire dose.

• *Dilute each milliliter of cyclosporine for I.V. infusion in 20 to 100 ml of normal saline or D_5W immediately before administration and infuse over 2 to 6 hours. Ensure that the solution is free of particulate matter and discoloration. If it is not, discard it and start over.*

• Administer I.V. ATG as an infusion, diluted in 250 to 1,000 ml of normal or 0.45% saline solution over 4 to 8 hours.

• *Refrigerate the ATG solution if it will not be given immediately. If refrigeration time plus infusion time exceeds 12 hours, do not use the solution.*

• *Administer the ATG solution into high-flow veins to decrease the risk of phlebitis and thrombosis. Always use an in-line filter and make sure the solution is free of particulate matter and discoloration.*

(Text continues on page 978.)

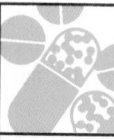

SELECTED MAJOR DRUGS

Corticosteroid and other immunosuppressant agents

This chart summarizes the major corticosteroid and other immunosuppressant agents currently in clinical use.

DRUG	MAJOR INDICATIONS	USUAL ADULT DOSAGES	CONTRAINDICATIONS AND PRECAUTIONS
Systemic glucocorticoids			
cortisone	Replacement therapy for adrenocortical insufficiency; anti-inflammatory conditions	25 to 300 mg P.O. daily or 20 to 300 mg I.M. daily	• Know that cortisone is contraindicated in a patient with a systemic fungal infection or known hypersensitivity to any component of the drug. • Administer with caution to a patient with gastrointestinal (GI) ulceration, renal disease, hypertension, osteoporosis, varicella, vaccinia, exanthema, diabetes mellitus, hypothyroidism, thromboembolic disorder, seizures, myasthenia gravis, congestive heart failure (CHF), tuberculosis, ocular herpes simplex, hypoalbuminemia, emotional instability, or psychosis.
dexamethasone sodium phosphate	Cerebral edema	Initially, 10 mg I.V., then 4 to 6 mg I.M. every 6 hours for 2 to 4 days, then tapered off	• Know that dexamethasone sodium phosphate is contraindicated in a patient with systemic fungal infection or known hypersensitivity to any component of the drug. • Administer with caution to a patient with GI ulceration, renal disease, hypertension, osteoporosis, varicella, vaccinia, exanthema, diabetes mellitus, hypothyroidism, thromboembolic disorders, seizures, myasthenia gravis, CHF, tuberculosis, ocular herpes simplex, hypoalbuminemia, emotional instability, or psychosis.
methylprednisolone	Inflammatory conditions and those requiring immunosuppression	Initially, 2 to 60 mg P.O. daily; further therapy must be individualized	• Know that methylprednisone is contraindicated in a patient with systemic fungal infection or known hypersensitivity to any component of the drug. • Administer with caution to a patient with GI ulceration, renal disease, hypertension, osteoporosis, varicella, vaccinia, exanthema, diabetes mellitus, hypothyroidism, thromboembolic disorder, seizures, myasthenia gravis, CHF, tuberculosis, ocular herpes simplex, hypoalbuminemia, emotional instability, or psychosis.
prednisone	Inflammatory conditions and those requiring immunosuppression	Initially, 5 to 60 mg P.O. daily; further therapy must be individualized	• Know that prednisone is contraindicated in a patient with systemic fungal infection or known hypersensitivity to any component of the drug. • Administer with caution to a patient with GI ulceration, renal disease, hypertension, osteoporosis, varicella, vaccinia, exanthema, diabetes mellitus, hypothyroidism, thromboembolic disorder, seizures, myasthenia gravis, CHF, tuberculosis, ocular herpes simplex, hypoalbuminemia, emotional instability, or psychosis.

Coricosteroid and other immunosuppressant agents (continued)

DRUG	MAJOR INDICATIONS	USUAL ADULT DOSAGES	CONTRAINDICATIONS AND PRECAUTIONS
Topical glucocorticoids			
betamethasone valerate	Inflammatory conditions such as corticosteroid-responsive dermatoses	0.1% cream, ointment, or lotion applied b.i.d. or t.i.d.	• Know that topical glucocorticoids are contraindicated in a patient with known hypersensitivity to any components of the drug.
fluocinolone	Inflammatory conditions such as corticosteroid-responsive dermatoses	0.01% to 0.2% cream, 0.025% ointment, or 0.01% solution applied b.i.d. to q.i.d	• Know that topical glucocorticoids are contraindicated in a patient with known hypersensitivity to any components of the drug.
flurandrenolide	Inflammatory conditions such as corticosteroid-responsive dermatoses	0.05% or 0.025% cream or ointment applied b.i.d. or t.i.d., or 4 mcg/cm² drug-impregnated tape applied daily or b.i.d.	• Know that topical glucocorticoids are contraindicated in a patient with known hypersensitivity to any components of the drug.
triamcinolone acetonide	Inflammatory conditions such as corticosteroid-responsive dermatoses	0.025% or 0.5% cream, ointment, or lotion applied b.i.d. to q.i.d.	• Know that topical glucocorticoids are contraindicated in a patient with known hypersensitivity to any components of the drug.
Mineralocorticoids			
desoxycorticosterone acetate, desoxycorticosterone pivalate	Adrenocortical insufficiency, salt-losing adrenogenital syndrome	1 to 5 mg (acetate) I.M. daily, or 1 pellet (125 mg) implanted S.C. for each 0.5 mg of the daily maintenance dosage; 25 to 100 mg (pivalate) I.M. every 4 weeks	• Know that desoxycorticosterone acetate and desoxycorticosterone pivalate are contraindicated in a patient with hypertension, CHF, cardiac disease, or known hypersensitivity to any components of these drugs. • Administer with caution to a patient with Addison's disease.
fludrocortisone	Adrenocortical insufficiency, salt-losing adrenogenital syndrome	0.1 to 0.2 mg P.O. daily with 10 to 37.5 mg cortisone P.O. daily or with 10 to 30 mg hydrocortisone P.O. daily in three or four divided doses	• Know that fludrocortisone is contraindicated in a patient with systemic fungal infection or known hypersensitivity to any components of the drug. • Administer with caution to a patient with GI ulceration, renal disease, hypertension, osteoporosis, varicella, vaccinia, exanthema, diabetes mellitus, cushingoid symptoms, thromboembolic disorder, myasthenia gravis, metastatic cancer, CHF, tuberculosis, ocular herpes simplex, hypoalbuminemia, emotional instability, or psychosis.
Immunosuppressants			
azathioprine	Prevention of kidney allograft rejection	3 to 5 mg/kg P.O. daily, starting on the day of transplantation or 1 to 3 days before; after transplantation, the same dosage I.V. until the patient can tolerate oral dosing	• Know that azathioprine is contraindicated in a pregnant or lactating patient, one with known hypersensitivity to the drug, or one who has received previous treatment with an alkylating agent. (continued)

SELECTED MAJOR DRUGS

Coricosteroid and other immunosuppressant agents *(continued)*

DRUG	MAJOR INDICATIONS	USUAL ADULT DOSAGES	CONTRAINDICATIONS AND PRECAUTIONS
Immunosuppressants *(continued)*			
lymphocyte immune globulin, antithymocyte globulin (ATG)	Prevention or delay of allograft rejection	15 mg/kg I.V. daily for 14 days, followed by alternate-day therapy with the same dosage for 14 more days	• Know that ATG is contraindicated in a pregnant patient or one who has had a severe systemic hypersensitivity reaction to the drug or other equine immunoglobulin G preparation. • Administer with extreme caution to a patient with a systemic hypersensitivity reaction to the skin test.
	Prevention of graft-versus-host disease after bone marrow allograft transplantation	7 to 10 mg/kg I.V. every other day for six doses	
	Management of acute allograft rejection	10 to 15 mg/kg I.V. daily for 14 days, followed by alternate-day therapy with the same dosage for up to 14 more days	
	Treatment of graft-versus-host disease after bone marrow allograft transplantation	7 mg/kg I.V. every other day for six doses	
muromonab-CD3	Treatment or "rescue" of allograft rejection unresponsive to other therapies; prevention of allograft rejection	5 mg I.V. daily for 10 to 14 days	• Know that muromonab-CD3 is contraindicated in a patient with fluid overload or known hypersensitivity to the drug or any other product of murine origin. • Administer with caution to a pregnant patient or one who previously received the drug.

• Administer a muromonab-CD3 I.V. bolus in less than 1 minute. Do not administer it as an infusion or with other solutions.

• Monitor the patient for drug interactions during concomitant therapy with an immunosuppressant.

• Notify the physician if adverse reactions or signs of organ or graft rejection occur.

• *Monitor the patient for signs and symptoms of infection during immunosuppressant therapy. Keep in mind that classic signs of infection maybe suppressed. However, the WBC count remains a reliable indicator.*

• Monitor the patient's WBC and differential counts regularly during immunosuppressant therapy.

• *Take infection control measures, such as maintaining reverse isolation.*

• Notify the physician immediately if the patient displays signs of infection. Prepare to begin appropriate treatment, such as antibiotic therapy, as prescribed.

Patient teaching
• Teach the patient and family the name, dose, frequency, action, and adverse effects of the prescribed immunosuppressant.

• Explain the therapeutic purpose of the immunosuppressant thoroughly.

• *Inform the patient that infection, which can be life-threatening, is the most common hazard associated with immunosuppressant therapy.*

• *Emphasize that preventing infection requires scrupulous oral and personal hygiene during immunosuppressant therapy.*

• *Advise the patient to avoid crowds and people who have infections while taking the immunosuppressant.*

• *Urge the patient to postpone immunizations until after cessation of immunosuppressant therapy.*

• *Urge a female patient to avoid conception during immunosuppressant therapy and for up to 4 months afterward.*

• Emphasize the importance of prescribed laboratory tests and periodic monitoring by the physician.

• *Teach the patient to take bleeding precautions if the platelet count falls below normal.*

• Instruct the patient receiving cyclosporine to notify the physician if paresthesia, tinnitus, or hearing loss occurs.

• Inform the diabetic patient that hyperglycemia may occur during cyclosporine therapy. Instruct such a patient to monitor the blood glucose level closely and adhere to the prescribed treatment regimen strictly.

• Prepare the patient for immunosuppressant-induced changes in appearance, such as alopecia, hirsutism, gynecomastia, or rashes.

• Instruct the patient to notify the physician if adverse reactions occur.

Evaluation

The following examples represent appropriate evaluation statements for a patient receiving an immunosuppressant.

• The patient has no conditions that contraindicate immunosuppressant therapy.

• The patient exhibits no signs of complications in the preexisting condition linked to the prescribed immunosuppressant.

• The patient experiences no adverse reactions to the prescribed immunosuppressant.

• The patient remains free from infection during immunosuppressant therapy.

• The patient and family express an accurate understanding of the points taught about the prescribed immunosuppressant.

• The patient adheres to infection-control measures.

CHAPTER SUMMARY

Chapter 57 discussed the systemic and topical corticosteroid and other immunosuppressant agents as they are used to suppress the inflammatory response and the allograft rejection response and to treat adrenocortical insufficiency. Here are the highlights of the chapter.

• Systemic and topical corticosteroids affect nearly every body system and have the potential to cause severe adverse reactions.

• Systemic glucocorticoids are synthetic analogues of natural corticosteroids secreted by the adrenal cortex.

• Because the systemic glucocorticoids are distributed throughout the body, they can cause widespread adverse reactions, some of which can be life-threatening. Cushingoid signs and symptoms are the best known adverse reactions.

• When caring for a patient receiving a systemic glucocorticoid, the nurse should monitor closely for adverse reactions and teach the patient about the correct timing and self-administration of doses as well as the signs and symptoms of adverse reactions.

• The anti-inflammatory and antiproliferative effects of the topical glucocorticoids make them useful in treating various skin disorders.

• Adverse reactions to the topical glucocorticoids are more pronounced with the use of fluorinated preparations and occlusive dressings.

• For a patient who is receiving a topical glucocorticoid, the nurse should understand which formulations to use for which types of lesions. The nurse also should teach the patient proper application techniques.

• Mineralocorticoids also are synthetic analogues of corticosteroids excreted by the adrenal cortex. They exert their principal effect on fluid and electrolyte balance and extracellular fluid volume. They are used chiefly for replacement therapy in patients with adrenocortical insufficiency.

• Nursing care related to mineralocorticoid therapy includes preparing the patient for long-term use of the drug.

• The major immunosuppressant drugs, used to prevent or treat allograft rejection, are highly potent and can cause severe—even life-threatening—adverse reactions.

• Nursing care for a patient receiving an immunosuppressant includes taking all possible measures to prevent infection, teaching the patient the importance of preventing infection, and stressing the need for the patient to report any change in health status because it may signal infection.

STUDY QUESTIONS

See Appendix 1 for answers.

1. Gordon Selfridge, age 50, has chronic obstructive pulmonary disease. In addition to his respiratory medications, he must take the systemic glucocorticoid prednisone 5 mg P.O. daily. During a patient-teaching session, the nurse instructs Mr. Selfridge to take prednisone exactly as prescribed. Which adverse reaction may occur if the drug is discontinued suddenly?
(a) hyperglycemia and glycosuria
(b) acute adrenocortical insufficiency
(c) posterior subcapsular cataracts
(d) restlessness and seizures

2. The nurse should advise Mr. Selfridge to take prednisone at what time?
(a) at bedtime to minimize adverse reactions
(b) in the morning to mimic normal hormone secretion
(c) on an empty stomach to enhance absorption
(d) in the evening when normal hormone secretion is low

3. Jim Quigley, age 63, develops psoriasis every winter. This year, however, it is worse than usual. His physician prescribes betamethasone valerate cream to be applied twice a day. When teaching Mr. Quigley how to apply this topical glucocorticoid cream, the nurse should include which instruction?

(a) Apply the smallest amount possible in a thin coat over the affected area.

(b) Apply a thick coat to ensure maximum therapeutic effects.

(c) Apply to nearby unaffected areas to prevent the spread of psoriasis.

(d) Apply an occlusive dressing over a thick coat on the affected area.

4. The nurse also should teach Mr. Quigley to avoid applying the cream to which area?

(a) wet lesions

(b) scalp only

(c) all hairy areas

(d) eye area

5. At age 18, Carla Gallen appears healthy and seems to have a deep bronze suntan. However, she complains of weakness, fatigue, weight loss, and GI disturbances. Laboratory findings indicate adrenal insufficiency. Her physician prescribes desoxycorticosterone acetate 5 mg I.M. daily. What is the mechanism of action of this mineralcorticoid agent?

(a) It increases sodium and chloride excretion and decreases potassium secretion.

(b) It increases sodium resorption and potassium and hydrogen secretion.

(c) It decreases potassium and hydrogen excretion.

(d) It decreases water absorption from the renal tubules.

6. The nurse monitors Ms. Gallen frequently. Which sign should alert the nurse to an adverse reaction to the mineralocorticoid?

(a) diarrhea

(b) stomatitis

(c) nausea and vomiting

(d) edema and weight gain

7. Lin Cheng, age 48, has just received a kidney transplant. To prevent transplant rejection, her physician prescribes corticosteroid and immunosuppressant therapy. Her current regimen includes cyclosporine 1,000 mg P.O. daily, azathioprine 100 mg P.O. daily, and prednisone 30 mg P.O. daily. When caring for Ms. Cheng, the nurse should assess for which primary adverse reaction to azathioprine?

(a) renal failure

(b) peptic ulcer

(c) severe pulmonary edema

(d) bone marrow depression

8. The nurse monitors serum electrolyte levels closely while Ms. Cheng is receiving cyclosporine. Which electrolyte imbalance may indicate an adverse reaction to cyclosporine?

(a) hyperkalemia

(b) hypernatremia

(c) hypercalcemia

(d) hypokalemia

SELECTED REFERENCES

AHFS drug information 90. (1990). Bethesda, MD: American Society of Hospital Pharmacists.

Baciewicz, A., and Baciewicz, F., Jr. (1989). Cyclosporine pharmacokinetic drug interactions. *American Journal of Surgery,* 157(2), 264-271.

Caudell, K., and Adams, J. (1990). Cyclosporine administration practices on bone marrow transplant units: A national survey. *Oncology Nursing Forum,* 17(4), 563-568.

Drug facts and comparisons. (1991). St. Louis: Facts and Comparisons Division, J.B. Lippincott.

Goodman and Gilman's the pharmacological basis of therapeutics (8th ed.; 1990). Elmsford, NY: Pergamon Press.

North American Nursing Diagnosis Association. (1990). *Taxonomy I - Revised, with official categories.* St. Louis: NANDA.

Sandimmune gel capsules. (1990). *Nurses Drug Alert,* 14(5), 40.

CHAPTER

58

URICOSURICS, OTHER ANTIGOUT AGENTS, AND GOLD SALTS

OBJECTIVES

After reading and studying this chapter, the student should be able to:

1. Describe the etiology and signs and symptoms of gout and rheumatoid arthritis.

2. Identify the specific clinical indications for the following drugs: probenecid, sulfinpyrazone, allopurinol, colchicine, auranofin, aurothioglucose, and gold sodium thiomalate.

3. Describe the mechanism of action of the uricosurics probenecid and sulfinpyrazone and the antigout agents allopurinol and colchicine.

4. Identify the pharmacotherapeutic advantages and disadvantages of the uricosurics, other antigout drugs, and gold salts.

5. Describe the adverse reactions to the major drugs used to treat acute gouty attacks and rheumatoid arthritis.

6. Differentiate between the pharmacokinetic properties of parenteral and oral gold salt preparations.

7. Describe how to apply the nursing process when caring for a patient who is receiving a uricosuric, other antigout agent, or gold salt.

INTRODUCTION

Joint inflammation can be treated with many drugs, depending on its etiology. For example, gout and rheumatoid arthritis produce joint inflammation that responds to quite different drug interventions. Gout, a hereditary disease involving an error in metabolism, leads to hyperuricemia and the formation of monosodium urate crystals. Deposition of the monosodium urate crystals in and around a joint causes the inflammation and resultant pain. Gout is best treated with uricosuric drugs, such as probenecid and sulfinpyrazone, or other antigout medications, such as allopurinol and colchicine. Indomethacin, naproxen, and phenylbutazone also are used to treat gout. (For more information

about these drugs, see Chapter 21, Nonnarcotic Analgesic, Antipyretic, and Nonsteroidal Anti-inflammatory Agents.)

In rheumatoid arthritis, inflammation and destruction occur primarily in the peripheral joints, producing pain. Treatment of rheumatoid arthritis, however, differs markedly from that of gout. The drugs of choice include auranofin, an oral gold salt, or aurothioglucose and gold sodium thiomalate, two parenteral forms of gold salt therapy. These drugs are used only after other drugs, such as nonsteroidal anti-inflammatory agents, have failed to work effectively.

For a summary of representative drugs, see *Selected major drugs: Uricosurics, other antigout agents, and gold salts,* page 994. For a listing of applicable nursing diagnoses that the nurse may formulate when caring for a patient receiving these agents, see *Selected nursing diagnoses: Uricosurics, other antigout agents, and gold salts,* page 982. For detailed information on applying the nursing process, see Chapter 6, The Nursing Process and Drug Therapy.

URICOSURICS

The two major uricosurics are probenecid and sulfinpyrazone, which act by increasing uric acid excretion in the urine. The primary goal in using the uricosurics is to prevent or control the frequency of gouty arthritis attacks.

PHARMACOKINETICS

Uricosurics are absorbed from the gastrointestinal (GI) tract and metabolized in the liver.

SELECTED NURSING DIAGNOSES

Uricosurics, other antigout agents, and gold salts

The following nursing diagnoses address representative problems and etiologies that a nurse may encounter when caring for a patient who is receiving a uricosuric, other antigout agent, or gold salt. Some of these nursing diagnoses contain generalized etiologies, which the nurse must individualize based on the patient's needs. (For some common nursing diagnoses and related interventions for each drug class, see the "Nursing Process Application" sections of this chapter.)

- Altered oral mucous membrane related to stomatitis caused by colchicine or a gold salt
- Altered protection related to the adverse hematologic effects of the prescribed uricosuric, other antigout agent, or gold salt
- Altered urinary elimination related to auranofin-induced renal dysfunction
- Altered urinary elimination related to probenecid-induced urinary frequency
- Body image disturbance related to the adverse dermatologic effects of allopurinol, colchicine, or a gold salt
- Diarrhea related to the adverse GI effects of allopurinol, colchicine, or auranofin
- Fluid volume excess related to sulfinpyrazone-induced edema
- Hyperthermia related to colchicine-induced fever
- Impaired physical mobility related to colchicine-induced muscle weakness
- Knowledge deficit related to the prescribed uricosuric, other antigout agent, or gold salt
- Noncompliance related to long-term use and adverse effects of auranofin

- Pain related to colchicine-induced intermittent abdominal pain or bladder spasms
- Pain related to probenecid-induced headache
- Potential activity intolerance related to anemia caused by a uricosuric or other antigout agent
- Potential fluid volume deficit related to the adverse GI effects of the prescribed uricosuric, other antigout agent, or gold salt
- Potential for injury related to a preexisting condition that contraindicates the use of a uricosuric, other antigout agent, or gold salt
- Potential for injury related to a preexisting condition that requires cautious use of a uricosuric, other antigout agent, or gold salt
- Potential for injury related to adverse drug reactions
- Potential for injury related to drug interactions
- Potential for trauma related to dizziness or vertigo caused by a uricosuric or drowsiness caused by allopurinol
- Sensory-perceptual alterations (auditory) related to sulfinpyrazone-induced tinnitus
- Sensory-perceptual alterations (tactile) related to peripheral neuritis caused by allopurinol or colchicine

Absorption, distribution, metabolism, excretion

After oral administration, probenecid and sulfinpyrazone are absorbed rapidly and completely from the GI tract. Distribution of the two drugs also is similar, with 75% to 95% of probenecid and 98% of sulfinpyrazone being protein bound. Metabolism of the drugs occurs in the liver; probenecid is metabolized slowly. Excretion takes place within the renal system, where small amounts of both drugs are filtered by the glomeruli. However, probenecid and sulfinpyrazone are secreted primarily at the proximal tubule. Only small amounts of these two drugs are excreted in the feces. Sulfinpyrazone is excreted primarily unchanged.

Onset, peak, duration

The onset of action for probenecid and sulfinpyrazone usually occurs rapidly—within 30 minutes after oral administration. Maximal renal clearance of uric acid also occurs within 30 minutes after administering probenecid. Peak plasma concentration levels of probenecid are reached in 2 to 4 hours, while the peak concentration for sulfinpyrazone is reached in 1 to 2 hours. The duration of action for both drugs usually ranges from 4 to 6 hours but may last as long as 10 hours. The half-life of probenecid ranges from 4 to 17 hours; that of sulfinpyrazone is only 3 hours.

(For a depiction of the onset, peak, and duration, see *Pharmacokinetics of the uricosurics.*)

PHARMACODYNAMICS

Probenecid and sulfinpyrazone competitively inhibit the active resorption of uric acid at the proximal convoluted tubules. This leads to urinary excretion of uric acid and a subsequent reduction of the serum urate level.

Probenecid and sulfinpyrazone produce minimal, if any, analgesic or anti-inflammatory effect. Instead, by promoting a decrease in the serum urate level, they reduce chronic joint destruction and tophi (sodium urate deposits around a joint) formation. The goal of using the uricosuric drugs is to reduce the frequency of gouty arthritis attacks.

PHARMACOTHERAPEUTICS

Probenecid and sulfinpyrazone, which lower the serum urate level, are indicated for patients with chronic gouty arthritis and tophaceous gout. An elevated serum urate level without symptoms of gouty arthritis usually is not considered an indication for uricosuric therapy. However, when the serum urate level exceeds 9 mg/dl, therapy sometimes

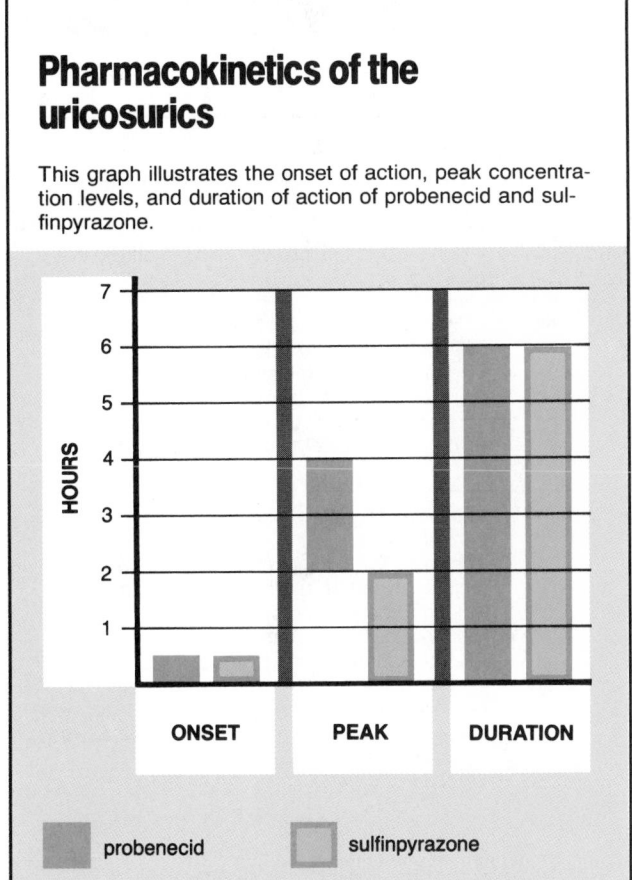

Pharmacokinetics of the uricosurics

This graph illustrates the onset of action, peak concentration levels, and duration of action of probenecid and sulfinpyrazone.

▨ probenecid   ▨ sulfinpyrazone

is started to prevent joint changes and renal impairment, which can occur above that level.

Uricosuric drugs also are used in patients with visible tophi, with a serum urate level above 8.5 to 9 mg/dl, and with a family history of tophi or decreased uric acid excretion. Probenecid and sulfinpyrazone are not indicated during an acute gouty attack. If taken at that time, the drugs only prolong inflammation.

Probenecid and sulfinpyrazone also are used to promote uric acid excretion in patients experiencing hyperuricemia secondary to thiazide and other related diuretics.

Both drugs work effectively when given with allopurinol. Although they promote excretion of the active metabolite of allopurinol, the uricosurics produce an additive effect and are of therapeutic value. Nonetheless, when a uricosuric is administered concomitantly with allopurinol, smaller dosages of each drug are advised.

The major disadvantage of the uricosurics is that they cannot be used to treat acute gouty attacks. Furthermore, uricosuric drugs prove ineffective in patients with a creatinine clearance of less than 30 ml/minute. Probenecid and sulfinpyrazone also may increase the chance of an acute gouty attack when therapy begins and whenever the serum urate level changes rapidly. To prevent this reaction, col-

chicine is administered in prophylactic doses during the first 3 to 6 months of probenecid or sulfinpyrazone therapy.

probenecid (Benemid). Used to treat chronic gouty arthritis and tophaceous gout, probenecid also is used to treat hyperuricemia secondary to thiazide diuretic use.
Usual adult dosage: 250 mg P.O. b.i.d. during the first week of therapy; then the dosage is increased to 500 mg b.i.d. If symptoms are not controlled, the dosage can be increased by 500 mg every 4 weeks, up to 2 grams daily. After 6 months of therapy, if no gouty attacks occur and the serum uric acid level falls within normal limits, the daily dosage may be decreased by 500 mg every 6 months.

sulfinpyrazone (Anturane). Used to treat chronic gouty arthritis, sulfinpyrazone also is used to treat tophaceous gout and hyperuricemia secondary to thiazide diuretic therapy.
Usual adult dosage: 100 to 200 mg P.O. b.i.d. during the first week of therapy; after the first week, the dosage is increased gradually until the full maintenance dosage of 200 to 400 mg b.i.d. is reached. The maximum dosage is 800 mg/day in divided doses.

Drug interactions
Numerous drugs interact with uricosurics. Although some of these interactions can be potentially harmful, others can prove beneficial. For example, probenecid elevates and prolongs the plasma level of penicillin. Although not used commonly, this dual therapy is indicated primarily to treat patients with sexually transmitted diseases requiring high plasma and tissue concentrations of the antibiotic. (For more information, see *Drug interactions: Uricosurics,* page 984.)

Uricosurics also may interact with Clinitest, a reactive agent used to test for urine glucose. This interaction produces a false-positive test result.

Interactions between uricosurics and food do not seem to present problems. In fact, the patient should take uricosurics with meals, milk, or antacids to prevent adverse GI reactions.

ADVERSE DRUG REACTIONS

Although the uricosurics usually are tolerated well, some adverse reactions can occur. Probenecid, which commonly is considered the preferred drug of the two uricosurics, produces less severe adverse GI and hematologic reactions than sulfinpyrazone. On the other hand, sulfinpyrazone produces fewer rashes and hypersensitivity reactions. If a patient is refractory to one uricosuric drug or cannot tolerate its adverse effects, the other drug can be used effectively.

When given in therapeutic dosages, probenecid usually is tolerated well by patients. Its most frequent adverse ef-

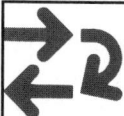

DRUG INTERACTIONS

Uricosurics

Some drug interactions involving the uricosurics represent potentially serious complications for the patient.

DRUG	INTERACTING DRUGS	POSSIBLE EFFECTS	NURSING IMPLICATIONS
probenecid	weak organic acid antibiotics	Increases the plasma level of the antibiotic	• Monitor the patient's serum antibiotic level as prescribed.
	salicylates	May antagonize the action of probenecid	• Explain to the patient that prolonged use of salicylates is contraindicated. • Administer acetaminophen as prescribed if an analgesic or antipyretic is needed.
	antineoplastic drugs	May increase the serum urate level	• Do not administer these drugs together.
	dapsone	Increases the serum dapsone level	• Monitor the patient's hemoglobin level and hematocrit. • Observe for signs of methemoglobinemia, such as cyanosis and shortness of breath. • Monitor the patient for peripheral neuropathy (pain or change in sensation in extremities). • Reduce the dapsone dosage, if prescribed.
	dyphylline	Increases the serum dyphylline level	• Monitor for signs and symptoms of theophylline toxicity, such as nausea, tachycardia, and nervousness. • Monitor the patient's serum theophylline level as prescribed. • Administer theophylline instead of dyphylline, if prescribed.
	ketoprofen	Increases the serum ketoprofen level	• Monitor for signs and symptoms of ketoprofen excess, such as nausea, abdominal pain, dizziness, drowsiness, headache, tinnitis, and impaired renal function. • Decrease the ketoprofen dosage, if prescribed.
	methotrexate	Increases the serum methotrexate level by inhibiting the drug's elimination	• Monitor for signs and symptoms of methotrexate toxicity, such as stomatitis, bone marrow suppression, and fatigue. • Decrease the methotrexate dosage, if prescribed.
sulfinpyrazone	warfarin	Increases hypoprothrombinemic response to warfarin as exhibited by increased prothrombin time (PT); increases risk of bleeding	• Monitor the patient's PT when beginning or discontinuing therapy with either drug. • Teach the patient the signs and symptoms of bleeding, such as epistaxis, hematuria, and easy bruising. • Monitor for changes in the patient's red blood cells, hemoglobin level, and hematocrit. • Assess for blood in the patient's urine, feces, and vomitus.
	salicylates	Inhibit the uricosuric effect of sulfinpyrazone	• Avoid the concomitant use of salicylates during uricosuric therapy.

fects are headache and GI distress, including anorexia, nausea, and vomiting. Other adverse reactions include flushing, dizziness, urinary frequency, sore gums, and anemia.

When given in therapeutic dosages, sulfinpyrazone usually is tolerated well. Nausea, dyspepsia, GI pain, and GI blood loss are the most commonly reported adverse reactions to sulfinpyrazone. Reactivation or aggravation of peptic ulcer disease also can occur. Other adverse reactions include dizziness, rash, vertigo, tinnitus, and edema. Blood dyscrasias, such as anemia, leukopenia, granulocytopenia, and thrombocytopenia, are reported, but rarely.

Some patients taking probenecid or sulfinpyrazone may form uric acid calculi. This usually occurs upon initiation of therapy. Acute gouty attacks also can occur in some patients during the first 6 to 12 months of therapy.

Hypersensitivity reactions can occur in some patients taking probenecid. Signs and symptoms of such reactions may include dermatitis, pruritus, fever, sweating, or hypotension. Rarely, a patient may experience an anaphylactic reaction, nephrotic syndrome, hepatic necrosis, or aplastic anemia. In some patients, discontinuation of sulfinpyrazone therapy has reversed renal dysfunction.

NURSING PROCESS APPLICATION

The following information assists the nurse in caring for a patient receiving a uricosuric.

Assessment
• Review the patient's history for a preexisting condition that contraindicates the use of a uricosuric, such as known hypersensitivity to the drug, blood dyscrasia, uric acid renal calculi, or the use of penicillin in a patient with renal impairment.
• Review the patient's history for a preexisting condition that requires cautious use of a uricosuric, such as a history of peptic ulcer.
• Assess the patient for adverse reactions to the prescribed uricosuric, such as hypersensitivity, GI, and hematologic reactions.
• Review the patient's medication history to identify the use of drugs that may interact with the prescribed uricosuric, such as penicillin, salicylates, or oral anticoagulants.
• Assess the effectiveness of the prescribed uricosuric periodically.
• Assess the patient's fluid balance if adverse GI reactions occur.
• Evaluate the patient's and family's knowledge about the prescribed uricosuric.

Nursing diagnoses
The following examples represent appropriate nursing diagnoses for a patient receiving a uricosuric.
• Potential for injury related to a preexisting condition that contraindicates the use of a uricosuric
• Potential for injury related to a preexisting condition that requires cautious use of a uricosuric agent
• Potential for injury related to adverse drug reactions
• Potential fluid volume deficit related to the adverse GI effects of the prescribed uricosuric
• Knowledge deficit related to the prescribed uricosuric

Planning and implementation
• Do not administer a uricosuric to a patient with a condition that contraindicates its use.
• Administer a uricosuric cautiously to a patient at risk because of a preexisting condition.
• Monitor the patient frequently for adverse reactions during uricosuric therapy.
• *Observe the patient closely for hypersensitivity reactions to probenecid, such as dermatitis, pruritus, fever, sweating, or hypotension. Keep standard emergency equipment nearby because anaphylaxis can occur.*
• Monitor appropriate laboratory values, including a complete blood count (CBC), urinalysis, and serum uric acid level. Monitor renal function tests and blood urea nitrogen regularly.
• Obtain a prescription for a mild analgesic, such as acetaminophen, if probenecid causes headaches. Avoid salicylate administration because it may prolong bleeding time.
• *Take safety precautions if the patient experiences dizziness or vertigo. For example, place the bed in the lowest position, keep the bed rails raised, and supervise ambulation.*
• Provide a soft diet if the patient develops sore gums from probenecid use.
• Stagger activities and provide frequent rest periods if the patient develops anemia.
• Place a bedpan or urinal within easy reach if probenecid causes frequent urination in a patient who requires assistance to the bathroom.
• Monitor the patient for signs of edema, such as ankle swelling, jugular vein distention, or crackles in the lungs.
• *Notify the physician if the patient has an acute gouty attack. Discuss temporary discontinuation of the uricosuric, because it may prolong inflammation in an acute gouty attack.*
• Administer colchicine, if prescribed, with the uricosuric to help prevent an acute attack of gouty arthritis, which can occur at the start of uricosuric therapy.
• Encourage the patient to drink between ten and twelve 8-oz (240-ml) glasses of water daily, unless contraindicated. Maintaining a high fluid intake minimizes calculus formation.

• Encourage the patient to ingest a high-vegetable diet to alkalinize the urine. Maintaining alkaline urine decreases the formation of uric acid calculi.

• Notify the physician if adverse reactions occur.

• Monitor hydration if the patient experiences adverse GI reactions, such as anorexia, nausea, or vomiting. Obtain a prescription for an antiemetic agent, as needed.

• Notify the physician if the patient cannot tolerate oral therapy.

• Administer the drug with food, milk, or an antacid to prevent GI distress, the most common adverse reaction to uricosurics.

Patient teaching

• Teach the patient and family the name, dose, frequency, action, and adverse effects of the prescribed uricosuric.

• *Instruct the patient to take the drug exactly as prescribed and not to stop the drug without consulting the physician because gout symptoms may reappear.*

• Advise the patient to notify the physician if GI distress persists.

• *Instruct the patient not to take aspirin during uricosuric therapy. If an analgesic or antipyretic is needed, the patient should take acetaminophen.*

• *Ensure that the patient understands that the uricosuric should not be taken during an acute attack of gout.* Explain that taking the drug at that time will prolong the inflammation and will not relieve the acute symptoms. Inform the patient that the drug usually is not started until 2 to 3 weeks after an acute attack.

• *Alert the diabetic patient who tests urine with Clinitest of the possibility of false-positive test results. Recommend that the patient use Clinistix or another urine glucose testing product.*

• *Advise the patient not to perform activities that require mental alertness if dizziness or vertigo occurs.*

• Emphasize the importance of having laboratory studies performed regularly as prescribed.

• Instruct the patient to notify the physician if adverse reactions occur.

Evaluation

The following examples represent appropriate evaluation statements for a patient receiving a uricosuric.

• The patient has no conditions that contraindicate uricosuric therapy.

• The patient exhibits no signs of complications in the preexisting condition linked to the prescribed uricosuric.

• The patient experiences no adverse reactions to the prescribed uricosuric.

• The patient maintains normal fluid balance during uricosuric therapy.

• The patient and family express an accurate understanding of the points taught about the prescribed uricosuric.

• The patient self-administers the prescribed uricosuric with meals, milk, or an antacid.

OTHER ANTIGOUT AGENTS

Two other drugs, allopurinol and colchicine, commonly are prescribed to treat gout. Allopurinol is used to inhibit uric acid synthesis, thereby reducing the metabolic pool of uric acid in the body and preventing gouty attacks. Colchicine has a relatively specific use: to treat acute gouty attacks.

PHARMACOKINETICS

After oral administration, allopurinol and colchicine are absorbed and metabolized in the liver. Allopurinol is excreted primarily in the urine; colchicine, in the feces.

Absorption, distribution, metabolism, excretion

Allopurinol is absorbed rapidly from the GI tract after oral administration and is metabolized in the liver. The drug and its inactive metabolite alloxanthine are distributed throughout the tissue fluid, with the exception of the brain, where its concentration is about one-third of that found in other tissues. Allopurinol is cleared rapidly from plasma, with small amounts excreted unchanged in the urine within 6 hours of ingestion. Small amounts also are excreted unabsorbed in the feces. Most of the drug, however, is excreted slowly in the urine as the metabolite alloxanthine.

After oral administration, colchicine is absorbed from the GI tract and then partially metabolized in the liver. The drug and its metabolites then reenter the intestinal tract via biliary secretions. After resorption from the intestines, colchicine is distributed to various tissues throughout the body, including the kidneys, liver, spleen, and intestinal tract. The highest concentration of colchicine, however, can be found in leukocytes. The drug is excreted primarily in the feces and to a lesser degree in the urine.

Onset, peak, duration

Allopurinol appears in plasma 30 to 60 minutes after oral administration. Its metabolite, alloxanthine, reaches a peak concentration level in 2 to 6 hours, with a duration of 2 to 3 days. At that time, serum and urine uric acid levels begin to fall. The half-life of allopurinol is 2 to 3 hours, during which time the drug is converted to alloxanthine. Alloxanthine, however, has a plasma half-life of 18 to 30 hours. The long half-life of alloxanthine contributes significantly to inhibition of xanthine oxidase, the enzyme responsible

Sites of allopurinol action

This diagram depicts allopurinol's mechanism of action. Alloxanthine, the primary metabolite, inhibits the enzyme xanthine oxidase, which converts hypoxanthine to xanthine and then acts on xanthine to form uric acid. By blocking xanthine oxidase, alloxanthine inhibits uric acid production.

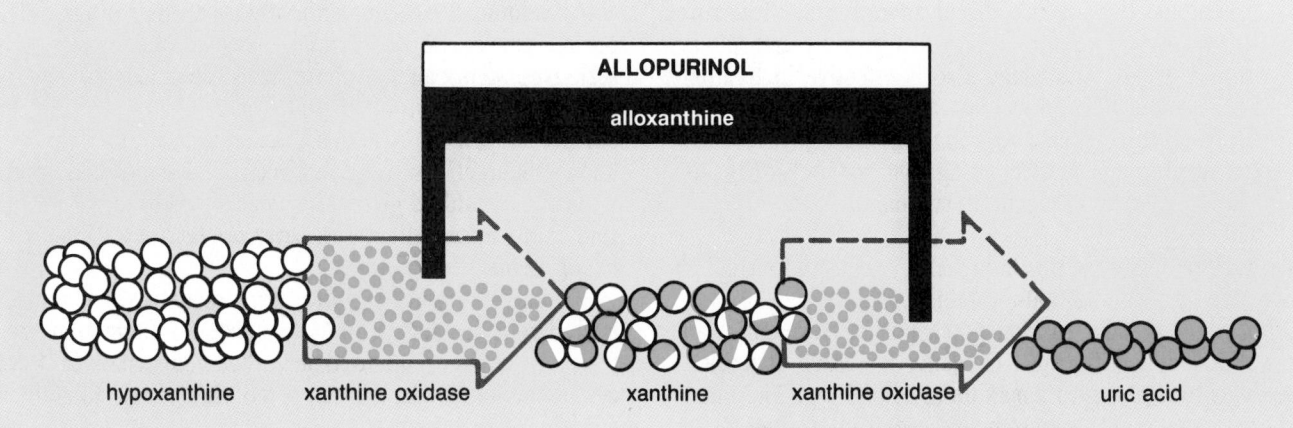

for converting hypoxanthine to xanthine as well as xanthine to uric acid.

Colchicine rapidly achieves a peak concentration in the plasma within ½ to 2 hours. The pain that accompanies an acute gouty attack is relieved 12 to 48 hours after oral administration and 4 to 12 hours after I.V. therapy. The duration of action for colchicine varies, as the plasma concentration declines 1 to 2 hours after ingestion and then rises as the drug recycles. After I.V. administration, the half-life of colchicine is 20 minutes. In leukocytes, however, where the highest concentration of colchicine exists, the half-life is 60 hours.

PHARMACODYNAMICS

Allopurinol lowers serum and urine uric acid levels in the treatment of primary gout. Allopurinol and its primary metabolite alloxanthine inhibit xanthine oxidase, which contributes to the pharmacologic effectiveness of allopurinol. (For more information, see *Sites of allopurinol action*.)

The mechanism of action of allopurinol is understood much better than that of colchicine, although colchicine has been in use longer. Colchicine, however, appears to reduce the inflammatory response to monosodium urate crystals deposited in joint tissues. Colchicine may produce its effects by interfering with the polymorphonuclear leukocyte activity that results when metabolism, mobility, chemotaxis, or other leukocyte functions become inhibited.

PHARMACOTHERAPEUTICS

Allopurinol is used to treat primary gout and gout associated with blood dyscrasias and related therapy. This drug is recommended for primary or secondary uric acid nephropathy, with or without the accompanying symptoms of gout, and for patients with recurrent uric acid calculus formation. Allopurinol also proves effective in patients who respond poorly to maximum dosages of uricosuric agents or who have allergic reactions or intolerance to uricosuric drugs. Allopurinol is useful in preventing hyperuricemia in patients who are receiving cancer chemotherapy for myeloproliferative disorders. It also is effective when given with uricosurics, where smaller dosages of each drug are used.

Allopurinol is the drug of choice for patients at risk for renal calculi, such as those who have renal disease or who excrete excessive uric acid in the urine. By reducing urinary uric acid formation, allopurinol eliminates the hazards of hyperuricuria.

The major disadvantage of using allopurinol is the acute attack of gouty arthritis that may occur initially. To prevent such attacks, concurrent use of colchicine may be prescribed.

Colchicine is used to relieve acute attacks of gouty arthritis. When initiated early enough and in adequate amounts, the drug proves especially effective in relieving the pain. Colchicine also is recommended for prevention of recurrent gouty arthritis. Also, colchicine administered during the first several months of allopurinol, probenecid, or sulfinpyrazone therapy may prevent the acute gouty attacks that sometimes accompany the use of these drugs.

Colchicine can be especially valuable in diagnosing gouty arthritis. When a small joint is involved, synovial fluid is unavailable for examination. If the condition is from gouty arthritis, therapeutic response occurs within 48 hours after oral administration of colchicine and within 12 hours after I.V. injection. This consistent response to colchicine occurs only with gouty arthritis.

Colchicine therapy has its advantages and disadvantages. The use of the drug in diagnosing gouty arthritis is of primary value. Colchicine also is effective in treating crystalline-induced arthropathies. Unfortunately, the drug produces several adverse reactions, especially in the GI tract. Colchicine is ineffective against nongouty arthritis and does not affect uric acid metabolism.

allopurinol (Zyloprim). Administered orally, allopurinol is available in 100- and 300-mg tablets.
Usual adult dosage: to treat gout and hyperuricemia, an initial dosage of 100 mg P.O. daily; increased at weekly intervals by 100 mg to a maximum of 800 mg. The maximum dosage never should be exceeded in an attempt to reach a normal serum uric acid level of 6 mg/dl or less. Daily dosages that exceed 300 mg should be given in divided doses.

Patients with renal failure require dosage adjustments. To estimate these adjustments, a serum creatinine level and a 12- or 24-hour urine creatinine level should be obtained to calculate a creatinine clearance. With a creatinine clearance of 10 to 20 ml/minute, the daily dosage is 200 mg. When the creatinine clearance is 3 to 10 ml/minute, the dosage is 100 mg. When renal impairment is severe, as indicated by a creatinine clearance of less than 3 ml/minute, the dosage schedule may need to be lengthened.

colchicine. Administered orally and intravenously, colchicine is used to treat acute attacks of gouty arthritis.
Usual adult dosage: for acute gouty arthritis, starting dose of 1 to 1.2 mg P.O.; followed by 0.5 to 0.6 mg every hour, or 1 to 1.2 mg every 2 hours until pain ceases or until nausea, vomiting, or diarrhea ensues. The total oral dosage in a course of therapy for acute gouty arthritis may range from 4 to 8 mg. Given I.V., the initial dose is 2 mg, followed by 0.5 mg every 6 hours until a satisfactory response is achieved. The daily dosage of I.V. colchicine should not exceed 4 mg.

As prophylactic or maintenance therapy for acute attacks of gout, the amount prescribed depends on the number of attacks a patient has. For a patient with fewer than one attack per year, the usual oral dosage is 0.5 to 0.6 mg one to four times a week; in a patient who has more than one attack per year, 0.5 to 0.6 mg/day. Some patients, however, may need up to 1.5 to 1.8 mg/day to achieve the benefit of prophylactic therapy. For I.V. prophylaxis, 0.5 to 1 mg

is given once or twice daily. However, oral administration is preferred.

To prevent an attack of gout in a patient with gouty arthritis who is undergoing surgery, the dosage is 0.5 to 0.6 mg P.O. t.i.d. for 3 days before and after surgery.

Drug interactions
When administered concomitantly with other drugs, allopurinol can create interactions that can affect the patient seriously. Anticoagulants, iron salts, angiotensin-converting enzyme inhibitors, theophylline, and certain cancer chemotherapeutic drugs can interact with allopurinol. No known interactions occur between allopurinol and food. The drug should be given after meals to prevent GI upset. (For more information, see *Drug interactions: Other antigout agents.*)

No drugs produce significant interactions when administered concomitantly with colchicine. No interactions between colchicine and food have been reported. In fact, colchicine should be administered with meals to reduce adverse GI reactions.

ADVERSE DRUG REACTIONS

The most common reaction to allopurinol is a skin rash, which usually is maculopapular. Adverse GI reactions include nausea, vomiting, diarrhea, and intermittent abdominal pain. Less common reactions include those that cause hematopoietic changes, such as granulocytopenia, anemia, aplastic anemia, and bone marrow depression. However, these reactions usually result from concomitant use of allopurinol and any drug known to cause such reactions. Peripheral neuritis and drowsiness also can occur. Rare instances of sensitivity reactions, such as alopecia and altered liver function test results, have occurred during allopurinol therapy.

The most common adverse reactions to orally administered colchicine include nausea, vomiting, abdominal discomfort, and diarrhea. These reactions usually occur with dosages used to achieve a therapeutic level of colchicine. However, they also indicate drug toxicity, and the colchicine should be discontinued. Therapy can be resumed after the symptoms have disappeared, usually within 24 to 48 hours. GI symptoms also can occur when colchicine is administered I.V., but these adverse reactions usually occur only when the recommended dosage is exceeded.

Other adverse reactions involving colchicine primarily affect the skin, vascular system, and central nervous system (CNS). The most common skin problems include dermatitis, urticaria, and alopecia. Prolonged administration may cause bone marrow depression and related hematologic problems, such as aplastic anemia, granulocytopenia, leukopenia, and thrombocytopenia. The only adverse CNS reaction is peripheral neuritis. Rare adverse reactions in-

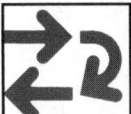

DRUG INTERACTIONS

Other antigout agents

When given with other drugs, allopurinol may cause interactions that affect the patient adversely. The nurse should exercise caution and monitor the patient closely.

DRUG	INTERACTING DRUGS	POSSIBLE EFFECTS	NURSING IMPLICATIONS
allopurinol	oral anticoagulants	May inhibit the metabolism of the anticoagulants, leading to a prolonged anticoagulant half-life	• Monitor the patient's prothrombin time. • Teach the patient the signs and symptoms of bleeding, such as spontaneous epistaxis, hematuria, and easy bruising. • Monitor the patient's urine, feces, and emesis for blood.
	mercaptopurine, azathioprine	Increases the antimetabolite effect of these drugs	• Expect to reduce the drug dosages as prescribed. • Monitor the patient for signs and symptoms of toxicity, such as additive bone marrow suppression and fatigue.
	angiotensin-converting enzyme inhibitors	Increase the risk of hypersensitivity reactions to allopurinol	• Monitor the patient for rash, fever, and arthralgia. • Avoid concomitant use of these drugs.
	theophylline	Increases the theophylline level	• Monitor the patient for signs and symptoms of theophylline toxicity, such as nervousness, nausea, and tachycardia. • Monitor the patient's theophylline blood level.

clude renal damage, muscle weakness, reversible azoospermia, and an increased serum level of alkaline phosphatase.

Although colchicine produces few hypersensitivity reactions, some have been reported. These include bladder spasms, paralytic ileus, stomatitis, hypothyroidism, and nonthrombocytopenic purpura. Fever, chills, leukopenia, eosinophilia, arthralgia, skin rash, and pruritus also may be present.

NURSING PROCESS APPLICATION

The following information assists the nurse in caring for a patient receiving an antigout agent.

Assessment
• Review the patient's history for a preexisting condition that contraindicates the use of an antigout agent, such as pregnancy, known hypersensitivity to the drug, or serious GI, renal, hepatic, or cardiac disease.
• Review the patient's history for a preexisting condition that requires cautious use of an antigout agent, such as lactation, advanced age, debilitation, or impaired renal function.
• Assess the patient for adverse reactions to the prescribed antigout agent, such as GI, dermatologic, and hypersensitivity reactions.

• Review the patient's medication history to identify the use of drugs that may interact with allopurinol, such as oral anticoagulants, mercaptopurine, azathioprine, angiotensin-converting enzyme inhibitors, or theophylline.
• Assess the effectiveness of the prescribed antigout agent periodically.
• Assess the patient for signs of fluid volume deficit, such as decreased blood pressure and dry mucous membranes, if adverse GI reactions occur.
• Evaluate the patient's and family's knowledge about the prescribed antigout agent.

Nursing diagnoses
The following examples represent appropriate nursing diagnoses for a patient receiving an antigout agent.
• Potential for injury related to a preexisting condition that contraindicates the use of an antigout agent
• Potential for injury related to a preexisting condition that requires cautious use of an antigout agent
• Potential for injury related to adverse drug reactions
• Potential fluid volume deficit related to the adverse GI effects of the prescribed antigout agent
• Knowledge deficit related to the prescribed antigout agent

Planning and implementation

• Do not administer an antigout agent to a patient with a condition that contraindicates its use.

• Administer an antigout agent cautiously to a patient at risk because of a preexisting condition.

• Monitor the patient closely for adverse reactions during antigout therapy.

• Monitor CBC, urinalysis, serum uric acid level, and liver and kidney function test results before and periodically during antigout therapy as instructed.

• *Inspect the patient's skin for adverse dermatologic reactions to allopurinol, such as a maculopapular rash, or to colchicine, such as dermatitis, urticaria, or alopecia. If the patient develops a rash, expect to discontinue allopurinol.*

• Monitor the patient for signs and symptoms of peripheral neuritis, such as pain or changes in sensation in the extremities.

• *Auscultate the patient's bowel sounds regularly during colchicine therapy to detect paralytic ileus.*

• Inspect the patient's mouth regularly during colchicine therapy for signs and symptoms of stomatitis, such as painful, bleeding ulcers. If stomatitis occurs, consult the physician to obtain a prescription for a topical anesthetic or other medication for symptomatic relief and to discuss placing the patient on a soft or pureed diet.

• Obtain a prescription for an antispasmodic agent if bladder spasms occur during colchicine therapy.

• Monitor the patient's vital signs regularly, particularly noting any signs of hypothyroidism, such as decreased temperature, pulse, respirations, or blood pressure.

• *Take safety measures if the patient experiences drowsiness during allopurinol therapy. For example, place the bed in the lowest position, keep the bed rails up, and supervise ambulation.*

• Administer allopurinol in divided doses as prescribed if the dosage exceeds 300 mg daily.

• Expect to adjust the allopurinol dosage as prescribed, based on a serum creatinine level and a 12 or 24 hour urine creatinine level for a patient with renal failure.

• *Do not give more than 4 mg/ml of colchicine I.V. during a 24-hour period. Parenteral colchicine is available in a strength of 0.5 mg/ml given I.V. by diluting the drug with normal saline solution.*

• *Prevent extravasation of colchicine into surrounding tissues during I.V. administration. During I.V. administration, properly position the needle in the vein and check for good blood return before injecting the drug. If extravasation occurs, apply heat or cold to relieve the discomfort and notify the physician. Analgesics also may be given.*

• *Do not give more than 12 tablets of oral colchicine for any single acute attack in a 24-hour period.*

• Notify the physician if adverse reactions occur.

• Monitor hydration if the patient experiences adverse GI reactions, such as nausea, vomiting, or diarrhea. Notify the physician and obtain a prescription for an antiemetic or antidiarrheal agent, as needed. Expect to discontinue colchicine until GI distress has subsided.

• Administer allopurinol after meals; oral colchicine with food or milk, to decrease GI distress.

• Inform the physician of the GI effects of the prescribed agent on the patient.

Patient teaching

• Teach the patient and family the name, dose, frequency, action, and adverse effects of the prescribed antigout agent.

• *Instruct the patient to keep colchicine readily available so that it can be taken as soon as symptoms of an acute gouty attack occur. Explain that a delay in taking the drug can impair its effectiveness.*

• Advise the patient to discontinue colchicine if nausea, vomiting, or diarrhea occurs and to notify the physician.

• *Instruct the patient to discontinue allopurinol and to notify the physician at the first sign of a skin rash because this reaction may precede a severe hypersensitivity reaction.*

• Instruct the patient to store allopurinol or colchicine in a tightly closed, light-resistant container.

• *Advise the patient to exercise caution when engaging in activities that require alertness because allopurinol can cause drowsiness.*

• Instruct the patient to notify the physician if adverse reactions occur.

Evaluation

The following examples represent appropriate evaluation statements for a patient receiving an antigout agent.

• The patient has no conditions that contraindicate antigout therapy.

• The patient exhibits no signs of complications in the preexisting condition linked to antigout therapy.

• The patient experiences no adverse reactions to the prescribed antigout agent.

• The patient maintains adequate hydration throughout antigout therapy.

• The patient and family express an accurate understanding of the points taught about the prescribed antigout agent.

• The patient keeps colchicine readily available and takes it as soon as symptoms of an acute gouty attack occur.

GOLD SALTS

Gold salts are administered orally and parenterally, primarily to treat rheumatoid arthritis. The oral gold salt is auranofin, and the parenteral forms are aurothioglucose and gold sodium thiomalate.

PHARMACOKINETICS

The pharmacokinetics of gold salts vary with the route of administration.

Absorption, distribution, metabolism, excretion

Absorption of auranofin takes place in the GI tract. Approximately 20% to 25% of auranofin is absorbed after an oral dose. Distribution of auranofin is related primarily to its binding with erythrocytes. Within an erythrocyte, 90% of auranofin is distributed intracellularly; the remaining 10% is membrane bound. The metabolic fate of auranofin is not understood completely. About 60% of the absorbed auranofin is excreted in the urine, with the remainder excreted in the feces. The unabsorbed auranofin is excreted primarily in the feces.

The parenteral gold salts aurothioglucose and gold sodium thiomalate differ in their ability to be absorbed. Aurothioglucose is absorbed more slowly and irregularly; gold sodium thiomalate, rapidly after I.M. administration. The parenteral gold salts are distributed throughout the body, with concentrations occurring in the kidneys, liver, spleen, bone marrow, and the reticuloendothelial cells of the lymph nodes. The metabolic fate of the parenteral gold salts remains obscure. They are excreted slowly from the body, with about 70% excreted in the urine and the remainder in the feces.

Onset, peak, duration

Gold salts exhibit a slow onset of action. Benefits usually occur about 8 to 12 weeks after the initiation of therapy, but may not occur for 6 months or longer in some patients. Peak serum concentration levels, however, are found within a couple of hours of administration.

The duration of action of gold salts increases with each dose. The half-life changes dramatically depending on the administration route. After 6 months of daily oral therapy, auranofin has a half-life ranging from 26 to 81 days. Parenteral gold salts have a half-life of 14 to 40 days after only 3 weeks of weekly injections. After the eleventh weekly dose of a parenteral gold salt, the half-life increases to 168 days.

PHARMACODYNAMICS

The complexity of the disease and the pharmacologic effects of gold salts makes understanding the mechanism of action of these drugs difficult. They may act by decreasing liposomal enzyme release and altering the immune response.

Like the uricosurics, gold salts do not provide a direct analgesic action. Pain relief occurs from the anti-inflammatory and antiarthritic effects they provide.

PHARMACOTHERAPEUTICS

Gold salts are one of a group of drugs referred to by rheumatologists as *remittive agents* — drugs that may block the inflammatory disease process rather than provide anti-inflammatory action and pain relief only.

Gold salts are prescribed only for patients who have an established diagnosis of rheumatoid arthritis and display an insufficient therapeutic response to an adequate trial of one or more nonsteroidal anti-inflammatory drugs (NSAIDs). NSAIDs are used primarily to decrease the number of painful, tender, swollen joints, to shorten the duration of morning stiffness, and to improve grip strength. Nondrug therapies, such as physical therapy, always accompany the use of gold salts.

Using gold salts to treat rheumatoid arthritis has advantages and disadvantages. When effective, these drugs can have dramatic effects. By slowing the progress of joint destruction, gold salts effectively can decrease the signs and symptoms that accompany rheumatoid arthritis. On the other hand, gold salts can be toxic — the primary reason why they are prescribed only after other treatments have failed.

A major benefit of auranofin is its oral administration. Auranofin also produces fewer toxic effects than parenteral gold. As a result, substantially fewer patients withdraw from therapy because of adverse reactions. Unfortunately, auranofin therapy usually proves slightly less effective than parenteral gold therapy, and the drug is likely to be discontinued because of the patient's poor or inadequate response.

Parenteral gold therapy is slightly more effective than auranofin, and fewer patients discontinue treatment because of poor therapeutic response. Parenteral gold also produces its therapeutic effects sooner and with more pronounced results than does oral gold. As a result, parenteral gold therapy is preferred to treat rheumatoid arthritis. It also is preferred in patients with severe or rapidly progressing arthritis and in patients for whom compliance with the daily dosing regimen presents problems. The numerous, severe adverse effects of parenteral gold represent the major disadvantage of this therapy. The patient also must make frequent office visits, which can be costly, to receive the parenteral administration of the drug. Because of the slow therapeutic response to gold salts, concomitant use of an NSAID or salicylate usually is prescribed until the patient begins to experience symptomatic relief. If cartilage and bone destruction also have occurred, gold salts cannot reverse the structural damage to the joints.

auranofin (Ridaura). Available in a 3-mg capsule, auranofin is used to treat active synovitis associated with classical or definite rheumatoid arthritis. Auranofin usually is given concomitantly with an NSAID.
Usual adult dosage: 6 mg P.O. daily as a single dose or in two divided doses. If adverse GI reactions occur, the dosage is reduced to 3 mg daily. If the patient's response is inadequate, the dosage is increased to 9 mg P.O. daily (3 mg t.i.d.). If the response remains inadequate after 3 months of 9 mg/day, therapy is discontinued.

aurothioglucose (Solganal). The oil-based form of injectable gold, aurothioglucose is available in a suspension of 50 mg/ml. Parenteral gold salts are administered initially at weekly intervals. During the first week, an initial test dose of 10 mg is given.
Usual adult dosage: initial test dose of 10 mg I.M. followed in the second and third weeks by a dose of 25 mg I.M.; thereafter, weekly injections of 50 mg I.M. until 0.8 to 1 gram has been administered. Therapy must be reevaluated when the patient has received 1 gram of parenteral gold salt. If the patient shows signs of improvement without any toxic effects with 25- to 50-mg injections every third or fourth week, therapy continues indefinitely. If the patient shows no clinical improvement after receiving the initial 1-gram dosage, therapy is discontinued.

gold sodium thiomalate (Myochrysine). The water-based form of injectable gold, gold sodium thiomalate is available in doses of 10, 25, and 50 mg/ml. The drug is administered initially at weekly intervals. During the first week, an initial test dose of 10 mg I.M. is given.
Usual adult dosage: initial dose of 10 mg followed in the second and third weeks by a dose of 25 mg I.M.; thereafter, weekly injections of 50 mg I.M. until 1 gram has been administered. The therapy is reevaluated when the patient has received 1 gram I.M. of parenteral gold salt. If the patient experiences a favorable response, continued maintenance therapy at 25 to 50 mg I.M. every 2 weeks for 2 to 20 weeks begins. Thereafter, if the patient's clinical course remains stable, injections of 25 to 50 mg I.M. are given every third to fourth week indefinitely. If the patient shows no clinical improvement after receiving the initial 1-gram dosage, therapy is discontinued.

Drug interactions
Gold salts produce no significant drug interactions.

ADVERSE DRUG REACTIONS

The numerous adverse reactions to gold salts explain why these drugs are not the first choice for treating rheumatoid arthritis.

Most adverse drug reactions involving the gold salts occur during the first 6 months of therapy. However, reactions can occur at any time, and the nurse continually should monitor the patient on maintenance therapy for reactions.

The most common adverse reactions to auranofin involve the GI system. More than 50% of patients taking auranofin experience diarrhea. Nausea, vomiting, anorexia, abdominal cramps, and flatulence also occur but less frequently. Ulcerative enterocolitis is a rare but serious adverse reaction.

Patients on oral gold therapy also experience mucocutaneous reactions. A rash, commonly preceded by pruritus, occurs in about 25% of patients taking auranofin. Other mucocutaneous reactions include conjunctivitis, glossitis, and stomatitis. Stomatitis occurs in about 13% of patients and produces shallow ulcers on the buccal membranes, palate, pharynx, and borders of the tongue. Alopecia, a dermatologic reaction, also can occur with gold salt therapy.

Other, less common, adverse reactions to auranofin involve the renal and hematologic systems. Renal effects include nephrotic syndrome and glomerulonephritis with proteinuria and hematuria. Blood dyscrasias, including leukopenia, thrombocytopenia, and anemia, have occurred.

Most adverse reactions to parenteral gold therapy occur during the second or third month of treatment after a total of 250 to 500 mg of the drug has been given. An estimated 25% to 30% of patients receiving parenteral gold discontinue therapy because of adverse reactions.

The most common adverse reactions involve mucocutaneous conditions, including stomatitis, gingivitis, glossitis, pharyngitis, tracheitis, and vaginitis. Parenteral gold salts also can produce severe blood dyscrasias, as well as renal and hepatic damage, which warrant immediate attention. Adverse GI reactions rarely develop.

Most hypersensitivity reactions seem to occur with the parenteral gold salts. Up to 5% of patients receiving gold sodium thiomalate experience a vasomotor reaction, commonly called the nitritoid reaction. This reaction is characterized by flushing, dizziness, nausea, weakness, tachycardia, and syncope. Having the patient lie down can alleviate the nitritoid reaction; then the patient should be changed to aurothioglucose.

Rare incidents of anaphylactic shock, syncope, bradycardia, difficulty swallowing, and angioedema have occurred with injectable gold. These reactions usually occur immediately or within 10 minutes of injection.

NURSING PROCESS APPLICATION

The following information assists the nurse in caring for a patient receiving a gold salt.

Assessment

• Review the patient's history for a preexisting condition that contraindicates the use of a gold salt, such as known hypersensitivity to the drug, a history of a gold-induced disorder, uncontrolled diabetes mellitus, severe debilitation, or systemic lupus erythematosus.

• Review the patient's history for a preexisting condition that requires cautious use of a gold salt, such as GI dysfunction or compromised cardiovascular or cerebral circulation.

• Assess the patient for adverse reactions to the prescribed gold salt, such as GI, mucocutaneous, or vasomotor disturbances.

• Assess the effectiveness of the prescribed gold salt periodically.

• Assess the patient's bowel status regularly.

• Assess the patient's compliance with oral gold salt therapy.

• Evaluate the patient's and family's knowledge about the prescribed gold salt.

Nursing diagnoses

The following examples represent appropriate nursing diagnoses for a patient receiving a gold salt.

• Potential for injury related to a preexisting condition that contraindicates the use of a gold salt

• Potential for injury related to a preexisting condition that requires cautious use of a gold salt

• Potential for injury related to adverse drug reactions

• Diarrhea related to the adverse GI effects of auranofin

• Noncompliance related to long-term use and adverse effects of auranofin

• Knowledge deficit related to the prescribed gold salt

Planning and implementation

• Do not administer a gold salt to a patient with a condition that contraindicates its use.

• Administer a gold salt cautiously to a patient at risk because of a preexisting condition.

• Monitor the patient closely for adverse reactions, especially during the first 6 months of therapy.

• Obtain a baseline urinalysis, CBC, and platelet count as instructed for later comparison with subsequent monthly laboratory values to assess the patient's response to therapy.

• *Assess the patient for anaphylactic shock, syncope, bradycardia, difficulty swallowing, and angioedema, which can occur up to 10 minutes after injection of a gold salt. Keep standard emergency equipment nearby.*

• *Monitor the patient for flushing, dizziness, nausea, weakness, tachycardia, and syncope during administration of gold sodium thiomalate. If such a vasomotor response occurs, have the patient lie down during and for 10 minutes after administration. Continue to observe the patient for adverse reactions for another 15 minutes. Expect to change the patient to aurothioglucose as prescribed if this response occurs.*

• Treat a patient's localized skin eruptions with topical corticosteroids as prescribed; more severe or generalized rashes may require oral antihistamines. Consider any skin eruption a reaction to the gold salt until proven otherwise.

• Inspect the patient's eyes for signs of conjunctivitis, such as redness, swelling, or discharge. Also inspect the mouth for evidence of glossitis or stomatitis, such as ulcerations and swollen, bleeding gums or tongue. Consult the physician to obtain appropriate symptomatic relief, as needed.

• Ensure that physical therapy accompanies gold salt therapy as prescribed to maximize the drug's beneficial effects. Schedule patient activities around the physical therapy sessions.

• *Administer auranofin orally; give aurothioglucose and gold sodium thiomalate I.M., preferably in the gluteal muscle.*

• Take special care to withdraw a uniform suspension of aurothioglucose from the vial because it is an oil-based suspension. To do this, immerse the vial in warm water and then remove the medication with a dry needle and syringe.

• Monitor for gold salt toxicity by asking the patient at each visit about any signs and symptoms that indicate an adverse reaction.

• *Ensure that the patient is reevaluated after receiving 1 gram of a parenteral gold salt.*

• Notify the physician if adverse reactions occur.

• Monitor hydration if the patient experiences diarrhea or other adverse GI effects, such as anorexia, nausea, or vomiting. If GI distress is present, notify the physician and obtain a prescription for an antidiarrheal or antiemetic agent, as needed.

• Expect to decrease the auranofin dosage, as prescribed, if adverse GI reactions occur. If auranofin is not tolerated at the reduced dosage, expect to change the patient to a parenteral gold salt.

• Question the patient regularly about compliance with auranofin therapy.

• Notify the physician if noncompliance occurs.

Patient teaching

• Teach the patient and family the name, dose, frequency, action, and adverse effects of the prescribed gold salt.

• Instruct the patient to report diarrhea that persists for more than 3 to 4 days or that interferes with normal daily activities.

SELECTED MAJOR DRUGS

Uricosurics, other antigout agents, and gold salts

The following chart lists the drugs most commonly used to treat gout and rheumatoid arthritis.

DRUG	MAJOR INDICATIONS	USUAL ADULT DOSAGES	CONTRAINDICATIONS AND PRECAUTIONS
Uricosurics			
probenecid	Chronic gouty arthritis and tophaceous gout	250 mg P.O. b.i.d. during the first week, then 500 mg b.i.d.; can be increased by 500 mg every 4 weeks until a maximum of 2 grams daily is achieved	• Know that probenecid is contraindicated in a patient with known hypersensitivity to the drug, blood dyscrasia, or uric acid renal calculi, or in one who takes penicillin and has renal impairment. • Administer with caution to a patient with a history of peptic ulcer.
Other antigout agents			
allopurinol	Gout and hyperuricemia	100 mg P.O. daily, increased at weekly intervals by 100 mg to a maximum of 800 mg	• Know that allopurinol is contraindicated in a patient with known hypersensitivity to the drug. • Administer with caution to a pregnant or lactating patient, one with impaired renal function, or one who takes a thiazide diuretic and has impaired renal function.
colchicine	Acute gouty arthritis	Starting dose of 1 to 1.2 mg P.O., then 0.5 to 0.6 mg every hour, or 1 to 1.2 mg every 2 hours; or 2 mg I.V. followed by 0.5 mg every 6 hours until a satisfactory response occurs	• Know that colchicine is contraindicated in a pregnant patient or one with a serious gastrointestinal (GI), renal, hepatic, or cardiac disease. • Administer with extreme caution to an elderly or debilitated patient. • Administer with caution to a lactating patient.
Gold salts			
auranofin	Rheumatoid arthritis	6 mg P.O. daily in single or divided doses	• Know that auranofin is contraindicated in a pregnant or lactating patient or one with a history of a gold-induced disorder, such as anaphylactic reaction, necrotizing enterocolitis, pulmonary fibrosis, exfoliative dermatitis, bone marrow aplasia, or other severe hematologic disorder. • Administer with caution to a patient with GI symptoms, such as nausea, vomiting, diarrhea, constipation, or abdominal pain.
aurothioglucose	Rheumatoid arthritis	10 mg I.M. during the first week, 25 mg I.M. during second and third weeks, then 50 mg I.M. weekly until 0.8 to 1 gram I.M. has been administered Maintenance dosage: 25 to 50 mg I.M. every 2 weeks for 2 to 20 weeks, then 25 to 50 mg I.M. every 3 to 4 weeks indefinitely	• Know that aurothioglucose is contraindicated in a pregnant or lactating patient; one with known hypersensitivity to the drug, uncontrolled diabetes mellitus, severe debilitation, systemic lupus erythematosus, renal disease, hepatic dysfunction, uncontrolled congestive heart failure, marked hypertension, granulocytopenia, other blood dyscrasias, hemorrhagic diathesis, history of infectious hepatitis, urticaria, eczema, or colitis; or one who has had recent radiation therapy. • Administer with caution to a patient with compromised cardiovascular or cerebral circulation.

• *Stress the importance of compliance with gold therapy. Explain to the patient that the therapeutic effects of the gold salt usually occur 8 to 12 weeks after treatment begins or may not occur for 6 months or longer.*

• Counsel the patient to keep follow-up appointments with the physician.

• *Explain that monthly platelet counts are needed, and teach the patient the signs and symptoms of a decreased platelet count, such as purpura, ecchymoses, petechiae, and bleeding gums. If the platelet count drops below 100,000/mm³, the drug may be discontinued.*

• Explain to the patient that rinsing the mouth with 1 teaspoon of salt in 8 oz (240 ml) of water can help treat symptomatic, mild mouth ulcers.

• Instruct the patient to store oral gold in a tight, light-resistant container and to use capsules before their expiration date, 4 years after the date of manufacture.

• Instruct the patient to notify the physician if adverse reactions occur.

Evaluation

The following examples represent appropriate evaluation statements for a patient receiving a gold salt.

• The patient has no conditions that contraindicate gold salt therapy.

• The patient exhibits no signs of complications in the preexisting condition linked to the prescribed gold salt.

• The patient experiences no adverse reactions to the prescribed gold salt.

• The patient's bowel status remains unchanged during auranofin therapy.

• The patient complies with auranofin therapy, as prescribed.

• The patient and family express an accurate understanding of the points taught about the prescribed gold salt.

• The patient stores oral gold in a tight, light-resistant container.

CHAPTER SUMMARY

Chapter 58 presented the uricosurics, other antigout agents, and gold salts. Here are the chapter highlights.

• Uricosurics and other antigout preparations are used to treat gout. The gold salts are used to treat rheumatoid arthritis. The antigout agents cannot be used to treat rheumatoid arthritis, nor can gold salts be used to treat gout.

• The drug administered to treat gout depends on the acuity of the disease. During an acute gout attack, colchicine is prescribed. The uricosurics and allopurinol are used only when a patient has chronic gouty arthritis or hyperuricemia, which places the patient at risk for an acute attack of gout.

• The use of gold salts can help a patient with rheumatoid arthritis achieve a remission. The effects of gold salts can be dramatic, but the drugs can be toxic.

• The uricosurics, antigout agents, and gold salts exert their effects through their anti-inflammatory actions; they are not analgesics.

• When caring for a patient receiving a uricosuric, antigout agent, or gold salt, the nurse should teach the patient about the risks and benefits of the prescribed treatment. The nurse also should monitor the patient closely for adverse reactions. Monitoring involves comparing periodic laboratory test results and discussing with the patient the response to drug therapy.

STUDY QUESTIONS

See Appendix 1 for answers.

1. Walter Owens, age 52, receives the uricosuric agent probenecid (Benemid) as maintenance therapy for chronic gouty arthritis. How does a uricosuric agent exert its therapeutic effect?
(a) It inhibits uric acid production in the body.
(b) It inhibits uric acid resorption at the proximal convoluted tubules.
(c) It inhibits the inflammatory response to deposited sodium urate crystals.
(d) It inhibits xanthine oxidase, an enzyme that converts xanthine to uric acid.

2. The nurse monitors Mr. Owens for adverse reactions. What is one of the most common adverse reactions to probenecid?
(a) edema
(b) vertigo
(c) tinnitus
(d) GI distress

3. Mr. Owens says he has had frequent headaches since he began taking probenecid. What should the nurse advise him to do?
(a) Discontinue the medication immediately.
(b) Take aspirin as needed to relieve any headache.
(c) Take acetaminophen to prevent bleeding problems linked with concomitant salicylate use.
(d) Notify the physician because headache is a sign of a toxic reactions to probenecid.

4. Lena Salvino, age 61, comes to the emergency department for treatment of an acute attack of gouty arthritis. What is the drug of choice for treating this problem?
(a) auranofin
(b) colchicine
(c) allopurinol
(d) aurothioglucose

5. The nurse assesses Ms. Salvino for adverse reactions to her antigout therapy. Which system is most likely to be adversely affected?
(a) respiratory
(b) cardiac
(c) CNS
(d) GI

6. Roberta Godwin, age 45, has chronic rheumatoid arthritis that is not responding well to NSAID therapy. Her physician prescribes the gold salt aurothioglucose. When should Ms. Godwin expect to see the benefits of gold salt therapy?
(a) immediately after administration
(b) 1 full week after administration
(c) up to 4 weeks after administration
(d) 8 to 12 weeks after administration

7. By which action may a gold salt relieve rheumatoid arthritis?
(a) It acts primarily as an analgesic.
(b) It provides anti-inflammatory effects.
(c) It decreases lipsomal enzyme release.
(d) It reverses rheumatoid arthritis deformation.

8. For Ms. Godwin, when are adverse reactions to parenteral gold therapy most likely to occur?
(a) during the first 10 minutes after treatment
(b) during the first week of treatment
(c) during the first month of treatment
(d) during the second month of treatment

SELECTED REFERENCES

AHFS drug information 90. (1990). Bethesda, MD: American Society of Hospital Pharmacists.

Drug facts and comparisons. (1990). St. Louis: Facts and Comparisons Division, J.B. Lippincott.

Dunbar, R. (1990). *Doctor discusses learning to cope with arthritis, rheumatism, and gout.* Chicago: Budlong Press.

Gillenwater, J. (1990). *Yearbook of urology 1990.* St. Louis: Year Book Medical Publishers.

Goodman and Gilman's the pharmacological basis of therapeutics (8th ed.; 1990). Elmsford, NY: Pergamon Press.

Hansten, P., and Horn, J. (1989). *Drug interactions* (6th ed.). Philadelphia: Lea & Febiger.

Kursh, E., and Resnick, M. (Eds.). (1987). *Urology* (Problems in patient care series). Oradell, NJ: Medical Economics Books.

North American Nursing Diagnosis Association. (1990). *Taxonomy I - Revised, with official categories.* St. Louis: NANDA.

Reichert, K. (1987). *Gold: Studies and uses in science and health.* Washington, DC: ABBE Pubs Association.

DRUGS TO PREVENT OR TREAT INFECTION

Attempts to treat systemic microbial infections with chemicals date back to the 16th century when mercury was used to treat syphilis. Other organometallic compounds, such as arsenic and bismuth, were introduced during the 1920s to treat syphilis, malaria, and other parasitic diseases. Compounds containing arsenic, an antimony, still are used to treat protozoa and other parasites. With the introduction of sulfonamides in 1936, a new era began in treating infectious diseases. In 1941, penicillin was introduced as the first antimicrobial that could be mass-produced, making it available to treat a wide patient population. Since then, numerous other antimicrobials have been introduced.

ANTIMICROBIAL SPECTRUM

The currently available antimicrobial drugs vary in their degree of effectiveness against different microorganisms. A drug's *spectrum of activity* refers to the number and type of organisms vulnerable to its action. Broad-spectrum antimicrobials affect a wide variety of pathogens, and narrow-spectrum drugs affect a few. Antimicrobials tend to affect pathogens with similar biochemical characteristics.

The most common method used to distinguish among various microorganisms is the Gram stain, which uses laboratory dyes to stain organisms; the reactions reveal chemical differences in the cell wall. Organisms that are stained by the Gram stain are called gram-positive; those that are not are called gram-negative.

For some bacteria, Gram staining is not a useful diagnostic tool. Some of these organisms, such as mycobacteria, can be stained with carbolfuchsin, then decolorized with ethyl alcohol and hydrochloric acid. They are classified as acid-fast if they retain the stain.

Spirochetes can be visualized only by special techniques, such as dark-field examination. Other important stains used to identify bacteria include Gimenez stain for

Rickettsia, Giemsa and Wright's stain for parasites and intracellular microorganisms, and fluorescent antibody for various organisms.

Organisms with similar staining properties tend to be susceptible to the same antimicrobial agents. Therefore, a drug's antimicrobial spectrum may be described by its activity against gram-negative, gram-positive, or acid-fast bacilli. (For examples of these organisms, see *Gram-negative and gram-positive bacteria and acid-fast bacilli,* page 1000.)

Organisms also are classified as aerobes—those that can live and grow in the presence of oxygen—or as anaerobes—those that can live or grow without oxygen.

DRUG SELECTION

Selecting an appropriate antimicrobial agent to treat a specific infection involves several important factors. First the microorganism must be isolated and identified. Then its susceptibility to various drugs must be determined. The lowest antimicrobial concentration that prevents visible growth after an 18- to 24-hour incubation is known as the minimal inhibitory concentration (MIC). The minimal bactericidal concentration (MBC) is defined as the lowest antimicrobial concentration that totally suppresses growth after overnight incubation. Because culture and sensitivity results take 48 hours, treatment usually is initiated on clinical assessment and then reevaluated when test results are complete.

Another important factor in choosing an antimicrobial is the infection site. For antimicrobial therapy to be effective, an adequate concentration of the drug must be delivered to the infection site. That means the local antimicrobial concentration should equal at least the MIC for the infecting organism. Other factors in selecting an antimicrobial are the relative cost of the drug, its potential adverse effects, and patient allergies.

Glossary

Acetylation: metabolic process that introduces an acetyl group into the molecule of an organic compound.

Acid fast: organism that retains carbolfuchsin stain after being decolorized with 95% ethyl alcohol and 3% hydrochloric acid—a unique characteristic of mycobacteria.

Aerobe: microorganism that can live and grow only in the presence of molecular oxygen.

Amoebicidal: pertaining to an agent that destroys amoebas.

Anaerobe: microorganism that can live and grow only in the complete, or almost complete, absence of molecular oxygen.

Anaphylaxis: life-threatening reaction of a person to a foreign protein or other substance.

Antibacterial: substance, derived from cultures or semi-synthetically produced, that inhibits bacterial growth or kills bacteria.

Antibiotic: substance, derived from cultures or semi-synthetically produced, that inhibits growth of or kills other organisms, such as parasites.

Antimicrobial: substance used to treat infection with pathogenic microorganisms.

Bacillus: any rod-shaped, gram-positive, spore-forming microorganism.

Bacteremia: presence of bacteria in the blood.

Bacteria: group of single-cell organisms, usually possessing a rigid cell wall, dividing by binary fission, and exhibiting either round, rodlike, or spiral form.

Bactericidal: pertaining to an agent that destroys bacteria.

Bacteriostatic: pertaining to an agent that inhibits growth or multiplication of bacteria.

Bacteriuria: presence of bacteria in the urine.

Cestode: tapeworm or platyhelminth that has a head, or scolex, and segmented joints, or proglottids.

Coccus: a spherical bacterial cell, usually slightly less than 1 micron in diameter.

Conjugation: chemical combination of a toxic product with a substance in the body to form a detoxified product that is then excreted.

Dermatophytosis: fungal skin infection.

Encephalitis: inflammation of the brain.

Fungicidal: pertaining to an agent that destroys fungi.

Fungistatic: pertaining to an agent that inhibits fungal growth.

Gram stain: laboratory dye used to differentiate organisms. An organism that retains the dye is classified as gram-positive; otherwise, the organism is gram-negative.

Hansen's disease: chronic communicable disease caused by *Mycobacterium leprae,* characterized by granulomatous lesions in the skin, mucous membranes, and peripheral nervous system; also called leprosy.

Helminth: worm or wormlike parasite.

Hydrolysis: splitting of a compound into fragments by adding water, with the hydroxyl group incorporated in one fragment and the hydrogen atom in the other.

Iatrogenic: caused by a treatment or diagnostic procedure.

Induction: stimulation of the hepatic microsomal enzyme system by one drug, which increases metabolism of another drug.

Infection: reactions of tissues to invading pathogenic microorganisms and the toxins they generate.

Malaria: infectious febrile disease caused by protozoa transmitted by the bites of infected mosquitoes; characterized by periodic attacks of chills, fever, and diaphoresis.

Meningitis: inflammation of the membranes that envelop the brain and spinal cord.

Microbial: pertaining to minute living organisms capable of producing diseases, including bacteria, protozoa, and fungi.

Microorganism: microscopic organism, including bacteria, spiral organisms, *Rickettsiae,* viruses, molds, yeasts, and protozoa.

Morphologic: pertaining to the science of the physical forms and structures of an organism.

Mycobacteria: slender, gram-positive, acid-fast, rod-shaped microorganisms.

Mycoses: diseases caused by fungi.

Nematode: multicellular parasite, such as a roundworm or threadworm.

Nosocomial: pertaining to a hospital.

Ototoxicity: quality or property of exerting a destructive or poisonous effect upon the eighth cranial nerve or the organs of hearing and balance.

Parasite: plant or animal that lives upon or within another living organism, at whose expense it obtains some advantage without return compensation.

Pathogen: disease-producing microorganism or material.

Phosphorylation: chemical process of introducing the trivalent phosphoryl group into an organic molecule.

Prophylaxis: disease prevention.

Protozoa: unicellular organisms constituting the lowest division of the animal kingdom.

Resistance: natural ability of an organism to ward off deleterious effects of noxious agents, such as toxins, poisons, irritants, or pathogenic microorganisms.

Ribosome: one of the minute granules composed of nucleic acid, attached to the membranes of the endoplasmic reticulum of a cell where cellular protein synthesis occurs.

Schistosome: blood fluke that is a type of trematode parasite.

Sepsis: poisoning from pathogenic organisms or their toxins.

Serum sickness: type of immune complex hypersensitivity occurring 6 to 14 days after injection with foreign serum; characterized by edema, fever, inflammation of the blood vessels and joints, and urticaria.

Spectrum: range of bacteria affected by an antibacterial agent.

Sterol: monohydroxyl alcohol of high molecular weight, commonly classified as a lipid.

Glossary (continued)

Superinfection: condition produced by the sudden overgrowth of resistant bacteria or fungi, which can occur in a patient on antibiotic therapy.

Thrush: fungal infection characterized by whitish spots and shallow ulcers in the oral cavity, fever, and gastrointestinal irritation; usually from superinfection.

Toxicity: quality of being poisonous.

Trematode: parasite resulting from ingestion of fluke-contaminated uncooked fish, crustaceans, or vegetation.

Trough levels: the lowest serum therapeutic concentration of a drug.

Tuberculosis: infectious disease caused by a species of *Mycobacterium,* characterized by small rounded nodules in the tissues, as well as fever, emaciation, and night sweats.

Virulence: degree of pathogenicity of a microorganism as indicated by case fatality rates or its ability to invade host tissues.

Virus: group of minute infectious agents characterized by a lack of independent metabolism and by ability to replicate within living host cells only.

Xanthine: white amorphous base formed by the oxidation of hypoxanthine and oxidized to uric acid.

Mixed infections (those caused by two or more organisms, each of which may be sensitive to different drugs) respond best to treatment with a selected combination of antimicrobial agents. Examples are peritoneal or pelvic infections caused by mixed bowel flora and diabetic foot infections.

The patient's clinical condition determines when antimicrobial therapy is started and how it is administered. If the patient is stable, therapy may be delayed until culture and sensitivity test results are available. Unstable patients usually are treated immediately with broad-spectrum agents. Patients with serious infections usually need higher and more predictable blood concentration levels, necessitating intravenous (I.V.) therapy. In less severe infections, intramuscular (I.M.) or oral therapy can be used.

PREVENTION OF RESISTANCE

One factor limits the usefulness of antimicrobial agents: Pathogens may develop resistance to a drug's action. *Resistance* is the ability of a microorganism to live and grow in the presence of an antibacterial agent that usually is bactericidal or bacteriostatic. Resistance usually results from genetic events that develop mutant strains of the microorganism. These mutant strains resist a drug's activity by enhancing the action of specific enzymes that break down the chemical structure of the drug, restricting uptake of the drug, or altering critical cellular target sites.

Antimicrobial drugs should not be used indiscriminately, because unnecessary exposure of organisms to these agents encourages resistant strains. The drugs should be reserved for patients with infections caused by susceptible organisms and should be used in high enough doses and for an appropriate duration to eradicate even the most resistant mutants. Administration of subtherapeutic dosages may allow resistant mutant strains to proliferate. New antimicrobial agents should be reserved for severely ill patients with serious infections that do not respond to conventional drugs.

ADVERSE REACTIONS TO ANTIMICROBIAL AGENTS

All antimicrobials can produce beneficial and adverse reactions in a patient. The adverse reactions can be classified as direct toxic effects on such organs as the gastrointestinal tract, kidneys, and liver or the auditory, optic, and peripheral nerves; allergic reactions and other kinds of hypersensitivity reactions affecting the skin and other organs and structures, including the bone marrow and blood; and superinfections resulting from drug-induced overgrowths of resistant bacterial strains or fungal organisms.

OVERVIEW OF CHAPTERS

The chapters in Unit Fourteen explore the agents used to prevent or treat infections and the nurse's responsibilities when administering them. It addresses antibacterial, antitubercular, antileprotic, antiviral, antimycotic (antifungal), anthelmintic, antimalarial, other antiprotozoal, and urinary antiseptic agents.

Chapter 59
Antibacterial Agents

Chapter 59 discusses agents used to treat systemic bacterial infections. It emphasizes the mechanisms of action and clinical indications for the aminoglycosides, penicillins, cephalosporins, tetracyclines, chloramphenicol, erythromycin, clindamycin, lincomycin, vancomycin, imipenem/cilastatin, and aztreonam. The chapter also provides the spectrum of activity, nursing implications, and patient teaching for each drug class.

Gram-negative, gram-positive, and acid-fast organisms

Knowing which organisms are gram-negative, gram-positive, or acid-fast helps the nurse understand the therapeutic use of selected agents. An antibacterial agent that is effective against one gram-negative bacterium may be effective against other bacteria in that group. The same principle applies to the gram-positive group. In contrast, the bacilli in the acid-fast group must be treated individually with drugs that are effective against that specific organism.

Gram-negative bacteria

Acinetobacter calcoaceticus	Calymmatobacterium granulomatis	Klebsiella pneumoniae	Salmonella sendai
Bacteroides asaccharolyticus	Campylobacter coli	Legionella micdadei	Salmonella typhimurium
Bacteroides fragilis	Campylobacter faecalis	Legionella pneumophila	Salmonella typhosa
Bartonella bacilliformis	Campylobacter fetus	Morganella morganii	Serratia marcescens
Bacteroides distasonis	Campylobacter jejuni	Mycoplasma pneumoniae	Shigella dysenteriae
Bacteroides gingivalis	Chlamydia trachomatis	Neisseria gonorrhoeae	Shigella boydii
Bacteroides melaninogenicus	Citrobacter diversus	Neisseria meningitidis	Shigella flexneri
Bacteroides ovatus	Citrobacter freundii	Pasteurella multocida	Shigella sonnei
Bacteroides thetaiotaomicron	Enterobacter aerogines	Proteus mirabilis	Spirillum minus
Bacteroides vulgatus	Enterobacter cloacae	Proteus morgani	Streptobacillus moniliformis
Bordetella pertussis	Escherichia coli	Proteus vulgaris	Ureaplasma urealyticum
Branhamella catarrhalis	Francisella tularensis	Providencia stuartii	Veillonella
Brucella abortus	Fusobacterium nucleatum	Providencia rettgeri	Vibrio alginolyticus
Brucella canis	Haemophilus ducreyi	Pseudomonas aeruginosa	Vibrio cholerae
Brucella melitensis	Haemophilus influenzae	Salmonella choleraesuis	Vibrio mimicus
Brucella rangiferi	Haemophilus parahemolyticus	Salmonella dublin	Vibrio parahaemolyticus
Brucella suis	Haemophilus parainfluenzae	Salmonella enteritidis	Vibrio vulnificus
			Yersinia enterocolitica

Gram-positive bacteria

Actinomyces israelii	Corynebacterium diphtheriae	Propionibacterium acnes
Arachnia propionica	Erysipelothrix insidiosa	Staphylococcus aureus
Bacillus anthracis	Erysipelothrix rhusiopathiae	Staphylococcus epidermidis
Bacillus cereus	Eubacterium alactolyticum	Streptococcus bovis
Clostridium botulinum	Listeria monocytogenes	Streptococcus faecalis
Clostridium butyricum	Nocardia asteroides	Streptococcus pneumoniae
Clostridium difficile	Peptococcus	Streptococcus pyogenes
Clostridium fusobacterium	Peptostreptococcus	Streptococcus sanguis
Clostridium perfringens		Streptococcus viridans
Clostridium septicum		
Clostridium sordellii		
Clostridium tetani		

Acid-fast bacilli

Mycobacterium avium

Mycobacterium bovis

Mycobacterium chelonei

Mycobacterium fortuitum

Mycobacterium intracellulare

Mycobacterium kansasii

Mycobacterium leprae

Mycobacterium marinum

Mycobacterium scrofulaceum

Mycobacterium tuberculosis

Mycobacterium xenopi

Chapter 60
Antitubercular and Antileprotic Agents
The anti-infective agents used to treat diseases caused by organisms of the genus *Mycobacterium* are the focus of Chapter 60. The two major diseases addressed are tuberculosis and Hansen's disease, or leprosy. The mechanisms of action of these drugs are delineated as well as their adverse effects. The nursing implications focus on patient teaching because of the necessary prolonged use of these drugs.

Chapter 61
Antiviral Agents
Chapter 61 begins with an overview of the difficulties inherent in developing antiviral agents that are not toxic to host cells. Then it explores the current major drugs—including acyclovir, ganciclovir, vidarabine, amantadine, ribavirin, and zidovudine. The chapter emphasizes the adverse reactions to these agents and use of the nursing process when administering them.

Chapter 62
Antimycotic (Antifungal) Agents
Chapter 62 discusses the various classes of antifungal agents used to treat diseases ranging from athlete's foot to exotic systemic infections. It delineates the mechanisms of action of the five major drugs—amphotericin, nystatin, flucytosine, ketoconazole, and fluconazole—and briefly describes other antimycotic agents. The chapter describes the clinical uses and adverse effects of these agents and presents related nursing care.

Chapter 63
Anthelmintic Agents
Chapter 63 discusses those agents used to treat helminthic infections. After providing an overview of the various types of helminths, including their site of entry into the host and infection site, the chapter explores the specific drugs, their mechanisms of action, clinical uses, and associated nursing implications.

Chapter 64
Antimalarial and Other Antiprotozoal Agents
Chapter 64 focuses on agents used to treat human protozoal diseases. After suggesting reasons for the increased number of protozoal diseases in the United States, the chapter provides details about the antimalarial agents and the agents used to manage other protozoal infections, such as amebiasis, *Pneumocystis carinii* pneumonia, and giardiasis. Along with the pharmacokinetics, pharmacodynamics, pharmacotherapeutics, and adverse drug reactions, the chapter delineates associated nursing care for these agents.

Chapter 65
Urinary Antiseptic Agents
Agents used to treat bacterial infections in the urine usually are not effective in treating systemic infections. Chapter 65 begins by reviewing those individuals at greatest risk for developing urinary tract infections. Then it presents the agents used to treat these infections (quinolones, sulfonamides, and nitrofurantoin), with an emphasis on the spectrum of antibacterial activity. For each drug class, the chapter highlights related nursing implications and patient teaching.

CHAPTER

59

ANTIBACTERIAL AGENTS

OBJECTIVES

After reading and studying this chapter, the student should be able to:

1. Identify the different types of antibacterial agents used to treat systemic bacterial infections.
2. Describe the adverse reactions associated with the aminoglycosides.
3. Discuss the reasons for ordering serum aminoglycoside peak and trough serum concentration levels.
4. Compare the antibacterial activity of the four types of penicillins: natural penicillins, penicillinase-resistant penicillins, aminopenicillins, and extended-spectrum penicillins.
5. Describe the differences among the first-, second-, and third-generation cephalosporins.
6. Identify the adverse reactions to tetracyclines.
7. Discuss the pharmacokinetics of chloramphenicol.
8. Explain the pharmacodynamics of lincomycin and clindamycin.
9. Discuss the pharmacotherapeutic uses of the various erythromycin preparations.
10. Describe the hypotension reaction associated with vancomycin administration.
11. Discuss why imipenem and cilastatin have been combined to make a new antibacterial drug.
12. Discuss the antibacterial spectrum of aztreonam.
13. Describe how to apply the nursing process when caring for a patient who is receiving an antibacterial agent.

INTRODUCTION

The discovery of drugs that prevent and treat infection from pathogenic microorganisms was one of the most important pharmacologic developments in modern medicine. The discovery and clinical use of penicillin and streptomycin began in the 1940s. Since the 1950s, a new antimicrobial agent has been introduced almost every year.

Some of the newly developed drugs act against antibiotic-resistant bacteria; others are more effective against a specific organism or are less toxic than older drugs. However, every antimicrobial agent that selectively kills pathogens also can inflict damage on the patient. Therefore, before prescribing and instituting antimicrobial drug therapy, the physician must identify the infecting organism and consider the appropriate pharmacologic and toxicologic characteristics of the drug. The physician also must consider the pharmacokinetic characteristics of the selected drug and its ability to diffuse into the infection site. (For information on topical antibacterial agents, see the appendix on Integumentary Agents.)

This chapter describes drugs used mainly to treat systemic bacterial infections. The antibacterial classes discussed include aminoglycosides, penicillins, cephalosporins, tetracyclines, chloramphenicol, clindamycin and lincomycin, erythromycin, vancomycin, carbapenems, and monobactams.

Because polymyxin B sulfate and spectinomycin hydrochloride have been replaced largely by more effective and less toxic antibiotics, they will not be covered in detail in this chapter. Polymyxin B is indicated only for treating urinary tract and meningeal infections caused by organisms that are resistant to other antibiotics. Spectinomycin is used to treat penicillinase-producing strains of *Neisseria gonorrhoeae*. It also is used to treat patients who are allergic to penicillin, cephalosporins, probenecid, and tetracycline and those who do not comply with multiple-dose tetracycline therapy.

For a summary of representative drugs, see *Selected major drugs: Antibacterial agents,* pages 1046 to 1048. For a listing of applicable nursing diagnoses that the nurse may formulate when caring for a patient receiving these agents, see *Selected nursing diagnoses: Antibacterial agents.* For detailed information on applying the nursing process, see Chapter 6, The Nursing Process and Drug Therapy.

SELECTED NURSING DIAGNOSES

Antibacterial agents

The following nursing diagnoses address representative problems and etiologies that a nurse may encounter when caring for a patient who is receiving an antibacterial agent. Some of these nursing diagnoses contain generalized etiologies, which the nurse must individualize based on the patient's needs. (For some common nursing diagnoses and related interventions for each drug class, see the "Nursing Process Application" sections of this chapter.)

- Altered health maintenance related to ineffectiveness of the prescribed antibacterial agent
- Altered oral mucous membrane related to stomatitis caused by an antibacterial agent
- Altered protection related to the adverse hematologic effects of an antibacterial agent
- Altered protection related to chloramphenicol-induced bone marrow suppression
- Altered protection related to development of superinfection caused by an antibacterial agent
- Altered thought processes related to aztreonam-induced confusion
- Altered thought processes related to penicillin G-induced coma
- Body image disturbance related to tooth discoloration caused by tetracycline use during tooth formation.
- Decreased tissue perfusion (systemic) related to hypotension caused by rapid I.V. administration of vancomycin or use of aztreonam
- Diarrhea related to the adverse GI effects of an antibacterial agent
- Fluid volume excess related to administration of the disodium salt form of an extended-spectrum penicillin
- Impaired physical mobility related to neuromuscular blockade caused by the prescribed aminoglycoside
- Impaired tissue integrity related to pseudomembranous colitis caused by an antibacterial agent
- Impaired tissue integrity related to thrombophlebitis caused by I.V. administration of an antibacterial agent
- Knowledge deficit related to the prescribed antibacterial agent

- Noncompliance related to adverse reactions to the prescribed antibacterial agent
- Pain related to parenteral administration of an antibacterial agent
- Potential fluid volume deficit related to the adverse GI effects of an antibacterial agent
- Potential for injury related to a preexisting condition that contraindicates the use of an antibacterial agent
- Potential for injury related to a preexisting condition that requires cautious use of an antibacterial agent
- Potential for injury related to adverse drug reactions
- Potential for injury related to chloramphenicol-induced gray syndrome
- Potential for injury related to drug interactions
- Potential for injury related to hypersensitivity reactions to the prescribed antibacterial agent
- Potential for injury related to the adverse hepatic effects of an antibacterial agent
- Potential for injury related to the adverse urinary effects of an antibacterial agent
- Potential for trauma related to seizures caused by an antibacterial agent
- Potential for trauma related to the adverse CNS effects of an antibiotic agent
- Potential impaired skin integrity related to perineal irritation caused by oral chloramphenicol
- Sensory-perceptual alterations (auditory) related to ototoxicity caused by an antibacterial agent
- Sensory-perceptual alterations (visual) related to photosensitivity caused by a tetracycline

AMINOGLYCOSIDES

The aminoglycosides primarily are used to treat gram-negative bacterial infections. They also are used with beta-lactam agents, such as penicillin and cephalosporins, to treat critically ill patients with peritonitis or pneumonia. The aminoglycosides provide effective bactericidal activity against aerobic gram-negative bacilli, some aerobic gram-positive bacteria, mycobacteria, and some protozoa. They all contain aminosugars in glycosidic linkage, and all display a similar antimicrobial spectrum of activity, a similar pharmacokinetic profile, and similar toxicities.

Although streptomycin sulfate at first was useful clinically, bacterial resistance to it developed rapidly. Subsequently, neomycin sulfate and kanamycin sulfate were introduced, but their usefulness was limited by their potential toxicity and by bacterial resistance to them. Currently, gentamicin sulfate, tobramycin sulfate, netilmicin sulfate, and amikacin sulfate are the most commonly prescribed aminoglycosides for serious gram-negative bacillary infections, although paromomycin sulfate occasionally may be prescribed to treat intestinal amebiasis and other parasitic infections.

Currently used aminoglycosides include amikacin, gentamicin, kanamycin, neomycin, netilmicin, paromomycin, streptomycin, and tobramycin.

PHARMACOKINETICS

The various aminoglycosides have similar pharmacokinetic properties. All are absorbed poorly after oral administration and are excreted almost entirely unchanged in the urine by glomerular filtration.

Absorption, distribution, metabolism, excretion

After oral administration, aminoglycosides are absorbed poorly from the gastrointestinal (GI) tract. However, after intravenous (I.V.) and intramuscular (I.M.) administration, aminoglycoside absorption is complete and rapid if impaired tissue perfusion does not exist. In patients with serious infections, I.V. administration is used to ensure optimal reliable serum concentrations.

The aminoglycosides are distributed widely in extracellular fluid. Small amounts are distributed to bile, sweat, tears, saliva, sputum, and breast milk. Concentrations in the renal cortex and the perilymph of the inner ear far exceed plasma concentrations. However, concentrations in bronchial secretions attain only about 20% of plasma concentrations. When administered in therapeutic doses, aminoglycosides readily cross the placenta. They do not cross the blood-brain barrier even in patients with inflamed meninges. As a result, intrathecal administration is proposed for gram-negative bacillary meningitis in adults. Drug concentrations in prostatic fluid and bile are significantly lower than plasma concentrations. In the urine, aminoglycoside concentrations exceed plasma concentrations by 25 to 100 times. Aminoglycosides are not metabolized.

Aminoglycosides are excreted primarily via the kidneys. From 40% to 97% of a single dose is excreted within 24 hours of administration. Complete urine recovery can be seen 20 to 30 days after administration of the last dose. Because aminoglycosides are excreted by the kidneys, decreased renal function can increase the serum half-life from the normal 2 to 3 hours to between 50 and 60 hours in uremic patients. In patients with diminished renal glomerular function, the daily dosage must be reduced. Less than 1% of a given dose appears in the feces.

Onset, peak, duration

After I.M. administration, the peak concentration level usually is achieved within 30 minutes to 2 hours. With I.V. administration, peak concentration occurs 30 minutes after the infusion ends. The recommended length of infusion to achieve peak concentration is 30 minutes. In the patient with impaired renal function, the dosage interval may be increased.

PHARMACODYNAMICS

The aminoglycosides act as bactericidal agents against susceptible organisms by binding irreversibly to their ribosomal subunits, thus inhibiting protein synthesis.

Mechanism of action

Aminoglycosides are transported across cell membranes to bind within the pathogen to ribosomes, which process genetically coded information. As a result, protein synthesis required for maintaining the structure and metabolic activity of the bacterial cell is inhibited.

Bacterial resistance to an aminoglycoside may be related to failure of the drug to cross the cell membrane, altered binding to ribosomes, or destruction of the drug by bacterial enzymes. Some gram-positive cocci (enterococci) resist aminoglycoside transport across the cell membrane. When penicillin is used with aminoglycoside therapy, the cell wall is altered, enabling the aminoglycoside to penetrate the bacterial cell.

PHARMACOTHERAPEUTICS

Aminoglycosides are most useful in treating infections caused by aerobic gram-negative bacilli. They also are valuable in treating serious nosocomial infections in critically ill patients, such as gram-negative bacteremia, peritonitis, and pneumonia. Urinary tract infections caused by enteric bacilli that are resistant to less toxic antibiotics, such as penicillins and cephalosporins, frequently respond to aminoglycosides. Infections of the central nervous system (CNS) and the eye require local instillation. Streptomycin is active against many strains of mycobacteria, including *Mycobacterium tuberculosis,* and against gram-positive bacteria *Nocardia* and *Erysipelothrix.* Amikacin, gentamicin, netilmicin, and tobramycin, are active against *Acinetobacter, Citrobacter, Enterobacter, Klebsiella, Proteus* (indole-positive and indole-negative), *Providencia, Serratia, Escherichia coli,* and *Pseudomonas aeruginosa.* Because susceptibility of these organisms to the particular aminoglycoside varies with time and clinical setting, a culture and sensitivity test should be performed before and periodically during therapy.

Against gram-positive organisms, aminoglycosides are used as synergistic combinations with penicillins to treat staphylococcal or enterococcal infections. Aminoglycosides are inactive against anaerobic bacteria.

Potentially serious toxicity limits the usefulness of the aminoglycosides; all display the same spectrum of toxicity, which can damage auditory, vestibular, and renal functions. Toxic and therapeutic effects can be monitored by assessing the aminoglycoside level. (For more information, see *Serum aminoglycoside levels.*)

amikacin sulfate (Amikin). Amikacin is active against many aminoglycoside-resistant gram-negative bacilli. With restricted use, bacterial resistance may be prevented.
Usual adult dosage: 7 to 7.5 mg/kg I.V. or I.M. every 12 hours; dosage adjustment is required for patients with renal impairment.
Usual pediatric dosage: same as adult.

gentamicin sulfate (Garamycin). The most widely prescribed aminoglycoside, gentamicin use has been limited

Serum aminoglycoside levels

Periodic assessment of aminoglycoside serum peak and trough concentration levels is needed to assess therapeutic efficacy and toxicity. That is especially important in patients with changing renal function and in those on concomitant therapy with an extended-spectrum penicillin. The goal is to obtain a peak serum concentration between 4 and 8 mcg/ml for gentamicin or tobramycin, 4 and 10 mcg/ml for netilmicin, or 15 and 30 mcg/ml for kanamycin or amikacin. These therapeutic peak concentrations will vary with the pathogen and the infection site. Serum trough concentrations for gentamicin, tobramycin, and netilmicin generally are lower than 2 mcg/ml; for amikacin and kanamycin, lower than 5 mcg/ml. High trough concentrations correlate with nephrotoxicity; high peak concentrations, with ototoxicity and nephrotoxicity.

Blood for serum aminoglycoside trough concentrations should be obtained within ½ hour before the next dose. Blood for peak concentrations should be obtained 1 hour after the administration of an I.M. dose and ½ hour after the end of a 30-minute infusion. Each specimen must be dated and timed.

by the increasing numbers of gentamicin-resistant gram-negative bacilli. It is the drug of choice for suspected infection from *P. aeruginosa, E. coli, Staphylococcus, Serratia, Citrobacter,* indole-positive and indole-negative *Proteus, Providencia, Klebsiella, Enterobacter,* and other gram-negative aerobic bacteria.

Usual adult dosage: 1 to 1.75 mg/kg I.V. or I.M. every 8 hours; dosage adjustment is required for patients with renal impairment.

Usual pediatric dosage: for children ages 6 weeks to 12 years, 2 to 2.5 mg/kg I.V. or I.M. every 8 hours, or 3 to 3.75 mg/kg I.M. or I.V. every 12 hours.

kanamycin sulfate (Kantrex). Kanamycin is effective against infections caused by *E. coli, Proteus* species, *Enterobacter aerogines, Serratia marcescens, Klebsiella pneumoniae,* and *Acinetobacter* species. It is ineffective against *P. aeruginosa.*

Usual adult dosage: 7.5 mg/kg I.M. or I.V. every 12 hours, not to exceed 1.5 grams/day; for inhalation therapy, 250 mg diluted in 3 ml of normal saline solution and nebulized b.i.d. to q.i.d.; for intraperitoneal therapy, 500 mg in 20 ml of sterile water instilled into the peritoneal cavity.

Usual pediatric dosage: 7.5 mg/kg I.M. or I.V. every 12 hours, not to exceed 30 mg/kg/day.

neomycin sulfate (Mycifradin, Neobiotic). Used as an adjunct to treat hepatic coma and as a bowel antiseptic before intestinal surgery, neomycin is administered orally.

Usual adult dosage: for hepatic encephalopathy, 4 to 12 grams P.O. daily in divided doses; for preoperative intes-

tinal antisepsis, 1 gram P.O. every hour for 4 doses, then 1 gram every 4 hours for the balance of the 24 hours. A saline cathartic should precede therapy.

Usual pediatric dosage: for preoperative intestinal antisepsis, 88 mg/kg P.O. daily divided into six equal doses and administered every 4 hours. The first dose should be preceded by a saline cathartic.

netilmicin sulfate (Netromycin). Netilmicin resembles gentamicin and tobramycin, but may be less likely to produce ototoxicity and nephrotoxicity.

Usual adult dosage: 1.5 to 2 mg/kg I.V. or I.M. every 8 to 12 hours; dosage adjustment is required for patients with renal insufficiency.

Usual pediatric dosage: for children ages 6 weeks to 12 years, 1.8 to 2.7 mg/kg 1 day every 8 hours I.V. or I.M. or 2.7 to 4 mg/kg every 12 hours I.M. or I.V.; for neonates under age 6 weeks, 2 to 3.25 mg/kg every 12 hours; dosage adjustment is required for patients with renal insufficiency.

paromomycin sulfate (Humatin). Paromomycin has been used as adjunctive therapy to treat hepatic coma, but is not used commonly today. Because paromomycin is amebicidal, it sometimes is used to treat intestinal amebiasis and other parasitic infections.

Usual adult dosage: for intestinal amebiasis, 25 to 35 mg/kg P.O. daily in three divided doses.

Usual pediatric dosage: 7.5 mg/kg I.M. or I.V. every 12 hours.

streptomycin sulfate. Used to treat plague, tularemia, and tuberculosis, streptomycin also is used with penicillin to treat bacterial endocarditis. The route of administration usually is intramuscular.

Usual adult dosage: 250 to 1,000 mg I.M. every 12 hours; dosage adjustment is required for elderly patients and those with renal impairment.

Usual pediatric dosage: 20 to 40 mg/kg I.M. daily in divided doses; dosage adjustment is required patients renal impairment.

tobramycin sulfate (Nebcin). The antimicrobial spectrum of tobramycin resembles that of gentamicin, with greater activity against *P. aeruginosa* demonstrated in vitro.

Usual adult dosage: 1 to 1.75 mg/kg I.V. or I.M. every 8 hours; dosage adjustment is required for patients with renal impairment.

Usual pediatric dosage: 1.5 to 1.9 mg/kg I.M. or I.V. every 8 hours.

Drug interactions
The use of various aminoglycosides with extended-spectrum penicillins (carbenicillin, ticarcillin, mezlocillin, piperacillin, and azlocillin) can inactivate the aminoglycosides

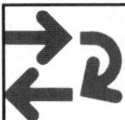

DRUG INTERACTIONS

Aminoglycosides

This chart summarizes significant interactions between aminoglycosides and other drugs. The nurse should be familiar with these interactions before administering an aminoglycoside.

DRUG	INTERACTING DRUGS	POSSIBLE EFFECTS	NURSING IMPLICATIONS
all aminoglycosides	antihistamines	Mask ototoxicity	• Monitor the patient for hearing loss.
	loop diuretics	Increase ototoxicity	• Monitor the patient for hearing loss.
	methoxyflurane	Produce additive nephrotoxicity and neurotoxicity	• Do not administer together.
amikacin, kanamycin, tobramycin, gentamicin, neomycin, streptomycin, netilmicin	neuromuscular blocking agents	Increase neuromuscular blockade	• Administer calcium and anticholinesterase agents as prescribed. • Administer the aminoglycoside cautiously during surgery and the postoperative period.
	carbenicillin, ticarcillin, azlocillin, mezlocillin, piperacillin	Inactivate the aminoglycoside	• Never mix these two types of antibacterials; if the patient must receive concomitant therapy, administer the doses at least 1 hour apart.
gentamicin, tobramycin	amphotericin B, cephalosporins, acyclovir	Produce additive nephrotoxicity	• Monitor renal function tests frequently for the patient on combination therapy.
	cyclosporines	Produce additive nephrotoxicity	• Do not administer an aminoglycoside to a patient receiving a cyclosporine. • Monitor the patient's blood urea nitrogen and creatinine levels.

when the drugs are mixed together or administered concomitantly. This interaction is clinically important for patients with impaired renal function or those receiving high doses of extended-spectrum penicillins. The serum aminoglycoside level should be monitored to ensure adequate therapy. (For more information, see *Drug interactions: Aminoglycosides*.)

ADVERSE DRUG REACTIONS

Serious adverse reactions limit the use of aminoglycosides, all of which display the same spectrum of toxicity. Careful patient monitoring using appropriate laboratory tests can help reduce the incidence of toxicity. The total dosage and duration of therapy contribute to toxicity.

The most notable adverse reactions to aminoglycosides are ototoxicity and nephrotoxicity. These most often occur in elderly patients, dehydrated patients, those with renal impairment, and those receiving concomitant therapy with an ototoxic or nephrotoxic drug.

Aminoglycosides can produce irreversible eighth cranial nerve damage. High-frequency tone loss usually occurs before clinical hearing loss. Audiometric testing can help prevent permanent hearing loss. These drugs can induce vestibular symptoms, such as dizziness, nystagmus, vertigo, and ataxia.

Aminoglycosides can produce renal tubular necrosis, resulting in elevated serum creatinine and blood urea nitrogen (BUN) levels. Nephrotoxicity is related to high drug concentrations that accumulate in the renal cortex. Renal tubular damage usually is reversible after discontinuation of the drug. Monitoring the patient's renal function and serum aminoglycoside level and making appropriate dosage adjustments may decrease the severity of nephrotoxicity and renal tubular damage.

Aminoglycosides can produce neuromuscular reactions that range from peripheral nerve toxicity to neuromuscular blockade. Reactions commonly occur after local, peritoneal, pleural, or wound instillation. Neuromuscular reactions also can occur when aminoglycosides are administered to patients immediately after surgery. Neomycin and netilmicin produce the most potent neuromuscular reactions.

The most common adverse reactions to orally administered aminoglycosides are nausea, vomiting, and diarrhea.

Allergic reactions to aminoglycosides are rare. Rash, urticaria, stomatitis, pruritus, generalized burning, fever, and eosinophilia occasionally occur.

NURSING PROCESS APPLICATION

The following information assists the nurse in caring for a patient who is receiving an aminoglycoside.

Assessment

• Review the patient's history for a preexisting condition that contraindicates the use of an aminoglycoside, such as known hypersensitivity to these agents.

• Review the patient's history for a preexisting condition that requires cautious use of an aminoglycoside, such as pregnancy, lactation, advanced age, a neuromuscular disorder, or renal impairment.

• Assess the patient for adverse reactions to the prescribed aminoglycoside, such as ototoxicity, nephrotoxicity, neuromuscular blockage, or GI dysfunction.

• Assess the patient for altered auditory sensory perception.

• Assess the effectiveness of the prescribed aminoglycoside regularly.

• Assess the patient's medication history to identify the use of drugs that may interact with the prescribed aminoglycoside, such as antihistamines, methoxyflurane, neuromuscular blocking agents, extended-spectrum penicillins, and other antibiotics.

• Evaluate the patient's and family's knowledge about the prescribed aminoglycoside.

Nursing diagnoses

The following examples represent appropriate nursing diagnoses for a patient receiving an aminoglycoside.

• Potential for injury related to a preexisting condition that contraindicates the use of an aminoglycoside

• Potential for injury related to a preexisting condition that requires cautious use of an aminoglycoside

• Potential for injury related to adverse drug reactions

• Sensory-perceptual alterations (auditory) related to ototoxicity caused by the adverse effects of the prescribed aminoglycoside on the eighth cranial nerve

• Knowledge deficit related to the prescribed aminoglycoside

Planning and implementation

• Do not administer an aminoglycoside to a patient with a condition that contraindicates its use.

• Administer an aminoglycoside cautiously to a patient at risk because of a preexisting condition.

• Monitor the patient closely for adverse reactions during aminoglycoside therapy.

• Monitor the serum aminoglycoside level regularly, especially in an elderly patient, a patient with altered renal function, or one receiving concomitant therapy with an extended-spectrum penicillin or cephalosporin. Immediately after drawing the serum sample, place it on ice and transport it to the laboratory to prevent inactivation of the aminoglycoside. Notify the physician if the peak or trough serum concentration does not fall within the expected range for the prescribed aminoglycoside.

• *Collect appropriate specimens (blood, urine, sputum, wound) for culture and sensitivity tests before beginning aminoglycoside therapy.*

• Ensure that the patient is well hydrated before therapy (unless contraindicated) to decrease the risk of nephrotoxicity.

• *Monitor the serum creatinine level to help detect changes in renal function. The serum creatinine level should be monitored every other day in a patient with unstable renal function and at least once weekly in a patient with normal renal function.*

• Notify the physician if routine urinalysis indicates casts or protein in the urine. These findings may indicate renal damage caused by the aminoglycoside.

• Monitor the respiratory rate and heart rhythm of a patient receiving an aminoglycoside to detect neuromuscular blockade, especially if neomycin or netilmicin is used. This is a particularly important intervention after surgery or after local, peritoneal, pleural, or wound instillation.

• Monitor the patient for signs and symptoms of vestibular toxicity, such as dizziness, nystagmus, vertigo, and ataxia. Notify the physician if these signs or symptoms occur, and take such safety precautions as supervising ambulation.

• Monitor hydration if the patient experiences nausea, vomiting, or diarrhea with during therapy with an oral aminoglycoside. Request a prescription for an antiemetic or antidiarrheal agent as needed.

• Refrigerate prepared I.V. aminoglycoside solution until use; infuse the drug over at least 30 minutes.

• Do not mix aminoglycosides in the same solution with extended-spectrum penicillins; the aminoglycosides may be inactivated.

• *Administer an aminoglycoside and an extended-spectrum penicillin or cephalosporin at least 2 hours apart to prevent a decrease in the aminoglycoside level and half-life in a patient with normal renal function.*

• Expect to adjust the dosage as prescribed when administering amikacin, gentamicin, netilmicin, streptomycin, or tobramycin to an elderly patient or one with renal impairment.

• Notify the physician if adverse reactions occur.

• *Monitor for ototoxicity in a patient receiving an aminoglycoside, especially if the patient is elderly or dehydrated, has renal impairment, or is receiving concomitant therapy with another ototoxic drug.*

• Prepare the patient for audiometric testing as indicated, because high frequency tone loss usually occurs before clinical hearing loss.

• Expect to discontinue the prescribed aminoglycoside and initiate another type of antibiotic therapy if ototoxicity is suspected.

Patient teaching
• Teach the patient and family the name, dose, frequency, action, and adverse effects of the prescribed aminoglycoside.
• Stress the importance of taking the aminoglycoside for the full amount of time prescribed.
• Instruct the female patient to alert the physician if pregnancy is suspected or confirmed during aminoglycoside therapy.
• *Stress the importance of having blood tests done as instructed to monitor the serum aminoglycoside level and renal function to determine the effectiveness of therapy or detect any increased risk of adverse drug reactions.*
• *Instruct the patient to notify the nurse immediately if breathing difficulty or irregular heartbeat occurs because neuromuscular blockade may be present.*
• Caution the patient with vestibular toxicity not to perform any activity that requires alertness. Also instruct the patient to notify the physician if dizziness, nystagmus, vertigo, or ataxia occur.
• Advise the patient receiving oral aminoglycoside therapy to notify the physician if nausea, vomiting, or diarrhea occurs and to request a prescription for an antiemetic or antidiarrheal agent if needed.
• *Instruct the patient to notify the physician at once if hearing changes occur.*
• Instruct the patient to notify the physician if other adverse reactions occur, if the infection does not improve, or or if it worsens.

Evaluation
The following examples represent appropriate evaluation statements for a patient receiving an aminoglycoside.
• The patient has no conditions that contraindicate aminoglycoside therapy.
• The patient exhibits no signs of complications in the preexisting condition linked to the prescribed aminoglycoside.
• The patient exhibits no signs of adverse reactions to the prescribed aminoglycoside.
• The patient maintains normal auditory function.
• The patient and family express an accurate understanding of the points taught about the prescribed aminoglycoside.
• The patient agrees to report hearing changes immediately.

PENICILLINS

The era of chemotherapy began with the development of penicillin during World War II. Penicillin remains one of the most important and useful antibacterials, despite the availability of numerous others. Since the discovery of penicillin, researchers have developed natural and semi-synthetic congeners. The penicillins can be divided into four groups: natural penicillins, penicillinase-resistant penicillins, aminopenicillins, and extended-spectrum penicillins. (For classification of penicillins according to their antimicrobial spectrum of activity, see *Penicillins and their uses.*)

PHARMACOKINETICS

Clinical use of penicillin G, the first penicillin introduced, has been limited because it is hydrolyzed readily by penicillinase and because many organisms have developed a resistance to it. Over the years, new forms superior to penicillin G have been developed.

Absorption, distribution, metabolism, excretion
After oral administration, the penicillins are absorbed mainly in the duodenum and the upper jejunum. Extent of absorption of oral dosage forms varies and depends on such factors as the particular penicillin, the patient's gastric and intestinal pH, and the presence of food. Penicillin G is inactivated rapidly within the acidic environment of the stomach, and only 15% to 30% of an orally administered dose is absorbed in healthy, fasting adults. The presence of food in the GI tract also contributes to penicillin G destruction. Because penicillin V, a phenoxymethyl derivative, resists acid hydrolysis, it is absorbed better after oral administration. From 60% to 70% of a dose of oral penicillin V is absorbed in an adult; food intake has minimal effect.

Methicillin, which is acid-labile, is inactivated by gastric contents after oral administration; it must be administered parenterally. Dicloxacillin sodium, cloxacillin sodium, nafcillin sodium, and oxacillin sodium are acid-stable but are absorbed incompletely and erratically after oral administration. In healthy, fasting adults, 37% to 60% of a cloxacillin dose, 35% to 76% of a dicloxacillin dose, and 30% to 35% of an oxacillin dose are absorbed after oral administration. The percentage of naficillin absorbed varies considerably among individuals.

Amoxicillin is stable in the presence of acidic gastric secretions and is absorbed well after oral administration. Ampicillin is 35% to 66% absorbed. Bacampicillin hydrochloride is a prodrug of ampicillin; it is absorbed rapidly and becomes effective when hydrolyzed to ampicillin after oral administration. Food decreases the rate and extent of ampicillin absorption. Food lowers and delays the peak concentration level of amoxicillin trihydrate; however, it does not affect the total amount of drug absorbed. Food does not alter the absorption of bacampicillin.

Azlocillin sodium, carbenicillin, mezlocillin sodium, piperacillin sodium, and ticarcillin disodium are not ab-

Penicillins and their uses

Natural or semisynthetic derivatives of the *Penicillium* fungus, penicillins are prepared by chemically modifying a natural penicillin. The resulting drugs are classified according to their antimicrobial spectrum of activity.

DRUG	ANTIMICROBIAL SPECTRUM
Natural penicillins	
penicillin G benzathine penicillin G potassium penicillin G procaine penicillin G sodium penicillin V potassium	Gram-positive organisms: *Actinomyces israelii* *Staphylococcus aureus* (non-penicillinase-producing strains) *Streptococci* (groups A,B,C, and D) *Streptococcus viridans* *Streptococcus faecalis* Beta-hemolytic streptococci *Streptococcus bovis* *Streptococcus (Diplococcus) pneumoniae* *Eubacterium* species *Bacillus anthracis* *Peptostreptococcus* species *Clostridium tetani* *Clostridium perfringens* *Listeria monocytogenes* Gram-negative organisms: *Bacteroides* (all species except for many strains of *B. fragilis*) *Neisseria gonorrhoeae* *Neisseria meningitidis* *Pasteurella multocida* *Spirillum minor* *Streptobacillus moniliformis* Anaerobic oganisms: *Treponema pallidum* *Treponema pertenue* *Borrelia recurrentis* *Leptospira icterohaemorrhagiae*

DRUG	ANTIMICROBIAL SPECTRUM
Penicillinase-resistant penicillins	
cloxacillin dicloxacillin methicillin nafcillin oxacillin	*Staphylococcus aureus* *Staphylococcus epidermidis* streptococci (some species)
Aminopenicillins	
amoxicillin ampicillin bacampicillin	Gram-positive organisms: staphylococci (non-penicillinase-producing streptococci (some species) Gram-negative organisms: *Escherichia coli* *Haemophilus influenzae* *Neisseria gonorrhoeae* *Proteus mirabilis* *Salmonella* species *Shigella* species
Extended-spectrum penicillins	
azlocillin carbenicillin mezlocillin piperacillin ticarcillin	Gram-positive and gram-negative organisms that natural penicillins and aminopenicillins are active against, plus: *Pseudomonas aeruginosa* *Proteus* species (indole-positive) *Providencia* species *Enterobacter* species *Citrobacter* species *Serratia* species *Acinetobacter* species *Veillonella* species

sorbed well from the GI tract and must be given parenterally. Only carbenicillin is available orally in ester form, which is acid-stable, allowing carbenicillin to be absorbed partially from the small intestine. After absorption, the ester is hydrolyzed, and free carbenicillin appears in the systemic circulation.

Intramuscular administration is indicated primarily when compliance with an oral regimen is inconvenient or questionable. Because long-acting preparations of penicillin G (penicillin G benzathine and penicillin G procaine) are relatively insoluble, they must be administered by the I.M. route. Penicillin G benzathine is absorbed slowly after I.M. administration and is detectable even after 28 days. Penicillin G procaine usually is preferred for I.M. administration because it provides more consistent steady-state levels for up to 24 hours. Also, penicillin G procaine provides

the local anesthetic properties of procaine, thereby reducing pain at the injection site.

Penicillins are distributed widely to most areas of the body, including the lungs, liver, kidneys, muscle, bone, and placenta. The highest concentrations occur in the plasma, where much of a dose is bound reversibly to plasma albumin. Because of their lipid insolubility, penicillins do not penetrate cell membranes well. Distribution to the eyes, cerebrospinal fluid, and prostate is poor in the absence of inflammation; inflammation alters normal barriers and enhances distribution. High concentrations appear in the urine, making penicillins useful in treating urinary tract infections.

Penicillins are metabolized to a limited extent in the liver to inactive metabolites. They are excreted 60% unchanged by the kidneys, largely by glomerular filtration and

Peak concentration levels and durations of action for penicillins

The following chart provides pharmacokinetic information about the different penicillins and their administration in fasting adults.

DRUG	ADMINISTRATION ROUTE	PEAK CONCENTRATION LEVEL	DURATION OF ACTION
penicillin G, penicillin V	Oral	½ to 1 hour	6 hours
penicillin G potassium, penicillin G sodium	I.M.	15 to 30 minutes	3 to 6 hours
penicillin G procaine	I.M.	1 to 3 hours	1 to 2 days
penicillin G benzathine	I.M.	13 to 24 hours	1 to 4 weeks
cloxacillin, dicloxacillin, nafcillin, oxacillin	Oral	½ to 2 hours	4 to 6 hours
methicillin, nafcillin, oxacillin	I.M.	½ to 1 hour	4 to 6 hours
methicillin, nafcillin, oxacillin (1 gram)	I.V.	Immediately after infusion	2 to 3 hours
amoxicillin, ampicillin	Oral	1 to 2 hours	6 to 8 hours
ampicillin	I.M.	1 hour	6 to 8 hours
ampicillin	I.V. (30 minutes)	Immediately after infusion	6 hours
bacampicillin	Oral	½ to 1½ hours	6 to 8 hours
carbenicillin, mezlocillin, piperacillin, ticarcillin	I.M.	½ to 2 hours	6 to 8 hours
azlocillin, carbenicillin, mezlocillin, piperacillin, ticarcillin	I.V.	Immediately after infusion	6 to 8 hours

active tubular secretion. Because excretion into the urine is rapid, they have a short half-life, ranging from less than 30 minutes for penicillin G to 72 minutes for carbenicillin. Biliary excretion is important for nafcillin only. Reduced renal function (creatinine clearance less than 30 to 40 ml/ minute) may require reduced doses of certain penicillins, such as penicillin G, carbenicillin, ticarcillin, azlocillin, mezlocillin, and piperacillin.

Onset, peak, duration

Peak concentration levels and durations of action for the penicillins vary, depending on the specific drug and the route of administration. (For specific data, see *Peak concentration levels and durations of action for penicillins.*)

PHARMACODYNAMICS

Penicillins usually are bactericidal in action. Traditionally, they have been thought to inhibit the last step of mucopeptide synthesis in the bacterial cell wall. Recent studies suggest a more complicated mechanism of action.

Mechanism of action

Although the exact mechanism of action of penicillins is not understood, research has shown that they bind reversibly to several enzymes outside the bacterial cytoplasmic membrane. These enzymes, known as penicillin-binding proteins (PBPs), are involved in cell-wall synthesis and cell division. Interference with these processes increases internal osmotic pressure and ruptures the cell.

The antibacterial activity of penicillins depends partly on their ability to bind to the target enzymes. The cell walls of gram-positive bacteria are relatively permeable to most penicillins, especially natural penicillins. However, gram-negative bacteria possess an outer membrane around the cell wall that decreases accessibility to the PBPs. The production of penicillinases (enzymes that convert penicillin to inactive penicilloic acid) by the bacteria also contributes to bacterial resistance. Aminopenicillins and extended-spectrum penicillins penetrate the outer membranes of gram-negative bacteria more readily than the natural penicillins, such as penicillin G, or penicillinase-resistant penicillins, such as cloxacillin, dicloxacillin, methicillin, nafcillin, and oxacillin. The greater ability of the penicillin derivatives to gain access to the PBPs may relate to their increased antibacterial activity against these gram-negative organisms.

PHARMACOTHERAPEUTICS

No other class of antibacterials provides as wide a spectrum of antimicrobial activity as the penicillins.

Natural penicillins and their derivatives are used to treat many common infections. Therapeutic indications include streptococcal pharyngitis, streptococcal endocarditis, staphylococcal infections, pneumococcal pneumonia, meningococcal meningitis, gonorrhea, syphilis, GI infections caused by *Shigella* and *Salmonella,* upper respiratory tract infections, otitis media, sinusitis caused by *Haemophilus influenzae,* and various gram-negative bacillary infections. (For more information, see *Penicillins and their uses,* page 1009.)

Concurrent administration of probenecid increases the penicillin serum concentration by 50% to 100%, because probenecid blocks tubular secretion of penicillin. Combined probenecid-penicillin therapy is used to treat bacterial endocarditis and acute gonorrhea.

penicillin G aqueous. Penicillin G is available for I.M. or I.V. administration in two salts—penicillin G potassium and penicillin G sodium. A natural penicillin and the prototype for all penicillins, aqueous penicillin G is used to treat such disorders as meningitis, septicemia, pericarditis, endocarditis, severe pneumonia, and other serious infections.
Usual adult dosage: 600,000 to 5 million units I.V. or I.M. every 4 to 6 hours.
Usual pediatric dosage: 100,000 to 250,000 units/kg I.V. or I.M. daily in divided doses every 4 hours.

penicillin G benzathine (Bicillin, Bicillin L-A). Penicillin G benzathine is used to manage streptococcal upper respiratory infection (URI) and syphilis, and to prevent rheumatic fever. It should not be used to treat gonorrhea because the peak concentration is too low for satisfactory results. The suspension form can be given I.M. only.
Usual adult dosage: for group A streptococcal URIs, 1.2 million units I.M. in a single injection or 400,000 to 600,000 units P.O. every 4 to 6 hours for 10 days; for prophylaxis of poststreptococcal rheumatic fever, 1.2 million units I.M. once a month, 600,000 units I.M. twice a month, or 200,000 units P.O. b.i.d.; for syphilis of less than 1 year's duration, 2.4 million units I.M. in a single dose; for syphilis of more than 1 year's duration, 2.4 million units I.M. weekly for 3 successive weeks.
Usual pediatric dosage: for congenital syphilis in children ages 2 and under, 50,000 units/kg I.M. as a single dose;

for group A streptococcal URIs, 25,000 to 90,000 units/ kg P.O. daily in three to six divided doses, or 900,000 units I.M. in a single injection for children over 27 kg, or 300,000 to 600,000 units I.M. in a single injection for children under 27 kg; for prophylaxis of poststreptococcal rheumatic fever, 1.2 million units I.M. once a month, 600,000 units I.M. twice a month, or 200,000 units P.O. b.i.d.

penicillin G potassium (Pentids). This oral form of penicillin G is used to treat mild to moderately severe bacterial infections, such as streptococcal URI, pneumococcal respiratory tract infection, or staphylococcal infection.
Usual adult dosage: for mild streptococcal URI, 200,000 to 250,000 units P.O. every 6 to 8 hours for 10 days; for moderately severe URI, 400,000 to 500,000 units P.O. every 8 hours for 10 days or 800,000 units every 12 hours P.O.; for mild to moderate pneumococcal respiratory tract infection, 400,000 to 500,000 units P.O. every 6 hours for at least 2 days; for staphylococcal infection, 200,000 to 500,000 units P.O. every 6 to 8 hours until therapy is effective.
Usual pediatric dosage: for the same indications as adults, 25,000 to 90,000 units/kg P.O. daily in three to six divided doses.

penicillin G procaine (Wycillin). Used when a long-acting preparation is preferred and high blood concentrations are not required to treat systemic bacterial infections that are penicillin G-sensitive, this suspension is administered I.M. only.
Usual adult and pediatric dosage: for moderately severe penicillin G-sensitive systemic infection, 600,000 to 1.2 million units I.M. daily.

penicillin V or **penicillin V potassium [phenoxymethyl penicillin]** (Pen-Vee K, V-Cillin K). This drug is acid-stable; when given orally, it provides a higher peak serum concentration than a similar dose of penicillin G does. Penicillin V is not a substitute for parenterally administered penicillin G. Penicillin V is used to treat mild infections of the throat, respiratory tract, or soft tissues.
Usual adult dosage: 125 to 500 mg P.O. every 6 hours.
Usual pediatric dosage: 25 to 50 mg/kg P.O. daily every 6 to 8 hours.

cloxacillin sodium (Tegopen). Used to treat infections caused by penicillinase-producing staphylococci, this penicillinase-resistant penicillin is not absorbed as well as dicloxacillin after oral administration.
Usual adult dosage: 250 to 500 mg P.O. every 6 hours.
Usual pediatric dosage: 50 to 100 mg/kg P.O. daily in divided doses every 6 hours.

dicloxacillin sodium (Dynapen). This penicillinase-resistant penicillin is the oral drug of choice against staphylococci because of its superior absorption and lower minimum inhibitory concentration levels.
Usual adult dosage: 125 to 250 mg P.O. every 6 hours.
Usual pediatric dosage: 12.5 to 25 mg/kg P.O. daily in equally divided doses every 6 hours.

methicillin sodium (Staphcillin). First of the semisynthetic penicillinase-resistant penicillins, methicillin is effective against *S. aureus.* Because it is inactivated by gastric acid, it must be administered parenterally. Methicillin seems to be associated with interstitial nephritis and currently is used less commonly than nafcillin or oxacillin.
Usual adult dosage: 1 gram I.M. every 4 to 6 hours, or 1 gram I.V. every 6 hours.
Usual pediatric dosage: 100 to 300 mg/kg I.M. or I.V. daily in divided doses every 4 to 6 hours.

nafcillin sodium (Unipen). Similar to oxacillin in its activity against *S. aureus,* nafcillin is a penicillinase-resistant penicillin. Nafcillin is excreted in bile; therefore, dosage adjustment is not required in patients with renal impairment.
Usual adult dosage: 2 to 4 grams P.O. daily in divided doses every 6 hours, or 2 to 12 grams I.M. or I.V. daily in divided doses every 4 to 6 hours.
Usual pediatric dosage: 50 to 100 mg/kg P.O. daily in divided doses every 4 to 6 hours or 100 to 200 mg/kg I.M. or I.V. daily in divided doses every 4 to 6 hours.

oxacillin sodium (Prostaphlin). A penicillinase-resistant penicillin, oxacillin is as effective as methicillin against staphylococcal infections and causes less interstitial nephritis. Orally administered oxacillin produces less predictable serum concentrations than does dicloxacillin.
Usual adult dosage: 2 to 4 grams P.O. daily in divided doses every 6 hours, or 2 to 12 grams I.M. or I.V. daily in divided doses every 4 to 6 hours.
Usual pediatric dosage: for children under 40 kg, 30 to 40 mg/kg P.O. daily in divided doses every 6 hours, or 50 to 200 mg/kg I.M. or I.V. daily in divided doses every 4 to 6 hours; for children over 40 kg, same as adult.

amoxicillin/clavulanate potassium (Augmentin). The clavulanic acid inhibits beta-lactamases that usually inactivate amoxicillin. This combination provides an antibacterial spectrum of activity similar to that of amoxicillin, with added coverage for *Staphylococcus aureus* and *Klebsiella.* It is used to treat skin infections caused by beta-lactamase-producing staphylococci, otitis caused by *H. influenzae,* and urinary tract infections (UTIs) caused by beta-lactamase-producing *E. coli* and *Klebsiella.*

Usual adult dosage: 250 mg of amoxicillin/125 mg of clavulanic acid P.O. every 8 hours; 250- and 500-mg tablets contain 125 mg of clavulanic acid.
Usual pediatric dosage: 20 to 40 mg/kg P.O. daily in divided doses every 8 hours.

amoxicillin trihydrate (Amoxil). An analogue of ampicillin similar in spectrum of activity and pharmacology, amoxicillin is an aminopenicillin. This drug is less effective against shigellosis.
Usual adult dosage: for systemic infections including acute and chronic UTIs caused by susceptible strains of gram-positive and gram-negative organisms, 750 mg to 1.5 grams P.O. daily in divided doses every 8 hours; for uncomplicated gonorrhea, 3 grams P.O. with 1 gram of probenecid as a single dose along with 500 mg of tetracycline P.O. q.i.d. for 7 days.
Usual pediatric dosage: 20 to 40 mg/kg P.O. daily in divided doses every 8 hours.

ampicillin (Omnipen). An aminopenicillin, ampicillin is acid-stable and penicillinase-sensitive. When it was introduced, most *E. coli, H. influenzae, N. gonorrhoeae,* and *Proteus mirabilis* strains were sensitive. Today, ampicillin-resistant strains have emerged.
Usual adult dosage: for respiratory tract infections, 250 to 500 mg P.O. every 6 hours, or 1 to 3 grams I.M. or I.V. every 6 hours.
Usual pediatric dosage: for acute and chronic UTIs or URIs caused by gram-positive or gram-negative organisms, 50 to 100 mg/kg P.O. daily in divided doses every 6 hours, or 100 to 200 mg/kg I.M. or I.V. daily in divided doses every 6 hours; for meningitis, up to 300 mg/kg I.V. daily in divided doses every 4 hours.

ampicillin sodium/sulbactam sodium (Unasyn). This parenteral antibacterial combination agent consists of the antibiotic ampicillin and the beta-lactamase inhibitor sulbactam. It is indicated to treat skin, intra-abdominal, and gynecologic infections and has a broader antibacterial spectrum of activity than ampicillin alone.
Usual adult dosage: 1.5 gram I.V. or I.M. (1 gram ampicillin and 0.5 gram sulbactam) to 3 gram (2 gram ampicillin and 1 gram sulbactam) every 6 hours, with daily dosage of sulbactam not to exceed 4 gram. The dosage should be adjusted for patients with impaired renal function.
Usual pediatric dosage: for children under age 12, the safety and efficacy of this drug has not been established.

bacampicillin hydrochloride (Spectrobid). This aminopenicillin is an ester of ampicillin and is hydrolyzed to ampicillin during absorption from the GI tract. It is used to treat upper and lower respiratory tract, urinary tract, and skin infections caused by susceptible organisms.

Usual adult dosage: 400 to 800 mg P.O. every 12 hours; for gonorrhea, 1.6 grams P.O. with 1 gram of probenecid as a single dose.

Usual pediatric dosage: in children under 25 kg, 12.5 to 25 mg/kg P.O. every 12 hours; for children 25 kg and over, same as adult.

azlocillin sodium (Azlin). An extended-spectrum penicillin, azlocillin is as active as piperacillin against *P. aeruginosa* but is less active against most Enterobacteriaceae and anaerobes. Azlocillin is used primarily with an aminoglycoside to treat *Pseudomonas* infections in patients with extensive burns or cystic fibrosis.

Usual adult dosage: 3 grams I.V. every 4 hours, or 4 grams I.V. every 6 hours.

Usual pediatric dosage: for acute exacerbation of cystic fibrosis, 75 mg/kg I.V. every 4 hours or 100 to 200 mg/kg I.V. every 8 hours; maximum daily dosage, 24 grams.

carbenicillin disodium (Geopen). An extended-spectrum penicillin, carbenicillin has an antibacterial spectrum of activity similar to that of ampicillin with important added activity against *P. aeruginosa,* the indole-positive *Proteus,* and *Enterobacter.* Large parenteral doses are necessary to treat serious *Pseudomonas* infections outside the urinary tract. With large doses of carbenicillin, the patient receives significant amounts of sodium, which can be problematic for patients with hypertension or congestive heart failure.

Usual adult dosage: for systemic infections caused by susceptible strains of gram-positive and especially gram-negative organisms (*Proteus, P. aeruginosa*), 30 to 40 grams I.V. infusion daily in divided doses every 4 to 6 hours; for UTIs, 200 mg/kg I.M. or I.V. infusion daily in divided doses every 4 to 6 hours.

Usual pediatric dosage: for systemic infections caused by susceptible strains of gram-positive and gram-negative organisms, 250 to 500 mg/kg I.V. infusion daily in divided doses every 4 to 6 hours; for UTIs, 50 to 200 mg/kg I.M. or I.V. infusion daily in divided doses every 4 to 6 hours.

carbenicillin indanyl sodium (Geocillin). As an extended-spectrum penicillin and oral form of carbenicillin, this drug is used only to treat certain UTIs and prostatitis caused by susceptible strains of gram-negative organisms. Carbenicillin indanyl sodium should not be used to treat systemic infections because the blood concentration remains too low. The drug is not recommended for pediatric use.

Usual adult dosage: for UTIs and prostatitis caused by susceptible strains of gram-negative organisms, 382 to 764 mg P.O. q.i.d.

mezlocillin sodium (Mezlin). An extended-spectrum penicillin, the activity of mezlocillin against *P. aeruginosa* is similar to that of ticarcillin. Mezlocillin has some activity against *K. pneumoniae;* however, it is used primarily with an aminoglycoside. Of all extended-spectrum penicillins, mezlocillin contains the least amount of sodium.

Usual adult dosage: 3 grams I.V. or I.M. every 4 hours, or 4 grams I.V. or I.M. every 6 hours.

Usual pediatric dosage: 50 mg/kg I.V. every 4 hours.

piperacillin sodium (Pipracil). The most active of the extended-spectrum penicillins against *P. aeruginosa,* piperacillin provides increased activity against *K. pneumoniae* in vitro. Clinical trials have not shown that piperacillin is more effective than carbenicillin or ticarcillin when used with an aminoglycoside. Piperacillin should be reserved for clinical situations in which a deleterious platelet dysfunction or salt loading may occur with carbenicillin or ticarcillin or for situations in which the infecting organism is sensitive to piperacillin only. This drug also can be used with amikacin as empiric therapy for the febrile neutropenic patient.

Usual adult dosage: 12 to 24 grams I.V. daily, 3 grams I.M. or I.V. every 4 hours, or 4 grams I.M. or I.V. every 6 hours; for prophylaxis against surgical infections, 2 grams I.V. 30 to 60 minutes before surgery; may be repeated during and after surgery.

Usual pediatric dosage: for ages 12 and older, same as adult; for under age 12, dosage has not been established.

ticarcillin disodium (Ticar). An extended-spectrum penicillin, ticarcillin is similar to carbenicillin but is more active against *P. aeruginosa.* Like carbenicillin, ticarcillin is synergistic with aminoglycosides against *P. aeruginosa.* Ticarcillin and carbenicillin have a similar sodium content; however, ticarcillin delivers less sodium because the daily dosage is smaller. No oral form is available.

Usual adult dosage: for uncomplicated UTIs, 1 gram I.V. or I.M. every 6 hours; for complicated UTIs, 3 grams I.V. every 4 to 6 hours; for septicemia, 3 grams I.V. every 3 to 6 hours.

Usual pediatric dosage: for neonates up to 2 kg, 100 mg/kg I.M. initially, then 75 mg/kg every 8 hours; for neonates 2 kg and over, 100 mg/kg I.M. initially, then 75 mg/kg every 4 to 6 hours; for children up to 40 kg, 25 to 75 mg/kg every 4 to 8 hours; for children over 40 kg, same as adult.

ticarcillin disodium/clavulanate potassium (Timentin). This combination contains 3 grams of ticarcillin and 100 mg of clavulanic acid. Its antibacterial spectrum resembles that of ticarcillin, with added coverage for *S. aureus* and *Klebsiella.*

Usual adult dosage: 3.1 grams I.V. every 4 to 6 hours.

Usual pediatric dosage: for ages 12 and older, same as adult; for under age 12, dosage has not been established.

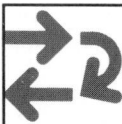

DRUG INTERACTIONS

Penicillins

This chart summarizes significant interactions between penicillins and other drugs. The nurse should be familiar with these interactions before administering any penicillin.

DRUG	INTERACTING DRUGS	POSSIBLE EFFECTS	NURSING IMPLICATIONS
penicillins	probenecid	Increases plasma penicillin concentration	• May be used to enhance antibiotic efficiency.
	methotrexate	Interfere with renal tubular secretion of methotrexate	• Monitor the patient for enhanced action and possible methotrexate toxicity.
	tetracyclines, chloramphenicol	Interfere with bactericidal action of penicillin	• Separate the doses of these drugs by several hours if they are used together.
penicillin G (high doses) and extended-spectrum penicillins: azlocillin, carbenicillin, mezlocillin, piperacillin, ticarcillin	aminoglycosides	Inactivate aminoglycosides	• Do not mix these drugs; separate doses by at least 1 hour.
penicillin V	neomycin	Decreases absorption of penicillin V	• Separate doses by at least 1 hour.
penicillin V, ampicillin	oral contraceptives	Alter GI flora, increasing the risk of decreased contraceptive efficacy and breakthrough bleeding	• Advise the patient to use an alternative contraceptive method during antibacterial therapy and for 1 week after therapy.

Drug interactions

High doses of penicillin G and extended-spectrum penicillins (azlocillin, carbenicillin, mezlocillin, piperacillin, and ticarcillin) inactivate aminoglycosides. This interaction is clinically relevant in patients with poor renal function because elevated blood concentrations of both agents may exist simultaneously. Penicillins should not be mixed in the same I.V. fluid with aminoglycosides.

Inactivation of aminoglycosides by penicillins depends on the penicillin concentration, the temperature of the blood sample, and the duration of contact between the two drugs. When the serum aminoglycoside level is measured, the sample should be kept on ice while being transported to the laboratory and should be stored in the laboratory until the assay can be made. The presence of penicillins in the serum samples may result in falsely decreased aminoglycoside concentrations. (For additional interactions, see *Drug interactions: Penicillins.*)

ADVERSE DRUG REACTIONS

The low incidence of serious toxicity and the relatively low cost make penicillins the drugs of choice for treating susceptible organisms in nonallergic patients. Toxic effects include hypersensitivity reactions, neurotoxicity, nephrotoxicity, electrolyte imbalances, and hematologic reactions.

Hypersensitivity reactions are the major adverse reactions to penicillins. Penicillin allergy occurs in 3% to 5% of the population and in up to 10% of those who have received penicillin previously. Large doses or prolonged therapy may lead to allergic reactions. Allergic reactions are less common when the drugs are administered orally and more common when given parenterally. Penicillin hypersensitivity may occur as anaphylactic reactions, serum sickness, drug fever, or various skin rashes.

Certain extended-spectrum penicillins (carbenicillin and ticarcillin) are administered as disodium salts. The increased sodium or potassium intake with these drugs may pose a therapeutic problem for patients with cardiac disease or decreased renal function.

Penicillins can produce hematologic reactions. A positive Coombs' test for hemolytic anemia (evidenced by a fall in hemoglobin concentration) can occur in patients receiving high doses of I.V. penicillin G (in excess of 10 million units a day in uremic patients, or 40 million units a day in patients with normal renal function). Withdrawing the penicillin usually returns the hemoglobin to the baseline normal value. Penicillins (especially carbenicillin and ticarcillin) may induce platelet dysfunction, causing prolonged bleeding time. This is significant in patients with uremia or hepatic disease. Platelet function returns to normal when the drug is discontinued.

Hepatotoxicity occasionally has developed during oxacillin therapy. Adverse GI reactions, such as glossitis, nausea, vomiting, and diarrhea, usually are associated with oral use. They occur most commonly with ampicillin. The aminopenicillins and extended-spectrum penicillins can produce pseudomembranous colitis.

Seizures or coma caused by direct central nervous system (CNS) irritation can occur with penicillin G doses greater than 20 million units daily in patients with decreased renal function.

Anaphylactic shock is a syndrome characterized by rapidly developing dyspnea and hypotension. Immediate treatment includes epinephrine, corticosteroids, antihistamines, and other resuscitative measures. Serum sickness may occur 7 to 10 days after penicillin treatment is initiated, but is uncommon. It may produce fever, urticaria (hives), joint pain, or angioneurotic edema. Patients with infectious mononucleosis may develop a macular or maculopapular erythematous skin rash when given ampicillin.

Renal failure and interstitial nephritis may occur in patients receiving large parenteral doses of penicillin G or methicillin. Usually, the reaction begins within 5 to 10 days after therapy begins. Signs and symptoms may include fever, eosinophilia, hematuria, proteinuria, or pyuria. Renal biopsy has revealed tubular damage and interstitial mononuclear cells and eosinophils, considered to be components of a hypersensitivity reaction. This reaction usually subsides when the penicillin is discontinued. In some cases, corticosteroids may be administered to improve renal function.

Some patients may experience an allergic reaction to tartrazine, a dye contained in certain penicillin preparations.

NURSING PROCESS APPLICATION

The following information assists the nurse in caring for a patient who is receiving a penicillin.

Assessment
• Review the patient's history for a preexisting condition that contraindicates the use of a penicillin, such as known hypersensitivity to any penicillin.
• Review the patient's history for a preexisting condition that requires cautious use of a penicillin, such as pregnancy, drug allergy, a history of asthma, mononucleosis, a hemorrhagic condition, or electrolyte imbalance.
• Assess the patient for adverse reactions to the prescribed penicillin, such as hypersensitivity reactions, neurotoxicity, nephrotoxicity, electrolyte imbalances, or hematologic reactions.
• Assess the patient for bleeding tendencies regularly.

• Review the patient's medication history to identify the use of drugs that may interact with the prescribed penicillin, such as aminoglycosides, probenecid, methotrexate, tetracyclines, chloramphenicol, neomycin, or oral contraceptives.
• Evaluate the effectiveness of the prescribed penicillin regularly.
• Evaluate the patient's and family's knowledge about the prescribed penicillin.

Nursing diagnoses
The following examples represent appropriate nursing diagnoses for a patient receiving a penicillin.
• Potential for injury related to a preexisting condition that contraindicates the use of a penicillin
• Potential for injury related to a preexisting condition that requires cautious use of a penicillin
• Potential for injury related to adverse drug reactions
• Altered protection related to platelet dysfunction caused by the prescribed penicillin
• Knowledge deficit related to the prescribed penicillin

Planning and implementation
• Do not administer a penicillin to a patient with a condition that contraindicates its use.
• Administer a penicillin cautiously to a patient at risk because of a preexisting condition.
• Monitor the patient closely for adverse reactions during penicillin therapy. Allergic reactions are the major adverse reactions to penicillin, especially large doses, parenteral administration, or prolonged therapy. Keep in mind that the patient may become sensitized to penicillin through exposure.
• *Obtain a complete patient history to assess the risk of allergic reaction whenever penicillin therapy is considered. Ask the patient about previous penicillin use (name of drug, route of administration, type of adverse reaction, and date of occurrence). If a patient is allergic to penicillin and its derivatives, alternative therapy should be considered.*
• *Discontinue the prescribed penicillin at once if the patient develops anaphylactic shock (exhibited by rapidly developing dyspnea and hypotension). Notify the physician and prepare to administer immediate treatment, such as epinephrine, corticosteroids, antihistamines, and other resuscitative measures as indicated.*
• Observe the patient for evidence of serum sickness (fever, urticaria, joint pain, or angioneurotic edema) for 7 to 10 days after penicillin therapy is initiated. If evidence of this rare form of penicillin hypersensitivity appears, notify the physician. Expect to discontinue the drug and administer symptomatic treatment, such as an antihistaminic and antipyretic agent.

• Inspect the patient's skin routinely for rash, another sign of penicillin hypersensitivity. For example, the patient with infectious mononucleosis will develop a macular or maculopapular erythematous rash when given ampicillin. Notify the physician and expect to discontinue the prescribed penicillin if skin rash occurs.

• Monitor the patient's temperature for a sudden elevation that may indicate drug fever. Notify the physician if a fever occurs.

• Monitor for decreased level of consciousness or seizures in a patient with decreased renal function who is receiving more than 20 million units of Penicillin G daily. Take seizure precautions upon initiation of drug therapy.

• Expect to administer a reduced dosage of penicillin G, carbenicillin, ticarcillin, azlocillin, mezlocillin, or piperacillin as prescribed for a patient with reduced renal function.

• Observe for signs of renal failure or interstitial nephritis, such as fever, eosinophilia, hematuria, proteinuria, or pyuria, which usually occur 5 to 10 days after therapy begins in a patient receiving large parenteral doses of penicillin G or methicillin. Notify the physician if any of these signs occur and expect to discontinue the drug. Corticosteroids may be required to improve renal function.

• Monitor the patient for signs of hemolytic anemia, such as a positive Coombs' test (a sudden fall in hemoglobin concentration level). This reaction is most common when the patient is receiving high doses of I.V. penicillin G (in excess of 10 million units a day in uremic patients or 40 million units a day in patients with normal renal function). Expect to discontinue the drug.

• Monitor electrolyte levels if the patient is receiving a penicillin that is high in sodium or potassium, such as carbenicillin or ticarcillin.

• Review liver function studies for the patient receiving oxacillin. Particularly note abnormalities that suggest hepatotoxicity.

• Observe for signs and symptoms of pseudomembranous colitis, such as abdominal pain or diarrhea, in a patient receiving an aminopenicillin or extended-spectrum penicillin. If signs or symptoms occur, notify the physician before giving the next dose.

• Monitor for adverse GI reactions in a patient receiving an oral penicillin, especially ampicillin. If nausea, vomiting, diarrhea, or glossitis occurs, monitor the patient's hydration and request a prescription for an antiemetic or antidiarrheal agent as needed. If the GI reactions are severe, expect the drug to be discontinued or replaced with a parenteral form.

• Do not mix an aminoglycoside with an extended-spectrum penicillin or a high dose of penicillin G. This prevents inactivation of the aminoglycoside.

• *Administer oral penicillin 1 hour before or 2 hours after meals to ensure an optimal serum concentration.*

• Administer penicillin G benzathine by the I.M. route only.

• Notify the physician if adverse reactions occur.

• Monitor the patient closely for bleeding tendencies, such as easy bruising, bleeding gums, or blood in the urine or stool.

• Monitor the patient's platelet count during penicillin therapy. Prolonged bleeding time is most likely to occur in a patient with uremic or hepatic disease who is receiving carbenicillin or ticarcillin. Expect to discontinue the drug if this occurs.

Patient teaching

• Teach the patient and family the name, dose, frequency, action, and adverse effects of the prescribed penicillin.

• Advise the patient to complete the course of penicillin therapy.

• *Advise the patient to take an oral penicillin 1 hour before or 2 hours after meals to ensure an optimal serum concentration.*

• *Review the signs and symptoms of allergic reactions with the patient. Instruct the patient to withhold the drug and notify the physician if such a reaction occurs. If an anaphylactic reaction occurs, instruct the family to seek emergency help immediately.*

• Advise the patient who is allergic to penicillins to wear a Medic Alert necklace or bracelet stating this information.

• Encourage the patient to have prescribed blood or urine tests done and to keep follow-up appointments.

• Instruct the patient to notify the physician if the infection does not subside, it it worsens, or if adverse reactions occur.

• Describe the risk of elevated sodium or potassium levels to a patient with cardiac disease or decreased renal function who is taking carbenicillin or ticarcillin. Teach the patient to recognize and report the signs and symptoms of sodium and potassium imbalances.

Evaluation

The following examples represent appropriate evaluation statements for a patient receiving a penicillin.

• The patient has no conditions that contraindicate penicillin therapy.

• The patient exhibits no signs of complications in the preexisting condition linked to the prescribed penicillin.

• The patient exhibits no adverse reactions to the prescribed penicillin.

• The patient's platelet count remains normal throughout penicillin therapy.

• The patient and family express an accurate understanding of the points taught about the prescribed penicillin.

• The patient completes the entire course of penicillin therapy as prescribed.

CEPHALOSPORINS

Most of the antibacterial agents introduced for clinical use in recent years have been cephalosporins. Because penicillins and cephalosporin molecules have a beta-lactam structure, some cross-sensitivity occurs. The pharmacokinetic properties and mechanisms of action of the cephalosporins resemble those of the penicillins. Cephalosporins are categorized into groups called generations, based on their antibacterial spectra of activity. (For the specific drugs in each generation, see *Antibacterial activity of cephalosporins.*)

PHARMACOKINETICS

A few cephalosporins are administered orally. Those that are not absorbed from the GI tract must be administered parenterally; I.M. injections may be painful. The degree of protein binding and renal excretion varies.

Absorption, distribution, metabolism, excretion

Cephradine, cephalexin monohydrate, cefadroxil monohydrate, cefaclor, cefuroxime axetil, and cefixime are absorbed from the GI tract and administered orally. Food usually delays the absorption of the oral cephalosporins, resulting in lower peak serum concentration levels. However, peak concentrations of cefadroxil are not affected by food. Many cephalosporins are administered I.M., although peak concentrations are higher when the drugs are administered I.V.

After absorption, the cephalosporins are distributed widely, although they are not distributed into the CNS. Most are distributed poorly into cerebrospinal fluid (CSF), even when meninges are inflamed, but some (cefuroxime sodium, cefotaxime sodium, moxalactam disodium, cefoperazone sodium, ceftizoxime sodium, ceftriaxone sodium, and ceftazidime) penetrate CSF sufficiently to be useful for treating meningitis.

The cephalosporins are distributed widely to tissues and fluids, including pleural, pericardial, and synovial fluids; bone; and the placenta. Biliary levels usually are high, especially after cefoperazone administration. (For an illustration of distribution sites, see *Distribution of cephalosporins,* page 1018.)

Many cephalosporins are not metabolized at all. Cephalothin sodium, cephapirin sodium, and cefotaxime are metabolized to the desacetyl forms and provide less antibacterial activity than the parent compounds do. Ceftriaxone is metabolized to a small extent in the intestines to inactive metabolites, which are excreted via the biliary system.

Antibacterial activity of cephalosporins

This chart shows the generations of cephalosporins and the basis for those generations—their antibacterial spectrum of activity.

CEPHALOSPORINS	ANTIBACTERIAL SPECTRUM OF ACTIVITY
First-generation	
cefadroxil cefazolin cephalexin cephalothin cephapirin cephradine	Gram-positive organisms: 　Most staphylococci 　Groups A and B hemolytic 　streptococci 　Most streptococci Gram-negative organisms: 　*Escherichia coli* 　*Klebsiella* species 　*Proteus mirabilis* 　*Haemophilus influenzae*
Second-generation	
cefaclor cefamandole cefmetazole cefonicid ceforanide cefoxitin cefuroxime	All of the above Gram-negative organisms: 　*Neisseria gonorroheae* 　*Neisseria meningitidis* 　Indole-positive *Proteus* 　species 　*Providencia* species 　*Enterobacter* species 　*Citrobacter* species Anaerobic organisms: 　*Clostridium* species 　*Peptococcus* species 　*Peptostreptococcus* species 　*Fusobacterium* species 　*Bacteroides* species
Third-generation	
cefixime cefoperazone cefotaxime cefotetan ceftazidime ceftizoxime ceftriaxone moxalactam	All of the above Gram-negative organisms: 　*Pseudomonas aeruginosa* 　*Serratia* species 　*Acinetobacter* species

All cephalosporins are excreted primarily unchanged by the kidneys with the exception of cefoperazone and ceftriaxone, which are excreted in the feces via bile. Renal elimination occurs via glomerular filtration and tubular secretion. Dosage adjustments are necessary in patients with renal insufficiency because the serum concentration will increase. Dosages need not be altered for cefoperazone or ceftriaxone in patients with impaired renal function unless hepatic impairment exists also.

Distribution of cephalosporins

Therapeutic levels of cephalosporins are achieved in most tissues, but some cephalosporins are more effective than others in treating infections in certain areas. This illustration shows which cephalosporins are distributed most effectively to specific body parts or systems.

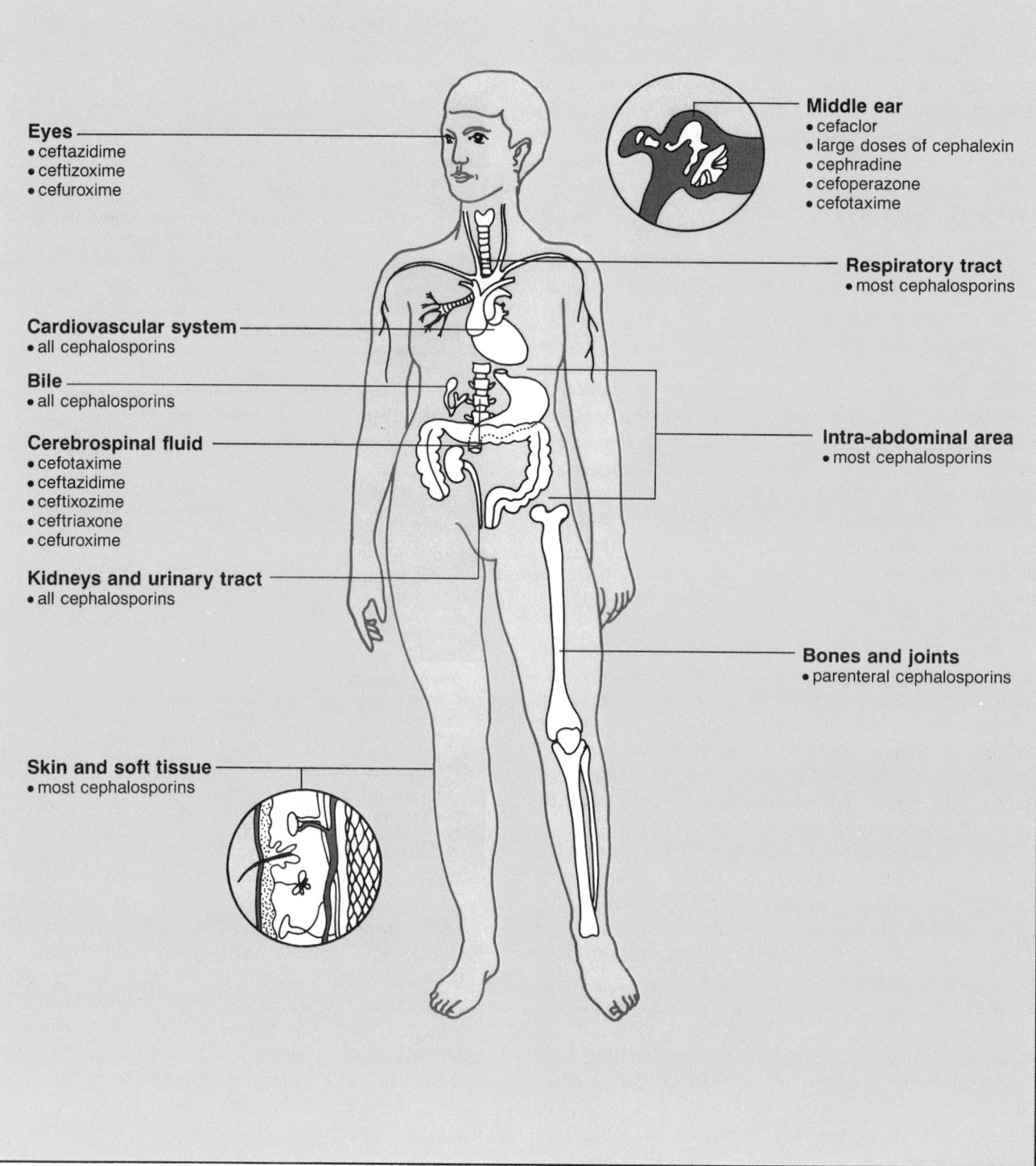

Eyes
• ceftazidime
• ceftizoxime
• cefuroxime

Middle ear
• cefaclor
• large doses of cephalexin
• cephradine
• cefoperazone
• cefotaxime

Respiratory tract
• most cephalosporins

Cardiovascular system
• all cephalosporins

Bile
• all cephalosporins

Cerebrospinal fluid
• cefotaxime
• ceftazidime
• ceftixozime
• ceftriaxone
• cefuroxime

Intra-abdominal area
• most cephalosporins

Kidneys and urinary tract
• all cephalosporins

Bones and joints
• parenteral cephalosporins

Skin and soft tissue
• most cephalosporins

Onset, peak, duration

Oral cephalosporins attain a peak concentration level within 1 to 2 hours after administration. After a 30-minute I.V. infusion, onset of action is rapid. Peak concentration usually is achieved within 1 hour. After I.V. administration of 1 gram, the peak concentration is 50 to 100 mcg/ml for most cephalosporins. The higher concentration of cefazolin sodium given I.V. or I.M. is a considerable advantage over other first-generation cephalosporins. After I.M. administration, the onset usually is delayed. The peak concentration achieved is about 50% of that achieved after I.V. administration.

The serum half-life of cephalosporins in adults with normal renal function ranges from 0.4 to 10.9 hours. Among first-generation cephalosporins, cefazolin has the longest half-life, 2.2 hours, which allows an every-8-hour dosage schedule. Cefonicid sodium is the longest-acting second-generation cephalosporin, with a serum half-life of nearly 6 hours and 90% to 98% of the drug bound to serum proteins. The drug normally is given once daily. In patients with renal impairment, the dosage and frequency of cefonicid administration depend on creatinine clearance. Among the third-generation cephalosporins, ceftriaxone displays the highest degree of plasma protein binding (85% to 95%) and the longest serum half-life (up to 10.9 hours). Ceftriaxone usually is administered once daily. Dosage adjustments of ceftriaxone usually are unnecessary in patients with impaired renal or hepatic function. The remaining cephalosporins have a serum half-life of 0.5 to 4 hours and are administered at 4- to 12-hour intervals in patients with normal renal function.

PHARMACODYNAMICS

The mechanism of action of the beta-lactam antibacterials is related to interference with cell-wall synthesis similar to penicillins. Rapidly growing organisms are more susceptible to these antibacterials.

Mechanism of action

Cephalosporins inhibit cell-wall synthesis by binding to bacterial enzymes located on the cell membrane. These enzymes, which have been classified as PBPs, are important for the biosynthesis of bacterial cell-wall components. The antibacterial action of cephalosporins depends on their ability to penetrate the bacterial cell wall and bind with proteins in the cytoplasmic membrane. Once the drug damages the cell wall by binding with the PBPs, the body's natural defense mechanisms destroy the bacteria. To produce a bactericidal effect on the cell, the cephalosporins must reach the PBPs in sufficient concentrations to inhibit cell-wall synthesis and must resist the destructive action of the beta-lactamases produced by some bacteria, which inactivate the drug by hydrolyzing its beta-lactam ring. (For

---

Mechanism of action of cephalosporins

An understanding of the mechanism of action of cephalosporins requires an understanding of the structure of a bacterial cell. Outside the *cytoplasmic membrane* lies a chemically complex, rigid cell wall that protects the cell against osmotic pressure and the outside environment. This cell wall contains a *mucocomplex layer,* which forms a sac around the bacterium. Acting as a filter, this layer prevents large molecules from passing through it. Gram-positive bacteria have a thick mucocomplex layer extending from the cytoplasmic membrane to the *teichoic acid layer* that coats the exterior of the cell. In contrast, the mucocomplex layer in gram-negative cells is thin and supported by a complex outer cell wall composed of polysaccharides, lipids, and proteins. The gram-negative cell also contains *periplasmic space,* which lies between the cytoplasmic membrane and the cell wall.

Gram-positive and gram-negative bacterial cell walls contain chemically similar *peptidoglycans,* the basic building blocks of the mucocomplex layer, which are necessary for cell-wall strength and rigidity. Cephalosporins inhibit the synthesis of these cell walls apparently by interfering with enzymatic action and preventing cross-linkage of these peptidoglycan chains.

---

more information, see *Mechanism of action of cephalosporins.*)

PHARMACOTHERAPEUTICS

Cephalosporins are classified into generations based on their spectra of activity. (For a listing, see *Antibacterial activity of cephalosporins,* page 1017.) All cephalosporins are ineffective against enterococci (such as *Streptococcus faecalis),* methicillin-resistant staphylococci, and beta-hemolytic streptococci. Toxicity and cost of the drugs increase from first-generation to third-generation cephalosporins.

Cephalosporins are among the most prescribed antibacterials. With or without aminoglycosides, they have been the drugs of choice to treat serious *Klebsiella* infections. They also are used widely in surgical prophylaxis. Cephalosporins are used to treat infections involving the respiratory tract, the skin and soft tissues, and the bones and joints as well as certain UTIs.

First-generation cephalosporins can be used as alternative therapy in patients allergic to penicillin. They also are used to treat staphylococcal and streptococcal infections, including pneumonia, cellulitis, and osteomyelitis. Second-generation cephalosporins are used to treat polymicrobial infections, such as diabetic foot ulcers, nosocomial aspiration pneumonias, and pelvic and intra-abdominal infections. Third-generation cephalosporins are the drugs of choice for infections caused by *Acinetobacter* and anaerobic organisms.

Oral cephalosporins are used to treat UTIs caused by organisms resistant to ampicillin, tetracycline, or the sulfonamides.

Cephalosporins are effective and well tolerated. Their major disadvantages are their cost and the emergence of gram-negative resistance.

cefaclor (Ceclor). Cefaclor is used to treat respiratory tract infections and otitis media. This second-generation cephalosporin is more active against *H. influenzae, E.coli,* and *P. mirabilis* than the first-generation oral cephalosporins.
Usual adult dosage: 250 to 500 mg P.O. every 8 hours.
Usual pediatric dosage: 20 mg/kg/day P.O. in divided doses every 8 hours.

cefadroxil monohydrate (Duricef, Ultracef). This first-generation cephalosporin is used to treat urinary tract, skin, and soft tissue infections caused primarily by gram-positive aerobic organisms.
Usual adult dosage: 1 to 2 grams in a single daily dose or in equally divided doses P.O. b.i.d.
Usual pediatric dosage: 30 mg/kg/day P.O. in two divided doses.

cefamandole nafate (Mandol). A second-generation cephalosporin, cefamandole is more active than first-generation cephalosporins against such gram-negative organisms as *H. influenzae, Enterobacter,* and indole-positive *Proteus;* it also is used for gram-positive cocci. Because cefamandole is not absorbed orally, it must be administered parenterally.
Usual adult dosage: 500 mg to 2 grams I.V. or I.M. every 4 to 8 hours.
Usual pediatric dosage: 50 to 100 mg/kg/day I.V. or I.M. in divided doses every 4 to 8 hours.

cefazolin sodium (Ancef, Kefzol). The antibacterial spectrum of activity for cefazolin resembles that of cephalothin. Because of its high serum concentration, this first-generation cephalosporin is more active than cephalothin against *E. coli* and *Klebsiella* species. It is the best-tolerated cephalosporin for I.M. administration. A 500-mg dose every 8 hours is equivalent to 1 gram of cephalothin every 6 hours.
Usual adult dosage: 0.25 to 1 gram I.V. or I.M. every 6 to 8 hours.
Usual pediatric dosage: for children over age 1 month, 6.25 to 25 mg/kg I.V. every 6 hours or 8.3 to 33.3 mg/kg I.V. every 8 hours.

cefixime (Suprax). A third-generation cephalosporin, cefixime is indicated to treat uncomplicated UTIs caused by *E. coli* and *P. mirabilis,* otitis media caused by *H. influenzae, Branhamella catarrhalis,* and *Streptococcus pyogenes;* pharyngitis and tonsillitis caused by *S. pyogenes;*

and bronchitis and acute exacerbations of chronic bronchitis caused by *Streptococcus pneumoniae* and *H. influenzae.*
Usual adult dosage: 400 mg P.O. daily as a single 400-mg tablet or 200 mg P.O. every 12 hours; maximum dosage 400 mg/day.
Usual pediatric dosage: 8 mg/kg/day of suspension P.O. as a single dose or in divided doses every 12 hours. Children over 50 kg or over age 12 should receive the adult dosage.

cefmetazole sodium (Zefazone). The spectrum of antibacterial activity for cefmetazole is similar to that of cefoxitin. It is used to treat UTIs caused by *E. coli,* lower respiratory tract infections caused by a variety of organisms, and in intra-abdominal infections caused by *E. coli* and *Bacteroides fragilis.* It is also indicated for the prophylaxis of patients undergoing various abdominal surgeries. Cefmetazole is administered I.V. and dosage adjustments must be made for patients with renal function impairment.
Usual adult dosage: 2 grams I.V. every 6 to 12 hours for 5 to 14 days.
Usual pediatric dosage: not established.

cefonicid sodium (Monocid). A second-generation cephalosporin, the spectrum of activity for cefonicid resembles that of cefamandole. Cefonicid is used in single-dose surgical prophylaxis and for patients in nursing home and home care programs who require antibiotic therapy.
Usual adult dosage: 1 gram I.V. or I.M. daily.
Usual pediatric dosage: not established.

cefoperazone sodium (Cefobid). Less active than cefotaxime against the Enterobacteriaceae, this third-generation cephalosporin has greater activity against *P. aeruginosa.* The dosage need not be adjusted in patients with renal impairment. Although it achieves adequate CNS levels, cefoperazone is not indicated to treat meningitis.
Usual adult dosage: 1 to 2 grams I.V. or I.M. every 12 hours.
Usual pediatric dosage: not established.

ceforanide (Precef). A second-generation cephalosporin, the structure and antibacterial spectrum of activity for ceforanide resemble those of cefamandole. However, ceforanide can be administered twice daily because its serum half-life is about 3 hours. It is used to treat pneumonia and soft-tissue and urinary tract infections.
Usual adult dosage: 0.5 to 1 gram I.V. or I.M. every 12 hours.
Usual pediatric dosage: 20 to 40 mg/kg/day I.M. or I.V. in divided doses every 12 hours.

cefotaxime sodium (Claforan). The first of the third-generation cephalosporins available in the United States, ce-

fotaxime has an enhanced spectrum of activity against all gram-negative aerobic organisms except *P. aeruginosa.* Used to treat gram-negative meningitis, cefotaxime provides effective activity against all gram-positive organisms except enterococci and exhibits poor activity against anaerobes, such as *B. fragilis.*
Usual adult dosage: 1 to 2 grams I.V. or I.M. every 4 to 8 hours.
Usual pediatric dosage: for neonates up to age 1 week, 50 mg/kg I.V. every 12 hours; for neonates ages 1 week to 4 weeks, 50 mg/kg I.V. every 8 hours; for children over age 4 weeks up to 50 kg, 8.3 to 30 mg/kg I.M. or I.V. every 4 hours or 12.5 to 45 mg/kg I.M. or I.V. every 6 hours; for children over 50 kg, same as adult.

cefotetan disodium (Cefotan). A semisynthetic parenteral cephamycin derivative, cefotetan has a spectrum of activity somewhere between the second- and third-generation cephalosporins. However, it usually is considered a third-generation cephalosporin. The in vitro activity against gram-negative bacilli resembles that of cefotaxime; however, cefotetan is less active against *Enterobacter* and *Serratia* species and has no useful activity against *P. aeruginosa.* Compared with cefoxitin, cefotetan is less active against *B. fragilis.*
Usual adult dosage: 1 to 2 grams I.V. or I.M. every 12 hours.
Usual pediatric dosage: not established.

cefoxitin sodium (Mefoxin). A derivative of cephamycin C, produced by *Streptomyces lactamdurans,* cefoxitin is highly beta-lactamase resistant and provides excellent activity against anaerobes, especially *B. fragilis.* This second-generation cephalosporin is somewhat less active than cefamandole and the first-generation cephalosporins against gram-positive organisms but is more active against gram-negative bacteria, such as indole-positive *Proteus,* penicillinase-producing *N. gonorrhoeae,* and some strains of *S. marcescens.* The special role of cefoxitin is to treat certain mixed anaerobic-aerobic infections, such as diabetic foot ulcers, pelvic inflammatory disease, lung abscess, and aspiration pneumonia. Because cefoxitin causes pain at the I.M. injection site, it usually is administered I.V.
Usual adult dosage: 1 to 2 grams I.V. or I.M. every 6 to 8 hours.
Usual pediatric dosage: 80 to 160 mg/kg/day I.V. or I.M. in divided doses every 4 to 6 hours.

ceftazidime (Fortaz, Tazicef, Tazidime). The spectrum of activity for ceftazidime is excellent against *P. aeruginosa* and good against the Enterobacteriaceae (resembling that of cefotaxime), but ceftazidime exhibits the poorest activity among all third-generation cephalosporins against gram-positive organisms and *B. fragilis.* Ceftazidime is used to

treat *P. aeruginosa* meningitis and CNS infections caused by *H. influenzae* and *Neisseria meningitidis.*
Usual adult dosage: 1 gram I.V. or I.M. every 8 to 12 hours.
Usual pediatric dosage: for neonates up to age 1 month, 30 mg/kg I.V. every 12 hours; for children ages 1 month to 12 years, 30 to 50 mg/kg I.V. every 8 hours.

ceftizoxime sodium (Cefizox). A third-generation cephalosporin, the spectrum of activity for ceftizoxime resembles that of cefotaxime. However, ceftizoxime has a longer serum half-life and can be administered every 8 to 12 hours instead of every 4 to 8 hours.
Usual adult dosage: 1 to 2 grams I.V. or I.M. every 8 to 12 hours.
Usual pediatric dosage: for children over age 6 months, 50 mg/kg I.V. every 6 to 8 hours.

ceftriaxone sodium (Rocephin). The antibacterial spectrum of activity for ceftriaxone is similar to that of ceftizoxime and cefotaxime. Ceftriaxone has the longest half-life of all the third-generation cephalosporins (about 9 hours), which allows for once-daily dosage. Ceftriaxone is used to treat meningitis caused by susceptible organisms and penicillinase-producing *N. gonorrhoeae.* Dosage adjustment is not necessary in patients with renal insufficiency.
Usual adult dosage: 1 to 2 grams I.V. or I.M. every 12 to 24 hours; for meningitis, 100 mg/kg I.V. or I.M. in divided doses every 12 hours; may administer 75 mg/kg as a loading dose. The total daily dosage should not exceed 4 grams.
Usual pediatric dosage: 25 to 37.5 mg/kg I.V. or I.M. every 12 hours.

cefuroxime axetil oral (Ceftin). This oral form of cefuroxime is used to treat pharyngitis, tonsillitis, otitis media, and lower respiratory tract, urinary tract, and skin infections caused by susceptible bacteria.
Usual adult dosage: 250 to 500 mg P.O. every 12 hours.
Usual pediatric dosage: for otitis media in children ages 2 to 12, 250 mg P.O. every 12 hours; for other indications in children ages 2 to 12, 125 mg P.O. every 12 hours; for other indications in children under age 2, 125 mg P.O. every 12 hours.

cefuroxime sodium (Zinacef). The antibacterial spectrum of activity for cefuroxime resembles that of cefamandole, but cefuroxime also can penetrate inflamed meninges. It is the only second-generation cephalosporin approved to treat bacterial meningitis *H. influenzae, N. meningitidis,* and *S. pneumoniae.*
Usual adult dosage: 750 mg to 1.5 grams I.V. or I.M. every 8 hours, usually for 5 to 10 days.

Usual pediatric dosage: 50 to 100 mg/kg/day I.M. or I.V. in divided doses every 6 to 8 hours; not for infants under age 3 months.

cephalexin monohydrate (Keflex). This first-generation cephalosporin is used to treat otitis media; acute prostatitis; and respiratory tract, skin, skin structure, bone, and urinary tract infections. Cephalexin is interchangeable with oral cephradine.
Usual adult dosage: 250 mg to 1 gram P.O. every 6 hours.
Usual pediatric dosage: 6 to 12 mg/kg P.O. every 6 hours; maximum dosage of 25 mg/kg/day.

cephalothin sodium (Keflin). The earliest available cephalosporin and the most stable against staphylococcal beta-lactamase, cephalothin is used to treat severe staphylococcal infections. This first-generation cephalosporin is not absorbed well after oral administration and is administered parenterally only. Cephalothin usually is administered I.V. because it causes pain at the I.M. injection site.
Usual adult dosage: 0.5 to 2 grams I.V. every 4 to 6 hours.
Usual pediatric dosage: 14 to 27 mg/kg I.V. every 4 hours or 20 to 40 mg/kg I.V. every 6 hours.

cephapirin sodium (Cefadyl). Pharmacologically, this first-generation cephalosporin resembles cephalothin. I.M. administration can cause pain at the injection site.
Usual adult dosage: 0.50 to 1 grams I.V. every 4 to 6 hours.
Usual pediatric dosage: for children over age 3 months, 10 to 20 mg/kg I.M. or I.V. every 6 hours.

cephradine (Anspor, Velosef). This first-generation agent is available in oral and parenteral forms. The antibacterial spectrum of activity of oral cephradine appears to be chemically interchangeable with cephalexin; that of the parenteral form resembles cefazolin.
Usual adult dosage: 250 to 500 mg P.O. every 6 to 12 hours, or 0.5 to 1 gram I.V. or I.M. every 6 to 12 hours.
Usual pediatric dosage: 6.25 to 25 mg/kg P.O. every 6 hours.

moxalactam disodium (Moxam). A semisynthetic 1-oxa-beta-lactam, moxalactam differs structurally from the other third-generation cephalosporins. This difference greatly enhances its antibacterial activity, particularly against gram-negative bacteria. Compared to cefotaxime, moxalactam is less active against staphylococci and enterococci but is equally effective against most of the Enterobacteriaceae.
Usual adult dosage: 1 to 4 grams I.V. or I.M. every 8 to 12 hours for up to 14 days.
Usual pediatric dosage: for children, 50 mg/kg I.M. or I.V. every 6 to 8 hours; for neonates, 50 mg/kg I.M. or I.V. every 8 to 12 hours.

Drug interactions

Patients receiving cefamandole, cefoperazone, or moxalactam who drink alcoholic beverages concurrently or up to 72 hours after drug administration may experience acute alcohol intolerance with signs and symptoms similar to a disulfiram (Antabuse) reaction. Patients may experience headache, flushing, dizziness, nausea, vomiting, or abdominal cramps within 30 minutes of alcohol ingestion.

Concomitant use of cephalosporins and imipenem/cilastatin can antagonize the antibacterial activity of the beta-lactam cephalosporins.

Uricosurics, such as probenecid and sulfinpyrazone, can block the renal tubular secretion of some cephalosporins. Probenecid is used therapeutically to increase and prolong cephalosporin plasma concentrations.

ADVERSE DRUG REACTIONS

Cephalosporins are relatively safe, but with the development of newer and more potent second- and third-generation cephalosporins, adverse reactions have increased.

Hypersensitivity reactions are the most common systemic adverse reactions to cephalosporins. Allergic reactions range in severity from mild to life-threatening. Usual allergic reactions appear as urticaria, pruritus or morbilliform eruptions, and serum sickness reactions. Anaphylaxis is rare.

Because of the similarities between penicillins and cephalosporins, a 5% to 10% cross-reactivity may occur. No cephalosporin skin test can predict whether a patient will have an allergic reaction. Patients with a history of mild penicillin reactions are at low risk for developing an allergic reaction to cephalosporins; however, patients who have had severe immediate reactions to penicillin are at high risk and should be monitored carefully when they are receiving a cephalosporin.

Intramuscular administration of cephalothin and cefoxitin commonly produces pain, induration, and tenderness at the injection site. Thrombophlebitis is associated most commonly with I.V. cephalothin. Frequent changes of I.V. sites may be necessary.

In patients with impaired renal function who are receiving high doses of cephalosporins, the most common reactions are confusion and seizures. Seizures associated with high doses of cefazolin also can occur.

Serious bleeding related to hypoprothrombinemia, thrombocytopenia, or platelet dysfunction can occur in patients receiving moxalactam or cefoperazone. This coagulation disorder is a problem in elderly and poorly nourished patients and in those with renal failure.

Orally administered cephalosporins commonly cause nausea, vomiting, and diarrhea. These reactions, which usually are mild and transient, may be alleviated by administering the drug with food. Antibiotic-associated pseudomembranous colitis caused by *Clostridium difficile* may occur during or after cephalosporin therapy, especially with the third-generation cephalosporins.

Cephalosporins may produce nephrotoxicity. High doses of cephalothin can lead to acute tubular necrosis, and usual dosages of 8 to 12 grams/day can be nephrotoxic in patients with renal disease. Cephalothin administered with an aminoglycoside, such as gentamicin, can be nephrotoxic.

Use of the cephalosporins may lead to superinfection, producing such problems as diarrhea, sore mouth (oral thrush), and vaginal itching.

All cephalosporins, except cetotaxime, can cause false-positive results on urine glucose tests using cupric sulfate solution, such as Benedict's reagent and Clinitest. However, they do not affect the results of glucose oxidase tests, such as Tes-Tape and Clinistix.

NURSING PROCESS APPLICATION

The following information assists the nurse in caring for a patient who is receiving a cephalosporin.

Assessment
• Review the patient's history for a preexisting condition that contraindicates the use of a cephalosporin, such as known hypersensitivity to the prescribed agent or other cephalosporins.
• Review the patient's history for a preexisting condition that requires cautious use of a cephalosporin, such as pregnancy, lactation, a history of allergies (especially to such drugs as penicillin), or GI disease (particularly colitis).
• Assess the patient for adverse reactions to the prescribed cephalosporin, such as hypersensitivity reactions, nephrotoxicity, GI distress, bleeding, seizures, or confusion.
• Review the patient's medication history to identify the use of drugs that may interact with the prescribed cephalosporin, such as alcohol, imipenem/cilastatin, and uricosurics.
• Assess the effectiveness of the prescribed cephalosporin regularly.
• Evaluate the patient's and family's knowledge about the prescribed cephalosporin.

Nursing diagnoses
The following examples represent appropriate nursing diagnoses for a patient receiving a cephalosporin.
• Potential for injury related to a preexisting condition that contraindicates the use of a cephalosporin
• Potential for injury related to a preexisting condition that requires cautious use of a cephalosporin
• Potential for injury related to adverse drug reactions
• Potential fluid volume deficit related to the adverse GI effects of an oral cephalosporin
• Knowledge deficit related to the prescribed cephalosporin

Planning and implementation
• Do not administer a cephalosporin to a patient with a condition that contraindicates its use.
• Administer a cephalosporin cautiously to a patient at risk because of a preexisting condition.
• Monitor the patient periodically for adverse reactions during cephalosporin therapy. Keep in mind that toxicity increases from the first to the third generation of cephalosporins.
• *Observe the patient for hypersensitivity reactions, such as urticaria, pruritus, morbilliform eruptions, serum sickness, or anaphylaxis. Keep standard emergency equipment readily available. If a hypersensitivity reaction occurs, withhold the drug and notify the physician. Expect the patient to be switched to a different antibacterial agent.*
• Avoid administering a cephalosporin to a patient who recently has experienced a severe, immediate reaction to a penicillin or cephalosporin. Obtain a thorough drug history, and screen the patient for possible allergy and cross-reactions with cephalosporins.
• *Monitor for confusion or seizures in the patient with impaired renal function who is receiving high doses of a cephalosporin. Seizures also may occur in the patient with normal renal function receiving high doses of cefazolin. Take seizure precautions at the start of therapy, and notify the physician if seizures occur. If the patient develops confusion, take safety precautions, such as supervising patient activities.*
• Take bleeding precautions in the patient receiving moxalactam or cefoperazone, especially if the patient is elderly, poorly nourished, or has renal failure.
• Monitor the patient for nephrotoxicity, reflected in rising blood urea nitrogen and creatinine levels, changes in urine output, proteinuria, and water retention. High doses of cephalothin, concomitant administration of cephalothin with an aminoglycoside, or administration of 8 to 12 grams/day in the patient with renal disease can be especially nephrotoxic.
• *Monitor the patient closely for signs and symptoms of superinfection, such as diarrhea, sore mouth (oral thrush), and vaginal itching.*
• Expect to adjust the dosage as prescribed in a patient with renal insufficiency who is receiving a cephalosporin (except for cefoperazone or ceftriaxone).
• *Infuse all I.V. cephalosporins over 30 minutes to prevent pain and irritation.*
• *Monitor the I.V. site routinely for signs of thrombophlebitis, such as localized redness, swelling, and pain.*
• Reconstitute cefoxitin and ceftriaxone with a 0.5% to 1% lidocaine injection, as prescribed, to decrease pain at the injection site during I.M. administration.
• Notify the physician if adverse reactions occur.
• Monitor for nausea, vomiting, and diarrhea in a patient receiving an oral cephalosporin.

• *Administer the prescribed cephalosporin with food to prevent or minimize GI upset.*
• Monitor hydration if the patient experiences nausea, vomiting, or diarrhea. If these adverse reactions persist or worsen, notify the physician, request a prescription for an antiemetic or antidiarrheal agent, and expect to change the oral form to a parenteral equivalent.
• Monitor the patient for signs of pseudomembranous colitis, such as abdominal pain and diarrhea, during and after cephalosporin therapy, especially with a third-generation cephalosporin.

Patient teaching
• Teach the patient and family the name, dose, frequency, action, and adverse effects of the prescribed cephalosporin.
• Teach the patient to recognize and immediately report the signs and symptoms of a hypersensitivity reaction.
• Review with the patient the signs and symptoms of a superinfection.
• Advise the patient to ingest yogurt or buttermilk, which replenishes normal GI flora, to prevent intestinal superinfection.
• Instruct the patient to take a prescribed oral cephalosporin with food to prevent GI upset.
• Inform the patient that an I.M. cephalosporin may cause pain, inflammation, or tenderness at the injection site.
• Advise the patient to avoid taking moxalactam, cefoperazone, cefamandole, or cefotetan with alcohol or medications that contain alcohol (elixirs).
• Advise the diabetic patient taking a cephalosporin to test urine glucose levels with Tes-Tape or Clinistix (not Clinitest).
• Instruct the patient to complete the entire course of cephalosporin therapy.
• Stress the importance of keeping follow-up appointments and having laboratory tests done as prescribed to evaluate drug effectiveness or detect adverse drug reactions.
• Advise the patient receiving moxalactam or cefoperazone to take bleeding precautions, such as using an electric razor, avoiding cuts and bruises, using a soft toothbrush, and wearing shoes at all times.
• Instruct the patient to notify the physician if adverse reactions occur or if the condition persists or worsens.

Evaluation
The following examples represent appropriate evaluation statements for a patient receiving a cephalosporin.
• The patient has no conditions that contraindicate cephalosporin therapy.
• The patient exhibits no signs of complications in the preexisting condition linked to the prescribed cephalosporin.
• The patient exhibits no adverse reactions to the prescribed cephalosporin.

• The patient maintains an adequate fluid balance throughout cephalosporin therapy.
• The patient and family express an accurate understanding of the points taught about the prescribed cephalosporin.
• The patient completes the entire course of cephalosporin therapy as prescribed.

TETRACYCLINES

Although among the most commonly prescribed antibacterials in the world, tetracyclines rarely are considered drugs of choice for most common bacterial infections. Overuse of tetracyclines has led to the emergence of tetracycline-resistant bacteria.

The tetracycline analogues are classified as (1) short-acting compounds (chlortetracycline, oxytetracycline, and tetracycline), (2) intermediate-acting compounds (demeclocycline hydrochloride and methacycline hydrochloride), and (3) long-acting compounds (doxycycline and minocycline). Doxycycline and minocycline provide an improved antibacterial spectrum of activity.

PHARMACOKINETICS

Tetracyclines are absorbed from the duodenum after oral administration, distributed widely into body tissues and fluids, concentrated in bile, and excreted primarily by the kidneys, except for doxycycline and minocycline. The onset, peak, and duration of action vary among the different tetracyclines.

Absorption, distribution, metabolism, excretion
After oral administration, tetracyclines are absorbed rapidly from the duodenum. Absorption is impaired by intake of dairy products; it is reduced drastically by iron preparations or the concomitant administration of antacids that contain calcium, magnesium, or aluminum salts. Food interferes little with doxycycline and minocycline absorption; both drugs usually are taken with food to minimize possible GI irritation. However, food does affect the absorption of other tetracyclines, which should be taken on an empty stomach (1 hour before or 2 hours after meals). Absorption of various tetracyclines differs: doxycycline and minocycline are absorbed well (90% to 100%); oxytetracycline and tetracycline are absorbed poorly. After I.M. administration, tetracyclines are absorbed poorly and erratically.

The tetracyclines are distributed widely into body tissues and fluids, including pleural fluid, synovial fluid, bronchial secretions, sputum, and prostatic fluid. Intravenous administration of a tetracycline results in a CSF concentration of approximately 25% of serum concentration levels. Oral or I.M. administration results in an even lower CSF concentration. Meningeal inflammation is not required for tetracycline penetration into the CSF. Because doxycycline and, to a greater extent, minocycline are more lipid-soluble than other tetracyclines, they penetrate most body tissues and fluids well. Relatively high concentrations of minocycline are found in tears and saliva, and minocycline is used as an alternative to rifampin to eradicate *N. meningitidis* from asymptomatic carriers. All tetracyclines are distributed into bile; the tetracyclines cross the placenta, and relatively high concentrations appear in breast milk.

The tetracyclines concentrate in bile with biliary concentrations 5 to 10 times higher than corresponding serum concentrations. Obstruction of the hepatobiliary tract decreases the biliary concentrations of tetracyclines. Minocycline is partially metabolized in the liver to at least six metabolites. Doxycycline is partially inactivated in the intestine. Demeclocycline, methacycline, oxytetracycline, and tetracycline are not metabolized in the liver.

With the exception of doxycycline and minocycline, tetracyclines are excreted primarily by the kidneys. Oxytetracycline and tetracycline are excreted almost entirely unchanged in urine. About 60% of the active drug is recovered in the urine; 40%, in the feces. Demeclocycline and methacycline also are excreted primarily by the kidneys; about 60% of methacycline and 40% of demeclocycline are excreted unchanged. Doxycycline is excreted independent of renal and hepatic function. Researchers believe that doxycycline is inactivated by chelate formation in the intestines and is excreted in the feces. Minocycline undergoes enterohepatic recirculation; only about 10% of the active drug is excreted in the urine. The metabolism and excretion of chlortetracycline is unknown.

Onset, peak, duration
Oral administration of the tetracyclines results in detectable serum concentrations in 30 minutes; peak concentration levels are reached in 1 to 4 hours. After oral administration of 500 mg of tetracycline or 100 mg of doxycycline or minocycline, peak serum concentration is reached in 2 hours. Peak serum concentration is reached 1 hour after I.V. administration of 500 mg of tetracycline or 100 mg of doxycycline or minocycline. Because of a prolonged serum half-life of about 20 hours, doxycycline and minocycline can maintain adequate serum concentrations with administration every 12 to 24 hours. The serum half-life of tetracycline is about 8.5 hours; the patient should receive a dose every 6 hours. After I.M. administration of oxytetracycline or tetracycline, peak serum concentration is reached in 30 minutes to 1 hour. With usual dosages, the serum concentration achieved after I.M. administration is lower than that after oral administration.

PHARMACODYNAMICS

All tetracyclines are primarily bacteriostatic. Like the aminoglycosides, they interfere with protein synthesis.

Mechanism of action
The tetracyclines penetrate the interior of the bacterial cell by an energy-dependent process. Once within the cell, the tetracyclines reversibly bind primarily to a subunit of the ribosome, thereby inhibiting access of transfer RNA-amino acid complexes to the messenger RNA-ribosome complex. This action prevents the addition of new amino acids to the peptide chain.

PHARMACOTHERAPEUTICS

The tetracyclines provide a broad spectrum of activity against gram-positive, gram-negative, aerobic, and anaerobic bacteria as well as spirochetes, mycoplasmas, rickettsiae, chlamydiae, and some protozoa. Doxycycline and minocycline typically provide more action against various organisms than the other tetracyclines do. Tetracyclines are used to treat Rocky Mountain spotted fever, Q fever, Lyme disease, brucellosis, and tularemia. They are the drugs of choice for treating nongonococcal urethritis caused by *Chlamydia* and *Ureaplasma urealyticum.*

Tetracycline or erythromycin is the drug of choice for treating *Mycoplasma pneumoniae* infections. Combination therapy with a tetracycline and streptomycin is the most effective treatment for brucellosis. The tetracyclines effectively treat acne because they can decrease the fatty acid content of sebum; low-dose tetracycline (250 mg b.i.d.) is used for this condition. Although the tetracyclines are active against many aerobic gram-positive cocci, they are not used to treat staphylococcal, group A beta-hemolytic streptococcal, or pneumococcal infections because of the tetracycline resistance displayed by these bacteria.

chlortetracycline hydrochloride (Aureomycin). Available as a 3% ointment for topical use, chlortetracycline is indicated for infection prophylaxis in minor skin abrasions and for treating superficial skin infections. The preparation may stain clothing. Chlortetracycline also is available as a 1% ophthalmic ointment, which is used to treat bacterial conjunctivitis. The safety and efficacy of this drug has not been established in children under age 11.
Usual adult dosage: for skin infections, applied to the affected area b.i.d. or t.i.d.; for conjunctivitis, approximately 1 cm of ointment applied to the conjunctival sac every 2 to 4 hours.

demeclocycline hydrochloride (Declomycin). Demeclocycline is used commonly to treat chronic syndrome of inappropriate antidiuretic hormone secretion (SIADH). It is used rarely to treat susceptible gram-negative and gram-positive infections.

Usual adult dosage: for SIADH, 600 mg to 1.2 grams P.O. daily in three or four divided doses; for infections caused by susceptible gram-negative and gram-positive organisms, *Chlamydia trachomatis,* and rickettsiae, 150 to 300 mg P.O. every 6 hours or 300 mg P.O. every 12 hours; for gonorrhea, 600 mg P.O. initially, then 300 mg P.O. every 12 hours for 4 days.

Usual pediatric dosage: for children over age 8, 6 to 12 mg/kg P.O. daily in divided doses every 6 to 12 hours.

doxycycline hyclate (Vibramycin). Doxycycline does not accumulate in patients with renal or hepatic dysfunction. It is effective as a prophylactic treatment for traveler's diarrhea caused by toxigenic strains of *E. coli* and commonly is used to treat pelvic inflammatory disease and cervicitis caused by *C. trachomatis.* Doxycycline and rifampin have been used as an alternative to erythromycin to treat pneumonia caused by *Legionella pneumophila.*

Usual adult dosage: for infections caused by sensitive gram-negative and gram-positive organisms, *C. trachomatis,* and rickettsiae, 100 mg P.O. every 12 hours on first day followed by 100 mg P.O. daily, or 200 mg I.V. on the first day in one or two infusions followed by 100 to 200 mg I.V. daily; administer the I.V. infusion slowly (minimum of 1 hour); complete the infusion within 12 hours (within 6 hours in lactated Ringer's solution or dextrose 5% in lactated Ringer's solution); for gonorrhea in patients allergic to penicillin, 200 mg P.O. initially, followed by 100 mg P.O. at bedtime and 100 mg P.O. b.i.d. for 3 days, or 300 mg P.O. initially with the dose repeated in 1 hour; for primary or secondary syphilis in patients allergic to penicillin, 200 mg P.O. daily in divided doses for 10 days; for uncomplicated urethral, endocervical, or rectal infections caused by *C. trachomatis* or *U. urealyticum,* 100 mg P.O. b.i.d. for at least 7 days; to prevent traveler's diarrhea caused by enterotoxigenic *E. coli,* 100 mg P.O. daily.

Usual pediatric dosage: for children 45 kg and under, 2.2 to 4.4 mg/kg P.O. or I.V. once daily or 1.1 to 2.2 mg/kg P.O. or I.V. every 12 hours; for children over 45 kg, same as adult.

methacycline hydrochloride (Rondomycin). Although methacycline is indicated to treat *M. pneumoniae,* uncomplicated gonorrhea, and syphilis, it is used rarely. Tetracycline and doxycycline have replaced methacycline because they are recommended by the Centers for Disease Control.

Usual adult dosage: 150 to 300 mg P.O. every 6 to 12 hours.

Usual pediatric dosage: for children ages 8 and over, 1.65 to 3.3 mg/kg P.O. every 6 hours or 3.3 to 6.6 mg/kg P.O. every 12 hours; not recommended for children under age 8.

minocycline hydrochloride (Minocin). Because it enters salivary secretions, minocycline is effective in treating asymptomatic carriers of *N. meningitidis.* Minocycline also is used to treat severe acne because of its high lipophilicity. The drug may require dosage adjustment in patients with renal insufficiency.

Usual adult dosage: for infections caused by sensitive gram-negative and gram-positive organisms, *C. trachomatis,* or amebiasis, 200 mg P.O. or I.V. initially, followed by 100 mg every 12 hours or 50 mg P.O. every 6 hours; for meningococcal carrier state, 100 to 200 mg P.O. every 12 hours for 5 days; for uncomplicated urethral, endocervical, or rectal infection caused by *C. trachomatis* or *U. urealyticum,* 100 mg P.O. b.i.d. for at least 7 days; for uncomplicated gonococcal urethritis in males, 100 mg P.O. b.i.d. for 7 days.

Usual pediatric dosage: for infections caused by sensitive gram-negative and gram-positive organisms, *C. trachomatis,* or amebiasis, for children over age 8, 4 mg/kg P.O. or I.V. initially, followed by 4 mg/kg P.O. daily in divided doses every 12 hours; administer I.V. in 500 to 1,000 ml of solution without calcium over 6 hours. Not recommended for children ages 8 and under.

oxytetracycline hydrochloride (Terramycin). Oral administration of oxytetracycline is preferred; I.M. administration produces pain and a lower serum concentration. Intravenous therapy may lead to thrombophlebitis. Because oxytetracycline is excreted in urine to a great degree, it is ideal for treating IUTs.

Usual adult dosage: for infections caused by sensitive gram-negative and gram-positive organisms, *C. trachomatis,* or rickettsiae, 250 mg P.O. every 6 hours, 100 mg I.M. every 8 to 12 hours, 250 mg I.M. every 12 hours, or 250 to 500 mg I.V. every 6 to 12 hours; for brucellosis, 500 mg P.O. q.i.d. for 3 weeks, given with 1 gram of streptomycin sulfate I.M. every 12 hours the first week and once daily the second week; for syphilis in patients sensitive to penicillin, a total of 30 to 50 grams P.O. divided equally over 10 to 15 days; for gonorrhea in patients sensitive to penicillin, 1.5 grams P.O. initially, followed by 0.5 gram q.i.d. for a total of 9 grams.

Usual pediatric dosage: for infections caused by sensitive gram-negative and gram-positive organisms, *C. trachomatis,* and rickettsiae in children over age 8, 25 to 50 mg/kg P.O. daily in divided doses every 6 hours, 15 to 25 mg/kg I.M. daily in divided doses every 8 to 12 hours, or 10 to 20 mg/kg I.V. daily in divided doses every 12 hours.

tetracycline hydrochloride (Achromycin, Sumycin). This drug commonly is used to treat acute exacerbations of chronic bronchitis, infections caused by *M. pneumoniae,* UTIs, Lyme disease, and syphilis in penicillin-allergic patients. Phlebitis and pain at the infusion site limit I.V. use to those situations in which oral administration is not feasible. Intramuscular injection is not recommended because of pain on injection.

Usual adult dosage: for infections caused by sensitive gram-negative and gram-positive organisms, rickettsiae, and *Mycoplasma,* 250 to 500 mg P.O. every 6 hours, 250 mg I.M. daily, 150 mg I.M. every 12 hours, or 250 to 500 mg I.V. every 8 to 12 hours (for I.M. and I.V., hydrochloride salt only); for uncomplicated urethral, endocervical, or rectal infection caused by *C. trachomatis,* 500 mg P.O. every 6 hours for at least 7 days; for brucellosis, 500 mg P.O. every 6 hours for 3 weeks with 1 gram of streptomycin I.M. every 12 hours the first week and daily the second week; for Lyme disease, 500 mg P.O. q.i.d. for 10 to 30 days; for syphilis in patients hypersensitive to penicillin, a total of 30 to 50 grams in equally divided doses over 10 to 15 days; for acne in adults and adolescents, 250 mg P.O. every 6 hours initially followed by 125 to 500 mg P.O. daily or every other day.

Usual pediatric dosage: for children over age 8, 25 to 50 mg/kg/day P.O. in divided doses every 6 hours, 15 to 25 mg/kg/day (maximum dosage of 250 mg) I.M. as a single dose or in divided doses every 8 to 12 hours, or 10 to 20 mg/kg/day I.V. in divided doses every 12 hours.

Drug interactions

The nurse should be aware of the numerous significant interactions between tetracyclines and other drugs. (For a summary, see *Drug interactions: Tetracyclines,* page 1028.) These drugs, except for doxycycline and minocycline, may interact with milk and mild products, which bind with the drugs and prevent their absorption.

ADVERSE DRUG REACTIONS

Tetracyclines produce many of the same adverse reactions that the other antibacterials do, such as superinfection (overgrowth of tetracycline-resistant organisms) and GI disturbances. Because these drugs can affect tooth enamel development significantly, they are not recommended for children under age 8 or for pregnant patients.

Adverse GI reactions resulting from oral administration include nausea, vomiting, abdominal distress and distention, and diarrhea. Diarrhea commonly is related to alterations in the enteric flora. Doxycycline affects GI flora less than tetracycline. The diarrhea usually subsides when the drug is stopped; prolonged symptoms from pseudomembranous colitis have occurred.

Photosensitivity reactions (red rash on areas exposed to sunlight) are most common in patients receiving demeclocycline and doxycycline. However, photosensitivity reactions can occur with any tetracycline.

The tetracyclines cause permanent gray-brown to yellow discoloration of the teeth when administered during tooth formation. Darkening of permanent teeth may be related to the total dosage of tetracycline. The tetracyclines should not be administered to pregnant patients or to children under age 8, the period when tooth enamel is forming. Bone deposition from a tetracycline temporarily halts bone growth.

Hepatotoxic reactions to tetracyclines include fatty infiltration of the liver associated primarily with I.V. tetracyclines. This reaction is most significant in patients with an excessive serum concentration caused by renal failure.

Nephrotoxicity develops in patients with renal failure; the antianabolic effects of tetracyclines may increase BUN and serum creatinine levels. Outdated or degraded tetracycline can produce a reversible Fanconi-like syndrome with renal tubular acidosis. However, because tetracycline preparations that have produced this syndrome have been reformulated, this complication is unlikely to occur.

Central nervous system toxicity, including vestibular disturbances, occurs primarily with minocycline. Lightheadedness, loss of balance, dizziness, and tinnitus usually begin on the second or third day of therapy and occur more commonly in women than men. Symptoms are reversible within several days after discontinuing the drug.

As with any antibiotic, superinfection commonly develops during tetracycline therapy. Overgrowth of yeast typically occurs, and oral or vaginal moniliasis requires specific therapy. Staphylococcal enterocolitis caused by tetracycline-resistant staphylococci can lead to severe diarrhea, dehydration, and possible circulatory collapse.

Although uncommon, hypersensitivity reactions to tetracyclines include anaphylaxis, urticaria, periorbital edema, fixed drug eruptions, and morbilliform rashes.

NURSING PROCESS APPLICATION

The following information assists the nurse in caring for a patient who is receiving a tetracycline.

Assessment
• Review the patient's history for a preexisting condition that contraindicates the use of a tetracycline, such as pregnancy, lactation, infancy, childhood up to age 8, or known hypersensitivity to any tetracycline.
• Review the patient's history for a preexisting condition that requires cautious use of a tetracycline, such as impaired renal or hepatic function.
• Assess the patient for adverse reactions to the prescribed tetracycline, such as GI dysfunction, dermatologic reactions, hepatotoxicity, nephrotoxicity, or CNS toxicity.
• Assess the patient for superinfection during tetracycline therapy.

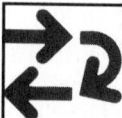

DRUG INTERACTIONS
Tetracyclines

This chart summarizes significant interactions between the tetracyclines and other drugs. The nurse should be familiar with these interactions before administering any tetracycline.

DRUG	INTERACTING DRUGS	POSSIBLE EFFECTS	NURSING IMPLICATIONS
chlortetracycline, demeclocycline, doxycycline, methacycline, minocycline, oxytetracycline, tetracycline	antacids with divalent or trivalent cations, such as aluminum and magnesium	Inhibit oral absorption of tetracyclines	• Separate doses by 1 to 2 hours.
	methoxyflurane	Produce nephrotoxicity	• Avoid tetracycline use in patients who are to receive anesthesia with methoxyflurane.
doxycycline, methacycline, oxytetracycline, tetracycline	iron salts, bismuth subsalicylate, zinc sulfate	Impair GI absorption of tetracyclines	• Administer these agents 3 hours before or 2 hours after tetracyclines.
doxycycline	barbiturates, carbamazepine, phenytoin	Enhance doxycycline metabolism	• Avoid concurrent use. • Use a tetracycline other than doxycycline if barbiturate, phenytoin, or carbamazepine therapy is required, or expect to increase the doxycycline dosage.
tetracycline	oral contraceptives	May alter GI bacterial flora, leading to decreased contraceptive efficacy and breakthrough bleeding	• Advise the patient to use an alternative contraceptive method during tetracycline therapy and for 1 week after tetracycline is discontinued.
all tetracyclines	penicillin	May interfere with bacteriocidal action of penicillin	• Separate doses by several hours.

• Review the patient's medication history to identify the use of drugs that may interfere with the prescribed tetracycline, such as antacids that contain aluminum or magnesium, iron salts, bismuth subsalicylate, zinc sulfate, or penicillin.
• Assess the effectiveness of the prescribed tetracycline periodically.
• Evaluate the patient's and family's knowledge about the prescribed tetracycline.

Nursing diagnoses
The following examples represent appropriate nursing diagnoses for a patient receiving a tetracycline.
• Potential for injury related to a preexisting condition that contraindicates the use of a tetracycline
• Potential for injury related to a preexisting condition that requires cautious use of a tetracycline
• Potential for injury related to adverse drug reactions
• Altered protection related to development of a superinfection caused by tetracycline therapy
• Knowledge deficit related to the prescribed tetracycline

Planning and implementation
• Do not administer a tetracycline to a patient with a condition that contraindicates its use.
• Administer a tetracycline cautiously to a patient at risk because of a preexisting condition.
• Monitor the patient periodically for adverse reactions during tetracycline therapy.
• Observe the patient closely for hypersensitivity reactions, such as anaphylaxis, urticaria, periorbital edema, fixed drug eruptions, or morbilliform rashes. Although anaphylaxis is rare, have standard emergency equipment nearby. If a hypersensitivity reaction occurs, notify the physician and expect to discontinue the drug.
• Monitor hydration if the patient experiences nausea, vomiting, or diarrhea. Request a prescription for an antiemetic or antidiarrheal agent, if needed. Expect to switch to a parenteral form of tetracycline or to a different antibiotic as prescribed.
• *Administer doxycycline or minocycline with food to minimize GI irritation. Administer any other tetracycline on an empty stomach, 1 hour before or 2 hours after meals.*
• Do not administer a tetracycline (except doxycycline or minocycline) with milk, milk products, or drugs that con-

tain calcium, magnesium, aluminum, or iron. These foods and drugs can bind with the tetracycline, preventing its absorption.
• Monitor liver function studies for abnormalities indicating a hepatotoxic reaction to the prescribed tetracycline, especially in a patient with an excessive serum concentration caused by renal failure.
• Monitor the BUN and creatinine levels for further elevations in the patient with renal failure.
• Monitor for symptoms of CNS toxicity, such as lightheadedness, loss of balance, dizziness, and tinnitus, particularly on the second or third day of therapy, in a patient receiving minocycline. If these symptoms occur, notify the physician and take safety measures, such as supervising ambulation. Expect to discontinue the agent.
• Dilute an I.V. preparation in a large volume of fluid and administer it by continuous slow drip.
• Monitor for thrombophlebitis at the I.V. site in a patient receiving parenteral tetracycline or oxytetracycline.
• *Check any prescription for I.M. injection because I.M. administration usually is not recommended. If I.M. injections must be administered, inject the drug deep into a large muscle.*
• Notify the physician if adverse reactions occur.
• Monitor the patient regularly for signs of superinfection, such as oral thrush, GI disturbance, or worsening of signs and symptoms of the systemic infection.
• *Inspect the patient's mouth regularly for signs of oral moniliasis, such as cream-colored or bluish-white pseudomembranous patches on the tongue, mouth, or pharynx. Encourage the female patient to report any unusual vaginal discharge.*
• Notify the physician if oral or vaginal moniliasis is suspected; specific therapy will be required.

Patient teaching
• Teach the patient and family the name, dose, frequency, action, and adverse effects of the prescribed tetracycline.
• Advise the patient experiencing a hypersensitivity reaction to withhold the drug until the physician is notified.
• *Advise the patient not to ingest milk, milk products, or drugs containing calcium, magnesium, aluminum, or iron at the same time as the prescribed tetracycline because these products prevent tetracycline absorption.*
• Advise the patient to take the prescribed tetracycline on an empty stomach (except for doxycycline or minocycline, which should be taken with food to minimize GI irritation).
• Advise the patient who experiences esophageal irritation to take tetracycline with 8 oz of water.
• Warn the patient receiving oxytetracycline I.M. that the injection will be painful.
• Inform the patient that chlortetracycline may stain clothing.

• Inform the patient with monocycline-induced CNS toxicity that the symptoms should disappear several days after the drug is discontinued.
• *Advise the patient to avoid direct sunlight, cover exposed skin, or use a sunscreen with an SPF of 15 or higher during tetracycline therapy.*
• Teach the patient the importance of completing the prescribed course of tetracycline therapy.
• *Advise the female patient taking an oral contraceptive to use an alternative means of contraception during tetracycline therapy and for 1 week after therapy is discontinued.*
• Instruct the patient to notify the physician if adverse reactions occur.

Evaluation
The following examples represent appropriate evaluation statements for a patient receiving a tetracycline.
• The patient has no conditions that contraindicate tetracycline therapy.
• The patient exhibits no signs of complications in the preexisting condition linked to the prescribed tetracycline.
• The patient exhibits no adverse reactions to the prescribed tetracycline.
• The patient remains free of superinfection during tetracycline therapy.
• The patient and family express an accurate understanding of the points taught about the prescribed tetracycline.
• The patient takes the tetracycline as instructed in related to food and other drugs.

CHLORAMPHENICOL

Chloramphenicol was released for clinical use in 1949. Soon afterward, drug-induced aplastic anemia limited its clinical usefulness. Today, chloramphenicol usually is reserved for treating serious infections and infections with ampicillin-resistant *H. influenzae*.

PHARMACOKINETICS

Chloramphenicol is available in capsules for oral treatment and in ointment for topical treatment of ophthalmic or otic infections. It also is available as chloramphenicol palmitate in oral suspensions and as chloramphenicol succinate for I.V. administration. Chloramphenicol salts must be hydrolyzed to free chloramphenicol before pharmacologic action can occur.

Absorption, distribution, metabolism, excretion

Chloramphenicol is absorbed rapidly and completely from the GI tract and is not impaired by the concomitant administration of food or antacids. Chloramphenicol salts are hydrolyzed slowly to free drug by pancreatic lipases in the duodenum; as a result, peak serum concentration levels are somewhat lower and delayed compared with those of chloramphenicol. Intravenous preparations also must be hydrolyzed before they can provide antibacterial activity. When chloramphenicol is administered orally, hydrolysis occurs in the GI tract; after I.V. administration, in the plasma.

After absorption, chloramphenicol is distributed widely to body fluids and tissue. The lipid solubility of the drug permits penetration across lipid barriers. The peak concentration is high in the CNS even without inflammation. Concentration in the CSF, with or without meningitis, usually is one-third to three-quarters of the peak serum concentration. Chloramphenicol crosses the blood-ocular barrier. Lipid solubility also accounts for increased uptake by alveolar macrophages. Chloramphenicol crosses the placenta to the fetal circulation but appears in negligible amounts in the amniotic fluid. Chloramphenicol is excreted in breast milk.

In patients with normal hepatic function, free chloramphenicol is metabolized primarily in the liver by glucuronide conjugation. The nontoxic glucuronide metabolite is excreted in inactive form by the kidneys. Glucuronyl transferase, the enzyme that metabolizes chloramphenicol, is not very active in neonates or in adults with serious hepatic dysfunction. Administering usual dosages of chloramphenicol to such patients can lead to increased serum concentrations of biologically active drug.

Only 5% to 10% of an administered dose is recovered in urine as biologically active chloramphenicol. The rest is metabolized by the liver. If the patient has no renal disease, concentrations of 150 to 200 mcg/ml of active drug are achieved, sufficient to treat UTIs. However, urine concentrations are decreased greatly in patients with renal failure.

Onset, peak, duration

Peak serum concentration levels occur 2 to 3 hours after oral administration. Peak concentrations occur 1 to 2 hours after I.V. infusion. Chloramphenicol is 50% to 60% bound to serum albumin. Plasma half-life in adults with normal liver function is 1.5 to 3.5 hours. The half-life is prolonged greatly in patients with immature or inadequate liver function, lasting 24 hours or longer in neonates.

Therapeutic peak concentrations are 10 to 25 mcg/ml. Levels exceeding 25 mcg/ml may lead to reversible bone marrow suppression; levels greater than 40 mcg/ml have been associated with gray syndrome in neonates, older children, and adults as well as encephalitis in adults.

PHARMACODYNAMICS

Chloramphenicol usually is bacteriostatic and may be bactericidal against some organisms.

Mechanism of action

Chloramphenicol, which inhibits protein synthesis of susceptible organisms, also inhibits protein synthesis in cells that proliferate rapidly, such as bone marrow cells. The inhibition can lead to bone marrow suppression. The major mechanism of resistance in gram-negative bacilli other than *P. aeruginosa* is enzymatic acetylation, which is plasmid-mediated. *P. aeruginosa* and some strains of *Proteus* and *Klebsiella* resist via nonenzymatic mechanisms, including an induced block that prevents chloramphenicol from entering the bacterial cell.

PHARMACOTHERAPEUTICS

Chloramphenicol is active against various organisms, including bacteria, spirochetes, rickettsiae, chlamydiae, and mycoplasmas. Easily reached serum concentrations of chloramphenicol inhibit most gram-positive and gram-negative aerobic bacteria, but more active and less toxic agents are available. Chloramphenicol is extremely active against anaerobic bacteria, including *B. fragilis*. It is the drug of choice for treating ampicillin-resistant typhoid fever and other systemic *Salmonella* infections. It also is effective for brain abscesses and certain types of bacterial meningitis. Because of the increasing resistance of *H. influenzae* to ampicillin, ampicillin given with chloramphenicol currently is the recommended regimen for initial treatment of *H. influenzae* meningitis. Topical chloramphenicol is used to treat eye and external ear infections. (For information about the use of topical chloramphenicol for these infections, see Chapter 71, Ophthalmic Agents, and Chapter 72, Otic Agents.)

chloramphenicol (Chloromycetin). The oral formulation has greater bioavailability than chloramphenicol sodium succinate, the I.V. form. Whenever possible, oral administration is preferable because it costs less. In vitro, the drug is active against many gram-positive aerobic bacteria, including *S. pneumoniae* and other streptococci, and many gram-negative aerobic bacteria, including *H. influenzae*, *N. meningitidis*, *Salmonella*, and *Shigella*. It also is active against many anaerobic bacteria, such as *B. melaninogenicus*, *B. fragilis*, *Clostridium fusobacterium*, *Veillonella*, *Rickettsia*, *Chlamydia*, and *Mycoplasma*. Because of potential toxicity, chloramphenicol should be reserved for serious infections in which the infection site and pathogen susceptibility indicate limited treatment alternatives. Careful monitoring of the serum concentration is essential.

Usual adult dosage: 50 to 100 mg/kg/day P.O. in divided doses every 6 hours.

Usual pediatric dosage: for neonates up to age 2 weeks, 6.25 mg/kg P.O. every 6 hours; for children over age 2 weeks, 12.5 mg/kg P.O. every 6 hours or 25 mg/kg P.O. every 12 hours.

chloramphenicol palmitate (Chloromycetin Palmitate). Oral suspension is available as 150 mg per 5 ml; it should be administered to patients who cannot swallow capsules.

Usual adult dosage: 50 to 100 mg/kg/day P.O. in divided doses every 6 hours.

Usual pediatric dosage: for neonates up to age 2 weeks, 6.25 mg/kg P.O. every 6 hours; for children over age 2 weeks, 12.5 mg/kg P.O. every 6 hours or 25 mg/kg P.O. every 12 hours.

chloramphenicol sodium succinate (Chloromycetin Sodium Succinate). This preparation is used for I.V. administration. Because the ester must be hydrolyzed to its active form, a time lag follows infusion before an adequate serum concentration is reached.

Usual adult dosage: 50 to 100 mg/kg/day I.V. in four divided doses every 6 hours.

Usual pediatric dosage: for neonates up to age 2 weeks, 6.25 mg/kg I.V. every 6 hours; for children over age 2 weeks, 12.5 mg/kg I.V. every 6 hours or 25 mg/kg I.V. every 12 hours.

Drug interactions

Chloramphenicol may inhibit the metabolism of oral hypoglycemic agents such as chlorpropamide and tolbutamide, anticonvulsants such as phenytoin, and oral anticoagulants such as dicumarol. This inhibited metabolism can lead to hypoglycemia, phenytoin toxicity, or hemorrhage. During concomitant therapy, the dosage of the oral hypoglycemic, anticonvulsant, or anticoagulant may need to be decreased.

Concomitant administration of chloramphenicol and other drugs causing bone marrow suppression should be avoided because additive toxicity can occur.

ADVERSE DRUG REACTIONS

The use of chloramphenicol is limited by its potential toxicities. When the drug is used, the nurse must recognize adverse reactions in the patient.

Adverse GI reactions to oral chloramphenicol may include nausea, vomiting, glossitis, unpleasant taste in the mouth, stomatitis, diarrhea, and perineal irritation.

Gray syndrome, a potentially fatal adverse reaction associated with excessive chloramphenicol serum concentrations, is most common in neonates. Initial manifestations include abdominal distention, vomiting, anorexia, tachy-pnea, cyanosis, green stools, lethargy, and an ashen color. These reactions are followed by circulatory collapse and death. Gray syndrome results from the neonate's decreased ability to conjugate chloramphenicol and to excrete the active form in urine, especially when the drug is given within the first 48 hours after birth. Gray syndrome also may occur in older children or adults receiving excessive chloramphenicol doses resulting in serum concentrations greater than 40 to 200 mcg/ml.

Bone marrow suppression is the most toxic reaction to chloramphenicol. Reversible bone marrow suppression results from inhibiting mitochondrial protein synthesis. Signs of bone marrow suppression include granulocytopenia, reticulocytopenia, anemia, leukopenia, and thrombocytopenia. These signs correlate with daily doses greater than 4 grams, duration of treatment, and serum concentrations exceeding 25 mcg/ml. Bone marrow suppression is reversible when chloramphenicol is discontinued.

Aplastic anemia, which usually is irreversible, may occur after chloramphenicol is discontinued. The peripheral blood shows pancytopenia. Aplastic anemia is produced by a different mechanism than the direct bone marrow suppression; it may be an allergic reaction. Aplastic anemia occurs in about 1 in 40,000 or more patients taking chloramphenicol. Mortality is greater than 50%.

Hypersensitivity reactions, including fever, macular and vesicular rashes, angioedema, urticaria, and anaphylaxis, have been reported.

NURSING PROCESS APPLICATION

The following information assists the nurse in caring for a patient who is receiving chloramphenicol.

Assessment

• Review the patient's history for a preexisting condition that contraindicates the use of chloramphenicol, such as known hypersensitivity or toxic reactions to the drug. It also is contraindicated in the treatment of trivial infections or conditions where it is not indicated (as in colds, influenza, or throat infections), or in the prevention of bacterial infection.

• Review the patient's history for a preexisting condition that requires cautious use of chloramphenicol, such as infancy, term pregnancy, labor, lactation, or impaired renal or hepatic function.

• Assess the patient for adverse reactions to chloramphenicol, such as GI upset, gray syndrome, bone marrow suppression, aplastic anemia, or hypersensitivity reactions.

• Review the patient's medication history to identify the use of drugs that may interact with chloramphenicol, such as oral hypoglycemic agents, anticonvulsants, and anticoagulants.

• Assess the effectiveness of chloramphenicol periodically.

• Evaluate the patient's and family's knowledge about chloramphenicol.

Nursing diagnoses

The following examples represent appropriate nursing diagnoses for a patient receiving chloramphenicol.
• Potential for injury related to a preexisting condition that contraindicates the use of chloramphenicol
• Potential for injury related to a preexisting condition that requires cautious use of chloramphenicol
• Potential for injury related to adverse drug reactions
• Altered protection related to bone marrow suppression caused by chloramphenicol
• Knowledge deficit related to chloramphenicol

Planning and implementation

• Do not administer chloramphenicol to a patient with a condition that contraindicates its use.
• Administer chloramphenicol cautiously to a patient at risk because of a preexisting condition.
• Monitor the patient periodically for adverse reactions during chloramphenicol therapy.
• Monitor the patient's chloramphenicol serum concentration for values greater than 40 mcg/ml.
• Observe the neonate, older child, or adult for signs of gray syndrome, such as abdominal distention, vomiting, anorexia, tachypnea, cyanosis, green stools, lethargy, and an ashen color, if the serum concentration is greater than 40 mcg/ml. Observe the adult patient for evidence of encephalitis, such as decresed level of consciousness, headache, fever, seizures, and nuchal rigidity.
• Continue to observe the patient for signs and symptoms of aplastic anemia, such as anemia, infection, or bleeding, after chloramphenicol therapy has been discontinued.
• Monitor the patient's complete blood counts regularly.
• *Screen the patient for a history of chloramphenicol hypersensitivity before initiating therapy. Throughout therapy, monitor the patient for hypersensitivity reactions, such as fever, macular and vesicular rashes, angioedema, urticaria, or anaphylaxis. Have standard emergency equipment nearby. If a hypersensitivity reaction occurs, withhold the drug and notify the physician.*
• Monitor hydration if the patient experiences nausea, vomiting, or diarrhea. Request a prescription for an antiemetic or antidiarrheal, if needed. If adverse GI reactons are severe, expect to discontinue chloramphenicol.
• *Inspect the patient's mouth regularly for evidence of stomatitis, such as pain, redness, and swollen mucous membranes. Notify the physician if stomatitis occurs.*
• Expect to decrease the chloramphenicol dosage as prescribed in a patient with serious hepatic dysfunction or renal failure or in a neonate to prevent bone marrow suppression, encephalitis, or gray syndrome.

• Notify the physician if adverse reactions occur.
• Monitor the patient's chloramphenicol serum concentration closely for values that exceed 25 mcg/ml. If the concentration exceeds 25 mcg/ml, take bleeding precautions and infection-control measures because bone marrow suppression can occur.
• *Consult the physician about decreasing the dosage or substituting another antibiotic if bone marrow suppression occurs.*

Patient teaching
• Teach the patient and family the name, dose, frequency, action, and adverse effects of chloramphenicol.
• Instruct the patient to withhold the chloramphenicol dose and notify the physician if a hypersensitivity reaction occurs.
• Advise the patient to notify the physician if fever, sore throat, fatigue, unusual bleeding, or bruising occurs.
• Teach the patient the importance of returning for regular blood tests as instructed to detect adverse reactions.
• Warn the patient about the unpleasant taste of oral chloramphenicol.
• Instruct the patient to notify the nurse or physician if any other adverse reactions occur.
• Instruct the patient to complete the entire course of chloramphenicol therapy.

Evaluation
The following examples represent appropriate evaluation statements for a patient receiving chloramphenicol.
• The patient has no conditions that contraindicate chloramphenicol therapy.
• The patient exhibits no signs of complications in the preexisting condition linked to chloraphenicol.
• The patient exhibits no adverse reactions to chloramphenicol.
• The patient's chloramphenicol serum concentration remains below 25 mcg/ml.
• The patient and family express an accurate understanding of the points taught about chloramphenicol.
• The patient returns for regular blood tests as instructed.

CLINDAMYCIN AND LINCOMYCIN

Clindamycin and lincomycin hydrochloride are lincosamide antibacterials with similar spectra of activity. Clindamycin usually is more effective than lincomycin, which remains particularly important in treating certain anaerobic infections. With its limited indications and greater incidence of adverse effects, lincomycin is used rarely.

PHARMACOKINETICS

Clindamycin and lincomycin can be administered orally, intramuscularly, or intravenously. After oral administration, clindamycin is absorbed well and distributed widely in the body. Lincomycin is absorbed more poorly. Clindamycin and lincomycin are eliminated primarily via hepatic metabolism and renal and biliary excretion.

Absorption, distribution, metabolism, excretion

Clindamycin hydrochloride is absorbed rapidly and almost completely (about 90%) from the GI tract. The presence of food slightly delays but does not decrease the absorption of the drug. Lincomycin is absorbed only 20% to 30% in the fasting state; the presence of food greatly decreases its absorption.

Clindamycin and lincomycin are distributed well to most body tissues with the exception of the CSF. Even when the meninges are inflamed, only small concentration levels of clindamycin are found in the CSF. The clindamycin concentration in bone is 60% to 80% that of the serum concentration. Clindamycin readily crosses the placenta and enters fetal blood and tissues.

Most of a clindamycin dose is metabolized in the liver to N-demethyl-clindamycin (more active than the parent compound) and clindamycin sulfoxide (less active than the parent compound). Both of these metabolites may appear in bile and urine but not in serum. Lincomycin is metabolized partially in the liver.

About 10% of active clindamycin is excreted unchanged in urine, and only small quantities are excreted in feces. However, excretion in feces is increased in patients with impaired renal function. About 40% of oral lincomycin is excreted unchanged in the feces. About 30% of I.V. or I.M. lincomycin is excreted in the urine. The normal half-life of clindamycin is 2.4 hours; the half-life of lincomycin is 4.5 hours. In patients with severe renal failure, the half-life of clindamycin increases to about 6 hours and lincomycin increases to 9 hours. Appreciable dosage adjustments should be made when a patient has severe renal and hepatic disease concomitantly.

Onset, peak, duration

After oral administration of clindamycin, the peak serum concentration level is reached earlier and is at least twice as high as that of lincomycin. The mean peak serum concentrations in adults after a single oral dose of clindamycin is reached in 1 hour; that of lincomycin, in 2 to 4 hours. However, after I.M. administration of lincomycin, the peak plasma concentration occurs in 30 minutes, compared to 3 hours for clindamycin given I.M. With I.V. infusion, the peak concentration is reached when the infusion is complete.

PHARMACODYNAMICS

Clindamycin and lincomycin have the same mechanism of action as chloramphenicol and erythromycin. Clindamycin and lincomycin may compete for the same binding sites on the ribosomes.

Mechanism of action

Clindamycin and lincomycin inhibit bacterial protein synthesis; they may inhibit the binding of bacterial ribosomes. At therapeutically attainable concentrations, clindamycin and lincomycin are primarily bacteriostatic against most organisms.

PHARMACOTHERAPEUTICS

Because of its greater activity, enhanced absorption properties, and smaller potential for toxicity, clindamycin is preferred over lincomycin. However, because of its potential for serious toxicity and pseudomembranous colitis, clindamycin is limited to a few clinical indications where safer alternative antibacterials are not available.

Clindamycin is more potent than lincomycin against most aerobic gram-positive organisms, including staphylococci, streptococci (except *S. faecalis*), and pneumococci. Clindamycin is effective against most of the clinically important anaerobes, particularly *B. fragilis.* However, resistance to clindamycin has been found in 5% to 15% of *B. fragilis* strains. Clindamycin and lincomycin are inactive against aerobic gram-negative bacilli.

Clindamycin is used primarily to treat anaerobic intraabdominal or pleuropulmonary infections caused by *B. fragilis.* It also is used as an alternative to penicillin in treating *Clostridium perfringens* infections. In addition, it may be used as an alternative to penicillin in treating staphylococcal infections; however, clindamycin is an unreliable bactericidal. It should not be used for deep-seated staphylococcal infections, particularly endocarditis.

clindamycin hydrochloride (Cleocin). Clindamycin hydrochloride is used to treat soft-tissue and respiratory tract infections.
Usual adult dosage: 150 to 450 mg P.O. every 6 hours.
Usual pediatric dosage: for children over age 1 month, 2 to 6.3 mg/kg P.O. every 6 hours or 2.7 to 8.3 mg/kg P.O. every 8 hours.

clindamycin palmitate hydrochloride (Cleocin Pediatric). This suspension preparation of flavored granules, at 75 mg of clindamycin per milliliter, is convenient for children and elderly patients who cannot swallow capsules. The

water-soluble clindamycin compound is hydrolyzed in vivo to the active drug and is used to treat soft-tissue and respiratory tract infections.
Usual adult dosage: 150 to 450 mg P.O. every 6 to 8 hours.
Usual pediatric dosage: for children over age 1 month, 2 to 6.3 mg/kg P.O. every 6 hours or 2.7 to 8.3 mg/kg P.O. every 8 hours.

clindamycin phosphate (Cleocin Phosphate). For treating serious infections caused by aerobic gram-positive cocci and anaerobes, this parenteral form of clindamycin should be administered initially.
Usual adult dosage: 300 to 600 mg I.V. or I.M. every 6 to 8 hours.
Usual pediatric dosage: for children over age 1 month, 3.75 to 10 mg I.M. or I.V. every 6 hours or 5 to 13.3 mg/kg I.M. or I.V. every 8 hours.

lincomycin hydrochloride (Lincocin). This agent is used to treat serious infections caused by most streptococcus pneumoniae and staphylocci and several anaerobic gram-negative and gram-positive organisms.
Usual adult dosage: 500 mg P.O. every 6 to 8 hours, 600 mg to 1 gram I.V. every 12 hours, or 600 mg I.M. every 12 to 24 hours.
Usual pediatric dosage: for children over age 1 month, 7.5 to 15 mg/kg P.O. every 6 hours or 10 to 20 mg/kg P.O. every 8 hours; 10 mg/kg I.M. every 12 to 24 hours, 3.3 to 6.7 mg/kg I.V. every 8 hours, or 5 to 10 mg/kg I.V. every 12 hours.

Drug interactions

Clindamycin and lincomycin may block neuromuscular transmission and may enhance the action of neuromuscular blocking agents. Clindamycin phosphate in solution is incompatible with ampicillin, aminophylline, calcium gluconate, and magnesium sulfate.

Concomitant use with kaolin preparations reduces lincomycin absorption by 90%. Food decreases the rate and extent of lincomycin absorption.

ADVERSE DRUG REACTIONS

Clindamycin and lincomycin can produce severe and even fatal toxicities. As a result, these drugs are reserved for serious infections for which less toxic antibacterial agents are unavailable.

During clindamycin therapy, diarrhea occurs in about 80% of patients, most commonly with oral administration. It may begin a few days after initiation of therapy or days to weeks after the drug is discontinued, and it can be severe. Persistent diarrhea also may occur with lincomycin.

Pseudomembranous colitis, characterized by severe diarrhea, abdominal pain, fever, and mucus and blood in the stools, can occur with clindamycin or lincomycin. This syndrome, which can be fatal, is caused by a toxin secreted by *C. difficile* that overgrows in the presence of clindamycin or lincomycin. Prompt discontinuation of the antibacterial is essential. Use of antiperistaltic drugs, which may aggravate the condition, should be avoided. The treatment of choice for pseudomembranous colitis is 125 to 500 mg vancomycin P.O., or 500 mg metronidazole P.O., every 6 hours for 5 to 10 days. Oral administration of clindamycin or lincomycin also can produce stomatitis, nausea, and vomiting.

When administered I.V., clindamycin can damage tissue. Intramuscular administration can produce pain, induration, and sterile abscess. Lincomycin can cause pain and phlebitis at the I.V. infusion site.

Hypersensitivity reactions in the form of skin rashes occur in approximately 10% of patients treated with clindamycin or lincomycin. The skin rashes resemble those seen in patients receiving ampicillin.

Stevens-Johnson syndrome has occurred rarely, and a few instances of anaphylactic reactions also have occurred.

NURSING PROCESS APPLICATION

The following information assists the nurse in caring for a patient who is receiving clindamycin or lincomycin.

Assessment
• Review the patient's history for a preexisting condition that contraindicates the use of clindamycin or lincomycin, such as pregnancy, lactation, or known hypersensitivity to either drug.
• Review the patient's history for a preexisting condition that requires cautious use of clindamycin or lincomycin, such as a history of GI disease, severe renal or hepatic impairment, or multiple allergies.
• Assess the patient for adverse reactions to clindamycin or lincomycin, such as GI upset (especially diarrhea), stomatitis, tissue damage at the injection or infusion site, hypersensitivity reactions, or Stevens-Johnson syndrome.
• Assess the patient periodically for pseudomembranous colitis.
• Review the patient's medication history to identify the use of drugs that may interact with clindamycin, such as neuromuscular blocking agents, ampicillin, aminophylline, calcium gluconate, and magnesium sulfate, and of drugs that may interact with lincomycin, such as kaolin preparations.
• Assess the effectiveness of clindamycin or lincomycin periodically.
• Evaluate the patient's and family's knowledge about clindamycin or lincomycin.

Nursing diagnoses

The following examples represent appropriate nursing diagnoses for a patient receiving clindamycin or lincomycin.

• Potential for injury related to a preexisting condition that contraindicates the use of clindamycin or lincomycin

• Potential for injury related to a preexisting condition that requires cautious use of clindamycin or lincomycin

• Potential for injury related to adverse drug reactions

• Impaired tissue integrity related to pseudomembranous colitis caused by clindamycin or lincomycin

• Knowledge deficit related to clindamycin or lincomycin

Planning and implementation

• Do not administer clindamycin or lincomycin to a patient with a condition that contraindicates its use.

• Administer clindamycin or lincomycin cautiously to a patient at risk because of a preexisting condition.

• Monitor the patient periodically for adverse reactions during clindamycin or lincomycin therapy.

• Inspect the patient's skin for rashes similar to those seen with ampicillin during clindamycin or lincomycin therapy.

• *Have standard emergency equipment nearby to treat anaphylactic reactions that may occur, although they are rare.*

• Monitor hydration closely if the patient experiences GI upset, especially severe diarrhea. Request a prescription for an antiemetic or antidiarrheal agent, if needed. If symptoms persist or worsen, expect to discontinue the drug as prescribed.

• Inspect the patient's mouth regularly for signs of stomatitis, such as red, swollen mucous membranes.

• *Inspect the infusion site regularly for signs and symptoms of thrombophlebitis, such as pain upon touch, color change, or swelling, when administering lincomycin or clindamycin I.V. If signs and symptoms occur, switch the infusion to another site.*

• Observe I.M. clindamycin injection sites regularly for signs of irritation, such as induration or sterile abscess.

• Expect to adjust the dosage appreciably, as prescribed, in a patient with severe, concomitant hepatic and renal disease.

• *Do not refrigerate reconstituted oral clindamycin palmitate hydrochloride solution because it thickens and becomes difficult to measure accurately. The solution remains stable for 2 weeks at room temperature.*

• Monitor the patient for signs and symptoms of Stevens-Johnson syndrome, such as acute onset of fever, bullae on the skin, and ulcers on the mucous membranes of the lips, eyes, mouth, nasal passages, and genitalia. If this occurs, notify the physician and expect to discontinue the drug and initiate appropriate treatment.

• Notify the physician if other adverse reactions occur.

• Monitor the patient for evidence of pseudomembranous colitis, such as severe diarrhea, abdominal pain, fever, and mucus and blood in the stools. If this occurs, promptly discontinue the drug and notify the physician.

• Do not administer an antiperistaltic drug because it can aggravate the colitis.

• Expect to administer vancomycin or metronidazole for 5 to 10 days to treat pseudomembranous colitis.

Patient teaching

• Teach the patient and family the name, dose, frequency, action, and adverse effects of clindamycin or lincomycin.

• Instruct the patient to complete the entire course of clindamycin or lincomycin therapy.

• Warn the patient receiving clindamycin I.M. that the injection may be painful.

• Instruct the patient receiving clindamycin I.V. to notify the nurse if discomfort is felt at the infusion site.

• Teach the patient the importance of notifying the nurse if adverse reactions occur, such as GI upset (especially diarrhea), pseudomembranous colitis, or hypersensitivity reactions.

Evaluation

The following examples represent appropriate evaluation statements for a patient receiving clindamycin or lincomycin.

• The patient has no conditions that contraindicate clindamycin or lincomycin therapy.

• The patient exhibits no signs of complications in the preexisting condition linked to clindamycin or lincomycin.

• The patient exhibits no adverse reactions to clindamycin or lincomycin.

• The patient exhibits no signs of pseudomembranous colitis.

• The patient and family express an accurate understanding of the points taught about clindamycin or lincomycin.

• The patient agrees to notify the nurse if discomfort is felt at the infusion site.

ERYTHROMYCIN

A macrolide antibacterial, erythromycin contains a large macrocyclic lactone ring. Erythromycin is used to treat a number of common infections. Because this highly effective drug is considered one of the safest antibiotics, clinical indications for erythromycin continue to increase.

PHARMACOKINETICS

Erythromycin, the unmodified drug, is a bitter, crystalline compound that dissolves poorly in water. It is inactivated rapidly by gastric acid. Investigators have modified the drug and its preparations to improve absorption and increase the serum concentration level.

Absorption, distribution, metabolism, excretion

Because gastric acid destroys erythromycin, preparations are made with an acid-resistant film coating that delays drug dissolution until it reaches the small intestine. Erythromycin esters and ester salts, which are more acid-stable and tasteless, form a stable suspension in water. Because of their characteristics, the esters and ester salts are used in liquid suspension for children.

Erythromycin is absorbed intact. The type of tablet and the patient's food intake affect absorption.

Erythromycin is distributed well to most tissues and body fluids except for the CSF. Limited data on CSF concentrations in patients with meningitis suggest that large parenteral doses may be effective against only highly susceptible organisms, such as the pneumococci. Protein binding varies from 70% to 90%. The drug persists longer in tissues than in serum.

Erythromycin has poor penetration into the synovial fluid. Concentrations achieved in the middle ear in otitis media and in the sputum and sinus secretions are adequate to treat infections caused by pneumococci and group A streptococci but are not adequate to eradicate *H. influenzae* consistently. Erythromycin is transported across the placenta and is excreted in breast milk.

Erythromycin is metabolized by the liver and excreted in bile in high concentrations. After oral administration, a high concentration of erythromycin, representing unabsorbed drug and some excreted by the biliary tract, appears in the stool.

Small amounts of erythromycin, ranging from about 2% of an oral dose to about 15% of a parenteral dose, are excreted in urine. Active transport and net tubular reabsorption of erythromycin may occur. The normal serum half-life of erythromycin is about 1.2 to 2.6 hours. In anuric patients, the serum half-life is increased to about 6 hours.

Onset, peak, duration

Peak serum concentration levels obtained after administration of various erythromycin preparations depend on several factors, including the chemical structure, coating, and number of doses of the drug, and whether the patient is fasting. Enteric-coated erythromycin provides excellent bioavailability. The mean peak serum concentration occurs 2 to 4 hours after a single 250-mg dose in the fasting patient.

PHARMACODYNAMICS

Erythromycin is a bacteriostatic antibacterial that inhibits protein synthesis similarly to chloramphenicol, clindamycin, and lincomycin. Acting on the ribosomal subunit, erythromycin inhibits RNA-dependent protein synthesis by blocking translocation of peptides. The antibacterial spectrum of activity of chloramphenicol, clindamycin, and lincomycin may be affected by erythromycin because of competition for common binding sites.

PHARMACOTHERAPEUTICS

Erythromycin provides a broad spectrum of antimicrobial activity against gram-positive and gram-negative bacteria, including *Acinetobacter* and mycobacteria, treponemas, mycoplasmas, rickettsiae, and chlamydiae. Erythromycin also is effective against pneumococci and group A streptococci. Most clinical isolates of *S. aureus* are sensitive to erythromycin; however, resistant strains may emerge during therapy. Erythromycin is the drug of choice for treating *M. pneumoniae* infections. It also is the preferred drug for treating pneumonia caused by *L. pneumophila*. In patients who are allergic to penicillin, erythromycin is effective for infections produced by group A beta-hemolytic streptococci or *S. pneumoniae*. It also may be used to treat gonorrhea and syphilis in patients who cannot tolerate penicillin G or the tetracyclines. Erythromycin also may be used to treat minor cutaneous staphylococcal infections, although the semisynthetic penicillins, cephalosporins, and vancomycin are used to treat serious staphylococcal infections.

erythromycin (E-Mycin, Ery-Tab, Ilotycin). No one oral preparation provides any clinical advantages over another. Erythromycin appears to be the best absorbed. It is available as enteric-coated and film-coated tablets.
Usual adult dosage: 250 mg P.O. every 6 hours.
Usual pediatric dosage: 7.5 to 25 mg/kg P.O. every 6 hours, 15 to 50 mg/kg P.O. every 12 hours, or 500 mg P.O. every 12 hours.

erythromycin estolate (Ilosone). Erythromycin estolate is available in tablet, capsule, and liquid forms. A higher incidence of hepatotoxicity is associated with erythromycin estolate than with other forms. The liquid form is absorbed well and used mostly for pediatric patients.
Usual adult dosage: 250 mg P.O. every 6 hours.
Usual pediatric dosage: 7.5 to 25 mg/kg P.O. every 6 hours or 15 to 50 mg/kg P.O. every 12 hours.

erythromycin ethylsuccinate (E.E.S., Pediamycin). This preparation is not affected by food. A 400-mg erythromycin ethylsuccinate dose produces the same free erythromycin

serum concentration as 250 mg of erythromycin stearate or estolate.
Usual adult dosage: 400 mg every 6 hours.
Usual pediatric dosage: 7.5 to 25 mg/kg P.O. every 6 hours or 15 to 50 mg/kg P.O. every 12 hours.

erythromycin gluceptate (Ilotycin). This preparation should be diluted in 100 to 200 ml of solution and infused intravenously over 30 to 60 minutes. The serum concentration achieved is much higher than that with any oral preparation.
Usual adult dosage: 250 to 500 mg I.V. every 6 hours.
Usual pediatric dosage: 3.75 to 5 mg/kg I.V. every 6 hours.

erythromycin lactobionate (Erythrocin Lactobionate). This preparation is the most common salt form used for I.V. administration.
Usual adult dosage: 250 to 500 mg I.V. every 6 hours.
Usual pediatric dosage: 3.75 to 5 mg/kg I.V. every 6 hours.

erythromycin stearate (Erythrocin). An acid-stable preparation available as film-coated tablets, erythromycin stearate should not be administered with food. After dissociation in the duodenum, it is absorbed as free erythromycin.
Usual adult dosage: 250 mg P.O. every 6 hours.
Usual pediatric dosage: 7.5 to 25 mg/kg P.O. every 6 hours or 15 to 50 mg/kg P.O. every 12 hours.

Drug interactions
Concurrent use of erythromycin in patients receiving high doses of theophylline can decrease theophylline clearance and increase theophylline concentrations. The theophylline dose may have to be decreased to avoid toxicity.

Erythromycin solution is incompatible with vitamins B complex and C, cephalothin, tetracycline, heparin, and chloramphenicol. When combined in a solution, the drugs form a precipitate, which renders both drugs ineffective.

ADVERSE DRUG REACTIONS

Few adverse reactions are associated with erythromycin. Dose-related GI reactions (epigastric distress, nausea, vomiting, and diarrhea) are most common, especially with large doses. Stomatitis, heartburn, anorexia, and melena also can occur.

Although rare, reversible sensorineural hearing loss can occur with I.V. erythromycin lactobionate. This reaction is most likely to occur in patients with renal failure who are receiving high doses of erythromycin. Venous irritation and thrombophlebitis can occur after I.V. administration of erythromycin gluceptate or erythromycin lactobionate.

Allergic reactions, including rashes, fever, eosinophilia, and anaphylaxis, also can occur with the use of erythromycin.

Although rare, the most serious toxicity is a characteristic syndrome of cholestatic hepatitis most commonly associated with erythromycin estolate and erythromycin ethylsuccinate. The syndrome consists of nausea, vomiting, and abdominal pain followed by jaundice, fever, and abnormal liver function test results that are consistent with cholestatic hepatitis. These reactions sometimes are accompanied by rash, leukocytosis, and eosinophilia. The syndrome may represent a hypersensitivity reaction to the specific structure of the estolate compound. The cholestatic jaundice and hepatocellular necrosis may resolve within days to a few weeks after discontinuing the drug.

NURSING PROCESS APPLICATION

The following information assists the nurse in caring for a patient who is receiving erythromycin.

Assessment
• Review the patient's history for a preexisting condition that contraindicates the use of erythromycin, such as known hypersensitivity to the drug.
• Review the patient's history for a preexisting condition that requires cautious use of erythromycin, such as lactation or impaired hepatic function or biliary excretion.
• Assess the patient for adverse reactions to erythromycin, such as GI distress, hearing loss, venous irritation, hypersensitivity reactions, or cholestatic hepatitis.
• Review the patient's medication history to identify the use of drugs that may interact with erythromycin, such as theophylline.
• Assess the effectiveness of erythromycin periodically.
• Evaluate the patient's and family's knowledge about erythromycin.

Nursing diagnoses
The following examples represent appropriate nursing diagnoses for a patient receiving erythromycin.
• Potential for injury related to a preexisting condition that contraindicates the use of erythromycin
• Potential for injury related to a preexisting condition that requires cautious use of erythromycin
• Potential for injury related to adverse drug reactions
• Potential for injury related to cholestatic hepatitis caused by erythromycin
• Knowledge deficit related to erythromycin

Planning and implementation
• Do not administer erythromycin to a patient with a condition that contraindicates its use.
• Administer erythromycin cautiously to a patient at risk because of a preexisting condition.
• Monitor the patient periodically for adverse reactions during erythromycin therapy.

• *Observe the patient for allergic reactions that may include rash, fever, eosinophilia, or anaphylaxis. Have standard emergency equipment nearby. Withhold further doses of erythromycin until the physician is notified.*

• Monitor hydration if the patient develops anorexia, nausea, vomiting, or diarrhea. Notify the physician and request a prescription for an antiemetic or antidiarrheal, if needed. If these GI reactions persist or worsen, expect to discontinue the erythromycin.

• Inspect the patient's mouth regularly for signs of stomatitis, such as red, swollen mucous membranes.

• *Monitor for hearing changes in a patient receiving I.V. erythromycin lactobionate, especially an elderly patient or one with renal insufficiency.*

• *Do not mix I.V. erythromycin with vitamins B complex and C, cephalothin, tetracycline, heparin, or chloramphenicol because they are incompatible.*

• Reconstitute erythromycin solutions in normal saline solution (0.9% sodium chloride) or dextrose 5% in water (D₅W) and administer the solution within 4 hours after preparation.

• Observe the I.V. site for thrombophlebitis when administering erythromycin gluceptate or erythromycin lactobionate.

• *Do not administer erythromycin stearate with food.*

• *Do not administer erythromycin by I.M. injection; the injection is painful and may cause abscess or local tissue necrosis.*

• Notify the physician if adverse reactions occur.

• *Monitor the patient for hepatic dysfunction. Patients on long-term therapy should undergo frequent liver function tests and physical assessment for signs of liver failure.*

• Monitor for signs of cholestatic hepatitis, such as nausea, vomiting, abdominal pain, jaundice, rash, leukocytosis, and eosinophilia, in a patient receiving erythromycin estolate or erythromycin ethyl succinate.

• Expect to discontinue erythromycin if cholestatic hepatitis occurs.

Patient teaching

• Teach the patient and family the name, dose, frequency, action, and adverse effects of erythromycin.

• Instruct the patient to complete the entire course of erythromycin therapy.

• *Instruct the patient not to take erythromycin stearate with food.*

• *Instruct the patient receiving I.V. erythromycin lactobionate to notify the nurse if hearing changes occur.*

• Review the signs and symptoms of cholestatic hepatitis with the patient receiving erythromycin estolate or erythromycin ethylsuccinate. Advise the patient to notify the physician if they appear.

• *Teach the patient on long-term erythromycin therapy the importance of having routine liver function studies as prescribed.*

• Instruct the patient to notify the physician if other adverse reactions occur.

Evaluation

The following examples represent appropriate evaluation statements for a patient receiving erythromycin.

• The patient has no conditions that contraindicate erythromycin therapy.

• The patient exhibits no signs of complications in the preexisting condition linked to erythromycin.

• The patient exhibits no adverse reactions to erythromycin.

• The patient does not develop cholestatic hepatitis during erythromycin therapy.

• The patient and family express an accurate understanding of the points taught about erythromycin.

• The patient states the importance of completing the course of erythromycin therapy.

VANCOMYCIN

Vancomycin hydrochloride is used increasingly to treat methicillin-resistant *S. aureus*, which has become a major concern in the United States and other parts of the world.

PHARMACOKINETICS

Vancomycin is absorbed poorly when administered orally. For systemic infections, vancomycin is administered intravenously. Intramuscular administration is not recommended because of injection pain and tissue necrosis.

Absorption, distribution, metabolism, excretion

Vancomycin is absorbed poorly from the GI tract and is used orally only to treat *C. difficile*-induced pseudomembranous colitis and staphylococcal enterocolitis. To treat systemic infections, vancomycin is administered by intermittent I.V. infusion over 30 to 60 minutes. Rapid or bolus administration is dangerous and can cause flushing and anaphylactic reactions.

Vancomycin diffuses well into pleural, pericardial, synovial, and ascitic fluids. Only small amounts are found in bile. Vancomycin is not found in normal CSF, but bactericidal levels have been found in patients with inflamed meninges. The metabolism of vancomycin is unknown.

Vancomycin is eliminated from the body almost exclusively by glomerular filtration. Approximately 85% of the dose is excreted unchanged in urine within 24 hours. A small amount may be eliminated via the liver and biliary tract. Peak serum concentration levels of vancomycin occur 1 to 2 hours after I.V. administration. The half-life of vancomycin is 4 to 6 hours in patients with normal renal function. In patients with anuria, half-life may be up to 10 days. In such patients, as little as 1 gram of vancomycin may be administered every 7 to 10 days. Because high and potentially toxic serum concentrations of vancomycin can occur in patients with renal insufficiency, dosage adjustments must be made. Vancomycin is not removed by hemodialysis or peritoneal dialysis.

PHARMACODYNAMICS

Vancomycin has a narrow spectrum of antibacterial activity.

Mechanism of action

Vancomycin is a complex soluble glycopolypeptide that is unrelated chemically to any other antibacterial agent. It inhibits biosynthesis of peptidoglycan, the major structural component of the bacterial cell wall. When the bacterial cell wall is damaged, the body's natural defenses can attack the organism.

PHARMACOTHERAPEUTICS

Vancomycin is active against gram-positive organisms, such as *S. aureus, Staphylococcus epidermidis, S. pyogenes,* and *S. pneumoniae.* Gram-negative organisms, fungi, and yeasts are resistant to vancomycin. Intravenous vancomycin is the therapy of choice for patients with serious staphylococcal infections; methicillin-, oxacillin-, nafcillin-, or cephalosporin-resistant organisms; or intolerance to those drugs.

Vancomycin, when used with an aminoglycoside, also is the treatment of choice for *S. faecalis* (enterococcal) endocarditis in patients who are allergic to penicillin. (Vancomycin alone is not a dependable bactericide against all the indicated streptococci.) Orally administered vancomycin is the drug of choice for treating seriously ill patients with antibiotic-associated *C. difficile* colitis. This organism is highly susceptible to vancomycin. Oral vancomycin also may be used to treat staphylococcal enterocolitis.

vancomycin hydrochloride (Vancocin). Available in 500-mg or 1-gram vials, vancomycin is administered I.V. to treat serious systemic infections.
Usual adult dosage: 500 mg I.V. every 6 hours or 1 gram I.V. every 12 hours; maximum dosage, 2 grams/day.
Usual pediatric dosage: 44 mg/kg I.V. daily in divided doses; for neonates, 10 mg/kg I.V. daily every 6 to 12 hours.

vancomycin hydrochloride pulvules (Vancocin). Administered orally, this vancomycin preparation is used to treat staphylococcal enterocolitis or antibiotic-associated pseudomembranous colitis caused by *C. difficile.* It is available as 125- or 250-mg capsules as well as 1- or 10-gram powder for oral solutions.
Usual adult dosage: 125 to 500 mg P.O. every 6 hours for 7 to 10 days.
Usual pediatric dosage: 44 mg/kg P.O. daily in divided doses every 6 hours.

Drug interactions

Vancomycin may enhance the possibility of additive toxicities when administered concurrently with such other nephrotoxic or ototoxic drugs as aminoglycosides, amphotericin B, cisplatin, bacitracin, colistin, and polymixin B.

ADVERSE DRUG REACTIONS

With purified vancomycin preparations now available and with clinicians more aware of the potential toxicity of the drug, adverse reactions are less common.

Ototoxicity is the most serious reaction to parenteral vancomycin. It is most likely to occur in patients with renal impairment and those receiving long-term, high-dose I.V. vancomycin. Vancomycin may damage the auditory branch of the eighth cranial nerve. Permanent deafness can occur. Tinnitus may precede deafness and necessitates drug discontinuation. Hearing loss occasionally improves when the drug is discontinued, but in many cases, deteriorates further.

Occasional mild hematuria, proteinuria, casts in the urine, and azotemia may occur. High doses of parenteral vancomycin should be avoided. The serum concentration should be monitored when other nephrotoxic drugs are administered concurrently. A higher incidence of nephrotoxicity occurs when vancomycin is administered concurrently with an aminoglycoside.

Parenteral vancomycin must be administered I.V. only, and care must be taken to avoid extravasation. Pain and thrombophlebitis may occur after I.V. administration.

Hypotensive reaction associated with rapid I.V. administration of vancomycin is characterized by a sudden blood pressure decrease, which can be severe and may be accompanied by a maculopapular or erythematous rash on the face, neck, chest, and arms. The reaction usually begins a few minutes after the infusion is started and resolves spontaneously several hours after the infusion is discontinued.

Hypersensitivity reactions occur in 5% to 10% of patients receiving vancomycin. Anaphylactic reactions, eosinophilia, and drug fever can occur. Neutropenia, which is rapidly reversible after discontinuation, also can occur.

NURSING PROCESS APPLICATION

The following information assists the nurse in caring for a patient who is receiving vancomycin.

Assessment
• Review the patient's history for a preexisting condition that contraindicates the use of vancomycin, such as pregnancy, known hypersensitivity to the drug, or impaired hearing.
• Review the patient's history for a preexisting condition that requires cautious use of vancomycin, such as lactation or impaired renal function.
• Assess the patient for adverse reactions to vancomycin, such as ototoxicity, nephrotoxicity, thrombophlebitis, hypotension, and hypersensitivity reactions.
• Review the patient's medication history to identify the use of drugs that may interact with vancomycin, such as aminoglycosides, amphotericin B, cisplatin, bacitracin, colistin, and polymixin B.
• Assess the effectiveness of vancomycin periodically.
• Assess the patient's hearing regularly.
• Evaluate the patient's and family's knowledge about vancomycin.

Nursing diagnoses
The following examples represent appropriate nursing diagnoses for a patient receiving vancomycin.
• Potential for injury related to a preexisting condition that contraindicates the use of vancomycin
• Potential for injury related to a preexisting condition that requires cautious use of vancomycin
• Potential for injury related to adverse drug reactions
• Sensory-perceptual alterations (auditory) related to vancomycin-induced ototoxicity
• Knowledge deficit related to vancomycin

Planning and implementation
• Do not administer vancomycin to a patient with a condition that contraindicates its use.
• Administer vancomycin cautiously to a patient at risk because of a preexisting condition.
• *Monitor the patient periodically for adverse reactions to vancomycin, especially ototoxicity, nephrotoxicity, and such hypersensitivity reactions as anaphylactic reactions, drug fever, and eosinophilia or neutropenia. Have standard emergency equipment nearby.*
• *Assess the patient's renal status before beginning vancomycin therapy. Monitor vancomycin serum concentrations (peak and trough levels) and the serum creatinine level if the patient is receiving another ototoxic or nephrotoxic drug concurrently.*

• Monitor the patient for thrombophlebitis at the infusion site.
• Administer vancomycin orally only if the patient has *C. difficile*-induced pseudomembranous colitis or staphylococcal enterocolitis. Question the physician if the oral form is prescribed for any other indication.
• *Do not administer vancomycin by I.M. injection because it is painful and can produce tissue necrosis.*
• *Do not administer vancomycin by rapid I.V. It should be infused slowly over 30 to 60 minutes in a large volume of fluid to avoid a hypotensive reaction.*
• Do not mix vancomycin with other drugs in the same I.V. solution.
• Notify the physician if adverse reactions occur.
• *Monitor closely for signs of ototoxicity, especially in a patient with renal impairment or one receiving long-term, high doses of I.V. vancomycin.*
• Request a baseline audiogram, if possible, before initiating vancomycin therapy. Ask the patient about tinnitus or hearing loss during vancomycin therapy. Notify the physician if the patient reports either problem.
• Withhold vancomycin and notify the physician if tinnitus or hearing loss occurs. Expect to discontinue vancomycin and initiate a different antibiotic as prescribed.

Patient teaching
• Teach the patient and family the name, dose, frequency, action, and adverse effects of vancomycin.
• *Instruct the patient to report tinnitus or hearing loss.*
• Teach the patient the importance of having laboratory studies performed regularly as instructed.
• *Instruct the patient to alert the nurse if pain is felt at the I.V. infusion site.*
• Advise the patient to notify the physician if other adverse reactions occur, if symptoms do not improve, or if they worsen.

Evaluation
The following examples represent appropriate evaluation statements for a patient receiving vancomycin.
• The patient has no conditions that contraindicate vancomycin therapy.
• The patient exhibits no signs of complications in the preexisting condition linked to vancomycin.
• The patient exhibits no adverse reactions to vancomycin.
• The patient maintains usual hearing level.
• The patient and family express an accurate understanding of the points taught about vancomycin.
• The patient agrees to report tinnitus or hearing loss immediately.

CARBAPENEMS

A fixed combination, imipenem/cilastatin sodium is the first of a new class of beta-lactam antibacterials called carbapenems. The antibacterial spectrum of activity for imipenem/cilastatin is broader than that of any other antibacterial studied to date and includes gram-positive, gram-negative, and anaerobic organisms. Imipenem/cilastatin has been used to treat many clinically important infections, especially those acquired nosocomially.

PHARMACOKINETICS

To be effective, imipenem must be given with cilastatin, otherwise, imipenem would be hydrolyzed rapidly in the brush border of the renal tubules, rendering it ineffective. After parenteral administration, imipenem/cilastatin is absorbed well and distributed widely. It is metabolized by several mechanisms and excreted primarily in the urine.

Absorption, distribution, metabolism, excretion

Imipenem/cilastatin is not absorbed after oral ingestion because of the instability of the molecule in gastric acid. It must be administered parenterally. Imipenem is absorbed incompletely after I.M. administration. The bioavailabilities of imipenem and cilastatin are 75% and 95%, respectively, after I.M. administration in healthy adults. The absorption of imipenem from the I.M. injection site continues for 6 to 8 hours, whereas that for cilastatin is essentially complete within 4 hours.

After I.V. or I.M. administration, imipenem is distributed widely to various body compartments, including sputum, bone, aqueous humor, and pleural and peritoneal fluids. In the absence of meningeal inflammation, only minor amounts of imipenem enter the CSF. With meningeal inflammation, the CSF concentration level usually is 1% to 10% of the concurrent serum concentration level. Imipenem is distributed into breast milk.

Imipenem is metabolized to some extent by a nonrenal mechanism unrelated to dehydropeptidase-I. About 25% of an imipenem dose is inactivated by nonspecific hydrolysis of the beta-lactam ring. Cilastatin is metabolized partially in the kidneys to N-acetyl cilastatin, which also is an effective inhibitor of dehydropeptidase-I. Less than 1% of an imipenem dose and less than 2% of a cilastatin dose are excreted in feces after I.V. administration.

Imipenem is excreted primarily by glomerular filtration. Tubular secretion also assists in drug elimination. Imipenem is metabolized by dehydropeptidase-I at the brush border of the renal tubular cells. Cilastatin, a dehydropeptidase-I inhibitor, blocks this peptidase in the renal tubular cells, increasing excretion of active imipenem into the luminal tubular urine. Cilastatin has no antibacterial activity, nor does it alter the antibacterial activity of imipenem. About 50% of an I.M. dose and 70% of an I.V. dose of imipenem is recovered in urine when imipenem is administered with cilastatin.

With I.V. administration, imipenem and cilastatin have a half-life of about 1 hour. With I.M. administration, imipenem/cilastatin results in an effective plasma half-life of imipenem and cilastatin of about 2 to 3 hours. In patients with decreased renal function, the serum half-life of the imipenem/cilastatin combination increases. Therefore, the imipenem/cilastatin dose should be reduced when the patient's creatinine clearance is below 30 ml/minute. The drug combination is hemodialyzable, and 40% to 82% of the I.V.-administered imipenem is removed in a dialysis session, depending on the technique used. However, the usefulness of this procedure in overdosage of I.M.-administered imipenem/cilastatin is questionable.

Onset, peak, duration

Within 25 minutes after a single dose of 500 mg of imipenem/cilastatin, the plasma concentration level of the I.V. form of the drug is 45.1 mcg/ml compared to 6.0 mcg/ml for the I.M. form. However, after 2 hours, the plasma concentration is approximately the same for both forms of the drug.

PHARMACODYNAMICS

Imipenem usually is bactericidal. It exerts antibacterial activity by inhibiting mucopeptide synthesis in the bacterial cell wall. Because of its spatial configuration, it is particularly resistant to beta-lactamase.

Mechanism of action

Imipenem binds to all of the PBPs, but most avidly and most importantly to penicillin-binding protein 2. The binding to penicillin-binding protein 2 of imipenem in the cell wall causes the bacterium to develop into a round, osmotically unstable form, which then lyses.

PHARMACOTHERAPEUTICS

Imipenem has a broader spectrum of activity than that of other currently available beta-lactam antibiotics. It displays excellent in vitro activity against aerobic gram-positive species such as the streptococci, *S. aureus,* and *S. epidermidis.* Most Enterobacteriaceae are inhibited by imipenem concentrations less than or equal to 1 mcg/ml. *P. aeruginosa,* including strains resistant to piperacillin and ceftazidime, is inhibited by imipenem. Imipenem inhibits most anaerobic species, including *B. fragilis.* The precise clinical role of imipenem/cilastatin is not clear. It may be used alone for mixed aerobic and anaerobic infections; as therapy for serious nosocomial infections or infections in immunocompromised hosts; and as treatment for those infections normally requiring combinations of antibiotics.

imipenem/cilastatin sodium (Primaxin). With its wide antibacterial spectrum of activity, imipenem/cilastatin is effective against gram-positive, gram-negative, and anaerobic organisms. It is especially useful against nosocomial infections. Before imipenem/cilastatin therapy begins, appropriate specimens must be obtained for culture and sensitivity testing. Because resistant strains of *P. aeruginosa* have developed during imipenem/cilastatin therapy, concomitant therapy with an aminoglycoside is recommended when treating infections caused by this organism.
Usual adult dosage: 250 mg imipenem/250 mg cilastatin or 500 mg imipenem/500 mg cilastatin for more serious infections, administered via intermittent I.V. every 6 hours, or 500 mg or 750 mg I.M. every 6 to 12 hours. (Dosage depends on the severity of the infection and the patient's renal function.)
Usual pediatric dosage: for children ages 12 and over, same as adult; not recommended for children under age 12.

Drug interactions

Only a few significant interactions occur between imipenem/cilastatin and other drugs. Concomitant administration of probenecid and imipenem/cilastatin produces a higher and prolonged serum concentration of cilastatin but only slightly higher serum concentration of imipenem. Consequently, concomitant use of these drugs is not recommended.

The combination of imipenem/cilastatin and an aminoglycoside acts synergistically against *S. faecalis* but is not effective against most strains of *P. aeruginosa*. Chloramphenicol can decrease the bactericidal activity of imipenem against *K. pneumoniae*.

ADVERSE DRUG REACTIONS

The adverse reactions associated with imipenem/cilastatin are neither common nor particularly serious.

Elderly patients and patients with a history of previous seizure activity, underlying CNS disease, or renal insufficiency may experience seizures. The most common adverse reactions are nausea, vomiting, and diarrhea. In some instances, nausea is related to rapid infusion and is reduced by increasing the administration time. Pseudomembranous colitis caused by *C. difficile* also can occur.

Phlebitis, thrombophlebitis, and pain at the infusion site can occur. Pain also can occur at the injection site when the drug is administered I.M. Transient elevations in liver function values (aspartate aminotransferase [AST, formerly SGOT], alanine aminotransferase [ALT, formerly SGPT], and lactic dehydrogenase [LDH]) may occur.

Hypersensitivity reactions, such as rashes, have occurred in clinical trials and have been reported in patients with a history of hypersensitivity to penicillins.

NURSING PROCESS APPLICATION

The following information assists the nurse in caring for a patient who is receiving imipenem/cilastatin.

Assessment
• Review the patient's history for a preexisting condition that contraindicates the use of imipenem/cilastatin, such as pregnancy or known hypersensitivity to these agents.
• Review the patient's history for a preexisting condition that requires cautious use of imipenem/cilastatin, such as lactation, impaired renal function, or a history of hypersensitivity reactions to penicillins.
• Assess the patient for adverse reactions to imipenem/cilastatin, such as seizures, GI upset, thrombophlebitis, or hypersensitivity reactions.
• Review the patient's medication history to identify the use of drugs that may interact with imipenem/cilastatin, such as probenecid, aminoglycosides, or chloramphenicol.
• Assess the effectiveness of imipenem/cilastatin periodically.
• Assess the patient for seizure activity during imipenem/cilastatin therapy.
• Evaluate the patient's and family's knowledge about imipenem/cilastatin.

Nursing diagnoses
The following examples represent appropriate nursing diagnoses for a patient receiving imipenem/cilastatin.
• Potential for injury related to a preexisting condition that contraindicates the use of imipenem/cilastatin
• Potential for injury related to a preexisting condition that requires cautious use of imipenem/cilastatin
• Potential for injury related to adverse drug reactions
• Potential for trauma related to imipenem/cilastatin-induced seizures
• Knowledge deficit related to imipenem/cilastatin

Planning and implementation
• Do not administer imipenem/cilastatin to a patient with a condition that contraindicates its use. Also do not administer this combination drug concomitantly with probenecid.
• Administer imipenem/cilastatin with caution to a patient at risk because of a preexisting condition.
• Monitor the patient periodically for adverse reactions during imipenem/cilastatin therapy. Be especially alert for hypersensitivity reactions in patients with a history of penicillin hypersensitivity.

• *Monitor the patient's I.V. infusion site regularly for signs of thrombophlebitis.*

• Monitor the patient's liver function studies regularly for transient elevations in AST, ALT, and LDH.

• Monitor hydration if the patient experiences nausea, vomiting, or diarrhea. Request a prescription for an antiemetic or antidiarrheal agent if needed and prolong the administration time of imipenem/cilastatin.

• *Verify that appropriate specimens have been obtained for culture and sensitivity testing before beginning imipenem/cilastatin therapy.*

• Expect to administer an aminoglycoside with imipenem/cilastatin as prescribed when treating a patient with *P. aeruginosa* infection to prevent resistant strains from developing.

• *Do not mix imipenem/cilastatin with, or add it to, other antibiotics.*

• Administer imipenem/cilastatin by intermittent I.V. infusion over 30 minutes. Administer I.M. imipenem/cilastatin by deep I.M. injection into a large muscle mass, such as the gluteal muscle or lateral part of the thigh.

• Notify the physician if adverse reactions occur.

• *Take seizure precautions throughout imipenem/cilastatin therapy. Be especially alert for seizure activity in an elderly patient or one with a history of previous seizure activity, underlying CNS disease, or renal insufficiency.*

• Alert the physician if seizures occur.

Patient teaching

• Teach the patient and family the name, dose, frequency, action, and adverse effects of imipenem/cilastatin.

• Instruct the patient receiving I.V. imipenem/cilastatin to alert the nurse if nausea is experienced.

• *Instruct the patient to inform the nurse if pain is felt at the I.V. infusion site.*

• Teach the patient and family to take seizure precautions during imipenem/cilastatic therapy, especially in an elderly patient or one with a history of seizures, an underlying CNS disease, or renal insufficency.

• Encourage the patient and family to express concerns or ask questions about imipenem/cilastatin therapy as they arise.

• Instruct the patient to notify the physician if adverse reactions occur.

Evaluation

The following examples represent appropriate evaluation statements for a patient receiving imipenem/cilastatin.

• The patient has no conditions that contraindicate imipenem/cilastatin therapy.

• The patient exhibits no signs of complications in the preexisting condition liked to imipenem/cilastatin.

• The patient exhibits no adverse reactions to imipenem/cilastatin.

• The patient has no seizures during imipenem/cilastatin therapy.

• The patient and family express an accurate understanding of the points taught about imipenem/cilastatin.

• The patient agrees to notify the nurse if nausea occurs during imipenem/cilastatin therapy.

MONOBACTAMS

Aztreonam is the first member of a new class of monobactam antibiotics. The monobactams have a unique monocyclic beta-lactam ring. The naturally occurring monobactams are produced by bacteria found in soil and have weak antibacterial activity. Aztreonam is a synthetic monobactam with a narrow spectrum of activity that includes many gram-negative aerobic bacteria. It has little or no activity against gram-positive aerobic and anaerobic bacteria and has no activity against *Chlamydia, Mycoplasma,* viruses, and fungi.

PHARMACOKINETICS

Aztreonam is absorbed completely and rapidly after parenteral administration, distributed widely, metabolized partially, and excreted primarily in the urine as an unchanged drug.

Absorption, distribution, metabolism, excretion

Aztreonam is absorbed poorly from the GI tract—less than 1% of the drug is absorbed after oral administration. It is absorbed completely and rapidly after I.M. administration and therefore is administered by the I.M. or I.V. route.

After parenteral administration, aztreonam is distributed widely into all body tissues and body fluids, including bile, breast milk, and CSF. Higher CSF concentrations are found in patients with inflamed meninges. Aztreonam crosses the placenta and is distributed into amniotic fluid. It is 46% to 60% bound to serum proteins in healthy adults.

Aztreonam is metabolized partially to inactive metabolites and is excreted primarily in the urine as unchanged drug by glomerular filtration and tubular secretion. A small amount of the drug is eliminated in the feces.

Onset, peak, duration

Peak serum concentration levels of aztreonam usually are attained within 1 hour after an I.M. injection. The serum half-life of aztreonam in patients with normal renal function ranges from 1.5 to 2 hours. In patients with impaired renal function, the half-life is prolonged, and dosage adjustments usually are necessary.

PHARMACODYNAMICS

Similar to the bicyclic beta-lactam antibiotics, aztreonam antibacterial activity results from inhibition of mucopeptide synthesis in the bacterial cell wall. It preferentially binds to the penicillin-binding protein of susceptible gram-negative bacteria. As a result, division of the cell wall is inhibited and lysis occurs.

PHARMACOTHERAPEUTICS

Aztreonam exhibits activity against a wide variety of gram-negative aerobic organisms, including *P. aeruginosa*. Aztreonam has shown activity in vitro and is effective in clinical infections against most strains of the following organisms: *E. coli, Enterobacter* species, *K. pneumoniae* and *Klebsiella oxytoca, P. mirabilis, S. marcescens, H. influenzae,* and *Citrobacter* species.

Aztreonam is used to treat complicated and uncomplicated UTIs, septicemia, and lower respiratory tract, skin and skin structure, intra-abdominal, and gynecologic infections caused by susceptible gram-negative aerobic bacteria. Aztreonam should not be used alone for empiric therapy in seriously ill patients if the infection may result from gram-positive bacteria or if a mixed aerobic-anaerobic bacterial infection is suspected. Aztreonam does not induce beta-lactamase activity and usually is active against gram-negative aerobic organisms that are resistant to antibiotics hydrolyzed by beta lactamases.

aztreonam (Azactam). Before beginning aztreonam therapy, appropriate cultures should be obtained for identification of the infecting organism and in vitro susceptibility testing. Therapy may be started before the susceptibility test results are known, but should be discontinued if the organism is found to be resistant.

Usual adult dosage: for UTIs, 500 mg to 1 gram I.M. or I.V. every 8 to 12 hours; for moderate to severe systemic infections, 1 to 2 grams I.M. or I.V. every 8 to 12 hours; for severe systemic or life-threatening infections, 2 grams I.V. every 6 to 8 hours. The maximum recommended dosage is 8 grams per day. The duration of therapy depends on the severity of the infection. Dosage adjustments are necessary for patients with renal impairment.

Drug interactions

When used concomitantly, probenecid may prolong the rate of tubular secretion of aztreonam. Synergistic or additive effects occur when the drug is used concomitantly with aminoglycosides or other beta-lactam antibiotics, including azlocillin, cefoperazone, cefotaxime, clindamycin, metronidazole, moxalactam, or piperacillin. Potent inducers of beta-lactamase production (cefoxitin, imipenem) may in-activate aztreonam. Chloramphenicol is antagonistic; the two preparations must be given several hours apart.

Use with clavulanic acid may be synergistic or antagonistic, depending on the organism involved. Furosemide increases the serum aztreonam concentration, but this is clinically insignificant.

ADVERSE DRUG REACTIONS

Adverse reactions to aztreonam are similar to the other beta-lactam antibiotics. The drug usually is tolerated well, with adverse reactions being reported in 7% or fewer patients.

The most common GI reactions include diarrhea, nausea, and vomiting. Less common GI reactions include GI bleeding, abdominal cramps, bloating, a transient unusual taste during or after I.V. infusion, numbness of the tongue, oral ulceration, and halitosis. *C. difficile* diarrhea also may occur.

Hematologic reactions from aztreonam use are varied and may include transient eosinophilia, leukopenia, neutropenia, thrombocytopenia, pancytopenia, anemia, leukocytosis, and thrombocytosis.

Transient increases in serum AST, ALT, and alkaline phosphatase concentrations may occur in 2% to 40% of patients receiving aztreonam. They return to pretreatment concentrations shortly after aztreonam is discontinued. Hepatitis, jaundice, and other manifestations of hepatotoxicity are rare.

Hypotension and transient electrocardiogram changes, including ventricular bigeminy and premature ventricular contractions, may occur. Seizures, confusion, insomnia, dizziness, paresthesia, weakness, fatigue, and headache also may occur as a result of adverse CNS effects. Aztreonam does not appear to be nephrotoxic in humans, although transient increases in BUN or serum creatinine level may occur.

Thrombophlebitis may occur in patients receiving aztreonam I.V. Discomfort, pain, and swelling at the injection site also may occur with patients receiving I.M. aztreonam, although the drug generally is tolerated well when administered by this route.

Dermatologic and hypersensitivity reactions also may occur and range from anaphylaxis, urticaria, and pruritus to erythema multiforme and exfoliative dermatitis.

NURSING PROCESS APPLICATION

The following information assists the nurse in caring for a patient who is receiving aztreonam.

Assessment

• Review the patient's history for a preexisting condition that contraindicates the use of aztreonam, such as known hypersensitivity to the drug.

• Review the patient's history for a preexisting condition that requires cautious use of aztreonam, such as impaired renal or hepatic function or a history of immediate type I hypersensitivity reactions to penicillins or cephalosporins.

• Assess the patient for adverse reactions to aztreonam, such as GI upset, hematologic abnormalities, hypotension, arrhythmias, CNS effects, and dermatologic or hypersensitivity reaction.

• Review the patient's medication history to identify the use of drugs that may interact with aztreonam, such as aminoglycosides, beta-lactam antibiotics, chloramphenicol, clavulanic acid, or probenecid.

• Assess the effectiveness of aztreonam periodically.

• Evaluate the patient's and family's knowledge about aztreonam.

Nursing diagnoses

The following examples represent appropriate nursing diagnoses for a patient receiving aztreonam.

• Potential for injury related to a preexisting condition that contraindicates the use of aztreonam

• Potential for injury related to a preexisting condition that requires cautious use of aztreonam

• Potential for injury related to adverse drug reactions

• Altered protection related to hematologic abnormalities caused by aztreonam

• Knowledge deficit related to aztreonam

Planning and implementation

• Do not administer aztreonam to a patient with a condition that contraindicates its use.

• Administer aztreonam cautiously to a patient at risk because of a preexisting condition.

• Monitor the patient periodically for adverse reactions during aztreonam therapy.

• Monitor the patient closely for hypersensitivity reactions, such as anaphylaxis, urticaria, pruritus, or skin rash. If a hypersensitivity reaction occurs, withhold aztreonam and notify the physician, and expect to switch the patient to a different antibiotic. Have standard emergency equipment nearby.

• *Obtain specimens for culture and sensitivity testing before administering the first dose of aztreonam. Notify the physician if results reveal organisms that are resistant to aztreonam.*

• Expect to adjust the dosage as prescribed if the patient has renal impairment.

• *Monitor the I.V. site closely for signs of thrombophlebitis, such as swelling and redness. Change the I.V. site as needed.*

• Observe the I.M. site for swelling. If swelling or pain occurs, consult the physician about changing to I.V. administration.

• Monitor hydration if the patient experiences nausea, vomiting, or diarrhea. Request a prescription for an antiemetic or antidiarrheal agent if needed. Test the patient's emesis and stools for occult blood.

• *Take seizure precautions throughout aztreonam therapy.*

• Take safety precautions if the patient experiences confusion, dizziness, or other adverse CNS reactions. For example, keep the bed rails raised and supervise ambulation.

• Administer a mild analgesic as prescribed if the patient develops a headache during aztreonam therapy.

• *Inspect the patient's mouth regularly for ulcers. Provide symptomatic relief, such as warm-water rinses and a soft diet, if ulceration occurs.*

• Notify the physician if adverse reactions occur.

• Monitor the patient's complete blood count and liver function studies for abnormalities.

• Take infection-control measures if leukocytopenia occurs.

• Take bleeding precautions if thrombocytopenia occurs.

• Stagger the patient's activities and provide frequent rest periods if anemia occurs.

• *Notify the physician if adverse hematologic or hepatic reactions occur. Prepare to treat the specific reaction as prescribed. If the reaction becomes severe, expect to discontinue aztreonam therapy.*

Patient teaching

• Teach the patient and family the name name, dose, frequency, action, and adverse effects of aztreonam.

• *Warn the patient receiving I.M. aztreonam that pain may occur. Advise the patient receiving I.V. aztreonam to report pain at the infusion site.*

• *Teach the patient the importance of having blood studies done periodically as instructed to detect adverse hematologic or hepatic reactions.*

• Instruct the patient to notify the nurse before getting out of bed if dizziness is present.

• *Teach the patient how to manage mouth ulcers and perform frequent mouth care.*

• Instruct the patient with thrombocytopenia to take bleeding precautions, such as avoiding cuts and bruises and using a soft toothbrush and electric razor.

• Review appropriate infection-control measures with the patient and family if leukopenia is present.

• Teach the patient with anemia to stagger activities and rest frequently.

• Instruct the patient to alert the nurse or physician if other adverse reactions occur.

(Text continues on page 1049.)

SELECTED MAJOR DRUGS

Antibacterial agents

This chart summarizes representative antibacterial agents currently in clinical use.

DRUG	MAJOR INDICATIONS	USUAL ADULT DOSAGES	CONTRAINDICATIONS AND PRECAUTIONS
Aminoglycosides			
gentamicin	Infections caused by sensitive *Pseudomonas aeruginosa, Escherichia coli,* indole-positive and indole-negative *Proteus, Providencia, Klebsiella, Serratia, Enterobacter, Citrobacter, Staphylococcus,* and other gram-negative aerobic bacteria	1 to 1.75 mg/kg I.V. or I.M. every 8 hours; dosage adjustment required for patients with renal impairment	• Know that gentamicin is contraindicated in a patient with known hypersensitivity to it or other aminoglycosides. • Administer with extreme caution to a pregnant, lactating, or elderly patient. • Administer with caution to a patient with a neuromuscular disorder or renal impairment.
Penicillins			
ampicillin	Respiratory tract infections	250 to 500 mg P.O. every 6 hours, or 1 to 3 grams I.M. or I.V. every 6 hours	• Know that ampicillin is contraindicated in a patient with known hypersensitivity to any penicillin. • Administer with caution to a lactating patient or one with allergies to other drugs (especially cephalosporins) or mononucleosis.
penicillin G aqueous	Infections such as meningitis, septicemia, pericarditis, endocarditis, severe pneumonia, and other serious infections	600,000 to 5 million units I.V. or I.M. every 4 to 6 hours	• Know that penicillin G aqueous is contraindicated in a lactating patient or one with known hypersensitivity to any penicillin. • Administer with caution to a pregnant patient or one with a history of significant allergies (such as to penicillins, related drugs, molds) or asthma.
ticarcillin	Uncomplicated urinary tract infections	1 gram I.M. or I.V. every 6 hours	• Know that ticarcillin is contraindicated in a patient with known hypersensitivity to any penicillin. • Administer with caution to a patient with allergies to drugs (especially cephalosporins), a hemorrhagic condition, hypokalemia, or sodium restriction.
	Complicated urinary tract infections	3 grams I.V. every 4 to 6 hours	
	Septicemia	3 grams I.V. every 3 to 6 hours	
Cephalosporins			
ceftizoxime	Infections caused by gram-negative aerobic organisms except *P. aeruginosa* and gram-positive organisms except enterococci and anaerobes, such as *B. fragilis*	1 to 2 grams I.V. or I.M. every 8 to 12 hours	• Know that ceftizoxime is contraindicated in a patient with hypersensitivity to any cephalosporin. • Administer with caution to a pregnant or lactating patient or one with a history of allergies (especially to such drugs as penicillin) or gastrointestinal (GI) disease (particularly colitis).
cefaclor	Respiratory tract infections and otitis media	250 to 500 mg P.O. every 8 hours	• Know that cefaclor is contraindicated in a patient with hypersensitivity to any cephalosporin. • Administer with caution to a pregnant or lactating patient or one with a history of allergies (especially to such drugs as penicillin) or GI disease (particularly colitis).

SELECTED MAJOR DRUGS

Antibacterial agents (continued)

DRUG	MAJOR INDICATIONS	USUAL ADULT DOSAGES	CONTRAINDICATIONS AND PRECAUTIONS
Tetracyclines			
minocycline	Infections caused by sensitive gram-negative and gram-positive organisms, *C. trachomatis,* amebiasis	200 mg P.O. or I.V. initially; then 100 mg every 12 hours or 50 mg P.O. every 6 hours	• Know that minocycline is contraindicated in an infant, child up to age 8, pregnant or lactating patient, or one with known hypersensitivity to any tetracycline. • Administer with extreme caution to a patient with impaired renal or hepatic function.
	Meningococcal carrier state	100 to 200 mg P.O. every 12 hours for 5 days	
	Uncomplicated urethral, endocervical, or rectal infection caused by *C. trachomatis* or *Ureaplasma urealyticum*	100 mg P.O. b.i.d. for at least 7 days	
	Uncomplicated gonococcal urethritis in males	100 mg P.O. b.i.d. for 7 days	
tetracycline	Infections caused by sensitive gram-negative and gram-positive organisms, rickettsiae, and *Mycoplasma*	250 to 500 mg P.O. every 6 hours, 250 mg I.M. daily, 150 mg I.M. every 12 hours, or 250 to 500 mg I.V. every 8 to 12 hours (I.M. and I.V., hydrochloride salt only)	• Know that tetracycline is contraindicated in an infant, child up to age 8, pregant or lactating patient, or one with hypersensitivity to any tetracycline. • Administer with extreme caution to a patient with impaired renal or hepatic function.
	Uncomplicated urethral, endocervical, or rectal infections caused by *C. trachomatis*	500 mg P.O. every 6 hours for at least 7 days	
	Brucellosis	500 mg P.O. every 6 hours for 3 weeks with 1 gram of streptomycin I.M. every 12 hours in week 1 and daily in week 2	
	Syphilis in a patient hypersensitive to penicillin	30 to 50 grams total in equally divided doses over 10 to 15 days	
	Acne	250 mg P.O. initially every 6 hours, then 125 to 500 mg P.O. daily or every other day	
	Lyme disease	500 mg P.O. b.i.d. for 10 to 30 days	
Chloramphenicol			
chloramphenicol	Serious infections caused by many gram-positive and gram-negative aerobic organisms and some anaerobic organisms	50 to 100 mg/kg/day P.O. in divided doses every 6 hours	• Know that chloramphenicol is contraindicated in a patient with known hypersensitivity or toxic reactions to it, in the treatment of trivial infections or in conditions where it is not indicated (as in colds, influenza, and infections of the throat), or in prevention of bacterial infection. • Administer with caution to an infant, a pregnant patient at term or during labor, a lactating patient, or one with impaired renal or hepatic function.

(continued)

SELECTED MAJOR DRUGS

Antibacterial agents *(continued)*

DRUG	MAJOR INDICATIONS	USUAL ADULT DOSAGES	CONTRAINDICATIONS AND PRECAUTIONS
Clindamycin			
clindamycin	Serious infections caused by aerobic gram-positive cocci and anaerobes	300 to 600 mg I.V. or I.M. every 6 to 8 hours	• Know that clindamycin is contraindicated in a pregnant or lactating patient or one with a known hypersensitivity to clindamycin or linco-mycin. • Administer with caution to a patient with a history of GI disease (particularly colitis), severe renal or hepatic impairment, or multiple allergies.
Erythromycin			
erythromycin	Infections caused by many gram-positive and gram-negative bacteria, including *Acinetobacter* and *Mycobacterium,* treponemas, mycoplasmas, rickettsiae, and chlamydiae	250 mg P.O. every 6 hours	• Know that erythromycin is contraindicated in a patient with known hypersensitivity to the drug. • Administer with caution to a lactating patient or one with impaired hepatic function or biliary excretion.
Vancomycin			
vancomycin hydro-chloride	Serious staphylococcal infections when other antibacterials are ineffective or contraindicated	500 mg I.V. every 6 hours, or 1 gram I.V. every 12 hours; daily dosage should not exceed 2 grams	• Know that vancomycin is contraindicated in a pregnant patient or one with known hypersensitivity to the drug or impaired hearing. • Administer with caution to a lactating patient or one with impaired renal function.
Carbapenems			
imipenem/cilastatin	Infections caused by gram-positive, gram-negative, and anaerobic organisms	250 mg imipenem and 250 mg cilastatin via intermittent I.V.; for more serious infections, 500 mg imipenem and 500 mg cilastatin via intermittent I.V.	• Know that imipenem/cilastatin is contraindicated in a pregnant patient or one with known hypersensitivity to any ingredient in the formulation. • Administer with caution to a lactating patient or one with impaired renal function or a history of hypersensitivity reactions to penicillins.
Monobactams			
aztreonam	Urinary tract infections	500 mg to 1 gram I.M. or I.V. every 8 to 12 hours	• Know that aztreonam is contraindicated in a patient with known hypersensitivity to the drug. • Administer with caution to a patient with impaired renal or hepatic function or a history of immediate type I hypersensitivity reactions to penicillins or cephalosporins.
	Moderate to severe systemic infections caused by a wide range of gram-negative aerobic organisms including *P. aeruginosa*	1 to 2 grams I.M. or I.V. every 8 to 12 hours	
	Severe systemic or life-threatening infections	2 grams I.V. every 6 to 8 hours	

Evaluation

The following examples represent appropriate evaluation statements for a patient receiving aztreonam.

• The patient has no conditions that contraindicate aztreonam therapy.

• The patient exhibits no signs of complications in the preexisting condition linked to aztreonam.

• The patient exhibits no adverse reactions to aztreonam.

• The patient's complete blood count and liver function tests remain normal throughout aztreonam therapy.

• The patient and family express an accurate understanding of the points taught about aztreonam.

• The patient correctly identifies measures to take if thrombocytopenia occurs.

CHAPTER SUMMARY

Chapter 59 described the clinically important antibacterial drugs used to treat systemic infections. Here are the chapter highlights.

• Aminoglycosides are used primarily to treat gram-negative bacterial infections. Currently, amikacin, gentamicin, netilmicin, and tobramycin are prescribed most commonly.

• In a patient with renal insufficiency, the aminoglycoside dosage must be adjusted to avoid serious toxicities and damage to the auditory, vestibular, and renal functions. Periodic assessment of peak and trough serum concentration levels is needed to assess therapeutic efficacy and toxicity.

• Penicillins remain one of the most important and useful antibacterial groups available for clinical use. No other antibacterial class has as wide a spectrum of activity as the penicillins, which are used to treat gram-positive and gram-negative aerobic bacteria as well as anaerobic bacteria and *Streptococcus viridans.* Because penicillins have a low incidence of serious toxicity and are relatively inexpensive, they are the drugs of choice to treat susceptible organisms in nonallergic patients.

• Cephalosporins are prescribed frequently. Many new cephalosporins have been introduced for clinical use recently. The available cephalosporins are classified into three generations based on their spectra of activity.

• A patient taking penicillins and cephalosporins concurrently may develop cross-sensitivities.

• Tetracyclines rarely are considered the drugs of choice to treat most common bacterial infections; however, they are among the most commonly prescribed antibacterials in the world. The tetracyclines are primarily bacteriostatic.

• Chloramphenicol-induced aplastic anemia has limited the use of this drug. This broad-spectrum antibacterial usually is reserved for treating serious infections.

• Clindamycin is more effective than lincomycin against susceptible bacteria. Clindamycin remains particularly important in treating certain anaerobic infections. Diarrhea occurs in 80% or more of patients receiving clindamycin (most commonly with oral administration).

• Erythromycin is used to treat a number of common infections. A bacteriostatic antibacterial, erythromycin inhibits protein synthesis, similar to chloramphenicol, clindamycin, and lincomycin. Erythromycin is the drug of choice to treat *Mycoplasma pneumoniae* infections as well as *Legionella pneumophila.* The adverse effects of the drug are few.

• Vancomycin is experiencing a resurgence in popularity because of increasing problems with methicillin-resistant *Staphylococcus aureus,* which has become a major concern in the United States and throughout the world.

• Imipenem/cilastatin is the first of a new class of beta-lactam antibacterials called carbapenems. The antibacterial spectrum of activity of imipenem/cilastatin is broader than that of any other antibacterial studied to date. Imipenem/cilastatin is used to treat many clinically important infections, especially nosocomial ones.

• Aztreonam is the first member of a new class of monobactams. It has a narrow spectrum of activity that includes many aerobic gram-negative bacteria. It must be administered parenterally and has an antibacterial activity that is similar to the other beta-lactam antibiotics. Because it is eliminated primarily by the kidneys, dosage adjustments are necessary in patients with renal disease.

• Before administering an antibacterial agent, the nurse should ensure that specimens have been obtained for culture and sensitivity testing. During antibacterial therapy, the nurse should monitor the patient closely for adverse reactions, especially hypersensitivity reactions.

STUDY QUESTIONS

See Appendix 1 for answers.

1. Gloria Franken, age 35, has a pelvic infection for which her physician has prescribed the aminoglycoside, gentamicin, and another antibacterial agent. To promote bacterial cell penetration, a drug from which class commonly is used with an aminoglycoside?

(a) penicillin

(b) cephalosporin

(c) erythromycin

(d) tetracycline

2. Patty Smith, age 40, has been diagnosed as having streptococcal pharyngitis (strep throat). To treat this condition the physician prescribes amoxicillin 250 mg P.O. every 8 hours. During penicillin therapy, the nurse should assess for which major adverse reaction?
(a) allergic reaction
(b) hepatotoxicity
(c) blood dyscrasia
(d) serum sickness

3. Daniel Brown, age 52, a diabetic, is admitted to the hospital with a foot ulcer. The physician prescribes cefoxitin sodium, a second generation cephalosporin, 1 gm I.V. every 6 hours. How should the nurse administer cefoxitin to Mr. Brown?
(a) I.V. bolus
(b) continuous I.V. infusion
(c) intermittent infusion over 30 minutes
(d) infusion with 1% lidocaine

4. After receiving cefoxitin for 5 days, Mr. Brown develops oral thrush. This probably is a sign of which reaction?
(a) allergic reaction
(b) superinfection
(c) cefoxitin toxicity
(d) uncontrolled diabetes

5. Katie Jones, age 16, is taking tetracycline 250 mg P.O. once daily to treat acne. This drug should not be administered to children under age 8. Why?
(a) It is metabolized poorly and may result in toxicity.
(b) It may darken permanent teeth and disrupt bone growth.
(c) It has a high incidence of adverse reactions.
(d) It is absorbed poorly from the GI tract.

6. Which instruction should the nurse give Katie about tetracycline administration?
(a) Take the drug with meals to minimize GI upset.
(b) Take the drug with milk to minimize GI upset.
(c) Take the drug with an antacid if GI upset occurs.
(d) Take the drug with 8 oz of water to prevent esophageal irritation.

7. Billy Grobowski, age 9, is receiving chloramphenicol (Chloromycetin) for *Haemophilus influenzae* meningitis. Which adverse reaction limits chloramphenicol to treating serious infections only?
(a) ototoxicity
(b) drug-induced aplastic anemia
(c) nephrotoxicity
(d) bone marrow suppression

8. Billy requires careful monitoring because chloramphenicol dosages that produce a serum concentration greater than 40 mcg/ml may cause which adverse reaction?
(a) hepatoxicity
(b) renal failure
(c) gray syndrome
(d) seizures and coma

9. Angela Drew, age 33, develops pneumonia caused by *Mycoplasma pneumoniae*. What is the drug of choice for treating this infection?
(a) penicillin
(b) chloramphenicol
(c) sulfamethoxazole
(d) erythromycin

SELECTED REFERENCES

AHFS drug information 90. (1990). Bethesda, MD: American Society of Hospital Pharmacists.

Cockerill, F., and Edson, R. (1987). Trimethoprim-sulfamethoxazole. *Mayo Clinic Proceedings, 62*(10), 921-929.

Conte, J., and Barriere, S. (1988). *Manual of antibiotics and infectious diseases* (6th ed.). Philadelphia: Lea & Febiger.

Donowitz, G., and Mandell, G. (1988). Beta lactam antibiotics. (Part I). *New England Journal of Medicine, 318*(7), 419-426.

Donowitz, G., and Mandell, G. (1988). Beta lactam antibiotics. (Part II). *New England Journal of Medicine, 318*(8), 490-500.

Drug facts and comparisons. (1991). St. Louis: Facts and Comparisons Division, Lippincott.

Edson, R., and Terrell, C. (1987). The aminoglycosides: Streptomycin, kanamycin, gentamicin, tobramycin, amikacin, metilmicin, sisomicin. *Mayo Clinic Proceedings, 62*(10), 916-920.

Goodman and Gilman's the pharmacological basis of therapeutics (8th ed.; 1990). Elmsford, NY: Pergamon Press.

Hansten, P., and Horn, J. (1989). *Drug interactions* (6th ed.). Philadelphia: Lea & Febiger.

Hermans, P., and Wilhelm, M. (1987). Vancomycin. *Mayo Clinic Proceedings, 62*(2), 901-905.

Kucers, A., and Bennett, N. (1987). *The use of antibiotics* (4th ed.). Philadelphia: J.B. Lippincott.

Mandell, G., et al. (Eds.). (1990). *Principles and practice of infectious diseases* (3rd ed.). New York: Churchill.

North American Nursing Diagnosis Association. (1990). *Taxonomy I-Revised, with official diagnostic categories.* St. Louis: NANDA.

Thompson, R. (1987). Cephalosporin, carbapenem, and monobactam antibiotics. *Mayo Clinic Proceedings, 62*(9), 821-834.

Wilson, W., and Cockerill, F. (1987). Tetracyclines, chloramphenicol, erythromycin, and clindamycin. *Mayo Clinic Proceedings, 62*(10), 906-015.

Wright, A., and Wilkowske, C. (1987). The penicillins. *Mayo Clinic Proceedings, 62*(9), 806-820.

ANTITUBERCULAR AND ANTILEPROTIC AGENTS

OBJECTIVES

After reading and studying this chapter, the student should be able to:
1. Identify the first-line agents employed in treating tuberculosis and Hansen's disease (leprosy).
2. Identify the genetic factors that can affect the actions of these agents.
3. Identify drug interactions associated with antitubercular and antileprotic agents.
4. Identify the major adverse reactions to these agents and intervene appropriately.
5. Teach the patient with a mycobacterial infection about the disease and its drug therapy.
6. Describe how to apply the nursing process when caring for a patient who is receiving an antitubercular or antileprotic agent.

INTRODUCTION

Antitubercular and antileprotic agents are used to treat mycobacterial infections: tuberculosis, which is caused by *Mycobacterium tuberculosis;* and Hansen's disease (previously called *leprosy*), which is caused by *M. leprae.* These agents also are effective against less common mycobacterial infections caused by *M. kansasii, M. avium, M. fortuitum, M. intracellulare,* and related organisms. Not always curative, these agents can halt the progression of a mycobacterial infection.

Unlike most antibiotics, antitubercular and antileprotic agents may need to be administered over many months, or even years. This creates problems, such as patient noncompliance, the development of bacterial resistance, and drug toxicity. To help the patient during long-term therapy, the nurse must be aware of these and other problems.

For a summary of representative drugs, see *Selected major drugs: Antitubercular and antileprotic agents,* page 1060. For a listing of applicable nursing diagnoses that the nurse may formulate when caring for a patient receiving these agents, see *Selected nursing diagnoses: Antitubercular and antileprotic agents*. For detailed information on applying the nursing process, see Chapter 6, The Nursing Process and Drug Therapy.

ANTITUBERCULAR AGENTS

Ethambutol hydrochloride, isoniazid (INH), and rifampin are the mainstays of tuberculosis therapy. Streptomycin sulfate, the first effective antitubercular agent, also is used, but not as commonly. Other antitubercular agents are used even less commonly because they are less effective and more toxic. These include aminosalicylic acid, capreomycin sulfate, cycloserine, ethionamide, and pyrazinamide. Usually, these agents are used only when hypersensitivity, intolerance, or bacterial resistance to a first-line agent exists. (For information about these secondary drugs, see "Other antitubercular agents" later in this chapter.)

PHARMACOKINETICS

Antitubercular agents almost exclusively are administered orally; only INH is commercially available parenterally. When administered orally, they are absorbed well from the gastrointestinal (GI) tract and distributed widely throughout the body. The drugs are metabolized primarily in the liver and excreted by the kidneys.

Absorption, distribution, metabolism, excretion
About 75% to 80% of an oral dose of ethambutol is absorbed rapidly from the GI tract. The drug is distributed widely into most body tissues and fluids; about twice as much appears in erythrocytes as appears in plasma. (The erythrocytes may serve as a reservoir, slowly releasing the drug into the circulation.) Ethambutol crosses the placenta. It appears in breast milk in concentrations roughly equal to those of plasma concentrations. The liver metabolizes up to 15% of ethambutol, and the kidneys excrete almost all of it, primarily as unchanged drug.

INH, readily absorbed from the GI tract and intramuscular (I.M.) injection sites, is distributed into all body tissues and fluids, readily crossing the blood-brain barrier and the placenta. It is distributed into breast milk in concentration levels similar to those of the maternal plasma. INH is metabolized almost completely by enzymatic acetylation and hydrolysis in the liver. The rate of acetylation,

however, is determined by race-linked genetic factors. Although these genetic factors can produce significant variations in the rate of INH elimination, the drug still is effective when administered two or three times a week. Its effectiveness is reduced for some patients (fast acetylators), however, when administered once weekly. From 75% to 95% of INH is excreted in the urine as metabolites and unchanged drug within 24 hours after administration. Small amounts are excreted in the saliva, sputum, and feces.

Rifampin also is absorbed well from the GI tract, although food in the stomach can reduce its rate and extent of absorption. The drug diffuses freely into most body tissues and fluids, including the cerebrospinal fluid, in concentrations that are 10% to 20% of plasma concentrations. It crosses the placenta and appears in breast milk. After metabolism in the liver, it is excreted primarily in the feces but also in urine and bile.

Onset, peak, duration
After an oral dose of ethambutol, the plasma concentration peaks in 2 to 4 hours in proportion to the size of the dose. The drug's half-life in a patient with normal renal function is about 3 hours; in a patient with renal impairment, the drug will have a longer half-life, and a dosage adjustment may be necessary.

After oral administration, INH reaches a peak plasma concentration in 1 to 2 hours. The half-life of this drug ranges from 1 to 4 hours, but it may be longer for a patient with renal or hepatic impairment.

Rifampin reaches a peak plasma concentration in 2 to 4 hours. Initially, its half-life ranges from 1.5 to 5 hours and averages 3 hours, but because biliary excretion of rifampin increases during the first 2 weeks of therapy, the half-life gradually decreases to about 2 hours. Plasma concentration of rifampin is higher and more prolonged in a patient with hepatic dysfunction but unaffected in a patient with renal dysfunction.

PHARMACODYNAMICS

Antitubercular agents are specific for mycobacteria. At usual doses, ethambutol and INH are tuberculostatic, inhibiting growth of *M. tuberculosis* bacteria. In contrast, rifampin is tuberculocidal, destroying the bacteria. Because bacterial resistance to INH and rifampin can develop rapidly, however, they usually are used with other antitubercular agents.

Mechanism of action
Ethambutol is most active against *M. tuberculosis* and *M. kansasii* but acts — to varying degrees — against all mycobacteria. Although mycobacteria rapidly take up ethambutol, the drug does not inhibit their growth significantly for approximately 24 hours. Its exact mechanism of action

remains unclear but may be related to inhibition of cell metabolism, arrest of multiplication, and cell death. Ethambutol acts only against replicating bacteria.

Although the exact mechanism of action of INH is not known, evidence suggests that the drug inhibits the synthesis of mycolic acids, important components of the mycobacterium cell wall. This inhibition alters the acid-fastness of the cell and disrupts the cell wall. Because mycolic acid synthesis is unique to mycobacteria, this mechanism explains the high degree of specificity of INH. Only INH-sensitive bacteria take up the drug, and only replicating, not resting, bacteria appear to be inhibited.

Rifampin inhibits ribonucleic acid (RNA) synthesis in susceptible organisms by acting on the beta subunit of the enzyme RNA polymerase. The drug is effective primarily in replicating bacteria but may have some effect on resting bacteria as well.

PHARMACOTHERAPEUTICS

INH usually is used with ethambutol, rifampin, or streptomycin. This is because combination therapy for tuberculosis and other mycobacterial infections can prevent or delay the development of bacterial resistance to the drug regimen.

ethambutol hydrochloride (Myambutol). Ethambutol is used with INH and rifampin to treat uncomplicated pulmonary tuberculosis in a patient who lives in a geographic area noted for a high incidence of bacterial resistance or who previously has been treated with antitubercular agents. The drug also is used to treat infections resulting from *M. bovis* and most strains of *M. kansasii.*
Usual adult dosage: for infections previously untreated with antitubercular agents, 15 mg/kg of body weight P.O. once daily; for previously treated infections, 25 mg/kg P.O. daily for 60 days, then decreased to 15 mg/kg P.O. once daily; for intermittent therapy, 50 mg/kg two or three times weekly. In a patient with renal impairment, the dosage may be reduced or the interval between doses may be increased. For instance, if the creatinine clearance is 10 to 50 ml/minute, the interval may be increased to 24 to 36 hours; if the creatinine clearance is less than 10 ml/minute, the interval may be increased to 48 hours.
Usual pediatric dosage: for children ages 6 and older, 10 to 15 mg/kg P.O. daily. Although the manufacturer does not recommend ethambutol for pediatric use, many clinicians use this drug dosage for pediatric patients.

isoniazid [INH] (Nydrazid, Laniazid). Although INH is the most important drug for treating tuberculosis, bacterial resistance develops rapidly if it is used alone. However, resistance does not pose a problem when INH is used alone to prevent tuberculosis in individuals who have been ex-

posed to the disease, and no evidence exists of cross-resistance between INH and other antitubercular agents. Although INH may be given I.M. or P.O., I.M. administration offers no special advantages. Experiments with continuous and intermittent therapy eventually may lead to revision of current dosages and regimens.
Usual adult dosage: for treating tuberculosis, 5 to 10 mg/kg of body weight P.O. or I.M. once daily, up to a maximum of 300 mg daily for at least 1 year; for preventing tuberculosis, 300 mg P.O. once daily for 6 to 12 months.
Usual pediatric dosage: 10 to 20 mg/kg P.O. or I.M. once daily, depending on the severity of the disease, up to a maximum of 500 mg daily.

rifampin (Rifadin, Rimactane). A first-line agent for treating pulmonary tuberculosis, rifampin is particularly effective when combined with INH or another antitubercular agent. This drug combats many gram-positive and some gram-negative bacteria but seldom is used for nonmycobacterial infections because bacterial resistance develops rapidly. It is used to treat asymptomatic carriers of *Neisseria meningitidis* when the risk of meningitis is high, but it is not used to treat *N. meningitidis* infections because of the potential for bacterial resistance. Rifampin usually is used with other drugs to treat Hansen's disease and is the drug of choice for treating dapsone-resistant Hansen's disease.
Usual adult dosage: for tuberculosis or Hansen's disease, 600 mg P.O. once daily 1 hour before or 2 hours after a meal; for asymptomatic carriers of *N. meningitidis,* 600 mg P.O. once daily 1 hour before or 2 hours after a meal for 4 days, or 600 mg b.i.d. for 2 days.
Usual pediatric dosage: for neonates under age 1 week, up to 10 mg/kg P.O. or I.V. once daily; for older children, 10 to 20 mg/kg P.O. or I.V. once daily, up to a maximum of 600 mg daily.

Drug interactions

Antacids that contain aluminum hydroxide or other aluminum salts may decrease the GI absorption of ethambutol slightly.

Some evidence suggests that INH, cycloserine, and ethionamide may produce additive central nervous system (CNS) effects, such as drowsiness, dizziness, headache, lethargy, depression, tremor, anxiety, confusion, and tinnitus. Therefore, these drugs should be administered cautiously in combination. INH increases plasma concentrations of phenytoin, increasing the likelihood of phenytoin toxicity in patients who are slow acetylators. Aluminum hydroxide, a common ingredient in antacids, significantly decreases INH absorption. INH should be administered at least one hour before aluminum antacids. INH administration with a corticosteroid decreases INH's effects and increases the corticosteroid's effects. Psychotic episodes and difficulty with coordination have occurred when INH has been given with disulfiram. Concomitant administration should be avoided.

Rifampin can increase the rate of metabolism — and consequently decrease the plasma concentration — of some drugs, including oral contraceptives, ketoconazole, quinidine, cyclosporine, chloramphenicol, estrogens, corticosteroids, methadone, oral hypoglycemics, warfarin, cardiac glycosides, and dapsone. The dosages of these agents may need to be increased during rifampin therapy. Aminosalicylic acid may inhibit rifampin absorption.

ADVERSE DRUG REACTIONS

Adverse reactions to antitubercular agents primarily occur in the GI tract, the peripheral nervous system, and the hepatic system. Fortunately, these reactions seldom are severe enough to necessitate interruption of tuberculosis therapy.

Optic neuritis is the only significant adverse reaction to ethambutol. Signs and symptoms include decreased visual acuity, loss of red-green color discrimination, visual field constriction, and central and peripheral scotomas (areas of depressed vision in the visual field). This adverse reaction occurs in only 0.8% of patients receiving 15 mg/ kg, but its incidence increases in patients who receive higher dosages or who have renal dysfunction. Discontinuing ethambutol usually reverses the optic neuritis — but if vision impairment is severe, recovery may be incomplete. Pruritus, joint pain, GI distress, malaise, headache, dizziness, and confusion also have been reported with ethambutol therapy. Occasionally, ethambutol therapy increases serum uric acid levels and precipitates an acute gout episode.

The most common hypersensitivity reactions to ethambutol are rash (in 10.5% of patients) and fever (in 0.3%). Hypersensitivity reactions occur rarely with ethambutol and tend to be mild. Leukopenia, anaphylaxis, and peripheral neuritis with paresthesia of the extremities have been reported.

Peripheral neuritis occurs in 20% of the patients receiving 6 mg/kg of INH daily, and higher doses increase the incidence of this reaction. Usually preceded by paresthesia of the feet and hands, peripheral neuritis is more likely to affect an alcoholic, diabetic, or malnourished individual, or one who is predisposed to peripheral neuritis. Typically, it produces muscle twitching, dizziness, ataxia, stupor, and paresthesia. Daily administration of 10 to 50 mg of pyridoxine (vitamin B_6) may prevent this reaction. During the first 6 months of therapy, transient elevations occur in levels of the enzymes alanine aminotransferase (ALT, formerly SGPT) and aspartate aminotransferase (AST, formerly SGOT); and in bilirubin concentrations in 10% to 20% of patients receiving INH. This drug also may produce hepatitis, especially in elderly patients and usually in the first 4 to 8 weeks of therapy. INH may precipitate seizures in a patient with a seizure disorder. It also may produce optic neuritis and atrophy, mental abnormalities (such as euphoria and memory impairment), and sedation or uncoordination.

Hypersensitivity reactions to INH occur rarely, producing fever, skin eruptions (morbilliform, maculopapular, purpuric, or exfoliative), lymphadenopathy, and vasculitis. These reactions usually appear 3 to 7 weeks after therapy begins.

The most common adverse reactions to rifampin include epigastric pain, nausea, vomiting, abdominal cramps, flatulence, anorexia, and diarrhea. Joint pain and muscle aches and cramps also may occur. All these reactions, which are most likely to occur during the first 2 weeks of therapy, may subside as biliary excretion of rifampin increases and its half-life decreases; interruption of therapy seldom is necessary. Rifampin can elevate ALT, AST, bilirubin, and alkaline phosphatase levels, possibly leading to eventual discontinuation of the drug. Transient asymptomatic jaundice and red-orange discoloration of sweat, tears, saliva, urine, and feces also may occur but do not necessitate discontinuation of drug therapy.

Large (900- to 1,200-mg) intermittent doses of rifampin produce hypersensitivity reactions in about 1% of patients so treated. This reaction appears as a flulike syndrome characterized by dyspnea with or without wheezing, purpura associated with thrombocytopenia, leukopenia, and, rarely, anaphylaxis. A patient with this reaction probably will be able to tolerate a reduced rifampin dosage (only 3% of all patients require discontinuation of this drug).

NURSING PROCESS APPLICATION

The following information assists the nurse in caring for a patient who is receiving an antitubercular agent.

Assessment

• Review the patient's history for a preexisting condition that contraindicates the use of an antitubercular agent, such as known hypersensitivity to the drug or optic neuritis.

• Review the patient's history for a preexisting condition that requires cautious use of an antitubercular agent, such as pregnancy, lactation, chronic liver disease, severe renal dysfunction, daily alcohol use, or concomitant phenytoid therapy.

• Assess the patient for adverse reactions to the prescribed antitubercular agent, such as GI distress, peripheral neuritis, hepatic dysfunction, optic neuritis, or hypersensitivity reactions.

• Review the patient's medication history to identify the use of drugs that may interact with the prescribed antitubercular agent, such as cycloserine, aluminum hydroxide, phenytoin, oral contraceptives, corticosteroids, or warfarin.

• Assess the effectiveness of the prescribed antitubercular agent periodically.
• Evaluate the patient's and family's knowledge about the prescribed antitubercular agent.

Nursing diagnoses

The following examples represent appropriate nursing diagnoses for a patient receiving an antitubercular agent.
• Potential for injury related to a preexisting condition that contraindicates the use of an antitubercular agent
• Potential for injury related to a preexisting condition that requires cautious use of an antitubercular agent
• Potential for injury related to adverse drug reactions
• Sensory-perceptual alterations (tactile, visual) related to peripheral or optic neuritis caused by INH or ethambutol
• Knowledge deficit related to the prescribed antitubercular agent

Planning and implementation

• Do not administer an antitubercular agent to a patient with a condition that contraindicates its use.
• Administer an antitubercular agent cautiously to a patient at risk because of a preexisting condition.
• Monitor the patient periodically for adverse reactions during therapy with an antitubercular agent.
• Assess the patient routinely for sensory deficits when administering ethambutol or INH.
• *Monitor the patient closely for hypersensitivity reactions. Keep standard emergency equipment nearby.*
• Monitor the patient's liver function tests for abnormalities with INH or rifampin therapy, serum uric acid levels with ethambutol therapy, and white blood count with rifampin and ethambutol therapy.
• Monitor hydration if the patient experiences nausea, vomiting, anorexia, or diarrhea during rifampin or ethambutol therapy. Obtain a prescription for an antiemetic or antidiarrheal agent, as needed.
• Administer an analgesic as prescribed if the patient experiences a headache during ethambutol therapy or joint pain or muscle aches or cramps during rifampin therapy.
• Take safety measures if the patient experiences adverse CNS reactions, such as confusion or uncoordination. For example, place the patient's bed in the lowest position, keep the bed rails raised, and supervise ambulation.
• Take seizure precautions when administering INH to a patient with a seizure disorder.
• *Administer rifampin 1 hour before or 2 hours after a meal because food affects the rate and extent of absorption.*
• *Administer INH at least 1 hour before administering an aluminum antacid to prevent a drug interaction.*

• Monitor the patient closely for additive CNS effects, such as drowsiness, dizziness, headache, lethargy, and depression, during concomitant therapy with INH and cycloserine or ethionamide.
• Expect to increase the dosage of such drugs as oral contraceptives, corticosteroids, and warfarin because rifampin is known to accelerate their metabolism.
• Notify the physician if adverse reactions or drug interactions occur.
• *Monitor the patient closely for peripheral neuritis (exhibited initially by paresthesia of the hands and feet followed by muscle twitching, dizziness, ataxia, and stupor) when administering 6 mg/kg of INH daily or higher.*
• Administer pyridoxine concurrently with INH, as prescribed, to prevent peripheral neuritis.
• *Monitor the patient closely for optic neuritis when administering INH or 15 mg/kg or higher of ethambutol.*
• Test the patient's visual acuity before INH or ethambutol therapy begins, and monthly thereafter, when the ethambutol dose exceeds 15 mg/kg and throughout INH therapy.
• Notify the physician if visual disturbances occur.

Patient teaching

• Teach the patient and family the name, dose, frequency, action, and adverse effects of the prescribed antitubercular agent.
• Instruct the patient taking INH to consult the physician if signs and symptoms of hepatic dysfunction appear, such as nausea, vomiting, fatigue, weakness, and anorexia.
• *Instruct the patient taking INH or ethambutol to report any visual changes immediately.*
• *Advise the patient that rifampin may produce red-orange urine, tears, sputum, sweat, and feces that stain clothes, linen, and soft contact lenses.*
• *Advise the female patient who is taking rifampin and an oral contraceptive to use an alternate form of birth control.*
• Reassure the patient who experiences adverse reactions early in rifampin therapy that most of them will subside with continued treatment.
• Teach the patient the importance of having periodic blood studies performed as instructed.
• Advise the patient to take a mild analgesic (unless contraindicated) for joint pain, muscle aches or cramps, or headache.
• Caution the patient not to perform activities that require mental alertness or motor coordination if adverse CNS reactions occur.
• *Teach the patient when to take rifampin in relation to meals and INH in relation to aluminum antacids if prescribed.*
• Instruct the patient to notify the physician if adverse reactions occur.

Evaluation

The following examples represent appropriate evaluation statements for a patient receiving an antitubercular agent.

• The patient has no conditions that contraindicate antitubercular agent therapy.

• The patient exhibits no signs of complications in the preexisting condition linked to the prescribed antitubercular agent.

• The patient exhibits no adverse reactions to the prescribed antitubercular agent.

• The patient does not experience peripheral or optic neuritis during INH or ethambutol therapy.

• The patient and family express an accurate understanding of the points taught about the prescribed antitubercular agent.

• The patient agrees to report paresthesia of the feet and hands or visual disturbances promptly.

OTHER ANTITUBERCULAR AGENTS

Several other drugs are used as antitubercular agents in combination with first-line agents. Because these drugs have a greater incidence of toxicity, they are used primarily when resistance or allergies to less toxic agents exist.

aminosalicylic acid (Para-Aminosalicytic Acid, P.A.S.). A tuberculostatic agent, aminosalicylic acid acts like a sulfonamide by decreasing bacterial synthesis of folic acid. The drug is absorbed readily, distributed widely, metabolized rapidly by the liver, and excreted by the kidneys. Its half-life is about 1 hour. The potential for severe GI disturbances limits the use of aminosalicylic acid.

capreomycin sulfate (Capastat Sulfate). Capreomycin is a polypeptide antibiotic whose mechanism of action is unknown. Because it is not absorbed well from the G.I. tract, it must be given I.M. Its half-life is 4 to 6 hours, and it is excreted primarily unchanged in the urine.

cycloserine (Seromycin). An antibiotic derived from the *Streptomyces* genus, cycloserine acts against many strains of mycobacteria by inhibiting cell wall synthesis. After oral administration, cycloserine is absorbed well, distributed widely, and excreted primarily by the kidneys. It has a half-life of 10 hours. It is used with other antitubercular agents, but its neurotoxicity and the rapid development of bacterial resistance limit its use.

ethionamide (Trecator-SC). A derivative of isonicotinic acid, ethionamide is used to treat tuberculosis and Hansen's disease and is especially useful in treating Hansen's disease produced by dapsone-resistant *M. leprae*. Its mechanism of action is unknown. Ethionamide is absorbed well after oral administration and is distributed widely. It is metabolized extensively and is excreted in the urine. The plasma half-life is approximately 3 hours. GI disturbances are the most common adverse reactions to the drug.

pyrazinamide. A niacinamide derivative, pyrazinamide is highly specific for *M. tuberculosis*. Its mechanism of action is unknown. Absorbed well and distributed widely, pyrazinamide is metabolized extensively by the liver and has a half-life of 9 to 10 hours. Because this drug commonly produces hepatotoxicity, a patient receiving it requires close monitoring.

streptomycin sulfate. The first agent recognized as effective in treating tuberculosis, streptomycin is administered I.M. only. It appears to enhance the activity of oral antitubercular agents and is of greatest value in the early weeks to months of therapy. However, I.M. administration limits its usefulness in long-term therapy. Rapidly absorbed from the I.M. injection site, streptomycin is excreted primarily by the kidneys as unchanged drug. Most patients tolerate streptomycin well, but those receiving large doses may exhibit eighth cranial nerve toxicity. (For information about the other uses of streptomycin, see Chapter 59, Antibacterial Agents.)

ANTILEPROTIC AGENTS

The primary agent used to treat Hansen's disease (leprosy) is dapsone, a sulfone drug; however, rifampin and clofazimine also are used. Clofazimine and dapsone are discussed in this section. Rifampin was discussed under "Antitubercular Agents" earlier in this chapter. Ethionamide, an antitubercular agent, is used to treat dapsone-resistant Hansen's disease and usually is combined with rifampin, or clofazimine and rifampin. (For more information, see the previous section on "Other Antitubercular Agents.")

PHARMACOKINETICS

Clofazimine and dapsone are administered orally. Clofazimine is distributed primarily to fatty tissues and the reticuloendothelial system and excreted primarily unchanged in the urine and feces. Dapsone is distributed into most body tissues and fluids, slowly metabolized in the liver, and excreted in the urine.

Absorption, distribution, metabolism, excretion

Clofazimine is absorbed incompletely after oral administration. The extent of absorption depends on several factors, including dose and the presence of food in the GI tract. Clofazimine is highly lipophilic and is distributed primarily to fatty tissues and the reticuloendothelial system. It crosses the placenta and is distributed into breast milk. Metabolism of clofazimine is unclear. It appears to accumulate in the body and is excreted primarily unchanged in the urine and feces. Small amounts are excreted in the sebaceous and sweat glands.

Administered orally, dapsone is absorbed slowly but completely from the GI tract and is distributed freely throughout the body. It appears in most tissues and fluids and is retained in the skin, muscles, liver, and kidneys. Dapsone is distributed into breast milk. Similar to INH, dapsone undergoes acetylation in the liver at a genetically determined rate. Approximately 20% of the drug is excreted unchanged in the urine, and the rest is excreted as metabolites.

Onset, peak, duration

In a healthy patient receiving a 200-mg dose of clofazimine, the peak plasma concentration level is reached in 4 to 12 hours. The steady state plasma concentration after multiple doses may not be achieved for 30 days. The half-life after repeated doses is approximately 70 days.

Dapsone reaches a peak serum concentration in 2 to 8 hours. The drug's half-life ranges from 10 to 83 hours, and averages 20 to 30 hours. Trace amounts may remain in the body 8 to 12 days after a single 200-mg dose or up to 35 days after discontinuation of repeated doses.

PHARMACODYNAMICS

Clofazimine is a phenazine dye whose mechanism of action against mycobacteria is not understood completely. It appears to bind to mycobacterial DNA and inhibit replication and growth. Clofazimine also has anti-inflammatory and immunosuppressive properties. The mechanisms of action for these properties remain unknown.

Dapsone is bacteriostatic for *M. leprae*. Although its antibacterial action is not understood fully, it may parallel that of the sulfonamides. Like those drugs, dapsone inhibits folic acid synthesis by bacteria.

PHARMACOTHERAPEUTICS

Clofazimine is used to treat lepromatous Hansen's disease, including dapsone-resistant and erythema nodosum leprosum. Dapsone is the drug of choice for treating Hansen's disease because it is effective, inexpensive, and relatively nontoxic. It also is used to treat dermatitis herpetiformis.

clofazimine (Lamprene). Clofazimine is used to treat lepromatous Hansen's disease, including dapsone-resistant and that which is complicated by erythema nodosum leprosum. Combination therapy has been recommended for initial treatment of multibacillary Hansen's disease to prevent the development of drug resistance.
Usual adult dosage: for lepromatous Hansen's disease, 50 to 100 mg P.O. once daily or 50 mg P.O. once daily plus an additional 300-mg dose given once monthly with other antileprotic drugs; for dapsone-resistant Hansen's disease, 50 to 100 mg P.O. once daily with other antileprotic drugs for 2 years, followed by single therapy with clofazimine 50 to 100 mg P.O. once daily for 10 or more years; for erythema nodosum leprosum, dosage depends on the severity of symptoms and must be individualized.

dapsone. Dapsone is used to treat all forms of Hansen's disease, and bacterial resistance to it develops by degrees. The drug is used alone only after intensive multi-drug treatment. Sulfone-sensitive infections usually require a combination of dapsone and rifampin; sulfone-resistant infections require combinations of rifampin and clofazimine or ethionamide. Treatment may continue for 6 months to life, depending on the severity of the disease.
Usual adult dosage: for Hansen's disease, 50 to 100 mg P.O. once daily, depending on the disease classification; for dermatitis herpetiformis, 25 to 400 mg P.O. daily.
Usual pediatric dosage: for Hansen's disease, 1 to 1.5 mg/kg P.O. daily.

Drug interactions

To date, no clinically significant drug interactions have been reported with clofazimine.

Probenecid may decrease urinary excretion of dapsone metabolites, increasing the drug's serum concentration. Rifampin may increase dapsone metabolism, lowering its serum concentration. However, the clinical significance of these interactions are unknown. Concurrent use of folic acid antagonists, such as pyrimethamine, may result in additive adverse hematologic effects. Patients should be monitored closely if concomitant administration occurs.

ADVERSE DRUG REACTIONS

Because clofazimine and dapsone produce relatively few adverse reactions, interruption of therapy seldom is required.

Clofazimine usually is tolerated well. Most adverse reactions are dose-related and reversible upon discontinuation of the drug. Discoloration, such as changes in skin pigmentation, are the most common adverse reactions and occur in 75% to 100% of patients. Other dermatologic reactions include ichthyosis, dryness, rash, and pruritus. The most common GI reactions include epigastric pain, diarrhea, nausea, and vomiting.

Hemolytic anemia and methemoglobinemia are the most common dose-related reactions to dapsone. Hemolysis can occur in varying degrees. It develops in almost every patient receiving 200 to 300 mg of dapsone daily but hardly ever affects those receiving 100 mg/day. Some degree of methemoglobinemia occurs in most patients receiving dapsone but usually does not necessitate discontinuation of therapy. Cyanosis may accompany mild methemoglobinemia. Although these adverse hematologic reactions pose no problems for most patients, dapsone may produce severe hemolysis and methemoglobinemia in a patient with glucose-6-phosphate dehydrogenase (G6PD) deficiency. (For more information, see *G6PD deficiency*.)

Serious complications of dapsone therapy are uncommon, but may include granulocytopenia and dapsone syndrome, which mimic infectious mononucleosis. Hypersensitivity to dapsone rarely produce adverse cutaneous reactions, such as exfoliative dermatitis, toxic erythema, erythema multiforme, urticaria, and erythema nodosum.

G6PD deficiency

Glucose-6-phosphate dehydrogenase (G6PD) deficiency affects many people, especially Blacks, Chinese, Thais, and Eastern Mediterranean peoples, such as Greeks, Sardinians, and Sephardic Jews. The more than 100 variants of this genetic chromosomal deficiency can produce varying degrees of erythrocyte hemolysis when affected individuals receive such drugs as dapsone, antimalarial agents, analgesics, sulfonamides, vitamin K, and probenecid. All these drugs should be administered cautiously to patients with G6PD deficiency. Complicating this risk, G6PD deficiency also may trigger erythrocyte hemolysis when an affected individual is subjected to the stress of metabolic acidosis, diabetic ketoacidosis, or a bacterial infection. Such stress shortens the erythrocyte life span, decreasing the hemoglobin level (especially in older erythrocytes) and increasing the reticulocyte count. Thus, an infection *and* the drug used to treat it pose special hazards for the person with G6PD deficiency.

NURSING PROCESS APPLICATION

The following information assists the nurse in caring for a patient who is receiving an antileprotic agent.

Assessment
• Review the patient's history for a preexisting condition that contraindicates the use of an antileprotic agent, such as known hypersensitivity to the drug.
• Review the patient's history for a preexisting condition that requires cautious use of an antileprotic agent, such as G6PD deficiency, methemoglobin reductase deficiency, GI problems, or lactation.
• Assess the patient for adverse reactions to the prescribed antileprotic agent, such as GI distress, and hypersensitivity, hematologic, or dermatologic reactions.
• Review the patient's medication history to identify the use of drugs that may interact with the prescribed antileprotic agent, such as probenecid, rifampin, or folic acid antagonists.
• Assess the effectiveness of the prescribed antileprotic drug periodically.
• Assess the patient's compliance with antileprotic therapy.
• Evaluate the patient's and family's knowledge about the prescribed antileprotic agent.

Nursing diagnoses
The following examples represent appropriate nursing diagnoses for a patient receiving an antileprotic agent.
• Potential for injury related to a preexisting condition that contraindicates the use of dapsone
• Potential for injury related to a preexisting condition that requires cautious use of an antileprotic agent
• Potential for injury related to adverse drug reactions
• Noncompliance related to long-term use of an antileprotic agent
• Knowledge deficit related to the prescribed antileprotic agent

Planning and implementation
• Do not administer dapsone to a patient with a condition that contraindicates its use. Clofazimine does not have any contraindications.
• Administer an antileprotic agent cautiously to a patient at risk because of a preexisting condition.
• Monitor the patient periodically for adverse reactions during antileprotic agent therapy.
• Monitor the patient's complete blood count weekly during the first 6 months of dapsone therapy and monthly thereafter. Notify the physician of any abnormality.
• *Observe the patient who is receiving 200 to 300 mg of dapsone daily or who has G6PD deficiency for signs and symptoms of hemolytic anemia (pallor, fatigue, dyspnea) or methemoglobinemia (cyanosis).*

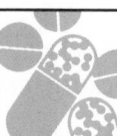

Antitubercular and antileprotic agents

This chart summarizes the first-line agents used to treat mycobacterial infections. Effective therapy usually combines these drugs with each other or with second-line agents.

DRUG	MAJOR INDICATIONS	USUAL ADULT DOSAGES	CONTRAINDICATIONS AND PRECAUTIONS
Antitubercular agents			
ethambutol	Uncomplicated pulmonary tuberculosis, infections caused by *Mycobacterium bovis* and most strains of *M. kansasii*	15 mg/kg P.O. once daily, if previously untreated; 25 mg/kg P.O. daily, for 60 days with dosage decreased to 15 mg/kg P.O. once daily, if previously treated	• Know that ethambutol is contraindicated in a patient with known optic neuritis or hypersitivity to the drug, unless clinical judgment determines that it may be used. • Administer with caution to a pregnant patient.
isoniazid (INH)	Treatment of tuberculosis	5 to 10 mg/kg P.O. or I.M. once daily, up to a maximum of 300 mg/day for at least 1 year	• Know that INH is contraindicated in a patient with known hypersensitivity to the drug; a history of severe adverse reactions to INH, such as drug fever, chills, or arthritis; or acute liver disease of any etiology. • Administer with caution to a pregnant or lactating patient, one with current chronic liver disease, severe renal dysfunction, or daily alcohol use; or one who is receiving phenytoin concurrently.
	Prevention of tuberculosis	300 mg P.O. once daily for 6 to 12 months	
rifampin	Tuberculosis or Hansen's disease	600 mg P.O. once daily, 1 hour before or 2 hours after a meal	• Know that rifampin is contraindicated in a lactating patient, one with a history of hypersensitivity to any of the rifamycins, or in the treatment of meningococcal disease. • Administer with extreme caution to a pregnant patient.
	Asymptomatic *Neisseria meningitidis* carriers	600 mg P.O. once daily 1 hour before or 2 hours after a meal for 4 days, or 600 mg P.O. b.i.d. for 2 days	
Antileprotic agents			
clofazimine	Dapsone-resistant Hansen's disease	50 to 100 mg P.O. once daily with one or more antileprotic drugs for 3 years, followed by single therapy with clofazimine 50 to 100 mg P.O. daily	• Administer with caution to a pregnant or lactating patient or one with gastrointestinal problems, such as abdominal pain or diarrhea.
dapsone	Hansen's disease caused by *M. leprae*	50 to 100 mg P.O. once daily	• Know that dapsone is contraindicated in a lactating patient or one with known hypersensitivity to the drug or any of its derivatives. • Administer with caution to a pregnant patient or one with glucose-6-phosphate dehydrogenase deficiency, methemoglobin reductase deficiency, or exposure to agents or conditions capable of producing hemolysis, such as diabetic ketosis.
	Dermatitis herpetiformis	25 to 400 mg P.O. daily	

• Monitor the patient receiving dapsone therapy for granulocytopenia and dapsone syndrome, exhibited by fever, sore throat, swollen lymph glands, and easy bruising.
• Administer dapsone cautiously in combination with nitrites, aniline derivatives, nitrofurantoin, primaquine, or other drugs that can induce hemolysis, particularly if the patient has G6PD deficiency.

• *Inspect the patient for changes in skin pigmentation, ichthyosis, dryness, rash, or evidence of pruritus, during clofazimine therapy.*
• Monitor hydration if the patient receiving clofazimine experiences nausea, vomiting, or diarrhea. Obtain a prescription for an antiemetic or antidiarrheal agent if needed
• Notify the physician if adverse reactions occur.

• *Determine the patient's degree of compliance with antileprotic therapy.*

• Attempt to identify psychosocial or physiological factors that may influence noncompliant behavior.

Patient teaching

• Teach the patient and family the name, dose, frequency, action, and adverse effects of the prescribed antileprotic agent.

• Instruct the patient to take clofazimine with meals to minimize adverse GI reactions.

• *Warn the patient that clofazimine may discolor the skin, conjunctivae, tears, sweat, sputum, urine, and feces, and that although this discoloration is reversible, it may take years or months to disappear.*

• Instruct the patient to report sore throat, fever, purpura, or jaundice during dapsone therapy.

• *Instruct the patient to have a complete blood count performed weekly for 6 months and monthly thereafter during dapsone therapy.*

• *Explain to the patient the importance of adhering to the prescribed antileprotic therapy.*

• Instruct the patient to notify the physician if adverse reactions occur.

Evaluation

The following examples represent appropriate evaluation statements for a patient receiving an antileprotic agent.

• The patient has no preexisting conditions that contraindicate antileprotic agent therapy.

• The patient exhibits no signs of complications in the preexisting condition linked to the prescribed antileprotic agent.

• The patient exhibits no adverse reactions to the prescribed antileprotic agent.

• The patient verifies compliance with antileprotic therapy as prescribed.

• The patient and family express an accurate understanding of the points taught about the prescribed antileprotic agent.

• The patient returns for blood tests weekly as instructed.

CHAPTER SUMMARY

Chapter 60 covered the antitubercular and antileprotic agents as they are used to treat various mycobacterial infections. Here are the chapter highlights.

• Various chemically unrelated agents are used to treat mycobacterial infections. Although these agents show relatively high mycobacterial specificity and inhibition, *M.*

tuberculosis and *M. leprae* infections typically require long-term treatment. In almost all compliant patients, however, combinations of antitubercular and antileprotic agents can control these diseases successfully.

• Ethambutol, INH, and rifampin serve as the first-line agents for treating tuberculosis. Although these drugs vary in terms of specific regimens and length of treatment required, they produce similar therapeutic results.

• Antitubercular agents have a favorable benefit-to-risk ratio. Significant adverse reactions do occur, however, usually producing neurotoxic or hepatotoxic effects.

• Although the development of bacterial resistance to these drugs is a constant threat, aggressive combination therapy can minimize it greatly.

• Clofazimine, dapsone, and rifamipin currently dominate the treatment of Hansen's disease, although ethionamide also may be used. Like most drugs used to treat mycobacterial infections, these antileprotic agents are used in combination to improve their effectiveness and reduce the likelihood of the development of bacterial resistance to them.

• Hematologic, immunologic, GI, and cutaneous disturbances can result from antileprotic therapy, but they seldom require interruption of therapy.

• The nurse must instruct the patient and family in the administration, effects of, and possible adverse reactions to antitubercular and antileprotic agents; monitor the patient throughout therapy; and notify the physician if adverse reactions occur.

STUDY QUESTIONS

See Appendix 1 for answers.

1. Bob Dixon, age 63, recently developed fatigue, night sweats, and a productive cough. A positive Mantoux test and abnormal chest X-ray suggested pulmonary tuberculosis; a positive acid-fast bacillus sputum culture confirmed the diagnosis. The physician prescribes a drug regimen of INH 300 mg P.O. once daily, rifampin 600 mg P.O. once daily, and pyradoxine 10 mg P.O. once daily. What is the rationale for administering INH and rifampin concurrently in treating active tuberculosis?

(a) They are second-line agents and only effective together.

(b) Rifampin increases the activity of INH.

(c) The drugs are bacteriostatic in usual doses.

(d) Combination therapy can prevent or delay bacterial resistance.

2. After taking INH and rifampin for several days, Mr. Dixon complains of GI upset. What information should the nurse give Mr. Dixon about using an antacid that contains aluminum hydroxide during antitubercular therapy?
(a) Aluminum hydroxide decreases INH absorption.
(b) Aluminum hydroxide may produce additive CNS effects.
(c) Aluminum hydroxide increases the risk of bacterial resistance.
(d) Aluminum hydroxide increases INH absorption and the risk of toxicity.

3. What is the rationale for prescribing pyradoxine with the antitubercular drugs?
(a) Pyradoxine enhances the effects of antitubercular drugs.
(b) Pyradoxine prevents bacterial resistance.
(c) Pyradoxine helps prevent the neurotoxic effects of INH.
(d) Pyradoxine minimizes GI distress associated with rifampin.

4. The nurse should prepare Mr. Dixon for which potential adverse urinary reaction to rifampin?
(a) oliguria
(b) red-orange urine
(c) polyuria
(d) hematuria

5. Mr. Dixon's GI distress persists, so the physician replaces rifampin with ethambutol. Which major adverse reaction is associated with ethambutol?
(a) optic neuritis
(b) hepatotoxicity
(c) renal failure
(d) peripheral neuritis

6. Anne Larkin, age 23, takes 50 mg of dapsone P.O. daily as prescribed for Hansen's disease. Which factor is most likely to influence Ms. Larkin's compliance with therapy?
(a) cost of medication
(b) frequency of adverse reactions
(c) duration of treatment
(d) administration schedule

7. When Ms. Larkin does not respond adequately after one week of dapsone therapy, the physician suspects that she has developed dapsone resistance. Which agent is most likely to be prescribed?
(a) probenicid
(b) INH
(c) clofazimine
(d) ethambutol

8. Which of the following is one of the most common dose-related adverse reaction to dapsone?
(a) peripheral neuritis
(b) hepatotoxicity
(c) hemolytic anemia
(d) hypersensitivity reaction

SELECTED REFERENCES

Abramowicz, M. (Ed.). (1988). Drugs for tuberculosis. *Medical Letter on Drugs and Therapeutics, 30,* 43.

AHFS drug information 90. (1990). Bethesda, MD: American Society of Hospital Pharmacists.

Goodman and Gilman's the pharmacological basis of therapeutics (8th ed.; 1990). Elmsford, NY: Pergamon Press.

Hansten, P., and Horn, J. (1989). *Drug interactions* (6th ed.). Philadelphia: Lea & Febiger.

Drug facts and comparisons. (1991). St. Louis: Facts and Comparisons Division, Lippincott.

North American Nursing Diagnosis Association (1990). *Taxonomy I - Revised, with official diagnostic categories.* St. Louis, NANDA.

Weintraub, M., and Evans, P. (1987). Clofazimine: An orphan drug approved for the treatment of leprosy that also has potential use in AIDS patients. *Hospital Formulary, 22*(9), 766-775.

CHAPTER

▽
61
△

ANTIVIRAL AGENTS

OBJECTIVES

After reading and studying this chapter, the student should be able to:
1. Discuss the pharmacokinetics and mechanisms of action of the antiviral agents acyclovir, ganciclovir, vidarabine, amantadine, ribavirin, and zidovudine.
2. Identify the indications for antiviral agents.
3. Discuss the adverse reactions associated with antiviral agents.
4. Describe the difficulties and dangers in administering parenteral antiviral agents.
5. Describe how to apply the nursing process when caring for a patient who is receiving an antiviral agent.

INTRODUCTION

Antiviral agents are drugs used to prevent or treat viral infections. They usually work by interfering with viral replication. The relatively few antiviral agents available for clinical use will kill a specific virus while leaving the host cell intact. Unlike other infecting organisms, viruses are intracellular parasites that survive and multiply through the metabolic processes of the invaded cell. Thus, any agent that kills the virus also may destroy the cells that harbor it. In fact, many experimental antiviral compounds are too toxic for human use. Although they inhibit viral deoxyribonucleic acid (DNA) or protein synthesis, they also inhibit these functions in host cells. Recently, significant progress has been made in producing antiviral agents with actions specific to viral function.

Chapter 61 discusses six major antiviral agents: acyclovir sodium, ganciclovir sodium, vidarabine monohydrate, amantadine hydrochloride, ribavirin, and zidovudine. For the most part, they are effective against herpes simplex virus (HSV) and influenza A and B viruses. Zidovudine is the first antiviral drug released by the Food and Drug Administration (FDA) for use against human immunodeficiency virus (HIV) in the treatment of acquired immunodeficiency syndrome (AIDS). Ganciclovir is the first

---

SELECTED NURSING DIAGNOSES

Antiviral agents

The following nursing diagnoses address representative problems and etiologies that a nurse may encounter when caring for a patient who is receiving an antiviral agent. Some of these nursing diagnoses contain generalized etiologies, which the nurse must individualize based on the patient's needs. (For some common nursing diagnoses and related interventions for each drug class, see the "Nursing Process Application" sections of this chapter.)

- Altered health maintenance related to drug interactions
- Altered protection related to the adverse hematologic effects of the prescribed antiviral agent
- Altered thought processes related to the adverse CNS effects of the prescribed antiviral agent
- Decreased cardiac output related to ganciclovir-induced arrhythmias
- Diarrhea related to the adverse GI effects of an antiviral agent
- Fluid volume excess related to vidarabine-induced fluid retention
- Impaired gas exchange related to worsening of respiratory function caused by ribavirin
- Impaired physical mobility related to the adverse CNS effects of an antiviral agent
- Impaired tissue integrity related to irritation or thrombophlebitis from parenteral antiviral therapy
- Knowledge deficit related to the prescribed antiviral agent
- Noncompliance related to adverse reactions to oral antiviral therapy
- Potential fluid volume deficit related to the adverse GI effects of an antiviral agent
- Potential for infection related to the adverse hematologic effects of an antiviral agent
- Potential for injury related to a preexisting condition that contraindicates the use of an antiviral agent
- Potential for injury related to a preexisting condition that requires cautious use of an antiviral agent
- Potential for injury related to adverse drug reactions
- Sensory-perceptual alterations (gustatory, visual) related to the adverse CNS effects of an antiviral agent

antiviral agent used to treat cytomegalovirus (CMV) disease. The primary emphasis is on systemic therapy. Topical therapy, including dermatologic and ophthalmologic routes, is covered in more detail in the appendix on Integumentary System Agents and in Chapter 71, Ophthalmic Agents.

For a summary of representative drugs, see *Selected major drugs: Antiviral agents,* page 1076. For a listing of applicable nursing diagnoses that the nurse may formulate when caring for a patient receiving one of these agents, see *Selected nursing diagnoses: Antiviral agents,* page 1063. For detailed information on applying the nursing process, see Chapter 6, The Nursing Process and Drug Therapy.

ACYCLOVIR AND GANCICLOVIR

The anti-herpesvirus agent, acyclovir, produces marked antiviral activity and minimal cellular toxicity. It is 300 to 3,000 times more toxic to herpesviruses than it is to mammalian cells. A derivative of acyclovir, ganciclovir has been shown to have potent antiviral activity against HSV and CMV.

PHARMACOKINETICS

Acyclovir is available in oral, intravenous (I.V.), and topical forms. The topical form of the drug is covered in the appendix on Integumentary System Agents. Ganciclovir is available as a parenteral agent for I.V. administration only.

Absorption, distribution, metabolism, excretion

Although gastrointestinal (GI) absorption of acyclovir is slow and only 15% to 30% complete, serum concentration levels of the drug are therapeutic. Acyclovir is distributed throughout the body and can be detected in the kidneys, brain, lungs, liver, intestines, spleen, uterus, muscles, vaginal mucosa and secretions, cerebrospinal fluid (CSF), and herpetic vesicular fluid. CSF concentration levels are approximately 50% of plasma concentrations. Acyclovir crosses the placenta. Data on breast milk distribution are lacking. The drug is 9% to 33% protein bound.

Metabolism of acyclovir is complex. The drug has five metabolites: two produced from hepatic metabolism and three produced by cells infected by herpesviruses. Infected cells produce the inactive monophosphate and diphosphate metabolites and the active triphosphate metabolite, which is the antiviral form of the drug.

Acyclovir is excreted primarily in the urine via glomerular filtration and renal tubular secretion.

Ganciclovir is administered I.V. because it is absorbed poorly from the GI tract. Distribution into human body tissues has not been elucidated fully. The drug is 1% to 2% bound to plasma proteins and is thought to cross the blood-brain barrier. More than 90% is excreted by the kidneys unchanged.

Onset, peak, duration

The onset of action, peak concentration level, and duration of action of acyclovir are related to the time the drug maintains a serum concentration higher than the minimal inhibitory concentration. Host defense mechanisms, such as white blood cell (WBC) activity, also contribute to the drug's effectiveness and can extend its duration. Usually, average peak concentrations of acyclovir are reached 1.5 to 2.5 hours after oral administration and immediately after I.V. administration.

Acyclovir's half-life in adults with normal renal function is between 2 and 3.5 hours. The half-life increases as renal function deteriorates, and anuria prolongs it to nearly 20 hours. Thus the dosage needs to be adjusted in patients with renal impairment.

Peak concentrations of ganciclovir occur immediately after I.V. administration. In patients with renal insufficiency, the plasma half-life of ganciclovir increases and renal excretion decreases.

PHARMACODYNAMICS

To be effective, acyclovir and ganciclovir must be metabolized to their active form in cells infected by the herpesvirus. Although metabolism to the active drug form also takes place in uninfected cells, it proceeds at a rate so slow and limited that it does not cause significant toxicity to uninfected cells.

Mechanism of action

Acyclovir enters virus-infected cells, where it is changed to an organic phosphate by a virus-specific enzyme called thymidine kinase. The resulting monophosphate metabolite of acyclovir is polarized and cannot diffuse readily out of the cell. This monophosphate form then is converted further by cellular enzymes to diphosphate and triphosphate forms. The latter—acyclovir triphosphate—is the effective antiviral compound that inhibits virus-specific DNA polymerase, an enzyme necessary for viral growth, and disrupts viral replication.

Ganciclovir is a synthetic nucleoside analogue of 2'-deoxyguanosine. Upon entry into host cells, ganciclovir is converted to its triphosphate by one or more cellular kinases. CMV-infected cells have about 10 times more ganciclovir-triphosphate than uninfected cells. Ganciclovir triphosphate is thought to produce its antiviral activity by inhibiting viral DNA synthesis.

PHARMACOTHERAPEUTICS

The antiviral activity of acyclovir is limited to the herpesviruses, including HSV types 1 and 2 and the varicella-zoster virus.

Oral acyclovir is used primarily to treat initial and recurrent genital HSV infections. Long-term use of oral acyclovir significantly decreases recurrence in patients with genital HSV infection, but all patients experience recurrent infection if acyclovir is discontinued.

Parenteral acyclovir has several clinical indications. It is used to treat severe initial genital HSV infections in patients with normal immune systems, initial and recurrent mucocutaneous herpes simplex (HSV-1 and HSV-2) infections in immunocompromised patients, herpes zoster (shingles) infections caused by the varicella-zoster virus in immunocompromised patients, disseminated varicella-zoster virus in immunocompromised patients, and varicella (chicken pox) infections caused by varicella-zoster virus in immunocompromised patients. Although parenteral acyclovir prevents new vesicle formation, it does not seem to reduce the frequency of recurrent genital herpes lesions. Use of parenteral acyclovir in primary (self-limiting, acute) genital HSV infections reduces viral shedding, shortens healing time, and limits the duration of symptoms.

Ganciclovir is used to treat CMV retinitis in immunocompromised patients, including those with AIDS.

Patients with renal dysfunction require dosage adjustments during therapy with acyclovir or ganciclovir. (For more information, see *Dosage adjustments in patients with renal dysfunction.*)

acyclovir sodium (Zovirax). Available in oral and parenteral forms, acyclovir is used to treat various HSV-1, HSV-2, varicella-zoster, and herpes zoster infections. The dosage must be reduced in patients with renal impairment (with a creatinine clearance below 50 ml/minute).
Usual adult dosage: for primary genital HSV infection in patients with a creatinine clearance greater than 50 ml/minute, 200 mg P.O. every 4 hours while awake five times a day for 10 days, or 5 mg/kg of body weight I.V. every 8 hours for 5 to 7 days; for recurrent genital HSV infection, 200 mg P.O. five times a day for 5 days; for prophylaxis of recurrent genital HSV infections, 200 mg P.O. t.i.d. for 6 months; for varicella-zoster infections in patients with normal renal function, 5 to 10 mg/kg of body weight I.V. every 8 hours for 5 days; for varicella-zoster infections in immunocompromised patients, 500 mg/m² I.V. every 8 hours for 7 days; for herpes simplex encephalitis, 10 mg/kg of body weight I.V. every 8 hours for at least 10 days; for acute herpes zoster infections in nonimmunocompromised patients, 800 mg P.O. every 4 hours (five times daily) for 7 to 10 days; for the initial episode of herpes simplex proctitis, 400 mg P.O. five times daily for 10 days.

Dosage adjustments in patients with renal dysfunction

Adults and children age 12 or older with acute or chronic renal impairment require a reduction in the dosage of acyclovir or ganciclovir, as summarized in this table.

CREATININE CLEARANCE (ml/min/1.73 m²)	DOSAGE INTERVALS (mg/kg)
Acyclovir	
50 or greater	5 mg/kg every 8 hours
25 to 50	5 mg/kg every 12 hours
10 to 25	5 mg/kg every 24 hours
less than 10	2.5 mg/kg every 24 hours
Ganciclovir	
80 or greater	5.0 mg/kg every 12 hours
50 to 79	2.5 mg/kg every 12 hours
25 to 49	2.5 mg/kg every 24 hours
less than 25	1.25 mg/kg every 24 hours

ganciclovir (Cytovene). Ganciclovir is indicated to treat CMV retinitis in immunocompromised patients, including those with AIDS. In patients with a creatinine clearance below 80 ml/minute, the dosage must be reduced.
Usual adult dosage: for initial treatment of patients with normal renal function, 5 mg/kg I.V. over 1 hour every 12 hours for 14 to 21 days; for maintenance, 5 mg/kg I.V. over 1 hour once daily or 6 mg/kg I.V. once daily for 5 out of 7 days a week. Patients in whom the disease progresses during maintenance therapy may need to return to the every-12-hour treatment.

Drug interactions

Acyclovir and ganciclovir may interact with probenecid and other drugs that inhibit renal tubular secretion or resorption. Concomitant administration of acyclovir with other nephrotoxic agents increases the risk of renal dysfunction and requires close monitoring of the patient's renal function. Ganciclovir has significant interactions with several other drugs, including cytotoxic agents, imipenem/cilastatin, and zidovudine. (For more information, see *Drug interactions: Acyclovir and ganciclovir,* page 1066.)

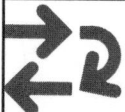

DRUG INTERACTIONS

Acyclovir and ganciclovir

Drug interactions with acyclovir and ganciclovir therapy are potentially serious.

DRUG	INTERACTING DRUGS	POSSIBLE EFFECTS	NURSING IMPLICATIONS
acyclovir, ganciclovir	probenecid and other drugs that inhibit renal tubular secretion or resorption	May reduce the renal clearance of ganciclovir and increase plasma concentration	• Monitor the patient's renal function. • Keep the patient well hydrated. • Watch for signs of drug toxicity.
acyclovir	nephrotoxic agents	Increase chance of renal dysfunction	• Monitor the patient's renal function. • Keep the patient well hydrated.
ganciclovir	cytotoxic drugs, such as dapsone, pentamidine, flucytosine, vincristine, vinblastine, doxorubicin, amphoteracin B, and trimethoprim-sulfa combinations	Inhibits replication of rapidly dividing cells in bone marrow, GI tract, skin, and spermatogonia; may produce additive toxicity	• Administer these drugs concomitantly only if the potential benefits are thought to outweigh the risks. • Monitor the patient closely for toxicity.
	imipenem/cilastatin	Increase frequency of seizures	• Avoid concomitant administration.
	zidovudine	May cause granulocytopenia	• Avoid concomitant administration.

ADVERSE DRUG REACTIONS

Adverse reactions to oral and parenteral acyclovir usually are minimal—primarily because the drug is inactive until metabolized by the virus-infected cell. However, those that occur are significant. Adverse reactions to ganciclovir may be significant, requiring discontinuation or interruption of therapy in about one-third of the patients receiving this drug.

Local reactions at the injection site, particularly with inadvertent extravasation, are the most common problems with parenteral acyclovir. These reactions include irritation, phlebitis, inflammation, and pain. Reversible renal impairment, demonstrated by transient rises in blood urea nitrogen (BUN) or serum creatinine levels and decreases in creatinine clearance, occurs in patients receiving parenteral acyclovir by rapid I.V. injection or infusion. Patients at greatest risk are dehydrated, have a low urine output, or have had a too-rapid infusion (less than 60 minutes).

Headache is common with oral acyclovir, as are such GI reactions as nausea, vomiting, and diarrhea. Other reactions include vertigo and hematuria.

Oral or parenteral acyclovir occasionally cause diaphoresis, fatigue, insomnia, irritability, depression, and hypotension. Rarely, patients report muscle cramps and leg pain.

Other rare reactions to acyclovir include thrombocytosis, thrombocytopenia, transient lymphopenia, transient leukopenia, and bone marrow hypoplasia. Fever, rash, arthralgia, sore throat, lymphadenopathy, and inguinal adenopathy indicate hypersensitivity responses to acyclovir.

During clinical trials, the most common adverse reactions to ganciclovir were granulocytopenia and thrombocytopenia. Anemia, fever, rash, and abnormal liver function tests also were reported. The following reactions occurred in fewer than 1% of patients: arrhythmias, hypertension, hypotension, abnormal thoughts and dreams, ataxia, headache, coma, confusion, dizziness, nervousness, paresthesia, psychosis, somnolence, tremor, nausea, vomiting, anorexia, diarrhea, hemorrhage, abdominal pain, alopecia, pruritus, urticaria, hematuria, increased serum creatinine and BUN levels, inflammation, pain and phlebitis at the injection site, decreased blood glucose level, chills, edema, infections, and malaise. In animals, ganciclovir has displayed mutagenic and carcinogenic effects. Although these effects have not been proven in humans, the manufacturer recommends that these potential risks be weighed against the drug's potential benefits.

NURSING PROCESS APPLICATION

The following information assists the nurse in caring for a patient who is receiving acyclovir or ganciclovir.

Assessment

• Review the patient's history for a preexisting condition that contraindicates the use of acyclovir or ganciclovir, such as known hypersensitivity to the drug or intolerance to any of the components in the formulation.

• Review the patient's history for a preexisting condition that requires cautious use of acyclovir or ganciclovir, such as pregnancy, lactation, or renal impairment.

• Assess the patient for adverse reactions to acyclovir or ganciclovir, such as local reactions at the injection site, reversible renal impairment, headache, GI distress, hematologic disorders, hypersensitivity reactions, or central nervous system (CNS) or cardiac dysfunction.

• Review the patient's medication history to identify the use of drugs that may interact with acyclovir or ganciclovir, such as nephrotoxic or cytotoxic drugs, probenecid, imipenem/cilastatin, or zidovudine.

• Assess the effectiveness of acyclovir or ganciclovir periodically.

• Assess the patient for signs of bleeding or infection throughout acyclovir or ganciclovir therapy.

• Evaluate the patient's and family's knowledge about acyclovir or ganciclovir.

Nursing diagnoses

The following examples represent appropriate nursing diagnoses for a patient receiving acyclovir or ganciclovir.

• Potential for injury related to a preexisting condition that contraindicates the use of acyclovir or ganciclovir

• Potential for injury related to a preexisting condition that requires cautious use of acyclovir or ganciclovir

• Potential for injury related to adverse drug reactions

• Altered protection related to the adverse hematologic effects of acyclovir or ganciclovir

• Knowledge deficit related to acyclovir or ganciclovir

Planning and implementation

• Do not administer acyclovir or ganciclovir to a patient with a condition that contraindicates its use.

• Administer acyclovir or ganciclovir cautiously to a patient at risk because of a preexisting condition.

• Monitor the patient periodically for adverse reactions during acyclovir or ganciclovir therapy.

• Monitor the patient closely for hypersensitivity to acyclovir, exhibited by fever, rash, arthralgia, sore throat, lymphadenopathy, and inguinal adenopathy.

• *Monitor the patient's renal function — especially the serum creatinine level — closely during parenteral acyclovir or ganciclovir therapy.*

• Expect to adjust the dosage as prescribed for a patient with decreased renal function, especially during parenteral therapy.

• Administer an I.V. infusion of acyclovir or ganciclovir slowly (over 60 minutes or as prescribed) to prevent drug crystals from precipitating in renal tubules.

• *Infuse prepared I.V. solution only into veins with adequate blood flow to avoid phlebitis; ganciclovir infusions have a high pH.*

• *Inspect the patient's I.V. infusion site regularly for signs of irritation, phlebitis, inflammation, and extravasation. Ask the patient about pain at the I.V. site. Rotate the patient's I.V. infusion sites regularly to help prevent irritation or phlebitis.*

• Keep the patient well hydrated during parenteral therapy to ensure good urine output.

• Administer a mild analgesic as prescribed if the patient develops a headache during acyclovir or ganciclovir therapy.

• Monitor hydration if the patient experiences nausea, vomiting, or diarrhea. Obtain a prescription for an antiemetic or antidiarrheal agent if needed.

• Take safety precautions if the patient experiences vertigo or other adverse CNS reactions. For example, place the bed in the low position, keep the bed rails raised, and supervise ambulation and other activities.

• Monitor the patient's blood pressure for changes, such as hypotension or hypertension.

• Avoid concomitant therapy with drugs that may interact with acyclovir or ganciclovir, whenever possible.

• Avoid inhalation or direct skin contact because of ganciclovir's carcinogenic potential.

• Notify the physician if adverse reactions occur.

• *Monitor the patient's complete blood count (CBC) regularly during acyclovir or ganciclovir therapy. Also monitor neutrophil and platelet counts every 2 days during twice-daily therapy and at least weekly thereafter when administering ganciclovir.*

• Monitor closely for signs of infection, such as fever, chills, cough, and purulent drainage, if the patient develops leukopenia. Take infection-control measures until the patient's WBC returns to normal.

• *Monitor closely for signs of bleeding, such as spontaneous epistaxis and easy bruising, if the patient develops thrombocytopenia, which is especially likely to occur with ganciclovir therapy. Test urine, feces, and emesis for occult blood. Take bleeding precautions until the thrombocyte level returns to normal.*

• Stagger the patient's activities and provide frequent rest periods if anemia occurs.

• Notify the physician of abnormal blood test results, especially the CBC.

Patient teaching
- Teach the patient and family the name, dose, frequency, action, and adverse effects of acyclovir or ganciclovir.
- Instruct the patient to report pain or discomfort at the I.V. infusion site to the nurse.
- Advise the patient to take a mild analgesic at home if acyclovir or ganciclovir causes a headache.
- *Advise a patient of childbearing age to use effective contraception during and for at least 90 days after ganciclovir treatment because of the drug's mutagenic potential.*
- *Advise the female patient to discontinue breast-feeding and not to resume for at least 72 hours after the last ganciclovir dose.*
- Caution the patient to avoid activities that require alertness if vertigo occurs.
- Teach the patient how to minimize adverse CNS reactions at home.
- Stress the importance of returning for regular blood tests as instructed. If the patient develops leukopenia, teach about infection-control measures; if the patient develops thrombocytopenia, teach bleeding precautions.
- Instruct the patient to notify the physician if adverse reactions occur.

Evaluation

The following examples represent appropriate evaluation statements for a patient receiving acyclovir or ganciclovir.
- The patient has no conditions that contraindicate acyclovir or ganciclovir therapy.
- The patient exhibits no signs of complications in the preexisting condition linked to acyclovir or ganciclovir.
- The patient exhibits no adverse reactions to acyclovir or ganciclovir.
- The patient's CBC remains normal during acyclovir or ganciclovir therapy.
- The patient and family express an accurate understanding of the points taught about acyclovir or ganciclovir.
- The patient returns for blood tests regularly as instructed.

VIDARABINE

Vidarabine was the first important anti-herpesvirus drug clinically available for parenteral use. It is used to treat patients with herpes simplex encephalitis.

PHARMACOKINETICS

Systemic vidarabine is administered by the I.V. route. The ophthalmic preparation is covered in more depth in Chapter 71, Ophthalmic Agents.

Absorption, distribution, metabolism, excretion

Vidarabine and its active metabolite ara-Hx (arabinosyl-hypoxanthine) are distributed widely in body fluids and tissues. Drug and metabolite readily cross the blood-brain barrier and achieve adequate CSF concentration levels. Vidarabine crosses the placenta. Its presence in breast milk is unverified. Vidarabine is 20% to 30% protein bound, whereas ara-Hx is up to 3% bound to plasma proteins.

Other than its change to ara-Hx, vidarabine does not undergo significant metabolism. The unchanged drug and ara-Hx are excreted primarily by the kidneys.

Onset, peak, duration

In adults with normal renal function, the half-life for vidarabine is 1.5 hours; for ara-Hx, 3.3 hours. Information is unavailable on the specific onset of action, peak concentration levels, and duration of action of vidarabine.

PHARMACODYNAMICS

Initially, vidarabine was produced as an antileukemic agent but was found to have antiviral activity.

The exact mechanism of action of vidarabine is unknown. It may be changed to an organic phosphate by cellular enzymes to its active form, vidarabine triphosphate, which blocks viral replication. Vidarabine and its metabolites appear to halt viral DNA synthesis by inhibiting viral DNA polymerase.

PHARMACOTHERAPEUTICS

Vidarabine is active against HSV-1, HSV-2, and varicella-zoster virus.

Intravenous vidarabine is indicated primarily to treat herpes simplex encephalitis and herpes zoster (shingles) caused by reactivated varicella-zoster infections in immunocompromised adults and children. Although vidarabine decreases mortality from herpes simplex encephalitis, it does not decrease the neurologic aftereffects of the disease. Vidarabine also is used to treat varicella (chicken pox) in immunocompromised patients. Sometimes, the drug is used to treat disseminated herpesvirus infections in neonates. The major drawback to I.V. vidarabine therapy is its poor solubility, which necessitates diluting it in large volumes of I.V. fluids. This may cause heart failure and hyponatremia.

vidarabine monohydrate (Vira-A). Available only as a slow I.V. infusion, vidarabine is used to treat HSV-1, HSV-2, and varicella-zoster viral infections. Dosages must be reduced in patients with renal impairment (with a creatinine clearance below 10 ml/minute). Specific guidelines have not been established, but a 25% reduction currently is recommended. Because vidarabine is removed by hemodialysis, a supplementary dose may be necessary after dialysis.

Usual adult dosage: for herpes simplex encephalitis, 15 mg/kg of body weight I.V. daily, infused over 12 to 24 hours for 10 days; for varicella-zoster infections, 10 mg/kg of body weight I.V. daily, infused over 12 to 24 hours for 5 days; for varicella-zoster infections in immunocompromised patients, 10 mg/kg of body weight I.V. daily, infused over 12 to 24 hours for 5 days or longer.

Drug interactions

Allopurinol interferes with the metabolism of vidarabine, resulting in tremor, anemia, nausea, pain, and pruritus.

ADVERSE DRUG REACTIONS

The primary adverse reactions of vidarabine involve the GI tract and CNS and usually are related to a high serum concentration of the drug.

Dose-related adverse GI reactions include nausea, vomiting, diarrhea, anorexia, and weight loss. These reactions usually are mild, occurring after 2 to 3 days of therapy and subsiding within 1 to 4 days while therapy continues. CNS problems include weakness, tremor, ataxia, hallucinations, malaise, and confusion. These subside once therapy is discontinued. GI and CNS reactions are more prevalent in patients receiving a vidarabine dose greater than 10 mg/kg/day and in patients with decreased renal function. Less common adverse reactions include local responses, such as pain and thrombophlebitis; transient elevations in liver function test results; and depressed leukocytes, platelets, and hemoglobin. Hyponatremia and the syndrome of inappropriate antidiuretic hormone (SIADH) occur rarely.

Hypersensitivity reactions, including rash and pruritus, may occur during vidarabine therapy.

NURSING PROCESS APPLICATION

The following information assists the nurse in caring for a patient who is receiving vidarabine.

Assessment

• Review the patient's history for a preexisting condition that contraindicates the use of vidarabine, such as lactation or known hypersensitivity to the drug.

• Review the patient's history for a preexisting condition that requires cautious use of vidarabine, such as pregnancy, CNS infection, or hepatic or renal impairment.

• Assess the patient for adverse reactions to vidarabine, such as GI distress, CNS dysfunction, or hypersensitivity reactions.

• Review the patient's medication history to identify the use of drugs that may interact with vidarabine, such as allopurinol.

• Assess the effectiveness of vidarabine periodically.

• Assess the patient for signs and symptoms of fluid overload during vidarabine therapy.

• Evaluate the patient's and family's knowledge about vidarabine.

Nursing diagnoses

The following examples represent appropriate nursing diagnoses for a patient receiving vidarabine.

• Potential for injury related to a preexisting condition that contraindicates the use of vidarabine

• Potential for injury related to a preexisting condition that requires cautious use of vidarabine

• Potential for injury related to adverse drug reactions

• Fluid volume excess related to vidarabine-induced fluid retention

• Knowledge deficit related to vidarabine

Planning and implementation

• Do not administer vidarabine to a patient with a condition that contraindicates its use.

• Administer vidarabine cautiously to a patient at risk because of a preexisting condition.

• Monitor the patient periodically for adverse reactions during vidarabine therapy.

• Inspect the patient's skin regularly for a rash and ask the patient about pruritus, which may indicate a hypersensitivity reaction. If a hypersensitivity reaction is suspected, withhold the drug and notify the physician.

• Monitor the patient's renal function, along with CBC, electrolyte levels, and hepatic function.

• Monitor hydration if the patient experiences nausea, vomiting, diarrhea, or anorexia. Obtain a prescription for an antiemetic or antidiarrheal agent as needed.

• Take safety measures if the patient experiences ataxia, hallucinations, or confusion. For example, place the bed in the low position, keep the bed rails raised, and supervise the patient's activities.

• Assist the patient with activities if weakness or malaise occurs.

• *Make sure the solution is clear before infusion, and use an in-line 0.45-micron (or smaller) filter for the infusion.*

• *Do not exceed the maximum of 450 mg of vidarabine in a liter of I.V. solution.*

• *Inspect the I.V. infusion site regularly for signs of thrombophlebitis, such as redness, swelling, and pain on touch. Change the I.V. infusion site regularly.*
• Expect to adjust the vidarabine dosage as prescribed in a patient with decreased renal function.
• Notify the physician if adverse reactions develop with vidarabine therapy.
• *Monitor the patient for signs of fluid volume excess, especially if patient has a cardiac disorder, because vidarabine must be diluted in large volumes of fluid for I.V. administration and can cause fluid overload.*
• *Weigh the patient daily and report a sudden weight gain of 2 lb or more in a 24-hour period.*
• Monitor the patient's fluid intake and output, noting if intake is significantly greater than output (a difference of 500 ml or more). Also monitor vital signs for abnormalities that suggest fluid retention or heart failure, such as elevated blood pressure, heart rate, or respiratory rate.
• *Auscultate the patient's lungs to detect crackles, and observe the patient for jugular vein distention or swollen ankles – all signs of fluid retention.*
• Notify the physician if fluid retention occurs.

Patient teaching
• Teach the patient and family the name, dose, frequency, action, and adverse effects of the prescribed vidarabine.
• Instruct the patient to report pruritus or pain at the I.V. infusion site.
• Advise the patient to stagger activities and to take frequent rest periods if weakness or malaise occurs.
• Encourage the patient and family to ask questions about vidarabine therapy and to report adverse reactions.

Evaluation
The following examples represent appropriate evaluation statements for a patient receiving vidarabine.
• The patient has no conditions that contraindicate vidarabine therapy.
• The patient exhibits no signs of complications in the preexisting condition linked to vidarabine.
• The patient exhibits no adverse reactions to vidarabine.
• The patient maintains normal hydration throughout vidarabine therapy.
• The patient and family express an accurate understanding of the points taught about vidarabine.
• The patient agrees to notify the nurse if adverse reactions occur.

AMANTADINE

Amantadine was the first oral antiviral drug available for clinical use. It is used to prevent or treat influenza A infections.

PHARMACOKINETICS

After oral administration, amantadine is absorbed well in the GI tract. Distribution is limited to saliva, CSF, nasal secretions, breast milk, and lung tissue. Amantadine is not metabolized and is eliminated primarily in the urine.

Amantadine reaches a peak concentration level in 1 to 4 hours after oral administration. Its half-life in adults with normal renal function averages 24 hours, and is prolonged in patients with renal impairment. Unlike vidarabine, amantadine is removed only minimally by hemodialysis.

PHARMACODYNAMICS

Although the exact mechanism of action of amantadine is unknown, it appears to inhibit an early stage of viral replication, such as prevention of virus penetration into the host cell or inhibition of the uncoating of the virus particle.

PHARMACOTHERAPEUTICS

Amantadine has no activity against influenza B virus, but is active against most strains of influenza A. Its effectiveness depends on the concentration of the virus and the drug and varies with the viral strain.

Used to prevent and treat respiratory tract infections caused by influenza A virus strains, amantadine is a fairly effective prophylactic during influenza A epidemics. It is particularly useful because it can be administered to patients undergoing immunization and can protect them during the 2 weeks needed for immunity to develop. It also is useful for patients who cannot take the influenza vaccine because of hypersensitivity. When used to treat patients with influenza A infections, amantadine reduces the severity and duration of fever and other symptoms.

Amantadine also is used to treat parkinsonism and drug-induced extrapyramidal reactions. These uses are described in Chapter 19, Antiparkinsonian Agents.

amantadine hydrochloride (Symmetrel). Amantadine is an oral drug effective in preventing and treating influenza A infections. Dosage must be reduced in patients with renal impairment. (For details, see *Dosage adjustments in patients with renal dysfunction.*) Dosage adjustments also are necessary for patients with a history of seizure disorders. For

Dosage adjustments in patients with renal dysfunction

Adults with impaired renal function require an adjustment in the dosage of amantadine, as summarized in this table.

CREATININE CLEARANCE (ml/min/1.73 m²)	DOSAGE INTERVALS
80 or greater	100 mg b.i.d.
60 to 79	200 mg once daily; 100 mg on alternate days
40 to 59	100 mg once daily
30 to 39	200 mg twice weekly
20 to 29	100 mg three times a week
10 to 19	200 mg; 100 mg alternating every 7 days

these patients, the usual adult dosage of 200 mg/day must be reduced by half.

Amantadine is contraindicated in a patient with known hypersensitivity to the drug. It should be used with caution in a patient with liver disease, a story of recurrent eczematoid rash, psychosis, or severe psychoneurosis not controlled by chemotherapeutic agents.

Usual adult dosage: 200 mg P.O. daily in a single dose or divided and given b.i.d.; to treat infection, the dosage should be started 24 to 48 hours after the onset of symptoms and continue for at least 2 days after symptoms resolve; to prevent infection, therapy should begin immediately after an outbreak and continue until the risk of infection is eliminated.

Drug interactions

Significant reactions result when amantadine is given with large doses of anticholinergic drugs. Because amantadine enhances adverse reactions to anticholinergic agents, the patient must be observed closely for excessive anticholinergic effects if the drugs are administered concomitantly.

ADVERSE DRUG REACTIONS

Amantadine usually is tolerated well, with mild adverse reactions occurring in approximately 5% of patients. The most common reactions are nausea, anorexia, nervousness, fatigue, depression, irritability, insomnia, psychosis, anxiety, confusion, forgetfulness, and hallucinations. Other CNS reactions include headache, dizziness, light-headed-ness, slurred speech, ataxia, tremor, and a sense of drunkenness. Patients with seizure disorders are more prone to seizures while using amantadine.

Other, less common, adverse reactions include congestive heart failure (CHF), orthostatic hypotension, edema, leukopenia, dermatitis, photosensitivity, dry mouth, rash, urine retention, constipation, and vomiting. Neutropenia, visual disturbances, and oculogyric events are rare. Amantadine also may cause hypersensitivity reactions.

NURSING PROCESS APPLICATION

The following information assists the nurse in caring for a patient who is receiving amantadine.

Assessment

• Review the patient's history for a preexisting condition that contraindicates the use of amantadine, such as known hypersensitivity to the drug.
• Review the patient's history for a preexisting condition that requires cautious use of amantadine, such as liver disease, history of recurrent eczematoid rash, psychosis, or severe psychoneurosis not controlled by chemotherapeutic agents.
• Assess the patient for adverse reactions to amantadine, such as GI distress, CNS disturbances, orthostatic hypotension, and CHF.
• Review the patient's medication history to identify the use of drugs that may interact with amantadine, such as anticholinergic agents.
• Assess the effectiveness of amantadine periodically.
• Assess the patient for excessive anticholinergic effects, such as dry mouth, blurred vision, constipation, and urine retention, during concomitant use of amantadine and an anticholinergic agent.
• Evaluate the patient's and family's knowledge about amantadine.

Nursing diagnoses

The following examples represent appropriate nursing diagnoses for a patient receiving amantadine.
• Potential for injury related to a preexisting condition that contraindicates the use of amantadine
• Potential for injury related to a preexisting condition that requires cautious use of amantadine
• Potential for injury related to adverse drug reactions
• Altered health maintenance related to drug interactions
• Knowledge deficit related to amantadine

Planning and implementation

• Do not administer amantadine to a patient with a condition that contraindicates its use.
• Administer amantadine cautiously to a patient at risk because of a preexisting condition.

• Monitor the patient periodically for adverse reactions during amantadine therapy.

• Inspect the patient's skin routinely for a rash.

• Monitor hydration if the patient experiences nausea, vomiting, or anorexia. Obtain a prescription for an antiemetic agent if needed.

• Stagger the patient's activities and provide frequent rest periods if fatigue occurs.

• Take safety measures if adverse CNS effects occur. For example, place the bed in the low position, keep the bed rails raised, and supervise ambulation.

• *Administer amantadine several hours before bedtime if insomnia occurs.*

• Administer a mild analgesic as prescribed if the patient experiences a headache.

• Take seizure precautions when administering amantadine to a patient with a history of seizures.

• *Monitor the patient with a history of CHF closely for exacerbation or recurrence of CHF, as evidenced by such signs as shortness of breath, tachycardia, jugular vein distention, or crackles in the lungs.*

• Provide symptomatic relief for such adverse reactions as dry mouth and constipation.

• Ask the patient about urine retention. If the patient complains of bladder fullness after voiding or inability to void, palpate and percuss the bladder. Notify the physician if bladder fullness is present and be prepared to catheterize the patient.

• *Expect to reduce the dosage as prescribed in a patient with renal impairment or a history of seizures.*

• Notify the physician if adverse reactions occur.

• *Administer amantadine cautiously to a patient receiving concomitant therapy with an anticholinergic agent.*

• Monitor the patient closely for excessive anticholinergic effects.

Patient teaching

• Teach the patient and family the name, dose, frequency, action, and adverse effects of amantadine.

• *Instruct the patient to take the drug after meals for best absorption.*

• Advise an elderly patient to take the drug in two daily doses rather than a single dose to avoid adverse neurologic reactions.

• *Instruct the patient with insomnia to take the drug several hours before bedtime.*

• Instruct the patient to stand or change positions slowly if orthostatic hypotension occurs.

• Instruct the patient to report adverse reactions, especially signs of CNS disturbance (dizziness, depression, anxiety, and nausea) and renal impairment (change in urine elimination pattern or characteristics).

• *Caution the patient not to perform activities that require alertness or physical coordination if adverse CNS reactions occur.*

• Teach the patient to use infection-control measures, such as staying away from crowds or people with infections, if leukopenia occurs.

• *Advise the patient to be alert for excessive anticholinergic effects during concomitant therapy with amantadine and an anticholinergic agent.*

• Teach the patient how to handle such adverse reactions as dry mouth or constipation.

• Instruct the patient to limit salt and fluid intake if fluid retention occurs.

• Instruct the patient to notify the physician if adverse reactions or drug interactions occur.

Evaluation

The following examples represent appropriate evaluation statements for a patient receiving amantadine.

• The patient has no conditions that contraindicate amantadine therapy.

• The patient exhibits no signs of complications in the preexisting condition linked to amantadine.

• The patient exhibits no adverse reactions to amantadine.

• The patient exhibits minimal anticholinergic effects when receiving amantadine and an anticholinergic agent concomitantly.

• The patient and family express an accurate understanding of the points taught about amantadine.

• The patient takes amantadine after meals as prescribed.

RIBAVIRIN

Ribavirin inhibits a number of ribonucleic acid (RNA) and DNA viruses, but currently is available only to treat respiratory syncytial virus (RSV) infections in children. It is administered by aerosol inhalation only.

PHARMACOKINETICS

Ribavirin is administered via nasal or oral inhalation and is absorbed well by these routes. After nasal or oral inhalation, the drug has limited, specific distribution, with the highest concentration level found in the pulmonary tract and erythrocytes. Ribavirin is metabolized in the liver and by erythrocytes. The main route of excretion is via the kidneys, with some excretion in the feces.

Onset of action and peak concentration of ribavirin are virtually simultaneous, occurring immediately after inhalation. The drug's half-life is 1.5 to 2.5 hours; the plasma half-life is approximately 9 hours.

PHARMACODYNAMICS

The mechanism of action of ribavirin is not known completely, but the drug probably becomes effective after it is converted to an active metabolite.

Mechanism of action
Ribavirin is transported rapidly into virus-infected cells, where it is metabolized by cellular enzymes to monophosphate, diphosphate, and triphosphate derivatives. All three metabolites inhibit viral DNA and RNA synthesis, subsequently halting viral replication. Ribavirin does not seem to have the same affinity for host DNA and RNA synthesis.

PHARMACOTHERAPEUTICS

Ribavirin therapy is indicated in infants and young children who have severe lower respiratory tract infections caused by RSV. The drug also has been used experimentally to treat respiratory infections with influenza viruses A and B in elderly patients. However, no clinical guidelines are available for this application.

ribavirin (Virazole). Ribavirin sterile powder is reconstituted with sterile water and administered by aerosol inhalation using a Viratek Small Particle Aerosol Generator (SPAG-2). It is contraindicated in a pregnant or lactating patient or in one with assisted ventilation. It should be administered with caution to an infant with decreased respiratory function or an adult with chronic obstructive pulmonary disease or asthma.
Usual pediatric dosage: 20 mg/ml solution administered via aerosol inhalant over 12 to 18 hours/day for 3 to 7 days; dosage depends on patient's lung pathology and ventilation.

Drug interactions
Ribavirin has been shown to antagonize the antiviral activity of zidovudine in vitro. The clinical importance of this interaction is unknown, but the patient should be monitored closely if both drugs are administered concomitantly. In addition, concomitant use of these drugs may cause hematologic toxicity. Therefore, blood counts should be monitored routinely during concomitant administration.

Concomitant use of ribavirin with a cardiac glycoside, such as digitoxin or digoxin, can cause cardiac glycoside intoxication, producing such effects as GI distress, CNS abnormalities, and cardiac arrhythmias.

ADVERSE DRUG REACTIONS

Adverse reactions to ribavirin therapy have been infrequent and, in many cases, uncertain. Reactions include worsening of respiratory function, ventilator dependence, pneumothorax, apnea, cardiac arrest, and hypotension. Reticulosis also has been reported. Other adverse reactions include rash, conjunctivitis, and erythema of the eyelids.

NURSING PROCESS APPLICATION

The following information assists the nurse in caring for a patient who is receiving ribavirin.

Assessment
• Review the patient's history for a preexisting condition that contraindicates the use of ribavirin, such as pregnancy, lactation, or assisted ventilation.
• Review the patient's history for a preexisting condition that requires cautious use of ribavirin, such as decreased respiratory function in an infant or chronic obstructive pulmonary disease or asthma in an adult.
• Assess the patient for adverse reactions to ribavirin, such as respiratory and cardiac dysfunction or rash.
• Review the patient's medication history to identify the use of drugs that may interact with ribavirin, such as zidovudine.
• Assess the effectiveness of ribavirin periodically.
• Assess the patient's respiratory status throughout ribavirin therapy.
• Evaluate the family's knowledge about ribavirin.

Nursing diagnoses
The following examples represent appropriate nursing diagnoses for a patient receiving ribavirin.
• Potential for injury related to a preexisting condition that contraindicates the use of ribavirin
• Potential for injury related to adverse drug reactions
• Impaired gas exchange related to worsening of respiratory function caused by ribavirin
• Knowledge deficit related to ribavirin

Planning and implementation
• Do not administer ribavirin to a patient with a condition that contraindicates its use.
• Do not administer ribavirin to a patient who requires mechanical ventilation; the drug can precipitate in the ventilatory apparatus, jeopardizing adequate ventilation.
• Monitor the patient closely for adverse reactions during ribavirin therapy.
• *Monitor the patient's cardiac status throughout ribavirin therapy. Report hypotension or cardiac dysfunction. Keep*

standard emergency equipment nearby and be prepared to begin cardiopulmonary resuscitation if cardiac arrest occurs.

• Observe the patient receiving concomitant therapy with a cardiac glycoside for signs of cardiac glycoside intoxication, such as GI distress, CNS abnormalities, or cardiac arrhythmias. If intoxication occurs, draw a serum blood sample for evaluation of the cardiac glycoside level, and expect to withhold or decrease the cardiac glycoside dose as prescribed.

• Monitor the CBC for evidence of reticulosis, especially if the patient has been receiving ribavirin therapy for longer than 1 week.

• Inspect the patient's skin for rash, the eyes for signs of conjunctivitis (redness, swelling, and drainage), and the eyelids for erythema.

• Ensure that ribavirin solution is prepared by diluting 6 grams of ribavirin powder in 50 to 100 ml of sterile water. The solution should be transferred to an Erlenmeyer flask (which serves as the reservoir for the SPAG-2) and diluted further to a volume of 300 ml.

• *Administer ribavirin with the SPAG-2. Do not use any other aerosol-generating device.*

• Use sterile USP water for injection, not bacteriostatic water, for reconstituting ribavirin powder that does not contain any antimicrobial agent.

• Discard solutions placed in the SPAG-2 unit at least every 24 hours before adding newly reconstituted solutions

• Store reconstituted solutions at room temperature for 24 hours.

• *Perform a complete respiratory assessment every hour throughout ribavirin therapy. Monitor arterial blood gases and be prepared to support the patient's ventilation if the respiratory condition worsens. Notify the physician immiedately of any change in the patient's respiratory status.*

Patient teaching

• Teach the family the name, dose, frequency, action, and adverse effects of ribavirin.

• Encourage the family to ask questions throughout ribavirin therapy.

Evaluation

The following examples represent appropriate evaluation statements for a patient receiving ribavirin.

• The patient has no conditions that contraindicate ribavirin therapy.

• The patient maintains an adequate gas exchange throughout ribavirin therapy.

• The family expresses an accurate understanding of the points taught about ribavirin.

• The family members ask appropriate questions about ribavirin therapy.

ZIDOVUDINE

Zidovudine is the first drug to receive FDA approval for treating AIDS or AIDS-related complex (ARC). The drug, also known as azidothymidine or AZT, was studied initially as an antineoplastic agent.

PHARMACOKINETICS

After oral administration, zidovudine is 63% to 95% absorbed from the GI tract. Zidovudine appears to be distributed widely, and 34% to 38% of the drug is protein bound. It undergoes rapid hepatic metabolism to inactive metabolites. The drug is renally excreted. Zidovudine reaches a peak concentration level in 0.5 to 1.5 hours and has a duration of action of 4 hours. Its half-life is approximately 1 hour.

PHARMACODYNAMICS

The mechanism of action of zidovudine is much like that of acyclovir. The drug is converted by cellular enzymes to an active form, zidovudine triphosphate. The metabolite inhibits RNA-dependent DNA polymerase produced by HIV, thus preventing viral DNA from replicating. The sensitivity of HIV to inhibition by zidovudine appears to depend on the duration of cell infection.

PHARMACOTHERAPEUTICS

Zidovudine has been used for patients with AIDS and ARC who have a history of *Pneumocystis carinii* pneumonia or a T-lymphocyte count lower than 200 mm^3. Clinical trials have demonstrated reduced mortality with the use of zidovudine. The drug also has reduced the incidence and severity of opportunistic infections.

zidovudine (Retrovir). Zidovudine is used to treat AIDS and ARC and has been successful in reducing opportunistic infections in these patients.
Usual adult dosage: 200 mg P.O. every 4 hours around the clock. Doses are adjusted in relation to the anemia and granulocytopenia that usually occur.

Drug interactions

Many drug interactions occur with zidovudine. (For specific information, see *Drug interactions: Zidovudine.*)

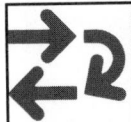

DRUG INTERACTIONS

Zidovudine

Zidovudine may interact with various drugs, producing toxic and other adverse effects.

DRUG	INTERACTING DRUGS	POSSIBLE EFFECTS	NURSING IMPLICATIONS
zidovudine	dapsone, pentamidine, flucytosine, vincristine, vinblastine, doxorubicin, interferon, ganciclovir	Increase nephrotoxic and cytotoxic effects	• Avoid concurrent administration if possible; if not, monitor the patient's blood count and renal function closely.
	probenecid, aspirin, acetaminophen, indomethacin, cimetidine, lorazepam,	Inhibit zidovudine metabolism; increase the risk of toxicity for either drug	• Avoid concurrent use if possible; if not, use with extreme caution.
	acyclovir	Causes profound drowsiness and lethargy	• Monitor the patient closely during concomitant therapy.

ADVERSE DRUG REACTIONS

The most common adverse reactions to zidovudine are hematologic. Significant anemia occurs 4 to 6 weeks after therapy has begun, and granulocytopenia appears within 6 to 8 weeks. When reductions in RBC and WBC counts occur, the dose usually is adjusted or stopped. Reducing or stopping therapy produces an immediate reversal of the abnormal blood cell counts.

Headache has been reported in up to 50% of patients receiving zidovudine. Other CNS reactions include dizziness, agitation, restlessness, and insomnia. Nausea, abdominal pain, diarrhea, dyspepsia, anorexia, and vomiting are the most common GI reactions. Other commonly reported adverse reactions include myalgia, diaphoresis, dyspnea, fever, rash, and taste perversion.

NURSING PROCESS APPLICATION

The following information assists the nurse in caring for a patient who is receiving zidovudine.

Assessment
• Review the patient's history for a preexisting condition that contraindicates the use of zidovudine, such as lactation or known hypersensitivity to the drug or any of the components of the formulation.
• Review the patient's history for a preexisting condition that requires cautious use of zidovudine, such as pregnancy or impaired hepatic or renal function.
• Assess the patient for adverse reactions to zidovudine, such as hematologic abnormalities, GI distress, or CNS dysfunction.

• Review the patient's medication history to identify the use of drugs that may interact with zidovudine, such as dapsone, ganciclovir, cimetidine, lorazepam, or acyclovir.
• Assess the effectiveness of zidovudine periodically.
• Evaluate the patient's and family's knowledge about zidovudine.

Nursing diagnoses
The following examples represent appropriate nursing diagnoses for a patient receiving zidovudine.
• Potential for injury related to a preexisting condition that contraindicates the use of zidovudine
• Potential for injury related to a preexisting condition that requires cautious use of zidovudine
• Potential for injury related to adverse drug reactions
• Knowledge deficit related to zidovudine

Planning and implementation
• Do not administer zidovudine to a patient with a condition that contraindicates its use.
• Administer zidovudine cautiously to a patient at risk because of a preexisting condition.
• Monitor the patient periodically for adverse reactions during zidovudine therapy.
• *Monitor the patient's RBC and WBC counts, as prescribed. Expect to decrease the dose or discontinue the drug as prescribed if reductions in blood counts occur. Take bleeding precautions, stagger the patient's activities, and provide frequent rest periods if anemia occurs.*

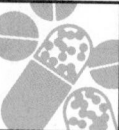

SELECTED MAJOR DRUGS

Antiviral agents

This chart summarizes the major antiviral agents currently in clinical use.

DRUG	MAJOR INDICATIONS	USUAL ADULT DOSAGES	CONTRAINDICATIONS AND PRECAUTIONS
acyclovir	Primary genital herpes simplex virus (HSV) infection	200 mg P.O. every 4 hours while awake, five times a day for 10 days; 5 mg/kg I.V. every 8 hours for 5 to 7 days in patients with creatinine clearance greater than 50 ml/minute	• Know that acyclovir is contraindicated in a patient with known hypersensitivity to the drug or intolerance to any of the components of the formulation. • Administer with caution to a pregnant or lactating patient or one with renal impairment.
	Recurrent genital HSV infection	200 mg P.O. five times a day for 5 days	
	Varicella-zoster infection	5 to 10 mg/kg I.V. every 8 hours for 5 days	
	Herpes simplex encephalitis	10 mg/kg I.V. every 8 hours for at least 10 days	
ganciclovir	Cytomegalovirus retinitis in immunocompromised patients, including those with acquired immunodeficiency syndrome (AIDS)	5 mg/kg I.V. over 1 hour every 12 hours for 14 to 21 days, followed by a maintenance dosage of 5 mg/kg I.V. over 1 hour once daily or 6 mg/kg I.V. once daily for 5 out of 7 days a week	• Know that ganciclovir is contraindicated in a patient with known hypersensitivity to the drug or intolerance to any of the components of the formulation. • Administer with caution to a pregnant or lactating patient or one with renal impairment.
vidarabine	Herpes simplex encephalitis	15 mg/kg I.V. daily, infused over 12 to 24 hours for 10 days	• Know that vidarabine is contraindicated in a lactating patient or one with known hypersensitivity to the drug. • Administer with caution to a pregnant patient or one with a central nervous system infection or hepatic or renal impairment.
	Varicella-zoster infection	10 mg/kg I.V. daily, infused over 12 to 24 hours for 5 days	
	Varicella-zoster infection in immunocompromised patients	10 mg/kg I.V. daily, infused over 12 to 24 hrs for 5 days or longer	
zidovudine	AIDS or ARC patients with a history of *Pneumocystis carinii* pneumonia or a T-lymphocyte count below 200 mm³	200 mg P.O. every 4 hours around the clock	• Know that zidovudine is contraindicated in a lactating patient or one with known hypersensitivity to the drug or any of the components of the formulation. • Administer with caution to a pregnant patient or one with impaired hepatic or renal function.

• Administer a mild analgesic, as prescribed, if the patient experiences a headache.
• Take safety precautions if the patient experiences adverse CNS reactions, such as dizziness.
• Administer a mild sedative for insomnia as prescribed.
• Monitor hydration if the patient experiences nausea, vomiting, anorexia, or diarrhea. Obtain a prescription for an antiemetic or antidiarrheal agent if needed.
• Monitor the patient's temperature for fever.
• Inspect the patient's skin regularly for a rash.
• Notify the physician if adverse reactions occur.

Patient teaching
• Teach patient and family the name, dose, frequency, action, and adverse effects of zidovudine.
• *Instruct the patient to take the drug every 4 hours around the clock, even though it means interrupting sleep.*
• *Inform the patient that zidovudine does not reduce the risk of transmitting the virus to others through sexual contact or blood contamination.*
• *Caution the patient to avoid over-the-counter medications without first checking with the physician, pharmacist, or nurse.*

• Stress the importance of returning regularly for blood tests as instructed.

• Caution the patient not to perform activities that require alertness if such adverse CNS reactions as dizziness occur.

• Instruct the patient to notify the physician if adverse reactions occur.

Evaluation

The following examples represent appropriate evaluation statements for a patient receiving zidovudine.

• The patient has no conditions that contraindicate zidovudine therapy.

• The patient exhibits no signs of complications in the preexisting condition linked to zidovudine.

• The patient exhibits no adverse reactions to zidovudine.

• The patient and family express an accurate understanding of the points taught about zidovudine.

• The patient returns regularly for blood tests as instructed.

CHAPTER SUMMARY

Chapter 61 presented the six antiviral agents available today: acyclovir, ganciclovir, vidarabine, amantadine, ribavirin, and zidovudine. Here are the chapter highlights.

• Few antiviral agents are available because of the difficulty of developing drugs that selectively kill viruses and do not harm their host cells.

• Acyclovir is used to treat herpesvirus infections. It is available in oral, topical, and parenteral forms.

• Ganciclovir is the only antiviral agent available for the treatment of CMV infection; it is available only in a parenteral dosage form.

• Acyclovir and ganciclovir are relatively safe, although they have the potential to be nephrotoxic. This danger can be reduced by infusing the drug slowly (over 60 minutes) and keeping the patient well hydrated.

• Vidarabine is used to treat herpes simplex encephalitis and herpes zoster caused by reactivated varicella-zoster infections in immunocompromised adults and children. A major problem with parenteral vidarabine is its poor solubility, requiring large amounts of fluid for dissolution and administration. The patient may experience fluid overload or electrolyte abnormalities.

• Amantadine is an oral antiviral drug used to prevent or treat influenza A viral infections. The drug must be used with caution in a patient with a seizure disorder, and it can cause other CNS disturbances.

• Ribavirin, the only chemotherapeutic agent available to treat RSV in children, is available in aerosol form only.

• Zidovudine is the first drug to receive FDA approval for treating AIDS or ARC.

• The nurse must monitor the patient closely for adverse reactions to the prescribed antiviral agent because reactions can be significant and potentially serious.

STUDY QUESTIONS

See Appendix 1 for answers.

1. Ted Califano, age 26, tells his physician that he has swollen, tender blisters on his genitals. His history, physical examination, and preliminary laboratory tests suggest a herpes simplex virus type 2 (HSV-2) infection. The physician prescribes the antiviral agent acyclovir (Zovirax). What is the mechanism of action of acyclovir?
(a) It interferes with viral RNA and DNA synthesis.
(b) It converts to an active metabolite that disrupts viral replication.
(c) It inhibits the uncoating of the virus, an early stage of replication.
(d) It disrupts the integrity of the viral cell membrane.

2. Before administering acyclovir to Mr. Califano, the nurse obtains a medical history. A dosage adjustment would be required for which disorder?
(a) cardiovascular disease
(b) hepatic disease
(c) renal disease
(d) pulmonary disease

3. To prevent drug crystals from precipitating in the renal tubules, how should I.V. acyclovir be administered?
(a) as an I.V. bolus
(b) slowly (over 60 minutes)
(c) as a continuous infusion over 24 hours
(d) as an intermittent infusion over 15 minutes

4. Nina Chavez, age 50, recently has been diagnosed with herpes simplex encephalitis. Her physician prescribes I.V. vidarabine. What is the major drawback to I.V. vidarabine therapy?
(a) high toxicity
(b) poor solubility
(c) short duration of action
(d) long half-life

5. Which of the following nursing measures would be appropriate when caring for Ms. Chavez?
(a) Monitor the patient's fluid balance closely.
(b) Encourage the patient to drink plenty of fluids.
(c) Monitor for signs and symptoms of bleeding.
(d) Assess for temperature changes.

6. Mr. Donner, age 60, teaches Sunday school class. Because many of his students recently have been sick with influenza A infections, he asks his physician if he can do anything to prevent contracting the infection himself. Which antiviral agent is the physician most likely to prescribe?
(a) amantadine
(b) ribavirin
(c) zidovudine
(d) vidarabine

7. Julie Dean brings her daughter Amy, age 2, to the pediatrician because she is coughing, wheezing, and complaining of a sore throat and tiredness. Clinical findings and laboratory tests show that Amy has a RSV infection. To treat this severe infection, the physician prescribes ribavirin. This drug is administered by which route?
(a) oral
(b) I.M.
(c) I.V.
(d) inhalation

8. Bob Cummings, age 39, is hospitalized with AIDS. To reduce opportunistic infections, his physician prescribes zidovudine 200 mg P.O. every 4 hours. Which instruction should the nurse give Mr. Cummings about zidovudine therapy?
(a) Take zidovudine with meals.
(b) Take the medication on an empty stomach.
(c) Take the drug every 4 hours around the clock.
(d) Take over-the-counter agents to treat minor adverse reactions.

SELECTED REFERENCES

AHFS drug information 90. (1990). Bethesda, MD: American Society of Hospital Pharmacists.

Galasso, G., Whitley, R., and Merigan, T. (Eds.). (1990). *Antiviral agents and viral diseases of man* (3rd ed.). New York: Raven Press.

Goodman and Gilman's the pharmacological basis of therapeutics (8th ed.; 1990) Elmsford, NY: Pergamon Press.

Hansten, P., and Horn, J. (1989). *Drug interactions* (6th ed.). Philadelphia: Lea & Febiger.

Hermans, P., and Cockerill, F. (1987). Antiviral agents. *Mayo Clinic Proceedings,* 62(12), 1108-1115.

Nahata, M. (1987). Clinical use of antiviral drugs. *Drug Intelligence and Clinical Pharmacy,* 5(4), 399.

North American Nursing Diagnosis Association (1990). *Taxonomy I - Revised, with official diagnostic categories.* St. Louis, NANDA.

Straus, S., et al. (1988). Acyclovir suppression of frequently recurring genital herpes. *Journal of the American Medical Association,* 260(15), 2227-2230.

USPDI. (1991). *Drug information for the health care professional* (vol. I; 11th ed.). Rockville, MD: United States Pharmacopeial Convention.

Weintraub, M., and Standish, R. (1987). Ganciclovir: An antiviral agent for AIDS and other immunocompromised patients. *Hospital Formulary,* 22(12), 1011-1016.

Wood, M., and Geddes, A. (1987). Antiviral therapy. *Lancet,* 2(8569), 1189-1193.

ANTIMYCOTIC (ANTIFUNGAL) AGENTS

OBJECTIVES

After reading and studying this chapter, the student should be able to:

1. Describe the types of fungal infections that can affect humans.

2. Describe the pharmacokinetics of systemic and topical antimycotic agents.

3. Explain the actions of various antimycotic agents on fungal cells.

4. Describe the antimycotic agents used to treat systemic fungal infections: amphotericin B, miconazole, ketoconazole, fluconazole, and flucytosine.

5. Describe the antimycotic agents used to treat topical fungal infections: nystatin, clotrimazole, griseofulvin, ketoconazole, and miconazole.

6. Explain how certain antimycotic agents can be used together for synergistic effects.

7. Identify significant interactions between the antimycotic agents and other drugs.

8. Identify the adverse reactions caused by these agents, and describe ways to prevent or treat them.

9. Describe how to apply the nursing process when caring for a patient who is receiving an antimycotic agent.

INTRODUCTION

Antimycotic, or antifungal, agents include many drugs that are used to treat fungal infections. In humans, fungal infections can range from the common, such as tinea pedis (athlete's foot), to the rare and exotic, such as sporotrichosis (agranulomatous disease). Two general types of fungal infections exist: topical (superficial) infections, affecting the skin and mucous membranes, and systemic infections, affecting such areas as the lungs, central nervous system (CNS), and blood. Treating either type of infection requires a topical, oral, or parenteral agent chosen according to the site and severity of the infection.

The patient's underlying condition usually determines the type of fungal infection the patient will acquire. For example, a severely immunocompromised patient is predisposed to develop a systemic infection, such as aspergillosis. In contrast, a patient who is receiving antibiotic therapy that eliminates the normal flora, has poor oral hygiene, or wears dentures is predisposed to develop a mucocutaneous infection, such as oral candidiasis (thrush). Thus, managing fungal infections not only calls for antimycotic drug therapy, but also requires modification or elimination of predisposing factors.

Of the two types, topical infections are more common and include candidiasis, tinea versicolor (pityriasis versicolor), and infections by dermatophytes (various skin fungi). Candidiasis affects certain mucosal sites, such as the mouth, gastrointestinal (GI) tract, and vagina. It commonly follows antibiotic therapy that disrupts the natural flora, a physiologic change in the host, or immunosuppressive therapy. Therapy usually involves topical antimycotic agents. Tinea versicolor produces hypopigmented or hyperpigmented skin patches and usually requires topical treatment. Dermatophytes cause many common infections, such as tinea pedis, tinea cruris (jock itch), tinea capitis (scalp ringworm), tinea corporis (body ringworm), and tinea unguium (onychomycosis, or nail infection). Most of these infections respond well to topical therapy; however, infected nail beds require long-term systemic treatment.

Systemic fungal infections can result from pathogenic fungi or from so-called opportunistic fungi—those that are normally nonpathogenic but that become pathogenic under certain circumstances, such as a decreased immune response. Opportunistic systemic fungal infections usually affect immunosuppressed or immunocompromised patients and may include systemic candidiasis and aspergillosis. Pathogenic systemic fungal infections can affect normal or immunocompromised patients and include histoplasmosis and coccidioidomycosis. Pathogenic fungi usually enter the host by the respiratory tract, but opportunistic fungi may invade the host through various other routes, including the

SELECTED NURSING DIAGNOSES

Antimycotic (antifungal) agents

The following nursing diagnoses address representative problems and etiologies that a nurse may encounter when caring for a patient who is receiving an antimycotic agent. Some of these nursing diagnoses contain generalized etiologies, which the nurse must individualize based on the patient's needs. (For some common nursing diagnoses and related interventions for each drug class, see the "Nursing Process Application" sections of this chapter.)

- Altered health maintenance related to ketoconazole-induced hepatotoxicity
- Altered health maintenance related to ineffectiveness of the prescribed antimycotic agent
- Altered nutrition: less than body requirements, related to the adverse GI effects of an antimycotic agent
- Altered protection related to hematologic abnormalities caused by an antimycotic agent
- Altered thought processes related to the adverse CNS effects of the antimycotic agent
- Altered urinary elimination related to amphotericin B-induced nephrotoxicity
- Body image disturbance related to potential for ketoconazole-induced gynecomastia
- Diarrhea related to the adverse GI effects of an antimycotic agent
- Hyperthermia related to fever caused by an antimycotic agent
- Impaired physical mobility related to extreme muscle weakness caused by amphotericin B-induced hypokalemia
- Impaired tissue integrity related to phlebitis caused by I.V. administration of amphotericin B
- Knowledge deficit related to the prescribed antimycotic agent
- Noncompliance related to adverse reactions to the prescribed antimycotic agent
- Pain related to the adverse neuromuscular effects of amphotericin B
- Pain related to headache caused by an antimycotic agent
- Potential fluid volume deficit related to the adverse GI effects of an antimycotic agent
- Potential for infection related to antimycotic-induced leukopenia
- Potential for injury related to a preexisting condition that contraindicates the use of an antimycotic agent
- Potential for injury related to a preexisting condition that requires cautious use of an antimycotic agent
- Potential for injury related to adverse drug reactions
- Potential for injury related to drug interactions
- Potential impaired skin integrity related to the adverse dermatologic effects of a topical antimycotic agent
- Sensory-perceptual alterations (auditory, tactile, visual) related to the adverse CNS effects of an antimycotic agent
- Sexual dysfunction caused by ketoconazole-induced impotence
- Sleep pattern disturbance related to ketoconazole-induced insomnia
- Urinary retention related to the adverse genitourinary effects of intrathecal administration of amphotericin B

GI tract and intravenous (I.V.) lines. Whether pathogenic or opportunistic, a systemic fungal infection almost always requires systemic antimycotic therapy.

Antimycotic agents are categorized in five basic groups: polyene antimycotics, which include amphotericin B and nystatin; the antimetabolite antimycotic agent, flucytosine; the bistriazole derivative, fluconazole; imidazole agents, which include miconazole, ketoconazole, and clotrimazole; and superficial antimycotic agents, which include griseofulvin and various topical drugs.

Because the pharmacotherapeutics and nursing implications of amphotericin B and nystatin are so different, this chapter discusses them separately. It covers the major systemic antimycotic agents and includes information on major topical antimycotic agents.

For a summary of representative drugs, see *Selected major drugs: Antimycotic agents,* page 1093. For a listing of applicable nursing diagnoses that the nurse may formulate when caring for a patient receiving these agents, see *Selected nursing diagnoses: Antimycotic agents.* For detailed information on applying the nursing process, see Chapter 6, The Nursing Process and Drug Therapy.

AMPHOTERICIN B

This drug's potency has made it the most widely used antimycotic agent for severe systemic fungal infections. Unfortunately, it also causes a wide range of adverse reactions, especially when administered parenterally.

PHARMACOKINETICS

After I.V. administration, amphotericin B is distributed throughout the body and excreted by the kidneys. Its metabolic fate has not been demonstrated conclusively.

Absorption, distribution, metabolism, excretion

Because amphotericin B is absorbed poorly from the GI tract, it usually is administered by I.V. infusion to bypass the absorption process. The drug essentially is insoluble in water, so a colloidal suspension must be used. It also may be administered intrathecally.

Information on the distribution of amphotericin B is limited. Low concentration levels of the drug appear in the aqueous humor and urine and in pleural, peritoneal, and synovial fluids; high concentrations occur in the kidneys, spleen, and lungs. It appears to cross the placenta. With I.V. administration, the amphotericin B concentration in the cerebrospinal fluid (CSF) usually is too low to inhibit fungal growth. With intrathecal administration, however, the concentration in CSF is much higher. Amphotericin B is 90% to 95% bound to serum proteins.

Researchers have not yet discovered the metabolic fate or major route of excretion of amphotericin B. Less than 5% of the drug is excreted in the urine.

Onset, peak, duration
After I.V. administration, the onset of action of amphotericin B occurs almost immediately. In a patient with normal renal function, the half-life of the drug usually is 24 hours. As therapy continues, however, the half-life seems to lengthen; it may reach 15 days with long-term administration, possibly because of slow release of amphotericin B from tissue compartments. After therapy is discontinued, amphotericin B appears in the blood for up to 4 weeks and in the urine for 7 to 8 weeks.

PHARMACODYNAMICS

Amphotericin B primarily acts on sterols in fungal cells, binding with them to produce antimycotic effects.

Mechanism of action
The irreversible binding of amphotericin B to sterols in the membranes of amphotericin B-sensitive fungal cells seems to produce pores or channels that increase cell membrane permeability. This permeability allows leakage of intracellular components, which prevents the fungal cell membrane from functioning normally as a barrier. Amphotericin B usually acts as a fungistatic agent but can become fungicidal if it reaches high concentrations in the fungi.

PHARMACOTHERAPEUTICS

Amphotericin B usually is administered to treat severe systemic fungal infections and meningitis caused by fungi sensitive to the drug. Because the drug is highly toxic, its use must be limited to patients who have a definitive diagnosis of life-threatening infections and who are under close medical supervision.

amphotericin B (Fungizone). This potent antimycotic agent usually is considered the drug of choice for severe infections caused by *Candida* species, *Paracoccidioides brasiliensis*, *Blastomyces dermatitidis*, *Coccidioides immitis*, *Cryptococ-* *cus neoformans*, and *Sporothrix schenckii*. It also is effective against *Aspergillus fumigatus*, *Histoplasma capsulatum*, *Microsporum audouini*, *Rhizopus* species, *Torulopsis glabrata*, *Trichophyton* species, and *Rhodotorula* species. It can be used to treat aspergillosis; North American blastomycosis; pulmonary, disseminated, or meningeal coccidioidomycosis; disseminated candidiasis; pulmonary or disseminated cryptococcosis; and pulmonary or disseminated histoplasmosis. Because of the synergistic effects between flucytosine and amphotericin B, these two drugs commonly are combined in therapy for candidal or cryptococcal infections, especially for cryptococcal meningitis.

Amphotericin B therapy usually begins with a test dose that is increased daily until the desired dosage is reached. The dosage may be increased more rapidly to treat a life-threatening infection, such as fulminating cryptococcal meningitis. Duration of therapy depends on the maturity and severity of the infection. Some patients may need months of therapy with total dosages ranging from 300 to 4,000 mg.

Usual adult dosage: as a test dose for infection, 1 mg in 250 ml of dextrose 5% in water (D_5W) infused over 2 to 4 hours initially, increased to 5 mg, 10 mg, 20 mg, and up each day; as a test dose for severe infections, 1 mg I.V. given over 30 to 60 minutes initially, increased to 0.25 mg/kg the same day. For systemic fungal infections and meningitis, 0.25 to 1.5 mg/kg/day I.V. is given — based on the organism present and the patient's drug tolerance — infused over 4 to 6 hours. For coccidioidal meningitis and cryptococcal meningitis, 0.025 to 1 mg is given intrathecally two to three times weekly. For coccidioidal arthritis or osteoarticular sporotrichosis, 5 to 15 mg is injected into the joint spaces. For candidal infections of the bladder, 50 mg in 1 liter of sterile water is instilled continuously or intermittently into the bladder. For topical application, 3% ointment, cream, or lotion is applied liberally and rubbed well into the affected area b.i.d. to q.i.d.

As an alternate method of I.V. administration, amphotericin B can be given every other day. To do this, the daily dosage is doubled gradually and administered every 48 hours. Under no circumstances, however, should the daily dosage exceed 1.5 mg/kg.

Drug interactions
Amphotericin B can have significant interactions with many drugs. Some drug combinations may be unavoidable, however, and the patient will require close monitoring. When given with amphotericin B, several drugs can alter renal function and electrolyte balance. Also, certain I.V. solutions can inactivate amphotericin B. (For details, see *Drug interactions: Amphotericin B,* page 1082.)

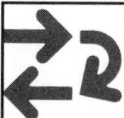

DRUG INTERACTIONS

Amphotericin B

When given with the drugs listed below, amphotericin B may cause significant drug interactions. Some may be severe, such as nephrotoxicity and hypokalemia. Thus, a patient receiving concomitant therapy will need to be monitored closely.

DRUG	INTERACTING DRUGS	POSSIBLE EFFECTS	NURSING IMPLICATIONS
amphotericin B	aminoglycosides, cyclosporine, acyclovir	Increase nephrotoxicity	• Monitor the patient's renal function by monitoring BUN and serum creatinine levels and intake and output patterns.
	corticosteroids	Increase hypokalemia, possibly leading to cardiac dysfunction	• Monitor the patient's serum potassium level. • Monitor the patient for signs and symptoms of cardiac dysfunction, such as palpitations, tachycardia, and hypotension.
	extended-spectrum penicillins	Increase hypokalemia	• Monitor the patient's serum potassium level.
	cardiac glycosides	Increase hypokalemia, which may cause digitalis toxicity	• Monitor the patient's serum potassium level. • Monitor the patient for signs and symptoms of hypokalemia, such as hypotension, muscle weakness, and confusion.
	nondepolarizing skeletal muscle relaxants (pancuronium bromide)	Increases muscle relaxant effects	• Monitor the patient's serum potassium level. • Monitor the patient for muscle weakness and respiratory insufficiency. • Have emergency equipment available.
	electrolyte solutions	Precipitate and inactivate amphotericin B colloid	• Do not dilute amphotericin B in electrolyte solutions; use only D$_5$W or sterile water without bacteriostatic agents.

ADVERSE DRUG REACTIONS

Amphotericin B probably is the most toxic antibiotic in use today. Adverse reactions to I.V. amphotericin B therapy may include nephrotoxicity and hypokalemia. Adverse reactions to other forms of amphotericin therapy tend to be less severe.

Almost all patients receiving I.V. amphotericin B experience chills, fever, nausea, vomiting, anorexia, muscle and joint pain, headache, abdominal pain, weight loss, and dyspepsia, especially at the beginning of therapy with low doses. As therapy continues and the dosage is increased to the optimum level, these reactions usually subside. Most patients also develop normochromic or normocytic anemia that significantly decreases the hematocrit.

Up to 80% of patients receiving amphotericin B develop some degree of nephrotoxicity. With this adverse reaction, blood urea nitrogen (BUN) and serum creatinine levels rise, and the kidneys lose their concentrating ability. The latter promotes renal losses of potassium, bicarbonate, water, and phosphate. Nephrotoxicity usually disappears within 3 months after the drug is discontinued, but it sometimes leads to permanent renal impairment. A direct relationship

may exist between the severity and permanency of the impairment and the total amphotericin B dosage. Permanent problems are more common in patients who receive a total of 5 grams or more.

Up to 25% of patients receiving amphotericin B may develop hypokalemia, which can be severe and lead to extreme muscle weakness and electrocardiographic changes. Distal renal tubular acidosis commonly occurs, contributing to the development of hypokalemia.

Other adverse reactions to I.V. amphotericin B therapy include phlebitis and thrombophlebitis. Hypotension, hypertension, flushing, paresthesia, and seizures occur rarely.

Intrathecal administration may cause headache, leg and back pain, paresthesia, peripheral neuropathies, sensory loss, and urine retention. Topical application may result in pruritus, skin thickening and discoloration, dry skin, erythema, and contact dermatitis. Uncommon reactions to amphotericin B include blurred or double vision, ventricular arrhythmias, thrombocytopenia, leukopenia, granulocytopenia, tinnitus, and hearing loss. Rarely, amphotericin B causes anaphylaxis or liver failure.

NURSING PROCESS APPLICATION

The following information assists the nurse in caring for a patient who is receiving amphotericin B.

Assessment

• Review the patient's history for a preexisting condition that contraindicates the use of amphotericin B, such as lactation or known hypersensitivity to the drug.

• Review the patient's history for a preexisting condition that requires cautious use of amphotericin B, such as pregnancy.

• Assess the patient for adverse reactions to amphotericin B, such as nephrotoxicity, hypokalemia, GI distress, chills, fever, muscle and joint pain, and hematologic abnormalities.

• Review the patient's medication history to identify the use of drugs that may interact with amphotericin B, such as aminoglycosides, cyclosporine, corticosteroids, cardiac glycosides, or electrolyte solutions.

• Assess the effectiveness of amphotericin B therapy periodically.

• Evaluate the patient's and family's knowledge about amphotericin B.

Nursing diagnoses

The following examples represent appropriate nursing diagnoses for a patient receiving amphotericin B.

• Potential for injury related to a preexisting condition that contraindicates the use of amphotericin B

• Potential for injury related to a preexisting condition that requires cautious use of amphotericin B

• Potential for injury related to adverse drug reactions

• Altered urinary elimination related to nephrotoxicity caused by amphotericin B

• Knowledge deficit related to amphotericin B

Planning and implementation

• Do not administer amphotericin B to a patient with a condition that contraindicates its use.

• Administer amphotericin B cautiously to a patient at risk because of a preexisting condition.

• Monitor the patient regularly for adverse reactions during amphotericin B therapy.

• *Monitor the patient for signs of an immediate hypersensitivity reaction, including dyspnea, wheezing, urticaria, pruritus, laryngeal edema, hypotension, and tachycardia.*

• Monitor the patient's serum electrolyte levels, particularly noting any changes in potassium, magnesium, calcium, and phosphorus levels. Potassium requires especially close monitoring in a patient who is receiving a cardiac glycoside or potassium-wasting drug, such as a diuretic or extended-spectrum penicillin, or who is losing potassium because of severe vomiting or diarrhea. Watch for muscle weakness, cramping, and fatigue, which may be the first signs of hypokalemia. Expect to administer potassium supplements, as prescribed.

• Monitor the patient's vital signs during I.V. infusion. Note that a fever may occur, but usually will subside within 4 hours after the infusion is discontinued. To relieve the fever and chills associated with the infusion, expect to administer an antihistamine or antipyretic as prescribed. Antiemetics sometimes are used to relieve other signs and symptoms, such as nausea and vomiting.

• *Check the I.V. site for phlebitis. To reduce phlebitis, rotate the site routinely and add small doses of heparin or corticosteroids to the infusion, as prescribed. Expect to use alternate-day therapy if phlebitis becomes severe. The patient may receive amphotericin B via a central line, which permits greater drug dilution in the blood and decreases the severity of the phlebitis.*

• Monitor for headache, leg and back pain, paresthesia, peripheral neuropathies, sensory loss, and urine retention in a patient receiving intrathecal amphotericin B.

• Monitor for pruritus, skin thickening and discoloration, dry skin, erythema, and contact dermatitis in a patient receiving topical amphotericin B.

• Refrigerate amphotericin B until it is used.

• *Dilute amphotericin B for infusion or injection in a D_5W solution with a pH greater than 4.2 or in sterile water. The drug is not compatible with any electrolyte solution.*

• Shake the vial vigorously for at least 3 minutes before administration to assure particle dispersion in the colloidal suspension.

• *Do not administer the solution if it contains precipitate.*

• Infuse I.V. amphotericin B over 4 to 6 hours, or as prescribed.

• Use an in-line filter with a mean pore diameter of 1 micron or greater for I.V. administration. Smaller filters will remove appreciable amounts of the drug from the solution.

• Infuse any other antibiotics separately; do not use the I.V. line for amphotericin B.

• Notify the physician if adverse reactions occur.

• *Monitor the patient's BUN and serum creatinine levels before therapy begins, every other day during initiation of therapy, and once a week after the optimal dosage is reached. Expect to administer a reduced dosage or to use alternate-day therapy as prescribed if the serum creatinine level approaches 3 mg/dl.*

• Monitor the patient's fluid intake and output, and observe for oliguria, hematuria, cloudy urine, or excessive urine output. These may be the first signs of nephrotoxicity.

• Notify the physician if abnormalities occur.

Patient teaching
• Teach the patient and family the name, dose, frequency, action, and adverse effects of amphotericin B.
• Stress the importance of returning for regular blood studies and follow-up appointments as instructed.
• Teach the patient how to apply topical amphotericin B.
• Instruct the patient using topical amphotericin B to report such adverse reactions as dry skin, erythema, pruritus, or skin discoloration. Warn the patient that the drug may stain clothing.
• *Inform the patient receiving I.V. amphotericin B that chills, fever, GI upset, muscle and joint pain, headache, abdominal pain, weight loss, and dyspepsia probably will occur, but that these reactions usually subside with continued therapy.*
• Teach the patient which adverse reactions may occur with intrathecal use of amphotericin B.
• Instruct the patient to report oliguria, hematuria, cloudy urine, lack of urine output, or other adverse reactions.

Evaluation

The following examples represent appropriate evaluation statements for a patient receiving amphotericin B.
• The patient has no conditions that contraindicate amphotericin B therapy.
• The patient exhibits no signs of complications in the preexisting condition linked to amphotericin B.
• The patient exhibits no adverse reactions to amphotericin B.
• The patient's renal function returns to normal after amphotericin B is discontinued.
• The patient and family express an accurate understanding of the points taught about amphotericin B.
• The patient correctly identifies the signs and symptoms of nephrotoxicity and agrees to report them to the physician.

NYSTATIN

Nystatin resembles amphotericin B in its chemical structure. Unlike amphotericin B, however, this drug usually is used only topically or orally to treat local infections because it is extremely toxic when administered parenterally.

PHARMACOKINETICS

Oral nystatin undergoes little or no absorption, distribution, or metabolism. It is excreted as unchanged drug in the feces.

Topical nystatin is not absorbed through the skin or mucous membranes, and the blood concentration level is not measurable at therapeutic doses.

Because nystatin is not systemically absorbed, its onset of action, peak concentration, and duration of action are not significant.

PHARMACODYNAMICS

Like amphotericin B, nystatin acts by binding to sterols in fungal cells.

Mechanism of action

Nystatin binds to sterols in fungal cell membranes and alters the permeability of the membranes, leading to loss of essential cell components. Nystatin can act as a fungicidal or fungistatic agent, depending on the organism present.

PHARMACOTHERAPEUTICS

Nystatin is used primarily to treat fungal skin infections. The drug is effective against *Candida albicans, Candida guilliermondii,* and other *Candida* species.

nystatin (Mycostatin, Nilstat). Different forms of nystatin are available for treating different types of candidal infections. Topical nystatin is used to treat cutaneous or mucocutaneous candidal infections, such as thrush, diaper rash, vulvovaginitis, and intertriginous candidiasis. Oral nystatin is used to treat intestinal candidiasis and may be used as an adjunct to vaginal application in treating vulvovaginitis. Oral nystatin also is used to prevent fungal infection in a neutropenic patient receiving immunosuppressive therapy.
Usual adult dosage: for oral or esophageal candidiasis, 500,000 units of oral suspension, gargled and then swallowed, t.i.d. or q.i.d., or 500,000 units of oral tablets, dissolved in the mouth t.i.d. or q.i.d. for 10 days or until 48 hours after overt symptoms have subsided; for intestinal candidiasis, 500,000 to 1 million units of oral tablets t.i.d. or q.i.d.; for vaginal candidiasis, 100,000 units (one vaginal tablet) inserted vaginally once or twice daily for 14 days or longer; for cutaneous candidiasis, topical cream, ointment, lotion, or powder applied to the affected area b.i.d. or as directed for 14 days or longer.

Drug interactions

No significant drug interactions occur with nystatin use.

ADVERSE DRUG REACTIONS

Reactions to nystatin, which rarely occur, usually are mild. The patient may experience diarrhea, nausea, vomiting, and abdominal pain, especially with high doses; some patients also report a bitter taste. Topical nystatin may cause skin irritation. A hypersensitivity reaction may occur with oral or topical nystatin administration.

NURSING PROCESS APPLICATION

The following information assists the nurse in caring for a patient who is receiving nystatin.

Assessment
• Review the patient's history for a preexisting condition that contraindicates the use of nystatin, such as known hypersensitivity to the drug.
• Assess the patient for adverse reactions to nystatin, such as GI distress, skin irritation, bitter taste, or hypersensitivity reactions.
• Assess the effectiveness of nystatin therapy periodically.
• Evaluate the patient's and family's knowledge about nystatin.

Nursing diagnoses
The following examples represent appropriate nursing diagnoses for a patient receiving nystatin.
• Potential for injury related to a preexisting condition that contraindicates the use of nystatin
• Potential for injury related to adverse drug reactions
• Knowledge deficit related to nystatin

Planning and implementation
• Do not administer nystatin to a patient with a condition that contraindicates its use.
• Monitor the patient periodically for adverse reactions during nystatin therapy.
• *Monitor for diarrhea, nausea, vomiting, and abdominal pain in a patient receiving high doses of nystatin. If GI distress becomes severe or is prolonged, monitor the patient's hydration status. Obtain a prescription for an antiemetic or antidiarrheal agent, as needed.*
• Inspect the patient's skin regularly for signs of irritation, such as a rash or redness, when administering topical nystatin. Expect to discontinue the drug if skin irritation occurs.
• Notify the physician if adverse reactions occur.

Patient teaching
• Teach the patient and family the name, dose, frequency, action, and adverse effects of nystatin.
• Instruct the patient taking nystatin in suspension form for oral candidiasis to divide the dose in half, place one half in each side of the mouth, swish the suspension in the mouth for as long as possible, and then swallow it.
• *Instruct the patient with oral candidiasis to dissolve the nystatin tablet in the mouth. Emphasize that the patient must not chew it or swallow it whole.*

• Advise the patient receiving topical nystatin to report any signs of a hypersensitivity reaction, such as redness or skin irritation.
• *Teach the patient how to apply topical nystatin properly. Also emphasize the importance of compliance and good hygiene.*
• Instruct the patient to insert the vaginal nystatin tablets high in the vagina. Also inform the patient that vaginal drainage from the tablets may stain clothing.
• *Instruct the patient to avoid using occlusive dressings during therapy with nystatin ointment or cream because they provide a favorable environment for fungal growth.*
• Advise the patient with a foot infection to apply nystatin topical powder to shoes and socks as a preventive measure.
• Instruct the patient to take the drug for the full length of time prescribed—usually 14 days—even though symptomatic relief may occur in 14 to 72 hours.
• Instruct the patient to notify the physician if adverse reactions occur.

Evaluation
The following examples represent appropriate evaluation statements for a patient receiving nystatin.
• The patient has no conditions that contraindicate nystatin therapy.
• The patient exhibits no adverse reactions to nystatin.
• The patient and family express an accurate understanding of the points taught about nystatin.
• The patient demonstrates the correct technique for applying topical nystatin.

FLUCYTOSINE

Flucytosine is the only antimetabolite with antimycotic activity. It is used primarily with another antimycotic agent, such as amphotericin B, to treat systemic fungal infections.

PHARMACOKINETICS

After oral administration, flucytosine is absorbed well and distributed widely. It usually undergoes little metabolism and is excreted primarily by the kidneys.

Absorption, distribution, metabolism, excretion
Flucytosine is absorbed rapidly and well from the GI tract. Although the presence of food in the stomach slows the rate of absorption, it does not affect its extent.

As a result of flucytosine's wide distribution throughout the body, it appears in the kidneys, liver, heart, spleen, aqueous humor, and bronchial secretions. It also reaches a high concentration level in the CSF. Distribution into breast milk is unknown. It is only 2% to 4% protein bound.

Because flucytosine is not metabolized significantly, about 90% of it is excreted unchanged in the urine. Unchanged, unabsorbed flucytosine also appears in feces.

Onset, peak, duration

Therapeutic serum concentrations of flucytosine range from 25 to 120 mcg/ml. The drug usually reaches a peak concentration 2 to 4 hours after administration unless the patient's renal function is impaired, in which case the drug will reach a peak concentration more slowly and will be prolonged. For a patient with normal renal function, flucytosine's half-life ranges from 2.5 to 8 hours. For a patient with renal impairment, the half-life can range from 1 to 10 days.

PHARMACODYNAMICS

Unlike the polyene antimycotic agents, flucytosine must be converted to its active metabolite within fungal cells.

Mechanism of action

Flucytosine penetrates fungal cells and there undergoes conversion to its active metabolite fluorouracil, a metabolic antagonist. Fluorouracil then is incorporated into the ribonucleic acid of the fungal cells, altering their protein synthesis and causing cell death. The drug displays selective toxicity against fungi. Most nonfungal cells do not take up and convert large quantities of flucytosine. Fungal resistance to flucytosine usually occurs when the drug is used alone to treat *Cryptococcus* infections; resistance also occurs, to a lesser degree, when the drug is used alone to treat *Candida, Torulopsis,* and *Cladosporium* infections.

PHARMACOTHERAPEUTICS

Some fungal species and strains are not susceptible to flucytosine. Therefore, susceptibility tests should be done before the drug is used. Also, because some fungi can develop a resistance to flucytosine when it is given alone, it usually is used with another antimycotic agent, such as amphotericin B. Flucytosine reaches a high concentration in the CSF and urinary tract, so it is effective against fungal meningitis and urinary candidiasis.

flucytosine (Ancobon). Administered orally, flucytosine is used in combination therapy to treat systemic fungal infections caused by *Candida* and *Cryptococcus.* Although amphotericin B is effective in treating candidal and cryptococcal meningitis, flucytosine usually is given with it to reduce the amphotericin B dosage and toxicity. This combination therapy is the treatment of choice for cryptococcal meningitis. Flucytosine can be used alone to treat lower

urinary tract *Candida* infections because it reaches a high urinary concentration. It also is used effectively to treat infections caused by *T. glabrata, Phialophora* species, and *Aspergillus* species.

Usual adult and pediatric dosage: for patients over 50 kg with normal renal function and fungal infections caused by *Candida* and *Cryptococcus,* 50 to 150 mg/kg P.O. daily, divided into four equal doses and administered every 6 hours; for patients under 50 kg with normal renal function, 1.5 to 4.5 grams/m² P.O. daily; for patients with impaired renal function, the dose and dosage interval should be altered as follows: 12.5 to 37.5 mg/kg every 12 hours for a patient with a creatinine clearance between 20 and 40 ml/minute; 12.5 to 37.5 mg/kg every 24 hours when the creatinine clearance ranges from 10 to 20 ml/minute; individualized doses based on the drug's serum concentration when the creatinine clearance falls below 10 ml/minute; and 20 to 50 mg/kg after each dialysis treatment (every 48 to 72 hours) for a patient on hemodialysis therapy.

Drug interactions

Flucytosine does not cause any significant drug interactions.

ADVERSE DRUG REACTIONS

Adverse reactions to flucytosine seem to involve rapidly proliferating cells in the bone marrow and the GI tract.

Bone marrow depression typically occurs when the flucytosine serum concentration exceeds 100 mcg/ml and may lead to leukopenia, thrombocytopenia, anemia, pancytopenia, or granulocytopenia. Most commonly it affects patients with renal failure who are undergoing combination therapy with amphotericin B or receiving large doses of flucytosine.

GI reactions also may occur with flucytosine therapy. They can be severe and may include nausea, vomiting, abdominal distention, diarrhea, and anorexia. Rarely, bowel perforation can occur, as can hepatotoxicity, manifested by elevated transaminase and alkaline phosphatase levels.

In the urinary system, flucytosine may cause azotemia, increased blood urea nitrogen (BUN) and creatinine levels, crystalluria, and renal failure. Because of these adverse urinary reactions, the drug must be used with extreme caution in a patient with impaired renal function.

Flucytosine may produce unpredictable adverse reactions, including confusion, headache, sedation, vertigo, hallucinations, dyspnea, respiratory arrest, and skin rash.

NURSING PROCESS APPLICATION

The following information assists the nurse in caring for a patient who is receiving flucytosine.

Assessment

• Review the patient's history for a preexisting condition that contraindicates the use of flucytosine, such as lactation or known hypersensitivity to the drug.

• Review the patient's history for a preexisting condition that requires cautious use of flucytosine, such as impaired renal function, bone marrow depression, or pregnancy.

• Assess the patient for adverse reactions to flucytosine, such as bone marrow depression, GI distress, urinary problems, CNS disturbances, and skin rash.

• Assess the effectiveness of flucytosine therapy periodically.

• Assess for fluid volume deficit if the patient experiences anorexia, nausea, vomiting, or diarrhea during flucytosine therapy.

• Evaluate the patient's and family's knowledge about flucytosine.

Nursing diagnoses

The following examples represent appropriate nursing diagnoses for a patient receiving flucytosine.

• Potential for injury related to a preexisting condition that contraindicates the use of flucytosine

• Potential for injury related to a preexisting condition that requires cautious use of flucytosine

• Potential for injury related to adverse drug reactions

• Potential fluid volume deficit related to the adverse GI effects of flucytosine

• Knowledge deficit related to flucytosine

Planning and implementation

• Do not administer flucytosine to a patient with a condition that contraindicates its use.

• Administer flucytosine cautiously to a patient at risk because of a preexisting condition.

• Monitor the patient periodically for adverse reactions during flucytosine therapy.

• *Monitor the patient's hematologic values, liver function tests, and BUN and creatinine levels during flucytosine therapy. Notify the physician if test results are abnormal.*

• *Monitor the patient for signs of infection, such as sore throat, fever, and productive cough, if leukopenia occurs. Take infection-control measures, such as keeping the patient away from others who have infections, until the white blood count returns to normal.*

• Monitor the patient for signs of bleeding, such as easy bruising and spontaneous epistaxis, if thrombocytopenia occurs. Test emesis and stool for occult blood and take bleeding precautions, such as having the patient use an electric razor and soft toothbrush, until the thrombocytes return to normal.

• *Monitor the patient's fluid intake and output. Notify the physician if the patient develops azotemia, crystalluria, or decreased urine output, which may indicate renal failure.*

• Take safety measures if the patient experiences adverse CNS reactions, such as confusion, sedation, vertigo, or hallucinations. For example, place the bed in the lowest position, keep the bed rails up, and supervise ambulation.

• Administer a mild analgesic if the patient develops a headache during flucytosine therapy.

• Inspect the patient's skin regularly for a rash, which may suggest a hypersensitivity reaction to flucytosine.

• *Monitor the flucytosine blood level regularly during long-term therapy. Therapeutic serum concentrations range from 25 to 120 mcg/ml.*

• Notify the physician if adverse reactions occur.

• Monitor for fluid volume deficit if the patient experiences anorexia, nausea, vomiting, or diarrhea during flucytosine therapy. Administer an antiemetic or antidiarrheal agent as prescribed.

• Notify the physician if GI symptoms persist or become severe.

Patient teaching

• Teach the patient and family the name, dose, frequency, action, and adverse effects of flucytosine.

• Emphasize to the patient the importance of compliance with therapy.

• Teach the patient the importance of returning for blood tests as instructed.

• Instruct the patient about infection control measures or bleeding precautions as needed.

• *Instruct the patient to report sore throat, fever, easy bruising, bleeding, unusual fatigue or weakness, changes in urine output, severe nausea, vomiting, or skin rash.*

• Advise the patient to take flucytosine capsules over 15 minutes to minimize nausea or vomiting.

• *Instruct the patient to take a missed dose as soon as possible, but not to take a double dose. Explain that missing a dose is safer than overmedicating with a double dose.*

• Caution the patient against performing activities that require mental alertness if adverse CNS reactions occur.

• Instruct the patient to notify the physician if adverse reactions occur.

Evalution

The following examples represent appropriate evaluation statements for a patient receiving flucytosine.

• The patient has no conditions that contraindicate flucytosine therapy.

• The patient exhibits no signs of complications in the preexisting condition linked to flucytosine.

• The patient exhibits no adverse reactions to flucytosine.

• The patient maintains adequate hydration throughout flucytosine therapy.

• The patient and family express an accurate understanding of the points taught about flucytosine.

• The patient correctly identifies adverse reactions and steps to take if they occur.

KETOCONAZOLE

The imidazole group includes ketoconazole, miconazole, clotrimazole, and griseofulvin. Ketoconazole and miconazole are used to treat systemic and topical fungal infections; clotrimazole and griseofulvin, only topical ones. (For more information about miconazole, clotrimazole, and griseofulvin, see "Other antimycotic agents," page 1092.) Because ketoconazole provides effective antimycotic activity with oral administration, its use overshadows that of miconazole, which is available only in parenteral and topical preparations. Considered an important advance in fungal infection therapy, ketoconazole is the first effective oral antimycotic agent with a broad spectrum of activity.

PHARMACOKINETICS

After oral administration, ketoconazole is absorbed variably and distributed widely. It undergoes extensive metabolism and is excreted through the bile and feces.

Absorption, distribution, metabolism, excretion
Ketoconazole usually is absorbed well from the GI tract. Its degree of absorption, however, depends on the pH of the GI tract. A normal acidic environment increases absorption; an alkaline environment, which may result from diseases, other drugs, or foods that reduce gastric acid, decreases absorption. The drug is absorbed best when the patient's stomach is empty.

Widely distributed throughout the body, ketoconazole appears in bile, saliva, serum, cerumen, feces, and the skin and soft tissues. It is distributed poorly in urine and CSF, however, where concentration levels usually are low. The drug crosses the placenta and appears in breast milk. Its protein binding—primarily to albumin—ranges from 84% to 99%.

Ketoconazole metabolism in the liver produces inactive metabolites; these metabolites and unchanged drug are excreted primarily in the feces.

Onset, peak, duration
When administered ½ to 1 hour after meals, ketoconazole reaches a peak plasma concentration level in 1 to 4 hours. The ensuing decline in plasma concentration appears to be biphasic. During the initial phase, the drug's half-life is about 2 hours; in the terminal phase, 8 hours.

PHARMACODYNAMICS

Like the polyene antimycotic agents, ketoconazole acts by affecting cell permeability. It usually produces fungistatic effects, but also can produce fungicidal effects under certain conditions.

Mechanism of action
Within the fungal cells, ketoconazole interferes with sterol synthesis, damaging the cell membrane and increasing its permeability. This leads to a loss of essential intracellular elements and inhibition of cell growth.

PHARMACOTHERAPEUTICS

Ketoconazole is used to treat topical and systemic infections caused by susceptible fungi, which include dermatophytes and most other fungi. However, it should not be used to treat fungal meningitis because it does not reach an adequate concentration in the CSF. Ketoconazole also is active against some gram-positive bacteria, including *Staphylococcus epidermis, Staphylococcus aureus, Nocardia* species, *Actinomadura* species, and enterococci.

ketoconazole (Nizoral). Administered orally, this antimycotic agent can treat topical and systemic fungal infections effectively, including chronic mucocutaneous candidiasis. Mucosal infections respond in days, skin infections in weeks, and nail infections in months.

Other clinical indications for ketoconazole therapy include pulmonary and disseminated blastomycosis caused by *B. dermatitidis,* chromomycosis caused by *Phialophora* species, pulmonary and disseminated coccidioidomycosis caused by *C. immitis,* pulmonary and disseminated histoplasmosis caused by *H. capsulatum,* oral candidiasis caused by *Candida* species, and paracoccidioidomycosis caused by *P. brasiliensis.*
Usual adult dosage: 200 mg P.O. daily, increased to 400 mg/day if the infection is severe or does not respond. The duration of therapy varies with the organism and infection site, as follows: 1 to 4 weeks for oral candidiasis; 1 to 2 months for most dermatophyte infections; 6 months for histoplasmosis; and 6 to 12 months for coccidioidomycosis, chromomycosis, chronic mucocutaneous candidiasis, and tinea unguium.

Drug interactions
Use of ketoconazole with drugs that decrease gastric acidity, such as cimetidine, ranitidine, famotidine, antacids, and anticholinergics, may decrease its absorption and antimycotic effects. Concomitant administration of ketoconazole and phenytoin may alter metabolism and blood levels of both drugs. Concomitant administration of ketoconazole and theophylline may decrease the serum theophylline level.

Use of ketoconazole with other hepatotoxic drugs may increase the risk of liver disease. Concomitant administration of ketoconazole with cyclosporine may increase cyclosporine and serum creatinine levels. Concomitant administration with an oral anticoagulant can cause hemorrhage from the increased anticoagulant effect.

ADVERSE DRUG REACTIONS

Although ketoconazole appears to be safer than amphotericin B and miconazole, it may produce adverse reactions primarily affecting the CNS, GI tract, and skin. The most common reactions to ketoconazole are nausea and vomiting.

Other reactions, which have been reported in less than 1% of patients, include pruritus, rash, dermatitis, urticaria, headache, insomnia, dizziness, vivid dreams, lethargy, paresthesia, diarrhea, flatulence, and abdominal pain. The patient also may experience endocrine effects, such as gynecomastia and breast pain. Hepatotoxicity, although rare, is reversible with drug discontinuation. Rarely, ketoconazole also can cause anaphylaxis, arthralgia, chills, fever, tinnitus, impotence, and photophobia.

NURSING PROCESS APPLICATION

The following information assists the nurse in caring for a patient who is receiving ketoconazole.

Assessment
• Review the patient's history for a preexisting condition that contraindicates the use of ketoconazole, such as lactation or known hypersensitivity to the drug.
• Review the patient's history for a preexisting condition that requires cautious use of ketoconazole, such as pregnancy.
• Assess the patient for adverse reactions to ketoconazole, such as GI, CNS, or skin disorders.
• Review the patient's medication history to identify the use of drugs that may interact with ketoconazole, such as cimetidine, antacids, phenytoin, theophylline, cyclosporine, hepatotoxic drugs, or an oral anticoagulant.
• Assess the effectiveness of ketoconazole periodically.
• Assess the patient for fluid volume deficit if nausea, vomiting, or diarrhea occur during ketoconazole therapy.
• Evaluate the patient's and family's knowledge about ketoconazole.

Nursing diagnoses
The following examples represent appropriate nursing diagnoses for a patient receiving ketoconazole.
• Potential for injury related to a preexisting condition that contraindicates the use of ketoconazole
• Potential for injury related to a preexisting condition that requires cautious use of ketoconazole

• Potential for injury related to adverse drug reactions
• Potential for fluid volume deficit related to the adverse GI effects of ketoconazole
• Knowledge deficit related to ketoconazole

Planning and implementation
• Do not administer ketoconazole to a patient with a condition that contraindicates its use.
• Administer ketoconazole cautiously to a patient at risk because of a preexisting condition.
• Monitor the patient periodically for adverse reactions during ketoconazole therapy.
• *Monitor the patient's liver function tests. Expect to discontinue the drug if test results show persistent elevations and the patient displays signs of hepatotoxicity, such as fatigue, jaundice, or right upper abdominal quadrant pain.*
• Monitor the serum level of phenytoin, theophylline, or cyclosporine administered concomitantly with ketoconazole. Expect to adjust the dosage as prescribed.
• Monitor the patient for signs and symptoms of hepatotoxicity if ketoconazole is administered concomitantly with another hepatotoxic drug.
• Administer a mild analgesic as prescribed if the patient experiences a headache.
• Help the patient relax before going to sleep if insomnia occurs. Review relaxation techniques with the patient and provide a warm beverage as desired. If insomnia persists, obtain a prescription for a sedative.
• Take safety measures if the patient experiences adverse CNS reactions, such as dizziness, lethargy, or paresthesia. For example, place the bed in the lowest position, keep the bed rails raised, and supervise ambulation.
• *Administer ketoconazole on an empty stomach, if possible, to promote absorption. If the patient experiences GI distress, however, administer the drug with food.*
• *Do not administer ketoconazole with drugs that decrease gastric acidity, such as antacids and anticholinergics. If these drugs must be used, administer ketoconazole at least 2 hours before administering them.*
• Notify the physician if adverse reactions or drug interactions occur.
• Monitor for fluid volume deficit if the patient experiences nausea, vomiting, or diarrhea during ketoconazole therapy.
• Administer an antiemetic or antidiarrheal agent as prescribed.
• Notify the physician if adverse GI reactions persist or worsen.

Patient teaching
• Teach the patient and family the name, dose, frequency, action, and adverse effects of ketoconazole.
• Inform the patient when to expect therapeutic results with ketoconazole therapy. Mucosal infections respond in days, skin infections in weeks, and nail infections in months.

• *Instruct the patient to notify the physician if signs and symptoms of hepatotoxicity develop during ketoconazole therapy, such as dark or amber-colored urine, pale stools, abdominal pain, unusual fatigue, or yellowing of the eyes or skin.*

• Advise the patient to report breast enlargement, breast pain, or a skin rash during ketoconazole therapy.

• Caution the patient not to perform activities that require mental alertness if dizziness or drowsiness occurs during ketoconazole therapy.

• *Advise the patient when to take ketoconazole in relation to any drugs that decrease gastric acidity.*

• Teach the patient relaxation techniques if insomnia occurs with ketoconazole therapy. Advise the patient with persistent insomnia to request a prescription for a sedative from the physician.

• Advise the patient to take ketoconazole on an empty stomach. However, instruct the patient experiencing adverse GI reactions to take ketoconazole with food and to notify the physician if the reactions persist or worsen.

• Instruct the patient to report any other adverse reactions to the physician.

Evaluation

The following examples represent appropriate evaluation statements for a patient receiving ketoconazole.

• The patient has no conditions that contraindicate ketoconazole therapy.

• The patient exhibits no signs of complications in the preexisting condition linked to ketoconazole.

• The patient exhibits no adverse reactions to ketoconazole.

• The patient maintains adequate hydration throughout ketoconazole therapy.

• The patient and family express an accurate understanding of the points taught about ketoconazole.

• The patient correctly describes when to take ketoconazole.

FLUCONAZOLE

Fluconazole is the first of a new class of synthetic, broad-spectrum bistriazole antifungal agents. It is used to treat oropharyngeal and esophageal candidiasis and serious systemic candidal infections, including urinary tract infections, peritonitis, pneumonia, and cryptococcal meningitis.

PHARMACOKINETICS

The pharmacokinetics of fluconazole are similar whether administered by the intravenous or oral route. After oral administration, fluconazole is about 90% absorbed. Fluconazole is distributed into all body fluids and is approximately 12% protein bound. Over 80% of the drug is excreted unchanged in the urine. Elimination may be reduced in patients with decreased renal function.

Peak plasma concentration levels occur 1 to 2 hours after oral administration. The half-life of fluconazole is about 30 hours, and steady-state plasma concentrations are reached within 5 to 10 days during daily administration.

PHARMACODYNAMICS

A selective inhibitor of fungal cytochrome P-450 and sterol C-14 alpha-demethylation, fluconazole causes fungal cells to lose normal sterol.

PHARMACOTHERAPEUTICS

The primary indications for fluconazole are treatment of specific candidal and cyryptococcal infections.

fluconazole (Diflucan). Fluconazole is used to treat oropharyngeal and esophageal candidiasis and serious systemic candidal infections, including urinary tract infections, peritonitis, and pneumonia. It also is used to treat cryptococcal meningitis. The recommended P.O. and I.V. doses are similar because the oral product is well-absorbed. For esophageal candidiasis and cryptococcal meningitis, dosages up to 400 mg daily may be used based on response.

Usual adult dosage: for oropharyngeal candidiasis, 200 mg P.O. or I.V. on the first day, followed by 100 mg daily for 2 weeks; for esophageal candidiasis, 200 mg P.O. or I.V. on the first day, followed by 100 mg daily for a minimum of 3 weeks and for at least 2 weeks after symptoms resolve; for systemic candidiasis, 400 mg P.O. or I.V. on the first day, followed by 200 mg daily for a minimum of 4 weeks and for at least 2 weeks after symptoms resolve; for cryptococcal meningitis, 400 mg P.O. or I.V. on the first day, followed by 200 mg daily for 10 to 12 weeks after the CSF culture becomes negative; for suppression of cryptococcal meningitis relapse in patients with acquired immunodeficiency syndrome (AIDS), 200 mg P.O. or I.V. daily.

Drug interactions

Administration of fluconazole with warfarin may increase prothrombin time; careful monitoring of prothrombin time is recommended. Fluconazole may increase levels of phenytoin and cyclosporine; blood levels of phenytoin and cyclosporine should be monitored carefully. Glyburide and glipizide metabolism may decrease, resulting in increased blood levels and hypoglycemia; blood glucose concentrations should be monitored closely. Rifampin enhances fluconazole metabolism, possibly requiring increased fluconazole dosage.

ADVERSE DRUG REACTIONS

In clinical trials, 5% to 7% of patients receiving fluconazole experienced transient elevations in aspartate aminotransferase (AST [formerly SGOT]), alanine aminotransferase (ALT [formerly SGPT]), alkaline phosphatase, and bilirubin levels. About 2% developed dizziness, and more than 1% experienced nausea, vomiting, abdominal pain, diarrhea, skin rash, and headache. Hypokalemia and increased BUN and creatinine levels also have been reported. All adverse drug reactions occur more commonly in patients infected with the human immunodeficiency virus (HIV).

Because fluconazole frequently is administered with other drugs in patients with a serious disorder, such as leukemia, cancer, and acquired immune deficiency syndrome (AIDS), adverse reactions to fluconazole may be difficult to distinguish from the effects of the disorder or from adverse reactions to the other drugs.

NURSING PROCESS APPLICATION

The following information assists the nurse in caring for a patient who is receiving fluconazole.

Assessment
• Review the patient's history for a preexisting condition that contraindicates the use of fluconazole, such as known hypersensitivity to the drug or any of its ingredients.
• Review the patient's history for a preexisting condition that requires cautious use of fluconazole, such as pregnancy or lactation.
• Assess the patient for adverse reactions to fluconazole, such as elevations in blood chemistry levels, dizziness, GI distress, skin rash, and headache.
• Review the patient's medication history to identify the use of drugs that may interact with fluconazole, such as warfarin, phenytoin, cyclosporine, glyburide, glipizide, or rifampin.
• Assess the effectiveness of fluconazole periodically.
• Assess the patient for fluid volume deficit if nausea, vomiting, or diarrhea occurs during fluconazole therapy.
• Evaluate the patient's and family's knowledge about fluconazole.

Nursing diagnoses
The following examples represent appropriate nursing diagnoses for a patient receiving fluconazole.
• Potential for injury related to a preexisting condition that contraindicates the use of fluconazole

• Potential for injury related to a preexisting condition that requires cautious use of fluconazole
• Potential for injury related to adverse drug reactions
• Potential fluid volume deficit related to the adverse GI effects of fluconazole
• Knowledge deficit related to fluconazole

Planning and implementation
• Do not administer fluconazole to a patient with a condition that contraindicates its use.
• Administer fluconazole cautiously to a patient at risk because of a preexisting condition.
• Monitor the patient periodically for adverse reactions during fluconazole therapy. Monitor for adverse reactions more frequently in a patient with a serious disorder, such as leukemia, cancer, or AIDS.
• Monitor the patient's laboratory test results to detect elevations in AST, ALT, alkaline phosphorous, bilirubin, BUN, and creatinine levels. Notify the physician of any abnormal results. *Adjust the dosage of one or both drugs as prescribed if the patient displays abnormal laboratory test results during concomitant administration of drugs known to interact with fluconazole.*
• Monitor the patient who develops a rash during fluconazole therapy. Be prepared to discontinue fluconazole if symptoms continue.
• Administer a mild analgesic as prescribed for a fluconazole-induced headache.
• *Expect to administer a low dose of fluconazole as prescribed to a patient with renal dysfunction.*
• *Do not administer an I.V. infusion of fluconazole greater than 200 mg/hr by continuous infusion.*
• Notify the physician if adverse reactions or drug interactions occur.
• Monitor hydration if the patient experiences nausea, vomiting, or diarrhea during fluconazole therapy. Administer an antiemetic or antidiarrheal agent as prescribed. Expect to switch from an oral to a parenteral form if nausea and vomiting prevents oral administration.
• Notify the physician if adverse GI reactions persist or worsen.

Patient teaching
• Teach the patient and family the name, dose, frequency, action, and adverse effects of fluconazole.
• Teach the patient the importance of having routine blood tests performed as instructed when taking drugs known to interact with fluconazole.
• *Instruct the patient on bleeding precautions during concomitant therapy with warfarin, which may increase the prothrombin time.*
• *Instruct the diabetic patient to monitor the blood glucose level regularly and to watch for signs and symptoms of hypoglycemia (profuse sweating, nervousness, irritability,*

headache) when taking glyburide or glipizide concomitantly with fluconazole.
• Teach the patient the importance of complying with drug therapy.
• Instruct the patient to report adverse reactions to the physician.

Evaluation

The following examples represent appropriate evaluation statements for a patient receiving fluconazole.
• The patient has no conditions that contraindicate fluconazole therapy.
• The patient exhibits no signs of complications in the preexisting condition linked to fluconazole.
• The patient exhibits no adverse reactions to fluconazole.
• The patient maintains adequate hydration throughout fluconazole therapy.
• The patient and family express an accurate understanding of the points taught about fluconazole.
• The patient correctly identifies the adverse reactions to report to the physician.

OTHER ANTIMYCOTIC AGENTS

Several other antimycotic agents offer alternative forms of treatment for topical fungal infections. These agents are effective against susceptible fungi and typically produce only mild, local adverse reactions.

Before ketoconazole was developed, griseofulvin was the only oral antimycotic agent available for effectively treating dermatophytic infections. In 1939, researchers isolated griseofulvin from *Penicillium griseofulvum.* Nearly 20 years later, physicians began to use the drug to treat fungal infections. Today, griseofulvin remains an important antimycotic agent for treating nonsystemic fungal infections. It is available in two oral forms—microsize and ultramicrosize—and is used to treat infections of the skin and nails.

Ciclopirox olamine, econazole nitrate, haloprogin, butoconazole, naftiline hydrochloride, tioconazole, terconazole, carbol-fushsin solution, tolnaftate, and undecylenic acid are available only as topical agents. (For information about these drugs, see the appendix on Integumentary Agents.) Agents briefly discussed here include griseofulvin, clotrimazole, and miconazole.

clotrimazole (Gyne-Lotrimin, Mycelex). An imidazole derivative, clotrimazole resembles miconazole and ketoconazole in chemical structure. It is used topically to treat dermatophyte and *C. albicans* infections, orally to treat oral candidiasis, and vaginally to treat vaginal candidiasis.

Adverse reactions to the oral troches are most common and may include elevated liver function test results, nausea, and vomiting. Adverse reactions to topical clotrimazole include localized blistering, stinging, pruritus, erythema, urticaria, and peeling.

griseofulvin. Available in microsize form (Fulvicin-U/F, Grifulvin V, Grisactin) and in ultramicrosize form (Fulvicin P/G, Grisactin-Ultra, Gris-PEG), griseofulvin is used to treat fungal infections of the skin on the body in general (tinea corporis), feet (tinea pedis), groin (tinea cruris), and beard area (tinea barbae), and infections of the nails (tinea unguium) and scalp (tinea capitis). However, it is less effective against nail infections than skin infections.

To prevent a relapse, griseofulvin therapy must continue until the fungus is eradicated completely and the infected skin or nails are replaced. Because the infected areas grow at different rates, the duration of therapy varies with the site of infection. For example, the duration of therapy is 4 to 6 weeks for tinea capitis, 4 to 8 weeks for tinea pedis, 4 months or more for tinea unguium of the fingernails, and 6 months or more for tinea unguium of the toenails.

Most patients tolerate griseofulvin well. When adverse reactions occur, they usually include nausea, vomiting, diarrhea, fatigue, confusion, and headaches. Headaches are common and can be severe, especially at the beginning of therapy, but they usually disappear as therapy continues. Other adverse reactions may include flatulence and excessive thirst.

Rarely, griseofulvin may cause such reactions as proteinuria, urticaria, rash, serum sickness (a hypersensitivity reaction), photosensitivity, hearing loss, paresthesia, dizziness, insomnia, and leukopenia. It even may cause oral candidiasis.

miconazole (Monistat) and **miconazole nitrate** (Micatin, Monistat 3, Monistat 7). An imidazole derivative, miconazole is used to treat systemic fungal infections, such as coccidioidomycosis, paracoccidioidomycosis, cryptococcosis, and candidiasis; local fungal infections, such as vulvovaginal candidiasis; and topical fungal infections, such as chronic mucocutaneous candidiasis. The drug may be administered I.V. or intrathecally to treat fungal meningitis, I.V. or in bladder irrigations to treat fungal bladder infections, locally to treat vaginal infections, and topically to treat topical infections.

In most cases, miconazole is less effective than amphotericin B for treating systemic fungal infections. Therefore, it usually is reserved for patients who cannot tolerate amphotericin B.

Miconazole may prolong prothrombin time in a patient receiving an oral anticoagulant. It also may antagonize the

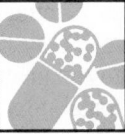

Antimycotic agents

The following chart summarizes the major antimycotic agents currently in clinical use.

DRUG	MAJOR INDICATIONS	USUAL ADULT DOSAGES	CONTRAINDICATIONS AND PRECAUTIONS
amphotericin B	Life-threatening systemic fungal infections and meningitis	0.25 to 1.5 mg/kg/day I.V. infused over 4 to 6 hours	• Know that amphotericin B is contraindicated in a lactating patient or one with known hypersensitivity to the drug. • Administer with caution to a pregnant patient.
	Candidal infection of the bladder	50 mg in 1 liter sterile water continuously or intermittently instilled into the bladder	
	Coccidioidal meningitis and cryptococcal meningitis	0.025 to 1 mg intrathecally two to three times weekly	
nystatin	Oral or esophageal candidiasis	500,000 units of oral suspension, gargled and then swallowed, t.i.d. or q.i.d., or 500,000 units of oral tablets, dissolved in the mouth, t.i.d. or q.i.d. for 10 days or until 48 hours after overt symptoms have subsided	• Know that nystatin is contraindicated in a patient with known hypersensitivity to the drug.
	Vaginal candidiasis	100,000 units inserted vaginally once or twice daily for 14 days or longer	
	Intestinal candidiasis	500,000 to 1 million units of oral tablets t.i.d. or q.i.d.	
ketoconazole	Systemic, subcutaneous, and superficial fungal infections	200 to 400 mg P.O. daily for 1 week to 12 months, depending on the organism and the infection site	• Know that ketoconazole is contraindicated in a lactating patient or one with known hypersensitivity to the drug. • Administer with caution to a pregnant patient.
flucytosine	Fungal infections caused by *Candida* or *Cryptococcus*; commonly used in combination with amphotericin B	50 to 150 mg/kg P.O. daily divided in four equal doses and administered every 6 hours	• Know that flucytosine is contraindicated in a lactating patient or one with known hypersensitivity to the drug. • Administer with extreme caution to a patient with impaired renal function or bone marrow depression. • Administer with caution to a pregnant patient.
fluconazole	Oropharyngeal candidiasis	200 mg P.O. or I.V. on the first day, followed by 100 mg daily for 2 weeks	• Know that fluconazole is contraindicated in a patient with known hypersensitivity to the drug or any of its ingredients. • Administer with caution to a pregnant or lactating patient.
	Esophageal candidiasis	200 mg P.O. or I.V. on the first day, followed by 100 mg for a minimum of 3 weeks and for at least 2 weeks following resolution of symptoms	
	Systemic candidiasis	400 mg P.O. or I.V. on the first day, followed by 200 mg daily for a minimum of 4 weeks	
	Cryptococcal meningitis	400 mg P.O. or I.V. on the first day, followed by 200 mg daily for 10 to 12 weeks after the cerebrospinal fluid culture becomes negative	

antimycotic effects of amphotericin B, contraindicating concomitant use of the two drugs.

The lipid vehicle in I.V. miconazole produces most of the significant adverse reactions to the drug, including phlebitis, pruritus, nausea, fever, chills, rash, and hyperlipidemia. These reactions, especially severe pruritus and hyperlipidemia, are more common in patients receiving high doses. When phlebitis occurs, it can be severe, and effective administration may require replacement of the peripheral line with a central venous catheter.

Other reactions to miconazole may include thrombocytopenia, anemia, hypersensitivity reactions, diarrhea, anorexia, and flushing. Intravenous administration of miconazole may produce cardiac arrhythmias, tachypnea, and cardiopulmonary arrest.

CHAPTER SUMMARY

Chapter 62 covered antimycotic (antifungal) agents as they are used to treat topical and systemic fungal infections. Here are the chapter highlights.

• The antimycotic agents used to treat systemic fungal infections include amphotericin B, miconazole, ketoconazole, flucytosine, and fluconazole. Nystatin, clotrimazole, and griseofulvin are used primarily to treat topical infections. Ketoconazole and miconazole also may be used for topical infections.

• Amphotericin B, a polyene antimycotic agent, is the most widely used antimycotic for severe systemic fungal infections. It usually is administered I.V. in D_5W or sterile water. Certain adverse reactions, however, limit its parenteral use. These include nephrotoxicity, phlebitis, hematologic effects, electrolyte imbalances, and immediate reactions, such as fever, chills, vomiting, muscle and joint pain, headache, weight loss, and dyspepsia. With long-term amphotericin B therapy, phlebitis may occur. Because of these adverse reactions and certain drug interactions, parenteral amphotericin B therapy requires close monitoring.

• Like amphotericin B, nystatin is a polyene antimycotic agent. Unlike amphotericin B, however, it cannot be given parenterally or used to treat systemic infections. Instead, it is administered as a tablet or suspension to treat oral,

vaginal, and intestinal candidiasis. Its adverse reactions may affect the GI tract and the skin.

• Flucytosine, an oral antimycotic agent, usually is given with amphotericin B to treat severe systemic fungal infections. Because this antimetabolite antimycotic increases the effects of amphotericin B, the patient can receive lower amphotericin B doses, decreasing the risk of adverse reactions. The most significant adverse reaction to flucytosine—bone marrow depression—can be severe enough to require drug discontinuation and usually occurs when the drug reaches a high serum concentration. A patient with renal impairment will need dosage adjustments to prevent a toxic serum concentration.

• Ketoconazole, an oral imidazole antimycotic agent, is used to treat topical and systemic fungal infections. Interactions between ketoconazole and other drugs may prevent ketoconazole absorption or alter the effectiveness of the other drug. A patient receiving ketoconazole as part of combination drug therapy requires close monitoring.

• Fluconazole is the first of a new class of synthetic, broad-spectrum bistriazole antifungal agents. It is used to treat oropharyngeal and esophageal candidiasis and serious systemic candidal infections, including urinary tract infections, peritonitis, pneumonia, and cryptococcal meningitis.

• Clotrimazole may be administered topically, orally, or vaginally to treat topical dermatophyte and candidal infections.

• Before the introduction of ketoconazole, griseofulvin was the only systemic antimycotic agent available for treating topical dermatophytic infections.

• For severe systemic fungal infections, miconazole offers one major advantage over amphotericin B: It does not cause nephrotoxicity. Infusion of I.V. miconazole can lead to significant adverse reactions, including phlebitis, pruritus, nausea, fever, chills, rash, or hyperlipidemia.

• When caring for a patient receiving antimycotic therapy, the nurse should monitor closely for adverse reactions, which may be severe. The nurse also should teach the patient how to administer the specific drug and form prescribed.

STUDY QUESTIONS

See Appendix 1 for answers.

1. Mark Hassam, age 45, is admitted with a tentative diagnosis of cryptococcosis. His physician prescribes an initial test dose of 1 mg of amphotericin B (Fungizone) in

250 ml of D₅W infused over 2 to 4 hours, followed by gradual dosage increases. Which factor limits the use of amphotericin B to life-threatening infections?
(a) high cost of the drug
(b) highly toxic effects
(c) large doses required to treat fungal infections
(d) high incidence of resistant infections

2. The nurse should assess Mr. Hassam for adverse reactions. Which of the following adverse reactions do most patients experience when receiving I.V. amphotericin B?
(a) anuria
(b) coagulation defects
(c) peripheral neuropathies
(d) normochromic or normocytic anemia

3. Which electrolyte disorder might Mr. Hassam develop during amphotericin B therapy?
(a) hypokalemia
(b) hypocalcemia
(c) hyponatremia
(d) hyperchloridemia

4. Which antimycotic agent may be administered with amphotericin B to reduce amphotericin B dosage and toxicity?
(a) nystatin
(b) flucytosine
(c) ketoconazole
(d) griseofulvin

5. After taking penicillin for strep throat, Ellen Brown, age 20, develops thrush (oral candidiasis). Her physician prescribes oral nystatin. Which instructions should the nurse give Ms. Brown about nystatin administration?
(a) Swallow the tablet whole.
(b) Chew the tablet thoroughly.
(c) Dissolve the tablet in the mouth.
(d) Dissolve the tablet in warm water and drink it.

6. Ms. Brown's symptoms abate after 72 hours of treatment. She asks the nurse if she still needs to take nystatin. How should the nurse respond?
(a) Stop taking the medication immediately.
(b) Continue the medication for the full length of time prescribed.
(c) Stop the medication, but resume treatment if symptoms recur.
(d) Halve the dosage and continue for the full length of time prescribed.

7. Glen Rubin is given ketoconazole for oral candidiasis. How long should Mr. Rubin take ketoconazole?
(a) 1 to 4 weeks
(b) 1 to 2 months
(c) 6 to 12 months
(d) indefinitely

8. Which new antimycotic agent could Mr. Rubin's physician prescribe instead of ketoconazole to treat oral candidiasis?
(a) fluconazole
(b) miconazole
(c) griseofulvin
(d) clotrimazole

SELECTED REFERENCES

AHFS drug information 90. (1990). Bethesda, MD: American Society of Hospital Pharmacists.

Conte, Jr., J., and Barriere, S. (1988). *Manual of antibiotics and infectious diseases* (6th ed.). Philadelphia: Lea & Febiger.

Drug facts and comparisons. (1991). St. Louis: Facts and Comparisons Division, Lippincott.

Farrington, E. (1990). Fluconazole. *Pediatric Nursing,* 16(4), 376-377.

Fluconazole certain to win FDA approval, researchers say. (1989). *AIDS Alert,* 4(5), 88-91.

Goodman and Gilman's the pharmacological basis of therapeutics (8th ed.; 1990). Elmsford, NY: Pergamon Press.

Holtzclaw, B., et al. (1990). Use of amphotericin B in immunosuppressed patients with cancer: Pharmacodynamics and nursing implications. *Oncology Nursing Forum,* 17(5), 737-742.

Kucers, A., and Bennett, N. (1987). *The use of antibiotics* (4th ed.). Philadelphia: J.B. Lippincott.

North American Nursing Diagnosis Association (1990). *Taxonomy I - Revised, with official diagnostic categories.* St. Louis, NANDA.

Rutledge, D., et al. (1990). Use of amphotericin B in immunosuppressed patients with cancer: Pharmacology and toxicities. *Oncology Nursing Forum,* 17(5), 731-736.

USPDI. (1991). *Drug information for the health care professional* (Vol. I, 11th ed.). Rockville, MD: United States Pharmacopeial Convention.

ANTHELMINTIC AGENTS

OBJECTIVES

After reading and studying this chapter, the student should be able to:

1. Explain the physiology of helminth infections, distinguishing among nematodes, cestodes, and trematodes.

2. Identify the antinematode, anticestode, and antitrematode agents.

3. Explain how the pharmacokinetics of these anthelmintic agents relates to their effectiveness.

4. Describe the mechanisms of action of the various anthelmintic agents.

5. Compare the indications and contraindications of the different classes of anthelmintic agents.

6. Discuss the common adverse reactions to anthelmintic agents.

7. Describe how to apply the nursing process when caring for a patient who is receiving an anthelmintic agent.

INTRODUCTION

Anthelmintic agents destroy helminths—parasitic worms that infect humans. They are divided into three groups: nematodes (roundworms); and two groups of flatworms, the cestodes (tapeworms) and the trematodes (flukes). Thus, the anthelmintic agents are classified as antinematode, anticestode, and antitrematode.

Although commonly believed to exist solely in tropic and subtropic areas, helminths are everywhere, and conservative estimates indicate that one-fourth of the world's population is infected with them. The most commonly encountered helminth infection in North America is childhood enterobiasis, or pinworm infection. Hookworm, whipworm, tapeworm, and threadworm infections occur occasionally in adults and children living in the southern United States. Helminth infections also are found in recent immigrants and tourists from areas of the world where such infections are endemic.

Anthelmintic agents are a varied group. Their only common link is their effectiveness against helminth infec-

tion. Many were discovered by chance; others were first used in veterinary medicine, then adapted for human use. Some anthelmintics are highly toxic, so positive helminth identification is imperative before treatment begins. Because of frequent patient reinfection and noncompliance, treatment must be repeated in many cases, usually with the same agent. (Secondary drugs commonly are less specific and more toxic than the drug of choice.)

Chapter 63 discusses anthelmintic agents currently used in North America, grouped according to the particular helminth group they combat most effectively. These agents include mebendazole, piperazine citrate, pyrantel pamoate, and thiabendazole (antinematode agents); mebendazole, niclosamide, paromomycin sulfate, and praziquantel (anticestode agents); and oxamniquine and praziquantel (antitrematode agents).

Physiology of helminth infection

Helminths are multicellular parasitic worms that vary in size from inches to yards. The nematodes, or roundworms, are cylindrical and elongated with tapered ends. The cestodes, or tapeworms, have heads with suckers and flattened bodies with distinct segments known as proglottides. The trematodes, or flukes, have flattened, unsegmented bodies that may be leaflike in shape. They are classified as blood, intestinal, lung, or liver flukes depending on their infection sites in the human host.

Helminths can infect humans by ingestion, skin penetration, or injection by insects. The means of infection has no particular relation to their classification. The life cycles of the helminths vary from simple to complex and are helpful in understanding the pathophysiology and treatment of infection. The signs and symptoms of helminth infection are specific for each helminth and infection site and reflect disturbances of the affected organ or body system including: tissue invasion and destruction, toxin production, obstruction, competition for host nutrients, and hypersensitivity.

For a summary of representative drugs, see *Selected major drugs: Anthelmintic agents,* page 1105. For a listing of applicable nursing diagnoses that the nurse may formulate when caring for a patient receiving these agents, see *Selected nursing diagnoses: Anthelmintic agents*. For detailed information on applying the nursing process, see Chapter 6, The Nursing Process and Drug Therapy.

ANTINEMATODE AGENTS

The four drugs with specific antiparasitic action against nematodes, or roundworms, are mebendazole, piperazine, pyrantel pamoate, and thiabendazole.

PHARMACOKINETICS

Antinematode agents have individually distinctive pharmacokinetic properties.

Absorption, distribution, metabolism, excretion

Less than 10% of an oral mebendazole dose is absorbed from the gastrointestinal (GI) tract; the remainder is excreted unchanged in the feces. The absorbed drug is metabolized by the liver and excreted unchanged in the urine. It is distributed well and crosses the placenta. Distribution into breast milk is unknown.

Like mebendazole, pyrantel pamoate is absorbed poorly from the GI tract. The absorbed drug is metabolized partially in the liver. Approximately 50% of an oral dose is excreted unchanged in the feces, and about 7% is excreted in the urine as the parent compound and its metabolites. Because these two drugs stay in the GI tract, they are particularly effective against roundworms that infect the intestines.

Piperazine is absorbed readily after oral administration and is distributed widely. Approximately 25% is metabolized in the liver, but most of a piperazine dose is excreted unchanged in the urine.

Thiabendazole is absorbed rapidly and almost completely from the GI tract. It is distributed widely in the body, metabolized rapidly by the liver, and excreted by the kidneys.

Onset, peak, duration

For anthelmintic agents, the onset of action varies and depends on when the agent comes in contact with the helminth. This in turn depends on the rate of drug uptake, which varies greatly between infected tissues, such as the lungs and liver.

The peak concentration level and duration of action have little effect on an agent's anthelmintic action. However, these pharmacokinetic processes affect the extent of systemic drug absorption, which determines whether toxic effects occur.

Peak plasma concentrations of the antinematode agents have a wider than usual range, particularly with oral mebendazole, which reaches peak plasma concentration in 0.5 to 7 hours after oral administration. Its half-life is 2.8 to 9 hours. Pyrantel pamoate achieves a peak plasma concentration in 1 to 3 hours. Because approximately 50% of pyrantel pamoate is eliminated unchanged in the feces, its elimination time depends on bowel transit time. Plasma concentration of piperazine after oral administration is unknown. The drug is excreted in the urine within 24 hours. Thiabendazole reaches a peak plasma concentration within 1 to 2 hours after oral administration, and has a half-life of 1.2 to 1.7 hours. About 90% of an oral dose is eliminated from the body within 24 to 48 hours.

PHARMACODYNAMICS

The pharmacodynamic effects of the antinematode agents are diverse and include several mechanisms of action, most not understood fully. Antinematode agents immobilize or kill roundworms by impairing their ability to use energy from available sources or by interfering with their nervous systems. Then the immobilized or dead roundworms are eliminated from the GI tract by peristalsis.

Mechanism of action

Mebendazole interferes with the microtubule system of the roundworm, preventing glucose uptake and distribution. As a result, the parasite depletes its energy stores and is immobilized or dies. It is expelled from the GI tract within several days. Piperazine paralyzes the roundworm by blocking the neurotransmitter acetylcholine at the myoneural junction, causing flaccid paralysis. Unable to counter peristalsis, the paralyzed roundworm is expelled from the GI tract. Pyrantel pamoate also acts by interfering with the neuromuscular transmission of the roundworm, causing spastic paralysis by a process similar to that of the depolarizing neuromuscular blocking agents. Like mebendazole, thiabendazole acts on microtubules; it inhibits the action of fumarate reductase, an enzyme critical to the anaerobic metabolism of the roundworm.

PHARMACOTHERAPEUTICS

The rule of thumb in treating nematode infection is to continue using the drug of choice for the particular invading organism until the organism is eradicated or the drug clearly has failed to eradicate it. Alternative choices are characteristically more toxic to the patient. Realistic cure rates range from 70% to 100%, depending on the drug and the type of roundworm. Repeat treatment commonly is necessary because of patient noncompliance or reinfection.

Mebendazole has broad anthelmintic activity and is the drug of choice against infection with *Trichuris trichiura* (whipworm), *Enterobius vermicularis* (pinworm), *Necator americanus* (hookworm), and *Ascaris lumbricoides* (giant intestinal roundworm). Mebendazole has been tried with some success in patients with hydatid disease (systemic infection) from *Echinococcus granulosus*, a liver tapeworm. Mebendazole's chief advantage is low systemic toxicity because of its limited absorption.

Piperazine no longer is recommended as a first-line drug for treating roundworm infections; other agents are more effective and less toxic. It is used primarily as an alternative mebendazole in patients with large *Ascaris* infections that cause intestinal blockage. Pyrantel pamoate is an alternative drug of choice for treating a number of nematode infections, including giant intestinal roundworm, hookworm, and pinworm infections. It has the advantage of one-time dosage for roundworm and pinworm infections.

Thiabendazole is the drug of choice to treat threadworm infection and also acts as an anti-inflammatory agent in trichinosis (caused by the nematode *Trichinella spiralis*).

mebendazole (Vermox). Available in 100-mg tablets, mebendazole may be administered before or after meals; tablets should be chewed to enhance the drug's efficacy. Mebendazole is used primarily to treat roundworm infections.
Usual adult and pediatric dosage: for *Ascaris* (giant intestinal roundworm), *Trichuris* (whipworm), and *Necator* (hookworm) infections, 100 mg P.O. b.i.d. for 3 days, may be repeated in 2 to 3 weeks; for *Enterobius* (pinworm) infection, one 100-mg tablet, repeated in 2 to 3 weeks. The dosage for children under age 2 has not been established.

piperazine citrate (Antepar). Piperazine is a secondary agent for all nematode infections, but principally for large *Ascaris* infections that cause intestinal blockage. It should be used cautiously in a patient with epilepsy.
Usual adult and pediatric dosage: for *Ascaris* infection, 75 mg/kg (up to a maximum of 3.5 grams/day) P.O. as a single dose for 2 days.

pyrantel pamoate (Antiminth). Available as an oral suspension, pyrantel pamoate is used as an alternative drug to treat nematode infections (hookworm, pinworm, and giant intestinal roundworm). It should be used cautiously in a patient with hepatic disease.
Usual adult and pediatric dosage: 11 mg/kg (up to a maximum 1 gram/day) P.O. as a one-time dose; may be repeated in 2 to 3 weeks if needed. The dosage for children under age 2 has not been established.

thiabendazole (Mintezol). Although effective against all nematodes, thiabendazole is highly toxic and therefore is the drug of choice for *Strongyloides stercoralis* (threadworm) infections only; it is used to treat other nematode infections only when the drug of choice clearly has failed.
Usual adult and pediatric dosage: for *S. stercoralis* infections, 25 mg/kg (up to a maximum of 3 grams/day) P.O. b.i.d. for 2 days, or 1.5 grams P.O. b.i.d for patients who weigh 155 lb (70 kg) or more; for trichinosis, 25 mg/kg (up to a maximum of 3 grams/day) P.O. b.i.d. for 2 to 5 days.

Drug interactions

As a group, antinematode agents are associated with few drug interactions. No special interactions between antinematode agents and food exist.

The most important potential interaction is between piperazine and pyrantel pamoate and relates to their mechanisms of action. Because piperazine causes flaccid paralysis and pyrantel pamoate causes spastic paralysis, the possibility exists that they could cancel each other's effect if administered together. In high concentrations, piperazine may increase extrapyramidal effects and the potential for seizures in patients also receiving phenothiazines. Carbamazepine and phenytoin may increase mebendazole metabolism. Use of alternative anticonvulsants should be considered for patients receiving mebendazole for extraintestinal infections. Thiabendazole may interfere with the hepatic metabolism of theophylline. The theophylline plasma concentration should be monitored if concomitant administration occurs.

ADVERSE DRUG REACTIONS

Almost all the antinematode agents cause adverse GI reactions ranging from abdominal pain to nausea, vomiting, and diarrhea. Other adverse reactions are less common. For example, mebendazole rarely may cause leukopenia, and piperazine occasionally causes headache, vertigo, and loss of coordination. Piperazine also may lower the seizure threshold, so it should not be used with phenothiazines or other drugs that have the same effect, particularly in patients with epilepsy. Pyrantel pamoate and thiabendazole sometimes cause headache, dizziness, drowsiness, and weakness; thiabendazole also may cause rash and hallucinations and rare occurrences of tinnitus and seizures.

NURSING PROCESS APPLICATION

The following information assists the nurse in caring for a patient who is receiving an antinematode agent.

Assessment
• Review the patient's history for a preexisting condition that contraindicates the use of an antinematode agent, such as known hypersensitivity to the drug.
• Review the patient's history for a preexisting condition that requires cautious use of an antinematode agent, such as hepatic or renal dysfunction or epilepsy.
• Assess the patient for adverse reactions to the prescribed antinematode agent, such as GI distress, central nervous system (CNS) disturbances, and rash.
• Review the patient's medication history to identify the use of drugs that may interact with the prescribed antinematode agent, such as phenothiazines, carbamazepine, phenytoin, or theophylline.
• Assess the effectiveness of the prescribed antinematode agent periodically.

• Assess the patient for fluid volume deficit if adverse GI reactions, such as nausea, vomiting, or diarrhea, occur with antinematode use.
• Evaluate the patient's and family's knowledge about the prescribed antinematode agent.

Nursing diagnoses
The following examples represent appropriate nursing diagnoses for a patient receiving an antinematode agent.
• Potential for injury related to a preexisting condition that contraindicates the use of an antinematode agent
• Potential for injury related to a preexisting condition that requires cautious use of an antinematode agent
• Potential for injury related to adverse drug reactions
• Potential fluid volume deficit related to the adverse GI effects of the prescribed antinematode agent
• Knowledge deficit related to the prescribed antinematode agent

Planning and implementation
• Do not administer an antinematode agent to a patient with a condition that contraindicates its use.
• Administer an antinematode agent cautiously to a patient at risk because of a preexisting condition.
• Monitor the patient periodically for adverse reactions during antinematode therapy.
• *Ensure that all family members are treated because pinworm and other nematode infections otherwise can recur.*
• Administer a mild analgesic as prescribed if the patient experiences a headache caused by antinematode therapy.
• Take safety measures if the patient experiences such CNS disturbances as vertigo, dizziness, drowsiness, or loss of coordination. For example, place the bed in the lowest position, keep the bed rails raised, and supervise the patient's activities.
• Inspect the patient's skin for a rash when administering thiabendazole.
• Monitor the patient's theophylline level if thiabendazole and theophylline are administered concomitantly.
• Monitor for increased extrapyramidal effects in a patient receiving a phenothiazene and piperazine concomitantly.
• Shake the container well before administering pyrantel pamoate or thiabendazole to ensure even dispersion of the agent in suspension.
• Notify the physician if adverse reactions or drug interactions occur.
• Monitor hydration if the patient experiences nausea, vomiting, or diarrhea during antinematode therapy. Obtain a prescription for an antiemetic or antidiarrheal agent as needed.
• Notify the physician if adverse GI reactions persist or worsen.

Patient teaching

• Teach the patient and family the name, dose, frequency, action, and adverse effects of the prescribed antinematode agent.

• *Instruct the patient receiving mebendazole or thiabendazole tablets to chew them for greatest effectiveness.*

• *Instruct the patient to change and wash underclothes and bedding daily until the nematodes are eradicated. Explain that washing the perineal area daily and the hands and fingernails after each bowel movement also will reduce the risk of reinfection.*

• Instruct the patient to take thiabendazole doses immediately after meals to minimize GI distress.

• Inform the patient that thiabendazole may make urine smell like asparagus but that the odor has no medical significance.

• *Teach the patient the importance of compliance with the antinematode regimen to prevent treatment failure.*

• Caution the patient not to perform any activity that requires mental alertness or physical coordination if adverse CNS reactions occur.

• Instruct the patient to notify the physician if adverse reactions occur.

Evaluation

The following examples represent appropriate evaluation statements for a patient receiving an antinematode agent.

• The patient has no conditions that contraindicate antinematode therapy.

• The patient exhibits no signs of complications in the preexisting condition linked to the prescribed antinematode.

• The patient exhibits no adverse reactions to the prescribed antinematode.

• The patient maintains normal hydration throughout antinematode therapy.

• The patient and family express an accurate understanding of the points taught about the prescribed antinematode.

• The patient correctly describes personal hygiene measures to use during antinematode therapy.

ANTICESTODE AGENTS

All cestode, or tapeworm, infections are acquired by ingestion and most are confined to the intestinal tract. The exception is *E. granulosus,* which causes hydatid disease with cystic lesions of the liver. If surgery, the treatment of choice, is not indicated, high-dose, long-term mebendazole therapy may cure or suppress the infection. Although its use for this disorder remains experimental in the United States, recent reports suggest that it is an effective treatment.

Two other agents, niclosamide and paromomycin sulfate, are used as anticestodes. Niclosamide acts specifically against tapeworm infection. Paromomycin, an aminoglycoside with antiamoebic action, also acts against tapeworms, although this use is considered experimental by the Food and Drug Administration (FDA). A fourth agent, praziquantel, currently is used to treat trematode (fluke) infections, but is gaining wider use for treating tapeworms. The FDA, however, considers this use investigational.

PHARMACOKINETICS

The pharmacokinetics of anticestode agents vary among the drugs. Less than 10% of an oral mebendazole dose is absorbed from the GI tract; the remainder is excreted unchanged in the feces. The absorbed drug is metabolized by the liver and excreted unchanged in the urine. It is distributed well and crosses the placenta. Oral mebendazole reaches a peak plasma concentration level from 0.5 to 7 hours after administration. Its half-life is 2.8 to 9 hours.

Niclosamide and paromomycin are absorbed negligibly from the GI tract. Therefore, their action against tapeworm infection remains confined to the intestinal tract. Because both drugs act locally in the GI tract, little systemic absorption occurs. Their onset of action, peak concentration, and duration of action vary greatly among individuals and indicate only the pharmacokinetics of the systemically absorbed drug. Neither drug is metabolized in the liver. Limited information suggests that niclosamide may be metabolized in the GI tract. Both drugs are excreted in the feces.

Praziquantel is absorbed readily (over 80%) after oral administration. It is distributed widely, crossing the blood-brain barrier. Praziquantel undergoes hepatic metabolism, and its metabolites are excreted in the urine. It reaches a peak concentration within 1 to 3 hours and has a plasma half-life of 0.8 to 1.5 hours for the parent compound.

PHARMACODYNAMICS

Mebendazole interferes with the microtubule system of the tapeworm, thus preventing glucose uptake and distribution. As a result, the tapeworm depletes its energy stores and is immobilized or dies.

Niclosamide and paromomycin have differing mechanisms of action. Niclosamide interferes with the tapeworm's ability to convert food into energy, either by inhibiting oxidative phosphorylation or by enhancing adenosine triphosphatase activity. Paromomycin is thought to inhibit the protein synthesis in the tapeworm by causing misreading of messenger ribonucleic acid.

Although the exact mechanism of praziquantel's activities against cestodes is unknown, the drug is thought to dislodge the worms from the intestines by impairing their suckers.

PHARMACOTHERAPEUTICS

Mebendazole is used experimentally to treat hydatid disease caused by *E. granulosus*. Niclosamide and praziquantel, the emerging drugs of choice, are similarly effective against all varieties of tapeworm infection. The adverse reactions they cause also are similar, however, so neither offers a clear advantage. Paromomycin is an alternative choice if the patient cannot tolerate niclosamide or praziquantel. However, it has a more complex dosage schedule and is considered experimental by the FDA for treating tapeworm infections.

mebendazole (Vermox). Primarily an antinematode agent, mebendazole also is used experimentally to treat hydatid disease caused by *E. granulosus* (liver tapeworm).
Usual adult and pediatric dosage: for liver tapeworm infection (hydatid disease), 40 mg/kg daily P.O. for 1 to 6 months or longer. The dosage for children under age 2 has not been established.

niclosamide (Niclocide). Active against all intestinal tapeworm species, niclosamide tablets should be chewed thoroughly and taken with water after a light meal.
Usual adult dosage: for *Hymenolepsis nana* (dwarf tapeworm) infection, 2 grams P.O. once daily for 7 days, or 2 grams P.O. for the first day and 1 gram P.O. for the next 6 days, repeated in 7 to 14 days, if needed; for *Taenia saginata* and *Taenia solium* infections, 2 grams P.O. as a single dose, repeated in 7 days if needed.
Usual pediatric dosage: for *H. nana,* 1 gram P.O. the first day and 500 mg P.O. the next 6 days for children who weigh from 11 to 34 kg, and 1.5 grams P.O. the first day and 1 gram P.O. the next 6 days (may be repeated in 7 to 14 days) for children who weigh more than 34 kg; for *T. saginata* or *T. solium* infections, 1 gram P.O. as a single dose for children who weigh from 11 to 34 kg, and 1.5 grams P.O. as a single dose (may be repeated in 7 days) for children who weigh more than 34 kg.

paromomycin sulfate (Humatin). The FDA considers paromomycin to be an investigational drug for treating tapeworm infections.
Usual adult dosage: for tapeworm infection, 1 gram P.O. every 15 minutes for 4 doses; for *H. nana* (dwarf tapeworm) infection, 45 mg/kg P.O. daily for 5 to 7 days.
Usual pediatric dosage: for tapeworm infection, 11 mg/kg P.O. every 15 minutes for 4 doses; for *H. nana* infection, 45 mg/kg P.O. daily for 5 to 7 days.

praziquantel (Biltricide). Primarily an antitrematode agent, praziquantel rapidly is becoming a drug of choice for treating tapeworm infections, although its use as such still is considered experimental by the FDA.
Usual adult and pediatric dosage: for *Taenia* infection, 10 to 20 mg/kg P.O. as a single dose; for *H. nana* infection, 25 mg/kg P.O. as a single dose that may be repeated in 1 to 2 weeks.

Drug interactions
No significant drug interactions involving niclosamide, praziquantel, or paromomycin are known to occur. Carbamazepine and phenytoin may increase mebendazole metabolism and decrease its efficacy.

ADVERSE DRUG REACTIONS

Adverse reactions to mebendazole include transient abdominal pain, diarrhea, and, rarely, neutropenia or leukopenia. Adverse reactions to niclosamide are uncommon. They include nausea and abdominal pain; rarely, a hypersensitivity-like reaction may occur, producing headache or vertigo.

The primary adverse reactions to paromomycin affect the GI tract and include anorexia, nausea, vomiting, cramps, and diarrhea. Secondary infection of the intestinal tract also may occur. Theoretically, paromomycin could cause aminoglycoside-like nephrotoxicity or ototoxicity in patients with renal impairment; however, this has not been reported.

Praziquantel causes transient dizziness, headache, malaise, abdominal pain or distention, and nausea in about 90% of patients. Drowsiness and fatigue also have been reported. In 3% to 27% of patients, praziquantel produces mild to moderate elevation of aspartate aminotransferase (AST, formerly SGOT) and alanine aminotransferase (ALT, formerly SGPT) levels. The drug also may cause macular rash with pruritus.

NURSING PROCESS APPLICATION

The following information assists the nurse in caring for a patient who is receiving an anticestode agent.

Assessment
• Review the patient's history for a preexisting condition that contraindicates the use of an anticestode agent, such as known hypersensitivity to the drug.
• Review the patient's history for a preexisting condition that requires cautious use of an anticestode agent, such as pregnancy.
• Assess the patient for adverse reactions to the prescribed anticestode agent, such as GI distress, secondary intestinal infection, or CNS disturbances.

• Review the patient's medication history to identify the use of drugs that may interact with mebendazole, such as carbamazepine and phenytoin.
• Assess the effectiveness of the prescribed anticestode agent periodically.
• Evaluate the patient's and family's knowledge about the prescribed anticestode agent.

Nursing diagnoses

The following examples represent appropriate nursing diagnoses for a patient receiving an anticestode agent.
• Potential for injury related to a preexisting condition that contraindicates the use of an anticestode agent
• Potential for injury related to a preexisting condition that requires cautious use of an anticestode agent
• Potential for injury related to adverse drug reactions
• Altered health maintenance related to ineffectiveness of the prescribed anticestode agent
• Knowledge deficit related to the prescribed anticestode agent

Planning and implementation

• Do not administer an anticestode agent to a patient with a condition that contraindicates its use.
• Administer an anticestode agent cautiously to a patient at risk because of a preexisting condition.
• Monitor the patient periodically for adverse reactions during anticestode therapy.
• *Monitor hydration if the patient experiences adverse GI reactions, such as nausea, vomiting, and diarrhea. Obtain a prescription for an antiemetic or antidiarrheal agent as needed. Notify the physician if adverse GI reactions persist or worsen.*
• Monitor the complete blood count regularly for a patient on high-dose mebendazole therapy to detect neutropenia.
• Inspect the patient's skin for a rash during niclosamide or praziquantel therapy. Notify the physician if a rash is present because it may indicate a hypersensitivity reaction that requires discontinuation of the prescribed anticestode agent.
• Administer a mild analgesic as prescribed if the patient experiences a headache during niclosamide or praziquantel therapy.
• Take safety measures if the patient experiences adverse CNS reactions, such as drowsiness or dizziness during praziquantel therapy. For example, place the bed in the lowest position, keep the bed rails raised, and supervise the patient's activities.
• Notify the physician if adverse reactions occur.
• Monitor the patient's response to the prescribed anticestode agent regularly.
• Expect to switch the patient to paromomycin as prescribed if praziquantel or niclosamide is ineffective.

• Notify the physician if the patient's symptoms persist or worsen.

Patient teaching

• Teach the patient and family the name, dose, frequency, action, and adverse effects of the prescribed anticestode agent.
• *Instruct the patient to chew niclosamide tablets thoroughly and then drink water.*
• *Instruct the patient to take praziquantel tablets with meals to minimize adverse GI reactions. Explain that the tablets are bitter and should be swallowed quickly to prevent gagging or vomiting.*
• *Teach the patient the importance of compliance with anticestode therapy to prevent treatment failure.*
• Caution the patient to not perform activities that require mental alertness if adverse CNS reactions, such as dizziness, drowsiness, or vertigo, occur.
• Instruct the patient to notify the physician if nausea, vomiting, abdominal pain, rash, or CNS reactions occur.
• Instruct the patient to alert the physician if symptoms persist or worsen despite treatment.

Evaluation

The following examples represent appropriate evaluation statements for a patient receiving an anticestode agent.
• The patient has no conditions that contraindicate anticestode therapy.
• The patient exhibits no signs of complications in the preexisting condition linked to the prescribed anticestode agent.
• The patient exhibits no adverse reactions to the prescribed anticestode agent.
• The patient displays no signs or symptoms of cestode infection upon completion of treatment.
• The patient and family express an accurate understanding of the points taught about the prescribed anticestode agent.
• The patient correctly describes the adverse reactions that should be reported to the physician.

ANTITREMATODE AGENTS

Trematode, or fluke, infections are characterized according to their anatomic location: the blood, lungs, or liver. In endemic areas, fluke infections can be devastating, giving rise to many seemingly unrelated disorders, such as hepatic cirrhosis, esophageal varices, pulmonary fibrosis, and cor pulmonale. The two drugs available to treat fluke infections are oxamniquine and praziquantel.

PHARMACOKINETICS

Administered orally, oxamniquine and praziquantel are effective against systemic fluke infections.

Absorption, distribution, metabolism, excretion

After oral administration, oxamniquine is absorbed well from the GI tract, although the presence of food in the stomach interferes with the rate and amount of absorption. Oxamniquine is metabolized primarily by the intestinal mucosa or lumen and is excreted by the kidneys. The distribution of oxamniquine into body tissues and fluids has not been determined.

Praziquantel also is absorbed readily (over 80%) after oral administration. It is distributed widely, crossing the blood-brain barrier. Praziquantel undergoes hepatic metabolism, and its metabolites are excreted in the urine.

Onset, peak, duration

Oxamniquine reaches a peak plasma concentration level within 3 hours after oral administration. Its plasma half-life is 1 to 2.5 hours. Praziquantel reaches a peak concentration within 1 to 3 hours and has a plasma half-life of 0.8 to 1.5 hours for the parent compound. The antitrematode agents act locally. Therefore, their onset of action, peak concentration, and duration of action, which relate to systemic absorption, do not indicate their therapeutic effect.

PHARMACODYNAMICS

Praziquantel has a known mechanism of action; oxamniquine's mechanism of action remains largely unknown.

Mechanism of action

Oxamniquine's known anticholinergic activity does not explain its antitrematode action. The drug is known, however, to induce schistosomes (adult blood flukes) to migrate from the mesenteric veins into the liver, where they eventually die. Like the antinematode agent pyrantel pamoate, praziquantel causes spastic paralysis of the fluke's musculature, which eventually leads to disintegration.

PHARMACOTHERAPEUTICS

Oxamniquine is no longer a drug of choice to treat fluke infections. It is effective against only one variety of blood fluke, *Schistosoma mansoni,* and its adverse reactions are significant, though rare. Praziquantel has become the drug of choice for all fluke infections because of its broad spectrum of action.

oxamniquine (Vansil). Available as a 250-mg capsule, oxamniquine is indicated for *S. mansoni;* it is ineffective against the other blood fluke species and fluke infections.

Usual adult dosage: for Western Hemisphere strains, 12 to 15 mg/kg P.O. as a one-time dose; for African and Middle Eastern strains, 15 mg/kg P.O. b.i.d. for 1 day.
Usual pediatric dosage: for children who have Western Hemisphere strains and who weigh less than 30 kg, 10 mg/kg P.O. for two doses given 2 to 8 hours apart (the adult dosage applies for children who weigh 30 kg or more); for African and Middle Eastern strains, 15 mg/kg P.O. b.i.d. for 1 to 2 days.

praziquantel (Biltricide). The first highly effective, broad-spectrum antitrematode agent, praziquantel is the drug of choice for treating all fluke infections.
Usual adult and pediatric dosage: for *Schistosoma* infections, 20 mg/kg P.O. t.i.d. for 1 day; for *Paragonimus* infections, 25 mg/kg P.O. t.i.d. for 2 days; for *Clonorchis* infections, 25 mg/kg P.O. t.i.d. for 2 days. The dosage for children under age 4 has not been established.

Drug interactions

The only significant drug interaction with this class of drugs involves interaction between the two antitrematode agents. One animal study indicated that concomitant administration of oxamniquine and praziquantel may enhance their effectiveness against *S. mansoni.* This is a preliminary finding, however; more studies are needed to determine its clinical relevance.

ADVERSE DRUG REACTIONS

Oxamniquine and praziquantel have low human toxicity compared to their effects on target flukes. However, some patients may experience a hypersensitivity reaction to the drugs.

Oxamniquine produces mild, transient dizziness, drowsiness, and headache in 30% to 50% of patients. It causes adverse GI reactions, such as nausea, vomiting, and abdominal pain, in a smaller percentage of patients. However, the most significant adverse reaction to oxamniquine is rare CNS stimulation that leads to behavioral changes, seizures, or hallucinations. (The seizures usually occur in patients with a history of epilepsy.) Oxamniquine also causes orange-red urine that has no clinical significance but may alarm the patient and interfere with laboratory tests based on spectrometry or color reactions.

Up to 90% of patients receiving praziquantel experience dizziness, headache, malaise, drowsiness, fatigue, and GI disturbances, such as nausea and abdominal pain or discomfort. From 3% to 27% of patients display a mild to moderate, transient increase in AST and ALT levels. Praziquantel also may cause macular rash with pruritus.

NURSING PROCESS APPLICATION

The following information assists the nurse in caring for a patient who is receiving an antitrematode agent.

Assessment
• Review the patient's history for a preexisting condition that contraindicates the use of an antitrematode agent, such as lactation, ocular cysticercosis, or known hypersensitivity to the drug.
• Review the patient's history for a preexisting condition that requires cautious use of an antitrematode agent, such as pregnancy.
• Assess the patient for adverse reactions to the prescribed antitrematode agent, such as GI distress or hypersensitivity reactions.
• Review the patient's medication history to identify whether both antitrematode drugs are being used concomitantly; they may interact with each other.
• Assess the effectiveness of the prescribed antitrematode agent peroidically.
• Assess the patient for adverse CNS reactions periodically.
• Evaluate the patient's and family's knowledge about the prescribed antitrematode agent.

Nursing diagnoses
The following examples represent appropriate nursing diagnoses for a patient receiving an antitrematode agent.
• Potential for injury related to a preexisting condition that contraindicates the use of an antitrematode agent
• Potential for injury related to a preexisting condition that requires cautious use of an antitrematode agent
• Potential for injury related to adverse drug reactions
• Potential for trauma related to the adverse CNS effects of the prescribed antitrematode agent
• Knowledge deficit related to the prescribed antitrematode agent

Planning and implementation
• Do not administer an antitrematode agent to a patient with a condition that contraindicates its use.
• Administer an antitrematode agent cautiously to a patient at risk because of a preexisting condition.
• Monitor the patient periodically for adverse reactions during antitrematode therapy.
• Monitor hydration if the patient experiences nausea or diarrhea. Obtain a prescription for an antiemetic or antidiarrheal agent as needed.
• Administer a mild analgesic as prescribed if the patient experiences headaches during antitrematode therapy.
• Inspect the patient's skin for a macular rash when administering praziquantel, and question the patient about pruritus.

• *Note on any laboratory slip for urine tests that the patient is receiving oxamniquine because the drug may interfere with laboratory tests based on spectrometry or color reactions.*
• *Give oxamniquine as a single dose after meals to help prevent adverse GI reactions.*
• Notify the physician if adverse reactions occur.
• Monitor for adverse CNS reactions, such as drowsiness, dizziness, behavioral changes, seizures, or hallucinations, in the patient receiving oxamniquine. In the patient receiving praziquantel, monitor for these adverse CNS reactions: dizziness, headache, malaise, drowsiness, and fatitue.
• Take safety measures if the patient experiences adverse CNS reactions. For example, place the bed in the lowest position, keep the bed rails raised, and supervise the patient's activities. Also take for a patient who is receiving oxamniquine and has a history of epilepsy.
• Notify the physician if adverse CNS reactions occur.

Patient teaching
• Teach the patient and family the name, dose, frequency, action, and adverse effects of the prescribed antitrematode agent.
• Inform the patient that oxamniquine may turn the urine a harmless orange-red.
• *Caution the patient taking oxamniquine or praziquantel that drowsiness and dizziness may occur, necessitating curtailment of activities on the day of and day after treatment.*
• *Instruct the patient to take praziquantel with meals to minimize adverse reactions. Explain that the tablet is bitter and should be swallowed rapidly to avoid gagging or vomiting.*
• Instruct the patient to report any adverse reactions to the physician.

Evaluation
The following examples represent appropriate evaluation statements for a patient receiving an antitrematode agent.
• The patient has no conditions that contraindicate antitrematode therapy.
• The patient exhibits no signs of complications in the preexisting condition linked to the prescribed antitrematode agent.
• The patient exhibits no adverse reactions to the prescribed antitrematode agent.
• The patient experiences no injury or trauma when adverse CNS reactions occur.
• The patient and family express an accurate understanding of the points taught about the prescribed antitrematode agent.
• The patient correctly states when to take praziquantel.

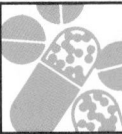

Anthelmintic agents

This chart summarizes the major anthelmintic agents currently in clinical use.

DRUG	MAJOR INDICATIONS	USUAL ADULT DOSAGES	CONTRAINDICATIONS AND PRECAUTIONS
Antinematode agents			
mebendazole	*Ascaris* (roundworm), *Trichuris* (whipworm), and *Necator* (hookworm) infections	100 mg P.O. b.i.d. for 3 days; may be repeated in 2 to 3 weeks	• Know that mebendazole is contraindicated in a pregnant patient or one with known hypersensitivity to the drug. • Administer with caution to a lactating patient.
	Enterobius (pinworm) infection	100 mg P.O. once; may be repeated in 2 to 3 weeks	
thiabendazole	*Strongyloides stercoralis* (threadworm) infection	25 mg/kg (maximum of 3 grams/day) P.O. b.i.d. for 2 days	• Know that thiabendazole is contraindicated in a lactating patient or one with known hypersensitivity to the drug. • Administer with caution to a pregnant patient or one with hepatic or renal dysfunction.
Anticestode agents			
niclosamide	*Hymenolepsis nana* infection	2 grams P.O. once daily for 7 days, or 2 grams P.O. for the first day and 1 gram P.O. for the next 6 days, repeated in 7 to 14 days, if needed.	• Know that niclosamide is contraindicated in a patient with known hypersensitivity to the drug. • Administer with caution to a pregnant patient.
	Taenia saginata and *Taenia solium* infections	2 grams P.O. as a single dose, repeated in 7 days if needed	
Antitrematode agents			
praziquantel	*Schistosoma* infections	20 mg/kg P.O. t.i.d. for 1 day	• Know that praziquantel is contraindicated in a lactating patient or one with ocular cystericercosis or known hypersensitivity to the drug. • Administer with caution to a pregnant patient.
	Paragonimus infections	25 mg/kg P.O. t.i.d. for 2 days	
	Clonorchis infections	25 mg/kg P.O. t.i.d. for 2 days	

CHAPTER SUMMARY

Chapter 63 discussed the anthelmintic agents as they are used to treat nematode (roundworm), cestode (tapeworm), and trematode (fluke) infections. Here are the chapter highlights.
• Anthelmintic agents are categorized according to the helminth groups they combat most effectively. The three major classes of anthelmintic agents are antinematode (antiroundworm), anticestode (antitapeworm), and antitrematode (antifluke) agents.

• Two anthelmintic agents are used to treat more than one type of helminth infection: mebendazole is used to treat roundworm infections and a systemic tapeworm infection (hydatid disease), and praziquantel is becoming the drug of choice for all tapeworm infections as well as trematode infections.
• The anthelmintic agents act primarily by disrupting the metabolic or neurologic systems of helminths.
• The toxicities of anthelmintic agents vary widely. Most of these agents cause adverse GI reactions. Adverse CNS and skin reactions also may occur. Some of the toxicity attributed to the anticestode agents actually may represent a reaction to the release of antigens when the tapeworms die.
• Patient noncompliance and reinfection are major factors in treatment failure.

• The nurse should instruct the patient and family in the administration, therapeutic effects, and possible adverse effects of anthelmintic agents, monitor the patient throughout therapy, and notify the physician if adverse reactions occur.

STUDY QUESTIONS

See Appendix 1 for answers.

1. Marcy Dixon brings her daughter Melissa, age 8, to the pediatrician because Melissa has perianal itching that keeps her awake at night and because she is irritable and has lost weight. Laboratory tests confirm the diagnosis of enterobiasis (pinworm). To treat this infection, the physician orders a single dose of mebendazole 100 mg P.O. What is the mechanism of action of mebendazole?
(a) It interferes with the microtubule system of the roundworm, preventing glucose uptake.
(b) It blocks the neurotransmitter acetylcholine, causing flaccid paralysis in the roundworm.
(c) It interferes with neuromuscular transmission, causing spastic paralysis in the roundworm.
(d) It inhibits an enzyme essential for the anaerobic metabolism of the roundworm.

2. Which instructions should the nurse give Ms. Dixon to prevent reinfection of Melissa and infection of other family members?
(a) Cook all pork products thoroughly.
(b) Change and launder underclothes and bedding daily.
(c) Drink bottled water to prevent ingestion of contaminated water.
(d) Wear shoes outdoors to prevent contact with contaminated ground.

3. Larry Swain, age 30, has just returned from Europe and is diagnosed as having a *Taenia solium* infection. His physician prescribes the anticestode agent niclosamide. Which agent has anticestode and antitrematode effects?
(a) praziquantel
(b) mebendazole
(c) oxamniquine
(d) thiabendazole

4. Which instructions should the nurse give Mr. Swain about niclosamide administration?
(a) Take the drug on an empty stomach.
(b) Swallow the tablet whole because its bitter taste may cause vomiting.
(c) Chew the tablet thoroughly and take it with water after a light meal.
(d) Dissolve the medication in water and take it on an empty stomach.

5. Upon returning from a vacation in Puerto Rico, Sara Hobbs develops fever, malaise, weakness, GI distress, and weight loss. A thorough examination and laboratory tests reveal that Ms. Hobbs has schistosomiasis, a trematode infection. Her physician prescribes oxamniquine. What is the most significant adverse reaction to oxamniquine?
(a) hepatotoxicity
(b) GI distress
(c) renal failure
(d) CNS stimulation

6. Which adverse urinary reaction might Ms. Hobbs experience during oxamniquine therapy?
(a) oliguria
(b) polyuria
(c) orange-red urine
(d) crystalluria

7. What should the nurse tell Ms. Hobbs about administering oxamniquine?
(a) Chew the tablet thoroughly.
(b) Take the medication with meals.
(c) Take the medication on an empty stomach.
(d) Swallow the tablet rapidly because its bitter taste may cause gagging or vomiting.

8. Praziquantel also may be used to treat schistosomiasis. What is the mechanism of action of praziquantel in treating a trematode infection?
(a) It causes blood flukes to migrate from the mesenteric vein into the liver.
(b) It produces anticholinergic effects that cause the flukes to disintegrate.
(c) It causes flaccid paralysis of the fluke musculature.
(d) It causes spastic paralysis of the fluke musculature.

SELECTED REFERENCES

AHFS drug information 90. (1990). Bethesda, MD: American Society of Hospital Pharmacists.

Conte, Jr., J., and Barriere, S. (1988). *Manual of antibiotics and infectious diseases* (6th ed.). Philadelphia: Lea & Febiger.

Drug facts and comparisons. (1991). St. Louis: Facts and Comparisons Division, J.B. Lippincott.

Goodman and Gilman's the pharmacological basis of therapeutics (8th ed.; 1990). Elmsford, NY: Pergamon Press.

Hansten, P., and Horn, J. (1990). *Drug interactions* (7th ed.). Philadelphia: Lea & Febiger.

Mandel, G., et al. (1990). *Principles and practice of infectious diseases* (3rd ed.). New York: John Wiley & Sons.

North American Nursing Diagnosis Association. (1990). *Taxonomy I - Revised, with official diagnostic categories.* St. Louis: NANDA.

ANTIMALARIAL AND OTHER ANTIPROTOZOAL AGENTS

OBJECTIVES

After reading and studying this chapter, the student should be able to:

1. Discuss the major prophylactic and therapeutic indications for antimalarial agents and the major therapeutic indications for other antiprotozoal agents.

2. Discuss why some antiprotozoal agents require dosage adjustments for a patient with hepatic or renal disease.

3. Identify alternative treatments if the antimalarial or antiprotozoal agent of choice is unavailable or contraindicated.

4. Describe potential interactions between antimalarial or antiprotozoal agents and other drugs.

5. Discuss the most common adverse effects of antimalarial and antiprotozoal agents, and explain how to minimize them during therapy.

6. Identify the contraindications for administering antiprotozoal agents.

7. Explain how to monitor the patient receiving antiprotozoal therapy.

8. Describe how to apply the nursing process when caring for a patient who is receiving an antimalarial or other antiprotozoal agent.

INTRODUCTION

Protozoal diseases, including malaria, have assumed critical importance in the United States for several reasons. An increase in the incidence and type of immune disorders that make the patient more susceptible to protozoal invasion, immigration from areas where protozoal diseases are endemic, and travel by Americans to those areas all have sharpened the focus of health care professionals on pro-

tozoal diseases and produced an increased need for effective antiprotozoal drugs. This chapter discusses the most frequently used antimalarial and antiprotozoal drugs and their indications.

For a summary of representative drugs, see *Selected major drugs: Antimalarial and other antiprotozoal agents,* pages 1121 and 1122. For a listing of applicable nursing diagnoses that the nurse may formulate when caring for a patient receiving these agents, see *Selected nursing diagnoses: Antimalarial and other antiprotozoal agents.* For detailed information on applying the nursing process, see Chapter 6, The Nursing Process and Drug Therapy.

ANTIMALARIAL AGENTS

The major agents used to prevent and treat malaria are the 4-aminoquinolones (chloroquine phosphate, chloroquine hydrochloride, and hydroxychloroquine sulfate) mefloquine, the 8-aminoquinolone primaquine phosphate, pyrimethamine,and quinine sulfate. The sulfonamides, sulfones, and tetracyclines also may be used in combination with these agents. (For information about these ancillary antimalarial agents, see Chapter 59, Antibacterial Agents.)

Four parasites can transmit malaria to humans: *Plasmodium falciparum, P. malariae, P. ovale,* and *P. vivax.* Although their life cycles vary, all four species transmit malaria in the same way. (For a description of this process, see *Malaria transmission cycle,* page 1110.) Because drug therapy and drug resistance vary among species, the development of more powerful antimalarials continues.

SELECTED NURSING DIAGNOSES

Antimalarial and other antiprotozoal agents

The following nursing diagnoses address representative problems and etiologies that a nurse may encounter when caring for a patient who is receiving an antimalarial or other antiprotozoal agent. Some of these nursing diagnoses contain generalized etiologies, which the nurse must individualize based on the patient's needs. (For some common nursing diagnoses and related interventions for each drug class, see the "Nursing Process Application" sections of this chapter.)

- Altered health maintenance related to quinine-induced cinchonism
- Altered oral mucous membrane related to metronidazole-induced furry tongue, glossitis, or stomatitis
- Altered protection related to the adverse hematologic effects of the prescribed antimalarial or antiprotozoal agent
- Altered sexuality patterns related to decreased libido caused by metronidazole
- Altered thought processes related to the adverse CNS effects of an antimalarial or antiprotozoal agent
- Altered urinary elimination related to pentamidine-induced nephrotoxicity
- Body image disturbance related to hair discoloration or loss caused by iodoquinol
- Constipation related to the adverse GI effects of an antiprotozoal agent
- Decreased cardiac output related to emetine-induced cardiotoxicity
- Diarrhea related to the adverse GI effects of an antimalarial or antiprotozoal agent
- Fatigue related to the adverse CNS effects of an antimalarial or antiprotozoal agent
- Impaired gas exchange related to bronchospasm caused by antimalarial agent hypersensitivity
- Impaired gas exchange related to pentamidine-induced bronchospasm with inhalation therapy
- Impaired physical mobility related to neuromuscular dysfunction caused by an antiprotozoal agent

- Impaired tissue integrity related to phlebitis at the pentamide infusion site
- Knowledge deficit related to the prescribed antimalarial and antiprotozoal agent
- Noncompliance related to adverse reactions to the prescribed antimalarial or antiprotozoal agent
- Pain related to neurotoxicity caused by iodoquinol
- Potential fluid volume deficit related to the adverse GI effects of the prescribed antimalarial or antiprotozoal agent
- Potential for injury related to a preexisting condition that contraindicates the use of an antimalarial or antiprotozoal agent
- Potential for injury related to a preexisting condition that requires cautious use of an antimalarial or antiprotozoal agent
- Potential for injury related to adverse drug reactions
- Potential for trauma related to the adverse CNS effects of an antimalarial or antiprotozoal agent
- Potential impaired skin integrity related to the adverse dermatologic effects of an antimalarial or antiprotozoal agent
- Sensory-perceptual alterations (auditory) related to the adverse effects of an antimalarial agent
- Sensory-perceptual alterations (kinesthetic) related to the adverse neuromuscular effects of an antimalarial or antiprotozoal agent
- Sexual dysfunction related to metronidazole-induced vaginal dryness or dyspareunia

PHARMACOKINETICS

After oral administration, the antimalarial agents are absorbed well and distributed widely throughout the body. The extent of metabolism among these agents varies, and excretion occurs primarily through the urine.

Absorption, distribution, metabolism, excretion

Chloroquine is absorbed well from the gastrointestinal (GI) tract, but only about 55% of it is serum protein bound. Widely distributed, chloroquine appears in high concentrations in the liver, spleen, kidneys, lungs, heart, brain, melanin-containing tissues, and erythrocytes. It binds to platelets and granulocytes. Serum and tissue concentrations of chloroquine are higher than those in plasma. Low concentrations are found in the central nervous system (CNS) and in breast milk, and it appears to cross the placenta. Chloroquine is metabolized partially in the liver and excreted slowly in the urine; up to 70% of an oral dose may be excreted as unchanged drug. The pharmacokinetics of

hydroxychloroquine are believed similar to those of chloroquine, except for metabolite formation.

Mefloquine is absorbed well from the GI tract. It is distributed widely and is approximately 98% bound to plasma proteins with high concentrations in the red blood cells. Mefloquine is metabolized partially in the liver and is excreted mainly in the bile and feces.

After oral administration, primaquine is absorbed well from the GI tract. Little is known about its pharmacokinetics, but the drug is thought to be distributed widely with small concentrations appearing in the liver, lungs, heart, and skeletal muscles. Primaquine is metabolized rapidly in the liver and excreted in urine. Only about 1% of an oral dose is excreted unchanged.

Pyrimethamine is absorbed almost completely from the GI tract after oral administration. Approximately 80% protein bound, this drug is distributed widely to the kidneys, lungs, liver, and spleen. It also appears in breast milk. Although its metabolism and excretion are not well defined,

Malaria transmission cycle

When the carrier mosquito (genus *Anopheles*) draws blood from an infected person, it picks up malarial parasites. The mosquito bites the next victim **(A)** and infects that person with the parasites, which enter the bloodstream and travel to the liver.

Each parasite invades a separate liver cell, then multiplies, rupturing the host cell **(B)**.

Ten to fourteen days later, the parasites leave the liver and invade the red blood cells, where they feed on hemoglobin **(C)**.

They multiply again and rupture the cells **(D)**. At this stage, the victim experiences the symptoms of malaria: backache, chills, fever, and severe headache.

Free parasites enter other red blood cells to multiply again. Any mosquito that feeds on the victim may become infected, beginning a new transmission cycle.

pyrimethamine appears to be metabolized partially in the liver and excreted in urine.

Quinine is absorbed almost completely from the GI tract. About 70% protein bound, it is distributed well throughout the body. It crosses the placenta readily and appears in breast milk. Quinine and its alkaloids are metabolized extensively in the liver and excreted in the urine.

Onset, peak, duration

Because chloroquine is absorbed rapidly into the bloodstream, peak plasma concentration occurs 1 to 2 hours after oral administration. The half-life of chloroquine ranges from 72 to 120 hours in a healthy adult. Hydroxychloroquine is thought to act in a similar manner.

The terminal half-life of mefloquine in healthy adults ranges from 13 to 24 days with a mean of 3 weeks; it appears to be shorter in patients with acute malaria.

After oral administration, the plasma concentration of primaquine usually peaks within 3 hours. The plasma half-life of the drug varies greatly, ranging from 3.7 to 9.6 hours.

The peak plasma concentration of pyrimethamine usually occurs within 2 hours of oral administration. Its half-life is approximately 4 days.

The peak plasma concentration of quinine usually occurs 1 to 3 hours after oral administration. When therapy is discontinued, the plasma concentration declines to a negligible level within 24 hours. The plasma concentration of the drug and its half-life may be prolonged in a patient with impaired hepatic function accompanying active malaria. The half-life of quinine varies from 8 to 21 hours in patients with active malaria, and from 4 to 12 hours in healthy adults.

PHARMACODYNAMICS

Although their exact mechanisms of action are not understood, antimalarial agents seem to work in differing ways to kill malarial parasites or inhibit their reproduction.

Mechanism of action

Chloroquine and hydroxychloroquine are thought to disrupt protein synthesis in the parasite. Also, the drugs may concentrate in the digestive vacuoles of the parasite, increasing pH and interfering with utilization of hemoglobin.

Primaquine appears to affect the parasite's mitochondria, eventually disrupting cellular metabolism.

Pyrimethamine selectively inhibits the enzyme dihydrofolate reductase, which impedes folic acid reduction and ultimately disrupts parasitic reproduction.

Quinine has diverse pharmacologic properties. Its antimalarial action may result from incorporation into the deoxyribonucleic acid (DNA) of the parasite, rendering it ineffective. Its action also may result from depression of oxygen uptake and carbohydrate metabolism in the parasite. In addition, quinine acts as a skeletal muscle relaxant, a local anesthetic, an antipyretic, and an analgesic, thus relieving malarial symptoms.

The exact mechanism of mefloquine's antimalarial effects remain unknown. Because it is a structural analogue of quinine, it may have similar pharmacodynamic effects.

PHARMACOTHERAPEUTICS

The prevention and treatment of malaria is continually changing, primarily because of the increasing resistance of *P. falciparum* to antimalarial drugs. Varying degrees of chloroquine resistance exist in parts of Africa, South America, Asia, India, and the South Pacific.

Chloroquine remains the drug of choice to prevent and treat all malaria strains, except chloroquine-resistant or multidrug-resistant strains of *P. falciparum*. Hydroxychloroquine serves as an alternative when chloroquine is not available.

For acute attacks of chloroquine-resistant or multidrug-resistant strains of *P. falciparum*, quinine is the drug of choice and is given with slower-acting antimalarial agents. Primaquine is the drug of choice to prevent *P. vivax* or *P. ovale* malaria relapse.

Mefloquine is used for acute attacks of mild to moderate malaria caused by susceptible strains of *P. falciparum* and *P. vivax*. It also is indicated to prevent malaria infections by *P. falciparum* and *P. vivax*, including chloroquine-resistant strains of *P. falciparum*.

Pyrimethamine is used with other antimalarial agents to treat chloroquine-resistant malaria. Pyrimethamine-sulfadoxine (Fansidar) combination should be used only with chloroquine prophylaxis for self-treatment of febrile illness when medical care is not immediately available in areas where chloroquine-resistant *P. falciprium* is found. Some fatalities have occurred with the use of this combination.

chloroquine hydrochloride and **chloroquine phosphate** (Aralen). Available in tablets as chloroquine phosphate or in injection form as chloroquine hydrochloride, chloroquine is the drug of choice to prevent and treat all types of malaria except for that caused by chloroquine-resistant *P. falciparum*. Chloroquine also serves as an adjunct in managing hepatic abscess caused by *Entamoeba histolytica*. The dosage may be expressed in terms of the drug base or its salt. To convert between dosage forms, keep in mind that 100 mg of chloroquine hydrochloride equals 80 mg of chloroquine base, and 100 mg of chloroquine phosphate equals 60 mg of chloroquine base.
Usual adult dosage: for preventing malaria in a person traveling to an area where chloroquine-resistant *P. falciparum* is not prevalent, 300 mg of chloroquine base P.O. once a week for 1 week before departure and for 6 weeks after returning; for preventing malaria in a person traveling to an area where chloroquine-resistant *P. falciparum* is found, 300 mg of chloroquine base P.O. once a week for 1 week before departure and for 6 weeks after returning; for self-treatment of febrile illness when medical care is not immediately available, add 3 tablets of 25 mg pyrimethamine and 500 mg sulfadoxine (Fansidar); for treating malaria caused by *P. malariae*, *P. ovale*, *P. vivax*, or susceptible strains of *P. falciparum*, 600 mg of chloroquine base P.O. initially, followed by 300 mg at 6, 24, and 48 hours (or 250 mg I.M. of chloroquine hydrochloride every 6 hours in a seriously ill patient). An infection caused by *P. vivax* or *P. ovale* will require concomitant or follow-up treatment with primaquine to prevent a relapse. For treating hepatic abscess caused by *E. histolytica* after emetine hydrochloride therapy, the dosage is 600 mg of chloroquine base P.O. daily for 2 days followed by 300 mg of chloroquine base P.O. daily for 2 to 3 weeks with iodoquinol (diiodohydroxyquin).
Usual pediatric dosage: for preventing and treating acute attacks of malaria caused by *P. malariae*, *P. ovale*, *P. vivax*, and susceptible strains of *P. falciparum*, 5 mg base/kg P.O. weekly, up to a maximum of 300 mg base.

hydroxychloroquine sulfate (Plaquenil Sulfate). When chloroquine is not available, this drug may be used to prevent and treat malaria caused by chloroquine-susceptible strains. A 200-mg dose of hydroxychloroquine sulfate equals 155 mg of hydroxychloroquine base.
Usual adult dosage: for preventing malaria in a person traveling to an endemic area, 310 mg of hydroxychloroquine base P.O. once a week for 1 week before departure and for 6 weeks after returning; for treating chloroquine-susceptible malaria, 620 mg of hydroxychloroquine base P.O. initially, followed by 310 mg of hydroxychloroquine base P.O. at 6, 24, and 48 hours.
Usual pediatric dosage: for preventing malaria in a child traveling to an endemic area, 5 mg base/kg weekly, up to the maximum adult dosage.

mefloquine hydrochloride (Lariam). Available as tablets, mefloquine is used to prevent malaria infections by *P. falciparum* and *P. vivax*, including chloroquine-resistant strains of *P. falciparum*, and to treat mild to moderate malaria caused by susceptible strains of *P. falciparum* and *P. vivax*.
Usual adult dosage: for preventing *P. falciparum* and *P. vivax* malaria, including chloroquine-resistant strains of *P. falciparum*, 250 mg P.O. once a week for 4 weeks, then 250 mg every other week. Begin 1 week before departure and continue for 4 weeks after returning from endemic area; for treating mild to moderate malaria caused by susceptible strains of *P. falciparum* and *P. vivax*, 1,250 mg (5 tablets) P.O. as a single dose. An infection caused by *P. vivax* will require follow-up treatment with primaquine to prevent a relapse.
Usual pediatric dosage: for preventing malaria caused by *P. falciparum* or *P. vivax*, 1/4 tablet P.O. for a child who weighs 15 to 19 kg, 1/2 tablet P.O. for a child who weighs 20 to 30 kg, 3/4 tablet P.O. for a child who weighs 31 to 45 kg, or 1 tablet P.O. for a child who weighs more than 45 kg. Prophylactic therapy should be given weekly, beginning 1 week before travel and continuing weekly during travel and for 4 weeks after returning from the endemic area.

primaquine phosphate. Available in tablets, primaquine is used to prevent *P. ovale* and *P. vivax* relapse.
Usual adult dosage: to prevent relapse, 79 mg P.O. once a week for 8 weeks or 26.3 mg P.O. daily for 14 days.
Usual pediatric dosage: 0.5 mg/kg/day P.O. for 14 days.

pyrimethamine (Daraprim). This drug is used to treat chloroquine-resistant malaria in combination with other antimalarial agents and to treat toxoplasmosis. It is available alone in tablet form or in combination with sulfadoxine.
Usual adult dosage: for treating chloroquine-resistant *P. falciparum* malaria, 25 mg P.O. b.i.d. for 3 days with 500 mg of sulfadiazine q.i.d. for 5 days with quinine sulfate; for self-treatment of febrile illness in areas of risk for chloroquine resistance, 3 tablets of 25 mg pyrimethamine and 500 mg sulfadoxine (Fansidar) in combination with standard chloroquine prophylaxis; for treating toxoplasmosis, 25 mg P.O. daily with 1 gram of sulfadiazine q.i.d. for 3 to 4 weeks.
Usual pediatric dosages: for preventing malaria, 6.25 mg P.O. once weekly in children under age 4, or 12.5 mg P.O. once weekly for children ages 4 to 10, continued for 6 to

10 weeks after exposure; for treating toxoplasmosis, 1 mg/kg/day P.O. divided into two equal doses, followed by half of this dosage after 2 to 4 days, and continued for about 1 month.

quinine sulfate (Quinamm, Strema) and **quinine dihydrochloride**. Available in tablets and capsules as quinine sulfate or in injection form as quinine dihydrochloride, quinine is the drug of choice for a patient with chloroquine-resistant or multidrug-resistant strains of *P. falciparum* malaria. If the patient cannot tolerate oral quinine sulfate, an I.V. preparation of quinine dihydrochloride may be obtained from the Centers for Disease Control (CDC). The I.V. form also is used for any patient with malaria who needs parenteral therapy.
Usual adult dosage: for treating chloroquine-resistant *P. falciparum* malaria, 650 mg P.O. t.i.d. for 3 days given with pyrimethamine and sulfadiazine. Tetracycline may be substituted for pyrimethamine and sulfadiazine; for parenteral treatment of all malarial infections, the dihydrochloride salt dosage is 600 mg I.V. in 300 ml of normal saline solution given over 2 to 4 hours and repeated every 8 hours until oral therapy can begin; the maximum daily I.V. dose is 1,800 mg.
Usual pediatric dosage: for treating chloroquine-resistant malaria, 25 mg/kg/day of quinine sulfate P.O. in divided doses every 8 hours for 5 to 7 days, or 25 mg/kg of quinine dihydrochloride (up to a maximum of 1.8 grams daily) divided into three doses and administered by slow I.V. infusion over 2 to 4 hours every 8 hours..

Drug interactions
Various interactions can occur between antimalarial agents and other drugs. Many result from decreased absorption from the GI tract, from concomitant administration of other drugs that cause similar adverse reactions, or protein-binding displacement that leads to elevated serum concentrations of the drug. (For more information, see *Drug interactions: Antimalarial agents.*)

ADVERSE DRUG REACTIONS

In the low dosages used to prevent or treat malaria, these agents usually produce few serious adverse reactions. (For information about other adverse reactions, see *Antimalarial agents: Summary of adverse reactions,* page 1114.)

Gastrointestinal complaints are the most common adverse reactions to the antimalarial agents. Adverse ocular effects have been reported for the 4-aminoquinolones, quinine, and primaquine. Cardiovascular reactions are most common with administration of I.V. quinine. Adverse CNS reactions have been attributed to all these agents, and a unique toxic syndrome known as cinchonism can be seen with quinine. This syndrome may produce mild to severe tinnitus, headache, vertigo, fever, light-headedness, and visual disturbances.

Granulocytopenia can occur, but it is rare. Reported hypersensitivity reactions, which can range from mild to life-threatening, include severe bronchospasm and skin reactions, such as exfoliative dermatitis, Stevens-Johnson syndrome, and toxic epidermal necrolysis.

NURSING PROCESS APPLICATION

The following information assists the nurse in caring for a patient who is receiving an antimalarial agent.

Assessment
• Review the patient's history for a preexisting condition that contraindicates the use of an antimalarial agent, such as pregnancy, thrombocytopenic purpura, tinnitus, blackwater fever, optic neuritis, psoriasis, porphyria, or known hypersensitivity to the drug.
• Review the patient's history for a preexisting condition that requires cautious use of an antimalarial agent, such as lactation, atrial fibrillation, a history of seizures, renal or hepatic dysfunction, folate deficiency, severe allergy, or bronchial asthma.
• Assess the patient for adverse reactions to the prescribed antimalarial agent, such as GI, cardiovascular, or CNS disturbances; ocular and auditory changes; and hypersensitivity reactions.
• Review the patient's medication history to identify the use of drugs that may interact with the prescribed antimalarial agent, such as an antacid, neuromuscular blocking agent, oral anticoagulant, cardiac glycoside, quinacrine, folic acid, beta-adrenergic blocker, or calcium channel blocker.
• Assess the effectiveness of the prescribed antimalarial agent periodically.
• Assess the patient receiving quinine for cinchonism throughout antimalarial therapy.
• Assess the patient for hematologic abnormalities throughout antimalarial therapy.
• Evaluate the patient's and family's knowledge about the prescribed antimalarial agent.

Nursing diagnoses
The following examples represent appropriate nursing diagnoses for a patient receiving an antimalarial agent.
• Potential for injury related to a preexisting condition that contraindicates the use of an antimalarial agent
• Potential for injury related to a preexisting condition that requires cautious use of an antimalarial agent

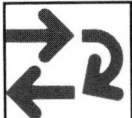

DRUG INTERACTIONS

Antimalarial agents

Antimalarial agents can produce a variety of interactions. The most serious are additive, occurring with concomitant administration of drugs that produce similar adverse reactions.

DRUG	INTERACTING DRUGS	POSSIBLE EFFECTS	NURSING IMPLICATIONS
chloroquine	oral antacids that contain magnesium trisilicate	Decrease chloroquine absorption	• Separate antacid doses as far as possible from chloroquine doses if these drugs must be used concomitantly.
hydroxychloroquine	digoxin	Elevates digoxin levels	• Monitor the patient's serum digoxin level when hydroxychloroquine therapy begins or ends.
mefloquine	beta-adrenergic blockers, calcium channel blockers, quinine and quinidine, and other drugs that may prolong cardiac conduction	May cause ECG abnormalities or cardiac arrest	• Avoid concomitant administration.
	chloroquine	Increases risk of seizure activity	• Monitor the patient closely if concomitant administration occurs.
	valproic acid	Decreases valproic acid blood levels; increases potential for seizures	• Monitor valproic acid blood levels; adjust the dosage if necessary.
primaquine	quinacrine	Increases toxicity of primaquine	• Monitor the patient for adverse reactions.
pyrimethamine	folic acid	Inhibits antimicrobial effect	• Monitor the patient for a decreased therapeutic effect.
quinine	antacids that contain aluminum	Delay or decrease quinine absorption	• Separate antacid doses as far as possible from quinine doses if these drugs must be used concomitantly.
	neuromuscular blocking agents (pancuronium, tubocurarine, succinylcholine)	Produce neuromuscular blockade, which may lead to respiratory arrest	• Monitor the patient's respirations. • Have emergency resuscitation equipment available. • Monitor the patient's arterial blood gases, as needed.
	oral anticoagulants (warfarin type)	Enhance hypoprothrombinemia	• Monitor the patient receiving an oral anticoagulant for altered anticoagulant effect when quinine therapy begins or ends.
	cardiac glycosides (digoxin, digitoxin)	Increases plasma levels of glycosides	• Monitor the patient's blood levels of cardiac glycosides, and adjust the dosages as prescribed.

• Potential for injury related to adverse drug reactions
• Altered health maintenance related to quinine-induced cinchonism
• Altered protection related to the adverse hematologic effects of the prescribed antimalarial agent
• Knowledge deficit related to the prescribed antimalarial agent

Planning and implementation

• Do not administer an antimalarial agent to a patient with a condition that contraindicates its use.
• Administer an antimalarial agent cautiously to a patient at risk because of a preexisting condition.
• Monitor the patient periodically for adverse reactions during therapy with an antimalarial agent. Be especially alert for hypersensitivity reactions that can range from mild to

Antimalarial agents: Summary of adverse reactions

This chart summarizes the adverse reactions to antimalarial agents, grouping them by frequency. Most of the adverse reactions result from high doses.

DRUG	COMMON	OCCASIONAL	RARE
chloroquine, hydroxychloroquine	Epigastric discomfort, anorexia, nausea, vomiting, abdominal cramps, diarrhea	Blurred vision, difficulty in focusing, corneal inclusions, corneal changes, skin rash, pruritus, changes in skin and mucosal pigment, hair bleaching, headache, fatigue, nervousness, anxiety, irritability, personality changes	Retinal changes, exfoliative dermatitis, psychotic episodes, seizures, hypotension, ECG changes, ototoxicity, tinnitus, neutropenia, granulocytopenia, aplastic anemia, thrombocytopenia, hemolytic anemia, neuropathy, neuromyopathy, hypersensitivity reaction
mefloquine	Vomiting, dizziness, myalgia, nausea, fever, headache, chills, diarrhea, skin rash, abdominal pain, fatigue, loss of appetite, tinnitus	Bradycardia, hair loss, emotional problems, pruritus, asthenia, transient emotional disturbance, seizures	Encephalopathy
primaquine	Nausea, vomiting, epigastric discomfort, abdominal cramps	Headache, difficulty in focusing, pruritus, hemolytic anemia, methemoglobinemia, mild anemia, leukocytosis, leukopenia	Hypertension, arrhythmias, granulocytopenia, extreme mental confusion, hypersensitivity reaction
pyrimethamine	Anorexia, vomiting, abdominal cramps	Megaloblastic anemia, leukopenia, thrombocytopenia, ataxia, tremor, hypersensitivity	Granulocytopenia, hemolytic anemia, seizures, respiratory failure, photosensitivity, malaise, fatigue, irritability, hypersensitivity reaction
quinine	Mild cinchonism	Moderate cinchonism, thrombocytopenic purpura, hypoprothrombinemia, hemolytic anemia, hearing disturbances, ventricular tachycardia, angina, fever, apprehension, hypothermia, restlessness, confusion, syncope, excitement, delirium	Severe cinchonism, granulocytopenia, optic atrophy, hepatitis, hypoglycemia, deafness, hypersensitivity reaction

life-threatening, including severe bronchospasm, exfoliative dermatitis, and Stevens-Johnson syndrome.

• Monitor hydration if the patient experiences anorexia, nausea, vomiting, or diarrhea. Obtain a prescription for an antiemetic or antidiarrheal agent if needed.

• *Administer chloroquine, primaquine, or quinine with food to minimize adverse GI reactions.*

• Inspect the patient's skin regularly for adverse reactions during therapy with an antimalarial agent.

• Administer a mild analgesic as prescribed for drug-induced headache or myalgia.

• *Monitor the patient's vital signs for abnormalities, such as fever, hypothermia, increased or decreased heart rate or blood pressure, or decreased respiratory rate. Also monitor the electrocardiogram (ECG) to detect arrhythmias or other ECG changes.*

• Take safety measures if the patient experiences adverse CNS reactions, such as dizziness, confusion, or delirium. For example, keep the bed rails raised and supervise the patient's activities.

• Observe the patient's behavior and emotional state for such changes as irritability, personality changes, or excitability during therapy with an antimalarial agent. If changes are observed, notify the physician to discuss changing the patient to a different agent.

• *Monitor the patient for visual or auditory changes when administering chloroquine, hydroxychloroquine, primaquine, or quinine. Ask the patient frequently about eye discomfort or hearing loss.*

• Monitor the patient's blood glucose level regularly and observe for signs of hypoglycemia (profuse sweating, nervousness, and headache) when administering quinine.

- *Take seizure precautions when administering chloroquine, hydroxychloroquine, mefloquine, or pyrimethamine.*
- Notify the physician if adverse reactions occur.
- *Monitor for cinchonism in a patient receiving quinine. This toxic reaction to cinchona alkaloids causes tinnitus, headache, vertigo, fever, light-headedness, and visual disturbances. Toxicity may occur after a single dose.*
- Notify the physician and expect to discontinue the drug if cinchonism occurs.
- *Monitor the patient's complete blood count (CBC) and liver and renal function studies for abnormalities throughout antimalarial therapy. Notify the physician if alterations occur.*
- Take bleeding precautions if thrombocytopenia occurs and observe the patient for signs of bleeding, such as spontaneous epistaxis, bruises, hematuria, and occult blood in the urine or feces, until the patient's platelet count returns to normal.
- Stagger the patient's activities and promote rest periods if anemia occurs.
- Notify the physician of any hematologic changes.

Patient teaching
- Teach the patient and family the name, dose, frequency, action, and adverse effects of the prescribed antimalarial agent.
- *Instruct the patient receiving primaquine or quinine to take the drug with food to minimize adverse GI reactions.*
- Instruct the patient to exercise caution while driving or operating hazardous machinery during antimalarial therapy.
- Inform the patient and family that the antimalarial agent may affect the patient's behavior and emotional state. Instruct them to report personality changes, confusion, or other alterations to the physician.
- Advise the patient to report any visual or auditory changes immediately to the physician and to have regular ophthalmic and auditory examinations.
- Teach the patient receiving quinine to recognize and report the signs and symptoms of hypoglycemia and cinchonism.
- *Warn a woman of childbearing age who is traveling to an area where malaria is endemic against becoming pregnant. Instruct her to continue contraceptive precautions for two months after the last dose of medication.*
- Explain to the patient that children are extremely sensitive to chloroquine and hydroxychloroquine and that accidental ingestion can cause death. Instruct the patient to keep these and all other medications out of the reach of children.
- Stress the importance of having a CBC and liver and renal function studies done as instructed. If thrombocytopenia occurs, teach the patient to use bleeding precautions.
- Instruct the patient to report any other adverse reactions.

Evaluation
The following examples represent appropriate evaluation statements for a patient receiving an antimalarial agent.
- The patient has no conditions that contraindicate antimalarial therapy.
- The patient exhibits no signs of complications in the preexisting condition linked to the prescribed antimalarial agent.
- The patient exhibits no adverse reactions to the prescribed antimalarial agent.
- The patient does not develop cinchonism during quinine therapy.
- The patient's CBC and liver and renal function studies remain normal throughout antimalarial therapy.
- The patient and family express an accurate understanding of the points taught about the prescribed antimalarial agent.
- The patient returns for laboratory tests as instructed.

OTHER ANTIPROTOZOAL AGENTS

Although many agents are used to treat protozoal infections, this section focuses on the readily obtainable antiprotozoal agents: emetine hydrochloride, furazolidone, iodoquinol, metronidazole, pentamidine isethionate, and quinacrine hydrochloride. Other antiprotozoal agents include investigational new drugs (INDs) that can be obtained only from the Centers for Disease Control (CDC), such as dehydroemetine (Meban), diloxanide furoate (Furamide), melarsoprol (Arsobal), nifurtimox (Lampit), stiboglucanate sodium (Pentostam), and suramin sodium (Germanin). Amphotericin B, paromomycin, and co-trimoxazole also are used sometimes as antiprotozoals. For information about these drugs, see Chapter 59, Antibacterial Agents, Chapter 65, Urinary Antiseptic Agents, and Chapter 62, Antimycotic (Antifungal) Agents.

PHARMACOKINETICS

The pharmacokinetic processes of the antiprotozoal agents vary widely and have not been defined completely.

Absorption, distribution, metabolism, excretion
The pharmacokinetics of emetine are unclear, but some facts are known. After administration by deep subcutaneous (S.C.) or intramuscular (I.M.) injection, high concentrations occur in the liver, kidneys, spleen, and lungs. Low concentrations occur in cardiac and striated muscle and in the intestinal lumen. It is eliminated primarily by the kidneys.

After oral administration, furazolidone is absorbed poorly and is inactivated in the intestine. About 5% of an oral dose of furazolidone is excreted in the urine as unchanged drug and metabolites.

Although little information exists about the pharmacokinetics of iodoquinol, researchers believe that only a small portion of an oral dose is absorbed from the GI tract and that most of it is excreted in the feces.

After oral administration, 80% to 90% of a metronidazole dose is absorbed. It is distributed widely and reaches therapeutic concentrations in vaginal tissue, bone, saliva, and bile; in seminal, pleural, peritoneal, and cerebrospinal fluids; and in hepatic and cerebral abscesses. Less than 20% of metronidazole is protein bound. It readily crosses the placenta and is distributed well in breast milk. Metronidazole is metabolized partially in the liver and excreted in the urine and, to a lesser degree, in the feces.

Little is known about the pharmacokinetics of pentamidine after intravenous (I.V.) and nebulized administration, although some evidence suggests that it is absorbed well after I.M. administration. Its distribution is not understood well, but research suggests that it is distributed well and highly protein bound. It probably is not metabolized but excreted unchanged in the urine and feces.

After oral administration, quinacrine is absorbed well from the GI tract and distributed widely. Highest concentrations appear in the pancreas, lungs, liver, bone marrow, spleen, erythrocytes, and skeletal muscles. The drug readily crosses the placenta, resulting in fetal tissue concentrations similar to those of the mother. Evidence suggests that quinacrine is metabolized slowly and eliminated primarily in the urine.

Onset, peak, duration

Little or no information exists about the onset of action, peak concentration levels, or duration of action of emetine, furazolidone, iodoquinol, and quinacrine. Some studies have detected small amounts of emetine in the urine 20 to 40 minutes after parenteral administration and for 40 to 60 days after discontinuation of therapy. Other research has determined that the peak plasma concentration of quinacrine occurs about 8 hours after oral administration.

Peak plasma concentration of metronidazole occurs about 1 hour after I.V. administration and up to 2 hours after oral administration with food. The plasma half-life is about 6 to 8 hours for healthy adults but longer for patients with hepatic failure.

Very little is known about pentamidine's onset, peak concentration, or duration. One study noted that the peak plasma concentration occurred about 1 hour after I.M. administration and did not vary much over 24 hours. The same study detected decreasing amounts of pentamidine in the urine up to 8 weeks after therapy was discontinued.

PHARMACODYNAMICS

The antiprotozoal agents act in very different ways, and many of their mechanisms of action are not understood well.

Mechanism of action

Emetine acts directly on *E. histolytica* by inhibiting its polypeptide elongation. This action blocks protein synthesis in parasitic cells.

Furazolidone may kill bacteria by interfering with their enzyme systems and by inhibiting monoamine oxidase.

Iodoquinol is a contact or luminal amebicide that acts directly on protozoa in the GI tract.

The bactericidal, amebicidal, and trichomonacidal properties of metronidazole may result from disruption of protozoal DNA and inhibition of nucleic acid synthesis, eventually causing cellular death.

Pentamidine may work by several mechanisms that may vary with the protozoa involved. These mechanisms include inhibition of dihydrofolate reductase, interference with aerobic glycolysis, and inhibition of oxidative phosphorylation and nucleic acid synthesis.

Quinacrine may act by coupling with DNA, which would make it unable to replicate or transcribe ribonucleic acid (RNA). This action would decrease protein synthesis and ultimately lead to ribosomal destruction.

PHARMACOTHERAPEUTICS

Antiprotozoal agents are used for a wide range of disorders, including *Pneumocystis carinii* infections, amebiasis, giardiasis, trichomoniasis, toxoplasmosis, African trypanosomiasis, and leishmaniasis.

emetine hydrochloride. Emetine is used to treat severe intestinal amebiasis and hepatic abscess, in combination with other antiparasitic drugs. It is contraindicated in children.
Usual adult dosage: to treat severe amoebic dysentery, 1 mg/kg/day up to 60 mg/day I.M. up to 5 days until symptoms of amebiasis are under control; for hepatic abscess, 1 mg/kg/day up to 60 mg/day I.M. for up to 5 days.

furazolidone (Furoxone). Furazolidone serves as an alternative drug for treating giardiasis.
Usual adult dosage: 100 mg P.O. q.i.d. for 7 to 10 days.
Usual pediatric dosage: for children ages 1 month to 1 year, 8 to 17 mg P.O. q.i.d.; for children ages 1 to 4, 17 to 25 mg P.O. q.i.d.; for children ages 5 and older, 25 to 50 mg P.O. q.i.d.

iodoquinol [diiodohydroxyquin] (Moebiquin, Yodoxin). The drug of choice for treating asymptomatic amebiasis, iodoquinol also can be used with metronidazole to treat mild, moderate, or severe intestinal amebiasis and hepatic abscess caused by *E. histolytica*.

Usual adult dosage: for asymptomatic amebiasis, 650 mg P.O. t.i.d. for 20 days; to treat mild, moderate, or severe intestinal amebiasis or hepatic abscess from *E. histolytica*, 650 mg P.O. t.i.d. for 20 days, after metronidazole.

Usual pediatric dosage: 30 to 40 mg/kg P.O. daily (up to a maximum of 1.95 grams daily) in two or three divided doses for 20 days.

metronidazole (Flagyl, Metryl, Satric). Metronidazole is the drug of choice for treating amoebic hepatic abscess and mild, moderate, or severe intestinal amebiasis. It also is used to treat bacterial infections caused by anaerobic microorganisms and is the drug of choice for vaginal trichomoniasis; it is under investigation for treatment of giardiasis. The metronidazole dosage should be decreased in a patient with severe hepatic impairment to avoid toxicity.

Usual adult dosage: for mild, moderate, and severe intestinal amebiasis or amoebic hepatic abscess, 750 mg P.O. t.i.d. for 10 days, followed by iodoquinol; for bacterial infections, a loading dose of 15 mg/kg I.V. infused over 1 hour, decreased to 7.5 mg/kg I.V. or P.O. every 6 hours (the maximum daily I.V. or P.O. adult dosage is 4 grams); for vaginal trichomoniasis, 2 grams P.O. once or 250 mg P.O. t.i.d. for 7 days given to the patient and her sexual contacts; for giardiasis, 250 mg P.O. t.i.d. for 5 days.

Usual pediatric dosage: for acute intestinal amebiasis, 35 to 50 mg/kg/day P.O. in three divided doses for 10 days.

pentamidine isethionate (Pentam 300, Nebupent). Pentamidine is becoming more widely used to prevent and treat *P. carinii* pneumonia (PCP) and can be administered by the parenteral or nebulized route. A patient with renal impairment may require lower parenteral doses of this potentially nephrotoxic drug. Pentamidine also is used to treat African trypanosomiasis and leishmaniasis.

Usual adult dosage: for treating PCP, 4 mg/kg I.V. or I.M. once daily for 14 days; for preventing PCP, 300 mg inhaled via a Respirgard II nebulizer every 4 weeks; for African trypanosomiasis, 4 mg/kg/day I.M. or I.V. for 10 days; for visceral leishmaniasis, 2 to 4 mg/kg/day I.M. or I.V. for up to 15 doses.

Usual pediatric dosage: for treating PCP, 4 mg/kg/day deep I.M. or I.V. for 14 days.

quinacrine hydrochloride (Atabrine). Quinacrine is the drug of choice for treating giardiasis caused by *Giardia lamblia*.

Usual adult dosage: 100 mg P.O. t.i.d. for 5 days.

Usual pediatric dosage: 2 mg/kg P.O. t.i.d. (up to a maximum of 300 mg daily) for 5 days.

Drug interactions

Emetine does not cause significant drug interactions. However, many interactions occur between the other antiprotozoal agents and other drugs. Some may result from interference of drug metabolism, concomitant administration of other drugs that cause similar adverse reactions, or protein-binding displacement leading to elevated plasma concentrations. Because most of these interactions are unpredictable, the nurse should monitor the patient closely if other medications are given concurrently. (For more information, see *Drug interactions: Other antiprotozoal agents,* page 1118.)

ADVERSE DRUG REACTIONS

Several antiprotozoal agents can produce severe, even life-threatening, adverse reactions. The recommended dosages and duration of therapy for these agents must not be exceeded. (For more details, see *Other antiprotozoal agents: Summary of adverse reactions,* page 1119.)

Adverse GI reactions have been reported with all of the antiprotozoal agents. Emetine and pentamidine produce adverse cardiovascular reactions, and pentamidine is associated with nephrotoxicity. Nebulized pentamidine has a high incidence of bronchospasm and cough. The most serious adverse reaction to iodoquinol is dose-related neurotoxicity. Emetine and metronidazole can produce adverse neuromuscular reactions, and all of the antiprotozoal agents can produce blood dyscrasias, although rare.

The following reactions occur very rarely. Furazolidone and quinacrine can provoke intravascular hemolysis in patients with G6PD deficiency. Aplastic anemia has occurred after quinacrine administration, and iodoquinol has produced granulocytopenia. Pentamidine has been associated with Stevens-Johnson syndrome and toxic epidermal necrolysis, and quinacrine has been implicated in exfoliative dermatitis.

NURSING PROCESS APPLICATION

The following information assists the nurse in caring for a patient who is receiving an antiprotozoal agent.

Assessment

• Review the patient's history for a preexisting condition that contraindicates the use of an antiprotozoal agent, such as first-trimester pregnancy, lactation, concomitant administration of primaquine, or known hypersensitivity to the drug.

• Review the patient's history for a preexisting condition that requires cautious use of an antiprotozoal agent, such as hepatic or renal dysfunction, blood pressure or blood glucose alterations, hematologic abnormalities, psoriasis,

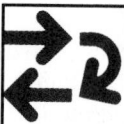

DRUG INTERACTIONS

Other antiprotozoal agents

Many interactions can occur between antiprotozoal agents and other drugs. Because most interactions are unpredictable, the nurse should monitor the patient closely.

DRUG	INTERACTING DRUGS	POSSIBLE EFFECTS	NURSING IMPLICATIONS
furazolidone	amphetamines, monoamine oxidase (MAO) inhibitors, levodopa, tyramine, phenylpropanolamine, ephedrine	Increases pressor effect caused by inhibition of MAO metabolism	• Instruct the patient to avoid amphetamines, MAO inhibitors, levodopa, cold preparations, anorexiants, and tyramine-rich foods, such as cheese, chocolate, and sausages. • Obtain a detailed patient drug history before administering furazolidone.
iodoquinol	preparations that contain iodine	Increase binding of iodine to protein, causing interference with thyroid function tests	• Explain to the patient that thyroid function tests may be abnormal for up to 6 months after iodoquinol therapy.
metronidazole	anticoagulants (warfarin type)	Enhance hypoprothrombinemia	• Monitor the patient receiving an oral anticoagulant for altered anticoagulant effect when metronidazole therapy begins or ends.
	disulfiram	Produces acute psychotic reaction and confusion	• Monitor the patient's psychological status for changes.
	alcohol	Produces disulfiram-like reactions, including flushing, headache, nausea, vomiting, abdominal cramps, and sweating	• Instruct the patient to avoid alcohol use during metronidazole therapy.
	phenobarbital	Increases metronidazole metabolism	• Expect to increase metronidazole dosage as prescribed.
pentamidine	aminoglycosides, cisplatin, amphotericin B	Increase nephrotoxic effects	• Reduce the doses or adjust the dose intervals, as prescribed, when these medications are used concomitantly. • Monitor the patient's renal function by measuring fluid intake and output and assessing the serum creatinine and blood urea nitrogen levels.
quinacrine	primaquine	Increases toxicity of primaquine	• Monitor the patient for adverse reactions.

G6PD deficiency, cardiac disease, alcoholism, or psychosis.
• Assess the patient for adverse reactions to the prescribed antiprotozoal agent, such as GI distress, nephrotoxicity, bronchospasm, cough, local reactions at the injection site, hypersensitivity reactions, and blood dyscrasias.
• Review the patient's medication history to identify the use of drugs that may interact with the prescribed antiprotozoal agent, such as amphetamines, iodine preparations, anticoagulants, aminoglycosides, or primaquine.
• Assess the effectiveness of the prescribed antiprotozoal agent periodically.
• Assess the patient for fluid volume deficit if adverse GI reactions occur during antiprotozoal therapy.

• Evaluate the patient's and family's knowledge about the prescribed antiprotozoal agent.

Nursing diagnoses
The following examples represent appropriate nursing diagnoses for a patient receiving an antiprotozoal agent.
• Potential for injury related to a preexisting condition that contraindicates the use of an antiprotozoal agent
• Potential for injury related to a preexisting condition that requires cautious use of an antiprotozoal agent
• Potential for injury related to adverse drug reactions
• Potential fluid volume deficit related to the adverse GI effects of the prescribed antiprotozoal agent

Other antiprotozoal agents: Summary of adverse reactions

This chart summarizes the adverse reactions to antiprotozoal agents, grouped by frequency.

DRUG	COMMON	OCCASIONAL	RARE
emetine	Diarrhea, abdominal cramps, nausea, vomiting, dizziness, headache; tenderness, aching, and muscle weakness at injection site	Cardiotoxicity, neuromuscular symptoms (weakness, aching, stiffness, tenderness, pain, tremor), generalized weakness; eczematous, urticarial, or purpuric lesions	Hypokalemia
furazolidone	Nausea, vomiting	Abdominal pain, diarrhea, headache, malaise	Hypersensitivity reaction, hypoglycemia, granulocytopenia, hemolytic anemia, disulfiram-like reaction
iodoquinol	Anorexia, vomiting, diarrhea, abdominal cramps, constipation, pruritus ani	Neurotoxicity, optic neuritis, optic atrophy, peripheral neuropathy, iodism, subacute myelo-opticoneuropathy (with muscle pain, weakness, optic atrophy, and ataxia), urticaria, pruritus, thyroid enlargement, fever, chills, headache, vertigo, malaise, discoloration of hair and nails	Agitation, amnesia, hair loss, granulocytopenia, hypersensitivity reaction
metronidazole	Nausea, headache, anorexia, dry mouth, metallic taste	Vomiting, diarrhea, epigastric distress, abdominal discomfort, constipation, dizziness, vertigo, uncoordination, ataxia, confusion, irritability, depression, weakness, insomnia, urethral burning, dysuria, vaginal dryness, dyspareunia, decreased libido	Pseudomembranous colitis, peripheral neuropathy, transient leukopenia, hypersensitivity reaction, furry tongue, glossitis, stomatitis, disulfiram-like reaction, flattening of T wave on ECG
pentamidine	Nephrotoxicity, pain or induration at the injection site, elevated liver function tests, leukopenia, nausea, anorexia, bronchospasm, cough with inhalation therapy	Hypotension, arrhythmias, phlebitis, pruritus, urticaria, hypoglycemia, hyperglycemia, thrombocytopenia, hypocalcemia, vomiting, sterile abscess	Stevens-Johnson syndrome, pancreatitis, anemia, neutropenia, thrombocytopenic purpura, toxic epidermal necrolysis
quinacrine	Headache, dizziness, diarrhea, abdominal cramps, discolored urine	Nervousness, skin eruptions, vertigo, irritability, emotional changes, nightmares, psychosis, corneal deposits	Seizures, aplastic anemia, exfoliative dermatitis, retinopathy, hepatitis, hemolytic anemia

• Knowledge deficit related to the prescribed antiprotozoal agent

Planning and implementation
• Do not administer an antiprotozoal agent to a patient with a condition that contraindicates its use.
• Administer an antiprotozoal agent cautiously to a patient at risk because of a preexisting condition.
• Monitor the patient periodically for adverse reactions during antiprotozoal therapy.

• Monitor the patient for a hypersensitivity reaction when administering an antiprotozoal agent.
• *Monitor the patient's blood pressure and ECG before, during, and after pentamidine administration. Infuse I.V. pentamidine over 1 hour with patient supine to minimize severe hypotension and arrhythmias. Keep emergency resuscitation equipment available.*
• *Monitor renal function closely for a patient receiving pentamidine by monitoring the blood urea nitrogen and serum creatinine concentrations before, during, and after*

therapy. Maintain adequate patient hydration to minimize the risk of nephrotoxicity.

• Monitor the blood glucose level for a patient receiving pentamidine during therapy and for several weeks afterward to detect hypoglycemia or hyperglycemia. Also monitor the patient's CBC, platelet count, liver function tests, and serum calcium level.

• Perform a respiratory assessment after administering nebulized pentamidine, particularly noting bronchospasm and cough.

• Dissolve nebulized pentamidine in sterile water and administer it via a Respirgard II nebulizer.

• *Inspect the injection site periodically for signs of induration or sterile abscess when administering pentamidine I.M. Inspect the I.V. infusion site for evidence of phlebitis when administering pentamidine I.V.*

• Expect to decrease the metronidazole dosage as prescribed in a patient with severe hepatic impairment to avoid toxicity.

• Take safety measures if the patient receiving metronidazole experiences adverse CNS reactions, such as dizziness, vertigo, uncoordination, ataxia, or confusion. For example, place the bed in the low position, keep the bed rails raised, and supervise the patient's activities.

• Inspect the patient's mouth regularly for signs of glossitis or stomatitis, such as ulcerations or swelling, during metronidazole therapy.

• Monitor for signs of neurotoxicity, such as pain or changes in sensation or function, in the patient receiving iodoquinol. Also monitor the patient for myelo-opticoneuropathy, exhibited by muscle pain, weakness, optic atrophy, weakness, or ataxia.

• Inspect the patient's skin for urticaria, hair for discoloration or loss, and nails for discoloration during iodoquinol therapy.

• Administer a mild analgesic or antipyretic agent if headache or fever occurs during furazolidone, iodoquinol, or quinacrine, use.

• *Be aware that emetine should be given only under direct medical supervision. Because the drug can be toxic, the patient should be hospitalized and confined to bed during therapy and for several days afterward. Closely monitor the patient's blood pressure, pulse rate, and ECG readings. If the patient experiences tachycardia, hypotension, neuromuscular reactions, marked GI reactions, or extreme weakness, notify the physician and expect to discontinue therapy.*

• Administer emetine only by deep I.M. injection.

• Stagger the patient's activities and provide frequent rest periods if the patient experiences generalized weakness during emetine therapy.

• Inspect the patient's skin for eczematous, urticarial, or purpuric lesions during emetine therapy.

• Monitor the patient's potassium level for hypokalemia during emetine therapy.

• *Monitor the CBC and liver function studies for abnormalities in a patient on prolonged quinacrine therapy.*

• Monitor for adverse CNS reactions, such as vertigo, emotional changes, psychosis, or seizures, in a patient receiving quinacrine. Take safety and seizure precautions as indicated.

• Inspect the patient's skin for skin eruptions or exfoliative dermatitis during quinacrine therapy.

• Observe the patient for signs of hypoglycemia, such as sweating, nervousness, and headache, during furazolidone or pentamidine therapy.

• Notify the physician if adverse reactions occur.

• Monitor hydration if the patient experiences anorexia, nausea, vomiting, or diarrhea. Obtain a prescription for an antiemetic or antidiarrheal agent if needed.

• Notify the physician if adverse GI reactions persist or worsen.

Patient teaching

• Teach the patient and family the name, dose, frequency, action, and adverse effects of the prescribed antiprotozoal agent.

• Inform the patient that pain may occur at the injection site with I.M. administration of pentamidine.

• *Advise the patient to alert the nurse or physician if a cough or shortness of breath occur after pentamidine inhalation therapy or if pruritus or skin changes occur with I.M. or I.V. pentamidine therapy. Review the signs and symptoms of hyperglycemia or hypoglycemia with the patient.*

• Advise the patient that metronidazole may darken the urine and cause dysuria and a lingering metallic taste in the mouth.

• Caution the patient to avoid activities that require mental alertness or physical coordination if adverse CNS reactions occur.

• Advise the patient to take a laxative if constipation occurs. Also, teach the patient how to prevent constipation.

• Inform the patient receiving metronidazole that decreased libido may occur. Inform the female patient that she may experience vaginal dryness and dyspareunia.

• Teach the patient how to manage metronidazole-induced insomnia through relaxation techniques and other nonpharmacologic measures.

• *Advise the patient to take metronidazole with food to minimize the risk of adverse GI reactions.* Also instruct the patient to avoid alcoholic beverages during therapy and for 48 hours after it is discontinued.

• Advise the patient to refrain from sexual intercourse during treatment for trichomoniasis, or to have her partner use a condom to avoid reinfection. Recommend that all sexual partners be evaluated for infection.

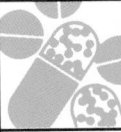

SELECTED MAJOR DRUGS

Antimalarial and other antiprotozoal agents

This table summarizes the major antimalarial and other antiprotozoal agents currently in clinical use.

DRUG	MAJOR INDICATIONS	USUAL ADULT DOSAGES	CONTRAINDICATIONS AND PRECAUTIONS
Antimalarial agents			
chloroquine hydrochloride, chloroquine phosphate	Malaria prevention in areas of low risk of exposure to chloroquine-resistant *Plasmodium falciparum* malaria	300 mg base P.O. once a week beginning 1 week before exposure and continuing 6 weeks after exposure	• Know that chloroquine is contraindicated in a pregnant patient or one with retinal or visual field changes or known hypersensitivity to the drug. • Administer with caution to a patient with hepatic disease, glucose 6-phosphate dehydrogenase (G6PD) deficiency, or a history of psoriasis or porphyria, or one who is taking another hepatotoxic agent.
	Malaria prevention in areas of risk of exposure to chloroquine-resistant *P. falciparum* malaria	300 mg base P.O. once a week beginning 1 week before exposure and continuing 6 weeks after exposure, plus pyrimethamine and sulfadoxine if necessary	
	Treatment of all malaria except chloroquine-resistant *P. falciparum* malaria	600 mg base P.O. initially, then 300 mg base at 6, 24, and 48 hours (or 250 mg I.M. of chloroquine hydrochloride every 6 hours in a seriously ill patient)	
pyrimethamine	Treatment of chloroquine-resistant *P. falciparum* malaria	25 mg P.O. b.i.d. for 3 days in combination with sulfadiazine and quinine	• Know that pyrimethamine is contraindicated in patient with severe renal insufficiency or known hypersensitivity to the drug. • Administer with caution to a pregnant or lactating patient or one with a history of seizures, impaired renal or hepatic function, folate deficiency, or bronchial asthma.
	Self treatment of febrile illness in areas of risk for chloroquine resistance	3 tablets of 25 mg of pyrimethamine and 500 mg of sulfadoxine once in combination with chloroquine prophylactic therapy	
quinine sulfate	Treatment of chloroquine-resistant *P. falciparum* malaria	650 mg P.O. t.i.d. for 3 days with pyrimethamine and sulfadiazine	• Know that quinine is contraindicated in a pregnant patient or one with G6PD deficiency, thrombocytopenic purpura, tinnitus, blackwater fever, optic neuritis, or known hypersensitivity to the drug. • Administer with caution to a lactating patient or one with atrial fibrillation.
quinine dihydrochloride	Parenteral treatment of all malarial infections	600 mg I.V. in 300 ml of normal saline solution over 2 to 4 hours, repeated every 8 hours, up to a maximum of 1,800 mg/day, until oral therapy can begin	
Other antiprotozoal agents			
metronidazole	Mild, moderate, or severe intestinal amebiasis or amoebic hepatic abscess	750 mg P.O. t.i.d. for 10 days followed by iodoquinol	• Know that metronidazole is contraindicated in a first-trimester pregnant or a lactating patient, or one with hypersensitivity to the drug or any nitroimidazole derivative. • Administer with caution to a patient with severe hepatic disease.
	Vaginal trichomoniasis	2 grams P.O. once or 250 mg P.O. t.i.d. for 7 days	

SELECTED MAJOR DRUGS

Antimalarial and other antiprotozoal agents (continued)

DRUG	MAJOR INDICATIONS	USUAL ADULT DOSAGES	CONTRAINDICATIONS AND PRECAUTIONS
Other antiprotozoal agents (continued)			
pentamidine ise-thionate	Treatment of *Pneumocystis carinii* pneumonia	4 mg/kg I.V. or I.M. once daily for 14 days	• Know that pentamidine isethionate has no known contraindications.
	Prevention of *P. carinii* pneumonia	300 mg inhaled via a Respiragard II nebulizer once every 4 weeks	• Administer with caution to a patient with hypotension, hypertension, hypoglycemia, hyperglycemia, hypocalcemia, leukopenia, thrombocytopenia, anemia, or hepatic or renal dysfunction.
	African trypanosomiasis	4 mg/kg/day I.M. or I.V. for 10 days	
	Visceral leishmaniasis	2 to 4 mg/kg/day I.M. or I.V. up to 15 doses	
quinacrine hydro-chloride	Giardiasis	100 mg P.O. t.i.d. for 5 days	• Know that quinacrine is contraindicated in a patient receiving primaquine.
			• Administer with caution to a patient who is over age 60 or to one with psoriasis, porphyria, G6PD deficiency, severe renal or cardiac disease, hepatic disease, alcoholism, or a history of psychosis.

• Instruct the patient to avoid drinking alcohol during furazolidone or metronidazole therapy because it can cause serious systemic adverse reactions.

• Teach the patient mouth care techniques if metronidazole causes glossitis or stomatitis.

• Inform the patient that iodoquinol can interfere with thyroid function tests.

• Inform the patient receiving iodoquinol that hair loss or nail and hair discoloration can occur.

• *Advise the patient that hospitalization and confinement to bed will be necessary during emetine therapy and for several days thereafter. Stress the importance of alerting the nurse immediately if chest pain, lightheadedness, or shortness of breath occur.*

• Warn the patient that emetine I.M. may cause tenderness and aching at the injection site and localized muscle weakness.

• *Advise the patient on long-term antiprotozoal therapy to have periodic ophthalmologic examinations and to report any vision disturbances to the physician.*

• Advise the patient that quinacrine may cause a harmless discoloration of the urine.

• Advise the patient to have periodic CBCs during long-term quinacrine therapy.

• Teach the patient about drug interactions that can occur with furazolidone. Advise the patient to avoid tyramine-rich foods, such as cheese, chocolate, and sausage, and over-the-counter medications containing sympathomimetics, such as cold capsules and anorexiants.

• Instruct the patient to report adverse reactions to the physician.

Evaluation

The following examples represent appropriate evaluation statements for a patient receiving an antiprotozoal agent.

• The patient has no conditions that contraindicate antiprotozoal therapy.

• The patient exhibits no signs of complications in the preexisting condition linked to the prescribed antiprotozoal agent.

• The patient exhibits no adverse reactions to the prescribed antiprotozoal agent.

• The patient maintains adequate hydration during antiprotozoal therapy.

• The patient and family express an accurate understanding of the points taught about the prescribed antiprotozoal agent.

• The patient correctly identifies adverse reactions that must be reported during antiprotozoal therapy.

CHAPTER SUMMARY

Chapter 64 discussed antimalarial and other antiprotozoal agents as they are used to prevent or treat malaria and other protozoal infections. Here are the chapter highlights.

• Four types of plasmodia cause malaria: *P. falciparum, P. malariae, P. ovale,* and *P. vivax.* In some areas of the world, strains of *P. falciparum* are chloroquine-resistant.

• The major agents used to prevent and treat malaria include the 4-aminoquinolones (chloroquine hydrochloride, chloroquine phosphate, and hydroxychloroquine), mefloquine, the 8-aminoquinolone primaquine, pyrimethamine, and quinine.

• Interactions occur when certain antimalarial drugs are used with antacids, neuromuscular blocking agents, oral anticoagulants, cardiac glycosides, quinacrine, beta-adrenergic blockers, calcium channel blockers, quinine and quinidine, chloroquine, valproic acid, and folic acid.

• Antimalarial drugs can produce a wide variety of adverse reactions. Quinine commonly produces cinchonism; the others typically produce adverse GI reactions. Less common adverse reactions range from blood disorders to deafness to psychotic episodes.

• Different antiprotozoal agents are used to manage amebiasis, giardiasis, leishmaniasis, *P. carinii* infections, toxoplasmosis, trichomoniasis, and African trypanosomiasis. These agents include emetine, furazolidone, iodoquinol, metronidazole, pentamidine, and quinacrine.

• Certain other antiprotozoal agents will interact with other drugs, including amphetamines, monoamine oxidase inhibitors, levodopa, tyramine, iodine preparations, anticoagulants, disulfiram, aminoglycosides, cisplatin, amphotericin B, phenylpropanolamine, ephedrine, ethanol, phenobarbital, and primaquine. Interactions can be severe and unpredictable and may include nephrotoxicity, acute psychosis, and increased drug toxicity.

• The other antiprotozoal drugs produce a range of adverse reactions, which include GI distress, CNS disturbances, and nephrotoxicity. More severe, but less common, adverse reactions affecting most body systems can occur.

• Because of the potential toxicity of the other antiprotozoal agents and their interactions with other drugs, a patient receiving an antiprotozoal agent requires close supervision during administration and regular monitoring for adverse reactions.

• The nurse should instruct the patient and family in the administration, therapeutic effects, and possible adverse effects of antimalarial and other antiprotozoal agents, monitor the patient throughout therapy, and notify the physician if adverse reactions occur.

STUDY QUESTIONS

See Appendix 1 for answers.

1. Ellen Hearst, age 22, is planning to go on a 3-week study tour of Southeast Asia. Because she knows that malaria is endemic in that part of the world, she asks her physician about antimalarial agents that are used to prevent infection. Her physician prescribes chloroquine. What is the mechanism of action of chloroquine?
(a) It disrupts the parasite's protein synthesis.
(b) It affects the parasite's mitochondria, disrupting cellular metabolism.
(c) It disrupts the parasite's reproduction.
(d) It affects the parasite's DNA, rendering it ineffective.

2. Chloroquine is effective against all types of malaria except which of the following?
(a) *Plasmodium malariae*
(b) *P. falciparum*
(c) *P. ovale*
(d) *P. vivax*

3. For chloroquine to prevent malaria effectively, when should Ms. Hearst take this medication?
(a) weekly from the day of departure until she returns
(b) weekly after departure and for 1 week after she returns
(c) weekly for 1 week before departure and for 6 weeks after she returns
(d) weekly for 8 weeks after she returns

4. Ms. Hearst reports GI distress since taking chloroquine. To minimize this adverse reaction, the nurse should give her which instructions?
(a) Take the medication with antacids.
(b) Take the medication with meals.
(c) Take the medication at bedtime.
(d) Take the medication before meals.

5. Cecilia Raymond, age 36, has a vaginal discharge, severe itching, tenderness, and dysuria. Laboratory tests confirm the diagnosis of vaginal trichomoniasis. Which agents is her physician most likely to prescribe?
(a) pentamidine
(b) metronidazole
(c) emetine
(d) iodoquinol

6. Mel Green, age 62, is admitted to the hospital with pleuritic chest pain, severe productive cough, chills, and fever. Laboratory tests confirm the diagnosis of *Pneumocystis carinii* pneumonia. The physician prescribes pentamidine. Concomitant use of an antibiotic from which class may increase pentamidine's nephrotoxic effects?
(a) penicillins
(b) aminoglycosides
(c) cephalosporins
(d) sulfonamides

7. During I.V. pentamidine therapy, the nurse should assess for which of the following adverse reactions?
(a) seizures
(b) nausea and vomiting
(c) hypotension and arrhythmias
(d) hypertensive crisis

8. Pentamidine also may be administered by inhalant nebulizer. Which adverse reaction is associated with inhalation administration of pentamidine?
(a) abdominal distention
(b) bronchospasm and cough
(c) cardiac arrythmias
(d) respiratory depression

SELECTED REFERENCES

Abramowicz, M. (Ed.). (January 26, 1990). Treatment of sexually transmitted diseases. *Medical Letter on Drugs and Therapeutics 32,* 5-10.

Abramowicz, M. (Ed.). (February 9, 1990). Mefloquine for malaria. *Medical Letter on Drugs and Therapeutics 32,* 13-14.

Abramowicz, M. (Ed.). (March 23, 1990). Drugs for parasitic infections. *Medical Letter on Drugs and Therapeutics 32,* 23-30.

AHFS drug information 90. (1990) Bethesda, MD: American Society of Hospital Pharmacists.

Drug facts and comparisons. (1991). St Louis: Facts and Comparisons Division, Lippincott.

Goodman and Gilman's the pharmacological basis of therapeutics (8th ed.; 1990). Elmsford, NY: Pergamon Press.

Hansten, P., and Horn, J. (1990). *Drug interactions* (7th ed.). Philadelphia: Lea & Febiger.

Herwaldt, B., Krogstad, D., and Schlesinger, P. (1988). Antimalarial agents: Specific chemoprophylaxis regimens. *Antimicrobial Agents and Chemotherapy, 32*(7), 953-956.

North American Nursing Diagnosis Association (1990). *Taxonomy I - Revised, with official diagnostic categories.* St. Louis: NANDA.

Rosenblatt, J., and Edson, R. (1987). Metronidazole. *Mayo Clinic Proceedings, 62*(11), 1013-1017.

CHAPTER

65

URINARY ANTISEPTIC AGENTS

OBJECTIVES

After reading and studying this chapter, the student should be able to:

1. Describe conditions that place patients at greater risk for developing urinary tract infections (UTIs).

2. Name the principal bacterial organism responsible for producing community-acquired UTIs.

3. Describe the mechanisms of action for the quinolones, nitrofurantoin, and sulfonamides.

4. Discuss drug interactions associated with urinary antiseptic agents.

5. Describe adverse reactions associated with quinolones, nitrofurantoin, and sulfonamides.

6. Describe how to apply the nursing process when caring for a patient who is receiving a urinary antiseptic agent.

INTRODUCTION

Urinary tract infections occur frequently in community and hospital environments. Certain patients—including females, diabetics, paraplegics, pregnant patients, elderly males, and those with Cushing's syndrome—run the greatest risk of developing UTIs. Surgery and other medical procedures involving the urinary tract, including catheter placement, also increase the patient's risk.

Urinary antiseptic agents provide antibacterial effects that are limited to the urine. As a rule, these agents are not used to treat systemic infections because safe doses of the drugs do not reach effective concentration levels in the plasma. Ciprofloxacin is the exception and is indicated for systemic infections. Urinary antiseptic agents do reach therapeutic concentrations in the urine, however, because they concentrate in the renal tubules during their excretion.

Before therapy with a urinary antiseptic agent is initiated, a diagnosis based on the patient's symptoms and urinalysis results is made. Although most community-acquired UTIs are caused by *Escherichia coli,* a urine culture and sensitivity test is necessary to confirm the infection, the specific organism, and appropriate antibiotics. More than 100,000 organisms per cubic milliliter cultured from a midstream urine specimen confirms the presence of a UTI. Treatment usually succeeds if an appropriate antimicrobial drug is administered at the proper dosage for an appropriate length of time and if the patient has no complications.

The most commonly used urinary antiseptics are the quinolones (ciprofloxacin, norfloxacin, and ofloxacin), sulfanomides (co-trimoxazole, sulfadiazine, sulfamethoxazole, and sulfisoxazole), and nitrofurantoin. These agents inhibit the growth of many species of bacteria in the urine and greatly diminish the symptoms of lower UTIs. Other, less commonly used urinary antiseptic agents include cinoxacin, methenamine, nalidixic acid, and trimethoprim.

For a summary of these agents. see *Selected major drugs: Urinary antiseptic agents,* page 1134. For a listing of applicable nursing diagnoses that the nurse may formulate when caring for a patient receiving these agents, see *Selected nursing diagnoses: Urinary antiseptic agents,* page 1125. For detailed information on applying the nursing process, see Chapter 6, The Nursing Process and Drug Therapy.

QUINOLONES

Ciprofloxacin, norfloxacin, and ofloxacin are structurally similar synthetic chemotherapeutic agents. They are administered orally to treat UTIs.

PHARMACOKINETICS

After oral administration, the quinolones are absorbed well, highly protein bound, metabolized in the liver, and excreted primarily by the kidneys in the urine.

Absorption, distribution, metabolism, excretion
After oral administration, about 70% of a ciprofloxacin dose is absorbed. Food in the stomach decreases the rate but not the extent of absorption. From 20% to 40% of a ciprofloxacin dose is protein bound in the plasma. Ciprofloxacin is distributed widely, with highest concentrations in the bile, lungs, kidneys, liver, gallbladder, uterus, seminal fluid, prostatic tissue, tonsils, endometrium, fallopian tubes, and ovaries. Researchers do not know if ciprofloxacin crosses the placenta or is distributed into breast milk. Ciprofloxacin is metabolized partially and is excreted in the urine and feces as the parent compound and its metabolites.

Orally administered norfloxacin is absorbed readily but incompletely from the gastrointestinal (GI) tract. Food in the stomach may decrease drug absorption. From 10% to 15% of a norfloxacin dose is protein bound in the plasma. A urine concentration level of 200 mcg/ml is attained in 2 to 3 hours after an oral dose of 400 mg. Concentration in prostatic tissue ranges from 1 to 3 mcg/ml. Norfloxacin crosses the placenta, but researchers do not know if it appears in breast milk. About 30% of a dose is excreted in the urine as unmetabolized norfloxacin, with an additional 5% to 8% excreted as six active metabolites of lesser activity. Another 30% of the norfloxacin dose is eliminated in the feces.

After oral administration, approximately 98% of ofloxacin is absorbed. The drug is distributed widely to body tissues and fluids and has been detected in blister fluid, cervix, lung tissue, ovaries, prostatic fluid and tissue, skin, and sputum. Researchers do not know if ofloxacin is distributed to cerebrospinal fluid or brain tissue. Most of an ofloxacin dose is excreted unchanged in the urine.

Onset, peak, duration
The onset of action for ciprofloxacin is about 30 minutes. The peak concentration level for ciprofloxacin increases in proportion to the dose over the oral dosage range. The peak plasma concentration of ciprofloxacin occurs 1 to 2 hours after administration. The serum half-life is about 4 hours and is longer in patients with reduced renal function.

The onset for norfloxacin is about 30 minutes. Norfloxacin's peak concentrations are 1.58 to 2.41 mcg/ml after 1 to 2 hours for doses of 400 mg and 800 mg. The plasma half-life of norfloxacin is 3 to 4 hours, increasing to 6.5 hours when the creatinine clearance is below 30 ml/min/ 1.73 m².

The maximum serum concentration of ofloxacin is reached 1 to 2 hours after an oral dose. Because ofloxacin has a biphasic elimination pattern, the half-lives are approximately 4 to 5 hours and 20 to 25 hours.

PHARMACODYNAMICS

The effectiveness of quinolones in treating UTIs relates to an affinity for enzymes within the bacterial cell. These drugs interrupt deoxyribonucleic acid (DNA) synthesis during bacterial replication.

PHARMACOTHERAPEUTICS

The quinolones can be used to treat a wide variety of UTIs. In addition, ciprofloxacin is used to treat lower respiratory tract infections; skin, bone, or joint infections; and infectious diarrhea. Ofloxacin also is used to treat selected sexually transmitted diseases, lower respiratory infections, skin and skin-structure infections, and prostatitis. All quinolones require dosage reductions when they are used to treat patients with renal dysfunction. They are contraindicated in pediatric patients.

ciprofloxacin (Cipro). This agent has a wide spectrum of antibacterial activity and is indicated to treat UTIs; lower respiratory tract, skin, bone, or joint infections; and infectious diarrhea caused by susceptible gram-negative and gram-positive aerobic bacteria. It is inactive against most anaerobic bacteria.

Usual adult dosage: for UTIs, 250 to 500 mg P.O. every 12 hours; for respiratory tract, skin, bone or joint infections, 500 to 750 mg P.O. every 12 hours; for infectious diarrhea, 500 mg P.O. every 12 hours.

norfloxacin (Noroxin). Indicated for treating complicated and uncomplicated UTIs, norfloxacin is 100 times more active than nalidixic acid, with a similar spectrum. Norfloxacin also is effective against *Pseudomonas aeruginosa*, *Staphylococcus aureus*, and enterococci.

Usual adult dosage: for uncomplicated UTIs, 400 mg P.O. b.i.d. for 7 to 10 days; for complicated UTIs, 400 mg P.O. b.i.d. for 10 to 21 days.

ofloxacin (Floxin). A new quinolone, ofloxacin is used to treat such UTIs as cystitis caused by *E. coli*, *Klebsiella pneumoniae*, or other organisms, and complicated UTIs. Ofloxacin, however, also is used to treat lower respiratory tract infections, mild to moderate skin and skinstructure infections, prostatitis, and such sexually transmitted diseases as acute, uncomplicated gonorrhea and cervicitis or urethritis caused by *Chlamydia trachomatis* or *Neisseria gonorrhoeae*.

Usual adult dosage: for UTIs, 200 mg P.O. every 12 hours for 3 to 10 days, depending on the organism present; for lower respiratory tract and mild to moderate skin and skinstructure infections, 400 mg P.O. every 12 hours for 10 days; for prostatitis, 300 mg P.O. every 12 hours for 6 weeks; for acute, uncomplicated gonorrhea, 400 mg P.O. as a single dose; for cervicitis or urethritis caused by *C. trachomatis* or *N. gonorrhoeae*, 300 mg P.O. every 12 hours for 7 days.

Drug interactions

Few drug interactions are associated with the quinolones. These agents interact with antacids that contain magnesium or aluminum hydroxide, resulting in decreased absorption of the quinolone agent. They also interact with xanthine derivatives, such as aminophylline or theophylline, increasing the plasma theophylline concentration and the risk of theophylline toxicity. Ciprofloxacin and norfloxacin interact with probenecid, resulting in decreased renal elimination of these quinolones—thus increasing their serum concentrations and half-lives.

ADVERSE DRUG REACTIONS

Well tolerated by most patients, the quinolones produce few adverse reactions. Any reactions that occur disappear with discontinuation of the drug. The most common reactions affect the GI tract and include nausea, vomiting, diarrhea, and abdominal pain. The affects 2% to 10% of patients receiving quinolones. About 1% of patients develop adverse central nervous system (CNS) reactions, such as headache, drowsiness, seizures, visual disturbances, hallucinations, depression, and agitation. Ofloxacin also may cause insomnia and dizziness. Less common adverse reactions affect the integumentary system.

In fewer than 1% of patients, the quinolones produce hypersensitivity reactions that include urticaria, nonspecific rashes, pruritus, and edema. Other rare reactions include hematologic problems, such as hemolytic anemia, that are associated with glucose-6-phosphate dehydrogenase (G6PD) deficiency.

NURSING PROCESS APPLICATION

The following information assists the nurse in caring for a patient who is receiving a quinolone.

Assessment
• Review the patient's history for a preexisting condition that contraindicates the use of a quinolone, such as pregnancy, lactation, or known hypersensitivity to the drug or other quinolones.
• Review the patient's history for a preexisting condition that requires cautious use of a quinolone, such as known or suspected CNS disorders or factors that predispose the patient to seizures.
• Assess the patient for adverse reactions to the prescribed quinolone, such as GI distress, CNS disturbances, skin disorders, and hypersensitivity reactions.
• Review the patient's medication history to identify the use of drugs that may interact with the prescribed quinolone, such as xanthine derivatives or antacids that contain magnesium or aluminum hydroxide.
• Assess the effectiveness of the prescribed quinolone periodically.
• Assess the patient for seizures.
• Evaluate the patient's and family's knowledge about the prescribed quinolone.

Nursing diagnoses
The following examples represent appropriate nursing diagnoses for a patient receiving a quinolone.
• Potential for injury related to a preexisting condition that contraindicates the use of a quinolone

• Potential for injury related to a preexisting condition that requires cautious use of a quinolone
• Potential for injury related to adverse drug reactions
• Potential for trauma related to quinolone-induced seizures
• Knowledge deficit related to the prescribed quinolone

Planning and implementation

• Do not administer a quinolone to a patient with a condition that contraindicates its use.
• Administer a quinolone cautiously to a patient at risk because of a preexisting condition.
• Monitor the patient periodically for adverse reactions during quinolone therapy.
• Monitor hydration if the patient experiences nausea, vomiting, or diarrhea. Request a prescription for an antiemetic or antidiarrheal agent if needed. Notify the physician if the patient cannot tolerate oral administration of the drug.
• Administer a mild analgesic as prescribed if the patient experiences a headache.
• *Take safety precautions if the patient experiences adverse CNS reactions, such as drowsiness, visual disturbances, or dizziness. For example, place the bed in the low position, keep the bed rails raised, and supervise ambulation.*
• Administer a sedative as prescribed if ofloxacin produces insomnia. Also use nonpharmacologic measures, such as a back rub or having the patient practice relaxation techniques.
• Adjust the dosage as prescribed for a patient with impaired renal function because the elimination rate will decrease and the serum half-life will increase.
• *Administer antacids, if prescribed, at least 2 hours after administering a quinolone.*
• Notify the physician if adverse reactions occur.
• Question the patient about any history of head trauma, seizures, or use of drugs known to cause seizures before administering a quinolone.
• Monitor the patient for seizures during quinolone therapy.
• Take seizure precautions, such as padding the bed rails, if needed.
• Notify the physician immediately if seizures occur.

Patient teaching

• Teach the patient and family the name, dose, frequency, action, and adverse effects of the prescribed quinolone.
• Advise the patient taking a quinolone to use extreme caution when driving or operating machinery because these drugs may cause dizziness, drowsiness, or other adverse CNS reactions.
• Advise the patient to take a mild analgesic if headache occurs.
• Teach the patient nonpharmacologic measures to use if ofloxacin causes insomnia. If these measures are ineffective, instruct the patient to request a prescription for a sedative from the physician.

• Instruct the patient to report any skin rash, urticaria, ankle swelling, or pruritus because these signs may indicate a quinolone hypersensitivity reaction.
• *Inform the patient when to take concomitantly prescribed antacids.*
• Instruct the patient to notify the physician of any other adverse reactions.

Evaluation

The following examples represent appropriate evaluation statements for a patient receiving a quinolone.
• The patient has no conditions that contraindicate quinolone therapy.
• The patient exhibits no signs of complications in the preexisting condition linked to the prescribed quinolone.
• The patient exhibits no adverse reactions to the prescribed quinolone.
• The patient experiences no seizures during quinolone therapy.
• The patient and family express an accurate understanding of the points taught about the prescribed quinolone.
• The patient takes the prescribed antacid dose at the appropriate time in relation to the quinolone dose.

SULFONAMIDES

The sulfonamides were the first effective systemic antibacterials. Today, they are less useful because resistant strains of bacteria have emerged. By modifying the sulfonamides, researchers have developed other useful drugs, including para-aminosalicylic acid (for treating tuberculosis), carbonic anhydrase inhibitor diuretics, sulfonylurea hypoglycemics, and thiouracil antithyroids.

PHARMACOKINETICS

Most sulfonamides are absorbed well and distributed widely in the body. They are metabolized in the liver to inactive metabolites.

Absorption, distribution, metabolism, excretion

The sulfonamides differ markedly in their absorption. Sulfonamides are absorbed well after oral administration. From 70% to 90% of an oral dose is absorbed from the GI tract. Food can delay but not reduce absorption.

Sulfonamides enter the cerebrospinal, synovial, pleural, and peritoneal fluids with concentration levels of 80% of serum concentration levels. These drugs cross the placenta readily; fetal plasma concentrations may exceed 50% of maternal plasma concentrations. They also are distributed into breast milk.

Most sulfonamides are metabolized in the liver by acetylation and glucuronidation. The metabolites lack antibacterial activity and usually are acetyl metabolites, which are less water-soluble than the parent sulfonamide.

Sulfonamides and their metabolites are excreted primarily by the kidneys via glomerular filtration. Partial reabsorption and active tubular secretion also are involved. The rates of excretion and solubility characteristics of the drugs vary widely with urine pH. Alkalinizing the urine increases renal excretion and decreases sulfonamide blood concentrations.

Onset, peak, duration

Sulfonamides are classified as short-acting, intermediate-acting, and long-acting, depending on their absorption and excretion rates. Sulfisoxazole is considered short-acting, with a plasma half-life of about 4 to 8 hours. Co-trimoxazole, sulfadiazine, and sulfamethoxazole are intermediate-acting, with plasma half-lives of about 7 to 17 hours. Sulfadoxine (in combination with pyrimethamine as Fansidar) is the only long-acting sulfonamide available in the United States. It has a half-life of 100 to 250 hours and is used for treatment and prevention of malaria caused by chloroquine-resistant *Plasmodium falciparum.* (For more information on this drug, see Chapter 64, Antimalarial and Other Antiprotozoal Agents.)

Peak plasma concentration levels usually are reached within 2 to 4 hours after oral administration of short-acting sulfonamides. Intermediate-acting sulfonamides are absorbed more slowly, with peak concentrations occurring within 3 to 17 hours, depending on the specific drug used.

Widely varying blood concentrations occur among patients receiving identical doses of the same sulfonamide. Blood concentrations are based on total sulfonamide concentration, even though only free (unmetabolized and unbound) sulfonamides are microbiologically active. Optimal blood concentrations of 60 to 150 mcg/ml have been reported. Those greater than 200 mcg/ml increase the incidence of toxicity.

PHARMACODYNAMICS

Sulfonamides are bacteriostatic agents that prevent the growth of microorganisms by inhibiting folic acid production.

Mechanism of action

Sulfonamides competitively inhibit the incorporation of para-aminobenzoic acid (PABA) into dihydropteroic acid and subsequently into dihydrofolic acid, thereby inhibiting folic acid synthesis. The decreased folic acid synthesis decreases bacterial nucleotides and inhibits bacterial growth.

PHARMACOTHERAPEUTICS

Sulfonamides are used primarily to treat acute UTIs. With recurrent or chronic UTIs, the infecting organism may or may not be susceptible to sulfonamides. The choice of therapy should be based on bacteria susceptibility tests. Sulfonamides also are used to treat infections caused by *Nocardia asteroides, Toxoplasma gondii,* and *C. trachomatis.* Sulfonamides exhibit a wide spectrum of activity against gram-positive and gram-negative bacteria. However, the increasing resistance of formerly susceptible bacteria has decreased the clinical usefulness of these drugs. Sulfonamides effectively prevent recurrent attacks of rheumatic fever caused by group A beta-hemolytic streptococcal infections, but are ineffective against established streptococcal pharyngitis. Sulfonamide prophylaxis against *Neisseria meningitidis* is variably effective.

co-trimoxazole (Bactrim, Septra). A combination of two drugs, co-trimoxazole is used to treat UTIs, shigellosis, otitis media in children, *Pneumocystis carinii* pneumonia, and chronic bronchitis. The co-trimoxazole dosage is expressed in terms of the amount of both drugs in a fixed combination that contains a ratio of 1 mg of trimethoprim to 5 mg of sulfamethoxazole.
Usual adult dosage: for UTIs, 160 mg trimethoprim and 800 mg sulfamethoxazole (double-strength tablet) P.O. every 12 hours for 10 to 14 days; for shigellosis, 160 mg trimethoprim and 800 mg sulfamethoxazole (double-strength tablet) P.O. every 12 hours for 5 days; for simple cystitis or acute urethral syndrome, one to three double-strength tablets as a single dose; for chronic bronchitis, 160 mg trimethoprim and 800 mg sulfamethoxazole every 12 hours for 10 to 14 days; for *P. carinii* pneumonia, 20 mg/kg trimethoprim and 100 mg/kg sulfamethoxazole daily, in equally divided doses every 6 hours for 14 days.
Usual pediatric dosage: for UTIs, 8 mg/kg trimethoprim and 40 mg/kg sulfamethoxazole daily in two divided doses every 12 hours for 10 days; for shigellosis, 8 mg/kg trimethoprim and 40 mg/kg sulfamethoxazole daily in two divided doses every 12 hours for 5 days; for otitis media, 8 mg/kg trimethoprim and 40 mg/kg sulfamethoxazole daily, in two divided doses every 12 hours for 10 days; for *P. carinii* pneumonia, 20 mg/kg trimethoprim and 100 mg/kg sulfamethoxazole daily, in equally divided doses every 6 hours for 14 days.

sulfadiazine (Microsulfon). An intermediate-acting sulfonamide, sulfadiazine is absorbed and excreted rapidly after oral administration. It may be used to prevent sul-

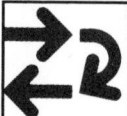

DRUG INTERACTIONS
Sulfonamides

The following chart summarizes the significant interactions between sulfonamides and other drugs.

DRUG	INTERACTING DRUGS	POSSIBLE EFFECTS	NURSING IMPLICATIONS
co-trimoxazole, sulfadiazine, sulfamethoxazole, sulfisoxazole	para-aminobenzoic acid	Decreases the antibacterial activity	• Avoid concurrent use.
	sulfonylurea hypoglycemic agents	Displace sulfonylurea from protein-binding site, increasing hypoglycemic effect	• Monitor the patient's blood glucose level more frequently. • Decrease the sulfonylurea dosage, if necessary.
	methenamine	May cause crystalluria	• Avoid concomitant use.
co-trimoxazole	coumarin anticoagulants	Displaces anticoagulant from protein-binding site, increasing the effect of anticoagulant	• Monitor the patient's prothrombin time frequently. • Decrease the anticoagulant dosage, if necessary.
	cyclosporine	Causes additive nephrotoxicity	• Monitor the patient's renal function closely.

fonamide-sensitive meningococcus and is the drug of choice for nocardiosis.

Usual adult dosage: for UTIs, initially, 2 to 4 grams P.O., then 500 mg to 1 gram P.O. every 6 hours; for adjunctive treatment in toxoplasmosis and sulfonamide-sensitive meningococcus, 2 to 8 grams P.O. in divided doses every 6 hours for 3 to 4 weeks, discontinued for 1 week, then administered with 25 mg of pyrimethamine P.O. daily for 3 to 4 weeks; for nocardiosis, 4 to 8 grams P.O. daily in divided doses for 6 weeks.

Usual pediatric dosage: for UTIs, initially, 75 mg/kg P.O., then 150 mg/kg P.O. in four to six divided doses daily; for rheumatic fever prophylaxis (as an alternative to penicillin), for children over 30 kg, 1 gram P.O. daily, and for children 30 kg and under, 500 mg P.O. daily; for adjunctive treatment of toxoplasmosis, 100 to 200 mg/kg P.O. in divided doses every 6 hours for 3 to 4 weeks, then administered with 2 mg/kg pyrimethamine daily for 3 days, then 1 mg/kg daily for 3 to 4 weeks.

sulfamethoxazole (Gantanol). An intermediate-acting sulfonamide, sulfamethoxazole is used to prevent acute and recurrent UTIs and to treat lymphogranuloma venereum.

Usual adult dosage: for UTIs, initially, 2 grams P.O., then 1 gram P.O. b.i.d. for severe infections; for lymphogranuloma venereum (genital, inguinal, or anorectal infections), 1 gram P.O. b.i.d. for at least 21 days.

Usual pediatric dosage: for UTIs in children over age 2 months, initially, 50 to 60 mg/kg P.O. every 12 hours, then 25 to 30 mg/kg P.O. every 12 hours.

sulfisoxazole (Gantrisin). Because of its low cost and high water-solubility, sulfisoxazole is considered the sulfonamide of choice. It commonly is used to treat UTIs.

Usual adult dosage: for UTIs, initially, 2 to 4 grams P.O., then 1 to 2 grams P.O. q.i.d.; or 4 to 5 grams P.O. of sustained-release suspension every 12 hours.

Usual pediatric dosage: for UTIs in children over age 2 months, initially, 75 mg/kg P.O. daily in divided doses every 6 hours, then 150 mg/kg P.O. daily in divided doses every 6 hours; for sustained-release suspension, 60 to 75 mg/kg P.O. every 12 hours, then 120 to 150 mg/kg P.O. daily in divided doses.

Drug interactions

All sulfonamides interact with PABA, sulfonylurea hypoglycemic agents, and methenamine. Co-trimoxazole also interacts with coumarin anticoagulants and cyclosporine. (For detailed information, see *Drug interactions: Sulfonamides.*)

ADVERSE DRUG REACTIONS

The sulfonamides cause numerous adverse reactions. Excessively high doses of less water-soluble sulfonamides can produce crystalluria and tubular deposits of sulfonamide crystals. These complications can be minimized by maintaining a high urine flow rate and alkalinized urine. With the newer water-soluble sulfonamides, these complications usually do not occur. Nausea, vomiting, and diarrhea are common.

The incidence of hypersensitivity reactions appears to increase as the dosage increases. Various dermatologic reactions, including rash, pruritus, erythema nodosum, erythema multiforme of the Stevens-Johnson type, and exfoliative dermatitis, can occur. Sulfonamides also can produce photosensitivity; the patient should avoid exposure to ultraviolet light or sunlight.

Fever may develop 7 to 10 days after the initial sulfonamide dose. Serum sickness-like reactions, including fever, joint pain, urticarial eruptions, bronchospasm, and leukopenia, can occur. Extremely rare reactions, such as, granulocytopenia, aplastic anemia, and hemolytic anemia, have been reported.

NURSING PROCESS APPLICATION

The following information assists the nurse in caring for a patient who is receiving a sulfonamide.

Assessment
• Review the patient's history for a preexisting condition that contraindicates the use of a sulfonamide, such as term pregnancy, lactation, and known hypersensitivity to the drug.
• Review the patient's history for a preexisting condition that requires cautious use of a sulfonamide, such as impaired renal or hepatic function, severe allergy, bronchial asthma, or G6PD deficiency.
• Assess the patient for adverse reactions to the prescribed sulfonamide, such as GI distress or hypersensitivity reactions.
• Review the patient's medication history to identify the use of drugs that may interact with the prescribed sulfonamide, such as PABA, sulfonylurea hypoglycemic agents, and methenamine.
• Assess the effectiveness of the prescribed sulfonamide periodically.
• Assess the patient for changes in the urine elimination pattern.
• Evaluate the patient's and family's knowledge about the prescribed sulfonamide.

Nursing diagnoses
The following examples represent appropriate nursing diagnoses for a patient receiving a sulfonamide.
• Potential for injury related to a preexisting condition that contraindicates the use of a sulfonamide
• Potential for injury related to a preexisting condition that requires cautious use of a sulfonamide
• Potential for injury related to adverse drug reactions
• Altered urinary elimination related to sulfonamide-induced crystalluria and tubular deposits of sulfonamide crystals
• Knowledge deficit related to the prescribed sulfonamide

Planning and implementation
• Do not administer a sulfonamide to a patient with a condition that contraindicates its use.
• Administer a sulfonamide cautiously to a patient at risk because of a preexisting condition.
• Monitor the patient periodically for adverse reactions during sulfonamide therapy.
• Monitor hydration if the patient experiences nausea, vomiting, or diarrhea. Notify the physician and request a prescription for an antiemetic or antidiarrheal agent if needed.
• Inspect the patient's skin regularly for evidence of dermatologic hypersensitivity reactions, such as rash, erythema nodosum, erythema multiforme, or exfoliative dermatitis. Ask the patient about pruritus. Withhold the prescribed sulfonamide dose and notify the physician if dermatologic reactions occur. Expect to provide dermatologic care to relieve discomfort caused by the reaction.
• Monitor the patient's temperature for an elevation that may develop 7 to 10 days after the initial sulfonamide dose. Also monitor the patient for other serum sickness-like reactions, such as joint pain, urticarial eruptions, bronchospasm, and leukopenia. Notify the physician if these symptoms occur and expect to administer a mild analgesic orantipyretic agent to reduce the temperature and promote comfort.
• Administer oral preparations of sulfonamides with ample fluids.
• Notify the physician if the adverse reactions occur.
• *Monitor the patient's urine elimination pattern for such changes as an increase or decrease in amount voided, urinary frequency, or dysuria.*
• *Monitor the patient's fluid intake and output. The urine output should be at least 1,500 ml per day to ensure proper hydration. Inadequate urine output can lead to crystalluria or tubular deposits of the sulfonamide.*
• *Notify the physician if the patient cannot consume adequate amounts of fluid or if the patient's urine elimination pattern changes for no apparent reason.*

Patient teaching
• Teach the patient and family the name, dose, frequency, action, and adverse effects of the prescribed sulfonamide.
• *Advise the patient to avoid direct sunlight to help prevent a photosensitivity reaction.*
• Advise calling the physician if the patient develops signs and symptoms of a hematologic reaction, such as sore throat, pallor, purpura, jaundice, or weakness, or of a dermatologic reaction, such as skin rash or pruritus.
• *Stress the importance of completing the prescribed sulfonamide regimen.*
• *Instruct the patient to consume at least eight 8-oz glasses (2 liters) of fluid daily while taking a sulfonamide.*
• Instruct the patient to notify the physician if any other adverse reactions occur.

Evaluation

The following examples represent appropriate evaluation statements for a patient receiving a sulfonamide.

• The patient has no conditions that contraindicate sulfonamide therapy.

• The patient exhibits no signs of complications in the preexisting condition linked to the prescribed sulfonamide.

• The patient exhibits no adverse reactions to the prescribed sulfonamide.

• The patient maintains a urine output of at least 1,500 ml daily throughout sulfonamide therapy.

• The patient and family express an accurate understanding of the points taught about the prescribed sulfonamide.

• The patient correctly identifies adverse reactions that must be reported to the physician.

NITROFURANTOIN

Nitrofurantoin is used primarily to treat acute and chronic UTIs.

PHARMACOKINETICS

After oral administration, nitrofurantoin is absorbed rapidly and well from the GI tract and excreted rapidly in the urine. The macrocrystalline form is absorbed and excreted more slowly than the microcrystalline.

Absorption, distribution, metabolism, excretion

Microcrystalline nitrofurantoin is absorbed rapidly and completely from the GI tract. Antibacterial activity in serum is low after oral doses. The macrocrystalline form, with its larger drug particles, delays absorption from the GI tract. Delaying the entrance of the drug into body fluids lowers the peak concentration level in serum and decreases the incidence and severity of nausea, without significantly affecting the peak concentration in the urinary tract.

Concomitant ingestion of food enhances the bioavailability of nitrofurantoin. Antibacterial activity is higher in acid urine. Nitrofurantoin crosses the placenta and appears in breast milk. It also is distributed in bile. Two-thirds of a nitrofurantoin dose is metabolized by the liver and one third is excreted unchanged in the urine. The presence of the drug in urine decreases as the creatinine clearance decreases.

Onset, peak, duration

Nitrofurantoin does not accumulate in the serum of patients with normal renal function because the serum half-life is 20 minutes. The drug is 20% to 60% protein bound. An average dose of nitrofurantoin yields a peak concentration level in the urine of about 200 mcg/ml. A urine concentration insufficient to inhibit common urinary tract pathogens occurs when the creatinine clearance is less than 40 ml/min.

PHARMACODYNAMICS

Usually bacteriostatic, nitrofurantoin may become bactericidal depending on its urinary concentration and the susceptibility of the infecting organisms. Although the exact mechanism of action has not been described, the drug appears to inhibit formation of acetyl coenzyme A from pyruvic acid, thereby inhibiting the energy production of the infecting organism. Nitrofurantoin also may disrupt bacterial cell wall formation.

PHARMACOTHERAPEUTICS

Nitrofurantoin is used to treat UTIs. It is not effective against systemic bacterial infections.

nitrofurantoin (Furadantin, Macrodantin). Used to treat initial or recurrent UTIs, nitrofurantoin is active against a wide spectrum of gram-positive and gram-negative bacteria, especially *E. coli, Klebsiella,* and *Enterobacter* and *Citrobacter* species. Most *Proteus* and *Serratia* species are moderately resistant and *P. aeruginosa* almost always is resistant. The drug also is effective against staphylococci and enterococci.

Usual adult dosage: for uncomplicated UTIs, 50 to 100 mg P.O. q.i.d. for 7 to 14 days and at least 3 days after sterility of urine is obtained; for suppression of recurrent UTIs, 50 to 100 mg P.O. daily at bedtime.

Drug interactions

Probenecid and sulfinpyrazone inhibit the renal excretion of nitrofurantoin, reduce its efficacy, and increase its toxic potential. Antacids can decrease the extent and rate of nitrofurantoin absorption. Nitrofurantoin may decrease the antibacterial activity of norfloxacin and nalidixic acid. It may produce false-positive results for urine glucose determinations when Benedict's solution (Clinitest) is used, but does not affect results when glucose oxidase methods (Clinistix, Tes-Tape) are used.

ADVERSE DRUG REACTIONS

GI irritation is the most common adverse reaction to nitrofurantoin. Anorexia, nausea, and vomiting occur frequently; diarrhea and abdominal pain, less often. GI intolerance is more common in patients receiving microcrystalline nitrofurantoin than in those receiving the macrocrystalline form. Some patients have experienced peripheral neuropathy, which usually begins with paresthesia and dysesthesia of the legs and can progress in severity to a debilitating state.

Hypersensitivity reactions occur occasionally and involve the skin, lungs, blood, and liver. Chills, fever, arthralgia (a lupus erythematosus syndrome), and anaphylaxis also can occur. Hypersensitivity dermatologic reactions include maculopapular, erythematous, or eczematous rashes; urticaria; angioneurotic edema; and pruritus. Pulmonary reactions include asthmatic attacks in patients with a history of asthma and acute pneumonitis. Acute pneumonitis is manifested by sudden fever, chills, cough, dyspnea, chest pain, eosinophilia, and pulmonary infiltration that may appear as consolidation or pleural effusion on X-rays. It is most common in elderly patients, with symptoms appearing within the first week of treatment.

Hematologic reactions are rare, but may include leukopenia, granulocytopenia, and megaloblastic anemia. In patients with G6PD deficiency, nitrofurantoin can precipitate an acute episode of hemolytic anemia, although this is rare. Non-dose-related hepatotoxicity occurs rarely, as well as chronic active hepatitis, cholestatic jaundice, and cholestatic hepatitis. Nitrofurantoin may color the urine dark yellow or brown.

NURSING PROCESS APPLICATION

The following information assists the nurse in caring for a patient who is receiving nitrofurantoin.

Assessment
• Review the patient's history for a preexisting condition that contraindicates the use of nitrofurantoin, such as term pregnancy, infancy under age 1 month, anuria, oliguria, significant renal impairment, or known hypersensitivity to the drug.
• Review the patient's history for a preexisting condition that requires cautious use of nitrofurantoin, such as lactation.
• Assess the patient for adverse reactions to nitrofurantoin, such as GI distress or peripheral neuropathy.
• Review the patient's medication history to identify the use of drugs that may interact with nitrofurantoin, such as probenecid, sulfinpyrazone, antacids, nalidixic acid, and norfloxacin.
• Assess the effectiveness of nitrofurantoin periodically.
• Assess the patient for hypersensitivity reactions involving the skin, lungs, blood, and liver.
• Evaluate the patient's and family's knowledge about nitrofurantoin.

Nursing diagnoses
The following examples represent appropriate nursing diagnoses for a patient receiving nitrofurantoin.
• Potential for injury related to a preexisting condition that contraindicates the use of nitrofurantoin
• Potential for injury related to a preexisting condition that requires cautious use of nitrofurantoin
• Potential for injury related to adverse drug reactions
• Altered health maintenance related to hypersensitivity reactions to nitrofurantoin
• Knowledge deficit related to nitrofurantoin

Planning and implementation
• Do not administer nitrofurantoin to a patient with a condition that contraindicates its use.
• Administer nitrofurantoin cautiously to a patient at risk because of a preexisting condition.
• Monitor the patient periodically for adverse reactions during nitrofuratoin therapy.
• *Monitor the patient for hypersensitivity reactions that may involve the skin, lungs, blood, and liver. Keep standard emergency equipment nearby because anaphylaxis can occur.*
• Inspect the patient's skin regularly for evidence of dermatologic hypersensitivity reactions, manifested as maculopapular, erythematous, or eczematous rashes; urticaria; or angioneurotic edema. Ask the patient about pruritus.
• Monitor the patient, especially the elderly patient, for pulmonary hypersensitivity reactions, manifested as asthmatic attacks in a patient with a history of asthma and acute pneumonitis (sudden fever, chills, cough, dyspnea, chest pain, eosinophilia, and pulmonary infiltration that may appear as consolidation or pleural effusion on X-rays).
• *Withhold the drug and notify the physician if any hypersensitivity reaction occurs during nitrofurantoin therapy. Provide symptomatic relief as prescribed.*
• Administer nitrofurantoin with food or milk to minimize adverse GI reactions.
• *Monitor hydration if the patient experiences anorexia, nausea, vomiting, or diarrhea. Request a prescription for an antiemetic or antidiarrheal agent if needed. If the patient displays adverse GI reactions during treatment with nitrofurantoin microcrystalline tablets, discuss with the physician changing the drug to nitrofurantoin macrocrystals, which are less likely to cause adverse GI reactions.*
• *Monitor the patient for peripheral neuropathy, which usually begins with paresthesia and dysesthesia of the legs. Because this condition can progress to a debilitating state if left unchecked, ask the patient regularly about sensory changes in the legs. If such changes are present, withhold nitrofurantoin and notify the physician.*
• *Obtain a urine culture and sensitivity test before beginning therapy and as prescribed to determine drug effec-*

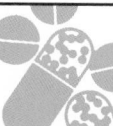

SELECTED MAJOR DRUGS

Urinary antiseptic agents

Urinary antiseptic agents are used in all types of clinical settings to treat urinary tract infections (UTIs). This chart summarizes the major urinary antiseptic agents currently in clinical use.

DRUG	MAJOR INDICATIONS	USUAL ADULT DOSAGES	CONTRAINDICATIONS AND PRECAUTIONS
Quinolones			
ciprofloxacin	UTIs	250 to 500 mg P.O. every 12 hours	• Know that ciprofloxacin is contraindicated in a pediatric, pregnant, or lactating patient or one with known hypersensitivity to it or other quinolones. • Administer with caution to a patient with known or suspected CNS disorders.
	Respiratory tract, skin, bone, or joint infections	500 to 750 mg P.O. every 12 hours	
	Infectious diarrhea	500 mg P.O. every 12 hours	
norfloxacin	Uncomplicated UTIs	400 mg P.O. b.i.d. for 7 to 10 days	• Know that norfloxacin is contraindicated in a pediatric, pregnant, or lactating patient or one with known hypersensitivity to it or other quinolones. • Administer with caution to a patient with factors that predispose the patient to seizures.
	Complicated UTIs	400 mg P.O. b.i.d. for 10 to 21 days	
Sulfonamides			
sulfamethoxazole	UTIs	2 grams P.O. initially, then 1 gram P.O. b.i.d. to t.i.d. for severe infections	• Know that sulfamethoxazole is contraindicated in a pregnant patient at term, a lactating patient, or one with known hypersensitivity to the drug. • Administer with caution to a patient with impaired renal or hepatic function, severe allergy to sulfa drugs, bronchial asthma, or glucose-6-phosphate dehydrogenase deficiency.
	Lymphogranuloma venereum (genital, inguinal, or anorectal infections)	1 gram P.O. b.i.d. for at least 21 days	
Nitrofurantoin			
nitrofurantoin	Uncomplicated UTIs	50 to 100 mg P.O. q.i.d. for 7 to 14 days	• Know that nitrofurantoin is contraindicated in an infant under age 1 month, a pregnant patient at term, or one with anuria, oliguria, significant renal impairment, or known hypersensitivity to the drug. • Administer with caution to a lactating patient.
	Suppression of recurrent UTIs	50 to 100 mg P.O. daily at bedtime	

tiveness. Nitrofurantoin should be continued for 3 days after urine sterility is ascertained.
• Avoid concomitant administration of nitrofurantoin with probenecid, sulfinpyrazone, antacids, nalidixic acid, and norfloxacin.
• Notify the physician if adverse reactions occur.

Patient teaching
• Teach the patient and family the name, dose, frequency, action, and adverse effects of nitrofurantoin.
• Stress the importance of taking the drug for the prescribed length of time.
• *Inform the patient that nitrofurantoin may turn urine brown or dark yellow.*

• Instruct the patient to take nitrofurantoin with food or milk.
• Advise the patient that GI upset is a common adverse reaction.
• Instruct the patient to stop taking nitrofurantoin and notify the physician if paresthesia, dysesthesia, or hypersensitivity reactions occur.
• Caution the patient against performing activities that require safety precautions, such as operating a motor vehicle or machinery, if paresthesia and dysesthesia occur.
• *Teach the patient the proper procedure for collecting a urine sample for culture and sensitivity testing.*

• Instruct the diabetic patient not to perform urine glucose determinations using Clinitest, because false-positive results may occur during nitrofurantoin therapy.
• Instruct the patient to notify the physician if any other adverse reactions occur.

Evaluation

The following examples represent appropriate evaluation statements for a patient receiving nitrofurantoin.
• The patient has no conditions that contraindicate nitrofurantoin therapy.
• The patient exhibits no signs of complications in the preexisting condition linked to nitrofurantoin.
• The patient exhibits no adverse reactions to nitrofurantoin.
• The patient does not develop a hypersensitivity reaction to nitrofurantoin.
• The patient and family express an accurate understanding of the points taught about nitrofurantoin.
• The patient takes nitrofurantoin with food or milk as prescribed.

OTHER URINARY ANTISEPTIC AGENTS

Less commonly used urinary antiseptic agents include cinoxacin, methenamine, nalidixic acid, and trimethoprim.

cinoxacin (Cinibac). Cinoxacin is a quinolone derivative indicated for acute and chronic uncomplicated UTIs. Its antibacterial spectrum is somewhat greater than that of nalidixic acid. It is effective against all *Proteus* species, *E. coli,* and most strains of *Klebsiella, Enterobacter, Citrobacter, Providencia,* and *Serratia* species. It is ineffective against *Pseudomonas, S. aureus,* and enterococci.

methenamine (Urised), **methenamine hippurate** (Hiprex, Urex), and **methenamine mandelate** (Mandelamine). Methenamine is prescribed to prevent recurrent UTIs, especially for long-term therapy. It is active against all gram-positive and gram-negative bacteria. However, UTIs caused by urea-splitting organisms, such as the *Proteus* species, may not respond, because acidifying the urine is difficult in the presence of these infections that increase urinary pH.

nalidixic acid (NegGram). Nalidixic acid is a quinolone derivative used to treat acute and chronic UTIs. It has a limited antibacterial spectrum. Although the development of resistance may limit the usefulness of this drug against *E. coli, Proteus mirabilis,* other *Proteus* species, *Klebsiella,* and *Enterobacter,* it is bactericidal at easily achieved concentrations in the urine of 16 mcg/ml or less. *Pseudomonas* species are resistant.

trimethoprim (Proloprim, Trimprex). Trimethoprim is used to treat initial episodes of acute uncomplicated UTIs caused by *E. coli, P. mirabilis, K. pneumoniae, Enterobacter,* or coagulase-negative staphylococci. The drug is active against most gram-positive cocci and most gram-negative rods. Using trimethoprim alone for acute uncomplicated UTIs may increase trimethoprim-resistant organisms.

CHAPTER SUMMARY

Chapter 65 presented the urinary antiseptic agents that can be used against UTIs. Here are the chapter highlights.
• Urinary antiseptic agents are used to treat acute, uncomplicated, symptomatic bacteriuria of the lower urinary tract.
• The quinolones, a major class of urinary antiseptic agents, include ciprofloxacin, norfloxacin, and ofloxacin.
• Ciprofloxacin also is used to treat lower respiratory tract infections; skin, bone, or joint infections; and infectious diarrhea.
• Ofloxacin also is indicated to treat lower respiratory infections, some sexually transmitted diseases, skin and skin structure infections, and prostatitis.
• The sulfonamides include co-trimoxazole, sulfadiazine, sulfamethoxazole, and sulfisoxazole. They are used primarily to treat acute UTIs. With recurrent or chronic UTIs, the infecting organism may or may not be susceptible to sulfonamides.
• Nitrofurantoin, another urinary antiseptic agent, is effective in acute UTIs and recurrent bacteriuria.
• Other, less commonly used urinary antiseptic agents include the quinolones, cinoxacin and nalidixic acid, and the antiinfective agents, methenamine and trimethoprim.
• The nurse should administer urinary antiseptic agents cautiously because various adverse reactions can occur. The nurse also must teach the patient and family about the importance of compliance with therapy to prevent recurrent UTIs.

STUDY QUESTIONS

See Appendix 1 for answers.

1. Maryann Stevens, age 32, is a diabetic and seeks treatment for a recurrent UTI. Her physician prescribes the quinolone ciprofloxacin. Before administering ciprofloxacin to Ms. Stevens, the nurse should obtain a complete medical history. Which of the following conditions would warrant cautious administration of a quinolone?
(a) cardiovascular disease
(b) CNS disorder
(c) GI disorder
(d) anemia

2. The nurse should monitor Ms. Stevens for which adverse drug reaction?
(a) bronchospasm
(b) tinnitus
(c) seizures
(d) constipation

3. Ms. Stevens states that she takes an antacid when she experiences heartburn. When should Ms. Stevens be instructed to take the antacid in relationship to the ciprofloxacin dose?
(a) 2 hours after the ciprofloxacin dose
(b) 2 hours before the ciprofloxacin dose
(c) immediately after the ciprofloxacin dose
(d) whenever the antacid is needed

4. Megan Thistle, age 20, has an acute lower UTI. Her physician prescribes the sulfonamide co-trimoxazole for 10 days. How do sulfonamides produce their bacteriostatic effects?
(a) They inhibit cell wall synthesis.
(b) They inhibit folic acid production.
(c) They inhibit protein synthesis.
(d) They alter bacterial cell wall permeability.

5. What instructions should the nurse give Ms. Thistle about co-trimoxazole administration?
(a) Take the medication with meals to minimize adverse GI reactions.
(b) Take the medication with an antacid.
(c) Drink at least eight 8-oz glasses of fluid daily.
(d) Limit the fluid intake to 1,000 ml/day

6. Over the past year, Althea Jones, age 45, has developed a recurrent UTI. Her physician prescribes nitrofurantoin. What is the usual dosage to treat a recurrent UTI?
(a) 50 to 100 mg P.O. daily at bedtime
(b) 100 to 150 mg P.O. b.i.d.
(c) 50 to 100 mg P.O. daily in the morning
(d) 100 to 150 mg P.O. daily

7. Ms. Jones, a diabetic, reports she tests her urine for glucose when she does not feel well. Which test produces a false-positive result for glucose during nitrofurantoin therapy?
(a) Clinistix
(b) Diastix
(c) Tes-Tape
(d) Clinitest

SELECTED REFERENCES

AHFS drug information 90. (1990). Bethesda, MD: American Society of Hospital Pharmacists.

Drug facts and comparisons. (1991). St. Louis: Facts and Comparisons Division, Lippincott.

Goodman and Gilman's the pharmacological basis of therapeutics (8th ed.; 1990). Elmsford, NY: Pergamon Press.

Hansten, P., and Horn, J. (1989). *Drug interactions* (6th ed.). Philadelphia: Lea & Febiger.

Mandell, G., et al. (Eds.). (1990). *Principles and practice of infectious diseases* (3rd ed.). New York: Churchill Livingston.

North American Nursing Diagnosis Association (1990). *Taxonomy I - Revised, with official diagnostic categories.* St. Louis, NANDA.

Walker, R., and Wright, A. (1987). The quinolones. *Mayo Clinic Proceedings,* 62(11), 1007-1012.

Wilhelm, M., and Edson, R. (1987). Antimicrobial agents in urinary tract infections. *Mayo Clinic Proceedings,* 62(11), 1025-1031.

DRUGS TO TREAT MALIGNANT NEOPLASMS

In the 1940s, antineoplastic, or chemotherapeutic, drugs were used to treat cancer when all other therapeutic measures failed for disseminated cancers that could not be treated by surgery or radiation therapy. Then, most antineoplastic drugs commonly had serious adverse effects. Today, many of these effects can be minimized so that they are not so devastating to the patient. In fact, many childhood cancers now are considered curable because of the advent of chemotherapeutic drugs. Many of these agents are the drugs of choice for different types of cancer and no longer are considered a last resort. Also, new agents, such as interferons, are being used to treat patients with cancer.

Nurses have participated actively in administering and evaluating more than 50 drugs to treat cancer. In caring for patients receiving these drugs, nurses have helped patients and their families understand chemotherapy and cope with its adverse effects.

CLINICAL USES

Antineoplastic agents may be used to cure, prevent, or relieve cancer symptoms. For patients with systemic cancer, such as leukemia, chemotherapy may be given as a curative treatment. In other patients, it may be given as an adjuvant treatment based on the premise that micrometastases, although undetectable, exist. In patients with advanced neoplastic disorders, chemotherapy may be palliative, reducing tumor size or relieving pain and other symptoms.

Chemotherapy commonly is combined with other cancer treatments. For example, it may be given preoperatively to reduce tumor size and allow less radical surgery.

CELL CYCLE

To understand the pharmacodynamics of antineoplastic agents, the nurse needs to know about the cell cycle. All animal cells follow a series of basic steps as they undergo division and replication. This series of steps is called the cell cycle; each step is a phase. During each phase, bio-chemical events that are necessary for cell division occur. (For a summary of these phases, see *Cell cycle,* page 1139.)

In the first phase, G_1 (G stands for gap), the cell manufactures the enzymes needed for deoxyribonucleic acid (DNA) synthesis. The time a cell spends in G_1 varies greatly but averages about 18 hours.

Next the cell enters the S phase (S stands for synthesis). In this phase, DNA replication occurs in preparation for mitosis (cell division). This phase lasts from 10 to 20 hours.

Then the cell enters the G_2 phase, when specialized DNA proteins and ribonucleic acid (RNA) are synthesized for later mitosis. This phase lasts about 3 hours.

Finally, the cell is ready to divide and enters the M phase (M stands for mitosis). During mitosis, the cell progresses through four subphases: *prophase,* when the chromosomes aggregate or clump; *metaphase,* when the chromosomes line up in the middle of the cell; *anaphase,* when the chromosomes segregate; and *telophase,* when the cell divides, producing two morphologically identical cells. The entire M phase lasts only 1 hour.

From the M phase, the cell may follow one of three paths. It may differentiate into a functional cell, enter the G_0 (resting) phase, or begin the cycle again by entering the G_1 phase. Resting cells in the G_0 phase may move on to the G_1 phase and progress through the cell cycle.

In different phases of the cycle, cells are susceptible to different drugs because the drugs interfere with specific biochemical events that occur in these phases.

MECHANISMS OF ACTION

Although not understood completely, cancer seems to occur when one cell undergoes a malignant transformation and produces an abnormal cell. Antineoplastic agents interfere with cell reproduction, leading to tumor destruction. (For details, see *Mechanisms and sites of action of selected antineoplastic agents,* page 1140.)

During administration of an antineoplastic agent, a fixed percentage of cells die. After treatment, the remaining cells

Glossary

Adenocarcinoma: malignant tumor that forms in a gland, infiltrates surrounding tissues, and leads to metastases.

Alkylation: linkage between a substance and deoxyribonucleic acid (DNA) that causes irreversible inhibition of the DNA molecule by enzyme modification.

Alopecia: loss of hair.

Anemia: blood disorder characterized by a decreased number of erythrocytes, amount of hemoglobin, or volume of packed red cells.

Benign: noncancerous, nonrecurring.

Cancer: general term for the many malignant neoplasms associated with infiltration, metastases, and fatality.

Carcinogenesis: cancer production.

Carcinoma: malignant neoplasm composed of epithelial cells, which tends to infiltrate surrounding tissues and lead to metastases.

Cell cycle: division pattern of cells characterized by five phases: nonproliferation, G_0; presynthesis, G_1; DNA synthesis, S; RNA production, G_2; and mitosis, M, cell division.

Cell-cycle-nonspecific: capable of acting during several or all cell-cycle stages.

Cell-cycle-specific: capable of acting during particular cell-cycle stages only.

Cytostatic: capable of halting cell growth and multiplication.

Cytotoxic: capable of destroying or poisoning cells.

Extravasation: escape of blood or solution from a vessel into surrounding tissues.

Granulocyte: leukocyte with granules in its cytoplasm; basophils, neutrophils, and eosinophils are granulocytes.

Granulocytopoiesis: granulocyte production.

Hepatotoxic: capable of destroying or poisoning liver cells.

Hodgkin's disease: malignant disorder that causes painless, progressive enlargement of the lymph nodes, spleen, and lymphoid tissues; also called malignant granuloma or lymphoma.

Intrathecal: within a sheath, as in the cerebrospinal fluid within the subarachnoid space.

Irritant: agent that produces undue sensitivity or tenderness.

Leukemia: malignant disorder of the blood-forming organs marked by increased leukocytes and leukocyte precursors in the blood and bone marrow.

Leukopenia: decreased leukocytes in the blood, usually under 5,000/mm³.

Lymphoblastic: pertaining to lymphoblasts (immature nucleolated lymphocytes).

Lymphocytic: pertaining to lymphocytes.

Lympholysis: lymphocyte destruction.

Lymphoma: neoplastic disorder of lymphoid tissue.

Malignancy: tendency to grow progressively worse and lead to death.

Melanoma: malignant neoplasm composed of melanin-pigmented cells.

Metastasis: disease transfer from one organ or part to distant parts of the body.

Mitosis: type of cell division that results in two morphologically identical cells.

Mucositis: mucous membrane inflammation.

Mutagenesis: induction of genetic mutation.

Myelocyte: immature white blood cell usually found in the bone marrow that becomes a granular leukocyte in the blood.

Myelogenous: pertaining to cells produced in the bone marrow.

Myeloma: neoplasm composed of cells that normally appear in the bone marrow.

Myeloproliferative: pertaining to or characterized by extramedullary and medullary proliferation of bone marrow constituents.

Nadir: lowest point on a scale or curve, often related to blood counts.

Neoplasm: new abnormal growth of tissue; may be benign or malignant.

Neuroblastoma: malignant tumor of the nervous system composed primarily of immature nerve cells (neuroblasts).

Palliative: providing relief but not cure.

Pancytopenia: deficiency of all cellular elements in the blood.

Phagocytosis: process of engulfing microorganisms, cells, and foreign particles by reticuloendothelial cells, monocytes, or polymorphonuclear leukocytes.

Pleiotropic: capable of having an affinity for several different types of tissue from different primary germ layers; also the ability of a gene to manifest itself in multiple ways.

Polycythemia vera: myeloproliferative disease characterized by increased red blood cells and total blood volume, accompanied in many cases by splenomegaly, leukocytosis, thrombocytosis, and bone marrow hyperactivity.

Remission: partial or complete disappearance of the clinical or subjective characteristics of a chronic or malignant disease.

Rhabdomyosarcoma: malignant neoplasm composed of striated muscle cells.

Sarcoma: malignant neoplasm composed of a substance similar to embryonic connective tissue.

Stomatitis: mouth inflammation that may affect the buccal mucosa, palate, tongue, floor of the mouth, and gingivae.

Thrombocytopenia: decrease in the number of blood platelets.

Tumor: new tissue growth marked by progressive, uncontrolled cell multiplication; neoplasm.

Tumorcidal: destructive to tumors.

Vesicant: agent that produces blisters.

Wilms' tumor: rapidly developing, malignant kidney tumor composed of embryonic elements, which usually affects children under age 5.

Cell cycle

Every cell progresses through a series of phases to replicate itself. During each phase, the cell is vulnerable to certain drugs that can interfere with its replication. This concept is the basis of antineoplastic therapy.

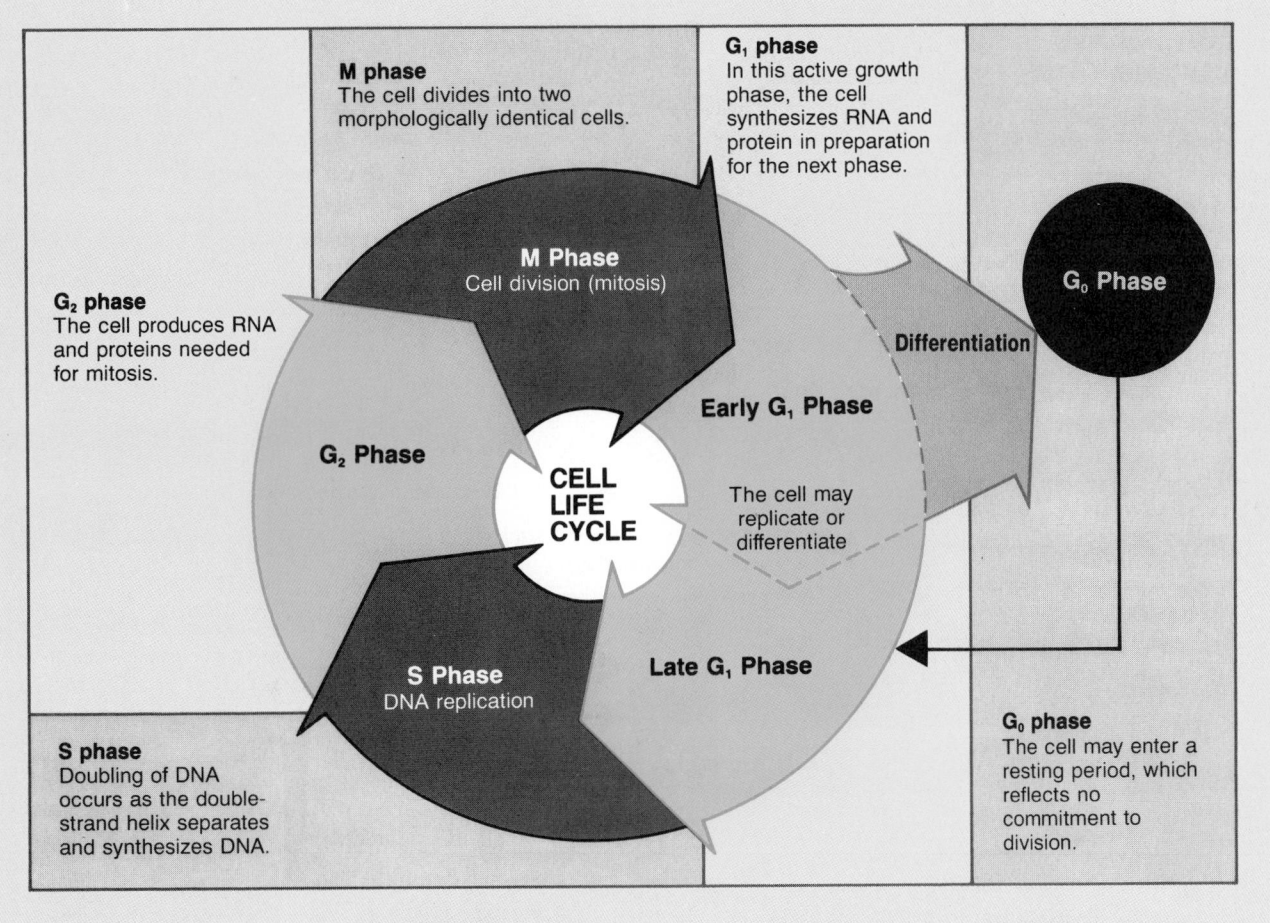

M phase
The cell divides into two morphologically identical cells.

G_1 phase
In this active growth phase, the cell synthesizes RNA and protein in preparation for the next phase.

G_2 phase
The cell produces RNA and proteins needed for mitosis.

S phase
Doubling of DNA occurs as the double-strand helix separates and synthesizes DNA.

G_0 phase
The cell may enter a resting period, which reflects no commitment to division.

M Phase
Cell division (mitosis)

G_2 Phase

CELL LIFE CYCLE

Early G_1 Phase

The cell may replicate or differentiate

Differentiation

G_0 Phase

S Phase
DNA replication

Late G_1 Phase

---

reproduce, and resting cells in the G_0 phase may return to a reproducing phase. (Cells in the G_0 phase are less sensitive to chemotherapy because they are not synthesizing DNA actively.) Total eradication of cancer cells, therefore, depends on repeated administration of the antineoplastic agent. An interval between treatments permits healthy cells to recover.

Because cancer cells are at various phases in the cell cycle, therapy commonly combines drugs that act on cells in different phases or that have different sites of action.

Although an antineoplastic agent kills cells as soon as they pass through a specific cell cycle, this action produces no immediate clinical response. Most patients need at least three treatments before a clinical response can be evaluated by physical examination, X-ray, computed tomography

(CT), magnetic resonance imaging (MRI), or biological marker determination.

Tumor regression depends on several factors, such as the percentage of cells killed, the rate of regrowth, and the development of resistant cells. Evaluation of chemotherapy is difficult, however, because the cancer may be undetected clinically but still may be present. Therefore, treatments may continue for a while after the disease no longer is detectable.

TUMOR RESISTANCE

Combination drug regimens may be used for patients with tumor resistance. Tumor cell populations are heterogeneous: Some cells are sensitive to antineoplastic agents; others are not. When an antineoplastic agent is adminis-

Mechanisms and sites of action of selected antineoplastic agents

During various phases in the cell cycle, antineoplastic agents act to halt cell growth or destroy it. Knowing where in the cycle these agents can act will help the nurse understand the basic principles of chemotherapy.

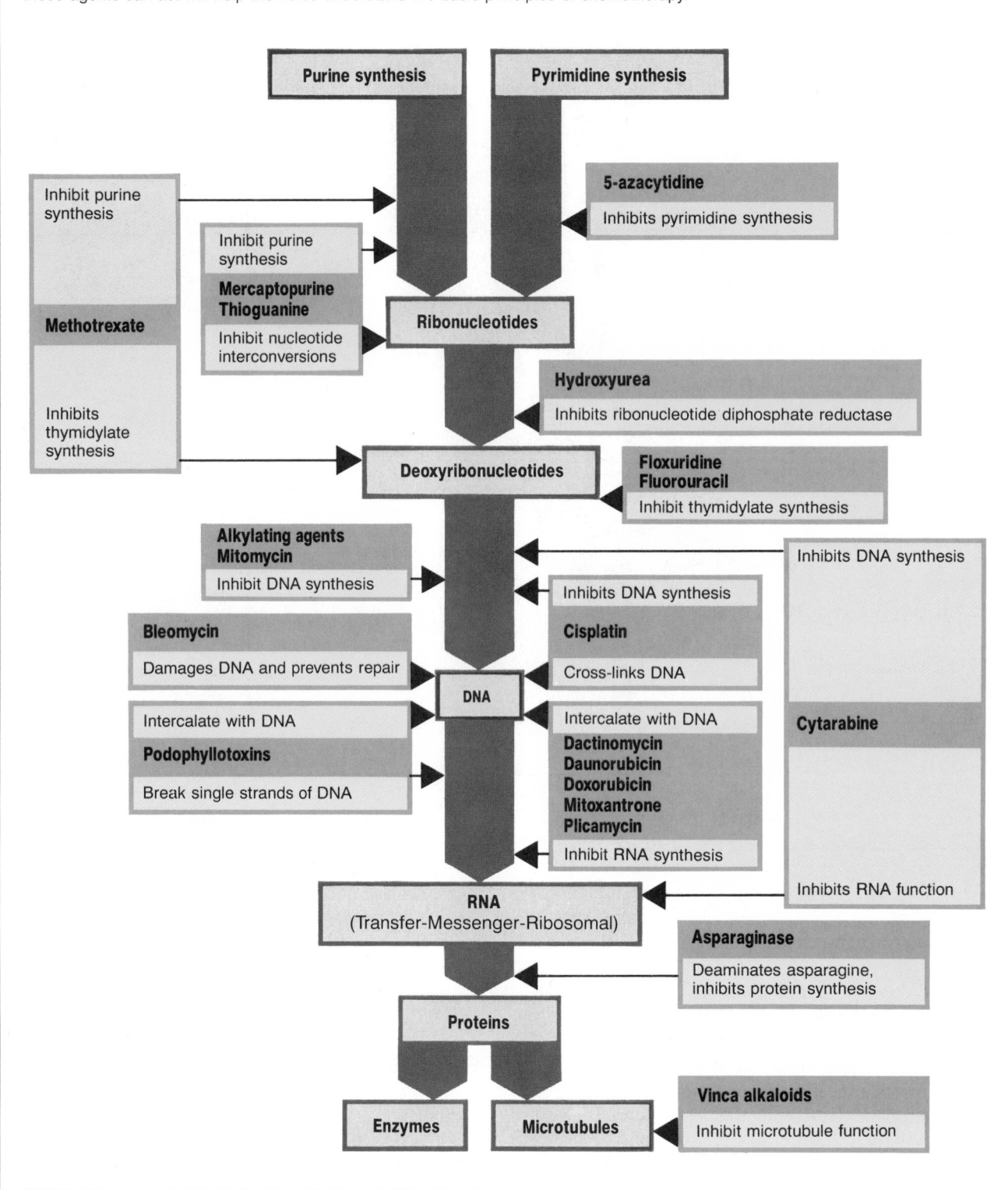

tered, it kills drug-sensitive cells initially. Repeated administration kills more drug-sensitive cells. Over time, however, tumor cells that are not drug-sensitive remain and replicate, producing a drug-resistant tumor. If these resistant cells are resistant to other drugs also, they will be even more difficult to kill.

Drug resistance may develop by one or more of the following mechanisms: decreased drug entry into the tumor cells, decreased drug-activating enzymes, increased drug-deactivating enzymes, increased levels of target enzymes, decreased target enzyme affinity for the drug, increased DNA repair, or development of alternate pathways that circumvent the action of the drug.

HANDLING ANTINEOPLASTIC AGENTS

Although the safe handling of antineoplastic agents remains controversial, most experts recommend conservative, protective methods. For maximum safety, the nurse should use the following techniques when handling antineoplastic agents.
• Mix antineoplastic agents in a Class II biological safety cabinet only.
• Wear powder-free, disposable, latex surgical gloves and a protective barrier garment with a closed front and long, cuffed sleeves to protect the body when mixing or administering antineoplastic agents. Some clinicians recommend wearing double gloves.
• Reconstitute and administer antineoplastic agents in syringes or intravenous (I.V.) sets with Luer-Lok connections.
• Use a closed delivery technique when administering these agents.
• Do not prime I.V. lines and syringes into a sink or waste basket; use sterile 2″ × 2″ gauze pads or alcohol wipes instead.
• After mixing and administering these agents, dispose of any waste in a leakproof, punctureproof container labeled "hazardous waste." Such containers must be disposed of by incineration or burial at a hazardous chemical waste site.
• If a spill occurs, follow the health care facility's policy for cleaning up hazardous materials.

ADMINISTERING ANTINEOPLASTIC AGENTS

Before administering an antineoplastic agent, the nurse should reinforce the information about the benefits and risks of treatment that the patient received from the physician. A patient who consents to investigational chemotherapy should receive additional information. Throughout the patient's therapy, the nurse should continue to teach and reinforce this information to promote patient safety and compliance.

To administer an antineoplastic agent safely, the nurse should select an appropriate site and vein, consider drug compatibilities, determine the vesicant potential of the agent, consider its sequencing and delivery, and prevent or treat extravasation as prescribed

For a patient who must receive several treatments with these potentially damaging agents, site and vein selection is especially important. To select an appropriate I.V. site, the nurse should begin with a distal spot, such as the hand, and proceed to proximal areas, such as up the forearm.

Before administering any antineoplastic agent, the nurse should consider drug compatibilities. As a rule, antineoplastic agents should not be mixed with any other medications. Although little research has been done to determine exact incompatibilities, the nature and toxicity of these agents usually prohibit mixing.

To choose the proper drug sequencing and delivery technique, the nurse needs to know the potential of the agent to act as a vesicant. (For a summary of vesicant, irritant, and nonvesicant drugs, see *Classifications of antineoplastic agents.*) For intermittent drug delivery, the nurse should administer a vesicant agent by direct push or delivery into the side port of an infusing I.V. line. For continuous infusion, a vesicant should be administered only via a cen-

Classifications of antineoplastic agents

To administer an antineoplastic agent safely, the nurse needs to know whether it is a vesicant (capable of producing blisters), an irritant (capable of producing undue sensitivity), or a nonvesicant drug.

Vesicant agents

• dacarbazine	• nitrogen mustards
• dactinomycin	• plicamycin
• daunorubicin	• vinblastine
• doxorubicin	• vincristine
• mitomycin	• vindesine
• mitoxantrone	

Irritant agents

• carmustine
• etoposide
• streptozocin

Nonvesicant agents

• asparaginase	• cytarabine
• bleomycin	• floxuridine
• carboplatin	• fluorouracil
• cisplatin	• ifosfamide
• cyclophosphamide	

tral line or vascular access device. Nonvesicant agents (including irritants) may be given by direct I.V. push, through the side port of an infusing I.V. line or as a continuous infusion. Some facilities require administration of the vesicant first because vein integrity decreases over time; others require administration of the vesicant last because it may increase vein fragility. Various venous access devices are available and are used when vesicants are administered. These venous access devices reduce patient discomfort by removing the necessity for multiple I.V. insertions.

During the administration of any I.V. antineoplastic agent, the patient's safety depends on the nurse's assessment of the infusion site during drug delivery. To ensure patency of the vein, the nurse must elicit a blood return before, during, and after drug administration.

To prevent extravasation, the nurse should use a splint to stabilize the needle and should check frequently for blood return. Although no definitive measures exist to treat extravasation of an antineoplastic agent, conservative measures include discontinuing the infusion, aspirating any residual drug from the tubing and needle, instilling an I.V. antidote, and removing the needle. After administering an antidote as prescribed, the nurse may apply heat or cold and may elevate the affected limb.

ADVERSE REACTIONS

The adverse reactions to antineoplastic agents result from the systemic effects of these drugs. Some reactions can be life-threatening, requiring modification of the drug dosage or treatment regimen. Others are less severe but may be stressful to the patient. (For a summary, see *Common adverse reactions and associated nursing implications.*)

Nausea and vomiting are common adverse reactions. Chemotherapy can cause nausea and vomiting by three basic mechanisms. Orally administered drugs can irritate the gastric mucosa directly, causing nausea and vomiting that is less severe than that caused by the other two mechanisms.

Other antineoplastic agents can stimulate the chemoreceptor trigger zone. The incidence of nausea and vomiting from this mechanism depends on the inherent emetic potential of the drug. (For more information, see *Emetic potential of antineoplastic agents.*)

Finally, chemotherapy can cause psychogenic nausea and vomiting, which originates in the cerebral cortex. Known as anticipatory emesis, this reaction can be disabling. A patient who remembers the unpleasantness of previous chemotherapy may feel nauseated or may vomit just by thinking about future treatments. This reaction may become so severe that sights, sounds, and smells associated with treatment may induce emesis, no matter how far removed the patient is from the actual treatment setting.

Chemotherapy-induced nausea and vomiting is of great concern because it can cause fluid and electrolyte imbalances, noncompliance with the treatment regimen, Mallory-Weiss syndrome (tears at the esophageal-gastric junction, leading to massive bleeding), wound dehiscence, and pathological fractures. It also can cause distress by limiting the patient's ability and motivation to take an active role in life.

To combat the nausea and vomiting caused by chemotherapy, nurses commonly administer antiemetic drugs, such as metoclopramide, lorazepam, dexamethasone, prochlorperazine, diphenhydramine, droperidol, and dronabinol. Usually, an antiemetic drug is given with several other antiemetics that act by different mechanisms. A combination regimen is more effective than a single drug, especially for a strong emetogenic agent, such as cisplatin. The nurse also can help control psychogenic factors related to nausea and vomiting by teaching the patient relaxation techniques that can help minimize feelings of isolation and anxiety, encouraging the patient to express anxieties, and helping the patient use relaxation techniques during chemotherapy.

Emetic potential of antineoplastic agents

Some antineoplastic agents are more likely than others to cause nausea and vomiting. Knowing the emetic potential of these agents will help the nurse plan patient care.

High (greater than 50% incidence)

• azacytidine	• daunorubicin
• carmustine	• doxorubicin
• cisplatin	• mechlorethamine
• cyclophosphamide	• mithramycin
• dacarbazine	• streptozocin
• dactinomycin	

Moderate (25% to 50% incidence)

• 5-azacytidine	• procarbazine
• cytarabine	• thiotepa
• etoposide	• vinblastine
• interferons	

Low (less than 25% incidence)

• asparaginase	• mercaptopurine
• bleomycin	• methotrexate
• busulfan	• plicamycin
• carboplatin	• thioguanine
• chlorambucil	• vincristine
• fluorouracil	
• hydroxyurea	

Common adverse reactions and associated nursing implications

The antineoplastic agents cause many of the same adverse reactions and have similar nursing implications. To provide quality patient care, the nurse must be aware of these reactions and implications.

ADVERSE REACTIONS	NURSING IMPLICATIONS
Bone marrow suppression	
Bone marrow suppression is the most common and potentially serious adverse reaction to the antineoplastic agents.	• Watch for the blood count nadir because that is when the patient is at greatest risk for the complications of leukopenia, thrombocytopenia, and anemia. • Plan a patient-teaching program about bone marrow suppression, including information about blood counts, potential sites of infection, and personal hygiene.
Leukopenia. This reaction increases the patient's risk of infection, especially if the granulocyte count is under 1,000/mm³.	• Provide information about good hygiene, and assess the patient frequently for signs and symptoms of infection. Keep in mind that a patient with leukopenia is subject to infections. • Teach the patient to recognize and report the signs and symptoms of infection, such as fever, cough, sore throat, or a burning sensation on urination. • Teach the patient how to take a temperature. • Caution the patient to avoid crowds and people with colds or the flu during the nadir. • Remember that the inflammatory response may be decreased and the complications of leukopenia more difficult to detect if the patient is receiving a corticosteroid.
Thrombocytopenia. This reaction occurs with leukopenia. When the platelet count is under 50,000/mm³, the patient is at risk for bleeding. When it is under 20,000/mm³, the patient is at severe risk and may require a platelet transfusion.	• Assess the patient for bleeding gums, increased bruising or petechiae, hypermenorrhea, tarry stools, hematuria, and coffee-ground emesis. • Advise the patient to avoid cuts and bruises and to use a soft toothbrush and an electric razor. • Instruct the patient to report sudden headaches, which could indicate potentially fatal intracranial bleeding. • Instruct the patient to use a stool softener, as prescribed, to prevent colonic irritation and bleeding. • Instruct the patient to avoid using a rectal thermometer and receiving I.M. injections, to prevent bleeding.
Anemia. This reaction develops slowly over several courses of treatment.	• Assess the patient for dizziness, fatigue, pallor, and shortness of breath on minimal exertion. • Monitor the patient's hematocrit, hemoglobin level, and red blood cell counts. Remember that a patient dehydrated from nausea, vomiting, or anorexia may exhibit a false-normal hematocrit. Once this patient is rehydrated, the hematocrit will decrease. • Be prepared to administer a blood transfusion to a symptomatic patient as prescribed. • Instruct the patient to rest more frequently and to increase the dietary intake of iron-rich foods. Advise the patient to take a multivitamin with iron, as prescribed.
Nausea and vomiting	
These reactions can result from gastric mucosal irritation, chemical irritation of the central nervous system, or psychogenic factors that may be activated by sensations, suggestions, or anxiety.	• Control the chemical irritation by administing combinations of antiemetics, as prescribed. • Monitor the patient for signs and symptoms of aspiration because most antiemetics sedate. • Control psychogenic factors by helping the patient perform relaxation techniques before chemotherapy to minimize feelings of isolation and anxiety. • Encourage the patient to express feelings of anxiety. • Encourage the patient to listen to music or to engage in relaxation exercises, meditation, or hypnosis to promote feelings of control and well-being. • Adjust the drug administration time to meet the patient's needs. Some patients prefer treatments in the evening when they find sedation comfortable. Patients who are employed may prefer their treatments on their days off.

(continued)

Common adverse reactions and associated nursing implications *(continued)*

ADVERSE REACTIONS	NURSING IMPLICATIONS
Stomatitis	
Although epithelial tissue damage can affect any mucous membrane, the most common site is the oral mucosa. Stomatitis is temporary and can range from mild and barely noticeable to severe and debilitating. (Debilitation may result from poor nutrition during acute stomatitis.)	• Initiate preventive mouth care before chemotherapy to provide comfort and decrease the severity of the stomatitis. • Provide therapeutic mouth care, including topical antibiotics, if prescribed.
Alopecia	
To the patient, alopecia may be the most distressing adverse reaction.	• Prepare the patient for alopecia. Inform the patient that hair loss usually is gradual and is reversible after treatment ends. • Inform the patient that alopecia may be partial or complete and that it affects men and women. • Inform the patient that alopecia may affect the scalp, eyebrows, eyelashes, and body hair.

OVERVIEW OF CHAPTERS

The chapters in Unit Fifteen present cell-cycle-specific and cell-cycle-nonspecific agents used to treat malignant neoplasms or to prevent or relieve their symptoms.

Chapter 66
Alkylating Agents

Chapter 66 discusses the cell-cycle-nonspecific alkylating agents used to treat malignant neoplasms: the nitrogen mustards, alkyl sulfonates, nitrosoureas, triazines, ethylenimines, and alkylating-like agents. It emphasizes pharmacokinetics, mechanisms of action, adverse reactions, and related care using the nursing process.

Chapter 67
Antimetabolite Agents

Chapter 67 focuses on the cell-cycle-specific antimetabolite antineoplastic agents: the folic acid, pyrimidine, and purine analogues. For each drug class, it explores mechanisms of action and clinical indications. It also discusses adverse reactions and leucovorin rescue therapy as well as nursing process application, including patient teaching.

Chapter 68
Antibiotic Antineoplastic Agents

Chapter 68 presents the cell-cycle-nonspecific antibiotic agents with tumoricidal action—dactinomycin, daunorubicin, doxorubicin, mitomycin, mitoxantrone, and plicamycin—and bleomycin, which is cell-cycle-specific. For these agents, the chapter discusses clinical indications. It also details their adverse reactions and associated nursing interventions—especially patient teaching—organized accoring to the steps of the nursing process.

Chapter 69
Hormonal Antineoplastic Agents

Chapter 69 highlights the hormonal antineoplastic agents, which include estrogens, antiestrogens, androgens, antiandrogens, adrenocortical suppressants, progestins, adrenocorticosteroids, and gonadotropin-releasing hormone analogues. The chapter describes the pharmacokinetics and pharmacotherapeutics of these cytostatic agents and emphasizes associated use of the nursing process.

Chapter 70
Other Antineoplastic Agents

Chapter 70 investigates the cell-cycle-specific vinca alkaloids and podophyllotoxins as well as these other unclassified antineoplastic agents: asparaginase, hydroxyurea, procarbazine, and the interferons. For these agents, the chapter discusses their mechanisms of action, clinical indications, and adverse reactions. It also features application of the nursing process when caring for a patient receiving one of these agents.

ALKYLATING AGENTS

OBJECTIVES

After reading and studying this chapter, the student should be able to:

1. Discuss the pharmacokinetics of the alkylating agents: nitrogen mustards, alkyl sulfonates, nitrosoureas, triazines, ethylenimines, and alkylating-like agents.

2. Explain the alkylation process and its role in the mechanism of action of alkylating agents.

3. Identify the clinical indications for each class of alkylating agent.

4. Describe the common adverse reactions to the alkylating agents.

5. Describe how to apply the nursing process when caring for a patient who is receiving an alkylating agent.

INTRODUCTION

Alkylating agents fall into one of six classes: nitrogen mustards, alkyl sulfonates, nitrosoureas, triazines, ethylenimines, and alkylating-like agents. (For a list of the specific drugs in each group, see *Alkylating agents by class*.)

Highly reactive drugs, alkylating agents enter the cell nuclei and disrupt the structure of deoxyribonucleic acid (DNA). These drugs exert cytotoxic activity in a cell-cycle-nonspecific manner but may act more effectively in the late G_1 phase and S phase. Interference with normal cell division in rapidly proliferating tissue explains the therapeutic and adverse effects of alkylating agents.

Alkylating agents, given alone or with other drugs, effectively act against various malignant neoplasms. The sensitive malignant neoplasms include chronic and acute leukemias, non-Hodgkin's lymphomas, multiple myeloma, melanoma, sarcoma, and cancers of the breast, ovaries,

Alkylating agents by class

This chart lists the different classes of alkylating agents as well as specific drugs in each class.

Nitrogen mustards

- chlorambucil (Leukeran)
- cyclophosphamide (Cytoxan)
- estramustine (Emcyt)
- ifosfamide (Ifex)
- mechlorethamine (Mustargen)
- melphalan (Alkeran)
- uracil mustard

Alkyl sulfonates

- busulfan (Myleran)

Nitrosoureas

- carmustine [BCNU] (BiCNU)
- lomustine [CCNU] (CeeNU)
- semustine [methyl-CCNU]
- streptozocin (Zanosar)

Triazines

- dacarbazine (DTIC-Dome)

Ethylenimines

- thiotepa (Thiotepa)

Alkylating-like agents

- carboplatin (Paraplatin)
- cisplatin [cis-platin] (Platinol)

SELECTED NURSING DIAGNOSES

Alkylating agents

The following nursing diagnoses address representative problems and etiologies that a nurse may encounter when caring for a patient who is receiving an alkylating agent. Some of these nursing diagnoses contain generalized etiologies, which the nurse must individualize based on the patient's needs. (For some common nursing diagnoses and related interventions for each drug class, see the "Nursing Process Application" sections of this chapter.)

- Altered health maintenance related to ineffectiveness of the administered alkylating-like agent
- Altered nutrition: less than body requirements, related to adverse GI effects of the alkylating agent
- Altered nutrition: less than body requirements, related to addisonian-like wasting syndrome from busulfan
- Altered oral mucous membrane related to stomatitis from alkylating agent therapy
- Altered protection related to hepatotoxicity from high-dose carmustine therapy
- Altered protection related to secondary malignancies from alkylating agent therapy
- Altered protection related to thrombocytopenia from the alkylating agent
- Altered urinary elimination related to nephrotoxicity from an alkylating agent therapy
- Body image disturbance related to alopecia from alkylating agent therapy
- Diarrhea related to the adverse GI effects of an alkylating agent
- Fatigue related to anemia caused by an alkylating agent
- Health seeking behaviors related to fertility changes caused by a nitrogen mustard agent
- Impaired gas exchange related to busulfan-induced interstitial pulmonary fibrosis

- Impaired gas exchange related to the adverse pulmonary effects of an alkylating agent
- Impaired tissue integrity related to extravasation of an alkylating agent infusion
- Impaired tissue integrity related to hemorrhagic cystitis from cyclophosphamide, ifosfamide, or thiotepa
- Knowledge deficit related to the administered alkylating agent
- Pain related to carmustine or dacarbazine infusion
- Pain related to the instillation of thiotepa into the bladder
- Potential activity intolerance related to anemia the alkylating agent
- Potential fluid volume deficit related to the adverse GI effects of the alkylating agent
- Potential for infection related to leukopenia from the alkylating agent
- Potential for injury related to a preexisting condition that contraindicates the use of an alkylating agent
- Potential for injury related to a preexisting condition that requires cautious use of an alkylating agent
- Potential for injury related to adverse drug reactions
- Sensory-perceptual alterations (auditory, gustatory, kinesthetic, tactile) related to neurotoxicity from the alkylating-like agent
- Sensory-perceptual alterations (visual) related to phototoxicity from dacarbazine

---

uterus, lung, brain, testes, bladder, prostate, and stomach. Protocols for administering these drugs vary from one health care facility to another.

The major adverse reactions produced by alkylating agents include bone marrow suppression, nausea, vomiting, alopecia, and damage to epithelial tissues. The severity of the adverse reactions depends on many variables, including drug dosage, prior chemotherapy, physical condition, and psychological factors. The reactions, which usually are reversible, may occur early or later in the therapeutic regimen.

For a summary of representative drugs, see *Selected major drugs: Alkylating agents,* pages 1163 and 1164. For a listing of applicable nursing diagnoses that the nurse may formulate when caring for a patient receiving these agents, see *Selected nursing diagnoses: Alkylating agents*. For detailed information on applying the nursing process, see Chapter 6, The Nursing Process and Drug Therapy.

NITROGEN MUSTARDS

The nitrogen mustards represent the largest group of alkylating agents. Mechlorethamine, which was the first nitrogen mustard introduced, also is the most rapid-acting of all these drugs. The other nitrogen mustards include chlorambucil, cyclophosphamide, estramustine, ifosfamide, melphalan, and uracil mustard.

PHARMACOKINETICS

The absorption and distribution of nitrogen mustards, as with most alkylating agents, vary widely. The nitrogen mustards are metabolized in the liver and excreted by the kidneys.

Absorption

The nitrogen mustards are administered intravenously (I.V.), orally, and topically, as well as by instillation. When administered I.V., the drugs are considered to be 100% bioavailable (available in the general circulation). Orally administered nitrogen mustards exhibit variable and incomplete absorption.

After oral administration, chlorambucil and cyclophosphamide are absorbed well, and about 75% of an estramustine dose is absorbed. Although ifosfamide is absorbed well after oral administration, an oral formulation is not commercially available. Absorption of melphalan is incomplete and variable; its bioavailability ranges from 25% to 89%. The absorption of uracil mustard is unknown.

Although rarely used today, mechlorethamine may be instilled into the pleural, pericardial, and peritoneal cavities to control malignant effusions. Although absorption is variable and incomplete, it may be sufficient to produce systemic toxicity. Systemic absorption from topically applied mechlorethamine for mycosis fungoides is minimal.

Distribution

Chlorambucil displays homogenous tissue distribution. Some is deposited in fatty tissue, which may explain the prolonged effect of the drug in some patients. Chlorambucil appears to be extensively bound to tissue and plasma proteins.

Cyclophosphamide exhibits limited entry into the central nervous system (CNS), breast milk, sweat, saliva, and synovial fluid. The moderate lipid and water solubility of the drug allows it and its metabolites to be distributed widely to extracellular fluid.

Estramustine is distributed widely into body tissues. Ifosfamide is lipid soluble and penetrates the blood-brain barrier. Mechlorethamine is highly reactive and is hydrolyzed rapidly after I.V. administration. Within a few minutes, less than 10% of the drug remains in the blood. Melphalan is not distributed well to fat because the volume of distribution approximates total body water at 44 liters. The distribution of uracil mustard is unknown.

Metabolism

Most nitrogen mustards undergo hepatic metabolism. Chlorambucil and estramustine are metabolized extensively in the liver. Cyclophosphamide is metabolized, then further oxidized to the inactive metabolites, phosphoramide mustard and acrolein, which are cytotoxic. About 50% of a ifosfamide dose is metabolized in the liver into ifosfamide mustard and acrolein. Mechlorethamine is inactivated rapidly as it undergoes chemical transformation in the plasma and other body tissues. Melphalan is metabolized in the plasma by spontaneous hydrolysis. The metabolism of uracil mustard is unknown.

Excretion

Chlorambucil, cyclophosphamide, ifosfamide, mechlorethamine, and melphalan are excreted in the urine. From 20% to 50% of melphalan also may be excreted in the feces. Estramustine is excreted primarily in feces. The excretion of uracil mustard is unknown. (For more information, see *Major administration and excretion routes for alkylating agents,* page 1148.)

Onset, peak, duration

Mechlorethamine undergoes metabolism in water and body fluids so rapidly that no active drug remains after a few minutes.

Most nitrogen mustards possess more intermediate half-lives than mechlorethamine. At 1 hour after an oral dose, the highest tissue concentration of chlorambucil occurs in the liver. Chlorambucil has a half-life of 2 hours.

Cyclophosphamide reaches a peak plasma concentration level about 1 hour after an oral dose, and has a plasma half-life of about 7 hours. However, the alkylating activity of the unbound metabolites lasts for at least 24 hours. The half-life of these alkylating metabolites is prolonged significantly in patients with renal failure.

The plasma half-life of ifosfamide is dose-dependent. High doses have a 15-hour half-life; low doses have a 7-hour half-life.

Melphalan reaches a peak plasma concentration about 2 hours after an oral dose, and has a plasma half-life of 90 minutes. The peak concentrations and half-lives of estramustine and uracil mustard have not been defined clearly.

PHARMACODYNAMICS

The nitrogen mustards form covalent bonds with DNA molecules in a chemical reaction known as alkylation. (For details, see *Mechanisms and sites of action of selected antineoplastic agents* in the introduction to this unit.) Alkylated DNA cannot replicate properly, resulting in cell death. Unfortunately, tumor cells may develop resistance to the cytotoxic effects of nitrogen mustards.

Mechanism of action

Researchers believe that most nitrogen mustards, like the other alkylating agents, enter cells via active transport systems. Once inside the cell, the drug undergoes strong electrophilic (having an affinity for electrons) chemical reactions with several substances, including phosphate, amino, sulfhydryl, carboxyl, and imidazole groups. These chemical reactions result in covalent bonds. The process is referred to as alkylation, and the alkylation of DNA inhibits its proper functioning. At pharmacologic dosages, the nitrogen mustards produce cytotoxic and other effects because of the DNA alkylation. (For a description of this reaction, see *DNA alkylation,* page 1149.)

Major administration and excretion routes for alkylating agents

The following chart summarizes the major administration and excretion routes of the alkylating agents, including approximate amounts of the drugs and metabolites excreted.

DRUG	ADMINISTRATION ROUTES	EXCRETION ROUTES	AMOUNT EXCRETED
Nitrogen mustards			
chlorambucil	Oral	Urinary	60% in 24 hours, mainly as metabolites
cyclophosphamide	Intravenous, oral	Urinary	60% in 24 hours, mainly as metabolites
estramustine	Oral	Fecal Urinary	Significant amount Small amount
ifosfamide	Intravenous	Urinary	70% to 86% as ifosfamide and metabolites
mechlorethamine	Intravenous	Urinary	>50% in 24 hours as metabolites
melphalan	Oral	Fecal Urinary	20% to 50% in 6 days with oral administration 50% in 24 hours
uracil mustard	Oral	Unknown	Unknown
Alkyl sulfonates			
busulfan	Oral	Urinary	10% to 50% in 24 hours as metabolites
Nitrosoureas			
carmustine	Intravenous	Urinary	30% in 24 hours as metabolites
lomustine	Oral	Urinary	50% in 12 hours as metabolites
semustine	Oral	Urinary	60% in 48 hours as metabolites
streptozocin	Intravenous	Urinary	60% to 70% in 24 hours as metabolites and 10% as parent compound
Triazines			
dacarbazine	Intravenous	Urinary	30% to 46%, half of this as metabolites
Ethylenimines			
thiotepa	Intravesicular, intravenous	Urinary	Unchanged in urine in 24 to 48 hours
Alkylating-like agents			
carboplatin	Intravenous	Urinary	71% in 24 hours
cisplatin	Intravenous	Urinary	23% in 24 hours and 27% to 45% in 5 days

Although nitrogen mustards are cell-cycle-nonspecific, they seem to be most effective against cells in the late G_1 phase or S phase. Alkylation becomes toxic when the cells enter the S phase, during which DNA synthesis occurs, and cell progression through the cycle is blocked at the G_2 phase. The alkylation reaction is nontoxic, however, if the cell repairs the DNA damage before cell division. In fact, DNA repair systems may play a key role in the relative resistance of nonproliferating tissue as well as in the selective action of the drugs against certain cell types and in the acquired resistance of tumors to the drugs. (For more information on how these drugs affect the cell cycle, see *Mechanisms and sites of action of selected antineoplastic agents* in the introduction to this unit.)

DNA alkylation

Alkylation of DNA can occur as a bifunctional or monofunctional reaction. Bifunctional reactions occur when one molecule of the alkylating agent undergoes two alkylation reactions. This may result in the cross-linking of two DNA molecules, the cross-linking of two strands of a single DNA molecule, or the linking of the DNA molecule to another protein. When bifunctional alkylation occurs, cytotoxic effects predominate.

Monofunctional reactions occur when a single molecule of the alkylating agent undergoes one alkylation reaction. This results in depurination and chain scission, which later may cause permanent damage, such as mutagenesis or carcinogenesis.

Resistance is an acquired phenomenon whereby previously sensitive tumors no longer are sensitive to the cytotoxic actions of alkylating agents. Resistance usually develops slowly and may result from several biochemical changes. Decreased drug permeation into the cell may occur, preventing the drug from reaching its site of action. The tumor cell also may increase production of nucleic substances that compete with DNA for alkylation. With the increased binding of the drug to these other substances, less drug remains to act on the DNA. The tumor cell also may increase DNA repair systems. If the damage caused by alkylation is repaired before the cell divides, cell death does not occur. Finally, increased metabolism of the active drug may occur, thereby decreasing the contact time between the drug and tumor cell. When resistance of a tumor to one alkylating agent occurs, the tumor cells usually become cross-resistant to other alkylating agents.

PHARMACOTHERAPEUTICS

The nitrogen mustards are indicated for various malignant neoplasms. Because they produce leukopenia, the nitrogen mustards are effective in treating malignant neoplasms, such as Hodgkin's disease and leukemias, that have an associated elevated white blood cell (WBC) count. Also, the nitrogen mustards prove effective against many solid tumors. These drugs can be given alone or with other classes of antineoplastic agents. The activity and effectiveness of each drug depend on many factors, including the type of cancer, the extent of disease, and the patient's condition. Furthermore, the toxicity of the nitrogen mustards depends to a large extent on the dosage and administration route. For instance, cyclophosphamide is given in low oral dosages and in high I.V. dosages, and toxicity is directly related to dosage. The nurse administering nitrogen mustards should be familiar not only with the specific pharmacologic data about the drug but also with the protocol being used for the patient.

chlorambucil (Leukeran). Administered orally, alone or as a combination agent, chlorambucil is used to treat chronic lymphocytic leukemia, non-Hodgkin's lymphomas, and advanced Hodgkin's disease.
Usual adult dosage: 4 to 10 mg P.O. daily for 3 to 6 weeks. As clinical improvement occurs and the WBC count decreases, a maintenance dosage of 2 to 4 mg/day is prescribed.

cyclophosphamide (Cytoxan). Alone or in combination therapies, cyclophosphamide is used to treat numerous hematologic and solid tumors. It is considered the drug of choice for treating chronic lymphocytic leukemia and neuroblastoma. When used alone, cyclophosphamide has produced a positive response in 30% of patients with multiple myeloma and in 90% of patients with Burkitt's lymphoma. Solid tumors treated with cyclophosphamide include ovarian, breast, and bronchogenic carcinoma and retinoblastoma. Cyclophosphamide is administered orally or by I.V. injection. It also is given intrapleurally and intraperitoneally.
Usual adult dosage: for patients with no hematologic deficiencies, from 2 to 3 mg/kg to as high as 100 mg/kg P.O. or I.V. Dosages vary for different types of cancer. Subsequent dosages are adjusted according to patient tolerance.

estramustine (Emcyt). A combination of an estrogen and nitrogen mustard, estramustine is used to treat advanced prostate cancer.
Usual adult dosage: 10 to 16 mg/kg P.O. in divided daily doses.

ifosfamide (Ifex). Ifosfamide is used with other antineoplastic agents for third-line chemotherapy of germ cell testicular cancer.
Usual adult dosage: 1.2 gm/m²/day I.V. for 5 consecutive days. Treatment usually is repeated every 3 weeks.

mechlorethamine (Mustargen). Administered I.V., mechlorethamine is used primarily to treat advanced Hodgkin's disease (Stages III and IV) in combination with other chemotherapeutic agents. The drug also is used to induce brief remissions in treating non-Hodgkin's lymphoma. The I.V. administration can be extremely irritating to the vein.

Although mechlorethamine should not be given intramuscularly or subcutaneously, it can be given by intracavitary administration to treat malignant pleural effusions. It also may used alone or in combination as adjunctive therapy for mycosis fungoides. For this indication, the drug is applied topically to skin lesions.
Usual adult dosage: for advanced Hodgkin's disease, non-Hodgkin's lymphoma, and mycosis fungoides, 0.4 mg/kg I.V. once every 3 to 6 weeks (depending on the protocol) for the course of therapy. Some patients being treated for

advanced Hodgkin's disease may receive higher dosages. For malignant pleural effusions, 0.2 to 0.4 mg/kg via intracavitary administration; for mycosis fungoides, topical application of sufficient lotion or ointment to cover lesion one to four times a day for 6 to 12 months after a complete response.

melphalan (Alkeran). Administered orally, melphalan is used primarily to treat multiple myeloma. Less commonly, it is used to treat non-resectable ovarian cancer.
Usual adult dosage: initially, 6 mg P.O. daily for 2 to 3 weeks followed by a rest period of at least 4 weeks to allow the leukocyte and platelet counts to rise. Subsequent dosages may be adjusted depending on the degree of leukopenia or thrombocytopenia induced. Usually, maintenance therapy is 2 to 4 mg P.O. daily to maintain the proper bone marrow suppression.

uracil mustard. Uracil mustard is used primarily in the palliative treatment of malignant neoplasms of the reticuloendothelial system, such as lymphomas and chronic myelogenous leukemia. However, it usually is not considered the drug of choice.
Usual adult dosage: 1 to 2 mg P.O. daily until the desired effect is obtained, usually 3 weeks, followed by a rest period of 1 week; then the protocol is repeated.

Drug interactions

Most drug interactions with antineoplastic agents, including the nitrogen mustards, are theoretically based on animal studies or basic chemical theory. (For more information, see the introduction to this unit.)

Human study data has revealed only two drug interactions. Cyclophosphamide interacts with succinylcholine, prolonging the neuromuscular blockade of succinylcholine. Cyclophosphamide also interacts with chloramphenicol, reducing the conversion of cyclophosphamide to active metabolites.

ADVERSE DRUG REACTIONS

Patients receiving nitrogen mustards may experience a wide range of adverse reactions, depending on which drug is given, the dosage, the patient's condition and morbidity, other drugs being used, and psychological factors. Pharmacologic or nonpharmacologic interventions can manage some reactions, such as nausea and vomiting. Others, such as bone marrow suppression, must resolve on their own. (For more information, see *Common adverse reactions and associated nursing implications* in the introduction to this unit.)

Bone marrow suppression, evidenced by severe leukopenia and thrombocytopenia, is an anticipated adverse reaction associated with the nitrogen mustards. Depending on the degree of the patient's bone marrow suppression, future drug dosages may be modified.

Nausea and vomiting from CNS irritation is another common adverse reaction to the nitrogen mustards. Nausea and vomiting may occur 30 minutes after drug administration, as happens with mechlorethamine, or may not begin for hours, as occurs with cyclophosphamide. If used in the right combination and in an effective dosing pattern, antiemetic drugs may control or lessen nausea and vomiting associated with nitrogen mustards.

Damage to rapidly proliferating cells produces stomatitis and alopecia. The swollen, inflamed mucous membranes that characterize stomatitis can lead to a nutritional problem because of pain associated with stomatitis. Alopecia, which is caused by hair follicle damage, results in thinning hair 2 to 3 weeks after the first administration of a nitrogen mustard. However, hair loss usually is not significant for two to three courses of treatment. Once treatment ends, hair growth resumes.

Many patients experience fatigue during nitrogen mustard therapy. Anemia from bone marrow suppression probably produces the fatigue. Some evidence suggests that circulating tumor breakdown products also may contribute to the fatigue. Many patients feel most fatigued immediately after treatment and have an increased energy level later in the interval between therapeutic courses. However, for patients on protocols that last for months, fatigue is persistent.

Because the nitrogen mustards are powerful local vesicants (blistering agents), direct contact with the drugs or their vapors can cause severe reactions, especially of the skin, eyes, and respiratory tract. Mechlorethamine extravasation may cause painful inflammation and induration.

Patients may experience alterations in fertility. After several courses of nitrogen mustard treatment, women may experience amenorrhea or irregular menses. Men may have decreased spermatogenesis. Many patients, however, experience no apparent alteration in fertility, and women treated with nitrogen mustards have conceived and given birth to normal children.

Hemorrhagic cystitis may develop within 48 hours of an I.V. dose of cyclophosphamide, or it may result after several months of oral administration of low doses of the drug. Cyclophosphamide metabolites in the urine irritate the bladder lining, producing this adverse reaction. Adequate hydration usually prevents hemorrhagic cystitis, and the nurse should encourage any patient receiving cyclophosphamide to consume at least eight 8-oz glasses (2 liters) of fluid daily.

Hemorrhagic cystitis is the dose-limiting toxicity for ifosfamide. However, administration with the uroprotectant mesna (Mesnex) may alleviate this adverse reaction. (For details, see Chapter 73, Uncategorized and Other Agents.) Ifosfamide also may cause adverse CNS reactions, such as somnolence, confusion, and hallucinations.

Chlorambucil may produce hepatotoxicity, but this reaction rarely occurs. Rarely, chlorambucil and cyclophosphamide may cause pulmonary reactions, such as interstitial pneumonitis or pulmonary fibrosis.

Like other alkylating agents, the nitrogen mustards have been implicated in producing hematologic and other malignancies, although this is rare. Anaphylaxis is another rare adverse reaction associated with the nitrogen mustards.

NURSING PROCESS APPLICATION

The following information assists the nurse in caring for a patient receiving a nitrogen mustard.

Assessment
• Review the patient's history for a preexisting condition that contraindicates the use of a nitrogen mustard, such as pregnancy, lactation, or known hypersensitivity to the drug.
• Review the patient's history for a preexisting condition that requires cautious use of a nitrogen mustard, such as leukopenia, thrombocytopenia, tumor cell infiltration of bone marrow, radiation therapy, or therapy with other cytotoxic agents.
• Assess the patient for adverse reactions to the prescribed nitrogen mustard, such as bone marrow suppression, nausea, vomiting, stomatitis, alopecia, and fatigue.
• Review the patient's medication history to identify the use of drugs that may interact with cyclophosphamide, such as succinylcholine or chloramphenicol.
• Assess the effectiveness of the prescribed nitrogen mustard regularly.
• Assess the patient with leukopenia for signs of infection, such as fever, malaise, and productive cough.
• Assess the patient with thrombocytopenia for signs of bleeding, such as spontaneous epistaxis, easy bruising, and hematuria.
• Evaluate the patient's and family's knowledge about the prescribed nitrogen mustard.

Nursing diagnoses
The following examples represent appropriate nursing diagnoses for a patient receiving a nitrogen mustard.
• Potential for injury related to a preexisting condition that contraindicates the use of a nitrogen mustard
• Potential for injury related to a preexisting condition that requires cautious use of a nitrogen mustard
• Potential for injury related to adverse drug reactions
• Potential for infection related to nitrogen mustard-induced leukopenia
• Altered protection related to nitrogen mustard-induced thrombocytopenia
• Knowledge deficit related to the prescribed nitrogen mustard

Planning and implementation
• Do not administer a nitrogen mustard to a patient with a condition that contraindicates its use.
• Administer a nitrogen mustard cautiously to a patient at risk because of a preexisting condition.
• Monitor the patient frequently for adverse reactions during nitrogen mustard therapy.
• Monitor hydration if the patient experiences nausea and vomiting from nitrogen mustard administration.
• Administer an antiemetic agent concomitantly as prescribed to control or lessen nausea and vomiting. If fluid intake is inadequate despite antiemetic use, expect to replace fluids I.V. as prescribed.
• Offer the patient frequent sips of iced beverages or ice chips to help relieve nausea.
• *Inspect the patient's oral cavity frequently for signs of stomatitis, such as swollen, inflamed mucous membranes. If stomatitis occurs, monitor the patient's nutritional status. A nutritional deficiency can result from decreased food consumption caused by the pain associated with stomatitis. To relieve stomatitis, provide frequent oral care, apply a topical medication for pain relief as prescribed, and provide a pureed or liquid diet.*
• Assist the patient with activities of daily living if fatigue occurs. Limit the patient's activities and stagger those that are necessary. Provide rest periods, especially after treatment—when the patient is most likely to feel fatigued.
• *Monitor all infusion sites for signs of extravasation, such as pain and swelling at the insertion site. Change infusion sites according to health care facility protocol and as needed.*
• *Monitor the patient for signs of hemorrhagic cystitis, such as hematuria and dysuria during cyclophosphamide or ifosfamide therapy.*
• Increase the fluid intake of the patient receiving I.V. cyclophosphamide. After treatment, instruct the patient to maintain increased fluids for 2 to 3 days.
• Administer cyclophosphamide or ifosfamide earlier in the day rather than at bedtime to prevent prolonged contact between the drug's metabolites and the bladder.
• Administer mesna with ifosfamide and 4 and 8 hours after treatment to help prevent hemorrhagic cystitis.
• *Take safety precautions if ifosfamide produces adverse CNS reactions, such as somnolence, confusion, or hallucinations. For example, place the bed in the low position, keep the side rails up, and supervise the patient's activities.*
• Assess the patient's respiratory status and monitor the results of prescribed chest X-ray results during chlorambucil or cyclophosphamide therapy to detect pulmonary reactions, such as interstitial pneumonitis or pulmonary fibrosis.
• *Wear gloves when administering the nitrogen mustard or as directed by health care facility policy and avoid inhaling the vapors. Direct contact with the drug or its*

vapors can cause severe reactions, especially of the skin, eyes, and respiratory tract.

• *Administer the nitrogen mustard exactly as directed in the manufacturer's guidelines.* (For more information about administration, see the introduction to this unit.)

• Administer mechlorethamine immediately after reconstitution because it is unstable in solution. Most other nitrogen mustards, which remain stable in solution, can be prepared well before administration.

• Reduce I.V. administration pain by altering the infusion rate or further diluting the drug if indicated, or by warming the injection site to distend the vein and increase blood flow.

• Notify the physician if adverse reactions occur.

• Monitor the patient's blood counts carefully, especially the complete blood count (CBC). Keep in mind that bone marrow suppression is the most common and potentially serious adverse reaction to alkylating agents.

• *Take infection control measures and monitor the patient for signs of infection if leukopenia occurs.*

• Notify the physician if an infection is suspected.

• Administer an antibiotic as prescribed if an infection occurs.

• *Take bleeding precautions if thrombocytopenia occurs. Avoid I.M. injections and venipunctures. When a venipuncture must be done, apply firm pressure to the site for at least 5 minutes afterwards. Monitor the patient for signs of bleeding and prepare to take emergency measures to stop bleeding if hemorrhage occurs. Assess the patient's CNS status to detect early signs and symptoms of intracranial hemorrhage.*

• Notify the physician if bleeding occurs.

• Use other appropriate interventions for a patient with bone marrow suppression, leukopenia, thrombocytopenia, anemia, nausea, vomiting, stomatitis, or alopecia. (For details, see the introduction to this unit.)

Patient teaching

• Teach the patient and family the name, dose, frequency, action, and adverse effects of the prescribed nitrogen mustard.

• Inform the patient that the nitrogen mustard can produce alopecia, which cannot be prevented. Explain that alopecia affects men and women and may include eyebrows, eyelashes, scalp hair, and other body hair. Reassure the patient that the hair loss is reversible when the treatment ends.

• Instruct the patient to increase oral fluid intake the day before cyclophosphamide or ifosfamide therapy to help prevent hemorrhagic cystitis. Advise the patient that fluid intake should not include caffeinated beverages, such as coffee or tea, because they have diuretic effects.

• Encourage the patient taking oral cyclophosphamide to take the medication earlier in the day, to maintain good fluid intake, and to void before going to bed.

• Discuss ways to relieve adverse reactions to the nitrogen mustard. For example, suggest dietary changes to relieve nausea, vomiting, or stomatitis; frequent oral care to help manage stomatitis, and activity restriction to help the patient manage fatigue.

• *Advise the patient not to perform activities that require mental alertness until the adverse CNS effects of ifosfamide are known.*

• *Teach the patient infection control measures and bleeding precautions to use during nitrogen mustard therapy.*

• Inform the patient that alterations in fertility may occur during nitrogen mustard therapy. Advise the female patient that amenorrhea or irregular menses also may occur.

• Stress the importance of returning for follow-up visits and blood tests as ordered.

• Instruct the patient to notify the physician if adverse reactions occur.

• *Advise the patient to notify the physician if any other symptoms appear because the nitrogen mustard may cause a secondary hematologic or other malignancy, such as leukemia.*

• Give the patient written materials about the prescribed nitrogen mustard for home reference.

Evaluation

The following examples represent appropriate evaluation statements for a patient receiving a nitrogen mustard.

• The patient has no conditions that contraindicate nitrogen mustard therapy.

• The patient exhibits no signs of complications in the preexisting condition linked to the prescribed nitrogen mustard.

• The patient experiences few adverse reactions to the prescribed nitrogen mustard.

• The patient remains free of infection during nitrogen mustard therapy.

• The patient maintains a a normal platelet count throughout nitrogen mustard therapy.

• The patient and family express an accurate understanding of the points taught about the prescribed nitrogen mustard.

• The patient correctly describes infection control and bleeding precautions to take during nitrogen mustard therapy.

ALKYL SULFONATES

The alkyl sulfonate, busulfan, commonly is used to treat chronic myelogenous leukemia and less commonly to treat polycythemia vera and other myeloproliferative disorders. Busulfan is not related chemically to the nitrogen mustards.

PHARMACOKINETICS

Busulfan is effective when administered orally.

Absorption, distribution, metabolism, excretion

Busulfan is absorbed rapidly and well from the gastrointestinal (GI) tract. The drug disappears from the plasma rapidly and has a half-life of 2 to 3 hours. Little is known about its distribution into the brain, cerebrospinal fluid, or breast milk. Busulfan is metabolized extensively in the liver before urinary excretion. Within 24 hours, 10% to 50% of busulfan metabolites are excreted in the urine. (For more information about the pharmacokinetics of this drug, see *Major administration and excretion routes for alkylating agents,* page 1148.)

Onset, peak, duration

Precise data concerning the onset of action, peak concentration level, and duration of action of busulfan are unavailable because analytical methods are insufficient. However, measurable blood concentrations are obtained within 0.5 to 2 hours after oral administration. The major effect of busulfan is myelosuppression, specifically granulocytopenia. The drug begins to reduce the WBC count about 10 days after the initiation of therapy. This effect lasts 2 weeks after the drug is discontinued.

PHARMACODYNAMICS

The alkyl sulfonate busulfan forms covalent bonds with the DNA molecules in a chemical reaction known as alkylation. (For more information, see *DNA alkylation,* page 1149, and *Mechanisms and sites of action of selected antineoplastic agents* in the introduction to this unit.)

Mechanism of action

Busulfan, in an aqueous medium, undergoes a wide range of nucleophilic substitution reactions, causing alkylation of DNA and leading to its cytotoxic effects.

PHARMACOTHERAPEUTICS

Busulfan, which is cell-cycle-nonspecific, affects primarily granulocytes and, to a lesser degree, platelets. Because of its action on granulocytes, it is the drug of choice for treating chronic myelogenous leukemia. This action also makes busulfan effective for polycythemia vera. However, other agents usually are used to treat polycythemia vera because busulfan can cause severe myelosuppression.

busulfan (Myleran). Administered orally, busulfan is the drug of choice to treat chronic myelogenous leukemia.

Usual adult dosage: 4 to 8 mg P.O. daily, until the WBC count falls between 10,000/mm^3 and 25,000/mm^3, depending on the prescriber's preference. Then the drug is stopped until the WBC count rises to 50,000/mm^3. Treatment is resumed to maintain the WBC count at 10,000 to 20,000/mm^3. The maintenance dosage is 1 to 4 mg P.O. daily for patients who do not remain in remission for more than 3 months.

Drug interactions

No significant drug interactions occur with busulfan.

ADVERSE DRUG REACTIONS

Busulfan can cause a wide range of adverse reactions, which may be mild or severe. The major adverse reaction is bone marrow suppression, which usually is dose-related and reversible. Bone marrow suppression produces severe leukopenia, anemia, and thrombocytopenia. Granulocytopenia occurs rarely and can progress to pancytopenia, which may be fatal.

Nausea, vomiting, and diarrhea are uncommon. Hyperuricemia occurs and is treated with hydration, allopurinol, or both. With long-term therapy, an addisonian-like wasting syndrome with hyperpigmentation and weight loss sometimes occurs. Busulfan also may produce irreversible interstitial pulmonary fibrosis (busulfan lung) after long-term use (1 to 3 years).

NURSING PROCESS APPLICATION

The following information assists the nurse in caring for a patient receiving busulfan.

Assessment

• Review the patient's history for a preexisting condition that contraindicates the use of busulfan, such as pregnancy, lactation, or previous resistance to the drug.
• Review the patient's history for a preexisting condition that requires cautious use of busulfan, such as prior radiation therapy or chemotherapy, or bone marrow suppression from prior cytotoxic therapy.
• Assess the patient for adverse reactions to busulfan, such as bone marrow suppression, nausea, vomiting, diarrhea, hyperuricemia, addisonian-like wasting syndrome, or interstitial pulmonary fibrosis.
• Assess the effectiveness of busulfan regularly.
• Assess the patient's respiratory status regularly during long-term busulfan therapy.
• Evaluate the patient's and family's knowledge about busulfan.

Nursing diagnoses

The following examples represent appropriate nursing diagnoses for a patient receiving busulfan.

- Potential for injury related to a preexisting condition that contraindicates the use of busulfan
- Potential for injury related to a preexisting condition that requires cautious use of busulfan
- Potential for injury related to adverse drug reactions
- Impaired gas exchange related to busulfan-induced interstitial pulmonary fibrosis
- Knowledge deficit related to busulfan

Planning and implementation

- Do not administer busulfan to a patient with a condition that contraindicates its use.
- Administer busulfan cautiously to a patient at risk because of a preexisting condition.
- Monitor the patient regularly for adverse reactions during busulfan therapy.
- Monitor the patient's CBC as prescribed to detect such abnormalities as leukopenia, thrombocytopenia, or anemia. If abnormalities occur, notify the physician before administering the next dose of busulfan.
- *Take infection control measures and bleeding precautions. If leukopenia occurs, monitor the patient for signs of infection, such as fever, malaise, sore throat, or productive cough. If thrombocytopenia occurs, monitor the patient for signs bleeding, such as spontaneous epistaxis, easy bruising, or hematuria. Also observe for early signs and symptoms of intracranial hemorrhage. Avoid I.M. injections and venipunctures when the patient's platelet count is low. When a venipuncture must be done, apply firm pressure to the site for at least 5 minutes afterward.*
- Expect to discontinue the drug as prescribed if CBC values decrease rapidly or significantly.
- *Use anticoagulants cautiously and observe for signs of bleeding during concomitant administration.*
- Stagger the patient's activities and provide frequent rest periods if anemia occurs.
- Monitor hydration if the patient experiences nausea, vomiting, or diarrhea. Administer an antiemetic or antidiarrheal agent as prescribed. If fluid intake is inadequate despite antiemetic use, expect to replace fluids I.V. as prescribed.
- Monitor the patient's uric acid level to detect hyperuricemia. If hyperuricemia occurs, expect to administer allopurinol as prescribed and ensure that the patient consumes at least 2 liters of fluid daily (unless contraindicated).
- Monitor the patient receiving long-term busulfan therapy for signs of addisonian-like wasting syndrome, such as hyperpigmentation and progressive weight loss.
- Use other appropriate interventions for a patient with bone marrow suppression, nausea, or vomiting. (For details, see the introduction to this unit.)
- Notify the physician if adverse reactions occur.

- *Monitor pulmonary function studies as prescribed for a patient receiving long-term busulfan therapy. Also monitor respiratory assessment findings regularly, particularly noting any changes in the quality of respirations, such as progressive dyspnea, or a persistent cough. Alert the physician if respiratory abnormalities occur.*

Patient teaching

- Teach the patient and family the name, dose, frequency, action, and adverse effects of busulfan.
- *Teach the patient infection control measures and bleeding precautions to use during busulfan therapy.*
- *Instruct the patient to notify the physician if fever, sore throat, unusual bleeding, bruising, or symptoms of anemia occur.*
- Stress the importance of returning for follow-up visits and regular CBC and other blood tests as ordered.
- Advise the patient with anemia to stagger activities and take frequent rests.
- Instruct the patient with hyperuricemia to drink at least eight 8-oz glasses of fluid a day (unless contraindicated).
- *Instruct the patient to notify the physician if hyperpigmentation, weight loss, persistent cough, progressive dyspnea, or any other adverse reactions occur.*

Evaluation

The following examples represent appropriate evaluation statements for a patient receiving busulfan.

- The patient has no conditions that contraindicate busulfan therapy.
- The patient exhibits no signs of complications in the preexisting condition linked to busulfan.
- The patient experiences few adverse reactions to busulfan.
- The patient maintains normal respiratory function throughout long-term busulfan therapy.
- The patient and family express an accurate understanding of the points taught about busulfan.
- The patient correctly identifies adverse reactions that must be reported.

NITROSOUREAS

The nitrosoureas in an aqueous medium are unstable and decompose to alkylating intermediates. The lethal effect of nitrosoureas on cells seems to result from inhibition of DNA synthesis. The nitrosoureas include carmustine, lomustine, semustine, and streptozocin.

PHARMACOKINETICS

Some nitrosoureas are absorbed well from the GI tract. These drugs are lipid-soluble and most of them readily cross the blood-brain barrier. They undergo significant metabolism in the liver. The metabolites of the nitrosoureas are excreted in the urine.

Absorption, distribution, metabolism, excretion

When administered topically for mycosis fungoides, carmustine provides systemic absorption of 5% to 28%. After oral administration, lomustine and semustine are absorbed adequately, although incompletely. Streptozocin, which is administered intravenously, does not undergo absorption.

All four nitrosoureas are lipophilic, distributing to fatty tissues and attaining significant cerebrospinal fluid (CSF) levels. Carmustine, lomustine, and semustine achieve CSF levels of 15% to 30% of plasma levels. Streptozocin does not appear to cross the blood-brain barrier; however, its metabolites enter the CSF to varying degrees. (For more information about the pharmacokinetics of these agents, see *Major administration and excretion routes for alkylating agents,* page 1148.)

The nitrosoureas are metabolized extensively before urinary excretion. Carmustine is metabolized rapidly by the liver, producing some active metabolites, and is excreted slowly in the urine. Within 24 hours, 30% of a carmustine dose appears in the urine as metabolites. Lomustine is metabolized rapidly and completely by the liver, and some of its metabolites are active. Up to 50% of a lomustine dose is excreted in the urine within 12 hours. Semustine also is metabolized by the liver to active metabolites. Up to 60% of a semustine dose is excreted in the urine as metabolites within 48 hours. Minor amounts of semustine are excreted in the feces and in the lungs as carbon dioxide. Although the metabolism of streptozocin is not established clearly, streptozocin is thought to be metabolized rapidly in the liver and kidneys. Within 24 hours, 60% to 70% of a streptozocin dose is excreted in the urine, principally as metabolites; about 10% is excreted as the parent compound. Less than 1% is excreted in the feces. A small amount of the drug also may be excreted in expired air.

Onset, peak, duration

The nitrosoureas vary in their peak concentration levels and half-lives. Carmustine peaks instantaneously with I.V. administration and disappears from the plasma, with a half-life of 15 to 30 minutes. The peak plasma concentration of lomustine metabolites is reached within 1 to 6 hours of oral administration. The half-life of the metabolites ranges from 24 to 48 hours. The peak plasma concentration of semustine occurs in 1 to 6 hours. Streptozocin has a plasma half-life of 35 minutes, with some streptozocin metabolites displaying a prolonged terminal half-life of more than 40 hours.

PHARMACODYNAMICS

The nitrosoureas display bifunctional alkylation of DNA. (For details, see *DNA alkylation,* page 1149.)

Mechanism of action

Like the mechanism of action of other alkylating agents, that of the nitrosoureas involves bifunctional alkylation of DNA. (For a more detailed discussion of this action, see the section on mechanism of action under nitrogen mustards on page 1147.)

PHARMACOTHERAPEUTICS

The nitrosoureas display a high degree of lipid solubility, which allows them or their metabolites to cross the blood-brain barrier easily. Because of this ability, nitrosoureas are used to treat brain tumors and meningeal leukemias.

carmustine [BCNU] (BiCNU). Carmustine is used to treat CNS tumors, multiple myeloma, refractory Hodgkin's disease, and non-Hodgkin's lymphoma. Administered I.V., carmustine irritates the vein and needs further dilution. The I.V. dose must be infused over 1 to 2 hours to decrease vein irritation. Two basic dosage schedules have been used for carmustine.
Usual adult dosage: first schedule, 75 to 100 mg/m² I.V. daily for 2 consecutive days, repeated every 6 to 8 weeks; the alternative schedule, up to 200 mg/m² in a single I.V. infusion, repeated every 6 to 8 weeks.

lomustine [CCNU] (CeeNU). This nitrosourea is used mainly to treat primary brain tumors or brain metastases from other malignant neoplasms.
Usual adult dosage: 100 to 130 mg/m² as a single oral dose, repeated about every 6 weeks.

semustine [methyl-CCNU]. Although semustine is an investigational drug that is not available commercially, it has been used effectively in combination treatment of advanced GI cancers in clinical research.
Usual adult dosage: 125 to 200 mg/m² P.O. no more than every 6 weeks.

streptozocin (Zanosar). The uses of streptozocin include the treatment of metastatic pancreatic islet cell tumor, malignant carcinoid tumors, and adenocarcinoma of the gallbladder.
Usual adult dosage: for a weekly regimen, 1 to 1.5 grams/m² I.V. for 6 consecutive weeks; for a consecutive-day

regimen, 500 mg/m² I.V. daily for 5 days, repeated every 6 weeks.

Drug interactions
When combined with cimetidine, carmustine seems to display an increased myelosuppressant effect, possibly because of inhibition of carmustine metabolism. Carmustine may reduce serum digoxin and phenytoin levels by altering their absorption. No significant interactions occur with lomustine, semustine, or streptozocin.

ADVERSE DRUG REACTIONS

The nitrosoureas, like all alkylating agents, can produce a range of mild to severe adverse reactions.

Carmustine and lomustine produce bone marrow depression that begins 4 to 6 weeks after treatment and lasts 1 to 2 weeks. The bone marrow suppression is cumulative — that is, it can become more severe and prolonged with repeated doses. Semustine also produces bone marrow depression, which begins 4 to 8 weeks after treatment and lasts up to 10 weeks. Severe nausea lasts 2 to 6 hours after carmustine, lomustine, or semustine administration. Lomustine and semustine also may cause anorexia for a few days after administration. The patient also may experience intense pain at the infusion site during carmustine administration. Renal dysfunction occurs in about two-thirds of patients receiving streptozocin and is dose-limiting. Severe nausea and vomiting also occur with this drug and may persist for more than 24 hours.

Nephrotoxicity and renal failure have occurred with the nitrosoureas. High-dose carmustine may produce reversible hepatotoxicity. Carmustine also may cause pulmonary toxicity characterized by pulmonary infiltrates or fibrosis. These pulmonary reactions are dose-related; their incidence is much higher in patients who receive cumulative doses of more than 1,400 mg/m². Hematologic toxicity and mild glucose intolerance are possible but are rare adverse reactions to streptozocin.

Streptozocin is irritating to tissues. If extravasated, it can cause necrosis. Carmustine may cause vein irritation.

NURSING PROCESS APPLICATION

The following information assists the nurse in caring for a patient receiving a nitrosourea.

Assessment
• Review the patient's history for a preexisting condition that contraindicates the use of a nitrosourea, such as pregnancy, lactation, or known hypersensitivity to the drug.
• Review the patient's history for a preexisting condition that requires cautious use of a nitrosourea, such as a depressed platelet, leukocyte, or erythrocyte count.

• Assess the patient for adverse reactions to the prescribed nitrosourea, such as bone marrow suppression, GI distress, and nephrotoxicity.
• Review the patient's medication history to identify the use of drugs that may interact with carmustine, such as cimetidine, digoxin, and phenytoin.
• Assess the effectiveness of the prescribed nitrosourea regularly.
• Assess the carmustine or streptozocin infusion site regularly for signs of irritation or necrosis.
• Evaluate the patient's and family's knowledge about the prescribed nitrosourea.

Nursing diagnoses
The following examples represent appropriate nursing diagnoses for a patient receiving a nitrosourea.
• Potential for injury related to a preexisting condition that contraindicates the use of a nitrosourea
• Potential for injury related to a preexisting condition that requires cautious use of a nitrosourea
• Potential for injury related to adverse drug reactions
• Impaired tissue integrity related to the adverse effects of carmustine or streptozocin at the infusion site
• Knowledge deficit related to the prescribed nitrosourea

Planning and implementation
• Do not administer a nitrosourea to a patient with a condition that contraindicates its use.
• Administer a nitrosourea cautiously to a patient at risk because of a preexisting condition.
• Monitor the patient regularly for adverse reactions throughout nitrosurea therapy.
• *Monitor the patient's CBC for abnormalities, such as delayed bone marrow suppression. Observe the patient for signs and symptoms of infection (fever, chills, sore throat, and malaise), bleeding (spontaneous epistaxis, easy bruising, and hematuria), or anemia (pallor and fatigue). Take infection control measures, bleeding precautions, or energy conservation measures as needed.*
• Monitor urinalysis, blood urea nitrogen (BUN), and creatinine levels for abnormalities that indicate nephrotoxicity and renal failure. Keep in mind that mild proteinuria is an early sign of nephrotoxicity.
• Monitor the patient's hepatic function studies as prescribed when administering high doses of carmustine. If abnormalities occur, lower the dose or change to a different agent as prescribed.
• Monitor hydration if the patient experiences nausea, vomiting, or anorexia. Administer an antiemetic as prescribed. If fluid intake is inadequate despite antiemetic use, expect to replace fluids I.V. as prescribed.
• *Monitor the patient's chest X-ray results and assess the patient's respiratory status regularly during carmustine therapy to detect signs and symptoms of pulmonary tox-*

icity, such as pulmonary infiltrates or fibrosis on the X-ray and shortness of breath. If pulmonary toxicity occurs, decrease the dosage or change to another agent as prescribed.

• Use other appropriate nursing interventions for a patient with bone marrow suppression, nausea, or vomiting. (For details, see the introduction to this unit.)

• Notify the physician if adverse reactions occur.

• Inspect the patient's I.V. site for signs of tissue damage or vein irritation, such as redness, swelling, or pain on touch, before administering each dose of carmustine or streptozocin. Change I.V. sites according to health care facility protocol and as needed.

• Dilute the carmustine infusion and administer it over 1 to 2 hours if vein irritation occurs. Also use warmth to dilate the veins and increase blood flow to further dilute the drug.

• *Stop the streptozocin infusion immediately and notify the physician if extravasation occurs. This agent is a vesicant and can cause tissue necrosis.*

Patient teaching

• Teach the patient and family the name, dose, frequency, action, and adverse effects of the prescribed nitrosourea.

• *Alert the patient to watch for signs of infection, bleeding, and anemia. If any occur, instruct the patient to notify the physician.*

• Stress the importance of returning for regular blood and urine studies as prescribed.

• *Teach the patient infection control measures, bleeding precautions, and energy conservation measures to use as needed.*

• Inform the patient that carmustine produces pain during administration and that appropriate measures will be taken to minimize discomfort.

• Instruct the patient with adverse GI reactions to sip fluids every hour. If nausea is severe or GI reactions persist, advise the patient to notify the physician.

• Instruct the patient to notify the physician if any other adverse reactions occur.

Evaluation

The following examples represent appropriate evaluation statements for a patient receiving a nitrosourea.

• The patient has no conditions that contraindicate nitrosourea therapy.

• The patient exhibits no signs of complications in the preexisting condition linked to the prescribed nitrosourea.

• The patient experiences few adverse reactions to the prescribed nitrosourea.

• The patient maintains normal tissue integrity at the infusion site during carmustine or streptozocin therapy.

• The patient and family express an accurate understanding of the points taught about the prescribed nitrosourea.

• The patient schedules follow-up visits for regular blood and urine tests as prescribed.

TRIAZINES

Dacarbazine, a triazine, functions as an alkylating agent after it has been metabolically activated in the liver. Dacarbazine is cell-cycle-nonspecific.

PHARMACOKINETICS

Dacarbazine is administered intravenously because oral administration results in variable, incomplete absorption.

Absorption, distribution, metabolism, excretion

After I.V. injection, dacarbazine is distributed throughout the body and minimally to the CSF. The CSF level is about 14% of the concurrent plasma level. After metabolism in the liver, cytotoxic metabolites are released. Within 6 hours, 30% to 46% of a dose is excreted renally; 50% is excreted unchanged, and 50% is excreted as one of the metabolites. (For more information, see *Major administration and excretion routes for alkylating agents,* page 1148.)

Onset, peak, duration

Dacarbazine reaches a peak plasma concentration rapidly after I.V. administration. It has a half-life of approximately 5 hours. In patients with renal and hepatic dysfunction, half-life may increase to 7 hours.

PHARMACODYNAMICS

Dacarbazine seems to inhibit ribonucleic acid (RNA) and protein synthesis. Like other alkylating agents, dacarbazine is cell-cycle-nonspecific.

Mechanism of action

Dacarbazine first must be metabolized in the liver to become an alkylating agent. Then the drug produces a greater effect on RNA synthesis than on DNA synthesis. This characteristic distinguishes dacarbazine from the other alkylating agents.

PHARMACOTHERAPEUTICS

Dacarbazine is used primarily to treat patients with malignant melanoma but also in combination with other drugs to treat patients with Hodgkin's disease.

dacarbazine (DTIC-Dome). This triazine agent acts most effectively against malignant melanoma and soft-tissue sarcomas. Dosage ranges vary greatly according to the protocol.

Usual adult dosage: 150 to 250 mg/m² I.V. daily for 5 days; treatment may be repeated in 3 to 4 weeks. Much higher dosages are used in some protocols, even as high as 850 mg/m² daily, for 1 day only.

Drug interactions

No significant drug interactions occur involving dacarbazine.

ADVERSE DRUG REACTIONS

Leukopenia and thrombocytopenia occur as a result of dacarbazine use. Nausea and vomiting begin within 1 to 3 hours of administration in most patients and may last up to 12 hours. Dacarbazine infusion typically causes pain at the infusion site, which may require further dilution or a slower infusion rate. If extravasation occurs, dacarbazine may cause severe tissue damage. Phototoxicity also occurs, as does a flulike syndrome and alopecia.

NURSING PROCESS APPLICATION

The following information assists the nurse in caring for a patient receiving dacarbazine.

Assessment
• Review the patient's history for a preexisting condition that contraindicates the use of dacarbazine, such as lactation or known hypersensitivity to the drug.
• Review the patient's history for a preexisting condition that requires cautious use of dacarbazine, such as pregnancy.
• Assess the patient for adverse reactions to dacarbazine, such as leukopenia, thrombocytopenia, nausea, vomiting, pain at the infusion site, phototoxicity, flulike syndrome, and alopecia.
• Assess the effectiveness of dacarbazine regularly.
• Assess the patient regularly for signs and symptoms of extravasation, such as redness, swelling, and pain at the dacarbazine infusion site.
• Evaluate the patient's and family's knowledge about dacarbazine.

Nursing diagnoses
The following examples represent appropriate nursing diagnoses for a patient receiving dacarbazine.
• Potential for injury related to a preexisting condition that contraindicates the use of dacarbazine
• Potential for injury related to a preexisting condition that requires cautious use of dacarbazine

• Potential for injury related to adverse drug reactions
• Impaired tissue integrity related to tissue damage caused by dacarbazine extravasation
• Knowledge deficit related to the dacarbazine

Planning and implementation
• Do not administer dacarbazine to a patient with a condition that contraindicates its use.
• Administer dacarbazine cautiously to a patient at risk because of a preexisting condition.
• Monitor the patient regularly for adverse reactions to dacarbazine therapy.
• *Monitor the patient's CBC regularly for abnormalities that indicate leukopenia or thrombocytopenia.*
• *Monitor the patient's temperature regularly, and observe for signs and symptoms of infection. Take infection control measures if leukopenia occurs.*
• *Monitor the patient for signs of bleeding, such as spontaneous epistaxis, hematuria, and easy bruising. Take bleeding precautions if thrombocytopenia occurs. Avoid I.M. injections and venipunctures in a patient with a low platelet count. When venipunctures must be done, apply firm pressure to the site for at least 5 minutes afterward. Use anticoagulants cautiously, and observe for signs and symptoms of bleeding during concomitant use.*
• Withhold food for 4 to 6 hours before dacarbazine therapy, and administer an antiemetic as prescribed to decrease nausea. Nausea and vomiting usually subside after 1 to 2 days of treatment.
• Discard refrigerated solution after 72 hours; discard room-temperature solution after 8 hours.
• Expect to administer a mild antipyretic agent as prescribed if flulike symptoms occur.
• Use other appropriate nursing interventions for a patient with leukopenia, thrombocytopenia, nausea, or vomiting. (For details, see the introduction to this unit.)
• Notify the physician if adverse reactions occur.
• *Inspect the patient's infusion site for signs of extravasation before and during dacarbazine administration. If extravasated, the drug may cause severe tissue damage.*
• Administer dacarbazine as an I.V. infusion in 50 to 100 ml of dextrose 5% in water or normal saline (0.9% sodium chloride) solution over 30 minutes. If pain occurs at the infusion site, dilute the infusion up to 250 ml, slow the rate of infusion, or apply warmth to the vein.
• *If extravasation occurs, stop the infusion immediately and notify the physician.*

Patient teaching
• Teach the patient and family the name, dose, frequency, action, and adverse effects of dacarbazine.
• Stress the importance of returning for CBC tests regularly as prescribed.

• *Teach the patient to recognize and report signs and symptoms of infection and bleeding. Review infection control measures and bleeding precautions to use if needed.*

• Advise the patient to avoid sunlight and sunlamps for the first 2 days after treatment.

• Instruct the patient to withhold food 4 to 6 hours before dacarbazine therapy to help decrease nausea.

• Reassure the patient that the flulike syndrome may be treated with a mild antipyretic, such as acetaminophen.

• Inform the patient that dacarbazine may cause alopecia. Discuss ways to cope with alopecia, such as wearing a wig or an attractive scarf.

• Instruct the patient to notify the physician if adverse reactions occur.

Evaluation

The following examples represent appropriate evaluation statements for a patient receiving dacarbazine.

• The patient has no conditions that contraindicate dacarbazine therapy.

• The patient exhibits no signs of complications in the preexisting condition linked to dacarbazine.

• The patient experiences few adverse reactions to dacarbazine.

• The patient maintains normal tissue integrity at the dacarbazine infusion site.

• The patient and family express an accurate understanding of the points taught about dacarbazine.

• The patient avoids food 4 to 6 hours before dacarbazine administration.

ETHYLENIMINES

The ethylenimine derivative thiotepa is a polyfunctional alkylating agent. Thiotepa is used to treat bladder cancer or as a palliative treatment for lymphomas and ovarian or breast carcinomas.

PHARMACOKINETICS

After I.V. administration, thiotepa is 100% bioavailable. Significant systemic absorption may occur when thiotepa is administered into pleural or peritoneal spaces to treat malignant effusions or is instilled into the bladder. Thiotepa crosses the blood-brain barrier and is metabolized extensively in the liver. Thiotepa and its metabolites are excreted in the urine. (For more information, see *Major administration and excretion routes for alkylating agents,* page 1148.)

The peak concentration level of thiotepa has not yet been quantified. However, the drug may have a half-life of 1 week or more.

PHARMACODYNAMICS

Thiotepa exerts its cytotoxic activity by interfering with DNA replication and RNA transcription. Ultimately, it disrupts nucleic acid function and causes cell death.

PHARMACOTHERAPEUTICS

This alkylating agent is used to treat bladder cancer. It also is prescribed for palliative treatment of lymphomas and ovarian or breast carcinomas.

thiotepa (Thiotepa). This drug may be instilled into the bladder to treat bladder cancer or administered parenterally in the palliative treatment of lymphomas and ovarian or breast carcinomas. Thiotepa also may be injected directly into the tumor mass or the pleural or peritoneal cavity. *Usual adult dosage:* for bladder instillation, 60 mg weekly for 4 weeks; for rapid I.V. administration, 0.3 to 0.4 mg/kg at 1- to 4-week intervals; for intratumor, intrapleural, or intraperitoneal administration, 0.6 to 0.8 mg/kg initially, followed by a maintenance dosage of 0.07 to 0.8 mg/kg at 1- to 4-week intervals.

Drug interactions

When used concomitantly with succinylcholine, thiotepa may cause prolonged respirations and apnea. Thiotepa appears to inhibit the activity of pseudocholinesterase, the enzyme that deactivates succinylcholine. Therefore, succinylcholine should be used with extreme caution in a patient receiving thiotepa.

ADVERSE DRUG REACTIONS

The major adverse reaction to thiotepa is hematologic toxicity, which usually is dose-related and cumulative. Adverse hematologic reactions include leukopenia, anemia, thrombocytopenia, and pancytopenia, which may be fatal.

Nausea, vomiting, and anorexia are uncommon after thiotepa administration. Stomatitis and ulceration of the intestinal mucosa been reported.

Other adverse reactions to thiotepa include pain at the injection site, alopecia, headache, dizziness, and throat tightness as well as hyperuricemia, febrile reactions, and exudation from subcutaneous lesions.

Hypersensitivity reactions are rare, but hives, rash, and pruritus occur occasionally. In some patients, thiotepa instillation has caused lower abdominal pain, bladder irritability, hematuria, and rarely hemorrhagic cystitis.

NURSING PROCESS APPLICATION

The following information assists the nurse in caring for a patient receiving thiotepa.

Assessment
• Review the patient's history for a preexisting condition that contraindicates the use of thiotepa, such as known hypersensitivity to the drug or hepatic, renal, or bone marrow damage.
• Review the patient's history for a preexisting condition that requires cautious use of thiotepa, such as previous therapy with other alkylating agents or radiation.
• Assess the patient for adverse reactions to thiotepa, such as hematologic toxicity, nausea, vomiting, anorexia, stomatitis, alopecia, pain at the injection site, dizziness, febrile reactions, and hypersensitivity reactions.
• Review the patient's medication history to identify the use of drugs that may interact with thiotepa, such as succinylcholine.
• Assess the effectiveness of thiotepa regularly.
• Assess the patient for signs and symptoms of infection, such as fever, malaise, sore throat, or productive cough, if thiotepa causes leukopenia.
• Evaluate the patient's and family's knowledge about thiotepa.

Nursing diagnoses
The following examples represent appropriate nursing diagnoses for a patient receiving thiotepa.
• Potential for injury related to a preexisting condition that contraindicates the use of thiotepa
• Potential for injury related to a preexisting condition that requires cautious use of thiotepa
• Potential for injury related to adverse drug reactions
• Potential for infection related to thiotepa-induced leukopenia
• Knowledge deficit related to the thiotepa

Planning and implementation
• Do not administer thiotepa to a patient with a condition that contraindicates its use.
• Administer thiotepa cautiously to a patient at risk because of a preexisting condition.
• Monitor the patient frequently for adverse reactions during thiotepa therapy.
• *Monitor the patient's CBC for abnormalities that indicate anemia, thrombocytopenia, or pancytopenia.*
• *Take bleeding precautions and monitor the patient for signs and symptoms of bleeding, such as spontaneous epistaxis, hematuria, and easy bruising, if thrombocytopenia occurs.*
• Stagger the patient's activities and provide frequent rest periods if the patient experiences anemia.

• *Notify the physician immediately if pancytopenia occurs.*
• Monitor hydration if the patient experiences nausea, vomiting, or anorexia. Administer an antiemetic as prescribed. If fluid intake is inadequate despite antiemetic use, expect to replace fluids I.V. as prescribed.
• Inspect the patient's mouth frequently for signs of stomatitis, such as red, swollen, ulcerated mucous membranes. Monitor the nutritional status of a patient with stomatitis. Minimize the effects of stomatitis by offering a pureed or liquid diet, providing frequent mouth care, and applying a local anesthetic agent as prescribed.
• Administer a mild analgesic or antipyretic as prescribed if the patient experiences a headache or febrile reaction during thiotepa therapy.
• *Take safety measures if the patient experiences dizziness. For example, place the bed in the low position, keep the side rails up, and supervise ambulation.*
• Monitor the patient's uric acid level; an elevation may indicate hyperuricemia.
• Inspect the patient's skin regularly for exudation from subcutaneous lesions. Keep these areas clean and minimize the risk of infection by placing a sterile dressing on the area if exudate is present.
• Monitor the patient for signs of a hypersensitivity reaction, such as hives, rash, and pruritus. Notify the physician if these signs occur.
• *Monitor the patient for hematuria and dysuria, which indicate hemorrhagic cystitis.*
• Use other appropriate nursing interventions as needed for leukopenia, thrombocytopenia, anemia, nausea, vomiting, and stomatitis. (For more informaton, see the introduction to this unit.)
• Notify the physician if adverse reactions occur.
• *Monitor the patient's CBC for abnormalities that suggest leukopenia. If leukopenia occurs, take infection control measures and monitor the patient for signs and symptoms of infection.*
• Notify the physician if leukopenia occurs.

Patient teaching
• Teach the patient the name, dose, frequency, action, and adverse effects of thiotepa.
• *Inform the patient that thiotepa instillation administration may cause lower abdominal pain, bladder irritability (with dysuria and frequent urination), and hematuria. Reassure the patient that these signs and symptoms will subside.*
• Inform the patient that thiotepa may cause alopecia. Reassure the patient that hair loss is reversible when the treatment ends.
• *Instruct the patient to inform the physician immediately if hives, rash, or pruritus occur. Any of these may indicate a hypersensitivity reaction.*

• *Caution the patient not to perform activities that require mental alertness if dizziness occurs.*

• Inform the patient that pain may occur at the injection site during infusion and that appropriate measures will be taken to minimize discomfort.

• *Advise the patient to notify the physician if throat tightness occurs during thiotepa therapy.*

• *Teach the patient infection control measures and bleeding precautions to use if needed.*

• Advise the patient with anemia to stagger activities and take frequent rests.

• Teach the patient how to handle troublesome adverse reactions, such as GI distress and stomatitis.

• Stress the importance of returning for follow-up visits and CBC tests as prescribed.

• Instruct the patient to notify the physician if adverse reactions occur.

Evaluation

The following examples represent appropriate evaluation statements for a patient receiving thiotepa.

• The patient has no conditions that contraindicate thiotepa therapy.

• The patient exhibits no signs of complications in the preexisting condition linked to thiotepa.

• The patient experiences few adverse reactions to thiotepa.

• The patient remains free of infection during thiotepa therapy.

• The patient and family express an accurate understanding of the points taught about thiotepa.

• The patient correctly identifies adverse drug reactions that must be reported to the physician.

ALKYLATING-LIKE AGENTS

Carboplatin and cisplatin are heavy metal complexes that contain platinum. Because their action resembles that of a bifunctional alkylating agent, the drugs are referred to as alkylating-like agents.

PHARMACOKINETICS

Administered intravenously, cisplatin is highly protein-bound in plasma; carboplatin is not. Both are ineffective when administered orally.

Absorption, distribution, metabolism, excretion

The distribution and metabolism of carboplatin are not defined clearly. Carboplatin is eliminated primarily by the kidneys. In patients with normal renal function, 71% of a dose is excreted within 24 hours.

Highly protein bound, cisplatin reaches high concentrations in the kidneys, liver, intestines, and testes, but displays poor CNS penetration. When administered intrapleurally or intraperitoneally, cisplatin may exhibit significant systemic absorption. The drug undergoes some hepatic metabolism, followed by renal excretion, with 15% to 50% of a dose being excreted in 1 to 2 days. Initially, cisplatin is excreted mainly as unchanged drug. As time passes, however, more of the excretion products contain platinum. (For more information about the pharmacokinetics of these drugs, see *Major administration and excretion routes for alkylating agents,* page 1148.)

Onset, peak, duration

The elimination of carboplatin is biphasic. It has an initial half-life of 1.1 to 2 hours and a terminal half-life of 2.5 to 6 hours.

The elimination of cisplatin also is biphasic. After rapid I.V. administration, the initial half-life is 25 to 50 minutes; however, the terminal half-life may extend to 70 hours. Platinum is detectable in tissue for at least 4 months after administration.

PHARMACODYNAMICS

Like other alkylating agents, carboplatin and cisplatin are cell-cycle-nonspecific and inhibit DNA synthesis.

Mechanism of action

Carboplatin and cisplatin act like bifunctional alkylating agents by cross-linking strands of DNA and inhibiting DNA synthesis. (For details, see the section on mechanism of action under nitrogen mustards on page 1147.)

PHARMACOTHERAPEUTICS

Carboplatin is used primarily to treat ovarian cancer. Unlike cisplatin, carboplatin does not require vigorous hydration therapy because it is less nephrotoxic.

Cisplatin is prescribed to treat bladder cancer and metastatic ovarian and testicular cancers. In fact, it is the drug of choice for testicular cancer. Cisplatin also may be used to treat head, neck, and lung cancer, although these indications are not approved by the Food and Drug Administration. Patients should be well hydrated before and for 24 hours after cisplatin administration to ensure good urine output. Solutions containing mannitol also may be administered before and during cisplatin administration to ensure adequate urine output.

carboplatin (Paraplatin). Carboplatin usually is used for the palliative treatment of recurrent ovarian cancer, even in patients previously treated with cisplatin. The carboplatin dosage depends on renal function; a creatinine clearance of less than 60 ml/minute requires a dosage adjustment. *Usual adult dosage:* single dose of 360 mg/m^2 I.V. once every 4 weeks.

cisplatin [cis-platin] (Platinol). Administered by I.V. infusion, cisplatin usually is combined with other antineoplastic agents to treat metastatic testicular cancer, metastatic ovarian tumors, and bladder, head, neck, and lung cancers. This drug also has been administered intra-arterially and intraperitoneally. The cisplatin dosage, which is highly dependent on renal function, must be reduced if renal dysfunction is indicated by elevations in BUN, creatinine, and serum uric acid levels and decreased creatinine clearance. *Usual adult dosage:* single dose of up to 120 mg/m^2 I.V. once every 3 to 4 weeks. In some protocols, lower dosages of 20 mg/m^2 are given daily for 3 to 5 days.

Drug interactions

When administered concomitantly with an aminoglycoside, carboplatin or cisplatin may result in nephrotoxicity and ototoxicity.

ADVERSE DRUG REACTIONS

Carboplatin or cisplatin produce many of the same adverse reactions as the alkylating agents. Carboplatin can produce bone marrow suppression that can limit the dose. Cisplatin usually does not cause severe leukopenia or thrombocytopenia; however, it can cause anemia.

Nephrotoxicity occurs in 28% to 36% of patients receiving cisplatin, usually after multiple courses of therapy. Carboplatin has less nephrotoxic potential. With long-term cisplatin therapy, neurotoxicity also can occur, producing sensory and motor peripheral neuropathies, loss of proprioception, loss of taste, and intestinal ileus. Neurotoxicity is less common with carboplatin.

Up to 30% of patients receiving cisplatin report tinnitus and hearing loss. These adverse reactions are much less common with carboplatin. Cisplatin also produces marked nausea and vomiting in almost all patients and requires prophylactic antiemetic therapy, usually with high doses of metoclopramide. Carboplatin usually produces less severe nausea and vomiting that is not as prolonged.

NURSING PROCESS APPLICATION

The following information assists the nurse in caring for a patient receiving an alkylating-like agent.

Assessment

• Review the patient's history for a preexisting condition that contraindicates the use of an alkylating-like agent, such as known hypersensitivity to the drug or other platinum-containing compounds, renal impairment, myelosuppression, or hearing impairment.

• Review the patient's history for a preexisting condition that requires cautious use of an alkylating agent, such as pregnancy.

• Assess the patient for adverse reactions to the administered alkylating-like agent, such as leukopenia, thrombocytopenia, anemia, nephrotoxicity, neurotoxicity, nausea, and vomiting.

• Review the patient's medication history to identify the use of drugs that may interact with the administered alkylating-like agent, such as aminoglycosides.

• Assess the effectiveness of the administered alkylating-like agent regularly.

• Assess the patient for altered urinary elimination during cisplatin therapy.

• Evaluate the patient's and family's knowledge about the prescribed alkylating-like agent.

Nursing diagnoses

The following examples represent appropriate nursing diagnoses for a patient receiving an alkylating-like agent.

• Potential for injury related to a preexisting condition that contraindicates the use of an alkylating-like agent

• Potential for injury related to a preexisting condition that requires cautious use of an alkylating-like agent

• Potential for injury related to adverse drug reactions

• Altered urinary elimination related to cisplatin-induced nephrotoxicity

• Knowledge deficit related to the prescribed alkylating-like agent

Planning and implementation

• Do not administer an alkylating-like agent to a patient with a condition that contraindicates its use.

• Administer an alkylating-like agent cautiously to a patient at risk because of a preexisting condition.

• Monitor the patient regularly for adverse reactions throughout the course of therapy.

• *Review the patient's CBC and platelet count before administering the initial dose and with each subsequent dose as prescribed.*

• *Monitor the patient for signs and symptoms of infection, such as fever, chills, malaise, and sore throat if leukopenia occurs. Take infection control measures until the patient's WBC count returns to normal.*

• *Monitor the patient for signs and symptoms of bleeding, such as spontaneous epistaxis, hematuria, and easy bruising, if thrombocytopenia occurs. Take bleeding precautions until the platelet count returns to normal. Avoid all*

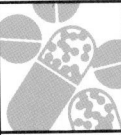

SELECTED MAJOR DRUGS

Alkylating agents

The following chart presents the major alkylating agents currently in clinical use. Keep in mind that dosages may vary greatly, depending on institutional protocol.

DRUG	MAJOR INDICATIONS	USUAL ADULT DOSAGES	CONTRAINDICATIONS AND PRECAUTIONS
Nitrogen mustards			
mechlorethamine	Hodgkin's disease, non-Hodgkin's lymphoma, mycosis fungoides Malignant pleural effusions	0.4 mg/kg I.V., once every 3 to 6 weeks 0.2 to 0.4 mg/kg intracavitary	• Know that mechlorethamine is contraindicated in a pregnant or lactating patient or one with a known infectious disease or a previous anaphylactic reaction to the drug. • Administer with extreme caution to a patient with chronic lymphatic leukemia. • Administer with caution to a patient undergoing radiation therapy or receiving other cytotoxic agents in alternating courses or one with leukopenia, thrombocytopenia, or anemia caused by tumor invasion of the bone marrow.
cyclophosphamide	Chronic lymphocytic leukemia; neuroblastoma; breast, ovarian, or lung cancer; multiple myeloma; Burkitt's lymphoma; retinoblastoma	2 to 3 mg/kg to 100 mg/kg P.O. or I.V.	• Know that cyclophosphamide is contraindicated in a pregnant or lactating patient or one with severely depressed bone marrow function or known hypersensitivity to the drug. • Administer with caution to a patient with leukopenia, thrombocytopenia, tumor cell infiltration of bone marrow, previous radiation therapy or therapy with other cytotoxic agents, or impaired hepatic or renal function.
Alkyl sulfonates			
busulfan	Chronic myelogenous leukemia	4 to 8 mg P.O. daily until the white blood cell (WBC) count falls between 10,000/mm³ and 25,000/mm³; resumed when the WBC count rises to 50,000/mm³ to maintain it between 10,000/mm³ and 20,000/mm³; 1 to 4 mg P.O. daily for maintenance	• Know that busulfan is contraindicated in a pregnant or lactating patient or one who has demonstrated resistance to the drug. • Administer with extreme caution to a patient whose bone marrow reserve may have been compromised by prior radiation therapy or chemotherapy or bone marrow suppression from prior cytotoxic therapy.
Nitrosoureas			
carmustine	Multiple myeloma, refractory Hodgkin's disease, non-Hodgkin's lymphoma	75 to 100 mg/m² I.V. for 2 days, or up to 200 mg/m² in a single I.V. infusion, repeated every 6 to 8 weeks	• Know that carmustine is contraindicated in a pregnant or lactating patient or one with known hypersensitivity to the drug. • Administer with caution to a patient with a depressed platelet, leukocyte, or erythrocyte count.
Triazines			
dacarbazine	Malignant melanoma, Hodgkin's disease, soft-tissue sarcoma	150 to 250 mg/m² I.V. daily for 5 days, repeated in 3 to 4 weeks. (Some protocols use much higher dosages.)	• Know that dacarbazine is contraindicated in a lactating patient or one with known hypersensitivity to the drug. • Administer with caution to a pregnant patient.

(continued)

SELECTED MAJOR DRUGS

Alkylating agents (continued)

DRUG	MAJOR INDICATIONS	USUAL ADULT DOSAGES	CONTRAINDICATIONS AND PRECAUTIONS
Ethylenimines			
thiotepa	Bladder cancer	60 mg via bladder instillation weekly for 4 weeks	• Know that thiotepa is contraindicated in a patient with hepatic, renal, or bone marrow damage or known hypersensitivity to the drug.
	Palliative treatment for ovarian or breast carcinoma or lymphoma	0.3 to 0.4 mg/kg by rapid I.V. infusion at 1- to 4- week intervals, or 0.6 to 0.8 mg/kg injected into the tumor intrapleurally or intraperitoreally; 0.07 to 0.8 mg/kg at 1- to 4-week intervals for maintenance	• Administer with caution to a patient who has been treated with other alkylating agents or radiation.
Alkylating-like agents			
cisplatin	Metastatic testicular cancer; lung, head, neck, bladder, or metastatic ovarian cancer	120 mg/m² I.V. every 3 to 4 weeks	• Know that cisplatin is contraindicated in a patient with renal impairment, hearing impairment, myelosuppression, or known hypersensitivity to the drug or other platinum-containing compounds. • Administer with extreme caution to a pregnant patient.

I.M. injections and venipunctures when the platelet count is low. When a venipuncture must be done, apply firm pressure to the site for at least 5 minutes afterward.

• Take energy conservation measures if anemia occurs. For example, stagger the patient's activities and provide frequent rest periods.

• *Monitor the patient for signs and symptoms of neurotoxicity, such as sensory or motor peripheral neuropathies, loss of proprioception or taste, intestinal ileus, tinnitus, and hearing loss.*

• Monitor hydration if the patient experiences nausea or vomiting. Nausea and vomiting may be severe and protracted (up to 24 hours); therefore, administer metoclopramide or other antiemetic before therapy, as prescribed.

• Maintain I.V. hydration as prescribed until the patient can tolerate adequate oral intake.

• Reconstitute cisplatin with sterile water for injection. Cisplatin remains stable for 24 hours in normal saline (0.9% sodium chloride) solution at room temperature; do not refrigerate solutions.

• *Do not use an aluminum needle for reconstituting or administering carboplatin or cisplatin because the drug will interact with the aluminum, forming a black precipitate.*

• Use other appropriate nursing interventions as needed for a patient with leukopenia, thrombocytopenia, anemia, nausea, or vomiting. (For more information, see the introduction to this unit.)

• Notify the physician if adverse reactions occur.

• Check the results of renal function studies as prescribed before administering the initial dose and with each subsequent dose.

• *Administer sufficient fluid to maintain the patient's urine output at 100 ml/hour for 4 consecutive hours before therapy and for 24 hours after therapy with cisplatin. Notify the physician if the urine output is less than 100 ml/hour during the first 24 hours.*

• Administer mannitol as prescribed, usually as a 12.5-gram I.V. bolus, before cisplatin infusion. Also administer a mannitol infusion as prescribed, usually up to 10 grams/hour, to maintain urine output during and for 6 to 24 hours after the cisplatin infusion.

Patient teaching

• Teach the patient and family the name, dose, frequency, action, and adverse effects of the prescribed alkylating-like agent.

• Stress the importance of returning for routine blood and urine tests as prescribed.

• *Teach the patient infection control measures, bleeding precautions, and energy conservation measures to use as needed.*

• *Instruct the patient to report tinnitus immediately to prevent permanent hearing loss.*

• *Caution the patient with neurotoxicity not to perform activities that require accurate perception and coordination, such as driving.*

• *Instruct the patient receiving cisplatin to consume sufficient fluid to produce a urine output of 100 ml/hour for 4 consecutive hours before therapy and for 24 hours after therapy.*

• Advise the patient that nausea and vomiting are possible, especially with cisplatin. Provide reassurance that an antiemetic usually is given before and after therapy to minimize these adverse reactions. Explain that I.V. therapy will be used to maintain hydration until oral fluids can be tolerated.

• Instruct the patient to report any adverse reactions.

Evaluation

The following examples represent appropriate evaluation statements for a patient receiving an alkylating-like agent.

• The patient has no conditions that contraindicate the use of an alkylating-like agent.

• The patient exhibits no signs of complications in the preexisting condition linked to the prescribed alkylating-like agent.

• The patient experiences few adverse reactions to the prescribed alkylating-like agent.

• The patient maintains a urinary output of 100 ml/hr for 4 consecutive hours before and 24 hours after cisplatin therapy.

• The patient and family express an accurate understanding of the points taught about the prescribed alkylating-like agent.

• The patient correctly describes infection control measures to use if leukopenia occurs.

CHAPTER SUMMARY

Chapter 66 discussed the alkylating agents, a class of antineoplastic drugs characterized by an ability to enter the cell nuclei and inhibit DNA synthesis. Here are the chapter highlights.

• The alkylating agents include nitrogen mustards, alkyl sulfonates, nitrosoureas, triazines, ethylenimines, and alkylating-like agents.

• With the exception of the triazine dacarbazine, the alkylating agents have the same mechanism of action. Most of these drugs enter the cell by active transport. Then they undergo alkylation, resulting in covalent bonds. The alkylation becomes toxic when the cell enters the S phase (during which DNA synthesis occurs) and blocks cell progression at the G_2 phase. Dacarbazine acts primarily on RNA synthesis.

• Used alone or with other antineoplastic drugs, alkylating agents are used to treat a wide variety of malignant neoplasms. Nitrogen mustards are indicated for Hodgkin's disease, certain leukemias, and many solid tumors. The alkyl sulfonate busulfan is used to treat chronic leukemia and other myeloproliferative disorders. Nitrosoureas are effective against brain tumors and meningeal leukemias. The triazine dacarbazine is used to treat malignant melanoma. Of the alkylating-like agents, carboplatin is used to treat ovarian cancer, and cisplatin is used primarily to treat metastatic ovarian and testicular cancers. The ethylenimine derivative thiotepa is prescribed to treat bladder cancer, ovarian or breast cancer, or lymphomas.

• The most common and potentially harmful adverse reaction to the alkylating agents is bone marrow suppression, resulting in leukopenia and thrombocytopenia. Other adverse reactions include nausea, vomiting, alopecia, and fatigue. Some of these reactions may be minimized through nursing interventions.

• During alkylating agent therapy, the nurse teaches the patient and family and minimizes adverse reactions.

STUDY QUESTIONS

See Appendix 1 for answers.

1. Jim Rogers, age 34, has Stage III Hodgkin's disease. For the first course of chemotherapy, he will receive a combined regimen of mechlorethamine (Mustargen), vincristine (Oncovin), procarbazine (Matulane), and prednisone (Deltasone) therapy. What are the major routes of administration and excretion of the nitrogen mustard mechlorethamine?

(a) oral administration; fecal excretion

(b) oral administration; urinary excretion

(c) intravenous administration; fecal excretion

(d) intravenous administration; urinary excretion

2. How does mechlorethamine, an alkylating agent, exert its therapeutic effects?

(a) It disrupts the structure of DNA.

(b) It damages the host's immune system.

(c) It resembles natural cell metabolites.

(d) It destroys the cell membrane, causing lysis.

3. Peter Huber, age 49, recently was diagnosed with chronic granulocytic (myelocytic) leukemia. His physician prescribes a course of chemotherapy that includes the alkylating agent busulfan. As with other alkylating agents, what is the *major* adverse reaction to busulfan?
(a) alopecia
(b) phototoxicity
(c) neurotoxicity
(d) bone marrow suppression

4. Which adverse respiratory reaction is associated with long-term busulfan therapy?
(a) asthma
(b) pulmonary fibrosis
(c) pulmonary hypertension
(d) chronic obstructive pulmonary disease

5. Rita Koons, age 40, has a brain tumor, for which the physician prescribes a course of treatment with the nitrosourea lomustine (CCNU). Nitrosoureas are used to treat brain tumors because they readily cross the blood-brain barrier. What percent of the plasma level does lomustine achieve in the CSF?
(a) 5% to 10%
(b) 10% to 15%
(c) 15% to 30%
(d) 30% to 50%

6. As with many other antineoplastic agents, lomustine may produce bone marrow suppression. When should the nurse expect to see signs of bone marrow suppression?
(a) immediately after treatment
(b) 2 to 4 weeks after treatment
(c) 4 to 6 weeks after treatment
(d) 6 to 8 weeks after treatment

7. Freida Johnson, age 60, is receiving dacarbazine (DTIC-Dome) to treat malignant melanoma. How does the action of dacarbazine differ from that of other alkylating agents?
(a) Dacarbazine produces a greater effect on RNA synthesis than DNA synthesis.
(b) Dacarbazine produces a greater effect on DNA synthesis than RNA synthesis.
(c) Dacarbazine is cell-cycle specific.
(d) Dacarbazine mainly affects protein synthesis.

8. Dorothy Black, age 72, is being treated for ovarian cancer with the nitrogen mustard cyclophosphamide (Cytoxan) and the alkylating-like agent carboplatin. The functioning of which body system determines the carboplatin dosage?
(a) urinary
(b) GI
(c) cardiovascular
(d) hematologic

SELECTED REFERENCES

AHFS drug information 90. (1990). Bethesda, MD: American Society of Hospital Pharmacists.

Betcher, D., and Burnham, N. (1990). Melphalan. *Journal of Pediatric Oncology Nursing, 7*(1), 35-36.

Drug facts and comparisons. (1991). St. Louis: Facts and Comparisons Division, Lippincott.

Freeman, E. (1990). Making sense of cytotoxic chemotherapy. *Nursing Times, 86*(31), 45-47.

Goodman and Gilman's the pharmacological basis of therapeutics (8th ed.; 1990). Elmsford, NY: Pergamon Press.

Hansten, P., and Horn, J. (1989). *Drug interactions* (6th ed.). Philadelphia: Lea & Febiger.

Harris, L., et al. (1989). Chemotherapy in head and neck cancer. *Seminars in Oncology Nursing, 5*(3), 174-181.

Higgs, D. (1990). The patient with testicular cancer: Nursing management of chemotherapy. *Oncology Nursing Forum, 17*(2), 243-249.

North American Nursing Diagnosis Association. (1990). *Taxonomy I - Revised, with official diagnostic categories.* St. Louis: NANDA.

Podack, E. (Ed.). (1988). *Cytotoxic effector mechanisms.* New York: Springer-Verlag.

Powis, G., & Hacker, M. (1990). *Mechanisms of toxicity of anticancer drugs.* Elmsford, NY: Pergamon Press.

Williams, D. (Ed.). (1990). *Chemistry of antitumour agents.* New York: Routledge Chapman & Hall.

C H A P T E R

67

ANTIMETABOLITE AGENTS

OBJECTIVES

After reading and studying this chapter, the student should be able to:

1. Describe the clinical uses of the antimetabolites.

2. Differentiate among the mechanisms of action of the folic acid, pyrimidine, and purine analogues.

3. Identify the common adverse reactions associated with methotrexate, cytarabine, 5-azacytidine, fluorouracil, floxuridine, mercaptopurine, and thioguanine.

4. Discuss the importance of oral care during antimetabolite therapy.

5. Explain the importance of monitoring the patient for leukopenia and thrombocytopenia during folic acid or pyrimidine analogue therapy.

6. Discuss the significance of jaundice in a patient receiving a purine analogue.

7. Describe how to apply the nursing process when caring for a patient who is receiving an antimetabolite agent.

INTRODUCTION

Because the antimetabolites structurally resemble natural metabolites, they can become involved in processes associated with the natural metabolites—that is, the synthesis of nucleic acids and proteins. However, the antimetabolites differ sufficiently from the natural metabolites to interfere with this synthesis. Because the antimetabolites are cell-cycle specific and primarily affect cells that actively synthesize deoxyribonucleic acid (DNA), they are referred to as S-phase specific. Normal cells that are reproducing actively, as well as the cancer cells, are affected by the antimetabolites. These drugs are subclassified further according to the metabolite affected. (For a list of the drugs in each antimetabolite class, see *Antimetabolites.*)

Malignancies that respond to the action of antimetabolites include acute leukemia, breast cancer, adenocarci-

---

Antimetabolites

The list below indicates the major classes of antimetabolites and the drugs that comprise each class.

Folic acid analogues
• methotrexate (Folex, Mexate)

Pyrimidine analogues
• 5-azacytidine (investigational) • cytarabine [ARA-C or cytosine arabinoside] (Cytosar-U) • floxuridine (FUDR) • fluorouracil [5-fluorouracil or 5-FU] (Adrucil, Efudex)

Purine analogues
• mercaptopurine [6-MP] (Purinethol) • thioguanine [6-thioguanine] (Tabloid)

---

noma of the gastrointestinal (GI) tract, non-Hodgkin's lymphomas, and squamous cell carcinoma of the head, neck, and cervix. The major adverse reactions occur in the bone marrow, mucosa, skin, and hair follicles. Adverse reactions usually are dose-related and reversible, and many patients may not experience any of these reactions.

For a summary of representative drugs, see *Selected major drugs: Antimetabolite agents,* page 1179. For a listing of applicable nursing diagnoses that the nurse may formulate when caring for a patient receiving these agents, see *Selected nursing diagnoses: Antimetabolite agents,* page 1168. For detailed information on applying the nursing process, see Chapter 6, The Nursing Process and Drug Therapy.

SELECTED NURSING DIAGNOSES

Antimetabolite agents

The following nursing diagnoses address representative problems and etiologies that a nurse may encounter when caring for a patient who is receiving an antimetabolite agent. Some of these nursing diagnoses contain generalized etiologies, which the nurse must individualize based on the patient's needs. (For some common nursing diagnoses and related interventions for each drug class, see the "Nursing Process Application" sections of this chapter.)

- Altered health maintenance related to the adverse CNS effects of intrathecal methotrexate administration
- Altered health maintenance related to purine catabolism
- Altered nutrition: less than body requirements, related to stomatitis or GI distress caused by the antimetabolite agent
- Altered oral mucous membrane related to antimetabolite-induced stomatitis
- Altered oral mucous membrane related to esophagopharyngitis caused by the pyrimidine analogue
- Altered protection related to antimetabolite-induced thrombocytopenia
- Body image disturbance related to alopecia caused by the antimetabolite agent
- Diarrhea related to the adverse GI effects of the antimetabolite agent
- Fatigue related to the adverse effects of the antimetabolite agent
- Hyperthermia related to fever caused by cytarabine or 5-azacytidine
- Impaired gas exchange related to methotrexate-induced pulmonary toxicity
- Knowledge deficit related to the prescribed antimetabolite agent
- Potential activity intolerance related to antimetabolite-induced anemia
- Potential fluid volume deficit related to the adverse GI effects of the antimetabolite agent
- Potential for infection related to bone marrow suppression caused by the antimetabolite agent
- Potential for injury related to a preexisting condition that contraindicates the use of an antimetabolite agent
- Potential for injury related to a preexisting condition that requires cautious use of an antimetabolite agent
- Potential for injury related to adverse drug reactions
- Potential for trauma related to hepatotoxicity caused by the antimetabolite agent
- Potential for trauma related to nephrotoxicity caused by the antimetabolite agent
- Potential impaired skin integrity related to the adverse dermatologic effects of the antimetabolite agent
- Sensory-perceptual alterations (tactile) related to photosensitivity caused by the antimetabolite agent

FOLIC ACID ANALOGUES

Although researchers have developed many folic acid analogues, the early compound methotrexate sodium remains the most commonly used.

PHARMACOKINETICS

Methotrexate is absorbed well and distributed throughout the body. At usual dosages, it does not enter the central nervous system (CNS) readily. Although methotrexate is metabolized partially, it is excreted primarily unchanged in the urine.

Absorption, distribution, metabolism, excretion

After oral administration, methotrexate is absorbed well and is distributed widely throughout the body. After I.M. or I.V. administration, the drug is absorbed almost completely. When administered intrathecally, it diffuses slowly into the plasma.

Methotrexate can remain in renal and hepatic tissue for weeks. It does not enter the cerebrospinal fluid (CSF) readily at normal dosages. The CSF levels are only 3% to 10% of concurrent plasma levels. Cytotoxic CNS levels are achieved with a high dose of intravenously administered methotrexate. Methotrexate may sequester (deposit) in pleural effusions or ascitic fluid; then the sequestered drug may be released slowly back into the plasma. About 50% plasma protein bound, methotrexate may be displaced from its plasma protein-binding sites by many drugs. The displacement increases the level of free methotrexate.

Methotrexate undergoes minimal metabolism. At high doses, however, metabolites—including a potentially nephrotoxic one—accumulate.

Methotrexate is excreted as a result of glomerular filtration and active tubular secretion. About 80% to 90% of a dose is excreted unchanged in the urine within 24 hours. Small amounts of the drug also are excreted in the feces and saliva. (For more information, see *Major administration and excretion routes for antimetabolite agents.*)

Onset, peak, duration

Methotrexate reaches a peak plasma concentration level 1 hour after an oral dose. This level is directly dose-related. The peak plasma concentration is achieved 30 minutes to 2 hours after parenteral administration. With intrathecal

Major administration and excretion routes for antimetabolite agents

This chart provides a quick reference for major routes of administration and excretion of the antimetabolite agents.

DRUG	ADMINISTRATION ROUTES	EXCRETION ROUTES	AMOUNT EXCRETED
Folic acid analogues			
methotrexate	Oral, intravenous, intramuscular, intrathecal	Kidneys	80% to 90% in 24 hours, unchanged
Pyrimidine analogues			
5-azacytidine	Intravenous	Kidneys	90% in 24 hours
cytarabine	Intravenous, subcutaneous, intrathecal	Kidneys	70% to 80% in 24 hours as metabolites
floxuridine	Intrahepatic	Kidneys	10% to 30% in 24 hours
fluorouracil	Intravenous, topical	Kidneys Lungs	15% in 6 hours, unchanged Up to 80% in 24 hours as CO_2
Purine analogues			
mercaptopurine	Oral	Kidneys	50% in 24 hours
thioguanine	Oral	Kidneys	40% in 24 hours as metabolites

administration, the peak concentration is reached in 3 to 12 hours. Methotrexate exhibits a three-compartment disappearance from plasma; the rapid distributive phase is followed by a second phase, which reflects renal clearance. The last phase, the terminal half-life, is 3 to 10 hours for a low dose and 8 to 15 hours for a high dose.

PHARMACODYNAMICS

Methotrexate reversibly inhibits the action of dihydrofolate reductase (DHFR), thereby blocking normal biochemical reactions and inhibiting DNA and ribonucleic acid (RNA) synthesis. The result is cell death.

Mechanism of action

Normally, DHFR reduces folic acid to tetrahydrofolic acid (FH_4). The FH_4 then serves as a cofactor in many metabolic reactions requiring the transfer of one-carbon units. Methotrexate enters cells via an active transport system and forms a competitive, high-affinity, noncovalent bond with DHFR. When all of the DHFR becomes bound with methotrexate, the DHFR no longer can reduce folic acid to FH_4. Without FH_4, thymidylate synthesis ceases and purine synthesis becomes inhibited. The blocking of thymidylate and purine synthesis leads to the inhibition of DNA and RNA synthesis

and cell death. Thus, methotrexate represents a cell-cycle, S-phase specific agent.

Tumor cells can develop resistance to the cytotoxic actions of methotrexate. Any one of several biochemical changes can result in resistance. The active transport system that carries methotrexate into the cells may become altered. With the impaired entry of methotrexate into the cells, lower intracellular levels of the drug become available for binding with DHFR, leading to resistance. Altered forms of DHFR also may be produced. The altered DHFR exhibits a decreased affinity for methotrexate and can function despite normal methotrexate levels. Finally, increased concentrations of DHFR may be produced so that at normal methotrexate levels, free DHFR is available to function normally.

High doses of methotrexate may be given to overcome resistance produced by increased DHFR concentrations or to achieve cytotoxic CNS levels. With very high doses of methotrexate, leucovorin is prescribed. This is known as a leucovorin rescue because leucovorin prevents the destruction of normal cells. Leucovorin, a fully reduced folate coenzyme, can function as a carrier of one-carbon units without being reduced by DHFR. By functioning in this way, leucovorin bypasses the biochemical block produced by methotrexate and allows the cell to synthesize DNA and RNA. (For details, see *Leucovorin rescue,* page 1170.)

Leucovorin rescue

Methotrexate interferes with cell division in the S phase of the cell cycle by inhibiting dihydrofolate reductase (DHFR), an enzyme involved in DNA synthesis. High-dose methotrexate is most effective against cells that have a high metabolic rate, such as leukemia cells. Used alone, high-dose methotrexate eventually will affect normal cells as well, producing toxicity.

To protect normal cells, methotrexate commonly is prescribed with leucovorin (folinic acid). Leucovorin rescues cells by bypassing the S phase, which methotrexate inhibits, as this schematic illustrates. It also acts by other mechanisms that are not understood completely. Leucovorin must be administered exactly on time, as prescribed, for the drug to work efficiently. When administered properly, leucovorin rescues cells before they begin active growth and division. Although leucovorin is considered a vitamin, doses must not be skipped because this drug plays an important role in preventing severe methotrexate toxicity.

Because leucovorin cannot prevent methotrexate toxicity completely, the nurse should closely monitor any patient on high-dose methotrexate therapy for bone marrow depression, stomatitis, pulmonary complications, and renal damage (from drug precipitation in tubules). The nurse also should maintain urine alkalinity to avoid precipitation in tubules and monitor the urine output closely.

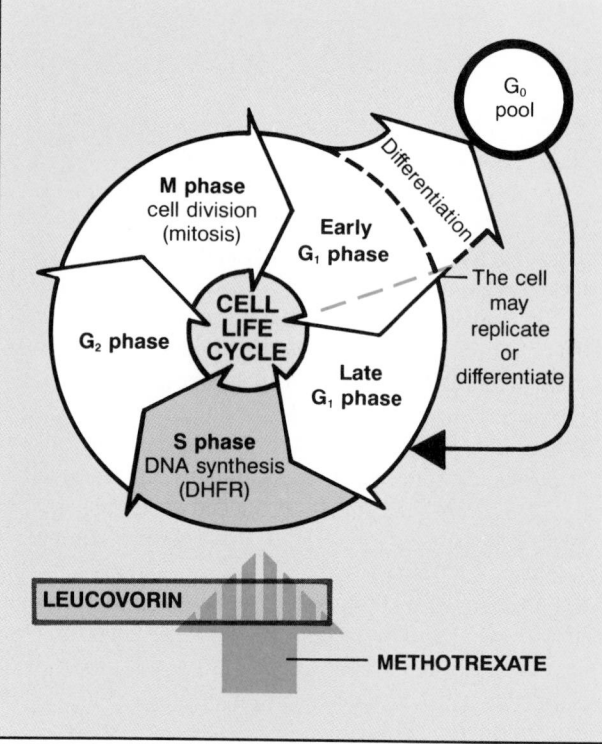

Leucovorin also enters the cells via the same active transport system as methotrexate. When this active transport system is occupied carrying leucovorin into the cell, less methotrexate enters and the intracellular methotrexate level falls.

PHARMACOTHERAPEUTICS

Methotrexate is especially useful in treating acute lymphoblastic leukemia in children, choriocarcinoma, osteogenic sarcoma, and non-Hodgkin's lymphomas, as well as carcinomas of the head, neck, bladder, testis, and breast. The drug also is prescribed in low doses to treat severe psoriasis and rheumatoid arthritis that resist conventional therapy.

methotrexate sodium (Folex, Mexate). This folic acid analogue may be administered orally, intravenously, intramuscularly, or intrathecally.
Usual adult dosage: to maintain remissions in acute lymphoblastic leukemia, 20 to 30 mg/m^2 of body-surface area P.O. or I.M. twice weekly or 2.5 mg/kg I.V. every 14 days; for choriocarcinoma, 15 mg/m^2 P.O. or I.M. daily for 5 days at 1- to 2-week intervals; for meningeal leukemia, 12 mg/m^2 to a maximum of 15 mg administered intrathecally at 2- to 5-day intervals; for osteogenic sarcoma, 12 to 15 grams/m^2 of methotrexate I.V. administered with leucovorin; for non-Hodgkin's lymphoma, 0.625 to 2.5 mg/kg daily P.O., I.M., or I.V.

Drug interactions
Because methotrexate is excreted as a result of glomerular filtration and active tubular secretion, other drugs excreted by tubular secretion may decrease methotrexate secretion. For example, salicylates and nonsteroidal anti-inflammatory drugs (NSAIDs) may increase methotrexate toxicity by decreasing its renal clearance or displacing it from plasma protein-binding sites. Probenecid also appears to decrease renal elimination of methotrexate, increasing its plasma levels and toxicity. (For more information, see *Drug interactions: Folic acid analogues.*)

ADVERSE DRUG REACTIONS

A patient receiving methotrexate may experience a wide range of adverse reactions depending on the dosage, the patient's condition, and other drugs the patient may be receiving.

Bone marrow suppression can occur with any dosage schedule. It is greatest 10 to 14 days after methotrexate administration. Stomatitis may develop 5 to 10 days after therapy begins. Patients receiving high-dose methotrexate are susceptible to severe stomatitis, which may result in a nutritional deficit. Fatigue, caused by combined factors,

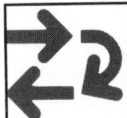

DRUG INTERACTIONS
Folic acid analogues

This chart lists drugs that interact with methotrexate, outlines possible effects for each, and presents selected nursing implications.

DRUG	INTERACTING DRUGS	POSSIBLE EFFECTS	NURSING IMPLICATIONS
methotrexate	probenecid	Inhibits methotrexate excretion, which increases the risk of methotrexate toxicity	• Monitor for increased adverse reactions, such as fatigue, bone marrow suppression, and stomatitis.
	salicylates and nonsteroidal anti-inflammatory agents, especially azopropazone, diclofinac, ketoprofen, indomethacin, phenylbutazone, and naproxen	May increase methotrexate toxicity by decreasing tubular secretion	• Avoid concomitant use when possible. • Monitor for increased adverse reactions, such as fatigue, bone marrow suppression, and stomatitis.
	cholestyramine	Reduces methotrexate absorption from GI tract	• Separate oral doses as much as possible if concomitant therapy is necessary.
	alcohol	Increases methotrexate hepatotoxicity	• Instruct the patient to avoid drinking alcohol.
	live vaccines	Increases the risk of infection by organism in live vaccine	• Avoid administration of live vaccines during methotrexate therapy.
	co-trimoxazole	May cause megaloblastic pancytopenia	• Avoid concomitant use.
	penicillins	Interfere with renal tubular secretion of methotrexate	• Monitor the patient for increased methotrexate toxicity.

such as bone marrow suppression and circulating products of tumor breakdown, may reduce a patient's stamina as well as participation in the drug therapy.

Although rare, two types of hepatotoxicity are associated with methotrexate: acute and chronic. Acute hepatotoxicity produces transient elevations in liver function tests 1 to 3 days after drug administration. Chronic hepatotoxicity may result in cirrhosis and, less commonly, acute liver atrophy. It is associated with high-dose, long-term methotrexate therapy and is related to the length and frequency of dosing and to a total dose of 1.5 grams or more.

Pulmonary toxicity, exhibited as pneumonitis or pulmonary fibrosis, may occur. With high doses, nephrotoxicity also can occur, raising blood urea nitrogen (BUN) and creatinine values. It may be minimized by maintaining urine alkalinization and encouraging the ingestion of large quantities of fluid, or by administering sodium bicarbonate I.V. to maintain urine alkalinization and infusing large quantities of fluid. Tumor cell destruction by methotrexate may increase the uric acid concentration, which may worsen

nephrotoxicity. In such cases, allopurinol may be prescribed to lower the urine and serum concentrations of uric acid.

Photosensitivity may occur in patients despite protection from the sun. A sunburnlike rash is the primary dermatologic reaction. Alopecia occurs in approximately 10% of patients receiving methotrexate.

Although rare, nausea and vomiting may be the first adverse reactions to high-dose methotrexate therapy. They typically occur less than 1 hour after administration.

Intrathecal administration of methotrexate warrants special attention because severe adverse reactions have occurred, including seizures, paresis, paralysis, and death. Other less severe adverse reactions may occur, such as headaches, fever, neck stiffness, confusion and irritability. Intrathecal administration also may produce systemic toxicity marked by tremor, ataxia, somnolence, and seizures. Rarely, systemic toxicity progresses to coma and death. Because methotrexate preparations that contain preservatives have caused more adverse reactions, only preservative-free methotrexate and diluents should be used for intrathecal drug administration.

NURSING PROCESS APPLICATION

The following information assists the nurse in caring for a patient receiving methotrexate.

Assessment

• Review the patient's history for a preexisting condition that contraindicates the use of methotrexate, such as pregnancy or a blood dyscrasia.
• Review the patient's history for a preexisting condition that requires cautious use of methotrexate, such as infection, peptic ulcer, ulcerative colitis, or extreme youth or age.
• Assess the patient for adverse reactions to methotrexate, such as bone marrow suppression, fatigue, hepatotoxicity, pulmonary toxicity, nephrotoxicity, photosensitivity, alopecia, nausea, and vomiting.
• Review the patient's medication history to identify the use of drugs that may interact with methotrexate, such as salicylates, NSAIDs, probenecid, cholestyramine, ethanol, live vaccines, co-trimoxazole, and penicillins.
• Assess the patient for stomatitis regularly.
• Assess the patient for adverse CNS reactions during intrathecal therapy.
• Evaluate the patient's and family's knowledge about methotrexate.

Nursing diagnoses

The following examples represent appropriate nursing diagnoses for a patient receiving methotrexate.
• Potential for injury related to a preexisting condition that contraindicates the use of methotrexate
• Potential for injury related to a preexisting condition that requires cautious use of methotrexate
• Potential for injury related to adverse drug reactions
• Altered oral mucous membrane related to methotrexate-induced stomatitis
• Altered health maintenance related to the adverse CNS effects of intrathecal methotrexate administration
• Knowledge deficit related to methotrexate

Planning and implementation

• Do not administer methotrexate to a patient with a condition that contraindicates its use.
• Administer methotrexate cautiously to a patient at risk because of a preexisting condition.
• Monitor the patient regularly for adverse reactions throughout methotrexate therapy.
• *Monitor the patient's BUN and creatinine values before each treatment to detect signs of nephrotoxicity. If values are abnormal, consult the physician for therapy modification.*
• Encourage fluid intake and administer I.V. fluids and sodium bicarbonate as prescribed to increase urine alka-

linity and volume and prevent nephrotoxicity in a patient receiving high-dose therapy.
• Document fluid intake and output accurately, and monitor urinary pH in a patient receiving high-dose therapy.
• *Monitor liver function test results regularly during methotrexate therapy to detect early changes in liver function that suggest hepatic cirrhosis or acute liver atrophy.*
• Avoid concomitant use of methotrexate and such drugs as salicylates, which may increase the risk of hepatotoxicity and cirrhosis.
• Monitor the patient for signs of liver dysfunction, such as jaundice, darkened urine, or clay-colored stools.
• *Monitor the patient's complete blood count (CBC) and platelet count regularly during methotrexate therapy to detect bone marrow suppression.*
• *Monitor the patient for signs of infection, such as fever, sore throat, malaise, and chills, if leukopenia occurs. Also take infection control measures until the white blood cell (WBC) count returns to normal.*
• *Observe the patient for signs and symptoms of bleeding, such as spontaneous epistaxis, hematuria, and easy bruising, if thrombocytopenia occurs. Take bleeding precautions until the platelet count returns to normal.*
• Monitor the patient for signs of anemia, such as fatigue and pallor. Take energy conservation measures until the anemia is corrected.
• *Monitor the patient's pulmonary function studies and chest X-ray results for abnormalities, such as patchy pulmonary infiltrates. Also assess the patient's respiratory status regularly to detect changes in respiratory function, such as shortness of breath and cough. Respiratory symptoms accompanied by fever may indicate pneumonitis, which requires prompt treatment.*
• Inspect the patient's skin regularly for a sunburnlike rash.
• Monitor hydration if the patient experiences nausea and vomiting. Request a prescription for an antiemetic agent, if needed.
• Monitor the serum methotrexate level as prescribed, especially during high-dose therapy.
• *Administer leucovorin with high doses of methotrexate, as prescribed.* (For more information, see *Leucovorin rescue,* page 1170.)
• Notify the physician if adverse reactions occur.
• Inspect the patient's oral cavity regularly. If stomatitis is present, provide appropriate care. (For details, see *Care of stomatitis.*)
• *Assess the patient receiving intrathecal methotrexate for adverse neurologic reactions, such as seizures or paresis, and take seizure precautions.*
• Monitor the CSF level of methotrexate as prescribed to help predict appropriate dosing of intrathecal methotrexate.
• Use only preservative-free methotrexate and diluents for intrathecal drug administration.
• Notify the physician if adverse CNS reactions occur.

Care of stomatitis

Stomatitis affects 30% to 60% of patients who receive antimetabolite agents, causing mucous membrane inflammation, local tissue breakdown, bleeding, oral hemorrhage, and infection. This adverse reaction not only disrupts the oral mucosa—a major first-line defense against infection—but also can compromise nutritional intake and patient comfort.

To help the patient minimize the effects of stomatitis during antimetabolite therapy, the nurse should follow these oral care guidelines.

Frequency of oral care	At least twice daily until a special program is required; then after each meal and at bedtime; for severe stomatitis, every 2 hours.
Aids to oral hygiene	Soft toothbrush, foam toothbrush (Toothette), normal saline rinse, lip moisturizer, Water Pik.
Recommendation for rinse	Isotonic solution of normal saline and sodium bicarbonate. Avoid hydrogen peroxide and mouthwash containing alcohol.
Recommendation for pain	Dyclonine hydrochloride (Dyclone), lidocaine (Xylocaine 2% Viscous Solution), or Benadryl and Maalox as a swish; systemic analgesics for severe pain.

• Use other appropriate nursing interventions for a patient with bone marrow suppression, nausea, vomiting, stomatitis, or alopecia. (For details, see the introduction to this unit.)

Patient teaching
• Teach the patient and family the name, dose, frequency, action, and adverse effects of methotrexate.
• Stress the importance of returning for blood and pulmonary function studies as prescribed.
• *Instruct the patient to notify the physician if a fever, nonproductive cough, shortness of breath, or other respiratory change occurs.*
• *Teach the patient to recognize the signs of liver dysfunction, such as yellowing skin or sclera, darkened urine, and clay-colored stools.*
• Advise the patient to drink at least eight 8-oz glasses of fluid daily to increase urine output and prevent methotrexate from precipitating in a renal tubule. Also instruct the patient to keep a record of fluid intake and output and to test the urine pH regularly.
• *Teach the patient to use infection control measures, bleeding precautions, and energy conservation measures, as needed.*
• Teach the patient how to manage stomatitis at home.

• Advise the patient to avoid sun exposure when possible or to use a sunscreen, hat, and sunglasses when sun exposure is unavoidable. Inform the patient a sunburnlike rash may occur even if these precautions are observed.
• Inform the patient that nausea and vomiting are most likely to occur up to 1 hour after methotrexate administration, if at all.
• Inform the patient that alopecia occurs in about 10% of all patients receiving methotrexate.
• *Teach the patient receiving intrathecal methotrexate to report immediately any of the following adverse neurologic reactions: paresis, seizures, loss of motor control, headache, neck stiffness, fever, confusion, or irritability.*
• Instruct the patient to notify the physician if adverse reactions occur.

Evaluation
The following examples represent appropriate evaluation statements for a patient receiving methotrexate.
• The patient has no conditions that contraindicate methotrexate therapy.
• The patient exhibits no signs of complications in the preexisting condition linked to methotrexate.
• The patient experiences no adverse reactions to methotrexate.
• The patient's oral mucous membrane remains normal throughout methotrexate therapy.
• The patient has no adverse CNS reactions to intrathecal methotrexate administration.
• The patient and family express an accurate understanding of the points taught about methotrexate.
• The patient demonstrates appropriate measures to care for stomatitis.

PYRIMIDINE ANALOGUES

The pyrimidine analogues include 5-azacytidine, cytarabine, floxuridine, and fluorouracil—a diverse group of drugs that inhibit the biosynthesis of pyrimidine nucleotides by mimicry.

PHARMACOKINETICS

Because the pyrimidine analogues are absorbed poorly when given orally, they usually are administered via other routes. With the exception of 5-azacytidine, the pyrimidine analogues are distributed well throughout the body, achieving CSF levels. They are metabolized extensively in the liver and are excreted in the urine. Pyrimidine analogues typically have short half-lives.

Absorption, distribution, metabolism, excretion

In most cases, no pyrimidine analogue is administered orally because of the resulting unpredictable and incomplete absorption. For example, only 20% of intact cytarabine reaches the circulation after oral administration. More cytarabine is absorbed from subcutaneous (S.C.) and intramuscular (I.M.) administration sites. However, the peak concentration is lower than that attained with I.V. administration. After S.C. administration, 5-azacytidine is absorbed well. Fluorouracil usually is administered I.V., but also can be injected into the pleural and peritoneal spaces or applied topically. These routes produce minimal systemic adverse reactions.

The pyrimidine analogues are distributed well throughout the body. Cytarabine is distributed widely, entering the CSF with levels approximately 50% of concurrent plasma levels. Higher CSF levels occur with continuous I.V. infusion than with I.V. bolus. Intrathecal doses of cytarabine diffuse into the plasma, but are metabolized rapidly. In contrast, 5-azacytidine is distributed less readily than the other pyrimidine analogues, with little of the drug entering the CSF. Fluorouracil is distributed to all areas of body water with a volume of distribution approximately 25% to 33% of body weight. It readily enters the CSF and effusions. Studies have found that fluorouracil concentrations are higher in tumors than in normal tissues. Although floxuridine has been studied less extensively, it is believed to enter the CSF also.

Cytarabine is metabolized rapidly and extensively in the liver by cytidine deaminase, producing the inactive metabolite uracil arabinoside. Within all body cells another enzyme, deoxycytidine kinase, converts cytarabine to the active metabolite cytarabine triphosphate. Fluorouracil is metabolized in the liver; its metabolites include carbon dioxide (CO_2), urea, and ammonia. Because floxuridine has a high hepatic extraction ratio, most of the drug administered via the hepatic artery is removed from the systemic circulation on the first pass through the liver. In the liver, floxuridine is metabolized to fluorouracil and its metabolites. Metabolism of floxuridine is less extensive with continuous I.V. infusions than with I.V. bolus injections.

Within the first 24 hours, about 70% to 80% of a cytarabine dose is excreted in urine, mainly as uracil arabinoside. More than 90% of 5-azacytidine is excreted in the urine in 24 hours. Within 24 hours, 10% to 30% of a floxuridine dose is excreted in the urine as floxuridine, fluorouracil, urea, and a number of other metabolites. Up to 80% of a fluorouracil dose is excreted from the lungs as CO_2 and 15% in the urine unchanged in 6 hours. (For more information, see *Major administration and excretion routes for antimetabolite agents,* page 1169.)

Onset, peak, duration

After S.C. administration, 5-azacytidine reaches a peak plasma concentration in 0.5 hours. It has a half-life of 3.5 to 4.5 hours. Continuous I.V. infusion of cytarabine produces a relatively constant plasma concentration level of the drug in 8 to 24 hours. Cytarabine has a plasma half-life of about 1 to 3 hours. After intrathecal administration, cytarabine has a half-life of 2 to 11 hours. The peak concentration time and half-life of floxuridine have not been quantified well. However, floxuridine's high hepatic extraction results in low systemic levels with a short half-life. After rapid I.V. bolus administration, fluorouracil reaches a peak plasma concentration of 0.1 to 1 mM. Fluorouracil has a rapid clearance, with a plasma half-life of only 10 to 20 minutes.

PHARMACODYNAMICS

The pyrimidine analogues exhibit their cytotoxic effects by interfering with the natural function of pyrimidine nucleotides. They interfere with the biosynthesis of natural pyrimidines or mimic the natural pyrimidines to the point where they interfere with cellular functions. The pyrimidine analogues are cell-cycle, S-phase specific.

Mechanism of action

The primary mechanism of action for 5-azacytidine has not been established. The drug may act as a false pyrimidine and become incorporated into DNA and RNA. It may inhibit the function of RNA, thus interfering with normal protein synthesis. Also, DNA incorporated with 5-azacytidine is more susceptible to breakage than normal DNA.

Cytarabine must be converted to cytarabine triphosphate to become active. Accumulation of the false nucleotide inhibits DNA synthesis and also may inhibit an enzyme involved in DNA repair. Researchers believe that cell death from cytarabine may result from unbalanced growth, which occurs when inhibition of DNA synthesis is accompanied by continued RNA and protein synthesis. Resistance to cytarabine may result from decreased intracellular drug levels, decreased activation of cytarabine, or increased levels of molecules that block cytarabine action.

The exact mechanism of action of floxuridine and fluorouracil has not been established fully. Fluorouracil and floxuridine, which is metabolized to fluorouracil, may act as antimetabolites in three different ways. First, they may inhibit the enzyme thymidylate synthetase, causing a thymidylate deficiency. This deficiency inhibits DNA, causing cell death—particularly of cells that grow rapidly. Second, fluorouracil may become incorporated in RNA, producing fraudulent RNA. Third, it may inhibit the use of uracil in RNA synthesis.

Numerous mechanisms may promote resistance to fluorouracil and floxuridine cytotoxicity. These mechanisms include decreased number or activity of enzymes activating fluorouracil, decreased enzymes incorporating the false nucleotide into RNA, and an alteration in thymidylate synthetase that prevents its inhibition by the false nucleotide.

PHARMACOTHERAPEUTICS

The pyrimidine analogues are used to treat many tumors. However, they are used mostly to treat acute leukemias, adenocarcinomas of the GI tract, carcinomas of the breast and ovaries, and non-Hodgkin's lymphomas.

5-azacytidine. 5-azacytidine is beneficial primarily against acute myelogenous leukemia. To a lesser extent, the drug acts against acute lymphocytic leukemia, but displays little activity against solid tumors. It may be administered by various schedules, depending on the protocol used for this investigational drug.
Usual adult dosage: 50 to 200 mg/m²/day by continuous infusion or divided I.V. bolus for 5 to 7 days, repeated every 14 to 28 days; or a single weekly dose of 750 mg/m² I.V.

cytarabine [ARA-C or cytosine arabinoside] (Cytosar-U). Cytarabine is used primarily to induce remission of acute myelogenous leukemia. Over 50% of patients using cytarabine with other drugs have achieved complete remission. Cytarabine also is used intrathecally to manage meningeal leukemia. It also acts effectively against Hodgkin's and other lymphomas.
Usual adult dosage: 100 mg/m² of body-surface area daily by I.V. bolus injections or continuous infusions for 5 to 7 days; for refractory acute myelogenous leukemia, high-dose therapy with 3 grams/m² I.V. every 12 hours for 4 to 12 doses, repeated every 2 to 3 weeks; for meningeal leukemia, 30 mg/m² intrathecally every 4 days.

floxuridine (FUDR). Administered by continuous infusion, usually intrahepatically (into the hepatic artery) or intra-arterially, floxuridine acts against adenocarcinomas of the GI tract, including oral, pancreatic, hepatic, and biliary tumors. Unfortunately, only 15% to 20% of the patients treated with floxuridine for these GI tumors demonstrate objective response.
Usual adult dosage: 0.1 to 0.6 mg/kg/day by continuous arterial infusion for 1 to 6 weeks until toxicity requires discontinuation.

fluorouracil [5-fluorouracil or 5-FU] (Adrucil, Efudex). Fluorouracil is active against many solid tumors, particularly carcinomas of the breast and GI tract, including oral, gastric, and colorectal tumors. Topically, fluorouracil acts against basal cell carcinomas and other malignant dermatologic entities. Various dosing schedules are used to administer fluorouracil.
Usual adult dosage: 12 mg/kg of body weight I.V. daily up to 800 mg/day for 4 successive days; if no toxicity occurs, then 6 mg/kg of body weight on the sixth, eighth, tenth, and twelfth days; for basal cell carcinomas and other malignant dermatologic entities, sufficient cream or lotion to cover lesions applied twice daily.

Drug interactions

No significant drug interactions occur involving the pyrimidine analogues.

ADVERSE DRUG REACTIONS

The adverse drug reactions to the pyrimidine analogues resemble those of the other antimetabolites.

Bone marrow suppression evidenced by neutropenia and thrombocytopenia is the major dose-limiting adverse reaction to the pyrimidine analogues. This reaction is noticeable 7 to 14 days after drug administration, with bone marrow recovery occurring 21 to 28 days after the drug is discontinued.

Stomatitis and esophagopharyngitis may occur 5 to 10 days after therapy begins. This adverse reaction can be particularly distressing to the patient because the oral cavity ulcerations and sloughing may be extremely painful and prevent eating.

Like most antineoplastic agents, the pyrimidine analogues can cause fatigue. Lack of energy can limit activities severely as well as the patient's involvement in therapy.

With the exception of 5-azacytidine, the pyrimidine analogues do not cause severe nausea and vomiting. About 70% of patients receiving 5-azacytidine experience moderate to severe nausea and vomiting 1½ to 3 hours after I.V. administration. Nausea and anorexia also may occur with fluorouracil or floxuridine therapy. Diarrhea also may occur with fluorouracil administration and may be severe enough to limit or discontinue therapy.

In most cases, fluorouracil is relatively well-tolerated. However, it can produce several hypersensitivity reactions, including mild to severe skin reactions. Such reactions may take the form of a pruritic rash on the extremities or less commonly on the trunk, photosensitivity with erythema or increased skin pigmentation, darkening of the veins with prolonged drug administration, or a rash on the hands and feet with prolonged high-dose infusions. Other hypersensitivity reactions may include increased lacrimation, nasal discharge, or epistaxis; these reactions disappear after therapy is discontinued. Alopecia commonly occurs with fluorouracil. Hepatic arterial infusion of floxuridine has been associated with bile duct sclerosis and liver cirrhosis.

Cytarabine and 5-azacytidine may precipitate a fever and flulike symptoms within 24 hours of therapy. Cytarabine also may produce a rash in 4% of patients. Intrathecal cytarabine usually does not cause systemic toxicity. It is more likely to cause nausea, vomiting, fever, and transient headaches.

NURSING PROCESS APPLICATION

The following information assists the nurse in caring for a patient receiving a pyrimidine analogue.

Assessment
• Review the patient's history for a preexisting condition that contraindicates the use of a pyrimidine analogue, such as pregnancy, lactation, or known hypersensitivity to the drug.
• Review the patient's history for a preexisting condition that requires cautious use of a pyrimidine analogue, such as drug-induced bone marrow suppression or impaired hepatic function.
• Assess the patient for adverse reactions to the prescribed pyrimidine analogue, such as bone marrow suppression, fatigue, nausea, vomiting, anorexia, and diarrhea.
• Assess the effectiveness of the prescribed pyrimidine analogue regularly.
• Assess the patient for signs and symptoms of stomatitis and esophagopharyngitis, such as ulcerations of the oral mucous membranes.
• Evaluate the patient's and family's knowledge about the prescribed pyrimidine analogue.

Nursing diagnoses
The following examples represent appropriate nursing diagnoses for a patient receiving a pyrimidine analogue.
• Potential for injury related to a preexisting condition that contraindicates the use of a pyrimidine analogue
• Potential for injury related to a preexisting condition that requires cautious use of a pyrimidine analogue
• Potential for injury related to adverse drug reactions
• Altered oral mucous membrane related to stomatitis and esophagopharyngitis caused by the pyrimidine analogue
• Knowledge deficit related to the prescribed pyrimidine analogue

Planning and implementation
• Do not administer a pyrimidine analogue to a patient with a condition that contraindicates its use.
• Administer a pyrimidine analogue cautiously to a patient at risk because of a preexisting condition.
• Monitor the patient regularly for adverse reactions to the prescribed pyrimidine analogue.
• *Monitor the patient's CBC to detect bone marrow suppression. If neutropenia occurs, monitor the patient*

for signs of infection, such as fever, chills, sore throat, and malaise. Also take infection control measures until the neutrophil count returns to normal. If thrombocytopenia occurs, monitor the patient for signs and symptoms of bleeding, such as spontaneous epistaxis, hematuria, and easy bruising. Also take bleeding precautions until the thrombocyte count returns to normal. Limit the pyrimidine analogue dosage, as prescribed, if hematologic abnormalities occur.
• Take energy conservation measures if the patient experiences fatigue. For example, assist the patient with activities of daily living, stagger activities, and encourage frequent rest periods.
• Monitor hydration if the patient experiences nausea, vomiting, anorexia, or diarrhea. Request a prescription for an antiemetic or antidiarrheal agent, if needed.
• Inspect the patient's skin regularly for a rash during fluorouracil or cytarabine therapy. For a patient on long-term fluorouracil therapy, also observe for other dermatologic reactions, such as pruritus, erythema, increased skin pigmentation, or darkening of the veins.
• *Review the results of the patient's liver function studies regularly throughout intra-arterial therapy with floxuridine.*
• Monitor for fever and flulike symptoms in a patient who is receiving cytarabine or 5-azacytidine. Administer a mild analgesic and antipyretic agent, as prescribed, to reduce the fever and ease the patient's discomfort.
• Store fluorouracil at room temperature and protect it from light.
• *Do not use a cloudy fluorouracil solution. If crystals form, redissolve the solution by warming.*
• Use plastic I.V. containers to administer continuous fluorouracil infusions because the solution is more stable in plastic I.V. bags than in glass bottles.
• Reconstitute floxuridine with sterile water for injection. For the actual infusion, dilute further in 5% dextrose in water or normal saline (0.9% sodium chloride) solution.
• Discard refrigerated floxuridine solution after 2 weeks because it becomes unstable after this time.
• *Use preservative-free normal saline solution for intrathecal cytarabine administration.*
• Discard any reconstituted cytarabine solution 48 hours after reconstitution because it becomes unstable after that time.
• Infuse 5-azacytidine using lactated Ringer's solution because the drug is unstable in other solutions.
• Discard reconstituted 5-azacytidine after 8 hours.
• Use other appropriate nursing interventions for a patient who develops bone marrow suppression, nausea, vomiting, or alopecia. (For details, see the introduction to this unit.)
• Notify the physician if adverse reactions occur.
• *Inspect the patient's mouth and throat regularly. If stomatitis or esophagopharyngitis is present, provide symp-*

tomatic care. (For details, see *Care of stomatitis,* page 1173.)
• Notify the physician if stomatitis or esophagopharyngitis becomes severe.

Patient teaching
• Teach the patient and family the name, dose, frequency, action, and adverse effects of the prescribed pyrimidine analogue.
• *Stress the importance of returning for follow-up blood tests.*
• *Teach the patient how to manage stomatitis and esophagopharyngitis at home.*
• Review energy conservation measures that the patient can use at home if fatigue occurs.
• *Teach the patient infection control measures and bleeding precautions to use as needed.*
• Teach the patient how to manage troublesome adverse GI reactions.
• Advise the patient receiving fluorouracil that photosensitivity may occur. Instruct the patient to avoid sun exposure or to wear a sun screen, hat, and sunglasses when sun exposure is unavoidable.
• Inform the patient that fluorouracil may cause increased lacrimation, nasal discharge, or epistaxis. Provide reassurance that these reactions disappear after therapy is discontinued.
• Inform the patient that cytarabine or 5-azacytidine may precipitate a fever and flulike symptoms up to 24 hours after therapy. Advise the patient to take an antipyretic and analgesic agent, as prescribed.
• Inform the patient that reversible alopecia may occur during fluorouracil therapy.
• Instruct the patient to notify the physician if adverse reactions occur.

Evaluation
The following examples represent appropriate evaluation statements for a patient receiving a pyrimidine analogue.
• The patient has no conditions that contraindicate pyrimidine analogue therapy.
• The patient exhibits no signs of complications in the preexisting condition linked to the prescribed pyrimidine analogue.
• The patient exhibits few adverse reactions to the prescribed pyrimidine analogue.
• The patient's oral mucous membrane remains normal throughout pyrimidine analogue therapy.
• The patient and family express an accurate understanding of the points taught about the prescribed pyrimidine analogue.
• The patient correctly describes how to manage stomatitis and esophagopharyngitis at home.

PURINE ANALOGUES

The purine analogues, mercaptopurine and thioguanine, are analogues of natural purine bases that must undergo enzymatic conversion to the nucleotide level before they become cytotoxic.

PHARMACOKINETICS

The absorption of the purine analogues is variable and incomplete. They are metabolized in the liver and excreted in the urine.

Absorption, distribution, metabolism, excretion
After oral administration, absorption of mercaptopurine and thioguanine is incomplete and variable. About 50% of a mercaptopurine dose is absorbed; only 30% of a thioguanine dose is absorbed.

Mercaptopurine and its metabolites are distributed throughout total body water. Although the drug is reported to cross the blood-brain barrier, CSF concentrations are not therapeutic. The distribution of thioguanine in humans has not been studied extensively.

Mercaptopurine is metabolized in the liver by two major pathways: methylation of the sulfhydryl group and oxidation by xanthine oxidase to inactive metabolites. Thioguanine is metabolized in the liver to several inactive products.

Within 24 hours, up to 50% of a mercaptopurine dose is excreted in the urine as active drug and metabolites. About 40% of an oral dose of thioguanine is excreted in the urine in 24 hours as metabolites. (For more information about the purine analogues, see *Major administration and excretion routes for antimetabolite agents,* page 1169.)

Onset, peak, duration
After oral administration, mercaptopurine achieves a peak serum concentration level within 2 hours. An oral dose of thioguanine reaches a peak concentration in 6 to 8 hours. Due to cellular uptake, renal excretion, and metabolic degradation, mercaptopurine has a short plasma half-life of 90 minutes. Thioguanine, however, has a plasma half-life of 11 hours.

PHARMACODYNAMICS

Mercaptopurine and thioguanine are analogues of the natural purine bases hypoxanthine and guanine. Because they resemble the natural bases, the purine analogues can enter into biochemical reactions in place of the natural bases.

However, because the analogues cannot function exactly like the natural bases, they cause cell death.

Mechanism of action

Like the other antimetabolites, mercaptopurine and thioguanine must first undergo conversion to the nucleotide level to be active. This conversion is facilitated by the enzyme hypoxanthine-guanine phosphoribosyltransferase (HGPRT). The resulting nucleotides then are incorporated into DNA, where they may inhibit DNA and RNA synthesis as well as other metabolic reactions necessary for proper cell growth. The purine analogues are cell-cycle, S-phase specific agents.

Cancer cells ultimately resist the cytotoxic effects of the purine analogues. Resistance may result from numerous mechanisms, including (1) a decreased quantity or complete lack of HGPRT, which converts mercaptopurine and thioguanine to the nucleotide level, (2) decreased affinity of HGPRT for the drugs, (3) decreased drug transport into the cells, and (4) increased degradation of the drugs or their corresponding nucleotides.

PHARMACOTHERAPEUTICS

The purine analogues are used to treat acute and chronic leukemias.

mercaptopurine [6-MP] (Purinethol). Mercaptopurine is especially useful in maintaining remission of acute leukemia in children. The results have been less impressive in adults with acute leukemia, although remissions sometimes are obtained. Mercaptopurine also is used to induce remission in acute lymphoblastic leukemia and chronic myelocytic leukemia.

Usual adult dosage: for induction, 2.5 mg/kg/day P.O. (range 100 to 200 mg/day); for maintenance after improvement, 1.5 to 2.5 mg/kg/day P.O. When administered concurrently with allopurinol, the mercaptopurine dosage should be reduced to 25% of the usual dosage because allopurinol interferes with mercaptopurine oxidation, potentiating its antineoplastic effect and increasing toxicity.

Usual pediatric dosage: same as the usual adult dosage.

thioguanine [6-thioguanine] (Tabloid). This purine analogue also is used to treat acute leukemia. When combined with cytarabine, thioguanine effectively induces remission in acute myelogenous leukemia.

Usual adult dosage: initially, 2 mg/kg P.O. daily; increased to 3 mg/kg/day after 4 weeks if the patient displays no clinical improvement or toxicity. Thioguanine can be administered concurrently with allopurinol without dosage reduction.

Usual pediatric dosage: same as the usual adult dosage.

Drug interactions

Concomitant administration of mercaptopurine and allopurinol may increase bone marrow suppression by decreasing mercaptopurine metabolism. No significant interactions occur with thioguanine.

ADVERSE DRUG REACTIONS

Mercaptopurine and thioguanine produce bone marrow suppression, which may not begin for 1 to 6 weeks. Leukopenia usually occurs first, followed by thrombocytopenia and anemia.

Many patients receiving mercaptopurine develop cholestatic jaundice after 1 to 2 months of therapy. This adverse reaction usually is associated with doses that exceed 2.5 mg/kg. The patient should report this reaction immediately because the jaundice may be reversible if the drug is discontinued. If the drug is not discontinued, the reaction may be fatal. Jaundice also has been reported with thioguanine use.

Nausea, vomiting, anorexia, mild diarrhea, and stomatitis occur in patients receiving mercaptopurine or thioguanine. Uric acid levels also may rise as a result of purine catabolism from cellular destruction. However, this reaction may be minimized by adequate hydration, urine alkalinization, or allopurinol administration.

NURSING PROCESS APPLICATION

The following information assists the nurse in caring for a patient receiving a purine analogue.

Assessment

• Review the patient's history for a preexisting condition that contraindicates the use of a purine analogue, such as pregnancy, lactation, or resistance to the drug.
• Review the patient's history for a preexisting condition that requires cautious use of a purine analogue, such as liver disease, concomitant therapy with another hepatotoxic drug, or continuous long-term therapy.
• Assess the patient for adverse reactions to the prescribed purine analogue, such as bone marrow suppression, cholestatic jaundice, GI distress, or stomatitis.
• Review the patient's medication history to identify the use of drugs that may interact with mercaptopurine, such as allopurinol.
• Assess the effectiveness of the prescribed purine analogue regularly.
• Assess the patient's uric acid level periodically.
• Evaluate the patient's and family's knowledge about the prescribed purine analogue.

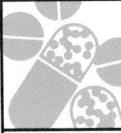

SELECTED MAJOR DRUGS

Antimetabolite agents

The following chart summarizes the major antimetabolites currently in clinical use.

DRUG	MAJOR INDICATIONS	USUAL ADULT DOSAGES	CONTRAINDICATIONS AND PRECAUTIONS
Folic acid analogues			
methotrexate	Maintenance of acute lymphoblastic leukemia remission	20 to 30 mg/m² P.O. or I.M. twice weekly or 2.5 mg/kg I.V. every 14 days	• Know that methotrexate is contraindicated in a pregnant patient or one with a blood dyscrasia.
	Choriocarcinoma	15 mg/m² P.O. or I.M. daily for 5 days at 1- to 2-week intervals	• Administer with extreme caution to a pediatric or elderly patient or any patient with an infection, peptic ulcer, or ulcerative colitis.
	Meningeal leukemia	12 mg/m² intrathecally at 2- to 5-day intervals	
	Osteogenic sarcoma	12 to 15 grams/m² I.V. with leucovorin	
Pyrimidine analogues			
cytarabine	Acute myelogenous leukemia	100 mg/m²/day for 5 to 7 days by I.V. bolus or continuous infusion	• Know that cytarabine is contraindicated in a pregnant or lactating patient or one with known hypersensitivity to the drug.
	Meningeal leukemia	30 mg/m² intrathecally every 4 days	• Administer with caution to a patient with drug-induced bone marrow suppression or impaired hepatic function.
fluorouracil	Solid tumors, such as carcinomas of the GI tract and breast	12 mg/kg I.V. daily, up to 800 mg daily, for 4 successive days; if no toxicity, give 6 mg/kg/day on the 6th, 8th, 10th, and 12th days.	• Know that fluorouracil is contraindicated in a patient with known hypersensitivity to the drug or any of its components.
	Basal cell carcinomas	Sufficient cream or lotion to cover lesions applied twice daily	
Purine analogues			
mercaptopurine	Acute lymphoblastic leukemia, chronic myelocytic leukemia	2.5 mg/kg/day P.O. (100 to 200 mg/day), decreased to 1.5 to 2.5 mg/kg/day for maintenance	• Know that mercaptopurine is contraindicated in a pregnant or lactating patient or one with acute lymphatic leukemia or prior resistance to the drug.
			• Administer with caution to a patient with liver disease or concomitant use of another hepatotoxic drug.
thioguanine	Acute myelogenous leukemia (used with cytarabine)	2 mg/kg/day P.O., increased to 3 mg/kg/day after 4 weeks if the patient displays no clinical improvement and no signs of toxicity	• Know that thioguanine is contraindicated in a pregnant or lactating patient or one who has demonstrated resistance to the drug.
			• Administer with caution to a patient receiving long-term, continuous therapy with thioguanine.

Nursing diagnoses

The following examples represent appropriate nursing diagnoses for a patient receiving a purine analogue.

• Potential for injury related to a preexisting condition that contraindicates the use of a purine analogue

• Potential for injury related to a preexisting condition that requires cautious use of a purine analogue

• Potential for injury related to adverse drug reactions

• Altered health maintenance related to purine catabolism

• Knowledge deficit related to the prescribed purine analogue

Planning and implementation

• Do not administer a purine analogue to a patient with a condition that contraindicates its use.

• Administer a purine analogue cautiously to a patient at risk because of a preexisting condition.

• Monitor the patient frequently for adverse reactions throughout purine analogue therapy.

• *Monitor the CBC weekly as prescribed, watching for a precipitous decrease.*

• *Observe the patient for signs of bleeding, such as spontaneous epistaxis, hematuria, and easy bruising, as well as signs of infection, such as fever, chills, and malaise.*

• *Take infection control measures and bleeding precautions if bone marrow suppression occurs.*

• Take energy conservation measures if anemia results from bone marrow suppression.

• *Monitor the patient for signs of cholestatic jaundice, such as pain in the right upper quadrant and elevated liver function enzymes. Cholestatic jaundice may progress to hepatic necrosis, which may reverse if the drug is stopped promptly.*

• Monitor hydration if the patient experiences nausea, vomiting, or diarrhea. Request a prescription for an antiemetic or antidiarrheal agent as needed.

• Inspect the patient's oral cavity regularly for signs of stomatitis, such as redness, ulceration, or bleeding of the oral mucous membrane. If stomatitis is present, provide symptomatic care. (For details, see *Care of stomatitis*, page 1173.)

• Use other appropriate nursing interventions for a patient who develops bone marrow suppression, nausea, vomiting, or stomatitis. (For more information, see the introduction to this unit.)

• Notify the physician if adverse reactions occur.

• Monitor the patient's serum uric acid level periodically.

• Document the patient's fluid intake and output accurately. To minimize the effects of uric acid level elevations, encourage the patient to drink at least 3 liters of fluids daily, and administer allopurinol as prescribed.

• Notify the physician if the uric acid level remains elevated.

Patient teaching

• Teach the patient and family the name, dose, frequency, action, and adverse effects of the prescribed purine analogue.

• *Stress the importance of returning regularly for follow-up blood tests.*

• *Review infection control measures, bleeding precautions, and energy conservation measures that the patient may use as needed.*

• *Instruct the patient to report any of the following to the physician immediately: yellowing of the skin or sclera, right upper quadrant pain, darkened urine, or clay-colored stools.*

• Teach the patient how to manage troublesome adverse reactions, such as GI distress and stomatitis.

• Advise the patient to drink at least 13 8-oz glasses of fluid daily to prevent renal damage.

• Instruct the patient to report any other adverse reactions to the physician.

Evaluation

The following examples represent appropriate evaluation statements for a patient receiving a purine analogue.

• The patient has no conditions that contraindicate purine analogue therapy.

• The patient exhibits no signs of complications in the preexisting condition linked to the prescribed purine analogue.

• The patient experiences few adverse reactions to the prescribed purine analogue.

• The patient's uric acid level remains normal during purine analogue therapy.

• The patient and family express an accurate understanding of the points taught about the prescribed purine analogue.

• The patient drinks at least 13 8-oz glasses of fluid daily.

CHAPTER SUMMARY

Chapter 67 discussed the three major classes of antimetabolite agents: the folic acid, pyrimidine, and purine analogues. Here are the chapter highlights.

• The antimetabolites are antineoplastic drugs that can interfere with the synthesis of nucleic acids and proteins.

• The antimetabolites, which are cell-cycle specific, are most active in the S phase.

• Antimetabolites are used to treat acute leukemia, breast cancer, adenocarcinomas of the GI tract, non-Hodgkin's lymphoma, and squamous cell carcinomas of the head, neck, and cervix.

- The most common adverse reactions to the antimetabolites include bone marrow suppression and stomatitis. During antimetabolite therapy, oral care can minimize injury to the mucosa, which is a first-line defense against infections.
- Other adverse reactions can include pulmonary or CNS toxicity with methotrexate, mild to severe skin reactions with fluorouracil, bile duct sclerosis with floxuridine, fever and flulike symptoms with 5-azacytidine and cytarabine, and cholestatic jaundice with any pyrimidine analogue.
- By applying the nursing process, the nurse helps the patient cope with chemotherapy. Specific interventions include monitoring the patient for signs and symptoms of adverse reactions and providing information about the drug and the patient's role in the therapy.

STUDY QUESTIONS

See Appendix 1 for answers.

1. Jeffrey Kane, age 60, has recently had a radical neck dissection for throat cancer. His physician prescribes chemotherapy with methotrexate. This antimetabolite agent is active during which phase of the cell cycle?
(a) G_0 phase
(b) G_1 phase
(c) M phase
(d) S phase

2. Methotrexate produces its therapeutic effects by which mechanism of action?
(a) It disrupts the DNA structure.
(b) It inhibits DNA and RNA synthesis.
(c) It inhibits hormone-mediated tumor cell growth.
(d) It intercalates between adjacent pairs of DNA molecules.

3. When high doses of methotrexate are administered, which drug should be prescribed to prevent severe methotrexate toxicity?
(a) leucovorin
(b) fluorouracil
(c) meclofenamate
(d) allopurinol

4. Joan MacGruder, age 57, has breast cancer and is admitted to the oncology unit for a course of chemotherapy with fluorouracil. After fluorouracil administration. Ms. MacGruder develops stomatitis. To help Ms. MacGruder deal with this problem, what should the nurse teach her?

(a) Limit oral care to once a day to avoid irritation.
(b) Brush her teeth vigorously to prevent bacterial overgrowth.
(c) Rinse regularly with saline and sodium bicarbonate solution.
(d) Rinse frequently with hydrogen peroxide solution.

5. In addition to stomatitis, which other adverse reaction is Ms. MacGruder likely to experience?
(a) pulmonary infiltrates
(b) renal failure
(c) congestive heart failure
(d) bone marrow suppression

6. Bobby Smith, age 10, has acute leukemia. He is receiving methotrexate with mercaptopurine for maintenance therapy. While Bobby is receiving mercaptopurine, the nurse should assess him for which adverse reaction?
(a) cholestatic jaundice
(b) renal failure
(c) pulmonary fibrosis
(d) CNS toxicity

7. Which instruction should the nurse give Bobby's parents regarding mercaptopurine?
(a) Provide high-acid foods to acidify the urine.
(b) Protect Bobby from exposure to the sun.
(c) Encourage him to drink 13 8-oz glasses of fluid daily.
(d) Limit Bobby's fluid intake to 4 8-oz glasses daily.

SELECTED REFERENCES

AHFS drug information 90. (1990). Bethesda, MD: American Society of Hospital Pharmacists.

Cunningham, M. (1990). Nonhematologic toxicities of selected chemotherapeutic agents used in the treatment of adult leukemia. *Seminars in Oncology Nursing,* 6(1), 67-75.

Drug facts and comparisons. (1991). St. Louis: Facts and Comparisons Division, Lippincott.

Fischetti, L. (1990). Interaction between nonsteroidal anti-inflammatory drugs and high-dose methotrexate: A literature review. *Journal of Pediatric Oncology Nursing,* 7(1), 14-16.

Goodman and Gilman's the pharmacological basis of therapeutics (8th ed.; 1990). Elmsford, NY: Pergamon Press.

Hansten, P., and Horn, J. (1989). *Drug interactions* (6th ed.). Philadelphia: Lea & Febiger.

Mitchell, M., and Higginbotham, P. (1990). Care of the elderly patient receiving continuous 5-fluorouracil at home. *Journal of Home Health Care Practice,* 2(4), 46-51.

North American Nursing Diagnosis Association. (1990). *Taxonomy I - Revised, with official diagnostic categories.* St. Louis: NANDA.

Podack, E. (Ed.). (1988). *Cytotoxic effector mechanisms.* New York: Springer-Verlag.

Powis, G., and Hacker, M. (1990). *Mechanisms of toxicity of anticancer drugs.* Elmsford, NY: Pergamon Press.

Wadler, S., Lyver, A., and Wiernik, P. (1989). Clinical toxicities of the combination of 5-fluorouracil and recombinant interferon alfa-2a: An unusual toxicity profile. *Oncology Nursing Forum,* 16(6), 12-15.

Walters, P. (1990). Chemo: A nurse's guide to action, administration, and side effects. *RN,* 53(2), 52-67.

Wilman, D. (Ed.). (1990). *Chemistry of antitumour agents.* New York: Routledge Chapman & Hall.

CHAPTER

68

ANTIBIOTIC ANTINEOPLASTIC AGENTS

OBJECTIVES

After reading and studying this chapter, the student should be able to:

1. Describe the primary mechanism of action by which the antibiotic antineoplastics inhibit deoxyribonucleic acid (DNA) and ribonucleic acid (RNA) synthesis.

2. Explain the mechanism of action of plicamycin in treating hypercalcemia.

3. Explain why maximum lifetime doses have been established for bleomycin, daunorubicin, doxorubicin, and mitoxantrone.

4. Identify the major adverse reactions to the antibiotic antineoplastics.

5. Discuss important information about antibiotic antineoplastic therapy that the nurse should include in patient teaching.

6. Describe how to apply the nursing process when caring for a patient who is receiving an antibiotic antineoplastic.

INTRODUCTION

Antibiotic antineoplastic agents are antimicrobial products that produce tumoricidal effects by binding with DNA. These drugs inhibit the cellular processes of normal and malignant cells and are cell-cycle-nonspecific, except for bleomycin, which is G_2-phase-specific.

Chapter 68 discusses the following antibiotic antineoplastics, which can be used alone or with other agents to inhibit the processes of malignant cells: bleomycin, dactinomycin, daunorubicin, doxorubicin, mitomycin, mitoxantrone, and plicamycin.

For a summary of representative drugs, see *Selected major drugs: Antibiotic antineoplastic agents,* page 1189. For a listing of applicable nursing diagnoses that the nurse may formulate when caring for a patient receiving these agents, see *Selected nursing diagnoses: Antibiotic antineoplastic agents*. For detailed information on applying the nursing process, see Chapter 6, The Nursing Process and Drug Therapy.

SELECTED NURSING DIAGNOSES

Antibiotic antineoplastic agents

The following nursing diagnoses address representative problems and etiologies that a nurse may encounter when caring for a patient who is receiving an antibiotic antineoplastic agent. Some of these nursing diagnoses contain generalized etiologies, which the nurse must individualize based on the patient's needs. (For some common nursing diagnoses and related interventions for each drug class, see the "Nursing Process Application" section of this chapter.)

- Altered nutrition: less than body requirements, related to the adverse GI effects of the antibiotic antineoplastic agent
- Altered oral mucous membrane related to stomatitis caused by the antibiotic antineoplastic agent
- Altered protection related to plicamycin-induced bleeding diathesis
- Altered protection related to thrombocytopenia caused by the antibiotic antineoplastic agent
- Body image disturbance related to alopecia caused by the antibiotic antineoplastic agent
- Decreased cardiac output related to cardiomyopathy caused by daunorubicin, doxorubicin, or mitoxantrone
- Hyperthermia related to bleomycin-induced fever
- Impaired gas exchange related to pulmonary toxicity caused by bleomycin or mitomycin
- Impaired tissue integrity related to tissue damage caused by extravasation of the antibiotic antineoplastic agent
- Knowledge deficit related to the prescribed antibiotic antineoplastic agent
- Potential fluid volume deficit related to the adverse GI effects of the antibiotic antineoplastic agent
- Potential for infection related to bone marrow suppression caused by the antibiotic antineoplastic
- Potential for injury related to a preexisting condition that contraindicates the use of an antibiotic antineoplastic agent
- Potential for injury related to a preexisting condition that requires cautious use of an antibiotic antineoplastic agent
- Potential for injury related to adverse drug reactions

MICROBIAL TUMORICIDAL AGENTS

The antibiotic antineoplastics (bleomycin, dactinomycin, daunorubicin, doxorubicin, mitomycin, mitoxantrone, and plicamycin) are prescribed to treat many malignant neoplasms.

PHARMACOKINETICS

The pharmacokinetics of the antibiotic antineoplastics vary widely. Some of these drugs enter the cerebrospinal fluid (CSF); others do not. The extent of metabolism and urinary elimination also varies. The half-lives of the antibiotic antineoplastics have a wide range.

Absorption, distribution, metabolism, excretion

Because the antibiotic antineoplastics usually are administered intravenously, no absorption need occur. They are considered 100% bioavailable. Some of the drugs also are administered via intracavitary routes. Bleomycin, doxorubicin, and mitomycin sometimes are given as topical bladder instillations. Significant systemic absorption, as assessed by blood concentration levels or systemic toxicity, does not occur. Bleomycin also has been injected into the pleural space for malignant effusions, with up to 50% of the dose absorbed via this route.

Distribution throughout the body of the antineoplastic antibiotics varies. Bleomycin is distributed rapidly, with a volume of distribution of 20 liters, approximating intracellular and extracellular fluid volume. Bleomycin concentrates in the skin and lungs, which may explain some of the toxicities of the drug. Its concentration in lung and skin tissue may result from the lack of inactivating enzymes in these tissues. The drug does not enter the CSF.

Dactinomycin is distributed rapidly to tissue-binding sites, with little drug remaining in the plasma 2 minutes after I.V. administration. The drug is distributed to nucleated (bone marrow) cells more than to non-nucleated (plasma) cells. Dactinomycin does not enter the CSF.

Daunorubicin and doxorubicin are distributed rapidly and widely to several organs in the body, including the heart, kidneys, lungs, liver, and spleen. Neither drug enters the CSF. Mitomycin is distributed widely throughout the body, but it does not enter the CSF. It concentrates in the nail beds, forming purple bands. Mitoxantrone distributes rapidly and extensively into tissues. It is 78% bound to plasma protein. Although little is known about the pharmacokinetics of plicamycin, the drug does enter the CSF.

The metabolism of the antibiotic antineoplastics varies widely. Bleomycin undergoes significant tissue inactivation, especially in the liver and kidneys. Dactinomycin undergoes minimal metabolism. Daunorubicin is metabolized in the liver, producing an active metabolite and some inactive ones. Doxorubicin is metabolized in the liver, producing a major metabolite with antineoplastic activity and several inactive metabolites. Its hepatic clearance approximates 60% of hepatic blood flow. Mitomycin is metabolized extensively and inactivated in the liver. Mitoxantrone is metabolized partially to two inactive metabolites. The metabolism of plicamycin has not been studied extensively.

The antibiotic antineoplastic agents vary in their excretion. Up to 50% of a bleomycin dose is excreted in the urine in 24 hours, 20% to 40% as active drug. Dactinomycin is excreted slowly in the feces and urine primarily as unchanged drug, with only 30% excreted in 1 week. Daunorubicin is excreted slowly, with 23% of a dose recovered in the urine in 5 days. It also is excreted (40%) via the biliary route. Doxorubicin (40%) also is excreted primarily via the biliary route, with only 4% to 5% of the intact drug being excreted in the urine within 5 days. From 40% to 50% of a dose of doxorubicin is excreted in the bile or feces within 7 days, with 50% of this as unchanged drug. Small amounts of mitomycin are excreted in bile and feces, while 10% to 30% is excreted in the urine. Mitoxantrone undergoes predominantly biliary excretion, with 25% of a dose being excreted in the feces in 5 days. Renal elimination of mitoxantrone is minimal, From 6% to 11% of a dose is recovered in the urine in 5 days, with 65% of this as unchanged drug. Up to 40% of a plicamycin dose is excreted in the urine within 15 hours. (For a summary, see *Major administration and excretion routes for antibiotic antineoplastic agents.*)

Onset, peak, duration

Bleomycin reaches a peak plasma concentration level in about 30 to 60 minutes. After an I.V. bolus, the drug has a half-life of about 2 hours, which extends to 9 hours with a continuous infusion. Dactinomycin concentration peaks immediately after an I.V. injection, with very little active drug remaining in the circulation after 2 minutes. With slow release from tissue-binding sites, the plasma half-life of dactinomycin is 36 hours.

Daunorubicin has a half-life of 18.5 hours. Its active metabolite has a half-life of about 27 hours. Doxorubicin has a multiphasic elimination pattern, with a half-life of 15 hours. Its active metabolite has a half-life of about 30 hours. Mitomycin reaches a peak plasma concentration of 1.5 mcg/ml after a dose of 20 mg. Its plasma half-life is 17 minutes. The terminal half-life of mitoxantrone is about 5.8 days. The peak concentration and half-life of plicamycin have not been determined.

Major administration and excretion routes for antibiotic antineoplastic agents

This chart provides a quick reference for major administration and excretion routes of the antibiotic antineoplastic agents. Because excretion amounts vary widely, the nurse who administers these agents should be familiar with the variations.

DRUG	ADMINISTRATION ROUTES	EXCRETION ROUTES	AMOUNT EXCRETED
bleomycin	Intravenous, intramuscular, subcutaneous	Urine	50% in 24 hours, mainly as metabolites
dactinomycin	Intravenous	Urine and feces	30% in 7 days
daunorubicin	Intravenous	Urine Bile	23% in 5 days 40%
doxorubicin	Intravenous	Urine Bile or feces	4% to 5% unchanged in 5 days 40% to 50% in 7 days
mitomycin	Intravenous	Urine	10% to 30%
mitoxantrone	Intravenous	Bile Urine	25% in 5 days 6% to 11% in 5 days
plicamycin	Intravenous	Urine	40% in 15 hours

PHARMACODYNAMICS

With the exception of mitomycin, the antibiotic antineoplastics intercalate, or insert themselves, between adjacent base pairs of a DNA molecule, physically separating them. When the DNA chain replicates, an extra base is inserted opposite the intercalated antibiotic, resulting in a mutant DNA molecule. The overall effect is cell death.

Mechanism of action

The cytotoxic action of bleomycin may result from copper-bleomycin and possibly iron-bleomycin complexes that form during intercalation with the DNA molecule. These complexes can generate highly reactive free radicals that cause chain scission (splitting) and fragmentation of DNA molecules. Bleomycin is a cell-cycle-specific drug that causes its major effects in the G_2 phase.

Dactinomycin intercalates between adjacent guanine-cytosine pairs in the DNA molecule, where it binds and inhibits the function of DNA-dependent RNA polymerase. This inhibiting action blocks transcription of the DNA molecule, which causes cell death. Dactinomycin is a cell-cycle-nonspecific drug.

Daunorubicin, doxorubicin, and mitoxantrone (the anthracycline antibiotics) also intercalate into DNA. This causes many cell changes that ultimately produce the cytotoxic effects of the drugs. The drugs inhibit DNA and RNA synthesis. Single- and double-strand breaks in the DNA occur, as does an information exchange between DNA strands known as sister chromatid exchange. These actions account for the mutagenic and carcinogenic actions of the anthracyclines. Finally, daunorubicin and doxorubicin can interfere with cell membrane function, an action that may contribute to cytotoxicity as well as to cardiotoxicity. These drugs are cell-cycle-nonspecific. However, they appear to be most active in the S phase.

Mitomycin is the one antibiotic antineoplastic that does not intercalate into DNA. Instead, it is activated intracellulary to a bifunctional or even trifunctional alkylating agent. Mitomycin produces single-strand breakage of DNA. It also cross-links DNA and inhibits DNA synthesis. The ability of the drug to cross-link DNA is related to the guanine and cytosine content of the DNA. Mitomycin is cell-cycle nonspecific, although its maximal action occurs in the late G_1 and early S phases.

Because mitoxantrone is a synthetic compound similar to doxorubicin, its mechanism of action probably is similar. Mitoxantrone is cell-cycle nonspecific.

Resembling dactinomycin, plicamycin intercalates between adjacent guanine-cytosine base pairs in the DNA molecule. Plicamycin inhibits RNA, DNA, and protein synthesis, and is cell-cycle nonspecific. When RNA synthesis is inhibited, osteoclasts cannot respond to parathyroid hormone, and bone destruction is inhibited. Plicamycin also can lower the serum calcium concentration.

PHARMACOTHERAPEUTICS

The antibiotic antineoplastics are products of microbial fermentation that exhibit antimicrobial activity. Their cytotoxic effects, however, preclude their antimicrobial use. These agents act against many tumors, including Hodgkin's disease and non-Hodgkin's lymphomas; testicular carcinoma; squamous cell carcinoma of the head, neck, and cervix; Wilms' tumor, osteogenic sarcoma, rhabdomyosarcoma; Ewing's tumor and other soft-tissue sarcomas; breast, ovarian, bladder, and bronchogenic carcinomas; acute leukemias; melanoma; carcinomas of the gastrointestinal (GI) tract; choriocarcinoma; and hypercalcemia.

bleomycin (Blenoxane). When combined with vinblastine and cisplatin, bleomycin acts effectively against testicular carcinoma, achieving response rates of over 90%, with complete remissions attained in many patients. Bleomycin also acts effectively against squamous cell carcinomas of the head, neck, esophagus, skin, and genitourinary tract; lung cancer; and Hodgkin's and non-Hodgkin's lymphomas. When combined with other agents, bleomycin may increase the activity of the regimen against the cancer without increased bone marrow toxicity.
Usual adult dosage: 10 to 20 units/m² I.V., I.M., or S.C. once or twice weekly. Bleomycin also may be given intra-arterially. A maximum lifetime dosage of 400 units is recommended because of the pulmonary toxicity associated with bleomycin. Dosage reductions should be made in patients with renal failure. Because 1% of lymphoma patients experience an anaphylactic reaction to bleomycin, all lymphoma patients should receive two test doses of 2 to 5 units before the initial dose.

dactinomycin [actinomycin D] (Cosmegen). Effective against rhabdomyosarcoma and Wilms' tumor in children, dactinomycin also acts against Ewing's sarcoma, gestational choriocarcinoma, and testicular carcinoma.
Usual adult dosage: 10 to 15 mcg/kg daily I.V. for 5 days repeated every 3 to 4 weeks. Usually, a total dosage of 2.5 to 5 mg is needed to produce antineoplastic effects.
Usual pediatric dosage: same as the usual adult dosage.

daunorubicin [daunomycin] (Cerubidine). When given with cytarabine, daunorubicin is the treatment of choice for acute nonlymphoblastic leukemia in adults. It also acts against numerous tumors in children, including Ewing's sarcoma, rhabdomyosarcoma, Wilms' tumor, and neuroblastoma. Daunorubicin can be given on various treatment schedules.
Usual adult dosage: 30 to 45 mg/m² daily I.V. for 1 to 3 days. A maximum lifetime dosage of 500 to 600 mg/m² is recommended to prevent cardiotoxicity. This maximum should be reduced to 400 to 450 mg/m² for patients re-

ceiving mediastinal radiation therapy. Cardiac problems usually preclude daunorubicin use. Dosage reduction is recommended in patients with impaired hepatic or renal function.

doxorubicin (Adriamycin). Effective against many hematologic and solid tumors, doxorubicin also is used in combination regimens against acute leukemias as well as non-Hodgkin's and Hodgkin's lymphomas. The solid tumors that are responsive to doxorubicin include breast, lung, ovarian, bladder, and thyroid carcinomas. Doxorubicin also is active against sarcomas, including osteogenic sarcoma, Ewing's tumor, and Wilms' tumor. Like daunorubicin, doxorubicin can be given using various dosing schedules.
Usual adult dosage: 60 to 75 mg/m² I.V. every 3 weeks; 20 to 30 mg/m² I.V. daily for 2 to 3 days, repeated every 4 weeks; or 20 mg/m² I.V. weekly. A maximum lifetime dosage of 550 mg/m² is recommended to avoid cardiotoxicity. Cardiac problems usually preclude doxorubicin use. The lifetime dose should be decreased to 400 mg/m² for patients receiving mediastinal radiation therapy. Patients with hepatic dysfunction should receive a dosage reduction based on the serum bilirubin level.

mitomycin [mitomycin-C] (Mutamycin). Active against various tumors, mitomycin is used particularly in the palliative treatment of metastatic adenocarcinoma of the stomach or pancreas. It also is active against carcinomas of the cervix, colon, rectum, breast, head, neck, and lungs. Mitomycin also exhibits topical activity against bladder carcinoma.
Usual adult dosage: 10 to 20 mg/m² as a single I.V. bolus, repeated in 6 to 8 weeks; for topical application for bladder carcinoma, 20- to 40-mg instillations once weekly, for 8 instillations per course.

mitoxantrone (Novantrone). When used with cytarabine, mitoxantrone is effective for induction and consolidation treatment of acute nonlymphocytic leukemia (ANLL). Evidence suggests that mitoxantrone may be beneficial in patients with breast cancer also. Mitoxantrone may be less cardiotoxic than other antibiotic antineoplastics. Therefore, higher maximum lifetime dosages may be given.
Usual adult dosage: for ANLL induction, 12 mg/m²/day by I.V. infusion on days 1 through 3; for ANLL consolidation, 12 mg/m²/day I.V. for days 1 and 2. A total lifetime dosage of 140 mg/m² is recommended.

plicamycin [mithramycin] (Mithracin). Although plicamycin exhibits its greatest antineoplastic activity against disseminated testicular cancer, its use for this tumor largely has been replaced by other drugs. Plicamycin is used primarily to treat hypercalcemia, especially that from cancer

Treating hypercalcemia

The normal serum calcium concentration is 8.5 to 10.5 mg/dl. Hypercalcemia occurs when the serum calcium concentration exceeds 10.5 mg/dl. This abnormal release of calcium occurs in 10% to 20% of all cancer patients and 40% to 50% of patients with multiple myeloma or metastatic breast cancer. The electrolyte imbalance is produced by several bone demineralization mechanisms, including bone destruction by metastases, prolonged immobilization, high concentrations of parathyroid hormone released by some tumors, and high levels of prostaglandin and osteoclast activating factor found in some cancer patients.

The signs and symptoms of hypercalcemia include anorexia, nausea, vomiting, polyuria, deep bone pain, fatigue, depression, loss of memory, stupor, coma, constipation, abdominal pain, arrhythmias, somnolence, lethargy, weakness, and confusion.

To treat severe hypercalcemia caused by malignancy, normal saline solution and diuretics are prescribed first. If these fail, then plicamycin, etidronate, or calcitonin may be used. Dosages of plicamycin for hypercalcemia range from 12.5 to 25 mcg/kg to inhibit bone resorption of calcium. Adverse reactions to this treatment include bone marrow suppression, hypotension, and nephrotoxicity.

that has metastasized to the bone. (For details, see *Treating hypercalcemia*.)

Usual adult dosage: for testicular cancer, 25 to 30 mcg/kg daily I.V. for 8 to 10 days; for hypercalcemia, 25 mcg/kg daily I.V., for 3 to 4 days, repeated weekly as necessary, or a single weekly dosage of 25 mcg/kg/day.

Drug interactions

No clinically significant drug interactions occur with the antibiotic antineoplastics.

ADVERSE DRUG REACTIONS

The antibiotic antineoplastics produce many of the same reactions as other drugs used to treat malignant neoplasms. The primary reaction is bone marrow suppression. All of these agents except bleomycin produce moderate to severe leukopenia and thrombocytopenia. The agents that produce the greatest bone marrow suppression are daunorubicin, doxorubicin, and mitomycin. Mitomycin causes delayed myelosuppression that requires 6 to 8 weeks for the bone marrow to recover.

Bone marrow suppression, stomatitis, and alopecia are produced by the effect of the antibiotic antineoplastics on rapidly proliferating tissues. Because bone marrow, epithelial tissue, and hair follicles have growth rates faster than many other body tissues, these cells are more vulnerable to antineoplastic agents.

Nausea and vomiting may result from the chemical irritation of the emetic center in the brain. Vomiting also may result from psychogenic factors and can be triggered by sights, sounds, and smells experienced during chemotherapy. This is known as anticipatory vomiting. (For more information, see the introduction to this unit.)

All antibiotic antineoplastic agents except bleomycin produce severe tissue damage if extravasated. Yet extravasation can occur with even the most careful administration. Bleomycin may produce fever and chills. If these effects become intense, the patient should receive immediate treatment with antihistamines and antipyretics. Patients who develop fever and chills with bleomycin therapy must receive premedication with antihistamines and antipyretics before each bleomycin administration. Bleomycin can result in irreversible pulmonary fibrosis, but this effect is uncommon, usually affecting patients over age 70 who have received more than the recommended lifetime dosage of 400 units. About 50% of patients receiving bleomycin develop a skin toxicity after receiving 150 to 200 units. Toxicity begins with urticaria and also may produce hyperpigmentation. Anaphylactoid reactions have been reported in 1% of patients receiving bleomycin for lymphoma. Therefore, test doses should be given.

The anthracycline antibiotic antineoplastics (daunorubicin, doxorubicin, and mitoxantrone) may cause irreversible cardiomyopathy. The potential for cardiomyopathy increases as the patient approaches the lifetime dosage. The anthracycline antibiotic antineoplastics also may produce acute electrocardiogram (ECG) changes. Dactinomycin and doxorubicin may potentiate the effects of radiation therapy and cause hyperpigmentation of the irradiated area or increased stomatitis or enteritis. Doxorubicin may color the urine red; mitoxantrone may color it blue-green.

Although uncommon, mitomycin may cause renal or pulmonary toxicity.

Plicamycin may produce bleeding diathesis, which may be dose-related. Bleeding diathesis may include epistaxis, hematemesis, hemoptysis, ecchymoses, and prolonged clotting and bleeding times. Plicamycin also may produce hypotension and nephrotoxicity.

NURSING PROCESS APPLICATION

The following information assists the nurse in caring for a patient receiving an antibiotic antineoplastic agent.

Assessment

• Review the patient's history for a preexisting condition that contraindicates the use of an antibiotic antineoplastic, such as pregnancy, myelosuppression, or known hypersensitivity to the drug.

• Review the patient's history for a preexisting condition that requires cautious use of an antibiotic antineoplastic, such as significant renal impairment, cardiovascular disease, concomitant anticancer therapy, mediastinal radiation therapy, or significant renal or hepatic impairment.

• Assess the patient for adverse reactions to the prescribed antibiotic antineoplastic, such as bone marrow suppression, stomatitis, alopecia, nausea, and vomiting.

• Assess the effectiveness of the prescribed antibiotic antineoplastic regularly.

• Assess for fever and chills in the patient receiving bleomycin.

• Evaluate the patient's and family's knowledge about the prescribed antibiotic antineoplastic.

Nursing diagnoses

The following examples represent appropriate nursing diagnoses for a patient receiving a antibiotic antineoplastic.

• Potential for injury related to a preexisting condition that contraindicates the use of an antibiotic antineoplastic

• Potential for injury related to a preexisting condition that requires cautious use of an antibiotic antineoplastic

• Potential for injury related to adverse drug reactions

• Hyperthermia related to bleomycin-induced fever

• Knowledge deficit related to the prescribed antibiotic antineoplastic agent

Planning and implementation

• Do not administer an antibiotic antineoplastic to a patient with a condition that contraindicates its use.

• Administer an antibiotic antineoplastic cautiously to a patient at risk because of a preexisting condition.

• Monitor the patient frequenty for adverse reactions during antibiotic antineoplastic therapy.

• *Monitor the patient for bone marrow suppression during treatment with any antibiotic antineoplastic except bleomycin.* Expect acute complications when the absolute granulocyte count is below 1,000/mm³. As the count declines, encourage the patient to maintain adequate nutritional and fluid intake. During the nadir, the patient should avoid crowds and anyone with an active contagious infection.

• *Monitor the hematocrit and the platelet count to detect anemia or thrombocytopenia from bone marrow suppression. Because red blood cells (RBCs) have a longer life than white blood cells and platelets, anemia usually does not occur unless the patient has an occult or overt blood loss. When the platelet count is lower than 50,000 mm³, take additional safety precautions, such as avoiding intramuscular (I.M.) injections, to prevent trauma. Supportive platelet transfusions and packed RBCs may be administered as prescribed.*

• *Use extreme caution when administering dactinomycin, daunorubicin, doxorubicin, mitomycin, mitoxantrone, and plicamycin because they are powerful vesicants. Vesicants are most safely given via intravenous (I.V.) push*

into the side port of a freely infusing I.V., which enables close supervision of the site throughout administration.

• *Stop the infusion immediately if infiltration or extravasation is suspected, and notify the physician. Apply cold compresses and elevate the affected extremity. To decrease tissue damage, instill hydrocortisone as prescribed into the affected site via an I.V. catheter, subcutaneous (S.C.) injection, or as indicated by health care facility protocol.*

• *Monitor the patient regularly for signs of stomatitis, such as erythema and ulceration of the oral mucosa, which may develop 7 to 10 days after therapy.* Use a Toothette for oral care at least every 4 hours. If the Toothette is too painful, provide normal saline solution rinses. Administer an antifungal agent, if prescribed, to prevent a candida infection.

• Administer an antiemetic agent with the antibiotic antineoplastic, if prescribed, to help prevent nausea and vomiting.

• Decrease the psychogenic factors of chemotherapy by helping the patient overcome feelings of isolation and anxiety; spend time with the patient, listen supportively, provide music, and use relaxation techniques.

• Consult the physician before initiating scalp hypothermia to decrease alopecia because the procedure is not appropriate for every patient. If appropriate, cool the scalp for 15 to 30 minutes before drug administration, and continue to cool it for 15 to 30 minutes after administration. The use of scalp hypothermia is indicated for a patient receiving a drug with an immediate onset of action, peak concentration, and short duration of action.

• *Monitor the patient closely during daunorubicin, doxorubicin, or mitoxantrone therapy for signs of congestive heart failure, such as dependent edema, tachycardia, dyspnea, decreased urine output, and unexplained weight gain. If the patient exhibits any of these signs, withhold the drug and notify the physician.*

• *Monitor the patient's ECG for changes when administering daunorubicin, doxorubicin, or mitoxantrone.*

• *Monitor the results of any prescribed pulmonary function studies and chest X-rays for evidence of pulmonary fibrosis in a patient receiving bleomycin (especially if the patient is over age 70 or has received more than 400 units) or mitomycin.*

• Inspect the patient's skin for urticaria and hyperpigmentation when administering bleomycin. Notify the physician if skin changes occur.

• *Ensure that the patient with lymphoma receives two test doses of 2 to 5 units before the initial dose of bleomycin to identify drug hypersensitivity, which can help prevent an anaphylactic reaction.*

• Monitor the results of renal function studies regularly during mitomycin therapy.

• *Observe the patient receiving plicamycin for signs of bleeding diathesis, such as epistaxis, hematemesis, he-*

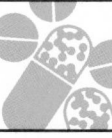

SELECTED MAJOR DRUGS
Antibiotic antineoplastic agents

This chart summarizes the major antineoplastic antibiotics currently in clinical use.

DRUG	MAJOR INDICATIONS	USUAL ADULT DOSAGES	CONTRAINDICATIONS AND PRECAUTIONS
bleomycin	Testicular carcinoma; squamous cell carcinomas of the head, neck, esophagus, skin, and genitourinary tract; lung cancer; Hodgkin's and non-Hodgkin's lymphomas	10 to 20 units/m² I.V., S.C., or I.M. one to two times weekly	• Know that bleomycin is contraindicated in a patient with a known hypersensitivity or idiosyncratic reactions to the drug. • Administer with extreme caution to a patient with significant renal impairment or compromised pulmonary function.
daunorubicin	Acute nonlymphoblastic leukemia (ANLL); childhood tumors, such as Ewing's sarcoma, rhabdomyosarcoma, Wilms' tumor, and neuroblastoma	30 to 45 mg/m² I.V. for 1 to 3 days	• Know that daunorubicin is contraindicated in a pregnant patient or one with drug-induced bone marrow suppression (unless the benefit of daunorubicin treatment warrants the risk). • Administer with extreme caution to a patient with heart disease.
doxorubicin	Solid tumors, such as breast, lung, ovarian, bladder, and thyroid carcinomas; acute leukemias; Hodgkin's and non-Hodgkin's lymphomas	60 to 75 mg/m² I.V. every 3 weeks; or 20 to 30 mg/m² I.V. for 2 to 3 days repeated every 4 weeks; or 20 mg/m² I.V. weekly	• Know that doxorubicin is contraindicated in a pregnant patient, one with marked myelosuppression or heart disease, or one who previously received a lifetime dose of daunorubicin, doxorubicin, or both. • Administer with caution to a patient receiving concomitant anticancer therapy.
mitoxantrone	ANLL	12 mg/m²/day I.V. on days 1 through 3 for ANLL induction; 12 mg/m²/day I.V. for days 1 and 2 for ANLL consolidation	• Know that mitoxantrane is contraindicated in a pregnant patient, one with myelosuppression or known hypersensitivity to the drug, or one who has received previous treatment with daunorubicin or doxorubicin (unless the potential benefits outweigh the risks). • Administer with caution to a patient with cardiovascular disease or one who is receiving mediastinal radiation therapy.
plicamycin	Hypercalcemia Testicular cancer	25 mcg/kg/day I.V. for 3 to 4 days, repeated weekly as necessary 25 to 30 mcg/kg/day I.V. for 8 to 10 days	• Know that plicamycin is contraindicated in a pregnant or lactating patient or one with thrombocytopenia, thrombocytopathy, coagulation disorder, increased susceptibility to bleeding from other causes, or impaired bone marrow function. • Administer with extreme caution to a patient with significant renal or hepatic impairment.

moptysis, and ecchymoses. Also monitor the patient's clotting and bleeding times if prescribed, which may become prolonged. Notify the physician if bleeding occurs and discuss dosage adjustment.
• Use other appropriate nursing interventions for a patient with bone marrow suppression, nausea, or vomiting. (For details, see the introduction to this unit.)
• Notify the physician if any other adverse reactions occur.
• Monitor for fever and chills during bleomycin therapy.
• Expect to administer antihistamine and antipyretic agents immediately as prescribed if fever and chills become severe.
• Premedicate with antihistamine and antipyretic agents before each bleomycin dose as prescribed if the patient has developed fever and chills with previous bleomycin therapy.

Patient teaching
• Teach the patient and family the name, dose, frequency, action, and adverse effects of the prescribed antibiotic antineoplastic.
• *Instruct the patient to watch for, recognize, and immediately report any signs or symptoms of infection, such as fever or sore throat. Also teach this to the hospitalized patient who is at risk for contracting an infection from altered skin integrity, hospital procedures such as I.V. punctures, or urinary drainage devices.*
• *Teach the patient bleeding precautions and energy conservation measures to use if needed.*
• *Instruct the patient to alert the nurse if pain or discomfort occurs at the infusion site during drug administration.*

- Teach the patient how to manage troublesome adverse reactions, such as nausea, vomiting, and stomatitis.
- Provide information and support for the patient with alopecia. Inform the patient that the hair loss is temporary, but that hair regrowth may be a different color or texture.
- *Teach the patient to recognize the signs and symptoms of pulmonary fibrosis and interstitial pneumonia, such as dry, unproductive cough and dyspnea.*
- Instruct the patient receiving bleomycin to take a temperature at home. Stress the importance of reporting fever and chills to the physician.
- Advise the patient receiving bleomycin to report urticaria or hyperpigmentation—possible signs of skin toxicity.
- *Teach the patient receiving daunorubicin, doxorubicin, or mitoxantrone to recognize and report the signs and symptoms of congestive heart failure.*
- Inform the patient that localized hyperpigmentation and increased stomatitis or enteritis may occur during concomitant therapy with dactinomycin or doxorubicin and radiation therapy.
- *Teach the patient receiving plicamycin to watch for—and immediately report—epistaxis, hematemesis, hemoptysis, or ecchymoses.*
- Stress the importance of returning for follow-up blood tests.
- Inform the patient that doxorubicin may cause a temporary red coloration of urine; mitoxantrone, a temporary blue-green coloration.
- Give the patient printed information about the prescribed antibiotic antineoplastic for home reference.
- Instruct the patient to report any adverse reaction to the physician.

Evaluation

The following examples represent appropriate evaluation statements for a patient receiving an antibiotic antineoplastic.
- The patient has no conditions that contraindicate antibiotic antineoplastic therapy.
- The patient exhibits no signs of complications in the preexisting condition linked to the prescribed antibiotic antineoplastic.
- The patient experiences few adverse reactions to the prescribed antibiotic antineoplastic.
- The patient's temperature remains normal throughout bleomycin therapy.
- The patient and family express an accurate understanding of the points taught about the prescribed antibiotic antineoplastic.
- The patient correctly identifies infection control measures to use at home during antibiotic antineoplastic therapy.

CHAPTER SUMMARY

Chapter 68 presented the antibiotic antineoplastics, agents that bind to DNA and prevent cellular reproduction. Here are the chapter highlights.
- The antibiotic antineoplastics dactinomycin, daunorubicin, doxorubicin, mitomycin, mitoxantrone, and plicamycin are cell-cycle-nonspecific. Bleomycin is G_2-phase-specific.
- Antibiotic antineoplastics are used alone or with other antineoplastic drugs to treat various malignant neoplasms, including Hodgkin's disease, non-Hodgkin's lymphoma, testicular carcinoma, Wilms' tumor, rhabdomyosarcoma, Ewing's sarcoma, acute leukemias, and breast, bladder, lung, and GI tract carcinomas.
- The most common adverse reactions to the antibiotic antineoplastics include bone marrow suppression, alopecia, nausea, and vomiting.
- Except for bleomycin, all antibiotic antineoplastics can cause severe tissue damage if extravasated.
- Daunorubicin and doxorubicin may cause cardiomyopathy; bleomycin may produce pulmonary fibrosis. These effects are cumulative, dose-related, and irreversible. Therefore, total lifetime dosages of these drugs are limited to prevent these effects.
- Using the nursing process, the nurse helps the patient cope with chemotherapy through careful drug administration, patient teaching, and interventions to minimize adverse reactions.

STUDY QUESTIONS

See Appendix 1 for answers.

1. Ralph Neill, age 30, has testicular cancer. His physician prescribes combination therapy with bleomycin, vinblastine, and cisplatin. What is the advantage of administering bleomycin with other antineoplastic agents?
(a) Bleomycin increases the regimen's therapeutic effectiveness, without increasing bone marrow toxicity.
(b) Bleomycin is cell-cycle nonspecific, thereby increasing the anticancer activity of the therapeutic regimen.
(c) When used with other antineoplastic agents, bleomycin has a synergistic effect, thereby increasing therapeutic response.
(d) When used with other antineoplastic agents, bleomycin has an additive effect, thus requiring lower dosages.

2. Before administering bleomycin to Mr. Neill, the physician prescribes an antihistamine and an antipyretic agent. Why?

(a) to prevent anaphylactic shock
(b) to prevent bone marrow suppression
(c) to sedate the patient
(d) to prevent fever and chills

3. What serious irreversible adverse reaction is associated with a bleomycin lifetime dosage that exceeds 400 units?

(a) renal failure
(b) cardiomyopathy
(c) pulmonary fibrosis
(d) hepatic failure

4. Mr. Thomas, age 52, is scheduled to begin radiation therapy and chemotherapy for lung cancer. His combination chemotherapy will include doxorubicin (Adramycin), cyclophosphamide (Cytoxan), and cisplatin (Platinol). How does doxorubicin exert its cytotoxic effects?

(a) It prevents DNA synthesis.
(b) It prevents RNA synthesis.
(c) It disrupts protein synthesis.
(d) It intercalates between DNA molecules.

5. Which risk limits the maximum lifetime dosage of doxorubicin to 550 mg/m^2?

(a) renal failure
(b) cardiac damage
(c) pulmonary fibrosis
(d) thrombocytopenia

6. During doxorubicin therapy, Mr. Thomas develops edema, tachycardia, dyspnea, and decreased urine output. How should the nurse intervene?

(a) Withhold the drug and notify the physician.
(b) Decrease the infusion rate and monitor the patient.
(c) Provide a fluid challenge and monitor the patient.
(d) Continue the treatment as prescribed and notify the physician.

7. The nurse administers doxorubicin with extreme care to Mr. Thomas. If infiltration or extravasation occurs, which step should the nurse take immediately?

(a) Stop the infusion.
(b) Apply a heat pack.
(c) Administer the antidote.
(d) Remove the I.V. catheter.

8. Molly Darnell, age 50, has hypercalcemia caused by metastatic breast cancer. So far, administration of normal saline solution and a diuretic has not lowered her serum calcium level. Which antibiotic antineoplastic agent may be prescribed for Ms. Smith to treat her hypercalcemia?

(a) bleomycin
(b) dactinomycin
(c) mitomycin
(d) plicamycin

SELECTED REFERENCES

AHFS drug information 90. (1990). Bethesda, MD: American Society of Hospital Pharmacists.

Cunningham, M. (1990). Nonhematologic toxicities of selected chemotherapeutic agents used in the treatment of adult leukemia. *Seminars in Oncology Nursing, 6*(1), 67-75.

Curran, C. (1990). Doxorubicin-associated flare reactions. *Oncology Nursing Forum, 17*(3), 387-389.

Drug facts and comparisons. (1991). St. Louis: Facts and Comparisons Division, Lippincott.

Goodman and Gilman's the pharmacological basis of therapeutics (8th ed.; 1990). Elmsford, NY: Pergamon Press.

Hansten, P., and Horn, J. (1989). *Drug interactions* (6th ed.) Philadelphia: Lea & Febiger.

North American Nursing Diagnosis Association. (1990). *Taxonomy I – Revised, with official diagnostic categories.* St. Louis: NANDA.

Podak, E. (Ed.). (1988). *Cytotoxic effector mechanisms.* New York: Springer-Verlag.

Powis, G., and Hacker, M. (1990). *Mechanisms of toxicity of anticancer drugs.* Elmsford, NY: Pergamon Press.

Schulmeister, L. (1989). Developing guidelines for bleomycin test dosing. *Oncology Nursing Forum, 16*(2), 205-207.

Wilman, D. (Ed.). (1990). *Chemistry of antitumour agents.* New York: Routledge, Chapman & Hall.

HORMONAL ANTINEOPLASTIC AGENTS

OBJECTIVES

After reading and studying this chapter, the student should be able to:

1. Describe the pharmacokinetic properties of the estrogens, antiestrogens, androgens, antiandrogens, adrenocortical suppressants, progestins, corticosteroids, and gonadotropin-releasing hormone analogues.

2. Describe how each group of hormonal antineoplastic agents works to inhibit malignant growth.

3. Differentiate among the specific indications for each group of hormonal antineoplastic agents.

4. Identify the major adverse reactions to each group of hormonal antineoplastic agents.

5. Describe how to apply the nursing process when caring for a patient who is receiving a hormonal antineoplastic agent.

INTRODUCTION

Hormonal antineoplastic agents are prescribed to alter the growth of malignant neoplasms or to manage and treat their physiologic effects. (For a list of these drugs, see *Hormonal antineoplastic agents*.) The mechanisms of action are not understood completely and, in fact, the early use of hormonal agents was largely empiric.

The use of hormonal agents as direct or indirect antagonists to inhibit hormonal influence began in 1939 with the use of androgens for breast cancer. However, the earliest therapy for endocrine-related tumors occurred in 1896 when Beatson performed an oophorectomy on a woman with breast cancer. Many advances occurred in the 1940s and 1950s as knowledge of the endocrine system grew rapidly. During that time, procedures that removed glands and eliminated stimulating hormones included orchiectomy in prostatic cancer, 1941; adrenalectomy in breast cancer, 1951; and hypophysectomy in breast cancer, 1952. More recent

Hormonal antineoplastic agents

This list summarizes hormonal antineoplastic agents used to alter the growth of malignant neoplasms or manage their effects.

Estrogens

- chlorotrianisene
- conjugated estrogens
- diethylstilbestrol
- diethylstilbestrol diphosphate
- ethinyl estradiol

Antiestrogens

- tamoxifen citrate

Androgens

- fluoxymesterone
- testolactone
- testosterone enanthate
- testosterone propionate

Antiandrogens

- flutamide

Adrenocorticol suppressants

- aminoglutethimide

Progestins

- hydroxyprogesterone caproate
- medroxyprogesterone acetate
- megestrol acetate

Corticosteroids

- dexamethasone
- hydrocortisone
- methylprednisolone
- prednisolone
- prednisone

Gonadotropin-releasing hormone analogues

- goserelin acetate
- leuprolide acetate

SELECTED NURSING DIAGNOSES

Hormonal antineoplastic agents

The following nursing diagnoses address representative problems and etiologies that a nurse may encounter when caring for a patient who is receiving a hormonal antineoplastic agent. Some of these nursing diagnoses contain generalized etiologies, which the nurse must individualize based on the patient's needs. (For some common nursing diagnoses and related interventions for each drug class, see the "Nursing Process Application" sections of this chapter.)

- Altered health maintenance related to endocrine and metabolic imbalances caused by a hormonal antineoplastic agent
- Altered health maintenance related to hypercalcemia caused by prolonged androgen therapy
- Altered nutrition: less than body requirements, related to stomatitis caused by a hormonal antineoplastic agent
- Altered nutrition: less than body requirements, related to the adverse GI effects of a hormonal antineoplastic agent
- Altered nutrition: more than body requirements, related to increased appetite caused by a corticosteroid
- Altered protection related to electrolyte imbalances caused by a hormonal antineoplastic agent
- Altered protection related to a local or systemic hypersensitivity reaction to an oil-based progestin injection
- Altered protection related to thrombocytopenia caused by a hormonal antineoplastic agent
- Altered thought processes related to the adverse CNS effects of a hormonal antineoplastic agent
- Altered urinary elimination related to frequent urination caused by estrogen therapy
- Anxiety related to the adverse effects of flutamide
- Body image disturbance related to estrogen-induced feminization in a male patient
- Body image disturbance related to virilization in a female patient caused by a hormonal antineoplastic agent
- Constipation related to the adverse GI effects of a gonadotropin-releasing hormone analogue
- Diarrhea related to the adverse GI effects of a hormonal antineoplastic agent

- Fatigue related to the adverse effects of a corticosteroid
- Fluid volume excess related to sodium and fluid retention caused by a hormonal antineoplastic agent
- Impaired cerebral, peripheral, or pulmonary tissue perfusion related to a thromboembolus caused by a hormonal antineoplastic agent
- Knowledge deficit related to the prescribed hormonal antineoplastic agent
- Pain related to tumor flare caused by a hormonal antineoplastic agent
- Potential activity intolerance related to flutamide-induced neuromuscular dysfunction
- Potential fluid volume deficit related to the adverse GI effects of a hormonal antineoplastic agent
- Potential for infection related to immunosuppression caused by a hormonal antineoplastic agent
- Potential for injury related to a preexisting condition that contraindicates the use of a hormonal antineoplastic agent
- Potential for injury related to a preexisting condition that requires cautious use of a hormonal antineoplastic agent
- Potential for injury related to adverse drug reactions
- Potential for trauma related to hepatotoxicity caused by a hormonal antineoplastic agent
- Sensory-perceptual alterations (visual) related to vision disturbances caused by a hormonal antineoplastic agent
- Sexual dysfunction related to the adverse genitourinary effects of a hormonal antineoplastic agent
- Sleep pattern disturbance related to corticosteroid-induced insomnia

advances in hormonal therapy include the role of estrogen and progesterone receptors in breast cancer treatment.

Although not cytotoxic, the hormonal antineoplastic agents can be cytostatic and prevent malignant neoplasm growth. Hormonal therapies prove effective against hormone-dependent tumors, such as cancers of the prostate, breast, and endometrium. Lymphomas and leukemias usually are treated with protocols that include corticosteroids because of their lympholytic potential. (For more information about hormonal agents, see Chapter 53, Androgenic and Anabolic Steroid Agents, and Chapter 54, Estrogens, Progestins, and Oral Contraceptive Agents.)

For a summary of representative drugs, see *Selected major drugs: Hormonal antineoplastic agents,* page 1210. For a listing of applicable nursing diagnoses that the nurse may formulate when caring for a patient receiving these agents, see *Selected nursing diagnoses: Hormonal antineo-*

plastic agents. For detailed information on applying the nursing process, see Chapter 6, The Nursing Process and Drug Therapy.

ESTROGENS

Estrogens include chlorotrianisene, conjugated estrogens, diethylstilbestrol, diethylstilbestrol diphosphate, and ethinyl estradiol. These drugs are prescribed as palliative therapy for metastatic breast cancer in postmenopausal women for whom antiestrogen therapy was ineffective. Estrogens also are prescribed for men with advanced prostate cancer.

PHARMACOKINETICS

The estrogens are absorbed readily and rapidly after oral and topical administration. They are distributed well throughout the body. Chlorotrianisene is distributed especially well and released slowly from fatty tissue, providing a prolonged duration of action. Metabolized in the liver, the estrogens undergo enterohepatic recirculation. Chlorotrianisene is metabolized to a more potent compound. After conjugation, the estrogens are excreted primarily in the urine.

Because estrogens have a slow onset of action, they must be administered for 2 to 3 months before they achieve maximum therapeutic effect.

PHARMACODYNAMICS

The estrogens act on tumor cells to inhibit hormone-mediated growth. However, the antitumor mechanism of action is not understood completely. The estrogen binds to a receptor on the cell membrane; then this complex is translocated to the nucleus, where it may modulate cell growth. In postmenopausal women with breast cancer, exogenous estrogens may displace endogenous growth-enhancing estrogens from their receptors. Researchers have not discovered how high doses of estrogens paradoxically inhibit estrogen production. In men with prostate cancer, estrogens act on the pituitary to suppress secretion of luteinizing hormone, which in turn decreases testicular androgen secretion.

PHARMACOTHERAPEUTICS

Estrogen therapy is used as a palliative treatment for metastatic breast cancer in postmenopausal women and for metastatic prostate cancer in men. Breast cancer tumor cells that are estrogen receptor-positive respond more to hormonal therapy than those that are not. The average duration of remission induced by hormonal therapy is 6 to 12 months.

chlorotrianisene (TACE). This drug is used to treat prostate cancer.
Usual adult dosage: 12 to 25 mg P.O. daily.

conjugated estrogens (Premarin). Given orally, conjugated estrogens are used to treat breast and prostate cancer.
Usual adult dosage: for breast cancer, 10 mg P.O. t.i.d. for at least 3 months; for prostate cancer, 1.25 to 2.5 mg P.O. t.i.d.

diethylstilbestrol [DES]. This drug is indicated for the palliative treatment of breast and prostate cancer.
Usual adult dosage: for breast cancer, 5 to 15 mg P.O. daily; for prostate cancer, 1 to 3 mg P.O. daily.

diethylstilbestrol diphosphate (Stilphostrol). Diethylstilbestrol diphosphate is used to treat prostate cancer. If oral therapy is ineffective, the drug may be administered intravenously.
Usual adult dosage: 50 to 200 mg P.O. t.i.d.; initially 500 mg I.V., then increased to 1,000 mg I.V. daily for 5 days, then 250 to 500 mg I.V. once or twice weekly.

ethinyl estradiol (Estinyl). Like DES, this estrogen is prescribed as a palliative treatment for breast and prostate cancer.
Usual adult dosage: for breast cancer, 1 mg P.O. t.i.d.; for prostate cancer, 0.15 to 2 mg P.O. daily.

Drug interactions
Few significant drug interactions occur with the estrogens.

ADVERSE DRUG REACTIONS

Estrogens are tolerated relatively well even in the large dosages usually prescribed for cancer treatment. Most adverse reactions to these agents are extensions of their natural hormonal activities.

Estrogen therapy may cause mild nausea, which is more pronounced in women, probably because of the higher dosages used for them. The nausea, which usually disappears after 2 or 3 weeks of therapy, is not severe enough to cause a nutritional deficit. Abdominal cramps, irritability, and frequent urination also occur.

Estrogen therapy causes feminization in men, primarily manifested by mammary gland development (gynecomastia) and impotence. Women may experience decreased libido and breast tenderness. Almost all patients display increased pigmentation of the nipples and areolae.

Estrogens may produce some adverse cardiovascular reactions, such as hypertension. High doses of estrogens predispose patients to an increased risk of thromboembolic complications, including pulmonary embolus, myocardial infarction, and cerebrovascular accident. Estrogens also may alter liver function tests.

Several endocrine and metabolic complications can develop during estrogen therapy. Patients may develop decreased glucose tolerance, increased serum triglycerides, or both. Sodium retention and resulting fluid retention can occur as dose-dependent adverse reactions. Fluid retention can prove extremely serious for patients with congestive heart failure. Patients, especially those with metastatic bone disease, also may develop hypercalcemia. Uterine breakthrough bleeding can occur in postmenopausal women. Patients with metastatic breast cancer may experience a flare of metastatic lesions, manifested by increased skin nodules or worsening bone pain.

NURSING PROCESS APPLICATION

The following information assists the nurse in caring for a patient receiving an estrogen.

Assessment

• Review the patient's history for a preexisting condition that contraindicates the use of an estrogen, such as known or suspected breast cancer (except in selected patients being treated for metastatic disease); estrogen-dependent neoplasia; pregnancy; undiagnosed abnormal genital bleeding; active thrombophlebitis or thromboembolic disorder; a history of thrombophlebitis, thrombosis, or thromboembolic disorder associated with previous use of estrogen (except when used to treat breast or prostate cancer).

• Review the patient's history for a preexisting condition that requires cautious use of an estrogen, such as epilepsy, migraine headaches, cardiac or renal dysfunction, depression, impaired liver function, or metabolic bone disease associated with hypercalcemia.

• Assess the patient for adverse reactions to the prescribed estrogen, such as nausea, abdominal cramps, irritability, frequent urination, feminization (in a male patient), sexual dysfunction, endocrine or metabolic complications, hypertension, and thromboembolic complications.

• Assess the effectiveness of the prescribed estrogen regularly.

• Assess the patient for signs and symptoms of fluid retention, such as sudden weight gain (greater than 2 pounds in one day), ankle swelling, puffy eyelids, swollen fingers, jugular vein distention, or elevated blood pressure, during estrogen therapy.

• Evaluate the patient's and family's knowledge about the prescribed estrogen.

Nursing diagnoses

The following examples represent appropriate nursing diagnoses for a patient receiving an estrogen.

• Potential for injury related to a preexisting condition that contraindicates the use of an estrogen

• Potential for injury related to a preexisting condition that requires cautious use of an estrogen

• Potential for injury related to adverse drug reactions

• Fluid volume excess related to sodium and fluid retention caused by estrogen therapy

• Knowledge deficit related to the prescribed estrogen

Planning and implementation

• Do not administer an estrogen to a patient with a condition that contraindicates its use.

• Administer an estrogen cautiously to a patient at risk because of a preexisting condition.

• Monitor the patient regularly for adverse reactions during estrogen therapy.

• Monitor hydration if the patient experiences nausea or frequent urination. Administer an antiemetic as prescribed. If nausea persists, expect a change in therapy. For a patient with frequent urination, provide sufficient liquids to replace fluid output.

• Monitor the patient's serum calcium level monthly if prescribed. Mobilize the patient and maintain adequate hydration. Limiting the patient's dietary calcium intake may have no significant effect on the serum calcium level.

• Monitor the patient's liver function studies and blood glucose and triglyceride levels if prescribed. Particularly note abnormalities that suggest an endocrine or metabolic disorder.

• Administer an analgesic as prescribed if bone pain worsens during estrogen therapy.

• *Monitor the patient for symptoms of thromboemboli, such as sudden onset of shortness of breath, partial or complete vision loss, headache, and local pain, tenderness, and swelling in the extremities.*

• Monitor the patient's blood pressure regularly to detect any elevation.

• Notify the physician if adverse reactions occur during estrogen therapy.

• *Monitor the patient for signs and symptoms of fluid retention, especially if the patient has congestive heart failure.*

• Weigh the patient daily at the same time with the same scale and the same amount of clothing to detect sudden weight gain.

• Document the patient's fluid intake and output.

• Restrict the patient's sodium intake as prescribed.

• *Monitor the patient's vital signs regularly to detect signs and symptoms of congestive heart failure, such as increased blood pressure, pulse rate, respiratory rate. Also auscultate the lungs to detect crackles.*

• Report fluid retention to the physician. If fluid retention is troublesome or severe, expect to treat it with such measures as diuretic administration and fluid restriction as prescribed.

Patient teaching

• Teach the patient and family the name, dose, frequency, action, and adverse effects of the prescribed estrogen.

• *Inform the patient of the possibility of fluid retention and explain how to observe for edema, especially of the hands, ankles, tibia, and sacrum. Advise the patient to restrict sodium intake and measure body weight daily. Instruct the patient to report sudden weight gain or signs of fluid retention.*

• *Inform a female patient that breakthrough uterine bleeding is not normal, and instruct her to report any uterine bleeding to the physician. Also explain that she may notice breast tenderness during therapy.*

• Provide emotional support for a male patient undergoing estrogen therapy, especially if it affects sexual characteristics. Reassure the patient that estrogen may cause temporary gynecomastia and impotence, which disappear after therapy ends.

• Inform a female patient that decreased libido may occur during estrogen therapy.

• Instruct the patient to report nausea so that symptomatic treatment may begin. Encourage the patient to eat frequent small meals and increase carbohydrate intake. Reassure the patient that nausea usually disappears after 2 to 3 weeks of therapy.

• Teach the patient and family to recognize the signs and symptoms of hypercalcemia, such as anorexia, nausea, vomiting, lethargy, and polyuria, because the combined effect of estrogen therapy and bone metastasis may produce this imbalance.

• *Advise the patient that thromboemboli may occur with long-term use of high-dose estrogens. Instruct the patient to avoid wearing restrictive clothing and sitting for long periods with the legs crossed.*

• Reassure the patient that increased pigmentation of the nipples and areolae may occur, but that it is harmless.

• Inform the patient with breast cancer that metastatic lesions may experience flare, causing increased skin nodules or bone pain. If this occurs, advise the patient to request additional analgesics to ease the pain.

• Instruct the patient to report any adverse reactions to the physician.

Evaluation

The following examples represent appropriate evaluation statements for a patient receiving an estrogen.

• The patient has no conditions that contraindicate estrogen therapy.

• The patient exhibits no signs of complications in the preexisting condition linked to the prescribed estrogen.

• The patient experiences no adverse reactions to the prescribed estrogen.

• The patient maintains normal body fluid balance.

• The patient and family express an accurate understanding of the points taught about the prescribed estrogen.

• The patient correctly identifies adverse drug reactions that must be reported.

ANTIESTROGENS

The antiestrogen tamoxifen citrate acts by competing with estradiol for receptor sites. Tamoxifen is the drug of choice for advanced breast cancer involving estrogen receptor-positive tumors in postmenopausal women.

PHARMACOKINETICS

After oral administration, tamoxifen is absorbed well and undergoes extensive hepatic metabolism before fecal excretion. Tamoxifen has a half-life of approximately 1 week.

Absorption, distribution, metabolism, excretion

Tamoxifen is absorbed well; however, its distribution has not been studied thoroughly. The drug is metabolized in the liver to various metabolites that display antiestrogenic and antitumor effects. Tamoxifen and its metabolites are excreted slowly in the feces, mainly as conjugates. Less than 30% of a dose is excreted as other metabolites or the parent compound. Minimal amounts are excreted in the urine.

Onset, peak, duration

The peak serum concentration level of tamoxifen occurs in 3 to 6 hours after an oral dose. The half-life of the drug is approximately 7 days. The steady state blood level is achieved in 4 weeks. Clinical responses usually appear in 1 to 2 months.

PHARMACODYNAMICS

Estrogen receptors, found in the cancer cells of 50% of premenopausal and 75% of postmenopausal women with breast cancer, respond to estrogenic influence to induce tumor growth. The antiestrogen, tamoxifen, binds to the estrogen receptors and inhibits estrogen-mediated tumor growth. The inhibition may result because tamoxifen binds to receptors at the nuclear level or because the binding reduces the number of free receptors in the cytoplasm. Ultimately, deoxyribonucleic acid (DNA) synthesis and cell growth are inhibited.

PHARMACOTHERAPEUTICS

The antiestrogen tamoxifen is the palliative treatment of choice for advanced breast cancer in postmenopausal women.

tamoxifen citrate (Nolvadex). This drug is indicated for palliative treatment of metastatic breast cancer that is estrogen receptor-positive. Tumors in postmenopausal women are more responsive to tamoxifen than those in premenopausal women. Tamoxifen also may be used as an adjunct to surgery in postmenopausal women with axillary lymph nodes that contain cancer cells and estrogen receptor-positive tumors. The drug may be used alone or with cytotoxic agents.

Usual adult dosage: 10 to 20 mg P.O. b.i.d.

Drug interactions

No drug interactions have been identified for tamoxifen.

ADVERSE DRUG REACTIONS

Tamoxifen is a relatively nontoxic drug. The most common adverse reactions are hot flashes, nausea, and vomiting. Transient mild leukopenia or thrombocytopenia occurs in about 4% of patients. In patients with bone metastases, hypercalcemia may occur.

About 1% of patients treated with tamoxifen may experience tumor flare, which may increase the number and size of lesions or increase bone pain. Patients receiving high doses of tamoxifen have experienced ocular lesions, retinopathy, and superficial corneal opacity, which reduce visual acuity.

NURSING PROCESS APPLICATION

The following information assists the nurse in caring for a patient receiving tamoxifen.

Assessment

• Review the patient's history for a preexisting condition that contraindicates the use of tamoxifen, such as pregnancy, lactation, or known hypersensitivity to the drug.
• Review the patient's history for a preexisting condition that requires cautious use of tamoxifen, such as leukopenia or thrombocytopenia.
• Assess the patient for adverse reactions to tamoxifen, such as hot flashes, nausea, vomiting, leukopenia, thrombocytopenia, hypercalcemia, and tumor flare.
• Assess the effectiveness of tamoxifen regularly.
• Assess the patient's vision regularly during tamoxifen therapy.
• Evaluate the patient's and family's knowledge about tamoxifen.

Nursing diagnoses

The following examples represent appropriate nursing diagnoses for a patient receiving tamoxifen.
• Potential for injury related to a preexisting condition that contraindicates the use of tamoxifen
• Potential for injury related to a preexisting condition that requires cautious use of tamoxifen

• Potential for injury related to adverse drug reactions
• Sensory-perceptual alterations (visual) related to vision disturbances caused by tamoxifen
• Knowledge deficit related to tamoxifen

Planning and implementation

• Do not administer tamoxifen to a patient with a condition that contraindicates its use.
• Administer tamoxifen cautiously to a patient at risk because of a preexisting condition.
• Monitor the patient regularly for adverse reactions during tamoxifen therapy.
• Monitor hydration the patient experiences nausea and vomiting during tamoxifen therapy. Administer an antiemetic as prescribed.
• *Monitor the patient's white blood cell (WBC) and platelet counts regularly for mild leukopenia or thrombocytopenia if prescribed. For a patient with bone metastasis, monitor the serum calcium level, if prescribed, to detect hypercalcemia.*
• *Observe the patient for signs of tamoxifen-induced tumor flare, such as increased lesion number and size or increased bone pain. Administer additional analgesics as prescribed.*
• Store tamoxifen tablets at room temperature and protect them from light.
• Notify the physician if adverse reactions occur.
• *Monitor the patient for decreased visual acuity. High doses of tamoxifen may produce ocular lesions, retinopathy, and superficial corneal opacity.*
• Schedule the patient for regular eye examinations by an ophthalmologist during tamoxifen therapy.
• Report any vision changes to the physician because the drug may need to be discontinued.

Patient teaching

• Teach the patient and family the name, dose, frequency, action, and adverse effects of tamoxifen.
• Inform the patient that hot flashes, nausea, and occasional vomiting are the most common adverse reactions to tamoxifen, and teach the patient how to manage them at home. Explain that tolerance to these symptoms usually develops rapidly.
• *Instruct the patient to report immediately to the physician any decreased visual acuity; it may be irreversible. Inform the patient of the need for routine eye examinations by an ophthalmologist, who should be told about the tamoxifen therapy.*
• *Assure the patient and family that tumor flare is an expected adverse reaction that will subside. Advise the patient to request increased analgesics in the meantime.*
• Instruct the patient to store tamoxifen at room temperature and protect it from light.

• *Stress the importance of having follow-up blood tests done.*

• Instruct the patient to inform the physician if adverse reactions occur.

Evaluation

The following examples represent appropriate evaluation statements for a patient receiving tamoxifen.

• The patient has no conditions that contraindicate tamoxifen therapy.

• The patient exhibits no signs of complications in the preexisting condition linked to tamoxifen.

• The patient demonstrates no adverse reactions to tamoxifen.

• The patient maintains normal visual acuity during tamoxifen therapy.

• The patient and family express an accurate understanding of the points taught about tamoxifen.

• The patient schedules regular eye examinations with an ophthalmologist during tamoxifen therapy.

ANDROGENS

The therapeutically useful androgens are synthetic derivatives of naturally occurring testosterone. They include fluoxymesterone, testolactone, testosterone enanthate, and testosterone propionate. Since 1939, androgens have been used to treat breast cancer in men and advanced breast cancer in women.

PHARMACOKINETICS

The pharmacokinetic properties of therapeutic androgens resemble those of naturally occurring testosterone. The oral androgens, fluoxymesterone and testolactone, are absorbed well. The parenteral ones, testosterone enanthate and testosterone propionate, are designed specifically for slow absorption. Androgens are distributed well throughout the body and metabolized extensively in the liver, conjugated primarily to the glucuronide. Androgens are excreted in the urine.

Because the onset of action of androgens is slow, a 2- to 3-month trial should be completed before a particular agent is considered a therapeutic failure. The oral agents have a short duration of action and require daily dosing. The duration of the parenteral forms is longer because the oil suspension is absorbed slowly. Parenteral androgens are administered one to three times weekly.

PHARMACODYNAMICS

Androgens probably act via one or more mechanisms. They may reduce the number of prolactin receptors or may bind competitively to those that are available. Also, the androgens may inhibit estrogen synthesis or competitively bind at estrogen receptors. These actions prevent estrogen from affecting estrogen-sensitive tumors.

PHARMACOTHERAPEUTICS

Androgens are indicated for the palliative treatment of advanced breast cancer, particularly in postmenopausal women with bone metastases. Because of their easy administration, the oral agents are used more commonly than the parenteral agents.

fluoxymesterone (Halotestin). Of all the androgens, fluoxymesterone is the most commonly prescribed.
Usual adult dosage: 10 to 40 mg P.O. daily in divided doses.

testolactone (Teslac). This androgen is administered orally.
Usual adult dosage: 250 mg P.O. q.i.d.

testosterone enanthate (Delatestryl). This drug is administered intramuscularly.
Usual adult dosage: 200 to 400 mg I.M. every 2 to 4 weeks.

testosterone propionate (Testex). This androgen also is administered intramuscularly.
Usual adult dosage: 50 to 100 mg I.M. three times weekly.

Drug interactions

No drug interactions have been identified for the androgens.

ADVERSE DRUG REACTIONS

Androgens usually are tolerated well. Dose-related nausea and vomiting are the most common adverse reactions. Fluid retention caused by sodium retention also may occur and should be monitored closely in a patient with compromised cardiovascular function. A female patient may develop masculine characteristics, including increased facial hair, acne, clitoral hypertrophy, increased libido, and voice deepening.

Prolonged high doses of androgens have produced jaundice, which may limit the use of these drugs in patients with liver dysfunction. Also, patients with bony metastases are at greater risk for developing hypercalcemia during prolonged androgen therapy.

NURSING PROCESS APPLICATION

The following information assists the nurse in caring for a patient receiving an androgen.

Assessment

• Review the patient's history for a preexisting condition that contraindicates the use of an androgen, such as pregnancy, lactation, breast or prostate cancer in a male patient, known hypersensitivity to the drug, or serious cardiac, hepatic, or renal disease.

• Review the patient's history for a preexisting condition that requires cautious use of an androgen, such as benign prostatic hypertrophy.

• Assess the patient for adverse reactions to the prescribed androgen, such as nausea, vomiting, fluid retention, masculinization in a female patient, and jaundice.

• Assess the effectiveness of the prescribed androgen regularly.

• Assess for hypercalcemia in a patient receiving prolonged androgen therapy.

• Evaluate the patient's and family's knowledge about the prescribed androgen.

Nursing diagnoses

The following examples represent appropriate nursing diagnoses for a patient receiving an androgen.

• Potential for injury related to a preexisting condition that contraindicates the use of an androgen

• Potential for injury related to a preexisting condition that requires cautious use of an androgen

• Potential for injury related to adverse drug reactions

• Altered health maintenance related to hypercalcemia caused by prolonged androgen therapy

• Knowledge deficit related to the prescribed androgen

Planning and implementation

• Do not administer an androgen to a patient with a condition that contraindicates its use.

• Administer an androgen cautiously to a patient at risk because of a preexisting condition.

• Monitor the patient regularly for adverse reactions during androgen therapy.

• Monitor hydration if the patient experiences nausea and vomiting during androgen therapy. Administer an antiemetic before meals as prescribed.

• *Monitor the patient for signs and symptoms of fluid retention, such as a sudden weight gain (more than 2 pounds per day), increased blood pressure, jugular vein distention, crackles in the lungs, or edema of the hands, ankles, tibia, or sacrum. Be especially alert for these signs in a patient with a history of congestive heart failure. If fluid retention occurs, restrict the patient's fluid intake to* about six 8-oz glasses daily and the sodium intake to 2 grams as prescribed.

• *Monitor the results of liver function studies for a patient receiving prolonged high doses of an androgen. Also monitor the patient for signs and symptoms of jaundice, such as yellow skin or sclera, darkened urine, clay-colored stools, and pruritus.*

• *Use extreme caution with I.M. injections to avoid inadvertent intravenous or subcutaneous injection. Because I.M. preparations are oil suspensions, serious oil embolism can occur if an I.M. androgen is administered into a vein.*

• *Use a 1½-inch (4-cm) needle to administer an androgen I.M., and inject the drug deep into muscle tissue. If irritation or inflammation develops, apply ice for comfort.*

• Notify the physician immediately if adverse reactions occur.

• Monitor the patient's serum calcium level monthly for hypercalcemia if prescribed. This adverse reaction is more common in patients with bone metastases receiving prolonged androgen therapy.

• Prevent hypercalcemia by mobilizing the patient as much as possible and maintaining adequate hydration. Limiting dietary calcium intake does not have a significant effect on the serum calcium level.

• Notify the physician if hypercalcemia occurs.

Patient teaching

• Teach the patient and family the name, dose, frequency, action, and adverse effects of the prescribed androgen.

• *Inform the patient that systemic reactions to the androgen include fluid retention, nausea, and vomiting.* Teach the patient to recognize signs and symptoms and to report them to the physician. Instruct the patient to measure body weight daily and to restrict sodium and fluid intake if fluid retention occurs. If nausea and vomiting occur, advise the patient to request an antiemetic and take it before meals as prescribed.

• *Inform the female patient well in advance about potential virilization and provide emotional support.* Prolonged androgen therapy can cause hirsutism, mild scalp hair loss, voice deepening, facial acne, clitoral enlargement, increased libido, and breast regression. If therapy is discontinued at the onset of virilization, the conditions may disappear. If therapy is continued, the conditions may become irreversible.

• *Teach the patient to recognize the signs and symptoms of jaundice, including yellowing of the skin or sclera, darkened urine, clay-colored stools, and pruritus, and to report any of these signs and symptoms immediately to the physician.*

• Teach the patient and family members to recognize and report the signs and symptoms of hypercalcemia, including anorexia, nausea, vomiting, lethargy, and polyuria. Explain that these signs and symptoms may be caused by a treatable complication.

• Instruct the patient to report adverse reactions to the physician.

Evaluation

The following examples represent appropriate evaluation statements for a patient receiving an androgen.

• The patient has no conditions that contraindicate androgen therapy.

• The patient exhibits no signs of complications in the preexisting condition linked to the prescribed androgen.

• The patient displays no adverse reactions to the prescribed androgen.

• The patient maintains a normal calcium level during androgen therapy.

• The patient and family express an accurate understanding of the points taught about the prescribed androgen.

• The patient limits sodium and fluid intake during androgen therapy.

ANTIANDROGENS

The antiandrogen flutamide is used as an adjunct to gonadotropin-releasing hormone analogues in treating advanced prostate cancer.

PHARMACOKINETICS

After oral administration, flutamide is absorbed rapidly and completely. It is metabolized rapidly and extensively to at least six metabolites, one of which is biologically active. Flutamide and its active metabolite are highly plasma protein bound. The drug is excreted primarily in the urine with only 4.2% of a dose excreted in the feces within 72 hours.

The active metabolite reaches a peak plasma concentration level in 2 hours and has a half-life of 6 hours.

PHARMACODYNAMICS

Flutamide exerts its antiandrogenic action by inhibiting androgen uptake or nuclear binding of androgen in target tissues. Prostate cancer cells are androgen-sensitive and respond to treatments that block androgen stimulation.

PHARMACOTHERAPEUTICS

Flutamide is used with a gonadotropin-releasing hormone analogue, such as leuprolide, to treat metastatic prostate cancer. Flutamide blocks testosterone at the cellular level while the gonadotropin-releasing hormone analogue decreases the circulating testosterone level. Concomitant administration of flutamide and a gonadotropin-releasing hormone analogue may help prevent the disease flare that occurs when the gonadotropin-releasing hormone analogue is used alone.

flutamide (Eulexin). This antiandrogen is used as an adjunct to manage metastatic prostate cancer. It is contraindicated in a patient with known hypersensitivity to the drug or any of its components. It should be used with caution in a patient with impaired liver function.

Usual adult dosage: 250 mg P.O. every 8 hours.

Drug interactions

No known interactions exist between flutamide and other drugs.

ADVERSE DRUG REACTIONS

When flutamide is used with a gonadotropin-releasing hormone analogue, the most common adverse reactions are hot flashes, decreased libido, impotence, diarrhea, nausea, vomiting, and gynecomastia. Other adverse reactions include drowsiness, confusion, depression, anxiety, nervousness, photosensitivity, neuromuscular dysfunction, and elevated liver enzyme and serum creatinine levels.

NURSING PROCESS APPLICATION

The following information assists the nurse in caring for a patient receiving flutamide.

Assessment

• Review the patient's history for a preexisting condition that contraindicates the use of flutamide, such as known hypersensitivity to the drug or its components.

• Review the patient's history for a preexisting condition that requires cautious use of flutamide, such as impaired liver function.

• Assess the patient for adverse reactions to flutamide, such as hot flashes, sexual dysfunction, and gynecomastia.

• Assess the effectiveness of flutamide regularly.

• Assess the patient for signs of dehydration, such as dry mucous membranes, decreased urine output, and concentrated urine.

• Evaluate the patient's and family's knowledge about flutamide.

Nursing diagnoses

The following examples represent appropriate nursing diagnoses for a patient receiving flutamide.

- Potential for injury related to a preexisting condition that contraindicates the use of flutamide
- Potential for injury related to a preexisting condition that requires cautious use of flutamide
- Potential for injury related to adverse drug reactions
- Potential fluid volume deficit related to the adverse gastrointestinal (GI) effects of flutamide
- Knowledge deficit related to flutamide

Planning and implementation

- Do not administer flutamide to a patient with a condition that contraindicates its use.
- Administer flutamide cautiously to a patient at risk because of a preexisting condition.
- Monitor the patient regularly for adverse reactions during flutamide therapy.
- *Administer flutamide concomitantly with a gonadotropin-releasing hormone analogue as prescribed for maximum effectiveness.*
- Ask the patient about decreased libido or impotence. If sexual dysfunction occurs and troubles the patient, refer the patient for sexual counseling.
- *Take safety precautions if the patient experiences drowsiness, confusion, or depression. For example, place the bed in a low position, keep the bed rails up, and supervise ambulation.*
- Assist the patient with activities of daily living if neuromuscular dysfunction occurs.
- *Monitor the patient's liver enzyme and serum creatinine levels regularly if prescribed throughout flutamide therapy.*
- Notify the physician if adverse reactions occur.
- Monitor hydration if the patient experiences nausea, vomiting, and diarrhea. Expect to administer an antiemetic or antidiarrheal agent as prescribed.
- Notify the physician if adverse GI reactions prevent flutamide administration.

Patient teaching

- Teach the patient and family the name, dose, frequency, action, and adverse effects of flutamide.
- Inform the patient that flutamide and the gonadotropin-releasing hormone analogue are taken together.
- Inform the patient of the potential for hot flashes and sexual dysfunction.
- Teach the patient how to manage troublesome adverse GI reactions at home.
- Advise the patient that gynecomastia may occur.
- *Caution the patient not to perform activities that require mental alertness if drowsiness or confusion occurs.*

- Inform the patient that anxiety and nervousness can occur and are drug-related.
- Advise the patient to avoid sun exposure whenever possible and to use a sun screen lotion, hat, and sunglasses if sun exposure cannot be avoided.
- *Stress the importance of returning for follow-up blood tests.*
- Instruct the patient to notify the physician if adverse reactions occur.

Evaluation

The following examples represent appropriate evaluation statements for a patient receiving flutamide.

- The patient has no conditions that contraindicate flutamide therapy.
- The patient exhibits no signs of complications in the preexisting condition linked to flutamide.
- The patient displays no adverse reactions to flutamide.
- The patient maintains adequate hydration throughout flutamide therapy.
- The patient and family express an accurate understanding of the points taught about flutamide.
- The patient correctly identifies sun precautions to take during flutamide therapy.

ADRENOCORTICAL SUPPRESSANTS

The adrenocortical suppressant aminoglutethimide has been proven to be as effective as surgical adrenalectomy in treating advanced breast cancer.

PHARMACOKINETICS

After oral administration, aminoglutethimide is absorbed adequately and distributed widely into body tissues. About 20% to 25% binds to plasma proteins. Aminoglutethimide is metabolized in the liver. Approximately 50% of a dose is excreted unchanged in the urine, and 20% to 50% is excreted as metabolites, four of which have been identified.

Data on the onset of action, peak concentration level, and duration of action of aminoglutethimide remain incomplete. The initial plasma half-life is 13 hours, decreasing to 7 hours 1 to 2 weeks after administration.

PHARMACODYNAMICS

Aminoglutethimide acts in the adrenal gland to block the production of cortisol, androgens, and estrogens. In extraadrenal tissues, it also inhibits the conversion of androgens to estrogens. These actions produce a reversible, chemical adrenalectomy.

Because of the compensatory increase in adrenocorticotropic hormone release after aminoglutethimide administration, a pituitary-suppressive glucocorticoid, such as hydrocortisone, must be administered concurrently. Patients treated with aminoglutethimide and hydrocortisone achieve a chemical adrenalectomy; the response is similar to that seen with surgical removal of the adrenal glands.

PHARMACOTHERAPEUTICS

The adrenocortical suppressant aminoglutethimide is used for the palliative treatment of hormonally responsive advanced breast and prostate cancers and Cushing's disease.

aminoglutethimide (Cytadren). Skin, soft tissue, and bone lesions have a higher response rate to aminoglutethimide therapy than lesions in other metastatic sites.
Usual adult dosage: 250 mg P.O. q.i.d.; may be increased in 250-mg increments daily every 1 to 2 weeks to a maximum dosage of 2 grams/day.

Drug interactions
Aminoglutethimide may decrease the efficacy of dexamethasone by inducing its metabolism. Therefore, aminoglutethimide should be administered with hydrocortisone rather than dexamethasone because higher-than-normal doses of dexamethasone may be required to achieve the same effect.

Aminoglutethimide also may increase the metabolism of warfarin and thereby reduce its effect. If concomitant therapy is required, the warfarin dosage may need to be increased.

ADVERSE DRUG REACTIONS

About 50% of patients taking aminoglutethimide experience an adverse reaction that usually is transient. The most common reaction is a rash that appears in the first weeks of treatment and usually disappears after 5 to 8 days. If the rash persists beyond 8 days, the drug should be discontinued. Fatigue, hypotension, drowsiness, and dizziness also can occur.

Rare reactions include leukopenia, thrombocytopenia, nausea, vomiting, and anorexia.

NURSING PROCESS APPLICATION

The following information assists the nurse in caring for a patient receiving aminoglutethimide.

Assessment
• Review the patient's history for a preexisting condition that contraindicates the use of aminoglutethimide, such as pregnancy, lactation, or known hypersensitivity to the drug or glutethimide.
• Assess the patient for adverse reactions to aminoglutethimide, such as rash, hypotension, drowsiness, dizziness, leukopenia, thrombocytopenia, and GI distress.
• Review the patient's medication history to identify the use of drugs that may interact with aminoglutethimide, such as dexamethasone and warfarin.
• Assess the effectiveness of aminoglutethimide periodically.
• Assess the patient for fatigue regularly.
• Evaluate the patient's and family's knowledge about aminoglutethimide.

Nursing diagnoses
The following examples represent appropriate nursing diagnoses for a patient receiving aminoglutethimide.
• Potential for injury related to a preexisting condition that contraindicates the use of aminoglutethimide
• Potential for injury related to adverse drug reactions
• Fatigue related to the adverse effects of aminoglutethimide
• Knowledge deficit related to aminoglutethimide

Planning and implementation
• Do not administer aminoglutethimide to a patient with a condition that contraindicates its use.
• Monitor the patient regularly for adverse reactions during aminoglutethimide therapy.
• Inspect the patient's skin for a rash, which may appear in the first weeks of therapy. Notify the physician if the rash does not clear after 8 days; the drug should be discontinued.
• *Monitor the patient's blood pressure regularly to detect hypotension.*
• *Take safety precautions if the patient experiences drowsiness or dizziness. For example, place the bed in a low position, keep the bed rails up, and supervise ambulation.*
• *Monitor the patient's WBC count regularly, if prescribed, to detect leukopenia. If leukopenia occurs, monitor the patient for signs of infection, such as fever, chills, malaise, and productive cough. Also take infection control measures until the WBC count returns to normal.*
• *Monitor the patient's platelet count regularly to detect thrombocytopenia. If thrombocytopenia occurs, observe the patient for signs and symptoms of bleeding, such as spontaneous epistaxis, hematuria, and easy bruising. Also take bleeding precautions until the platelet count returns to normal.*

• Monitor hydration if the patient experiences anorexia, nausea, or vomiting. Administer an antiemetic as prescribed.
• Notify the physician if adverse reactions occur.
• Monitor the patient for fatigue. If fatigue occurs, stagger the patient's activities and encourage frequent rest periods.
• Notify the physician if fatigue becomes severe.
• *Monitor the patient's prothrombin time regularly during concomitant therapy with aminoglutethimide and warfarin.*

Patient teaching

• Teach the patient and family the name, dose, frequency, action, and adverse effects of aminoglutethimide.
• Inform the patient that a rash will occur in the first weeks of aminoglutethimide therapy. Advise the patient to notify the physician if it does not disappear or begin to clear within 8 days.
• Teach the patient how to manage troublesome adverse reactions, such as GI distress and fatigue.
• *Caution the patient to avoid activities that require mental alertness if drowsiness or dizziness occurs.*
• *Instruct the patient to return for follow-up blood tests. Review infection control measures and bleeding precautions as needed.*
• Instruct the patient to notify the physician if adverse reactions occur.

Evaluation

The following examples represent appropriate evaluation statements for a patient receiving aminoglutethimide.
• The patient has no conditions that contraindicate aminoglutethimide therapy.
• The patient experiences no adverse reactions to aminoglutethimide.
• The patient experiences minimal fatigue during aminoglutethimide therapy.
• The patient and family express an accurate understanding of the points taught about aminoglutethimide.
• The patient expresses an understanding of the importance of reporting a skin rash that does not clear in 8 days.

PROGESTINS

Progestins are used as palliative treatment of advanced endometrial, breast, and renal cancers. They include hydroxyprogesterone caproate, medroxyprogesterone acetate, and megestrol acetate.

PHARMACOKINETICS

The pharmacokinetic properties of progestins resemble those of natural progesterone. Oil-based I.M. injections provide an extended duration of action.

After oral administration, megestrol acetate is absorbed well. After I.M. injection in aqueous or oil suspension, hydroxyprogesterone caproate and medroxyprogesterone are absorbed slowly from their deposit sites. These drugs are distributed well throughout the body and may sequester into fatty tissue. Progestins are metabolized in the liver, with a high first-pass extraction. After conjugation in the liver, the progestins are excreted as metabolites in the urine.

Two to three months of progestin therapy may pass before objective responses are observed. These drugs provide varying durations of action, ranging from 1 to 3 days for megestrol, 8 to 14 days for hydroxyprogesterone, and 4 to 6 weeks for medroxyprogesterone.

PHARMACODYNAMICS

The antitumor mechanism of action of the progestins is not understood completely. Researchers believe the drugs bind to a specific receptor to act on hormonally sensitive cells. Because the progestins do not exhibit a cytotoxic activity, they are considered cytostatic.

PHARMACOTHERAPEUTICS

The progestins are used for the palliative treatment of advanced endometrial, breast, and renal cancers. Of these agents, megestrol is used most often. Up to 30% of patients with advanced endometrial and breast cancers respond to progestin therapy.

hydroxyprogesterone caproate (Delalutin). This drug is given intramuscularly.
Usual adult dosage: 1 gram or more I.M.; repeated one or more times weekly up to 7 grams/week.

medroxyprogesterone acetate (Depo-Provera). This progestin is given intramuscularly.
Usual adult dosage: 400 to 1,000 mg I.M. weekly.

megestrol acetate (Megace). Megestrol is given orally.
Usual adult dosage: 40 mg P.O. daily, up to 40 mg P.O. q.i.d.

Drug interactions

No drug interactions have been identified for the progestins.

ADVERSE DRUG REACTIONS

Progestins usually are tolerated well. Patients using megestrol have the lowest incidence of adverse reactions.

Mild fluid retention with resulting weight gain is probably the most common reaction to progestins. Thromboemboli can develop with the use of progestins and may cause a cerebrovascular accident, pulmonary dysfunction, blocked blood flow to an extremity, and local, superficial tenderness or swelling. Breakthrough bleeding, spotting, changes in menstrual flow, and breast tenderness also occur with progestins. Because liver function abnormalities have occurred rarely with progestin use, patients with hepatic dysfunction should receive reduced dosages.

Oil in the injectable forms can cause oil embolus if the agent inadvertently is injected intravenously. With high doses of injected progestins, gluteal abscesses also can occur. Patients who are hypersensitive to the oil carrier used for injection (usually sesame or castor oil) may have a local or systemic hypersensitivity reaction.

NURSING PROCESS APPLICATION

The following information assists the nurse in caring for a patient receiving a progestin.

Assessment

• Review the patient's history for a preexisting condition that contraindicates the use of a progestin, such as known hypersensitivity to the drug, thrombophlebitis, thromboembolic disorder, cerebral apoplexy, breast cancer (except for palliative therapy), undiagnosed vaginal bleeding, or missed abortion.
• Review the patient's history for a preexisting condition that requires cautious use of a progestin, such as epilepsy, migraine headache, asthma, cardiac dysfunction, renal dysfunction (except for palliative therapy for renal cancer), depression, or diabetes mellitus.
• Assess the patient for adverse reactions to the prescribed progestin, such as fluid retention, thromboembolus, menstrual irregularities, breast tenderness, or gluteal abscess.
• Assess the effectiveness of the prescribed progestin periodically.
• Assess the patient for a local or systemic hypersensitivity reactions after injection of an oil-based progestin.
• Evaluate the patient's and family's knowledge about the prescribed progestin.

Nursing diagnoses

The following examples represent appropriate nursing diagnoses for a patient receiving a progestin.
• Potential for injury related to a preexisting condition that contraindicates the use of a progestin

• Potential for injury related to a preexisting condition that requires cautious use of a progestin
• Potential for injury related to adverse drug reactions
• Altered protection related to a local or systemic hypersensitivity reaction to an oil-based progestin injection
• Knowledge deficit related to the prescribed progestin

Planning and implementation

• Do not administer a progestin to a patient with a condition that contraindicates its use.
• Administer a progestin cautiously to a patient at risk because of a preexisting condition.
• Monitor the patient regularly for adverse reactions during progestin therapy.
• Monitor the patient for mild fluid retention characterized by edema and weight gain, especially in a patient with cardiac insufficiency. If fluid retention occurs, restrict the patient's daily fluid intake to four 8-oz glasses and sodium intake to 2 grams as prescribed. Weigh the patient at the same time every day on the same scale with similar clothing.
• *Do not administer an injectable progestin intravenously. The oil in the formulation can cause an oil embolus.*
• Inspect the gluteal injection sites of a parenteral progestin regularly for signs and symptoms of abscess, such as swelling, a fluid-filled sac, and localized pain. If an abscess occurs, avoid injecting the drug into the area, provide symptomatic relief such as frequent application of warm compresses, and encourage the patient not to put pressure on the site.
• *Monitor liver function studies regularly and observe the patient for signs and symptoms of hepatotoxicity, such as jaundice, dark-colored urine, clay-colored stools, and pruritus.*
• *Monitor the patient for signs and symptoms of thromboembolism, such as sudden onset of shortness of breath, loss of vision, severe headache, paresis, or local inflammation and tenderness in an extremity. Notify the physician immediately if thromboembolism is suspected. Expect to begin emergency treatment and anticoagulation therapy as prescribed.*
• Notify the physician if any other adverse reactions occur.
• *Monitor the patient for local and systemic hypersensitivity reactions regularly. Keep standard emergency equipment nearby. Notify the physician immediately if such reactions occur.*
• Avoid local adverse reactions to I.M. progestin by injecting the drug deeply and applying pressure and ice after the injection to lessen pain and irritation.

Patient teaching

- Teach the patient and family the name, dose, frequency, action, and adverse effects of the prescribed progestin.
- Explain the probability of fluid retention to the patient and how to recognize it. Inform the patient that fluid retention from progestin therapy usually is mild and not clinically significant.
- *Teach the patient to recognize and immediately report the signs and symptoms of thromboembolism.*
- *Explain that jaundice may indicate hepatotoxicity. Instruct the patient to report immediately any skin yellowing, dark-colored urine, clay-colored stools, or pruritus.*
- Inform the female patient that menstrual irregularities and breast tenderness may occur with progestin therapy.
- *Teach the patient to recognize the signs and symptoms of a local or systemic hypersensitivity reaction and to notify the physician promptly if they occur.*
- Advise the patient that the injections will be painful. Provide reassurance that measures will be taken to make injections less painful.
- Instruct the patient to notify the physician if adverse reactions occur.

Evaluation

The following examples represent appropriate evaluation statements for a patient receiving a progestin.

- The patient has no conditions that contraindicate progestin therapy.
- The patient exhibits no signs of complications in the preexisting condition linked to the prescribed progestin.
- The patient develops no adverse reactions to the prescribed progestin.
- The patient displays no local or systemic hypersensitivity reactions during progestin therapy.
- The patient and family express an accurate understanding of the points taught about the prescribed progestin.
- The patient correctly identifies adverse reactions to the prescribed progestin and describes what to do if they occur.

CORTICOSTEROIDS

Corticosteroids are naturally occurring hormones secreted by the adrenal cortex or synthetic analogues of these hormones. They include dexamethasone, hydrocortisone, methylprednisolone, prednisolone, and prednisone.

The corticosteroids target many different cells. The physiologic effects of these drugs vary widely, depending on the type of cells they act on.

PHARMACOKINETICS

When administered orally, the corticosteroids are absorbed rapidly and distributed throughout the body, including the central nervous system. These drugs are metabolized extensively in the liver and then excreted as conjugated metabolites in the urine. Prednisone must be metabolically activated in the liver.

The corticosteroids have a rapid onset of action and reach peak concentration within 1 hour of administration. They provide varying durations of action: hydrocortisone, 8 to 12 hours; prednisone, 24 hours; prednisolone and methylprednisolone, 36 hours; and dexamethasone, 3 days.

PHARMACODYNAMICS

The antitumor mechanisms of action of the corticosteroids are not understood fully. The drugs may inhibit glucose transportation and phosphorylation, two processes that supply cell energy. Without appropriate energy supplies, lymphoid proliferation is inhibited, lymphocytic mitosis is impaired, and cell lysis soon results. Leukemic lymphocyte cells may have specific receptors that selectively bind the corticosteroids, thereby targeting the drugs to the tumor cells.

Corticosteroids are prescribed for edema from metastatic cancer because the drugs are anti-inflammatory. (For more information about this action, see Chapter 57, Corticosteroid and Other Immunosuppressant Agents.)

Corticosteroids are contraindicated in a patient with a systemic fungal infection or known hypersensitivity to any component of the drug. They must be used with caution in a patient with GI ulceration, renal disease, hypertension, osteoporosis, varicella, vaccinia, exanthema, diabetes mellitus, hypothyroidism, thromboembolic disorders, seizures, myasthenia gravis, congestive heart failure, tuberculosis, ocular herpes simplex, hypoalbuminemia, emotional instability, or psychosis.

PHARMACOTHERAPEUTICS

The corticosteroids have a lympholytic action that makes them useful in treating lymphocytic leukemias, myeloma, and malignant lymphomas. For these indications, these drugs usually are used with cytotoxic agents to induce remissions.

dexamethasone (Decadron). Dexamethasone is used primarily for its anti-inflammatory properties in patients with intracranial metastases and spinal cord compression.
Usual adult dosage: for intracranial metastases, 3 to 6 mg I.V. or P.O. every 6 hours; for spinal cord compression, 4 to 10 mg I.V. or P.O. immediately, then every 6 hours. (Dosages are extremely individualized and may be higher.)

hydrocortisone (Cortef). Hydrocortisone is used in combination with aminoglutethimide or as replacement therapy after an adrenalectomy.

Usual adult dosage: for postadrenalectomy patients or those receiving aminoglutethimide therapy, 20 to 30 mg P.O. daily as replacement therapy.

methylprednisolone (Medrol, Solu-Medrol). In injectable form, methylprednisolone is prescribed to induce leukemia remission and to treat Hodgkin's disease, hypercalcemia, and the edema caused by intracranial metastases. It may be used instead of prednisone when the patient cannot tolerate oral therapy.

Usual adult dosage: 4 mg I.M. or I.V. of methylprednisolone for 5 mg of prednisone; requires dosage adjustments.

prednisolone (Delta-Cortef). Prednisolone is used for the same indications as methylprednisolone. It may be used interchangeably with prednisone.

Usual adult dosage: to induce leukemia remission, 40 to 50 mg/m^2/day P.O.; for Hodgkin's disease, 20 to 30 mg P.O. daily or 40 to 100 mg/m^2/day P.O. in patients with resistant disease; for hypercalcemia and edema from intracranial metastases, 60 to 80 mg P.O. daily.

prednisone (Deltasone). Prednisone is used for the same indications as methylprednisolone. The dosage varies according to the protocol used.

Usual adult dosage: to induce leukemia remission, 40 to 50 mg/m^2/day P.O.; for Hodgkin's disease, 20 to 30 mg P.O. daily or 40 to 100 mg/m^2/day P.O. in patients with resistant disease; for hypercalcemia and edema from intracranial metastases, 60 to 80 mg P.O. daily.

Drug interactions

Many drug interactions of clinical significance are identified with the corticosteroids. (For more information, see Chapter 57, Corticosteroid and Other Immunosuppressant Agents.)

ADVERSE DRUG REACTIONS

Most adverse reactions to synthetic corticosteroids are similar to those of natural corticosteroids. The large doses required for cancer therapy account for the possible enhanced toxicities.

Patients with cardiovascular disease, peptic ulcer, diabetes, and psychological disturbances are more likely to have adverse reactions to the corticosteroids, including fluid and sodium retention and increased potassium and calcium excretion. These may complicate the care of a patient with congestive heart failure. The corticosteroids also can disturb glucose metabolism and promote gluconeogenesis and anti-insulin effects that cause hyperglycemia. Epigastric distress may occur because corticosteroids increase gastric hydrochloric acid secretion and decrease gastric mucus secretion.

Behavioral changes commonly caused by the corticosteroids include mood swings, insomnia, nervousness, euphoria, sense of well-being, and psychosis. These reactions may occur with any dosage change. Increased appetite also is common.

Because of their lympholytic effects and their ability to suppress mitosis in lymphocytes, the corticosteroids can cause immunosuppression. They also may mask signs of infection, such as fever and inflammation. During prolonged therapy, patients may develop cataracts, glaucoma, or ocular infections.

Patients risk the complete suppression of the adrenal hormones. Many patients on long-term therapy develop some cushingoid symptoms, such as moon face, truncal obesity, purpura, buffalo hump, and acne. Patients withdrawn from long-term corticosteroid therapy may develop depression. The symptoms include fatigue, psychosomatic complaints, crying spells, and insomnia.

NURSING PROCESS APPLICATION

The following information assists the nurse in caring for a patient receiving a corticosteroid.

Assessment

• Review the patient's history for a preexisting condition that contraindicates the use of a corticosteroid, such as systemic fungal infections or known hypersensitivity to any component of the drug.
• Review the patient's history for a preexisting condition that requires cautious use of a corticosteroid, such as GI ulceration, renal disease, hypertension, osteoporosis, varicella, vaccinia, exanthema, diabetes mellitus, hypothyroidism, thromboembolic disorders, seizures, myasthenia gravis, congestive heart failure, tuberculosis, ocular herpes simplex, hypoalbuminemia, emotional instability, or psychosis.
• Assess the patient for adverse reactions to the prescribed corticosteroid, such as fluid and electrolyte imbalances, hyperglycemia, GI distress, behavioral changes, immunosuppression, ocular disorders, and cushingoid symptoms.
• Review the patient's medication history to identify the use of drugs that may interact with the prescribed corticosteroid, such as barbiturates, salicylates, oral contraceptives, cholestyramine, or antihypertensive agents.
• Assess the effectiveness of the prescribed corticosteroid regularly.
• Assess the patient for signs of infection regularly.
• Evaluate the patient's and family's knowledge about the prescribed corticosteroid.

Nursing diagnoses

The following examples represent appropriate nursing diagnoses for a patient receiving a corticosteroid.

• Potential for injury related to a preexisting condition that contraindicates the use of a corticosteroid

• Potential for injury related to a preexisting condition that requires cautious use of a corticosteroid

• Potential for injury related to adverse drug reactions

• Potential for infection related to immunosuppression caused by a corticosteroid

• Knowledge deficit related to the prescribed corticosteroid

Planning and implementation

• Do not administer a corticosteroid to a patient with a condition that contraindicates its use.

• Administer a corticosteroid cautiously to a patient at risk because of a preexisting condition.

• Monitor the patient regularly for adverse reactions during corticosteroid therapy, especially if the patient has cardiovascular disease, peptic ulcer, diabetes mellitus, or a psychological disturbance.

• *Monitor the patient for signs of fluid retention.* Weigh the patient daily at the same time, with the same scale, and with similar clothing to detect a sudden weight gain, auscultate the lungs for crackles, and observe for ankle swelling, puffy eyelids, swollen fingers, and other signs of edema. If fluid retention occurs, notify the physician and restrict the patient's daily fluid intake to four 8-oz glasses and sodium intake to 2 grams as prescribed.

• *Monitor the patient's serum sodium, potassium, and calcium levels for abnormalities (hypernatremia, hypokalemia, or hypocalcemia).* If a potassium supplement has not been prescribed, provide potassium-rich foods, such as bananas, oranges, raisins, prunes, and cranberry juice. Also provide calcium-rich foods, such as milk, cheese, and yogurt. If hypernatremia occurs, restrict the patient's sodium intake.

• *Monitor the fasting blood glucose level periodically to detect steroid-induced diabetes, which may occur in a patient on long-term therapy, or loss of blood glucose control in a diabetic patient.*

• Minimize GI distress by administering an oral agent with meals and avoiding concomitant use of aspirin or any other nonsteroidal anti-inflammatory drug.

• Provide additional snacks to the patient with an increased appetite.

• Assess the patient routinely for vision disturbances or eye discomfort. Ensure that the patient is scheduled for routine eye examinations to detect cataracts, glaucoma, or ocular infections.

• *Monitor the patient for signs of adrenal hormone suppression, such as hypotension, dehydration, fatigue, hyponatremia, diarrhea, and anorexia, during and after*

corticosteroid therapy. Administer additional corticosteroids as prescribed during times of stress.

• Monitor the patient for cushingoid symptoms, such as moon face, truncal obesity, purpura, buffalo hump, and acne.

• *Assess the patient for depression when tapering off the corticosteroid dosage after prolonged therapy. Particularly note fatigue, psychosomatic complaints, crying spells, and insomnia. Provide symptomatic support as needed.*

• Administer parenteral dexamathasone or methylprednisolone by slow I.V. push, or give methylprednisolone by I.M. injection, as prescribed.

• Notify the physician if adverse reactions occur.

• *Monitor the patient's WBC count for leukopenia, which indicates immunosuppression. If leukopenia occurs, monitor the patient for signs of infection, such as delayed wound healing, chills, malaise, or productive cough. Corticosteroids may mask other signs of infection, such as fever and inflammation.*

• *Use aseptic technique when handling or dressing all wounds, injection sites, tubes, and catheters.*

• *Take infection control measures. For example, keep the patient away from others with infections, promote adequate rest for the patient, and ensure that the patient remains well hydrated.*

• Notify the physician if leukopenia or signs of infection occur. Expect to administer an antibiotic as prescribed.

Patient teaching

• Teach the patient and family the name, dose, frequency, action, and adverse effects of the prescribed corticosteroid.

• Instruct the patient to obtain a daily weight. Also advise the patient to observe for edema and notify the physician if it occurs.

• *Teach the patient to recognize the signs and symptoms of hypocalcemia and hypokalemia. Advise the patient to consume more potassium-rich and calcium-rich foods.*

• *Instruct the patient to recognize the signs and symptoms of hyperglycemia, such as polyuria and polydipsia. Advise the diabetic patient to test blood glucose regularly and adjust the usual treatment according to the glucose level as prescribed.*

• Teach the patient when and how to take an oral corticosteroid to minimize GI distress.

• *Instruct the patient to contact the physician about missed doses.*

• Be aware that the behavioral changes associated with corticosteroid therapy may benefit the cancer patient initially. Euphoria and a sense of well-being combined with increased appetite temporarily may improve the patient's life-style. Advise the patient and family that such effects

may change negatively to mood swings, nervousness, or psychosis. These negative behavioral changes are reversible with drug discontinuation.
• Stress the importance of having routine blood studies done throughout corticosteroid therapy to detect adverse reactions.
• *Teach the patient to use infection control measures during corticosteroid therapy.*
• *Advise the patient to report vision changes or eye discomfort immediately and to have regular eye examinations by an ophthalmologist.*
• Inform the patient that corticosteroid therapy may increase the appetite. Encourage the use of nutritious snacks to meet appetite demands.
• Advise the patient who is taking the drug for more than 1 week not to discontinue it abruptly. Explain that the dosage must be decreased gradually.
• Inform the patient that cushingoid symptoms may change the appearance. Reassure the patient that these changes are drug-related.
• *Teach the patient to recognize and immediately report the signs and symptoms of adrenal insufficiency. These effects may require a dosage increase. Also advise the patient to notify the physician if illness, injury, or other stress occurs because a dosage increase may be needed.*
• *Advise the patient to wear or carry medical identification at all times. Also instruct the patient to notify any health care professional about corticosteroid therapy before undergoing other treatments.*
• Instruct the patient to notify the physician if adverse reactions occur.

Evaluation

The following examples represent appropriate evaluation statements for a patient receiving a corticosteroid.
• The patient has no conditions that contraindicate corticosteroid therapy.
• The patient exhibits no signs of complications in the preexisting condition linked to the prescribed corticosteroid.
• The patient experiences no adverse reactions to the prescribed corticosteroid.
• The patient remains free of infection throughout corticosteroid therapy.
• The patient and family express an accurate understanding of the points taught about the prescribed corticosteroid.
• The patient correctly identifies infection control measures to use during corticosteroid therapy.

GONADOTROPIN-RELEASING HORMONE ANALOGUES

The gonadotropin-releasing hormone analogues goserelin acetate and leuprolide acetate are indicated for advanced prostate cancer.

PHARMACOKINETICS

Not active orally, goserelin and leuprolide are administered by injection.

Absorption, distribution, metabolism, excretion

Goserelin acetate is absorbed slowly for the first 8 days, and rapidly and continuously thereafter. Its distribution, metabolism, and excretion are not defined clearly.

After S.C. injection, leuprolide is absorbed well, but its distribution, metabolism, and excretion have not been determined. After I.M. administration of leuprolide suspension, the drug is released slowly and gradually from a biodegradable copolymer titus, providing a prolonged duration of action and allowing monthly administration.

Onset, peak, duration

Goserelin achieves a peak concentration level after 12 to 15 days. Its serum half-life is about 4.2 hours in patients with normal renal function.

With daily leuprolide injections, the patient's testosterone level initially rises but falls to castration level in 2 to 4 weeks. The plasma half-life of leuprolide is about 3 hours.

PHARMACODYNAMICS

Goserelin and leuprolide act on a man's pituitary gland to increase luteinizing hormone (LH) secretion, which stimulates testosterone production. The peak testosterone level is reached about 72 hours after daily administration. However, with long-term administration, goserelin and leuprolide inhibit LH release from the pituitary and subsequently inhibit testicular release of testosterone. Because prostate tumor cells are stimulated by testosterone, the reduced testosterone level inhibits tumor growth.

PHARMACOTHERAPEUTICS

Goserelin and leuprolide are used for the palliative treatment of metastatic prostate cancer. The drugs lower the testosterone level without the adverse psychological effects of castration or the adverse cardiovascular effects of diethylstilbestrol.

goserelin acetate (Zoladex). Used to manage advanced prostate cancer, goserelin is administered subcutaneously. For this indication, it has no significant contraindications or precautions.

Usual adult dosage: 3.6 mg S.C. every 28 days.

leuprolide acetate (Lupron). Used to manage advanced prostate cancer, leuprolide may be administered subcutaneously or intramuscularly. Although leuprolide has no contraindications, it should be used with caution in a patient with hypersensitivity to benzyl alcohol, a preservative used in some formulations.

Usual adult dosage: 1 mg S.C. daily or 7.5 mg I.M. monthly.

Drug interactions

No drug interactions have been identified with goserelin or leuprolide.

ADVERSE DRUG REACTIONS

Generally well-tolerated, goserelin and leuprolide cause fewer adverse reactions than diethylstilbestrol. Hot flashes are the most commonly reported reactions to goserelin and leuprolide, ranging in severity from mild flushing to frequent sweating for 40% to 70% of patients. Impotence and decreased libido also are common. Disease symptoms and pain may worsen or flare during the first 2 weeks of goserelin or leuprolide therapy. The flare can be fatal in patients with bony vertebral metastases because it can increase nerve compression.

Peripheral edema occurs in about 8% of patients. Nausea, vomiting, constipation, or anorexia occur in about 2%. Thromboembolic complications are uncommon; gynecomastia and breast tenderness are rare.

NURSING PROCESS APPLICATION

The following information assists the nurse in caring for a patient receiving a gonadotropin-releasing hormone analogue.

Assessment

• Review the patient's history for a preexisting condition that requires cautious use of leuprolide, such as hypersensitivity to benzyl alcohol.

• Assess the patient for adverse reactions to the prescribed gonadotropin-releasing hormone analogue, such as hot flashes, sexual dysfunction, peripheral edema, GI distress, thromboembolic complications, gynecomastia, and breast tenderness.

• Assess the effectiveness of the prescribed gonadotropin-releasing hormone analogue regularly.

• Assess the patient for tumor flare during the first 2 weeks of gonadotropin-releasing hormone analogue therapy.

• Evaluate the patient's and family's knowledge about the prescribed gonadotropin-releasing hormone analogue.

Nursing diagnoses

The following examples represent appropriate nursing diagnoses for a patient receiving a gonadotropin-releasing hormone analogue.

• Potential for injury related to a preexisting condition that requires cautious use of leuprolide

• Potential for injury related to adverse drug reactions

• Pain related to tumor flare caused by a gonadotropin-releasing hormone analogue

• Knowledge deficit related to the prescribed gonadotropin-releasing hormone analogue

Planning and implementation

• Administer leuprolide cautiously to a patient at risk because of a preexisting condition.

• Monitor the patient regularly for adverse reactions during therapy.

• Assess the patient for signs of peripheral edema, such as ankle swelling.

• Monitor hydration if the patient experiences anorexia, nausea, or vomiting. Administer an antiemetic as prescribed.

• Increase the patient's fluid and fiber intake (unless contraindicated) to prevent constipation. If constipation occurs, administer a laxative as prescribed.

• *Monitor the patient for signs of thromboembolic complications, such as sudden onset of shortness of breath, vision loss, severe headache, paresis, or local inflammation and tenderness in an extremity. If any of these signs occur, notify the physician immediately and prepare to administer emergency treatment.*

• Notify the physician if any other adverse reactions occur.

• Monitor the patient for tumor flare, which is exhibited by an increase in disease symptoms and pain during the first 2 weeks of gonadotropin-releasing hormone analogue therapy.

• Increase the analgesic dosage as prescribed to control pain.

• *Notify the physician immediately at the first sign of tumor flare. This reaction can be fatal in a patient with bony vertebral metastasis.*

Patient teaching

• Teach the patient and family the name, dose, frequency, action, and adverse effects of the prescribed gonadotropin-releasing hormone analogue.

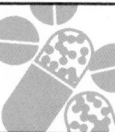

SELECTED MAJOR DRUGS

Hormonal antineoplastic agents

This chart summarizes the major hormonal antineoplastic agents currently in clinical use.

DRUG	MAJOR INDICATIONS	USUAL ADULT DOSAGES	CONTRAINDICATIONS AND PRECAUTIONS
Estrogens			
diethylstilbestrol (DES)	Breast cancer in post-menopausal women	5 to 15 mg P.O. daily	• Know that DES is contraindicated in a pregnant patient or one with known or suspected breast cancer (except in selected patients being treated for metastatic disease); estrogen-dependent neoplasia; undiagnosed abnormal genital bleeding; active thrombophlebitis or thromboembolic disorder; a history of thrombophlebitis, thrombosis, or thromboembolic disorder associated with previous use of estrogen (except when used to treat breast or prostate cancer).
	Prostate cancer	1 to 3 mg P.O. daily	• Administer with caution to a patient with epilepsy, migraine headache, cardiac or renal dysfunction, depression, impaired liver function, or metabolic bone disease associated with hypercalcemia.
Antiestrogens			
tamoxifen	Metastatic breast cancer that is estrogen receptor-positive, especially in post-menopausal women; adjunct to surgery in post-menopausal women whose axillary lymph nodes harbor cancer cells, and estrogen receptor-positive tumors	10 to 20 mg P.O. b.i.d.	• Know that tamoxifen is contraindicated in a pregnant or lactating patient or one with known hypersensitivity to the drug. • Administer with caution to a patient with leukopenia or thrombocytopenia.
Androgens			
fluoxymesterone	Metastatic breast cancer in postmenopausal women	10 to 40 mg P.O. daily in divided doses	• Know that fluoxymesterone is contraindicated in a pregnant or lactating patient, a male with breast or prostate cancer, or any patient with known hypersensitivity to the drug or serious cardiac, hepatic, or renal disease. • Administer with caution to a patient with benign prostatic hypertrophy.
Adrenocortical suppressants			
aminoglutethimide	Hormonally responsive skin, soft tissue, and bone lesions	250 mg P.O. q.i.d., may be increased to a maximum of 2 grams/day	• Know that aminoglutethimide is contraindicated in a pregnant or lactating patient or one with known hypersensitivity to the drug or glutethimide.
Progestins			
medroxyprogesterone	Advanced endometrial or renal cancer	400 to 1,000 mg I.M. weekly	• Know that medroxyprogesterone is contraindicated in a patient with known hypersensitivity to the drug, thrombophlebitis, thromboembolic disorder, cerebral apoplexy, breast cancer (except for palliative therapy), undiagnosed vaginal bleeding, or missed abortion. • Administer with caution to a patient with epilepsy, migraine headache, asthma, cardiac dysfunction, renal dysfunction (except for palliative therapy for renal cancer), depression, or diabetes mellitus.

- *Teach the patient and family how to prepare and administer S.C. injections of goserelin or leuprolide and how to rotate injection sites. The manufacturer provides the syringes and needles for injection.*
- *Instruct the patient to keep an accurate record of the doses administered and the injection sites.*
- Inform the patient of the risk of hot flashes, impotence, decreased libido, and tumor flare.
- Encourage the patient to consult with the physician about increasing the analgesic dosage to control pain.
- Teach the patient how to manage troublesome adverse GI reactions. For example, advise a patient with anorexia to eat smaller but more frequent meals or counsel a patient with constipation to increase fluid and dietary fiber intake.
- *Review the signs and symptoms of thromboembolic complications and instruct the patient to notify the physician immediately if any occur.*
- Inform the patient that gynecomastia and breast tenderness may occur.
- Instruct the patient to notify the physician if any other adverse reactions occur.

Evaluation

The following examples represent appropriate evaluation statements for a patient receiving a gonadotropin-releasing hormone analogue.

- The patient exhibits no signs of complications in the preexisting condition linked to leuprolide.
- The patient demonstrates no adverse reactions to the prescribed gonadotropin-releasing hormone analogue.
- The patient reports adequate pain relief during tumor flare.
- The patient and family express an accurate understanding of the points taught about the prescribed gonadotropin-releasing hormone analogue.
- The patient correctly demonstrates how to administer the prescribed gonadotropin-releasing hormone analogue.

CHAPTER SUMMARY

Chapter 69 discussed the hormonal agents used to treat malignant tumors. Here are the chapter highlights.
- The hormonal antineoplastic agents are not cytotoxic, but inhibit malignant growth by altering the hormonal environment of the tumor.
- Most hormonal antineoplastic agents have a slow onset of action and require a therapeutic trial of 2 to 3 months.
- Estrogen therapy is used as a palliative treatment for metastatic breast cancer in postmenopausal women and for metastatic prostate cancer.

- The nurse should inform male patients that estrogen therapy may cause feminization and female patients that it may cause decreased libido and breast tenderness.
- The antiestrogen tamoxifen is the drug of choice for treating advanced breast cancer of estrogen receptor-positive tumors in postmenopausal women. The drug can cause tumor flare.
- Usually administered orally, androgens prove effective in treating breast cancer in men and advanced breast cancer in women. Androgen therapy causes virilization and fluid retention.
- The antiandrogen flutamide is used with a gonadotropin-releasing hormone analogue to treat advanced prostate cancer.
- About 50% of patients taking the adrenocortical suppressant aminoglutethimide experience rash, hypotension, fatigue, drowsiness, and dizziness.
- The duration of action for progestins varies widely from 1 to 3 days for megestrol to 4 to 6 weeks for I.M. medroxyprogesterone. When giving an I.M. progestin injection, the nurse must be careful to avoid inadvertent I.V. injection.
- The corticosteroids are indicated for lymphocytic leukemias, myeloma, and malignant lymphomas.
- Patients taking corticosteroids may experience fluid and sodium retention, behavioral changes, immunosuppression, and cushingoid symptoms.
- The gonadotropin-releasing hormone analogues goserelin and leuprolide treat advanced prostate cancer by decreasing testosterone levels.
- By applying the nursing process, the nurse can help the patient cope with hormonal antineoplastic treatment. Nursing care includes teaching about potential adverse reactions and using specific interventions to minimize them.

STUDY QUESTIONS

See Appendix 1 for answers.

1. Joel Mayer, age 55, has advanced prostate cancer. Along with surgery, his physician prescribes the estrogen chlorotrianisene (TACE) 12 mg P.O. daily. Therapeutic effects are likely to be seen how long after estrogen therapy begins?
(a) immediately
(b) 2 to 3 weeks
(c) 1 to 2 months
(d) 2 to 3 months

2. How does chlorotrianisene exert its therapeutic effects in treating prostate cancer?
(a) It increases luteinizing hormone (LH) secretion by a negative feedback mechanism.
(b) It suppresses LH secretion, which decreases testicular androgen secretion.
(c) It inhibits androgen uptake in target tissue.
(d) It competes with testosterone by binding to receptor sites.

3. Because Irene McKenna, age 42, does not tolerate estrogen therapy, her physician prescribes tamoxifen 10 mg P.O. b.i.d. What is the mechanism of action of this antiestrogen agent?
(a) It alters the structure of cancer cells.
(b) It binds to estrogen receptors and inhibits estrogen-mediated tumor growth.
(c) It interrupts DNA synthesis in estrogen-receptor positive tumors.
(d) It inhibits estrogen synthesis in estrogen-dependent tumors.

4. After initial treatment with tamoxifen, Ms. McKenna develops an increase in lesion number and size. What may account for this reaction?
(a) tumor flare
(b) metastasis to bone
(c) resistance to therapy
(d) tamoxifen hypersensitivity

5. The physician could have prescribed an androgen for palliative treatment of Ms. McKenna's advanced breast cancer. Which adverse reaction is associated with androgen therapy?
(a) decreased libido
(b) breast enlargement
(c) breakthrough bleeding
(d) increased facial hair

6. The physician considers surgical adrenalectomy for Ms. McKenna. Because she is a poor surgical candidate, however, the physician decides to use the adrenocortical suppressant aminoglutethimide to produce a reversible chemical adrenalectomy. The physician should prescribe which other drug for Ms. McKenna along with aminoglutethimide?
(a) an anabolic steroid
(b) a synthetic progesterone derivative
(c) a pituitary-suppressive glucocorticoid
(d) a gonadotropin-releasing hormone analogue

7. Judy Miller, age 49, has advanced endometrial cancer. For palliative treatment, her physician is likely to prescribe which type of hormonal antineoplastic agent?
(a) estrogen
(b) androgen
(c) progestin
(d) corticosteroid

8. Leo Jarvis, age 50, has lung cancer with brain metastasis. The physician is most likely to prescribe which type of hormonal agent to reduce edema from intracranial metastasis?
(a) estrogen
(b) androgen
(c) corticosteroid
(d) adrenocortical suppressant

9. Tim Holloway, age 78, has advanced prostate cancer. His physician has prescribed leuprolide 1 mg S.C. daily. During the first 2 weeks of leuprolide therapy, the nurse should be particularly alert for which adverse reaction?
(a) tumor flare
(b) constipation
(c) peripheral edema
(d) thromboembolic complications

10. Which other hormonal antineoplastic agent should the physician prescribe for Mr. Holloway?
(a) flutamide
(b) tamoxifen
(c) prednisone
(d) aminoglutethimide

SELECTED REFERENCES

AHFS drug information 90. (1990). Bethesda, MD: American Society of Hospital Pharmacists.

Cawley, M. (1990). Recent advances in chemotherapy: Administration and nursing implications. *Nursing Clinics of North America, 25*(2), 377-391.

Drug facts and comparisons. (1991). St. Louis: Facts and Comparisons Division, Lippincott.

Goodman and Gilman's the pharmacological basis of therapeutics (8th ed.; 1990). Elmsford, NY: Pergamon Press.

Hankins, W., and Puett, D. (Eds.). *Hormones, cell biology, and cancer: Perspectives and potentials.* New York: John Wiley & Sons.

Hansten, P., and Horn, J. (1989). *Drug interactions* (6th ed.). Philadelphia: Lea & Febiger.

Hoffken, K. (Ed.). (1988). *Agonists in oncology.* New York: Springer-Verlag.

Jordan, V. (Ed.). (1986). *Estrogen antiestrogen action and breast cancer therapy.* Madison, WI: University of Wisconsin Press.

North American Nursing Diagnosis Association (1990). *Taxonomy I - Revised, with official diagnostic categories.* St. Louis: NANDA.

Payne, S. (1990). Coping with palliative chemotherapy. *Journal of Advanced Nursing,* 15(6), 652-658.

Walters, P. (1990). Chemo: A nurse's guide to action, administration, and side effects. *RN* 53(2), 52-67.

OTHER ANTINEOPLASTIC AGENTS

OBJECTIVES

After reading and studying this chapter, the student should be able to:
1. Describe the mechanisms of action for the vinca alkaloids, the podophyllotoxins, asparaginase, procarbazine, hydroxyurea, and interferons.
2. Discuss the indications for the vinca alkaloids, podophyllotoxins, asparaginase, procarbazine, hydroxyurea, and interferons.
3. Compare the major adverse reactions to the vinca alkaloids and the podophyllotoxins.
4. Describe how to apply the nursing process when caring for a patient receiving an antineoplastic agent.

INTRODUCTION

This chapter presents a subclass of antineoplastic agents, known as natural products, that includes the vinca alkaloids and the podophyllotoxins. It also discusses other antineoplastic agents that cannot be included in existing classifications, including asparaginase, procarbazine, hydroxyurea, and interferons. For a summary of representative drugs, see *Selected major drugs: Other antineoplastic agents,* pages 1230 and 1231. For a listing of applicable nursing diagnoses that the nurse may formulate when caring for a patient receiving one of these agents, see *Selected nursing diagnoses: Other antineoplastic agents*. For detailed information on applying the nursing process, see Chapter 6, The Nursing Process and Drug Therapy.

SELECTED NURSING DIAGNOSES

Other antineoplastic agents

The following nursing diagnoses address representative problems and etiologies that a nurse may encounter when caring for a patient who is receiving an other antineoplastic agent. Some of these nursing diagnoses contain generalized etiologies, which the nurse must individualize based on the patient's needs. (For some common nursing diagnoses and related interventions for each drug class, see the "Nursing Process Application" sections of this chapter.)

- Altered health maintenance related to flulike syndrome caused by an antineoplastic agent
- Altered health maintenance related to procarbazine-induced hypertensive crisis
- Altered oral mucous membrane related to stomatitis caused by an antineoplastic agent
- Altered protection related to an acute hypersensitivity reaction to the antineoplastic agent
- Body image disturbance related to alopecia caused by an antineoplastic agent
- Diarrhea related to the adverse GI effects of an antineoplastic agent
- Fluid volume excess related to vincristine-induced syndrome of inappropriate antidiuretic hormone secretion
- Fluid volume excess related to interferon-induced congestive heart failure
- Hyperthermia related to fever caused by an antineoplastic agent

- Impaired gas exchange related to pulmonary changes caused by an antineoplastic agent
- Impaired tissue integrity related to necrosis at the I.V. site caused by extravasation of an antineoplastic agent
- Knowledge deficit related to the prescribed antineoplastic agent
- Pain at the tumor site related to vinblastine administration
- Potential for infection related to bone marrow suppression caused by the antineoplastic agent
- Potential for injury related to a preexisting condition that contraindicates the use of an antineoplastic agent
- Potential for injury related to a preexisting condition that requires cautious use of an antineoplastic agent
- Potential for injury related to adverse drug reactions
- Potential for trauma related to antineoplastic agent-induced nephrotoxicity
- Potential for trauma related to hydroxyurea-induced uric acid nephropathy

VINCA ALKALOIDS

The vinca alkaloids (vinblastine, vincristine, and vindesine) are nitrogenous bases derived from the periwinkle plant. These drugs are cell-cycle-specific for the M phase. (For an explanation, see *Cell cycle* in the introduction to this unit.) They are used to treat various cancers, including Hodgkin's disease, non-Hodgkin's lymphoma, testicular cancer, lymphosarcoma, breast cancer, acute lymphocytic leukemia, Wilms' tumor, rhabdomyosarcoma, and neuroblastoma.

PHARMACOKINETICS

After I.V. administration, the vinca alkaloids are distributed well throughout the body. They undergo moderate hepatic metabolism before being eliminated, primarily in feces; a small percentage is eliminated in urine.

Absorption, distribution, metabolism, excretion

Because the vinca alkaloids are absorbed unpredictably after oral administration, they all are administered intravenously (I.V.). After I.V. administration, the drugs are distributed extensively throughout the body. Vinblastine and vincristine concentrate in platelets and, to a lesser extent, in leukocytes and erythrocytes. Vindesine may be bound extensively in tissue. Neither vinblastine nor vincristine enters the cerebrospinal fluid (CSF) in significant quantities. The extent of CSF penetration by vindesine remains unclear.

The vinca alkaloids are metabolized by the liver. Vinblastine is metabolized to an active metabolite, whereas vincristine is metabolized to inactive metabolites. The drugs then undergo biliary and urinary elimination. Within 72 hours after administration, up to 21% of a vinblastine dose is recovered in the feces and 30% in the urine. Up to 70% of a vincristine dose is recovered in the feces within 72 hours, and 12% in the urine. More than 50% of the vincristine dose is excreted unchanged. Vindesine is eliminated primarily via the biliary route, but its elimination has not been quantified completely. Because of their biliary elimination, the vinca alkaloids may cause toxicity in patients with obstructive liver disease. (For a summary, see *Major administration and excretion routes: Other antineoplastic agents.*)

Major administration and excretion routes: Other antineoplastic agents

This chart clarifies the routes of administration and excretion for the other antineoplastic agents.

DRUG	ADMINISTRATION ROUTES	EXCRETION ROUTES	AMOUNT EXCRETED
vinblastine	Intravenous	Urine Feces	30% within 72 hours 20% within 72 hours
vincristine	Intravenous	Urine, feces	50% unchanged
vindesine	Intravenous	Feces	Unknown
etoposide	Intravenous	Urine Feces	40% to 60% in 72 hours 2% to 16% in 72 hours
teniposide	Intravenous	Urine	40% in 72 hours primarily as metabolites
asparaginase	Intravenous, intramuscular	Unknown	Unknown
procarbazine	Oral	Urine	Less than 5% unchanged; 70% as metabolites within 24 hours
hydroxyurea	Oral	Urine, lungs	50% unchanged; 50% as urea and carbon dioxide
alpha interferons	Intramuscular, subcutaneous	Urine	Unknown

Onset, peak, duration

The vinca alkaloids have multiphasic elimination rates. The terminal half-life is about 25 hours for vinblastine, 85 hours for vincristine, and 24 hours for vindesine.

PHARMACODYNAMICS

The vinca alkaloids are cell-cycle-specific, inhibiting mitosis and causing cell death. These drugs are structurally similar but vary in their ability to enter specific cells. As a rule, a lack of cross-resistance appears among the vinca alkaloids. However, resistance to the vinca alkaloids may result from tubulin protein mutations, which affect drug binding, decrease uptake, and increase the capacity for the drug to flow out of the cell. Drug cross-resistance may include the podophyllotoxins, anthracyclines, and dactinomycin as well as the vinca alkaloids.

Mechanism of action

The vinca alkaloids may disrupt the normal function of the microtubules by binding to the protein tubulin in the microtubules. With the microtubules unable to separate chromosomes properly, the chromosomes are dispersed throughout the cytoplasm or arranged in unusual groupings. As a result, formation of the mitotic spindle is prevented, and the cells cannot complete mitosis. Cell division is arrested in metaphase, causing cell death. Therefore, vinca alkaloids are cell-cycle M-phase-specific. Interruption of the microtubule function also may impair some types of cellular movement, phagocytosis, and central nervous system (CNS) functions.

PHARMACOTHERAPEUTICS

Vinblastine and vincristine have been studied the most extensively. Both display various activities. Vinblastine is used to treat metastatic testicular carcinoma, lymphomas, Kaposi's sarcoma, neuroblastoma, breast carcinoma, and choriocarcinoma. Vincristine is used in combination therapy to treat Hodgkin's disease, non-Hodgkin's lymphoma, Wilms' tumor, rhabdomyosarcoma, and acute lymphocytic leukemia. Vindesine acts effectively against neoplasms that are resistant to vincristine.

vinblastine sulfate (Velban). Vinblastine is most effective when administered with bleomycin and cisplatin to treat metastatic testicular carcinoma. This combined treatment has produced a significant number of complete remissions. Also, when vinblastine is used to treat lymphomas, up to 90% of the patients show significant improvement. Vinblastine also is effective against Kaposi's sarcoma, neuroblastoma, breast carcinoma, and choriocarcinoma. Vinblastine dosing varies significantly, depending on protocol.

Usual adult dosage: initially, 0.1 mg/kg or 3.7 mg/m^2 I.V. with weekly increases in increments of 0.05 mg/kg or 1.8 mg/m^2 until the leukocyte count falls below 3,000/mm^3, the tumor size decreases, or the maximum dose of 0.5 mg/kg or 18.5 mg/m^2 is reached. For maintenance therapy, 0.05 mg/kg or 1.8 mg/m^2 I.V. less than the final dosage is given every 7 to 14 days. A 50% dosage reduction is recommended for patients with a direct serum bilirubin level that exceeds 3 mg/ml.

vincristine sulfate (Oncovin). Vincristine's activity resembles that of vinblastine, with important differences. Because the drug does not cause severe bone marrow suppression, it commonly is used in combination therapy. Vincristine is highly effective in the MOPP (mechlorethamine, vincristine [Oncovin], procarbazine, and prednisone) regimen used to treat Hodgkin's disease. It also is used to treat non-Hodgkin's lymphoma, Wilms' tumor, rhabdomyosarcoma, and acute lymphocytic leukemia in children. It is more effective than vinblastine against lymphocytic leukemia. The dosing schedules vary.
Usual adult dosage: 1.4 mg/m^2 I.V. in a single dose, no more frequently than once weekly. The total single dose for adults should not exceed 2 mg. A 50% dosage reduction is recommended for patients with a direct serum bilirubin level that exceeds 3 mg/ml.
Usual pediatric dosage: for inducing remission in childhood leukemias, dosage not to exceed 2 mg/m^2 I.V. weekly. For children who weigh 10 kg or less or have a body-surface area of less than 1 m^2, 0.05 mg/kg once a week. A 50% dosage reduction is recommended for patients with a direct serum bilirubin level that exceeds 3 mg/ml.

vindesine (Eldisine). Researchers continue to study the clinical usefulness of vindesine. The drug is effective against lymphomas and chronic granulocytic leukemia in a blastocyte crisis. Vindesine is effective against vincristine-resistant tumors.
Usual adult dosage: 3 to 4 mg/m^2 I.V. weekly.

Drug interactions

Researchers have identified no significant drug interactions with the vinca alkaloids.

ADVERSE DRUG REACTIONS

Minor differences in the chemical structure of the vinca alkaloids cause significant differences in toxicity. Vinblastine and vindesine toxicities occur primarily as bone marrow suppression, manifested by leukopenia and slight thrombocytopenia. Leukopenia increases the patient's risk of infection, especially if the absolute granulocyte count is less than 1,000 mm^3. In patients receiving corticosteroids, the inflammatory response may be decreased, and the signs and symptoms of infection may be difficult to detect.

Alopecia occurs in up to 50% of patients receiving vinca alkaloids, with hair loss more likely with vincristine than vinblastine. Many patients experience partial alopecia; others, total. Men are as affected as women by alopecia of the scalp, eyebrows, eyelashes, and body. Alopecia is reversible when the drugs are discontinued, and hair may begin to regrow during therapy. Although scalp tourniquets and ice caps have been used to decrease scalp circulation and limit the drug's effect on hair cells, results have been insignificant, and these methods may provide a sanctuary for cancer cells. (For more information, see the introduction to this unit.)

Neuromuscular abnormalities frequently occur with vincristine and occasionally with vinblastine. Peripheral neuropathies, which usually are dose-limiting with vincristine and vindesine, may include loss of deep tendon reflexes, paresthesia, numbness, pain, and tingling. Other neurotoxicities with vincristine include encephalopathies and cranial nerve dysfunction, such as vocal cord paralysis, ptosis (upper eyelid drooping), and jaw pain.

Vinca alkaloids may cause severe local necrosis if extravasation occurs. Vindesine may produce pain and phlebitis even without infiltration.

Stomatitis may occur with the vinca alkaloids. Nausea and vomiting that may occur can be controlled with antiemetics. Prophylactic laxatives sometimes can prevent constipation from vincristine.

Vinblastine may produce tumor pain described as an intense stinging or burning in the tumor bed, with an abrupt onset 1 to 3 minutes after drug administration. The pain usually lasts 20 minutes to 3 hours. Vincristine may induce the syndrome of inappropriate antidiuretic hormone (SIADH) secretion.

NURSING PROCESS APPLICATION

The following information assists the nurse in caring for a patient receiving a vinca alkaloid.

Assessment
• Review the patient's history for a preexisting condition that contraindicates the use of a vinca alkaloid, such as pregnancy, lactation, significant granulocytopenia (unless it results from the disease being treated), bacterial infection, or the demyelinating form of Charcot-Marie-Tooth syndrome.
• Review the patient's history for a preexisting condition that requires cautious use of a vinca alkaloid, such as acute uric acid nephropathy or neuromuscular disease.
• Assess the patient for adverse reactions to the prescribed vinca alkaloid, such as bone marrow suppression, alopecia,

neuromuscular abnormalities, local necrosis, stomatitis, nausea, vomiting, or SIADH.
• Assess the effectiveness of the prescribed vinca alkaloid regularly.
• Assess the patient for tumor pain after vinblastine administration.
• Evaluate the patient's and family's knowledge about the prescribed vinca alkaloid.

Nursing diagnoses
The following examples represent appropriate nursing diagnoses for a patient receiving a vinca alkaloid.
• Potential for injury related to a preexisting condition that contraindicates the use of a vinca alkaloid
• Potential for injury related to a preexisting condition that requires cautious use of a vinca alkaloid
• Potential for injury related to adverse drug reactions
• Pain at the tumor site related to vinblastine administration
• Knowledge deficit related to the prescribed vinca alkaloid

Planning and implementation
• Do not administer a vinca alkaloid to a patient with a condition that contraindicates its use.
• Administer a vinca alkaloid cautiously to a patient at risk because of a preexisting condition.
• Monitor the patient regularly for adverse reactions throughout vinca alkaloid therapy.
• *Monitor the patient's complete blood count (CBC) and platelet count regularly.* Note the CBC nadir when caring for a patient with bone marrow suppression. At the nadir, which usually occurs 4 to 10 days after drug administration, the patient is at the greatest risk for problems associated with leukopenia and thrombocytopenia.
• *Monitor the patient for signs and symptoms of infection, such as fever, chills, malaise, and sore throat, if leukopenia occurs. Also take infection control measures until the white blood cell count (WBC) returns to normal.*
• *Monitor the patient with leukopenia for thrombocytopenia because the two occur sequentially. When the platelet count is under 50,000 mm³, the patient is at risk for bleeding. When the count drops below 20,000 mm³, the patient is at severe risk and probably will need a platelet transfusion. Monitor the patient with thrombocytopenia for bleeding gums, increased bruising or petechiae, hypermenorrhea, tarry stools, hematuria, and coffee-ground emesis. Take bleeding precautions until the platelet count returns to normal. Rectal temperatures and intramuscular (I.M.) injections are contraindicated in the patient with thrombocytopenia or leukopenia.*
• *Monitor the patient routinely for dizziness, fatigue, pallor, and shortness of breath with minimal exertion; also monitor laboratory values that would indicate anemia.* The patient who is dehydrated from nausea, vomiting, or anorexia may have a normal hematocrit. Once rehydrated,

the hematocrit will fall, revealing anemia. A patient with a history of myocardial infarction may be at an increased risk for further coronary ischemia. If the patient is not experiencing symptoms related to anemia, transfusions may not be ordered; however, the symptomatic patient will receive a transfusion. Instruct the patient to rest more frequently and to be attentive to diet.

• Monitor the serum uric acid level, if prescribed, periodically throughout therapy to detect rapid cell lysis. If the level becomes elevated, administer allopurinol as prescribed. This drug prevents the rapid accumulation of uric acid.

• *Monitor the patient for neuromuscular abnormalities when administering vinblastine or vincristine.* To detect peripheral neuropathies, assess deep tendon reflexes and ask the patient about paresthesia, numbness, pain, and tingling. During vincristine therapy, observe for signs of other neurotoxicities, such as encephalopathy (drowsiness or decreased level of consciousness) and cranial nerve dysfunction (vocal cord paralysis, jaw pain, or ptosis). Notify the physician if neuromuscular abnormalities occur.

• Increase the patient's fluid and fiber intake during vincristine therapy to prevent constipation. A patient who also is receiving a narcotic for pain may be at increased risk for constipation and require a bowel regimen that includes stool softeners.

• Inspect the patient's mouth regularly for signs of stomatitis, such as redness, swelling, or ulceration of the mucous membrane. If stomatitis is present, provide symptomatic relief. (For more information, see the introduction to this unit.)

• *Examine the I.V. infusion site for evidence of extravasation, such as redness, swelling, or pain on touch, before administering a vinca alkaloid. If extravasation is suspected, change the infusion site to prevent severe local necrosis. Because vindesine may produce pain and phlebitis without infiltration, use a different infusion site for each dose.*

• Monitor hydration if the patient experiences nausea or vomiting. Be aware that antiemetics may be administered in combinations, using various delivery routes. Because most antiemetics have a sedative effect, monitor the patient for vomitus aspiration and hypotension.

• Monitor the patient's fluid intake and output and evaluate the electrolyte levels and urinalysis results when administering vincristine. Particularly note signs of SIADH, such as output less than intake, hyponatremia, increased urine osmolality, and decreased plasma osmolality.

• Consider the time of drug administration when encouraging patient compliance. Some patients prefer treatments in the evening; patients who are employed may prefer treatments on their days off.

• *Handle vinca alkaloids carefully.* (For more information, see the introduction to this unit.) *Administer the prescribed drug directly into the vein or into the injection port in the tubing of a freely infusing I.V. solution. These methods allow for direct observation of the injection site.*

• Use additional appropriate nursing interventions for a patient who experiences bone marrow suppression, nausea, vomiting, stomatitis, or alopecia. (For more information, see the introduction to this unit.)

• Notify the physician if adverse reactions occur.

• *Monitor the patient for intense stinging or burning in the tumor bed that begins abruptly 1 to 3 minutes after vinblastine administration. Relieve pain with an analgesic as prescribed, because the pain may last up to 3 hours.*

Patient teaching

• Teach the patient the name, dose, frequency, action, and adverse effects of the prescribed vinca alkaloid.

• Prepare the patient for alopecia by explaining when hair loss usually begins and that it is gradual and reversible once treatment ends.

• *Explain to the patient that burning or stinging pain commonly occurs at the tumor site after I.V. administration of vinblastine. Reassure the patient that this pain is not caused by a worsening of the tumor, but by cellular destruction that causes tissue swelling.*

• Teach the patient and family the signs and symptoms of neurotoxicity.

• *Plan an effective teaching program about bone marrow suppression that includes the patient's blood counts, potential sites of infection, and personal habits.*

• *Advise the patient with leukopenia to maintain proper hygiene and report signs and symptoms of infection, including fever, cough, sore throat, and a burning sensation during urination.*

• *Instruct the patient at risk for developing leukopenia and thrombocytopenia to avoid cuts and bruises and to use a sponge toothbrush and an electric razor.*

• Instruct the patient to report a sudden headache, which may indicate potentially lethal intracranial bleeding.

• Prevent colonic irritation and bleeding from vincristin-induced constipation by recommending a bowel program that includes prophylactic stool softeners as prescribed.

• Stress the importance of returning for follow-up blood tests.

• *Caution the patient not to engage in activities that require mental alertness if neurotoxicity occurs.*

• Teach the patient how to manage troublesome adverse gastrointestinal (GI) reactions.

• *Advise the patient to alert the nurse immediately if discomfort occurs at the infusion site during drug administration.*

• Instruct the patient to report any adverse reactions to the physician.

• Give the patient written materials about the prescribed vinca alkaloid for home reference.

Evaluation

The following examples represent appropriate evaluation statements for a patient receiving a vinca alkaloid.
• The patient has no conditions that contraindicate the use of a vinca alkaloid.
• The patient exhibits no signs of complications in the preexisting condition linked to the prescribed vinca alkaloid.
• The patient exhibits few adverse reactions to the prescribed vinca alkaloid.
• The patient remains comfortable throughout vincristine administration.
• The patient and family express an accurate understanding of the points taught about the prescribed vinca alkaloid.
• The patient states the importance of alerting the nurse immediately if discomfort occurs at the I.V. infusion site.

PODOPHYLLOTOXINS

The podophyllotoxins etoposide and teniposide are semisynthetic glycosides that are cell-cycle-specific. Teniposide, still an investigational agent, has demonstrated some activity in treating Hodgkin's disease, lymphomas, and brain tumors.

PHARMACOKINETICS

With oral administration, the podophyllotoxins are absorbed incompletely. Although the drugs are distributed widely throughout the body, they achieve poor CSF levels. The podophyllotoxins are excreted primarily in the urine.

Absorption, distribution, metabolism, excretion

After oral administration, about 50% of an etoposide dose is absorbed. The amount of absorption for teniposide has not been quantified. After intravesicular administration of teniposide, systemic toxicity does not seem to occur, which probably indicates minimal systemic absorption. When administered I.V., etoposide and teniposide are 100% bioavailable.

Distribution of both drugs into human body tissues and fluids has not been characterized fully. The drugs are bound extensively to plasma proteins; etoposide is 94% bound and teniposide is 99% bound. They do not appear to penetrate the CNS readily because etoposide achieves CSF levels of less than 5%, and teniposide reaches less than 1%. Drug distribution into breast milk is unknown.

The podophyllotoxins undergo hepatic metabolism. Etoposide is eliminated in urine (as unchanged drug and metabolites) and in the feces. Teniposide is excreted in urine, primarily as metabolites; less than 10% is recovered in feces. (For details, see *Major administration and excretion routes: Other antineoplastic agents,* page 1215.)

Onset, peak, duration

After oral administration, etoposide typically reaches a peak plasma concentration level in 1 to 1.5 hours. The peak plasma concentration after oral administration usually is 50% of that achieved after I.V. administration. The terminal half-life of etoposide ranges from 5 to 11 hours.

After an I.V. dose of 30 mg/m², teniposide attains a peak plasma concentration of 10 mcg/ml. The half-life of teniposide ranges from 10 to 40 hours.

PHARMACODYNAMICS

Although their mechanism of action is understood incompletely, the podophyllotoxins produce several biochemical changes in tumor cells. At low concentrations, these drugs block cells at the late S or G_2 phase. At higher concentrations, they arrest the cells in the G_2 phase. (For more information, see *Cell cycle* in the introduction to this unit.) Etoposide and teniposide can cause single-strand breaks of deoxyribonucleic acid (DNA), possibly by inhibiting topoisomerase II. These drugs also can inhibit nucleoside transport and incorporation into nucleic acids.

PHARMACOTHERAPEUTICS

Podophyllotoxins are prescribed to treat various tumors. Etoposide is used to treat testicular cancer and small-cell lung cancer. It also may be used to treat various lymphomas and leukemias, although these indications have not been approved by the Food and Drug Administration yet. An investigational drug, teniposide is used to treat acute lymphoblastic leukemia.

etoposide [VP-16] (VePesid). Used primarily to treat testicular cancer that fails to respond completely to vinblastine, bleomycin, and cisplatin, etoposide also is used with cisplatin for treating small-cell lung cancer. This podophyllotoxin should be administered over 30 to 60 minutes to minimize hypotensive reactions.
Usual adult dosage: for testicular cancer, 50 to 100 mg/m² I.V. daily for 5 days, or 100 mg/m² I.V. daily on days 1, 3, and 5, repeated every 3 to 4 weeks; for lymphomas and leukemias, individualized dosage based on the patient's response; for small-cell lung cancer, 35 mg/m² I.V. daily for 4 days up to 50 mg/m² I.V. daily for 5 days, repeated every 3 to 4 weeks. As an alternative, oral treatment for small-cell lung cancer is twice the I.V. dosage.

teniposide [VM-26]. Available as an investigational agent, the activity and toxicity of teniposide seem similar to those of etoposide. Teniposide is used with cytarabine to treat acute lymphoblastic leukemia in patients who do not respond to conventional therapy or who have relapsed for the first time. Various dosage regimens have been used for teniposide.

Usual adult dosage: the most common regimens are 100 mg/m^2 I.V. once a week or 50 mg/m^2 I.V. twice a week for 4 to 6 weeks; or 50 mg/m^2 I.V. for 5 days, repeated monthly.

Drug interactions

Researchers have identified no significant drug interactions with etoposide or teniposide.

ADVERSE DRUG REACTIONS

The podophyllotoxins and the vinca alkaloids produce similar adverse reactions. The podophyllotoxins suppress bone marrow with nadirs occurring in 7 to 14 days. These drugs can cause leukopenia and, less commonly, thrombocytopenia; leukopenia resolves in about 3 weeks. About 90% of patients receiving podophyllotoxins experience alopecia, which may resolve as the treatment continues.

About one-third of patients receiving podophyllotoxins develop nausea and vomiting, which lasts 2 to 6 hours. Anorexia is another common reaction. Stomatitis occurs in 5% of patients.

Acute hypotension may result if a podophyllotoxin is infused too rapidly. Slow administration and close patient monitoring can prevent this adverse reaction. Pain and burning at the injection site also have been reported.

Several rare reactions also can occur during podophyllotoxin therapy: acute hypersensitivity, which may be signaled by chills, fever, generalized erythema, pruritus, wheezing, bronchospasm, or tachycardia; transient liver function abnormalities; an elevated alkaline phosphatase level, which indicates impending hepatotoxicity; and peripheral neuropathy.

NURSING PROCESS APPLICATION

The following information assists the nurse in caring for a patient receiving a podophyllotoxin.

Assessment

• Review the patient's history for a preexisting condition that contraindicates the use of a podophyllotoxin, such as pregnancy, lactation, or known hypersensitivity to the drug.
• Assess the patient for adverse reactions to the prescribed podophyllotoxin, such as leukopenia, thrombocytopenia, alopecia, GI distress, hypotension, and acute hypersensitivity reactions.
• Assess the effectiveness of the prescribed podophyllotoxin regularly.

• Assess the patient regularly for signs of stomatitis, such as red, swollen, or ulcerated oral mucosa.
• Evaluate the patient's and family's knowledge about the prescribed podophyllotoxin.

Nursing diagnoses

The following examples represent appropriate nursing diagnoses for a patient receiving a podophyllotoxin.
• Potential for injury related to a preexisting condition that contraindicates the use of a podophyllotoxin
• Potential for injury related to adverse drug reactions
• Altered oral mucous membrane related to podophyllotoxin-induced stomatitis
• Knowledge deficit related to the prescribed podophyllotoxin

Planning and implementation

• Do not administer a podophyllotoxin to a patient with a condition that contraindicates its use.
• Monitor the patient regularly for adverse reactions during podophyllotoxin therapy.
• *Monitor the patient's WBC and platelet counts closely, especially during the expected nadir (days 7 to 14 for the WBC count and days 9 to 16 for the platelet count).* At the nadir, the patient is at the greatest risk for problems associated with leukopenia and thrombocytopenia. Acute complications occur when the absolute granulocyte count is less than 1,000/mm^3 and the platelet count is less than 20,000/mm^3.
• *Monitor the patient with leukopenia for signs of infection, such as fever, sore throat, or chills. Take infection control measures until the WBC count returns to normal.*
• *Monitor the patient with thrombocytopenia for signs of bleeding, such as spontaneous epistaxis, hematuria, or easy bruising. Take bleeding precautions until the platelet count has returned to normal.*
• Administer an antiemetic agent as prescribed before administering the podophyllotoxin, and every 2 to 4 hours, as needed, to prevent or control nausea and vomiting. Light snacks, such as dry crackers or toast and carbonated soda, also may alleviate nausea.
• *Administer I.V. etoposide and teniposide slowly over 30 to 60 minutes to prevent hypotension. Monitor the patient's blood pressure before the infusion and during treatment.*
• *Monitor the patient for signs of an acute hypersensitivity reaction, such as chills, fever, generalized erythema, pruritus, wheezing, bronchospasm, or tachycardia. If a hypersensitivity reaction occurs, stop the infusion and notify the physician immediately. During podophyllotoxin therapy, have standard emergency equipment, diphenhydramine hydrochloride, and epinephrine available.*

• Monitor the patient's liver function studies and alkaline phosphatase level if prescribed. Abnormalities may indicate impending hepatotoxicity.
• Use other appropriate nursing interventions for a patient with bone marrow suppression, nausea, vomiting, or stomatitis. (For details, see the introduction to this unit.)
• Notify the physician if adverse reactions occur.
• Inspect the patient's mouth regularly for signs of stomatitis, which is temporary. Prophylactic mouth care before chemotherapy may decrease stomatitis severity and provide patient comfort. Therapeutic mouth care, including topical antibiotics and analgesics, may be required, depending on the degree of stomatitis.
• Notify the physician if stomatitis persists or worsens.

Patient teaching
• Teach the patient the name, dose, frequency, action, and adverse effects of the prescribed podophyllotoxin.
• Inform the patient that burning or pain may be felt at the infusion site during podophyllotoxin administration.
• *Advise the patient to avoid people with active contagious infections, to watch for signs of infection, and to report them immediately to the physician.*
• *Explain to the patient that acute hypersensitivity reactions may occur with podophyllotoxin therapy. Instruct the patient to report any signs or symptoms promptly.*
• Prepare the patient for possible alopecia by explaining the timing and speed of hair loss and noting that it may affect the scalp, eyebrows, eyelashes, or body hair.
• Teach the patient how to manage troublesome adverse reactions, such as nausea and stomatitis, at home.
• Give the patient written materials about the possible effects of antineoplastic agents for home reference.
• Instruct the patient to notify the physician if adverse reactions persist or worsen.

Evaluation
The following examples represent appropriate evaluation statements for a patient receiving a podophyllotoxin.
• The patient has no conditions that contraindicate podophyllotoxin therapy.
• The patient demonstrates few adverse reactions to the prescribed podophyllotoxin.
• The patient maintains normal integrity of the oral mucous membrane.
• The patient and family express an accurate understanding of the points taught about the prescribed podophyllotoxin.
• The patient correctly identifies signs and symptoms of infection that must be reported.

ASPARAGINASE

Asparaginase, a cell-cycle-specific enzyme, exerts its effect by hydrolyzing exogenous asparagine, which leukemic cells need for survival. Nonleukemic cells can synthesize asparagine and are affected less by asparaginase treatment.

PHARMACOKINETICS

Asparaginase is administered parenterally and is considered 100% bioavailable when administered I.V. and about 50% bioavailable when administered I.M. After administration, it remains in the vascular compartment, with minimal distribution elsewhere. The metabolic route of asparaginase is unknown. Only trace amounts appear in urine.

The peak plasma concentration level relates to the dose and administration route. The half-life of asparaginase varies from 8 to 30 hours. A cumulative plasma concentration may occur with daily dosing, and active enzyme may appear in the blood up to 3 weeks after administration.

PHARMACODYNAMICS

Asparaginase capitalizes on the biochemical differences between normal cells and tumor cells; most normal cells can synthesize asparagine, but some tumor cells depend on exogenous sources. Asparaginase acts as a catalyst in the degradation of asparagine to aspartic acid and ammonia. Deprived of their supply of asparagine, the tumor cells die. Asparaginase is cell-cycle-specific in the G_1 phase.

PHARMACOTHERAPEUTICS

Asparaginase has not proved effective against solid tumors. It is used primarily to induce remission in patients with acute lymphocytic leukemia.

asparaginase [L-asparaginase] (Elspar). Administered I.V. or I.M., asparaginase is used primarily in combination therapies to induce remission in acute lymphocytic leukemia in children. Before administration, an intradermal dose should be given to test for hypersensitivity.
Usual adult dosage: 200 IU/kg I.V. or I.M. daily for 28 days; alternately to avoid anaphylaxis, 1,000 IU/kg I.V. daily for up to 10 days.
Usual pediatric dosage: same as the usual adult dosage.

Drug interactions
Researchers have identified no significant drug interactions with asparaginase.

ADVERSE DRUG REACTIONS

Asparaginase can cause several potentially serious toxicities, which are more severe in adults than in children. Anaphylaxis, the most serious reaction, is more likely to occur with intermittent I.V. dosing than with daily I.V. dosing or I.M. injections.

Many patients receiving asparaginase develop nausea and vomiting shortly after drug administration. Fever, headache, and abdominal pain also may occur. Hepatotoxicity commonly occurs and is manifested by transient and mild liver enzyme elevations, which peak in the second week of therapy.

Hypersensitivity reactions occur in 20% to 35% of patients receiving asparaginase. Anaphylaxis also occurs, with the risk for a reaction rising with successive treatment. Pancreatitis, evidenced by epigastric pain, vomiting, and a high serum amylase level, has appeared in 5% of patients receiving asparaginase. Consequently, patients with a history of pancreatitis should not receive this drug. Patients also may become hyperglycemic due to decreased insulin production. CNS toxicity also may occur in 25% of patients. Personality changes, seizures, and abnormal electroencephalogram (EEG) tracings have been reported. Renal impairment and coagulation abnormalities, such as hypofibrinogenemia and depression of other coagulation factors, also can occur.

NURSING PROCESS APPLICATION

The following information assists the nurse in caring for a patient receiving asparaginase.

Assessment
• Review the patient's history for a preexisting condition that contraindicates the use of asparaginase, such as lactation, pancreatitis or a history of it, or known hypersensitivity to the drug.
• Review the patient's history for a preexisting condition that requires cautious use of asparaginase, such as pregnancy.
• Assess the patient for adverse reactions to asparaginase, such as GI distress, fever, headache, abdominal pain, hepatotoxicity, nephrotoxicity, pancreatitis, hyperglycemia, CNS toxicity, and bleeding.
• Assess the effectiveness of asparaginase regularly.
• Assess the patient for signs of hypersensitivity reactions, such as urticaria, dyspnea, or a sudden change in vital signs.
• Evaluate the patient's and family's knowledge about asparaginase.

Nursing diagnoses
The following examples represent appropriate nursing diagnoses for a patient receiving asparaginase.
• Potential for injury related to a preexisting condition that contraindicates the use of asparaginase
• Potential for injury related to a preexisting condition that requires cautious use of asparaginase
• Potential for injury related to adverse drug reactions
• Altered protection related to an acute hypersensitivity reaction to asparaginase
• Knowledge deficit related to asparaginase

Planning and implementation
• Do not administer asparaginase to a patient with a condition that contraindicates its use.
• Administer asparaginase cautiously to a patient at risk because of a preexisting condition.
• Monitor the patient regularly for adverse reactions throughout asparaginase therapy.
• Administer an antiemetic with asparaginase as prescribed because nausea and vomiting are particularly noxious adverse reactions to asparaginase. If an antiemetic is not prescribed, consult with the physician. Use other appropriate nursing interventions for a patient with nausea or vomiting. (For details, see the introduction to this unit.)
• Administer a mild antipyretic-analgesic agent as prescribed if fever or headache occurs.
• Monitor the patient's liver and renal renal function studies and amylase and blood glucose levels if prescribed. Notify the physician of any abnormal results.
• *Take seizure precautions during asparaginase therapy. Stop the infusion immediately and notify the physician if seizures occur.*
• *Report personality changes to the physician. Such changes may indicate CNS toxicity from asparaginase.*
• *Note asparaginase treatment on any EEG request slip because it can cause abnormal EEG tracings.*
• *Monitor the patient's plasma coagulation factors. Withhold asparaginase and administer fresh frozen plasma, if prescribed. Take bleeding precautions until the patient's plasma coagulation factors return to normal.*
• *Handle I.V. preparations of asparaginase cautiously.* (For more information, see the introduction to this unit.)
• Refrigerate reconstituted asparaginase if the preparation is not used immediately. Use the solution only if it is clear.
• Notify the physician if adverse reactions persist or worsen.
• *Administer asparaginase in the hospital setting only with a physician present because of the potential for anaphylaxis. Keep available any drugs and equipment necessary to treat cardiac arrest.*
• Monitor the patient's baseline vital signs before and during asparaginase administration.

• *Stop the asparaginase infusion immediately if a hypersensitivity reaction occurs and be prepared to begin emergency treatment. Keep in mind that the risk of anaphylaxis increases with each successive treatment and is more likely to occur with intermittent therapy.*

Patient teaching
• Teach the patient and family the name, dose, frequency, action, and adverse effects of asparaginase.
• *Inform the patient of the potential for cardiac arrest, and provide support and reassurance. Instruct the patient to report immediately any signs or symptoms of hypersensitivity, including restlessness, wheezing, facial flushing or edema, urticaria, pruritus, tachycardia, hypotension, fever, or dyspnea.*
• *Teach the patient to recognize the signs and symptoms of CNS toxicity, such as personality changes and seizures, and of pancreatitis, such as abdominal tenderness, midepigastric pain, and vomiting. The CNS changes usually disappear when asparaginase is discontinued, but may persist. Inform the patient that CNS toxicity or pancreatitis may cause discontinuation of asparaginase therapy.*
• *Teach the patient to recognize and report the signs and symptoms of liver damage, such as yellowing of the skin or eyes, dark-colored urine, clay-colored stools, or pruritus.*
• Advise the patient to take a mild antipyretic-analgesic as prescribed if a fever or headache occurs after asparaginase therapy.
• *Teach the patient bleeding precautions to use if coagulation abnormalities occur.*
• Give the patient written materials about the possible effects of antineoplastic agents for home reference.
• Instruct the patient to notify the physician if adverse reactions persist or worsen.

Evaluation
The following examples represent appropriate evaluation statements for a patient receiving asparaginase.
• The patient has no conditions that contraindicate asparaginase therapy.
• The patient exhibits no signs of complications in the preexisting condition linked to asparaginase.
• The patient exhibits few adverse reactions to asparaginase.
• The patient does not experience a hypersensitivity reaction to asparaginase.
• The patient and family express an accurate understanding of the points taught about asparaginase.
• The patient correctly identifies the signs and symptoms of asparaginase hypersensitivity, which must be reported immediately.

PROCARBAZINE

Procarbazine hydrochloride, a methylhydrazine derivative with monoamine oxidase (MAO) inhibitory properties, is used to treat Hodgkin's disease. Because it is lipophilic (having an affinity for fat) and readily enters cells by diffusion, the drug also is used to treat primary and metastatic brain tumors. Procarbazine causes various cellular changes and is thought to be cell-cycle-nonspecific.

PHARMACOKINETICS

After oral administration, procarbazine is absorbed well. As a lipophilic molecule, it readily crosses the blood-brain barrier and is distributed well into the CSF. It is metabolized rapidly in the liver and must be activated metabolically by microsomal enzymes. Procarbazine is excreted in urine, primarily as metabolites. (For details, see *Major administration and excretion routes: Other antineoplastic agents,* page 1215.) Respiratory excretion of the drug occurs as methane and carbon dioxide. Procarbazine achieves a peak plasma concentration level within 1 hour; its half-life is 7 minutes.

PHARMACODYNAMICS

An inert drug, procarbazine must be activated metabolically in the liver. Then it can produce various cell changes. It can cause chromosomal damage, including chromatid breaks and translocation, produce antimitotic activity, and inhibit DNA, ribonucleic acid (RNA), and protein synthesis. Cancer cells can develop procarbazine resistance quickly, but that mechanism is not understood completely.

PHARMACOTHERAPEUTICS

Procarbazine usually is given with other antineoplastic agents to treat Hodgkin's disease. Its lipophilicity also makes it useful in treating CNS tumors.

procarbazine (Matulane). Used with other antineoplastic agents, procarbazine is most effective in the MOPP regimen for Hodgkin's disease. The drug also may be useful against small-cell lung cancer, non-Hodgkin's lymphoma, myeloma, melanoma, and CNS tumors.
Usual adult dosage: initially, 2 to 4 mg/kg P.O. daily for 1 week; increased to 4 to 6 mg/kg/day, as tolerated, until maximum response is achieved; maintenance dosage, 1 to 2 mg/kg P.O. daily.

Drug interactions

Concurrent use of alcohol and procarbazine may produce a disulfiram-like reaction (headache, nausea, vomiting, and sweating). Procarbazine produces an additive effect when administered with CNS depressants. Hypertensive reactions may occur when procarbazine is administered concurrently with sympathomimetics, antidepressants, and tyramine-rich foods because of its MAO inhibition.

ADVERSE DRUG REACTIONS

Procarbazine is administered orally. However, a crystalline powder for injection is available for investigational use. The following adverse reactions are those associated with oral administration.

Late-onset bone marrow suppression is the most common dose-limiting toxicity associated with procarbazine. The platelet count nadir occurs after about 4 weeks, followed by the leukocyte count nadir. Complete recovery occurs at about 6 weeks.

Nausea and vomiting occur in 50% of patients. Stomatitis and diarrhea also may occur. Initial procarbazine therapy may induce a flulike syndrome, including fever, chills, sweating, lethargy, and myalgia. High-dose procarbazine therapy can induce azoospermia or cessation of menses. Because procarbazine may be teratogenic, the patient should avoid pregnancy during treatment.

Dermatologic reactions have occurred in about 3% of patients. These reactions include pruritus, acneiform rash, and hyperpigmentation.

Procarbazine may produce CNS toxicity marked by such varied reactions as confusion, depression, psychosis, neuropathies, fingertip paresthesia, footdrop, and lack of muscle coordination. Because procarbazine exhibits MAO-inhibiting properties, a tyramine-rich diet during procarbazine therapy may trigger an acute hypertensive episode. Interstitial pneumonitis and pulmonary fibrosis can occur. Orthostatic hypotension occurs rarely.

NURSING PROCESS APPLICATION

The following information assists the nurse in caring for a patient receiving procarbazine.

Assessment

• Review the patient's history for a preexisting condition that contraindicates the use of procarbazine, such as pregnancy, lactation, inadequate bone marrow reserve, or known hypersensitivity to the drug.
• Review the patient's history for a preexisting condition that requires cautious use of procarbazine, such as impaired renal or hepatic function.
• Assess the patient for adverse reactions to procarbazine, such as bone marrow suppression, GI distress, stomatitis,

flulike syndrome, dermatologic reactions, CNS abnormalities, respiratory dysfunction, and orthostatic hypotension.
• Review the patient's medication history to identify the use of drugs that may interact with procarbazine, such as alcohol, CNS depressants, sympathomimetics, and antidepressants.
• Assess the effectiveness of procarbazine regularly.
• Assess the patient's blood pressure regularly throughout procarbazine therapy.
• Evaluate the patient's and family's knowledge about procarbazine.

Nursing diagnoses

The following examples represent appropriate nursing diagnoses for a patient receiving procarbazine.
• Potential for injury related to a preexisting condition that contraindicates the use of procarbazine
• Potential for injury related to a preexisting condition that requires cautious use of procarbazine
• Potential for injury related to adverse drug reactions
• Altered health maintenance related to procarbazine-induced hypertensive crisis
• Knowledge deficit related to procarbazine

Planning and implementation

• Do not administer procarbazine to a patient with a condition that contraindicates its use.
• Administer procarbazine cautiously to a patient at risk because of a preexisting condition.
• Monitor the patient regularly for adverse reactions throughout procarbazine therapy.
• *Monitor the patient's CBC and platelet counts for evidence of leukopenia, thrombocytopenia, or anemia.* Typically, the nadir of bone marrow suppression occurs at 4 weeks; recovery, at 6 weeks. Because RBCs have a longer life than WBCs and platelets, anemia is less of a problem than thrombocytopenia or leukopenia unless the patient has occult or overt blood loss.
• *Monitor the patient with leukopenia for signs of infection, such as fever, sore throat, chills, and malaise. Also take infection control measures until the patient's WBC count returns to normal.*
• *Take bleeding precautions when the platelet count is below 50,000/mm³. Expect to administer platelet transfusions and packed red blood cells (RBCs) as prescribed during times of severe bleeding.*
• Take energy conservation measures for a patient with anemia. For example, stagger the patient's activities, help with tasks, and arrange for frequent rest periods.
• Minimize procarbazine-induced nausea and vomiting by administering the drug in divided daily doses and at bedtime. If nausea and vomiting become severe, expect to administer a nonphenothiazine antiemetic as prescribed.

• Request a prescription for an antidiarrheal agent if the patient develops diarrhea.

• Inspect the patient's mouth regularly for signs of stomatitis, such as red, swollen, or ulcerated oral mucosa. Provide symptomatic relief, such as a bland soft diet and a topical anesthetic as prescribed.

• Monitor the patient for a flulike syndrome of fever, chills, sweating, lethargy, and myalgia. Administer a mild antipyretic-analgesic agent as prescribed.

• Assess the patient regularly for dermatologic reactions, such as an acneiform rash, hyperpigmentation, or pruritus.

• *Monitor the patient for signs of CNS toxicity, such as fingertip paresthesia, footdrop, lack of muscle coordination, confusion, and depression. Immediately report any of these signs and symptoms to the physician.*

• *Monitor the patient for signs and symptoms of orthostatic hypotension, such as lightheadedness or dizziness upon arising. Advise the patient to avoid sudden position changes.*

• *Monitor the patient's respiratory status and review reports of chest X-rays, if prescribed, for evidence of interstitial pneumonitis and pulmonary fibrosis.*

• Use other appropriate nursing interventions for a patient with bone marrow suppression, nausea, vomiting, or stomatitis. (For details, see the introduction to this unit.)

• Notify the physician if adverse reactions occur.

• *Place the patient on a tyramine-free diet as prescribed because procarbazine can interact with tyramines, producing hypertension.*

• *Monitor the patient's blood pressure regularly during procarbazine therapy to detect an impending acute hypertensive episode. If the patient displays a sudden elevation of blood pressure, stop the infusion and notify the physician. Keep standard emergency equipment nearby and be prepared to begin emergency measures to manage a hypertensive crisis.*

• Reevaluate compliance with the tyramine-free diet if the patient experiences a hypertensive crisis.

Patient teaching

• Teach the patient and family the name, dose, frequency, action, and adverse effects of procarbazine.

• *Stress the importance of returning for follow-up blood tests.*

• *Teach the patient to consume a tyramine-free diet to help prevent a drug and food interaction.* The patient should avoid such foods as pickled herring, chicken or beef liver, ripe or aged cheese, beer, Chianti, chocolate, coffee, and cola drinks.

• Instruct the patient to consult the pharmacist or physician before using any over-the-counter medication. Such a medication may contain alcohol or a CNS depressant, which can interact with procarbazine.

• Advise the patient to stagger activities and take frequent rests if anemia occurs.

• *Advise the patient with leukopenia to avoid people with active contagious infections. Also instruct the patient to watch for signs and symptoms of infection and to report them immediately to the physician.*

• *Teach the patient with thrombocytopenia to take bleeding precautions.*

• *Inform the patient and family about the potential for CNS toxicity.*

• *Advise the patient to avoid pregnancy during procarbazine therapy because the drug may be teratogenic. This is particularly important because procarbazine commonly is used to treat Hodgkin's disease, which predominantly affects young adults.*

• Inform the female patient receiving high doses of procarbazine that cessation of menses may occur and is drug related.

• *Instruct the patient to avoid driving and similar activities if adverse CNS reactions occur.*

• Teach the patient how to manage troublesome adverse reactions, such as GI distress, stomatitis, and flulike syndrome.

• Give the patient written materials about the possible effects of antineoplastic agents for home reference.

• Instruct the patient to notify the physician if adverse reactions occur.

Evaluation

The following examples represent appropriate evaluation statements for a patient receiving procarbazine.

• The patient has no conditions that contraindicate procarbazine therapy.

• The patient exhibits no signs of complications in the preexisting condition linked to procarbazine.

• The patient exhibits few adverse reactions to procarbazine.

• The patient maintains blood pressure within normal limits during procarbazine therapy.

• The patient and family express an accurate understanding of the points taught about procarbazine.

• The patient correctly identifies which foods to avoid during procarbazine therapy.

HYDROXYUREA

Although hydroxyurea has been used to treat tumors since the 1960s, it is not prescribed widely even though it enters the CSF. The drug is used most commonly for patients with chronic myelogenous leukemia.

PHARMACOKINETICS

Hydroxyurea is absorbed readily and distributed well into the CSF after oral administration. It reaches a peak CSF concentration level 3 hours after administration. About 50% of a dose is metabolized by the liver to carbon dioxide, which is excreted by the lungs, or urea, which is excreted by the kidneys. The remaining 50% is excreted unchanged in urine. Up to 80% of a dose is recovered in urine in 12 hours. (For a summary, see *Major administration and excretion routes: Other antineoplastic agents,* page 1215.)

Hydroxyurea achieves a peak plasma concentration 1 to 2 hours after administration. Its plasma half-life is 2 hours. Treatment should continue for at least 6 weeks before assessing the drug's clinical effectiveness.

PHARMACODYNAMICS

Hydroxyurea may act as a DNA-selective antimetabolite. The drug exerts its cytotoxic effect by inhibiting the enzyme ribonucleotide reductase, which causes ribonucleotides to convert to deoxyribonucleotides. Without deoxyribonucleotides, DNA synthesis cannot occur. In vitro, hydroxyurea kills cells in the S phase of the cell cycle and holds other cells in the G_1 phase, where they are most susceptible to irradiation.

Cancer cells may develop resistance to hydroxyurea, resulting from an increased quantity of ribonucleotide reductase or a decreased sensitivity of the enzyme to hydroxyurea. Gene amplification may change the enzyme.

PHARMACOTHERAPEUTICS

Hydroxyurea is used to treat selected myeloproliferative disorders. It also is used in combination therapy with radiation to treat carcinomas of the head, neck, and lung. It may produce temporary remissions in some patients with metastatic malignant melanomas.

hydroxyurea (Hydrea). Hydroxyurea primarily is used to manage myeloproliferative disorders, such as acute refractory and chronic granulocytic leukemia. The drug also has demonstrated slight activity against such solid tumors as malignant melanoma; carcinomas of the head, neck, and lung; renal cell carcinoma; and ovarian and advanced prostate carcinomas.
Usual adult dosage: 80 mg/kg P.O. every third day, or 20 to 30 mg/kg P.O. daily. Treatment should be continued for 6 weeks.

Drug interactions

Researchers have identified no significant drug interactions with hydroxyurea.

ADVERSE DRUG REACTIONS

Hydroxyurea causes dose-related bone marrow suppression characterized primarily by leukopenia. Patients also may experience drowsiness, headache, nausea, vomiting, or anorexia. These adverse reactions usually are dose-related. Mild dermatologic reactions may include pruritus, facial erythema, and a maculopapular rash.

Rarely, a patient receiving radiation will experience exacerbated radiation erythema when taking hydroxyurea. Stomatitis and alopecia also may occur but are rare. Patients taking hydroxyurea may need to take allopurinol to prevent uric acid nephropathy and its resultant renal damage.

NURSING PROCESS APPLICATION

The following information assists the nurse in caring for a patient receiving hydroxyurea.

Assessment

• Review the patient's history for a preexisting condition that contraindicates the use of hydroxyurea, such as pregnancy, marked bone marrow depression, or severe anemia.
• Review the patient's history for a preexisting condition that requires cautious use of hydroxyurea, such as marked renal dysfunction or previous radiation therapy or cytotoxic cancer chemotherapy.
• Assess the patient for adverse reactions to hydroxyurea, such as leukopenia, drowsiness, headache, GI distress, dermatologic reactions, stomatitis, and alopecia.
• Assess the effectiveness of hydroxyurea regularly.
• Monitor the results of renal function studies regularly, if prescribed, throughout hydroxyurea therapy.
• Evaluate the patient's and family's knowledge about hydroxyurea.

Nursing diagnoses

The following examples represent appropriate nursing diagnoses for a patient receiving hydroxyurea.
• Potential for injury related to a preexisting condition that contraindicates the use of hydroxyurea
• Potential for injury related to a preexisting condition that requires cautious use of hydroxyurea
• Potential for injury related to adverse drug reactions
• Potential for trauma related to hydroxyurea-induced uric acid nephropathy
• Knowledge deficit related to hydroxyurea

Planning and implementation

• Do not administer hydroxyurea to a patient with a condition that contraindicates its use.
• Administer hydroxyurea cautiously to a patient at risk because of a preexisting condition.

• Monitor the patient regularly for adverse reactions throughout hydroxyurea therapy.

• *Monitor the patient's WBC count regularly for leukopenia. If leukopenia occurs, monitor the patient for signs of infection, such as fever, chills, malaise, and sore throat. Also take infection control measures until the WBC count returns to normal.*

• *Take safety precautions if the patient experiences drowsiness. For example, place the bed in a low position, keep the side rails up, and supervise ambulation.*

• Monitor hydration if the patient experiences anorexia, nausea, or vomiting. Request a prescription for an antiemetic agent as needed.

• Administer a mild analgesic as prescribed to relieve hydroxyurea-induced headache.

• Inspect the patient's mouth for signs of stomatitis, such as red, swollen, or ulcerated oral mucosa. Provide symptomatic relief, for example, by providing bland, soft food and applying a topical anesthetic to the area, as prescribed.

• Observe the patient's skin for dermatologic changes, such as facial erythema, maculopapular rash, or, if the patient has received radiation therapy, exacerbated radiation erythema.

• *Administer oral hydroxyurea on a daily or every-third-day schedule, as prescribed, giving a large single dosage rather than divided doses to attain higher blood levels. If the patient has trouble swallowing capsules, dissolve the capsule contents in water and administer immediately.*

• Use other appropriate nursing interventions for a patient with leukopenia, nausea, vomiting, stomatitis, or alopecia. (For details, see the introduction to this unit.)

• Notify the physician if adverse reactions occur.

• *Monitor uric acid, blood urea nitrogen (BUN), and creatinine levels, if prescribed, throughout therapy to detect signs of uric acid nephropathy, such as rising uric acid, BUN, and creatinine levels.*

• Encourage the patient who exhibits signs of nephropathy to drink at least eight 8-oz glasses of fluid a day. Also expect to administer allopurinol as prescribed.

• Notify the physician if uric acid nephropathy occurs.

Patient teaching

• Teach the patient and family the name, dose, frequency, action, and adverse effects of hydroxyurea.

• *Stress the importance of returning for follow-up blood tests.*

• *Instruct the patient to watch for signs and symptoms of infection and to report them immediately to the physician.*

• *Advise the patient to avoid people with contagious infections.*

• Teach the patient about using an oral or suppository antiemetic agent, as prescribed, if nausea and vomiting occur during hydroxyurea therapy.

• Explain to the patient that mild, reversible dermatologic reactions, such as pruritus, maculopapular rash, and facial erythema, can occur. Instruct the patient to keep previously irradiated skin clean, dry, and protected from sunlight. Also instruct the patient to report erythema exacerbation of an irradiated site to the physician.

• *Caution the patient to avoid activities that require mental alertness if drowsiness occurs.*

• Teach the patient how to manage stomatitis at home.

• Inform the patient that alopecia may occur. Prepare the patient by explaining the timing and speed of hair loss, noting that it may affect the scalp, eyebrows, eyelashes, or other body hair.

• *Stress the importance of taking hydroxyurea exactly as prescribed to maximize therapeutic effects and minimize adverse ones.*

• Instruct the patient to drink at least eight 8-oz glasses of fluid daily during hydroxyurea therapy.

• Give the patient written materials about hydroxyurea therapy for home reference.

• Instruct the patient to notify the physician if adverse reactions occur.

Evaluation

The following examples represent appropriate evaluation statements for a patient receiving hydroxyurea.

• The patient has no conditions that contraindicate hydroxyurea therapy.

• The patient exhibits no signs of complications in the preexisting condition linked to hydroxyurea.

• The patient exhibits few adverse reactions to hydroxyurea.

• The patient maintains normal renal function throughout hydroxyurea therapy.

• The patient and family express an accurate understanding of the points taught about hydroxyurea.

• The patient correctly describes infection control measures to use if leukopenia occurs.

INTERFERONS

A family of naturally occurring glycoproteins, interferons are so named because of their ability to interfere with viral replication. These drugs have anticancer activity as well as activity against condylomata acuminata (soft, wartlike growths on the skin and mucous membrane of the genitalia caused by a virus).

Originally, interferons were purified from leukocytes and fibroblasts. Now they are produced by recombinant DNA technology, which yields larger quantities for clinical use. Three types of interferons exist, according to their cell source: alpha interferons, which are derived from leukocytes; beta interferons, from fibroblasts; and gamma interferons, from fibroblasts and lymphocytes. Currently, only alpha interferons (alpha-2A, alpha-2B, and alpha-n-3) are available commercially. The beta and gamma interferons are limited to investigational use.

Alpha interferons have minimal activity against solid tumors. However, they are effective against hairy cell leukemia and acquired immunodeficiency syndrome (AIDS)-related Kaposi's sarcoma, condylomata acuminata, and show promise in chronic myelogenous leukemia, non-Hodgkin's lymphoma, multiple myeloma, melanoma, and renal cell carcinoma.

PHARMACOKINETICS

After I.M. or S.C. administration, alpha interferons usually are absorbed well. They achieve a peak concentration level about 4 hours after I.M. or 7 hours after S.C. administration. Information about their distribution is unavailable. Alpha interferons are filtered by the kidneys, where they are degraded. Hepatic metabolism and biliary excretion of interferons are negligible. The half-life of these agents ranges from 2 to 8.5 hours.

PHARMACODYNAMICS

Interferons are naturally occurring molecules that are produced and secreted by human cells in response to viral infection. Although their exact mechanism of action is unknown, they have been shown to bind to specific membrane receptors on the cell surface. Once bound, they initiate a sequence of intracellular events that includes the induction of certain enzymes. This process may account for the ability of interferons to inhibit viral replication, suppress cell proliferation, enhance macrophage activity, and increase lymphocyte cytotoxicity.

PHARMACOTHERAPEUTICS

Alpha interferons have shown their most promising activity in treating hematologic malignancies, especially hairy cell leukemia. Their approved indications currently include hairy cell leukemia, AIDS-related Kaposi's sarcoma, and condylomata acuminata. However, alpha interferons also demonstrate some activity against chronic myelogenous leukemia, non-Hodgkin's lymphoma, multiple myeloma, melanoma, and renal cell carcinoma.

Three alpha interferons are available commercially. Two are manufactured by recombinant DNA technology: interferon alpha-2A and interferon alpha-2B. The third, interferon alpha-n-3, is derived from human leukocytes.

Different brands of interferon may contain different amounts of the drug.

interferon alpha-2A (Roferon-A). This drug is used to treat hairy cell leukemia and AIDS-related Kaposi's sarcoma. Patients with hairy cell leukemia should be treated for about 6 months before determining a response.
Usual adult dosage: for hairy cell leukemia, 3 million IU S.C. or I.M. daily for 16 to 24 weeks, followed by 3 million IU S.C. or I.M. three times a week; for AIDS-related Kaposi's sarcoma, 36 million IU I.M. or S.C. daily for 10 to 12 weeks, followed by 36 million IU I.M. or S.C. three times a week.

interferon alpha-2B (Intron A). This drug is used to treat hairy cell leukemia, AIDS-related Kaposi's sarcoma, and condylomata acuminata. A patient with hairy cell leukemia may require treatment for 6 months or longer before improvement occurs.
Usual adult dosage: for hairy cell leukemia, 2 million IU/m^2 I.M. or S.C. three times a week; for AIDS-related Kaposi's sarcoma, 30 million IU I.M. or S.C. three times a week; for condylomata acuminata, 1 million IU per lesion, injected directly into the lesion, three times a week for 3 weeks. The maximum response usually occurs in 4 to 8 weeks. If results are not satisfactory after 12 to 16 weeks, a second course may be given. A tuberculin syringe with a 25- to 30-gauge needle should be used for injection into the lesion.

interferon alpha-n-3. This drug is used to treat condylomata acuminata.
Usual adult dosage: 250,000 IU per wart, injected at the base of the wart, 2 times a week for up to 8 weeks. The maximum recommended dose per treatment session is 2.5 million IU. Injections should be made with a 30-gauge needle.

Drug interactions
Interferons may enhance the CNS effects of CNS depressants and substantially increase the half-life of methylxanthines (including theophylline and aminophylline), perhaps by interfering with the cytochrome P-450 drug metabolizing enzymes.

Concurrent use of an interferon with a live virus vaccine may potentiate replication of vaccine virus, increasing the adverse effects of the vaccine and decreasing the patient's antibody response.

Bone marrow suppression may be increased when an interferon is used concomitantly with radiation therapy or a drug that causes blood dyscrasias or bone marrow suppression. A dosage reduction for both drugs may be required.

ADVERSE REACTIONS

Adverse reactions to alpha interferons are dose-related. If severe adverse reactions occur, the dosage may be reduced by 50% and the patient may tolerate therapy better.

The most common adverse reaction is a flulike syndrome that may produce fever, fatigue, myalgia, headache, chills, and arthralgia. To minimize these problems, the drug may be administered in the evening or the patient may receive premedication with acetaminophen. Many patients develop a tolerance to these symptoms, which tend to diminish with continued therapy.

Hematologic toxicity occurs in up to 50% of patients and may produce leukopenia, neutropenia, thrombocytopenia, and anemia. Adverse GI reactions, such as anorexia, nausea, and diarrhea, occur in about 30% to 50% of patients receiving interferon. CNS disturbances can occur in 10% to 20% of patients and may include dizziness, confusion, paresthesia, numbness, lethargy, and depression.

Coughing and dyspnea also have been associated with interferon therapy, as have hypotension, edema, chest pain, and congestive heart failure. Adverse dermatologic reactions may include alopecia, rash, and dry skin. Interferon also may cause an elevation in the liver transaminase level and abnormalities in renal function tests.

NURSING PROCESS APPLICATION

The following information assists the nurse in caring for a patient receiving an interferon.

Assessment

• Review the patient's history for a preexisting condition that contraindicates the use of an interferon, such as lactation or known hypersensitivity to the drug.
• Review the patient's history for a preexisting condition that requires cautious use of an interferon, such as pregnancy, recent myocardial infarction, or a previous or recurrent arrhythmic disorder.
• Assess the patient for adverse reactions to the prescribed interferon, such as GI distress, CNS disturbances, cardiovascular dysfunction, skin reactions, and hematologic reactions.
• Review the patient's medication history to identify the use of drugs that may interact with the prescribed interferon, such as CNS depressants, methylxanthines, and live virus vaccines.
• Assess the effectiveness of the prescribed interferon regularly.
• Assess the patient for flulike syndrome during interferon therapy.
• Evaluate the patient's and family's knowledge about the prescribed interferon.

Nursing diagnoses

The following examples represent appropriate nursing diagnoses for a patient receiving an interferon.
• Potential for injury related to a preexisting condition that contraindicates the use of an interferon
• Potential for injury related to a preexisting condition that requires cautious use of an interferon
• Potential for injury related to adverse drug reactions
• Altered health maintenance related to flulike syndrome caused by the prescribed interferon
• Knowledge deficit related to the prescribed interferon

Planning and implementation

• Do not administer an interferon to a patient with a condition that contraindicates its use.
• Administer an interferon cautiously to a patient at risk because of a preexisting condition.
• Monitor the patient regularly for adverse reactions during interferon therapy.
• Monitor hydration if the patient experiences anorexia, nausea, or diarrhea. Obtain a prescription for an antiemetic or antidiarrheal agent as needed.
• *Take safety precautions if the patient experiences adverse CNS reactions, such as dizziness, confusion, paresthesia, numbness, lethargy, or depression. For example, place the bed in a low position, keep the side rails up, and supervise the patient's activities.*
• Monitor the patient for coughing and dyspnea. If these adverse reactions persist or become severe, notify the physician because a dosage reduction may be necessary.
• *Monitor the patient's blood pressure to detect hypotension. Regularly inquire about chest pain. Monitor for signs and symptoms of congestive heart failure. For example, auscultate the lungs for crackles and the heart for tachycardia, inspect the jugular veins for distention, and observe the ankles for swelling. Notify the physician if assessments reveal hypotension or signs of congestive heart failure.*
• *Monitor the patient's CBC and platelet count for evidence of leukopenia, neutropenia, thrombocytopenia, or anemia. Observe the patient with leukopenia for signs of infection, such as fever, chills, malaise, and sore throat. Take infection control measures until the WBC count returns to normal. Observe the patient with thrombocytopenia for signs of bleeding, such as spontaneous epistaxis, hematuria, and easy bruising. Also take bleeding precautions until the platelet count returns to normal. If the patient becomes anemic, take energy conservation measures until the RBC count returns to normal.*
• Monitor the results of the patient's liver transaminase level for elevations and renal function studies if prescribed. Abnormal results may require a dosage reduction.

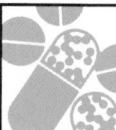

Other antineoplastic agents

This table summarizes the other major antineoplastic agents currently in clinical use.

DRUG	MAJOR INDICATIONS	USUAL ADULT DOSAGES	CONTRAINDICATIONS AND PRECAUTIONS
Vinca alkaloids			
vinblastine	Breast carcinoma, neuro-blastoma, metastatic testicular cancer, lymphomas, Kaposi's sarcoma, choriocarcinoma	0.1 mg/kg or 3.7 mg/m² I.V. increased weekly by increments of 0.05 mg/kg or 1.8 mg/m² to a maximum of 0.5 mg or 18.5 mg/m²; for maintenance therapy, 0.05 mg/kg or 1.8 mg/m² I.V. less than the final dosage every 7 to 14 days	• Know that vinblastine is contraindicated in a pregnant or lactating patient or one with significant granulocytopenia (unless it results from the disease being treated) or bacterial infection.
vincristine	Hodgkin's disease, non-Hodgkin's lymphoma, acute lymphocytic leukemia	1.4 mg/m² I.V. in a single dose, no more frequently than once weekly; not to exceed 2 mg per dose	• Know that vincristine is contraindicated in a pregnant or lactating patient or one with the demyelinating form of Charcot-Marie-Tooth syndrome. • Administer with caution to a patient with acute uric acid nephropathy or neuromuscular disease.
Podophyllotoxins			
etoposide	Testicular cancer	50 to 100 mg/m² I.V. daily for 5 days, or 100 mg/m² I.V. daily on days 1, 3, and 5, repeated every 3 to 4 weeks	• Know that etoposide is contraindicated in a pregnant or lactating patient or one with known hypersensitivity to the drug.
	Small-cell lung cancer	35 mg/m² I.V. daily for 4 days up to 50 mg/m² I.V. daily for 5 days, repeated every 3 to 4 weeks	
Asparaginase			
asparaginase	Acute lymphocytic leukemia	200 IU/kg I.V. daily for 28 days, or 1,000 IU/kg I.V. daily for 10 days	• Know that asparaginase is contraindicated in a lactating patient or one with pancreatitis, a history of pancreatitis, or known hypersensitivity to the drug. • Administer with caution to a pregnant patient.
Procarbazine			
procarbazine	Hodgkin's disease, small-cell lung cancer, non-Hodgkin's lymphoma, myeloma, melanoma, and central nervous system tumors	2 to 4 mg/kg P.O. daily for 1 week, then increased to 4 to 6 mg/kg P.O. daily; for maintenance therapy, 1 to 2 mg/kg P.O. daily	• Know that procarbazine is contraindicated in a pregnant or lactating patient or one with inadequate bone marrow reserve or known hypersensitivity to the drug. • Administer with caution to a patient with impaired renal or hepatic function.

SELECTED MAJOR DRUGS

Other antineoplastic agents (continued)

DRUG	MAJOR INDICATIONS	USUAL ADULT DOSAGES	CONTRAINDICATIONS AND PRECAUTIONS
Hydroxyurea			
hydroxyurea	Selected myeloproliferative disorders	80 mg/kg P.O. every third day, or 20 to 30 mg/kg P.O. daily	• Know that hydroxyurea is contraindicated in a pregnant patient or one with marked bone marrow depression or severe anemia. • Administer with caution to a patient with marked renal dysfunction or one who has had radiation therapy or cytotoxic cancer chemotherapy.
Interferons			
interferon alpha-2A	Hairy cell leukemia	3 million IU S.C. or I.M. daily for 16 to 24 weeks followed by 3 million IU S.C. or I.M. three times a week	• Know that interferon is contraindicated in a lactating patient or one with known hypersensitivity to the drug. • Administer with caution to a pregnant patient or one with a recent myocardial infarction or a previous or recurrent arrhythmic disorder.
	AIDS-related Kaposi's sarcoma	36 million IU I.M. or S.C. daily for 10 to 12 weeks followed by 36 million IU I.M. or S.C. three times a week	

• Use other appropriate nursing interventions for a patient with leukopenia, thrombocytopenia, anemia, nausea, or alopecia. (For details, see the introduction to this unit.)
• Notify the physician if adverse reactions occur.
• Monitor the patient for flulike symptoms, such as fever, headache, fatigue, myalgia, chills, and arthralgia.
• Administer interferon in the evening if prescribed to minimize troublesome flulike symptoms during the day.
• Consult with the physician about premedicating the patient with acetaminophen to help relieve flulike symptoms.
• Notify the physician if flulike symptoms become intolerable.

Patient teaching
• Teach the patient and family the name, dose, frequency, action, and adverse effects of the prescribed interferon.
• *Instruct the patient not to change to a different brand of interferon because this may result in an unintended dosage change.*
• Inform the patient about the likelihood and management of flulike symptoms. Reassure the patient that most people develop a tolerance to these symptoms, which tend to diminish with continued therapy.
• Teach the patient or family member how to administer the drug properly.
• Teach the patient how to manage troublesome GI reactions.

• *Caution the patient not to perform activities that require mental alertness if CNS disturbances occur.*
• *Instruct the patient to report cough, dyspnea, chest pain, lightheadedness, or ankle swelling because these signs and symptoms may suggest congestive heart failure, hypotension, or a respiratory disturbance.*
• Teach the patient infection control measures, bleeding precautions, and energy conservation measures to use, as needed.
• Stress the importance of returning for follow-up blood tests.
• Instruct the patient to report any other adverse reactions.

Evaluation
The following examples represent appropriate evaluation statements for a patient receiving an interferon.
• The patient has no conditions that contraindicate interferon therapy.
• The patient exhibits no signs of complications in the preexisting condition linked to the prescribed interferon.
• The patient exhibits few adverse reactions to the prescribed interferon.
• The patient manages flulike symptoms effectively.
• The patient and family express an accurate understanding of the points taught about the prescribed interferon.
• The patient correctly demonstrates how to self-administer the interferon as prescribed.

CHAPTER SUMMARY

Chapter 70 discussed various antineoplastic agents, including the vinca alkaloids, podophyllotoxins, asparaginase, procarbazine, hydroxyurea, and interferons. Here are the chapter highlights.

• The vinca alkaloids and podophyllotoxins are cell-cycle-specific.

• The vinca alkaloids, vesicants that must be administered carefully to prevent extravasation, are used to treat Hodgkin's disease, non-Hodgkin's lymphoma, testicular cancer, Kaposi's sarcoma, neuroblastoma, choriocarcinoma, breast cancer, acute lymphocytic leukemia, rhabdomyosarcoma, and Wilms' tumor. The podophyllotoxins are used to treat various tumors, including lymphomas, leukemias, small-cell lung carcinoma, and testicular carcinoma. Most vinca alkaloids and podophyllotoxins can produce bone marrow suppression, nausea, vomiting, and stomatitis.

• Asparaginase is a cell-cycle-specific enzyme used primarily to induce remission in acute lymphocytic leukemia. Because asparaginase increases the patient's risk of anaphylaxis, it should be administered with a physician present.

• Procarbazine and hydroxyurea are oral agents that distribute well into the CSF.

• Procarbazine is used to treat Hodgkin's disease and primary and metastatic brain tumors. Hydroxyurea inhibits DNA synthesis; the drug is used primarily to treat chronic myelogenous leukemia.

• Because procarbazine has MAO-inhibitory properties, it interacts with tyramine-rich foods, which can cause severe hypertension. Therefore, a patient taking procarbazine should avoid eating tyramine-rich foods.

• Interferons are naturally occurring molecules that inhibit viral replication, suppress cell proliferation, enhance macrophage activity, and increase lymphocyte cytotoxicity. They are used to treat hairy cell leukemia, AIDS-related Kaposi's sarcoma, and condylomata acuminata.

• The nurse should administer antineoplastic agents with extreme caution because they can produce many serious adverse reactions. For a patient receiving one of these agents, the nurse follows the steps of the nursing process to provide care that helps minimize such reactions.

STUDY QUESTIONS

See Appendix 1 for answers.

1. Alan Bolton, age 25, is receiving MOPP therapy for Hodgkin's disease. Like the other vinca alkaloids, vincristine (Oncovin) is cell-cycle specific for which phase?
(a) G_1 phase
(b) G_2 phase
(c) M phase
(d) S phase

2. Vincristine commonly produces which adverse reaction?
(a) fever
(b) alopecia
(c) hypotension
(d) photophobia

3. Because Mr. Bolton also is receiving procarbazine, the nurse assesses him closely for signs and symptoms of bone marrow suppression. When is this adverse reaction most likely to occur?
(a) immediately after treatment
(b) 2 weeks after treatment
(c) 4 weeks after treatment
(d) 6 weeks after treatment

4. Which dietary instructions should the nurse give Mr. Bolton while he is receiving procarbazine?
(a) Avoid tyramine-rich foods, such as coffee, chocolate, and aged cheese.
(b) Avoid calcium-rich foods, such as milk, yogurt, and other dairy products.
(c) Increase the fluid intake to 13 8-oz glasses daily, unless contraindicated.
(d) Increase the vitamin and mineral intake with supplements.

5. Keith Glenn, age 30, has testicular cancer that has not responded to vinblastine, bleomycin, and cisplatin therapy. His physician prescribes the podophyllotoxin etoposide. The nurse administers I.V. etoposide slowly over 60 minutes to prevent which adverse reaction?
(a) hypotension
(b) bronchospasm
(c) cardiac arrhythmia
(d) injection site pain

6. Justin Adler, age 4, suddenly develops high fever and epistaxis. Blood tests reveal thrombocytopenia, and bone marrow studies confirm acute lymphocytic leukemia. Part of his chemotherapy includes asparaginase. After receiving asparaginase, Justin develops midepigastric pain and vomiting. What probably accounts for this reaction?
(a) pancreatitis
(b) liver failure
(c) splenomegaly
(d) leukopenia

7. Alfred Brown, age 50, is receiving hydroxyurea to treat chronic granulocytic leukemia. Which other drug is most likely to be added to Mr. Brown's therapeutic regimen?
(a) prochlorperizine
(b) metoclopramide
(c) acetaminophen
(d) allopurinol

8. An AIDS patient, Ken Simpson, age 35, has Kaposi's sarcoma, for which his physician has prescribed interferon alpha-2A. Which adverse reaction commonly is associated with interferon therapy?
(a) stomatitis
(b) flulike syndrome
(c) alopecia
(d) photosensitivity

SELECTED REFERENCES

AHFS drug information 90. (1990). Bethesda, MD: American Society of Hospital Pharmacists.

Cawley, M. (1990). Recent advances in chemotherapy: Administration and nursing implications. *Nursing Clinics of North America,* 25(2), 377-391.

Drug facts and comparisons. (1991). St. Louis: Facts and Comparisons Division, Lippincott.

Goodman and Gilman's the pharmacological basis of therapeutics (8th ed.; 1990). Elmsford, NY: Pergamon Press.

Habermann, T. (1989). Alpha interferon: Progress and perspectives in the biotherapy of chronic myelogenous leukemia. *Oncology Nursing Forum,* 16(6), 8-11.

Hansten, P., and Horn, J. (1989). *Drug interactions* (6th ed.). Philadelphia: Lea & Febiger.

Mitsuyasu, R. (1989). The enhanced potential use of recombinant alpha interferon in the treatment of AIDS-related Kaposi's sarcoma. *Oncology Nursing Forum,* 16(6), 5-7.

North American Nursing Diagnosis Association. (1990). *Taxonomy I - Revised, with official diagnostic categories.* St. Louis: NANDA.

Okita, K., and Kaneko, T. (1990). The potential of interferons in malignant disease. *Drugs,* 39(1), 1-6.

Walters, P. (1990). Chemo: A nurse's guide to action, administration, and side effects. *RN,* 53(2), 52-67.

OTHER MAJOR DRUGS

Although oral and parenteral agents may be used to treat certain sensory system disorders, this unit emphasizes the topical agents used to manage disorders of the eyes and ears. It also includes uncategorized agents and new agents that are used to treat rare and other disorders.

OPHTHALMIC AGENTS

In ophthalmology, eye drops and ointments are used to relieve inflammation, reduce intraocular pressure and corneal edema, remove opacified corneal epithelium, and replace tears in dry eyes. They also are used for diagnostic procedures.

Many factors influence the ability of a drug to penetrate the eye. When administered topically, ophthalmic preparations are absorbed through the cornea, conjunctiva, and sclera. Because lipid-soluble agents readily penetrate the corneal epithelium and endothelium, and water-soluble agents penetrate the stroma, agents that are lipid- and water-soluble penetrate the cornea best. Wetting agents such as benzalkonium chloride, a preservative in many ophthalmic preparations, can improve corneal drug absorption. Limited absorption into the posterior eye, however, usually restricts the use of topical agents there. For posterior eye disorders, systemic agents usually are required.

OTIC AGENTS

Disorders of the external ear include fungal infections, impacted cerumen, acute edematous external otitis (swimmer's ear), and malignant external otitis. These disorders usually require treatment with the same agents that are used to manage dermatitis. Therapy also involves thorough cleansing, restoration of an acidic surface pH, reduction of swelling, elimination of infection, and control of predisposing factors.

Disorders of the middle ear include acute and chronic otitis media. Both disorders usually require a systemic agent to control the infection and possibly a systemic decongestant to restore eustachian tube function and permit fluid drainage from the middle ear.

UNCATEGORIZED AND OTHER AGENTS

This group of drugs includes uncategorized agents, which do not fall into any pharmacologic classification in this text, and other agents, which are used to treat rare disorders or disorders that differ from those treated by the other drugs in the classification. Most of the drugs in this group are new drugs approved for clinical use within the past few years. Some are used to treat uncommon conditions, such as severe homozygous cystinurea and urea cycle enzymopathies. Others are indicated for more familiar conditions, such as strabismus, gallstones, and cancer.

OVERVIEW OF CHAPTERS

Unit Sixteen provides information about agents that are used to treat eye and ear disorders as well as a variety of uncategorized and other agents.

Chapter 71
Ophthalmic Agents
Chapter 71 investigates the agents used to diagnose and treat eye disorders. It emphasizes the indications and pharmacodynamics of mydriatics, cycloplegics, miotics, agents that lower intraocular pressure, anesthetics, anti-inflammatory agents, and anti-infectives. It also details administration techniques and appropriate nursing care using the nursing process.

Chapter 72
Otic Agents
Chapter 72 discusses the anti-infective, anti-inflammatory, local anesthetic, and ceruminolytic agents used to treat ear disorders. Besides the clinical uses for these agents, the chapter includes information about combination products and administration techniques. For each drug class, it uses the nursing process as a framework to demonstrate related nursing care.

Glossary

Accommodation: adjustment of the eyes for vision at various distances.

Adnexa oculi: lacrimal apparatus, eyelids, and related structures of the eye.

Alpha₁-proteinase inhibitor: agent that inactivates several proteases, including trypsin, chymotrypsin, coagulation factor XI, plasmin, thrombin, and neutrophil elastase.

Amblyopia: reduced vision in an eye that appears structurally normal when examined with an ophthalmoscope.

Anisometropia: difference in the refractive power of the eyes.

Cerumen: waxlike secretion in the external opening of the ear; earwax.

Conjunctivitis: inflammation of the conjunctiva.

Cycloplegia: ciliary muscle paralysis.

Diplopia: double vision caused by defective function of the intraocular muscles or the nerves that innervate them.

Esotropia: type of strabismus with inward deviation of one eye in relation to the other eye; also called convergent strabismus.

Exotropia: type of strabismus with outward deviation of one eye in relation to the other eye; also called divergent strabismus.

Glaucoma: eye disorder characterized by increased intraocular pressure.

Immunomodulator: substance that alters the immune response by augmenting or reducing the ability of the immune system to produce antibodies or sensitized cells that recognize and react with antigens.

Iridectomy: surgical excision of part of the iris.

Iridocyclitis: inflammation of the iris and ciliary body.

Iritis: inflammation of the iris.

Keratitis: inflammation of the cornea.

Miosis: contraction of the pupil.

Mydriasis: extreme dilation of the pupil.

Otitis: inflammation of the ear.

Otitis externa: inflammation of the external ear.

Otitis media: inflammation of the middle ear.

Ototoxic: having a deleterious effect to the eighth cranial nerve or the organs of hearing and balance.

Strabismus: misalignment of the optic axis of each eye.

Synechia: adhesion of the iris to the cornea or lens.

Tonometry: indirect measurement of intraocular pressure by determining the resistance of the eyeball to indentation by an applied force.

Trachoma: infectious disease of the conjunctiva and cornea characterized by redness, inflammation, photophobia, and lacrimation.

Uveitis: inflammation of the iris, ciliary body, and choroid.

Chapter 73
Uncategorized and Other Agents

Chapter 73 explores 20 uncategorized and other agents used to treat a variety of disorders that range from rare conditions, such as congenital deficiency of alpha₁-antitrypsin, to well-known disorders, such as ulcerative colitis. The chapter presents the pharmacokinetics, pharmacodynamics, pharmacotherapeutics, drug interactions, and adverse reactions for each drug. It concludes with nursing implications and selected nursing diagnoses related to the use of each drug.

OPHTHALMIC AGENTS

OBJECTIVES

After reading and studying this chapter, the student should be able to:
1. Describe the clinical indications for mydriatic, cycloplegic, and miotic agents.
2. Compare the different types of glaucoma and the therapies used to treat them.
3. Describe the mechanism of action of ophthalmic drugs to lower intraocular pressure.
4. Explain the adverse reactions to ophthalmic anesthetic agents and how to prevent them.
5. Discuss the clinical indications for ophthalmic anti-inflammatory agents.
6. Differentiate the ophthalmic conditions that are treated with topical anti-infectives from those that are treated with systemic anti-infectives.
7. Explain how to instill eye drops and apply eye ointments.
8. Describe how to apply the nursing process when caring for a patient receiving an ophthalmic agent.

INTRODUCTION

Many ophthalmic agents mimic the action of the autonomic nervous system, which is divided into the sympathetic and parasympathetic nervous systems. (For an additional review of the autonomic nervous system, see the introduction to Unit Three.) Agents that mimic the actions of the sympathetic nervous system are called adrenergic, or sympathomimetic, agents; those that mimic the parasympathetic nervous system are called cholinergic, or parasympathomimetic, agents; those that inhibit the sympathetic nervous system are called adrenergic blockers, or sympatholytic agents; those that inhibit the parasympathetic nervous system are called cholinergic blockers, or parasympatholytic agents.

Adrenergic agents act directly on end-organ (eye) tissues. One example is phenylephrine, used to dilate the pupil. Cholinergic agents act on the eye directly in a manner similar to that of acetylcholine or indirectly by interfering with the action of the enzyme acetylcholinesterase.

The ophthalmic agents discussed in this chapter are instilled primarily as drops or applied as ointments. Mydriatics, cycloplegics, and miotics are the three groups of ophthalmic agents that most commonly are used. Besides these three groups, ophthalmic agents that lower intraocular pressure, anesthetic agents, anti-inflammatory agents, and anti-infective preparations also are discussed in this chapter.

For a summary of representative drugs, see *Selected major drugs: Ophthalmic agents,* pages 1255 and 1256. For a listing of applicable nursing diagnoses that the nurse may formulate when caring for a patient receiving these agents, see *Selected nursing diagnoses: Ophthalmic agents.* For detailed information on applying the nursing process, see Chapter 6, The Nursing Process and Drug Therapy.

MYDRIATICS AND CYCLOPLEGICS

Mydriatics are used to dilate the pupil for intraocular examinations and to facilitate refraction. Cycloplegics, which have a wide range of uses in ophthalmic diagnosis, also are used to paralyze the accommodative muscle of the ciliary body in patients before refraction. In postoperative patients or patients with intraocular inflammation, mydriatics and cycloplegics are used to dilate the pupils and to paralyze the accommodative muscle of the ciliary body. Some mydriatic agents also are used to lower intraocular pressure.

Mydriatics and cycloplegics include atropine sulfate, cyclopentolate hydrochloride, dipivefrin, epinephrine bitartrate, epinephrine hydrochloride, epinephryl borate, homatropine hydrobromide, phenylephrine hydrochloride, scopolamine hydrobromide, and tropicamide. Of these, di-

---

SELECTED NURSING DIAGNOSES

Ophthalmic agents

The following nursing diagnoses address representative problems and etiologies that a nurse may encounter when caring for a patient who is receiving an ophthalmic agent. Some of these nursing diagnoses contain generalized etiologies, which the nurse must individualize based on the patient's needs. (For some common nursing diagnoses and related interventions for each drug class, see the "Nursing Process Application" sections of this chapter.)

- Altered health maintenance related to development of an eye disorder caused by an ophthalmic agent
- Altered health maintenance related to hypokalemia caused by a carbonic anhydrase inhibitor
- Altered protection related to adrenal suppression caused by excessive or long-term use of an anti-inflammatory suspension
- Altered protection related to drug interaction between sulfacetamide and a local anesthetic
- Body image disturbance related to changes in the eyes or surrounding structures caused by an ophthalmic agent
- Decreased cardiac output related to altered heart rate caused by an ophthalmic agent
- Diarrhea related to the adverse GI effects of a miotic
- Fatigue related to the adverse effects of an adrenergic blocking agent
- Fluid volume excess caused by miotic-induced pulmonary edema
- Impaired gas exchange related to bronchoconstriction and bronchospasm caused by an ophthalmic agent
- Knowledge deficit related to the prescribed ophthalmic agent
- Pain related to application of an ophthalmic agent
- Pain related to headache caused by an adrenergic blocking agent

- Potential activity intolerance related to anemia caused by a carbonic anhydrase inhibitor
- Potential fluid volume deficit related to the adverse GI effects of an ophthalmic agent
- Potential for infection related to increased susceptibility to viral or fungal corneal infection caused by an anti-inflammatory agent
- Potential for infection related to leukopenia caused by a carbonic anhydrase inhibitor
- Potential for injury related to a hypersensitivity reaction to a sulfonamide anti-infective agent
- Potential for injury related to a preexisting condition that contraindicates the use of an ophthalmic agent
- Potential for injury related to a preexisting condition that requires cautious use of an ophthalmic agent
- Potential for injury related to adverse drug reactions
- Potential for injury related to the adverse ocular effects of an ophthalmic agent
- Potential for trauma related to the adverse CNS effects of an ophthalmic agent
- Potential for trauma related to visual disturbances caused by an ophthalmic agent
- Sensory-perceptual alterations (visual) related to the adverse ocular effects of an ophthalmic agent

---

pivefrin, epinephrine bitartrate, epinephrine hydrochloride, epinephryl borate, hydroxyamphetamine, and phenylephrine act only as mydriatics, and the rest have combined mydriatic-cycloplegic effects. Dipivefrin, epinephrine bitartrate, epinephrine hydrochloride, and epinephryl borate, also lower intraocular pressure.

PHARMACOKINETICS

Atropine, cyclopentolate, epinephrine, phenylephrine, and scopolamine may be absorbed systemically, which may cause adverse reactions especially in pediatric and geriatric patients. Systemic absorption may occur through the conjunctiva or through the gastrointestinal (GI) tract after a drug drains into the nasal sinuses and is swallowed. Absorption is enhanced during surgical procedures and treatment of traumatized eyes.

Onset, peak, duration

The onset of action of the adrenergic agents (dipivefrin, epinephrine, epinephryl, and phenylephrine) occurs within 10 to 15 minutes. The drugs achieve peak concentration levels 20 to 40 minutes after instillation, and have a duration

of action (pupil dilation) of 2 to 3 hours. When used to lower intraocular pressure, dipivefrin and epinephrine have a duration of about 12 hours.

The cholinergic-blocking mydriatics and cycloplegics (atropine, cyclopentolate, homatropine, scopolamine, and tropicamide) have an onset of 10 to 30 minutes for mydriatic effects and of 15 minutes to several hours for cycloplegic effects. Their duration is longer than that of the sympathomimetic drugs. The action of atropine, for example, may last for days.

PHARMACODYNAMICS

Mydriatic drops act on the iris to dilate the pupil. Cycloplegic drops act on the ciliary body to paralyze the fine-focusing muscles, thereby preventing accommodation for near vision.

Mechanism of action

The adrenergic mydriatics and cycloplegics stimulate mydriasis by contracting the dilator muscle of the pupil. Topical use of adrenergic drugs also constricts the arterioles and capillaries, thereby producing a whitening (decongesting) of the eye. Intraocular pressure decreases because of decreased production of aqueous humor and increased outflow of aqueous through the meshwork.

The cholinergic-blocking mydriatics and cycloplegics prevent acetylcholine action. With these drugs, mydriasis results from paralysis of the sphincter muscle of the iris and contraction of the dilator muscle. Cycloplegia results from ciliary muscle relaxation, which allows the lens to flatten.

PHARMACOTHERAPEUTICS

Mydriatics are used primarily to dilate the pupils for intraocular examinations. Cycloplegics are essential for performing refraction in children; they also are used before and after ophthalmic surgery and as adjunctive treatment for conditions involving the iris.

Pupil dilation in diabetic patients or in those with darkly pigmented irises requires stronger concentrations and repeated instillations of both types of drugs.

atropine sulfate (Atropisol, Isopto Atropine). This cholinergic blocker is used to treat acute iris inflammation (iritis) and to facilitate refraction.
Usual adult dosage: for acute iritis, 1 to 2 drops of 0.5% to 2% solution or a small amount of ointment b.i.d. or t.i.d.; for refraction, 1 to 2 drops of 1% solution 1 hour before eye examination.
Usual pediatric dosage: for acute iritis, 1 to 2 drops of 0.5% solution b.i.d. or t.i.d.; for refraction in children under age 5, 1 to 2 drops of 0.5% solution instilled in each eye for 1 to 3 days before eye examination and again 1 hour before refraction.

cyclopentolate hydrochloride (Cyclogyl). This cholinergic blocker is used for diagnostic procedures that require mydriatic and cycloplegic effects.
Usual adult dosage: 1 drop of 1% solution (2% solution for patients with heavily pigmented irises), then 1 drop 5 minutes later.
Usual pediatric dosage: 1 drop of 1% solution; if needed, 1 drop of 1% solution 5 minutes later. For infants under age 1, a 0.5% solution should be used.

dipivefrin (Propine). A topical adrenergic, dipivefrin is used to reduce intraocular pressure in patients with chronic open-angle glaucoma.
Usual adult dosage: 1 drop of 0.1% solution every 12 hours.

epinephrine bitartrate (Epitrate). A topical adrenergic, this drug is used to treat chronic open-angle glaucoma.

Usual adult and pediatric dosage: 1 to 2 drops of 2% solution (equivalent to 1.1% epinephrine) one to four times daily every 2 to 4 days.

epinephrine hydrochloride (Epifrin, Glaucon). An adrenergic agent, epinephrine hydrochloride is administered by intraocular injection during surgery to control bleeding or produce mydriasis. As a topical agent applied to the conjunctiva, epinephrine also is used to treat chronic open-angle glaucoma and to produce mydriasis before ophthalmologic examination.
Usual adult and pediatric dosage: for chronic open-angle glaucoma, 1 drop of 0.25%, 0.5%, 1%, or 2% solution one or two times daily; during surgery, 1 or more drops of 0.1% solution instilled up to three times or as needed, or 0.01% to 0.1% injected during surgery; for mydriasis before ophthalmologic examination, tip of filter paper moistened with 1% or 2% solution inserted in the inferior cul-de-sac for 1 to 3 minutes.

epinephryl borate (Epinal, Eppyl/N). A topical adrenergic, epinephryl is used to treat chronic open-angle glaucoma.
Usual adult and pediatric dosage: 1 drop of 0.5% or 1% solution b.i.d.

homatropine hydrobromide (Homatrocel Ophthalmic, Isopto Homatropine). Used to facilitate refraction, this cholinergic blocker also is used to treat uveitis.
Usual adult dosage: for refraction, 1 drop of 2% or 5% solution, repeated in 5 to 10 minutes; for uveitis, 1 drop of 2% or 5% solution b.i.d. or t.i.d.

phenylephrine hydrochloride (Mydfrin, NeoSynephrine). This adrenergic agent is used to achieve mydriasis without cycloplegia.
Usual adult and pediatric dosage: for mydriasis, 1 drop of 2.5% solution before examination.

scopolamine hydrobromide (Isopto Hyoscine). A cholinergic blocker, scopolamine is used to achieve postoperative mydriasis, to treat anterior uveitis, and occasionally to facilitate refraction before examination in children.
Usual adult dosage: for postoperative mydriasis, 1 drop of 0.25% solution daily; for anterior uveitis, 1 drop of 0.25% solution once daily or more frequently for severe inflammation.
Usual pediatric dosage: for refraction, 1 drop of 0.25% solution or a thin ribbon of 0.25% ointment b.i.d. for 2 days before refraction.

tropicamide (Mydriacyl). This cholinergic blocker is used to facilitate refraction and funduscopic examination.

Usual adult and pediatric dosage: for refraction, 1 drop of 1% solution 20 minutes before examination (an additional drop may be instilled in 20 to 30 minutes); for funduscopic examination, 1 drop of 0.5% solution 15 to 20 minutes before examination.

Drug interactions

Mydriatrics and cycloplegics do not cause significant drug interactions.

ADVERSE DRUG REACTIONS

Many local adverse reactions occur with the mydriatics and cycloplegics, which can include irritation, blurred vision, and transient burning sensations and stinging. With prolonged use, some of these drugs can increase intraocular pressure and cause ocular congestion, conjunctivitis, contact dermatitis, and eye dryness.

Systemic reactions include tachycardia, palpitations, flushing, dry skin, ataxia, and confusion. Dry mouth and tachycardia commonly occur after instillation of atropine, cyclopentolate, or scopolamine. Atropine, cyclopentolate, homatropine, and scopolamine can cause photophobia.

NURSING PROCESS APPLICATION

The following information assists the nurse in caring for a patient receiving a mydriatic or cycloplegic.

Assessment

• Review the patient's history for a preexisting condition that contraindicates the use of a mydriatic or cycloplegic, such as known or suspected closed-angle glaucoma or known hypersensitivity to the drug.
• Review the patient's history for a preexisting condition that requires cautious use of a mydriatic or cycloplegic, such as pregnancy, infancy, old age, predisposition to increased intraocular pressure, or spastic paralysis or brain damage in a child.
• Assess the patient for systemic adverse reactions to the prescribed mydriatic or cycloplegic, such as tachycardia, palpitations, flushing, dry skin, dry mouth, ataxia, or confusion.
• Assess the effectiveness of the prescribed mydriatic or cycloplegic periodically.
• Assess the patient for adverse ocular reactions, such as irritation, blurred vision, discomfort, increased intraocular pressure, contact dermatitis, conjunctivitis, and eye dryness.
• Evaluate the patient's and family's knowledge about the prescribed mydriatic or cycloplegic.

Nursing diagnoses

The following examples represent appropriate nursing diagnoses for a patient receiving a mydriatic or cycloplegic.
• Potential for injury related to a preexisting condition that contraindicates the use of a mydriatic or cycloplegic
• Potential for injury related to a preexisting condition that requires cautious use of a mydriatic or cycloplegic
• Potential for injury related to adverse drug reactions
• Sensory-perceptual alterations (visual) related to the adverse ocular effects of a mydriatic or cycloplegic
• Knowledge deficit related to the prescribed mydriatic or cycloplegic

Planning and implementation

• Do not administer a mydriatic or cycloplegic to a patient with a condition that contraindicates its use.
• Administ a mydriatic or cycloplegic cautiously to a patient at risk because of a preexisting condition.
• Monitor the patient closely for adverse reactions during therapy.
• *Monitor the patient's heart rate to detect tachycardia; ask the patient about palpitations.*
• Observe the patient's gait for ataxia.
• Monitor the patient regularly for confusion.
• Take safety precautions if the patient experiences ataxia or confusion. For example, keep the bed rails raised and supervise ambulation.
• Offer the patient frequent sips of water, ice chips, or sugarless hard candy to relieve dry mouth.
• *Minimize systemic absorption by applying digital pressure over the punctum at the inner canthus for 2 to 3 minutes after instilling the drops.*
• Ask the patient about photophobia during atropine, cyclopentolate, homatropine, or scopolamine therapy.
• Notify the physician if systemic adverse reactions occur.
• *Inspect the patient's eyes regularly for signs of irritation (redness), dryness, conjunctivitis (drainage), or contact dermatitis (redness and tearing).*
• Ask the patient about ocular disturbances, such as blurred vision and eye pain or itching.
• Ensure that eye examinations, including tonometric readings, are performed regularly.
• Notify the physician if adverse ocular reactions occur.

Patient teaching

• Teach the patient and family the name, dose, frequency, action, and adverse effects of the prescribed mydriatic or cycloplegic.
• *Warn the patient that eye irritation, blurred vision, and transient burning and stinging sensations may occur with mydriatic and cycloplegic administration.*

• Instruct the patient to wear dark glasses after administration and to avoid operating machinery until blurred vision disappears. Also advise the patient receiving atropine, cyclopentolate, homatropine, or scopolamine to wear dark glasses if photophobia occurs.
• *Teach the patient the proper method of instillation, including hand washing before and after administering the drops, and remind the patient not to touch the dropper to the eye or surrounding tissue.* (For more information, see *Ophthalmic agent administration.*)
• *Advise the patient to discard any discolored epinephrine solution.*
• Stress the importance of regular follow-up visits and ophthalmic examinations.
• Teach the patient to recognize and report systemic adverse reactions to the prescribed mydriatric or cycloplegic.
• *Instruct the patient to report sudden visual changes or pain or any eye drainage to the physician at once.*

Evaluation
The following examples represent appropriate evaluation statements for a patient receiving a mydriatic or cycloplegic.
• The patient has no conditions that contraindicate mydriatic or cycloplegic therapy
• The patient exhibits no signs of complications in the preexisting condition linked to the prescribed mydriatic or cycloplegic.
• The patient experiences no systemic adverse reactions to the prescribed mydriatic or cycloplegic.
• The patient displays no adverse ocular reactions to the prescribed mydriatic or cycloplegic.
• The patient and family express an accurate understanding of the points taught about the prescribed mydriatic or cycloplegic.
• The patient demonstrates proper administration of the prescribed mydriatic or cycloplegic.

MIOTICS

Miotics constrict the pupils and are used primarily to treat glaucoma and to manage accommodative esotropia. Miotics include direct-acting cholinergics (carbachol, pilocarpine hydrochloride, and pilocarpine nitrate), short-acting anticholinesterases (physostigmine salicylate and physostigmine sulfate), and long-acting anticholinesterases (demecarium bromide, echothiophate iodide, and isoflurophate).

PHARMACOKINETICS
Some systemic absorption is possible with all miotics but seldom occurs.

Onset, peak, duration
Pilocarpine, available in hydrochloride and nitrate forms, has an onset of action of 15 to 30 minutes, reaches a peak concentration level in 2 hours, and has a duration of action of 4 to 8 hours.

Carbachol has a similar duration—4 to 8 hours. However, it is absorbed poorly through the cornea and is used only if pilocarpine is ineffective or if the patient is hypersensitive to pilocarpine.

Physostigmine, the short-acting anticholinesterase available in salicylate and sulfate forms, has an onset of 10 minutes, reaches peak concentration in 3 to 4 hours, and has a duration of 12 to 36 hours. The long-acting anticholinesterases, demecarium, echothiophate, and isoflurophate, are potent miotics with a duration of days to weeks.

PHARMACODYNAMICS
Miotics stimulate and contract the sphincter muscle of the iris, thereby constricting the pupil. This action is called miosis.

Mechanism of action
Miotics are used to treat chronic open-angle glaucoma because they improve aqueous outflow from the anterior chamber of the eye by decreasing resistance to the outflow of aqueous humor. Miotics also are used to treat acute and chronic closed-angle glaucoma. (For description, see *Types of glaucoma,* page 1242. For an illustration, see *Normal flow of aqueous humor,* page 1242.)

The direct-acting cholinergic miotics constrict the pupil by contracting the sphincter muscles of the iris, contract the ciliary muscle, and widen the trabecular meshwork. These actions open the outflow channels, increasing aqueous outflow. The anticholinesterase miotics inactivate the enzyme cholinesterase, allowing acetylcholine to flow freely and exert its effects, which include pupil constriction and accommodative spasm. Long-acting anticholinesterases combine chemically and irreversibly with cholinesterase for intensified and prolonged action: marked miosis and vasodilation and strong accommodative spasm.

PHARMACOTHERAPEUTICS
The miotics are used to treat chronic open-angle glaucoma, acute and chronic closed-angle glaucoma, and certain cases of secondary glaucoma from disease- or injury-induced increases in intraocular pressure. However, if inflammation

Ophthalmic agent administration

Many ophthalmic agents come in two forms: eye drops for instillation and ointments for application. The form of an agent determines how it is administered, as shown below. With either form, hand washing is essential before administration to prevent infection and after administration to prevent self-mydriasis.

Applying eye ointment

Place the patient in a supine position or sitting with the neck hyperextended. Clean the eyelashes with saline solution and swabs to remove any secretions. Have the patient look upward; then pull down the lower lid with the finger. As the patient continues to look up, apply a thin ribbon of ointment (approximately ¼″) directly into the conjunctival sac, beginning at the inner canthus.

To avoid contamination, do not let the tube touch the eye or conjunctiva. At the outer canthus, rotate the tube to detach the ointment.

Instruct the patient to close the eye gently, but not to squeeze it closed.

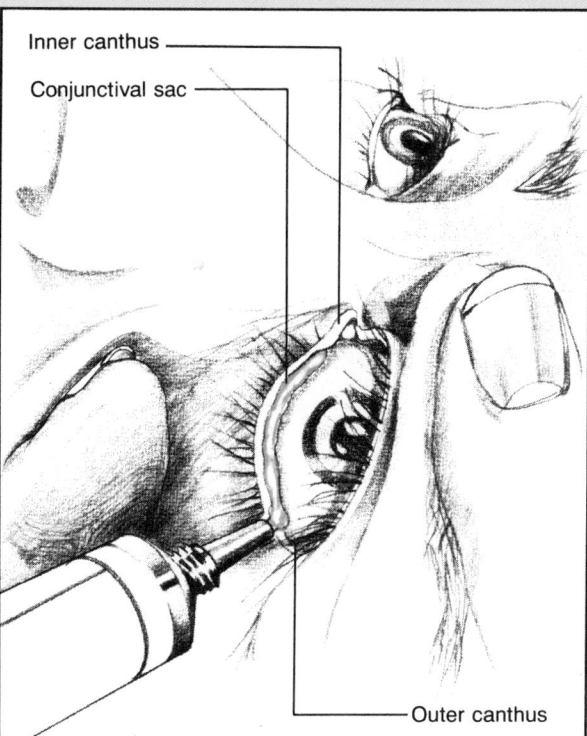

Inner canthus

Conjunctival sac

Outer canthus

Instilling eye drops

Place the patient in a supine or sitting position with the neck hyperextended, looking toward the ceiling. With the finger, pull down firmly on the lower lid while the patient continues to look upward. This movement exposes the lower conjunctival sac by relaxing the upper tarsal plate as it is retracted into the orbit.

Instill 1 drop of medication into the lower conjunctival sac. Instruct the patient to close the eye gently, but not to squeeze it closed. Wipe away excess tears with a cotton ball or tissue.

The eye can hold only 1 drop. When instilling more than 1 drop, wait 2 to 3 minutes between drops to avoid losing a drop from tearing or blinking.

After instilling drops, apply digital pressure over the punctum at the inner canthus for 2 to 3 minutes, and have the patient close the eyelids gently for 2 to 3 minutes to prevent drainage through the nasolacrimal duct. Stopping drainage through the nasolacrimal duct when instilling eye drops helps prevent systemic absorption. It also prevents the patient from tasting the drops.

To avoid contamination, do not allow the tip of the dropper to touch the lid or eyelashes.

Discard discolored solutions or solutions with floating particles.

When instilling a mydriatic or cycloplegic, pay special attention during administration to prevent accidental instillation into the unaffected eye.

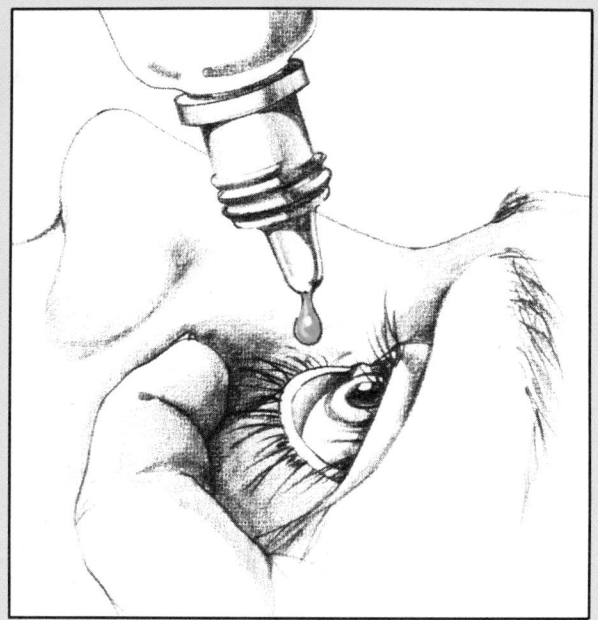

Types of glaucoma

Chronic open-angle (wide-angle) glaucoma results from overproduction of aqueous humor or obstruction of its outflow through the trabecular meshwork, the canal of Schlemm, or aqueous veins.

Acute closed-angle (narrow-angle) glaucoma results from obstruction of aqueous humor outflow because of anatomically narrow angles between the anterior iris and the posterior corneal surface; shallow anterior chambers; a thickened iris that causes angle closure on pupil dilation; or a bulging iris that presses on the trabeculae, thereby closing the angle.

Chronic closed-angle glaucoma follows an untreated episode of acute closed-angle glaucoma or mild recurring acute episodes that create increased synechiae in the trabecular meshwork.

Normal flow of aqueous humor

Aqueous humor, a transparent fluid produced by the ciliary epithelium of the ciliary body, flows from the posterior chamber to the anterior chamber through the pupil. Here it flows peripherally and filters through the trabecular meshwork to the canal of Schlemm. The fluid ultimately enters the venous circulation.

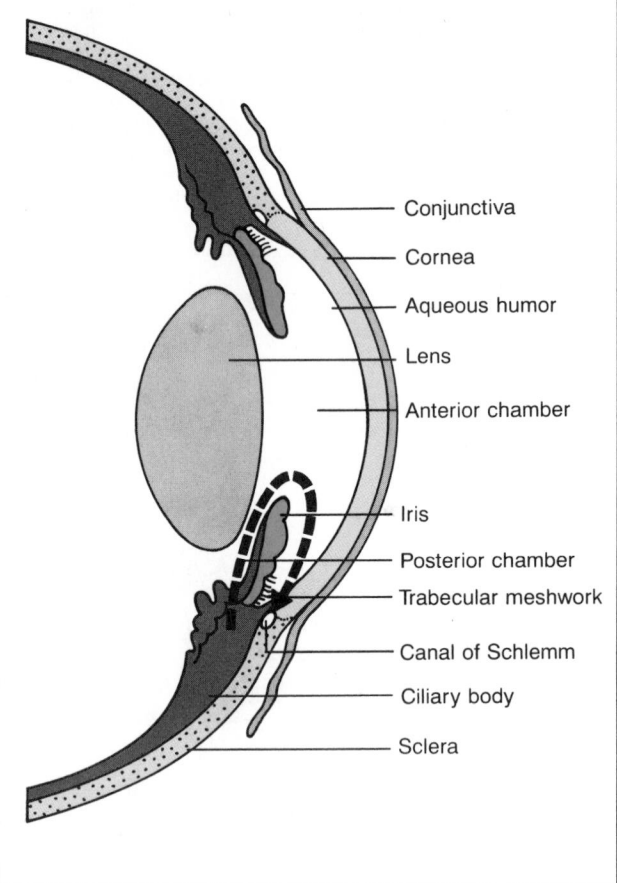

- Conjunctiva
- Cornea
- Aqueous humor
- Lens
- Anterior chamber
- Iris
- Posterior chamber
- Trabecular meshwork
- Canal of Schlemm
- Ciliary body
- Sclera

such as iritis is present, miotics should not be used because they may increase the inflammation.

Controlling intraocular pressure is the cornerstone of glaucoma therapy, and direct-acting miotics such as pilocarpine usually are the drugs of choice. Long-acting miotics such as isoflurophate, which can be toxic, are used only in patients refractory to direct- or short-acting agents.

carbachol (Carbacel, Isopto Carbachol). A cholinergic drug, intraocular carbachol is used to achieve miosis for ocular surgery; topical carbachol is used to treat open-angle and closed-angle glaucomas.
Usual adult dosage: for miosis, 0.5 ml of 0.01% solution into the anterior chamber; for open-angle or closed-angle glaucoma, 1 drop of 0.75% to 3% solution instilled into the conjunctival sac every 4 to 8 hours.

demecarium bromide (Humorsol). This long-acting anticholinesterase is used to treat glaucoma in adults and accommodative esotropia in children.
Usual adult dosage: for glaucoma, 1 drop of 0.125% or 0.25% solution every 12 to 48 hours.
Usual pediatric dosage: for esotropia, 1 drop of 0.125% solution daily for 2 to 3 weeks, then 1 drop every other day for 3 to 4 weeks, and, if improved, 1 drop twice weekly; therapy should be discontinued after 4 months if condition still requires therapy every other day or if the patient shows no response.

echothiophate iodide (Phospholine Iodide). A long-acting anticholinesterase, echothiophate is used to treat open-angle glaucoma, conditions obstructing aqueous outflow, and accommodative esotropia.
Usual adult and pediatric dosage: 1 drop of 0.03% to 0.06% solution in the conjunctival sac every 12 to 48 hours. A

stronger solution of 0.125% to 0.25% may be required in patients with highly pigmented irises.

isoflurophate (Floropryl). A long-acting anticholinesterase, isoflurophate is used to treat glaucoma and esotropia.
Usual adult and pediatric dosage: for open-angle glaucoma, ¼″ of 0.025% ointment in the conjunctival sac every 8 to 72 hours; for esotropia uncomplicated by amblyopia (loss of vision unrelated to poor refraction) or anisometropia (a difference in refraction between the two eyes), ¼″ of 0.025% ointment every night for 2 weeks.

physostigmine salicylate (Eserine Salicylate, Isopto Eserine) and **physostigmine sulfate** (Eserine Sulfate). These short-acting anticholinesterases are used to treat open-angle glaucoma.

Usual adult and pediatric dosage: ¼" of 0.25% ointment in the conjunctival sac or 1 to 2 drops 0.25% or 0.5% solution in the conjunctival sac every 4 to 8 hours.

pilocarpine hydrochloride (Isopto Carpine, Pilocar) and **pilocarpine nitrate** (P.V. Carpine). These cholinergics, considered reliable and highly effective, are two of the most commonly used drugs to treat chronic open-angle glaucoma and, before surgery, to treat acute closed-angle glaucoma.

Usual adult and pediatric dosage: for chronic open-angle glaucoma, 1 to 2 drops of 1% to 2% solution every 4 to 8 hours; for acute closed-angle glaucoma, 1 drop of a 2% solution instilled three to six times over a 30-minute period before surgery. A stronger solution of pilocarpine may be required in patients with highly pigmented irises.

pilocarpine ocuserts (Ocusert Pilo-20, Ocusert Pilo-40). This form of pilocarpine, an ocular insert, has the same indications as pilocarpine hydrochloride and pilocarpine nitrate and delivers 20 mg/hour or 40 mg/hour for 7 days.

Usual adult dosage: one ocular insert placed in the conjunctival sac every 7 days.

Drug interactions

Echothiophate, isoflurophate, and physostigmine may interact with succinylcholine, resulting in respiratory or cardiovascular collapse. Therefore, these agents should not be administered concomitantly. Pilocarpine interacts with carbachol, causing additive effects, and with phenylephrine, decreasing phenylephrine-induced mydriasis. These interactions prohibit concomitant use of these drugs.

ADVERSE DRUG REACTIONS

Miotics commonly cause blurred vision and eye and brow pain. Reversible iris cysts, lid pain, photosensitivity, and cataract formation also can occur. Although uncommon, systemic absorption can lead to abdominal cramps, diarrhea, and increased salivation.

The miotics also can cause bronchial constriction and spasm as well as pulmonary edema. In dark-skinned patients, hypersensitivity reactions to physostigmine can lead to reversible depigmentation of eyelid skin.

NURSING PROCESS APPLICATION

The following information assists the nurse in caring for a patient receiving a miotic.

Assessment

• Review the patient's history for a preexisting condition that contraindicates the use of a miotic, such as a history of or predisposition to retinal detachment, glaucoma associated with acute inflammation, or known hypersensitivity to the drug.

• Review the patient's history for a preexisting condition that requires cautious use of a miotic, such as corneal abrasions.

• Assess the patient for systemic adverse reactions to the prescribed miotic, such as abdominal cramps, diarrhea, increased salivation, bronchial constriction or spasm, pulmonary edema, or hypersensitivity reactions.

• Review the patient's medication history to identify the use of drugs that may interact with the prescribed miotic, such as succinylcholine, carbachol and phenylephrine.

• Assess the effectiveness of the prescribed miotics regularly.

• Assess the patient for adverse ocular reactions, such as blurred vision, eyelid and brow pain, iris cysts, photosensitivity, and cataract formation.

• Evaluate the patient's and family's knowledge about the prescribed miotic.

Nursing diagnoses

The following examples represent appropriate nursing diagnoses for a patient receiving a miotic.

• Potential for injury related to a preexisting condition that contraindicates the use of a miotic

• Potential for injury related to a preexisting condition that requires cautious use of a miotic

• Potential for injury related to adverse drug reactions

• Sensory-perceptual alterations (visual) related to the adverse ocular effects of the miotic

• Knowledge deficit related to the prescribed miotic

Planning and implementation

• Do not administer a miotic to a patient with a condition that contraindicates its use.

• Administer a miotic cautiously to a patient at risk because of a preexisting condition.

• Monitor the patient closely for adverse reactions during miotic therapy.

• Monitor hydration if the patient experiences diarrhea. Request a prescription for an antidiarrheal agent if needed.

• *Monitor the patient for signs of bronchial constriction or spasm and pulmonary edema, such as wheezing, crackles, jugular vein distention, and shortness of breath. Notify the physician if respiratory dysfunction occurs. Expect to administer a bronchodilator, diuretic, or other emergency treatments as prescribed.*

• Observe the dark-skinned patient for depigmentation of eyelid skin, a hypersensitivity reaction to physostigmine.

• *Minimize systemic absorption of the miotic by applying digital pressure over the punctum at the inner canthus for 2 to 3 minutes after instilling drops.*
• Notify the physician if systemic adverse reactions occur.
• Ask the patient about blurred vision during miotic therapy. Take safety precautions until vision returns to normal. For example, keep the bed rails raised and supervise ambulation.
• Ask the patient about eye, brow, or eyelid pain and photosensitivity.
• Ensure that routine ophthalmic examinations are performed to detect iris cysts or cataracts.
• Notify the physician if adverse ocular effects occur.

Patient teaching
• Teach the patient and family the name, dose, frequency, action, and adverse effects of the prescribed miotic.
• *Explain to the patient that blurred vision will occur after administration; instruct the patient to instill drops at bedtime, if possible, to minimize problems resulting from blurring.*
• Inform patient that eye, brow, or lid pain commonly occurs with miotic therapy. If pain persists or worsens, advise the patient to notify the physician.
• Advise the patient to wear dark glasses if photosensitivity occurs.
• Stress the importance of regular follow-up visits and ophthalmologic examinations to detect adverse ocular reactions and assess the drugs's effectiveness.
• *Teach the patient or a family member how to administer the prescribed miotic correctly.* (For more information, see *Ophthalmic agent administration,* page 1241.)
• Teach the patient how to reconstitute echothiophate with the enclosed diluent. Reconstituted echothiophate will remain stable for 1 month at room temperature or 6 months under refrigeration.
• Instruct the patient to notify the physician if adverse ocular reactions occur.
• Reassure the dark-skinned patient that depigmentation of eyelid skin is reversible.
• *Teach the patient to recognize the signs and symptoms of pulmonary edema and bronchoconstriction and to seek emergency care if they occur.*
• Advise the patient that abdominal cramps, diarrhea, and increased salivation may occur during miotic therapy.
• Instruct the patient to notify the physician if any systemic adverse reactions occur.

Evaluation
The following examples represent appropriate evaluation statements for a patient receiving a miotic.
• The patient has no conditions that contraindicate miotic therapy.

• The patient exhibits no signs of complications in the preexisting condition linked to the prescribed miotic.
• The patient experiences no systemic adverse reactions to the prescribed miotic.
• The patient experiences no visual disturbances caused by the prescribed miotic.
• The patient and family express an accurate understanding of the points taught about the prescribed miotic.
• The patient demonstrates correct administration of the prescribed miotic.

DRUGS THAT LOWER INTRAOCULAR PRESSURE

Topical adrenergic-blocking agents, hyperosmotic agents, and carbonic anhydrase inhibitors are used to lower intraocular pressure. These drugs lower intraocular pressure by reducing or blocking aqueous humor formation and increasing aqueous humor outflow. Topical adrenergic-blocking agents include apraclonidine hydrochloride (a selective alpha-adrenergic blocker), betaxolol hydrochloride (a cardioselective receptor blocking agent), levobunolol hydrochloride (a nonselective beta-adrenergic blocker), and timolol maleate (a nonselective adrenergic blocker).

Hyperosmotic agents include glycerin, glycerin (anhydrous), isosorbide, mannitol, and urea. The carbonic anhydrase inhibitors are acetazolamide, acetazolamide sodium, dichlorphenamide, and methazolamide.

PHARMACOKINETICS

The pharmacokinetics of drugs used to lower intraocular pressure varies with the route of administration.

Absorption, distribution, metabolism, excretion
The extent of ocular and systemic absorption of apraclonidine and betaxolol has not been elucidated. Levobunolol and timolol are absorbed systemically.

After oral administration, glycerin and isosorbide are absorbed rapidly. Their action begins within 30 minutes. Both drugs are distributed widely and excreted unchanged in the kidneys.

The distribution, metabolism, and excretion of the adrenergic blocking agents varies. (For more information, see Chapter 16, Adrenergic Blocking Agents.)

The hyperosmotic agents mannitol and urea are administered I.V. and distributed immediately. The carbonic anhydrase inhibitors are administered by various routes, so their pharmacokinetics differ accordingly. (For more information about the pharmacokinetics of hyperosmotic agents and carbonic anhydrase inhibitors, see Chapter 33, Diuretic Agents.)

Onset, peak, duration
The onset of action of the topical adrenergic-blocking agents occurs 20 minutes after administration, with peak concentration levels usually occurring within 1 to 2 hours. The duration of action of these drugs can range up to 24 hours.

The hyperosmotic agents have an onset within 15 minutes and a duration of 5 to 8 hours.

The onset of the carbonic anhydrase inhibitors varies. The effects of acetazolamide sodium appear within 2 minutes of injection, whereas the onset of oral acetazolamide is 60 to 90 minutes. Oral dichlorphenamide produces effects within 30 to 60 minutes. The effects of methazolamide do not appear until 2 hours after administration. The duration of the carbonic anhydrase inhibitors ranges from 4 hours to 24 hours for sustained-release acetazolamide.

PHARMACODYNAMICS

Each group of drugs lowers intraocular pressure by a different mechanism of action.

Mechanism of action
The adrenergic-blocking agent timolol decreases intraocular pressure without affecting pupil size or accommodation. Although its action is not understood well, timolol primarily may reduce aqueous humor formation and slightly increase aqueous humor outflow. The action of apraclonidine, betaxalol, and levobunolol in reducing intraocular pressure has not been established. However, it may be similar to that of timolol.

Hyperosmotic agents, which are reserved for emergencies, increase the absorption of water in the eye into the general circulation, thus lowering intraocular pressure.

The enzyme carbonic anhydrase is involved in aqueous humor production in the eye, so drugs that inhibit the action of carbonic anhydrase decrease aqueous production—by 30% to 60%—without affecting aqueous outflow. As less aqueous fluid enters the eye, intraocular pressure decreases.

PHARMACOTHERAPEUTICS

The indications for topical adrenergic-blocking agents varies. Apraclonidine is used to prevent or control elevated intraocular pressure after argon laser trabeculoplasty or iridotomy. Betaxolol and levobunolol are used to treat chronic open-angle glaucoma. Timolol is used to treat some secondary glaucoma.

The hyperosmotic agents are used to treat acute closed-angle glaucoma; they also are used before and after ocular surgery.

The carbonic anhydrase inhibitors are used to treat chronic open-angle glaucoma, acute angle-closure episodes, and secondary glaucoma.

apraclonidine hydrochloride (Iopidine). This selective alpha-adrenergic blocking agent is used to prevent or control elevated intraocular pressure after argon laser trabeculoplasty or iridotomy.
Usual adult dosage: 1 drop of 1% solution instilled 1 hour before anterior segment laser surgery and 1 drop of 1% solution instilled immediately after surgery.

betaxolol hydrochloride (Betoptic). This beta$_1$-adrenergic blocking agent is used to treat chronic open-angle glaucoma and increased intraocular pressure.
Usual adult dosage: 1 drop of 0.5% solution b.i.d.

levobunolol hydrochloride (Betagan). A long-acting, nonselective beta-adrenergic blocking agent, levobunolol is used to treat chronic open-angle glaucoma and increased intraocular pressure.
Usual adult dosage: 1 drop of 0.5% solution once or twice daily.

timolol maleate (Timoptic). A beta$_1$- and beta$_2$-adrenergic blocking agent, timolol is used to treat chronic open-angle glaucoma, aphakic glaucoma (occurring in an eye with no lens), and increased intraocular pressure.
Usual adult dosage: initially, 1 drop of 0.25% solution b.i.d., reduced to once daily for maintenance; if the patient does not respond, 1 drop of 0.5% solution b.i.d.

glycerin (Osmoglyn). This oral hyperosmotic agent is administered to reduce intraocular pressure, especially in patients with acute closed-angle glaucoma before iridectomy.
Usual adult dosage: 1 to 1.8 grams/kg P.O. every 5 hours; for preoperative use, 1 to 1.8 grams/kg P.O. 60 to 90 minutes before surgery.

glycerin, anhydrous (Ophthalgan). This topical hyperosmotic agent is used to treat corneal edema and to prepare for ophthalmoscopy or gonioscopy. It also is used to differentiate superficial edema from deep corneal edema because it is ineffective in patients with deep corneal edema.
Usual adult dosage: to facilitate ophthalmoscopic or gonioscopic examination, 1 or 2 drops instilled before examination; to reduce corneal edema caused by trauma or disease, 1 or 2 drops every 3 or 4 hours.

isosorbide (Ismotic). This oral hyperosmotic agent is used for short-term reduction of increased intraocular pressure from glaucoma and for preoperative reduction of intraocular pressure.

Usual adult dosage: 1.5 grams/kg P.O. up to four times per day.

mannitol (Osmitrol). A hyperosmotic agent, mannitol is used to reduce increased intraocular pressure during an episode of acute closed-angle glaucoma.
Usual adult dosage: 0.5 to 2 grams/kg of a 20% solution administered I.V. over 30 to 60 minutes.

urea (Ureaphil). This hyperosmotic agent is used to reduce increased intraocular pressure during an episode of acute closed-angle glaucoma.
Usual adult dosage: 1 to 1.5 grams/kg of 30% solution administered I.V. over 1½ to 2 hours.
Usual pediatric dosage: 0.5 to 1.5 grams/kg of 30% solution administered I.V. over 1½ to 2 hours for children over age 2.

acetazolamide (Ak-Zol, Diamox, Diamox Sequels) and **acetazolamide sodium** (Diamox Parenteral, Diamox Sodium). A carbonic anhydrase inhibitor, acetazolamide and acetazolamide sodium (the long-acting form of acetazolamide) are used primarily to treat chronic open-angle glaucoma.
Usual adult dosage: 250 mg P.O. of acetazolamide daily to q.i.d., or 500 mg P.O. of acetazolamide sodium every 12 hours. For rapid lowering of intraocular pressure, 500 mg I.M. or I.V. initially (may be repeated in 2 to 4 hours).

dichlorphenamide (Daranide, Oratrol). This carbonic anhydrase inhibitor is used as adjunctive therapy for patients with chronic open-angle glaucoma.
Usual adult dosage: initially, 100 to 200 mg P.O., followed by 100 mg every 12 hours until therapeutic response occurs; maintenance dosage, 25 to 50 mg P.O. b.i.d. or t.i.d.

methazolamide (Neptazane). This carbonic anhydrase inhibitor is used to treat chronic open-angle glaucoma. Methazolamide also is used preoperatively in patients with acute closed-angle glaucoma.
Usual adult dosage: 50 to 100 mg P.O. b.i.d. or t.i.d.

Drug interactions
No significant interactions occur between hyperosmotic agents and other drugs. Interactions between timolol and such oral beta-adrenergic blocking agents as propranolol increase ocular and systemic effects; caution is required with concomitant use of these drugs. The adrenergic-blocking agents also should be used cautiously with monoamine oxidase (MAO) inhibitors. Patients using acetazolamide with a salicylate may need a reduction in salicylate dosage.

ADVERSE DRUG REACTIONS

Adverse reactions vary among the topical adrenergic agents, hyperosmotic agents, and carbonic anhydrase inhibitors. The adrenergic-blocking agents can reduce heart rate, causing headaches and fatigue, and the beta blockade effects from systemic timolol absorption may lead to bradycardia and bronchospasm. Apraclonidine may cause upper eyelid elevation, conjunctival blanching, and mydriasis.

The hyperosmotic agents can cause stinging when administered. Use of a topical anesthetic is recommended with glycerin administration. (For adverse reactions to mannitol and urea, see Chapter 33, Diuretic Agents.)

Carbonic anhydrase inhibitors, such as acetazolamide, can cause drowsiness, hypokalemia, nausea, vomiting, leukopenia, hemolytic anemia, and aplastic anemia.

NURSING PROCESS APPLICATION

The following information assists the nurse in caring for a patient receiving a drug that lowers intraocular pressure.

Assessment
• Review the patient's history for a preexisting condition that contraindicates the use of a drug that lowers intraocular pressure, such as sinus bradycardia, greater-than-first-degree atrioventricular block, cardiogenic shock, overt cardiac failure, bronchial asthma, severe chronic obstructive pulmonary disease, or known hypersensitivity to the drug.
• Review the patient's history for a preexisting condition that requires cautious use of a drug that lowers intraocular pressure, such as pregnancy, lactation, diabetes, hyperthyroidism, pulmonary dysfunction, or cerebral vascular insufficiency.
• Assess the patient for systemic adverse reactions to the prescribed drug that lowers intraocular pressure, such as bradycardia, headaches, fatigue, bronchospasm, drowsiness, hypokalemia, nausea, vomiting, and blood disorders.
• Review the patient's medication history to identify the use of drugs that may interact with the prescribed drug that lowers intraocular pressure, such as oral beta-adrenergic blocking agents, MAO inhibitors, and salicylates.
• Assess the effectiveness of the prescribed drug that lowers intraocular pressure.
• Assess the patient for adverse ocular reactions to the prescribed drug that lowers intraocular pressure, such as transient stinging, upper eyelid elevation, conjunctival blanching, and mydriasis.
• Evaluate the patient's and family's knowledge about the prescribed drug that lowers intraocular pressure.

Nursing diagnoses

The following examples represent appropriate diagnoses for a patient receiving a drug that lowers intraocular pressure.

• Potential for injury related to a preexisting condition that contraindicates the use of a drug that lowers intraocular pressure

• Potential for injury related to a preexisting condition that requires cautious use of a drug that lowers intraocular pressure

• Potential for injury related to adverse drug reactions

• Potential for injury related to the adverse ocular effects of a drug that lowers intraocular pressure

• Knowledge deficit related to the prescribed drug that lowers intraocular pressure

Planning and implementation

• Do not administer a drug that lowers intraocular pressure to a patient with a condition that contraindicates its use.

• Administer a drug that lowers intraocular pressure cautiously to a patient at risk because of a preexisting condition.

• Monitor the patient closely for adverse reactions throughout the course of therapy.

• *Monitor the heart rate to detect bradycardia in a patient receiving an adrenergic-blocking agent. If the heart rate falls below 60 beats/minute, notify the physician and expect to administer a different drug as prescribed.*

• Administer a mild analgesic as prescribed if the patient experiences headache.

• Assist the patient with activities and provide frequent rest periods if fatigue occurs.

• *Auscultate the patient's lungs frequently during timolol therapy to detect bronchospasm. If bronchospasm occurs, notify the physician and expect to administer a bronchodilator and discontinue timolol as prescribed.*

• Take safety precautions if acetazolamide causes drowsiness. For example, keep the bed rails raised and supervise the patient's activities.

• Monitor the patient's serum potassium level for hypokalemia during treatment with a carbonic anhydrase inhibitor.

• Monitor hydration if the patient experiences nausea and vomiting. Request a prescription for an antiemetic if needed.

• Monitor the patient's complete blood count (CBC) regularly to detect leukopenia or anemia. If leukopenia occurs, monitor the patient for signs of infection, such as sore throat, malaise, and fever, and take infection control measures until the white blood count returns to normal. If anemia occurs, take energy conservation measures.

• Notify the physician if systemic adverse reactions occur.

• Observe for upper eyelid elevation, conjunctival blanching, and mydriasis in a patient receiving apraclonidine for laser surgery.

• Administer a topical anesthetic with glycerin to help prevent stinging during administration.

• Notify the physician if adverse ocular reactions occur.

Patient teaching

• Teach the patient the name, dose, frequency, action, and adverse effects of the prescribed drug that lowers intraocular pressure.

• *Instruct the patient in self-instillation of eye drops, if appropriate.* (For more information, see *Ophthalmic agent administration,* page 1241.) *Explain the importance of not touching the eyedropper to the eye and of hand washing before and after self-instillation.*

• Inform the patient that apraclonidine may cause upper eyelid elevation, conjunctival blanching, and mydriasis. Teach the patient how to manage these adverse reactions.

• Advise the patient that administration of a hyperosmotic agent may cause stinging, but that an anesthetic agent can be used concomitantly to promote comfort.

• *Instruct the patient to report to the physician a pulse rate below 60 beats/minute or wheezing.*

• Advise the patient to take a mild analgesic if headache occurs.

• Warn the patient not to perform activities that require alertness if drowsiness occurs.

• Teach the patient to use energy conservation measures if fatigue or anemia occurs and infection control measures if leukopenia occurs.

• Stress the importance of returning as instructed for blood tests, such as CBC and serum potassium determination, to detect adverse reactions.

• Instruct the patient to notify the physician if adverse reactions occur.

Evaluation

The following examples represent appropriate evaluation statements for a patient receiving a drug that lowers intraocular pressure.

• The patient has no conditions that contraindicate the use of a drug that lowers intraocular pressure.

• The patient exhibits no signs of complications in the preexisting condition linked to the prescribed drug that lowers intraocular pressure.

• The patient experiences no systemic adverse reactions to the prescribed drug that lowers intraocular pressure.

• The patient experiences no adverse ocular reactions to the drug that lowers intraocular pressure.

• The patient and family express an accurate understanding of the points taught about the prescribed drug that lowers intraocular pressure.

• The patient demonstrates proper administration of the prescribed drug that lowers intraocular pressure.

ANESTHETIC AGENTS

Because the cornea and the conjunctiva contain delicate sensory nerves, surgical (and some diagnostic) procedures involving the eye would be impossible without anesthetics. Topical ophthalmic anesthetics anesthetize the corneal surface so that instruments can be applied to measure intraocular pressure or to remove foreign bodies. Local ophthalmic anesthetics of the globe and eyelid are used to anesthetize and to paralyze muscles in the eye, eyelid, and face.

This section covers these topical ophthalmic anesthetics: proparacaine hydrochloride, tetracaine, and tetracaine hydrochloride. (For information on other local [regional] anesthetics, such as bupivacaine hydrochloride, etidocaine hydrochloride, lidocaine hydrochloride, mepivacaine hydrochloride, prilocaine hydrochloride, and procaine hydrochloride, see Chapter 24, Local and Topical Anesthetic Agents.)

Topical cocaine is a natural compound. Because of its corneal toxicity and adverse central nervous system (CNS) reactions, it has been replaced by synthetic anesthetics and is not covered here.

PHARMACOKINETICS

Most of these anesthetics have an onset of action of 1 minute.

PHARMACODYNAMICS

Proparacaine and tetracaine act by interfering with cell activity. More drops may be required to anesthetize an inflamed eye because the blood vessels carry the anesthetic away.

PHARMACOTHERAPEUTICS

Besides anesthetizing the cornea to allow application of instruments for measuring intraocular pressure or removing foreign bodies, topical ophthalmic anesthetics are used for suture removal, for conjunctival or corneal scraping, and for lacrimal canal manipulation.

proparacaine hydrochloride (Alcaine, Ophthaine). This topical anesthetic is used for tonometry, gonioscopy, corneal suture removal, and removal of corneal foreign bodies.
Usual adult dosage: 1 to 2 drops of 0.5% solution just before the procedure; for anesthesia for cataract extraction or glaucoma surgery, 1 drop of 0.5% solution every 5 to 10 minutes for five to seven doses; for suture or foreign body removal, 1 drop of 0.5% solution 2 to 3 minutes before the procedure.

tetracaine (Pontocaine) and **tetracaine hydrochloride** (Pontocaine Hydrochloride). These topical anesthetics are used for tonometry, gonioscopy, removal of corneal foreign bodies, corneal suture removal, and other diagnostic and minor surgical procedures. Tetracaine is a 0.5% ointment; tetracaine hydrochloride, a 0.5% solution.
Usual adult and pediatric dosage: 1 to 2 drops of 0.5% solution or a ½" to 1" ribbon of 0.5% ointment just before the procedure.

Drug interactions

The only significant interaction involving the topical ophthalmic anesthetics occurs with tetracaine, which interferes with the antibacterial action of sulfonamides. They should be administered ½ hour apart to prevent this interaction.

ADVERSE DRUG REACTIONS

All three topical ophthalmic anesthetics can cause transient eye pain and redness. Prolonged use can cause keratitis, corneal opacities, scarring, loss of visual acuity, and delayed corneal healing.

NURSING PROCESS APPLICATION

The following information assists the nurse in caring for a patient receiving an ophthalmic anesthetic agent.

Assessment
• Review the patient's history for a preexisting condition that contraindicates the use of an ophthalmic anesthetic, such as known hypersensitivity to the drug.
• Review the patient's history for a preexisting condition that requires cautious use of an ophthalmic anesthetic, such as cardiac disease, hyperthyroidism, or known allergies.
• Review the patient's medication history to identify the use of drugs that may interact with tetracaine, such as sulfonamides.
• Assess the effectiveness of the prescribed ophthalmic anesthetic regularly.
• Assess the patient for adverse ocular reactions, such as transient eye pain and redness, keratitis, corneal opacities, scarring, loss of visual acuity, or delayed corneal healing.
• Evaluate the patient's and family's knowledge about the prescribed ophthalmic anesthetic.

Nursing diagnoses
The following examples represent appropriate nursing diagnoses for a patient receiving an ophthalmic anesthetic.
• Potential for injury related to a preexisting condition that contraindicates the use of an ophthalmic anesthetic

• Potential for injury related to a preexisting condition that requires cautious use of an ophthalmic anesthetic
• Sensory-perceptual alterations (visual) related to the adverse ocular effects of the ophthalmic anesthetic
• Knowledge deficit related to the prescribed ophthalmic anesthetic

Planning and implementation
• Do not administer an ophthalmic anesthetic to a patient with a condition that contraindicates its use.
• Administer an ophthalmic anesthetic cautiously to a patient at risk because of a preexisting condition.
• Monitor the patient closely for adverse reactions to the ophthalmic anesthetic.
• *Apply digital pressure over the punctum at the inner canthus for 2 to 3 minutes after anesthetic administration to prevent systemic absorption.*
• Observe the patient for eye redness during ophthalmic anesthetic use. Ask the patient about eye pain.
• *Ensure that regular ophthalmic examinations are performed to detect keratitis, corneal opacities, scarring, or delayed corneal healing in a patient receiving an ophthalmic anesthetic agent over a prolonged time.*
• Monitor the patient's visual acuity regularly.
• Provide the patient with a protective eye patch, if necessary, to be worn while the eye is anesthetized.
• Notify the physician if adverse ocular reactions occur.

Patient teaching
• Teach the patient and family the name, dose, frequency, action, and adverse effects of the prescribed ophthalmic anesthetic.
• *Advise the patient receiving a topical anesthetic not to rub the eyes; explain that corneal abrasion may occur because the usual pain signal is absent. Also explain that the anesthetic will cause transient blurred vision.*
• Stress the importance of regular follow-up visits and ophthalmic examinations during prolonged therapy with an ophthalmic anesthetic.
• Instruct the patient to report any visual disturbances or discomfort to the physician.

Evaluation
The following examples represent appropriate evaluation statements for a patient receiving an ophthalmic anesthetic.
• The patient has no conditions that contraindicate ophthalmic anesthetic therapy.
• The patient exhibits no signs of complications in the preexisting condition linked to the prescribed ophthalmic anesthetic.
• The patient experiences no vision disturbances caused by the prescribed ophthalmic anesthetic.

• The patient and family express an accurate understanding of the points taught about the prescribed ophthalmic anesthetic.
• The patient correctly identifies adverse reactions that must be reported during ophthalmic anesthetic therapy.

ANTI-INFLAMMATORY AGENTS

Corticosteroids, hormones secreted by the adrenal glands, are produced synthetically for pharmacologic, including ophthalmic, use. Ophthalmic anti-inflammatory agents are corticosteroid solutions or suspensions that decrease leukocyte infiltration at the site of ocular inflammation.

Investigators used to believe that corticosteroids were contraindicated in patients with infectious diseases. Today, however, corticosteroids may be used cautiously with antimicrobial and antiviral agents when the causative organism has been identified to help prevent serious eye damage caused by inflammation. The topical agents include dexamethasone, fluorometholone, medrysone, prednisolone acetate, and prednisolone sodium phosphate.

PHARMACOKINETICS

Absorption of topical anti-inflammatory agents through the intact cornea is minimal. Suspensions, such as dexamethasone, usually are absorbed more completely than solutions, such as prednisolone sodium phosphate. Onset and duration of action vary among these anti-inflammatory agents; specific information is unavailable.

PHARMACODYNAMICS

The ophthalmic anti-inflammatory agents decrease leukocyte infiltration at inflammation sites. This reduces the exudative reaction of diseased tissue, leading to reduced edema, redness, and scarring.

PHARMACOTHERAPEUTICS

Corticosteroids are used to treat inflammatory disorders and hypersensitivity-related conditions of the cornea, iris, conjunctiva, sclera, and anterior uvea.

dexamethasone (Maxidex Ophthalmic Suspension). Dexamethasone is used to treat uveitis; iridocyclitis; inflammatory conditions of the eyelid, conjunctiva, cornea, and anterior segment; corneal injury from chemical or thermal burns; penetration of foreign bodies; and allergic conjunctivitis.

Usual adult and pediatric dosage: 1 to 2 drops of 0.1% solution instilled into the conjunctival sac; for severe disease, drops may be used hourly, tapering off to discontinuation as the condition improves; in mild conditions, drops may be used up to six times daily; treatment may extend from a few days to several weeks.

fluorometholone (Fluor-Op, FML, FML Forte). Fluorometholone is used to treat inflammatory and hypersensitivity-related conditions of the cornea, conjunctiva, sclera, and anterior uvea. It is available as an ointment and as a suspension.

Usual adult and pediatric dosage: 1 to 2 drops of 0.1% or 0.25% suspension every hour for the first 24 to 48 hours, then 1 to 2 drops of suspension b.i.d. to q.i.d.; or ½″ (1.25 cm) of ointment every six hours for 24 to 48 hours, then b.i.d. to daily.

medrysone (HMS Liquifilm Ophthalmic). This anti-inflammatory agent is used to treat allergic conjunctivitis, vernal conjunctivitis, episcleritis, and ophthalmic epinephrine reaction.

Usual adult and pediatric dosage: 1 drop of 1% solution instilled in the conjunctival sac b.i.d. to q.i.d.; may be used every hour during initial 1 to 2 days, if needed.

prednisolone acetate (Econopred, Econopred Plus, Pred Forte, Pred Mild) and **prednisolone sodium phosphate** (Ak-Pred, Metreton Ophthalmic). Prednisolone is used to treat inflammation of the palpebral and bulbar conjunctiva, the cornea, and the anterior segment.

Usual adult and pediatric dosage: 1 to 2 drops of 0.12% to 1% suspension; for severe conditions, may be used hourly, tapering to discontinuation; for mild conditions, may be used up to six times daily.

Drug interactions

No significant interactions occur between ophthalmic corticosteroid anti-inflammatory agents and other drugs.

ADVERSE DRUG REACTIONS

These drugs can increase intraocular pressure. Corneal thinning or ulceration, interference with corneal wound healing, and increased susceptibility to viral or fungal corneal infection also can occur. Long-term or excessive use of these drugs can lead to glaucoma exacerbation, cataracts, reduced visual acuity, and optic nerve damage. Excessive or long-term use of suspensions, which are absorbed more readily, can lead to adrenal suppression.

NURSING PROCESS APPLICATION

The following information assists the nurse in caring for a patient receiving an ophthalmic anti-inflammatory agent.

Assessment

• Review the patient's history for a preexisting condition that contraindicates the use of an anti-inflammatory agent, such as acute, untreated, purulent bacterial, viral, or fungal eye infections; acute, superficial herpes simplex keratitis; vaccina, varicella, and most other viral diseases of the cornea or conjunctiva; or known hypersensitivity to the drug.
• Review the patient's history for a preexisting condition that requires cautious use of an anti-inflammatory agent, such as pregnancy, lactation, or corneal abrasions.
• Assess the patient for adverse ocular reactions to the prescribed anti-inflammatory agent, such as increased intraocular pressure, corneal thinning or ulceration, delayed corneal wound healing, and viral or fungal corneal infection.
• Assess the effectiveness of the prescribed anti-inflammatory agent regularly.
• Assess for adrenal suppression in a patient receiving high dose or long-term therapy with an anti-inflammatory agent suspension.
• Evaluate the patient's and family's knowledge about the prescribed anti-inflammatory agent.

Nursing diagnoses

The following examples represent appropriate nursing diagnoses for a patient receiving an anti-inflammatory agent.
• Potential for injury related to a preexisting condition that contraindicates the use of an anti-inflammatory agent
• Potential for injury related to a preexisting condition that requires cautious use of an anti-inflammatory agent
• Potential for injury related to adverse drug reactions
• Altered protection related to adrenal suppression caused by excessive or long-term use of an anti-inflammatory suspension
• Knowledge deficit related to the prescribed anti-inflammatory agent

Planning and implementation

• Do not administer an anti-inflammatory agent to a patient with a condition that contraindicates its use.
• Administer an anti-inflammatory agent cautiously to a patient at risk because of a preexisting condition.
• Monitor the patient closely for adverse reactions during anti-inflammatory therapy.
• Ask the patient frequently about visual disturbances or eye discomfort.

• *Inspect the patient's eyes regularly for signs of infection (such as purulent drainage, redness, or swollen areas), corneal ulceration, or delayed corneal wound healing.*

• *Ensure that regular ophthalmic examinations are performed to detect adverse ocular reactions, such as glaucoma exacerbation, cataracts, reduced visual acuity, and optic nerve damage.*

• Notify the physician if adverse ocular reactions occur.

• Monitor for signs of adrenal suppression, such as dehydration and weakness, in a patient receiving high dose or long-term therapy with an anti-inflammatory suspension. Monitor the patient's electrolyte levels regularly to detect other signs of adrenal suppression, such as hyponatremia and hyperkalemia. If adrenal suppression is suspected, prepare the patient for adrenal function tests.

• Notify the physician if adrenal suppression is suspected. Expect to provide oral steroids and discontinue the anti-inflammatory suspension as prescribed.

Patient teaching

• Teach the patient and family the name, dose, frequency, action, and adverse effects of the prescribed ophthalmic anti-inflammatory agent.

• Instruct the patient to notify the physician if eye discomfort or any change in visual acuity occurs.

• *Teach the patient how to instill the drug.* (For more information, see *Ophthalmic agent administration,* page 1241.) *Instruct the patient to shake the suspension well before instillation. Also advise the patient to apply digital pressure on the punctum at the inner canthus for 2 to 3 minutes after instillation to minimize systemic absorption.*

• Stress the importance of regular ophthalmic examinations.

• Review the signs and symptoms of adrenal suppression with a patient who must receive high-dose or long-term therapy with an anti-inflammatory suspension. Instruct the patient to report such signs and symptoms to the physician at once.

• Advise the patient to wear a Medic Alert tag or carry identification that describes the use of an ophthalmic anti-inflammatory agent that may suppress adrenal function.

• Instruct the patient to notify the physician if adverse reactions occur.

Evaluation

The following examples represent appropriate evaluation statements for a patient receiving an anti-inflammatory agent.

• The patient has no conditions that contraindicate anti-inflammatory therapy.

• The patient exhibits no signs of complications in the preexisting condition linked to the prescribed anti-inflammatory agent.

• The patient experiences no adverse reactions to the prescribed anti-inflammatory agent.

• The patient's adrenal function remains intact throughout high dose or long-term therapy with an anti-inflammatory suspension.

• The patient and family express an accurate understanding of the points taught about the prescribed anti-inflammatory agent.

• The patient demonstrates proper administration of the prescribed anti-inflammatory agent.

OPHTHALMIC ANTI-INFECTIVE AGENTS

Ophthalmic anti-infective agents include antibacterial, antiseptic, and antiviral agents. To treat eye diseases, anti-infective agents may be injected beneath the conjunctiva, administered orally, or instilled into the eye. However, this section covers only topical anti-infective therapy.

Applied as solution or ointment, topical anti-infective agents include bacitracin, boric acid, chloramphenicol, chlortetracycline hydrochloride, erythromycin, gentamicin sulfate, idoxuridine, natamycin, polymyxin B sulfate, silver nitrate 1%, sulfacetamide sodium, tetracycline hydrochloride, tobramycin, trifluridine, and vidarabine. These drugs usually are sufficient to treat superficial infections of the conjunctiva, cornea, or eyelids. However, systemic antibacterials may be used along with topical anti-infective agents to treat some patients with conjunctivitis, endophthalmitis, or infections of the ocular adnexa (eyelids and lacrimal apparatus). (For information on systemic antibacterials that achieve therapeutic levels in the eye, see Chapter 59, Antibacterial Agents.)

PHARMACOKINETICS

The pharmacokinetics of the ophthalmic anti-infective agents vary greatly. A specific agent is prescribed based on its spectrum and mechanism of action.

Absorption, distribution, metabolism, excretion

Bacitracin, chloramphenicol, polymyxin B sulfate, and tobramycin penetrate the cornea and conjunctiva; chloramphenicol and tobramycin also penetrate aqueous humor. Silver nitrate does not penetrate intraocularly. Topical boric acid and idoxuridine are absorbed poorly. Erythromycin, gentamicin sulfate, polymyxin B, and the tetracyclines penetrate poorly through an intact cornea but well through corneal abrasions. Natamycin does not reach measurable levels in the deeper corneal layers unless a defect in the epithelium is present. Sulfacetamide's intraocular penetration varies. Trifluridine and vidarabine are found in trace amounts in the aqueous humor after topical application to a cornea with an epithelial defect or inflammation, but neither drug displays significant systemic absorption.

Bacitracin, chloramphenicol, gentamicin, and polymyxin B are excreted via the nasolacrimal system. Excretion of the other anti-infective agents is unknown.

Onset, peak, duration

As a rule, ophthalmic anti-infective agents are administered in frequent doses—as often as every 2 hours. Their onset and duration of action vary according to the patient's disorder and response.

PHARMACODYNAMICS

Antibacterials are chemical substances that inhibit the growth of, or directly kill, bacteria. Antibacterials are selected after the infecting organism is identified; however, withholding therapy until cultures are made is impractical. As a result, most ophthalmologists use broad-spectrum antibacterials until sensitivity has been determined. Broad-spectrum antibacterials provide complete coverage and minimize hypersensitivity reactions. (For more information, see Chapter 59, Antibacterial Agents, and Chapter 61, Antiviral Agents.)

Mechanism of action

Bacitracin, chloramphenicol, chlortetracycline, erythromycin, gentamicin, polymyxin B, and the tetracyclines inhibit protein synthesis in susceptible microorganisms. Boric acid's mechanism of action is unknown. Idoxuridine, trifluridine, and vidarabine interfere with deoxyribonucleic acid (DNA) synthesis in susceptible organisms. Natamycin increases fungal cell membrane permeability. Silver nitrate, instilled in the eyes of neonates, causes protein denaturation that prevents gonorrheal ophthalmia neonatorum. Sulfacetamide prevents uptake of para-aminobenzoic acid, a metabolite of bacterial folic acid synthesis. Tobramycin's mechanism of action is unknown, but it may inhibit protein synthesis.

PHARMACOTHERAPEUTICS

Bacitracin is effective against infections with gram-positive organisms. An antiseptic agent, boric acid is used to irrigate the eye after ocular procedures and to soothe and cleanse the eye, especially in connection with contact lens use. Chloramphenicol and gentamicin are used to treat gram-positive and gram-negative bacterial infections. Chlortetracycline is prescribed for superficial ocular infections. Erythromycin is used to fight infections with gram-positive cocci and gram-positive bacilli. The earliest developed an-

tiviral agent, idoxuridine is invaluable in treating herpes simplex of the cornea, because it prevents the herpes virus from feeding off the cells of the corneal epithelium. Natamycin is used to treat fungal infections. Polymyxin B is effective against infections with gram-negative organisms.

Silver nitrate 1% is an antiseptic agent used to prevent gonorrheal ophthalmia neonatorum. Sulfacetamide provides a wide spectrum of activity and effectiveness against some gram-positive and gram-negative bacterial infections. Tetracycline is used to treat superficial ocular infections, inclusion conjunctivitis, and trachoma. Tobramycin is used to treat external ocular infections from susceptible gram-negative bacteria. Trifluridine, an antiviral solution, also is used to treat herpes simplex infections, primary keratoconjunctivitis, and recurrent epithelial keratitis. The antiviral ophthalmic ointment vidarabine also is used to treat corneal herpes simplex, particularly in early stages.

bacitracin (AK-Tracin). This antibacterial agent is used to treat ocular infections. It is contraindicated in a patient with known hypersensitivity to the drug.
Usual adult and pediatric dosage: apply a ½" ribbon of ointment into the conjunctival sac several times a day or p.r.n. until a favorable response is achieved.

boric acid (Blinx, Collyrium). This antiseptic is used for eye irrigation after tonometry, gonioscopy, foreign body removal, or fluorescein use. It also is used to soothe and cleanse the eyes and in connection with contact lens use. It is contraindicated in a patient with corneal abrasions or known hypersensitivity to the drug.
Usual adult dosage: eye irrigation with 2% solution or 5% or 10% ointment, applied two or three times daily.

chloramphenicol (Chloromycetin Ophthalmic, Chloroptic, Chloroptic S.O.P., Econochlor Ophthalmic). As a solution or an ointment, chloramphenicol is used to treat surface bacterial infections involving the conjunctiva or cornea. It is contraindicated in a patient with known hypersensitivity to the drug and must be used cautiously in a patient with hepatic or renal dysfunction.
Usual adult and pediatric dosage: 2 drops of 0.5% solution instilled every hour until the condition improves or q.i.d., depending on the severity of the infection, or a small amount of 1% ointment applied to the lower conjunctival sac at bedtime as a supplement to drops; ointment may be used alone by applying a small amount to the lower conjunctival sac every 3 to 6 hours or more frequently, if necessary, until the condition improves.

chlortetracycline hydrochloride (Aureomycin). This antibacterial agent is used to treat superficial ocular infections. It is contraindicated in a patient with known

hypersensitivity to the drug and must be used cautiously during long-term therapy in any patient.
Usual adult and pediatric dosage: 1% ointment or 1 to 2 drops of 1% solution applied or instilled every 3 to 4 hours or b.i.d. or t.i.d., depending on the severity of the infection.

erythromycin (Ilotycin Ophthalmic). This antibacterial agent is used to treat acute and chronic conjunctivitis, trachoma, and other eye infections. It is contraindicated in a patient with known hypersensitivity to the drug.
Usual adult and pediatric dosage: 0.5% ointment applied one or more times daily, depending on the severity of the infection.

gentamicin sulfate (Garamycin Ophthalmic, Genoptic). This antibacterial agent is used to treat external ocular infections (conjunctivitis, keratoconjunctivitis, corneal ulcers, blepharitis, blepharoconjunctivitis, meibomianitis, and dacryocystitis) from susceptible organisms, especially *Pseudomonas aeruginosa, Proteus, Klebsiella pneumoniae, Escherichia coli,* and other gram-negative organisms. It is contraindicated in a patient with known hypersensitivity to the drug and must be used cautiously in a patient with hepatic or renal dysfunction.
Usual adult and pediatric dosage: 1 to 2 drops of 0.3% solution instilled every 4 hours; for severe infections, up to 2 drops every hour or 0.3% ointment applied to the lower conjunctival sac b.i.d. or t.i.d.

idoxuridine (Herplex, Stoxil). This antiviral agent is used to treat herpes simplex keratitis. It is contraindicated in a patient with known hypersensitivity to the drug.
Usual adult and pediatric dosage: 1 drop of 0.1% solution instilled into the conjunctival sac every hour during the day and every 2 hours at night, or 0.5% ointment applied to the conjunctival sac every 4 hours or five times daily, with the last dose at bedtime; response should occur within 7 days, or therapy should be discontinued and alternative therapy begun; therapy should not be continued longer than 21 days.

natamycin (Natacyn). This antifungal agent is used to treat fungal keratitis, conjunctivitis, and blepharitis. It is contraindicated in a patient with known hypersensitivity to the drug.
Usual adult dosage: initially, 1 drop of 5% suspension instilled in the conjunctival sac every 1 to 2 hours; after 3 to 4 days, dosage is reduced to 1 drop six to eight times daily.

polymyxin B sulfate (Neosporin Ophthalmic). This antibacterial agent is used alone or with other agents to treat corneal ulcers from *Pseudomonas* as well as other gram-negative organism infections. It is contraindicated in a pa-

tient with known hypersensitivity to the drug and must be used cautiously in a patient with neuromuscular disease.
Usual adult and pediatric dosage: 1 to 3 drops of 0.1% to 0.25% (10,000 to 25,000 units/ml) solution instilled every hour or 0.5% ointment placed in the conjunctival sac every 3 to 4 hours; interval is increased as prescribed, according to patient response.

silver nitrate 1%. This antiseptic agent is used to prevent gonorrheal ophthalmia neonatorum. It is contraindicated in a patient with known hypersensitivity to the drug.
Usual pediatric dosage: for neonates, 1 drop of 1% solution after the eyelids are cleaned.

sulfacetamide sodium 10% (Bleph-10 Liquifilm Ophthalmic, Cetamide Ophthalmic, Sulamyd Sodium 10% Ophthalmic), **sulfacetamide sodium 15%** (Isopto Cetamide Ophthalmic, Sulfair-15 Ophthalmic), and **sulfacetamide sodium 30%** (Sulamyd Sodium 30% Ophthalmic). Sulfacetamide sodium (a sulfonamide antibacterial) is used to treat inclusion conjunctivitis, corneal ulcers, and trachoma. It also is used to prevent ocular infection after foreign body removal or eye injury. It is contraindicated in a patient with known hypersensitivity to the drug and must be used cautiously during long-term therapy in any patient.
Usual adult and pediatric dosage: 1 to 2 drops of 10% solution instilled into the lower conjunctival sac every 2 to 3 hours during the day, less often at night; or, initially, 1 to 2 drops of 15% solution instilled into the lower conjunctival sac every 1 to 2 hours, then at increasing intervals as the patient responds; or 1 drop of 30% solution instilled into the lower conjunctival sac every 2 hours; ½″ to 1″ of 10% ointment applied to the conjunctival sac q.i.d. and at bedtime (ointment may be used at night and drops during the day).

tetracycline hydrochloride (Achromycin Ophthalmic). This anti-infective agent is used to treat superficial ocular infections, inclusion conjunctivitis, and trachoma. It is contraindicated in a patient with known hypersensitivity to the drug and must be used cautiously in a patient with hepatic or renal dysfunction.
Usual adult and pediatric dosage: for superficial ocular infections and inclusion conjunctivitis, a small amount of 1% ointment or 1 to 2 drops of 1% solution instilled b.i.d. to q.i.d. or more often, depending on severity; for trachoma, 2 drops instilled b.i.d. to q.i.d., continued for 3 weeks along with oral therapy.

tobramycin (Tobrex). This anti-infective agent is used to treat external ocular infections from susceptible gram-negative bacteria. It is contraindicated in a patient with known

hypersensitivity to the drug and must be used cautiously in a patient with hepatic or renal dysfunction.
Usual adult and pediatric dosage: for mild to moderate infections, a 0.4″ (1-cm) ribbon of 0.3% ointment or 1 to 2 drops of 0.3% solution instilled every 4 hours; for severe infections, 2 drops instilled hourly.

trifluridine (Viroptic Ophthalmic Solution). This antiviral agent is used to treat primary keratoconjunctivitis and recurrent epithelial keratitis resulting from herpes simplex virus, Types I and II. It is contraindicated in a patient with known hypersensitivity to the drug and must be used cautiously during long-term therapy in any patient.
Usual adult dosage: 1 drop of 1% solution every 2 hours while the patient is awake to a maximum of 9 drops daily until reepithelialization of the corneal ulcer occurs, then 1 drop every 4 hours (minimum 5 drops daily) for an additional 7 days.

vidarabine (Vira-A Ophthalmic). This antiviral agent is used to treat acute keratoconjunctivitis, superficial keratitis, and recurrent epithelial keratitis resulting from herpes simplex virus, Types I and II. It is contraindicated in a patient with known hypersensitivity to the drug and must be used cautiously in a patient with hepatic or renal dysfunction.
Usual adult and pediatric dosage: ½″ (1.25-cm) ribbon of 3% ointment applied to the lower conjunctival sac five times daily at 3-hour intervals.

Drug interactions

No significant interactions occur between most anti-infectives and other drugs. However, combined use of bacitracin and silver nitrate inactivates bacitracin. Sulfacetamide action will be decreased if it is used with a local anesthetic, such as procaine, tetracaine, or a para-aminobenzoic acid derivative. This interaction can be prevented by waiting 30 to 60 minutes after anesthetic instillation before instilling sulfacetamide.

ADVERSE DRUG REACTIONS

Hypersensitivity reactions to sulfonamides may occur; reactions may be severe. Secondary eye infections may occur with prolonged use of an anti-infective agent.

NURSING PROCESS APPLICATION

The following information assists the nurse in caring for a patient receiving an ophthalmic anti-infective agent.

Assessment

• Review the patient's history for a preexisting condition that contraindicates the use of an ophthalmic anti-infective agent, such as corneal abrasions or known hypersensitivity to the drug.
• Review the patient's history for a preexisting condition that requires cautious use of an ophthalmic anti-infective agent, such as neuromuscular disease, hepatic or renal dysfunction, or long-term therapy.
• Assess the patient for adverse reactions to the prescribed anti-infective agent, such as hypersensitivity reactions.
• Review the patient's medication history to identify the use of drugs that may interact with the prescribed ophthalmic anti-infective agent, such as other anti-infectives, procaine, tetracaine, para-aminobenzoic acid derivatives, and other local anesthetics.
• Assess the effectiveness of the prescribed ophthalmic anti-infective agent.
• Evaluate the patient's and family's knowledge about the prescribed ophthalmic anti-infective agent.

Nursing diagnoses

The following examples represent appropriate nursing diagnoses for a patient receiving an ophthalmic anti-infective agent.
• Potential for injury related to a preexisting condition that contraindicates the use of an ophthalmic anti-infective agent
• Potential for injury related to a preexisting condition that requires cautious use of an ophthalmic anti-infective agent
• Potential for injury related to a hypersensitivity reaction to a sulfonamide anti-infective agent
• Altered protection related to drug interaction between sulfacetamide and a local anesthetic
• Knowledge deficit related to the prescribed ophthalmic anti-infective agent

Planning and implementation

• Do not administer an ophthalmic anti-infective agent to a patient with a condition that contraindicates its use.
• Administer an ophthalmic anti-infective agent cautiously to a patient at risk because of a preexisting condition.
• Monitor the patient closely for adverse reactions to the anti-infective agent.
• Document the patient's history of allergy if sulfacetamide is prescribed. Hypersensitivity reactions to sulfonamides can be severe.
• *Monitor for hypersensitivity reactions in a patient receiving a sulfonamide anti-infective agent. Keep standard emergency equipment nearby.*
• Notify the physician immediately if a hypersensitivity reaction occurs and withhold the prescribed ophthalmic anti-infective agent.
• *Administer sulfacetamide 30 to 60 minutes after local anesthetic instillation to avoid a drug interaction.*

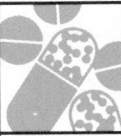

SELECTED MAJOR DRUGS

Ophthalmic agents

The following chart summarizes the major ophthalmic agents currently in clinical use.

DRUG	MAJOR INDICATIONS	USUAL ADULT DOSAGES	CONTRAINDICATIONS AND PRECAUTIONS
Mydriatics and cycloplegics			
atropine	Acute iritis	1 to 2 drops of 0.5% to 2% solution b.i.d. or t.i.d.	• Know that atropine is contraindicated in a patient with known or suspected closed-angle glaucoma or known hypersensitivity to the drug. • Administer with extreme caution to an infant or small child and to any child with spastic paralysis or brain damage.
	Refraction	1 to 2 drops of 1% solution 1 hour before examination	
cyclopentolate	Mydriasis and cycloplegia	1 drop of 1% solution followed by 1 drop 5 minutes later; use 2% solution in patients with heavily pigmented irises	• Know that cyclopentolate is contraindicated in a patient with closed-angle glaucoma. • Administer with caution to a geriatric patient or any other patient who is predisposed to increased intraocular pressure.
tropicamide	Refraction	1 drop of 1% solution 20 minutes before examination, repeated in 20 to 30 minutes if needed	• Know that tropicamide is contraindicated in a patient with known or suspected closed-angle glaucoma or known hypersensitivity to the drug. • Administer with caution to a pregnant patient.
	Funduscopic examination	1 drop of 0.5% solution 15 to 20 minutes before examination	
Miotics			
carbachol	Miosis	0.5 ml of 0.01% solution into the anterior chamber	• Be aware that carbachol has no contraindications when applied intraocularly. • Administer with caution to a patient with corneal abrasions.
	Open-angle or closed-angle glaucoma	1 drop of 0.75% to 3% solution instilled into the conjunctival sac every 4 to 8 hours	
pilocarpine	Chronic open-angle glaucoma	1 to 2 drops of 1% to 2% solution every 4 to 8 hours	• Know that pilocarpine is contraindicated in a patient with a history of or predisposition to retinal detachment, glaucoma associated with acute inflammation, or known hypersensitivity to the drug. • Administer with caution to a patient with corneal abrasions.
	Before surgery to treat acute closed-angle glaucoma	1 drop of 2% solution instilled three to six times over a 30-minute period before surgery	
Drugs that lower intraocular pressure			
betaxolol	Chronic open-angle glaucoma	1 drop of 0.5% solution b.i.d.	• Know that betaxolol is contraindicated in a patient with sinus bradycardia, greater-than-first-degree atrioventricular block, cardiogenic shock, overt cardiac failure, or known hypersensitivity to the drug. • Administer with caution to a pregnant or lactating patient or one with diabetes, hyperthyroidism, or pulmonary dysfunction.
glycerin, anhydrous	Reduction of superficial corneal edema	1 or 2 drops every 3 or 4 hours	• Know that glycerin, anhydrous is contraindicated in a patient with known hypersensitivity to the drug. • Be aware that glycerin, anhydrous has no major precautions.
	Preparation for ophthalmoscopic or gonioscopic examination	1 or 2 drops instilled into the eye before the examination	*(continued)*

SELECTED MAJOR DRUGS

Ophthalmic agents (continued)

DRUG	MAJOR INDICATIONS	USUAL ADULT DOSAGES	CONTRAINDICATIONS AND PRECAUTIONS
timolol	Chronic open-angle glaucoma, aphakic glaucoma, increased intraocular pressure	1 drop of 0.25% solution b.i.d., initially; may be increased to 1 drop of 0.5% solution b.i.d.	• Know that timolol is contraindicated in a lactating patient or one with bronchial asthma, a history of bronchial asthma, or severe chronic obstructive pulmonary disease. • Administer with caution to a pregnant patient or one with diabetes mellitus, hyperthyroidism, or cerebral vascular insufficiency.
Anesthetic agents			
tetracaine	Tonometry, gonioscopy, removal of corneal foreign bodies, corneal suture removal, and other diagnostic and minor surgical procedures	1 or 2 drops of 0.5% solution or ½" to 1" ribbon of 0.5% ointment just before the procedure	• Know that tetracaine is contraindicated in a patient with known hypersensitivity to the drug. • Administer with caution to a patient with allergies, cardiac disease, or hyperthyroidism.
Anti-inflammatory agents			
medrysone	Allergic conjunctivitis, vernal conjunctivities, episcleritis, and ophthalmic epinephrine reaction	1 drop of 1% solution instilled in the conjunctival sac b.i.d. to q.i.d.; may be used every hour during the first 1 to 2 days, if needed	• Know that medrysone is contraindicated in a patient with an acute, untreated, purulent bacterial, viral, or fungal eye infection; acute, superficial herpes simplex keratitis; vaccina, varicella, or other viral disease of the cornea or conjunctiva; or known hypersensitivity to the drug. • Administer with caution to a pregnant or lactating patient or one with corneal abrasions.
Ophthalmic anti-infective agents			
polymyxin B sulfate	Corneal ulcers from infections with *Pseudomonas* or other gram-negative organisms	1 to 3 drops of 0.1% to 0.25% solution every hour or 0.5% ointment placed in the conjunctival sac every 3 to 4 hours	• Know that polymyxin B sulfate is contraindicated in a patient with known hypersensitivity to the drug. • Administer with caution to a patient with neuromuscular disease.

Patient teaching

• Teach the patient and family the name, dose, frequency, action, and adverse effects of the prescribed anti-infective agent.

• Advise the patient against indiscriminate or prolonged use of anti-infectives; hypersensitivity or bacterial resistance may develop.

• Encourage the patient to see an ophthalmologist if a secondary eye infection occurs and to notify the ophthalmologist if the condition does not improve within 48 hours of initial treatment.

• Teach the patient with herpes simplex infection about the course of this disease. Explain that herpes will recur and that, at the first sign of recurrence, the patient should contact the ophthalmologist and start the prescribed medication.

• *Teach the patient how to administer the prescribed ophthalmic anti-infective agent.* (For more information, see *Ophthalmic agent administration,* page 1241.)

• Instruct the patient to withhold the drug and notify the physician if a hypersensitivity reaction occurs.

Evaluation

The following examples represent appropriate evaluation statements for a patient receiving an ophthalmic anti-infective agent.

• The patient has no conditions that contraindicate ophthalmic anti-infective agent therapy.

• The patient exhibits no signs of complications in the preexisting condition linked to the prescribed ophthalmic anti-infective agent.

• The patient experiences no hypersensitivity reactions to the sulfonamide anti-infective agent.

- The patient experiences no drug interaction between sulfacetamide and a local anesthetic.
- The patient and family express an accurate understanding of the points taught about the prescribed ophthalmic anti-infective agent.
- The patient demonstrates proper administration of the prescribed ophthalmic anti-infective agent.

- The nurse should teach the patient or family how to administer the prescribed ophthalmic agent and should teach the patient to recognize and report systemic and ocular adverse reactions.

CHAPTER SUMMARY

Chapter 71 discussed ophthalmic agents as they are used to achieve mydriasis, cycloplegia, miosis, and anesthesia; to lower intraocular pressure; and to treat ocular inflammation and infection. Here are the chapter highlights.

- Ophthalmic agents include mydriatics and cycloplegics, miotics, drugs that lower intraocular pressure, anesthetic agents, anti-inflammatory agents, and anti-infective agents.
- Mydriatics dilate the pupil; cycloplegics paralyze the accommodative muscle of the ciliary body of the eye. Mydriatics and cycloplegics are used primarily for intraocular examinations and refractions. Some mydriatics also are used to treat open-angle glaucoma.
- The nurse should not administer a mydriatic or cycloplegic to a patient with closed-angle glaucoma—pupil dilation can lead to an acute glaucoma episode. Digital pressure over the punctum at the inner canthus helps prevent systemic absorption and decreases the risk of adverse reactions.
- Miotics—including direct-acting cholinergics, short-acting anticholinesterases, and long-acting anticholinesterases—are used primarily to treat glaucoma and to manage accommodative esotropia.
- Pilocarpine is a drug of choice to treat glaucoma. It can be used for prolonged periods of time, and it causes minimal adverse reactions.
- Drugs that lower intraocular pressure include topical adrenergic blocking agents, hyperosmotic agents, and carbonic anhydrase inhibitors.
- The carbonic anhydrase inhibitors decrease aqueous production by inhibiting the action of carbonic anhydrase. When less fluid enters the eye, intraocular pressure decreases.
- Topical ophthalmic anesthetics anesthetize the corneal surface so that instruments can be applied to measure intraocular pressure or to remove foreign bodies.
- Corticosteroid anti-inflammatory agents reduce ocular edema, redness, and scarring.
- Ophthalmic anti-infective agents include antibacterial, antiseptic, and antiviral agents.

STUDY QUESTIONS

See Appendix 1 for answers.

1. Hal Johnson, age 50, visits his ophthalmologist for a routine eye examination. To prepare Mr. Johnson for an intraocular examination, the nurse instills cyclopentolate (Cyclogyl) eye drops to produce mydriatic and cycloplegic effects. How does cyclopentolate produce these effects?
(a) It paralyzes the sphincter muscle of the iris and contracts the dilator muscle.
(b) It relaxes the dilator muscle of the pupil.
(c) It paralyzes the dilator muscle and stimulates the sphincter muscle of the iris.
(d) It directly contracts the dilator muscle of the pupil.

2. Alice Kepler, age 57, has chronic open-angle glaucoma, for which she takes the miotic pilocarpine (Pilocar), 1 drop every 8 hours. If Ms. Kepler were to develop iritis, the physician would discontinue pilocarpine temporarily. Why?
(a) Pilocarpine is inactivated by inflammation.
(b) Pilocarpine may increase the inflammation.
(c) Pilocarpine is absorbed systemically with inflammation.
(d) Pilocarpine produces extreme miosis with inflammation.

3. When teaching Ms. Kepler how to administer pilocarpine eye drops, the nurse should instruct her to instill them in which location?
(a) on the iris
(b) on the cornea
(c) on the sclera
(d) in the lower conjunctival sac

4. To prevent systemic absorption of pilocarpine through the nasolacrimal duct, which instruction should the nurse give Ms. Kepler?
(a) Apply digital pressure over the punctum at the inner canthus for 2 to 3 minutes.
(b) Hold the head down for 2 to 3 minutes after instilling the eye drops.
(c) Apply digital pressure over the outer canthus for 1 to 2 minutes.
(d) Rub the eyes gently for about 1 minute after instilling the eye drops.

5. The physician could have prescribed a carbonic anhydrase inhibitor, such as acetazolamide, to treat chronic open-angle glaucoma. How do carbonic anhydrase inhibitors exert their therapeutic effects?
(a) They increase aqueous fluid outflow.
(b) They decrease aqueous fluid production.
(c) They prevent aqueous flow from the posterior chamber.
(d) They increase aqueous fluid absorption.

6. While refinishing an old desk, Emma Mann gets a small splinter lodged in her cornea. Her husband brings her to the emergency department, where the physician orders the topical anesthetic proparacaine before removal of the corneal foreign body. After the foreign body is removed, the nurse advises Ms. Mann not to rub her eyes. Why?
(a) It may result in redness.
(b) It may increase systemic absorption.
(c) It may cause excessive tearing, which would wash away the anesthetic.
(d) It may cause corneal abrasion because the pain signal is absent.

7. Which ophthalmic agent is likely to be prescribed after removal of the corneal foreign body?
(a) boric acid, an anti-infective agent
(b) tetracaine, an anesthetic agent
(c) carbachol, a miotic agent
(d) atropine, a mydriatic agent

8. Kelley Alvin, age 20, visits her physician because of moderate eye pain, conjunctival injection, and photophobia. After examining Ms. Alvin, the physician diagnoses the problem as an anterior uveitis and prescribes the mydriatic scopalamine and the corticosteroid dexamethasone. In Ms. Alvin's case, why is a corticosteroid prescribed?
(a) to paralyze the eye muscles
(b) to decrease inflammation
(c) to reduce photophobia
(d) to reduce eye pain

SELECTED REFERENCES

AHFS drug information 90. (1990). Bethesda, MD: American Hospital Formulary Service.

Goodman and Gilman's the pharmacological basis of therapeutics (8th ed.; 1990). Elmsford, NY: Pergamon Press.

Hansten, P., and Horn, J. (1988). Drug interactions: Clinical significance of drug-drug interactions (6th ed.). Philadelphia: Lea & Febiger.

Krieglstein, G. (1987). Glaucoma update III. New York: Springer-Verlag.

Krupin, T. (Ed.). (1988). Manual of glaucoma: Diagnosis and management. New York: Churchill Livingstone, Inc.

North American Nursing Diagnosis Association. (1990). Taxonomy I - Revised, with official diagnostic categories. St. Louis: NANDA.

Nursing91 drug handbook. (1991). Springhouse, PA: Springhouse Corporation.

Perry, J., and Tullo, A. (Eds.). (1990). Care of the ophthalmic patient: A guide for nurses and health professionals. New York: Routledge Chapman & Hall.

Systemic effects of glaucoma medications. (1990). Nurse's Drug Alert, 14(3), 24.

USPDI. (1991). Drug information for the health care professional (Vol. I, 11th ed.). Rockville, MD: United States Pharmacopeial Convention.

USPDI. (1991). Advice for the patient (Vol. II, 11th ed.). Rockville, MD: United States Pharmacopeial Convention.

CHAPTER

72

OTIC AGENTS

OBJECTIVES

After reading and studying this chapter, the student should be able to:

1. Identify the indications for the different classes of otic agents, including anti-infective, anti-inflammatory, local anesthestic, and ceruminolytic agents.

2. Describe the administration techniques for the various types of otic agents.

3. Identify the adverse reactions to the anti-infective otic agents and describe nursing interventions that can help prevent them.

4. Identify the possible adverse reactions to anti-inflammatory otic agents.

5. Explain how benzocaine produces analgesia.

6. Describe the mechanism of action for the ceruminolytic agent carbamide peroxide.

7. Describe how to apply the nursing process when caring for a patient receiving an otic agent.

INTRODUCTION

Otic agents are prescribed to treat ear infection, inflammation, and pain, and to soften cerumen (earwax). These drugs are categorized as anti-infective (single and compound), anti-inflammatory, local anesthetic, and ceruminolytic agents. Otic agents are administered via eardrops, ear irrigations, or ear wicks. Several combination products that contain anti-infective and anti-inflammatory agents are available.

For a summary of representative drugs, see *Selected major drugs: Otic agents,* page 1267. For a listing of applicable nursing diagnoses that the nurse may formulate when caring for a patient receiving these agents, see *Selected nursing diagnoses: Otic agents.* For detailed information on applying the nursing process, see Chapter 6, The Nursing Process and Drug Therapy.

SELECTED NURSING DIAGNOSES

Otic agents

The following nursing diagnoses address representative problems and etiologies that a nurse may encounter when caring for a patient who is receiving an otic agent. Some of these nursing diagnoses contain generalized etiologies, which the nurse must individualize based on the patient's needs. (For some common nursing diagnoses and related interventions for each drug class, see the "Nursing Process Application" sections of this chapter.)

- Altered health maintenance related to neurotoxicity caused by polymyxin B sulfate
- Altered protection related to hypersensitivity reactions to the prescribed otic agent
- Altered urinary elimination related to nephrotoxicity caused by concomitant therapy with otic and systemic polymyxin B sulfate
- Impaired tissue integrity related to the local effects of benzocaine or a ceruminolytic agent
- Knowledge deficit related to the prescribed otic agent
- Pain related to a stinging or burning sensation during application of an anti-inflammatory otic agent
- Potential for infection related to a superinfection caused by an anti-infective otic agent
- Potential for infection related to the masking of signs of a bacterial, fungal, or viral infection by a topical steroid
- Potential for infection related to the masking of symptoms of a fulminating middle ear infection by benzocaine
- Potential for injury related to a preexisting condition that contraindicates the use of an otic agent
- Potential for injury related to a preexisting condition that requires cautious use of an otic agent
- Potential for injury related to adverse drug reactions
- Potential impaired skin integrity related to triethanolamine-induced eczema

ANTI-INFECTIVE AGENTS

The anti-infective otic agents represent natural antibiotics or synthetic antibiotic derivatives. Used to treat ear infections, these agents also may be combined with systemic anti-infective therapy. This section discusses the following anti-infective agents: acetic acid, boric acid, chloramphenicol, colistin sulfate, and polymyxin B sulfate.

The antimicrobial activity of these drugs varies. Most anti-infective otic agents exhibit a broad spectrum of activity against gram-positive and gram-negative organisms. A few of the agents have a narrow spectrum.

PHARMACOKINETICS

Most anti-infective otics begin to act within 1 hour and have a 4-hour duration of action. The full therapeutic effect of these drugs may not be seen for 2 to 3 days.

PHARMACODYNAMICS

Anti-infective otics are bactericidal (kill bacteria) or bacteriostatic (inhibit bacterial growth). Boric acid and acetic acid possess weak bacteriostatic properties and also are fungistatic (inhibit fungal growth).

Mechanism of action

The anti-infective otics kill or inhibit bacterial growth by interfering with the metabolic functions of bacteria. Chloramphenicol primarily inhibits peptide bond formation and protein synthesis in susceptible bacteria. Colistin and polymyxin B alter the osmotic barrier of the bacterial membrane, enabling essential cellular metabolites to leak out.

Before the administration of an anti-infective otic, culture and sensitivity tests should be conducted to identify the causative organism and its drug susceptibility. An anti-infective is selected before the test results are known based on clinical findings. The test results confirm selection of an appropriate drug or guide the selection of a more effective agent. Culture and sensitivity test may be repeated during therapy. The anti-infective otic should be discontinued if the causative organism becomes resistant to it.

PHARMACOTHERAPEUTICS

Anti-infective otics are prescribed for otitis externa caused by various bacteria. Colistin and polymyxin B also prove effective in treating otitis media. Many combination products treat a wide range of microorganisms as well as ear pain and inflammation.

acetic acid (Domeboro Otic, VoSol Otic). Used in superficial infections of the external auditory canal, acetic acid provides antibacterial, antifungal, and hydrophilic actions. Acetic acid with hydrocortisone has anti-inflammatory and antipruritic actions as well.
Usual adult and pediatric dosage: 5 drops into the ear canal t.i.d., q.i.d., or every 2 to 3 hours, if needed; an ear wick can be inserted for the first 24 hours.

boric acid (Ear-Dry, Swim-Ear). A weak anti-infective agent with fungistatic and bacteriostatic properties, boric acid is indicated in otitis externa.
Usual adult and pediatric dosage: 4 to 6 drops in each ear, then plug with cotton, t.i.d. or q.i.d.

chloramphenicol (Chloromycetin Otic). A broad-spectrum, bacteriostatic antibiotic, chloramphenicol proves effective against a number of gram-positive and gram-negative bacteria, including rickettsiae and chlamydiae. It is used to treat otitis externa.
Usual adult and pediatric dosage: 2 to 3 drops into the external auditory canal t.i.d.

colistin sulfate. Closely related to polymyxin B sulfate, colistin acts against certain gram-negative organisms. When combined with neomycin, hydrocortisone, and thonzonium (Coly-Mycin S Otic), it is used to treat otitis externa and otitis media.
Usual adult dosage: 4 drops into the external auditory canal t.i.d. or q.i.d.
Usual pediatric dosage: 3 drops into the external auditory canal t.i.d. or q.i.d.

polymyxin B sulfate. One of several polymyxin antibiotics active against gram-negative organisms, polymyxin B sulfate appears in several combination products used to treat bacterial infections of the external auditory canal and otitis media. A common product combines polymyxin B sulfate with neomycin sulfate and hydrocortisone (Cortisporin Otic). Polymyxin B sulfate may be administered as an otic solution or suspension.
Usual adult dosage: 4 drops into the external auditory canal t.i.d. or q.i.d.
Usual pediatric dosage: 3 drops into external auditory canal t.i.d. or q.i.d.

Drug interactions

When administered concomitantly with an anti-infective otic, a topical steroid may mask the clinical signs of bacterial, fungal, or viral infections and may suppress hypersensitivity.

Boric acid is incompatible with alkali carbonates, hydroxides, and benzalkonium chloride. It precipitates in combination with salicylic acid. Cumulative nephrotoxicity and neurotoxicity can occur if polymyxin B sulfate is administered topically along with systemic polymyxin B therapy.

ADVERSE DRUG REACTIONS

Superinfections sometimes occur with use of anti-infective otics, resulting in overgrowth of nonsusceptible organisms. Hypersensitivity reactions, such as ear pruritus or burning, urticaria, and vesicular or maculopapular dermatitis, may occur with use of any anti-infective otic.

NURSING PROCESS APPLICATION

The following information assists the nurse in caring for a patient receiving an anti-infective otic agent.

Assessment
• Review the patient's history for a preexisting condition that contraindicates the use of an anti-infective otic agent, such as perforated tympanic membrane or known hypersensitivity to the drug.
• Review the patient's history for a preexisting condition that requires cautious use of an anti-infective otic agent, such as long-term use of the drug.
• Assess the patient for adverse reactions to the prescribed anti-infective otic agent, such as superinfections and hypersensitivity reactions.
• Review the patient's medication history to identify use of drugs that may interact with the prescribed anti-infective otic agent, such as topical steroids, alkali carbonates, hydroxides, benzalkonium chloride, salicylic acid, and systemic polymyxin B.
• Assess the effectiveness of the anti-infective otic agent periodically.
• Evaluate the patient's and family's knowledge about the prescribed anti-infective otic agent.

Nursing diagnoses
The following examples represent appropriate nursing diagnoses for a patient receiving an anti-infective otic agent.
• Potential for injury related to a preexisting condition that contraindicates the use of an anti-infective otic agent
• Potential for injury related to a preexisting condition that requires cautious use of an anti-infective otic agent
• Potential for injury related to adverse drug reactions
• Knowledge deficit related to the prescribed anti-infective otic agent

Planning and implementation
• Do not administer an anti-infective otic agent to a patient with a condition that contraindicates its use.

• Administer an anti-infective otic agent cautiously to a patient at risk because of a preexisting condition.
• Monitor the patient closely for adverse reactions during anti-infective otic therapy.
• Monitor the patient for evidence of superinfection, such as continued ear pain, inflammation, and fever. If superinfection is suspected, notify the physician.
• *Monitor the patient closely for signs of nephrotoxicity, such as altered urine elimination patterns, abnormal urinalysis results, and increased serum creatinine and blood urea nitrogen levels. Also monitor for signs of neurotoxicity, such as tinnitus, decreased hearing acuity, dizziness, and unsteady gait, when polymyxin B sulfate is administered with systemic polymyxin B therapy. If neurotoxicity or nephrotoxicity is suspected, withhold the drug and notify the physician.*
• Monitor the patient for signs and symptoms of a hypersensitivity reaction to the anti-infective otic, such as ear pruritus or burning, urticaria, and vesicular or maculopapular dermatitis. If such findings are detected, notify the physician because a different drug may be needed.
• Perform a patch test to assess for allergic contact dermatitis before administering an anti-infective otic to a patient who is sensitive to other agents. To perform this test, apply the otic agent onto the flexor surface of the patient's arm. Cover the area with a small sterile bandage and wait 24 hours before observing for erythema and urticaria.
• Clean and dry the ear canal before administering an anti-infective otic solution or suspension.
• *Warm the anti-infective otic to room temperature before instillation. To do this, roll the bottle between the hands or allow it to stand at room temperature for about 30 minutes. A solution that is too hot or cold may stimulate the central nervous system, possibly causing vertigo or nausea.*
• Notify the physician if adverse reactions occur.

Patient teaching
• Teach the patient and family the name, dose, frequency, action, and adverse effects of the prescribed anti-infective otic agent.
• *Instruct the patient to contact the physician immediately upon experiencing tinnitus, decreased hearing acuity, dizziness, or unsteady gait.*
• Advise the patient to discontinue the anti-infective otic and contact the physician if an allergic reaction occurs.
• Teach the patient (or parents of the pediatric patient) how to instill eardrops. (For an illustration of this procedure, see *Eardrop administration,* page 1262.)
• *Instruct the patient not to wash the dropper after use.*

Eardrop administration

The nurse should administer eardrops appropriately for the adult or pediatric patient, as described below.

Adult patient
• Shake the bottle if directed, and open it. Fill the dropper and place the bottle within reach.
• Tilt the patient's head so that the affected ear is up. Then gently pull the top of the ear up and back to straighten the ear canal.
• Position the dropper above but not touching the ear, and release the prescribed number of drops.
• Keep the patient's head tilted for 10 minutes. If desired, plug the ear with cotton moistened with the eardrops. Do not use dry cotton, because it will absorb the drops.
• Repeat the procedure for the other ear, if prescribed.

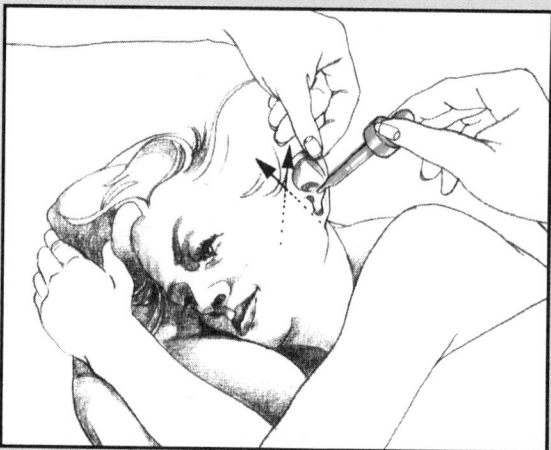

Pediatric patient
• Lay the child on the side so that the affected ear is turned up.
• Gently pull the ear down and back, then slowly release the prescribed number of drops. (Note the difference in the direction the ear is moved for a child. That is because the child's ear cartilage is immature.)
• Notify the physician if the child experiences any pain after instillation.

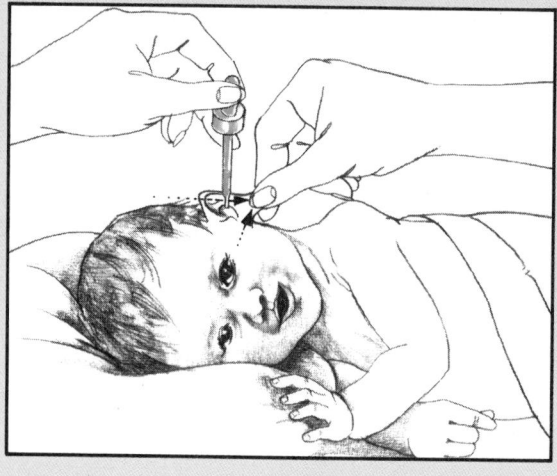

• Demonstrate how to gently insert a cotton pledget moistened with the eardrops into the ear canal. Inform the patient that the placement of the cotton pledget may impair hearing.
• Instruct the patient or parent to notify the physician if adverse reactions occur.

Evaluation
The following examples represent appropriate evaluation statements for a patient receiving an anti-infective otic agent.
• The patient has no conditions that contraindicate the use of an anti-infective otic agent.
• The patient exhibits no signs of complications in the preexisting condition linked to the prescribed anti-infective otic agent.
• The patient experiences no adverse reactions to the prescribed anti-infective otic agent.
• The patient and family express an accurate understanding of the points taught about the prescribed anti-infective otic agent.
• The patient demonstrates proper administration of the prescribed anti-infective otic agent.

ANTI-INFLAMMATORY AGENTS

Anti-inflammatory otic agents are administered to the auditory canal to produce anti-inflammatory, antipruritic, and vasoconstrictor effects. These agents include hydrocortisone and its synthetic derivative dexamethasone. Hydrocortisone is a corticosteroid, a hormone secreted by the adrenal cortex.

PHARMACOKINETICS

Long-term use of anti-inflammatory otics may cause some systemic absorption, although no clinical effects of the absorption have been noted. Anti-inflammatory otics begin to act within 1 hour, and effects last about 4 hours.

PHARMACODYNAMICS

In an acute inflammatory reaction, anti-inflammatory otics inhibit edema, capillary dilatation, fibrin deposition, and the migration of phagocytes and leukocytes. These drugs also reduce capillary and fibroblast proliferation, collagen deposition, and scar formation. Researchers have not determined the exact mechanisms for these responses. Some anti-inflammatory agents are fluorinated, which enhances their anti-inflammatory action.

PHARMACOTHERAPEUTICS

Anti-inflammatory otics are used for inflammatory conditions of the external ear canal and are administered with a dropper, via an ear wick, or as a cream or ointment.

dexamethasone sodium phosphate (Ak-dex with benzalkonium chloride in otic solution, Decadron phosphate cream). A fluorinated corticosteroid, dexamethasone sodium phosphate is used to treat inflammatory conditions of the external auditory canal.
Usual adult and pediatric dosage: 3 to 4 drops of solution into the external auditory canal b.i.d. or t.i.d.; thin film of cream applied with a cotton-tipped applicator t.i.d. or q.i.d.; when using a gauze wick, first insert the wick into the swollen ear canal, then saturate it with the medication and leave it in place for 12 to 24 hours. The wick should be kept moistened with medication while it is in the ear canal.

hydrocortisone and **hydrocortisone acetate**. For inflammatory conditions of the external auditory canal, hydrocortisone and hydrocortisone acetate are given by dropper or with an ear wick. Both forms of hydrocortisone commonly appear in combination products, such as Acetasol HC (hydrocortisone with acetic acid) and Coly-Mycin S Otic (hydrocortisone acetate with colistin sulfate, neomycin sulfate, and thonzonium bromide).
Usual adult dosage: 4 to 5 drops into the external auditory canal t.i.d. or q.i.d.; if using a gauze wick, first insert the wick into the ear canal, then saturate it with medication and leave it in place for 12 to 24 hours. The wick should be kept moistened with solution while it is in the ear. The length of treatment will vary from a few days to several weeks.
Usual pediatric dosage: for infants and children, 3 drops t.i.d. or q.i.d.

Drug interactions

No significant interactions occur between the anti-inflammatory otics and other drugs.

ADVERSE DRUG REACTIONS

Common adverse reactions to anti-inflammatory otics are transient, local stinging or burning sensations. These agents also may mask or exacerbate an underlying otic infection. Although rare, a hypersensitivity reaction can occur, producing such effects as ear itching or burning, urticaria, and vesicular or maculopapular dermatitis.

NURSING PROCESS APPLICATION

The following information assists the nurse in caring for a patient receiving an anti-inflammatory otic agent.

Assessment
• Review the patient's history for a preexisting condition that contraindicates the use of an anti-inflammatory otic agent, such as an acute purulent bacterial, viral, or fungal otic infection; perforated tympanic membrane; or known hypersensitivity to the drug.
• Assess the patient for adverse reactions to the prescribed anti-inflammatory otic agent, such as a stinging or burning sensation, exacerbation of infection, or hypersensitivity reactions.
• Assess the effectiveness of the prescribed anti-inflammatory otic agent periodically.
• Evaluate the patient's and family's knowledge about the prescribed anti-inflammatory otic agent.

Nursing diagnoses
The following examples represent appropriate nursing diagnoses for a patient receiving an anti-inflammatory otic agent.
• Potential for injury related to a preexisting condition that contraindicates the use of an anti-inflammatory otic agent
• Potential for injury related to adverse drug reactions
• Knowledge deficit related to the prescribed anti-inflammatory otic agent

Planning and implementation
• Do not administer an anti-inflammatory otic agent to a patient with a condition that contraindicates its use.
• Monitor the patient closely for adverse reactions during anti-inflammatory otic therapy.
• Observe the patient for signs and symptoms of a hypersensitivity reaction, such as ear pruritus or burning, urticaria, and vesicular or maculopapular dermatitis. If a hypersensitivity reaction occurs, notify the physician.
• Clean and dry the ear canal before administering an anti-inflammatory otic agent.
• Do not administer the anti-inflammatory otic with an anti-infective otic when the anti-inflammatory agent is prescribed to treat allergic otitis externa.
• Administer the anti-inflammatory otic sparingly to prevent debris accumulation in the ear canal.
• Expect to administer the anti-inflammatory otic with an anti-infective otic as prescribed to treat bacterial otitis externa.
• *Monitor the patient for worsening of symptoms, which may indicate exacerbation of the infection. Notify the physician if the patient's ear infection persists or worsens during anti-inflammatory otic therapy.*

Patient teaching

• Teach the patient and family the name, dose, frequency, action, and adverse effects of the prescribed anti-inflammatory otic agent.
• Instruct the patient to discontinue the medication and contact the physician if signs of an allergic reaction occur.
• Teach the patient (or parents of the pediatric patient) how to instill eardrops. (For a description and illustration, see *Eardrop administration,* page 1262.)
• *Show the patient how to insert a gauze wick into the ear canal, allowing the loose end of the wick to hang out of the ear canal.*
• Instruct the patient or parent to notify the physician if other adverse reactions occur or if the ear infection persists or worsens.

Evaluation

The following examples represent appropriate evaluation statements for a patient receiving an anti-inflammatory otic agent.
• The patient has no conditions that contraindicate the use of an anti-inflammatory otic agent.
• The patient experiences no adverse reactions to the prescribed anti-inflammatory otic agent.
• The patient and family express an accurate understanding of the points taught about the prescribed anti-inflammatory otic agent.
• The patient demonstrates proper administration of the prescribed anti-inflammatory otic agent.

LOCAL ANESTHETIC AGENTS

Local anesthetic agents block nerve conduction at and around the application site to produce an analgesic effect. These drugs affect sensory, motor, and autonomic nerve fibers and act on small nerve fibers more than on large nerve fibers. The only local anesthetic approved for otic use is benzocaine. It is administered topically as a solution or a gel.

PHARMACOKINETICS

Benzocaine is not absorbed systemically. Its onset of action occurs within minutes, and its duration of action is only 1 to 2 hours.

PHARMACODYNAMICS

Local anesthetic agents temporarily interrupt the conduction of nerve impulses, reducing the permeability of the nerve cell membrane to sodium and potassium ions. This action interferes with the ability of the nerve membrane to depolarize when stimulated.

In an area of mixed nerve fibers, local anesthetics initially affect autonomic nerve fibers, first blocking the small, nonmyelinated C fibers that mediate pain and produce vasoconstrictor responses, then the myelinated A-delta fibers that mediate pain and temperature. Then the local anesthetics block the large fibers that carry sensory impulses, thereby blocking impulse conduction in the motor nerves.

PHARMACOTHERAPEUTICS

Benzocaine is used for temporary relief of ear pain. It may be used with an anti-infective otic agent if an ear infection is present.

benzocaine (Americaine Otic, Auralgan Otic, Tympagesic). Ear pain, commonly caused by infection, can be relieved by instilling benzocaine.
Usual adult dosage: for pain relief, 4 to 5 drops t.i.d. or q.i.d.; benzocaine may be repeated as frequently as 1 to 2 hours. After instilling the drug, insert a cotton pledget moistened with benzocaine into the ear.

Drug interactions

No significant interactions occur between benzocaine and other drugs.

ADVERSE DRUG REACTIONS

Benzocaine may cause ear irritation, pruritus, and edema. It may mask the symptoms of a fulminating middle ear infection, although hearing loss, dizziness, or a sensation of fullness in the ear may remain. It also may cause urticaria, a hypersensitivity reaction.

NURSING PROCESS APPLICATION

The following information assists the nurse in caring for a patient receiving benzocaine.

Assessment

• Review the patient's history for a preexisting condition that contraindicates the use of benzocaine, such as perforated tympanic membrane, or known hypersensitivity to the drug.
• Assess the patient for adverse reactions to benzocaine, such as ear irritation, pruritus, and edema; urticaria; or masking of a fulminating middle ear infection.

• Assess the effectiveness of benzocaine periodically.
• Evaluate the patient's and family's knowledge about benzocaine.

Nursing diagnoses

The following examples represent appropriate nursing diagnoses for a patient receiving benzocaine.
• Potential for injury related to a preexisting condition that contraindicates the use of benzocaine
• Potential for injury related to adverse drug reactions
• Knowledge deficit related to benzocaine

Planning and implementation

• Do not administer benzocaine to a patient with a condition that contraindicates its use.
• Monitor the patient closely for adverse reactions during benzocaine therapy.
• *Inspect the patient's ear canal for signs of irritation or edema before each application of benzocaine. If inspection reveals either reaction, withhold benzocaine and notify the physician.*
• Irrigate the ear gently before administration to clear it of debris and impacted cerumen.
• Monitor the patient for early signs of an allergic reaction, such as urticaria. Discontinue the drug immediately and notify the physician if an allergic reaction is suspected.
• *Monitor the patient for signs of middle ear infection, such as hearing loss and dizziness. Notify the physician if either occurs.*
• *Avoid touching the patient's ear with the dropper; do not rinse the dropper.*
• Notify the physician if ear pain persists or worsens.

Patient teaching

• Teach the patient or family the name, dose, frequency, action, and adverse effects of benzocaine.
• *Instruct the patient not to use benzocaine for a prolonged time and to contact the physician if the ear problem persists or worsens.*
• Teach the patient (or parent of a pediatric patient) how to instill eardrops. (For a description and illustration, see *Eardrop administration,* page 1262.)
• *Instruct the patient to report hearing loss, dizziness, or ear irritation, pruritus, or fullness to the physician.*
• Instruct the patient to stop the drug and notify the physician if urticaria occurs.

Evaluation

The following examples represent appropriate evaluation statements for a patient receiving benzocaine.
• The patient has no conditions that contraindicate benzocaine therapy.
• The patient experiences no adverse reactions to benzocaine.

• The patient and family express an accurate understanding of the points taught about benzocaine.
• The patient demonstrates proper administration of benzocaine eardrops.

CERUMINOLYTIC AGENTS

Ceruminolytic agents emulsify hardened or impacted cerumen, or earwax. They also prevent ceruminosis (excessive cerumen) accumulation. Ceruminolytic agents discussed in this section include carbamide peroxide and triethanolamine polypeptide oleate-condensate.

PHARMACOKINETICS

Ceruminolytics are not absorbed systemically. Therapeutic effect occurs in 2 to 4 days.

PHARMACODYNAMICS

Ceruminolytics reduce hardened cerumen by emulsifying and mechanically loosening it. Carbamide peroxide is combined with anhydrous glycerin to soften cerumen. Exposing the carbamide peroxide to moisture releases oxygen and hydrogen peroxide, which produces an effervescence that mechanically removes cerumen. Carbamide peroxide also acts to deodorize odor-causing bacteria.

PHARMACOTHERAPEUTICS

Carbamide peroxide is used to loosen hardened or impacted cerumen and to prevent ceruminosis. Triethanolamine may be used to remove excess or impacted cerumen and to clear the ear canal before an ear examination or procedure. Nonetheless, the patient's ear should be irrigated after therapy to remove debris.

carbamide peroxide (Debrox, Murine). An equimolar compound of hydrogen peroxide and urea that releases hydrogen peroxide when moistened, carbamide peroxide is used to loosen hardened or impacted cerumen and to prevent ceruminosis.
Usual adult dosage: for adults and children ages 12 and older, 5 to 10 drops into the external auditory canal b.i.d. for 4 days, then irrigate gently.
Usual pediatric dosage: for children under age 12, individualized dosage under a physician's supervision.

triethanolamine polypeptide oleate-condensate (Cerumenex). Effective with a single 15- to 30-minute treatment,

triethanolamine is used to remove excess or impacted cerumen. It also may be used to clear the ear canal before an ear examination, otologic therapy, or audiometry.
Usual adult dosage: fill the patient's ear canal with solution and plug it with cotton for 15 to 30 minutes; then irrigate gently.

Drug interactions

No significant interactions occur between ceruminolytics and other drugs.

ADVERSE DRUG REACTIONS

Adverse reactions to ceruminolytics usually are insignificant. Mild, localized erythema and pruritus may occur with triethanolamine or carbamide peroxide. Some patients using triethanolamine experience hypersensitivity reactions, such as severe eczema.

NURSING PROCESS APPLICATION

The following information assists the nurse in caring for a patient receiving a ceruminolytic agent.

Assessment
• Review the patient's history for a preexisting condition that contraindicates the use of a ceruminolytic agent, such as perforated tympanic membrane or known hypersensitivity to the drug.
• Review the patient's history for a preexisting condition that requires cautious use of triethanolamine, such as a history of dermatologic disorders and allergic reactions.
• Assess the patient for adverse reactions to the prescribed ceruminolytic agent, such as localized erythema, pruritus, or severe eczema.
• Assess the effectiveness of the ceruminolytic agent after each application.
• Evaluate the patient's and family's knowledge about the prescribed ceruminolytic agent.

Nursing diagnoses
The following examples represent appropriate nursing diagnoses for a patient receiving a ceruminolytic agent.
• Potential for injury related to a preexisting condition that contraindicates the use of a ceruminolytic agent
• Potential for injury related to a preexisting condition that requires cautious use of triethanolamine
• Potential for injury related to adverse drug reactions
• Knowledge deficit related to the prescribed ceruminolytic agent

Planning and implementation
• Do not administer a ceruminolytic agent to a patient with a condition that contraindicates its use.
• Administer triethanolamine cautiously to a patient at risk because of a preexisting condition.
• Monitor the patient closely for adverse reactions to the prescribed ceruminolytic agent.
• Perform a patch test before administering triethanolamine to determine the possibility of an allergic reaction. To do this, drop the ceruminolytic agent onto the flexor surface of the arm. Then cover the area with a small sterile bandage and observe it, usually after 24 hours, for erythema and swelling.
• Inspect the patient's skin for eczema (patchy, scaly, red blotches) when administering triethanolamine. If eczema is present, withhold the drug and notify the physician because this may be a hypersensitivity reaction.
• *Inspect the ear canal for erythema before administering each dose of the ceruminolytic agent. Ask the patient about pruritus. Notify the physician if erythema or pruritus occurs.*
• Do not touch the patient's ear with the dropper.
• Keep the medication in a tightly closed, light-resistant container away from heat.
• *Irrigate the affected ear gently with warm water after administering the ceruminolytic agent. Avoid excessive pressure. Irrigation will help remove the cerumen loosened by the ceruminolytic agent.*
• Notify the physician if adverse reactions occur or if the ceruminolytic agent is ineffective.

Patient teaching
• Teach the patient and family the name, dose, frequency, action, and adverse effects of the prescribed ceruminolytic agent.
• Instruct the patient to contact the physician if an allergic reaction occurs.
• *Instruct the patient not to use carbamide peroxide for more than 4 days unless supervised by a physician, and not to use triethanolamine for more than 15 to 30 minutes unless instructed otherwise by the physician.*
• *Instruct the patient to allow the ceruminolytic solution to remain in the ear canal for at least 15 minutes.*
• Instruct the patient to store the ceruminolytic agent in a light-resistant container away from high temperatures.
• Teach the patient (or parent of a pediatric patient) how to administer eardrops. (For an illustration and description, see *Eardrop administration,* page 1262.)
• *Teach the patient how to irrigate the ear. Show how to tilt the head with the affected ear upward. Explain that the tip of the irrigating device is placed inside the meatus and directed toward the roof of the ear canal. Then warm water is allowed to flow into the ear canal. Explain that a basin should be positioned below the ear to collect the*

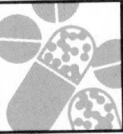

SELECTED MAJOR DRUGS

Otic agents

This chart summarizes the major otic agents currently in clinical use.

DRUG	MAJOR INDICATIONS	USUAL ADULT DOSAGES	CONTRAINDICATIONS AND PRECAUTIONS
Anti-infective agents			
boric acid	Otitis externa	4 to 6 drops in each ear, then plug with cotton t.i.d. or q.i.d.	• Know that boric acid is contraindicated as the sole treatment for earache in any patient. • Be aware that boric acid has no precautions.
chloramphenicol	Otitis externa	2 to 3 drops t.i.d.	• Know that chloramphenicol is contraindicated in a patient with a perforated tympanic membrane or known hypersensitivity to the drug. • Administer with caution to any patient who has received the drug for a prolonged time.
Anti-inflammatory agents			
dexamethasone sodium phosphate	External auditory canal inflammation	3 to 4 drops b.i.d. or t.i.d.	• Know that dexamethasone sodium phosphate is contraindicated in a patient with acute purulent bacterial, viral, or fungal otic infection; a perforated tympanic membrane; or known hypersensitivity to the drug. • Be aware that dexamethasone sodium phosphate has no precautions.
hydrocortisone	External auditory canal inflammation	4 to 5 drops t.i.d. or q.i.d.	• Know that hydrocortisone is contraindicated in a patient with acute purulent bacterial, viral, or fungal otic infection; a perforated tympanic membrane; or known hypersensitivity to the drug. • Be aware that hydrocortisone has no precautions.
Local anesthetic agents			
benzocaine	Ear pain from ear infection or other ear conditions	4 to 5 drops t.i.d. or q.i.d., every 1 to 2 hours as needed	• Know that benzocaine is contraindicated in a patient with a perforated tympanic membrane, or known hypersensitivity to the drug. • Be aware that benzocaine has no precautions.
Ceruminolytic agents			
carbamide peroxide	Hardened or impacted cerumen; prevention of ceruminosis	5 to 10 drops b.i.d. for 4 days, then irrigate gently	• Know that carbamide peroxide is contraindicated in a patient with perforated tympanic membrane; ear drainage, pain, irritation, or rash; dizziness; or known hypersensitivity to the drug. • Be aware that carbamide peroxide has no precautions.
triethanolamine polypeptide oleate-condensate	Removal of hardened or impacted cerumen; ear canal clearance before examinations, otologic therapy, or audiometry	Fill ear canal with solution and plug it with cotton for 15 to 30 minutes; then irrigate	• Know that triethanolamine is contraindicated in a patient with a perforated tympanic membrane, a history of otitis media, or known hypersensitivity to the drug. • Administer with caution to a patient with a history of dermatologic disorders and allergic reactions.

irrigating fluid as it flows out of the ear. Instruct the patient to lie on the affected side after irrigation to allow the irrigating solution to flow out.
• Inform the patient that a fizzing sound is normal during ceruminolytic agent application.
• Instruct the patient not to use cotton swabs in an attempt to remove cerumen. This prevents accidental perforation of the tympanic membrane.
• Instruct the patient to notify the physician if adverse reactions occur.

Evaluation
The following examples represent appropriate evaluation statements for a patient receiving a ceruminolytic agent.
• The patient has no conditions that contraindicate ceruminolytic agent therapy.
• The patient exhibits no signs of complications in the preexisting condition linked to triethanolamine.
• The patient experiences no adverse reactions to the prescribed ceruminolytic agent.
• The patient and family express an accurate understanding of the points taught about the prescribed ceruminolytic agent.
• The patient demonstrates the proper technique for ear irrigation.

CHAPTER SUMMARY

Chapter 72 presented information on four classes of otic drugs: anti-infective, anti-inflammatory, local anesthetic, and ceruminolytic agents. For each drug class, the chapter covered the mechanisms of action, therapeutic uses, dosage, administration, drug interactions, adverse reactions, and nursing process application. Here are the chapter highlights.
• Otic agents are used to treat external auditory canal infections (otitis externa), middle ear infections (otitis media), and ear inflammation and pain. They also are used to soften cerumen.
• Otic drugs are instilled topically via drops, irrigations, creams, ointments, and ear wicks.
• Anti-infective otics are bactericidal (kill bacteria) or bacteriostatic (inhibit bacterial growth). Acetic acid and boric acid are also fungistatic (inhibit fungal growth).
• Anti-infective otic agents include acetic acid, boric acid, chloramphenicol, colistin, and polymyxin B sulfate.

• Before administering an anti-infective otic agent, culture and sensitivity tests should be performed to identify the causative organism and its susceptibility to the agent.
• Adverse reactions to anti-infective otics include hypersensitivity reactions and superinfection.
• Anti-inflammatory otics produce anti-inflammatory, antipruritic, and vasoconstrictor effects. These agents include dexamethasone sodium phosphate, and hydrocortisone.
• Anti-inflammatory otics may precipitate a hypersensitivity reaction and may mask or exacerbate an underlying otic infection.
• Local anesthetics produce analgesia by blocking nerve impulse propagation in a given area. Benzocaine is the local anesthetic approved for otic use.
• Ceruminolytic agents emulsify hardened or impacted cerumen. They also deodorize odor-causing bacteria.
• As needed, the nurse should teach the patient or parent how to instill eardrops, irrigate the ear (when a ceruminolytic is used), or use an ear wick for drug administration. The nurse also should teach the patient or parent to recognize and report important adverse reactions.

STUDY QUESTIONS

See Appendix 1 for answers.

1. Alan Fontaine, age 23, seeks care for left ear pain and hearing loss that have occured for the past 3 days. Physical examination reveals cerumen impaction with otitis externa. The physician prescribes the anti-infective agent chloramphenicol, 2 to 3 drops into the external auditory canal t.i.d. The nurse instructs Mr. Fontaine to warm the drug to room temperature before administration. What may occur if the solution is too hot or too cold?
(a) tinnitus
(b) vertigo or nausea
(c) complete hearing loss
(d) tympanic membrane perforation

2. The nurse also teaches Mr. Fontaine how to instill the anti-infective agent properly. How should Mr. Fontaine straighten the ear canal for instillation?
(a) Pull the ear up and back.
(b) Pull the ear down and back.
(c) Pull the ear up and forward.
(d) Pull the ear down and forward.

3. The physician also prescribes an anti-inflammatory agent for Mr. Fontaine. Which statement accurately characterizes anti-inflammatory otic agents?
(a) They are more likely to exacerbate an otic infection than anti-infective otic agents.
(b) They are more likely to cause superinfection than anti-infective otic agents.
(c) They decrease the effectiveness of anti-infective otic agents.
(d) They exhibit greater systemic absorption than anti-infective otic agents.

4. The physician also prescribes the ceruminolytic agent carbamide peroxide for Mr. Fontaine. Which condition would contraindicate carbamide peroxide administration?
(a) vertigo
(b) tinnitus
(c) otitis media
(d) perforated tympanic membrane

5. Which instruction should the nurse give Mr. Fontaine about administering the ceruminolytic agent?
(a) Instill the solution and irrigate the ear canal immediately.
(b) Let the solution remain in the ear canal for at least 15 minutes.
(c) Instill the solution and apply a dry cotton plug.
(d) Instill the solution and use a cotton swab to remove cerumen.

6. Sandy Davis brings her daughter Katie, age 4, to the pediatrician with right ear pain, irritability, and low-grade fever. When the physical examination reveals otitis media, the physician prescribes an oral antibiotic and the local anesthetic benzocaine. Which instruction should Ms. Davis receive about administering benzocaine ear drops to Katie?
(a) Lay the child on the unaffected side, gently pull the ear down and back, and instill the drops.
(b) With the child seated, gently pull the ear up and back and instill drops.
(c) Lay the child on the affected side and gently instill the drops.
(d) With the child seated, tilt the head to the unaffected side and gently instill the drops.

7. When should Katie obtain pain relief after benzocaine administration?
(a) within minutes
(b) within 1 to 2 hours
(c) within 4 to 6 hours
(d) within 1 day

8. What instructions should the nurse give Ms. Davis about benzocaine therapy?
(a) Rinse the benzocaine dropper thoroughly after each use.
(b) Use benzocaine for as long as Katie must take the antibiotic.
(c) Contact the physician if ear pain persists despite benzocaine use.
(d) Administer benzocaine as frequently as needed.

SELECTED REFERENCES

AHFS drug information 90. (1990). Bethesda, MD: American Society of Hospital Pharmacists.

Britton, P. (1991) *Common problems in otology.* St. Louis: Mosby Year Book, Inc.

Cunha, B. (1988). Case studies in infectious disease: Otitis media, part 4. *Emergency medicine, 20*(9), 164-172.

Goodman and Gilman's the pharmacological basis of therapeutics (8th ed.; 1990). Elmsford, NY: Pergamon Press.

Hansten, P., and Horn, J. (1988). *Drug interactions: Clinical significance of drug-drug interactions* (6th ed.). Philadelphia: Lea & Febiger.

Hawke, M. (1987). *Clinical pocket guide to ear disease.* Philadelphia: Lea & Febiger.

North American Nursing Diagnosis Association. (1990). *Taxonomy I - Revised, with official diagnostic categories.* St. Louis: NANDA.

Patiak, M. (1987). Children's all-too-common ear infections. *FDA Consumer, 21*(10), 28-31.

USPDI. (1991). *Drug information for the health care professional* (Vol. I, 11th ed.). Rockville, MD: United States Pharmacopeial Convention.

USPDI. (1991). *Advice for the patient* (Vol. II, 11th ed.). Rockville, MD: United States Pharmacopeial Convention.

UNCATEGORIZED AND OTHER AGENTS

OBJECTIVES

After reading and studying this chapter, the student should be able to:

1. Discuss the pharmacokinetics of the fertility drugs described in this chapter.

2. Identify the drugs used to treat uncommon or rare conditions discussed in this chapter.

3. Describe the drug interactions that occur with levamisole hydrochloride, nafarelin acetate, nimodipine, octreotide acetate, pegademase bovine, pentoxifylline, sodium benzoate 10% and sodium phenylacetate 10%, sulfasalazine, and ursodiol.

4. Discuss the nursing implications of botulinum toxin type A, mesalamine, olsalazine sodium, colfosceril palmitate, ethanolamine oleate, and mesna.

INTRODUCTION

Chapter 73 discusses 20 uncategorized and other agents, most of which are new drugs approved for clinical use within the past several years. Some are used to treat uncommon or rare conditions, such as congenital deficiency of alpha$_1$-antitrypsin (alpha$_1$-proteinase inhibitor), severe combined immunodeficiency disease associated with adenosine deaminase (ADA) deficiency (pegademase bovine), urea cycle enzymopathies (sodium benzoate 10% and sodium phenylacetate 10%), and severe homozygous cystinuria (tiopronin).

Other agents are indicated for more familiar conditions, such as strabismus and blepharospasm (botulinum toxin type A), ulcerative colitis (mesalamine, olsalazine sodium, and sulfasalazine), intermittent claudication (pentoxifylline), gallstones (ursodiol), and cancer (levamisole hydrochloride and octreotide acetate).

Several agents discussed in Chapter 73 are prescribed to treat reproductive disorders (clomiphene citrate, human chorionic gonadotropin, human menopausal gonadotropin, and nafarelin acetate) or for prophylaxis of a specific body-system disorder (colfosceril palmitate and ethanolamine oleate). This chapter also discusses mesna, a detoxifying agent used to prevent ifosfamide-induced hemorrhagic cystitis, and nimodipine, a calcium channel blocker prescribed to reduce neurologic deficits caused by spasms after subarachnoid hemorrhage from a ruptured congenital intracranial aneurysm.

For each drug, Chapter 73 discusses pharmacokinetics, pharmacodynamics, and pharmacotherapeutics as well as known drug interactions and adverse reactions. The chapter includes a chart that highlights important nursing implications for each drug and presents selected nursing diagnoses that may be used when administering these drugs. (For details, see *Nursing considerations for uncategorized and other agents,* pages 1282 to 1287.)

ALPHA$_1$-PROTEINASE INHIBITOR

An orphan drug, purified human alpha$_1$-proteinase inhibitor is classified as an enzyme inhibitor.

PHARMACOKINETICS

Information on the pharmacokinetics of alpha$_1$-proteinase inhibitor is unavailable.

PHARMACODYNAMICS

Alpha$_1$-proteinase inhibitor is a protease inhibitor that inactivates several proteases, including trypsin, chymotrypsin, coagulation factor XI, plasmin, thrombin, and neutrophil elastase. Without such inactivation, a person with congenital alpha$_1$-antitrypsin deficiency develops emphysema from chronic degradation of elastin tissue.

PHARMACOTHERAPEUTICS

Alpha₁-proteinase inhibitor is prescribed to replace alpha₁-antitrypsin in patients with congenital deficiency of this substance who show signs of panacinar emphysema.

alpha₁-proteinase inhibitor (Prolastin). This drug is used for chronic replacement therapy in patients with congenital deficiency of alpha₁-antitrypsin and clinically demonstrable chronic degradation of elastin tissue (panacinar emphysema).
Usual adult dosage: 60 mg/kg I.V. once weekly.

Drug interactions
No known interactions exist.

ADVERSE DRUG REACTIONS

Alpha₁-proteinase inhibitor may cause delayed fever, lightheadedness, dizziness, and mild leukocytosis.

BOTULINUM TOXIN TYPE A

Botulinum toxin type A is a new ophthalmic agent used to treat selected disorders involving the eye muscles.

PHARMACOKINETICS

The pharmacokinetics of botulinum toxin type A are unknown. However, patients who received this drug for blepharospasm did not require retreatment for an average of 12.5 weeks after injection. More than half of patients who received it for strabismus maintained improvement over 6 months.

PHARMACODYNAMICS

Botulinum toxin type A causes neuromuscular paralysis by binding to acetylcholine receptors on the motor end plate. It also may inhibit release of acetylcholine from presynaptic nerve endings.

PHARMACOTHERAPEUTICS

Botulinum toxin type A is a muscle relaxant used to treat strabismus and blepharospasm.

botulinum toxin type A (Oculinum). This agent is used correct various degrees of strabismus and blepharospasm.

Usual adult dosage: for strabismus, the dosage varies with the degree of deviation (lower dosages are used for milder deviations). For vertical muscles and for horizontal strabismus of <20 prism diopters, 1.25 to 2.5 units injected into any one muscle; for horizontal strabismus of 20 to 50 prism diopters, 2.5 to 5 units injected into any one muscle. For persistent palsy of the seventh cranial nerve lasting more than 1 month, 1.25 to 2.5 units injected into the medial rectus muscle. Maximum single dosage for any one muscle is 25 units. For blepharospasm, initially 1.25 to 2.5 units injected into the medial and lateral pretarsal orbicularis oculi of the upper and lower lids; for subsequent treatments, the dosage may be doubled if inadequate paralysis is achieved (however, exceeding 5 units per site has no apparent benefit). The effects of each treatment last about 3 months. Treatment can be repeated indefinitely.

Drug interactions
No drug interactions have been reported.

ADVERSE DRUG REACTIONS

Adverse reactions are limited to the ocular area. They include double vision, blurred vision, spatial disorientation, ptosis, vertical deviation (after treatment of strabismus), irritation (after treatment of blepharospasm), a local diffuse rash, eyelid swelling, and ecchymosis.

CLOMIPHENE CITRATE

Clomiphene citrate is a fertility agent used to stimulate ovulation in females.

PHARMACOKINETICS

After oral administration, clomiphene is absorbed readily from the gastrointestinal (GI) tract. The distribution is not clear. The drug may undergo enterohepatic recirculation or may be stored in body fat. Clomiphene is metabolized in the liver and excreted primarily in the feces via bile elimination. Its half-life is 5 days; however, the drug can be found in the feces up to 6 weeks after administration.

PHARMACODYNAMICS

Clomiphene is an antiestrogenic agent that occupies estrogen receptor sites in the hypothalamus, preventing estrogen from binding to these sites. In turn, the hypothalamus stimulates the pituitary gland to release greater amounts of follicle-stimulating hormone (FSH) and luteinizing hormone (LH); these hormones then initiate and enhance the growth of an ovarian follicle in females.

PHARMACOTHERAPEUTICS

Clomiphene is a fertility agent used to correct reproductive disorders associated with ovulatory dysfunction.

clomiphene citrate (Clomid, Serophene). Clomiphene is prescribed to treat anovulation and oligo-ovulation and to regulate ovulatory cycles that are shorter than 23 days or longer than 37 days.
Usual adult dosage: 50 mg P.O. daily from day 5 to day 9 of the cycle; if the patient has not had recent uterine bleeding, the drug can be started at any time after a negative pregnancy test. If ovulation does not occur, the dosage may be increased by 50-mg increments each cycle until ovulation occurs or a daily dosage of 200 mg is reached.

Drug interactions
No significant drug interactions are associated with clomiphene.

ADVERSE DRUG REACTIONS

Adverse reactions to clomiphene include insomnia, hypertension, blurred vision, nausea, vomiting, bloating, photophobia, urinary frequency, polyuria, and ovarian enlargement and cyst formation (both of which regress spontaneously when the drug is discontinued). Occasionally, hyperglycemia occurs. Other adverse reactions include hot flashes, reversible alopecia, breast discomfort, and multiple fetuses. Sensitivity reactions to clomiphene include urticaria, rash, and dermatitis.

COLFOSCERIL PALMITATE

Colfosceril palmitate is a respiratory agent used exclusively to prevent or treat neonatal respiratory distress syndrome (RDS).

PHARMACOKINETICS

Absorbed from the alveoli into lung tissue after endotracheal administration, colfosceril is metabolized extensively. Its by-products are incorporated into alveolar phospholipid synthesis and secretion.

PHARMACODYNAMICS

An artificial surfactant, colfosceril reduces the surface tension of alveolar tissue. By replacing insufficient respiratory surfactant, it may reduce the risk and severity of RDS.

PHARMACOTHERAPEUTICS

A respiratory surfactant agent, colfosceril is used to reduce the surface tension of alveolar tissue in neonates with RDS.

colfosceril palmitate (Exosurf Neonatal). Colfosceril is used for the prophylaxis and rescue treatment of neonatal RDS.
Usual pediatric dosage: 5 ml/kg administered through the side port of an endotracheal tube adaptor; each dose is divided in half and given over 1 to 2 minutes with the neonate in the midline position. After the first half-dose is administered, the neonate is held for 30 seconds at a 45-degree angle to the right; after the second half-dose, at a 45-degree angle to the left. For prophylaxis against RDS, the drug is administered as soon as possible after delivery, with the second and third doses given at 12 and 24 hours if the neonate remains on mechanical ventilation. For rescue treatment, the first dose is administered as soon as RDS is identified; the second dose at 12 hours if the neonate remains on mechanical ventilation.

Drug interactions
No known interactions exist.

ADVERSE DRUG REACTIONS

During clinical trials, neonates who received colfosceril had a higher incidence of pulmonary hemorrhage and apnea than those who received a placebo. They also were more likely to require use of a methylxanthine, such as theophylline.

ETHANOLAMINE OLEATE

Ethanolamine oleate is a vascular agent used to treat esophageal varices.

PHARMACOKINETICS

When injected locally, ethanolamine is cleared via the portal vein within 5 minutes. Other information on the pharmacokinetics of ethanolamine is unknown.

PHARMACODYNAMICS

A mild sclerosing agent, ethanolamine irritates the intimal endothelium of the vein, causing a sterile inflammatory response that leads to fibrosis and occlusion.

PHARMACOTHERAPEUTICS

Ethanolamine is used to prevent further bleeding in patients who have had a recent bleeding episode from esophageal varices.

ethanolamine oleate (Ethamolin). Used to prevent new bleeding in patients with recent bleeding of esophageal varices, ethanolamine is a mild sclerosing agent. It should be administered by a gastroenterologist or other specialist because it must be instilled via gastroscope or endoscope directly into the esophageal area.
Usual adult dosage: 1.5 to 5 ml injected locally into each varix. The maximum dosage per treatment should not exceed 20 ml or 0.4 ml/kg. Subsequent injections usually follow at intervals of 1 week, 6 weeks, 3 months, and 6 months.

Drug interactions
No known interactions exist.

ADVERSE DRUG REACTIONS

Adverse reactions to ethanolamine include GI reactions, such as esophagitis, local mucosal sloughing or necrosis, and esophageal ulcer, stricture, or tearing; genitourinary reactions, such as acute renal failure; and respiratory reactions, such as pleural effusion or infiltration, pneumonia, and aspiration pneumonia. Other adverse reactions include pyrexia, retrosternal pain, and anaphylaxis.

HUMAN CHORIONIC GONADOTROPIN

Human chorionic gonadotropin (HCG) is a fertility agent used to treat male and female infertility.

PHARMACOKINETICS

Because HCG is destroyed by the GI tract, it is administered parenterally. After intramuscular (I.M.) administration, the drug is distributed primarily to the ovaries and testes. Smaller amounts are distributed to the proximal tubules of the kidneys. HCG reaches a peak concentration level in 5 to 6 hours; its half-life is 12 hours. Within 24 hours after I.M. administration of a therapeutic dose, 10% to 12% of the dose is excreted in the urine. Detectable amounts may continue to be excreted in the urine for up to 4 days.

PHARMACODYNAMICS

In females, HCG mimics the action of LH and allows ovarian follicle rupture. It also stimulates the corpus luteum to produce progesterone, needed to sustain the fertilized ovum. In males, HCG stimulates Leydig's cells in the testes to secrete testosterone, a hormone needed for spermatogenesis.

PHARMACOTHERAPEUTICS

HCG is a hormone used to treat infertility disorders by inducing ovulation in females and stimulating spermatogenesis in males.

human chorionic gonadotropin [HCG] (Follutein, Pregnyl). In females, HCG is prescribed to promote ovulation after follicular stimulation; in males, to stimulate spermatogenesis. The dosage varies with the indication, the patient's age and weight, and physician preference.
Usual adult dosage: for females, 5,000 to 10,000 IU I.M. at the time of ovulation or on the day after discontinuing human menopausal gonadotropin (HMG). For males, 4,000 IU I.M. three times weekly for 3 weeks, 5,000 IU I.M. every other day for 4 doses, 500 to 1,000 IU I.M. for 15 doses over 6 weeks, or 500 IU I.M. three times weekly for 6 to 9 months. If the testosterone level does not rise significantly, the dosage may be changed to 2,000 IU I.M. twice weekly with HMG for 6 to 12 weeks.

Drug interactions
No significant drug interactions exist.

ADVERSE DRUG REACTIONS

Adverse reactions associated with HCG are dose-related. They include headache, irritability, fatigue, depression, weight gain (from fluid retention), and gynecomastia. HCG also may cause ovarian hyperstimulation and multiple fetuses. Pain may occur at the injection site.

HUMAN MENOPAUSAL GONADOTROPIN

Human menopausal gonadotropin (HMG) is a fertility agent used to treat male and female infertility.

PHARMACOKINETICS

Because HMG is destroyed by the GI tract, it is administered I.M. The drug is distributed to the ovaries and testes. Its metabolism is unknown; however, about 8% of the dose is excreted unchanged in the urine. HMG has a half-life of several hours.

PHARMACODYNAMICS

HMG produces the physiologic effects of FSH by stimulating development and maturation of the ovarian follicle. HMG also mimics LH, causing ovulation and stimulating development of the corpus luteum in females. In males, HMG stimulates spermatogenesis.

PHARMACOTHERAPEUTICS

HMG is used to induce ovulation in females and to treat selected reproductive disorders in males.

human menopausal gonadotropin [HMG] (Pergonal). In females, HMG is prescribed mainly to initiate ovulation; it also is used to stimulate ovulation for special procedures (such as an in vitro fertilization, gamete intrafallopian transfer, or egg donation). In males, HMG is prescribed for hypogonadotropic hypogonadism and prepubertal cryptorchidism.
Usual adult dosage: for females, the dosage depends on whether the drug is used to induce ovulation or to stimulate ovulation for a special procedure. The usual initial dosage is one ampule (containing 75 IU of FSH and 75 IU of LH) I.M. once a day for 9 to 12 days, followed on the day after the last dose by 5,000 to 10,000 IU I.M. of HCG. For males, pretreatment consists of 5,000 IU of HCG three times weekly until normal testosterone levels are achieved; then one ampule of HMG (containing 75 IU of FSH and 75 IU of LH) I.M. three times weekly with 2,000 IU I.M. of HCG twice a week for 4 months.

Drug interactions
No significant drug interactions exist.

ADVERSE DRUG REACTIONS

The most common adverse reaction to HMG is ovarian enlargement, which may be accompanied by lower abdominal pain and distention. Ovarian hyperstimulation syndrome (OHSS), a life-threatening disorder, is much less common — and only when HMG is administered with HCG. In severe cases, OHSS may involve ovarian enlargement, ascites, and pleural effusion. Electrolyte imbalance, increased capillary permeability, and hypercoagulability sometimes accompany the syndrome.

Other adverse reactions to HMG include hemoperitoneum (from ruptured ovarian cyst) and arterial thromboembolism.

LEVAMISOLE HYDROCHLORIDE

Levamisole hydrochloride is an antineoplastic agent used to treat a specific type of colon cancer.

PHARMACOKINETICS

After oral administration, levamisole is absorbed well and achieves a peak plasma concentration level within 2 hours. The drug undergoes extensive metabolism in the liver and is excreted primarily in the urine. The plasma half-life is approximately 3.5 hours.

PHARMACODYNAMICS

An immunomodulator with a complex mechanism of action, levamisole restores depressed immune function rather than stimulates the immune response. Its mechanism of action in combination with fluorouracil, with which it is administered, is unknown.

PHARMACOTHERAPEUTICS

Levamisole is a chemotherapeutic agent used with fluorouracil to treat Duke's Stage C colon cancer.

levamisole (Ergamisol). In combination with fluorouracil, levamisole is prescribed as adjuvant therapy after surgical resection of Duke's Stage C colon cancer.
Usual adult dosage: for initial therapy, 50 mg P.O. every 8 hours for 3 days starting 7 to 30 days after surgery; for maintenance therapy, 50 mg P.O. every 8 hours for 3 days, administered every 2 weeks.

Drug interactions

Levamisole may increase the plasma phenytoin level. If taken with alcohol, it may cause a disulfiram-like reaction, producing such effects as facial flushing, optic neuritis, psychotic reactions, drowsiness, headache, and rash.

ADVERSE DRUG REACTIONS

Adverse reactions reported in more than 5% of patients in clinical trials include nausea, diarrhea, vomiting, taste changes, dermatitis, fatigue, arthralgia, and infection. Adverse reactions reported in more than 2% of patients include leukopenia, alopecia, fever, rigors, stomatitis, myalgia, dizziness, headache, and somnolence. Combination therapy with fluorouracil increased some adverse reactions.

Drug interactions

Concomitant administration with sulfasalazine and other oral products that liberate mesalamine may result in renal dysfunction.

ADVERSE DRUG REACTIONS

Mesalamine primarily causes adverse GI reactions, such as abdominal pain, cramps, and discomfort; flatulence; nausea; diarrhea; hemorrhoids; and constipation. Other adverse reactions include leg and joint pain, headache, dizziness, insomnia, weakness, malaise, fatigue, fever, rash, sore throat, flulike symptoms, back pain, hair loss, peripheral edema, urinary tract infection, and urinary burning.

MESALAMINE

Mesalamine is an anti-inflammatory agent used to treat selected inflammatory disorders.

PHARMACOKINETICS

Administered as a rectal enema, mesalamine is absorbed poorly through the bowel wall. Absorption varies from 10% to 30%, depending on retention time and individual variation. Unabsorbed mesalamine is excreted primarily in the feces. Absorbed mesalamine is metabolized at an unknown site and excreted in the urine. The plasma half-life of mesalamine ranges from 0.5 to 1.5 hours.

PHARMACODYNAMICS

Although the exact mechanism of action is unknown, mesalamine may act locally to decrease inflammation by blocking cyclooxygenase and inhibiting prostaglandin in the colon.

PHARMACOTHERAPEUTICS

Mesalamine is used to treat inflammatory bowel disease and ulcerative proctitis.

mesalamine (Rowasa). As a suspension enema, mesalamine is prescribed to treat mild to moderate distal ulcerative colitis, proctosigmoiditis, or proctitis.
Usual adult dosage: 60 ml (4 grams) given rectally once a day (preferably at bedtime) and retained for about 8 hours.

MESNA

A thiol derivative, mesna is used as a detoxifying agent in conjunction with ifosfamide therapy.

PHARMACOKINETICS

After I.V. administration, mesna remains in the vascular compartment and is metabolized to mesna disulfide. It is eliminated by the kidneys. After an 800-mg I.V. dose, the half-lives of mesna and mesna disulfide are 0.36 hours and 1.17 hours, respectively.

PHARMACODYNAMICS

In the kidneys, mesna disulfide is reduced to a free thiol compound that reacts chemically with urotoxic ifosfamide metabolites to detoxify them, preventing ifosfamide-induced hemorrhagic cystitis.

PHARMACOTHERAPEUTICS

Mesna is a detoxifying agent used to prevent hemorrhagic cystitis caused by ifosfamide therapy.

mesna (Mesnex). Mesna is prescribed prophylactically to reduce the risk of ifosfamide-induced hemorrhagic cystitis.
Usual adult dosage: equivalent to 20% of each ifosfamide dosage on a weight-per-weight basis, given by I.V. bolus injection t.i.d. The first dose is given with ifosfamide; the next two doses are given 4 and 8 hours after each ifosfamide dose, for a daily dosage equivalent to 60% of the ifosfamide dosage.

Drug interactions

No known drug interactions exist.

ADVERSE DRUG REACTIONS

Because mesna is administered with ifosfamide and other antineoplastic agents, its adverse reactions are difficult to isolate. The following reactions were reported during clinical trials in a limited number of patients: bad taste in the mouth, soft stools, diarrhea, limb pain, headache, fatigue, nausea, vomiting, hypotension, and allergy.

NAFARELIN ACETATE

Nafarelin acetate is a gonadotropin-releasing hormone (GnRH) agonist used to treat endometriosis.

PHARMACOKINETICS

After intranasal administration, nafarelin is absorbed rapidly into the bloodstream, with the peak plasma concentration level occurring between 10 and 40 minutes. The drug is approximately 80% plasma protein bound; its half-life is approximately 3 hours. After extensive metabolism, the drug is eliminated in the urine and feces.

PHARMACODYNAMICS

A GnRH agonist, nafarelin decreases the secretion of gonadal steroids and suppresses their physiologic effects during long-term administration.

PHARMACOTHERAPEUTICS

Nafarelin is used to treat endometriosis.

nafarelin acetate (Synarel). Nafarelin is prescribed to reduce endometric lesions and relieve pain in the management of endometriosis.
Usual adult dosage: 400 mcg daily as one spray (200 mcg) into oné nostril in the morning and one spray into the other nostril in the evening, beginning between days 2 and 4 of the menstrual cycle. For persistent regular menstruation after months of treatment, 800 mcg daily as one spray into each nostril in the morning and evening. Therapy should not exceed 6 months.

Drug interactions

No significant drug interactions have been reported. However, use of a nasal decongestant may interfere with nafarelin absorption. A patient should delay using such a decongestant for at least 30 minutes after taking nafarelin and should consult the physician to determine if a dosage adjustment is required.

ADVERSE DRUG REACTIONS

Adverse reactions reported in more than 5% of patients during clinical trials include hot flashes, decreased libido, vaginal dryness, headache, emotional lability, acne, myalgia, reduced breast size, edema, seborrhea, weight gain, and nasal irritation.

NIMODIPINE

Nimodipine is a calcium channel blocker used to induce cerebral vasodilation in certain patients.

PHARMACOKINETICS

After oral administration, nimodipine is absorbed rapidly, with the peak concentration level usually occurring within 1 hour. Approximately 95% protein bound, the drug is metabolized in the liver and eliminated by the kidneys. Its half-life is 1 to 2 hours.

PHARMACODYNAMICS

Nimodipine is a calcium channel blocker that inhibits contraction of vascular smooth muscle.

PHARMACOTHERAPEUTICS

Nimodipine is used to treat neurologic deficits caused by cerebral spasms resulting from a ruptured congenital aneurysm.

nimodipine (Nimotop). Nimodipine is prescribed to reduce neurologic deficits caused by spasms after subarachnoid hemorrhage resulting from ruptured congenital intracranial aneurysm in patients who otherwise are neurologically healthy. Therapy should begin within 96 hours of the hemorrhage and continue for 21 days.
Usual adult dosage: 60 mg P.O. every 4 hours for 21 days. For patients with severe liver disease, 30 mg P.O. every 4 hours.

Drug interactions

Concomitant administration with other calcium channel blockers may cause additive cardiovascular effects.

ADVERSE DRUG REACTIONS

Adverse reactions reported during clinical trials include hypotension, abnormal liver function test results, edema, diarrhea, rash, headache, nausea and other GI symptoms, dyspnea, electrocardiographic abnormalities, tachycardia, bradycardia, muscle pain or cramps, acne, and depression.

OCTREOTIDE ACETATE

Octreotide acetate is a long-acting octapeptide used to treat selected metastatic tumors.

PHARMACOKINETICS

Octreotide is absorbed into the circulation rapidly and completely after subcutaneous injection. It achieves a peak concentration level 24 minutes after a 100-mcg dose. The drug is bound approximately 65% to lipoproteins and albumin. Its elimination half-life is approximately 1.5 hours. Duration of action varies and may be as long as 12 hours under certain conditions. Approximately 32% of a dose is excreted unchanged in the urine.

PHARMACODYNAMICS

The pharmacologic properties of octreotide resemble those of the natural hormone somatostatin. Normally, somatostatin suppresses secretion of serotonin, gastrin, vasoactive intestinal peptide, insulin, glucagon, secretin motilin, and pancreatic polypeptide. Octreotide also may suppress growth hormone and decrease splanchnic blood flow.

PHARMACOTHERAPEUTICS

Octreotide is used to relieve symptoms of metastatic carcinoma and vasoactive intestinal peptide-secreting tumors (VIPomas).

octreotide acetate (Sandostatin). Octreotide is prescribed to control symptoms in patients with metastatic carcinoid or VIPomas.
Usual adult dosage: for carcinoid tumors, 100 to 600 mcg S.C. in two, three, or four divided doses for the first 2 weeks of therapy. (During clinical trials, the median daily maintenance dosage was approximately 450 mcg. Experience with maintenance dosages higher than 750 mcg/day

is limited.) For VIPomas, the recommended daily dosage is 200 to 300 mcg S.C. in two, three, or four divided doses during the first 2 weeks of therapy, then adjusted according to patient response and symptom control. Daily maintenance dosages above 450 mcg rarely are required.

Drug interactions

Octreotide may decrease the plasma level of cyclosporine. Concomitant use with insulin, an oral hypoglycemic agent, or oral diazoxide may require dosage adjustment. Octreotide therapy may necessitate dosage adjustment of other drugs used to control disease symptoms, such as beta blockers.

ADVERSE DRUG REACTIONS

Adverse reactions reported in 3% to 10% of patients during clinical trials include nausea, pain at the injection site, diarrhea, abdominal pain or discomfort, and vomiting. Adverse reactions reported in 1% to 2% of patients include headache, fat malabsorption, dizziness, light-headedness, fatigue, flushing, hypoglycemia or hyperglycemia, edema, weakness, and wheal or erythema at the injection site.

OLSALAZINE SODIUM

Olsalazine sodium is a salicylate derivative used to treat ulcerative colitis.

PHARMACOKINETICS

After oral administration, approximately 2.4% of a single 1-gram oral dose is absorbed. Olsalazine is more than 99% bound to plasma proteins. Approximately 0.1% of an oral dose is metabolized in the liver to olsalazine-0-sulfate, which has a half-life of 7 days and accumulates to a steady state within 2 to 3 weeks. The drug is excreted primarily in the feces.

PHARMACODYNAMICS

The mechanism of action is unknown but appears to be topical rather than systemic. Converted to S-amino salicylic acid, olsalazine may reduce colonic inflammation by blocking cyclooxygenase and inhibiting prostaglandin production in the bowel mucosa.

PHARMACOTHERAPEUTICS

Olsalazine is used to treat ulcerative colitis in patients who cannot tolerate sulfasalazine.

olsalazine sodium (Dipentum). Prescribed for sulfasalazine-intolerant patients, olsalazine is used to maintain remission of ulcerative colitis.
Usual adult dosage: 1 gram P.O. daily in two divided doses with food.

Drug interactions
No known drug interactions exist.

ADVERSE DRUG REACTIONS

The most common adverse reaction to olsalazine is diarrhea; approximately 17% of patients develop diarrhea during therapy. Other common adverse reactions include abdominal pain and cramps, headache, and arthralgia. Less common reactions include fatigue, drowsiness, lethargy, depression, vertigo, nausea, dyspepsia, bloating, anorexia, vomiting, stomatitis, rash, and pruritus.

PEGADEMASE BOVINE

Pegademase bovine is a modified enzyme used for enzyme replacement therapy in patients with ADA deficiency.

PHARMACOKINETICS

Information on the pharmacokinetics of pegademase bovine is unavailable.

PHARMACODYNAMICS

Pegademase bovine provides specific replacement of the deficient enzyme ADA. When ADA is absent, the purine substrates adenosine and 2'-deoxyadenosine accumulate, causing metabolic abnormalities that are directly toxic to lymphocytes. Pegademase bovine acts directly to correct these metabolic abnormalities. A lag time exists between correction of metabolic abnormalities and improved immune function; this interval varies from a few weeks to 6 months.

PHARMACOTHERAPEUTICS

Pegademase bovine is used to replace ADA in patients with severe combined immunodeficiency disease.

pegademase bovine (Adagen). As enzyme replacement therapy for ADA deficiency, pegademase bovine is prescribed for patients with severe combined immunodeficiency disease who are not suitable candidates for bone marrow transplantation or for whom that procedure has failed. It is recommended for use in neonates and children of any age.
Usual pediatric dosage: 10 U/kg I.M. as a single dose followed by a second dose of 15 U/kg I.M. after 7 days and a third dose of 20 U/kg I.M. after 7 more days; for maintenance, 20 U/kg I.M. once a week. Further increases of 5 U/kg/week may be necessary; however, the maximum single dosage should not exceed 30 U/kg. Preferably, the dosage is tailored according to plasma ADA activity levels.

Drug interactions
Because vidarabine is a substrate for ADA and 2'-deoxycoformycin is a potent ADA inhibitor, the activities of these drugs and pegademase bovine could be altered significantly if used concomitantly.

ADVERSE DRUG REACTIONS

Clinical experience with pegademase bovine is limited. Headache occurred in one patient and pain at the injection site in two patients.

PENTOXIFYLLINE

Pentoxifylline is a xanthine derivative used to treat intermittent claudication in selected patients.

PHARMACOKINETICS

After oral administration, pentoxifylline is absorbed extensively from the GI tract. However, its distribution is unknown. The drug is metabolized extensively by erythrocytes and the liver during first-pass hepatic metabolism. Pentoxifylline and its metabolites are excreted primarily in the urine; less than 4% of the drug is excreted in the feces. The half-life of the unchanged drug is approximately 30 to 45 minutes; the half-life of its metabolites is approximately 1 to 1.5 hours. The peak concentration level occurs in 2 to 4 hours; however, clinical effect requires 2 to 4 weeks of continuous therapy.

PHARMACODYNAMICS

Pentoxifylline and its metabolites improve capillary blood flow by increasing erythrocyte flexibility and reducing blood viscosity.

PHARMACOTHERAPEUTICS

Pentoxifylline is used to treat chronic occlusive peripheral vascular disease in the management of intermittent claudication.

pentoxifylline (Trental). This drug is prescribed for intermittent claudication associated with chronic occlusive peripheral vascular disease.
Usual adult dosage: 400 mg P.O. t.i.d. with meals.

Drug interactions

Concomitant use of pentoxifylline and antihypertensives may cause an increased hypotensive response. Bleeding abnormalities may occur in patients taking pentoxifylline concomitantly with oral anticoagulants or drugs that inhibit platelet aggregation, although a causal relationship has not been proven.

ADVERSE DRUG REACTIONS

The most common adverse reactions to pentoxifylline involve the GI tract and central nervous system (CNS). GI complaints include dyspepsia, nausea, and vomiting (1% to 3% of patients). Belching, flatus, and bloating also have been reported. Adverse CNS reactions include dizziness (2% of patients), headache, and tremor. Infrequent cardiovascular reactions also have been reported, although a causal relationship has not been established. Such reactions include chest pain, arrhythmias, tachycardia, palpitations, flushing, dyspnea, edema, and hypotension.

If adverse reactions occur, the dosage should be reduced; if adverse reactions persist after dosage reduction, pentoxifylline should be discontinued.

SODIUM BENZOATE 10% AND SODIUM PHENYLACETATE 10%

A combination drug, sodium benzoate 10% and sodium phenylacetate 10% is a blood ammonia reducing agent.

PHARMACOKINETICS

Pharmacokinetic data on sodium benzoate and sodium phenylacetate and their metabolites are limited. After oral administration of a single dose, the peak plasma concentration level occurs within 1 hour. Distribution is unknown. Most of the compound is metabolized by the liver and kidneys. Within 24 hours of administration, 80% to 100% of the compound is excreted via the kidneys.

PHARMACODYNAMICS

Sodium benzoate and sodium phenylacetate are metabolically active substances that decrease elevated serum ammonia concentrations in patients with inborn errors of ureagenesis. Their action results from acylation of amino acids, which decreases ammonia production. Benzoate and phenylacetate first activate enzymatic pathways, then act as a substitute in the defective ureagenic pathways in patients with urea cycle enzymopathies (UCE), preventing ammonia accumulation.

PHARMACOTHERAPEUTICS

Sodium benzoate 10% and sodium phenylacetate 10% is used to prevent or treat hyperammonemia in infants.

sodium benzoate 10% and sodium phenylacetate 10% (Ucephan). This agent is prescribed as adjunctive therapy to prevent and treat hyperammonemia in the long-term management of UCE in infants.
Usual pediatric dosage: 2.5 ml/kg P.O. (250 mg sodium benzoate and 250 mg sodium phenylacetate) in 3 to 6 equally divided doses daily; daily dosage not to exceed 100 ml.

Drug interactions

Concomitant administration of sodium benzoate and sodium phenylacetate with penicillin should be avoided because both drugs may compete for active secretion by the renal tubules, causing an altered renal excretion rate. Probenecid inhibits renal transport of many organic compounds and may alter renal elimination of sodium benzoate and sodium phenylacetate.

ADVERSE DRUG REACTIONS

Reported adverse reactions to sodium benzoate and sodium phenylacetate include nausea and vomiting. Certain adverse reactions associated with salicylate administration (such as peptic ulcer exacerbation, mild hyperventilation, and mild respiratory alkalosis) also may occur because of similarities between benzoate and salicylates.

SULFASALAZINE

Sulfasalazine is a sulfonamide used to treat ulcerative colitis.

PHARMACOKINETICS

Sulfasalazine is absorbed poorly from the GI tract after oral administration. About 80% is transported to the colon, where intestinal flora metabolize the drug to its active ingredients, sulfapyridine (an antibacterial) and 5-aminosalicylic acid (an anti-inflammatory), which exert their effects locally. Sulfapyridine is absorbed from the colon, but 5-aminosalicylic acid is not. Sulfasalazine is excreted chiefly in the urine. Its plasma half-life is approximately 6 to 8 hours.

PHARMACODYNAMICS

The exact mechanism of action of sulfasalazine in ulcerative colitis is unknown.

PHARMACOTHERAPEUTICS

Sulfasalazine is used to treat mild to moderate ulcerative colitis and, as adjunctive therapy, to treat severe ulcerative colitis.

sulfasalazine (Azulfidine). Administered for local effect in the gut, this short-acting sulfonamide is used to treat ulcerative colitis.
Usual adult dosage: for mild to moderate ulcerative colitis and as adjunctive therapy in severe ulcerative colitis, initially 3 to 4 grams P.O. daily in evenly divided doses; for maintenance, 1.5 to 2 grams P.O. daily in divided doses every 6 hours. To minimize adverse reactions, the dosage may start at 1 to 2 grams and be increased gradually.
Usual pediatric dosage: for children over age 2, initially 40 to 60 mg/kg P.O. daily in 3 to 6 divided doses, then 30 mg/kg daily in 4 doses. If GI intolerance occurs, a lower dosage may be used initially.

DRUG INTERACTIONS

Sulfasalazine may inhibit hepatic metabolism of oral anticoagulants, displacing them from binding sites and enhancing anticoagulant effects. Concomitant use with oral hypoglycemic agents enhances hypoglycemic effects, probably by displacing sulfonylureas from protein-binding sites. Sulfasalazine may reduce GI absorption of digoxin and folic acid. Concomitant use of urine-acidifying agents, such as ammonium chloride and ascorbic acid, decreases urine pH and sulfonamide solubility, increasing the risk of crystalluria. Concomitant use with antibiotics that alter intestinal flora may impede conversion of sulfasalazine to sulfapyridine and 5-aminosalicylic acid, decreasing the drug's effectiveness. Concomitant antacid use may cause premature dissolution of enteric-coated tablets, enhancing their systemic absorption and increasing the risk of toxicity.

ADVERSE DRUG REACTIONS

Adverse reactions associated with sulfasalazine involve various body systems. Adverse CNS reactions include headache, depression, seizures, hallucinations, and tinnitus. Adverse GI reactions include nausea, vomiting, diarrhea, abdominal pain, anorexia, and stomatitis. Adverse genitourinary reactions include general toxic nephrosis with oliguria and anuria, crystalluria, hematuria, oligospermia, and infertility. Hematologic reactions include aplastic anemia, megaloblastic anemia, thrombocytopenia, leukopenia, and hemolytic anemia. Other adverse reactions include jaundice, hypersensitivity, serum sickness, drug fever, anaphylaxis, and bacterial and fungal superinfections.

TIOPRONIN

Tiopronin is a urinary cystine reducing agent used prophylactically in selected patients.

PHARMACOKINETICS

Tiopronin is absorbed rapidly after oral administration. Its distribution and metabolism are not known fully. The drug is excreted in the urine; up to 48% of a dose appears in the urine after 4 hours, 78% after 3 days.

PHARMACODYNAMICS

Tiopronin forms a water-soluble chemical complex with cystine in the urine. This decreases cystine concentration and prevents formation of urinary cystine calculi in patients with severe homozygous cystinuria.

PHARMACOTHERAPEUTICS

Tiopronin is used to manage severe homozygous cystinuria.

tiopronin (Thiola). Tiopronin is prescribed to prevent urinary cystine calculi formation in patients with severe homozygous cystinuria (defined as urinary cystine excretion exceeding 500 mg daily) that has not responded to other therapies.

Usual adult dosage: initially 800 mg P.O. daily in three divided doses, then adjusted to control urinary cystine levels.

Usual pediatric dosage: 15 mg/kg P.O. daily in three divided doses.

Drug interactions

No interactions have been reported.

ADVERSE DRUG REACTIONS

Fatal complications from aplastic anemia, granulocytopenia, thrombocytopenia, or myasthenia gravis are possible, although these reactions have not been reported. Granulocytic leukopenia without eosinophilia and immunologic thrombocytopenia may occur. Membranous glomerulopathy may lead to severe proteinuria and nephrotic syndrome. A lupus erythematous-like reaction may occur; this may be associated with a positive antinuclear antibody test. Fever, arthralgia, and lymphadenopathy may be accompanied by nephropathy.

Drug fever may develop, especially during the first month of therapy. Tiopronin should be discontinued until the fever subsides, then reinstituted at lower dosages; subsequently, the dosage is increased gradually, as tolerated.

A generalized rash with mild pruritus may arise during the first few months of therapy. This reaction may be controlled by antihistamines and disappears after drug discontinuation. A less common rash occurring after at least 6 months of therapy appears on the trunk and is accompanied by intense pruritus. It disappears slowly after drug discontinuation.

The effects of tiopronin on collagen may cause skin wrinkling and friability. Chelation of trace metals by the drug can cause hypogeusia (diminished taste sensitivity).

Rare reactions to tiopronin include Goodpasture's syndrome (indicated by abnormal urinary findings, pulmonary infiltrates, and hemoptysis), myasthenic syndrome (indicated by severe muscle weakness), and pemphigus-like reactions (indicated by bullous skin eruptions).

URSODIOL

Ursodiol is a gallstone-solubilizing agent used to manage gallstones in selected patients.

PHARMACOKINETICS

After oral administration, approximately 90% of the dose is absorbed in the small intestine. After absorption, most of the drug enters the portal vein and is extracted by the liver, with only small amounts entering the systemic circulation. In the liver, ursodiol is conjugated and secreted into the hepatic bile ducts. It is excreted primarily in the feces after it is metabolized by the liver.

PHARMACODYNAMICS

A naturally occurring bile acid, ursodiol apparently suppresses cholesterol synthesis and secretion and inhibits intestinal resorption of cholesterol.

PHARMACOTHERAPEUTICS

Ursodiol is used to solubilize radiolucent, noncalcified gallstones in patients predisposed to these stones.

ursodiol (Actigall). Ursodiol is used to dissolve radiolucent, noncalcified gallstones less than 20 mm in diameter in patients for whom elective cholecystectomy carries an increased surgical risk (because of systemic disease, advanced age, or idiosyncratic reaction to general anesthesia) and in patients who refuse surgery. Gallstone dissolution with ursodiol requires months of therapy.

Usual adult dosage: 8 to 10 mg/kg P.O. daily in 2 or 3 divided doses.

Drug interactions

Concomitant administration of bile-sequestering agents (cholestyramine and colestipol) and aluminum-based antacids may decrease ursodiol absorption. Drugs that increase hepatic cholesterol secretion, such as estrogen, oral contraceptives, and clofibrate, may encourage gallstone formation, counteracting the effects of ursodiol.

ADVERSE DRUG REACTIONS

Adverse reactions noted during clinical trials include pruritus, urticaria, dry skin, diaphoresis, thinning hair, nausea, vomiting, dyspepsia, metallic taste, abdominal pain, biliary pain, cholecystitis, diarrhea, constipation, stomatitis, flatulence, headache, fatigue, anxiety, depression, sleep disorders, arthralgia, myalgia, back pain, cough, and rhinitis.

(Text continues on page 1288.)

Nursing considerations for uncategorized and other agents

This table presents nursing implications and selected nursing diagnoses for the uncategorized and other agents discussed in this chapter.

DRUG	NURSING IMPLICATIONS	SELECTED NURSING DIAGNOSES
alpha₁-proteinase inhibitor	• Administer with caution to a patient at risk for circulatory overload. • *Recommend that the patient be immunized against hepatitis B before beginning alpha₁-proteinase inhibitor therapy because this drug is made from donated human plasma and may contain the hepatitis virus.* • Administer the drug I.V. only within 3 hours after reconstitution with sterile water. Do not mix with other agents or diluting solutions.	• Altered tissue perfusion (cerebral) related to light-headedness caused by alpha₁-proteinase inhibitor • Fluid volume excess related to fluid retention caused by alpha₁-proteinase inhibitor • Hyperthermia related to fever caused by alpha₁-proteinase inhibitor • Potential for trauma related to the adverse central nervous system (CNS) effects of alpha₁-proteinase inhibitor
botulinum toxin type A	• Do not administer to a patient with known hypersensitivity to any ingredient in the formulation. • Administer with caution to a lactating patient. Administer to a pregnant patient only when clearly indicated because drug effects on the fetus are unknown. • *Take appropriate emergency measures if the patient develops an anaphylactic reaction to this drug.* • Caution a sedentary patient with blepharospasm to resume activity slowly and carefully after drug administration. • Administer several drops of a local anesthetic and an ocular decongestant, as prescribed, several minutes before injection. • *Reconstitute the drug using 0.9% sodium chloride (normal saline) solution as the diluent; inject the diluent into the vial gently because the drug is denatured by bubbling or similar violent agitation.* • Administer within 4 hours of reconstitution; during those 4 hours, keep the drug refrigerated.	• Altered health maintenance related to drug ineffectiveness caused by denaturing from improper mixing • Body image disturbance related to transient ocular changes caused by botulinum toxin type A • Fluid volume excess related to eyelid swelling caused by botulinum toxin type A • Sensory-perceptual alterations (visual) related to visual disturbances caused by botulinum toxin type A
clomiphene citrate	• Do not administer to a pregnant patient or one with liver disease, abnormal uterine bleeding, or cancer of the breast or reproductive organs. • Caution the patient to avoid activities that require alertness or physical coordination because this drug can cause visual disturbances, dizziness, and light-headedness. • *Teach the patient how and when to take her basal body temperature and how to calculate the length of her menstrual cycle (using the first day of flow as the first day of the new cycle).* • *Inform the patient that maximum fertility usually occurs 10 to 12 days after taking the last clomiphene tablet.* • Encourage the patient to have sexual intercourse every 36 to 40 hours during the maximum fertility period. • *Stress the importance of getting a pregnancy test if menses does not occur after 16 days from the last clomiphene tablet.* • Teach the patient about the proper timing for administering human chorionic gonadotropin if this agent is combined with clomiphene. • *Instruct the patient to stop the drug and call the physician immediately if abdominal pain occurs because this may indicate ovarian enlargement or ovarian cyst.*	• Altered sexuality patterns related to sex requirements during the maximum fertility time • Knowledge deficit related to taking basal body temperature and calculating the length of the menstrual cycle • Pain related to ovarian enlargement or cyst caused by clomiphene • Potential for trauma related to the adverse CNS effects of clomiphene

Nursing considerations for uncategorized and other agents *(continued)*

DRUG	NURSING IMPLICATIONS	SELECTED NURSING DIAGNOSES
colfosceril palmitate	• Expect this drug to be administered directly into the trachea (by trained medical personnel only). • *Obtain an accurate birth weight to calculate the dose.* • Reconstitute colfosceril with the accompanying diluent just before administering. • *Suction the neonate before administering this drug to decrease the incidence of mucus plugs in the endotracheal tube. Do not suction for 2 hours after administration unless medically necessary.* • Monitor pulmonary function closely during administration because colfosceril can affect oxygenation and lung compliance. • *Watch for signs of pulmonary hemorrhage, such as bloody sputum or secretions.* • Monitor the electrocardiogram (ECG) and transcutaneous oxygen saturation results continuously during administration.	• Altered tissue perfusion (cardiopulmonary) related to pulmonary hemorrhage caused by colfosceril • Impaired gas exchange related to the effects of colfosceril on oxygenation • Ineffective airway clearance related to the delay in suctioning required by colfosceril administration • Sleep pattern disturbance related to colfosceril administration
ethanolamine oleate	• Do not administer to a patient with known hypersensitivity to this drug or esophageal varices that have not bled. • Expect to administer smaller doses to a patient with concomitant cardiopulmonary disease to minimize adverse reactions. • Avoid submucosal injection because this is more likely to cause mucosal ulceration. • Explain the administration technique to the patient and stress the need for several follow-up visits to ensure successful sclerotherapy. • *Instruct the patient to report chest pain, shortness of breath, or bleeding immediately.* • *Be prepared to take measures against anaphylaxis in a patient undergoing sclerotherapy with this drug. Have epinephrine 1:1,000 available and control allergic reactions with antihistamines, as prescribed.*	• Altered protection related to ineffectiveness of ethanolamine in preventing rebleeding • Impaired tissue integrity related to adverse tissue changes at injection sites • Noncompliance related to the need for several follow-up visits • Potential for injury related to ethanolamine-induced hypersensitivity reaction
human chorionic gonadotropin (HCG)	• Administer with caution to a patient with asthma, seizure disorder, migraine headache, or cardiac or renal disease because androgen secretion may cause fluid retention. • *Teach the patient about HCG administration and explain how to time sexual intercourse relative to administration (usually 24 to 36 hours after injection).* • Instruct the female patient to continue recording basal body temperature and to test for pregnancy if menses does not occur within 16 days of injection.	• Altered sexuality patterns related to sex requirements required by HCG administration • Anxiety related to the need to self-administer HCG • Fluid volume excess related to HCG-induced fluid retention • Knowledge deficit related to HCG administration
human menopausal gonadotropin (HMG)	• *Do not administer to a pregnant patient, a patient who is receiving an anticoagulant, or one with thyroid or adrenal dysfunction, pituitary tumor, abnormal uterine bleeding, ovarian cyst, testicular enlargement, or a history of thrombophlebitis.* • Explain to the patient that HMG therapy is expensive, warrants close monitoring by an infertility specialist, and commonly requires travel to a facility offering the treatment. Also explain that HCG injections are needed to initiate ovulation. • *Instruct the patient when and how to administer HMG and HCG, as indicated, and teach the patient how to time sexual intercourse relative to HCG administration (usually 24 to 36 hours after injection).*	• Fear related to potential discomfort from parenteral administration of HMG • Ineffective family coping (compromised) related to the time, expense, and travel that HMG therapy may require • Knowledge deficit related to HMG administration • Pain related to HMG-induced ovarian enlargement

(continued)

Nursing considerations for uncategorized and other agents *(continued)*

DRUG	NURSING IMPLICATIONS	SELECTED NURSING DIAGNOSES
levamisole hydrochloride	• Do not administer to a pregnant or lactating patient or one with known hypersensitivity to the drug. • *Monitor the patient for anemia, neutropenia, and thrombocytopenia because combination therapy with fluorouracil is associated with a high incidence of these disorders.* • Ensure that the patient undergoes a complete laboratory workup on the first day of combination therapy. The workup should include a complete blood count (CBC) with differential and platelet count, electrolyte levels, and liver function tests. CBC with differential and platelet counts should be repeated weekly; electrolyte levels and liver function tests should be done every 3 months for 1 year. • Administer with caution to a patient receiving phenytoin; monitor the plasma drug level closely. • *Warn the patient to avoid alcohol to prevent disulfiram-like reactions, such as facial flushing, optic neuritis, psychotic reaction, drowsiness, headache, and rash.* • Instruct the patient to report sore throat, fever, and other signs of infection because this drug may cause leukopenia, which increases the infection risk.	• Activity intolerance related to the adverse effects of levamisole • Anxiety related to potential ineffectiveness of levamisole in combination with fluorouracil as cancer treatment • Knowledge deficit related to the effects of alcohol combined with levamisole • Potential for infection related to levamisole-induced leukopenia
mesalamine	• Do not administer to a patient with known hypersensitivity to mesalamine, its components, or sulfites. • Know that the safety and efficacy of mesalamine in children have not been established. • Administer to a pregnant pregnant only if the benefits outweigh the risks because the effects of this on the fetus are not known. • *Administer with caution to a patient with renal disease or one receiving an oral product that liberates mesalamine (such as sulfasalazine) because renal dysfunction may occur. Monitor urinalysis and blood urea nitrogen and serum creatinine levels in such a patient.* • *Discontinue mesalamine and notify the physician if a rash or fever develops.*	• Constipation related to the adverse gastrointestinal (GI) effects of mesalamine • Fatigue related to the adverse effects of mesalamine • Pain related to the adverse effects of mesalamine • Sleep pattern disturbance related to mesalamine-induced insomnia
mesna	• Do not administer to a lactating patient or one with known hypersensitivity to mesna or other thiol compounds. • Administer to a pregnant patient only if the potential benefits to the patient outweigh the potential risks to the fetus. • Expect to administer concurrently with ifosfamide as prescribed for maximal effectiveness. • *Inform the patient that mesna does not prevent ifosfamide-induced hemorrhagic cystitis in every case and does not reduce other toxicities associated with ifosfamide.*	• Altered protection related to ineffectiveness of mesna • Diarrhea related to the adverse GI effects of mesna • Fatigue related to the adverse CNS effects of mesna • Pain related to mesna-induced limb pain or headache
nafarelin acetate	• Do not administer to a pregnant or lactating patient, one with known hypersensitivity to gonadotropin-releasing hormone (GnRH) or GnRH-agonist analogs, or one with undiagnosed abnormal vaginal bleeding. • Inform a patient receiving long-term therapy that the drug may cause a slight loss in bone density, some of which may be irreversible; warn the patient that this increases the risk for fracture during injury.	• Body image disturbance related to the adverse dermatologic effects of nafarelin • Fluid volume excess related to nafarelin-induced edema • Impaired tissue integrity related to nasal irritation caused by nafarelin administration

Nursing considerations for uncategorized and other agents *(continued)*

DRUG	NURSING IMPLICATIONS	SELECTED NURSING DIAGNOSES
nafarelin acetate *(continued)*	• *Instruct the patient to notify her physician if regular menstruation persists during therapy; the dosage may have to be increased.* • *Instruct the patient to consult her physician if she uses a nasal decongestant; to reduce interference with drug absorption, she will have to delay using the decongestant for at least 30 minutes after taking nafarelin.* • Inform the patient that retreatment is not recommended because no safety data are available beyond 6 months.	• Sexual dysfunction related to the adverse genitourinary effects of nafarelin
nimodipine	• Do not administer to a lactating patient. • Administer to a pregnant patient only if the potential benefits to the patient justifies the potential risks to the fetus. • *Administer with caution to a patient taking other calcium channel blockers.* • *Monitor the patient's blood pressure and pulse closely because calcium channel blockers have known cardiovascular effects.* • Expect to decrease the dosage in a patient with severe liver disease. • Assist the patient who cannot swallow the capsule by extracting the contents with an 18G needle and administering through a nasogastric tube; follow this with 30 ml of normal saline solution.	• Altered protection related to nimodipine-induced liver dysfunction • Altered thought processes related to nimodipine-induced depression • Decreased cardiac output related to ECG abnormalities caused by nimodipine • Fluid volume excess related to edema caused by nimodipine
octreotide acetate	• Do not administer to a patient with known hypersensitivity to octreotide or any of its components. • Administer with caution to a lactating patient. • Monitor the patient for signs of gallbladder disease because octreotide is associated with cholelithiasis. • *Monitor the patient closely for signs and symptoms of hypoglycemia or hyperglycemia because octreotide may alter the balance among insulin, glucagon, and growth hormone.* • Ensure that the patient undergoes baseline and periodic thyroid function tests because the effects of chronic octreotide administration on hypothalamic-pituitary function are unknown. • *Expect the patient with insulin-dependent diabetes mellitus to require changes in the insulin dosage during octreotide therapy.* • Arrange for periodic measurements of fecal fat and serum carotene levels because octreotide may decrease dietary fat absorption. • Know that the half-life of octreotide may increase in a patient with severe renal dysfunction who is undergoing dialysis, and that this may necessitate dosage adjustment. • *Do not administer if the vial contains particulate matter or if the contents are discolored.*	• Altered health maintenance related to glucose abnormalities caused by octreotide • Altered nutrition: less than body requirements, related to the adverse GI effects of octreotide • Diarrhea related to the adverse GI effects of octreotide • Pain related to octreotide administration

(continued)

Nursing considerations for uncategorized and other agents (continued)

DRUG	NURSING IMPLICATIONS	SELECTED NURSING DIAGNOSES
olsalazine sodium	• Do not administer to a patient with known hypersensitivity to salicylates. • Administer with caution to a pregnant or lactating patient. • Monitor urinalysis results and blood urea nitrogen and creatinine levels regularly for renal abnormalities, especially in a patient with preexisting renal disease, because olsalazine may damage the renal tubules. (However, this effect has not been reported in clinical trials.) • *Inform the patient that diarrhea is the most common adverse reaction to olsalazine; instruct the patient to notify the physician if diarrhea occurs.* • *Teach the patient to take this drug in evenly divided doses with food.*	• Altered oral mucous membrane related to olsalazine-induced stomatitis • Diarrhea related to the adverse GI effects of olsalazine • Pain related to olsalazine-induced headache or arthralgia • Potential for injury related to the adverse CNS effects of olsalazine
pegademase bovine	• Administer with caution to a pregnant or lactating patient or one with thrombocytopenia. • Maintain appropriate care to protect an immune-deficient patient until improved immune function is documented. • *Monitor plasma adenosine deaminase activity and red blood cell and adenosine triphosphate levels before treatment begins and regularly during treatment.* • *Do not dilute or mix this drug with any other drug before administering.* • Refrigerate but do not freeze this drug; do not use if any evidence suggests it may have been frozen.	• Altered health maintenance related to drug interaction between vidarabine or 2'-deoxycoformycin and pegademase • Knowledge deficit related to pegademase therapy • Pain related to pegademase-induced headache • Potential for infection related to lag time between correction of metabolic abnormalities by pegademase and improved immune function
pentoxifylline	• Monitor a patient with chronic occlusive peripheral disease frequently for other evidence of arteriosclerotic disease, such as episodes of angina, hypotension, and arrhythmias. • *Monitor systemic blood pressure when starting pentoxifylline therapy, especially in a patient receiving concomitant antihypertensives.* • Monitor the prothrombin time when pentoxifylline therapy begins in a patient receiving warfarin. • *Do not split or crush tablets to administer because this will destroy the controlled-release properties.* • Expect to decrease administration frequency to twice daily if adverse GI or CNS reactions occur. • Inform the patient that therapy must continue for at least 8 weeks and that the drug must not be discontinued during this time without medical approval. • *Advise the patient to take pentoxifylline with meals to minimize GI distress.*	• Altered protection related to bleeding abnormalities caused by pentoxifylline • Noncompliance related to long-term therapy required for drug effectiveness • Potential fluid volume deficit related to the adverse GI effects of pentoxifylline • Potential for injury related to pentoxifylline-induced dizziness
sodium benzoate 10% and sodium phenylacetate 10%	• Do not administer to a patient with known hypersensitivity to either agent. • Administer with caution to a patient with congestive heart failure, renal insufficiency, or other condition that may increase the risk of sodium retention and edema. • Administer with caution to a neonate with hyperbilirubinemia because benzoate may compete with bilirubin for albumin-binding sites. Dilute the solution before administering. • *Avoid concomitant administration with penicillin and probenecid.* • Discontinue therapy and notify the physician if an adverse reaction occurs.	• Potential fluid volume deficit related to the adverse GI effects of sodium benzoate 10% and sodium phenylacetate 10% • Potential for injury related to drug interactions between sodium benzoate 10% and sodium phenylacetate 10% and a salicylate that leads to peptic ulcer disease or respiratory alkalosis • Potential for poisoning related to drug interactions between metabolites of sodium benzoate 10% and sodium phenylacetate 10% and drugs excreted by the kidneys, such as penicillin and probenecid

Nursing considerations for uncategorized and other agents *(continued)*

DRUG	NURSING IMPLICATIONS	SELECTED NURSING DIAGNOSES
sulfasalazine	• Do not administer to a patient with known hypersensitivity to sulfonamides or any other sulfa-containing drug, such as thiazides, furosemide, or oral sulfonylureas. • Do not administer to a pregnant patient at term; a lactating patient; or one with porphyria, known hypersensitivity to salicylates, or severe renal or hepatic dysfunction. • Administer with caution to a patient with mild to moderate renal or hepatic impairment, severe allergies, asthma, blood dyscrasias, or glucose-6-phosphate dehydrogenase deficiency. • *Space doses evenly and administer sulfasalazine after food to minimize adverse reactions and aid drug absorption.* • *Do not administer antacids concomitantly with enteric-coated sulfasalazine because antacids may alter drug absorption.* • Inform the patient that sulfasalazine normally discolors the urine orange-yellow and may discolor the skin orange-yellow. • *Teach the patient to take this drug after meals and to avoid taking antacids concomitantly.*	• Altered oral mucous membrane related to sulfasalazine-induced stomatitis • Altered thought processes related to mental changes caused by sulfasalazine • Altered urinary elimination related to sulfasalazine-induced renal dysfunction • Body image disturbance related to skin color change caused by sulfasalazine
tiopronin	• Do not administer to a patient with a history of granulocytopenia, aplastic anemia, or thrombocytopenia. • Expect to adjust the dosage to keep the urine cystine level below 250 mg/liter. • *Administer at least 1 hour before or 2 hours after a meal.* • Expect routine monitoring tests at 3- to 6-month intervals during therapy; these tests include CBC, platelet, hemoglobin, serum albumin, liver function, 24-hour urinary protein, and routine urinalysis. • Monitor the patient's urinary cystine level frequently during the first 6 months of therapy to assess therapeutic response, then at least every 6 months. • Expect the physician to order an abdominal X-ray annually to assess for renal calculi. • Instruct the patient to report signs and symptoms of hematologic abnormalities, such as fever, sore throat, bleeding, bruising, and chills, because blood dyscrasias have been reported in patients receiving other drugs for cystinuria. • Monitor the patient for these rare complications: Goodpasture's syndrome (indicated by abnormal urinary findings, pulmonary infiltrates, and hemoptysis), myasthenic syndrome (indicated by severe muscle weakness), and pemphigus-like reactions (indicated by bullous skin eruptions).	• Altered protection related to the adverse hematologic effects of tiopronin • Altered urinary elimination related to tiopronin-induced renal dysfunction • Body image disturbance related to the adverse dermatologic effects of tiopronin • Hyperthermia related to drug fever during the first month of tiopronin therapy
ursodiol	• Do not administer to a patient with known hypersensitivity to bile salts or chronic liver disease or to one who requires cholecystectomy for such reasons as unremitting acute cholecystitis, cholangitis, biliary obstruction, gallstones, pancreatitis, or biliary-GI fistula. • Do not administer to a patient with calcified cholesterol, radiopaque, or radiolucent bile pigment stones because the drug does not dissolve these stones. • *Administer with caution to a patient taking bile-sequestering agents (cholestyramine and colestipol), aluminum-based antacids, estrogen, oral contraceptives, or clofibrate.* • *Make sure that a patient receiving this drug undergoes liver function tests when therapy begins, after 1 month and 3 months of therapy, and every 6 months thereafter.*	• Altered oral mucous membrane related to ursodiol-induced stomatitis • Anxiety related to adverse reactions to ursodiol • Pain related to GI disturbances caused by ursodiol • Sleep pattern disturbance related to the adverse CNS effects of ursodiol

CHAPTER SUMMARY

Chapter 73 discussed uncategorized and other agents. Here are the chapter highlights.

• Agents used to treat uncommon or rare conditions include alpha$_1$-proteinase inhibitor, pegademase bovine, sodium benzoate 10% and sodium phenylacetate 10%, and tiopronin.

• Botulinum toxin type A, an ophthalmic agent, is a muscle relaxant used to treat strabismus and blepharospasm.

• New agents used to manage ulcerative colitis include mesalamine, olsalazine, and sulfasalazine.

• The most common adverse reactions to pentoxifylline in patients with intermittent claudication involve the GI tract and CNS.

• The antineoplastic agents levamisole and octreotide cause significant interactions with selected drugs.

• Agents used to treat reproductive disorders discussed in this chapter include clomiphene, HCG, HMG, and nafarelin.

• Colfosceril is a respiratory surfactant agent used to reduce alveolar surface tension associated with neonatal RDS.

• Ethanolamine is a mild sclerosing agent whose successful use requires several follow-up treatments.

• The detoxifying agent mesna is administered concomitantly with ifosfamide to prevent ifosfamide-induced hemorrhagic cystitis.

• Nimodipine, a new calcium channel blocker, is used to reduce neurologic deficits caused by spasms after a subarachnoid hemorrhage from a ruptured congenital intracranial aneurysm. For maximal effectiveness, therapy should begin within 96 hours of hemorrhage.

• Many of the drugs discussed in this chapter are new or have limited clinical use, and their associated reactions and interactions may not be known fully. Therefore, when administering these agents, the nurse should monitor the patient closely for adverse reactions and drug interactions.

STUDY QUESTIONS

See Appendix 1 for answers.

1. Virginia Lawson, age 36, develops palsy of the seventh cranial nerve that persists for more than 1 month. Her physician injects 1.25 units of botulinum toxin type A into her left medial rectus muscle. What is the mechanism of action of botulinum toxin type A?

(a) It binds to acetylcholine receptors on the motor end plate.

(b) It breaks down acetylcholine into an inactive substance.

(c) It stimulates the release of acetylcholine from presynaptic nerve endings.

(d) It enhances neurotransmission of acetylcholine from one muscle cell to another.

2. The nurse should observe Ms. Lawson for which adverse reaction associated with botulinum toxin type A?

(a) local diffuse skin rash

(b) color blindness

(c) local bleeding

(d) muscle pain

3. After trying for 1 year to get pregnant, Joanna Jones, age 27, decides to consult a fertility specialist. After an initial evaluation, the physician requests that her husband Stephen, age 29, undergo a sperm count. Results indicate that Mr. Jones has a low sperm count. To increase the testosterone level and stimulate spermatogenesis, the physician prescribes human chorionic gonadotropin (HCG) 4,000 IU I.M. three times weekly for 3 weeks. When providing Mr. Jones with instructions on HCG, the nurse should mention that HCG is associated with which of these adverse reactions?

(a) nausea, vomiting, diarrhea

(b) sterile abscess at the injection site

(c) weight loss

(d) gynecomastia

4. After 3 weeks of therapy, Mr. Jones's testosterone level does not rise significantly. Which other agent might the physician prescribe for Mr. Jones in conjunction with HCG for 6 to 12 weeks?

(a) HMG

(b) clomiphene

(c) nafarelin

(d) colfosceril

5. Edward Swartz, age 52, receives ifosfamide 1,000 mg/m^2/day I.V. for 5 days every 3 weeks to treat testicular cancer. To prevent ifosfamide-induced hemorrhagic cystitis, the physician prescribes mesna to be given concurrently. How is the mesna dosage determined?

(a) The daily mesna dosage equals 60% of the ifosfamide dosage.

(b) The daily mesna dosage is based on body weight alone.

(c) The daily mesna dosage is based on the number of red blood cells in the urine before each ifosfamide treatment.

(d) The daily mesna dosage should equal the ifosfamide dosage.

6. Carole Smith, age 21, has had ulcerative colitis since age 13. She takes sulfasalazine 2 grams P.O. daily every 6 hours for maintenance. Which agent can be prescribed for patients with ulcerative colitis who cannot tolerate sulfasalazine?
(a) mesalamine
(b) mesna
(c) olsalazine
(d) octreotide

7. When teaching Ms. Smith about sulfasalazine therapy, the nurse should mention that this drug may cause which adverse reaction?
(a) orange-yellow discoloration of the skin and urine
(b) seizures
(c) blurred vision
(d) polyuria

SELECTED REFERENCES

AHFS drug information 90. (1990). Bethesda MD: American Society of Hospital Pharmacists.

Drug facts and comparisons. (1991). St. Louis: Facts and Comparisons Division, Lippincott.

Goodman and Gilman's the pharmacological basis of therapeutics (8th ed.; 1990). Elmsford, NY: Pergamon Press.

Hansten, P., and Horn, J. (1989). *Drug interactions* (6th ed.). Philadelphia: Lea & Febiger.

Mutch, R., and Hutson, P. (1991). Levamisole in the adjuvant treatment of colon cancer. *Clinical Pharmacology,* 10(2), 95-109.

Physician's desk reference (45th ed.; 1991). Oradell, NJ: Medical Economics Company.

Saltiel, E., and Garabedian-Ruffalo, S. (1991). Pharmacologic management of endometriosis. *Clinical Pharmacology,* 10(7), 518-531.

USPDI. (1990). *Drug information for the health care professional* (Vol. I, 11th ed.). Rockville, MD: United States Pharmacopeial Convention.

USPDI. (1990). *Advice for the patient* (Vol. II, 11th ed.). Rockville, MD: United States Pharmacopeial Convention.

APPENDICES AND INDEX

APPENDICES

Answers to study questions

Unit One: General Pharmacology

Chapter 1: Introduction to Pharmacology

1. (a) pharmacokinetics
2. (b) Controlled drugs may lead to drug abuse or dependence.
3. (a) generic name
4. (c) 19th century
5. (a) study of natural drug sources
6. (c) phase III
7. (d) Controlled Substances Act
8. (d) purity

Chapter 2: Pharmacokinetics

1. (d) intravenous
2. (c) active transport
3. (b) absorption rate
4. (d) remain unbound
5. (a) It produces a low volume of distribution and high blood level.
6. (d) to transform the drug for renal and biliary elimination
7. (a) drug half-life

Chapter 3: Pharmacodynamics

1. (a) the interaction between a drug and cellular components
2. (b) modification of cell function
3. (a) by physically modifying the cell environment
4. (d) agonist
5. (b) tolerance
6. (b) Adverse reactions may occur with therapeutic doses.
7. (a) the amount of drug needed to produce the desired response
8. (c) therapeutic index

Chapter 4: Pharmacotherapeutics

1. (b) supportive therapy
2. (d) supplemental therapy
3. (a) hepatitis B immune globulin
4. (a) cumulative effect
5. (a) renal
6. (c) synergistic interaction
7. (b) distribution
8. (c) Drug incompatibility may cause a physical reaction.

Chapter 5: Adverse Drug Reactions

1. (a) rashes
2. (a) genetic variation
3. (d) drug dosage
4. (c) intravenous
5. (a) iatrogenic effect
6. (d) allergic response

Unit Two: The Nursing Process and Drug Administration

Chapter 6: The Nursing Process and Drug Therapy

1. (a) noncompliance related to misunderstanding the importance of prescribed drug regimen
2. (b) The patient states the importance of taking insulin as prescribed.
3. (a) interdependent
4. (c) assessment findings
5. (b) if the outcome criteria have been met
6. (a) dose-related reaction
7. (d) direct observation

Chapter 7: Responsibilities in Drug Administration

1. (c) MOM 30 ml h.s. p.r.n.
2. (c) immediately
3. (b) as needed
4. (b) two
5. (a) Check the identification bracelet and ask the patient his name.
6. (d) standing orders
7. (d) Consult with the physician about an alternative drug.
8. (c) autonomy

Chapter 8: Dosage Measurements and Calculations

1. (c) It may alter the pharmacokinetics—and dosage—of his drugs.
2. (b) metric system
3. (c) 1 ml
4. (c) $\frac{\text{total no. of ml} \times \text{drip factor}}{\text{total no. of minutes}} = \text{drip rate}$
5. (c) 30 ml
6. (a) grains
7. (a) 2 tsp : X ml :: 1 tsp : 5 ml
8. (b) no more than 10%

Chapter 9: Routes and Techniques of Administration

1. (c) in the intestine
2. (b) An elixir contains a sweetener; a tincture does not.
3. (c) Place the tablet under the tongue.
4. (d) at least 30 minutes
5. (a) 1 ml
6. (b) when the drug is extremely irritating to tissue
7. (c) intramuscular
8. (c) 30 minutes

Chapter 10: The Pediatric Patient

1. (a) on an empty stomach
2. (a) her higher percentage of water
3. (a) Use a syringe without a needle to give the medication.
4. (c) liver
5. (d) kidneys
6. (a) fluid overload
7. (b) vastus lateralis
8. (c) Pull the pinna down and back.

Answers to study questions *(continued)*

Chapter 11: The Geriatric Patient

1. (d) decreased pain perception
2. (a) drug toxicity
3. (a) decreased gastric acid secretion
4. (a) decreased total body water
5. (a) decreased albumin
6. (a) Bill Johnson, age 80, is malnourished and has hypertension, diabetes, and coronary artery disease. He takes multiple medications and lives alone.
7. (b) Simplify the medication schedule according to her routine.

Chapter 12: The Pregnant or Lactating Patient

1. (c) Category C
2. (d) increased blood volume
3. (b) They may speed excretion.
4. (a) first
5. (d) Tell her to increase her fluid and fiber intake.
6. (b) about 1% to 2% of the maternal dose
7. (b) Take the drug immediately after a feeding.

Unit Three: Drugs Affecting the Autonomic Nervous System

Chapter 13: Cholinergic Agents

1. (a) 5 to 15 minutes
2. (a) Have atropine readily available.
3. (c) nausea, vomiting, diarrhea, and abdominal cramps
4. (d) It inhibits the action of acetylcholinesterase, which usually inactivates acetylcholine.
5. (b) edrophonium
6. (d) blurred vision
7. (b) Increase the neostigmine dosage.

Chapter 14: Cholinergic Blocking Agents

1. (b) narrow-angle glaucoma
2. (a) GI tract
3. (b) It competes with acetylcholine at the muscarinic receptor sites.
4. (a) It has a greater effect on the CNS than any other drug in this class.
5. (d) physostigmine
6. (c) dry mouth and pupillary dilation
7. (b) Increase the patient's fluid and fiber intake.

Chapter 15: Adrenergic Agents

1. (b) It acts directly on sympathetically innervated organs and tissue.
2. (a) vasoconstriction, cardiac stimulation, and bronchodilation
3. (a) They are inactivated in the GI tract and liver.
4. (d) adverse reaction to catecholamine
5. (c) Catecholamines are not effective when given orally; most noncatecholamines are.
6. (b) It is a direct-acting beta$_2$-selective agent.
7. (a) MAO inhibitors

Chapter 16: Adrenergic Blocking Agents

1. (a) reduction of peripheral vascular resistance
2. (b) reflex tachycardia
3. (a) They act as competitive adrenergic antagonists at beta-receptor sites.
4. (a) Propranolol may cause bronchospasms.
5. (d) Do not discontinue the medication abruptly.
6. (d) broad, somewhat unpredictable effects
7. (d) They compete with acetylcholine at postganglionic synapses in the autonomic nervous system.

Chapter 17: Neuromuscular Blocking Agents

1. (a) It competes with acetylcholine at cholinergic receptor sites in the skeletal muscle.
2. (d) face, arms, and diaphragm
3. (b) Pancuronium does not cross the blood-brain barrier.
4. (c) ineffective breathing pattern
5. (b) to provide short-term muscle relaxation
6. (a) action of succinylcholine in Phase I

Unit Four: Drugs to Treat Neurologic and Neuromuscular System Disorders

Chapter 18: Skeletal Muscle Relaxing Agents

1. (a) It produces an atropine-like central action.
2. (b) drug toxicity
3. (c) It inhibits calcium release from the sarcoplasmic reticulum.
4. (a) muscle weakness
5. (d) exacerbation of spasticity
6. (b) Baclofen produces less sedation than diazepam.
7. (d) tolerance

Chapter 19: Antiparkinsonian Agents

1. (b) narrow-angle glaucoma
2. (a) It inhibits cerebral motor centers.
3. (c) Substitute the new agent and gradually discontinue benztropine.
4. (b) diphenhydramine
5. (a) in the brain
6. (a) carbidopa
7. (b) hypertensive crisis

Chapter 20: Anticonvulsant Agents

1. (b) slow
2. (a) by altering ion movement
3. (b) Addiction is unlikely because the dosage is at subhypnotic levels.
4. (b) tricyclic antidepressants
5. (c) Be alert for signs of hematologic problems, such as fever and bleeding.
6. (c) status epilepticus
7. (d) absence seizure
8. (b) hepatotoxicity

Unit Five: Drugs to Prevent and Treat Pain

Chapter 21: Nonnarcotic Analgesic, Antipyretic, and Nonsteroidal Anti-Inflammatory Agents

1. (c) nausea, vomiting, and GI distress
2. (a) bleeding
3. (a) Salicylates may cause Reye's syndrome.
4. (d) osteoarthritis
5. (b) hepatotoxicity
6. (a) Most NSAIDs are highly protein bound.
7. (d) GI disturbances
8. (b) Take the drug with milk or food.

Answers to study questions *(continued)*

Chapter 22: Narcotic Agonist and Antagonist Agents

1. (d) It alters the perception of, and response to, pain.
2. (d) codeine
3. (a) severe respiratory depression
4. (b) Narcotic agonists mask changes in the level of consciousness.
5. (d) A mixed narcotic agonist-antagonist is less likely to cause respiratory depression.
6. (d) withdrawal symptoms
7. (a) naloxone
8. (c) Narcotic antagonist effects seldom last as long as the overdose effects.

Chapter 23: General Anesthetic Agents

1. (b) stage 2
2. (d) the drug's solubility in blood
3. (b) the drug concentration that crosses the blood-brain barrier
4. (b) Inhalation anesthetics produce more precise and rapid control of anesthesia depth.
5. (d) exaggerated response to a normal dose
6. (a) injection anesthesia
7. (a) high blood pressure
8. (c) It allows easy arousal of the patient.

Chapter 24: Local and Topical Anesthetic Agents

1. (a) into the subarachnoid space
2. (b) Amide anesthetics are metabolized in the liver; esther anesthetics are metabolized in the plasma and liver.
3. (b) patient's position
4. (a) It inhibits nerve cell depolarization.
5. (d) Topical anesthetics are applied to the skin or mucous membranes, local anesthetics are injected.
6. (c) It blocks nerve impulse transmission by preventing nerve cell depolarization.
7. (d) decreased gag reflex

Unit Six: Drugs to Alter Psychogenic Behavior and Promote Sleep

Chapter 25: Sedative and Hypnotic Agents

1. (a) Sedatives reduce activity and excitement; hypnotics induce sleep.
2. (c) I.M. injections are absorbed erratically.
3. (a) high potential for drug dependence
4. (d) adverse reaction to barbiturates
5. (c) They lose their effectiveness by the end of the second week.
6. (d) GI symptoms and hangover effects
7. (c) with juice to disguise the taste and odor

Chapter 26: Antidepressant and Antimanic Agents

1. (b) an MAO inhibitor
2. (a) aged cheese
3. (d) hypertensive crisis
4. (a) It increases neurotransmitter concentration levels.
5. (b) Arise gradually from a supine position.
6. (c) They cause fewer adverse reactions.
7. (c) Monitor the lithium concentration regularly.

Chapter 27: Antianxiety Agents

1. (b) Elderly patients have a higher percentage of fatty tissue, which prolongs the drug's half-life.
2. (a) 1 to 2 mg P.O. b.i.d.
3. (c) enhancement of GABA activity
4. (d) sedation
5. (c) Buspirone does not affect GABA receptors.
6. (c) Buspirone does not interact with alcohol or other CNS depressants.
7. (b) in fatty tissue
8. (d) pulmonary disease

Chapter 28: Antipsychotic Agents

1. (d) several weeks after administration
2. (c) Phenothiazines produce a calming effect from which the patient is easily aroused.
3. (b) anticholinergic
4. (b) Take the drug exactly as prescribed, even if symptoms disappear.
5. (a) Administer the medication; a slightly yellow color is acceptable.
6. (b) neurologic effects of haloperidol
7. (c) clozapine

Unit Seven: Drugs to Improve Cardiovascular Function

Chapter 29: Cardiac Glycoside Agents and Bipyridines

1. (d) renal failure
2. (b) Digitoxin has a longer half-life than digoxin.
3. (c) 0.5 to 2.0 ng/ml
4. (b) A loading dose provides an immediate drug effect.
5. (c) digoxin-immune Fab
6. (a) pulse rate measurement
7. (d) if she does not respond adequately to digoxin therapy

Chapter 30: Antiarrhythmic Agents

1. (a) It alters the myocardial cell membrane, interfering with control of pacemaker cells.
2. (b) quinidine-related adverse reactions, such as tinnitus and visual disturbances
3. (a) phenytoin
4. (d) lidocaine
5. (c) bretylium
6. (d) They cause serious adverse reactions.
7. (a) It blocks beta-adrenergic receptors.
8. (b) It blocks calcium influx into myocardial cells.

Chapter 31: Antianginal Agents

1. (a) 1 to 3 minutes
2. (c) It acts directly on vascular smooth muscle, producing relaxation and vessel dilation.
3. (b) headache
4. (a) decreased heart rate
5. (c) systolic blood pressure less than 70 mm Hg
6. (d) It decreases contractility.
7. (d) Prinzmetal's angina
8. (b) congestive heart failure

Chapter 32: Antihypertensive Agents

1. (a) weight control, sodium restriction, and aerobic exercise
2. (c) It competes with epinephrine for receptor sites, thereby blocking sympathetic stimulation.

(continued)

Answers to study questions *(continued)*

Chapter 32: Antihypertensive Agents *(continued)*

3. (b) It may mask the signs of hypoglycemia.
4. (a) It directly relaxes arterial and venous smooth muscle.
5. (a) hypotension and bradycardia
6. (c) ACE-inhibiting agents
7. (d) thiazide diuretic
8. (d) Take the medication 1 hour before meals.

Chapter 33: Diuretic Agents

1. (a) by inhibiting sodium resorption in the distal renal tubule
2. (c) hypokalemia
3. (d) loop diuretic
4. (b) hyperglycemia
5. (b) It acts as an aldosterone antagonist.
6. (a) hyperkalemia
7. (a) Warm and shake the bottle to dissolve the crystals.
8. (d) rebound effect

Chapter 34: Antilipemic Agents

1. (b) GI tract
2. (c) Mix the powder in a liquid or semi-liquid food.
3. (b) Take the thiazide diuretic 1 hour before or 6 hours after taking cholestyramine.
4. (b) fibric acid derivative
5. (d) oral anticoagulant
6. (b) They cause fewer significant drug interactions.
7. (a) liver function test results
8. (c) It causes serious adverse reactions.

Unit Eight: Drugs Affecting the Hematologic System

Chapter 35: Hematinic Agents

1. (b) 1 week
2. (c) to prevent skin discoloration
3. (d) Increase fluid and fiber intake.
4. (a) Lack of intrinsic factor prevents absorption of oral cyanocobalamin.
5. (d) neurologic damage
6. (b) 100 to 400 mcg/day
7. (b) leucovorin calcium

Chapter 36: Anticoagulant Agents

1. (c) by accelerating the interaction between antithrombin III and thrombin
2. (d) activated partial thromboplastin time (APTT)
3. (c) protamine sulfate
4. (a) Warfarin's therapeutic effects do not occur until clotting factors are depleted.
5. (a) It acts as a vitamin K antagonist.
6. (d) PT
7. (a) It prevents platelet aggregation.
8. (b) GI distress

Chapter 37: Thrombolytic Agents

1. (c) cerebrovascular accident in the past 2 months
2. (a) to dissolve already formed clots
3. (b) They cause a systemic thrombolytic state.
4. (d) allergic reaction
5. (b) aminocaproic acid
6. (c) I.M.
7. (d) acetaminophen

Unit Nine: Drugs to Improve Respiratory Function

Chapter 38: Methylxanthine Agents

1. (b) weight
2. (d) 10 to 20 mcg/ml
3. (a) It increases the central respiratory center's sensitivity to carbon dioxide and stimulates the patient's respiratory drive.
4. (a) when the oral administration begins
5. (b) They may increase theophylline elimination.
6. (a) nausea, vomiting, and diarrhea

Chapter 39: Expectorant, Antitussive, and Mucolytic Agents

1. (d) promotion of mucus removal
2. (a) potential for toxic effects
3. (d) thyroid gland
4. (c) persistent cough that is exhausting
5. (b) Centrally acting antitussives depress the cough center in the medulla; peripherally acting antitussives do not.
6. (a) It alters the molecular composition of mucus, which decreases its viscosity.
7. (c) It may produce bronchospasm.
8. (a) acetaminophen overdose

Chapter 40: Decongestant Agents

1. (a) It stimulates alpha-adrenergic receptors, resulting in vasoconstriction and nasal decongestion.
2. (d) rebound hyperemia of nasal mucosa
3. (c) It produces fewer adverse reactions.
4. (b) fewer adverse reactions
5. (a) rebound nasal congestion
6. (d) Discontinue the decongestant and consult the physician.
7. (b) Lie supine with the head supported by a pillow during and for 5 minutes after instillation.

Unit Ten: Drugs to Improve Gastrointestinal Function

Chapter 41: Adsorbent, Antiflatulent, and Digestive Agents

1. (d) by attracting and binding with toxins, preventing their absorption in the GI tract
2. (c) 5 to 10 times the weight of the drug ingested
3. (d) a laxative
4. (a) It disperses and prevents gas pocket formation.
5. (c) Take one tablet after each meal and one at bedtime.
6. (d) Increase activity and exercise.
7. (a) after meals
8. (b) diarrhea

Chapter 42: Antidiarrheal and Laxative Agents

1. (b) history of asthma
2. (c) the intestines
3. (d) Take it up to eight times a day, as needed.
4. (a) docusate sodium
5. (d) electrolyte imbalance
6. (c) Drink plenty of fluids every day.
7. (b) bisacodyl
8. (a) abdominal cramping

Chapter 43: Emetic and Antiemetic Agents

1. (c) when a caustic substance has been ingested
2. (b) ipecac syrup
3. (d) dimenhydrinate

Answers to study questions *(continued)*

Chapter 43: Emetic and Antiemetic Agents *(continued)*

4. (b) 30 to 60 minutes before traveling
5. (d) transdermal
6. (d) dopaminergic receptor blockade in the CTZ
7. (a) sedation
8. (c) metoclopramide hydrochloride

Chapter 44: Peptic Ulcer Agents

1. (a) They increase gastric pH and neutralize stomach contents.
2. (a) to relieve epigastric pain and discomfort
3. (d) 1 to 2 hours before or after the antacid
4. (d) by blocking the stimulant action of histamine on acid-secreting cells in the stomach
5. (a) cimetidine
6. (b) It binds to the ulcer, forming a protective barrier.
7. (a) They stimulate mucus and bicarbonate secretion and suppress acid secretion.
8. (c) It affects the uterus in childbearing women.

Unit Eleven: Drugs for Fluid, Electrolyte, and Nutritional Balance

Chapter 45: Vitamin, Mineral, and Other Nutritional Agents

1. (d) to improve vision in dim light
2. (d) calcium and phosphorus balance
3. (a) phytonadione
4. (a) thiamine
5. (c) Long-term use of chewable vitamin C may cause dental erosion.
6. (b) Toxicity may occur because minerals have a narrow margin of safety.
7. (c) Take the mineral preparation with meals to minimize GI distress.
8. (a) vomiting and diarrhea

Chapter 46: Electrolyte Replacement Agents

1. (c) The body cannot store potassium.
2. (b) 10 mEq/hour by I.V. infusion
3. (a) paresthesia, weakness, and confusion
4. (d) prolonged PR interval and tall, tented T waves
5. (c) to strengthen myocardial tissue
6. (b) digitoxin
7. (b) magnesium

Chapter 47: Alkalinizing and Acidifying Agents

1. (a) by decreasing the hydrogen ion concentration
2. (b) metabolic alkalosis
3. (b) It avoids the high sodium load that can occur with other alkalinizing agents.
4. (c) Severe adverse reactions occur with longer use.
5. (d) to alkalinize urine, promoting phenobarbital excretion
6. (a) It is safer and easier to prepare.
7. (c) hypokalemia

Chapter 48: Cation-Exchange Resin and Ammonia-Detoxicating Agents

1. (d) GI tract
2. (b) rectal
3. (a) It exchanges sodium for hydrogen, which is exchanged for potassium.
4. (a) sorbitol
5. (b) It acidifies the colon, which prevents ammonia absorption.

6. (a) Neomycin may cause toxicity when absorbed systemically.
7. (c) diabetes mellitus
8. (a) increased level of consciousness

Unit Twelve: Drugs to Treat Endocrine System Disorders

Chapter 49: Hypoglycemic Agents and Glucagon

1. (c) It promotes glucose storage as glycogen and inhibits glycogen breakdown.
2. (a) Regular insulin is rapid-acting; NPH insulin is intermediate-acting.
3. (d) human insulin
4. (b) nervousness, diaphoresis, and confusion
5. (b) It stimulates pancreatic beta-cell production of insulin.
6. (d) 30 minutes before breakfast
7. (a) It promotes glycogenolysis and gluconeogenesis.
8. (c) It would be destroyed by the GI tract.

Chapter 50: Thyroid and Antithyroid Agents

1. (a) oral
2. (b) liothyronine
3. (d) by acting as the essential hormones that are lacking
4. (a) myxedema coma
5. (a) It inhibits thyroid hormone synthesis.
6. (b) Notify the physician immediately.
7. (c) Take full radiation precautions for 24 hours.
8. (b) thyroid crisis

Chapter 51: Parathyroid Agents

1. (a) It reduces bone resorption and increases renal calcium clearance.
2. (d) sodium
3. (c) development of resistance to calcitonin
4. (b) It increases GI absorption and bone resorption of calcium.
5. (b) weakness, fatigue, nausea, and vomiting
6. (a) Take seizure precautions.
7. (b) 70

Chapter 52: Pituitary Agents

1. (d) oral route
2. (a) 5 minutes
3. (d) iatrogenic Cushing's syndrome
4. (b) ADH
5. (d) water intoxication
6. (a) oxytocin
7. (c) Stop the medication immediately and notify the physician.

Chapter 53: Androgenic and Anabolic Steroid Agents

1. (a) Androgenic steroids produce masculinizing effects; anabolic steroids stimulate tissue building.
2. (c) testosterone
3. (b) voice deepening
4. (b) liver failure
5. (a) It may increase serum cholesterol and decrease high-density lipoprotein (HDL) levels.
6. (d) weight gain and edema
7. (d) Anabolic steroids should not be used to enhance performance because the risks outweigh the benefits.

Answers to study questions *(continued)*

Chapter 54: Estrogens, Progestins, and Oral Contraceptive Agents

1. (b) thromboembolic disorder
2. (a) endometrial
3. (c) leg cramps
4. (c) It prevents menstruation for several months, allowing ectopic endometrial growths to regress.
5. (a) Conception should be avoided because progestin may cause congenital defects.
6. (d) two consecutive missed menstrual cycles
7. (c) Take the missed dose as soon as she remembers or take two pills the next day.
8. (d) after at least three menstrual cycles

Chapter 55: Uterine Motility Agents

1. (c) carboprost
2. (a) fever
3. (d) methylergonovine
4. (a) It acts as a beta-receptor agonist.
5. (a) seizures in preeclampsia or eclampsia
6. (b) 4 to 6 mEq/liter
7. (c) absent deep tendon reflexes and hypotension

Unit Thirteen: Drugs to Control Inflammation, Allergy, and Organ Rejection

Chapter 56: Antihistaminic Agents

1. (c) IgE antibodies sensitize mast cells and basophils.
2. (b) It acts as a competitive H₁-receptor antagonist to prevent further response to histamine.
3. (c) CNS depression
4. (c) diphenhydramine hydrochloride
5. (b) profound CNS depression
6. (d) drug fever

Chapter 57: Corticosteroid and Other Immunosuppressant Agents

1. (b) acute adrenocortical insufficiency
2. (b) in the morning to mimic normal hormone secretion
3. (a) Apply the smallest amount possible in a thin coat over the affected area.
4. (d) eye area
5. (b) It increases sodium resorption and potassium and hydrogen secretion.
6. (d) edema and weight gain
7. (d) bone marrow depression
8. (a) hyperkalemia

Chapter 58: Uricosurics, Other Antigout Agents, and Gold Salts

1. (b) It inhibits uric acid resorption at the proximal convoluted tubules.
2. (d) GI distress
3. (c) Take acetaminophen to prevent bleeding problems linked with concomitant salicylate use.
4. (b) colchicine
5. (d) GI
6. (d) 8 to 12 weeks after administration
7. (c) It decreases liposomal enzyme release.
8. (d) during the second month of treatment

Unit Fourteen: Drugs to Prevent or Treat Infection

Chapter 59: Antibacterial Agents

1. (a) penicillin
2. (a) allergic reaction
3. (c) intermittent infusion over 30 minutes
4. (b) superinfection
5. (b) It may darken permanent teeth and disrupt bone growth.
6. (d) Take the drug with 8 oz of water to prevent esophageal irritation.
7. (b) drug-induced aplastic anemia
8. (c) gray syndrome
9. (d) erythromycin

Chapter 60: Antitubercular and Antileprotic Agents

1. (d) Combination therapy can prevent or delay bacterial resistance.
2. (a) Aluminum hydroxide decreases INH absorption.
3. (c) Pyradoxine helps prevent the neurotoxic effects of INH.
4. (b) red-orange urine
5. (a) optic neuritis
6. (c) duration of treatment
7. (c) clofazamine
8. (c) hemolytic anemia

Chapter 61: Antiviral Agents

1. (b) It converts to an active metabolite that disrupts viral replication.
2. (c) renal disease
3. (b) slowly (over 60 minutes)
4. (b) poor solubility
5. (a) Monitor the patient's fluid balance closely.
6. (a) amantadine
7. (d) inhalation
8. (c) Take the drug every 4 hours around the clock.

Chapter 62: Antimycotic (Antifungal) Agents

1. (b) highly toxic effects
2. (d) normochromic or normocytic anemia
3. (a) hypokalemia
4. (b) flucytosine
5. (c) Dissolve the tablet in the mouth.
6. (b) Continue the medication for the full length of time as prescribed.
7. (a) 1 to 4 weeks
8. (a) fluconazole

Chapter 63: Anthelmintic Agents

1. (a) It interferes with the microtubule system of the roundworm, preventing glucose uptake.
2. (b) Change and launder underclothes and bedding daily.
3. (a) praziquantel
4. (c) Chew the tablet thoroughly and take it with water after a light meal.
5. (d) CNS stimulation
6. (c) orange-red urine
7. (d) Swallow the tablet rapidly because its bitter taste may cause gagging or vomiting.
8. (d) It causes spastic paralysis of the fluke musculature.

Answers to study questions *(continued)*

Chapter 64: Antimalarial and Other Antiprotozoal Agents

1. (a) It disrupts the parasite's protein synthesis.
2. (b) *P. falciparum*
3. (c) weekly for 1 week before departure and for 6 weeks after she returns
4. (b) Take the medication with meals.
5. (b) metronidazole
6. (b) aminoglycosides
7. (c) hypotension and arrhythmias
8. (b) bronchospasm and cough

Chapter 65: Urinary Antiseptic Agents

1. (b) CNS disorder
2. (c) seizures
3. (a) 2 hours after the ciprofloxacin dose
4. (b) They inhibit folic acid production.
5. (c) Drink at least eight 8-oz glasses of fluid daily.
6. (a) 50 to 100 mg P.O. daily at bedtime
7. (d) Clinitest

Unit Fifteen: Drugs to Treat Malignant Neoplasms

Chapter 66: Alkylating Agents

1. (d) intravenous administration; urinary excretion
2. (a) It disrupts the structure of DNA.
3. (d) bone marrow suppression
4. (b) pulmonary fibrosis
5. (c) 15% to 30%
6. (c) 4 to 6 weeks after treatment
7. (a) Dacarbazine produces a greater effect on RNA synthesis than DNA synthesis.
8. (a) urinary

Chapter 67: Antimetabolite Agents

1. (d) S phase
2. (b) It inhibits DNA and RNA synthesis.
3. (a) leucovorin
4. (c) Rinse regularly with saline and sodium bicarbonate solution.
5. (d) bone marrow suppression
6. (a) cholestatic jaundice
7. (c) Encourage him to drink 13 8-oz glasses of fluid daily.

Chapter 68: Antibiotic Antineoplastic Agents

1. (a) Bleomycin increases the regimen's therapeutic effectiveness, without increasing bone marrow toxicity.
2. (d) to prevent fever and chills
3. (c) pulmonary fibrosis
4. (d) It intercalates between DNA molecules.
5. (b) cardiac damage
6. (a) Withhold the drug and notify the physician.
7. (a) Stop the infusion.
8. (d) plicamycin

Chapter 69: Hormonal Antineoplastic Agents

1. (d) 2 to 3 months
2. (b) It suppresses LH secretion, which decreases testicular androgen secretion.
3. (b) It binds to estrogen receptors and inhibits estrogen-mediated tumor growth.
4. (a) tumor flare
5. (d) increased facial hair
6. (c) a pituitary-suppressive glucocorticoid
7. (c) progestin
8. (c) corticosteroid
9. (a) tumor flare
10. (a) flutamide

Chapter 70: Other Antineoplastic Agents

1. (c) M phase
2. (b) alopecia
3. (c) 4 weeks after treatment
4. (a) Avoid tyramine-rich foods, such as coffee, chocolate, and aged cheese.
5. (a) hypotension
6. (a) pancreatitis
7. (d) allopurinol
8. (b) flulike syndrome

Unit Sixteen: Other Major Drugs

Chapter 71: Ophthalmic Agents

1. (a) It paralyzes the sphincter muscle of the iris and contracts the dilator muscle.
2. (b) Pilocarpine may increase the inflammation.
3. (d) in the lower conjunctival sac
4. (a) Apply digital pressure over the punctum at the inner canthus for 2 to 3 minutes.
5. (b) They decrease aqueous fluid production.
6. (d) It may cause corneal abrasion because the pain signal is absent.
7. (a) boric acid, an anti-infective agent
8. (b) to decrease inflammation

Chapter 72: Otic Agents

1. (b) vertigo or nausea
2. (a) Pull the ear up and back.
3. (a) They are more likely to exacerbate an otic infection than anti-infective otic agents.
4. (d) perforated tympanic membrane
5. (b) Let the solution remain in the ear canal for at least 15 minutes.
6. (a) Lay the child on the unaffected side, gently pull the ear down and back, and instill the drops.
7. (a) within minutes
8. (c) Contact the physician if ear pain persists despite benzocaine use.

Chapter 73: Uncategorized and Other Agents

1. (a) It binds to acetylcholine receptors on the motor end plate.
2. (a) local diffuse skin rash
3. (d) gynecomastia
4. (a) HMG
5. (a) The daily mesna dosage equals 60% of the ifosfamide dosage.
6. (c) olsalazine
7. (a) orange-yellow discoloration of the skin and urine

Commonly used abbreviations in drug therapy

In health care facilities that approve them, these abbreviations may be used in transcribing medication orders and documenting drug administration.

$\overline{aa}$	of each		g, gm, or GM	gram (quantity usually expressed in Arabic numerals)
a.c.	before meals		gr	grain (quantity usually expressed in Roman numerals)
A.D.	right ear			
ad lib	as desired		gtt	drop
A.M. or a.m.	morning		h or hr	hour
A.S.	left ear		h.s.	at bedtime
A.U.	each ear		I.M.	intramuscular
b.i.d.	twice a day		in or "	inch
$\overline{c}$	with		I.V.	intravenous
caps	capsules		IVPB	intravenous "piggyback"
cc	cubic centimeter		kg	kilogram
cm	centimeter		Ⓛ	left
comp	compound		L	liter
/d	per day		LA	long acting
D/C or dc	discontinue		lb or #	pound
disp	dispensary		M_x or ℳ	minim
DS	double strength		mcg	microgram
D_5W	dextrose 5% in water		mEq	milliequivalent
EC	enteric coated		mg	milligram
elix	elixir		ml	milliliter
ext	extract		mm	millimeter
fl or fld	fluid		N.P.O.	nothing by mouth

Commonly used abbreviations in drug therapy *(continued)*

NR	no refills		Rx	treatment, prescription
NS or N/S	normal saline (0.9%)		s̄	without
¼NS	¼ normal saline (0.225%)		s̄s̄	one-half
½NS	½ normal saline (0.45%)		sat	saturated
O.D.	right eye		S.C. or SQ	subcutaneous
os	mouth		sec	second
O.S.	left eye		Sig.	write on label
OTC	over the counter		SL or sl	sublingual
O.U.	each eye		sp.	spirits
p̄	after		SR	sustained release
p.c.	after meals		stat	immediately
per	by or through		supp	suppository
P.O. or p.o.	by mouth		syr.	syrup
p.r.n.	as needed		T, Tbs., or tbsp.	tablespoon
pt	pint		t or tsp.	teaspoon
q	every		tab	tablet
q a.m. or Q.M.	every morning		t.i.d.	three times a day
q.d.	every day		tinct or tr	tincture
q.h.	every hour		U	unit
q.i.d.	four times a day		ung.	ointment
q3h, q4h, etc.	every 3 hours, every 4 hours, etc.		vag	vaginal
q.o.d.	every other day		VO	verbal order
qt	quart		×	times, multiply
®R	right		ℨ	dram
R or PR	by rectum		℥ or oz	ounce

Commonly misinterpreted abbreviations in drug therapy

Physicians and nurses should use only approved abbreviations, writing each clearly and avoiding those that a patient or pharmacist might misinterpret, even if they are approved. Here are some commonly misinterpreted abbreviations.

ABBREVIATION	INTENDED MEANING	MISINTERPRETATION
A.U.	*auris uterque* (each ear)	Has been mistaken for "O.U." (*oculus uterque* — each eye).
Chemical symbol Na	sodium	Not understood or misread.
D/C	discharge discontinue	Patients' medications have been prematurely discontinued when D/C, intended to mean "discharge," was misinterpreted as "discontinue" when followed by list of drugs.
♏	minim	Not understood or misread.
Drug names MTX CPZ HCl DIG MVI HCTZ ARA-A	methotrexate Compazine (prochlorperazine) hydrochloric acid digoxin multivitamins *without* fat-soluble vitamins hydrochlorothiazide vidarabine	Mustargen (mechlorethamine HCl) chlorpromazine potassium chloride (The "H" is misinterpreted as "K.") digitoxin multivitamins *with* fat-soluble vitamins hydrocortisone (HCT) cytarabine (ARA-C)
μg	microgram	When handwritten, this easily can be mistaken for "mg."
o.d.	once daily	Frequently misinterpreted as "right eye" (O.D. — *oculus dexter*), so that oral medication is administered in a patient's right eye.
OJ	orange juice	Has been mistaken for "O.D." (*oculus dexter* — right eye) or "O.S." (*oculus sinister* — left eye). Medications that were meant to be diluted in orange juice and given orally have been given in a patient's right or left eye.
i/d	once daily	Mistaken as "t.i.d."
per os	orally	The "os" can be mistaken for left eye.
q.d.	every day	The period after the "q" sometimes has been mistaken for an "i," and the drug has been given q.i.d. rather than daily.
qn	nightly or at bedtime	Misinterpreted as "every hour" when poorly written.
q.o.d.	every other day	Misinterpreted as "q.d." or "q.i.d." if the "o" is poorly written.
sub q	subcutaneous	The "q" has been mistaken for "every." In the example, a prophylactic heparin dose meant to be given 2 hours before surgery was given every 2 hours before surgery.
U or u	unit	Seen as a "zero" or a "four," causing a tenfold or greater overdose.

EXAMPLE	CORRECTION
Colymycin gtts iii ou tid	Write clearly.
Na coumadin 5 mg today	Write it out.
D/c meds *Digoxin 0.25mg* *Lasix 40 mg*	Write out "discharge" and "discontinue."
Elixophyllin 3T tid *Tr opium 10 mx*	Use the metric system or write out "minim."
	Use the complete spelling for drug names.
Vit B₁₂ 1 mg IM Now	Use "mcg."
KCl 15 mEq OD	Don't abbreviate "daily." Write it out.
Lugol's sol'n gtts x̄ in OJ	Write out "orange juice."
Diabinese 250 mg/d	Write it out.
Lugol's sol'a gtts x̄ per os	Use "P.O.," "by mouth," or "orally."
Digoxin 0.25mg qd.	Write it out.
Librium 10 mg qh	Use "h.s." or "nightly."
digoxin 0.25 mg q.i.d.	Use "q other day" or "every other day."
Heparin 5000 units Sub q 2hrs before surgery	Use "S.C.," "SQ," or write out "subcutaneous."
NPH 6u Now SC *NPH 4u now SC*	Write it out.

NANDA Taxonomy of Nursing Diagnoses

A taxonomy for classifying nursing diagnoses has evolved over several years. The following list is grouped around nine human response patterns endorsed by the North American Nursing Diagnosis Association, as of summer 1990.

PATTERN 1. Exchanging: A human response pattern involving mutual giving and receiving

1.1.2.1. Altered nutrition: more than body requirements

1.1.2.2. Altered nutrition: less than body requirements

1.1.2.3. Altered nutrition: potential for more than body requirements

1.2.1.1. Potential for infection

1.2.2.1. Potential altered body temperature

1.2.2.2. Hypothermia

1.2.2.3. Hyperthermia

1.2.2.4. Ineffective thermoregulation

1.2.3.1. Dysreflexia

1.3.1.1. Constipation

1.3.1.1.1. Perceived constipation

1.3.1.1.2. Colonic constipation

1.3.1.2. Diarrhea

1.3.1.3. Bowel incontinence

1.3.2. Altered urinary elimination

1.3.2.1.1. Stress incontinence

1.3.2.1.2. Reflex incontinence

1.3.2.1.3. Urge incontinence

1.3.2.1.4. Functional incontinence

1.3.2.1.5. Total incontinence

1.3.2.2. Urinary retention

1.4.1.1. Altered (specify type) tissue perfusion (renal, cerebral, cardiopulmonary, gastrointestinal, peripheral)

1.4.1.2.1. Fluid volume excess

1.4.1.2.2.1. Fluid volume deficit

1.4.1.2.2.2. Potential fluid volume deficit

1.4.2.1. Decreased cardiac output

1.5.1.1. Impaired gas exchange

1.5.1.2. Ineffective airway clearance

1.5.1.3. Ineffective breathing pattern

1.6.1. Potential for injury

1.6.1.1. Potential for suffocation

1.6.1.2. Potential for poisoning

1.6.1.3. Potential for trauma

1.6.1.4. Potential for aspiration

1.6.1.5. Potential for disuse syndrome

1.6.2. Altered protection

1.6.2.1. Impaired tissue integrity

1.6.2.1.1. Altered oral mucous membrane

1.6.2.1.2.1. Impaired skin integrity

1.6.2.1.2.2. Potential impaired skin integrity

PATTERN 2. Communicating: A human response pattern involving sending messages

2.1.1.1. Impaired verbal communication

PATTERN 3. Relating: A human response pattern involving establishing bonds

3.1.1. Impaired social interaction

3.1.2. Social isolation

3.2.1. Altered role performance

3.2.1.1.1. Altered parenting

3.2.1.1.2. Potential altered parenting

3.2.1.2.1. Sexual dysfunction

3.2.2. Altered family processes

3.2.3.1. Parental role conflict

3.3. Altered sexuality patterns

PATTERN 4. Valuing: A human response pattern involving the assigning of relative worth

4.1.1. Spiritual distress (distress of the human spirit)

PATTERN 5. Choosing: A human response pattern involving the selection of alternatives

5.1.1.1. Ineffective individual coping

5.1.1.1.1. Impaired adjustment

5.1.1.1.2. Defensive coping

5.1.1.1.3. Ineffective denial

5.1.2.1.1. Ineffective family coping: disabling

5.1.2.1.2. Ineffective family coping: compromised

5.1.2.2. Family coping: potential for growth

5.2.1.1. Noncompliance (specify)

5.3.1.1. Decisional conflict (specify)

5.4. Health-seeking behaviors (specify)

NANDA Taxonomy of Nursing Diagnoses *(continued)*

PATTERN 6. Moving: A human response pattern involving activity
6.1.1.1. Impaired physical mobility
6.1.1.2. Activity intolerance
6.1.1.2.1. Fatigue
6.1.1.3. Potential activity intolerance
6.2.1. Sleep pattern disturbance
6.3.1.1. Diversional activity deficit
6.4.1.1. Impaired home maintenance management
6.4.2. Altered health maintenance
6.5.1. Feeding self-care deficit
6.5.1.1. Impaired swallowing
6.5.1.2. Ineffective breast-feeding
6.5.1.3. Effective breast-feeding
6.5.2. Bathing or hygiene self-care deficit
6.5.3. Dressing or grooming self-care deficit
6.5.4. Toileting self-care deficit
6.6. Altered growth and development

PATTERN 7. Perceiving: A human response pattern involving the reception of information
7.1.1. Body image disturbance
7.1.2. Self-esteem disturbance
7.1.2.1. Chronic low self-esteem
7.1.2.2. Situational low self-esteem
7.1.3. Personal identify disturbance
7.2. Sensory-perceptual alterations (specify — visual, auditory, kinesthetic, gustatory, tactile, olfactory)
7.2.1.1. Unilateral neglect
7.3.1. Hopelessness
7.3.2. Powerlessness

PATTERN 8. Knowing: A human response pattern involving the meaning associated with information
8.1.1. Knowledge deficit (specify)
8.3. Altered thought processes

PATTERN 9. Feeling: A human response pattern involving the subjective awareness of information
9.1.1. Pain
9.1.1.1. Chronic pain
9.2.1.1. Dysfunctional grieving
9.2.1.2. Anticipatory grieving
9.2.2. Potential for violence: self-directed or directed at others
9.2.3. Post-trauma response
9.2.3.1. Rape-trauma syndrome
9.2.3.1.1. Rape-trauma syndrome: compound reaction
9.2.3.1.2. Rape-trauma syndrome: silent reaction
9.3.1. Anxiety
9.3.2. Fear

APPENDIX

5

Emergency drugs

The following summarizes the indications, dosages, administration routes, and nursing implications for selected emergency drugs.

DRUG	INDICATIONS	DOSAGE AND ROUTE	NURSING IMPLICATIONS
aminophylline	Status asthmaticus	Loading dose: 5 to 6 mg/kg I.V. over 20 to 30 minutes (if patient is not on regular oral theophylline therapy) Maintenance dosage: 0.4 to 0.7 mg/kg/hour I.V. by continuous infusion	• Use an infusion pump to administer I.V. aminophylline as a constant infusion. • Determine the hourly infusion rate by dividing the daily dosage by 24 hours for a patient who has been receiving long-term oral theophylline therapy.
atropine	Cardiac arrest	I.V. bolus: for asystole, 1 mg I.V. push, repeated in 5 minutes if asystole persists; for bradycardia, 0.5 mg I.V. push Endotracheal: 1 mg followed by 2 to 3 ml of sterile saline solution	• Prepare all I.V. infusions using minidrip or microdrip tubing.
	Muscarinic toxicity	1 to 2 mg I.M. or I.V. every 20 to 30 minutes until muscarinic symptoms disappear	• Administer the first dose I.V. and subsequent doses I.M. or I.V.
bretylium	Cardiac arrest	I.V. bolus: 250 to 500 mg or 5 mg/kg I.V. push; may double-dose (10 mg/kg) and repeat every 15 to 30 minutes to a maximum dosage of 30 mg/kg I.V. infusion: 1 to 2 mg/minute; add 5 to 10 mg/kg to 50 ml of D$_5$W	• Know that bretylium may take 2 minutes to reach the central circulation. • Prepare all I.V. infusions using minidrip or microdrip tubing.
calcium gluceptate	Cardiac arrest	I.V. bolus: 5 to 7 ml of 22% solution given over 1 to 2 minutes	• Administer I.V. into a large vein. • Know that calcium gluceptate is not a first-line drug.
calcium gluconate	Cardiac arrest	I.V. bolus: 5 to 8 ml of 10% solution given at 1 to 2 ml/minute	• Administer I.V. into a large vein, although this drug is less irritating than calcium chloride. • Know that calcium gluconate is not a first-line drug.
diazepam	Status epilepticus	5 to 10 mg I.V. at a rate not to exceed 5 mg/minute; repeated at 10- to 15-minute intervals as needed up to a maximum dosage of 30 mg per seizure episode	• Repeat the regimen in 2 to 4 hours if necessary, but do not exceed the total dosage of 100 mg within a 24-hour period.
dobutamine	Cardiac arrest, cardiogenic shock	I.V. infusion: 2.5 to 10 mcg/kg/minute	• Add 250 mg of dobutamine to 500 ml of D$_5$W; this provides 500 mcg/ml. • Do not mix with sodium bicarbonate because dobutamine is inactivated by alkaline solutions. • Know that doses greater than 20 mcg/kg/minute increase the risk of tachycardia, arrhythmias, and worsening myocardial ischemia. • Prepare all I.V. infusions using minidrip or microdrip tubing.

Emergency drugs (continued)

DRUG	INDICATIONS	DOSAGE AND ROUTE	NURSING IMPLICATIONS
dopamine	Cardiac arrest	I.V. infusion: 2 to 5 mcg/kg/minute	• Add 400 mg of dopamine to 500 ml of D_5W; this provides 800 mcg/ml. • Do not mix with sodium bicarbonate because dopamine is inactivated by alkaline solutions. • Prepare all I.V. infusions using minidrip or microdrip tubing. • Increase the dosage gradually, if needed, in increments of 5 to 10 mcg/kg/minute until the optimum response is achieved.
	Cardiogenic shock	I.V. infusion: 5 to 10 mcg/kg/minute	
edrophonium chloride	Myasthenic crisis	1 mg I.V. followed by an additional 1 mg I.V. in 1 minute if no response	• Use a tuberculin syringe with an I.V. needle for easier administration.
epinephrine	Cardiac arrest	I.V. bolus: 0.1 to 1 mg (1 to 10 ml of a 1:10,000 solution) I.V. push, repeated every 5 minutes until myocardial contractility is restored Endotracheal: 1 mg (10 ml of a 1:10,000 solution) followed by 2 to 3 ml of sterile saline solution I.V. infusion: 1 to 4 mcg/minute, titrated according to the effect	• Do not mix epinephrine with alkaline solutions. • Add 1 mg of epinephrine to 250 ml of D_5W; this provides 4 mcg/ml.
	Status asthmaticus, severe anaphylaxis	Initially, 0.1 to 0.5 mg (0.1 to 0.5 ml of a 1:1,000 solution) S.C. or I.M., repeated at 10- to 15-minute intervals if needed; or 0.1 to 0.25 mg (1 to 2.5 ml of a 1:10,000 solution) I.V. slowly over 5 to 10 minutes, repeated every 5 to 15 minutes as needed or followed by a 1 to 4 mcg/minute I.V. infusion	• Do not mix epinephrine with alkaline solutions. • Add 1 mg of epinephrine to 250 ml of D_5W; this provides 4 mcg/ml.
glucagon	Insulin shock	0.5 to 1 mg S.C., I.M., or I.V., repeated once or twice if patient does not awaken within 5 to 20 minutes of the first injection.	• Do not mix the glucagon I.V. solution with solutions containing calcium, potassium, or sodium chloride because precipitation may occur. Glucagon does not precipitate in dextrose solution. • Monitor the patient's blood glucose level before, during, and after glucagon administration.
labetalol	Hypertensive crisis	I.V. bolus: 10 to 20 mg I.V. push over 2 minutes, repeated every 10 minutes if needed until a total of 300 mg is reached	• Monitor the patient's blood pressure frequently during and after labetalol administration. • Do not mix labetalol with 5% sodium bicarbonate injection because they are incompatible.
lidocaine	Life-threatening arrhythmias	I.V. bolus: 1 mg/kg I.V. push, followed by additional 0.5 mg/kg boluses every 8 to 10 minutes, if needed, until a total of 3 mg/kg is reached I.V. infusion: after successful resuscitation, 2 to 4 mg/minute	• Prepare all I.V. infusions using minidrip or microdrip tubing. • Add 1 gram of lidocaine to 250 ml of D_5W; this provides 4 mg/ml.
naloxone	Opiate drug overdose	0.4 mg I.V., S.C., or I.M., repeated every 2 to 3 minutes for three doses	• Dilute naloxone in D_5W or normal saline solution for I.V. administration; use it within 24 hours of mixing or discard it.

Emergency drugs (continued)

DRUG	INDICATIONS	DOSAGE AND ROUTE	NURSING IMPLICATIONS
nifedipine	Hypertensive crisis	Sublingual: 10 to 20 mg initially, repeated in 20 to 30 minutes if needed; then 10 to 20 mg every 2 hours Oral: 10 to 20 mg P.O. every 8 hours	• Administer the drug by cutting off the top of the capsule or using a sterile needle to make a hole in one end and then squeezing the liquid center under the patient's tongue. As an alternative, have the patient bite the capsule and then swallow it. • Monitor the patient's blood pressure frequently after nifedipine administration.
nitroprusside	Hypertensive crisis	I.V. infusion: 0.5 to 10 mcg/kg/minute	• Monitor the patient's blood pressure continuously to detect a rapid, profound decrease in blood pressure. • Do not piggyback nitroprusside into another I.V. • Protect I.V. solution from light by wrapping the I.V. bag in opaque material. • Know that cyanide toxicity can occur after rapid infusion of high doses. • Administer nitroprusside using minidrip tubing and an infusion pump. • Reconstitute the drug in D_5W only. • Discard any remaining nitroprusside 24 hours after reconstitution.
norepinephrine	Cardiac arrest, cardiogenic shock	I.V. infusion: 8 to 12 mcg/minute then 1 to 5 mcg/minute, titrated to effect; maintenance dosage, 2 to 4 mcg/minute	• Do not mix with sodium bicarbonate because norepinephrine is inactivated by alkaline solutions. • Avoid extravasation, which results in tissue ischemia, necrosis, and sloughing. • Prepare all I.V. infusions using minidrip or microdrip tubing. • Add 4 mg of norepinephrine to 500 ml of D_5W; this provides 8 mcg/minute.
procainamide	Cardiac arrest	I.V. bolus: 100 mg I.V. push over 5 minutes, repeated every 5 minutes, if needed, to a maximum dosage of 500 mg I.V. infusion: 1 to 5 mg/minute	• Decrease the dosage as prescribed for a patient with renal dysfunction. • Monitor the blood concentration levels; continued dosages are based on these levels. • Prepare all I.V. infusions using minidrip or microdrip tubing. • Add 1 gram of procainamide to 250 ml of D_5W; this provides 4 mg/ml.
sodium bicarbonate	Cardiac or respiratory arrest	I.V. bolus: 1 mEq/kg I.V. push; then 0.5 mEq/kg every 10 minutes according to arterial blood gas values	• Prepare all I.V. infusions using minidrip or microdrip tubing. • Base repeated doses on arterial blood pH or laboratory values.

Integumentary system agents

Many drugs are used to treat dermatologic diseases, but topical agents are the mainstay of treatment.

The skin has the lowest water permeability index of any biological membrane. This property, combined with the complex protein keratin in the stratum corneum, allows the skin to function as a barrier that does not block drug absorption. Because the skin is not an absolute barrier, percutaneous absorption may occur.

Most drugs that pass through the stratum corneum to the epidermis are metabolized there; this action may decrease the pharmacologic or toxicologic activity of a drug. Drugs not metabolized in the epidermis pass unchanged into the systemic circulation.

When applying topical integumentary agents, the nurse should begin at the midline and apply with long, even strokes outward and downward in the direction of hair growth. This pattern reduces the risk of follicle irritation and skin inflammation.

Numerous integumentary system agents are available. The chart below presents information on commonly used agents from the following categories: antibacterials; antifungals; antivirals; scabicides and pediculicides; keratolytics and caustics; antineoplastics; corticosteroids; antiseptics and disinfectants; astringents; emollients, demulcents, and protectants; and other integumentary system agents.

DRUG	MAJOR INDICATIONS	USUAL ADULT DOSAGES	NURSING IMPLICATIONS
Antibacterials			
bacitracin (Baciguent)	Gram-positive bacterial skin infections	Apply in a thin film b.i.d. or t.i.d.	• Clean the affected area before applying the medication.
chloramphenicol (Chloromycetin)	Superficial bacterial skin infections	Apply t.i.d. or q.i.d.	• Clean the affected area before applying the medication. • Be aware that chloramphenicol is available as a 1% cream.
chlortetracycline hydrochloride (Aureomycin)	Superficial bacterial skin infections	Apply b.i.d. or t.i.d.	• Rub into the affected area.
clindamycin phosphate (Cleocin T)	Inflammatory acne vulgaris	Apply b.i.d.	• Clean the affected area before applying the medication. • Be aware that clindamycin is available as a 1% solution.
erythromycin (A/T/S, EryDerm, Staticin)	Acne vulgaris	Apply b.i.d., morning and evening.	• Clean the affected area before applying the medication. • Be aware that erythromycin is available as a 2% ointment or 1.5% or 2% solution.
gentamicin sulfate (Garamycin)	Aerobic gram-negative and some gram-positive bacterial skin infections; secondary infections, including infectious eczematoid dermatitis, pustular acne, pustular psoriasis, and infected contact dermatitis	Apply t.i.d. or q.i.d.	• Clean the affected area before applying the medication. • Cover the area with a gauze dressing, if desired. • Be aware that gentamicin sulfate is available as a 0.1% cream or ointment.
mafenide acetate (Sulfamylon Acetate)	Adjunctive therapy in second- and third-degree burns	Apply 1/16″ thickness by sterile technique once daily or b.i.d. to debrided wounds.	• Clean the wounds before applying the medication. • Be aware that mafenide acetate is available as an 8.5% cream.

Integumentary system agents *(continued)*

DRUG	MAJOR INDICATIONS	USUAL ADULT DOSAGES	NURSING IMPLICATIONS
Antibacterials *(continued)*			
meclocycline sulfosalicylate (Meclan)	Acne vulgaris	Apply b.i.d., morning and evening.	• Be aware that meclocycline sulfosalicylate is available as a 1% cream.
metronidazole (MetroGel)	Inflammatory papules, pustules, and erythema of rosacea	Apply b.i.d., morning and evening.	• Inform the patient that significant results should occur within 3 weeks and that improvement should continue for another 6 weeks.
mupirocin (Bactroban)	Impetigo caused by *Staphylococcus aureus,* beta-hemolytic *Streptococcus,* and *Streptococcus pyogenes*	Apply t.i.d.	• Be aware that mupirocin is available as a 2% ointment.
neomycin sulfate (Myciguent)	Aerobic gram-negative and some aerobic gram-positive bacterial skin infections; secondary infections of dermatoses; traumatic lesions that are inflamed or suppurated from bacterial infection	Apply once daily, b.i.d., or t.i.d. by gently rubbing a small quantity into the affected area.	• Clean the affected area before applying the medication. • Be aware that neomycin sulfate is available as a 0.5% cream or ointment.
nitrofurazone (Furacin)	Surface infections, adjunct therapy in second- or third-degree burns, prevention of skin allograft rejection	Apply directly to the affected area and reapply once daily or as indicated.	• Be aware that nitrofurazone is available as a 0.2% cream, ointment, or solution.
silver sulfadiazine (Silvadene)	Many gram-negative and gram-positive bacterial infections; prophylaxis or adjunctive therapy for second- or third-degree burns in patients at risk for wound infection	Apply once or twice daily to a thickness of 1/16″, using a sterile glove.	• Keep the burned area covered with the cream at all times.
sulfapyridine (Dagenan)	Dermatitis herpetiformis	Initially, 500 mg P.O. q.i.d.; when improvement occurs, reduced to 500 mg P.O. daily at 2- or 3-day intervals until the minimum effective dosage is reached; if symptoms recur, the dosage may be increased.	• Monitor the patient carefully to ensure adequate fluid intake and avoid concomitant use of urine acidifiers, which increase the risk of crystalluria from this poorly soluble sulfonamide. • Be aware that sulfapyridine is available in Canada only.
tetracycline hydrochloride (Topicycline)	Inflammatory acne vulgaris	Apply generously b.i.d. to the affected area.	• Cover the entire affected area.
Antifungals			
amphotericin B (Fungizone)	Cutaneous and mucocutaneous candidal infections	Apply liberally to lesions b.i.d. to q.i.d., usually for 1 to 3 weeks.	• Be aware that amphotericin B is available as a 3% cream, lotion, or ointment.
butoconazole nitrate (Femstat)	Vulvovaginal candidiasis (moniliasis)	For non-pregnant adult: one applicatorful intravaginally at bedtime for 3 days. For pregnant adult: one applicatorful intravaginally at bedtime for 6 days.	• Be aware that butoconazole nitrate is available as a 2% vaginal cream. • Advise the patient that the drug should be used only during the second or third trimester.

Integumentary system agents *(continued)*

DRUG	MAJOR INDICATIONS	USUAL ADULT DOSAGES	NURSING IMPLICATIONS
Antifungals *(continued)*			
carbol-fuchsin solution (Castellani Paint, Castel Plus)	Tinea pedis and tinea cruris	Apply as a thin coat once or twice daily.	• Apply the drug more frequently as prescribed, depending on the severity of the condition.
ciclopirox olamine (Loprox)	Tinea pedis, tinea corporis, tinea cruris, tinea versicolor, and cutaneous candidiasis (moniliasis)	Apply b.i.d., morning and evening, to affected areas and surrounding skin.	• Advise the patient that treatment may be required for up to 4 weeks. • Be aware that ciclopirox olamine is available as a 1% cream.
clotrimazole (Lotrimin)	Tinea pedis, tinea cruris, tinea corporis, tinea versicolor, and cutaneous candidiasis	Apply b.i.d., morning and evening, and massage into the affected and surrounding skin.	• Be aware that clotrimazole is available as a 1% cream, lotion, or solution.
econazole nitrate (Spectazole)	Tinea cruris, tinea corporis, tinea pedis, and cutaneous candidiasis Tinea versicolor	Apply b.i.d., morning and evening. Apply once daily.	• Be aware that econazole nitrate is available as a 1% cream.
haloprogin (Halotex)	Tinea pedis, tinea cruris, tinea corporis, tinea manuum, and tinea versicolor	Apply liberally to affected area b.i.d. for 2 to 3 weeks.	• Be aware that haloprogin is available as 1% cream or solution.
ketoconazole (Nizoral)	Cutaneous candidiasis Seborrheic dermatitis	Apply daily. Apply b.i.d.	• Be aware that ketoconazole is available as a 2% cream.
miconazole nitrate (Micatin, Monistat-Derm)	Tinea pedis, tinea cruris, tinea corporis, tinea versicolor, and cutaneous candidiasis	Apply sparingly to affected areas b.i.d., morning and evening.	• Be aware that miconazole nitrate is available as a 2% cream, lotion, or powder and as an aerosol powder or solution.
naftifine hydrochloride (Naftin)	Tinea cruris and tinea corporis caused by *Trichophyton mentographytes, T. rubrum, T. verrucosum, T. violaceum, Epidermophyton floccosum,* or *Microsporum canis*	Apply cream once daily; apply gel b.i.d., morning and evening.	• Be aware that naftifine hydrochloride is available as a 1% cream or gel. • Wash hands before applying the cream or gel. • Avoid contact with the eyes, nose, mouth, and other mucous membranes. • Do not use with an occlusive dressing or wrapping.
nystatin (Mycostatin)	Cutaneous candidiasis	Apply b.i.d., morning and evening, by rubbing into or dusting the affected area.	• Be aware that nystatin is available as a cream, ointment, or powder.
oxiconazole (Oxistat)	Tinea pedis, tinea cruris, and tinea corporis caused by *T. rubrum* and *T. mentagrophytes*	Apply once daily in the evening.	• Teach the patient that treatment must continue for 2 weeks for tinea cruris or corporis or 1 month for tinea pedis to prevent recurrence.

Integumentary system agents *(continued)*

DRUG	MAJOR INDICATIONS	USUAL ADULT DOSAGES	NURSING IMPLICATIONS
Antifungals *(continued)*			
sulconazole nitrate (Exelderm)	Tinea versicolor, tinea cruris, and tinea corporis caused by *T. mentagrophytes, E. floccosum,* and *M. canis*	Apply once or twice daily, gently massaging into the affected area and surrounding skin.	• Be aware that sulconazole nitrate is available as a 1% solution. • Advise the patient to expect symptomatic relief in a few days.
terconazole (Terazol 7)	Vulvovaginal candidiasis	Apply one applicatorful (5 grams) intravaginally once daily at bedtime for 7 consecutive days.	• Be aware that terconazole is available as a 0.4% cream.
tioconazole (Vagistat)	Vulvovaginal candidiasis	Apply one applicatorful (4.6 grams) intravaginally once daily at bedtime).	• Be aware that tioconazole is available as a 6.5% vaginal ointment.
tolnaftate (Aftate, Tinactin)	Tinea cruris, tinea corporis, tinea manuum, tinea pedis, and tinea versicolor	Apply b.i.d. to affected area and massage into the skin, for 2 to 3 weeks.	• Inform the patient that treatment may need to continue for 4 to 6 weeks. • Be aware that tolnaftate is available as a 1% cream, gel, powder, solution, or aerosol.
undecylenic acid and zinc undecylenate (Cruex, Desenex, Quinsana Plus, Ting)	Minor skin rashes, such as diaper rash, prickly heat, chafing, tinea pedis, tinea cruris, and tinea corporis	Apply b.i.d. or as needed to affected areas.	• Be aware that undecylenic acid and zinc undecylenate are available as a cream, ointment, powder, or aerosol.
Antivirals			
acyclovir (Zovirax)	Primary herpes genitalis, limited non-life-threatening mucocutaneous herpes simplex virus infections in immunocompromised patients	Apply in sufficient quantities to cover all lesions every 3 hours, six times daily for 7 days.	• Begin therapy as soon as possible after the onset of signs and symptoms. • Be aware that acyclovir is available as a 5% ointment.
Scabicides and pediculicides			
benzyl benzoate	Scabies and pediculosis	Apply undiluted lotion to damp skin over the entire body from the neck down, let dry, reapply to the most affected area, then bathe the patient after 24 to 48 hours; for scalp treatment, apply lotion to the patient's scalp at night and shampoo in the morning, repeat one more night if necessary.	• Bathe the patient with soap and water before applying the medication. • Be aware that benzyl benzoate is available as a 28% lotion.
crotamiton (Eurax)	Scabies	Massage thoroughly into all skin surfaces from the neck down; reapply in 24 hours, and bathe the patient in 48 hours after the last application.	• Bathe the patient with soap and water before applying the medication. • Be aware that crotamiton is available as a 10% cream or lotion.

Integumentary system agents *(continued)*

DRUG	MAJOR INDICATIONS	USUAL ADULT DOSAGES	NURSING IMPLICATIONS
Scabicides and pediculicides *(continued)*			
lindane (Kwell, Kwildane, Scabene)	Scabies and pediculosis	Apply cream or lotion to dry skin in a thin layer over the entire body from the neck down, rub it in thoroughly, leave it on for 8 to 12 hours, then remove it thoroughly by bathing; alternatively, shampoo the affected area for 4 to 5 minutes, rinse and dry hair, then comb hair with a fine-tooth comb to remove remaining nits.	• Bathe the patient with soap and water and dry thoroughly before applying the medication. • Be aware that lindane is available as a 1% cream, lotion, or shampoo.
permethrin (Elimite)	Scabies	Apply in sufficient quantities to cover or saturate the hair and scalp; leave on the hair for 10 minutes before rinsing.	• Be aware that permethrin is available as a 5% cream or 1% solution.
pyrethrins with piperonyl butoxide (RID)	Pediculosis	Apply undiluted to the patient's hair, scalp, and any other infested areas until entirely wet; leave on the body for 10 minutes; wash thoroughly with warm water, soap, or shampoo as appropriate; comb the hair with a fine-tooth comb.	• Advise the patient that treatment must be repeated in 7 to 10 days. • Be aware that pyrethrins with piperonyl butoxide is available as a gel, shampoo, or solution. • Avoid applying to the patient's eyelashes and eyebrows.
Keratolytics and caustics			
anthralin (AntraDerm, Drithocreme, Lasan)	Psoriasis and other hyperkeratotic conditions	Apply as directed, using a short-contact regimen (apply petrolatum to normal skin around affected area, then apply anthralin directly on lesions, leave it on for 20 to 30 minutes, and then remove with mineral oil and a washcloth), beginning with the lowest concentration (0.1%), and gradually increasing the concentration until therapeutic effects are achieved.	• Apply a lubricant or prescribed medication after each anthralin treatment.
cantharidin (Cantharone)	Removal of *Molluscum contagiosum*	Apply to each lesion and cover with tape for 4 to 6 hours; repeat in 1 week.	• Be aware that cantharidin is available as a 0.7% solution.
	Plantar warts	Apply to each lesion and cover with tape for 4 to 6 hours; repeat in 1 week.	• Pare down keratin before applying to each lesion.
	Benign epithelial growths and periungual warts	Apply to each lesion and cover with tape for 4 to 6 hours; repeat in 1 week.	• Apply directly to the lesion (no cutting is required).

Integumentary system agents (continued)

DRUG	MAJOR INDICATIONS	USUAL ADULT DOSAGES	NURSING IMPLICATIONS
Keratolytics and caustics (continued)			
podophyllum resin (Podoben)	Benign epithelial growths, such as warts, fibroids, and papillomas	Apply to the lesion for the prescribed period (usually 1 to 6 hours), then wash off; repeat as needed once or twice weekly for up to four applications.	• Use petrolatum to protect the patient's surrounding normal skin. • Clean the area with soap and water thoroughly after therapy to ensure that all the drug has been removed.
resorcinol	Inflammatory skin diseases, such as eczema, urticaria, acne, seborrhea, psoriasis, and acne scarring	Apply to the affected area as directed.	• None.
salicylic acid (Occlusal, Keralyt Gel, Salacid)	Hyperkeratotic skin disorders, such as verrucae and various ichthyoses, keratosis palmaris and plantaris, keratosis pilaris, pityriasis rubra pilaris, and psoriasis	Apply thoroughly to the affected skin that has been hydrated for 5 minutes, occlude overnight, and wash off the medication in the morning.	• Apply more frequently to areas where occlusion is not possible.
silver nitrate	Indolent warts, exuberant granulations, freshening of the edges of ulcers and fissures, touching of the basis of vesicular, bullous, or aphthous lesions, and cauterization	Apply ointment to the affected area for up to 5 days or as needed; apply solution to the affected area 2 or 3 times a week for 2 or 3 weeks as needed.	• Do not apply the solution to wounds, cuts, or broken skin.
sulfur (Fostex, Sebulex, Sulfacet-R)	Acne	Apply to the skin once daily to t.i.d. or as directed.	• Clean the skin thoroughly with soap and water before applying the medication.
	Dandruff	Apply to wet hair, massage vigorously into the scalp, rinse, and then repeat application and rinse.	• None.
Antineoplastics			
fluorouracil (Efudex, Fluoroplex)	Multiple actinic (solar) keratoses	Apply 1% to 5% cream or solution b.i.d. for 2 to 6 weeks or until erosion occurs.	• Avoid applying the drug to normal skin. • Advise the patient to avoid exposure to strong sunlight and other sources of ultraviolet rays because such exposure intensifies skin reactions to the drug.
	Superficial basal cell carcinoma	Apply 5% cream or solution to the lesion b.i.d. for 3 to 6 weeks or until erosion occurs.	
Corticosteroids			
fluticasone propionate (Cutivate)	Inflammation and pruritus associated with corticosteroid-responsive dermatoses	Apply to the affected area b.i.d.	• Be aware that fluticasone propionate is available as a 0.005% ointment or 0.05% cream.

Integumentary system agents (continued)

DRUG	MAJOR INDICATIONS	USUAL ADULT DOSAGES	NURSING IMPLICATIONS
Corticosteroids (continued)			
halobetasol propionate (Ultravate)	Inflammation and pruritus associated with corticosteroid-responsive dermatoses	Apply to the affected area as prescribed.	• Be aware that halobetasol propionate is available as a 0.05% ointment.
mometasone (Elocon)	Inflammation and pruritus associated with corticosteroid-responsive dermatoses	Apply to the affected area once daily.	• Be aware that mometasone is available as a cream or ointment.
Antiseptics and disinfectants			
benzalkonium	Prevention of infection	Clean unbroken skin, mucous membranes, and denuded skin preoperatively as prescribed.	• Be aware that benzalkonium is used primarily as a preoperative skin cleaner. It also may be used to disinfect surgical equipment and other articles, such as thermometers.
chlorhexidine gluconate (Hibiclens, Hibistat)	Prevention of infection	Apply to skin, hands, or wound as indicated.	• Be aware that chlorhexidine gluconate is used as a surgical scrub, hand cleaner, preoperative skin cleaner, and wound cleaner.
ethyl alcohol and isopropyl alcohol	Prevention of infection	Rub on the skin before a procedure that breaks the skin, such as venipuncture or hypodermic injection.	• Be aware that ethyl alcohol and isopropyl alcohol are used as skin antiseptics. • Allow these drugs to remain on the skin for at least 2 minutes to ensure effectiveness.
hexachlorophene (pHisoHex)	Prevention of infection	Apply to skin or hands and rub vigorously as indicated.	• Be aware that hexachlorophene is used as an antibacterial skin cleaner and surgical hand scrub. • Use hexachlorophene for preoperative skin cleaning at least 3 days before the procedure to ensure its effectiveness. • Know that hexachlorophene is contraindicated in an infant.
hydrogen peroxide	Prevention of infection	Apply directly to wounds and ulcers as prescribed, or administer as a mouthwash or gargle for cleaning oral mucous membranes.	• Be aware that hydrogen peroxide is used as a cleaner for superficial wounds, ulcers, and oral mucous membranes. • Be aware that the drug is available in a 1.5% solution.

Integumentary system agents *(continued)*

DRUG	MAJOR INDICATIONS	USUAL ADULT DOSAGES	NURSING IMPLICATIONS
Antiseptics and disinfectants *(continued)*			
iodine (Iodine Tincture, Iodine Topical Solution) and iodine compounds (Betadine)	Prevention of infection	Apply directly to the affected area as indicated.	• Be aware that iodine and iodine compounds are used as skin cleaners and as a treatment for minor, superficial skin wounds. • Inform the patient that the solution can stain clothing.
potassium permanganate	Prevention of infection	Apply directly to the affected area as indicated.	• Be aware that potassium permanganate is used as a skin antiseptic and as a treatment for athlete's foot and intertriginous candidiasis. • Inform the patient that the solution may stain clothing and skin but that the stains may be removed with a dilute acid.
Astringents			
aluminum acetate solution (Burow's solution)	Inflammatory skin conditions, such as insect bites, poison ivy, and athlete's foot	Apply as a wet dressing to the affected area as indicated.	• None.
aluminum sulfate (Bluboro Powder, Domeboro Powder and Tablets)	Inflammatory skin conditions, such as insect bites, poison ivy, and athlete's foot	Apply to the affected area for 15 to 30 minutes every 4 to 8 hours.	• Mix aluminum sulfate in 1 pint of water before administering it.
hamamelis water [Witch hazel] (Tucks)	Anal or perineal discomfort	Apply locally t.i.d. or q.i.d.	• None.
Emollients, demulcents, and protectants			
compound benzoin tincture (Benzoin spray)	Cutaneous ulcers, pressure ulcers, cracked nipples, and fissures of the lips or anus	Spray directly onto the affected area as indicated.	• Inform the patient that the preparation may stain clothing.
glycerin (Corn Husker's lotion)	Dry skin	Apply to the affected area as often as needed to keep skin soft.	• None.
oatmeal (Aveeno)	Dry or irritated skin	Apply directly to the affected area or mix with bath water as needed.	• Be aware that oatmeal is available as a lotion or powder.
para-aminobenzoic acid [PABA] (Pabanol)	Sunscreen; skin irritation	Apply directly to the skin as needed.	• Advise the patient to apply PABA before sun exposure to prevent sunburn.
petrolatum (Vaseline) and liquid petrolatum (Mineral oil)	Dry skin	Apply directly to the skin as needed.	• Inform the patient that the preparation may stain clothing.
vitamin A and D ointment (Clocream, Desitin)	Superficial burns, abrasions, slow-healing lesions, chapped skin, and diaper rash	Apply directly to the affected area as indicated.	• None.
zinc oxide gelatin (Dome-Paste, Unna's Boot)	Lesions or injuries of the lower arms or legs	Apply as a bandage to the affected area.	• Instruct the patient the zinc oxide gelatin must be worn for about 1 week.

Integumentary system agents *(continued)*

DRUG	MAJOR INDICATIONS	USUAL ADULT DOSAGES	NURSING IMPLICATIONS
Other integumentary system agents			
minoxidil (Rogaine)	Alopecia androgenetica	Apply 1 ml to the affected area b.i.d.	• Be aware that minoxidil is available as a 2% solution. • Ensure that the hair and scalp are dry before application. • Wash the hands after applying the drug with the fingertips.
tretinoin (Retin-A)	Acne vulgaris	Apply nightly to the affected area.	• Wash the skin and allow it to dry for 15 to 30 minutes before applying the medication. • Inform patient that mild erythema and peeling of the area can be expected. Also explain that exposure to sunlight or use of a keratolytic or abrasive soap can aggravate this response.

Active immunity agents

Vaccines and toxoids provide active immunity. This chart presents indications, usual dosages, and nursing implications for the major active immunity agents.

DRUG	MAJOR INDICATIONS	USUAL DOSAGES	NURSING IMPLICATIONS
diphtheria and tetanus toxoids and pertussis vaccine (DTP)	Immunity to diphtheria, tetanus, and pertussis	0.5 ml I.M. for children at ages 2, 4, 6, and 15 to 18 months, followed by a booster before school entry (ages 4 to 6)	• Do not administer a live attenuated virus to an immunocompromised patient because the virus can cause the disease; wait until immunotherapy has been discontinued for 3 months. • Be aware that DTP should be withheld in a patient with an acute febrile illness to avoid the problem of differentiating signs and symptoms of illness from those of reaction; children should return for DTP as soon as they are well. • Document the patient's history of administration of plasma, whole blood, and immune serum globulin; immunization should be administered 3 months after plasma, whole blood, and immune globulin.
measles, mumps, and rubella virus vaccine, live (MMR)	Prevention of measles, mumps, and rubella	0.5 ml S.C. for children at age 15 months, followed by a second MMR at age 11 or older for children who have not had measles	• Know that MMR is contraindicated in a patient with severe febrile illness and after the administration of antimetabolites, steroids, or steroidlike medications. • Do not administer MMR if the patient is allergic to eggs or neomycin. • Do not administer to an immunocompromised patient. MMR may be given after chemotherapy has been discontinued for 3 months. • Do not administer to a woman of childbearing age; if the vaccine is given, the woman must not become pregnant for 3 months. • Be aware that children ages 6 months and older can be immunized during a measles outbreak, but must be reimmunized at age 15 months. • Administer live-virus vaccines on the same day. If this is not possible, wait at least 1 month before administering another live-virus vaccine. • Have epinephrine (1:1,000) available to treat anaphylactic reactions should they occur. • Do not administer MMR intravenously. • Refrigerate MMR vaccine at 39° F (4° C). • Protect the vaccine from heat and light.

Active immunity agents *(continued)*

DRUG	MAJOR INDICATIONS	USUAL DOSAGES	NURSING IMPLICATIONS
poliovirus vaccine, live, oral, trivalent (OPV)	Immunity to poliovirus	0.5 ml P.O.; primary series is administered in three doses. The first two doses are given 6 to 8 weeks apart, and a third dose is given 12 months later. If given to infants, the first dose is given at age 2 months, the second dose at 4 months, the third dose at 15 to 18 months, and the fourth dose at 4 to 6 years.	• Know that OPV is contraindicated in an immunocompromised patient; administer the inactivated form. • Avoid administering OPV in a pregnant patient or one with diarrhea, vomiting, or an acute illness. • Administer by mouth only. • Administer live-virus vaccines on the same day. If this is not possible, wait at least 1 month before administering another live-virus vaccine. • Store frozen OPV at 7° F (-13° C). Once thawed, store it at 36° to 46° F (2° to 8° C) and use within 30 days.
pneumococcal vaccine, polyvalent	Prevention of pneumococcal diseases, such as pneumonia and meningitis	0.5 ml I.M. or S.C. for adults and children ages 2 and older	• Do not administer if the patient has known hypersensitivity to a portion of the vaccine. • Do not administer to a patient receiving immunosuppressive therapy. • Be aware that the influenza and pneumococcal vaccines can be administered to children at the same time in different sites without increased adverse effects.
influenza virus vaccine, trivalent types A and B (whole or split virus)	Prevention of influenza virus	For adults and children over age 12: 0.5 ml of whole or split virus vaccine I.M. in the deltoid For children ages 9 to 12: 0.5 ml of split virus vaccine I.M. For children ages 3 to 8: 0.5 ml of split virus vaccine I.M. repeated in 4 weeks For children ages 6 to 35 months: 0.25 ml of split virus vaccine I.M. repeated in 4 weeks	• Do not administer if the patient is allergic to eggs. • Defer or delay immunization if the patient has an acute respiratory illness. • Be aware that the influenza and pneumococcal vaccines can be administered to children at the same time in different sites without increased adverse effects.
haemophilus influenzae and type b conjugate vaccine (HbOC and PRP-OMP)	Prevention of *Haemophilus influenzae* infections	For children ages 2 to 6 months: 0.5 mg I.M. The HbOC vaccine is given in three doses at 2-month intervals followed by a fourth dose at age 15 months; the PRP-OMP vaccine is given in two doses at 2-month intervals followed by a third dose at age 12 months.	• Administer in the outer aspect area of the vastus lateralis or deltoid muscle. • Do not inject via I.V. • Follow the initial dose of HbOC with two doses of HbOC. The fourth dose may be HbOC or PRP-OMP. • Follow the initial dose of PRP-OMP with two doses of PRP-OMP; do not substitute HbOC.

Active immunity agents *(continued)*

DRUG	MAJOR INDICATIONS	USUAL DOSAGES	NURSING IMPLICATIONS
hepatitis B vaccine	Immunity to hepatitis B and subtypes of hepatitis B	For adults and children over age 10: 1 ml I.M., followed by another 1-ml dose 1 month later, and a third 1-ml dose 6 months after the first dose For neonates and children up to age 10: 0.5 ml I.M., followed by another 0.5-ml dose 1 month later, and a third 0.5-ml dose 6 months after the first dose For dialysis and immuno-compromised patients: 2 ml I.M., followed by another 2-ml dose 1 month later, and a third 2-ml dose 6 months after the first dose. (The 2-ml doses should be divided into two 1-ml doses and administered at different sites.)	• Administer cautiously to a patient with a serious, active infection or compromised cardiac or pulmonary status; or one for whom a febrile or systemic reaction could pose a serious risk. • Administer the hepatitis B vaccine in the arm rather than the buttock. The Centers for Disease Control reports that administration in the arm produces a significantly better response to the vaccine. • Administer the vaccine subcutaneously *only* to patients who are at risk for hemorrhage, such as hemophiliacs. • Agitate the vial thoroughly just before administration to restore suspension. • Store opened and unopened vials in the refrigerator. Do not freeze the vaccine.

APPENDIX

8

Passive immunity agents

This chart presents indications, usual dosages, and nursing implications for the major passive immunity agents.

DRUG	MAJOR INDICATIONS	USUAL ADULT DOSAGES	NURSING IMPLICATIONS
hepatitis B immune globulin (HBIG)	Exposure to hepatitis B; post-hepatitis exposure prophylaxis	For postexposure prophylaxis, 0.06 ml/kg I.M. (most adults will receive a dose of 3 to 5 ml) within 7 days after exposure; a second injection is given 28 to 30 days later. For neonates whose mothers are HBsAg-positive: 0.5 ml I.M. as soon as possible after birth and no later than 24 hours after birth; this dose is repeated at ages 3 months and 6 months	• Administer HBIG cautiously to a patient who has experienced previous systemic allergic reactions to other human immunoglobulins. • Administer HBIG to a pregnant woman only when clearly indicated and ordered. • Administer HBIG I.M.; always aspirate to be sure the injection is not inadvertently administered I.V. • Administer the medication I.M., preferably into the deltoid in adults and older children; inject it into the vastus lateralis in infants and young children. • Store HBIG at 36° to 46° F (2° to 8° C); do not freeze. • Teach an adult patient the importance of receiving the second dose. Inform parents about the importance of obtaining the second and third doses for their child.
rabies immune globulin (RIG)	Exposure to rabies; post-rabies prophylaxis	20 IU/kg; about half the dose should be used to infiltrate the wound and the remainder administered I.M.	• Administer RIG cautiously to a patient with a history of systemic hypersensitivity reactions to immunoglobulins or known allergy to thimerosal. • Be aware of the risks and benefits of RIG for patients with isolated immunoglobulin A (IgA) deficiency, because hypersensitivity can develop from increased antibodies to IgA. Anaphylaxis can occur with subsequent administration of products that contain IgA. • Teach the patient about the predictable adverse reactions. • Administer the medication I.M. into the deltoid in adults and older children; inject it into the vastus lateralis in infants and young children. • Store RIG at 36° to 46° F; do not freeze. • Expect RIG and human diploid cell rabies vaccine to be administered if treatment against rabies is necessary. Do not administer these medications at the same site or in the same syringe.

Passive immunity agents (continued)

DRUG	MAJOR INDICATIONS	USUAL ADULT DOSAGES	NURSING IMPLICATIONS
tetanus immune globulin (TIG)	Susceptible wounds in nonimmunized patients, post-tetanus prophylaxis, treatment of tetanus	For post-tetanus prophylaxis, 250 to 500 units I.M.; for treatment of tetanus, 3,000 to 6,000 units	• Know that TIG is contraindicated in a patient with known hypersensitivity to immune globulin (IG) or thimerosal. • Do not perform a skin test with TIG because an area of inflammation after the injection may be interpreted as a positive skin reaction when actually it is a chemical irritation of the tissues. • Administer TIG I.M. to decrease the risk of anaphylaxis. • Monitor closely for anaphylaxis and a sharp decrease in blood pressure if TIG must be administered I.V. • Store TIG at 36° to 46° F. If the TIG has been frozen, do not use it. • Encourage the patient to schedule follow-up visits if the wound necessitates them.
varicella-zoster immune globulin (VZIG)	Exposure to chicken pox of immunocompromised children	For children weighing up to 10 kg, 125 units I.M.; 10.1 to 20 kg, 250 units I.M.; 20.1 to 30 kg, 375 units I.M.; 30.1 to 40 kg, 500 units I.M.; over 40 kg, 625 units I.M.	• Know that VZIG is contraindicated in a patient with a history of severe hypersensitivity reactions to IG and in patients with severe thrombocytopenia. • VZIG is not recommended during pregnancy. The pregnant patient and her physician should determine if the benefits outweight the risks. • Administer VZIG I.M. to avoid anaphylaxis, which may occur with I.V. injection. • Help the family plan a bland diet if the child experiences GI distress.

Poisons

Despite an extensive campaign against it, poisoning remains a serious problem in the United States. The National Clearinghouse for Poison Control Centers estimates that 2 to 3 million poisonings occur annually, resulting in approximately 5,000 deaths.

Although some poisonings result from the intentional ingestion of toxic substances and others from homicidal actions, most incidents are accidental. Drug ingestion, often in conjunction with alcohol, commonly causes accidental poisoning as does the ingestion of household substances used for cleaning and maintenance. Industrial poisonings from environmental pollutants, pesticides, and radioactive substances pose a growing threat.

Treating acute poisoning usually is complex because specific systemic antidotes are available for only a small number of drugs and toxic substances, as shown in the chart below. To treat acute poisoning most effectively, the physician or nurse should obtain the following information as soon as possible: the drug or substance ingested, the amount and time of ingestion, and any significant medical problem that the patient had before the poisoning. If this information is not available, the physician or nurse must assume that the patient may have ingested multiple substances.

Treatment goals for the poisoned patient typically include:
• administering the appropriate antidote, if available
• supporting vital functions
• decreasing further absorption of the toxic substance
• promoting excretion of the toxin
• managing complications.

The most common complications of poisoning are central nervous system depression and coma. Other complications may include toxic delirium, seizures, blood pressure alterations, arrhythmias, and tissue damage.

Antidotes for selected poisons

This chart outlines potential poisons, their antidotes, and how each antidote works to remove or neutralize the poison.

POISON	ANTIDOTE	TYPE AND EFFECT OF ANTIDOTE
acetaminophen	acetylcysteine	Dispositional antagonist: hastens detoxification
anticholinergics	physostigmine	Receptor antidote: blocks receptors
anticholinesterases (organophosphates)	atropine	Receptor antidote: blocks muscarinic receptors
	pralidoxime	Dispositional antagonist: reactivates cholinesterase
carbon monoxide	oxygen	Dispositional antagonist: hastens carboxyhemoglobin breakdown
fluoride	calcium	Chemical antidote: precipitates fluoride
iron	sodium bicarbonate (before absorption)	Chemical antidote: forms insoluble iron carbonate
lead	succimer	Chemical antidote: forms water-soluble lead chelate that is excreted in urine
methanol	ethanol	Dispositional antidote: slows formation of toxic products
	sodium bicarbonate	Physiologic antagonist: offsets acidosis
narcotics and derivatives	naloxone	Receptor antidote: displaces narcotic from receptor
strychnine	diazepam, barbiturates	Physiologic antagonists: offset central nervous system stimulation

Substance abuse

Substance abuse is a maladaptive pattern of substance use marked by continuation despite knowledge of impaired social, occupational, psychological, or physical functioning caused or exacerbated by that use. The abused substance may be nicotine, alcohol, or an over-the-counter, prescription, or illegal drug.

Behaviors that indicate abuse
According to the American Psychiatric Association, any three or more of the following behaviors indicate abuse:
• ingesting the substance more frequently or in larger amounts than prescribed
• persistently desiring to quit or reduce use, or unsuccessfully attempting to quit or reduce use
• spending an inordinate amount of time seeking, taking, or recovering from the substance
• neglecting obligations because of intoxication or withdrawal symptoms
• reducing important occupational or social activities because of substance use
• continuing substance use despite knowledge of adverse effects
• developing a tolerance to the effects of the substance
• manifesting characteristic withdrawal symptoms when not taking the substance
• taking the substance to relieve or prevent withdrawal symptoms.

Addiction
The nurse who cares for a substance abuser should keep the following points in mind:
• Addictive substances act on the brain, engaging brain circuits related to emotion, motivation, and behavior.
• Addictive behavior is motivated by the pleasure or reward the substance gives.
• Susceptibility to addictive drugs and the capacity to recover from addiction vary greatly among individuals.
• No single addictive personality exists, although personality traits may play a role in addiction.

Addictive drugs include alcohol, cocaine, marijuana, opiates, barbiturates, amphetamines, hallucinogens, tranquilizers, and sedatives. (For more information about these drugs, see *Commonly abused substances,* pages 1323 and 1324.)

Defense mechanisms in substance abuse
A substance abuser typically uses two key defense mechanisms: denial and isolation. With denial, the abuser rejects the notion that the abused substance is causing a problem, thus impeding treatment and recovery. With isolation, the abuser separates himself or herself from people, situations, information, or feelings that challenge the denial. Use of denial may prevent recovery or promote a relapse in a former substance abuser.

The denial-isolation pattern that enables the user to continue substance abuse also may induce guilt, shame, low self-esteem, and loneliness. The abuser may rationalize the dependence or project emotions onto others, resulting in dependence on others, lying about or making excuses for continued substance abuse, extreme withdrawal symptoms, social isolation, or loss of responsibility.

Nursing implications
When obtaining a drug history, the nurse should ask the patient about all drug use and should be aware that a substance abuse problem may be complicated by polypharmacy (simultaneous use of several drugs). Polypharmacy is a major cause of drug-related deaths.

During the drug history, the nurse should ask about illegal drug use. When providing this information, the patient may use street names to refer to particular drugs or drug classes rather than the correct pharmacologic names. Therefore, the nurse should be familiar with commonly used names for street drugs. (For a list, see *Glossary of street drug names,* page 1325.)

After identifying a substance abuse problem, the nurse can intervene by teaching the patient about treatment and rehabilitation measures, making referrals for substance abuse programs, and helping family members identify and cope with their feelings about the problem.

Commonly abused substances

When caring for a patient who abuses alcohol or drugs, the nurse should be familiar with the incidence, signs and symptoms, and treatment of abuse for each substance.

SUBSTANCE AND INCIDENCE	SIGNS AND SYMPTOMS	TREATMENT
Alcohol		
About 42 million people in the United States drink alcoholic beverages at least once a week*	• Depressed brain activity and respirations • Blood vessel dilation resulting in flushed skin, sweating, and clammy palms • Alcohol-related medical complications, such as cirrhosis, gastritis, pancreatitis, polyneuropathy, heart muscle disease, heart failure, and coronary artery disease • Alcoholic blackouts (amnesia of the time period when drinking) • Drinking bouts of 48 hours or more • Alcohol-related problems, such as arrests for drunken driving, work problems, drinking before breakfast, or controlling the alcohol craving by drinking mouthwash, antifreeze, or other forms of nonbeverage alcohol *Withdrawal symptoms* • Mild symptoms, including agitation, tremulousness, anorexia, disturbed sleep, and occasional hallucinations and seizures • Severe symptoms, including seizures, hallucinations, and delirium tremens (acute psychotic reaction to alcohol withdrawal)	• Detoxification (process of freeing the patient from alcohol dependency by lowering the blood alcohol level and controlling withdrawal symptoms) • Withdrawal over 3 or more days • Treatment of withdrawal symptoms with medications and support from a health care professional, friend, or family member • Total avoidance of alcohol and reliance on a supportive network after detoxification • Referral to an alcoholic rehabilitation program, such as Alcoholics Anonymous • Referral to a family support group
Cocaine		
In the United States, 6.2 million people used cocaine once a week or more during 1990*	• Vasoconstriction, tachycardia, increased blood pressure • Euphoria, hallucinations, feelings of increased mental and physical prowess • Gaunt appearance • Maladaptive behavior, impaired judgment and social or occupational functioning • Postcocaine crash lasting several hours or days after drug binge, producing severe depression, anxiety, irritability, and migrainelike headaches *Withdrawal symptoms* • Drug craving, irritability, shaking • Anorexia or hunger and nausea • Irregular sleep patterns • Lack of motivation, intense subjective feelings, depression, suicidal urges	• Detoxification • Withdrawal over 3 or more days • Treatment of withdrawal symptoms with medications and support from a health care professional, friend, or family member • Strict control over or total avoidance of cocaine use • Replacement of the cocaine addiction with activities that support positive human relationships and increase self-esteem • Referral to a drug rehabilitation program
Marijuana (cannabis sativa)		
Approximately 66.5 million U.S. citizens have tried marijuana at least once in their lives; about 5.5 million use the drug once a week or more*	• Dreamlike state, sense of contentment, improved social interaction, loss of inhibitions • Damage to nasal mucosa, alveolar cells, bronchioles, and airways *Acute panic reactions* • Flashback phenomenon, acute psychosis, paranoia • Abdominal discomfort, headache *Acute toxicity* • Impaired reflexes, short-term memory, and depth perception	• Treatment to improve disturbed interpersonal relationships (particularly helpful in adolescents, who may use marijuana to defy authority) • Time to outgrow the habit • Establishment of permanent relationships with nondrug users to help decrease drug use

*National Institute on Drug Abuse. (1990). *NIDA capsules: Summary of findings from the 1990 National Household Survey on Drug Abuse.* Rockville, MD.

Commonly abused substances (continued)

SUBSTANCE AND INCIDENCE	SIGNS AND SYMPTOMS	TREATMENT
Opiates		
Use probably is high because opiates are readily available on the street.	• Lethargy, nodding, warm, flushed skin • Lower abdominal sensation of intense pleasure • Sensation of pleasure lasting 2 or more hours *Withdrawal symptoms 8 to 12 hours after the last dose of heroin or morphine* • Dilated pupils, rhinorrhea, and lacrimation • Sweating, slight temperature elevation *Withdrawal symptoms 2 to 14 days after the last dose of heroin or morphine* • Insomnia • Nausea, vomiting, and diarrhea • Tachycardia and hypertension • Muscle weakness, twitches, joint pain, piloerection	• Correction of opiate overdose with naloxone or naltrexone • Detoxification with methadone • Referral to a specific drug treatment center
Barbiturates		
Use is unknown because barbiturates are obtained easily by prescription.	• Slurred speech, unsteady gait • Vertical or horizontal nystagmus *Barbiturate overdose* • Respiratory depression, death *Withdrawal symptoms* • Seizures	• Detoxification with decreasing doses of pentobarbital until the drug is metabolized to prevent seizures associated with a rapid drop in barbiturate blood level
Amphetamines		
Amphetamine use is estimated to be higher than opiate use in the United States.	• Rapid speech • Headache, anorexia, or nausea • Elevated pulse and blood pressure • Fine tremor of the extremities • Dilated pupils with decreased light reactivity *Withdrawal symptoms* • Lethargy, severe depression	• Detoxification with the benzodiazepine diazepam (Valium) to promote sedation and propranolol (Inderal) to counteract severe adrenergic hyperactivity • Hospitalization to control suicidal impulses if post-amphetamine depression persists
Hallucinogens		
Use is probably high because hallucinogens are the easiest and least expensive to manufacture.	• Kaleidoscopic hallucinations • Tactile, visual, and auditory images • Strong feelings of introspection and disengagement • Feelings of superhuman powers • Extreme excitement, unpredictable destructive behavior, frightening hallucinations • Severe panic reaction or psychotic behavior with overdose (uncommon)	• Supportive management for undesirable adverse reactions • Hospitalization for severe panic reactions or prolonged psychotic episodes
Tranquilizers and sedatives		
Use probably is very high because tranquilizers (especially diazepam [Valium]) and sedatives are obtained easily by prescription.	• Drowsiness, fatigue, dizziness • Impaired motor coordination, reaction time, and cognitive reasoning • Dysarthria, slurred speech, tremor *Drug overdose* • Confusion, coma, diminished reflexes • Hypotension and depression *Withdrawal symptoms* • Hyperreflexia, seizures, hallucinations	• Gradual withdrawal under medical supervision • Rehabilitation to prevent recurrence of drug abuse

*National Institute on Drug Abuse. (1990). *NIDA capsules: Summary of findings from the 1990 National Household Survey on Drug Abuse.* Rockville, MD.

Glossary of street drug names

CNS stimulants*

Bennies
Blue angels
Chris
Christine
Christmas trees
Coast to coast
Coke (cocaine)
Copilot
Crisscross
Crossroads
Crystal (I.V. metham-
   phetamine)†
Dexies
Double cross
Flake (cocaine)
Footballs
Glass (metham-
   phetamine)
Gold dust (cocaine)
Green and clears
Hearts
Ice (methamphetamine)
Lip poppers
Meth
Oranges
Peaches
Pep pills
Pinks
Roses
Snow (cocaine)
Speed
Speedball (heroin plus
   cocaine)
Truck drivers
Uppers
Ups
Wake-ups
Whites

Phencyclidine (PCP)

Angel dust
Aurora
Bust bee
Cheap cocaine
Cosmos
Criptal
Dummy mist
Goon
Green
Guerilla
Hot
Jet
K
Lovely
Mauve
Mist
Mumm dust
Peace pill
Purple
Rocket fuel
Shermans
Sherms
Special L.A. coke
Superacid
Supercoke
Supergrass
Superjoint
Tranq†
Whack

Heroin

Brown
H
H and stuff
Horse
Junk
Scat
Shit
Skag
Smack

Other analgesics

Black (opium)
Blue velvet (paregoric
   plus amphetamine)
Dollies (methadone)
M (morphine)
Microdots (morphine)
PG or PO (paregoric)
Pinks and grays (Propox-
   yphene hydrochloride)
Poppy (opium)
Tar (opium)
Terp (terpin hydrate or
   cough syrup with co-
   deine)

CNS depressants‡

Blue birds
Blue devil
Blue heaven
Blues
Bullets
Dolls
Double trouble
Downs
Goofballs
Green and whites
   (chlordiazepoxide)
Greenies
Nembies
Peanuts
Peter (chloral hydrate)
Rainbows
Red devils
Roaches (chlordiaze-
   poxide)†
Seccy
Seggy
Sleepers
T-birds
Toolies
Tranqs†
Yellow jackets
Yellows

Hallucinogens

Acid (LSD)
Blue dots (LSD)
Cactus (mescaline)
Crystal†
Cube (LSD)
D (LSD)
Mescal (mescaline)
Owsleys (LSD)
Pearly gates (morning
   glory seeds)

Cannabinols

Acapulco gold
Bhang
Brick
Charas
Gage
Ganja
Grass
Hash
Hay
Hemp
Jive
Joint
Key or kee
Lid
Locoweed
Mary Jane
MJ
Muggles
Pot
Reefer
Roach†
Rope
Sativa
Stick
Sweet Lucy
Tea
Texas tea
Weed
Yesca

Solvents and inhalants

Huffing
Jac aroma
Kicks
Locker room
Poppers
Rush
Snappers
Sniffers

* A form of amphetamine unless otherwise stated.
† Many drugs have the same name.
‡ Moderate length of action like secobarbital unless otherwise noted.
Source: Schuckit, M.A. (1989). *Drug and alcohol abuse* (3rd ed.). New York: Plenum Publishing Corp. Reprinted with permission of the publisher.

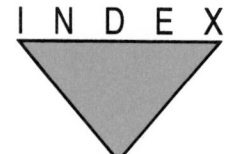

INDEX

---

i refers to an illustration; t refers to a table

Butoconazole nitrate, 1308t
Butorphanol tartrate, 357. *See also* Mixed
    narcotic agonist-antagonists.
    action of, 356
    dosage, 357
    equianalgesic dosage of, 356t
    pharmacokinetics of, 356

C

Cafergot, 235. *See also* Ergotamine tar-
    trate.
Cafergot P-B, 235. *See also* Ergotamine
    tartrate.
Cafetrate, 235. *See also* Ergotamine tar-
    trate.
Caffeine, 662. *See also* Methylxanthine
    agents.
    action of, 659
    administration considerations for, 665
    dosage, 662
    interaction of, with drugs, 662
    in lactating patient, 658
    for neonatal apnea, 662
    in neonate, 658
    pharmacokinetics of, 657-658
    in pregnant patient, 176t, 657-658
Caladryl, 946. *See also* Diphenhydramine
    hydrochloride.
Calan, 509, 528, 552. *See also* Verapamil
    hydrochloride.
Calan SR, 552. *See also* Verapamil hydro-
    chloride.
Calcifediol, 876. *See also* Calcium regula-
    tors.
    action of, 876
    adverse reactions to, 878, 878t
    dosage, 876
    interaction of, with drugs, 877t
    patient teaching for, 881
    pharmacokinetics of, 875
Calciferol, 780. *See also* Vitamin D.
Calcilac, 757. *See also* Calcium carbonate.
Calcimar, 876. *See also* Calcitonin-
    salmon.
Calcitonin. *See also* Calcitonin-salmon.
    synthetic analogues of, 874
    as thyroid hormone, 833, 835i
Calcitonin-human, 876. *See also* Calciton-
    in-salmon.
Calcitonin-salmon. *See also* Calcium regu-
    lators.
    action of, 875
    adverse reactions to, 877-878, 878t
    dosage, 876
    interaction of, with drugs, 877, 877t
    nursing process application for, 878-881
    pharmacokinetics of, 874, 875
    vs. porcine calcitonin, 874
Calcitriol, 877. *See also* Calcium regula-
    tors.
    action of, 875
    administration considerations for, 880
    adverse reactions to, 878, 878t
    dosage, 877
    patient teaching for, 881
    pharmacokinetics of, 875

Calcium, 803-806
    action of, 804
    adverse reactions to, 805
    concentration levels of, in fluid com-
        partments, 771t
    dosage, 804
    foods that interfere with absorption of,
        804
    homeostasis of, 872-873
    interaction of, with drugs, 804, 805t
    nursing process applications for,
        805-806
    pharmacokinetics of, 804
    in pregnant or lactating patient, 804
    therapeutic uses of, 804
Calcium carbonate, 757, 804. *See also*
    Antacids *and* Calcium.
    administration considerations for, 759
    adverse reactions to, 758-759
    as antacid, 757
    as dietary supplement, 804
    dosage, 757, 804
    effectiveness of, 757
    interaction of, with drugs, 758t, 805t
    pharmacokinetics of, 756
Calcium channel blockers
    adverse reactions to, 529
    as antianginals, 527-531
    as antihypertensive agents, 550, 552
    interaction of, with drugs, 528-529,
        530t
    mechanism of action of, 528
    nursing process applications for,
        529-531
    pharmacokinetics of, 527-528
    therapeutic uses of, 528
Calcium chloride, 804. *See also* Calcium.
    for cardiac arrest, 804
    dosages, 804
    for hypocalcemia, 804
Calcium citrate, 804. *See also* Calcium.
Calcium glubionate, 804. *See also* Cal-
    cium.
Calcium gluceptate, 1304t
Calcium gluconate, 804. *See also* Cal-
    cium.
    for cardiac arrest, 1304t
Calcium lactate, 804. *See also* Calcium.
Calcium regulators, 874-881
    adverse reactions to, 877-878
    interaction of, with drugs, 877t; with
        foods, 877t
    major drugs in class of, 880t
    mechanism of action of, 875-876
    nursing process application for, 878-881
    pharmacokinetics of, 874-875
    therapeutic uses of, 876-877
Calderol, 876. *See also* Calcifediol.
Camphorated opium tincture, 711-713.
    See also Paregoric.
Canadian drug control, 14
Canadian Food and Drugs Act, 14
Canadian Narcotic Control Act, 14
Candidiasis, 1079
Cannabis abuse, 1323t

Cantharidin, 1311t
Cantharone, 1311t
Capastat Sulfate, 1057
Capoten, 555. *See also* Captopril.
Capreomycin sulfate as antitubercular
    agent, 1057
Capsules
    administration of, 124-125
        gastric tube and, 125, 126
    difficulty swallowing, 125
    as solid drug form, 123
Captopril, 555. *See also* Angiotensin-con-
    verting enzyme inhibitors.
    administration considerations for, 556
    adverse reactions to, 555
    dosage, 555
    in lactating patient, 555
    patient teaching for, 556, 559
    pharmacokinetics of, 554-555
Carafate, 766. *See also* Sucralfate.
Carbacel, 191, 1242. *See also* Carbachol.
Carbachol, 191, 1242. *See also* Choliner-
    gic agonists *and* Ophthalmic
    agents.
    dosage, 1242
    for glaucoma, 1242
    interaction of, with drugs, 193t
    for miosis, 1242
    pharmacokinetics of, 191, 1240
    sites of action of, 192t
Carbamazepine, 308-311
    action of, 308
    adverse reactions to, 310
    blood concentration levels of, 60t
    dosage, 308
    interaction of, with drugs, 308, 309t
    oral contraceptives and, 310
    pharmacokinetics of, 308
    for seizure disorders, 308
    therapeutic use of, 308
Carbamide, 577. *See also* Urea.
Carbamide peroxide, 1265. *See also* Ceru-
    minolytic agents.
    action of, 1265
    adverse reactions to, 1265
    patient teaching for, 1266
Carbapenems, 1041-1043. *See also* Imipe-
    nem/cilastatin sodium.
Carbenicillin disodium, 1013. *See also*
    Penicillins.
    administration considerations for, 1016
    adverse reactions to, 1014-1015
    dosage, 1013
    interaction of, with drugs, 1014t
    organisms susceptible to, 1009t
    patient teaching for, 1016
    peak concentration levels of, 1010t
    pharmacokinetics of, 1008-1009, 1010,
        1010t
Carbenicillin indanyl sodium, 1013. *See*
    also Penicillins.
    adverse reactions to, 1014-1015
    dosage, 1013
    interaction of, with drugs, 1014t
    organisms susceptible to, 1009t
    pharmacokinetics of, 1008-1009, 1010,
        1010t

---

i refers to an illustration; t refers to a table

Dexchlor, 947. *See also* Dexchlorpheniramine maleate.
Dexchlorpheniramine maleate, 947. *See
also* Antihistaminic agents.
dosage, 947
effects of, 945t
interaction of, with drugs, 949t
Dexedrine, 230. *See also* Dextroamphetamine sulfate.
Dextrans as antiplatelet drugs, 635
Dextroamphetamine sulfate, 230
Dextromethorphan hydrobromide, 676.
See also Antitussives.
action of, 675, 675i
administration considerations for, 678
adverse reactions to, 676
characteristics of, 676t
dosage, 676
interaction of, with drugs, 676, 677t
pharmacokinetics of, 674, 675
Dextrothyroxine sodium, 597
Dey-Lute, 224. *See also* Isoetharine hydrochloride.
Dezocine, 357. *See also* Narcotic agonist-
antagonists, mixed.
action of, 356
dosage, 357
equianalgesic dosage for, 356t
pharmacokinetics of, 356
DHT Intensol, 877. *See also* Dihydrotachysterol.
DHT Oral Solution, 877. *See also* Dihydrotachysterol.
DiaBeta, 849. *See also* Glyburide.
Diabetes mellitus
adverse beta-adrenergic blocker reaction
in, 244t
characteristics of, 839t
treatment of, 838-851
types of, 837-838
Diabinese, 848. *See also* Chlorpropamide.
Diagnostic agents, 51-52, 52t
Dialose, 724. *See also* Emollient laxatives.
Diamox, 319, 813, 1246. *See also* Acetazolamide.
Diamox Parenteral, 1246. *See also* Acetazolamide sodium.
Diamox Sequels, 1246. *See also* Acetazolamide.
Diamox Sodium, 1246. *See also* Acetazolamide sodium.
Diapid Nasal Spray, 891. *See also* Lypressin.
Diarrhea, 710
disorders involving, 710
drug absorption and, 23, 25
drugs to relieve, 711-717
Diazepam, 312, 440. *See also* Benzodiazepines, as antianxiety agents; as anticonvulsants *and* Injection
anesthetics.
as adjunct to anesthetic agents, 373
administration considerations for, 312,
442

Diazepam *(continued)*
adverse reactions to, 441
for anxiety, 440
dosage, 311, 440
in geriatric patient, 165
I.V. administration of, 312
as parent drug, 29t
in patient with liver disease, 439
pharmacokinetics of, 311, 373, 439
as preoperative medication, 368t
as skeletal muscle relaxant, 275
for status epilepticus, 312, 1304t
Diazoxide, 551. *See also* Vasodilating
agents.
action of, 550
administration considerations for, 553,
554
adverse reactions to, 552
as antihypertensive, 551
dosage, 551
pharmacokinetics of, 550, 551t
Dibenzyline, 235. *See also* Phenoxybenzamine hydrochloride.
Dibucaine hydrochloride, 391. *See also*
Topical anesthetics.
action of, 390
dosage, 391
patient teaching for, 394
pharmacokinetics of, 390
Dicarbosil, 757. *See also* Calcium carbonate.
Dichlorphenamide, 1246
dosage, 1246
as ophthalmic agent, 1246
pharmacokinetics of, 1245
Diclofenac, 336. *See also* Nonsteroidal anti-inflammatory drugs.
dosage, 336
interaction of, with drugs, 339t
Dicloxacillin sodium, 1012. *See also* Penicillins.
action of, 1010
dosage, 1012
organisms susceptible to, 1009t
peak concentration levels of, 1010t
pharmacokinetics of, 1008, 1010t
Dicumarol, 631. *See also* Oral anticoagulants.
dosage, 631
interaction of, with drugs, 633t
pharmacokinetics of, 630, 631
Dicumarol Pulvules, 631. *See also* Dicumarol.
Dicyclomine hydrochloride, 204. *See also*
Cholinergic blockers.
dosage, 204
interaction of, with drugs, 206t
pharmacokinetics of, 202, 203
Didronel, 876. *See also* Etidronate disodium.
Dienestrol, 910. *See also* Estrogens.
Dietary factors predisposing to adverse reactions, 66

Dietary fiber laxatives, 721-723
administration considerations for, 723
adverse reactions to, 722
daily requirement of, 722
laxative effect of, 722
patient teaching for, 712
pharmacokinetics of, 722
therapeutic uses of, 722
Dietary habits as component of drug history, 74
Diethylstilbestrol, 910. *See also* Estrogens.
for breast and prostate cancer, 1194
Diethylstilbestrol diphosphate, 910. *See
also* Estrogens.
dosage, 1194
for prostate cancer, 1194
Difenoxin hydrochloride, 713, 714
action of, 714
adverse reactions to, 714-715
dosage, 714
interaction of, with drugs, 714
nursing process application for, 715-716
pharmacokinetics of, 714
Diffusion, drug absorption and, 21, 22t
Diflorasone diacetate, 967. *See also* Topical glucocorticoids.
Diflucan, 1090. *See also* Fluconazole.
Diflunisal, 328. *See also* Salicylates.
administration considerations for, 330,
331
blood concentration levels of, 328
dosage, 328
interaction of, with drugs, 329-330t
patient teaching for, 332
Digestalin, 701. *See also* Activated charcoal.
Digestive agents, 701, 704-708
adverse reactions to, 706
interaction of, with drugs, 706
mechanism of action of, 705
nursing diagnoses related to use of, 701
nursing process application for, 706-708
pharmacokinetics of, 704-705
therapeutic uses of, 705-706
Digestive enzymes, 699-700, 700t. *See
also* Digestive hormones.
sites of formation of, 705i
Digestive hormones, 699, 700t. *See also*
Digestive enzymes.
sites of formation of, 705i
Digibind, 477
Digitalis, 470. *See also* Digoxin *and* Digitoxin.
Digitalis toxicity, 475-476
ECG changes in, 476
phenytoin for, 495
predisposing factors for, 475-476
signs and symptoms of, 476
treatment of, 477

Hormonal antineoplastic agents *(continued)*
    estrogens as, 1193-1196
    gonadotropin-releasing hormone analogues as, 1208-1209, 1211
    major drugs in class of, 1210t
    nursing diagnoses related to use of, 1193
    progestins as, 1203-1205
Hospitalized patient, medication orders for, 90-92,91i
Household system of weights and measure, 107-108, 108i
H.P. Acthar Gel, 886. *See also* Corticotropin repository.
Human chorionic gonadotropin, 1273
    nursing considerations for, 1283t
Human menopausal gonadotropin, 1274
    nursing considerations for, 1283t
Humatin, 1005, 1101. *See also* Paromomycin sulfate.
Humoral response, 938, 939i
Humorsol, 1242. *See also* Demecarium bromide.
Humulin L, 841t
Humulin N, 841t
Humulin R, 841t
Hycodan, 676. *See also* Hydrocodone bitartrate.
Hydantoins, 294-303
    adverse reactions to, 299
    blood glucose levels and, 303
    interaction of, with drugs, 299, 300-302t
    mechanism of action of, 298
    nursing process application for, 299, 302-303
    oral contraceptives and, 302
    pharmacokinetics of, 295-298
    in pregnant or lactating patient, 299
Hydeltrasol, 960. *See also* Systemic glucocorticoids.
Hydeltra-TBA, 960. *See also* Systemic glucocorticoids.
Hydergine, 234. *See also* Ergoloid mesylates.
Hydralazine hydrochloride, 551. *See also* Vasodilating agents.
    action of, 550
    administration considerations for, 553, 554
    adverse reactions to, 552
    dosage, 551
        as predisposing factor in adverse reactions, 65
    interaction of, with drugs, 552
    pharmacokinetics of, 550, 551t
    slow acetylation rate as risk factor for, 55
Hydrea, 1226. *See also* Hydroxyurea.
Hydrochloric acid, dilute, 817. *See also* Acidifying agents *and* Digestive agents.
    action of, 705, 816
    administration considerations for, 707, 818
    adverse reactions to, 706, 817
    as digestive aid, 706

Hydrochloric acid *(continued)*
    dosage, 706, 817
    for metabolic acidosis, 817
    patient teaching for, 707, 818
    pharmacokinetics of, 704, 816
Hydrochlorothiazide, 565. *See also* Thiazide andthiazide-like diuretics.
    dosage, 565
    interaction of, with drugs, 567t
    pharmacokinetics of, 564, 564t
    potency of, 45
Hydrocodone bitartrate, 676. *See also* Antitussives.
    action of, 675, 675i
    administration considerations for, 677
    adverse reactions to, 676
    characteristics of, 676t
    dosage, 676
    interaction of, with drugs, 677t
    pharmacokinetics of, 674, 675
    in pregnant or lactating patient, 674
Hydrocodone bitartrate and acetaminophen, 350. *See also* Narcotic agonists.
    dosage, 350
Hydrocodone and phenyltoloxamine, 350. *See also* Narcotic agonists.
    dosage, 350
Hydrocortisone, 959, 967, 1263. *See also* Systemic glucocorticoids *and* Topical glucocorticoids.
    as antineoplastic agent, 1206
    dosage, 959, 967, 1206
    as otic anti-inflammatory agent, 1263
    pharmacokinetics of, 1205
    as systemic glucocorticoids, 959
    as topical glucocorticoids, 967
Hydrocortisone acetate, 959, 1263. *See also* Systemic glucocorticoids.
    as otic anti-inflammatory agent, 1263
    for severe inflammation, 959
Hydrocortisone sodium phosphate, 959. *See also* Systemic glucocorticoids.
Hydrocortisone sodium succinate, 959. *See also* Systemic glucocorticoids.
Hydrocortone, 959. *See also* Systemic glucocorticoids.
Hydrocortone Acetate, 959. *See also* Systemic glucocorticoids.
Hydrocortone Phosphate, 959. *See also* Systemic glucocorticoids.
HydroDiuril, 565. *See also* Hydrochlorothiazide.
Hydroflumethiazide, 565. *See also* Thiazide and thiazide-like diuretics.
    dosage, 565
    interaction of, with drugs, 567t
    pharmacokinetics of, 564t
Hydrogen peroxide, 1313t
Hydromorphone hydrochloride, 350. *See also* Narcotic agonists.
    dosage, 350
    equianalgesic dosage of, 351t
    interaction of, with drugs, 353t
    pharmacokinetics of, 348t
Hydromox, 566. *See also* Quinethazone.

Hydroxocobalamin, 616. *See also* Vitamin B₁₂.
    dosage, 616
    patient teaching for, 617
    pharmacokinetics of, 615
Hydroxychloroquine sulfate, 111. *See also* Antimalarial agents.
    action of, 1110
    adverse reactions to, 1114t
    dosage, 1111
    interaction of, with drugs, 1113t
    pharmacokinetics of, 1109, 1110
Hydroxyprogesterone caproate, 915. *See also* Progestins.
    as antineoplastic agent, 1203
    pharmacokinetics of, 1203
4-Hydroxypropranolol, 32t
Hydroxyurea, 1225-1227
    action of, 1226
    adverse reactions to, 1226
    dosage, 1226
    emetic potential of, 1142t
    mechanism and sites of action of, 1140t
    nursing process application for, 1226-1227
    pharmacokinetics of, 1226
Hydroxyzine hydrochloride, 741, 948. *See also* Antihistamine antiemetics *and* Antihistaminic agents.
    as antiemetic, 741
    dosage, 741
    effects of, 945t
    interaction of, with drugs, 949t
    pharmacokinetics of, 739
    as preoperative medication, 368t
    for pruritus, 948
Hydroxyzine pamoate, 741, 948. *See also* Antihistamine antiemetics.
    dosage, 741, 948
    effects of, 945t
    interaction of, with drugs, 742t, 948
    pharmacokinetics of, 742
Hygroton, 566. *See also* Chlorthalidone.
Hylorel, 544. *See also* Guanadrel sulfate.
Hyoscyamine sulfate, 204. *See also* Cholinergic blockers.
    dosage, 204
    interaction of, with drugs, 206t
    pharmacokinetics of, 202, 203
    therapeutic uses of, 203
Hyperbaric anesthetic solution, 384
Hypercalcemia
    signs of, 805
    treatment of, 1187
Hypercholesterolemia, 586
    treatment of, 588
Hyperglycemia, treatment of, 837-847. *See also* Diabetes mellitus.
Hyperkalemia, signs of, 802
Hyperlipidemia, 586
Hyperlipoproteinemia, 586
    treatment of, 588, 592, 595, 597-598
    types of, 586t
Hypermagnesemia
    antacids and, 756, 758
    signs of, 719c

Metronidazole, 1117. *See also* Antiprotozoal agents.
  action of, 1116
  administration considerations for, 1120
  adverse reactions to, 1117, 1119t
  dosage, 1117
  interaction of with alcohol, 1118t; with drugs, 1118t
  patient teaching for, 1120, 1122
  pharmacokinetics of, 1116
  in pregnant or lactating patient, 1116
  for skin infections, 1308t
Metryl, 1117. *See also* Metronidazole.
Metubine, 255. *See also* Metocurine iodide.
Mevacor, 596. *See also* Lovastatin.
Mexate, 1170. *See also* Methotrexate sodium.
Mexiletine hydrochloride, 495-496. *See also* Class IB antiarrhythmics.
  administration considerations for, 496
  adverse reactions to, 496
  interaction of, with drugs, 496
  patient teaching for, 497
  pharmacokinetics of, 494, 495
Mexitil, 495-496. *See also* Mexiletine hydrochloride.
Mezlin, 1013. *See also* Mezlocillin sodium.
Mezlocillin sodium, 1013. *See also* Penicillins.
  dosage, 1013
  interaction of, with drugs, 1014t
  organisms susceptible to, 1009t
  peak concentration levels of, 1010t
  pharmacokinetics of, 1008-1009, 1010, 1010t
Micatin, 1092, 1309t
Miconazole, 1092, 1094
Miconazole nitrate, 1309t
Microbial tumorcidal agents, 1184-1191
  adverse reactions to, 1187
  mechanism of action of, 1185
  nursing process application for, 1187-1190
  pharmacokinetics of, 1184, 1185t
  therapeutic uses of, 1186-1187
Microcytic anemia, 609. *See also* Iron-deficiency anemia.
Microfibrillar collagen hemostat, 605t
Micronase, 849. *See also* Glyburide.
Micronor, 919. *See also* Oral contraceptives.
Microsulfon, 1129-1130. *See also* Sulfadiazine.
Midamor, 574. *See also* Amiloride hydrochloride.
Midazolam hydrochloride, 374. *See also* Injection anesthetics.
  dosage, 374
  as preoperative medication, 368t
Milk of Magnesia, 719. *See also* Magnesium salts.
Milliequivalents, 109
Milontin, 314. *See also* Phensuximide.
Miltown, 447. *See also* Meprobamate.

Mineralocorticoids, 969-971
  adverse reactions to, 970
  effect of stress on, 956
  interaction of, with drugs, 961-962t
  major drugs in class of, 977t
  mechanism of action of, 969
  nursing process application for, 970-971
  pharmacokinetics of, 969
  synthesis of, 956
  therapeutic uses of, 970
Mineral oil, 727-728, 731
  action of, 728
  adverse reactions to, 728
  dosage, 728
  for dry skin, 1314t
  interaction of, with drugs, 728; with food, 59
  nursing process application for, 728, 731
  pharmacokinetics of, 727
  in pregnant patient, 176
  therapeutic uses of, 728
Minerals, 775-776, 790-793
  adverse reactions to, 792
  food sources of, 790t
  mechanism of action of, 791
  nursing diagnoses related to use of, 776
  nursing process application for, 792-793
  pharmacokinetics of, 790-791
  therapeutic uses of, 791-792
Mineral sources of drugs, 10
Minimal bactericidal concentration, 997
Minimal inhibitory concentration of microorganisms, 997
Minimum alveolar concentration, 369
Minimum toxic concentration, 34t, 35
Minipres, 543-544. *See also* Prazosin hydrochloride.
Minocin, 1026. *See also* Minocycline hydrochloride.
Minocycline hydrochloride, 1026. *See also* Tetracyclines.
  administration considerations for, 1028, 1029
  adverse reactions to, 1027
  dosage, 1026
  interaction of, with drugs, 1028t
  organisms susceptible to, 1025, 1026
  patient teaching for, 1029
  pharmacokinetics of, 1024, 1025
Minodyl, 551. *See also* Minoxidil.
Minoxidil, 551. *See also* Vasodilating agents.
  action of, 550
  adverse reactions to, 552
  dosage, 551
  for hair loss, 1315t
  interaction of, with drugs, 552
  patient teaching for, 554
  pharmacokinetics of, 550, 551t
  as vasodilator, 551
Mintezol, 1098. *See also* Thiabendazole.
Miostat, 191. *See also* Carbachol.
Miotics, 1240-1244
  adverse reactions to, 1243
  interaction of, with drugs, 1243
  mechanism of action of, 1240
  nursing process application for, 1243-1244
  pharmacokinetics of, 1240
  therapeutic uses of, 1240, 1242

Misoprostol, 765
  action of, 765
  administration considerations for, 768
  adverse reactions to, 766
  dosage, 765
  interaction of, with drugs, 766
  patient teaching for, 768
  pharmacokinetics of, 764
  in pregnant patient, 768
Mithracin, 1186. *See also* Plicamycin.
Mithramycin, emetic potential of, 1142t. *See also* Plicamycin.
Mitomycin, 1186. *See also* Microbial tumorcidal agents.
  administration considerations for, 1188
  adverse reactions to, 1187
  dosage, 1186
  mechanism and sites of action of, 1140t, 1185
  pharmacokinetics of, 1184, 1185t
Mitomycin C, 1186. *See also* Mitomycin.
Mitoxantrone, 1186. *See also* Microbial tumorcidal agents.
  administration considerations for, 1188
  adverse reactions to, 1187
  dosage, 1186
  mechanism and sites of action of, 1140t, 1185
  patient teaching for, 1190
  pharmacokinetics of, 1184, 1156
Mitrolan, 722. *See also* Bulk-forming laxatives.
Mixed alpha- and beta-adrenergic blocking agents, 538. *See also* Alpha- and beta-adrenergic blocking agents, mixed, as antihypertensives.
Mixed narcotic agonists-antagonists, 346, 356-359. *See also* Narcotic agonist--antagonists, mixed.
Moban, 459. *See also* Molindone hydrochloride.
Modicon, 918. *See also* Oral contraceptives.
Moebiquin, 1116. *See also* Iodoquinol.
Molindone hydrochloride, 459. *See also* Nonphenothiazines.
  dosage, 459
  relative effects of, 460t
Molybdenum, 792. *See also* Minerals.
  action of, 791
  adverse reactions to, 792
  dosage, 792
  food sources of, 790t
  pharmacokinetics of, 791
Molypale, 792. *See also* Molybdenum.
Molypen, 792. *See also* Molybdenum.
Mometasone, 1313t
Monistat, 1092
Monistat-Derm, 1309t
Monitoring response, 60-61
Monoamine oxidase inhibitors, 421-425. *See also* MAO inhibitors.
Monobactams, 1043-1045, 1049. *See also* Aztreonam.
Monocid, 1020. *See also* Cefonicid sodium.
Monoclate, 604t

Mono-Gesic, 328. *See also* Salsalate.
Monostat 3, 1092
Monostat 7, 1092
Moral principles, application of, to patient care, 102
Moricizine hydrochloride, 487-489
    action of, 487
    adverse reactions to, 487
    dosage, 487
    interaction of, with drugs, 487
    nursing process application for, 488-489
    pharmacokinetics of, 487
    therapeutic uses of, 487
Morning sickness, treatment of, 736
Morphine sulfate, 351. *See also* Injection anesthetics *and* Narcotic agonists.
    action of, 349
    as adjunct to general anesthesia, 374
    adverse reactions to, 353
    dosage, 351, 374
    dose-response correlation of, 44
    efficacy of, 45
    as enzyme inhibitor, 29, 30t
    equianalgesic dosage of, 351t
    as first-pass effect drug, 25, 348
    interaction of, with drugs, 353t
    for obstetric anesthesia, 374
    pharmacokinetics of, 348, 348t
    as preoperative medication, 368t, 374
    as standard, 347
    therapeutic uses of, 349
Morphine sulfate intensified oral solution, 352. *See also* Narcotic agonists.
Morphine sulfate sustained-release tablets, 351-352. *See also* Narcotic agonists.
    administration considerations for, 355
    dosage, 352
    patient teaching for, 355
Motion sickness, 735
    prevention of, 748, 749i
    treatment of, 739-744
Motofen, 714. *See also* Difenoxin hydrochloride.
Motor end plate, 253i
    physiology of, 253
Motrin, 336. *See also* Ibuprofen.
Moxalactam disodium, 1022. *See also* Cephalosporins.
    adverse reactions to, 1022
    dosage, 1022
    interaction of, with alcohol, 1022
    organisms susceptible to, 1017t
    patient teaching for, 1024
    pharmacokinetics of, 1017, 1018i
Moxam, 1022. *See also* Moxalactam disodium.
6-MP, 1178. *See also* Mercaptopurine.
MS Contin, 351-352. *See also* Narcotic agonists.
Mucociliary clearance mechanism, 669
Mucokinesis, drug therapy to enhance, 670-672
Mucolytics, 679-682. *See also* Acetylcysteine.
    nursing diagnoses related to use of, 670
Mucomyst, 680. *See also* Acetylcysteine.

Mucus, 669
Mupirocin, 1308t
Muromonab-CD3, 973. *See also* Immunosuppressants.
    action of, 972
    administration considerations for, 975, 978
    adverse reactions to, 973
    dosage, 973
    interaction of, with drugs, 974t
    pharmacokinetics of, 971, 972
Muscarinic receptor, physiology of, 201-202
Muscle mass as factor in dosage, 55-56
Musculoskeletal spasms, acute, cause and effect of, 267
Musculoskeletal system, effects of aging on, 168
Mustargen, 1149-1150. *See also* Mechlorethamine.
Mutamycin, 1185. *See also* Mitomycin.
Myambutol, 1054. *See also* Ethambutol hydrochloride.
Myasthenia gravis, drugs used for diagnosis of, 195
Mycelex, 1092
Mycifradin, 1005. *See also* Neomycin.
Mycifradin Sulfate, 827. *See also* Neomycin.
Myciguent, 1308t. *See also* Neomycin.
Mycostatin, 1084, 1309t. *See also* Nystatin.
Mydfrin, 1238. *See also* Phenylephrine hydrochloride.
Mydriacyl, 1239. *See also* Mydriatics.
Mydriatics, 1236-1240
    adverse reactions to, 1239
    mechanism of action of, 1237-1238
    nursing process application for, 1239-1240
    pharmacokinetics of, 1237
    therapeutic uses of, 1238-1239
Mylanta, 757t. *See also* Antacids.
Mylanta II, 757t, 758. *See also* Antacids.
Myleran, 1153. *See also* Busulfan.
Mylicon, 703. *See also* Simethicone.
Myochrysine, 992. *See also* Gold sodium thiomalate.
Myotonachol, 191. *See also* Bethanechol chloride.
Mysoline, 304. *See also* Primidone.
Mytelase, 195. *See also* Ambenonium.
Myxedema coma, 863

N

Nadolol, 241, 524, 543. *See also* Beta-adrenergic blockers *and* Sympatholytic agents.
    administration considerations for, 548
    adverse reactions to, 525
    for angina, 524
    as antihypertensive, 241
    dosage, 241, 524, 543
    interaction of, with drugs, 243t, 526t, 545-546t
    patient teaching for, 527
    pharmacokinetics of, 238, 239t, 524, 538, 539, 540t

Nafarelin acetate, 1276
    nursing considerations for, 1284-1285t
Nafcillin sodium, 1012. *See also* Penicillins.
    action of, 1010-1011
    dosage, 1012
    organisms susceptible to, 1009t
    peak concentration levels of, 1010t
    in pediatric patient, 151
    pharmacokinetics of, 1008, 1010t
Naftifine hydrochloride, 1309t
Naftin, 1309t
Nalbuphine hydrochloride, 357. *See also* Narcotic agonist-antagonists, mixed.
    administration considerations for, 358
    adverse reactions to, 357
    dosage, 357
    equianalgesic dosage of, 356t
    interaction of, with drugs, 357
    pharmacokinetics of, 356
Naldecon, 946. *See also* Phenyltoloxamine citrate.
Nalfon, 336. *See also* Fenoprofen calcium.
Nalidixic acid, 1135
Naloxone challenge test, 360
Naloxone hydrochloride, 360. *See also* Narcotic antagonists.
    administration considerations for, 361
    adverse reactions to, 360
    dosage, 360
    for opiate overdose, 42, 58, 1305t
    patient teaching for, 361
    pharmacokinetics of, 359
    therapeutic uses of, 359-360
Naltrexone hydrochloride, 360. *See also* Narcotic antagonists.
    administration considerations for, 361
    adverse reactions to, 360
    dosage, 360
    interaction of, with drugs, 360
    patient teaching for, 361
    pharmacokinetics of, 359
Nandrolone decanoate, 900. *See also* Anabolic steroids.
    dosage, 900
    pharmacokinetics of, 898
Nandrolone phenproprionate, 900. *See also* Anabolic steroids.
    dosage, 900
    pharmacokinetics of, 898
Naphazoline, 690. *See also* Topical decongestants.
    dosage, 690
    interaction of, with drugs, 691t
Naprosyn, 337. *See also* Naproxen.
Naproxen, 337. *See also* Nonsteroidal anti-inflammatory drugs.
    administration considerations for, 340
    dosage, 337
    interaction of, with drugs, 57-58, 339t
    patient teaching for, 341
    pharmacokinetics of, 335
    therapeutic uses of, 336

i refers to an illustration; t refers to a table

---

i refers to an illustration; t refers to a table

S

Saddle block, 381
Safety as drug standard, 14
Salacid, 1312t
Salicylates, 326-332. *See also* Salicylate toxicity.
  adverse reactions to, 64t, 328, 330
  as cause of Reye's syndrome, 330
  interaction of, with drugs, 328, 329-330t
  interference of, with glucose testing, 328
  mechanism of action of, 326
  nursing process application for, 330-332
  pharmacokinetics of, 326
  role of, in prostaglandin inhibition, 326, 327i
  therapeutic levels of, 326
  therapeutic uses of, 327-328
Salicylate toxicity, signs and symptoms of, 328, 329, 331
Salicylic acid, 1312t
Salicylism, 328, 329, 331
Salsalate, 328. *See also* Salicylates.
  dosage, 328
  interaction of, with drugs, 329-330t
Saluron, 565. *See also* Hydroflumethiazide.
Sandimmune, 972. *See also* Cyclosporine.
Sandostatin, 1277
Sanorex, 230. *See* Mazindol.
Satric, 1117. *See also* Metronidazole.
Scabene, 1311t
Scabicides, 1310-1311t
Schedules of controlled drugs, 15-16t
School-age child
  administration of medication to, 55, 156t. *See also* Pediatric administration techniques.
  I.M. injection for, 158
  I.V. administration in, 158
Scopolamine hydrobromide, 204-205, 1238. *See also* Cholinergic blockers.
  administration considerations for, 1239
  adverse reactions to, 205, 743t, 1239
  as antiemetic, 748
  compared with antihistamine antiemetics, 740
  dosage, 205, 1238
  effect of, on GI motility, 23
  interaction of, with drugs, 206t
  as mydriatic, 1238
  patient teaching for, 1240
  pharmacokinetics of, 202, 203, 1237
  as preoperative medication, 368t
  therapeutic uses of, 203
  transdermal patches, 749i
Sebulex, 1312
Secobarbital sodium, 408. *See also* Barbiturates.
  administration considerations for, 411
  dosage, 408
  interaction of, with drugs, 409-410t
  pharmacokinetics of, 405
  as preoperative medication, 368t
Seconal, 408. *See also* Secobarbital sodium.
Secondary reactions, 66
Second-generation antidepressants, 426-432
  adverse reactions to, 431
  interaction of, with drugs, 431
  mechanism of action of, 430
  nursing process application for, 431-432
  pharmacokinetics of, 429-430
  therapeutic uses of, 430
Secretin, 699, 700t
  site of formation of, 705i
Sectral, 239, 502, 542. *See also* Acebutolol hydrochloride.
Sedative and hypnotic agents, 398-419
  adverse reactions to, 64t. *See also specific groups of drugs in class.*
  barbiturates as, 405-408, 410-412
  benzodiazepines as, 400-405
  in geriatric patient, 167
  in lactating patient, 176t
  major drugs in class of, 416-418t
  nonbenzodiazepines-nonbarbiturates as, 412-415
  nursing diagnoses related to use of, 399
  patient teaching for, 404
Sedatives, 398. *See also* Sedative and hypnotic agents.
  abuse of, 1324t
Seizures
  diagnoses of, 294
  epileptic, international classification of, 296t
  therapy for, 294-320
Seldane, 948. *See also* Terfenadine.
Selegiline, 288. *See also* Dopaminergic agents.
  action of, 287
  adverse reactions to, 288, 290
  dosage, 288
  interaction of, with drugs, 289t
  pharmacokinetics of, 286, 287
Selenitrace, 792. *See also* Selenium.
Selenium, 792. *See also* Minerals.
  action of, 791
  administration considerations for, 793
  adverse reactions to, 792
  dosage, 792
  food sources of, 790t
  pharmacokinetics of, 791
Self-contained system of drug packaging, 124
Semilente Iletin I, 841t
Semilente Insulin, 841t
Semilente Purified Pork Prompt Insulin Zinc Suspension, 841t
Semustine, 1155. *See also* Nitrosureas.
  adverse reactions to, 1156
  dosage, 1155
  pharmacokinetics of, 1148t, 1155
Senna, 726. *See also* Stimulant laxatives.
  adverse reactions to, 726
  dosage, 726
  patient teaching for, 727
  pharmacokinetics of, 725
  in pregnant patient, 176
Senokot, 726. *See also* Senna.
Sensitivity-related adverse reactions, 67
  evaluating, 86
Sensory deficits, as component of drug history, 75
Septra, 1129. *See also* Co-trimoxazole.
Serax, 441. *See also* Oxazepam.
Serentil, 453. *See also* Mesoridazine besylate.
Seromycin, 1057
Serophene, 1272
Serpasil, 544. *See also* Reserpine.
Serum albumin, normal, 606-607
Serum sickness, 1015
Sex, as factor in clinical response, 55
Sherley Amendment, 12t, 13
Shock, as factor in drug absorption, 54
Shol's solution, 813. *See also* Sodium citrate.
  adverse reactions to, 813
Sialorrhea, controlling, 281
Side effect, 63. *See also* Adverse reactions.
Silvadene, 1308t
Silver nitrate, 1253, 1312t. *See also* Keratolytics *and* Ophthalmic anti-infective agents.
  interaction of, with drugs, 1254
  for neonates, 1253
Silver sulfadiazine, 1308t
Simethicone, 703. *See also* Antiflatulents.
  action of, 703
  dosage, 703
  nursing process application for, 703-704
  pharmacokinetics of, 703
Sinemet, 287. *See also* Carbidopa-levodopa.
Sinequan, 426. *See also* Doxepin hydrochloride.
Sinex, 690. *See also* Phenylephrine hydrochloride.
Single orders for medications, 92
Sinus drops, patient positioning for, 692i. *See also* Topical decongestants.
Size as factor in drug dosage, 105-106
SK-Bamate, 447. *See also* Meprobamate.
SK-Chloral Hydrate, 412. *See also* Chloral hydrate.
Skelaxin, 269. *See also* Metaxalone.
Skeletal muscle contraction, physiology of, 267
Skeletal muscle relaxing agents, 267-279
  centrally acting, 268-272
  major drugs in class of, 277t
  nursing diagnoses related to use of, 268
  peripherally acting, 272-275

i refers to an illustration; t refers to a table

---

i refers to an illustration; t refers to a table

---

i refers to an illustration; t refers to a table